Jennie Fenstermacher

Handbook of Speech Pathology and Audiology

CONTRIBUTING AUTHORS

STANLEY H. AINSWORTH, PH.D., *Alumni Foundation Distinguished Professor of Speech Correction and Associate Dean, Research and Graduate Studies, College of Education, University of Georgia*

CLAYTON L. BENNETT, PH.D., *Special Education Coordinator, Department of Education, San Diego County, California*

H. HARLAN BLOOMER, PH.D., *Professor of Speech and Director, Speech and Hearing Clinic, University of Michigan*

ISAAC P. BRACKETT, PH.D., *Professor of Speech Pathology and Audiology, and System Vice President, Southern Illinois University*

DAVID J. BROAD, PH.D., *Associate Director, Speech Communications Research Laboratory, Inc., Santa Barbara*

BRYNG BRYNGELSON, PH.D., *Professor Emeritus, Speech Pathology and Clinical Professor of Pediatrics, University of Minnesota*

GENE J. BRUTTEN, PH.D., *Research Professor of Speech Pathology and Professor of Psychology, Southern Illinois University*

COURTNEY B. CAZDEN, PH.D., *Associate Professor of Education, Harvard University*

MORTON COOPER, PH.D., *Private Practice, West Los Angeles*

ROBERT M. DEU PREE, M.D., *U.S. Public Health Service DFEH, Los Angeles*

JON EISENSON, PH.D., *Professor, Hearing and Speech Sciences, Stanford School of Medicine*

ROBERT GILLEN, PH.D., *Associate Professor of Speech, California State College, Los Angeles*

VICTOR GOODHILL, M.D., *Professor of Surgery (Otology), School of Medicine, University of California, Los Angeles*

GILES WILKESON GRAY, PH.D., *Professor Emeritus of Speech, Louisiana State University*

PAUL GUGGENHEIM, M.D., *Assistant Clinical Professor (Otology), School of Medicine, University of California, Los Angeles*

H. RUSSELL HANEY, PH.D., *Associate Professor of Speech, University of Southern California*

T. D. HANLEY, PH.D., *Professor of Speech, University of California, Santa Barbara*

DONALD B. KINSTLER, PH.D., *Professor of Audiology and Director, Hearing Clinic, California State College, Los Angeles*

HERBERT KOEPP-BAKER, PH.D., *Research Professor and Chairman, Department of Speech Pathology and Audiology, Southern Illinois University*

MERLE LAWRENCE, PH.D., *Professor of Otorhinolaryngology and Director, Kresge Hearing Research Institute, University of Michigan Medical School*

JACK MATTHEWS, PH.D., *Professor and Chairman, Speech Department and Theatre Arts, University of Pittsburgh*

JOHN MICHEL, PH.D., *Research Associate, Bureau of Child Research, University of Kansas*

ROBERT MILISEN, PH.D., *Professor of Speech Pathology, Indiana University*

G. PAUL MOORE, PH.D., *Professor and Chairman, Department of Speech, University of Florida*

HELMER R. MYKLEBUST, PH.D., *Research Professor of Special Education, Northern Illinois University*

EDWARD D. MYSAK, PH.D., *Professor and Chairman, Department of Speech Pathology and Audiology, Teachers College, Columbia University*

HAYES A. NEWBY, PH.D., *Professor and Director of Division of Speech and Hearing Science, University of Maryland*

WILLIAM PERKINS, PH.D., *Professor of Communicative Disorders, University of Southern California*

ROBERT W. PETERS, PH.D., *Professor of Speech and Hearing Sciences and Director, Institute of Speech and Hearing Sciences, University of North Carolina*

GORDON E. PETERSON, PH.D. (*deceased*)

MARGARET HALL POWERS, PH.D., *Private Consultant, Services for Handicapped Children, Chicago*

CLYDE LEE ROUSEY, PH.D., *Speech Pathology and Audiology, Menninger Foundation*

THOMAS H. SHRINER, PH.D., *Associate Professor of Speech and Research Associate Professor, Children's Research Center, University of Illinois*

DONALD J. SHOEMAKER, PH.D., *Professor of Psychology and Speech Pathology and Coordinator of Psychological Services, Southern Illinois University*

S. RICHARD SILVERMAN, PH.D., *Director, Central Institute for the Deaf, and Professor of Audiology, Washington University*

JOHN SNIDECOR, PH.D., *Professor of Speech Pathology, Speech and Hearing Center, University of California, Santa Barbara*

LAVERNE DEEL SUTHERLAND, M.A., *Speech and Hearing Specialist, Los Angeles City Unified School District*

LEE EDWARD TRAVIS, PH.D., *Professor and Dean, Graduate School of Psychology, Fuller Theological Seminary, Pasadena*

CHARLES VAN RIPER, PH.D., *Distinguished Professor, Western Michigan University*

RONALD W. WENDAHL, PH.D., *Professor of Speech and Hearing Sciences, University of Houston and Adjunct Professor of Audiology and Speech Pathology, Baylor College of Medicine*

ROBERT WILLIAM WEST, PH.D. (*deceased*)

DEAN E. WILLIAMS, PH.D., *Professor of Speech Pathology and Audiology, Wendell Johnson Speech and Hearing Center, University of Iowa*

HARRIS WINITZ, PH.D., *Professor of Speech and Hearing Science, University of Missouri, Kansas City*

KENNETH SCOTT WOOD, PH.D., *Professor and Director, Speech Pathology and Audiology, University of Oregon*

Handbook of Speech Pathology and Audiology

edited by

Lee Edward Travis
GRADUATE SCHOOL OF PSYCHOLOGY
FULLER THEOLOGICAL SEMINARY

Prentice-Hall, Inc., Englewood Cliffs, N. J.

Printed in the United States of America

ISBN: 0-13-381764-4

Library of Congress Catalog Card Number: 74-146360

10 9 8 7 6 5 4

PRENTICE-HALL INTERNATIONAL, INC., *London*
PRENTICE-HALL OF AUSTRALIA, PTY. LTD., *Sydney*
PRENTICE-HALL OF CANADA, LTD., *Toronto*
PRENTICE-HALL OF INDIA PRIVATE LIMITED, *New Delhi*
PRENTICE-HALL OF JAPAN, INC., *Tokyo*

Preface

In the nineteen-fifties in the preface to the *Handbook of Speech Pathology* I wrote that no one man could react authoritatively to the subject matter of communication disorders. That statement is even more appropriate in this preface to the new work, the *Handbook of Speech Pathology and Audiology*, which has fifty chapters in place of the older handbook's thirty-three, forty-four authors rather than twenty-seven, and five parts instead of four.

Part I includes nine chapters dealing with concepts and factors common to all disorders of communication, such as terminology, phonetics, acoustics, personality, diagnosis, and therapy.

Part II, with seven chapters, deals with hearing. The person with a hearing loss and his organs of hearing are considered together in anatomy, physiology, pathology, psychology, speech, diagnosis, and treatment.

Part III has seven chapters telling of the origin, nature, uses, troubles, and means of modification of the voice in the communication process.

The largest single portion of the book is contained in Part IV, which deals with speech. Nineteen chapters reveal the nature of speech itself and note the multiple factors that operate in its pathologies. Diagnosis and treatment of the troubled speaker are approached from a wide range of viewpoints. Medicine, dentistry, psychiatry, psychology, sociology, and education are all sampled in the most comprehensive understanding possible of speech disorders.

Part V gives an exposition of language and its disorders. Eight chapters cover the development, nature, and disturbances of language. Aphasia in both childhood and in adults is fully considered diagnostically and therapeutically.

We have tried to structure this work in order to reveal the ground plan as well as the articulation of various areas of specialization. We hope that the tremendous scope of the research, theory, and practice portrayed here will prove useful not only to students majoring in some phase of the communicative disorders but also to many other professionals in the social and behavioral sciences as well.

Conceivably, the only true and unique disorder of man as man is a disorder in his language, spoken or written or perceived. Man, and man alone, can communicate cognitive information and not merely an emotion or a signal, can endow an utterance with universal reference, and can paraphrase a message to make poetry as well as science.

These three features of language are the projections of the whole human personality, and any kind of trouble with any one of them results ineluctably in a troubled human being. In this sense then this book should have relatively universal appeal—in college and university classes and laboratories, in public and private schools, and in hospitals and schools for the handicapped.

Speech pathology and audiology are young and vigorous fields of endeavor. They challenge the theoretician, the philosopher, the researcher, the teacher, the practitioner, the young scholar, and the old professional. Every year increasing numbers of students are trained, a growing number of significant publications appear in a large number of journals, and national and local professional meetings find their registrations on the rise. Although borrowings from other disciplines remain high, original contributions are now so sound and ample that loans can be made to others.

I have been richly blessed in serving as the editor of this large and impressive volume. Forty-four outstanding members of our profession have sacrificed time and energy in bringing it to fruition. My gratitude to them is great. My pain is sharp over the passing of Robert West, Wendell Johnson, Gordon Peterson, and Clarence Simon who were associated with this book and/or its predecessor. The passing of these great minds is a severe loss to all of us and a demand that we close the ranks of competence thus impaired.

I acknowledge with grateful appreciation the support and encouragement of many colleagues and friends. I am all the more in debt to my wife, Lysa Virginia Travis, for again she has edited the bibliographies and made them conform to a chosen system of citation. Her help to me also included cutting, typing, and pasting manuscript for many tireless hours. Happily, I thank Dr. and Mrs. Robert M. Deu Pree, Jennifer Weyerhaeuser, and my loyal secretary Marnie Frederickson for all they have done in helping me with this book.

L. E. T.

Graduate School of Psychology
Fuller Theological Seminary

Contents

PART IV

SPEECH

PART V

LANGUAGE

PART 1

Basic Considerations

1

Terminology and Nomenclature

Kenneth Scott Wood

GENERAL PROBLEMS

All areas of scientific study are afflicted with a certain amount of ambiguity, duplication, inappropriateness, and disagreement in the use of terms. Like other sciences, speech pathology, audiology, and the entire cluster of studies associated with the production and perception of speech have been developing over the years a terminology and nomenclature that leave much to be desired in logic and stability. Many terms and their meanings are not well crystallized because the subject matter is always changing; concepts themselves are often tentative and fluid, and many writers have liberally coined new terms whenever they felt a need to do so. The growth of speech pathology and audiology, stimulated as it has been by so many different workers, has generated hundreds of terms, some of which are interchangeable, some of which have different meanings to different people, some of which are now rare or obsolete, and some of which for various reasons have had only a short literary life.

Hammond and Allen (1953) in an exploratory study asked a number of psychiatric social workers, graduate students in psychology, and practicing clinical psychologists to define 61 terms that are often used in clinical reports. They found a relatively high percentage of the words inadequately, vaguely, and even absolutely incorrectly, defined.

When the graduate student is required to read a great quantity of technical literature in a limited time, many of the words he encounters at first sight are unfamiliar to him. He may look these words up, but usually he does not because his time is limited and the context frequently makes the word intelligible. As he continues his reading, he encounters these words again and again, and they become familiar to him. Consequently, even though the words are imperfectly understood, or their meanings only guessed at, the student assumes that he knows their full meanings. He thus fails to form habits of verbal accuracy. When the meanings of some technical words are still not agreed upon and different authorities use the same term to mean different things, the whole problem of accuracy is aggravated.

To take another example from psychology, Grayson and Tolman (1950) studied the possibility of semantic differences in the use of psychological terms as an obstacle to interprofessional understanding. They selected 50 words appearing with greatest frequency in psychological reports and analyzed the definitions returned by 20 psychologists and 17 psychiatrists together with definitions of the same words appearing in six authoritative sources. The definitions of the first 20 words were analyzed by establishing the number of words used in each definition and by placing each definition in the conceptual response category into which each fell.

In the quantitative analysis, the psychologists were found to be more verbose and circuitous in their definitions than were the psychiatrists. This was true whether the terms were psychological, psychiatric, or psychoanalytical ones. Further analysis showed that only rarely did as many as 75 percent of the definition responses for each term fall into a single category. Grayson and Tolman concluded that although a central core of meaning tended to prevail, wide variations occurred. The most striking finding of this study was the looseness and ambiguity of the definitions of most of the terms. Verbalization and conceptualization have clearly lagged behind the useful application of psychological terms, and the lack of verbal precision seems to stem from theoretical confusion in the face of complexity and logical inconsistency of psychological phenomena. Grayson and Tolman believe that verbal discrepancies can only be reconciled by deeper understanding and by many years of psychological experience.

Johnson and Wilson (1945) found a low degree of agreement among 20 psychologists as to the applicability of three words—*hypothesis*, *theory*, and *law*—to a group of 20 statements each of which had been labeled in one of three ways by the original author of the statement. This study concludes that lack of such basic agreement might well account for a considerable portion of the controversy existing in the field of psychology.

The problems in the terminology of psychology and psychiatry probably apply equally to speech pathology and audiology, since all deal with aspects of persons and their behavior. When confusions threaten adequate communication among those who are interested in the nature and correction of failures in the communication process itself, it is important to give direct attention to terminology. The student should keep in mind, however, that he will always encounter a considerable number of irreducible ambiguities and confusions, which he will just have to learn to tolerate. He should try to understand in each instance the nature of the ambiguity and the reasons why it exists. Improving terminology is not so simple a task as getting "a definition-cutter with his logical scissors" to straighten matters out once and for all. It is not the function of glossaries or dictionaries to create terms or to assign meanings; they should clarify and reflect, insofar as possible, the usages among the professional members of the field.

LEARNING TERMS AND NAMES

The acquisition of terms together with the things, processes, and concepts for which they stand is an important part of securing a working knowledge in speech pathology and audiology; the student entering this field, however, cannot acquire his terminology in advance of his basic knowledge. The real meanings of terms are never learned first. They are acquired simultaneously with concepts, or they come later. In a sense, all speech pathologists and audiologists are continually enriching, expanding, and qualifying the terms they know. The real meanings and implications of terms are learned not so much from linguistic context or from dictionaries and glossaries as they are learned from experience and observation. Defining terms by circumlocution with a generic vocabulary may help some, but a term like *aphasia*, for example, can never really be comprehended until the student encounters *aphasia* and relates himself to persons with *aphasic* symptoms. On the other hand, the student can learn something about certain terms in advance of direct experience with the subject matter itself. For example, if he knows that striated muscles are often named by their points of attachment, the meanings of terms such as *thyroarytenoid* and *cricothyroid* are more readily understood.

If the student will acquaint himself with some of the Greek and Latin roots, prefixes, and suffixes, he may be able to formulate central meanings of many terms even though the current meanings may have twisted away from the significance of the roots. The etymology or history of a term often yields a good beginning clue to its meaning and lends semantic reinforcement to it. For example, if one learns that *thyro-* comes from a Greek word meaning "shield" and that *-oid* is a suffix meaning "form," he may visualize the *thyroid cartilage* as having the shape of a shield, thus enriching his concept. It is possible to learn terms by rote without ever seeing any logical relationship between the terms and their meanings, but they are probably less easily remembered. It is much easier to remember the location of the *adrenal glands* when it is known that *ad-* means "near" and *-renal* means "kidney." As a further example, it will serve the student to know at the beginning that the prefix *para-* carries the meaning of "faulty" and "disordered" and that *dys-* means "bad" or "ill." From this he will have a better start on such words as *paralalia*, *parasigmatism*, *dyslexia*, and *dysphasia*. Many prefixes, roots, and suffixes have more than one meaning, such as *para-*, which also means "beside" and "secondary"; thus, the word *paramedical* means "having a medical aspect."

It should, of course, be remembered that the

acquisition of terminology in any field is always related to the general vocabulary of the student. In many cases, when the student has difficulty with the technical vocabulary, his real tr0uble is traceable to the fact that he does not know the meanings of more commonly used words.

The glossaries of earlier works in speech pathology include terms which properly belong to such fields as antomy, psychology, orthopedics, neurology, physics, and medicine; some of them are included, however, because they are commonly referred to in speech pathology and audiology. The name of every muscle, nerve, and sense organ related to the speech and hearing process is necessarily part of the terminology of this field. The terms which speech pathology and audiology have borrowed from other fields are evidence that it is closely related to these many fields. They are signs of a natural eclecticism. It makes little difference as to which field a term originally belonged —if there is a need for it in speech pathology and audiology, it becomes part of the terminology of this field.

Because there is no limit to the acquisition of terms from other fields, the first and central concern of the student should be to master as soon as possible a core terminology which represents specific speech defects as symptoms, as collections of symptoms, and as having predominating psychological or somatic causes. It should be learned early that some terms designating speech defects refer to symptoms, as in the case of *aphonia;* others refer to cause, as in the case of *cleft-palate speech;* and still other terms refer to both symptoms and cause, as in the case of *deaf-mutism.* Meanings of the core terms may often be acquired first from the general definitions; these then become more and more specific in context. Often it will be helpful to have a means of referring to the general definitions when terms are found in contexts which do not adequately clarify them.

The student or professional worker will be involved continually in three types of communication: He will be reading the literature in the field; he will be talking about speech pathology and audiology in various situations; and he will be writing clinical reports for professional purposes or writing for publication. In all of these communication functions, his ability to use and understand appropriate terminology and nomenclature is of signal importance. It is important enough to warrant a direct approach to the development of a technical vocabulary.

ANATOMICAL TERMS

For many years, the designation of body parts and diseases by names of persons has been popular among clinical workers and medical specialists, but it has been accompanied by a growing resistance against the practice, especially when other terms are available. The main problem is that there is no logical connection except an historical one when an anomaly, syndrome, or body part is named after an individual who first observed or described it. To know or remember the term in such instances is a matter of rote learning; but the student must take terminology as it is and not as it perhaps ought to be. Recently the term Hz has been adopted to stand for wave frequency and *cycles per second* in recognition of Heinrich Hertz and his work with electromagnetic waves. As far as sound waves are concerned, the term Hz could well stand for Helmholtz, who contributed much more than Hertz to the understanding of acoustics and the human perception of sound.

In 1895 the Anatomical Society, meeting in international convention in Basle, Switzerland, adopted a list of nearly 5,000 anatomical terms which are known today as the B.N.A. (Basle Nomina Anatomica). This is the basic system of terminology now used in anatomy, although it has been under revision for some time in an attempt to decrease the number of terms and to simplify them. Many muscles of the body have two names, one in Latin and one in English. Some muscles have more than one Latin name, and some have Anglicized versions of the B.N.A. names.

Muscles are named on the basis of several characteristics: 1) their shape, such as the *orbicularis oris* which is circular; 2) their location, such as the *buccinator* which is situated in the cheek; 3) the direction in which their fibers run, such as the *transversus linguae* with fibers running across the tongue; 4) the number of their divisions, such as the *quadriceps femoris* consisting of four muscles attached to a common tendon; 5) their action, such as the *levator palati* which raises the soft palate; and 6) their points of attachment, such as the *glossopalatinus* with one end attached to the tongue and the other to the soft palate. Nerves are similarly named according to their locations, the structures they serve, their arrangement, and their functions.

A GLOSSARY OF TERMS USED IN SPEECH PATHOLOGY AND AUDIOLOGY

AAAS: American Association for the Advancement of Science.

AAOO: American Academy of Ophthalmology and Otolaryngology.

abdominal wall muscles: the anterolateral muscles of the abdomen consisting of the obliquus externus abdominis, obliquus internus abdominis, transversus abdominis, rectus abdominis, and pyramidalis; important in controlled exhalation because their contraction forces the intestinal mass inward and upward in opposition to the descent of the diaphragm.

abducent n.: VIth Cranial nerve; innervates the lateral rectus muscle of the eye.

abduct: to draw away from the axis of the body; to move away from the midline or from a neighboring part or limb. Opp. to *adduct.*

aberration: deviation from the usual course; a disordered mental state.

ABESPA: American Board of Examiners in Speech Pathology and Audiology; a board functioning under the auspices of the American Speech and Hearing Association for the purpose of certifying members.

ablate: to remove, especially by cutting.

abreaction: the process of acting off, working off, or discharging original, repressed feelings by living through them again in speech or action, usually in the presence of the psychoanalyst.

abscissa: the horizontal axis of reference in a two-dimensional graph. Dist. from *ordinate.*

acalculia: loss of the ability to do simple arithmetic, often as the result of a brain lesion.

accent: an articulative effort giving prominence, stress, or increased sonority to one syllable of a word or group of words over adjacent syllables; sometimes used to designate the retention of foreign language characteristics in spoken English.

accessory n.: Same as *spinal accessory nerve.*

acoustic n.: the sensory nerve for hearing and equilibrium; the VIIIth Cranial nerve having two roots, the vestibular branch originating in the vestibule and the semicircular canals and the cochlear branch originating in the cochlea.

acoustic spectrum: the distribution of the intensity levels of the various frequency components of a sound.

acoustics: the science of sound including the origin, transmission, and effects of mechanical vibrations in any medium, whether audible or not.

adduct: to draw toward the midline or toward the axis of the body. Opp. to *abduct.*

adenoids: an enlargement of the phargyneal tonsil, a mass of lymphoid tissue located in about the center of the posterior wall of the nasopharynx.

adiadochokinesis: inability to perform rapid, repetitive movements. See *diadochokinesis.*

aditus: an entrance or approach; for example, the *aditus laryngis*, the entrance of the larynx.

adrenal gland: a ductless gland located at the upper end of each kidney. Same as *suprarenal gland.*

adventitious deafness: deafness acquired through illness or accident; not congenital.

aerophagia: spasmodic swallowing of air followed by belching.

aerotitis: malfunction of the Eustachian tube; used in reference to flyers in World War II.

affective: an adjective connoting any variety of feeling, emotional experience, or emotional accompaniment.

afferent: conducting toward the brain or spinal cord; refers to nerves which convey sensory impulses from the periphery to the central nervous system. Opp. to *efferent.*

affricate: a fricative speech sound initiated by a plosive. Examples are [tʃ] as in *chew* and [dʒ] as in *jam.*

agitographia: extremely rapid writing with unconscious omission and distortion of letters, words, or parts of words.

agitophasia: extremely rapid speech in which sounds, words, or parts of words are unconsciously omitted or distorted. Same as *agitolalia.*

agnosia: loss of the function of recognition of individual sensory stimuli; varieties correspond with the several senses.

agonist: a contracting muscle opposed in action by another muscle called the *antagonist.*

agrammalogia: inability to produce words in their correct sequence; impairment of the power to speak grammatically and syntactically. Same as *agrammatalogia*, *agrammatica*, and *agrammatism.*

agraphia: inability to express thoughts in writing due to a lesion in the central nervous system.

air blade: descriptive of friction sounds emitted through an opening that is wide horizontally and very narrow vertically, as in the sound of [f].

air-bone gap: the differences between a patient's bone conduction hearing thresholds and his air conduction hearing thresholds as shown on his audiogram. See *Carhart notch.*

air conduction: the normal process of conducting sound waves through the ear canal to the drum membrane. Dist. from *bone conduction.*

alalia: inability to speak due to impairment or absence of one or more of the peripheral speech organs, that is, impairment of muscles and sense organs involved in speech.

alexia: complete inability to read, characterized by an associative learning disability. See *dyslexia.*

alogia: inability to speak due to a lesion in the central nervous system or to mental impairment.

alpha wave: a type of brain wave registered by an electroencephalograph representing about 10 major discharges of cortical cells per second. Alpha rhythm is relatively low in frequency and high in voltage and is associated with reduced levels of consciousness. Dist. from *beta wave.*

alternate binaural loudness-balance test: a test of recruitment used in diagnosis of sensorineural hearing impairment when hearing loss is primarily monaural; a comparison is made among hearing levels at which pure tones sound equally loud to the patient.

alveolar ridge: the upper or lower gum ridge containing the row of sockets which enclose the teeth.

alveolus: tooth socket; also, an air sac of the lung.

AMA: American Medical Association.

ambidextrous: able to use either hand effectively.

ambivalence: the simultaneous existence of contradictory and contrasting emotions toward the same person; Bleuler's term for the tendency of some patients to give expression equally to opposing impulses.

amentia: a permanent form of mental retardation with a wide variety of clinical manifestations; mental deficiency based on congenital or developmental factors which retard the rate of maturing and reduce the ultimate level of behavior. Dist. from *dementia.*

amnesia: a disorder characterized by partial or total inability to recall or to identify past experiences; lack or loss of memory.

amplitude: largeness; wideness, breadth of range or extent; the distance through space a vibrating body moves; directly related to intensity of sound and sometimes used synonymously with *intensity* and *volume.*

amusia: inability to produce or to comprehend musical sounds.

anacusis: total deafness. Same as *anakusis.*

anarthria: inability to articulate due to brain lesion or damage to peripheral nerves which innervate the articulatory muscles.

anesthesia: loss of feeling or sensation.

aneurysm: a sac formed by the dilation of the walls of an artery or vein and filled with blood.

angular gyrus: a convolution of the cerebral cortex continuous anteriorly with the supramarginal gyrus; in the left hemisphere a probable center for some of the functions of speech.

ankylosis: the stiffening of a joint which impairs articulation of the bones at the joint.

annular: shaped like a ring.

anomaly: a structure or function which deviates from the normal.

anomia: loss of the power to name objects or to recall and recognize names.

anorexia: lack or loss of appetite for food.

anoxemia: deficiency in the oxygen content of the blood.

antagonist: a muscle which acts in opposition to another muscle. Opp. to *agonist.*

anterior: stituated in front of or in the forward part of; toward the head end of the body; also, toward the ventral side. Opp. to *posterior.*

anthelix: the inner curved ridge of the pinna.

antitragus: a prominence on the pinna opposite the tragus.

antitropy: a condition in which an organ forms a symmetrical pair with another; such as the cerebral hemispheres.

APA: American Psychological Association; American Psychoanalytic Association; American Psychiatric Association.

aphasia: loss of symbolic formulation and expression due to brain lesion. See *dysphasia.*

aphemia: inability to speak due to a lesion of the central nervous system; term originally used by Broca and later supplanted by the term *aphasia.*

aphonia: loss or absence of voice as a result of the failure of the vocal cords to vibrate properly.

aphrasia: inability to speak in phrases or to understand words arranged in phrases.

aplasia: incomplete or defective development of tissue.

apperception: focused perception, as exhibited in the relative clearness or prominence of certain of the data in perception.

apraxia: loss of the ability to execute simple voluntary acts; especially loss of the ability to perform elementary units of action in the expression of language.

articulation: literally the state of being united by a joint or joints; in speech, the production of individual sounds in connected discourse; the movement and placement during speech of the organs which serve to interrupt or modify the voiced or unvoiced air stream into meaningful sounds; the speech function performed largely through the movements of the lower jaw, lips, tongue, and soft palate. In an older sense, the term articulation refers to the intelligibility of a speech sample in relation to some variable dimension of its production such as amplification.

articulation curve: one plotted from the increases of PB words that are intelligible and the increases of the intensity levels at which they are presented to the subject.

artificial ear: a metered device for calibrating the output of a pure-tone audiometer by coupling the audiometer headphones to a microphone of known characteristics; the coupling device is constructed so that its dimensions approximate those of the average ear canal.

artificial larynx: any external device which produces a substitute sound for a lost vocal function; a battery-powered device which generates a sound resembling laryngeal vibrations and which is held against the outside of the throat so that the sounds thus transferred to the pharyngeal cavity may be articulated.

aryepiglottic: pertaining to the arytenoid cartilage and to the epiglottis.

arytenoid: shaped like a pitcher; one of a pair of

cartilages mounted on the cricoid cartilage and attached to the vocal band at the posterior end. The movement of the arytenoids approximate the vocal bands.

ASA: American Standards Association.

ASHA: American Speech and Hearing Association; also the name of the monthly journal dealing with news, announcements, and professional matters.

aspirate: a phonetic unit whose identifying characteristic is the sound generated by the passage of air through a relatively open channel; the sound of [h]; a sound followed by or combined with the sound of [h].

assimilation: a process of adaptive change in speech sounds uttered in close sequence. When two sounds become contiguous, one or both may undergo changes which make each more like its neighbor.

atavism: the reappearance of long-absent or dormant characteristics after one or more generations.

ataxia: a disorder characterized by marked disturbance in muscular coordination; irregularity of muscular action.

athetosis: a recurring series of slow, twisting movements of the skeletal musculature due principally to brain lesion.

atresia: absence or closure of an opening.

atrophy: a wasting away or diminution in the size of cell, tissue, organ, or part.

attenuate: to reduce in intensity or amount.

audiogram: a graphic summary of the measurements of hearing loss showing number of decibels loss at each frequency tested.

audiology: the study of the entire field of hearing, normal and disordered; it is concerned with the nature of hearing, conservation of hearing, identification of hearing loss in the population, assessment of hearing loss in the individual, and the rehabilitation of all those with hearing impairment; within the field of study and practice there are specialities consisting of diagnostic work, rehabilitation, research, and teaching.

audiometer: a device for the testing of hearing; it is calibrated to register hearing loss in terms of decibels.

audiometric zero: the zero reference setting for the tone-intensity control at each selected frequency on a pure-tone audiometer; the tone intensity obtained at zero is presumed to represent the average normal hearing threshold at each frequency used for testing; recently the sound pressure level of audiometric zero in the U.S. has been reduced from that set by the American Standards Association to that set by the International Organization for Standardization on the basis that the contour of average normal hearing at the usual frequencies tested is six to 15 decibels better than that established by the earlier American hearing surveys.

auditory aphasia: defect, loss, or nondevelopment of the ability to comprehend spoken words, due to disease, injury, or maldevelopment of the hearing centers of the brain; word deafness. Same as *receptive aphasia.*

auditory discrimination: ability to discriminate between sounds of different frequency, intensity, and pressure-pattern components; ability to distinguish one speech sound from another.

auditory feedback: hearing one's own speech; part of the control system of the speaking act in which output is fed back to the ear producing a self-monitoring regulation of speech. See *delayed auditory feedback* and *side-tone.*

auditory memory span: the number of related or unrelated items that can be recalled immediately after hearing them presented.

auditory n.: Same as *acoustic n.*

auditory perception: mental awareness of sound.

auditory training: any method applied to a hearing-impaired child or adult which has the purpose of teaching him to use more effectively his remaining hearing with or without a hearing aid.

aural: pertaining to the ear or to the sensation of hearing. Same as *auditory.*

auricle: the portion of the external ear not contained within the head. Same as *pinna.*

auscultation: the act of listening for sounds within the body.

autism: a psychological aspect of schizophrenia; in childhood the chief symptoms of autism are withdrawal behavior, reduction or absence of socialization, bizarre play activity, echolalia, lack of verbal communication, purposeless activity, and perseveration.

automatic audiometry: testing hearing by means of audiometers operated by the person tested. See *Békésy audiometer.*

automatic speech: inappropriate words or phrases produced without voluntary control as characteristic of aphasic adults; also, words such as consecutive numbers, days of the week, expletives, and various kinds of accessory expressions.

autonomic nervous system: the efferent system of peripheral nerves, ganglia, and plexuses which innervate smooth muscles, gland cells, and the heart. Same as visceral system. Dist. from *central nervous system.*

azygous: having no fellow; said of an unpaired muscle.

babbling: a stage in the acquisition of speech during which the child carries on vocal play with its random production of different speech sounds.

baby-talk: a speech defect characterized by substitution of speech sounds similar to those used by the normal-speaking child in the early stages of speech development. Same as *lalling* and *infantile speech.*

barbaralalia: habitual use of the speech sounds and rhythmo-melody of a native language when learning to speak another. Same as *foreign accent.*

basal ganglia: the collection or mass of nerve cells below the cortex of the brain connecting the cerebrum with the lower centers and comprising the thalami, corpora striata, corpora quadrigemina, tuber cinerum, and geniculate bodies.

basilar membrane: the lower boundary of the scala media or middle passage of the cochlear canal in the internal ear.

beats: the pulsations heard when two tones of different frequencies are perceived at the same time; the periodic increases in intensity due to phase differences of two tones produced simultaneously and in which there are as many beats per second as there are differences in Hz.

Békésy audiometer: one first developed by Georg von Békésy (1947) with which the patient makes his own audiogram tracings by pushing and releasing a button to indicate whether or not he hears pure tones at changing intensity levels.

Bell's palsy: paralysis of the facial muscles due to lesion of the VIIth Cranial or facial nerve resulting in a characteristic distortion of facial symmetry.

beta wave: a type of brain wave registered by an electroencephalograph representing about 20–30 discharges of cortical cells per second. Beta rhythm is relatively high in frequency and low in voltage and is associated with heightened states of attention. Dist. from *alpha wave.*

bicuspid: having two cusps or points; one of eight premolar teeth in man, two on each side, upper and lower, located between the cuspid and first molar.

bifurcation: division into two branches like a fork.

bilabial: used to describe a consonant sound formed with the aid of both lips as in [p], [b], and [m].

bilingual: having two native languages; being reared in a two-language environment.

binaural: pertaining to both ears.

BNA *system:* scientific anatomical terminology adopted by international convention at Basle, Switzerland in 1895; Basle Nomina Anatomica. See BR, NK, INA, and PNA systems.

bone conduction: the transmission of sound waves through the head bones to the inner ear. Dist. from *air conduction.*

BR *system:* British revision of the BNA *system* of anatomical terminology adopted in 1933. See BNA, NK, INA, and PNA *systems.*

brain stem: all of the brain except the cerebellum and the cerebral hemispheres. Same as *segmental apparatus.*

brain waves: See *alpha wave* and *beta wave.*

Broca's area: the inferior frontal gyrus in the left cerebral hemisphere of right-handed persons identified by Broca in 1861 as the cortical association center for motor speech. Same as *Broca's convolution* or *center.*

bronchus: one of two main branches of the trachea.

buccal: pertaining to the mouth cavity and the cheeks.

buccinator: the flat muscle of the cheek which controls compression and distention of the cheek wall.

bulbar: pertaining to the medulla oblongata, the bulb of nervous tissue continuous above with the pons and below with the spinal cord.

bulbar paralysis: paralysis due to changes in the motor centers of the medulla oblongata or bulb usually marked by paralysis and atrophy of the muscles of the lips, tongue, mouth, pharynx, and larynx.

ca.: L. *circa,* approximately.

canine: the single cuspid tooth between the lateral incisor and the premolar. Same as *cuspid.*

caninus m.: a muscle originating in the fossa of the maxilla and inserted in the orbicularis oris; innervated by the facial (VIIth Cranial) nerve and acts to raise the corners of the mouth.

Carhart notch: a loss in bone-conduction hearing acuity at 500, 1,000, 2,000, and 4,000 Hz observed by Raymond Carhart in otosclerotic patients and not attributable to cochlear impairment but due to the blockage of cochlear fluid movement by the fixated stapes; used as a correction for more accurate assessment of preoperative bone-conduction hearing loss.

catalogia: the insane repetition of meaningless words and sentences. Same as *verbigeration.*

catarrhal deafness: hearing loss caused by inflammation of the mucous membrane of the air passages in the head and throat with blockage of the Eustachian tube.

catharsis: see *psychocatharsis.*

caudal: toward the tail; in a posterior direction. Opp. to *cephalic.*

caudate nucleus: a pear-shaped mass of nerve cells, the largest component of the corpus striatum in the brain; it lies in contact with the cephalic end of the thalamus and has relation to the production of voluntary activity.

central deafness: impairment of hearing as a result of damage to auditory nerve pathways in the brain stem, in on-relaying pathways, or in the centers of hearing in the cerebral cortex; may be caused by brain tumor, brain injury, kernicterus, or vascular changes in the brain.

central nervous system: the brain and the spinal cord; abbreviated C.N.S.

central tendon: the heart-shaped fibrous cord of connective tissue in which the muscle fibers of the diaphragm end.

cephalic: pertaining to the head or directed toward the head end of the body. Opp. to *caudal.*

cerebellum: a main division of the brain situated behind the cerebrum and above the pons; it is concerned with the coordination of muscular activity.

cerebral dominance: a condition in which one cerebral hemisphere leads the other in the initiation and control of bodily movement.

cerebral palsy: paralysis or muscular incoordination due to intracranial lesion; the term is applied to a group of cerebral afflictions in children including Little's disease, spastic paralysis, and many others.

cerebrospinal fluid: the fluid contained within the cerebral ventricles, subarachnoid sinus, and the central canal of the spinal cord.

cerebrum: the main portion of the brain consisting of two equal hemispheres united at the bottom by a band of connective tissue called the corpus callosum.

cerumen: waxlike secretion found in the external canal of the ear.
cervical: pertaining to the region of the neck; the term is applied to the vertebrae and to the nerves distributed in this region.
cf.: L. *confer*, compare.
CGS *system:* the centimeter-gram-second system of measuring distance, weight, and time in the metric system.
chorditis tuberosa: a small whitish node on one or both vocal bands.
chorea: a convulsive nervous disease characterized by involuntary and irregular jerking movements.
chronic: long-continued; not sharp, severe, or acute.
CID: Central Institute for the Deaf, St. Louis.
cleft palate: congenital fissure of the soft palate and roof of the mouth, sometimes extending through the premaxilla and upper lip.
clinic: an establishment where patients are admitted for special study and treatment usually by a group of specialists in different areas.
clinical: literally, pertaining to the bedside; pertaining to or founded on actual observation and treatment of cases as distinguished from theoretical or experimental; pertaining to individual diagnosis and treatment on the basis of individual symptoms and not on the basis of membership in a stereotyped group.
clonus: muscular spasm in which there is an alternation of rigidity and relaxation.
cluttering: rapid, nervous speech marked by omission of sounds or syllables.
cochlea: the auditory part of the internal ear; it is shaped like a snail shell and contains the basilar membrane upon which are situated the hair cells or end organs of the cochlear branch of the VIIIth Cranial nerve.
communication: the process of imparting to one another ideas, thoughts, feelings or opinions by means of signs, signals, and symbols expressed consciously or unconsciously; a broader and more inclusive term than *language* and *speech.*
communication network: a pattern organized formally or informally through which thoughts or feelings are transmitted among members of a group.
communication theory: a body of more or less plausible or scientifically acceptable principles offered to describe and explain the sociopsychological nature of communication among human beings; a loosely defined field of study which draws together from other disciplines those observations and research which bear upon various aspects of communication.
concha: a structure resembling a shell in shape as the hollow of the external ear or the turbinate bones in the nose.
conditioned response: a response, simple or elaborated, aroused in a subject by some stimulus other than the original or biologically adequate one as a result of the two stimuli having been presented simultaneously or in some time relationship. Same as *substitute response.*
conditioned stimulus: an originally ineffective stimulus which, when presented simultaneously or in some time relationship with an effective stimulus, brings about by itself the same response as the effective stimulus. Same as *substitute stimulus.*
conduction deafness: an impairment of hearing due to damage or obstruction of the ear canal, drum membrane, or the ossicular chain in the middle ear; a failure of air vibrations to be adequately conducted to the cochlea.
consonant: a conventional speech sound produced, with or without laryngeal vibration, by certain successive contractions of the articulatory muscles which modify, interrupt, or obstruct the expired air stream to the extent that its pressure is raised.
continuant: a speech sound in which the speech organs are held relatively fixed during the period of production. Examples are [s], [m], [f], and the vowels.
contralateral: associated with a part on the opposite side.
conversion: a psychoanalytical term referring to the transformation of repressed emotions into a physical manifestation as in hysterical deafness or hysterical aphonia.
conversion deafness: See *hysterical deafness.*
corniculate cartilage: a small nodule at the apex of each arytenoid cartilage in the larynx.
corpus callosum: an arched band of white matter whose transverse fibers connect the two cerebral hemispheres at the bottom below the longitudinal fissure.
cortex: the outer layers of an organ as distinguished from its inner substance; the cerebral cortex is the ashen-gray matter making up the outer layers of the cerebrum.
cps: cycles per second. See Hz.
CR: conditioned response.
Cranial nerve: a nerve which originates or terminates within the cranium; there are 12 pairs numbered I–XII. Dist. from *spinal nerve.*
cretinism: a congenital condition due to thyroid deficiency and characterized by physical and mental retardation.
cricoarytenoid m.: an intrinsic muscle of the larynx originating in the side and back of the cricoid cartilage and inserted at the base of the arytenoid cartilages; the lateral pair closes the glottis and the posterior pair opens the glottis; all are innervated by the recurrent laryngeal nerve.
cricoid cartilage: a ringlike cartilage forming the lower and back part of the laryngeal cavity.
cricothyroid m.: an intrinsic muscle of the larynx originating on the front side of the cricoid cartilage and inserted at the lower border of the thyroid cartilage; it is innervated by the superior laryngeal nerve and acts to tense the vocal bands.
cuneiform cartilage: a wedge-shaped cartilage on either side of the aryepiglottic fold in the larynx.
cuspid: a tooth having one cusp or point. Same as *canine.*
cutaneous: pertaining to the skin.

CVA: cerebral vascular accident; a stroke.
cyanosis: blueness of the skin due to insufficient oxygenation of the blood; usually the result of heart malformation.
cybernetics: studies involving the analogous functioning of the nervous system and electromechanical control systems such as computing machines.

DAF: delayed auditory feedback.
damping effect: diminution of the amplitude of vibrations because of the absorption of energy by the surrounding medium.
dB: decibel; capitalization is in honor of Alexander G. Bell.
deaf: pertaining to congenital loss of all usable hearing.
deafened: pertaining to adventitious loss of all usable hearing.
deaf-mute: a person who can neither hear nor speak; usually one who is born deaf.
decibel: a logarithmic ratio unit indicating by what proportion one intensity level differs from another; the decibel is equal to approximately one just-noticeable difference of loudness under certain conditions; sometimes inaccurately called a *sensation unit*.
decussation: the crossing of nerve tracts in their course to or from lower centers of the central nervous system.
delayed auditory feedback: an experimentally imposed electronic delay of speech signals returning to the speaker's ears by way of headphones when he talks.
delayed speech: failure of speech to develop at the expected age; usually due to slow maturation, hearing impairment, brain injury, mental retardation, or emotional disturbance.
denasality: pertains to the quality of the voice when the nasal passages are obstructed to prevent adequate nasal resonance during speech.
dental: a speech sound made by tongue or lip contact with the teeth; pertaining to teeth.
dextral: pertaining to or located on the right side of the body. Opp. to *sinistral*.
diadochokinesis: the performance of rapid, alternating and repetitive bodily movements such as opening and closing the jaws or lips, raising and lowering the eyebrows, or tapping the finger.
diagnosis: the study of the nature of a disorder, its origin, development, and symptoms; also the identification of a disorder by such procedure.
diaphragm: the muscular and tendonous partition which separates the abdominal and thoracic cavities; the chief muscle in breathing.
diathesis: an inherited tendency or predisposition to certain diseases or disorders.
diphthong: a speech sound gliding continuously from one vowel to another in the same syllable such as [ɑʊ], [ɔɪ], and [aɪ].
diplacusis: the hearing of one sound as two; the difference between the apparent frequency of the same sound as heard by each of the two ears.
diplegia: paralysis affecting like parts on either side of the body; bilateral paralysis.
DL: difference limen; the degree of change in any stimulus required to produce a just-noticeable difference in perception on the part of a subject. See *jnd*.
Doerfler-Stewart test: an auditory test to determine functional or psychogenic hearing loss by examining a patient's ability to respond to spondee words spoken in the presence of a masking noise through earphones; in cases of functional hearing loss the masking noise prevents the patient from being consistent in his responses to the word stimuli at varying intensity levels.
dorsal: the back side; pertains to any part which corresponds to the back in position. Opp. to *ventral*.
drum membrane: the eardrum or membrane which separates the external ear from the middle ear. Same as *tympanic membrane*.
dsh Abstracts; a quarterly publication containing short summaries of current articles related to deafness, speech, and hearing from professional journals throughout the world; published jointly by ASHA and Gallaudet College.
dyne: the force required to accelerate one gram of mass at the rate of one centimeter per second per second; in measuring sound pressure the reference level is a pressure of .0002 dyne/cm^2, the force exerted against a field of one square centimeter. See *microbar*.
dysarthria: a disorder of articulation due to impairment of the part of the central nervous system which directly controls the muscles of articulation.
dyslalia: defective articulation due to faulty learning or to abnormality of the external speech organs and not to lesions of the central nervous system.
dyslexia: partial inability to read characterized by associative learning difficulty; a form of dysphasia. See *alexia*.
dyslogia: defective speech associated with mental impairment.
dysphasia; partial or complete loss of the ability to speak or to comprehend the spoken word due to injury, disease, or maldevelopment of the brain. Same as *aphasia*.
dysphemia; a nervous disorder of speech arising from psychological disturbance; includes stuttering.
dysphonia: a disturbance of vocalization; any defect of phonation.
dysrhythmia: abnormality in speech rhythm characterized by defects of stress placement, defects of breath-grouping, or defects of inflection.

E: examiner or experimenter.
ear canal: See *external auditory meatus*.
eardrum: commonly used to mean *tympanic membrane*, but technically represents the entire *middle ear* or *tympanum*.
echolalia: automatic reiteration of words or phrases, usually those which have just been heard.
EDA: electrodermal audiometry. See GSR.

EDR: electrodermal response. See GSR.

EEG: electroencephalography. See *brain waves*.

EEG *audiometry:* the use of electroencephalography to obtain gross measures of hearing sensitivity by studying changes in brain-wave patterns when sound stimuli are introduced at levels above the patient's threshold.

efferent: conducting from a central region to a peripheral region; refers to nerves which convey motor impulses from the central nervous system to the muscles. Opp. to *afferent*.

e.g.: L. *exempli gratia*, for example.

elasticity: the capacity of a body to return to its original form or position after deformation by some applied force.

electroencephalograph: an instrument for graphically recording electrical currents developed in the cerebral cortex during brain functioning; often abbreviated EEG.

emphasis: a prominence of utterance given to one or more words or syllables.

encephalitis: inflammation of the brain or its membranous envelopes.

endolymph: the fluid contained in the labyrinth of the inner ear.

enuresis: involuntary discharge of urine.

epiglottis: a lidlike cartilage, shaped like a bicycle seat, which covers the entrance to the laryngeal cavity.

epilepsy: a chronic functional disease characterized by convulsions and loss of consciousness for short periods; the mild form is called *petit mal* and the severe form *grand mal*.

epileptiform: refers to behavior which resembles manifestations of epilepsy.

erythroblastosis fetalis: a congenital disease of the red blood cells resulting from blood-group incompatibilities of mother and fetus.

esophageal voice: low-frequency vibrations produced by the upper narrow portion of the esophagus when swallowed air bubbles are belched out.

et al.: L. *et alii*, and others.

ethmoid bone: the sievelike bone which forms a roof for the nasal hollows and a portion of the floor of the anterior fossa of the cranium.

etiology: the study of causes of a given condition.

euphoria: bodily comfort; well-being; sometimes a pathological mental state characterized by unfounded feelings of optimism, strength, or health.

Eustachian tube: a channel about 35 mm. long connecting the tympanic cavity with the nasopharynx and serving to adjust air pressure within the tympanic cavity to that of the air on the external side of the drum membrane.

experimental phonetics: a laboratory science concerned with measurement, description, and analysis of speech signals, their production, and the processes by which they are perceived and interpreted; sometimes the same as *voice science*.

expiration: the act of breathing out and expelling air from the lungs.

expressive aphasia: a disturbance of speech due to brain lesion and in which the major difficulty is inability to remember the pattern of movements required to produce words even though the patient knows what he wants to say.

extensor: any muscle which functions to extend the organ to which it is attached. Opp. to *flexor*.

external auditory meatus: the passage through the temporal bone from the external ear to the tympanic cavity of the middle ear where it is sealed by the drum membrane.

extrapyramidal tract: outside the pyramidal tracts.

extrinsic muscle: a muscle whose origin and insertion are not in the same organ or part; a muscle which connects an organ to the bony skeleton or to other organs or parts. Dist. from *intrinsic muscle*.

facial n.: the VIIth Cranial nerve, motor to the muscles of the face.

falsetto: the artificial voice of the male lying above his natural range of pitch.

fauces: the passage between the mouth and the pharynx.

febrile: pertaining to fever.

fenestra ovalis: an oval opening in the inner wall of the middle ear into which the footplate of the stapes is inserted. Same as *oval window*.

fenestra rotunda: a round opening in the inner wall of the middle ear below the oval window and covered by a membrane permitting accommodation of pressure on the fluid in the cochlea. Same as *round window*.

fenestration: the act of perforation; specifically, the operation for improvement of hearing in otosclerotic conditions in which a substitute "window" is formed in the bony wall of the middle ear and into the horizontal semicircular canal in order to enable sound waves to excite the cochlea.

finger spelling: the use of the manual alphabet to spell out words for the deaf.

flaccid paralysis: paralysis with loss of tonus and absence of reflexes in the affected parts producing a weak, flabby, and relaxed condition. Dist. from *spastic paralysis*.

flat hearing loss: one in which the loss is observed to be about the same at all important frequencies.

flexor: any muscle which flexes or bends a joint. Opp. to *extensor*.

foreign accent: the influence of speech sounds of a native language on those of a later learned second language.

formant: a natural mode of air vibration in the vocal tract characterized on a spectrogram by a dark area indicating a relatively high intensity of a group of frequency components.

fossa: a pit, depression, hollow, or trench.

Fourier analysis: application of a mathematical principle according to which any complex sound may be represented as the sum of a series of pure tones whose frequencies increase in the ratio of the natural numbers 1, 2, 3, 4, 5, etc.; resolving complex vibrations into single components.

free association: a psychoanalytic process in which the patient verbalizes everything that enters his mind, without selection, without reacting to external stimuli, and without preexamination or censorship of his utterances.

free field testing: a method of measuring auditory sensitivity by reducing sound intensity to the threshold of perception and measuring the actual intensity of the sound after the subject has been removed from the field in order to eliminate the effect of absorption, reflection, and diffraction by the body.

frenum: a fold of the skin or mucous membrane which checks or limits the movements of an organ or part; usually the lingual frenum under the tongue.

frequency: the number of cycles per second of a wave or other periodic phenomenon.

fricative: any speech sound produced by forcing an air stream through a narrow opening and resulting in audible high-frequency vibrations. Examples are [f], [ʃ], and [v].

frontal lobe: that part of either hemisphere of the cerebrum which lies above the Sylvian fissure and in front of the Rolandic fissure.

functional defect: any defect in which structural alteration can be neither demonstrated nor inferred. Dist. from *organic defect.*

fundamental tone: the lowest tone in a complex tone. Dist. from *overtone.*

Gallaudet College: a college exclusively for the deaf located in Washington, D.C. and supported by the federal government.

general semantics: an adaptation of the science of meaning developed by Alfred Korzybski and applied to human problems; a collection of such doctrines aimed at improving interpersonal adjustment by securing better orientational adequacy of word-fact relationship.

genioglossus m.: a muscle originating in the mental spine of the mandible and inserted in the under surface of the tongue and in the hyoid bone; it is innervated by the hypoglossal nerve and acts to depress, retract, and protrude the tongue.

geriatrics: the branch of medicine which treats the clinical problems of old age.

German measles: See *rubella.*

gerontology: study of the aging process and its diseases.

glossal: pertaining to the tongue.

glossopalatinus m.: a muscle originating in the under surface of the soft palate and inserted in the side of the tongue; it lifts the back of the tongue and narrows the fauces.

glossopharyngeal n.: the IXth Cranial nerve; distributed to the middle ear, pharynx, meninges, tonsils, and tongue; serves the taste receptors in the back of the tongue and motor functions of the throat.

glottis: the opening between the vocal bands.

GSR: galvanic skin response; used as a method of testing hearing in which the patient receives a pure-tone stimulus from an audiometer and an electric shock at nearly the same time; the patient is conditioned to respond to the tone as an emotion-producing stimulus, and when conditioning has been achieved, the patient responds emotionally to the tone alone if he is able to hear it; results of the testing are read on the basis of whether or not the skin resistance decreases as an indication of momentary emotional response.

gutturophonia: a form of dysphonia characterized by a throaty or guttural voice.

gyrus: a fold or convolution of the cerebral cortex bounded by fissures and sulci.

hard-of-hearing: applied to those whose hearing is impaired but who have enough hearing left for practical use.

hard palate: the bony anterior part of the roof of the mouth.

harelip: a congenital cleft of one or both of the lips, usually the upper lip.

harmonic: a partial tone or overtone whose frequency is an exact multiple of the lowest or fundamental tone.

hearing aid: any device which amplifies or focuses sound waves in the listener's ear; usually refers to the various types of wearable amplifiers which operate with miniature loudspeakers in the ear or oscillators on the head.

hearing center: a nonprofit agency with professionally qualified personnel which offers diagnosis, advice, and rehabilitation services to hard-of-hearing people.

hearing conservation: any program undertaken to preserve hearing and to prevent hearing loss through public education, through screening programs to identify persons needing attention, and through reduction of occupational hazards that pose a threat to a worker's hearing.

helicotrema: a small opening in the basilar membrane at the apex of the cochlear canal through which the scala tympani communicates with the scala vestibuli.

helix: the margin or curved border of the pinna or outer ear.

hemiatrophy: atrophy or wasting away of one side of the body, organ, or part. See *atrophy.*

hemorrhage: escape of blood from ruptured vessels.

high-pass filter: an electronic device which allows all frequency components of a sound wave to pass through except those below a certain cut-off frequency. See *low-pass filter.*

homophenous: a term applied to words which look alike to a person who is lip-reading.

hyoglossus m.: an extrinsic tongue muscle; it is innervated by the hypoglossal nerve and acts to depress the sides of the tongue and retract the tongue.

hyoid bone: a horseshoe-shaped bone situated at the base of the tongue and above the thyroid cartilage.

hypacusis: Same as *hard-of-hearing.*

hyperacusis: an abnormally acute sense of hearing.

hypernasality: a vowel quality characterized by the presence of excessive resonance of the voice in the nasal cavity usually due to varying degrees of functional or structural inadequacy of the velopharyngeal mechanism; a voice quality frequently perceived in cases of cleft palate.

hypertonicity: excessive tonus, tension, or activity. Same as *hypertonia.*

hypertrophy: the morbid enlargement or overgrowth of an organ or part due to increase in its tissue elements.

hypnosis: an artificially induced state resembling sleep but physiologically distinct from it and characterized by increased suggestibility.

hypochondria: morbid anxiety about health and pessimistic interpretation of bodily discomfort.

hypoglossal n.: the XIIth Cranial nerve; it innervates the hypoglossus muscle of the tongue.

hypophonia: a form of dysphonia characterized by a whispered voice.

hypoplasia: defective or incomplete development.

hysterical deafness: psychogenic hearing loss; a functional hearing impairment developed under emotional stress as an unconscious means of escape from intolerable situations. Same as *conversion deafness.*

Hz: a unit of vibration frequency adopted internationally to replace the term *cycles per second*; named after Heinrich Rudolf Hertz, German physicist.

ibid.: L. *ibidem*, in the place cited.

identification audiometry: methods used to discover or identify children or adults with hearing problems by screening large numbers to select those who need to be given more exact tests on an individual basis. See *Johnston test*, *Massachusetts test*, and *sweep-check test.*

idioglossia: omission, substitution, distortion, and transposition of so many sounds that speech is unintelligible and appears to be an invented language; often associated with mental retardation. Same as *idiolalia.*

idiolalia: See *idioglossia.*

idiopathic: pertains to a pathological condition of spontaneous origin; that is, not the result of some other disorder or injury.

i.e.: L. *id est*, that is.

implosion: the process of building up internal pressure in the air tract immediately prior to its explosive release in the production of plosive speech sounds.

in situ: L. in position.

INA *system:* Jena Nomina Anatomica, a revision of the anatomical classification system adopted in 1937. See BNA, NK, and PNA *systems.*

incisor: any one of the four front teeth in either the upper or lower jaw.

incus: the anvil-shaped middle bone of the three ossicles in the middle ear.

infantile speech: See *baby-talk.*

inferior: situated below.

information theory: a broad theory of communication which treats quantitatively the probability and accuracy of events in the transmission and translation of messages composed of symbols.

inner ear: the labyrinth; the end organ for hearing and balance consisting of the vestibule, saccule, utricle, the three semicircular canals, and the cochlea.

inner speech: the mental image of words in terms of visual, auditory, and kinesthetic sensations.

innervation: the supplying of any organ with efferent nerve impulses.

insertion: the place of attachment of a muscle to the bone it moves.

insight: a sudden apprehension of meaning without reference to previous experience.

intensity: the magnitude or degree of tension, activity, or energy; refers to the measure of the energy flow acting to produce a sound wave.

intercostal: situated between the ribs.

interdental sigmatism: substitution of [θ] and [ð] for [s] and [z]. See *lisping.*

internal acoustic meatus: a passage in the temporal bone for the facial and auditory nerves.

intrinsic muscle: a muscle whose origin and insertion are in the same organ; any muscle which lies wholly within a given organ. Dist. from *extrinsic muscle.*

introjection: the mental process of absorbing or appropriating the attributes of others into one's own personality system.

IPA: International Phonetic Alphabet established by the International Phonetic Association.

ipsilateral: situated on the same side. Opp. to *contralateral.*

IQ: intelligence quotient; the mental age divided by the chronological age and multiplied by 100.

ISO: International Organization for Standardization. See *audiometric zero.*

ITA: initial teaching alphabet; a reorganized set of aphabetical characters designed to facilitate the teaching of reading.

Jena method: a system of teaching lipreading developed by Karl Brauckmann in Jena, Germany; the method focuses attention on the syllable and rhythm patterns in speech.

jnd: just-noticeable difference; the smallest difference between two stimuli perceived by a subject 50 percent of the time. See DL.

John Tracy Clinic: a clinic in Los Angeles which specializes in deaf children of preschool age and concentrates on training parents to help their own deaf children.

Johnston test: a group pure-tone screening test for children in kindergarten through the second grade. See *Massachusetts test* and *sweep-check test.*

JSHD: *Journal of Speech and Hearing Disorders* published quarterly by the American Speech and Hearing Association.

JSHR: *Journal of Speech and Hearing Research* published quarterly by the American Speech and Hearing Association.

kernicterus: jaundiced areas of the brain brought about by destruction of red blood cells in the newborn; a cause of athetoid cerebral palsy, mental retardation, and central deafness. See *erythroblastosis fetalis*.

kinesthetic: pertaining to the sense by which muscular motion, position, or weight are perceived.

kymograph: an instrument used to record variations in any phsyiological or muscular process.

labial: pertaining to the lips; a speech sound produced with the aid of the lips. Examples are [p], [b], and [m].

labiodental: a speech sound produced by the contact of the lips with the teeth. Examples are [f] and [v].

labyrinth: the ramified passages of the internal ear made up of the cochlea, vestibule, and semicircular canals.

lalling: a babbling, infantile form of speech.

lalopathy: any form of speech disorder.

laminography: a system of taking x-ray pictures which show flat surfaces of various bodily sections.

language: any means, vocal or other, of expressing or communicating thought or feeling.

laryngectomy: surgical removal of the larynx, usually because of cancer.

laryngitis: inflammation of the larynx often resulting in hoarseness or loss of voice.

laryngology: the study and treatment of the throat, pharynx, larynx, nasopharynx, trachea, and bronchial tree.

laryngopharynx: the lower portion of the pharynx lying between the larynx and oropharynx.

laryngoscope: an apparatus used for visual examination of the larynx.

larynx: the cartilaginous and muscular structure situated at the top of the trachea and below the tongue roots and hyoid bone; the organ of voice consisting of nine cartilages connected by ligaments.

lateral: pertaining to a side.

lateral lisping: defective production of the sibilant sounds due to excessive escape of air over or around the sides of the tongue.

laterality: sidedness; handedness.

lesion: an injury or wound in any part of the body; deficit of tissue.

levator: any muscle concerned with lifting an organ or part.

levator veli palatini m.: a muscle which raises the soft palate.

ligament: a tough, fibrous band of tissue connecting bones or cartilages.

ligate: to tie or bind.

linguadental: a speech sound produced with the aid of the tongue and teeth. Examples are [θ] and [ð].

lingual: pertaining to the tongue.

linguistics: the study of the origin, structure, and modifications of speech; it includes phonetics, morphology, and semantics.

lipreading: the art of comprehending the speech of another through the visual interpretation of gestures, facial movements, and especially lip movements. Same as *speechreading*.

lisping: defective production of the sibilant sounds, caused by improper tongue placement or by abnormalities of the articulatory mechanism.

loc. cit.: L. *in loco citato*, in the place cited.

logopedics: the study and treatment of speech defects.

logorrhea: a mental aberration characterized by continuous, incoherent talking.

Lombard test: a special test for functional hearing loss in which masking sounds are introduced into the ears while the subject talks; the test is positive if the subject raises the intensity level of his voice in order to hear himself above the masking sound, and negative if his voice remains at a fixed level. Same as *voice-reflex test*.

longitudinal: lengthwise, running in the direction of the long axis of the body, organ, or part.

longitudinalis inferior m.: a muscle originating in the under surface of the tongue at its base and inserted in the tip; it is innervated by the *chorda tympani* and acts to shorten the tongue.

longitudinalis superior m.: a muscle originating in the submucosa and septum of the tongue and inserted in the edges of the tongue; it is innervated by the hypoglossal (XIIth Cranial) nerve and acts to shorten the tongue and to raise its edges and tip.

loudness: the intensity factor in sound.

low-pass filter: an electronic device which allows all frequency components of a sound wave to pass through except those above a certain cut-off frequency. See *high-pass filter*.

lumen: the area of the interior cross section of a tube.

macroglossia: an abnormally large tongue.

malingering: the pretending of illness or disability.

malleus: the first of the ossicles in the middle ear joining the drum membrane to the incus.

malocclusion: a condition in which the teeth do not come together properly due to malformation.

mand: Skinner's term for a verbal operant which specifies the reinforcement behavior of a listener; a term coined from *demand*, *command*, and *countermand* representing a functional linguistic expression and not a formal one. Examples are *wait! stop! listen!*

mandible: the lower jaw.

manualism: a method of instruction for the deaf in which the chief element is communication by means of finger spelling and sign language.

manubrium: handle; the uppermost piece of the sternum; the inferior process or handle of the malleus.

masking: a partial or complete obscuring of a tone by the simultaneous presentation in one or both ears of another sound.

Massachusetts test: a group pure-tone hearing test which enables an audiometrist to screen 40 school children simultaneously by presenting pure tones of 500, 4,000, and 6,000 Hz at 20, 25, and 30 dB respectively. See *Johnston test* and *sweep-check test*.

masseter m.: the large chewing muscle; it originates in the upper maxilla and is inserted in the lower jaw; it is innervated by the mandibular branch of the trigeminal nerve.

mastoid: pertaining to the mastoid process located just behind the ear.
mastoidectomy: an operation to cut away or take out infected mastoid cells in the mastoid bone in order to prevent the spread of disease within the skull.
maxilla: the irregularly shaped bone articulated with the ethmoid bone and forming the upper jaw.
MCL: most comfortable loudness level.
meatus: a canal. Same as *external auditory meatus.*
medial: pertaining to the middle; near the median plane.
medulla oblongata: the portion of the brain which is continuous with the spinal cord below and the pons above; it lies ventral to the cerebellum and its back forms the floor of the fourth ventricle.
melancholia: a form of mental disorder marked by depressed and painful emotional states with inhibited mental and bodily activity.
Ménière's disease: a sudden impairment of the inner ear producing a combination of tinnitus, dizziness, nausea, and hearing loss probably caused by an increased pressure in the endolymph.
meninges: the three membranes which envelop the brain and spinal cord; the *dura mater*, *pia mater*, and *arachnoid mater*.
meningitis: inflammation of the meninges.
mental: pertaining to the chin, from *mentum;* also pertaining to the mind, from *mens.*
mentalis m.: a muscle originating in the mandible and inserted in the skin of the chin; it is innervated by the facial (VIIth Cranial) nerve and acts to raise the lower lip and wrinkle the skin of the chin.
microbar: a unit of pressure used to measure the intensity of sound; one microbar equals the force of one dyne exerted against a field of one square centimeter. See *dyne.*
microglossia: an abnormally small tongue.
middle ear: the tympanic cavity containing the ossicular chain, the *stapedius* and *tensor tympani* muscles, the opening to the Eustachian tube, and the *chorda tympani* nerve passing through.
mirror writing: the tendency to write mirrored forms of letters, words, and numbers so that they are read correctly when seen in a mirror.
modiolus: the central column or pillar of the cochlea.
molar: one of the back grinding teeth of which there are three on each side in both jaws.
monaural: pertaining to one ear. Dist. from *binaural.*
mongolism: congenital mental defection marked by hyperactivity, imitativeness, malformation of the skull, oblique eyeslits, and shortness of thumbs and little finger.
Moro's reflex: a startle reflex in response to sound seen in newborn infants consisting of general muscle contraction and often eye-blinks.
motokinesthetic method: a method for developing speech in which the therapist manually manipulates some of the speech muscles of the patient or touches parts to suggest movement at that point.
motor aphasia: See *expressive aphasia.*
MR: mentally retarded.
mucous membrane: a membrane which secretes a viscid, watery substance called mucus.
musculus uvulae: an unpaired muscle originating in the posterior nasal spine and forming the greater part of the uvula; it acts to raise and shrivel the uvula.
mutism: inability to speak due to hysteria, abnormal inhibition, or deafness.
myotatic reflex: a reflex contraction of a muscle by suddenly stretching it longitudinally.
myringoplasty: a surgical restoration of the tympanic membrane.
myringotomy: making an incision in the drum membrane to allow drainage of the middle ear in cases of otitis media.

nares: the nostrils, both anterior and posterior.
nasal: pertaining to the nose; also a voiced continuant speech sound having nasal resonance as its distinctive acoustic characteristic. Examples are [m], [n], and [ŋ].
nasal emission: the escape of air through the nose preventing normal production of most consonant sounds due to deficit or malfunction of the soft palate.
nasal septum: the partition in the midplane which separates the two nasal cavities.
nasality: the quality of speech sounds when the nasal cavity is used as a resonator; especially when there is too much nasal resonance.
nasopharynx: the portion of the pharynx above the level of the soft palate.
nasoscope: an instrument used to inspect the nasal cavity.
n.b.: L. *nota bene*, note well.
negative practice: the deliberate and voluntary practicing of errors in order to break habits which have become automatic.
neologism: a new word; also a meaningless word spoken by a psychotic patient.
neonate: newborn.
neurasthenia: nervous exhaustion; a psychoneurosis characterized by abnormal fatigue.
neurogram: an automatic response; a habit.
neurosis: a relatively minor functional nervous disorder in which the personality system remains for the most part intact.
NK *system:* German revision of the system of anatomical nomenclature adopted in 1935 by the Nomenklatur-Komission report. See BNA, BR, INA, and PNA systems.
noise: psychologically, an unwanted sound; physically, an erratic, nonperiodic, intermittent, and statistically random vibratory activity.
nominal aphasia: aphasia marked by inability to recall names of objects. See *aphasia.*

O: observer.
obturator: an artificial disc, plate, or bulb used to partially or completely close an opening; used especially in cleft-palate cases.
occipital lobe: a cerebral lobe in the back part of the brain corresponding to the occipital bone.

occlude: to close tightly; to fit together.

occulomotor n.: the IIIrd Cranial nerve; it is motor to all muscles of the eye except the external rectus and superior oblique muscles.

olfactory n.: the Ist Cranial nerve; the sensory nerve of smell originating in the olfactory lobe and distributed to the nasal mucous membrane.

omohyoid m.: a muscle originating in the border of the scapula and inserted in the hyoid bone; it retracts and depresses the hyoid.

ontogeny: the developmental history of the individual.

op. cit.: L. *opere citato*, in the work cited.

operant: a unit of *operant behavior.*

operant behavior: a form or kind of behavior which has an effect on the environment which then has a return effect upon the individual; often used interchangeably with the term *response* except that the latter traditionally refers to an instance of behavior rather than a form or kind of behavior as designated by B. F. Skinner.

optic n.: the IInd Cranial nerve; the sensory nerve of vision originating in the occipital cortex and distributed to the retina.

oralism: a method of instruction for the deaf in which the chief means of communication is lipreading and talking.

orbicularis oris m.: the sphincter muscle which closes the mouth and wrinkles the lips; it is supplied by the VIIth Cranial or facial nerve.

ordinate: the vertical axis of reference in a two-dimensional graph. Dist. from *abscissa.*

organ of Corti: the spiral apparatus in the internal ear lying on the basilar membrane in the cochlear canal.

organic defect: a defect in which structural alteration is an important contributing cause. Dist. from *functional defect.*

orifice: an aperture or opening.

origin: the more-fixed end or attachment of a muscle as distinguished from insertion; also the point at which a Cranial nerve emerges from the brain.

oropharynx: that portion of the pharynx extending from the level of the hyoid bone to the soft palate.

oscillograph: an instrument for recording oscillations.

ossicle: a small bone; one of the three bones in the middle ear.

otitis media: inflammation of the middle ear.

otolaryngology: the single specialty of *otology* and *laryngology.*

otology: the study and treatment of the ear.

otosclerosis: the formation of spongy bone in the labyrinth of the ear; especially such growth around the footplate of the stapes impeding its movements in the oval window.

outer ear: the pinna and the ear canal. Same as *external ear.*

oval window: See *fenestra ovalis.*

overtone: any partial in a complex tone except the fundamental tone; when the frequency of an overtone is an exact multiple of the fundamental tone, it is called a harmonic. Dist. from *fundamental tone.*

palatogram: an imprint on a thin, artificial hard palate made by contact of the tongue when a given sound is produced.

palatopharyngeus m.: a muscle originating in the soft palate and inserted in the posterior border of the thyroid cartilage and in the pharynx; it acts to narrow the fauces and shut off the nasopharynx. Same as *pharyngopalatinus muscle.*

palpation: the act of feeling with the hand or fingers.

paracusis willisiana: the ability to hear speech better in a noisy surrounding; after Thomas Willis (1670).

paragrammatism: See *agrammalogia.*

paralalia: the substitution of one speech sound for another; sometimes any speech disturbance.

paralambdacism: faulty production of the sound [l].

paramedical: having medical aspects; sometimes secondary or subsidiary to medicine.

paraplegia: paralysis of the legs and lower part of the body.

pararhoticism: faulty production of the sound [r].

parasigmatism: faulty production of the sounds [s] or [z].

parasympathetic nervous system: that part of the autonomic nervous system which is made up of the ocular, bulbar, and sacral divisions.

parathyroid gland: any one of the two small glands on each lobe of the thyroid gland.

parietal lobe: a cerebral lobe in the upper center of the cerebrum corresponding to the parietal bone.

Parkinsonism: a degenerative and progressive central nervous system disease of late life characterized by tremors, a masklike face, slowing of voluntary movements, peculiar posture, and general muscular weakness. Same as *paralysis agitans.*

partial: one of the frequency components of a complex tone.

Passavant's ridge: a ridge projecting from the posterior and lateral walls of the pharynx at the level of the soft palate; it acts with the palate in closing the opening to the nasopharynx.

patellar reflex: the knee jerk elicited by striking the tense patellar tendon and bringing about a contraction of the quadriceps extensors.

pathology: the study of the nature of disease and its resulting structural and functional changes.

PB *words:* a phonetically balanced list of words for articulation tests in hearing; so-called because the words include speech sounds in approximately the same relative frequency of occurrence as in the stream of ordinary speech.

pediatrics: the study and treatment of children and their care.

peripheral: situated more or less in the outward part or surface of the body as distinguished from the central mechanism consisting of the brain and spinal cord; muscles and sense organs.

pertussis: whooping cough.

PGSR: psychogalvanic skin response. Same as GSR and EDR.

pH: a symbol representing the hydrogen ion concentration in liquids; a low pH indicates acidity, and a high pH alkalinity.

pharyngeal constrictors: three muscles in the pharynx, *superior*, *middle*, and *inferior*, which contract the pharynx as in swallowing.

pharyngeal tonsil: See *adenoids*.

pharyngopalatinus m.: See *palatopharyngeus muscle*.

pharyngoplasty: surgical procedures used to reduce the size of the pharynx in cases where there is impairment of the soft palate.

pharynx: the muscular and membranous sac between the mouth and nares and the esophagus; it consists of three main divisions, the laryngopharynx, oropharynx, and the nasopharynx.

phenylketonuria: a congenital faulty metabolism resulting from the absence of an enzyme necessary for the conversion of phenylalanine; clinical symptoms include mental deficiency, neuromuscular abnormalities, lack of pigmentation, and low resistance to infection.

phi phenomenon: the apparent motion of stationary stimuli when they are presented successively in neighboring positions.

philtrum: the groove in the middle of the upper lip.

phobia: pathological fear of some specific stimulus or situation.

phon: a unit of loudness level.

phonation: the production of voiced sound by means of vocal cord vibrations.

phoneme: a group or family of closely related speech sounds all of which have the same distinctive acoustic characteristics in spite of their differences; often used in place of the term *speech sound*.

phonetic method: an approach to the treatment of articulation difficulties in which the therapist directs attention to the specific movements and placements of the articulatory structures.

phonetics: the study of the production and perception of speech sounds including individual and group variations as to their use in speech.

phonics: the study of speech sounds with special reference to reading.

phonophobia: an extreme sense of discomfort caused by sounds above the threshold of hearing; a morbid fear of speaking aloud.

phrase: a word or group of words uttered without perceptible pause and set aside as a group by pauses of sufficient duration to perform this function.

physiogenic: originating from physiological causes. Dist. from *psychogenic*.

Pierre Robin syndrome: micrognathia, or underdeveloped lower jaw, sometimes associated with cleft palate and characterized by the retropositioning of the tongue causing respiratory difficulty shortly after birth when the tongue intrudes into the pharyngeal airway.

pinna: Same as *auricle*.

PKN: See *phenylketonuria*.

platysma m.: the platsyma myoides, a muscle which depresses the mouth and lower lip.

play therapy: a process of examination and treatment by observing the child as he plays freely with a selected inventory; the role of the therapist is usually a passive one.

plosive: any speech sound made by creating air pressure in the air tract and suddenly releasing it. Examples are [p], [d], and [t].

PNA *system:* Paris Nomina Anatomica; a revised system of anatomical nomenclature adopted by the Fifth International Congress of Anatomists in Paris, 1955. See BNA, BR, NK, and INA systems.

pneumogastric n.: Same as *vagus nerve*.

pneumograph: a device for recording the rate and extent of breathing movements.

pneumophonia: a form of dysphonia; voice characterized by breathiness.

polylogia: Same as *logorrhea*.

pons: the pons Varolii; a large transverse band of nerve fibers in the hindbrain which forms the cerebellar stem and encircles the medulla oblongata.

posterior: pertaining to or located in the rear. Opp. to *anterior*.

presbycusis: the diminution of hearing acuity associated with old age.

primary stuttering: the neuromuscular spasms in the early speech of children about which there is an absence of awareness and anxiety and an absence of irrelevant movement of distant parts.

prognathism: a marked projection of the jaw, usually the upper jaw.

prognosis: prediction or judgment concerning the course, duration, termination, and recovery from a pathological condition.

projection: the tendency of a person to attribute to the external world repressed mental complexes which are his own.

pseudobulbar paralysis: paralysis which appears to be a result of bulbar lesion, but is not.

psychasthenia: a neurosis marked by morbid anxiety, obsessions, feelings of inadequacy, self-condemnation, and fixed ideas.

psychiatry: that branch of medicine which deals with mental disorders.

psychoanalysis: a dynamic system of psychology, developed by Freud, which attributes behavior to repressed factors in the subconscious and which has a specialized technique for the investigation and treatment of such factors.

psychocatharsis: Freud's treatment of neurosis in which the patient relates everything that is associated with a given train of thought; it is closely related to *abreaction*. Same as *catharsis*.

psychogenic: originating in the mind. Dist. from *physiogenic*.

psycholinguistics: a loosely used term representing an amorphous field of study which in the main attempts to interrelate all aspects of human behavior and culture with all aspects of human language function.

psychometry: the broad field of mental measurement.

psychotherapy: the treatment of disorders by any of a wide variety of psychological methods.

pterygoid m.: external and internal pterygoid muscles which raise the lower jaw and draw it forward.

pure tone: periodic sound wave of the sinusoidal type which has no partial or overtone.

quadratus labii inferioris m.: a muscle innervated by the facial (VIIth Cranial) nerve and which acts to depress the lower lip.

quadriplegia: paralysis of all four limbs.

quality: when applied to voice, the acoustic characteristics of vowels resulting from their overtone structure or the relative intensities of their frequency components.

q.v.: L. *quod vide*, which see.

raphe: a ridge which marks the line of union between halves of symmetrical parts.

rapport: a relationship of ease, harmony, and accord between the subject and examiner or therapist.

receptive aphasia: a disturbance of speech due to brain lesion in which the major difficulty is inability to comprehend the meaning of words heard. Same as *auditory aphasia.*

recruitment: when applied to hearing, the condition in which the patient cannot hear sounds of moderate intensity but experiences no loss of his sense of loudness for loud tones; it is associated with sensorineural deafness.

recurrent laryngeal n.: the branch of the Vagus (Xth Cranial) nerve which innervates all intrinsic muscles of the larynx except the cricothyroid muscle; also called *inferior laryngeal.*

reflex: a movement performed involuntarily as a result of the stimulation of a sensory nerve which sends an impulse through a connecting nerve to a nerve center and thence to a motor nerve; this functional unit of the nervous system is called a *reflex arc.*

refractory period: the brief elapse of time following excitation of a nerve or muscle fiber before it can be excited again.

Reissner's membrane: a thin membrane between the cochlear canal and the scala vestibuli.

relaxed palate: functional failure of palatal movement, not due to paralysis or muscular weakness.

resonance: the vibratory response of a body or air-filled cavity to a frequency imposed upon it.

retarded speech: slowness in speech development in which intelligibility is severely impaired; often preceded by late or delayed emergence of speech.

retrocochlear lesion: a type of lesion causing sensorineural hearing impairment that is located in the auditory nerve and not in the cochlea.

Rh factor: Rhesus factor; an agglutinogen first found in the blood of Rhesus monkeys and normally present in 85 percent of the Caucasian population; those who have this blood factor are Rh positive, and those who do not are Rh negative.

rhinolalia: speech characterized by abnormal nasal resonance.

rhythm: the serial recurrence of stress, sounds, or organic movement.

rima glottidis: See *glottis.*

Rinné test: a tuning-fork test used to aid in differentiating conduction from sensorineural deafness.

risorius m.: a muscle originating in the fascia over the masseter muscle and inserted in the angle of the mouth; it is innervated by the buccal branch of the facial (VIIth Cranial) nerve; it acts to draw the angle of the mouth out and to compress the cheeks.

round window: See *fenestra rotunda.*

rubella: German measles, a disease which if occurring in the first four months of pregnancy is known to harm the embryo producing combinations of deafness, blindness, cleft palate, cerebral palsy, mental deficiency, and other anomalies.

rugal: pertaining to a ridge, fold, or furrow; especially the transverse ridges extending outward on both sides of the raphe of the hard palate.

S: subject.

SAA: Speech Association of America.

saccule: a little sac in the vestibular apparatus of the inner ear.

sagittal: shaped like an arrow; running in a plane parallel to the long axis of the body.

SAI: social adequacy index; a measure of the degree to which a person is handicapped in hearing and understanding speech; it is computed from the results of speech reception thresholds and speech discrimination tests.

SAL: sensorineural acuity level; a method of testing bone-conduction hearing by using a bone-conduction vibrator to deliver a masking noise at the midline of the skull and noting threshold shifts caused by the masking noise in pure-tone air-conduction hearing.

salpingopharyngeus m.: a muscle originating in the Eustachian tube near the nasopharynx and inserted in the posterior part of the palatopharyngeus muscle; it is innervated by the accessory (XIth Cranial) nerve and acts to raise the pharynx.

scala tympani: the spiral canal in the cochlea situated below the basilar membrane.

scala vestibuli: the spiral canal in the cochlea situated above the basilar membrane.

Schwabach test: a test of bone-conduction hearing by comparing a patient's ability to hear a tuning fork on his mastoid process with that of an examiner; when the patient no longer hears the fork it is transferred to the mastoid process of the examiner, who then counts the number of seconds he can hear it; the score is reported as minus seconds for the patient; the test assumes normal hearing on the part of the examiner.

secondary stuttering: neuromuscular spasms of the speech mechanism accompanied by anxiety about nonfluency and accompanied by habitual irrelevant movements used as devices to break up or conceal speech blockages.

segmental apparatus: See *brain stem.*

semantics: the study of the history and evolution of word meanings. Dist. from *general semantics.*

semicircular canals: three bony canals lying at right

angles to one another at the posterior end of the vestibule of the inner ear; they are filled with a fluid and serve as the sense organs of equilibrium.

sensorineural: a term applied to that type of hearing loss which is due to pathology in the inner ear, in the VIIIth Cranial nerve, or both.

sensorium: the entire sensory mechanism; sometimes the part of the cerebral cortex concerned with the reception of sensory nerve impulses.

serous otitis media: presence of fluid in the middle ear which impedes the movements of the ossicular chain, thus reducing hearing acuity.

sibilant: accompanied by a hissing sound; especially a type of fricative speech sound called a sibilant. Examples are [s], [z], [ʒ], [ʃ], [tʃ], and [dʒ].

side-tone: the auditory signal which gives a speaker information concerning his own speech performance.

sigma: when spelled out, one-thousandth of a second.

sign language: a system of communication among the deaf through conventional hand or body movements which represent ideas, objects, action, etc. Dist. from *finger spelling.*

signal-to-noise ratio: the relationship between the intensity of speech and the intensity of noise in a particular communicative situation. Same as S/N.

singer's nodule: See *chorditis tuberosa.*

sinistral: pertaining to or located on the left side of the body. Opp. to *dextral.*

sinus: a recess, cavity, or hollow space in the bone or other tissue.

SISI: short increment sensitivity index; a test used for differential diagnosis of auditory disorders; the subject is asked to detect increments of one dB introduced for a very short interval every five seconds in steady tones; subjects with purely conductive loss usually have difficulty in detecting these small intensity increments, and those with cochlear disturbance exhibit extremely high recognition scores.

slurring: passing over speech sounds so lightly during utterance that they are obscured, suppressed, omitted, or only partially produced.

S/N: See *signal-to-noise ratio.*

soft palate: a fibromuscular, movable muscular sheet which is attached to the posterior margin of the hard palate; it helps to separate the oral cavity from the pharynx and, when elevated, closes off the nasopharynx. Same as *velum.*

somatic: pertaining to the body substance in general.

sonant: a voiced sound. Opp. to *surd.*

sound intensity: the power or energy of a sound wave measured per unit area; usually measured in fractions of a watt per square centimeter; a just-audible sound has an intensity of about 10^{-16} watt/cm^2; sound intensity is usually inferred from sound pressure, which is easier to measure; sound intensity is proportional to the square of sound pressure.

sound pressure: the force exerted by a sound wave over a unit area of surface; measured in dynes per square centimeter; the smallest pressure variation sufficient to produce an audible sound is approximately .0002 dyne/cm^2.

sound spectrograph: an instrument for graphically recording the continually changing intensity levels of the frequency components in a complex sound wave accomplished by means of filter analyzers; a commercial instrument known as the Sonagraph. See *formant.*

sound spectrum: See *acoustic spectrum.*

spasm: a convulsive involuntary contraction of a muscle or group of muscles.

spasmophemia: a disturbance in the rhythm of speech; a blocking or convulsive repetition of sounds. Same as *stuttering.*

spastic paralysis: paralysis marked by rigidity and heightened tendon reflexes. Dist. from *flaccid paralysis.*

speech: communication through conventional vocal and oral symbols.

speech audiometry: the measurement of hearing in terms of the reception of spoken words presented at controlled levels of intensity.

speech correction: the professional field which deals with the elimination and alleviation of speech defects or with the development and improvement of speaking intelligibility; sometimes dist. from *speech improvement.*

speech defect: any deviation of speech which is outside the range of acceptable variation in a given environment.

speech discrimination: the degree to which one is able to hear and recognize acoustic differences among all the phonemes in speech segments to the extent that the speech perceived is intelligible; same as the audiological meaning of *articulation.* See PB *words.*

speech disorder: a deviation of speech together with the underlying conditions causing such a deviation; often the same as *speech defect.*

speech education: the broad field dealing with the training of the person to speak and listen more effectively.

speech frequencies: the pure-tone frequencies in audiometric testing which give the best prediction for the level at which speech can be understood; they are 500, 1,000, and 2,000 Hz.

speech improvement: the betterment of poor or average speech; sometimes distinguished from *speech correction.*

speech pathology: the study and treatment of all aspects of functional and organic speech defects and disorders; often the same as *speech correction.*

speech science: the broad field dealing with the study, analysis, and measurement of all the components of the processes involved in the production and reception of speech; sometimes the same as *voice science.*

speechreading: see *lipreading.*

speech reeducation: the process of restoring a lost speech function by means of an appropriate form of training; same as *speech rehabilitation.*

sphincter: a ring-shaped muscle which, on contracting, wholly or partly closes a natural opening.

spinal accessory n.: the XIth Cranial nerve; partly

united with the Vagus nerve, it originates in the medulla and spinal cord and is motor to the larynx and pharynx; same as *accessory nerve*.

spirometer: an instrument used to measure the air capacity of the lungs.

SPL: sound pressure level; the ratio expressed in decibels between the pressure exerted by any sound and the standard reference level of .0002 dyne/cm^2.

spondee words: words of two syllables with about the same stress on each syllable. Examples are *baseball*, *airplane*, and *birthday*.

SRT: speech reception threshold; usually determined by presenting spondee words to the subject and finding the amplification level which will enable him to repeat correctly approximately half of the words.

staffing: an interdisciplinary conference bringing together several professional experts, each of whom has examined a given patient, for the purpose of combining diagnostic knowledge in order to arrive at a decision concerning the nature, the initiation, or the continuation of treatment.

stammering: Same as *stuttering*.

stapedectomy: surgical removal of the stapes in otosclerotic patients followed by the insertion of a synthetic strut between the incus and the oval window.

stapedius m.: a tiny muscle originating in the inner wall of the middle ear and inserted in the neck of the stapes; it is innervated by the VIIth Cranial nerve (facial) and acts to retract the stapes.

stapes: the stirrup-shaped third bone in the chain of ossicles in the middle ear; its footplate is inserted in the oval window of the cochlea.

stapes mobilization: a surgical operation to restore movement to the footplate of the stapes which has become fixated in the oval window in otosclerotic patients.

Stenger test: a test for functional hearing impairment; both ears are stimulated by the same frequency but at different intensities; used to assess a person's claim of monaural hearing loss.

sternohyoid m.: a muscle originating in the clavicle and inserted in the body of the hyoid bone; it acts to depress the hyoid and the larynx.

sternothyroid m.: a muscle originating in the sternum and inserted in the thyroid cartilage; it acts to depress the larynx.

stimulation method: an approach to the treatment of speech defects in which major emphasis is placed upon the development of auditory concepts; teaching speech sounds by having the subject listen to them.

stop: a speech sound produced when the air stream is blocked. See *plosive*.

stress: in speech, the relatively increased force of breath in the production of some syllables as compared with others.

stretch reflex: See *myotatic reflex*.

stridor: a harsh, shrill, high-pitched sound.

stuttering: a disturbance of rhythm and fluency of speech by an intermittent blocking, a convulsive repetition, or prolongation of sounds, syllables, words, phrases, or posture of the speech organs.

styloglossus m.: a muscle originating in the styloid process and inserted in the side of the tongue; it is innervated by the hypoglossal (XIIth Cranial) nerve and acts to raise and retract the tongue.

stylopharyngeus m.: a muscle originating in the styloid process of the temporal bone and inserted in the side of the pharynx; it raises and dilates the pharynx.

sulcus: a depression or furrow in the surface of the brain; same as *fissure*.

superior: situated above.

superior laryngeal n.: the branch of the Xth Cranial nerve (Vagus) which innervates the cricothyroid muscles and supplies sensory fibers to the mucous membrane of the larynx.

surd: a voiceless sound. Opp. to *sonant*.

SWAMI: speech with alternating masking index; a discrimination test.

sweep-check test: an audiometric method of screening out possible hearing-loss cases by testing for auditory response to different frequencies presented at a constant intensity level. See *Johnston test* and *Massachusetts test*.

sympathetic nervous system: the system of ganglia lying outside the spinal cord in the lumbar and thoracic regions and the peripheral nerves which serve the viscera. Same as *autonomic nervous system*.

symptom: a structural or functional change or peculiarity which indicates the presence of a disease or disorder in a given individual; the answer given by an organism to demands of the environment which it cannot meet.

symptomatology: the systematic study of symptoms; the combined symptoms of a disorder.

synapse: the region of contact between one nerve cell and another in a neural chain.

syndrome: a complex of symptoms; a set of symptoms which occur together.

synergy: the combining of elementary motor processes into a complex, coordinate movement.

T *and* A: tonsillectomy and adenoidectomy.

tachyphemia: speech characterized by great rapidity and volubility, especially in nervous patients.

tact: Skinner's term coined from the word *contact* to represent a verbal operant in which a response of given form is evoked or strengthened by the presence of a particular object or event.

temporal lobe: a major division of each cerebral hemisphere; it lies on the undersurface and side of the brain and contains the hearing centers.

temporalis m.: a muscle originating in the temporal fossa and side of the head and inserted in the mandibular process; it is innervated by the mandibular branch of the trigeminal (Vth Cranial) nerve and acts to shut the mouth and retract the jaw.

tendon: a fibrous cord of nonelastic connective tissue in which muscle fibers end and by which they are attached to a bone.

tensor tympani: a muscle originating in the temporal

bone and inserted in the handle of the malleus; it is innervated by the otic ganglion and acts to keep the drum membrane taut.

tensor veli palatini m.: a muscle which renders the soft palate tense.

thalamus: a mass of grey matter situated at the base of the cerebrum projecting into and bounding the third ventricle.

therapy: the science which deals with the treatment or application of remedies for the cure, alleviation, or prevention of disorders.

thoracic cavity: the chest; the portion of the body between the neck and the abdomen; it contains the bronchi, lungs, and heart; sometimes called the thoracic cage.

thyrohyoid m.: a muscle originating on the side of the thyroid cartilage and inserted in the greater horn of the hyoid bone; it is innervated by the upper cervical nerves and acts to raise and change the shape of the larynx.

thyroid cartilage: the large cartilage of the larynx shaped like a shield in front and forming the eminence known as Adam's apple.

thyroid gland: one of a pair of endocrine glands situated on either side of the larynx; it secretes hormones which maintain basal metabolism rate and is important for normal growth and development.

timbre: a qualitative aspect of a complex tone dependent upon the number and relative intensities of partial tones present. Same as *quality.*

tinnitus: head noises; ringing in the ears; often associated with hearing impairment.

tongue-tie: limited movement of the tongue due to abnormal shortness of the lingual frenum.

tonsil: a small, almond-shaped mass between the faucial pillars on either side; it is mainly composed of lymphoid tissue and is covered with a mucous membrane.

tonus: a condition of tension in muscles which exists independently of voluntary innervation.

trachea: the windpipe; the cartilaginous and membranous tube descending from the larynx to the bronchi.

tracheostomy: cutting an opening into the trachea through the neck to allow the patient to breathe when the air tract above is blocked.

tracheotomy: any operation of cutting into the trachea; usually the same as *tracheostomy.*

trachyphonia: roughness or hoarseness of the voice.

tragus: a small cartilaginous projection in the pinna near the opening of the ear canal.

transference: development of positive or negative emotional attitudes toward a person, usually the psychoanalyst, when such attitudes are derived from earlier relationships between the patient and his parents.

transverse: lying or moving across; crosswise.

transversus linguae m.: a muscle originating in the median septum of the tongue and inserted in the edges; it is innervated by the hypoglossal (XIIth Cranial) nerve and acts to narrow and stretch the tongue as well as to raise its edges.

trauma: any wound or injury, especially an organic injury.

Trends: an employment bulletin published monthly by the American Speech and Hearing Association.

triangularis m.: a muscle originating in the lower border of the mandible and inserted in the lower lip; it is innervated by the facial (VIIth Cranial) nerve and acts to pull down the corners of the mouth.

trigeminal n.: the Vth Cranial nerve; it is sensory and motor with three main branches, the *ophthalmic, maxillary,* and *mandibular.*

trochlear n.: the IVth Cranial nerve; it is motor to the superior oblique muscle of the eyeball.

TTS: temporary threshold shift.

tuning fork: a two-pronged instrument of highly tempered metal alloy constructed to vibrate at a constant frequency when struck.

turbinate bone: the *concha nasalis;* one of three small shell-like bones in the nose.

tympanic cavity: an air-filled cavity in the temporal bone which communicates with the nasopharynx by means of the Eustacian tube; it is bounded laterally by the tympanic membrane and contains the ossicular chain; known also as the middle ear.

tympanic membrane: Same as drum membrane.

tympanoplasty: Same as *myringoplasty.*

UCL: uncomfortable loudness level.

ulcer: an open sore other than a wound; loss of substance on a cutaneous surface causing disintegration of tissue.

unilateral: pertaining to one side of the body.

uraniscolalia: speech difficulty due to a cleft palate.

uranoschisis: Same as *cleft palate.*

utricle: a small sac in the vestibule of the inner ear.

uvula: the appendage which hangs from the free margin of the soft palate.

vagus n.: the Xth Cranial nerve; it is a motor and sensory nerve sending fibers to the larynx, lungs, heart, esophagus, stomach, and most of the abdominal viscera; sometimes called the *pneumogastric nerve.*

vegetative: pertaining to nutrition and growth.

velum: Same as *soft palate.*

ventral: located on the belly side; opp. to *dorsal.*

ventricle: one of the cavities in the brain; any cavity or hollow organ of the body.

verbigeration: See *catalogia.*

vermillion ridge: the red external portion of the lips.

verticalis linguae m.: a muscle originating in the upper surface of the tongue near the sides and inserted under the surface; it is innervated by the hypoglossal (XIIth Cranial) nerve and acts to flatten the tip of the tongue.

vertigo: a sensation of whirling or dizziness from overstimulation of the semicircular canal receptors; often associated with disease of the ear and deafness.

vestibule: a portion of the labyrinth of the inner ear; it is situated between the cochlea and the semicircular canals.

vibrato: periodic variations in pitch or loudness of a tone.
viscera: the large internal organs of the body.
visible speech: audible speech patterns which have been transformed by electronic apparatus into visual patterns which may be read by the deaf.
vital capacity: the maximum amount of air which may be exhaled following a maximal inhalation.
viz.: L. *videlicet*, namely.
vocal cords: the thyroarytenoid ligaments which produce sound when set into vibration; same as *vocal bands.*
vocalization: Same as *phonation.*
voice: sound produced primarily by the vibration of the vocal bands.
voice-reflex test: Same as *Lombard test.*
voice science: See *speech science.*
volume: the loudness of a tone.
vomer: the bone which forms the inferior and posterior portion of the nasal septum; from L. meaning *plowshare.*
vowel: a conventional vocal sound produced by certain positions of the speech organs which offer little obstruction to the air stream and which form a series of resonators above the level of the larynx in the vocal tracts. Dist. from *consonant.*
vowel glide: a speech sound in which the speech mechanism moves from the position for one vowel to that of another without interruption and accompanied by continuous voicing. Examples are [aɪ], [ɪu], and [eɪ].
VU: volume units.

Waardenburg syndrome: a congenital abnormality consisting of displacement of the medial angles of the eyelid slits, diversity of coloration in the iris of the eye, partial albinism with a white forelock and white skin, and deafness.
WAIS: Wechsler Adult Intelligence Scale.
watt: unit of power or energy; intensity of sound may be measured in decibels with a small fraction of a watt as the reference level, namely, 10^{-16} watt per square centimeter.
wave length: the distance between any one particle in a wave and the particle in the next wave which is moving in a corresponding fashion; the wave length of a sound is equal to the velocity of the sound in feet per second divided by the frequency of the sound in cycles per second; thus, the higher the frequency the shorter the wave length.
Weber test: a tuning-fork test in cases of unilateral hearing loss to differentiate conduction from sensorineural deafness.
Wernicke's area: a region in the superior convolution of the temporal lobe of the cerebrum identified as the center for understanding speech heard.
white noise: a noise containing a wide distribution of audible frequencies and used for masking purposes in audiometry; so called because it is somewhat analogous to white light.
WISC: Wechsler Intelligence Scale for Children.
word-deafness: Same as *auditory aphasia.*

zygomaticus m.: major and minor zygomaticus muscles innervated by the facial (VIIth Cranial) nerve and which act to draw the upper lip upward, outward, and backward.

ROOTS, PREFIXES, AND SUFFIXES

a-, (an-): Gr. not; without
ab-: L. away from
acro-: Gr. tip or extremities; highest
ad-: L. toward
ambi-: L. both
amphi-: Gr. both; around
ana-: Gr. up; upward
ante-: L. before
antero-: L. in front
anthrop-: Gr. human being; man
anti-: Gr. against
apo-: Gr. from; away from; off
arch-: Gr. first; chief; principal; great
arthro-: Gr. joint
aryten-: Gr. pitcher
auto-: Gr. self

bari-: Gr. heavy
bene-: L. well; good
bi-: L. two
biblio-: Gr. book
brachy-: Gr. abnormally short
brady-: Gr. slow
bucco-: L. cheek

capit-: L. head
cardio-: Gr. heart
cata-: Gr. downward
ced-: L. move; yield
centi-: L. hundred; hundredth
cephalo-: Gr. head
chrom-: Gr. color
chron-: Gr. time
circum-: L. round about
com-: L. with; together
contra-: L. against; in opposition
corp-: L. body
costo-: L. rib
cresc-: L. rise; grow
crypto-: Gr. hidden; covered
cut-: L. skin
cycl-: Gr. ring; circle; cycle

de-: L. reversal; undoing
dec-: Gr. ten
demi-: L. half
dent-: L. tooth
derm-: Gr. skin
di-: Gr. twice
dia-: Gr. through; between; across
dic-: L. say
dis-: L. apart; separated from
dolicho-: Gr. long
duc-: L. lead
dyna-: Gr. power
dys-: Gr. ill; bad; hard

ec-: Gr. out of
ecto-: Gr. outside; external
-ectomy: Gr. surgical removal
embolo-: Gr. wedge; stopper
en-: Gr. in
endo-: Gr. inside
epi-: Gr. on; upon
eso-: Gr. inner
eu-: Gr. good; advantageous
ex-: L. out of; from
extero:- L. outside
extra-: L. beyond; outside of

fac-: L. make; do
fin-: L. end
flu-: L. flow
fort-: L. strong

gastro-: Gr. stomach
gen-: Gr. origin
gingiv-: L. gum
glosso-: Gr. tongue
gnath-: Gr. jaw
-gnosis: Gr. knowing; recognition
-gram: Gr. something drawn or written
-graph: Gr. writing

helio-: Gr. sun
hemi-: Gr. half
hepta-: Gr. seven
hetero-: Gr. unlike; different
hexa-: Gr. six
histo-: Gr. tissue
homo-: Gr. same; similar
hydro-: Gr. water
hyper-: Gr. excess; over; superiority
hypno-: Gr. sleep
hypo-: Gr. under; less than ordinary; inferior

idio-: Gr. personal; separate; distinct
infra-: L. below; lower
inter-: L. among; between; together
intro-: L. directed inward
-ism: Gr. state; condition
iso-: Gr. equal
-itis: Gr. inflammatory disease

juxta-: L. close to

kata-: See *cata-*
kilo-: Gr. thousand
kine-: Gr. movement

labio-: L. lip
-lalia: Gr. speech
lalo-: Gr. speech
loc-: L. place
log-: Gr. words; reasoning
luc-: L. light

macro-: Gr. large
mal-: L. defect; bad
man-: L. hand
medio-: L. middle
mega-: Gr. great; powerful
meningo-: Gr. membrane
ment-: L. chin
meso-: Gr. in the middle
meta-: Gr. after; change
-meter: Gr. measure
micro-: Gr. small
milli-: L. thousand; one thousandth
mis-: L. and AS. wrong
mono-: Gr. one; single
-morph: Gr. characterized by a specific form
multi-: L. many
myo-: Gr. muscle

neo-: Gr. new; recent
-nomy: Gr. a system of laws
non-: L. absence

oculo-: L. eye
odonto-: Gr. tooth
-oid: Gr. like; resembling
-oma: Gr. growth; tumor
omni-: L. all
onto-: Gr. existing
-onym: Gr. name
-opia: Gr. related to the eye
oro-: L. mouth
ortho-: Gr. straight; correct
-osis: Gr. diseased condition
oto-: Gr. ear

palato-: L. palate
pan-: Gr. all
para-: Gr. faulty or disordered condition; subsidiary
path-: Gr. suffering; disease
-pathy: Gr. feeling; disease; treatment
ped-: L. foot
pedo- (ped-): Gr. child
penta-: Gr. five
peri-: Gr. around
phil-: Gr. love
-phobia: Gr. morbid fear
phon-: Gr. sound
photo-: Gr. light

phren-: Gr. diaphragm; mind
pneumato-: Gr. air; respiration
pneumono-: Gr. lung
-pod: Gr. footed
poly-: Gr. many; manifold
post-: L. later; after
pre-: L. before
pro-: L. in front of; in place of
prosthe-: Gr. to add.
proto-: Gr. first in time or status
pseudo-: Gr. false; erroneous
psycho-: Gr. mind
pyro-: Gr. fire

quadr-: L. four
quasi-: L. seemingly
quinque-: L. five

re-: L. again
rect-: L. straight
ren-: L. kidney
retro-: L. backward; situated behind
rhino-: Gr. nose

-scope: Gr. instrument for observing
scoto-: Gr. darkness
-sect: L. cut; divided
semi-: L. half
sept-: L. seven
sex-: L. six
somno-: L. sleep
son-: L. sound
sphygmo-: Gr. pulse
spiro-: L. respiration
stereo-: Gr. a solid body
stomato-: Gr. mouth or mouthlike opening
sub-: L. beneath; of lower order
super-: L. above; of higher order
supra-: L. above in position
syn-: Gr. together

tachy-: Gr. quick; swift
tele-: Gr. far
tetra-: Gr. four
thermo-: Gr. heat
thyro-: Gr. shield
-tomy: Gr. a cutting
trachy-: Gr. rough
trans-: L. across
tri-: L. three

ultra-: L. extreme; beyond
uni-: L. one

zo-: Gr. animal

BIBLIOGRAPHY

Brunner, T., and Berkowitz, L. 1967. The elements of scientific and specialized terminology. Minneapolis: Burgess.

Coats-Longerich, M., and Longerich, E. 1945. German-English speech terminology. *J. Speech Disorders*, 10, 39–46.

DeVries, L. 1946. German-English science dictionary. New York: McGraw-Hill.

———. 1951. French-English science dictionary. New York: McGraw-Hill.

Dorland, W. 1951. The American illustrated medical dictionary. Philadelphia: Saunders.

Drever, J. 1952. A dictionary of psychology. Baltimore: Penguin.

Fairchild, H. 1944. Dictionary of sociology. New York: Philosophical.

Fodor, N., and Gaynor, F. 1950. Freud: dictionary of psychoanalysis. New York: Philosophical.

Good, C. 1945. Dictionary of education. New York: McGraw-Hill.

Gray, H. 1963. Anatomy of the human body (27th ed.). Philadelphia: Lea & Febiger.

Grayson, H., and Tolman, R. 1950. A semantic study of clinical concepts. *J. abnorm. soc. Psychol.*, 45, 216–231.

Hammond, K., and Allen, J. 1953. Writing clinical reports. Englewood Cliffs, N.J.: Prentice-Hall.

Henderson, I., and Henderson, W. 1949. Dictionary of scientific terms: pronunciation, derivation, and definition of terms in biology, botany, zoology, anatomy, cytology, embryology, physiology. New York: Van Nostrand.

Hinsie, L., and Shatzky, J. 1940. Psychiatric dictionary with encyclopedic treatment of modern terms. London: Oxford.

Hutchings, R. 1943. A psychiatric word book: a lexicon of terms employed in psychiatry, and psychoanalysis designed for students of medicine and nursing, and psychiatric social workers. Utica, N.Y.: State Hospitals Press.

Johnson, W., and Wilson, J. 1945. The degree of extensional agreement among twenty psychologists in their use of the labels, hypothesis, theory, and law. Proceedings of the Iowa academy of science, 52, 255–259.

Jones, H., Hoerr, N., and Osol, A. 1949. Blakiston's new Gould medical dictionary. Philadelphia: Blakiston.

Judson, L., and Weaver, A. 1965. Voice science. New York: Appleton-Century-Crofts. Pp. 396–414.

Kahn, S. 1940. Psychological and neurological definitions and the unconscious. Boston: Meador.

Longerich, E., and Longerich, M. 1946. French-English speech terminology, *J. Speech Disorders*, 11, 193–196.

Ogilvie, M. 1942. Terminology and definitions of speech defects. New York: Columbia.

Robbins, S. 1947. Principles of nomenclature and of classification of speech and voice disorders. *J. Speech Disorders*, 12, 17–22.

———. 1951. A dictionary of speech pathology and therapy. Cambridge, Mass.: Sci-Art Publishers.

———, and Stinchfield, S. 1931. Dictionary of speech terms dealing with disorders of speech. Boston: Expression Co.

Stedman, T., and Stanley, T. 1946. Stedman's medical dictionary. Baltimore: Williams & Wilkins.

Warren, H. 1934. Dictionary of psychology. Boston: Houghton Mifflin.

West, R., and Ansberry, M. 1968. The rehabilitation of speech. New York: Harper & Row. Pp. 453–508.

Wise, H. 1946. A revised classification of disorders of speech. *J. Speech Disorders*, 11, 327–334.

Zemlin, W. 1968. Speech and hearing science: anatomy and physiology. Englewood Cliffs, N.J.: Prentice-Hall. Pp. 536–551.

2

The Muscles of Voice and Speech

*Robert M. DeuPree**

SCOPE AND IMPORTANCE

It took Man about five years to build the atom bomb after he started seriously. It took Man about 10 years to hurl a couple of tons of metal into space after he decided he could do it. It has taken Man and nature several million years to develop the human voice and speech to the current point of personal communication. The mechanism does not work perfectly all of the time, and because of this fact other authorities in this volume have presented many possibilities and involvements. Whatever the cause of the overlays, however, when the mechanism does not perform to our standards of excellence, the trouble is manifested simply by dyskinesis, or distorted movement.

Our bodies are composed of many types of tissue: bone, cartilage, epithelium, and nerve, to list a few. Tissue is defined as a collection of cells with a specific function, and muscle tissue has the unique characteristic of producing movement. Speech is the skilled, willful, and elaborate movement of muscles used for initiating vocal sounds, plus the molding of these sounds into meaningful oral communication. It matters little if the cortex, basal ganglia, or association fibers of the brain are intact; it means little if the efferent nerve pathways or if the cartilages of the larynx have developed properly. Of what importance are psychological or sociological influences if the muscles of breathing, voice, and articulation are distorted, diseased, incapacitated, or absent to some point of dyskinesis? In every such case the resultant speech pattern will be aberrant.

Compared to the mechanism of human speech, the hardware of an atom bomb or a space missile is simple engineering work. Voluntary modification of the outgoing breath stream that we call "speech" is covered from a developmental standpoint by Shriner in Chapter 44 and with considerations of the nervous system by West in Chapter 3. This chapter is concerned with some of the anatomical and physiological phenomena which participate in the function of muscles used for respiration, phonation, and articulation, together with some of the biochemical and biophysical activities necessary for muscle contraction in general any place in the body.

In nature, structure determines function. Anatomy determines physiology and it changes amutationally only in response to physiological demands from one millenia to the next. Anatomical structures used in human oral communication are marvels of evolutionary development and selective physiological enrichment through the ages. Probably none of the anatomical units which make up the voice and speech mechanism has escaped change. Equally probably none was originally used for more than a primitive action. For example, the vocal cords or folds close the glottis (the opening between them) airtight to enable abdominal muscles to contract and assist micturation and defecation, probably a far more "primitive" act in any species than phonation. Or consider the action

* This article was written by Robert M. DeuPree, M.D., in his private capacity. No official support or endorsement by the U.S. Public Health Service is intended or should be inferred.

of the epiglottis, which folds firmly over the laryngeal opening to prevent a bolus of food from entering the upper part of the respiratory tract during swallowing. The action of this epiglottis in assisting with the glottal stop so prevalent in Arabic languages is of much later development.

Any listing or tabulation of muscles used in voice and speech is far from exact. The classic *Gray's Anatomy* (1966) names 240 muscles in the entire body; Dorland (1957) names 290; and Stedman (1966) names 442. This is not caprice. It comes from the difference in criteria of different anatomists. For example, the Basioglossus is not found in Gray. Dorland, on the other hand, considers it sufficiently separated from some fibers of the Hyoglossus to deserve its own identity.

Method of Muscle Classification

The purpose of any anatomical classification must be kept in mind because of the orientation of those for whom it is intended. *Gray's Anatomy* is used primarily by medical students and practising physicians. On the other hand, Dorland's listing is more cyclopedic, less detailed, and is intended for quick reference or recall.

The author's classification in this chapter is intended for study by students of speech pathology, and the included content and arrangement of the muscles are expected to serve as orientation and reference for problems encountered in the study of voice and speech mechanisms. Dorland's tabulation of "muscles" served as the starting point, and the following protocol was observed:

1. use of Latin spelling, which is standard throughout the world.
2. bibliographic verification of such muscle by its inclusion in two standard English language reference works.
3. identification in actual head and neck surgery (Rappaport, 1963) or in the author's postmortem dissections from 1962 to 1963 on no less than 20 subjects with the muscle in question noted in no less than 90 percent of these subjects.

The standard English language reference works were Toldt (1919), Truex and Kellner (1948), Gould (1956), Dorland (1957), Saunders (1964), Taber (1965), Stedman (1966), and *Gray's Anatomy* (1966).

Activity of single muscles and groups of muscles in the production of phonemes is entirely deductive and is based upon the author's experience as an actor, a physician, and a speech pathologist.

Human anatomy has changed little since daVinci, Vesalius, Morgagni, or Valsalva. Techniques of observation, evaluation, and reporting of the function of any part of the body improve with each generation, but the structure of our physical organism is essentially the same now as it was several thousand years ago.

VOCAL SOUND FORMATION

Sounds made in speech or song are produced by vibration of the vocal cords, which lengthen or shorten or become thick or thin as the result of muscle movements. These changes in turn produce oscillations of pressure of the expired air. Vibrations thus produced are a series of rhythmic condensations and rarefactions of air, and they are accentuated or suppressed further by the everchanging resonating qualities of the nose and mouth as well as by molding of the sounds through the articulating muscles of the tongue, palate, lips, jaw, and possibly the pharynx itself.

The vocal cords[1] produce alternating rarefactions and condensations of air by vibrating laterally, allowing the expired air to escape through the glottis in little puffs. Changes in pitch (Hz) are thus produced by the vocal cords continually altering in response to changes in tension brought about by laryngeal muscle contraction.

A cavity containing air will accentuate tones having a certain vibration rate while suppressing others. Above the larynx we find the hypopharynx, pharynx, nasopharynx, and mouth, all serving as resonating cavities that assist in modification of the vocalized air which has been given regulated periodicity upon leaving the larynx during expiration. The extrinsic laryngeal muscles, which elevate the hyoid bone, cause the larynx to move progressively upward as higher tones are produced and thus modify laryngeal vibratory tones in still another way. This shortens the posterior pharynx at the same time so that higher pitches with shorter wavelengths will be resonated.

ANATOMICAL CONSIDERATIONS OF MUSCLE CONTRACTION

There are three types of muscle tissue in the body: 1) cardiac muscle, a highly specialized type found in the heart only; 2) smooth, nonstriated, or involuntary muscle, found in the walls of viscera and blood vessels

[1] Anatomically speaking, "vocal folds" is correct but so much of the lexicon today dictates that they be called "vocal cords."

and which is activated principally through the autonomic nervous system; and 3) voluntary, skeletal, striated, or peripheral muscle which can be controlled entirely through some process of volition. This chapter is concerned only with voluntary muscle action because it is the only type found in the muscles of voice and speech.

Gross Action

When a muscle contracts, it acts upon movable parts to bring about certain movements. These movements should be considered from three points of view: individual action, group action, and action correlated with the nerve supply and its engramic feedback. The individual action is closely associated with the anatomy of a muscle because, mechanically, the action is the direct result of the spatial attachment of its ends. As *Gray's Anatomy* (1966) points out, it is not necessarily true that the action in the living body is the same as that deduced from observing its attachments or even from pulling on it in a dead subject, because incidental actions may not be utilized or may be suppressed in the lifestate of the body. This has been substantiated by DeuPree and Rappaport (1963). It is seldom possible for a person to make a single muscle, whether within or without the vocal mechanism, contract at will. The movements, not the muscles, are represented within the central nervous system at any one point in time. A muscle may be associated with one group for one action and a different group for another, possibly even antagonistic action. Correlation of the knowledge of the action of a muscle with its nerve supply is mandatory, as is the recognition that instantaneous circuitry through the association fibers functions as an overlay.

Practically every muscle of speech has another muscle with an opposing action. For example, the Geniohyoideus, Digastricus, and Stylohyoideus raise the larynx; their opposing group members, the Sternohyoideus, Sternothyroideus, and Omohyoideus lower the larynx. The cartilages of the larynx which give it identity as an organ do not fall by gravity, as do the arms, for instance, when the elevators are relaxed. Instead the cartilages need to be lowered by the contraction of muscles.

Individual muscles cannot always be treated as single mechanical units with regard to their actions. Different parts of the same muscle may have different or even antagonistic actions. For example, the anterior belly of the Digastricus moves the hyoid bone forward while the posterior belly of the same muscle moves the bone backward. Both, however, effect an upward movement at the same time. Or again, consider the action of several parts of the Cricothyroideus; its anterior fibers move the cricoid cartilage upward while more posterior fibers have a somewhat backward pull on the posterior aspect of the cricoid.

The typical voluntary muscle is a reddish mass of tissue attached to a bone or other structure by means of a fibrous white tendon which, if flattened, is called an aponeurosis. In anatomical nomenclature the origin of a muscle forms the first part of the name given to it and the insertion forms the last part of the term. If there is more than one origin, both of them precede the insertion, as in the Sternocleidomastoideus, i.e., origin in both the sternum and clavicle and insertion into the mastoid process. One usually only has to look at the name of a muscle to know where it originates, where it is inserted, and many times the action as well. There are a few exceptions: Uvulae, Vocalis, and Stapedius, for example; they are rare, however, and when they are encountered some anatomists precede the name with the Latin *Musculus*. For example, muscle contracts. The Styloglossus originates in the styloid process of the temporal bone, which is more fixed, and it ends in the tongue, which is more movable. Looking at the name "Styloglossus" we know that the muscle moves the tongue. Remembering that the origin is above and behind the insertion it is clear that the Styloglossus elevates and retracts the tongue.

Another point to bear in mind is that with some muscles which have equally movable attachments at both ends the two syllables in the name may be reversed. The Glossopalatinus in some books may be listed as the Palatoglossus. Whenever this occurs both names are usually given.

A muscle may extend from bone to bone as in the case of the Geniohyoideus, from cartilage to bone as does the Thyrohyoideus, from cartilage to cartilage as does the Thyroepiglotticus, or from bone to muscle itself as is the case of the Constrictores pharyngis inferior and medius where muscle fibers from each side of the bony attachments of the pharynx interlace with those of the opposite side to form the median raphe, thus narrowing, slightly elevating, and shortening the tubular pharynx when they contract.

While some of the muscles used in breathing, voice, and speech are single, such as the Orbicularis oris, most of them are paired, which means they have a mirror image of themselves on the opposite side of the midline. In this chapter the single muscles will be so designated and the absence of any such designation indicates that the muscle is paired.

Microscopic Action

Skeletal muscle consists of long, cylindrical muscle fibers which vary in length from 1–40 mm and in thickness from 50–100 μ or more (Kelle and Neil, 1961). These muscle fibers are distinguished microscopically by transverse bands of alternating light and dark shades, or sarcomeres. They are in turn enclosed in a structureless membrane called the sarcolemma. Each muscle fiber contains many myofibrils of 1–2 μ in diameter and which lie parallel to one another among the sarcoplasm. Both are enclosed by a sheath called the sarcolemma.

A number of noncontractile connective tissue elements are necessary for the organization of contractile components of the muscle (muscle fibers) into mechanically functioning units. The fibers are thus bound together into fasciculi by the fibroelastic perimyseum, and the ends of the muscle, whatever their size or shape, are attached by means of tendons or flat fibrous aponeuroses to the various parts of the skeleton.

THE MOTOR UNIT

Skeletal muscles receive their motor nerve supply from the ventral horn cells of the spinal cord, or from the corresponding cells in the cranial motor nucleii. Each ventral horn cell, or cranial equivalent, supplies a considerable number of muscle fibers varying with the individual muscle, from 5–150 μ (Kelle and Neil, 1961). A ventral horn cell with its efferent fiber is called a motor neurone, and because it is more peripheral than the cells of the cortex the designation "lower" is appended. A lower motor neurone together with the group of muscle fibers which it innervates is called a motor unit, and the point of attachment of the nerve cell ending to the muscle is termed the end plate.

PHYSIOLOGY OF MUSCLE CONTRACTION

Efferent nerve fibers passing to a skeletal muscle are excitory: they produce contraction of the muscle fibers which, working as a group, shorten the distance between origin and insertion of the muscle. The nerve impulse is a physico-chemical change which is transmitted by the nerve fiber ends to the end plate. Activity extends from the nerve endings across the motor units into the muscle fibers by the release of chemical transmitters either acetylcholine or noradrenalin, the same chemical substances released through synapses of parasympathetic and sympathetic nerve fibers respectively. According to Kelle and Neil (1961), Hanson and Huxley (1955), and Palay and Palade (1955), the sequence of events in the neuromuscular junction is probably as follows:[2]

1. Arrival of an impulse at the motor nerve terminal.
2. Release of acetylcholine from the nerve terminal and its diffusion to the motor end plate.
3. Attachment of acetylcholine to the end plate receptors and production of local end plate bioelectric potential (depolarization).
4. When the end plate potential reaches a certain critical magnitude it depolarizes the surface membrane of the muscle fiber and sets up a propagated muscle action potential.
5. Depolarization leads to the development of mechanical tension (contraction); to a complicated exchange of hydrogen, potassium, and sodium ions; and to the production of lactic acid, CO_2, and heat.

An understanding of the biophysical and biochemical phenomena of initiatory nerve impulses at the end plate is of more than passing interest to the speech pathologist because there is a strange disease called myasthenia gravis, which is characterized by rapid fatiguability and loss of strength of the muscles of speech. This appears quite early in the manifestation of the clinical condition and is followed by the same loss of strength in extraocular and then in other groups of muscles. There is no recognizable change in the nerves or in the muscles themselves. The abnormality appears to reside in the motor end plate. Neuromuscular transmission is probably blocked by choline, the hydrolysis product of acetylcholine. Administration of an acetylcholine inhibitor such as neostigmine effects striking clinical improvement in all of the muscles involved, and while not curative it keeps the symptoms at a minimum (Grog, Johns, and Harvey, 1955).

The All-or-None Phenomena

A fascinating aspect of both muscle cells and nerve cells is the "all-or-none law." When skeletal muscle

[2] This mechanism is not completely understood. Like so many other phenomena of science we know *what* happens but not yet *why* it happens.

is stimulated it displays the all-or-none relationship in the sense defined elsewhere for nerve (Chapter 3). The individual muscle fiber does not respond at all if the stimulus is too weak; it responds maximally (for the prevailing environmental conditions) when the stimulus rises to threshold. The contraction is not increased if the stimulus strength is further raised. Stronger stimuli, however, progressively bring *more* muscle fibers into action and thus the tension of a muscle increases as the strength of the stimulus applied to it increases.

This explains how a "muscle" which is actually a group of thousands of muscle cells (and motor units attached to many of them) can seem to become fatigued and work at less than capacity as may be seen in the condition the speech pathologist may diagnose as "vocal fatigue." As a total muscle the collective cells in this condition are responding with much individual variability: tiring, resting, and becoming rejuvenated in a continually overlapping pattern. As one part of the motor unit, however, the muscle cell, like the neurone which energizes it, responds in conformity to the all-or-none "law."

PHYSIOLOGY AND ANATOMY OF RESPIRATION

Any consideration of the muscles of voice and speech must include some investigation of the muscles of respiration as well as those of phonation and articulation. Breathing for speech is essentially the same process as breathing for life. It consists of two cycles: inhalation or active respiration by which the air flows into the lungs, and exhalation or passive respiration during which the air flows outward from the lungs and upward through the larynx, pharynx, nose, and mouth (Gray and Wise, 1959).

Physical Phenomena

The physical process of this exchange of air is simple and is based on the law of physics which states that a gas (in this case air) in a closed container exhibits equal pressure upon all the walls of the container, and that if the pressure in the container is greater than the ambient air pressure outside the container the air will move from the greater to the lesser pressure. Conversely, if the air pressure inside is greater than the ambient pressure outside, the air will move in the opposite direction.

This is what happens 18 or 20 times per minute during our lives. As the thorax (a container for the elastic lungs and their contained air) enlarges, air within the lungs decreases in pressure because it has a larger cavity to fill and the higher pressured, ambient air from the outside rushes in to neutralize the situation. When the thorax contracts, pressure of the air within the elastic lungs is raised and this air in turn hurries out into the less dense atmosphere.

Physiological Phenomena

The physiology of this exchange of air is complex. It has three contributing mechanisms: nervous, chemical, and muscular. The nervous and chemical factors will be considered here and the muscular mechanism will be explained later in the section on antomy of the respiratory apparatus.

NERVOUS MECHANISM

Respiration is under voluntary cortical and involuntary reflex control. The pacemaker is the nucleus of the respiratory center in the medulla. It calls upon the external supply of air to meet the internal needs of the body. In the respiratory center, inspiratory stimuli are received by afferent nerves and expiratory stimuli are transmitted to the muscles by efferent nerves.

Reflex afferent impulses are derived from the lungs, the carotid sinus, and the aortic arch, and possibly the larynx itself through the laryngeal branches of the vagus nerve (Xth Cranial), which, it will be recalled, has some afferent fibers. Other impulses arrive at the respiratory center through fibers from the nasopharynx in the trigeminal nerve (Vth Cranial) from the oropharynx and hypopharynx in the glossopharyngeal (IXth Cranial) and from the anterior and lateral abdominal and thoracic muscles in afferent fibers of the intercostal nerves (Thoracic 1–13). Impulses from the diaphragm arrive at the medulla through sensory fibers of the phrenic nerve into Cervical 3, 4, and 5. From the lungs a succession of impulses is set up in the vagus nerve (Xth Cranial) from receptors in the delicate alveolar walls, which are particularly sensitive to pressure changes. The nerve impulses discharged at the respiratory center in the medulla induce shortening of inspiratory action of the muscles of breathing and initiate their expiratory action. The receptors in the cardioaortic and carotid sinuses act as a result of both pressure and chemical changes in the blood. Increased arterial pressure induces reflex inhibition of the respiratory center; lowering of the arterial pressure stimulates the center and causes hyperpnea. The reverse is true with venous pressure changes. The pressosensitive nerve endings are situated mainly in the arteries, in the dilated portion of the internal carotid (Kelle and Neil, 1961; Roughton, 1954; Heymans, 1938; Liljestrand, 1958; Netter, 1948; Whitteridge, 1948).

It must be remembered that in addition to the reflex nervous control of respiration there is a purely voluntary cortical control of the process, and this is probably of more interest to students of speech than is the reflex mechanism. In speech, the willful influences of breathing are called upon more frequently than the purely automatic inspiration and expiration. This does not imply that respiration during speech changes from medullary to cortical control. If we accept the postulate that speech itself is entirely cortical then it is safe to assume at least some part of the outgoing breath stream has been affected by cortical control of the respirators as well as the phonators and articulators. This issue is less practical than academic and awaits further study.

To the point where the chemical factors considered below block out voluntary control, breathing can be controlled at will through impulses originating in the precentral gyrus and ending in association fibers in the medullary basal ganglia (*Gray's Anatomy*, 1966).

Efferent nerve impulses, whether originating in the cortex voluntarily or in the respiratory center through reflex action, are transmitted to all of the muscles of inspiration through the facial nerve (VIIth Cranial), vagus (Xth Cranial), accessory (XIth Cranial), the phrenic (Cervical 3, 4, and 5), and the intercostal nerves (Thoracic 1–13).

CHEMICAL MECHANISM

Carbon dioxide and to a much lesser extent lactic acid, by increasing the hydrogen ion concentration in the blood, are the chief chemical regulators of respiration. An increase of the carbon dioxide content of the air in the lung alveoli of as little as 0.2 percent stimulates increased respiratory action by direct influence on the respiratory center, and also reflexly by stimulation of the nerve endings (sensory) in the region of the carotid sinus and in the aortic arch. Within fairly wide limits ventilation is not influenced by the amount of oxygen inhaled. In rarified atmosphere or high altitudes, when the O_2 pressure in the air is greatly reduced, increased ventilatory effort is required both reflexly and voluntarily to compensate for the lack of oxygen (Johnson, 1966; Roughton, 1954). This is due more to increased CO_2 than to decreased oxygen.

The Muscles of Respiration

In considering the muscles involved in respiration one should remember that there are several types of breathing and that while some muscles are constant to all types, each of the following types of breathing probably calls into play additional muscles, singly or in groups:

1. involuntary breathing such as occurs the vast majority of the moments of our lives from the first slap on the buttocks of a newborn to the last gasp of the Hippocratic death rattle. As we have seen, this is medullary in nervous control.
2. forced involuntary breathing, exemplified by a more violent, deeper, and sometimes more rapid respiratory cycle during sleep and sometimes during waking hours, but in which there is no feedback from the respiratory center to the cognitive cortical areas.
3. voluntary breathing of the type when we deliberately let the cortex take over and set out to inhale and exhale somewhat more or less than the normal 16 to 20 times per minute, and which is influenced little, if at all, by any of the chemical regulating factors previously discussed.
4. voluntary forced breathing, as when a swimmer aerates his lungs to their maximum capacity before plunging beneath the surface, and which as in 3) above is not effected by any chemical change in the blood.

The muscles of breathing thus fall into one of two classes: obligatory respirators, or those used at all times in any of the four types of breathing, and facultative respirators, or those activated by either cortical or brain stem impulses and which bring into use muscles or groups not necessary to, but which assist in, speeding or deepening the process of respiration in one of several ways.[3]

Muscles of the Thorax

Diaphragm (Single)
Intercostales externi
Intercostales interni

[3] Some of the muscles, as for example the Levatores costarum which also extend the vertebral column, have an additional action but the student should remember that their respiratory activity is principally described in this Chapter.

Subcostales
Levatores costarum
Serratus posterior superior
Serratus posterior inferior
Transversus thoracis (Single)

Muscles of the Neck
Scalanus anterior
Scalanus medius
Scalanus posterior
Sternocleidomastoideus

Intrinsic Laryngeal Muscle
Cricoarytenoideus posterior
Cricoarytenoideus lateralis

The Cricoarytenoideus posterior, while classified as a Phonator elsewhere with the intrinsic muscles of the larynx must be considered here, and first, because **it is the single, most important muscle of the entire body** (except for the heart).

This muscle (paired) arises from the broad depression on the corresponding half of the posterior surface of the lamina of the cricoid cartilage; its fibers run cranialward and lateralward and converge to be inserted into the back of the muscular process of the arytenoid cartilage. The uppermost fibers are nearly horizontal, the middle oblique, and the lowest almost vertical. This muscle, and this muscle alone, *opens the glottis* and permits the column of air to move in and out of the lungs. Other intrinsic laryngeal muscles, as we shall see, close, elevate, and shorten the opening between the vocal folds, but the Cricoarytenoidei posterior (possibly assisted by a few lower fibers from the Cricopharyngeus which some anatomists term the inferior portion of the Constrictor pharyngis inferior) separate the vocal folds and consequently open the glottis by rotating the arytenoid cartilages outward around a vertical axis passing through the cricoarytenoid joints, so that their vocal processes and the vocal folds attached to them become widely separated (Figs. 2-2 and 2-3).

This is the muscle that, in cases of laryngospasm brought on through infection or the edema of a severe allergy, and at times during early stages of anesthesia, contracts to the degree that a tracheotomy is necessary to save life. Nearly all the other muscles of the body have some assistance from other muscles or groups, but the Cricoarytenoideus posterior is frighteningly alone in its action, 60 seconds of every minute and 60 minutes of every hour during our entire life span.

The Diaphragm is a single, dome-shaped musculofibrous septum which separates the thoracic from the abdominal cavity, its convex upper surface forming the floor of the former and its concave undersurface forming the roof of the latter. Its muscular fibers arise from the xiphoid process of the sternum, from the inner surfaces of the lower six ribs, and as the crura from the lumbar vertebrae and arcuate ligaments to converge on the domed central tendon. The muscle fibers sweep upwards from their origin along the inner part of the thoracic cage and then arch toward the midline. Contraction of the fibers of the muscle draws the central tendon downwards. Radiologically it can be demonstrated that the vertical movement of the diaphragm is about 1.5 cm. during quiet breathing and that it can descend as much as seven cm. during forced inspiration. The movements of the diaphragm, though responsible for some 75 percent of tidal respiration, are not essential to respiration. This is shown by conditions of bilateral diaphragmatic paralysis not involving other obligatory respirators and providing the lungs are not diseased (*Gray's Anatomy*, 1966). The Diaphragm is, however, included with the obligatory respirators in this listing because we are concerned with normal and not with pathological breathing conditions. Innervation of the Diaphragm is through the phrenic nerve (Cervical 3, 4, and 5).

The Intercostales externi are 11 in number on each side. They arise from the tubercles of the ribs and slope obliquely downwards and forwards to the costochondral junctions and are inserted into the upper borders of the ribs below. In the case of the two lower muscles they extend to the ends of the cartilages.

The Intercostales interni, also 11 in number on each side, extend from the anterior end of the intercostal space to the angles of the ribs posteriorly, the fibers sloping obliquely downward and backwards from the upper rib to the one below. They can be subdivided into a posterior interosseous portion where the ribs slope downwards and forwards and an interior intercartilaginous portion where the costal cartilages slope upward and forward.

Both the internal and external intercostals raise the ribs and thereby increase the anteroposterior diameter of the thorax. Nerve supply is from the intercostals (Thoracic 1–11).

The Subcostales are better developed in the lower part of the thorax. Each arises from the inner surface of one rib near its angle and is inserted into the inner surface of the second or third rib below; their fibers run in the same direction as those of the internal intercostals. The action of the Subcostales is to draw adjacent ribs together, and with the last rib fixed by the Quadratus lumborum they lower the ribs and decrease the volume of the thoracic cavity. Nerve supply is from the intercostals (Thoracis 1–11).

The Levatores costarum are small and 12 in number on each side. They arise from the ends of the transverse processes of the seventh cervical and upper 11 thoracic vertebrae, pass obliquely downward and lateralward, and each is inserted into the outer surface of the rib immediately below the vertebra from which it takes origin. Each of the four lower muscles is divided into a brevis and longus fasciculus to which it gives a descriptive addition to its name. The action of these muscles is to raise the ribs, thus increasing the thoracic cavity. Nerve supply is from the intercostals (Thoracic 1–11).

The Serratus posterior superior arises from the lower part of the ligamentum nuchae at the base of the cervical vertebrae and from the seventh cervical and upper two or three thoracic vertebrae. The fibers move downward and lateralward and are inserted by digitations into the upper borders of the second, third, fourth, and fifth ribs. Their action is to raise these ribs. They are innervated by branches from Thoracic 1–4.

The Serratus posterior inferior arises from the lower two thoracic and upper two or three lumbar vertebrae and their supraspinal ligaments. It is divided into four digitations which are inserted into the inferior borders of the lower four ribs.

The action of this muscle is to draw the ribs to which it is attached outward and downward, thus counteracting the inward pull of the diaphragm and assisting in stopping the process of inspiration. Nerve supply is from divisions of Thoracic 9–12.

The Transversus thoracis is a single plane of muscular fibers on the inner surface of either side of the front wall of the thorax. It arises from the body of the sternum and from the sternal ends of the costal cartilages. Its fibers sweep upward and lateralward and are inserted into the lower borders and inner surfaces of the costal cartilages of the second, third, fourth, fifth, and sixth ribs. Its action is to draw the ribs downward, thus decreasing the size ot the thoracic cavity. Its nerve supply is from the second, third, fourth, fifth, and sixth branches of the intercostals.

The Scaleni anterior, medius, and posterior are long muscles on either side of the neck arising from the transverse processes of the third, fourth, fifth, sixth, and seventh cervical vertebrae and are inserted into the first and second ribs. Their action is to raise these ribs, thereby increasing the size of the thoracic cavity. They are innervated from the second, third, fourth, fifth, sixth, and seventh cervicals.

The Sternocleidomastoideus arises from the outer, lateral aspect of the sternum and from the inner third of the clavicle on either side. Its fibers extend upward to be inserted into the mastoid process and posteriorly to the lateral aspect of the occipital bone. In respiration the action of this muscle appears to be one of fixation of the clavicle, and through the sternal origin of the muscle, to elevate the sternum. Nerve supply is from branches of the accessory (XIth Cranial) and from anterior rami of the second and third cervical nerves.

FACULTATIVE RESPIRATORS

It would be specious to list all the muscles of the body which could be voluntarily called upon to assist in the process of inspiration and expiration because such a list conceivably would include every body muscle except those of the extremities. Ordinarily when we think about "forced breathing" we consider only those muscles which raise the shoulders and tense the abdomen. But by no means are the levatores of the shoulder girdle and the strong abdominal muscles the only ones making such forced breathing possible.

Consider what happens on forced inspiration: the abdominal muscles are tightened and drawn backwards which, in association with the diaphragm descending, makes the abdominal cavity smaller. In order for this increased intra-abdominal tension not to effect a simultaneous expulsion of the contents of the bladder and lower colon the entire lower pelvic and perineal muscles contract and together prevent contained material from being expressed.

If we accept the premise that forced breathing cannot be accomplished without an increased extension of the vertebral column we then know that such action calls into work some eight pairs of deep back muscles, plus the Erector spinae which is subclassified into nine distinct muscles, and we include four paired suboccipital muscles, all the anterior and lateral muscles of the abdominal wall and trunk, those of the low back and the iliac region as well.

Thus we see that breathing in general as well as breathing for voice or speech is not the uninvolved process it appears to be; the very automatism makes it seem simple.

THE MUSCLES OF PHONATION

Before considering in detail the anatomy and physiology of individual muscles or groups responsible for sound formation we should take a general look at the total structure of the larynx.

General Anatomy of the Larynx

The voice box is placed astride the upper part of the air passage between the trachea and the root of the tongue. It consists of a framework of cartilages held in position by an intrinsic and an extrinsic musculature.

Cartilage, any where in the body, is a fibroelastic substance, considered a part of the skeleton, attached to articular or nonarticular bone surface and its purpose is to lend rigidity intermediate between the extensile properties of the muscles and completely sessile bone. Cartilages of the larynx are lined with mucous membrane continuous with that above and below. The organ has an average measurement as follows (*Gray's Anatomy*, 1966).[4]

	MALES	FEMALES
Length	44 mm	36 mm
Transverse diameter	43 mm	41 mm[5]
Anteroposterior diameter	36 mm	26 mm
Circumference	136 mm	112 mm

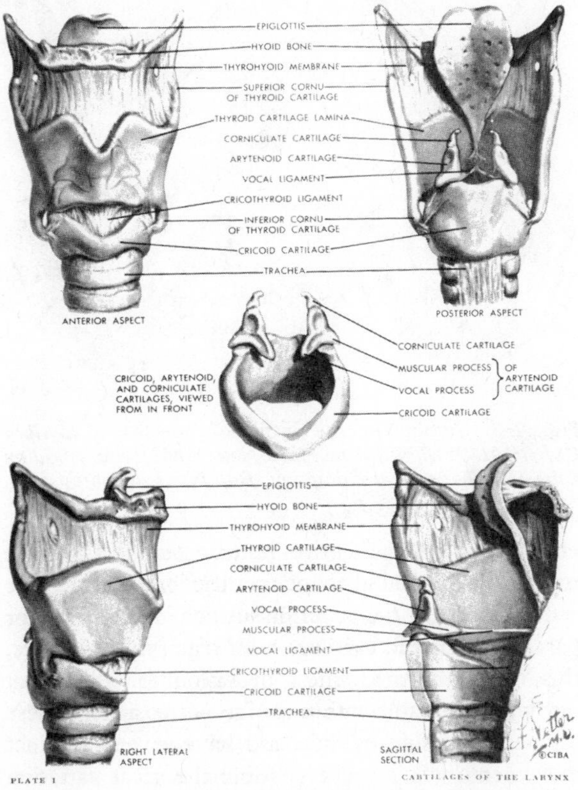

Fig. 2-1. Cartilages of the larynx. *Copyright CLINICAL SYMPOSIA by Frank Netter, M.D. Published by Ciba Pharmaceutical Company. Reprinted by permission.*

CARTILAGES OF THE LARYNX (Fig. 2-1)

All body cartilages are whitish-grey in color and are made up of tough fibrous bands usually running lengthwise within the cartilage. While somewhat movable with force, in the living state within the body they do not extend and contract to any appreciable degree.

The laryngeal cartilages are nine in number, three single and three paired:

- Thyroid
- Cricoid
- Two Arytenoid
- Two Corniculate
- Two Cuneiform
- Epiglottis

Their location and action will be discussed together with that of the intrinsic muscles of the organ.

THE INTRINSIC MUSCLES OF THE LARYNX (Figs. 2-2 and 2-3)

These are four paired and one single muscle:

- Cricothyroideus
- Cricoarytenoideus posterior
- Cricoarytenoideus lateralis
- Thyroarytenoideus
- Arytenoideus (Single)

ACTION OF THE INTRINSIC MUSCLES ON THE CARTILAGES

The largest and most sturdy of the cartilages is the thyroid. It is composed grossly of two alae or wings

[4] In dissection of many larynges the author has noted that both male and female members of the black race exceed these measurements with a degree greater than the variation found in Caucasoids. It was noted further that the cartilages of blacks were heavier and the intrinsic muscles appeared somewhat larger and apparently stronger.

[5] A search of the literature to date has not revealed why the difference between the male and the female for the transverse diameter is less than the difference between the two sexes for each of the other measurements. One would think that the greater laterality in the female might make for a deeper rather than higher voice quality.

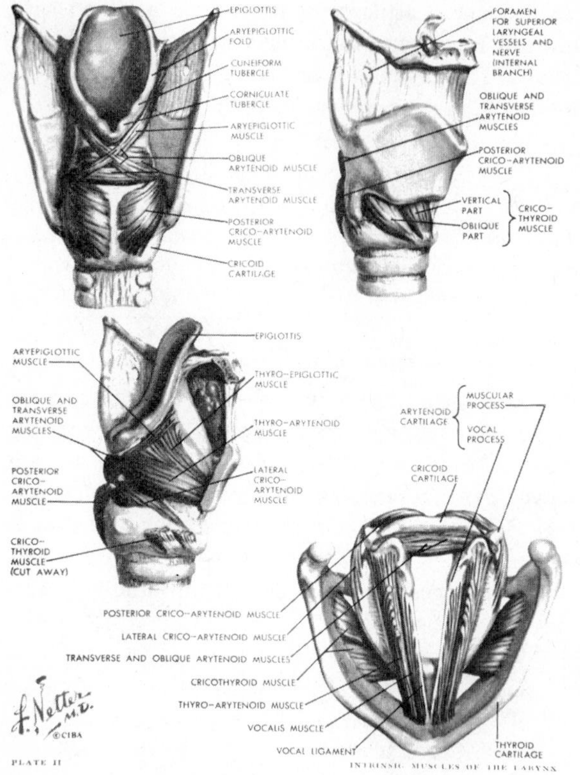

Fig. 2-2. Intrinsic Muscles of the larynx. *Copyright CLINICAL SYMPOSIA by Frank Netter, M.D. Published by Ciba Pharmaceutical Company. Reprinted by permission.*

which meet anteriorly and dip down from above to form the thyroid notch before meeting at the prominence known as "Adam's Apple." Each wing has a superior cornu posteriorly which extends upward and a much shorter inferior cornu which articulates with the cricoid cartilage below. The purpose of the thyroid cartilage is to form a solid anterior wall for the larynx and to prevent damage to its delicate contents. (Remember the Cricoarytenoideus posterior muscle and how quickly injury to it could shut off one's air supply. Perhaps that is why it is placed on the most protected part of the exterior of the organ.) In addition, it serves as a posterior attachment of great strength for the vocal bands.

The Cricoid cartilage lies directly below the thyroid cartilage and forms a complete ring around the larynx below the vocal cords. The cricoid is thicker and wider in the posterior, thus resembling a signet ring. The cricoid cartilage articulates posteriorly and laterally with the inferior cornu of the thyroid cartilage. These joints permit a slight anteroposterior sliding motion and a rocking action of the cricoid on the thyroid. The thyroid and cricoid cartilages are connected anteriorly by a heavy fibrous membrane, the cricothyroid ligament, and it is through this area that laryngotomy is sometimes performed in preference to the lower tracheotomy. It is more difficult to locate in a hurry, but lies much closer to the surface and in an emergency closing of the glottis, a much smaller cannula will suffice for life-giving air.

On its posteriosuperior aspect the cricoid cartilage supports the two arytenoid cartilages, the most charmingly delicate, durable, and ingenious piece of

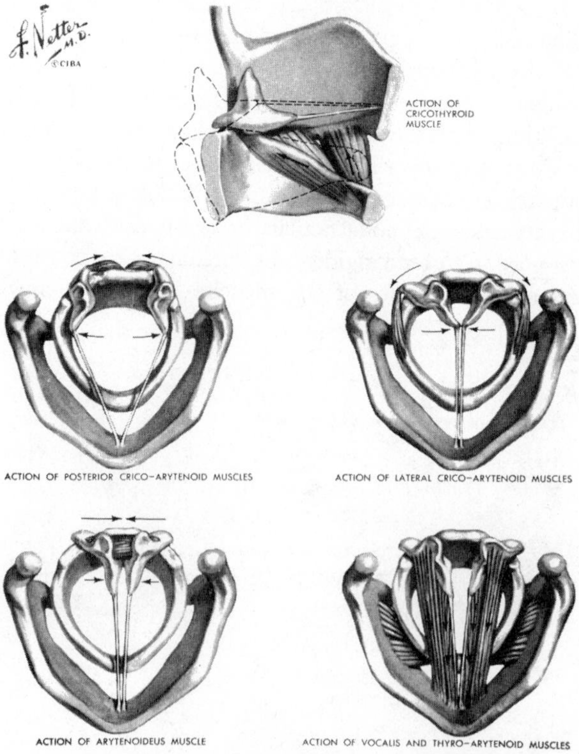

Fig. 2-3. Action of the intrinsic muscles. *Copyright CLINICAL SYMPOSIA by Frank Netter, M.D. Published by Ciba Pharmaceutical Company. Reprinted by permission.*

engineering in the entire human body. They are roughly pyramidal in shape on their long axis and are articulated with the superior surface of the posterior part of the cricoid cartilage with true synovial joints, this being the anatomical provision for the freest movement possible within confines of position. These cartilages lie side by side and have several distinct movements which make possible the great variation of vocal sounds. They *rotate* on a vertical axis and they *slide* at the same time on the cricoid. The posterior ends of the vocal cords are attached to the bases of the arytenoid cartilages. The muscular processes of the arytenoids to which the Cricoarytenoidei muscles on each side are attached lie on the posterolateral angles of these cartilages.

As the muscular processes of the arytenoid cartilages are pulled backward and somewhat medialward by the posterior cricoarytenoid muscles the cartilages are rotated in addition so that the vocal processes with their attached cords are abducted or pulled laterally, thus, as we have seen, opening the glottis. Opposing this action the forward pull of the lateral Cricoarytenoideus on the muscular process will adduct the vocal processes with their attached cords so that they meet in the midline during phonation, thus temporarily arresting or modifying the outgoing breath stream. The single Arytenoideus muscle which joins the arytenoid cartilages posteriorly, adducts the cartilages and slides them together to firm approximation. The two vocal folds thus have a movable posterior attachment which is closed principally by the Cricoarytenoidei laterales and the Arytenoideus, but their anterior fibers meet in an immovable commissure which is attached to the perichondrium of the thyroid (Fig. 2-3).

Within each vocal fold there are found some fibers of the Thyroarytenoideus muscle which are considered by some anatomists to be a separate muscle, the Vocalis. This Thyroarytenoideus muscle passes from the inside of the thyroid cartilage anteriorly to the base of the arytenoid cartilage posteriorly and tension upon this muscle, acting against its antagonist, the Cricothyroideus firms and tenses the cords. Acting without any antagonism from the Cricothyroideus, the Thyroarytenoideus passes from a simple tension to an actual shortening of the vocal cords (Fig. 2-3).

The Cricothyroideus (paired) arises from the lateral aspect of the cricoid cartilage, sweeps medialward and upward in a triangular shape, to be attached to the mediolateral aspect of the thyroid cartilage. This muscle has two functions, both of which lengthen, stretch, and tense the vocal bands, and this action is absolutely necessary to the production of tones of higher pitch. The anterior portion of this muscle shortens the distance between the cricoid and thyroid cartilages anteriorly. Because of the posterolateral position of the articulations between these two cartilages, this action depresses the posterior portion of the cricoid cartilage with its attached arytenoids, thus increasing the distance between the posterior attachment of the cords and their anterior commissure. The lateral, oblique portion of the Cricothyroideus slides the cricoid posterior to some extent, also lengthening the cords (Saunders, 1964) (Fig. 2-2).

Stretching action of the cricothyroid muscles tends to bring the vocal bands into approximation in the midline position. Saunders (1964) says about them: "thus they may be considered auxiliary adductors if the cords are in the lateral or intermediate position; auxiliary abductors if they are in the midline."

The "false cords" are two thick folds of mucous membrane each enclosing a narrow band of fibrous tissue and a few fibers of muscle, named Musculus Vocalis. These folds are attached to the inside of the thyroid cartilage anteriorly and the arytenoid cartilages posteriorly. Except under pathological conditions the false cords do not contract or shorten during sound formation.

A lateral invagination of mucosa known as the laryngeal ventricle lies between the true and false cords on each side. The only function that can be deduced for the laryngeal ventricle is possible provision for an additional amount of trapped air after even forced exhalation. After the lungs forcibly expel all the air possible an amount termed reserve air remains within them, as well as in the trachea, larynx, and oropharynx. The air that remains within the speech mechanism some of the time is equal in pressure to that within the lungs and outside the body. It can assume importance in phonation and singing where this isopressured air does not escape from the area but is merely set into vibration by the phonating mechanism. These structures are also important in certain pathologies that the student of speech should find interesting, particularly vocal abuse and laryngitis. Structurally, mucous membrane is the one body tissue most capable of edema or swelling with contained fluid. Since the vocal folds are principally mucous membrane they enlarge greatly in response to allergy, abuse, infection, or irritation. The edematous condition can be reversible, however, and when no longer congested the folds return to their normal state.

Below the true cords the Conus Elasticus, a part of the submucosal tissue, sweeps outward and around to enclose the full circumference of the trachea just above its uppermost cartilaginous ring.

The epiglottis is a thin lamella of yellow elastic cartilage, shaped like a leaf, which projects obliquely upward behind the root of the tongue and ventral to the entrance of the larynx. The free extremity is broad and rounded; the attached part of the stem is long, narrow, and connected by the thyroepiglottic ligament to the inner, upper, aspect of the thyroid cartilage. To its sides below, the aryepiglottic folds are attached. This structure must close tightly over the upper part of the larynx during swallowing to prevent any food reaching the respiratory tree. Apparently the only muscle involved in this closure is the Thyroepiglotticus which some anatomists consider to be just a part of the Thyroarytenoideus. The epiglottis returns to the open position, where it remains most of the time, through relaxation of these muscles and the inherent elasticity of the stem and its attachments.

Laterally, folds of mucous membrane sweep downward and backward from the epiglottis. This membrane merges into an X-shaped mass, the single Arytenoideus muscle, filling up the posterior concave surfaces of the arytenoid cartilages. It arises from the posterior surfaces and lateral border of one arytenoid cartilage and is inserted into the corresponding parts of the opposite cartilage. It consists of a transverse part and an oblique part (sometimes the additional designation A. Transversus and Obliquus is used); the latter, more superficial, forms two fasciculi which pass from the base of one cartilage to the apex of the other one of the opposite side, therefore crossing each other like the limbs of an X. A few fibers are continued around the lateral margin of the cartilage, and are prolonged into the aryepiglottic fold; they are sometimes described as a separate muscle, the Aryepiglotticus. The transverse part of the muscle crosses the midline and extends to the outer border of the two cartilages.

Nerve supply to all of the intrinsic muscles of the larynx is by way of the internal and external branches of the superior laryngeal nerve and from the recurrent laryngeal nerve. These are all part of the vagus nerve (Xth Cranial). Afferent sensory fibers are also carried in the internal laryngeal branch.

THE EXTRINSIC LARYNGEAL MUSCLES

The Suprahyoid Group

Digastricus
Mylohyoideus
Stylohyoideus
Geniohyoideus

The Infrahyoid Group

Sternohyoideus
Sternothyroideus
Thyrohyoideus
Omohyoideus

The larynx lies in a vertical slideway of loose areolar tissue through which it may be quickly elevated during swallowing, or raised and lowered to adjust the resonating characteristics of the posterior pharynx during phonation. The hyoid bone forms the division point and is the fulcrum on which vertical or tilting movements of the larynx as a whole depend (Fig. 2-4).

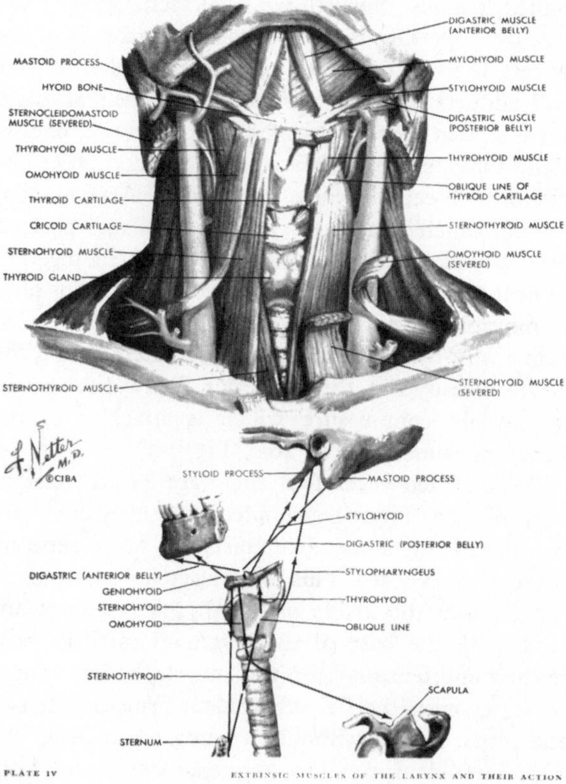

Fig. 2-4. Extrinsic muscles of the larynx and their action. *Copyright CLINICAL SYMPOSIA by Frank Netter, M.D. Published by Ciba Pharmaceutical Company. Reprinted by permission.*

The action of these muscles, which probably work most of the time as groups rather than as individual muscles, is very simple. The suprahyoid group, by contracting, raises the hyoid bone. In addition the Stylohyoideus and posterior belly of the Digastricus tend to pull the hyoid bone posteriorward; the Geniohyoideus and anterior belly of the Digastricus tend to pull the bone forward. (Because of some of its action in tending to elevate the lower part of the pharynx, the Stylopharyngeus muscle is occasionally placed in the suprahyoid listing.) The infrahyoid group pulls the hyoid bone downward.

Nerves to the suprahyoid group are from branches of the trigeminal (Vth Cranial), the facial (VIIth Cranial), and the hypoglossal (XIIth Cranial). The infrahyoid group is supplied by branches of the first three cervicals and the ansa hypoglossi.

From the standpoint of speech it can be stated simply that the entire group of phonatory muscles initiates the vowels. The articulators, as we shall see, are charged with the responsibility of molding some of these sounds further into the consonants.

THE MUSCLES OF ARTICULATION

As a group, the muscles of articulation participate in the formation of speech sounds by structuring the consonants. Thus they are of undoubted later phylogenetic origin than the phonators which form the more primitive sounds.

Because so many tiny fibrils of so many different muscles are, at any one point in time, assisting, neutralizing, or opposing each other, detailed evaluation of the role of each single muscle in the articulation of any particular phoneme, much more in running speech, must be looked at critically.

One muscle was studied in a unique and sophisticated way (it was not named but from its action it could be assumed to be the Constrictor pharyngis superioris) by the promising technique of ultrasound profiling, and it is far from revealing the movements to any degree of scientific satisfaction (Kelsey et al., 1968). A critical survey, however, of the anatomy and function of each of the muscles that could possibly be used in articulation is revealing and hopefully of value to the speech pathologist as well as to the surgeon, who is called upon from time to time to insult or remove some muscle and when there is an option what might the exercise of such option do to the speech mechanism.[6]

It is conceivable that there are times, initiated by stress or emotion, when almost every one of the voluntary muscles of the body could be called upon in the process of speech. Look at a voluble Frenchman, for instance. Are his hands a part of his "speech?" He would undoubtedly say so. But in America and many other cultures these occasions are not so usual. Consideration of the muscles which effect a modulation of the outgoing breath stream as articulators is therefore limited in this chapter to "normal" (nonpathological) general American, day-to-day working speech. What muscles or groups that are found with any consistency to be used in any one speech aberration will have to await further research and be as of now of academic interest only.

Some of the muscles that are classified here as articulators are called upon to serve as "resonators," but there is no need for the additional classification because it is unlikely that any of them would not also be involved in articulation, and most of the articulators are only secondarily involved in resonating the air stream.

It should be mentioned here that the important resonators are three tubes, the cavities of which contain columns of air more, less, or in isopressure with that in the lungs and outside the body at any one point in time. By their vibration, the air they contain can continue to effect audible sounds for 15, 20, or even 40 seconds after maximum expulsion of air appears to have been reached. These tubes are, of course, the pharynx, the mouth, and the double tube which is the nose. Possibly, according to Gray and Wise (1959), the larynx itself, the trachea, and even the bronchi and accessory nasal sinuses might play some role as resonators by muscular alteration of such of those as have any muscle fibers at all in their walls.[7]

As the air stream is propelled upward from the larynx it enters the pharynx, about 12 cm. in length, conical in form with the base upward, and extending from the level of the cricoid cartilage in front to the under surface of the skull. There are six pairs of muscles arising from bony structures laterally, and in the case of the Constrictor pharyngis superior, from the base of the calivarum. The fibers sweep laterally and downward and unite with those of the other side in a fibrous band, the median raphe.

Muscles of the Pharynx

Constrictor pharyngis superior
Constrictor pharyngis medius

[6] The author did just such a study at Long Beach State College and the VA Hospital in 1962–1963. It was found that insofar as surgical technique was concerned, and whether a muscle was left intact, insulted, or removed in its entirety during laryngectomy, the abilities to develop intelligible esophageal speech must be due to other factors.

[7] The author once had as a patient, a professional radio announcer whose severe, chronic, and intractable pansinusitis necessitated surgery to enlarge the ostia of the frontal, sphenoidal, and maxillary sinuses to establish drainage. Prior to surgery, they had been completely stenosed. Following surgery, there was no difference in his voice or speech or in any of its components as evaluated by himself, his associates, or any of the physicians who attended him. This might lead us to believe the role of the paranasal sinuses as resonators is greatly overrated.

Constrictor pharyngis inferior
Stylopharyngeus
Salpingopharyngeus
Pharyngopalatinus or Palatopharyngeus

Detailed description of the origin and insertion of these muscles is best left to standard anatomy textbooks. We will concentrate here on their actions principally in swallowing and secondarily in speech.

When deglutition is about to be performed, the pharynx is drawn upward and dilated in different directions to receive the food propelled into it from the mouth. The Stylopharyngei, which are much farther removed from one another at their origin than at their insertion, draw the sides of the pharynx upward and lateralward, and so increase its transverse diameter; its breadth in the anteroposterior direction is increased by the larynx and tongue being carried forward in their ascent. As soon as the bolus of food is received in the pharynx, the elevator muscles relax, the pharynx descends, and the Constrictores contract upon the bolus, and convey it downward into the esophagus. Students of speech pathology should understand this mechanism because it can be a part of the activity in "tongue-thrust."

From the standpoint of speech sounds, by contracting more than relaxing, they assist in the formation of the plosives /b/, /p/, /d/, /t/, /g/, and /k/, and, this time by relaxing more than contracting, in the nasals /m/, /n/, and /ŋ/.

This latter activity is accomplished partly in this way: man has an important reflex, the pharyngeal, which causes the act of swallowing whenever the velum is sufficiently stimulated. (Of course this act can also be accomplished through voluntary cortical impulses in addition to reflex control.) The velum is not discriminatory in its reception of impulses, however. Whenever it is stimulated and the stimulation is of sufficient magnitude and lasts for about one second the process of deglutition continues. If the stimulation is less than one second, however, the only part of the activity which takes place is momentary dilation of the pharynx through relaxation (it has no muscles to accomplish this) followed shortly by constriction of the three muscles forming its walls, thus forcing the bolus of food downward.

This time factor of about one second explains why we do not continue to swallow whenever, in the formation of the nasals, the velum approximates the tongue. All of the nasal sounds in running speech are of less than one second duration and the brief stimulation of the velum by the tongue results in the dilation of the Constrictores. This also enlarges the air cavity which is within the pharynx and contributes to the particularly resonant sounds of the nasal phonemes. The entire process is easily demonstrated by coating the appropriate surfaces with a mixture of barium in boroglyceride of glycerine and observing the subject under fluroscopy.

Another unique mechanism is worthy of mention here. During the process of swallowing, at whatever the point it is initiated, the inspiratory and expiratory action of the muscles of respiration ceases. This is brought about again by the pharyngeal reflex sending the impulses to the medulla and association fibers carrying the message to the initiatory-inhibitory nuclei of the breaching apparatus.

So far as nerve supply is concerned, the Constrictores and Salpingopharyngeus are supplied by branches from the pharyngeal plexus, the Constrictor pharyngis inferior by additional branches from the external laryngeal and recurrent nerves, and the Stylopharyngeus by the glossopharyngeal nerve (IXth Cranial). It should be recalled that within the pharyngeal plexus there are branches of the sympathetic portion of the autonomic system in addition to fibers from the central nervous system.

The Palatine Muscles

Levator veli palatini
Tensor veli palatini
Glossopalatinus (Palatoglossus)
Pharyngopalatinus (Palatopharyngeus)
Musculus uvulae (Single)

The Levator veli palatini originates from the apex of the petrous portion of the temporal bone and the cartilaginous Eustachian tube. The Tensor veli palatini arises from the scaphoid fossa of the sphenoid bone as well as the walls of the tube. Both are inserted in the aponeurosis of the soft palate and together they tense and close the soft palate as well as open the Eustachian tube. The Glossopalatinus arises from the under surface of the soft palate and is inserted into the lateral side of the tongue. The Pharyngopalatinus arises in the soft palate and is inserted in the midline raphe.

The Glossopalatinus muscle elevates the root of the tongue, or, if the tongue remains fixed, depresses the velum. The Pharyngopalatinus probably depresses and tightens the palate in the open position. The Musculus uvulae arises from the palatine bones and loses itself in the delicate mucous membrane of the midline uvula suspended from the soft palate. The muscle is of little value in the speech process.

The nerve supply of the Tensor veli palatini is from a branch of the mandibular division of the trigeminal (Vth Cranial) while all the others in this group are innervated from branches of the accessory nerve (XIth Cranial) and the pharyngeal plexus.

The palatine tonsils lie in a fossa between the palatoglossal arch anteriorly and the palatopharyngeal arch posteriorly. These structures derive their names from the respective muscles. Many speech therapists express great concern, somewhat unnecessarily, when a tonsillectomy has to be done on one of their small patients, or, if they get the child after some destructive tonsillar surgery, they put too much emphasis on any degree of accompanying muscular desecration. The author, in many years first as a resident then as a consultant on the Los Angeles PTA Tonsil Service, had a chance to evaluate several thousand children and saw few who had a noticeable alteration in the speech following a T and A (Tonsillectomy and Adenoidectomy) except for the improvement in physiological nasality which resulted from the removal of some occluding pharyngeal tonsils or adenoids.

The tonsils and adenoids, together with the lingual tonsils, form what is known as "Waldeyer's Ring," a circle of lymphoid tissue which in the newborn and young children completely surrounds the posterior of the oral cavity which is also the opening of both the respiratory and digestive systems. Lymphoid tissue acts as a physiological filter between the outside bacteria-laden environment and the sterility of the inside of the body so necessary to its continued life. As the child progresses through the first few years these lymphoid tissues are called upon to screen out much of the bacteria (or hold and permit the body to develop immunity against it). As with many things in nature, however, the process is not always controlled to our satisfaction. Nature fully intended most of the adenoid tissue in Waldeyer's ring to atrophy, and become if not extinct at least very fibrosclerotic, within the first half to two-thirds of the first decade of life. In the majority of children this is what happens. In many, however, too many, the infective process is so overwhelming within the lymphoid tissue that it becomes hypertrophic to the point of occlusion. The author once saw an 11-month-old baby who had to have a tracheotomy because the oropharynx was completely occluded by lymphoid tissue.

This presents another problem besides mechanical obstruction. The infective process can remain within the tonsils and adenoids and serve as a focus of infection for, particularly, all the diseases which have a bacterial etiology. These can be meningitis, pneumonia, rheumatic fever, carditis, nephritis, and abcesses any place in the body. More frequently, however, this smouldering infection calls upon so much of the body's resistive mechanism that the general health of the child is depleted and it is prey to many other conditions it should be able to ward off.

Thus speech therapists can be reassured on two points; even if one of their young subjects presents itself with a complete absence of both tonsil pillars and the uvula too, or if the youngster under therapy needs a T and A the matter will be of minimal influence in the process of speech. This is because the human body has a magnificent process of adaptation. The worst thing to be feared would be hypernasality, and even with the most destructive surgery that could be imagined in removal of this lymphoid tissue (providing of course it is not malignant) the root and upper dorsal portion of the tongue could effect a velar closure with only a little instruction.

The palatine muscles, by opening and tensing the velum, assist in the formation of many speech sounds, particularly the voiced /g/, /n/, /m/, and /ŋ/, and the voiceless /k/. With the velum closed, the voiced /b/, /d/, /g/, /l/, /r/, /v/, /z/, /w/, /i/, /ð/, and /ʒ/ and the voiceless /p/, /t/, /k/, /f/, /h/, /θ/, /ʃ/, /ʍ/, and the glottal stop /ʔ/ are influenced. This is reported by Wise (1959), who also believes that the voiced vowels /i/, /u/, /ɪ/, /ʊ/, /e/, /o/, /!/, /ɝ/, /ð/, /ʒ/, /ə/, /ɛ/, /ʌ/, /ɔ/, /æ/, /ɑ/, /ɑ/, and /a/ as well as the diphthongs /ɪ/, /ʊ/, /e/, /o/, /ɔ/, and /a/ are produced with the velum closed. This may well be so. If it is, it leaves few English speech sounds that are not produced with the velum in some state of activity. It is possible, however, that this could be more accurate in evaluation of individual phonemes than it is in running speech.

Muscles of the Mouth

An intricate, interwoven, yet distinct group of muscles surrounds the mouth. It is possible that in articulation there is such an instantaneous opposition or assistance given by any one muscle to any other muscle that no clear-cut, single action could be attributed to any one of them. That no single one, or possibly groups, of muscles of the mouth would be necessary to intelligible speech is demonstrated by the skill of theatrical ventriloquists. Observe either Edgar Bergen or Paul Winchell. Their entire articulation seems, even in a critical huge closeup, to be accomplished without use of any oral muscles except possibly the formation of the plosives and a few of the glides. Granted the speech is distinctive, but it is not unpleasant and is highly intelligible to most listeners.

The Elevators of the Mouth

Levator labii superioris
Levator labii superioris alaeque nasi
Zygomaticus major
Zygomaticus minor
Risorius
Caninus (Levator anguli oris)

The Depressors of the Mouth

Depressor labii inferioris
Depressor anguli oris
Mentalis
Buccinator
Transversus menti (Single)

Not strictly muscles of the mouth, but classified here because of their action in the speech process, are the following:

Orbicularis oris (Single) (This is considered a muscle of the lips)
Platysma

The elevators of the mouth originate from some part of the maxillary bone and are inserted into and beneath the fibers of the Orbicularis. Working together they all either raise or advance the upper lip. Their nerve supply is from the mandibular branch of the facial nerve (VIIth Cranial).

The depressors of the mouth all arise from the mandible but the Buccinator has some fibers originating from the maxilla. They depress and thrust the lower lip forward. Their nerve supply, too, is from the mandibular branch of the facial nerve (VIIth Cranial).

The Mentalis is small, weak, and situated lateral to the frenulum of the lower lip. It assists in depressing the lower lip.

The Buccinator is the principal muscle of the cheek and forms the lateral wall of the oral cavity. Its two heads originate from the maxilla above and from the mandible below to be inserted by blending with the deeper strata of muscle fibers from the corresponding lips. It is supplied by branches of the facial nerve (VIIth Cranial).

The Transversus menti is single and the least important of the depressors of the mouth and it is not found in all cadavers. It firms the tissues of the chin, thus forming a resistance to other muscles more active and larger in pulling down the lower lip.

The Orbicularis oris, however, is of great importance in articulation. It is not a simple sphincter like that surrounding the eye or the anus. It consists of numerous strata of muscular fibers surrounding the entire orifice of the mouth but having different directions. It consists in part of the fibers derived from the other facial muscles; those which are inserted into the lips and those proper to the lips alone. Of those fibers inserted into the lips a considerable number are derived from the Buccinator and form the deeper strata of the Orbicularis oris. Fibers from one side will cross over the midline to the other side, and at the corners of the mouth fibers from the upper lip cross a transverse plane to be inserted into the lower lip, and those from the lower lip cross the same plane to be inserted into the upper lip. In its ordinary action the Orbicularis oris effects direct closure of the lips; by its deep fibers, assisted by the oblique ones, it closely applies the lips to the alveolar arch. The superficial fibers of this muscle bring the lips together and assist in thrusting them forward or pursing them. Branches of the facial nerve (VIIth Cranial) activate it.

The Platysma is actually a superficial muscle; large, flat, and somewhat triangular with the base down. It arises from parts of the Pectoralis major on the chest and Deltoideus on the upper arm. Its fibers cross the clavicle and proceed obliquely upward and medialward across the side of the neck. The anterior fibers interlace below and behind the symphysis of the mandible with the fibers of the opposite side. The posterior fibers cross the mandible with insertion into it and into the skin and subcutaneous tissue. Many of them blend with the muscles at the angle and lower part of the mouth.

The action of the Platysma is to draw the outer part of the lower lip downward and backward, widening the corners of the mouth. It also assists in opening the jaws, but to a small degree only. Nerve supply is from a branch of the facial nerve (VIIth Cranial).

From the action of the depressors of the mouth and the Orbicularis oris and Platysma it can be seen that they effect principally the formation of the articular activity necessary to the plosives /b/, /p/, /d/, /t/, /k/, and /g/, the nasal /m/, the glide /w/, and the fricative /ʍ/. They also play a part in the sound from the high vowels /ʊ/ and /U/ and the midvowels /m/, /ɔ/, and /α/.

The Muscles of the Jaw

Temporalis
Masseter
Pterygoideus internus (medialis)
Pterygoideus externalis (lateralis)

Close your mouth and try to speak. You cannot. Some kind of an unintelligible grunt is all that emerges. This establishes that a mouth open to some degree is absolutely necessary for speech. Because the jaw muscles are primarily for mastication and probably only lately in our evolution adapted to assist in oral communication, they are relatively large and strong in comparison with some of the extrinsic muscles of the larynx, those of the pharynx, and the lips which we have just considered. Many authorities refer to this group as Muscles of Mastication.

Their work is to close the mandible against the maxilla. The Masseter and the Pterygoideus internus are so placed that they suspend the angle of the mandible in a sling. They form a functional apparatus to move the temporomandibular joint which acts as a guide. When the mouth is opened and closed the mandible moves about a center of rotation established by the sling and the sphenomandibular ligament.

The Temporalis, largest of this group, is a broad, fan-shaped muscle situated at the side of the head. It arises from the temporal fossa and temporal fascia. The fibers converge and descend to form a tendon which passes deep into the arch under the zygomatic process of the temporal bone. It ends in the coronoid process and the ramus of the mandible nearly as far forward as the last molar tooth.

The Masseter consists of a superficial portion which arises from the zygomatic process and zygomatic arch. Its fibers are inserted into the ramus of the mandible. The deep portion, much smaller, arises from the medial surface of the zygomatic arch and is inserted into the coronoid process of the mandible.

The Pterygoideus internus occupies a position on the inside of the ramus of the mandible and similar to that of the Masseter on the outside. It arises from the lateral pterygoid plate and the tuberosity of the maxilla and is inserted in the medial surface of the ramus of the mandible.

The Pterygoideus externus originates by an upper head from the great wing of the sphenoid bone and from the infratemporal crest; a lower head originates from the lateral surface of the lateral pterygoid plate (*Gray's Anatomy*, 1966).

The first three of these muscles, as we have seen, close the jaw while the Pterygoideus externus assists in opening the mouth by dropping the jaw. In this it is aided by the Mylohyoideus, Digastricus, and Geniohyoideus which have been discussed. The nerve supply of this group of four muscles is from the mandibular branch of the facial nerve (VIIth Cranial).

By altering the size and shape of the oral cavity the principle articulatory action of this group is assistance in forming the plosives. Of course they play a more active role whenever the sounds call for more closure of the mouth at any given point in time.

Of course it can be argued that all of the muscles which open and close the jaws participate in all speech, for an open mouth is mandatory to organized modification of the outgoing breath stream. If the lips function normally but the jaw remains fixed in the open position (as in the case of a fractured mandible which has been wired to the maxilla to prevent any movement) many intelligible sounds can be produced. But with the lips *and* the jaws closed only animal grunts can emerge regardless of how or under what condition of genetics, development, neuro-integrity, or psychological integration the phonators originate the sounds.

Muscles of the Tongue

Extrinsic
Genioglossus
Hyoglossus
Chondroglossus
Styloglossus
Glossopalatinus (also listed as a muscle of the palate)

Intrinsic
Longitudinalis superior
Longitudinalis inferior
Transversus
Verticalis

The human tongue is a multipurposed organ. It is of great importance not only in speech; it is also the principal organ of the sense of taste. It assists strongly in mastication and, by propelling a bolus of food backward and downward, aids in deglutition. It is situated in the floor of the mouth within the curve of the body of the mandible and is much larger and more powerful than it appears when one "sticks out his tongue" or in the phenomenon of "tongue-thrust" so well known to speech therapists.

The Genioglossus arises from the mental spine of the mandible (genu) and is inserted into the hyoid bone and under surface of the tongue.

The Hyoglossus originates in the body and greater cornu of the hyoid bone and is inserted in the side of the tongue.

The Chondroglossus is considered by some anatomists to be a part of the Hyoglossus but is actually a distinct muscle because it is separated from the Hyoglossus by fibers of the Genioglossus. It originates from the lesser cornu of the hyoid bone and is inserted into the lateral side of the tongue.

The Styloglossus originates from the styloid process of the temporal bone and is inserted in the side of the tongue throughout its entire length, right to the tip.

Of the intrinsic muscles of the tongue, the Longitudinalis superior originates in the septum and submucosa of the tongue and is inserted into the edges of the organ.

The Longitudinalis inferior arises from the under surface of the tongue at its base and is inserted into the tip of the tongue.

The Transversus arises from the median septum of the tongue and is inserted into the dorsum and lateral margins of the tongue.

The Verticalis originates in the dorsal fascia of the organ and is inserted into the sides and base of the tongue.

Nerve supply of both the intrinsic and extrinsic groups of lingual muscles is from branches of the hypoglossal nerve (XIIth Cranial).

The following is the explanation of the action of the muscle groups as adapted from *Gray's Anatomy* (1966) and confirmed or added to by the author's studies:

> Movements of the tongue are complicated and numerous and may be best understood by carefully considering the direction of the fibers of its muscles. The Genioglossi, by means of their posterior fibers, draw the root of the organ anteriorly and protrude the apex from the mouth. The anterior fibers draw the tongue back into the mouth. Acting in their entirety the two parts draw the tongue downward so as to make its superior surface concave from side to side and forming a channel along which fluids may pass toward the pharynx, as in sucking. The Hyoglossi depress the tongue and draw down its sides. The Styloglossi draw the tongue upward and backward. The Glossopalatini draw the root of the tongue upward.
>
> The intrinsic muscles are mainly concerned in altering the shape of the tongue whereby it becomes shortened, narrowed, or curved in different directions; thus the Longitudinalis superior and inferior tend to shorten the tongue, but the former, in addition, turns the tip and sides upward so as to render the dorsum concave, while the latter pulls the tip downward and renders the dorsum convex. The Transversus narrows and elongates the tongue, and the Verticalis broadens and flattens it.
>
> The complex arrangement of the muscular fibers of the tongue and the various directions in which they run, give to this organ the power of assuming the forms necessary for the enunciation of the different consonantal sounds.

The most prominent of the consonantal sounds which bring the tongue muscles into use would be the fricatives /ʍ/, /v/, /f/, /ð/, /θ/, /z/, /s/, /ʒ/, and /f/. It also participates actively in the production of the plosives /b/, /p/, /d/, /t/, /g/, and /k/. It assists greatly in formation of the nasals /m/, /n/, and /n/, and of course in all of the /r/ sounds, particularly where there is a trill.

Most anatomists feel there is reason to believe that the musculature of the tongue varies in different races owing to the hereditary practice and habitual use of certain motions required for enunciating the several vernacular languages and their many dialects.

SUMMARY

In living organisms only the contraction of one type of tissue we call muscle can produce motion to move the animal or its parts. This is a complex biophysical and biochemical response to nerve impulses reaching the junction of nerve fibers with muscle fibers at the motor end plate, and at this junction initiating a change in bioelectric potential of the muscle cells causing them to contract and pull some two parts of movable structures closer together, thus causing movement.

The muscles in humans which effect the production of speech are arbitrarily classified as respirators, phonators, or articulators. These muscles provide movement to effect an outgoing breath stream, to form it into sounds, and to mold those sounds into phonemes.

Breathing is a structural modification of body cavities to permit air under varying changes of pressure to enter and leave the lungs. It is under chemical, neurological, and muscular control: 11 paired and two single muscles are specifically designated as obligatory respirators because their contraction is necessary to accomplish any one of several types of breathing we do each day of our lives. There is another group of muscles termed facultative respirators which may be called upon to assist in forced inspiration, and this group includes the entire musculature of the thorax, abdomen, back, flanks, and pelvis.

The larynx sits astride this outgoing breath stream and modifies it by motion initiated in the nine cartilages and contiguous soft tissues which form the "voice box." Such motion is effected by four pairs and one single muscle forming the intrinsic group, and eight pairs (four suprahyoid and four infrahyoid) forming the extrinsic group sometimes designated as "strap muscles." The intrinsic and extrinsic muscles of the larynx are classified as *phonators* because their action initiate the periodicity of the outgoing breath stream that we know as "voice."

The emerging sounds are further modified by the muscles of articulation. These are comprised of six muscles of the pharynx, five palatine muscles, five elevators of the mouth, six depressors of the mouth, four muscles of the jaw, four extrinsic muscles of the tongue, and four intrinsic muscles of the tongue.

With the exception of those which open the lips, no one muscle or group is absolutely essential to articulation, but the absence, paresis, or aberration of any single muscle or group gives the emerging voice a peculiarly distorted speech pattern.

Table I gives an alphabetical listing of the muscles of speech together with their origin, insertion, nerve supply, and action. This listing affords more complete descriptions than those given in the text.

TABLE 2-I

DeuPree-Rappaport Classification
Origin, Insertion, Nerve Supply, and the Action of Muscles of Speech

O—Origin I—Insertion N—Nerve Supply A—Action
PH: muscles used for phonation or initiation of voice sounds
AR: muscles for articulation or the further molding of these sounds into speech

REFERENCE NUMBER OF MUSCLE	PHONATOR OR ARTICULATOR	NAME OF MUSCLE, ORIGIN INSERTION, NERVE SUPPLY, AND ACTION
1	AR	AMYGDALOGLOSSUS O—Pharyngeal aponeurosis of the tonsil I—Continuous with palatoglossus N—Pharyngeal plexus A—Assists in lifting edge of tongue and rendering dorsum concave
2	PH	ARYTENOIDEUS OBLIQUUS O—Posterior of arytenoid cartilage I—Corniculuum laryngis N—Recurrent laryngeal A—Probably shortens the larynx
3	PH	ARYTENOIDEUS TRANSVERSUS O—Base and outer border of arytenoid cartilage I—Apex of the outer arytenoid cartilage N—Recurrent laryngeal A—Closes the posterior part of the glottis
4	AR	BASIOGLOSSUS O—Some fibres of hyglossus muscle arising from base of hyoid bone I—Intrinsic muscles of the tongue N—Hypoglossal A—Depresses the sides of the tongue
5	AR	BUCCINATOR O—Ridge of the mandible, alveolar process of maxilla, pterygomaxillary ligament I—Orbicularis oris muscle N—Buccal branch of the facial nerve A—Compresses the cheeks and retracts the angles of the mouth
6	AR	BUCCOPHARYNGEUS (the part of the constrictor pharyngis superior which arises from the pterygomandibular ligament)
7	AR	CANINUS O—Canine fossa of the maxillary bone I—Orbicularis oris, and the skin at the angle of the mouth N—Facial

REFERENCE NUMBER OF MUSCLE	PHONATOR OR ARTICULATOR	NAME OF MUSCLE, ORIGIN, INSERTION, NERVE SUPPLY, AND ACTION
		A—Raises the angle of the mouth
8	AR	CHONDROGLOSSUS (occasional) O—Medial side and base of lesser cornu of hyoid bone I—Intrinsic muscles of the tongue N—Hypoglossal A—Depresses and retracts the tongue
9	AR	CONSTRICTOR PHARYNGIS INFERIOR O—Cricoid and thyroid cartilages I—Posterior-median raphe of the pharynx N—Glossopharyngeal, pharyngeal plexus, and external and recurrent laryngeal A—Contracts the pharynx
10	AR	CONSTRICTOR PHARYNGIS MEDIUS O—Cornua of the hyoid bone, and the stylohyoid ligament I—Posterior-median raphe of the pharynx N—Glossopharyngeal, and pharyngeal plexus A—Contracts the pharynx
11	AR	CONSTRICTOR PHARYNGIS SUPERIOR O—Internal pterygoid plate, pterygomaxillary ligament, palate bone, alveolar process of the jaw and the sides of the tongue I—Posteriormedian raphe of the pharynx N—Pharyngeal plexus A—Contracts the pharynx
12	PH	CRICOARYTENOIDEUS LATERALIS O—Side of cricoid cartilage I—Outer angle and base of the arytenoid cartilage N—Recurrent laryngeal A—Closes the glottis
13	PH	CRICOARYTENOIDEUS POSTERIOR O—Posterior and cricoid cartilage I—Outer angle and base of the arytenoid cartilage N—Recurrent laryngeal A—Opens the glottis
14	PH	CRICOPHARYNGEUS O—Portion of constrictor pharyngis inferior arising from the cricoid cartilage I—Outer angle and base of arytenoid cartilage N—Recurrent laryngeal A—Opens the glottis
15	PH	CRICOTHYROIDEUS O—Anterior-lateral surfaces of cricoid cartilage I—Thyroid cartilage at lower, inner border N—Superior laryngeal A—Tenses the vocal cords
16	PH	DEPRESSOR EPIGLOTTIDIS O—A portion of the throepiglottideus I—Epiglottis N—Recurrent laryngeal A—Depresses epiglottis
17	AR	DIGASTRICUS (Anterior Belly) O—Intermediate tendon and hyoid bone I—Inner surface of mandible near symphysis N—Mylohyoid branch of inferior dental A—Elevates and retracts hyoid bone (Posterior Belly) O—Digastric groove of mastoid process I—Hyoid bone and intermediate tendon N—Facial A—Elevates and retracts hyoid bone and tongue
18	AR	GENIOGLOSSUS O—Mental spine of mandible near genu I—Hyoid bone and under surface of tongue N—Hypoglossal

REFERENCE NUMBER OF MUSCLE	PHONATOR OR ARTICULATOR	NAME OF MUSCLE, ORIGIN, INSERTION, NERVE SUPPLY, AND ACTION
		A—Retracts, depresses, and protrudes tongue: raises hyoid bone
19	AR	GENIOHYOIDEUS O—Mental spine of mandible I—Body of hyoid bone N—Hypoglossal A—Lifts and advances hyoid: aids in depressing jaw
20	AR	GLOSSOPALATINUS O—Under surface of soft palate I—Side of tongue N—Pharyngeal plexus A—Lifts back of tongue and narrows fauces
21	AR	GLOSSOPHARYNGEUS O—The part of the constrictor pharyngis superior arising from floor of mouth I—Posterior median raphe of the pharynx N—Pharyngeal plexus A—Contracts the pharynx
22	AR	HYOGLOSSUS O—Body of cornua and hyoid bone I—Side of tongue N—Hypoglossal A—Depresses side of tongue and retracts tongue
23	AR	LEVATOR LABII INFERIORIS (same as mentalis)
24	AR	LEVATOR LABII SUPERIORIS O—Inferior margin of orbit I—Upper lip N—Facial A—Lifts and protrudes upper lip
25	AR	LEVATOR LABII SUPERIORIS ALAE QUE NASI O—Nasal process of maxilla I—Upper lip, cartilage of ala nasi N—Facial A—Raises upper lip: dilates nostril
26	AR	LEVATOR VELI PALATINI O—Temporal bone, and cartilaginous part of Eustachian tube I—Aponeurosis of soft palate N—Pharyngeal plexus A—Raises soft palate
27	AR	LINGUALIS INFERIOR O—Under surface of tongue at base I—Tip of tongue N—Chorda tympani A—Shortens the tongue
28	AR	LINGUALIS SUPERIOR O—Submucosa and septum of the tongue I—Edges of the tongue N—Hypoglossal A—Shortens tongue: raises edges and tip of tongue
29	AR	LINGUALIS TRANSVERSUS O—Median septum of the tongue I—Edges of the tongue N—Hypoglossal A—Narrows and stretches tongue and lifts its edges
30	AR	LINGUALIS VERTICALIS O—Upper surface of tongue near sides of tip I—Under surface of tongue N—Hypoglossal A—Flattens tip of tongue
31	AR	MASSETER O—Zygomatic arch and malar process I—Angle and ramus of mandible N—Mandibular division of trigeminal A—Assists in closing the mouth
32	AR	MENTALIS O—Mandible I—Skin of chin N—Facial A—Raises lower lip and wrinkles skin of chin
33	AR	MYLOHYOIDEUS O—Mylohoid ridge of mandible

REFERENCE NUMBER OF MUSCLE	PHONATOR OR ARTICULATOR	NAME OF MUSCLE, ORIGIN, INSERTION, NERVE SUPPLY, AND ACTION
		I—Hyoid bone and median raphe N—Branch of trigeminal A—Raises hyoid: helps depress jaw
34	AR	NASOLABIALIS O—Septum of the nose I—Upper lip N—Buccal branch of facial A—Raises the upper lip
35	AR	OMOHYOIDEUS O—Superior border of the scapula I—Hyoid bone N—Upper cervical through ansa hypoglossi A—Retracts and depresses hyoid. Contracts cervical fascia
36	AR	ORBICULARIS ORIS O—Nasal septum and canine fossa of mandible I—Angle of the mouth N—Facial A—Closes mouth: wrinkles puckers lips
37	AR	PHARYNGOPALATINUS O—Soft palate I—APONEUROSIS of pharynx N—Pharyngeal plexus A—Narrows fauces and shuts off nasopharynx
38	AR	PLATYSMA MYOIDES O—Clavicle and scapula I—Lower border of mandible: muscles of cheek; angle of mouth N—Facial and cervical plexus A—Wrinkles skin, depresses mouth and lower lip
39	AR	PTERYGOIDUS EXTERNUS O—External pterygoid plate; great wing of sphenoid bone I—Condyle of mandible N—External pterygoid A—Draws lower jaw forward
40	AR	PTERYGOIDUS INTERNUS O—Pterygoid fossa of sphenoid bone; tuberosity maxilla I—Inner surface of ramus and angle of mandible N—Internal pterygoid A—Raises and juts forward the lower jaw
41	AR	QUADRATUS LABII INFERIORIS O—Anterior portion of lower border of the mandible I—Orbicularis oris and skin of lower lip N—Facial A—Depresses the lower lip
		QUADRATUS LABII SUPERIORIS composed of three muscles: LEVATOR LABII SUPERIORIS LEVATOR LABII SUPERIORIS ALAE QUE NASI ZYGOMATICUS MINOR (each as listed elsewhere)
42	AR	RISORIUS O—Fascia over masseter I—Angle of the mouth N—Buccal branch of facial nerve A—Draws angle of the mouth out; compresses cheek
43	AR	SALPINGOPHARYNGEUS O—Eustachian tube near nasopharynx I—Posterior part of palatopharyngeus N—Internal branch of spinal accessory A—Raises nasopharynx
44	AR	STERNOHYOIDEUS O—Sternum and clavicle I—Body of hyoid bone N—Upper cervical A—Depresses the hyoid and larynx
45	PH	STERNOTHYROIDEUS

REFERENCE NUMBER OF MUSCLE	PHONATOR OR ARTICULATOR	NAME OF MUSCLE, ORIGIN, INSERTION, NERVE SUPPLY, AND ACTION
		O—Sternum and first rib I—Ala of thyroid cartilage N—Upper cervical A—Depresses the larynx
46	AR	STYLOGLOSSUS O—Styloid process and stylomaxillary ligament I—Side of tongue N—Hypoglossal A—Raises and retracts tongue
47	AR	STYLOHYOIDEUS O—Styloid process of temporal bone I—Body of hyoid bone N—Facial A—Draws hyoid bone and the tongue upward and backward
48	AR	STYLOPHARYNGEUS O—Styloid process of temporal bone I—Lateral side of pharynx N—Pharyngeal plexus: Glossopharyngeal A—Raises and dilates the pharynx
49	AR	TEMPORALIS O—Temporal fossa and fascia on side of head I—Coronoid process of mandible N—Mandibular branch of trigeminal A—Shuts mouth and retracts the jaw
50	AR	TENSOR VELI PALATINI O—Scaphoid fossa, spine or sphenoid, and the temporal bone I—Palatine aponeurosis and the palatum durum N—Otic ganglion A—Tenses the soft palate
51	PH	THYROARYTENOIDEUS O—Thyroid cartilage and cricothyroid membrane I—Arytenoid cartilage N—Recurrent laryngeal A—Relaxes and shortens vocal cords
52	PH	THYROEPIGLOTTICUS O—Thyroid cartilage I—Sacculus laryngis and aryteno-epiglottidean folds N—Recurrent laryngeal A—Depresses epiglottis and compresses bacculus
53	PH	THYROHYOIDEUS O—Side of thyroid cartilage I—Greater horn and body of hyoid bone N—Upper cervical A—Raises and changes the form of the larynx
54	AR	TRIANGULARIS O—Lower border of mandible I—Lower lip near angle of mouth N—Facial A—Pulls down corners of the mouth
55	AR	UVULAE O—Posterior nasal spine I—Greater part of the uvula N—Pharyngeal plexus A—Raises uvula
56	PH	VOCALIS O—Thyroid cartilage, internal surfaces I—Vocal process of arytenoid cartilages N—Recurrent laryngeal A—Shortens and relaxes vocal cords
57	AR	ZYGOMATICUS MAJOR O—Malar bone before zygomatic suture I—Angle of mouth N—Facial A—Draws angle of mouth upward and backward
58	AR	ZYGOMATICUS MINOR O—Malar bone behind zygomatic suture I—Orbicularis oris and levator labii superioris N—Facial A—Draws upper lip upward and outward

BIBLIOGRAPHY

Blakiston's New Gould Medical Dictionary. 1956. Hoerr, N., and Osol, A., eds. (2nd. ed.). New York: McGraw-Hill.

DeuPree, R. 1963. A comparative study of laryngectomy procedures and their effect on the intelligibility of esophageal speech. Long Beach: Calif. State. Master's thesis.

———, and Rappaport, I. 1963. Origin, insertion, nerve supply and action of some muscles of speech. *Research report to VA Hosp.* Long Beach, Calif.

Deweese, D., and Saunders, W. 1964. Textbook of otolaryngology (2nd. ed.). St. Louis: Mosby. Pp. 115–127.

Dolowitz, D. 1964. Basic otolaryngology. New York: McGraw-Hill. Pp. 239–242.

Dorland's illustrated medical dictionary. 1957 (23rd. ed.). Philadelphia: Saunders.

Grant, J. 1962. Atlas of anatomy (5th. ed.). Baltimore: Williams & Wilkins. Pp. 458–475; Pp. 540–558; Pp. 572–579; Pp. 584–588; Pp. 591–600.

Gray, G., and Wise, C. 1959. The bases of speech (3rd. ed.). New York: Harper and Row. Pp. 135–199.

Gray, H. 1966. Anatomy of the human body (28th. ed.), Goss, C., ed. Philadelphia: Lea & Febiger. Pp. 382–448; Pp. 907–965; Pp. 1185–1206.

Grog, D., Johns, R., and Harvey, A. 1955. Symposium on myasthenia gravis. *JAMA*, 19, 694.

Hamm, A., and Leeson, T. 1961. Histology. (4th. ed.). Philadelphia: Lippincott. Pp. 431–436.

Hanson, J., and Huxley, H. 1955. The structural bases of contraction in striated muscle. *Symp. soc. exper. biol.*, 9, 228–264.

Heymans, C. 1938. Role of the cardioaortic and carotid sinus nerves in the reflex control of the respiratory center. *New Eng. J. Med.*, 219, 157.

Hoops, R. 1960. Speech science. Springfield, Ill.: Thomas. Pp. 33–34.

Johnson, P. 1966. In Physiology. (2nd. ed.). Selkirk, E., ed. The dynamics of respiratory structures. Nervous and chemical control of respiration. Boston: Little, Brown. Pp. 427–443; Pp. 471–487.

Katz, B., and Miledi, R. 1965. Propagation of electric activity in motor nerve terminals *Proc. roy. soc. (biol.)*, 161, 453–503.

Kelsey, C., Wanowski, S., Hixton, T., and Minifie, F. 1968. Determination of lateral pharyngeal wall motion during connected speech by use of pulsed ultrasound. *Science.* 161, 1259–1260.

Liljestrand, A. 1958. Mechanism of respiration. *Physiol. Rev.*, 38, 691.

Lindsay, J. 1968. ed. Yearbook of the ear, nose, and throat. Chicago: Year Book Med. Pub. Pp. 135–187.

Meano, C. 1967. The human voice in speech and song. *Trans. by* Khoury, A. Springfield, Ill.: Thomas. Pp. 3–150.

Morris' Human Anatomy. 1966. Anson, B., ed. Pharynx, nasal, and oral cavities. Pp. 1261–1279; Larynx, Pp. 1409–1427. New York: McGraw-Hill.

Myerson, M. 1964. The human larynx. Springfield, Ill.: Thomas. Pp. 11–48.

Netter, F. 1948. The ciba collection of medical illustrations. Summit, N.J.: Ciba Phar. Co., P. 20. (Out of print.)

Ochs, S. 1966. In Physiology (2nd. ed.). Selkirk, E., ed. Receptors and effectors. Boston: Little, Brown. Pp. 60–63.

Palay, S. and Palade, G. 1955. Muscle contraction. *J. Biophys. and Biochem. Cytol.*, 1, 69.

Patton, H. 1965. Physiology and biophysica, Ruch, T., and Patton, H., ed. (19th. ed.). Philadelphia: Saunders. Pp. 73–110.

Rappaport, I. 1962. Address before the tumor board, VA Hosp. Long Beach, Calif.

Roughton, F. 1954. Respiratory physiology in aviation. Boothby, W. M., ed. San Antonio: USAF School of Aviation Medicine. P. 51.

Ruch, T. 1961. Neurophysiology. Philadelphia: Saunders. P. 390.

Sansom Wright's Applied Physiology. 1961. Muscle and the nervous system, Keele, C. and Neill, E., eds. (10th. ed.). London: Oxford. Pp. 227–238.

Saunders, W. 1964. The larynx. *Clin. Symp.*, 16–3, 67–99.

Stedman's Medical Dictionary. 1966. Baltimore: Williams & Wilkins.

Taber, C. 1965. Taber's cyclopedic medical dictionary. Philadelphia: Davis.

Toldt, C. 1919. An atlas of human anatomy. New York: MacMillan. Vol. 2, Pp. 260–262; Pp. 412–436.

Truex, R., and Kellner, C. 1948. Detailed atlas of the head and neck. London: Oxford. P. 67.

Whitteridge, D. 1948. Afferent nerve fibers from the heart and lungs in the cervical vagus. *J. Physiol.*, 107, 496–512.

Wise, C. 1960. Introduction to phonetics. Englewood Cliffs, N.J.: Prentice-Hall. Pp. 46–47.

Woodbury, J., Gordon, A., and Conrad, J. 1965. Physiology and biophysics. Ruch, T., and Patton, H. eds. (19th. ed.). Philadelphia: Saunders. Pp. 113–146.

3

The Neurophysiology of Speech

Robert West

The neurophysiology of speech is as complex as speech itself. Speech is produced by many coordinating factors. To analyze the neurophysiology of speech it is necessary to study separately each of these factors.

BREATHING

The underlying basis of speech is voice, and voice is basically a respiratory function. Breathing is managed by a complicated respiratory reflex involving the two vagus nerves (Xth Cranial nerves) and the two phrenic nerves from the cervical section of the cord. In this reflex the vagus nerves carry inhibitory, sensory impulses from the lungs to the respiratory center of the medulla; and the phrenic nerves carry excitatory impulses from the medulla to the muscles of the diaphragm. Thus the two sets of nerves function as reciprocating antagonists in the in-and-out processes of breathing. This reflex process begins at birth and is coterminous with life itself. Breathing is automatic (not autonomic). This automatism is based upon the respiratory center of the medulla, and is an inborn function of the brain stem. It is modifiable, within limits, by at least three cerebral automatisms:

1. emotional mechanisms subtended by the basal ganglia under the floor of the cerebrum. It is a commonly known fact that emotional reactions modify breathing.
2. learned processes of utterance, such as the acts of counting aloud, saying one's prayers, or reciting or singing poetry. These acts involve the breaking up of the basic respiratory reflexes.
3. the conscious and deliberate spacing, timing, and checking of the respiratory reflex such as in voluntary speech. Here the reflex of breathing is consciously made subservient to the needs of speech utterance.

An essential part of the breathing mechanism is the valve that controls the entrance and exit of the air through the bronchus, viz., the larynx. The impulses that control this valve come via branches from the motor portions of the vagus nerve, which are designated the inferior and superior laryngeal nerves; the greater control of the valve comes via the inferior nerves. As with breathing, the control is reflexive and automatic, but the automatism is subject to higher centers. The fundamental difference between *come* and *gum*, for example, is not a difference between modes of articulation of the tongue, but a difference in the laryngeal positions at the beginnings of the two words. Speech changes are often laryngeal, rather than lingual, that is, phonatory rather than articulatory. Two British Tommies were startled by a voice in the night and one said to the other: "wat's that?" The other said "that's a owl." Then the first said: "Yes, I know it'a a owl, but oo the ell is owling?" Here the failure of communication is due to the fact they simply did not understand each other's laryngeal neurophysiology. In the evolution of language the neurophysiological modification of the laryngeal reflexes may take on real discriminatory meanings, such as *price* vs. *prize*, *safe* vs. *save*, *loose* vs. *lose*, *sheath* vs. *sheathe*. The *h* sound, and all voiceless consonants, require the momentary opening of the larynx. Whispering requires voluntary inhibition of the laryngeal abductors for all sounds, even vowels.

ARTICULATION

The musculature of articulation receives impulses from several branches of the Cranial nerves. In speech these impulses are completely voluntary. The important controls are as follows:

1. the right and left hypoglossal, the XII Cranial nerves. They carry impulses for the movements of the blade of the tongue. These movements are essential aspects of certain speech sounds, such as *n*, *l*, *r*, *s*, *z*, *t*, *d*, ʃ, ʒ, *θ*, and ð in which the tongue tip is raised or pointed or shaped. This does not mean that the hypoglossals are the only Cranial nerves involved in these sounds, but rather that there is a commonality in control, and that commonality is via the hypoglossals. Failure of hypoglossal control characteristically disturbs them all.
2. the pharyngeal plexus. This nucleus is made up of fibers from the IXth, Xth and XIth Cranial nerves, the glossopharyngeal, the vagus, and the spinal accessory nerves. Impulses from this plexus characteristically control in the production of *p*, *b*, *t*, *d*, *k*, and *g*; also *s*, *z*, *θ*, ð, ʃ, ʒ; and to some extent they control the vowel sounds and the consonants *f* and *v*.
3. the right and left glossopharyngeal nerves, the IXth Cranials. Impulses from these nerves control the production of the vowels, especially those that are made with the back of the tongue, such as *u*, *v*, ɔ, and ð.
4. the right and left auditory nerves, the VIIIth Cranials. Impulses from these sensory nerves serve as monitors in the servosystem that is involved in the learning and control of speech. Every sound of speech is thus partially under control of the auditory nerves.
5. the right and left facial nerves, the VIIth Cranials. Impulses from these nerves characteristically control the production of the consonants *f*, *v*, *p*, *b*, *m*, and *w*, also the vowels *u*, *v*, and ð. One branch of each facial nerve serves to control the stapedius muscle on its side of the body. The stapedius muscle functions as the antagonist of the tensor tympani, balancing the muscular pressure and adjusting it to the changes of acoustic intensity that impinge upon the ear. The proprioceptive fibers of the stapedius nerve carry impulses to the auditory center of the brain by which one judges the intensity of a sound striking the ear.
6. the right and left trigeminals, the Vth pair of Cranial nerves. Those articulatory movements that involve the opening and closing of the jaws are controlled by impulses from that pair. These impulses are purely voluntary. Proprioceptive impulses are carried by the trigeminals to help monitor the articulatory movements of the lips. Thus vowels *æ*, *a*, ɔ are in part controlled by the trigeminals, as well as the consonants *f*, *v*, *m*, *p*, and *b*. A branch of each trigeminal nerve enters the ear to control automatically the movements of the tensor tympani muscles. This mechanism serves as the antagonist of the muscular adjustments of the stapedius. When impulses are sent via the Vth nerves to increase the tonus of the tensor tympani muscles, they serve to balance the impulses sent via the VIIth nerves to decrease the tension of the stapedius muscles. Proprioceptive impulses, carried by the Vth nerve, from the tensor tympani muscles are interpreted in the brain as changes of pressure on the outer membrane of the tympanum and give a sense of the loudness, or faintness, of the sound entering the outer meatus of the ear.

THE RETICULAR FORMATION

All sensory inputs enter the brain proper via the thalamus, where the nerves that carry the incoming stimuli synapse with the cerebral connections. Parallel with the sensory nerves via the thalamus is a series of reticulate structures through which the incoming stimuli pass and in which they are sorted out. Those impulses that are meaningful to the individual are relayed to the cerebral centers in which they can produce appropriate reactions. Those impulses that are relatively meaningless are shunted out of the cerebral circuits. Were it not for this sorting mechanism, called the reticular formation, the process of sensory reception would be a melange of stimulations of all sensory areas of the cerebrum. The individual would react to unrelated stimuli, and to stimuli that might be antagonistic to each other. Apparently this reticular formation normally develops in babyhood and early childhood. Before the development of this formation the baby is prevented from overstimulation by the functioning of the sleep brain, which quiets reactions to all stimulation.

In cooperation with the sensory areas of the cerebrum, the reticular formation serves as an arousal mechanism to alert the individual to meaningful patterns of stimulation. Sound patterns in particular are reacted to when such patterns are either harbingers of danger or signals of pleasant stimulation. Thus the processes of attention and alarm are negotiated by the cooperation between the reticular formation and the auditory center of the left cortex. Not only is the auditory center made sensitive to bells, whistles, sirens, and musical patterns, but to spoken words of special significance. Any of these acoustic effects may be signals of alarm or of pleasant stimulations to follow, depending upon the training of the cooperating mechanisms involved. The reaction, moreover, to countless other sounds and words may be obscured, such as miscellaneous conversations, television programs, street noises, etc.

THE BASAL GANGLIA

So far as the neurophysiology of speech is concerned, the basal ganglia are emotional centers that color, and sometimes block, speech. These ganglia, or nuclei, are located deep within the cerebrum on either side of the midline. They are arranged, as though in line, with the thalamus first. This organ is largely sensory. Next is the caudate nucleus, an associative instrument in which some primitive and unconscious interpretations are made of the sensations that have been received in the thalamus. Next in the line is the putamen, a center where are "stored" innate patterns for motor responses appropriate to the interpretations made by the caudate nucleus. Last is the globus pallidus, a body made up largely of efferent neurones that are immediately responsible for activating impulses that will result in reactions of the body—in speech the emotional accompaniments of the words spoken and heard, and sometimes the actual inhibiting of language.

The caudate nucleus, putamen, and globus pallidus are by some referred to as the corpora striata, or striate bodies, though some limit the term to the putamen and the globus pallidus. The globus pallidus and the putamen are physically intimately related and are together often referred to as the lenticular nucleus or lentiform body. The globus pallidus alone is often referred to as the paleostriatum, in contrast to the neostriatum, consisting of the putamen and the caudate nucleus. To help the student to move with ease among the organs and ideas here mentioned, Fig. 3-1 has been prepared.

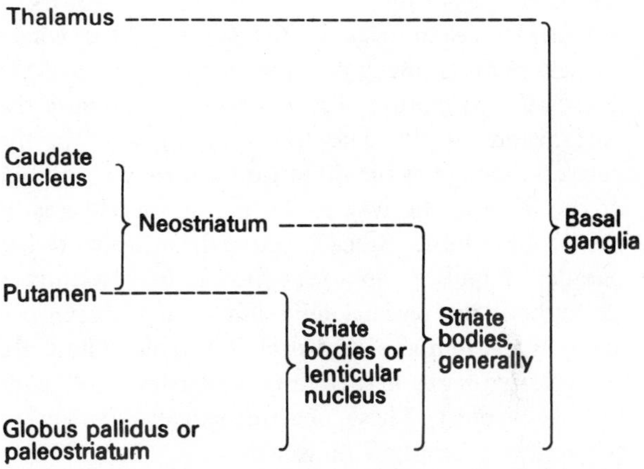

Fig. 3-1. The relation of the basal ganglia to one another.

LINGUISTIC MECHANISMS

The unit of language is a word. This word in neurophysiology begins with a sensory pattern made up of stimulations from audition, vision, touch, proprioception, etc. This sensory pattern is transferred to the parietal lobe (usually in the left hemisphere of the cerebrum). Here the miracle of *conscious recognition* takes place. (In the meantime the sorting-out process by means of the reticular formation has taken place.) If the situation involves the speaking of the word standing for the thing recognized, impulses issue from this parietal lobe and travel to the left motor cortex of the frontal lobe. Here the second miracle takes place, the conscious will to speak the word. This is in the famous convolution of Broca. Now impulses are sent to the special motor cells on the posterior border of the left frontal lobe (on the bank of the fissure of Rolando). At the same instant, impulses are sent by way of the corpus callosum to the motor cells of the right frontal lobe. The motor areas of the right lobe that are stimulated are those that are analogical to the ones stimulated on the left.

Thus the first movement of the word to be spoken is initiated. As soon as the muscular movement is undertaken, sensations are received to report the fact. These sensations are by way of the auditory area and via the proprioceptive area on the anterior border of the parietal lobe. These sensations trigger the next movement involved in the sound to be spoken. The motor process is repeated and the next movement in the word is uttered, and the next, and the next, in very rapid succession. This is, in simple terms (perhaps overly simple), the utterance of a word.

Now let us go back to the parietal lobe where miracle number one is performed, the miracle of the conscious recognition of a unit word. Seldom is the recognition simple. The travel of impulses in the parietal lobe is not the direct, into, through, and out of the lobe on the way to the motor speech area of the frontal lobe, Broca's convolution, but rather parallel impulses are sent in circular pathways throughout the parietal lobe and even into sensory areas in the temporal and occipital lobes. These are complicated *nerve nets* (more about nerve nets later in the chapter). These nets furnish enrichment to the simple concept of the word.

Let us take, as a simple illustration, the word *cat*. One may enrich the concept by a net circuit by way of the occipital lobe in which the picture of his own cat is exhibited, or one may think of catlike animals, or the spelling of the word *cat*. Or on a trip through the temporal lobe one may think of the sound of the cat's cry—all these in addition to the network circuits in the parietal lobe itself, involving the concepts of pain (the cat's scratch and bite), the texture of her fur, the weight of the animal, and the feel of her body against one's leg.

After this complicated concept of *cat* has been built up, then one says about a person, "She is a real cat," then other cricuits are involved, circuits that must be traveled before the command is issued to the convolution of Broca. Although the actual motor patterns for the utterance of the word *cat* may be the same as for the simple, uncomplicated utterance of the word, the conscious experience mediated by the parietal lobe will be vastly different. There is little outward evidence of this activity but, unless we completely discount our introspections, we must accept the reality of this and other hidden mental processes. Worry, recurrent fears, dreams, and so on, are to most of us incontrovertible realities. We know that we have experienced them; and we know that, for the most part, we can conceal these processes from the observer. We assume, however, that others have similar experiences; and that, without a recounting by the dreamer of the plot of his dreams, we can have little, if any, knowledge of what he is dreaming. These inner experiences are processed by feedback mechanisms. All contemplations, imaginings, plannings, calculations, considered decisions, and the like, are similarly processed. Accompanying all speech except the most mechanical processes of reading and reciting is a great deal of reverberating, circular cerebration employing feedback nets.

An illustration: You are asked to introduce one of your friends to another. You look at each to recall his name. Your memory of the name of each is immediate, but you are dismayed to discover that only the first name of each "comes to your mind." The more you struggle to recall the last names, the more you are disconcerted, and the more loudly these first names ring out in your auditory memory. There is no use in struggling with the problem. To wrestle with a reverberating nerve net is futile. All you can say is, "If I had not wanted to speak his name, it would have come to me instantly; but never mind, don't tell me; it will come to me later." Then, after a change of association, the "reverberations" will stop and you will interrupt a conversation with, "I have it now: Your name is Williams." If instead of trying to introduce your friends you had sat alone in the quiet of your home and had called each on the telephone, you would have had no difficulty in finding their numbers in an alphabetical listing of their last names. There is probably a good deal of this type of reverberation in stuttering.

It is obvious that many mental fixations, compulsions, and recurring fantasies of psychopathologies are also viewable as the result of complex reverberating circuits. In fact, the rationale frequently offered for electroshock therapy is to break up such nerve nets in which the patient's personality is ensnared. One such resonant circuit is particularly significant in the understanding of the speech failures of young children. Speech depends for its initial motivation upon an instinct, or appetence, for gregarious relations. The child who is completely indifferent to his human environment does not develop speech. Antisocial attitudes are more productive of speech than the asocial.Asocial attitudes in a child potentially normal in intellectual equipment involve preoccupation with his fantasy life. Such a child learns to derive great psychic income from inner experiences unrelated to the social world of reality. The child whose mental mechanisms are prompted by the attitudes, remarks, and deeds of persons around him is not so likely to develop self-stimulating nerve circuits as the one whose promptings are from within his own system. In limiting his reactions to those triggered from within, the variety of response is restricted, until finally the repertoire of these responses is reduced to those few mental mechanisms that characterize his special and particular aberrations. These mechanisms have very aptly been labeled autistic. There is in this label a definitely *double entendre*: *autistic* signifies, *psychologically*, a preoccupation with self and a rejection of the psychosocial environment, and, *physiologically*, a lowering of the threshold of stimulation of the nerve nets of the brain by impulses from other nets and a raising of the threshold to stimulations brought over exteroceptor pathways.

THE BINARY NATURE OF NEUROMUSCULAR ACTIVITY

Inasmuch as all mental processes are, in the last analysis, the result of activity of nerve fibers, so mental functions, as well as simple muscle responses, follow the law of all-or-none reaction. Since there are only two states of a living nerve fiber: 1) that of activity or discharge, and 2) that of rest and recharge, all mental activity can be reduced to formulas of binary numbers.[1]

Binary:	0	1	10	11	100	101	110	111	1000	1001
Decimal:	0	1	2	3	4	5	6	7	8	9

In the body there are two major systems of internal communication, the nervous and the endocrine. In terms of quantitative values, the former may better be represented by binary and the latter by decimal numbers. The strength of contraction of a given muscle at a given instant depends, among other factors, upon the amount of the stimulation by the nerve supplying the muscle. This amount is the measure of the number of nerve fibers firing at the instant in question, each fiber functioning at maximum intensity. The amount is, therefore, expressible in binary numbers. The strength of contraction of a given muscle is also, in part, dependent upon the hormonic conditioning of the muscle by catalysts carried from the endocrine gland, through the blood stream, into the cells of the muscle itself. The amount of hormonic effect is a linear function of the amount of the catalyst brought to the muscle, and can best be represented in degrees, percentage, proportions, or other values expressed decimally. The picture of a functioning motor nerve is like a halftone, its surface being made up of black dots on a white background. None of the dots, even on the areas that seem gray, are anything but black, each as black as the rest. The picture, however, of the hormonic effect of the endocrine gland is like that of a colored photograph in which the color consists of dyes. The color of any one area, no matter how small, can be expressed in shades and tints of primary colors. Thus, we listen, and think, and speak in terms of either-or-, plus-minus, 1–0 process; but the thresholds at which these intellectual phenomena appear are determined by more-less, stronger-weaker, acid-basic, combinations and relations.

CYBERNETIC REACTIONS OF THE C.N.S.[2]

An electronic calculating machine makes use of the all-or-none principle and the binary system of numbers. Such an instrument seems functionally analogous to the human central nervous system. Just as the calculating machine receives and stores information to use later in solving problems, stating overall values, and making predictions, so the human being receives and stores information and later, sometimes decades later, makes linguistic pronouncements on the basis of the information received.

Just as the accuracy and validity of the record that issues from the calculating machine are dependent upon the material that was punched upon the tapes

[1] The binary number system is one in which there is only one digit (instead of nine) and the zero. In this system every number is an expression of a selection between one value or another, or one series or another, of a series of such selections. In this system 0 (decimal system)=0 (binary system), and 1 (*d*)=1 (*b*). The choice here is between whether something *is* or *is not*. 0 (*b*) means *is not*. The number 2 (*d*) is in last analysis two choices as to whether two things are or are not, with the decision being "are" in both cases. This doubling of the positive decision is in the binary system indicated by placing the figure 1 in the first space to the left, as is done in a decimal system to indicate ten. Thus if "one-zero" (10) equals ten in a system of 10 digits, "one-zero" (10) equals two in a system of 2 digits. 3 (*d*) is really the result of the decisions involved in 2 (*d*) with one more decision as to whether an additional thing *is* or *is not*. 4 (*d*) involves two decisions such as in 2 (*d*). 5 (*d*), the same as 4 (*d*), plus the additional decision as to an extra unit, etc.

[2] *Cybernetics* (Greek *kubernētēs*=steersman) is a word adapted by Norbert Wiener to generalize his study of communication and control in the theory of messages. Hence *cybernetic*, used adjectivally as here.

making up the creature's experience, so the accuracy and validity of this record that you are now following with your eye are dependent upon the author's experience. What you are now reading is like the tapes that your electronic cousin scans with his electric eye. You can respond to this "tape" by reading it, either silently or aloud, or by copying it in your notebook; or you can respond to it as it becomes one of a great many tapes you have experienced in the past. Just as the reliability of the calculating machine suffers when a condenser is shorted or a tube is blown, so the reliability of your machine is disturbed by defects of structure. A single bullet may destroy either machine, or it may cause either to function erratically.

It is obvious that all automatisms subtended by the central nervous system, both innate and acquired, are developed, stored, and "played back," much as are the routine reactions of any man-made cybernetic device. Following this figure a little further, we can say the C.N.S. is not one cybernetic instrument but several interlocking automatic devices employing many of the same mechanical effectors. It is true that in the cerebellum the vermis is an automatic integrator of the various, often conflicting, machines; yet this clearing-house center leaves unresolved many of the conflicts among the acquired automatisms, and, in clearing the demands of conflicting cybernetic instruments, gives precedence to those whose functions are vital and vegetative, to the detriment of the intellectual and linguistic instrumentalities. In short, the automatic talking machine often is the last cleared.

Cybernetics helps us to understand not only the acquired automatisms already described in this chapter but also most of our intellectual processes. Practically all that we call *mind* can be conceived in part as being the product of an electronic calculating machine or of a binary system or of both. The center of it all is the parietal lobe and related cortical parts.

Cybernetic processes

1. Association of ideas
2. Conditioned reflexes
3. Mathematical processes
4. Prediction of future events
5. Intuition
6. Recall and imagination
7. Rote memory
8. Immediate memory span and positive after-image
9. Hypnosis and suggestion
10. Analogical thinking and figures of speech

Binary processes

1. If a word has both a synonym and an antonym the utterance of that word will by free association call forth the antonym rather than the synonym: *boy-girl*, rather than *boy-lad; bad-good*, rather than *bad-evil; yes-no*, rather than *yes-O.K.*

2. Negative questions and answers. Illustration: Suppose you ask someone about the weather today. If you really want information, you inquire, "*Is it nice today or isn't it?*" In terms of the binary system you are asking for 1 or 0. If you have already discovered the weather to be pleasant you say, "*Isn't it nice?*" You ask for an answer exactly opposite to what you expect. You virtually say "*Is it foul out today?*" The answer to "*Isn't it nice?*" is "*yes.*" The informer is agreeing, not to the question as stated, but as implied. His answer is equivalent to "*Yes, we have no bananas.*" If you have discovered the weather to be unpleasant, you say, "*It isn't nice today, is it?*" Again the answer is illogical, but still clear by negative implication or association. The reply is "*no.*"

3. Antonyms made by change of sign (like changing the 1 to 0): like-dislike, like-unlike, behave-misbehave, polite-impolite, typical-atypical, thing-nothing, encode-decode, can-can't, where-nowhere, body-nobody. We even have double reverses of meaning like: encouraged-discouraged-undiscouraged. One perfect example of the binary system is the antonymous pair *one-none* (*one-no-one* or 1–0).

On a higher level of experience we polarize our reactions to many aspects of an environment. The room is either "hot" or "cold," seldom "just right" (and never "just right" for the whole party). "Love" and "hate" are notoriously identified as related polarizations of romantic attachments. We and our allies are noble: our enemies are evil: and we have no difficulty in switching our opinion from "bad" to "good," when an enemy changes sides and becomes our ally. All the characters in the Western thriller may be placed in two simple categories, the "good ones" and the "bad ones." Most opinions about individuals from social, racial, political, and religious groups other than our own are drawn from generalizations in which various qualities of character and sundry physical aspects are listed as being either present or absent. Hence our first question about such a person, to whom we have just been introduced, is not a decimal calculation of "to what degree?" but a binary question of "is he, or isn't he?" Delusions of persecution are but overextensions, or oversimplifications, of these "black or white" polarizations. The Whigs won the last election. Our party lost. Now we can expect a depression, high taxes, and severe drought.

Much of our problem solving, mathematical or otherwise, is by binary processes. "If one dozen oranges costs 30 cents, how much would 18 cost?" The child who first encounters such a problem in his "oral arithmetic" does not move at once to the correct method of solution. He tries many methods, rejecting each in turn until he finds one that satisfies him. He has in this simple problem the numbers, ½, 1, 2, 3, 6, 12, 18, and 30. Shall he add, subtract, multiply, or divide? Several right, and many wrong, combinations are available. The question always comes to him: Is this right or wrong? Seldom does he list all the possibilities and then make a selection. He employs binary judgements of random suggestions. Even an experienced adult employs some binary processes in the solution of the problem. He has several correct methods to try and, if he wishes, reject. For example, he tries the logical method of finding the cost of one orange, but rejects the method when he discovers that the cost would not be even money. Then, "on second thought," he may see that the cost of one orange could be expressed as 30/12 of one cent; and thus one solution would require the multiplication of 30 by 18, followed by division by 12. This seems too big a project to solve without paper and pencil. Then he starts again and finds that he can easily discover the cost of six oranges, and that 18 is exactly three sixes. This flitting from method to method is done with such great speed that it is only by dint of sharp introspection that one can discover his binary calculator at work.

Another example of perceptive binary processes is that of proofreading. The proofreader makes rapid judgements as to whether what he hears the copyreader say is, or is not, the same as what he sees on the proof sheet. Whenever the general pattern of one agrees with the other, the judgement is "same." His mistakes consist of letting what he sees influence what he hears or vice versa. Advertisers exploit this propensity to binary error by making meaningless claims that seem to have definite meaning. "After a national survey of the dentifrice used by 50,000 dentists it was found that more dentists chose Scratcho than any other dentifrice." What the average reader understands this to say is that "dentists use more Scratcho than any other dentifrice." His error arises from the fact that he tries to fit a meaning to the overall pattern of the sentence, not noticing that the word *more* modifies *dentists* rather than *Scratcho*. No meaning fits the sentence as a whole, but he accepts his version just as the proofreader accepts *house* for *horse* in the sentence, "He put spurs to his house."

The binary and cybernetic illustrations seem even more cogent when one considers what happens to an individual's mental processes when the machinery back of those processes is damaged. Just as a damaged card-sorting machine will make errors in assembling cards in predetermined categories, so a lesion in the C.N.S. will manifest itself in one or more of the following:

1. bizarre association of ideas, or a paucity of association.
2. failure to apply measures consistently in solving problems involving counting or other numerical processes.
3. failure to employ past experiences in anticipation of future situations.
4. degeneration of intuition into impulsive, unrealistic rationalization.
5. inability to construct in imagery that which is not presently sensed.
6. inability to learn such stereotypes of expression as poems, musical compositions, prayers, and dance routines, or the inability to change a stereotype once learned.
7. a perseveration of pattern of immediate response, such as verbal iterations.
8. tendency of the patient to respond to conflicting suggestions (ambivalent reactions).
9. inability of the patient to make any but the most literal interpretations of what he hears or reads; or the tendency to invest literal language with absurd figurative meanings.

Just as a person inexperienced in the manipulations of the binary number system will be slow, clumsy, and inaccurate in his calculations in the 0–1 notation, so will the damaged brain show binary errors. The patient will record 0 instead of 1 for two quite different reasons:

1) The loss of the concept of *opposite*. Associations are all of one sign: *good, evil, bad, kind* are all responses to either of the following questions: what words mean the same as *nice?* What words mean the opposite of *nice?* In spite of this failure the patient usually knows what each of these words means. He has but lost the concept of the relationship between ideas.

2) The uncertainty of response involving words having well-known opposites. He may say *yes* when he means *no*. He knows that *yes* and *no* are opposite, but he is not sure of which is which. He often chooses 1 instead of 0, or vice versa.

NERVE NETS

One of the all-pervasive mechanisms of the cerebrospinal nervous system is that of the "feedback circuit." Again a close analogy can be drawn from the realm of electronics. If the microphone into which a person is talking—such as the microphone of the hearing aid—be brought too close to the earpiece of the instrument, a squeal results. The electrical output of the amplifier is converted into acoustic energy, a part of which finds its way to the diaphragm of the microphone. This increases the flow of electrons from the cathode of the microphone tube, thus causing an extra discharge across the amplifier with increased output to the ear piece. The frequency, or pitch, of the discharge and the feedback will be that to which the entire circuit is most resonant. The simplest feedback circuits of the cerebrospinal system are much like the circuit described above. A contracting muscle pinches, and thus stimulates, the kinesthetic end organs in the tendon of the muscle. The afferent fibers thus stimulated start impulses across association neurones of the cord. These neurones synapse with fibers that stimulate the muscle. Hence the muscle by its contraction furnishes its own ever-increasing stimulation. A severe muscle cramp results.

To prevent such a neuromuscular feedback, another purely nervous feedback checks it. This circuit is like the automatic volume control (AVC) of the audio amplifier. In such a circuit a small part of the electrical output of one of the tubes in line is fed back into a special grid of the tube. Before it passes to the grid, however, its voltage is reversed from + to −. Thus, when the output of the tube reaches a predetermined level it checks itself through the inhibiting feedback to the AVC grid. In the neuromuscular circuit described above, the cramp is prevented in a similar manner. At the point where the impulses enter the cord, to synapse with the across-the-cord association neurones, synapses are also made with ascending neurones, which carry relatively weak impulses to association fibers on a higher level of the C.N.S. These fibers synapse with descending neurones, which in turn end in the synaptic field of the lower neurones supplying the muscle. We thus have two parallel bridges from the primary afferent neurone to the final motor neurone. The upper bridge, however, transmits impulses that, though they may be weaker, are opposite in sign to those from the lower, more direct, bridge. Since the impulses are opposite in sign they serve to check the effects of the neuromuscular feedback.

Another interesting feedback is that which enters the thalamus by way of fibers that originate in the globus pallidus, so that a part of the output of the basal ganglia is fed back into the ganglia at the opposite end of the chain (Fig. 3-2). Thus when the basal ganglia are allowed to escape from inhibitory control by the cerebrum, a circular reaction is set up, so reinforcing itself that the cerebrum has difficulty in reestablishing its checks. Thus, crying spells occur, and temper tantrums, and hysterical laughter.

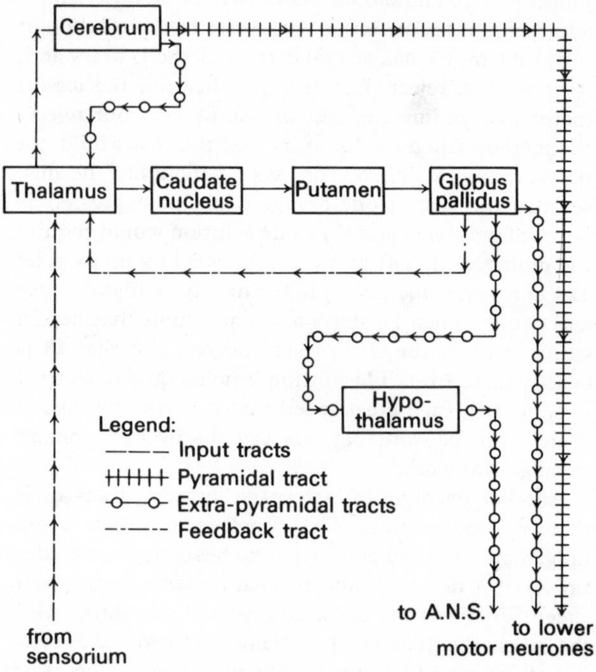

Fig. 3-2. The basal ganglia and their connections.

The nervous system is made up of a complicated maze of such closed circuits, interconnected and interacting. They are variously designated: feedback circuits, reverberating circuits, nerve nets, resonant circuits. The maintenance of body tonus is largely brought about by such a circular reflex; so is postural balance. Breathing, walking, and suckling and similar reciprocating reactions are negotiated through nerve nets that intermittently restrain other nerve nets.

From the point of view of the student of speech, however, the most interesting of the nerve nets are those in the parietal lobe, and other areas of the cerebrum, which are involved in the intellectual activity that (apparently) takes place there.

BIBLIOGRAPHY

Brazier, M. 1951. The electrical activity of the nervous system. New York: Macmillan.

Eisenson, J., Auer, J., and Irwin, J. 1963. The psychology of communication. New York: Appleton-Century-Crofts.

Fairbanks, G. 1954. A theory of the speech mechanism as a servo-system. *J. Speech Hearing Disorders*, 19, 133.

Gasser, H. 1935. Nerve potentials produced by rapidly repeated stimuli and their relation to responsiveness of nerve stimulation. *Amer. J. Physiol.*, III, 35.

Lorente de No, R. 1935. Facilitation of motoneurones. *Amer. J. Physiol.*, 113, 505.

Luchsinger, R., and Arnold, G. 1965. Voice-speech-language. Belmont, Calif.: Wadsworth.

Magoun, H. 1958. The waking brain. Springfield, Ill.: Thomas.

Patterns of organization in the central nervous system. 1952. Proceedings of the Assn. for Res. in Ner. and and Ment. Dis. (New York session, 1950). Baltimore: Williams & Wilkins.

Penfield, W., and Roberts, L. 1959. Speech and brain mechanisms. Princeton, N.J.: Princeton.

West, R., and Ansberry, M. 1967. The rehabilitation of speech (4th. ed.). New York: Harper & Row.

Wiener, N. 1948. Cybernetics or control and communication in the animal and in the machine. New York: Wiley.

4

Speech-Sound Formation

Giles Wilkeson Gray

GENERAL CONSIDERATIONS

Any attempt to describe completely and accurately the manner in which the sounds of speech are formed must necessarily take into consideration a number of possible contributing factors. Contrary to earlier theory, physiologists now generally agree that one of the distinguishing characteristics of speech-sound formation is that it consists not of fixed, static positions of the organs of articulation, but rather of dynamic, functional activity, of movements of those organs, though generally about some fairly consistent and uniform pattern. These movements are themselves, moreover, highly complicated and extremely variable. They are modified by their phonetic context, that is, by the influence of the preceding and following sounds, if any are present. They are further modified, in continuous speech, by both the logical content of the utterance and the emotional attitude of the speaker at the moment, but the formality or informality of the speaking situation, by the immediately desired precision of the articulation, and, at times, by the demands of utmost intelligibility.

Still further, since the same speaker will not always utter a given sound in the same combination of context, ideational content, and emotional attitude, his articular movements will never follow identical successive patterns, a fact that adds to the variability of the formation itself. Added to these bases for individual variation is the fact that no two persons' oral configurations are identical; for the differences among them give rise to significant differences in the manner in which the "same" sounds are formed by different people. These differences are observable in the ease with which our friends' voice and speech patterns are identifiable, even over the telephone.

At least one other factor will influence a full and complete description of the manner in which speech sounds are formed, namely, the use which is to be made of that description. Few will have use for such minute detail as Jesperson (1889) developed in his analphabetic system; furthermore, his descriptions were based on a static rather than a dynamic theory of the processes of articulation. Perhaps as an indication of what might be in the production of a single, isolated sound his analysis might be helpful to the phonologist; but to the teacher, who is interested in helping her students to speak more distinctly in the ordinary, everyday speaking situation, it offers little that is useful. Accurate and detailed descriptions may in some instances be highly desirable; in other situations they would be so cumbersome as to be useless. Most of us, including speech pathologists, and therapists, who are dealing with everyday problems involving articulation and pronunciation, are probably interested first of all in developing speech of acceptable intelligibility, after which it may be possible to add the more delicate shadings that may contribute significantly to speech over and above bare understanding.

It may sometimes make a significant difference in one's description of a given speech sound, *in what particular linguistic context* that description is likely to be useful. No two languages, even though phonemically the sound systems are similar, will employ the same descriptions for all the cognate allophones of those particular languages. For example, one would not give identical descriptions of all the sounds in the English word *dough* and the French *dot*.

To attempt to apply any description of the formation of any sound of any two people, and to expect that detailed description to fit exactly the speech of those two people, or that of either of them, or to the speech of any one person on two or more different occasions, is equivalent to trying to describe two snowflakes and make them appear as exactly alike. A written language implies oral identities that do not always exist.

The purpose of the present chapter is not, therefore, to develop a complete phonetic theory with respect to the formation of the sounds of speech. Rather it is to present as concisely and as directly as possible the minimum essentials of speech-sound formation which will be of value to the therapist in developing a practically functional degree of intelligibility in the use of the English language, even more specifically that dialectal branch of spoken English as heard primarily in Midland America, that is, the "General American." Much as Daniel Jones, a half-century ago, chose the speech of South England to describe in his *Introduction to Phonetics* (1922), because that was the variety of British speech with which he was most familiar, so, in the interests of simplicity of treatment, I have based my descriptions in this chapter on the speech of Midland America: it happens, through no conniving of my own, that that is the variety of American pronunciation, of speech-sound formation, with which I am most familiar.

In the production of any sound of speech, whether in isolation or in context, four essentials must be observed.[1] First, the sound must be correctly formed; second, it must be adequately formed; third, it must be supported by sufficient breath; and fourth, the "release," or the movement into the next sound formation, whichever is called for in the context, must be clean, sharp, and positive.[2]

[1] As an indication that these essentials are also involved in normal speech, see G. W. Gray and W. W. Braden, 1963, pp. 548ff.

[2] See also Pierre Jean Rousselot and Fauste Laclotte, 1913, p. 25.: Sound formation consists of three acts: ". . . prendre à la position volée, maintenir celle-ci quelques instants et ensuite l'abandonner."

Correct Formation

Although an essential aspect of sound formation consists of movements, as was pointed out in the first paragraph of this chapter, at the same time these movements are generally around some fairly consistent position. Unless there were some common elements in the production there could be no consistency in the product, and oral language itself would be impossible. Although it is true that many factors influence the essential movements, the positions about which those movements center are what give the sounds their identifying individuality. An attempted *s*-sound, for instance, formed with the tip of the tongue between the teeth, is incorrectly formed; the sound will not a characteristic [s]. Whatever the context may be in which a [b] occurs, at some time in its formation the lips must come together if the [b] is to be correctly produced. My laryngologist sometimes insists on my using the vowel [e] whenever he wants to examine my vocal bands. I tell him, "You can't do that": the [e], if it is to be a good one, cannot be formed with the tongue held down far enough for an adequate examination of the larynx. Now that I understand that he is more interested in the position of the epiglottis than in the quality of the resultant vowel, I follow his instruction as best I can, and raise no protest.

Movement in the articulation of speech sounds is important; but instruction in the production of those sounds will more profitably focus on the positions about which those movements center. The [k] in *beak* and *book* is not the same, it is true; nor in *keel* and *cool*. Nor is the [l] identical in the last two words. In teaching either the [k] or the [l] in these and other contexts, however, the emphasis should be laid on the consistency with which the tongue rises to the palate at approximately the same places every time the sounds are produced.

In using the term and the concept of *correctness* in speech usage, we are not here concerned with the linguist's insistence that there is no justification, in the study of language, to postulate any comparative evaluation of one form or another as "right" or "wrong," "correct" or "incorrect," except as usage has somehow placed a stamp of "acceptable" or "unacceptable." What we are concerned with here is intelligibility. It should require no profound philosophy of language to recognize that a sound system based on Swahili would be of little or no use in a culture maintained and propagated in English or any other of the current languages of present-day Western civilizations.

Adequate Formation

It is not enough that the articulatory organs move about some distinguishing position and do it correctly; the movement must be positive and the position definite. When the tongue is brought to the palate in a [t], the movement and the position that the tongue takes must have adequate strength to produce the sound cleanly and without confusion. This demands both flexibility and agility of all the organs involved in articulation, if the resulting speech is to be readily intelligible. A major problem in voice training consists in strengthening and invigorating the musculature of articulation sufficiently to produce the required sounds with adequate distinctness. Inadequacy of formation, whether resulting from careless habits or from malformations, results in indistinct, inarticulate speech that interferes seriously with the effectiveness of the communication. The movements and the positions may be, so far as the general *place* of articulation is concerned, entirely correct; but if they are so indefinite, so weak, that many of the sounds themselves are unidentifiable, the inevitable result is unintelligibility, partial or complete.

Adequate Breath Support

One may close and open one's lips repeatedly without producing a sound that would have, alone or in context, meaningful significance. With strong support from the breath, however, creating a pressure against each separate occlusion, a series of [p]s will result. Except for certain abnormal or unusual conditions, breath is essential in the production of voice and of voiceless sounds, that is, those in which the vocal bands are vibrating. Even under these extreme conditions, such as esophageal speech, some stream of air must be provided to produce the vibrations necessary for any sound at all. Actually, it takes little pressure of breath to produce the sounds of speech, and little breath in the utterance of an average single phrase. Unless that adequate little pressure is present, however, either the sounds will lack positiveness or the utterance will be entirely inaudible. In fact, there may not be any sounds at all, in which case resort may be had to what is known as lipreading, or "speechreading."

Definite Ending

Sometimes the peculiar nature of the sound itself, or of its phonetic context, calls for a definite finish. In such instances, as in the case of a final vowel or a final continuing consonant, as in *see*, *will*, *rare*, *sing*, the sound is ended either by stopping the flow of breath, or by opening the glottis, so that no further vibration is produced. In other instances, the articulatory organs move directly from the characteristic position of the sound being produced to that of the next. In still others the organs move sharply away from the sound position, as in final plosives, providing a "release" or a positive ending to the sound itself. In no case, however, should the significant sound be permitted to fade out indefinitely, or to glide so vaguely into the next that most of the distinctness, and hence the intelligibility, is lost.

The [t] provides a good illustration of the second and third cases. When appearing as a final sound, as in *get*, the tongue pulls sharply away from the palate, so that a slight aspiration, or escape of breath, follows, giving a finish to the sound and to the entire word. Without this "release" *cat* and *cap* may be indistinguishable: the difference in the sound of the aspiration, however, contributes to the two words as they are heard. In combination, as in *aptly*, the tongue pulls away from the palate (as also in this last word, *partly*) leaving the tip in position for the following [l]. Two common errors here consist, first, of insisting on the aspiration before forming the [l], and second, of omitting the [t] altogether, taking away part of the word's distinctiveness.

For the maximum correctness and distinctness of utterance, the organs of articulation, especially the tongue and lips, must be exercised to develop precision and strength of movement and definiteness of position. Overprecise, pedantically meticulous articulation is not the goal; however, consistent and persistent drill on tongue and lip movements and position will contribute immeasurably to the effectiveness of communication.

Sound Clusters

Many if not most of the writers on, and teachers of, the vocal aspects of speech (for example, those of the mid-nineteenth century) placed much stress on the articulation of what may be termed sound clusters, such as the *tl* and *ptl* mentioned in the paragraph second above. Their published books contain pages of exercises on a large number of different combinations, and the student was supposed to practice diligently on all of them, especially the most complicated and difficult. Such teaching inevitably led to all sorts of exaggerated utterances, which were a far cry from a normal, everyday utterance which sounded anything but natural. It produced a pedantic, overmeticulous speech which could make the speaker sound as if he were much more interested in the mechanics of utterance than in the meanings he was trying to communicate.

What we have been saying heretofore might be taken to indicate that in our judgment speech consists of a succession of well-formed, intelligible but separate *sounds*, whether they meant anything or not. Actually, we speak in *sound sequences* which comprise what are known as words, phrases, sentences, to formulate intelligent intercourse between and among people. The basic sounds and their sequences may be thought of as the "building blocks" of speech. It is not enough, therefore, that the basic sounds be intelligible when put into their proper contexts; the total patterns of sequences must also meet the requirements of intelligibility. Whether these patterns, as they are used in sequences to make sense, actually do contribute to the intelligibility of the communication depends on the manner in which the sounds themselves are adequately produced, plus the manner in which those sounds themselves are combined into intelligible sequences in which each sound is given its proper emphasis and quality for *that particular context*.

Attention must be paid, therefore, to the adequate, intelligible production of the sounds in sequence and in "clusters" as well as to the individual, separate sounds themselves, if acceptable speech is to be learned. A careful study of the later sections in which the specific formations of the various individual sounds of speech are described, will suggest what is further required to produce most of the more common sound combinations as well as the separate sounds themselves. Notice must be taken of the fact that many if not most of these individual sounds vary in formation according to the contexts in which they are used. Some of the references mentioned in the bibliography describe in detail just what these variations may be. They are introduced at this point to direct attention to their presence in speech, and to the necessity of including them in whatever course of training may be adopted for distinct, readily intelligible speech.

BASES OF CLASSIFICATION

Speech sounds may be classified on a number of bases. One such basis is the mode of production. According to this classification, the sounds of speech are formed: 1. by the modification of vocal tones produced in the larynx, and shaped into their variant forms in the resonating cavities of the throat, mouth, and nose; 2. by a partial or complete obstruction to the emission of breath by the vocal folds, by most of the palate, the tongue, or the lips; 3. by a combination of these two.

They may be classified on bases other than that of the manner of their production, however. They may be differentiated according to the position around which the movements heretofore indicated take place, and the customary designations of the sounds include references to these positions. For example, a sound described in part as *bilabial* would be produced by specific movement or juxtaposition of the two lips. Similarly, a sound indicated as *labiodental* would be produced by interaction of the lips and teeth—in all sounds in English so described, the upper teeth and lower lip. An alveolar sound would be one in the formation of which the tongue touches or approximates the ridge of the hard palate just slightly back of the upper teeth. Other sounds are similarly designated.

Speech sounds are further classified according to the degree of obstruction or occlusion set up against the outgoing breath stream. In certain sounds, for instance, the closure is complete; and is usually followed in English speech by a fairly sharp aspiration, as already described, immediately following the "release." Such sounds are appropriately called "plosives"; if the fact of the closure rather than of the release is to be emphasized, they may be designated as "stops." They are of necessity of short duration, as contrasted with many other sounds in which the obstruction is only partial, or so slight as hardly to constitute any obstruction at all, and which may be continued for as long as desirable, or as long as the breath holds out. Those sounds which may be held indefinitely are known as continuants.

THE VOWELS

Let us first consider those sounds with which most of us are familiar, and which are commonly known as the *vowels*. They consist entirely of vocal tones modified by positions and movements, and thereby in the harmonic structure of the sounds themselves. Other laryngeal structures, such as the epiglottis, are also involved; since we have no conscious control over them, however, they are not included in the present descriptions. Since the actual positions and movements are not readily or positively defined, the descriptions of the formations themselves are therefore less specific and somewhat more difficult than those of the consonants. Furthermore, since the formation constantly shifts from the beginning of a vowel to its ending (Black, 1937), any description must take only that portion of the movement, or that position, which seems to be most positively characteristic of that vowel. This shifting varies in degree from the barely perceptible, and that by a trained ear, to the readily identifiable diphthongs.

So far as conscious control is involved, the different vowels are produced chiefly by varying movements and positions of the tongue and lips, together with varying degrees of tenseness of the muscles involved. Actually, as Heffner points out, none of the so-called organs of articulation are absolutely essential to the production of identifiable sounds (1952, p. 90). In most cases, however, their absence is likely to be the exception and requires highly specialized techniques in order to develop acceptable and intelligible speech. For the most part, the tongue is the most important organ, not excepting the larynx itself.

With respect to the part played by the tongue itself, the vowels may be classified as front, central, and back; high, mid, and low; tense and lax; closed or open; the lips may be narrow or wide (referring to the opening between them), rounded or unrounded (Heffner, 1952, p. 96).

The Basic Positions

The four basic positions, as indicated by Heffner (pp. 88 f.), are the high front, the high back, the low front, and low back. If one raises the blade of the tongue, at about C on Fig. 4-1, so that it is very close to the hard palate at about 5 on the figure, providing a narrow slit between tongue and palate, and then produces a vocal tone, the resulting sound will be the "high front" vowel [i]. The spaces both in front and back of the position of closest approximation form resonance cavities which give the [i] its characteristic timbre. One may get much the same result from raising the tongue to whistle the highest note possible, and then without moving the tongue, producing a vocal tone, which should be close to an [i].

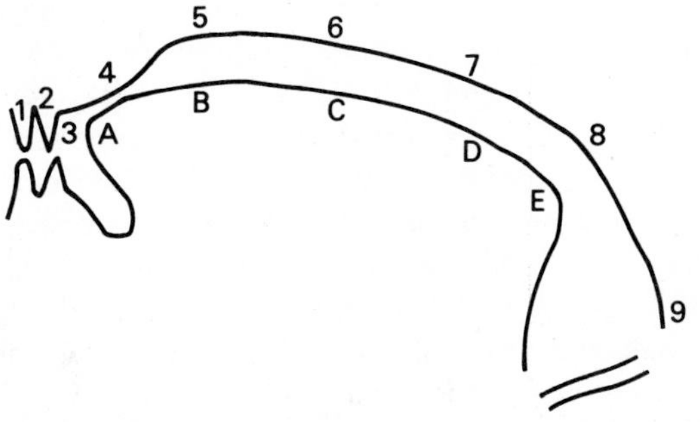

Fig. 4-1. Relative positions of closest approximations of tongue and palate in the formation of the various sounds of speech. See text for details of descriptions.

If, now, one raises the back of the tongue, at about E, to approximately the point 7 (Fig. 4-1), where the hard and soft palates are joined, so that a narrow slit is formed between the tongue and palate at that point, and then produces a vocal tone, the resultant sound will be the "high back" vowel approaching a [u]. Rounding and protruding the lips slightly at the same time will aid in producing a more definite vowel. Producing a vocal tone with the lips and tongue in position to whistle the lowest tone possible should give much the same effect.

With the tongue lowered as far as it will go without forcing, and drawn slightly back toward the pharynx (Heffner, 1952, p. 104), the vocal sound should be the "low back" [α]. The entire resonating cavity above the larynx, with the exception of the nasal passages, seems to be functioning as a single resonator. In these and all other English vowels the nasal cavities are closed off from the oral by means of the soft palate, which rises to close against the back wall of the oral pharynx, except as hereinafter noted.

The remaining front and back vowels are characteristically produced by successively lowering the tongue through positions from the high front [i] to the low front [a], and from the high back [u] to the low back [α]. The familiar vowel diagram (Gray and Wise, 1959, p. 241), which represents graphically these positions, will help to clarify these relationships. The left side, indicating the front of the tongue, begins with [i] at the extreme high point, representing the "high front" vowel, then goes downward successively through [ɪ], [e], [ɛ], and [æ], to [a], the "low front" vowel. The right side, indicating the back of the tongue, drops successively from [u] at the extreme high position—the "high back" vowel—through [ʊ], [o], and [ɔ], to [ɑ], the "low back" vowel.

When the lips are brought into play in the formation of these successive vowels they characteristically, though not necessarily, exhibit a fairly definite progression. In producing the [ɑ] the lips are normally open, relaxed, and "unrounded." As one advances through the series of back vowels, from [ɑ] progressively to [u], the corners of the mouth draw in, the lips become more and more rounded, and tend to protrude slightly. Because of this progression the back vowels are also classified as "rounded."

If, on the other hand, one advances through the front vowels, from [a] through the gamut to [i], the corners of the lips are progressively drawn back fairly widely, so that for the highest vowel, [i], the opening between them becomes narrow and elongated. It is difficult to produce an [i] with the teeth as far apart as the width of two fingers. These are the "unrounded" vowels.

These positions are all relative; and while helpful for instructional purposes, they are not absolutely essential in the formation of the vowels. It is possible to produce readily distinguishable front vowels with only a slight spreading of the lips, or even with none at all; or one may produce the back vowels with the lips completely relaxed. Labial agility is not a basic requirement in the formation of the vowels.

The Central Vowels

The central vowels are so called because of the fact that in their formation neither the front nor the back of the tongue is elevated other than as it is influenced by the movements of the central portion. In the lowest of these, [ʌ], the tongue is raised only slightly more than for [ɑ] and is perhaps a bit more forward; it is lax and the lips are unrounded. The vowel occurs in such words as *but*, *come*, *tub*, *enough*, *mother*, *touch*, *bug*, but rarely if ever in unaccented syllables. Closely related to this sound is the [ɜ], which occurs syllabically or in stressed syllables when the "r is dropped," in such words as *her*, *bird*, *world*, *first*, *colonel*. In this central vowel the midportion of the tongue is elevated slightly higher than for [ʌ], with the sides curving up to touch lightly the molar teeth. Whereas in [ʌ] the tongue is lax, in [ɜ] it is tense. In a third of these central vowels, [ɝ], used characteristically syllabically or in stressed syllables (as in the *her* words listed above in this paragraph) by those speakers who "retain their r's," the fore part of the tongue is raised still higher, narrowing the opening between the tongue and the palate (about D-6 in Fig. 4-1). According to most descriptions of this sound, the tip of the tongue tends to curl backward, giving rise to its description as a retroflex movement, of position. Although it is true that an extreme sound can be made by such curving back, it is doubtful if retroflexion is an essential aspect of the formation of [ɝ].

The fourth of these central vowels is known as the "schwa," a name said to be derivative of the Hebrew *sh'wa*. It is represented by the symbol [ə]. The tongue and lips are completely relaxed, and the sound itself is so short in duration that it is difficult to identify its characteristic timbre, if indeed it has one. It seems to resemble as closely as may be a completely unstressed [ʌ]. The sound is used in two ways, both of them in unstressed syllables. It serves for the "er" syllable (with its various spellings) in such words as *mother*, *sailor*, *forward*, and so on, by speakers who do not use the [ɝ] in stressed syllables, that is, by those who habitually "drop their r's." Again, it is used by all speakers in the unstressed syllables of such words as *sofa*, *Illinois*, *Iowa*, *formative*, *vowel*, where there is no indication of an *r*-sound in the spelling. In this connection it has no relation to the *r*-sounds.

The *schwa* [ə], as a substitute for the unstressed "er" syllables, has its counterpart in [ɚ], for those speakers who commonly retain their *r*'s in these words, and who use the [ɝ] in stressed syllables. With respect to the use of the *r*-sounds, the usage of these four central vowels may be shown in the following:

	STRESSED SYLLABLES	UNSTRESSED SYLLABLES
For those who "retain their *r*'s"	ɝ	ɚ
For those who "drop their *r*'s"	ɜ	ə

Further discussion of the consonantal *r*-sounds will be presented in a later section.

The Diphthongs

It is well known that none of the vowels remains constant through its duration (Black, 1937; Stetson, 1951, p. 37). Gemelli and Pastori (1934) point out that in every instance there is a period during which the sound is being built up, so to speak, either from the initiation of the sound itself or through a transition from the preceding sound. Following this formative period come a few sound waves, the number depending on the duration of the total vowel, which exhibit the "typical" wave form, and presumably the characteristic timbre of that particular vowel. Finally comes the ending, occurring either by a "dying-out" of the typical waves or by a transition into the following sound. These changes are normal; since they are ordinarily imperceptible to the ear, they do not affect the identification of the vowels. They can be isolated only through the most careful observation of a highly trained ear or by instrumental analysis. In some of the vowels, notably [e] and [o], the final shift in characteristic timbre is considered by most phoneticians to be so marked as to warrant identifying the sounds themselves as diphthongs, which are defined by Thomas (1947, p. 104) as a "vocalic glide within the limits of a single syllable." According to Heffner (1952, p. 112), they consist of "a syllabic element, which begins with one sound and shifts to another. . . ." This shift is exclusive of "those brief build-up and dying-out stages which characterize every speech sound."

The identification of the various diphthongs themselves will serve to indicate the direction and the degree of shifting. In the words *try*, *fine*, *sigh*, *my*, in which the diphthong [aɪ] occurs, the shift is from low front [a] to the high front lax [ɪ]. In words such as *now*, *house*, *found*, *plow*, in which the diphthong [aʊ] is found, the shift is from [a] up and back to the mid-back lax [ʊ]. In the diphthong [ɔɪ], as it is heard in *boy*, *noise*, *employ*, the shift is from the low back lax [ɔ] forward and up to the high front lax [ɪ].

Theoretically, diphthongs can be formed from almost any combination of two vowels; indeed, when an intermediate vowel is distinctly recognizable or where there is a pronounced glide consonant mixed in, we may even have a triphthong, as in an occasional southern [hæjand] for [hænd] *hand*. In the typical diphthong, however, the shift is from one of the lower to one of the higher vowels, with the one exception of [ju], both elements of which are high.

THE CONSONANTS

The sounds of speech commonly known as consonants are characteristically produced by interposing some sort of partial or complete obstruction to the passage of breath as it is forced from the lungs. In some of these, the vibrations set up by the passage of the breath as it is forced past the obstruction produces the only sound heard; in others it is the sudden stoppage in the emission by a complete occlusion, followed by a "release," that produces the only sound, as in a completely voiceless final *t*. In still others the consonant is a combination of the two. To these ways in which such sounds are formed is added, in many instances, the effect from the vibration of the vocal folds; and in some of these instances it is the sound from this vocal fold vibration that is modified in the oral and nasal passages, much as are the vowels. In fact, in some instances the obstruction is so slight that the sound itself takes on something of the characteristics of a vowel.

Two other means of identifying the consonants as differentiated from the vowels which may be useful, are first, the fact that generally before words beginning with a consonant sound we use the article *a*, as *a building*, *a dream*, *a flower*, *a paper*, *a train*, and so on, whereas before words beginning with a vowel (the *sound* rather than the *letter*, as *an hour*, *an able man*) we characteristically use the article *an*. Thus, if one uses the *sound h* in the word *hotel*, or *humble*, the preceding article would be *a*, whereas if one does not use the *h*-sound, the preceding article is *an*. Either pronunciation of either word is acceptable, by the way.

Although this difference does not describe the essential nature of the two classes of sounds, it may serve to distinguish them as they are used. Second, whenever a sound, usually a continuant and characteristically a consonant, can be used syllabically, without the aid of any other sound to complete the syllable, it has in that situation the characteristics of a vowel rather than a consonant. For instance, in button [bʌtn], when the [t] explodes directly into the [n], without an intervening [ə], the [n] stands alone, forming a syllable by itself; hence it is essentially a vowel, and designated as syllabic. Similarly, when *bottle* is so pronounced that the [t] explodes directly into the [l], the [l] becomes vocalic rather than consonantal, and hence it is also designated as syllable.

The Plosives

If a complete obstruction is set up in the oral passage so that no breath can escape, and some additional pressure is built up against this dam, there is created the basis of a prominent group of consonants known as *plosives*. A further essential aspect of this complete closure is that the velum (or soft palate) be pressed firmly against the back wall of the oral pharynx, so that none of the breath escapes through the nasal passages. Like most other consonants, these plosives may be accompanied by vibration of the vocal folds, the former being "voiced" and the latter "unvoiced." The plosive consonant is completed when the tongue is pulled sharply from its position against the palate, and a slight aspiration may be heard, particularly if the sound is made by itself, with no following or attached sound (another consonant, for instance).

It should be noted that for the best production of these plosives, to insure that all the conditions mentioned in the early pages of this chapter be met, the obstruction must be in the right place. *Care* must not be mistaken for *dare*; *pawl* for *ball*; *tack* for *tag* nor *pack* for *back*. Many such pairs can be found, practice on which will aid in fixing the proper positions for the respective plosives.

The obstruction must be firm and definite, so that the breath pressure can be built up behind it; and finally, the "release" must be sharp and positive. If any of these are lacking or inadequately achieved, the resulting sounds will be indistinct and some of the intelligibility may be lost.

The first of the positions where these plosives may be produced is at the two lips: hence the term applied to them, *bilabial*. The formation is simple: press the lips firmly together, build up the breath pressure back of them, and suddenly separate them. The only sound that can be produced in this manner is a [p]. If to this sound is added the vibration of the vocal folds, the sound must be a [b]. It is probable that the pressure is greater for a voiceless plosive than for a voiced; the distinction for present purposes is not important. Both [p] and [b] are bilabial plosives, unvoiced and voiced respectively.

Neither of these plosives, nor indeed any of the others, ever stands alone in our language. They are not prolonged except briefly in such expressions as *cap pistol*, *top pile*, *tub bath*, *mad dancer*, *book keeper* (or *bookkeeper*), and the like. The difference between *some ice* and *some mice* should cause no difficulty. In such cases as those offered here, although there are two *letters* juxtaposed in the two successive words, suggesting two sounds, actually there is only one stop, and one plosive. The *stop* phase of the sound, that is, the closure, is merely prolonged and finally released into the following sound, usually a vowel. (Jones, 1922, pp. 36 f.) The pronunciation of two separate and distinct consonants in such instances—frequently heard in speakers who have been told that they must articulate distinctly—is probably the result of overcompensation. It smacks highly of objectionable pedantry.

The second place where plosives may be produced is at the alveolar ridge in the hard palate, about 4 on Fig. 1. If you will slide the tip of your tongue back from the base of the upper teeth, you will notice a smooth ridge from a quarter to a half inch back of the teeth. This is called the *alveolar ridge*. Now if the tip of the tongue is pressed firmly against this ridge (the velum being closed), and then if the pressure is built up against this closure, and finally if the tongue is then pulled sharply down from the palate, the only possible resulting sound is a [t]. When voice is added the result is a [d]. The terms designating these two sounds are derived from the point of occlusion; hence the voiceless and voiced alveolar plosives.

A readily identifiable [t] and [d] can be formed at various positions in the general area of the alveolar ridge; but in English the formation of these consonants is characteristically as here described.

A third place where plosives can be formed is at the back of the oral cavity. If the back of the tongue is brought into firm contact with the palate, about where the hard and soft palate are joined, and as before the breath pressure increased, and finally the tongue is drawn down from the palate allowing usually an audible escape of breath, the resulting sound will be a [k]. If voice is added it will be a [g]. Since these are formed at the soft palate, or the velum, they are called *velar plosives*, voiceless and voiced respectively.

It was said that lingual agility is not required for the production of adequate vowels. The same cannot be said for the production of most of the consonants, for in these sounds the lips and tongue must move rapidly and positively indeed. Drills to develop the ability to produce sharp, distinct consonants in rapid succession are of great value in the development of intelligible speech. On the other hand, care must be taken to avoid utterance that is too rapid either for understanding at all or for retaining much of what one is able to grasp. Radio newscasters often err in this direction. They speak so rapidly into the microphone that the listener cannot remember at the close of the broadcast what he heard at the beginning, or much of anything in between. It is not true that the faster one talks the more he can say.

The Fricatives

Many of the sounds of speech are produced not by complete, but by partial obstruction of the breath emission, so that what is heard is the friction or hissing as the breath passes through the narrow opening: hence the term *fricative*. Each sound so produced, with only the friction of the outward rushing, however gentle or strong, has its counterpart in another produced in the same manner, but with the addition of the voice. Like the plosives, the fricatives can be produced at various positions of the oral cavity.

The first pair of these sounds to occur in American English speech consists of the *labiodentals*, so called from the fact that they are produced by placing the inner surface of the lower lip lightly against the tips of the upper teeth, forming a narrow slit, and forcing the breath through the opening so provided. The voiceless *labiodental fricative* is [f], the voiced [v]. Since they can be maintained as long as the breath holds out, they are also designated as continuants.

A second fricative in English is that produced by placing the tip of the tongue against the back of the upper teeth, sometimes even protruding between the upper and lower teeth, and forcing the breath through the narrow slit thus formed. An attempted [s] formed with the tongue too far forward often approaches this sound; when substituted for an [s] the sound is often called a lisp. Because the tongue is so often placed between the teeth, with or without protrusion, these sounds are sometimes designated as *interdentals;* because the tongue is often placed directly behind the teeth, they are sometimes thought of as *postdentals*. Heffner (1952, p. 158) calls them *dental spirants*. The voiceless interdental fricative continuant, as in *thin*, is represented by the Greek *theta* [θ], while the voiced counterpart, as in *this*, is represented by a [ð], which was the old "crossed *d*" of Anglo-Saxon.

If the fore surface of the tongue at about B (Fig. 1) is brought into close contact with the alveolar ridge, so that only a narrow opening is left along the median line of the palate and tongue, and breath is forced through the narrow passage, the friction will produce a hissing sound readily identified as [s]. The correct formation of this fricative does not permit much latitude; if the tongue is too far forward the resulting sound will approach a [θ]; if too far back, or if the opening is too wide, it will take on some of the characteristics of a [ʃ]. If the sound is permitted to escape over one or both sides of the tongue, instead of past the middle, the result will be a particular kind of deviation from the normal known as a *lateral s*, which may be unilateral or bilateral.

The voiced cognate of the [s] is of course [z], incorrect formations of which may produce either [ð] or [ʒ], or a lateral. In the formation of these sounds [s] and [z] it is necessary that the occlusion between the tongue and the palate be complete except for the narrow opening at the median line of the alveolar ridge.

The sounds formed next to the [s] and [z] are [ʃ] and [ʒ], voiceless and voiced respectively. In these the tongue is brought to the palate just slightly back of the alveolar ridge, and the opening is somewhat wider than for those sounds formed on the ridge. The lips are sometimes slightly protruded, but not always; a slight protrusion seems to help in the production of the sound. Apparently the small space thus provided serves somewhat as a resonator for the characteristic high frequencies present; at any rate, it is difficult if not impossible to produce a good [ʃ] or a [ʒ] with the lips spread widely and drawn back at the corners.

No other fricative consonants produced by linguadental or palatal action at points farther back are heard in English speech. The sound combination [hju], in such words as *Hugh*, *huge*, *humor*, *Huron*, and the like, may sometimes be produced as a palatal fricative. This sound, known as the *ichlaut* [ç], is represented in German spelling by *ch* when followed by a front vowel. In its formation the blade of the tongue at about D is brought close to the hard palate at about 6 (Fig. 1) to form a close, fairly narrow opening. When the breath is forced through the passage a hissing sound of a peculiar character is produced, much as if one were clearing a small bit of mucus from the palate. The result is a pronunciation of the words represented above as [çu], [çudz], [çumɚ], [çurən].

As in the case of the plosives, the fricatives must be made with the articulatory organs in the right places; there must be an adequate firmness in the constriction set up for the restricted passage of the breath; and there must be an adequate pressure to force the breath through the narrow openings. Finally, the release, or the movement into the next sound, whichever is called for in the context, must be positive and clean.

The Affricates

Partaking somewhat of the nature of both plosives and fricatives are pairs of sounds known as the affricates. These are sounds represented in English by such spellings as *ch* for the voiceless form, and j or *g* respectively. In these sounds the first element, consisting essentially of an alveolar stop (sometimes postalveolar) very similar to a [t], is generally produced at position 4, but sometimes nearer to 5 (Fig. 1). It releases relatively gradually into [ʃ] rather than suddenly into the aspirate as is usual for the plosives. The formation for [dʒ] is the same, with the addition of voice.

There has been some question as to whether these affricates are to be considered a single sound, or as no more than a [t] plus [ʃ], or [d] plus [ʒ]. There are many instances in our speech of stops followed by fricatives; these two, however, are so often used together phonemically that it seems justifiable to consider them as an integrated unit, at the same time recognizing that, somewhat like the diphthongs, they consist of at least two elements.

It may be well at this point to reemphasize the definite distinction that must be made between the voiceless and the voiced consonants. The difference was suggested above, in another connection. It should be stressed in teaching the formation of the sounds of speech, for it is one of the bases on which such sounds are classified. The very meanings of the words often depend on whether certain of the sounds therein are voiced or voiceless. Path, bath, and badge are all different words, whatever the context, although a *patch* may also be a *badge*. Their difference, however, lies in the voicing or unvoicing of the consonants. Similarly, *pig*, *big*, and *pick*, though one may on occasion *pick* a *big pig*, depend for their identification on whether the consonants are voiced or unvoiced. Insistence on this difference will result in cleaner, more distinct, more intelligible speech.

The Nasal Consonants

In English three distinct sounds are used which are generally known as nasals. These are [m], [n], and [ŋ]. In formation they are somewhat similar to certain of the plosives, in that the oral occlusions are in the same places as for the latter, [p], [t], and [k] respectively. They differ in two respects: they are voiced continuants rather than plosives, and as such have some of the characteristics of the vowels. Moreover, they can be used syllabically; that is, they can form syllables by themselves, without the aid of other sounds, as in [bʌtn], [opm], [θɪŋkŋ].

The second way in which the nasals differ from the plosives is that whereas in the latter the obstruction to the breath emission is complete, with the velum being closed, in the former the occlusion occurs only in the oral passage. Since the sounds are continuants, there must be some passage for the breath and the voice to be emitted. This passage is provided by dropping the velum, which ordinarily is pressed against the back wall of the oral pharynx to close off the nasal passages, and forcing the breath and/or voice through the oral cavities. When the velum is dropped and the oral occlusion maintained, the nasal cavities are opened up so that the breath and voice go out through them. The addition of these cavities to the resonating chambers gives to the nasal sounds their peculiar character.

It is not generally recognized, although it seems quite obvious, that the effect of the nasal consonants, more particularly, the effect of opening the nasal passages (the dropping of the velum) for the nasal consonants is to anticipate, so to speak the preceding vowels, so that the velum is open for them too, making them also nasalized. My French teacher at college, in teaching the nasal vowels, would say, for example, "To produce the French nasal *o* [õ] pronounce the word *home, but don't close your lips*. It is an instance of what is termed "regressive assimilation," which is characterized by the anticipation of an approaching sound in such a way that the sound being uttered is modified by the approaching sound (Gray and Wise, 1959, p. 357). In moderation the phenomenon should cause no concern, since it is a normal linguistic phenomenon. Nasality is offensive when excessively strong, when accompanied by much tension of the resonator walls, or when occurring in sounds which neither by assimilation nor otherwise should be nasalized at all. The "nasal" voice is nasal even in the absence of nasal consonants.

The r-Sounds

It is incorrect to speak of the *r* as if there were but one *r*-sound, although in the English language most of the sounds of this group center about approximately the same position. There are many variations in other languages, which are described in current texts; but since they are rare in our own language, they need not be discussed here. Perhaps a brief discussion of the various uses of the sound group may have some significance.

The vocalic *r*-sounds (that is, when used as vowels, or syllabically), have been discussed in the section on the vowels. Consonantal [r] may be found in two basic types of phonetic context: a prevocalic and a postvocalic position, with variants of each of these. The prevocalic [r] occurs in such words as *run*, *wreck*, *rare*, *real*, *recede;* the postvocalic [r] occurs in *heart*, *here*, *horse*, *their*, and the like. A variant of the former is found in the consonant combinations in which the [r], as part of the combination (as in *strong*, *bring*, *fresh*, *shred*, *pride*, and so on, still precedes the vowel. When following the voiceless consonants in such contexts, the [r] is likely to be also unvoiced through at least the first part of its duration, and to take on something of the character of a fricative. The intervocalic [r] (as in *far away*, *character*), though it is postvocalic it is at the same time prevocalic, and takes on the character of the voiced vowel.

In usage, the prevocalic [r] is, or should be, always pronounced in all American dialects; and since the [r] is influenced more by the following than by the preceding vowel, the intervocalic sound is also, correctly always pronounced. The postvocalic [r] may or may not be heard, depending on the particular dialect in which it may occur. In General American it is, at least theoretically, heard wherever it is indicated by the spelling. Also theoretically, it is characteristically omitted in Eastern and Southern speech; actually, it is becoming more and more common in all phonetic contexts, in all of the major American dialects.

The central position about which the movements are focused in producing the consonantal [r] in any context is basically similar to that in the formation of the vocalic [r], or the central /ɝ/, as it is used in General American speech. That is, the sides of the tongue curve up to touch lightly the molar teeth. The agreeableness or disagreeableness of the sound depends largely on the degree of tenseness in the tongue itself, and perhaps on the nonessential retroflexion of the tongue tip, which demands additional tension. In the initial, or prevocalic [r], the movement of the tongue is away from its characteristic position; in the postvocalic, when the [r] is used at all, the movement is toward that characteristic position. In the intervocalic position the tongue approaches the palate to form the [r], and then moves quickly into position for the next sound. In these movements the [r] may be thought of as a "glide consonant."

One more variant may be heard among those speakers who characteristically omit the postvocalic [r]. When used finally, as in *here*, *bare*, *fire*, *door*, *your*, or *poor*, the vowel often becomes in effect a diphthong, the final element being [ə].

The l-Sounds

In some respects the *l*-sounds resemble in their functioning the *r*-sounds. They may be used syllabically, as in *bottle*, *meddle*, *little;* consonantally in initial, medial, or final positions, or in consonant combinations such as *black*, *flight*, *slender*, and so on, following voiceless plosives or voiceless fricatives. The [l] is not heard as a vowel, as are the vocalic *r*-sounds in *were*, *heard*, *further*, and the like. When occurring prevocally the organs move away from the l-position; when occurring postvocally they move toward it. In the intervocalic [l] the tongue moves first into, and then away from, the characteristic position.

In the normal [l] the tip of the tongue is raised to the roof of the mouth at the alveolar ridge, so that it touches the palate *only* at the median line, the sound going off over the sides. If one simply places the tongue tip against the ridge and utters a vocal sound, the result will be an [l]. This position, however, is not critical; actually, the tip of the tongue can touch the palate at any point from the base of the teeth as far back as it will reach, and a readily recognizable sound will be produced, so long as only the tip is touching, and the sound goes out over the sides. As the tongue lies normally in the mouth, the tip as it rises will probably touch the palate at or near the alveolar ridge.

The [l] following a voiceless consonant in combination in the same syllable will tend to be voiceless itself, at least through a part of its duration, as in *play*, *fly*, *slack*, *cling* (Jones, 1950, p. 90). Intervocalic [l], like the [r], may be thought of as a glide consonant. Syllabic [l] is produced primarily by releasing a plosive directly into the *l*-position without going through an intervening vowel, as in *buckle*, *bugle*, *mettle*, *medal*, *apple*, *bobble*. In these the tongue may form an *l*-position even before the release of the plosive, or so close thereafter that no vowel can be formed. The syllabic [l] is much less frequent following other consonants, although it can hardly be said that it never occurs in such context.

The Glide Consonants

It will be helpful to consider the so-called glide consonants [j] and [w] together, since they follow much the same principles. In their formation they resemble somewhat the diphthongs in that they consist essentially of two elements, an initial followed by a rapid but smooth glide into the second or following sound. They differ from the diphthongs in at least two respects: first, they are always used consonantally, the consonant itself consisting of the initial element and the glide. Second, whereas the final element of a given diphthong is always the same, or of the same phoneme, the final element of the glide consonant may be any following vowel or diphthong.

Consider, for instance, the glide [j] in the words *ye*, *yip*, *yes*, *yap*, *yard*, *yo-yo*, *eunuch*, *your*, *use*, *eulogy*, *Europe*, *Euxine*. In each case there is a constriction of the tongue close to the palate at about the position for [j] (Jones, 1922, p. 66; Thomas, 1947, p. 54ff; Heffner, 1952, p. 154). This constriction may be held for an appreciable time, although such a hold is not essential. In fact, so long as the position is held the [j]-glide cannot be completed. What is important is the release from the constriction to the following sound. Apparently, the higher the vowel into which the glide moves, the more tense the constriction. The release may move into any of the vowel positions, however, and thence often into a diphthong, as in *yipe*, *yowl*, *yoicks*, although these are not common words.

The initial element is sometimes thought of as a fricative; Heffner (1952, pp. 150f.) insists that the friction is an essential characteristic of the sound itself. Probably the nearest sound to the voiceless counterpart is heard in certain dialectal pronunciations, at one time advocated by the lexicographer and elocutionist, John Walker, as giving a certain "elegance" to the pronunciation of *card* as *kyard*, *cow* *kyow*, *garden* as *gyarden*, in which the [j] follows the plosive, voiced or voiceless. The [ç] described above (the *ich-laut*) as heard in some pronunciations of *huge*, *humor*, *human*, also approaches the voiceless palatal glide consonant.

The [w] consists of a glide from a lip and tongue position similar to that for a [u] or [ʊ] into the position for the following vowel or diphthong. It is often called a bilabial semivowel, often a bilabial glide vowel. It functions as a consonant, however, in somewhat the same manner as does the [j] glide. In such words as *we*, *will*, *way*, *wet*, *wag*, *watt*, *wall*, *woke*, *wood*, *woo*, the tongue tends to take the position for the following vowel while the lips are forming the initial bilabial construction. The release is into the vowel or diphthong which has been forming. *Wide and wound* (pret. of *wind* [waɪnd]) represent perhaps the principal diphthongs preceded by the bilabial glide consonant.

The voiceless counterpart of [w]—[ʍ]—is heard in General American *wheat*, *which*, *whey*, *whet*, *wham*, *what*, *whoa* (often if not usually [wo], *whup* (an old rustic pronunciation of *whip*), *whoop* (often simply [hʉp]), and *whirl*. The formation is essentially the same as for the voiced [w]; voicing, however, does not normally begin until the initiation of the following vowel. The expulsion of breath is considerably stronger than for [w], since the chief audible element is dependent on that expulsion, and not on the following vowel. Like [j] and [w], [ʍ] is a glide consonant, with as many variations as there are sounds which may follow it.

The Glottal Fricative

About the only characteristic of [h] is that it consists of a forcible emission of breath through an open or partially open glottis, and through pharyngeal and oral cavities formed to produce a following vowel or diphthong (Jones, 1922, p. 61; Thomas, 1947, p. 101; Heffner, 1952, p. 150 f.). From another point of view, since the [h] rarely if ever occurs without a following vowel, it may be thought of as a strongly aspirated voiceless vowel immediately preceding the voiced vowel. A still further approach may be to consider the [h] as a particular manner of attaching a vowel. When the articulatory mechanism is in position for the following vowel the friction of breath as it is forced through the glottis and oral passages produces a whispered sound readily identified as the approaching vowel. It is this sound which in English normally constitutes the [h] in any given phonetic context (Heffner, 1952, p. 151).

The descriptions given above are intended to present only the minimum essentials of speech sound formation for the production of speech of socially adequate intelligibility. They will not, obviously, satisfy the phonetician or the linguist; on the other hand, it is thought that they will be found sufficient for the correction of many if not most of the common articulation errors, for both the therapist and the classroom teacher of "normal" speech. For those who would like to pursue the study still further, a thorough familiarity with the sources listed in the bibliography will give as complete information as is presently available for an understanding of the manner in which the sounds of speech are formed. There still remains much to be discovered; the search for yet more complete understanding is a fruitful field of inquiry.

BIBLIOGRAPHY

Black, J. 1937. The quality of a spoken vowel. *Arch. Speech*, 2, 7–27.

Gemelli, A., and Pastori, G. 1934. La durata minima di un fonema sufficiente par la sua percezione. *In* L'analisi e'elettroacustica del linguaggio. Milano: Universita Cattolica del Sacro Cuore. Pp. 149–163.

Gray, G., and Braden, W. 1951. Public speaking: principles and practice. New York: Harper.

———, and Wise, C. 1946. The bases of speech (rev. ed.). New York: Harper.

Heffner, R. 1952. General phonetics. Madison: Univ. Wis. Press.

Jespersen, O. 1889. The articulation of speech sounds represented by means of analphabetic symbols. Marburg in Hessen: N. G. Elwert.

Jones, D. 1922. An outline of English phonetics. New York: G. W. Stechert.

———. 1950. The pronunciation of English. Cambridge: Univ. Press.

Rousselot, P., and Laclotte, F. 1913. Précis de prononciation. Paris: H. Welter.

Stetson, R. 1951. Motor phonetics. Amsterdam: North Holland Pub.

Thomas, C. 1947. An introduction to the phonetics of American English. New York: Ronald.

5

The Speech and Hearing Laboratory

Theodore D. Hanley and Robert Peters

In the *Handbook of Speech Pathology*, the chapter on instrumentation was entitled "Instruments of Diagnosis, Therapy, and Research." In the present chapter the focus is not so much on individual instruments as it is on circuits that involve instrument systems found in speech and hearing laboratories. This evolution of instrumentation is in keeping with trends in both the physical and social sciences. Clinical and research procedures utilized in laboratories today are more sophisticated than in previous years, for researchers are increasingly zealous to isolate relevant variables that pertain to speech or hearing and to control or measure these variables. This new focus in research does not mean that a single instrument (e.g., an audiometer) is infrequently the only requirement for a clinical test or an experiment; neither should it be inferred from the foregoing discussion that separate devices will not, in this chapter, receive individual attention. Where this chapter does depart from the pattern of the previous one is in an attempt to concentrate attention on patterns of instrumentation by describing a series of laboratories that have produced distinguished work reported regularly in speech and hearing and other journals. Because such distinguished laboratories are numerous it was necessary to choose a limited number for inclusion in this chapter on instrumentation. We recognize that some laboratories of acknowledged eminence have not been included. The discussion of instrumentation in the major kinds of laboratories should be sufficient, however, so that the reader will not miss too keenly comments on specific laboratories.

The speech and hearing laboratories that have been visited by the authors of this chapter have certain elements in common, even though each laboratory bears a stamp of individuality that stems from clinical or research enthusiasms of personnel and from the environmental and financial conditions under which each functions. The plan of this chapter is, first, to present a section on basic instrumentation that is common to a wide variety of laboratories; secondly, to describe selected laboratories; and to conclude by presenting, as an appendix, a list of all instrumentation mentioned in the *Journal of Speech and Hearing Research* within this decade. Throughout the chapter, whenever possible and appropriate, when a specific item of major instrumentation is mentioned, references will be made to articles in which these instruments were used.

Although attention in this chapter is on instruments and instrument systems, the rightful place of instrumentation in laboratories must be observed. Instruments obviously are adjunctive rather than central to clinical and research laboratory work. To devise a study to fit an instrument rather than to seek and use an instrument appropriate to a study is an unfortunate inversion of the normal cart and horse relationship. The most elaborate instrumentation, however, has the basic purpose of facilitating the fundamental goals of the therapist or researcher.

These goals are the modification or measurement of speech or hearing behavior or the formulation, testing, and verification or rejection of hypotheses. In the speech and/or hearing laboratories these hypotheses usually concern aspects of speech production and perception or language and hearing behavior. The laboratory provides a facility where speech, hearing, and language behavior, both normal and anomalous, may be measured and recorded.

In the laboratory or through the utilization of laboratory techniques, clinical diagnoses of speech disorders are made. For example, the simple act of examining an individual's dental structure for proper occlusion is a laboratory method; the tongue depressor is a laboratory tool.

In clinical speech therapy as well as in diagnosis, on the other hand, great reliance is placed on laboratory methods and instrumentation. The tape recorder is an aid in the teaching of sound discrimination by auditory means, while the cathode-ray oscilloscope can fill the same function as a visual aid in the course of therapy.

Although much of the instrumentation discussed in this chapter is within the framework of laboratory settings, the use of instruments has permeated both the teaching and clinical aspects of speech, hearing, and language. The role of the speech and hearing scientist, who conducts investigations in his laboratory, is that of testing hypotheses with observations and data in order to derive laws or generalizations about normal and abnormal speech, hearing, and language. These generalizations, in addition to providing fundamental knowledge, can provide information useful for the therapist who is concerned with modification of anomalous speech, hearing, and language.

Since the original chapter was written, a number of changes in instrumentation have occurred; these include not only advances in the technical capabilities of devices but also the ways in which instruments are used. Primary advances in the automation of experimental procedures include control of stimuli presented to observers and the storing and recovery of responses made to the stimuli. Automation now extends to therapeutic procedures as well as to research. Computers are increasingly a part of instrumentation in speech and hearing, not only for data control and analysis but also for such uses as speech synthesis and dynamic modeling of vocal tract function. It must be anticipated that further advances in instrumentation and their uses will increase the ease with which both the investigator and clinician can study or modify speech, hearing, and language behavior.

BASIC INSTRUMENTATION

Basic instrumentation for speech and hearing includes a wide variety of devices that, in one way or another, control, store, produce, measure, or modify sounds. One group of instruments, microphones, amplifiers, and loudspeakers, convert sounds into electrical waves, amplify the waves, and convert the waves again to sounds. Oscillators, function generators, audiometers, noise generators, and speech synthesizers are instruments used to produce sound. Sounds are stored either by magnetic-tape recorders or disc recorders. Instruments used for the measurement of a sound include digital and analog voltmeters, sound-level meters, frequency counters, and analyzers.

In order to study speech and man's response to sound in both clinical and research settings, an acoustic signal must often be modified in a particular way. Attenuators, frequency filters, and electronic switches are some of the devices employed to modify levels, frequency bandwidths, and durations of sounds. Interval timers with associated electronic switches, pulse generators, and signal-activated relays are utilized for temporal control procedures. A number of instruments are utilized for measurement of basic parameters of sound: oscilloscopes and power-level recorders display amplitude in time data, whereas spectral analyzers and electronic counters give information about the frequency characteristics of sound.

In addition to those instruments used primarily for the production, control, and measurement of sound, other apparatus is widely used to measure physiological aspects of behavior relative to speech and hearing. For example, an impedance bridge is used to measure middle-ear function; evoked-response audiometry systems average electroencephalographic responses to acoustic stimuli; the psychogalvanometer measures electrodermal changes in response to conditioned sounds; and the spirometer assesses breath functions.

Microphones, Amplifiers, Loudspeakers, and Receivers

The use of microphones, amplifiers, and loudspeakers is universal in speech and hearing settings. Microphones and loudspeakers are transducers that convert acoustic to electrical energy or, conversely, electrical to acoustic energy. An amplifier is an instrument wherein an input signal controls an output signal of greater power resulting in a gain of energy. Applications of amplifiers in speech and hearing are primarily for driving either loudspeakers or receivers to provide the appropriate level of an acoustic signal at the listener's ear.

MICROPHONES

A microphone is an electroacoustic transducer that is used to convert changes in acoustic pressure or particle velocity into electrical energy where the variations in the resultant voltage or current correspond to the variations in the acoustical energy. Microphones can be classified in various ways that include whether or not the response of the microphone is to acoustic pressure or to particle velocity; whether or not the acoustic source supplies the energy generated by the microphone or the sound source controls the flow of energy that is provided by a source other than the acoustic one; and according to the kinds of materials used to construct the microphone or the design of the microphone. When considerations are given to the selection of a particular microphone for use in a laboratory or clinical setting, such matters as the fidelity of response, sensitivity, directionality, durability, and cost enter into decisions as to the appropriate instrument. Condenser microphones, for example, maintain the fidelity of the acoustic wave well but have the disadvantage of requiring an adjacent coupled preamplifier and a polarizing voltage source for operation of the microphone. Condenser microphones for this reason are well suited for laboratory and precision work, such as calibration of instruments, but are not well suited for situations that require high output voltages and constant rugged use. Functional characteristics of microphones are summarized in Fig. 5-1.

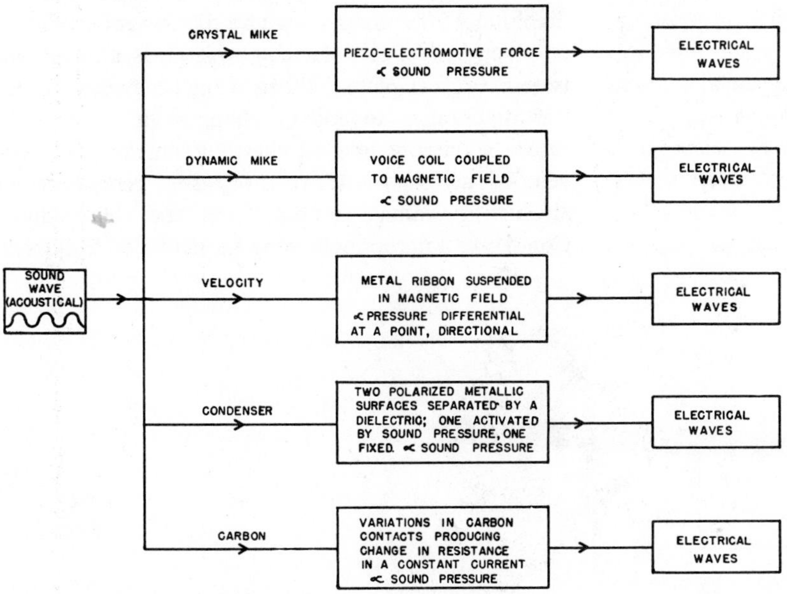

Fig. 5-1. Functional characteristics of microphones.

The carbon microphone is the oldest type and is characteristically used where high sensitivity and durability are required. Carbon microphones consist of a metal diaphragm attached to an enclosure, called the carbon button, which contains carbon granules. Movement of the diaphragm in response to sound increases and decreases pressure on the carbon button. These changes produce proportional fluctuations in the resistance of the granules that correspond in a linear manner to the acoustic pressure. The variation in resistance produces changes in current so that the resultant alternating voltage can be amplified and used as a signal source. Carbon microphones can be manufactured at low cost and, where the fidelity requirements are not high, can function with little or no maintenance. Carbon microphones respond to pressure and require a voltage source other than that produced by the carbon particles.

The crystal microphone also responds to sound pressure. In this instance, sound pressure distorts a crystal, most often Rochelle salts, and a varying voltage is produced between opposite faces of the crystal. The action of the sound wave is to produce a piezoelectric electromotive force. In crystal microphones, sound waves activate a diaphragm that is mechanically attached to a crystal. In the manufacture of these microphones, metal electrodes are attached to the crystal substance. The advantages of crystal microphones are that their cost is low and their output is high with a reasonably good quality signal. These microphones, however, are sensitive to extremes of heat and moisture and cannot tolerate mechanical shock.

A third type of microphone that also responds to sound pressure is the electrodynamic microphone that consists of a voice coil attached to a diaphragm. The coil is suspended between the poles of a permanent magnet. Sound waves impinging upon the diaphragm cause the coil to move back and forth in a radial field of the magnet generating an alternating voltage that is proportional to the applied sound.

The dynamic microphone, Fig. 5-2, is similar to the dynamic loudspeaker in its action except that it converts acoustic into electric energy, whereas the loudspeaker converts electric into acoustic energy. The dynamic microphone generates less voltage than either the carbon or crystal microphones and, as a result, greater amplification of the output of the microphone is necessary.

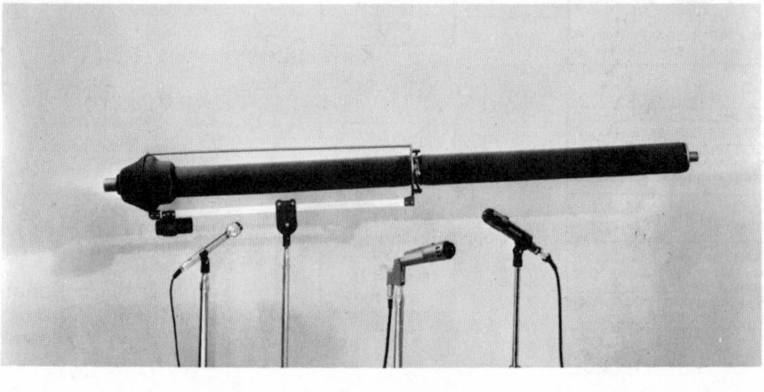

Fig. 5-2. Dynamic microphones; all are unidirectional. *Photo courtesy Electro-Voice, Inc.*

The carbon, crystal, and dynamic microphones are classified as pressure microphones in that acoustic pressure impinges upon one side of a movable diaphragm, resulting in a movement that is proportional to and in phase with the pressure. Another kind of microphone is the pressure-gradient microphone. Pressure-gradient or velocity microphones are those where the driving force corresponds to the differences in pressures that act on the opposing side of a moving element. The velocity-ribbon microphone is a pressure-gradient microphone where a thin, corrugated, metallic ribbon is suspended between the poles of a permanent magnet. When the ribbon is set in motion by acoustic energy, the lines of force between the two poles are cut and an alternating voltage is generated. Because of its construction, the velocity microphone tends to be directional in its response. Velocity microphones tend to have good low-frequency responses, but the response drops off at higher frequencies.

Another variety of pressure microphone, and one with widespread use in speech and hearing laboratories and clinics, is the condenser microphone. This microphone is constructed with a fixed plate and a closely adjacent, tightly stretched metal disc or diaphragm. The fixed plate and diaphragm are plates of a condenser. A polarizing voltage is applied between the two plates. When acoustic energy causes the diaphragm to move, changes in capacitance result. Charging and discharging currents are developed across a load resistor, thus generating an alternating voltage output from the microphone. Condenser microphones tend to have flat frequency responses in the auditory range and have stability in time and under temperature changes. High-quality condenser microphones for special purposes are available, and for this reason they are frequently the appropriate ones for precision laboratory uses.

AMPLIFIERS

Amplifiers are instruments that increase weak signals to a desired level by a process whereby a small amount of force controls a large amount of energy. Amplifiers are also used to isolate one circuit from another. There are various ways in which amplifiers can be classified. One of these is to classify them as either voltage or power amplifiers. Voltage amplifiers deliver maximum voltage, whereas a power amplifier delivers maximum power. The gain in energy results in a vacuum tube amplifier, for example, when a small voltage variation on a control electrode or grid produces a large voltage or power variation at the output or plate circuit of the tube. Although in the past the vacuum tube amplifier has been the most common type, the transistor is now used extensively for amplification. The transistor controls electrons in a solid, whereas the vacuum tube amplifier controls electrons in a vacuum. The process of amplification in the transistor is similar to that of the vacuum tube in that a small amount of energy can control a large amount of energy at the output. Amplifiers used in speech and hearing laboratories are increasingly solid-state ones, and they have the advantages of small size, low power consumption, and relatively trouble-free operation as compared to vacuum tube amplifiers. Although in the past audio amplifiers that covered the frequency range of 20 to 20,000 Hz were those of primary interest for speech and hearing, other kinds of amplifiers for control circuitry, such as programming of stimuli and the recovery of responses, are increasingly useful for work in this area. When amplifiers are used for audio signals, there may be two sections to the amplifier, a preamplifier and a power amplifier. The preamplifier is a voltage amplifier that raises the input signal to the point at which it can drive a power amplifier. The power amplifier is necessary to drive transducers such as earphones and loudspeakers. The condenser microphone is a good example of a weak signal source that requires a preamplifier as part of its circuit in order to deliver a signal of sufficient magnitude for subsequent amplification.

LOUDSPEAKERS AND RECEIVERS

Loudspeakers and receivers are transducers that change electrical voltage or current into sound. Loudspeaker functions can be divided for convenience into two aspects. The first of these is the conversion of electrical energy into mechanical motion. The second aspect involves changing these mechanical motions into movements of air particles that constitute sound. When these two functions are considered with respect to the techniques necessary to achieve them, a variety of loudspeaker and receiver designs is possible. The most basic and common principle applied to loudspeaker design is the electrodynamic one. The electrodynamic principle specifies that when there is a flow of current through a coil suspended in a constant magnetic field, fluctuations in the current will be reflected in coil movements. Variations of this phenomenon are the most common methods of converting electrical to mechanical energy. In one variation the magnetic field varies instead of the coil. Transducers of this latter type are referred to as magnetic. Changes in the flow of current through the coil result in fluctuations in the magnetic field that cause a diaphragm to move back and forth.

Electrostatic elements are another design used for loudspeakers based on repulsion and attraction between electrical charges. Electrostatic loudspeakers have two conductive surfaces separated to form a condenser. One surface is rigid and the other flexible. Fluctuations in a direct current voltage applied between the two surfaces result in movement of the flexible plate that is transmitted to air particles. Other principles used for loudspeaker and receiver elements include piezoelectric, where an electric voltage applied across the material results in changes in its shape that can be transmitted to air particles. Most of the principles that can be applied to microphone construction can be applied in reverse to loudspeaker and receiver construction, although the functional designs will be different to obtain optimal performance as either a loudspeaker or a receiver.

The second aspect of loudspeaker or receiver function is the conversion of mechanical energy to sound. Usually the element in a loudspeaker or receiver that converts electrical to mechanical energy is small and is not well coupled to the surrounding air. The matching of mechanical energy to air is usually accomplished in one of two ways. One of these is the direct-radiator loudspeaker in which a large-area cone of either paper or cloth is rigidly attached to the unit that transduces electrical energy to mechanical energy. A large volume of air can be displaced by small movements of the cone. A second type is a horn loudspeaker in which mechanical movement is transmitted by a small piston source coupled to a large volume of air by means of a flared horn. The horn in this case is an acoustic transformer that allows the air to be impedance matched to the vibrating piston. For most applications in speech and hearing, the direct-radiator loudspeaker is more commonly used.

In order that the loudspeaker or receiver may reproduce audio signals faithfully, several techniques are possible in loudspeaker and receiver construction. One procedure involves placing the speaker in an enclosure in order to baffle sounds that are produced by the back side of the loudspeaker cone and tailoring the size and shape of the enclosures to either attenuate or accentuate the particular frequencies. Other installations utilize different speakers in both kind and shape adequately to handle various frequencies. Low- and high-frequency speakers, tweeters, and woofers can be combined into a single unit for efficient sound radiation. For example, some loudspeakers incorporate both direct-radiation and horn features by means of concentric mounted speakers. The woofer provides for the lower frequencies and the multicellular horn for the higher frequencies with resulting uniform frequency response in the audio range.

In many applications, for both research and clinical purposes, it is desirable that headsets be used. The use of headsets provides better control of the signal at an individual's ear than does a loudspeaker used free field; it also permits simultaneous presentation of a different signal to each ear. In addition to good frequency responses required for headset receivers, it is important that the earphones attenuate external sound and can be worn comfortably for a period of time. Some uses such as aural rehabilitation, for example, also require that a high-level signal be delivered to the ears without distortion. The Koss headset, PRO-4A, for example, utilizes fluid-filled ear cushions for comfort and sound attenuation and provides a good frequency response through the radio range.

Oscillators and Signal Generators

Many instruments that emit signals of various waveforms are used as signal sources and also as control devices. These include oscillators, function generators, noise generators, waveform generators, sawtooth generators, square-wave generators, and similar devices. An oscillator is a device that generates sine-wave signals of known frequency and amplitude. Some of the signal generators listed above are oscillators with an additional capability for modulation.

OSCILLATORS

The audio oscillator, perhaps one of the most basic units in speech and hearing settings, is usually of the RC Wein-bridge type, although beat-frequency oscillators are still constructed. In the RC oscillators, frequency is determined by passive resistors and capacitors. Frequency changes are provided by a variable air capacitor, and frequency ranges are determined by fixed resistances that change frequency in discrete steps. Examples of audio-frequency oscillators that are of the RC design are the General Radio 1310-A oscillator and the Hewlett-Packard model 200 series. (Model 200CD is shown in Fig. 5-3.) Most oscillators used today are solid-state devices that provide considerable stability of operation. An exception to RC oscillators is the beat-frequency type 1304-B oscillators manufactured by General Radio. Audio oscillators are basic components for many aspects of tests and experimentation, particularly in the area of hearing. Various pure-tone audiometers, including both manual and automatic, have oscillators as signal sources. A wide variety of audiological tests from pure-tone thresholds to the detection of difference limen are dependent upon oscillators for the generation of sine waves. The use of transistors has reduced the size of oscillators and increased their stability. The oscillator remains one of the most dependable and necessary units for speech and hearing, whether it be for providing signal sources for auditory responses, the testing of response characteristics of various pieces of equipment, or providing calibration and timing tones for experimental purposes.

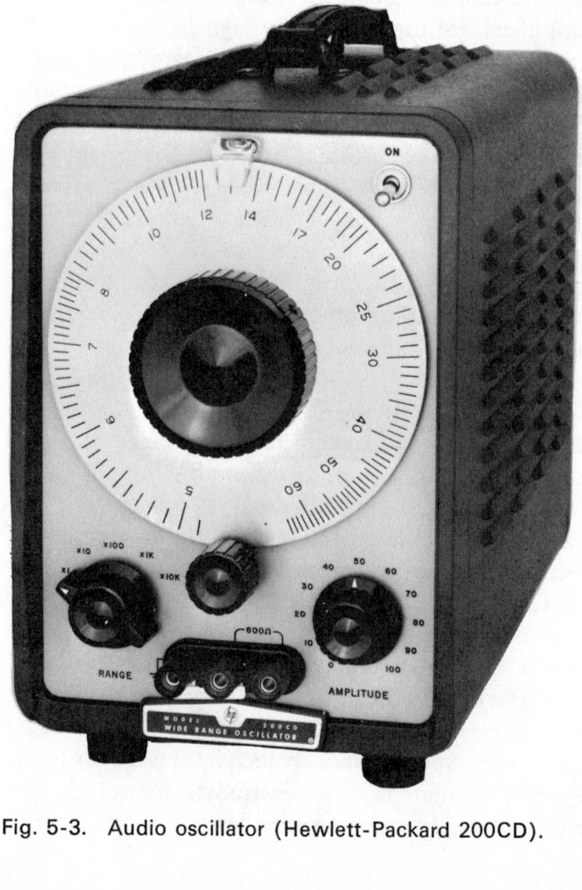

Fig. 5-3. Audio oscillator (Hewlett-Packard 200CD).

FUNCTION AND WAVEFORM GENERATORS

Function and waveform generators are units that provide a number of different waveforms over a wide frequency range. Function generators are available that produce sine, sawtooth, square, and triangular waves. The Hewlett-Packard function generator model 3300A, shown in Fig. 5-4, produces three types of calibrated output waveforms: sinusoidal, square, and triangular. Function generators are extremely versatile instruments for speech and hearing settings, including the classroom, clinics, and laboratories, because a number of auditory and speech phenomena can be demonstrated, tested, and investigated using these instruments. A waveform generator, for example, with associated pulse generators can be used for triggering electronic switches to obtain a wide variety of on-off signal patterns with excellent accuracy in milliseconds or better. Temporal integrating times of the auditory system can be explored with this kind of equipment, as also can temporal aspects of speech behavior. Function generators used in association either with other generators or oscillators can be used to produce a wide variety of waveforms. Control of waveforms opens many possibilities for the study of auditory perception, as, for example, an increased pitch perception efficiency was found for highly modulated tone bursts as compared to rectangular tone bursts (Mahaffey, 1967).

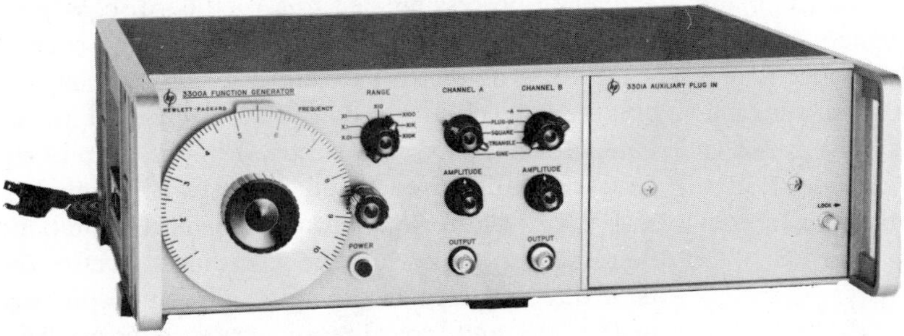

Fig. 5-4. Function generator (Hewlett-Packard 3300A).

NOISE GENERATORS

Random-noise generators are used both clinically and experimentally for many aspects of speech and hearing. Initially, the noise generator was used in the laboratory to simulate aircraft noises in order to study the effects of noise on speech communication (Licklider and Miller, 1951). The effects of noise on speech were systematically studied relative to the listener, the equipment that constituted the channel, and the talker (Black, 1957). Noise generators have been employed in studies of other auditory phenomena such as masking (Bilger, 1958), binaural fusion (Cherry, 1961), and the effects of correlated and uncorrelated noise on speech intelligibility (Licklider, 1948). Random noise is also employed for testing the performance of equipment by obtaining response curves for noise of known characteristics. An example of a noise generator is the Grason-Stadler Model 901B shown in Fig. 5-5. Two kinds of spectra are provided, white and speech-masking noise. A clinical application of noise generators is the narrow band masking used in conventional audiometry (Newby, 1964).

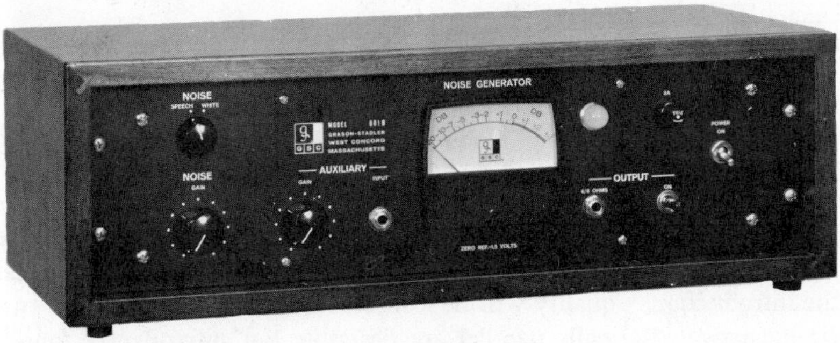

Fig. 5-5. Noise generator (Grason-Stadler 901B). *Photo courtesy Grason-Stadler.*

Although speech synthesis represents a specific example of waveform generation, because of its considerable importance for speech and hearing, it will be discussed in a subsequent section.

Disc and Magnetic-Tape Recording

A basic tool in speech and hearing settings in both the laboratory and the clinic is a device for the recording, storage, and reproduction of speech, sounds, or electrical signals. There are two major types of recording devices, disc and magnetic tape. Disc recorders are used primarily for recording and playback of speech, whereas the magnetic-tape recorder is considerably more versatile in that it may be used not only for speech and other sounds but also as a data recorder. The principle of operation of both disc and analog magnetic-tape recorders is the same in that any time varying event that can be converted into an electrical signal can be recorded.

DISC RECORDING

In his excellent brief history of the disc recorder, Windesheim (1938) gives credit for its invention to Thomas Edison in 1877. From its crude beginnings as a sound-powered engraver of tin foil, many improvements have been made. The names of Bell and Tainter, Berliner, and Masfield and Harrison are associated, respectively, with the substitution of stylus cutting for stylus indentation, the substitution of the lateral for the vertical cut, and the introduction of microphone, amplifier, and electrically activated cutting stylus.

Today, phonograph disc recording is obtained by converting sound to electricity and back to sound again. This is accomplished by transforming mechanical energy into electrical energy (microphone), then using an amplifier to enlarge the small electrical variations from the microphone and a device for transforming electrical energy back into mechanical vibrations (recording head). Typical types of microphones have already been discussed. The mechanical action of the recording head and stylus results in an engraving process applied to a rotating disc. Reproduction is accomplished by converting the sound-wave patterns on the acetate disc into mechanical vibrations (pick-up needle). The mechanical vibrations are converted into electrical impulses (pick-up head), magnified into useful proportions (amplifier), and then transformed into mechanical vibrations (loudspeaker) as sound. The recording processes for both disc and tape recording are shown graphically in Fig. 5-6, and typical reproducer systems are likewise shown graphically in Fig. 5-7.

Fidelity of recording and reproduction is a function of the acoustics of the recording studio, the disc employed, and the frequency-response characteristics of the recording and reproducing apparatus. The recording chamber should be free from excessive reverberation and peculiarities of resonance. The room should not be too "dead," or brilliance of tonal quality will be lost. Rooms constructed with no two walls parallel are desirable but infrequently found. Square rooms are usually bad for recording purposes

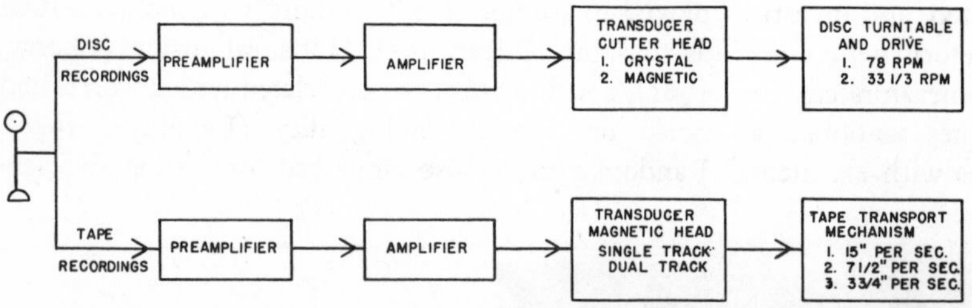

Fig. 5-6. Recording systems.

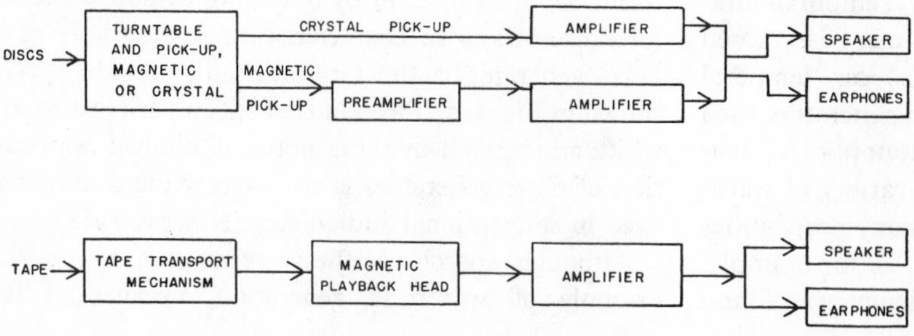

Fig. 5-7. Reproducer systems.

unless acoustic treatment affords compensation. Reverberant rooms, having poor acoustical qualities, can be improved by placing monk's cloth or other sound-absorbing material on three or more walls and the ceiling, and a heavy carpet on the floor. Commercial acoustical materials are available and should be used for permanent installations. Frequency-response characteristics of the apparatus are determined by the nature of the component elements of the equipment and the proper matching of the components to each other. A high-quality amplifier will not yield high-fidelity recordings if the microphone and/or the recording head is of poor quality. Likewise, when all the components are of high quality, recordings may still lack fidelity if the elements are mismatched.

In making a laboratory disc recording, microphone technique is important. Usually adequate results may be obtained by facing the microphone at a distance of 18 to 24 inches. Speaking into a microphone from a distance of six inches or less often increases the bass response of the instrument and causes distortion. Lip and tongue noises and breathing noises are usually objectionable at close operating distances. Greater distances usually result in too weak a voice signal in relation to room noise. A "conversational level" of voice should be adequate in all but unusual circumstances.

Before the actual cutting of the disc, the operator should check the cutting action of the stylus on a practice disc. The chip (portion of the disc removed by the stylus) should be about the diameter of a coarse human hair and should fall away from the stylus. The groove should be shiny and a little more than twice as wide as the uncut portion between grooves and land (ratio 70/30). Adjustments for depth of groove can be made on the tension of the spring supporting the cutting head during this checking operation.

Another preliminary checking operation which should be performed is a testing of the electrical components: responsiveness of the instrument to microphone-channel gain controls and of the stylus to an input signal. The former is observed by inspection of the VU meter (or other volume indicator) when the gain control is manipulated with a constant signal entering the microphone. The presence of stylus action is verified by a finger touch on the stylus when a signal is transmitted to it; the stylus should be felt to vibrate.

The uses to which the disc recorder may be put are many and varied. The discs provide, for the clinician, excellent evidence of the results of therapy. For the client they provide both opportunity for learning sound discrimination and a strong motivating influence for improvement (Henkrikson and Irwin, 1949; Williamson, 1935). The researcher finds the disc a most convenient means of preserving, presenting, and re-presenting auditory stimuli to the subjects of his investigations (Henkrikson, 1943) or to analyzing instruments. Many other uses of disc recorders undoubtedly will suggest themselves to the reader.

MAGNETIC-TAPE RECORDING

A more recent development than the disc recorder is the magnetic-tape recorder that probably dates back to the Telegraphone of Poulsen in Denmark developed in 1898. Even earlier, Marconi was reported to have experimented with this type of recording in his investigations of electromagnetic radiation. The evolution of the primitive wire recorder was slow until World War II, when the demands of the military brought about rapid advances in mechanical and electronic perfection of this type of recording instrument (LeBel, 1951). Tape have superseded wire recorders, and the following discussion of magnetic recording refers to magnetic-tape instruments. A block diagram showing basic components is shown in Fig. 5-8.

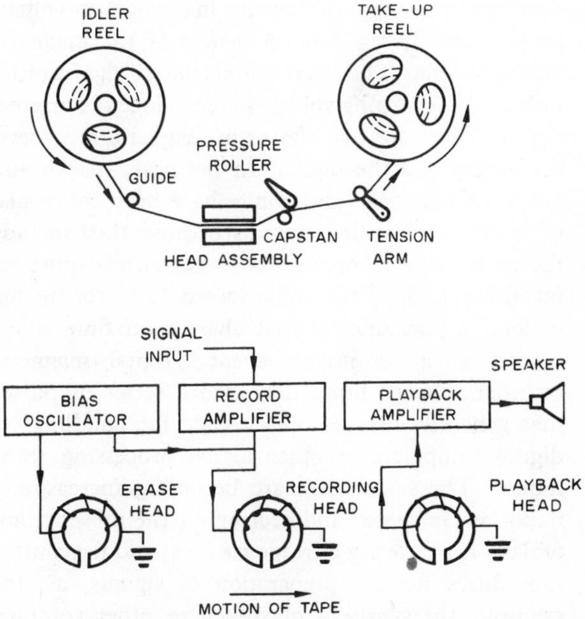

Fig. 5-8. Mechanical and electronic systems of a tape recorder.

The principle of magnetic recording is that signals can be impressed upon a moving magnetizable tape by fluctuations in current flow through a coil. The recording depends on inducing a magnetic pattern in a semipermanent magnet that is usually material treated with metal oxide. There are three basic parts for the recorder. These include the electronics of the system, the head assembly, and tape transport. The electronic portion of the system transduces and delivers the input signals in the appropriate form to the record head and, vice versa, recovers data from the playback head and delivers it in the necessary form for output. The head portion of the recorder includes both the record and the reproduce sections. The head assembly also includes an erase section that demagnetizes the tape before it passes the record head. The recording head is an electromagnet that has a small gap in the core across which the tape is moved. The magnetic tape shunts this gap; and, when the tape is in motion, the tape that has just passed the gap is left permanently magnetized in the direction of the head magnetization at that moment. The intensity of the magnetization is controlled by the magnitude of the signal when this portion of tape passed the gap. The reproduce head of a recorder is similar to the record head and performs a function that is the reverse of the record head. It is also an electromagnet with the gap in the core. When the magnetic tape is moved across this gap, a flux develops in the core that results in changes in voltage proportional to the rate of change of the magnetic field at the gap. The electronic section of the recorder utilizes this changing voltage to reproduce the original signal. There are two classes of magnetic recorders, the analog and the digital. In the past, speech and hearing laboratories and clinics have been concerned primarily with analog systems because they include the audio tape recorders and other special-purpose recorders, such as the video recorder. In the analog system, a phenomenon that changes in time is recorded as a continuous event. Digital magnetic recorders change input data into a series of pulses that generally fits the binary code for handling by digital computers or other digital processing techniques. These recorders are becoming increasingly important in speech and hearing for the presentation of data, the recovery of response data, and for control procedures for the preparation of signals, as, for example, the synthesis of speech or other complex signals.

In the selection of a magnetic-tape instrument, the faithfulness of reproduction of signals necessary for anticipated uses will govern the particular instrument chosen. There are a number of technical factors that need to be taken into account relative to high-fidelity recording and reproduction. One of these relates to tape speed, because this governs how many oscillations are recorded on a particular space on the tape. Each oscillation requires a certain minimum amount of space, and at slower tape speeds fidelity of reproduction, particularly the higher frequencies, is lost. Another requirement for good recording and reproduction is constant tape speed. In some professional quality tape recorders there will be three motors: one for the supply reel, one for the take-up reel, and the third to drive the tape. Console-type tape recorders are illustrated in Fig. 5-9, and a portable, battery-powered tape recorder is shown in Fig. 5-10.

There are some instruments that utilize the principles of magnetic-tape recording for special purposes. Three of these are the delayed-feedback recorder, the time compressor-expander, and the Language Master.

DELAYED FEEDBACK (SIDETONE)

The disturbing influence of reverberations in large auditoria upon public speakers has been casually

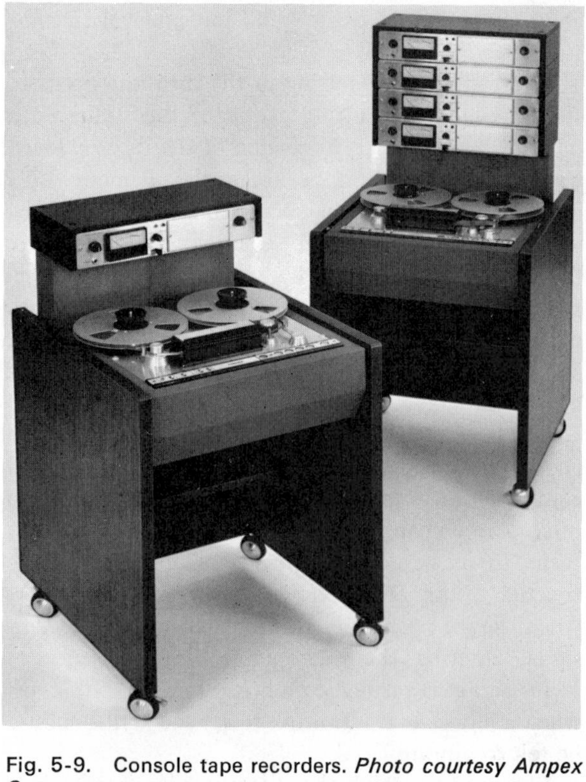

Fig. 5-9. Console tape recorders. *Photo courtesy Ampex Corp.*

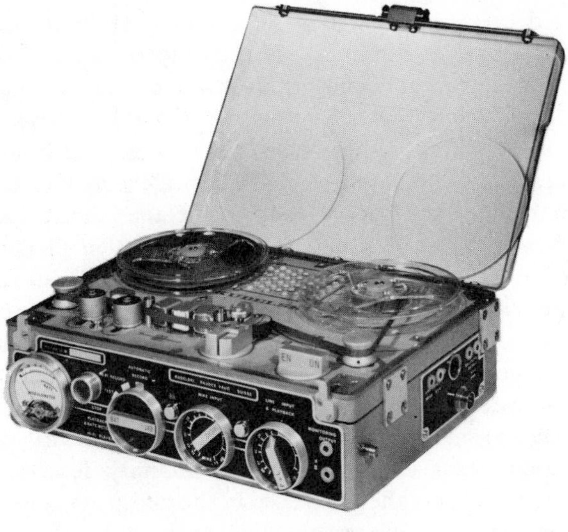

Fig. 5-10. Portable, battery-powered tape recorder.

observed, over hundreds of years, by the individuals affected. However, not until this century have there been formal attempts to identify the mechanism or mechanisms involved in partial speech breakdown under these conditions—when the speaker's voice is returned to his ear an appreciable time after the sounds have been produced. A name—delayed feedback or delayed sidetone—has been given to the precipitating phenomenon; instruments have been developed or modified in order to induce and control it, and many investigations have been performed to test its effects under various conditions. Perhaps more importantly, the results of sidetone research have been incorporated into, and in some cases have formed, the basis for theoretical formulations concerning initiation, control, and breakdown in speech.

Typical of the instruments developed or modified to provide for a controlled delay in returning a subject's speech signals to his auditory mechanism is the delayed-feedback tape recorder-reproducer illustrated in Fig. 5-11. The recorder is equipped with a standard roll of recording tape, which passes first over an erase-head that removes all previous signals from the tape. The heart of the delay mechanism is a recording head, mounted in a slotted track, that permits the head to be displaced from .6 to 3.0 inches from the reproduce head, providing for continuous delay from 0.08 to 0.40 seconds. An external amplifying and switching unit makes it possible for the experimenter to direct the recorded signal into the subject's earphones either synchronously (no-delay condition) from the monitor circuit in the recording head, or delayed by a predetermined time fraction from the normal output circuit associated with the fixed-position reproducing head.

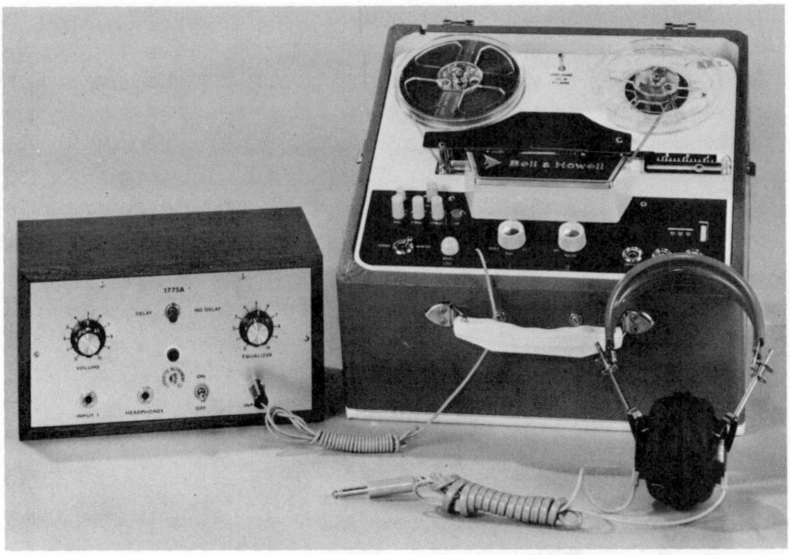

Fig. 5-11. Delayed feedback recorder. *Photo courtesy Lafayette Instrument Co.*

To illustrate the delay procedure: the recorder is started and record switch depressed; the tape is wiped clean as it moves over the erase-head; the message being spoken by the subject is impressed on the tape by the recording head; the tape then moves, at seven and one-half inches per second, on to the reproduce head, which may be, for example, one and one-half inches beyond the recording head. At this setting the elapsed time between a spoken syllable and perception of it in the ear would be just slightly more than .2 second, sufficient to create a considerable vocal disturbance in the speaker.

Early investigations making use of delayed sidetone were designed to establish critical delay times related to maximum disruption of the subjects' normal speech patterns. Lee (1951) and Black (1951) contributed basic information on this point. Spilka (1952) investigated relationships between measured personality traits and degree of speech breakdown under delay conditions, and Atkinson (1953) tested for adaptation to delay. Tiffany and C. N. Hanley (1952) have used delayed feedback as an adjunct to conventional audiometry, finding it a useful technique for the detection of malingering and hysterical deafness. Fairbanks (1954) has incorporated feedback implications into an operational theory of the speech mechanism. He, with many of the other writers on speech theory, acknowledges the important contributions made by Wiener (1950) in *Cybernetics*.

Since delayed-speech feedback was suggested as an adjunct to conventional audiometry (Tiffany and Hanley, 1952), it has been incorporated as a speech test for auditory malingering. Because many individuals experience difficulty with their speech under a delay of approximately 200 milliseconds, an individual is suspected of malingering when there is evidence of speech difficulty with the level of the delayed speech at his ear below that produced by his pure-tone audiogram.

The development of the delayed-feedback device and prediction about its effects were based on the theory of cybernetics (Wiener, 1950) under the hypothesis that organisms break into oscillation when control or servomechanisms are disturbed. Perhaps more than any other one instrument in speech and hearing, the delayed-feedback device exemplifies the interaction of theory and predictable data. The principle has been extended to articulation therapy (Van Riper and Irwin, 1958) and employed in theories concerning speech and sensory-feedback control (Chase, 1958). Yeni-Komshian, Chase, and Mobley (1968) have studied sensory-feedback control for speech and the development of speech-feedback mechanisms in children. Yates (1963), in reviewing studies that employed delayed auditory feedback, suggested that the difference in the effects on speech may relate to personality differences in individuals. This suggestion is certainly in accord with other psychoacoustic data where the kind of response is found to relate to the kind of individual who is making the response.

TIME COMPRESSOR-EXPANDER

It has long been observed that compression and expansion of signals along a time axis, with accompanying rise or fall of frequency, may be accomplished by means of accelerating or retarding playback speeds on a tape or disc reproducer. Fairbanks, Everett, and Jaeger (1954) described an important instrument which makes possible the compression-expansion of either time or frequency, with the alternate variable held constant. A device with this capability (see Fig. 5-12) opens up a large area of perceptual phenomenology for controlled investigation. In presenting

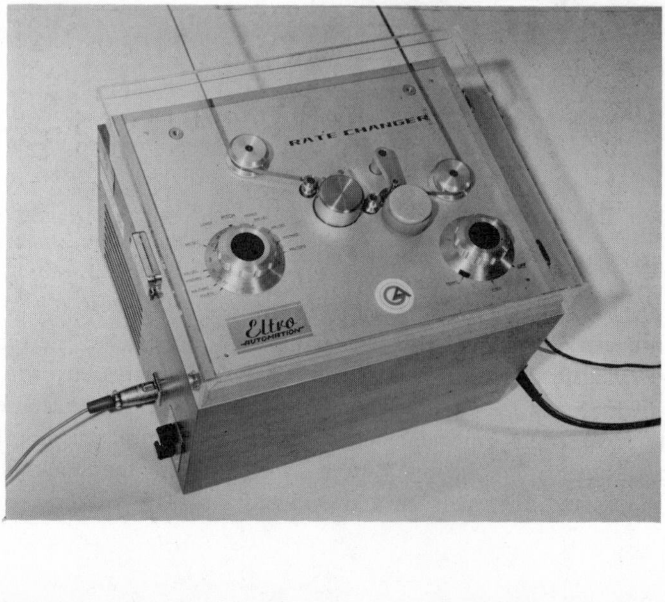

Fig. 5-12. Device for compression–expansion on time axis or rise–fall on pitch axis of recorded signals. *Photo courtesy Gotham Audio Corp.*

the operational characteristics of the compressor-expander, the writers acknowledged the similarity in theory and design of their method of approach to the same problem made independently by other investigators. Several of these are summarized by Gabor (1946, 1947, 1948).

In playback of the stored samplings in this instrument, the operator is able to duplicate the original frequency and also to modify the time aspect in the fractional or multiplicative manner. Conversely, he may play back the modified signal so that the original time values are retained, but frequency is fractionated or multiplied. Control of record and reproduce speeds being continuous, rather than in discrete steps, the operator may elect to compress original signals by any desired fraction. Similarly, expansion is under a wide range of continuous control.

Many voice scientists have engaged in research problems involving temporal aspects of speech. Basic among these studies are those of Darley (1940) and Franke (1939), which provided normative information about oral reading rate, and an investigation by Kelly and Steer (1949) which revealed important relationships between perception of speaking rate and various methods of expressing rate. Relations between time measures and speech skills have been reported by Murray and Tiffin (1933), and durational characteristics of voice during emotional expression have been reported by Fairbanks and Hoaglin (1941). Irwin and Becklund (1953) have published some preliminary findings with respect to diadochokinetic rate revealed by the sylrater. Tiffany (1953), in a study involving arbitrary compression and expansion of vowel sounds, has presented evidence of the importance of duration for phonemic identification. Duration also is a significant contributor to emphasis, according to the findings of Tiffin and Steer (1937). The duration of individual phonemes, measured sonagraphically, appears to be related to regional dialect, according to evidence presented by Hanley (1951). Draegert's (1951) findings indicate that of all voice variables tested, syllable duration was most highly related to speech intelligibility in high-level noise.

The use of instrumentation for time measurement in the speech clinic, in contrast to the laboratory, has been relatively restricted. However, there is some evidence of increased attention being paid by clinicians to the time variable. The significance of rate and duration, revealed in the studies noted above and in many others, has impressed many clinicians with the desirability of teaching control over time values to some of the clients of the clinic. Among those who have received benefit from this type of therapy have been stutterers, cerebral-palsied individuals, and people with foreign-language speech backgrounds.

A series of studies have examined the effects of time compression upon comprehension of connected speech (Fairbanks, Everett, and Jeager, 1954; Fairbanks, Guttman, and Miron, 1957) and word intelligibility as a function of time compression (Fairbanks, Guttman, and Miron, 1957). Comprehension for connected speech was found to be good at 50 percent compression. Word intelligibility remained close to 100 percent even when words were shortened to 20 percent of their original durations.

THE LANGUAGE MASTER

This instrument is a special-purpose magnetic-tape recorder that records on and plays back from magnetic tape that is mounted on a card. The drive mechanism of this instrument moves a card past the head mechanism. The advantages of the Language Master are that in addition to the material recorded on the card the same material may also be printed and/or shown pictorially. Because recording is on a short segment of tape, material does not have to be

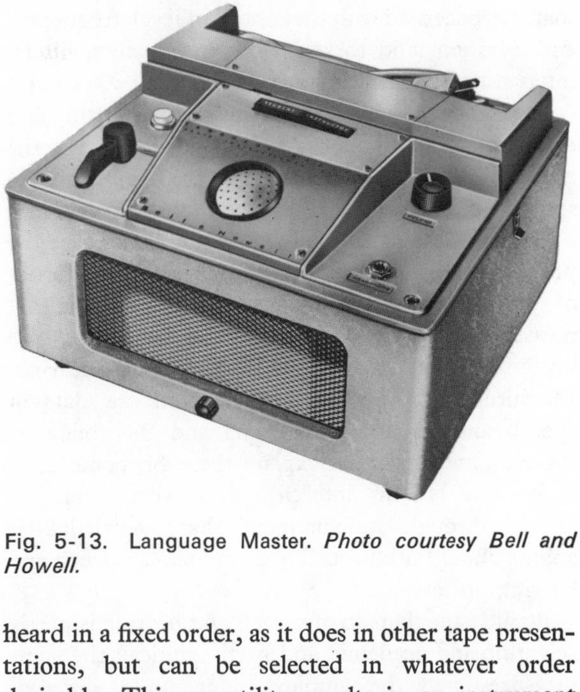

Fig. 5-13. Language Master. *Photo courtesy Bell and Howell.*

heard in a fixed order, as it does in other tape presentations, but can be selected in whatever order desirable. This versatility results in an instrument that has many clinical applications and, where high-frequency response is not critical, can be used in investigations where random presentations of short stimuli are required. The Language Master is shown in Fig. 5-13. Instruments that utilize a magnetic drum and multiple record and playback heads can also perform some of the functions that are achieved by the Language Master. The simplicity of operation and moderate cost of the Language Master in comparison, however, to these instruments makes it valuable for speech and hearing settings.

Instruments for the Measurement of Fundamental Physical Properties of Sound

Measurement in speech and hearing, whether it be that of the signal at the ear or the vocal output at the mouth, is primarily concerned with specifying the amount, the form, and the duration of the acoustic event. Measurements of amount or level, form or spectra, and time or duration constitute fundamental measures of sounds; instruments employed for these measurements are the ones discussed in this section. Included are such instruments as voltmeters and sound-level meters concerned with measurement of amplitude, spectral or wave analyzers concerned with frequency determinations, and electronic counters and signal-activated units concerned with temporal measures. Also included are some of the instruments that are concerned with the control of level, frequency, and duration, and these include attenuators, filters, interval timers, and electronic switches.

Instruments that measure intensity, spectra, and duration of sound in combinations often form the more complex measuring devices that are utilized in speech and hearing. When new instruments are developed, it is usually in an attempt to increase the precision in measuring these fundamental properties of sound. This fact emphasizes the essential role that measurement plays in an academic, scientific, and professional area such as speech and hearing. Measurement forms the link between raw data of speech and hearing phenomena and the concepts, theories, and laws that explain these phenomena. It is because of this interchange between data and theory through measurement that knowledge is gained about both normal and anomalous speech and hearing processes.

Because the domain of speech and hearing is partly scientific and academic and partly clinical, the same measures may be employed for quite different purposes. The measurement of the level of the signal that can barely be heard by normal ears on the one hand provides knowledge about sensitivity of the system and, on the other hand, normative data against which the sensitivity of a pathological ear may be evaluated. This exemplifies a phenomenon that is true with respect to measurement and instrumentation throughout the field of speech and hearing. Measurement samples raw data for scientific and knowledge purposes; these measurements are then applied as normative data for the definition of anomalous speech and hearing.

In the field of speech and hearing, workers are also concerned with behavioral scales of measurement as well as physical measures of sound. Although there are instruments that are modeled on behavioral units, such as the measurement of loudness, most of the instruments employed are those that are used to measure physical properties of sound.

In general, sounds including speech can be described in terms of either their waveform or their spectra. Waveform refers to amplitude of a sound as a function of time, whereas spectra show amplitude and phase relationships as a function of frequency. Some instruments, such as the Sona-Graph, described in a subsequent section, combine waveform and spectra and show spectral data as a function of time. Most of the instruments employed in speech and hearing derive the physical measures for a sound from the electrical form of the sound, either after an airborne sound has been transduced to an electrical state or before an electrical signal has been changed to sound. The first class of instruments discussed are those concerned with the measurement of intensity.

VOLTMETERS AND SOUND-LEVEL MEASURING DEVICES

According to Fletcher (1953) it was the minuteness of speech power that made measurement of the voice variable difficult until the discovery of the vacuum tube. Modern speech and hearing laboratories are equipped with calibrated microphones, amplifiers, and voltmeters, as well as with instruments designed specifically for the analysis of speech and other signals. Early studies in the analysis of speech utilizing electronic circuitry include Dunn (1930) and Sivian, Dunn, and White (1931) where an electrical circuit was employed for measuring the average power-frequency distribution of speech sounds. Tiffin (1932) described a technique where a vacuum tube voltmeter was used as a high-speed output-level indicator. A photographic record was obtained by means of a Westinghouse supersensitive oscillograph element. The deflections of the oscillograph were photographed on moving film on which decibel lines were automatically traced. A voice was considered variable or flexible in intensity to the extent that the maximum excursions of the curves for different syllables spread over a wide range. The average deviation of amplitude values from the mean was used to indicate mean deviation in syllabic power. Typical of published research studies employing this technique were those of Murray and Tiffin (1933), Lewis and Tiffin (1934), and Steer and Tiffin (1934).

Voltmeters form an essential part, either as isolated instruments, components of more complex instruments, or as part of instrumental systems, of speech and hearing laboratories and clinical settings. Voltmeters, instruments for the measurement of voltage, current, and resistance, utilize rectifiers, amplifiers, and/or thermocouples within their circuits to generate an electrical quantity that is proportional to the amplitude of the signal that is being measured. Voltmeters can be either analog, that depict continuous quantities, or digital, that display measurement in discrete units. Although analog voltmeters have been those most frequently employed in speech and hearing, digital units are becoming increasingly useful for data acquisition and as components in a wide range of applications. This aspect will be discussed in a subsequent section that treats automation and digital-to-analog and analog-to-digital conversions as applied to speech and hearing. Although current and resistance measures obtained from voltmeters are necessary and important, particularly in testing, maintaining, and fabricating instruments, the measure that is most frequently used in acoustical and speech and hearing applications is that of voltage or, more particularly, its complement, the decibel. The amplitude or level of sound, in speech and hearing, is most commonly measured in sound-pressure level (SPL) and, since voltage is analogous to and the complement of pressure, the voltage reading can be directly in decibels. Many voltmeters show both voltage and decibel (dB) scales. An electronic voltmeter is shown in Fig. 5-14. Because voltmeters are the level-measuring devices incorporated in a number of instruments used in speech and hearing, such as sound-level meters, audiometers, and spectrum analyzers, where the decibel is employed as a basic unit, it is necessary to specify the particular unit of the decibel that is applicable. The decibel is a logarithmic number that expresses the ratio of the measured level of a signal to a reference level. When the intensity level (IL) of a sound is given, the measurement is in watts, units of power, and the referent level is 10^{-16} watts/cm^2. As was previously indicated, sound pressure level is the most frequently used measure for speech and hearing purposes. When the measurement is in pressure, the referent is 0.0002 dyne/cm^2. Another decibel unit, hearing level, is that shown on audiometers and refers to the sensitivity of the normal ear at various frequencies. Sensation level (SL) is another measure given in decibels and refers to the level of a sound above a particular individual's threshold; the reference in this case is the individual's own hearing.

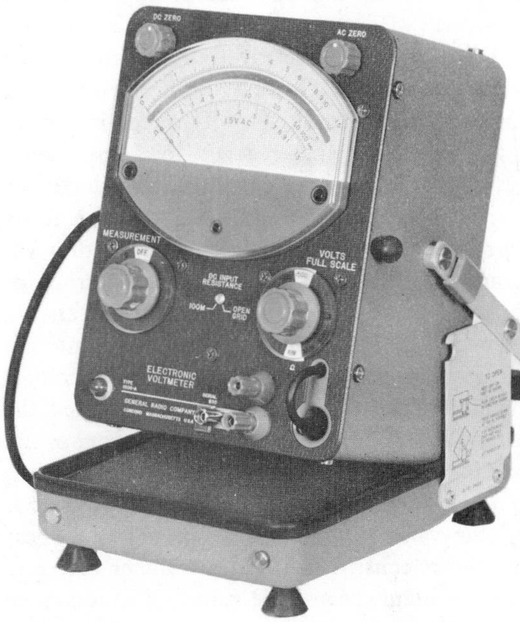

Fig. 5-14. Electronic voltmeter (General Radio Type 1806-A).

A considerable range of characteristics exists with respect to the design and measurement properties of voltmeters. In the selection of a particular unit, the kinds of signals that are to be measured, the situation under which the signals are to be sampled, and the accuracy necessary are determining factors. In general, there are three kinds of voltmeters of particular importance for speech and hearing measurement. These include those that show an average value of the measured voltage, those that indicate peak values, and those that provide a root-mean-square (rms) value. Instruments of the latter type have the highest degree of accuracy for signals like speech that depart markedly from a sinusoidal waveform.

Many instruments used in speech and hearing, particularly magnetic-tape recorders, employ a volume-level (VU) meter as an amplitude indicator. The VU meter provides relative rather than absolute dB values except when it is used in calibrated circuits. By virtue of the fact that the VU meter is a component of recorders, speech levels for both clinical and research purposes are frequently calibrated using this meter. Levitt and Bricker (1967), recognizing that speech-level measurements obtained with a VU meter are subject to sources of variability, proposed an objective procedure for reading VU meters. In their suggested procedure, the meter pointer is visible only during brief intervals because of control illumination. Each time the dial is illuminated the meter reader is required to determine whether or not the pointer exceeds a given value. If the pointer is above this value, the signal is attenuated; if it is below this value, attenuation is decreased. These authors report consistency from one meter reader to another and highly repeatable values. The increased accuracy obtained by this meter-reading procedure demonstrates possible sources of variability that are always present when an investigator or a clinician is part of the measurement system.

The sound-level meter, although not specifically designed for speech and hearing clinics and laboratories, is a useful instrument for measurement of level in both clinical and research settings. Fig. 5-15

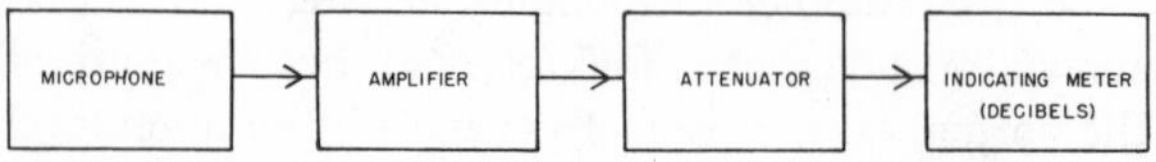

Fig. 5-15. Sound-level meter components.

is a block diagram indicating the basic components of a sound-level-meter circuit. The sound-level meter usually includes a microphone, an amplifier, a calibrated attenuator, an output meter, and frequency-weighting networks for the measurement of noise and sound. The apparent loudness attributed to sounds varies not only with sound pressure but also with the frequency of the sounds. The way it varies with frequency depends on the sound pressure, and to some extent provision is made for this phenomenon by the inclusion of the weighting networks (Peterson and Beranek, 1953). Some sound-level meters are designed specifically for portability, such as the General Radio Company types 1565-A and 1551-C illustrated in Figs. 5-16 and 5-17, respectively. These

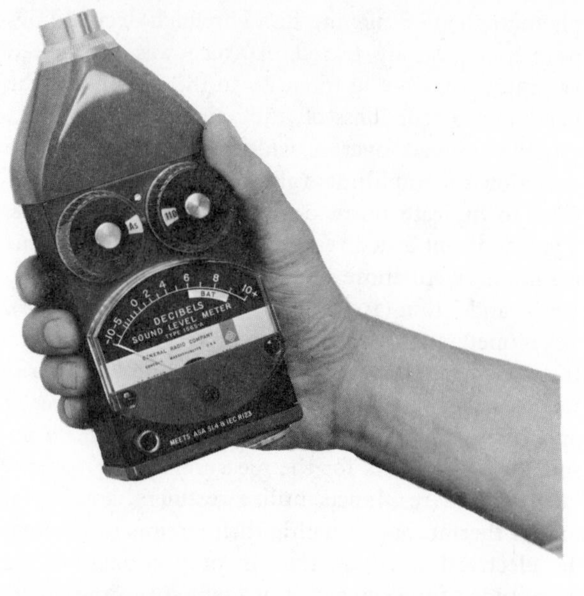

Fig. 5-16. Sound-level meter (General Radio Type 1565-A). *Photo courtesy General Radio Co.*

instruments are especially useful to the clinician when the maintenance of steady-state vocal-intensity levels is an important aspect of the therapeutic method or when range of speech intensity is required to satisfy a differential diagnosis. To the speech scientist, these instruments provide a means of visual metering of the pressure level of speech stimuli and the sound level in the research environment.

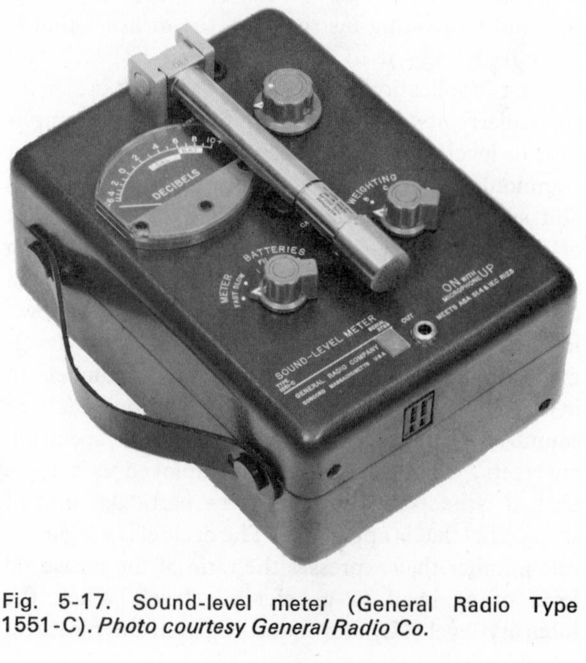

Fig. 5-17. Sound-level meter (General Radio Type 1551-C). *Photo courtesy General Radio Co.*

X-Y Recorders, Graphic Level Recorders, and Oscilloscopes

Speech and hearing data can frequently be portrayed on a Cartesian coordinate graph. Speech, for example, is a quasi-continuous signal that is defined by amplitude changes in time that can well be depicted by time and amplitude coordinates. X-Y recorders used in speech and hearing usually show time on the X or horizontal axis and amplitude on the Y or vertical axis. There are a number of instruments in the class of X-Y recorders including sound-level recorders, graphic level recorders, oscilloscopes, and oscillographs.

Graphic level recorders are designed to convert sound-signal inputs to permanent sound-pressure indications on a time basis. The final record is in the form of tracings plotted on a calibrated decibel scale. Basically, the sound-level recorder consists of an electromechanical feedback system in which the signal to be measured is amplified and then coupled to a square-law rectifier, where the intensity of the signal is converted to a d-c signal. The d-c output is balanced against a reference d-c voltage. Differences in these two voltages reflect known amounts of variation in the signal being measured. This is achieved by coupling the difference voltage through a feedback circuit to an electromechanical recording element. Circuits are available to have the indication reflect logarithmic or linear measurements. Examples of sound-level recorders found in laboratories include the Bruel and Kjaer level recorder type 2305 and the General Radio graphic level recorder type 1521-B. Both of these instruments and similar instruments provided by other manufacturers record signal levels as a function of time with considerable accuracy. Insofar as speech-intensity level is one of the basic voice variables, the sound-level recorder has high priority among instruments required in a well-equipped speech laboratory. The amplitude display unit of the Kay Sona-Graph, discussed in more detail in a subsequent section, also can be used to provide a graphic level record of level versus time for speech signals.

The oscilloscope, probably the most versatile instrument for speech and hearing applications, is an X-Y device that portrays one signal versus another signal. Usually the X-axis on the oscilloscope represents time and the Y-axis, amplitude. Whereas other X-Y instruments write with a mechanical stylus, the the stylus is the oscilloscope is a luminous spot that moves from left to right across the face of a cathode-ray tube. Oscilloscopes offer many possibilities for applications in speech and hearing. Extremely accurate time measurements can be made by examining the duration of a signal on the X-axis and, in a similar manner, levels can be determined from the voltages shown on the Y-axis. The waveform information is also of extreme importance. Shown in Fig. 5-18

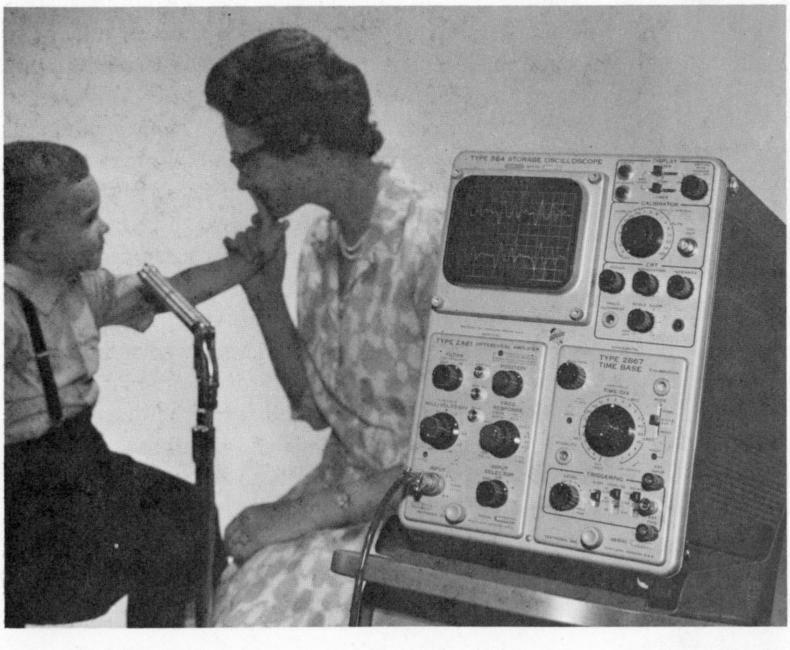

Fig. 5-18. Storage oscilloscope (Tektronix Type 564). *Photo courtesy Tektronix, Inc.*

is a Tektronix type 564 storage oscilloscope where a standard signal can be stored for over an hour for comparison to an incoming sound. The storage aspects of oscilloscopes suggest clinical applications in the field of speech and hearing. Dual-beam oscilloscopes are useful for monitoring simultaneous signals, a situation that frequently occurs in both research and clinical procedures. Many investigators and clinicians prefer to monitor oscilloscopic tracings during either investigations or diagnostic procedures.

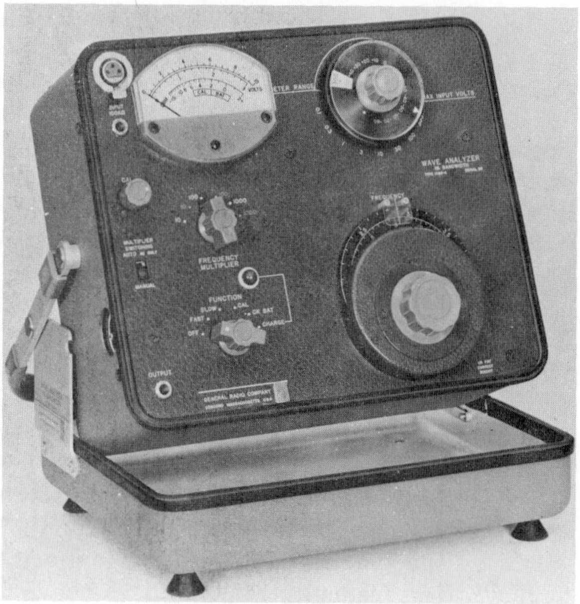

Fig. 5-20. Wave analyzer (General Radio Type 1568-A).

Spectrum and Wave Analyzers

Graphic and sound-level meters provide information about the level of a sound but do not provide knowledge about the waveform. Oscilloscopes do show waveform, and the display on the cathode-ray tube can be photographed to provide a permanent record.

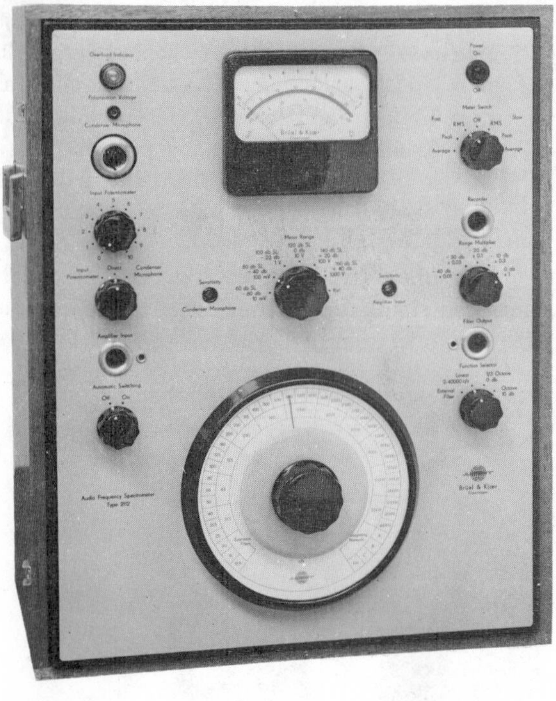

Fig. 5-19. Audio frequency spectrometer (Bruel and Kjaer Type 2112).

Another measure of importance with respect to complex sounds is the distribution of energy over the frequency spectrum. For speech and hearing it is usually the human audio spectrum that is of interest, and this measure of energy is called a spectrum analysis. Spectrum or wave analyzers consist of a set of filters and a precision voltmeter that indicates the energy within a specified frequency bandwidth. In the case where steady-state sound signals are to be analyzed, a number of commercial instruments are available. The Bruel and Kjaer type 2112 audio-frequency spectrometer (Fig. 5-19) is able to perform analyses in the frequency range from 22 to 45,000 Hz for either one-third octave or octave analyses. In conjunction with the Bruel and Kjaer level recorder type 2305, automatic recording of spectrograms for complex signals can be completed. Two other instruments for frequency analyses are the General Radio wave analyzer type 1568-A and the General Radio sound and vibration analyzer type 1564-A, shown in Figs. 5-20 and 5-21, respectively. The wave analyzer covers a frequency range from 20 Hz to 20 kHz with a bandwidth of one percent of the selected frequency. This instrument in conjunction with the General Radio type 1521 graphic level recorder can provide automatic and continuous spectrum plotting. The sound and vibration analyzer type 1564-A has a similar frequency range, from 2.5 Hz to 25 kHz, with bandwidths of either one-third or one-tenth octave. This system is also available with the drive mechanisms to provide automatic and continuous spectrum analysis. For speech signals to depict their ongoing characteristics, patterns of acoustic change in time, the spectrum and wave analyzers are not capable of meaningfully portraying these kinds of events, because they treat spectrum and amplitude and not

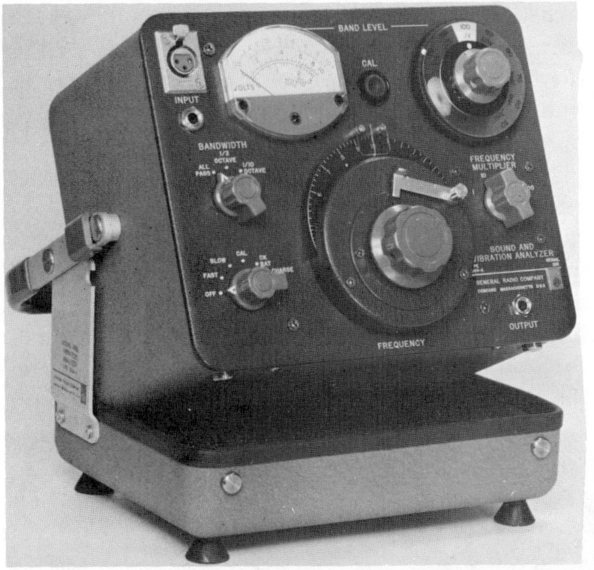

Fig. 5-21. Sound and vibration analyzer (General Radio Type 1564-A).

time. Spectral analyses of ongoing speech need to include time as well as spectral energies. Vocoders and similar devices provide this kind of analysis; these instruments are discussed in a subsequent section.

In the previous discussion, it can be observed that filters were an integral part of instrumentation for analysis. Both acoustic and electronic filters are relevant to many aspects of speech and hearing. For speech production, the speech wave has been described as the response of the vocal tract filter systems to one or more sound sources (Fant, 1960), and electronic filter analogs have been employed to depict the vocal tract (Stevens and House, 1955). Filters employ coils, capacitors, and resistors in various combinations and values to provide the desired characteristics. Filters are designated as low-pass if they pass signals of a frequency lower than the cutoff frequency, and are called high-pass if they pass signals higher than the cutoff frequency. Band-pass filters are defined by the frequencies between the high-pass cutoff and the low-pass cutoff points. A band-pass filter set, Bruel and Kjaer type 1612, is shown in Fig. 5-22 along with a special-purpose filter, the spectrum shaper model 123. Filters can also be classified as either active or passive. When an amplifier is part of the filter circuit and the response is dependent upon the gain of the amplifier, it is referred to as an active filter. Passive filters do not include an amplifier as a part of their circuit and are dependent upon resistors, inductors, and capacitors for their performance. Although the ideal filter is assumed to pass frequencies within the desired range and to have no response beyond the limits of this range, for actual filters, frequencies beyond the range are attenuated rather than eliminated. The frequency response characteristics for a particular instrument indicate how much attenuation is accomplished by the filter.

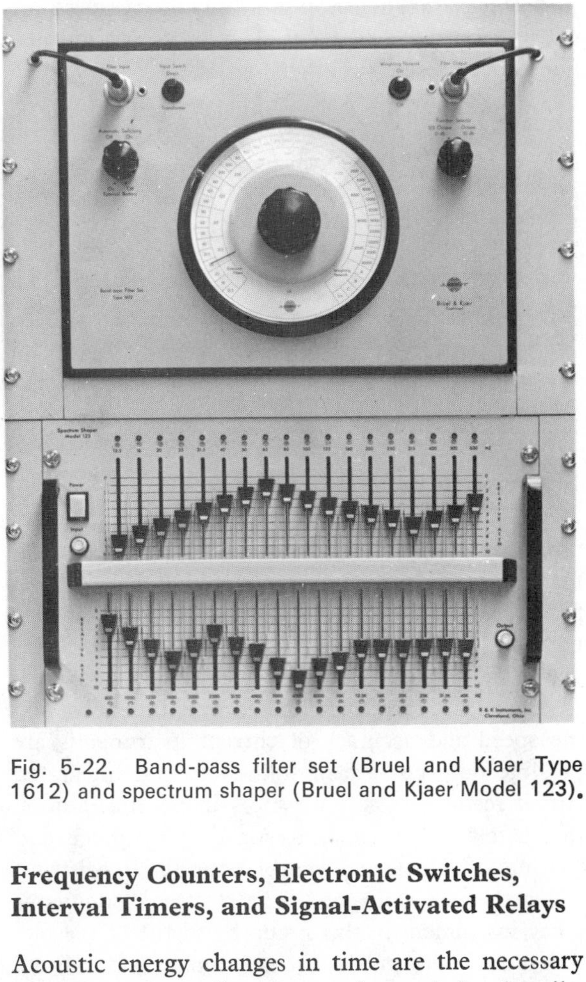

Fig. 5-22. Band-pass filter set (Bruel and Kjaer Type 1612) and spectrum shaper (Bruel and Kjaer Model 123).

Frequency Counters, Electronic Switches, Interval Timers, and Signal-Activated Relays

Acoustic energy changes in time are the necessary ingredients for auditory perception and also describe speech. The measurements of these changes are crucial to the understanding of both speech and hearing phenomena. The time required for the integration of energy for either loudness or pitch perception, the duration of a speech clue required for identification by a listener, and the amount of time required between events for reliable judgments of order are examples of problems that, in part, are dependent upon accurate time measurements of speech and other signals. Liberman (1957) summarized the importance of formant transitions on the perception of consonants, and Lisker (1957) found that durations of silence within a word determined the medial consonant heard. That time is an important dimension in the perception of temporal order has been well demonstrated by Hirsh (1959) and Hirsh and Sherrick (1961). Although some of the instruments previously discussed, including graphic and sound-level recorders, can be used to indicate such things as phonation time, these measures are not sufficiently detailed to provide necessary information about speech and other signals.

A group of instruments that deal specifically with time measurements and the control of temporal parameters of sound are electronic counters, switches, timers, and signal-activated devices. Precision temporal measures and control of sounds were difficult before the advent of the vacuum tube. Vacuum tube circuitry itself inherently limited time functions, and the speed and accuracy of current instruments are possible only because of solid-state and integrated circuit features. These advances in instrumentation fortunately will permit investigators in speech and hearing to evaluate and control better the signals with which they are concerned. The electronic counter is a key instrument in this group by virtue of the fact that it can count pulses, average signals, and indicate durations as well as other functions. The General Radio type 1191 frequency counter and the Hewlett-Packard model 5245L electronic counter are examples of instruments that perform such functions as measuring frequency, period, period average, frequency ratio, and time interval. An electronic counter, in conjunction with other instruments, can provide a number of accurate measures that deal with temporal parameters of speech and hearing. These include response-time values, phonation time, durations of signals and intervals between signals, calibration of stimuli, and the summation of responses as well as the reduction and display of other data that can be transformed into an appropriate form to be processed by a counter.

An electronic switch is another instrument that has many speech and hearing applications. Fig. 5-23 shows the Grason-Stadler model 829C. This instrument turns signals on and off at specified rise and decay times and, when used in conjunction with an interval timer, can provide variable on and off times that can by synchronized with a particular point on the waveform of a recurring stimulus. The timer, switch, and counter offer many possibilities for temporal control and measurement of signals. For example, when used with a voice-operated relay, temporal patterns of speech can be extracted or phonation times obtained.

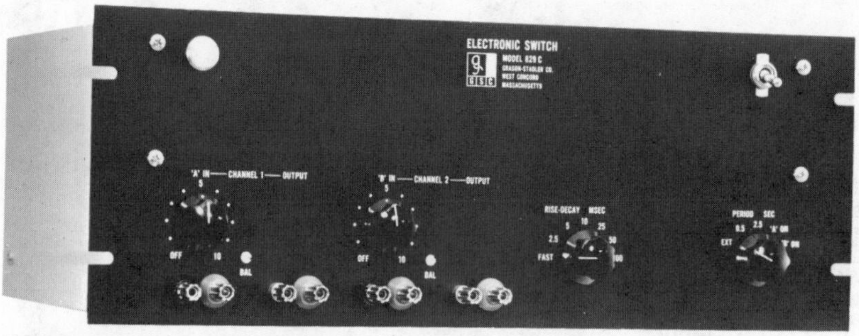

Fig. 5-23. Electronic switch (Grason-Stadler Model 829C).

INSTITUTE OF LARYNGOLOGY

We have chosen to exemplify laboratories having a primary focus on physiological aspects of voice production with the Laryngeal Research Laboratory of the Institute of Laryngology and Voice Disorders. This Laboratory is located in a medical office building on Wilshire Boulevard in the Westwood district of Los Angeles. The Institute in its present and previous locations, the Medical Center of UCLA and an office building on the near north side of Chicago, has produced significant research contributions and teaching materials in the form of films and models of laryngeal phenomena, as well as related subjects. Many noteworthy scientists, mentioned in this chapter and elsewhere in the present work, are, or at one time have been, associated with the work of this laboratory.

The floor plan of the Institute (Fig. 5-24) is an

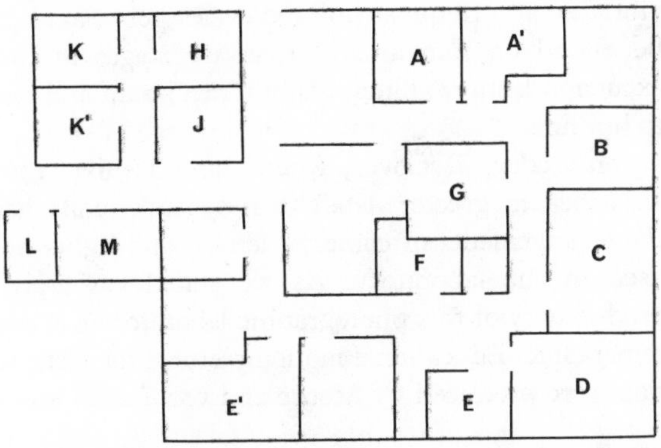

Fig. 5-24. Floor plan, Institute of Laryngology. See text for legend.

efficient arrangement serving the dual functions of clinical service to the patients and the research interests of the staff. A subject, whether clinical or normal, enters the waiting room (top center in the plan), is met by the receptionist, and taken by appointment to one of the examining rooms, A and A^1. The convenient location of the central office, below the waiting room, affording easy access to all other areas, is to be noted. The examining rooms contain standard equipment and medical supplies such as are normally found in a laryngologist's office. Many of the smaller instruments are shelved in the nearby supply room, G, where routine sterilization of them is performed in an autoclave. Fig. 5-25 depicts a few

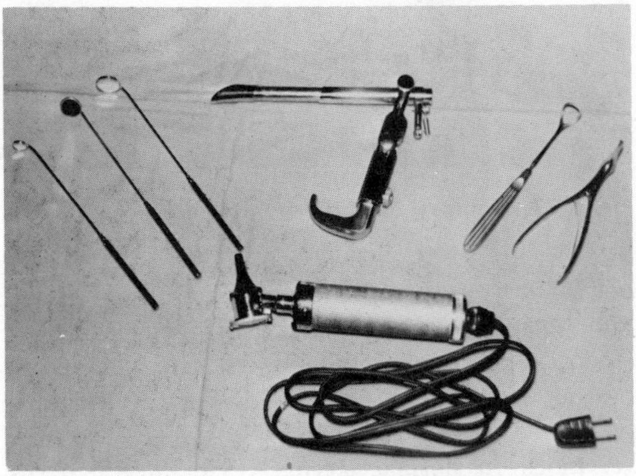

Fig. 5-25. Instruments for laryngeal, oral, nasal, and aural examinations.

of these instruments. Viewed from left to right across the top row, they are: a small mirror for indirect examination of the nasopharynx, a slightly larger mirror for indirect examination of a child's larynx, and a still larger mirror for an adult larynx. An external light source is directed by these mirrors onto the area under observation and the image is reflected outward to the eye of the examiner. Top row center is an instrument used for direct laryngoscopy, with its own internal light source. Next, to the right, is a metal tongue depressor whose curved surfaces facilitate manipulation of the tongue, affording the laryngologist a better field of view. On the extreme right is a nasal speculum, the function of which is to spread the nostrils for viewing of the anterior nasal passages. Centered below is an otoscope, containing a light source and magnifying lens for examination of the external auditory canal and tympanic membrane.

The chamber labeled B on the floor plan is the second stage in the laryngeal examination. Here vocal fold function can be observed with the aid of an Electronic Synchron-Stroboscope (Timcke), developed originally for use in the Institute. Described in detail by von Leden (1961), this strobolaryngoscope makes possible the focusing of a pulsating beam of light from a Xenon lamp upon a laryngeal mirror, whence it is reflected onto the vocal cords. The frequency of pulsations of the lamp corresponds exactly to the fundamental frequency of cord vibration, accomplished by means of a contact microphone placed at the larynx and connected to a frequency-analyzing electronic circuit the output of which controls the power supply to the lamp. Accessory controls permit the examiner to modify the phase angle of the light flashes in relation to the input source. Thus the cords may be "stopped" at any position in their cycle, or their image may be viewed in slow motion. The advantage to the clinician or researcher of being able to observe an action, one complete cycle of vocal cord vibration, that normally may be completed in 1/100 or 1/500 second, slowed down to once per second or even slower, is obvious. If normal laryngeal vibratory patterns are revealed by stroboscopic examination, motion picture photography of clinical patients is not performed.

Prior to the examination described above, the subject is interviewed in the Director's office, C on the floor plan. A detailed medical history is taken and the subject is informed about later stages in the data collection process.

Although located at the corner of the laboratory, the chamber labeled D on the chart is, in the minds of many, the heart of the Institute. Here are mounted the motion picture cameras that have photographed hundreds of larynges and provided objective data about normal and pathological vocal function of great clinical and research significance. Figs. 5-26 and 5-27 show one of the two photo units housed in room D. In the first, representing the equipment without subject or operators, the light source (top), camera housing, and viewing element are seen above subject's and operator's seats to left and right, respectively. A magnasync magnetic-film recorder for correlation of tone with photograph is seen in the background. Fig. 5-27 demonstrates the photo unit in use. One examiner, standing left, controls the camera focus and advises the second, seated right, as to placement of the laryngeal mirror in the oropharynx of the subject, center, obscured from view by the camera housing. These pictures depict the normal speed photo unit on which most of the color photography of the Institute is performed. The second, similar unit, not shown, contains the high-speed Fastax camera that permits exposure of black and white film up to 4,000 frames per second. Photography at or near this speed and subsequent projection at the normal rate accomplishes slow motion by a factor of 250 : 1. Vocal cords vibrating at a frequency of 200 cycles per second can be placed on film at 20 successive stages in their excursion from midline to lateral maximum and back to midline.

von Leden, LeCover, Ringel, and Isshiki (1966) described in greater detail than space permits here the arrangements of cameras, lenses, and lights now used in the laboratory. As we stated earlier, the productivity of this photographic laboratory has been remarkable. Educational motion pictures for distribution were produced by Moore and von Leden on the normal larynx (1956), the physiology of the larynx under daily stress (1958), and the pathological larynx (1960). Hollien and Moore (1960) have reported on measurements of the vocal folds during changes in pitch, and Moore and von Leden (1958) described variations in normal laryngeal vibratory patterns, while von Leden and Moore (1961) reported similar data for unilateral laryngeal paralysis. Even the mechanism of the cough has been explored by von Leden and Isshiki (1965). In a recent investigation reported from the laboratory, von Leden, Yanagihara, and Werner-Kukuk (1967) described the use and

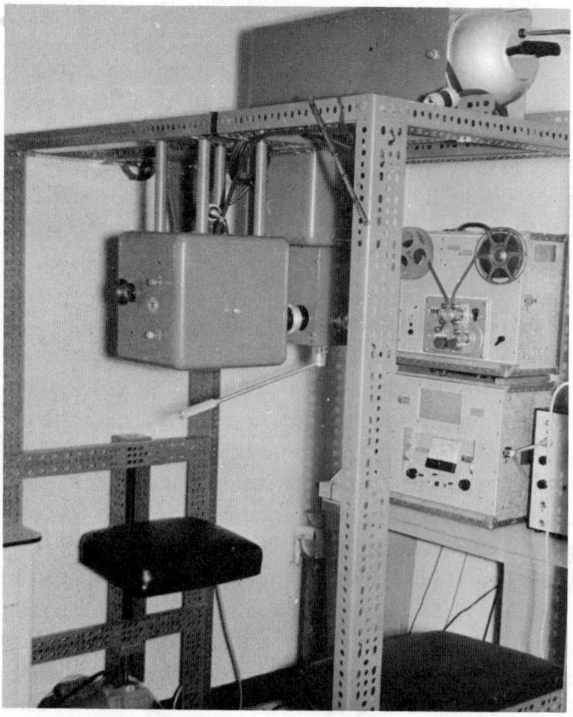

Fig. 5-26. Laryngoscopic photo unit.

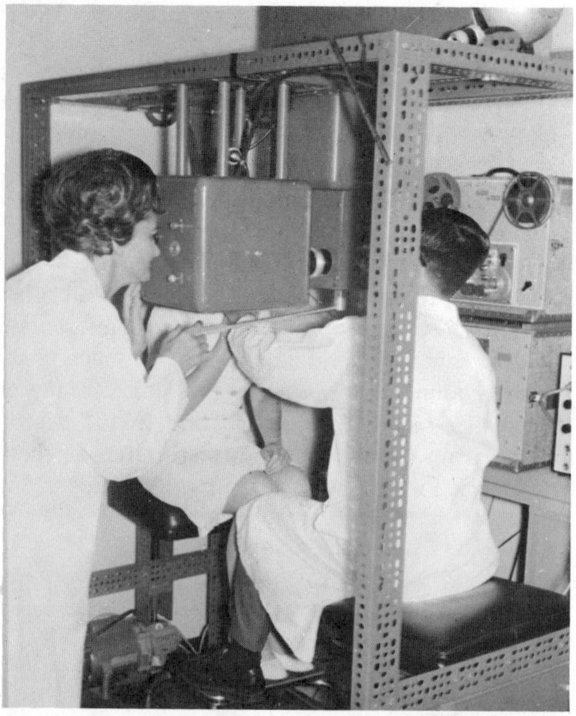

Fig. 5-27. Laryngeal motion picture photography.

effect of teflon injections in unilateral vocal cord paralysis, a study in which the photographic technique was used in assessment of the results of this procedure. Similar use was made of the technique in a study of effects of radium therapy on laryngeal physiology (Werner-Kukuk, von Leden, and Yanagihara, 1968).

Adjacent to the motion picture area, in room E, is the darkroom, suitably equipped for such developing and enlarging as required for reports by the laboratory. The high-speed and color movies are developed commercially. Across the corridor, in room F, is the electronic shop, with the standard test and calibration instruments and a useful array of small tools. On either side of the shop and in several other locations on the floor plan are unmarked rooms. These are offices, storage spaces, and rest rooms.

Room E[1] is a library-seminar room, much used in staff conferences for the design and interpretation of research and for informal seminars with visiting scientists.

Returning to the top of the plan, room H is the aerodynamic laboratory. On the right of the entry is a recording spirometer, shown in Fig. 5-28, a type of gasometer used for measuring and recording certain aspects of breathing. The device consists of a metal tank containing a movable piston with a water seal, input line for air, exhaust valve for resetting, ink stylus, and revolving cylinder on which is mounted chart paper calibrated in cubic centimeters. As the subject breathes into the mouthpiece, air replaces water in the inner piston which then rises by an amount proportional to the exhaled air. When a subject is given appropriate instructions, certain breathing functions associated with speech production can be measured that include vital capacity and tidal, supplemental, and complemental air. *Vital capacity* is the total volume of air which the individual can expel from his lungs after they have been filled to the greatest extent possible. *Tidal air* is the quantity of air which is inhaled or exhaled in normal relaxed breathing. *Supplemental air* is the quantity of

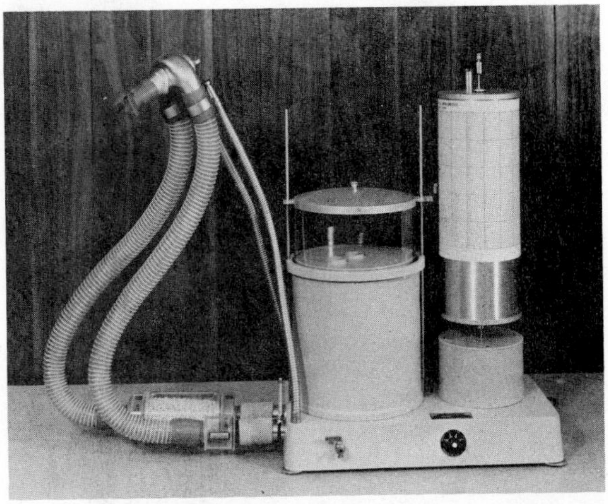

Fig. 5-28. Respirometer. *Photo courtesy Collins, Inc.*

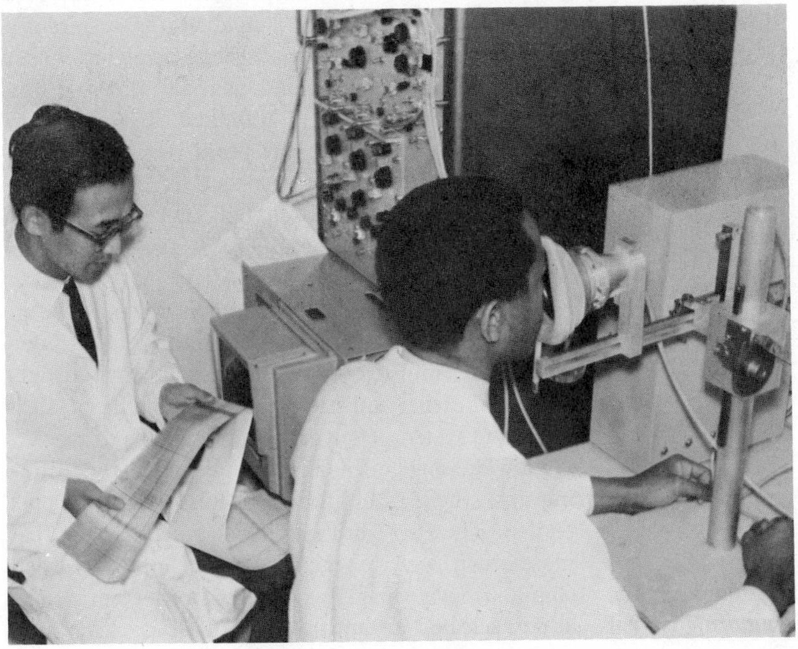

Fig. 5-29. Air flow measurement.

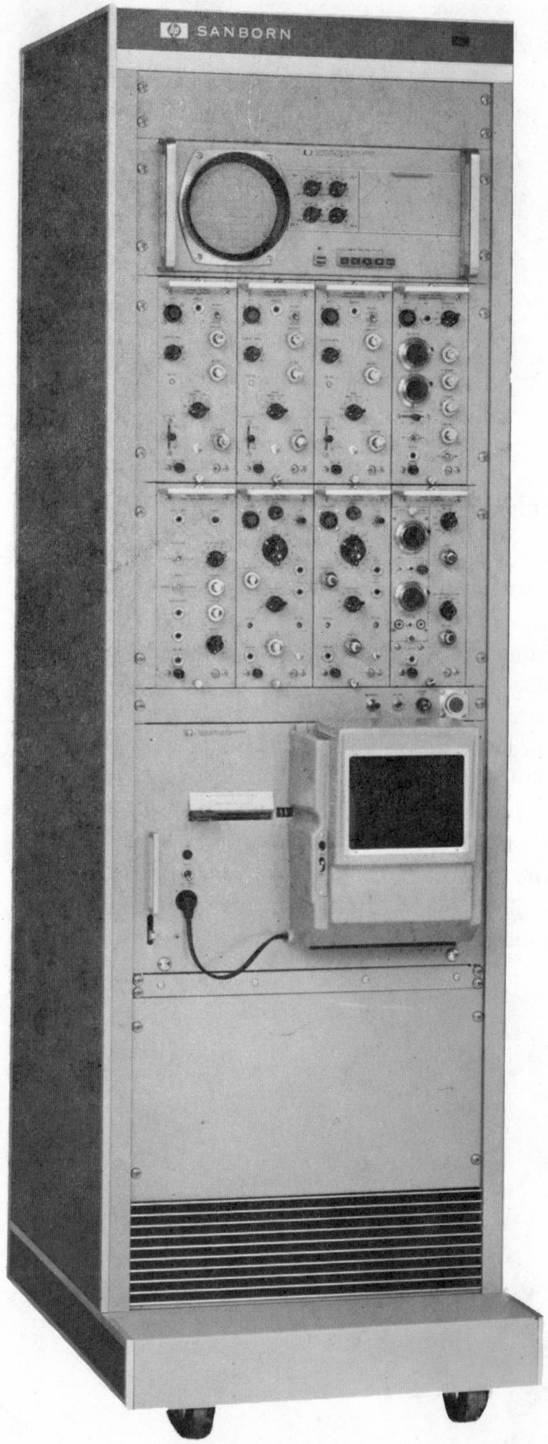

Fig. 5-30. Poly-beam oscillographic recording device. *Photo courtesy Hewlett-Packard.*

air which can be expelled from the lungs after the tidal air has been expelled. *Complemental air* is that quantity of air which can still be inhaled after the peak of a normal relaxed inhalation.

The respirometer illustrated in Fig. 5-28 is commonly referred to as a wet spirometer. Another device, used for the same measurement, is a dry spirometer, a miniature anemometer contained within a bakelite case. The volume of air exhaled, causing the vanes of the device to rotate, is registered by a needle on a calibrated dial. While much less cumbersome and space-consuming than the wet spirometer, the dry model appears to be less reliable and more dependent upon the force with which the breath is exhaled.

Across the room from the respirometer is the instrument complex developed in the Institute for its data collection of aerodynamic phenomena associated with phonation, shown in Fig. 5-29. On the right side of the photograph is the heart of the system, a pneumotachograph. In the assembly are a respiratory mask, a laminar flow resistor (pneumotach screen), and bidirectional, differential gas-pressure transducer (Sanborn 270). The output of this unit is recorded on the poly-beam recorder described below. In use, the subject places his face against the cushioned surfaces of the mask and performs as specified by the experimenter: breathing normally or maximally, phonating a vowel with specified inflections or rise-fall intensity characteristics, reading a phrase or longer syntactic unit, coughing, etc. The flow of air through the screen is converted to electrical current, amplified, and recorded. Derived measurements are air flow rate and volume. On the stand holding the respiratory mask also is mounted a condenser microphone, which serves to pick up the audio signal and direct it to a tape recorder from which, amplified, it is carried to another channel of the poly-beam recorder. Sometimes a second microphone-tape recorder unit is added to the system, this microphone being placed in surface contact with the subject at the level of the larynx.

On the left of the photograph is the poly-beam oscillographic recording device, similar to the one reproduced in Fig. 5-30. This instrument, an outgrowth of earlier and still commonly used mechanical recording systems (polygraphs), is capable of recording a wide range of biophysical phenomena, depending upon the preamplifier and accessory instruments chosen. The versatility of the instrument is such that more than one phenomenon may be recorded simultaneously, making possible direct comparisons at any selected instant in time. In either system the amount of movement (in the case of measurements having to do with, for example, changes in the diameter of thoracic or abdominal walls) or the amount of air flow (in aerodynamic studies) or electrical conductivity (in the galvanic skin response) is reflected proportionally by movements of a recording stylus or deflections of a light beam on suitable recording paper driven at a constant speed past the stylus or beam. Another variation of the device, the Oscillomink (Fig. 5-31), makes use of an extremely fine jet of pressure-driven ink, its deflections proportional to the strength of the input signal, on the recording chart paper. As suggested earlier, all of these devices normally have provision for the simultaneous recording of two, four, eight, or even more concurrent events.

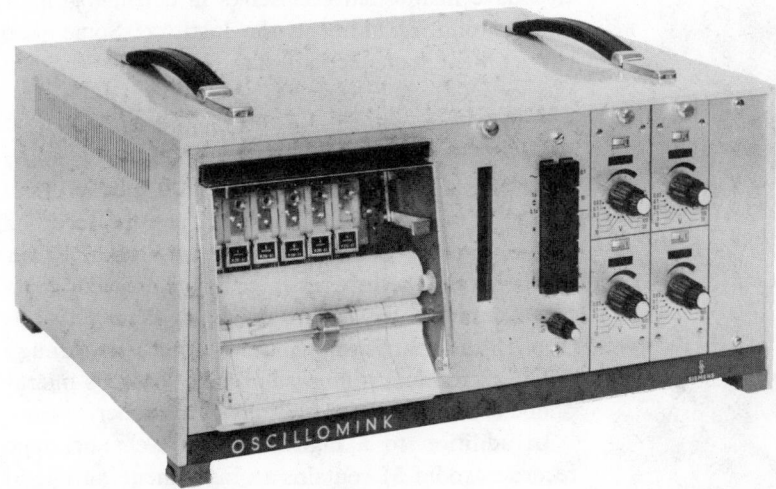

Fig. 5-31. Ink-stream recording device. *Photo courtesy Siemens America.*

One of the accessories frequently used with recorders of the type just described is a pneumograph, conventionally consisting of a helical spring and rubber tube attached to end plates. Straps or chains from the end plates permit the pneumograph to be held taut around the chest or abdomen. A second, smaller rubber tube leads from one of the end plates to the polygraph, thus completing an airtight system. When the pneumograph is stretched by expansion of the area which it encircles, a partial vacuum is created. This vacuum is communicated by means of the recording tambour to the recording instrument. More recent variations of the pneumograph substitute electrical and photoelectric systems for the air-pressure system described above.

A wide variety of studies has been reported from the Institute in which the aerodynamic assembly alone, or in combination with other measuring and recording devices, was used. Yanagihara, Koike, and von Leden (1966) sought to discover relationships between phonation volume (total volume available for maximally sustained phonation) and vital capacity, and between phonation volume and maximum duration of phonation. Yanagihara, von Leden, and Werner-Kukuk (1966) presented results of an investigation of physical parameters of the cough, in which air flow rate, air volume, subglottic pressure, and the acoustic signal were concurrently recorded and later compared. Snidecor and Isshiki (1965) examined air flow and acoustic data for a superior esophageal speaker. A cross-comparison of aerodynamic, acoustic, and electromyographic data was used by Yanagihara and von Leden (1966) in an examination of the role of the cricothyroid muscle during phonation. Interactions among air flow rate, air volume, duration of phonation, vocal intensity, and fundamental vocal frequency were reported by Yanagihara and Koike (1967). This list is representative of the articles published, but not a complete listing of them.

Adjacent to the aerodynamic laboratory, in room J, the instrumentation used for electromyography (EMG) is concentrated. Facing the door, along the back wall, is a standard physician's examining table, necessary because, in studies requiring the recording of the minute electrical discharges of discrete muscles, relaxation of the subject is essential. On the left wall is a console model tape recorder and on the right wall a Meditron Multi-Channel Electromyographic Recorder, Research Model P-1. A second, portable tape recorder is placed next to the EMG unit. Linked to the EMG recorder is a two-channel oscilloscope, the Memo-Scope (Fig. 5-32), an attractive feature of which is the ability of the operator to lock on to the oscilloscope screen any desired transient phenomenon, such as the waveform of a muscle discharge, for detailed examination. The dual-channel feature also is useful, enabling the experimenter to view two phenomena simultaneously.

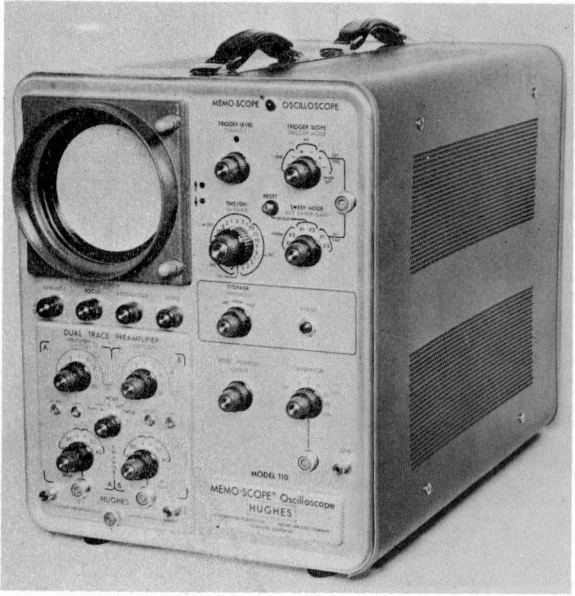

Fig. 5-32. Memo-Scope (Hughes Model 110).

Great flexibility and another research dimension are added to the Institute's research and clinical potential by this room and its equipment. In a previously mentioned article, for example, Yanagihara and von Leden (1966) used EMG recordings in association with other instrumentation to demonstrate a close correlation between electrical activity in the cricothyroid muscle and glottal resistance. Another close correlation was revealed between electrical activity and pitch rise, pointing to the role of the cricothyroid muscle in varying the tension of the vocal cords. Similar findings were reported by Faaborg-Andersen, Yanagihara, and von Leden (1967), whereas the relation between cricothyroid activity and vocal intensity appeared to be more complex, an interaction with air flow rate accounting for inconsistencies in the data.

The chief feature of room K, the photo editing room, is a custom-made bench and tracing table. On the underside of the bench, motion picture film is threaded into a Photo-Optical Data Analyzer (L. W. Photo, Inc., model 224A), a reconstructed Kodak Analyst projector. The film image is reflected onto a mirror and thence upward onto a ruled translucent grid, set into the bench. Use of this arrangement affords a 12 : 1 magnification of structures in the film. The projector will advance or reverse the film on a frame-by-frame basis, at slow or normal speed. Room K also is used for film storage.

Room K^1 is used for the display of models constructed to reveal certain physiological relationships that have manifested themselves in cinematographic and anatomical studies in the Institute. Some 5000 slides of histologic sections of the larynx also are filed in room K.

A two-room suite, L and M, completes the Institute of Laryngology. The smaller of the two rooms is a sound-isolated chamber (Industrial Acoustics Corp. Model 401-A), in which a subject may be recorded with no ambient noise to compete with vocal signals on the tape. The experimenter in the adjacent room may communicate with the subject by manual signals through the connecting window, or verbally through an intercommunication system. The subject's microphone is suspended in the isolation chamber.

In addition to a high-fidelity two-channel tape recorder, room M contains an instrument console in which are rack-mounted a variable filter (Krohn-Hite Model 315AR), an electronic counter (Hewlett-Packard 5223L), a speech-time analyzer (Grason-Stadler E4446A), a sine-random generator (Bruel and Kjaer 1024, Fig. 5-33), and paired speakers. This instrument array makes possible application of a variety of auditory stimuli to the subject in room L, or analyses of vocal signals from that chamber. For example, the output of the sine-random generator, at the experimenter's choice, is a pure tone at any frequency within the auditory range, or narrow- or wide-band random noise. The incoming signal may be shaped by filtering out low- or high-frequency components on the variable filter, or certain relationships in the time domain may be explored with the speech-time analyzer, which accumulates on one counter time segments when the signal strength exceeds a preset level and on another counter segments when there is silence or signals below the preset level. Vocal signals appropriately filtered through the variable filter may be assessed for fundamental frequency level on the electronic counter. Either incoming or output signals may be monitored with the loudspeakers.

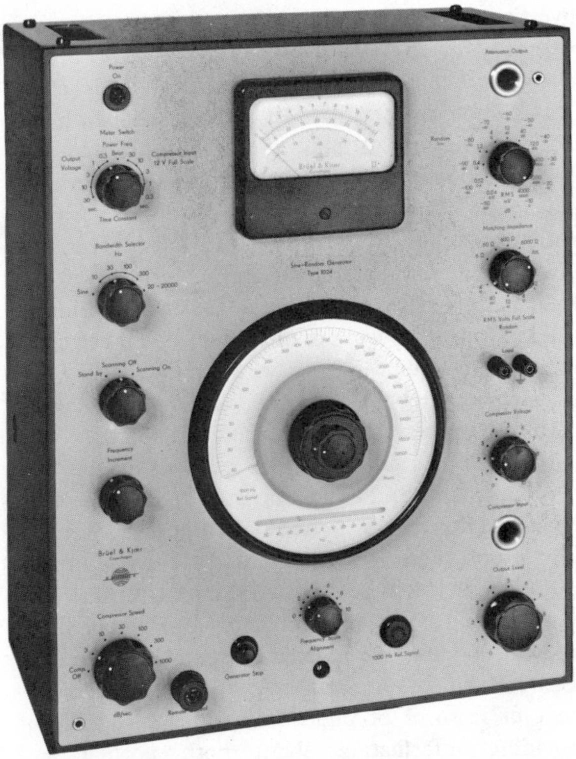

Fig. 5-33. Sine-random generator. *Photo courtesy Bruel and Kjaer Instruments, Inc.*

Beneath the viewing window in room M is a standard audiometer and adjacent to it a sound-spectrum analyzer (Sona-Graph 6061-A, Fig. 5-34), to be described in greater detail in a later section.

Finally, on the near wall is a combination spectrum analyzer and power-level recorder (Bruel and Kjaer model 2112 and 2305, respectively). A more recent version of this combination, the model 3329, is shown in Fig. 5-35. A later model of the same instrument, 3335, consisting of sine and narrow-band random-noise generator, spectrometer, and graphic level recorder, is similar in appearance to the model illustrated here. Acoustic energy (sound-pressure level) within narrow frequency bands or in the whole signal may be analyzed and recorded on this device, either from a live source or a prerecorded tape. The strength of the signal in decibels above a selected level is traced on the chart paper by a moving stylus. An advantage of the level recorder, and of the Sona-Graph as well, is that the record is linear on the horizontal axis with respect to time. Hence, the exact duration of identifiable speech units—paragraphs, phrases, even phonemes—may be determined.

Acoustic analyses of normal and pathological voices are performed as standard procedures in the Institute and are reported in research articles written by staff members and visiting scientists. In the Snidecor-Isshiki (1965) analysis of vocal characteristics of an esophageal speaker, for example, pitch (fundamental vocal frequency) was measured on the Sona-Graph, the sound-pressure level on the level recorder, and a ratio of phonated to total speaking time was derived from the speech-time analyzer. Similar analyses were performed in the Yanagihara, Koike, and von Leden (1966) analysis of phonation and respiration in normal subjects. Vennard and von Leden (1967) used the Sona-Graph to examine characteristics of the vocal trill in arias sung by four outstanding sopranos. Isshiki (1965) investigated relations between air flow rate and vocal intensity in one study, and flow rate, subglottic pressure, glottal resistance, and intensity in another (1964), making use of the instrumentation described above.

The reader will recognize, in this and other descriptions of speech laboratories, that selectivity with respect to instrumentation and published research has been necessary. Despite the exclusion of significant detail, the writers are hopeful that a sense of the variety in instrumentation and flexibility of research approach has been conveyed.

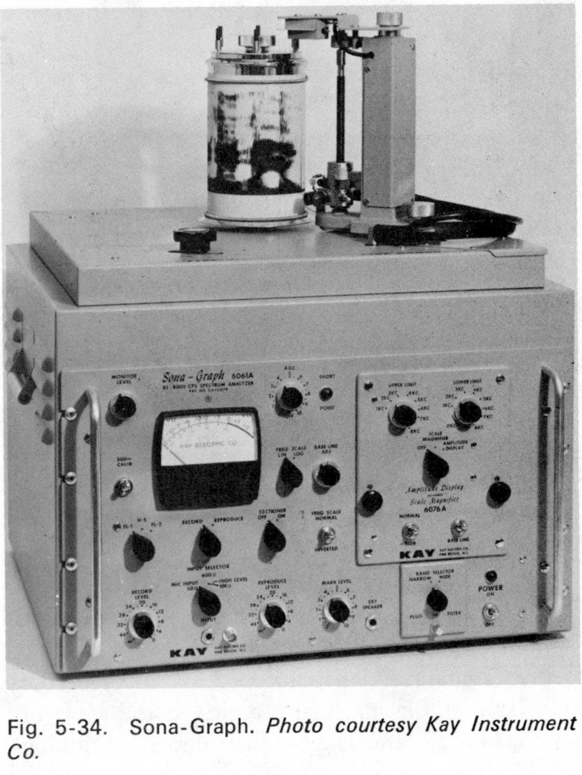

Fig. 5-34. Sona-Graph. *Photo courtesy Kay Instrument Co.*

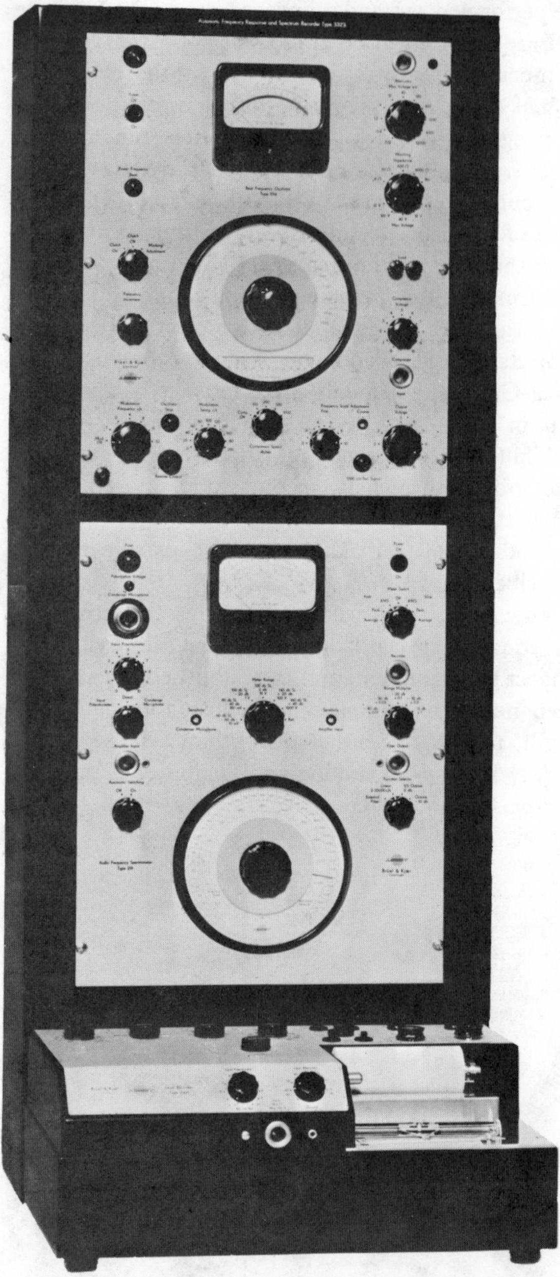

Fig. 5-35. Spectrum and power level analyzer. *Photo courtesy Bruel and Kjaer Instruments, Inc.*

COMMUNICATION SCIENCES LABORATORY

At the Communication Sciences Laboratory of the University of Florida, many topics in the areas of speech, hearing, and language are under continuing investigation. As an indication of the range and versatility of the laboratory, one project concerns diver-communication research programs, an effort that amounts essentially to an underwater speech and hearing laboratory. Another project is concerned with the development of group hearing tests for children and adults. This test will be discussed later in the section on audiology. Dr. G. Paul Moore, Founding Director of the laboratory and chairman of the department of speech at the University of Florida, is well known for his work in ultra-high-speed laryngeal photography. Some of this work by Dr. Moore and his associates on both the normal and the pathological larynx was reviewed in the preceding section.

Although a sizable number of instruments and methodologies could be reported advantageously within the framework of the Communication Sciences Laboratory, there are two instruments in use at this laboratory that will be reported upon in considerable detail, because of their uniqueness and potential for studying a particular aspect of speech production. Both instruments are concerned with the measurement of features of phonation and are capable of providing information about both normal and anomalous speech functions. Dr. Harry Hollien, Director of the laboratory and professor of speech, has been largely responsible for the development of these two instruments. The first instrument to be discussed is concerned with examination of vocal fold movements by stroboscopic laminagraphy and the second with measurement of fundamental frequency of phonation.

Stroboscopic laminagraphy (STROL) is a methodology that was developed to provide a series of laminagraphic x-ray photographs that show coronal views of the vocal folds at each of several phases throughout the vibratory cycle. Each x-ray picture is a composite of several short exposures obtained from a number of vibratory cycles. This is the result of x-ray firings occurring when the folds are almost in exactly the same position. Following this procedure, photographs are obtained in several positions, usually 10, throughout the vibratory cycle. When coronal cross-sectional area and thickness measurements are desired, x-rays of the folds in their closed phase are also obtained. For studies of the vibratory action of the folds, another series of photographs is utilized. Hollien and Curtis (1960) report that although the technique of laminagraphic x-ray had been used as a medical diagnostic tool before they began their work in 1954, only Griesman (1943) had used the procedure for the study of laryngeal function. Hollien and Curtis (1960) employed this methodology to compare coronal cross-sectional dimensions and thickness of the vocal folds to the fundamental frequency of voice. From the data obtained, they concluded that individuals with low pitch exhibit larger, more massive vocal folds than do individuals with higher pitch, that as the fundamental frequency of the voice is raised, the vocal folds are reduced in cross-sectional area and become thinner, and cross-sectional dimensions of vocal folds seem to be correlated with absolute frequency level rather than with relative level. Hollien (1962), in a subsequent study, further substantiated that vocal fold thickness is an important determinant of fundamental frequency of voice.

high-voltage transformer, a pulse-forming network that converts either an experimental subject's phonating frequency or a 60 Hz signal into sharp pulses that are amplified to provide sufficient power to pulse the x-ray tube, the x-ray tube, a five-inch image intensifier tube, and a brightness indicator that is associated with the intensifier tube. Two cameras are included in the STROL system. One, a 35 mm camera, for photographing the x-ray image, the other a television camera for monitoring purposes. The voice and phase system has as its purpose the providing of an input to the pulse circuit that is connected to the x-ray tube firing network. This allows the stroboscopic mode of the STROL operation to be triggered by the subject's voice. The Technic select relay

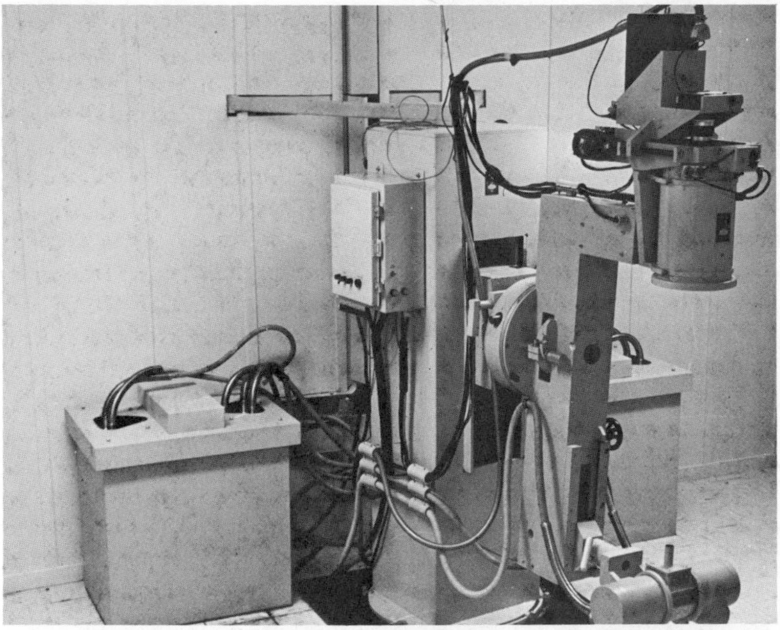

Fig. 5-36. Stroboscopic laminagraphy.

Stroboscopic laminagraphy (STROL) is shown in Fig. 5-36. This includes the laminagraphic drive, the x-ray, and the optical system of STROL. The specific components pictured are the x-ray tube, the image intensifier tube, a 35 mm camera, a television camera, a yoke drive, and a yoke stand. In Fig. 5-37 is shown the normal x-ray control console and the STROL control console. The components of STROL are shown in Fig. 5-38 in block diagram form. These components include the x-ray source, a camera system, a voice and phase shift system, a Technic select and relay control, and laminagraphic drive system. The x-ray source includes, as shown in Fig. 5-38, the power source for the x-ray tube, the

control system is the master control for all other subsystems and is the primary master control for the STROL operation. The laminagraphic drive system includes the x-ray tube yoke, stand, and associated mechanical components. The ability of the system to move on both the horizontal and vertical planes is necessary to locate the precise plane desired within the structures to be x-rayed.

In a typical operation of the STROL, a subject is first screened to determine his vocal range and whether or not he can maintain a relatively steady-state fundamental frequency for a period of from 15 to 20 seconds. If he is able to accomplish this, he is trained to monitor his vocal fundamental and sound-pressure level by the use of frequency and sound-level meters. Fluoroscopic techniques are used to place and periodically check the position of the subject's larynx. The desired laminagraph x-ray plane is determined by the adjustment of the yoke assembly of STROL, and the subject hears the experimental frequency through earphones for matching by the fundamental of his phonation. If the subject's vocalization is adequate, a stroboscopic laminagraph series is made. In Fig. 5-39 is shown a sequence of stroboscopic laminagrams for a subject phonating at a fundamental frequency of 124 Hz at a moderate loudness level. Inspection of the photographs indicates that the folds appear to be blown slightly upward as they open and appear to be thrust back to a horizontal plane as they close.

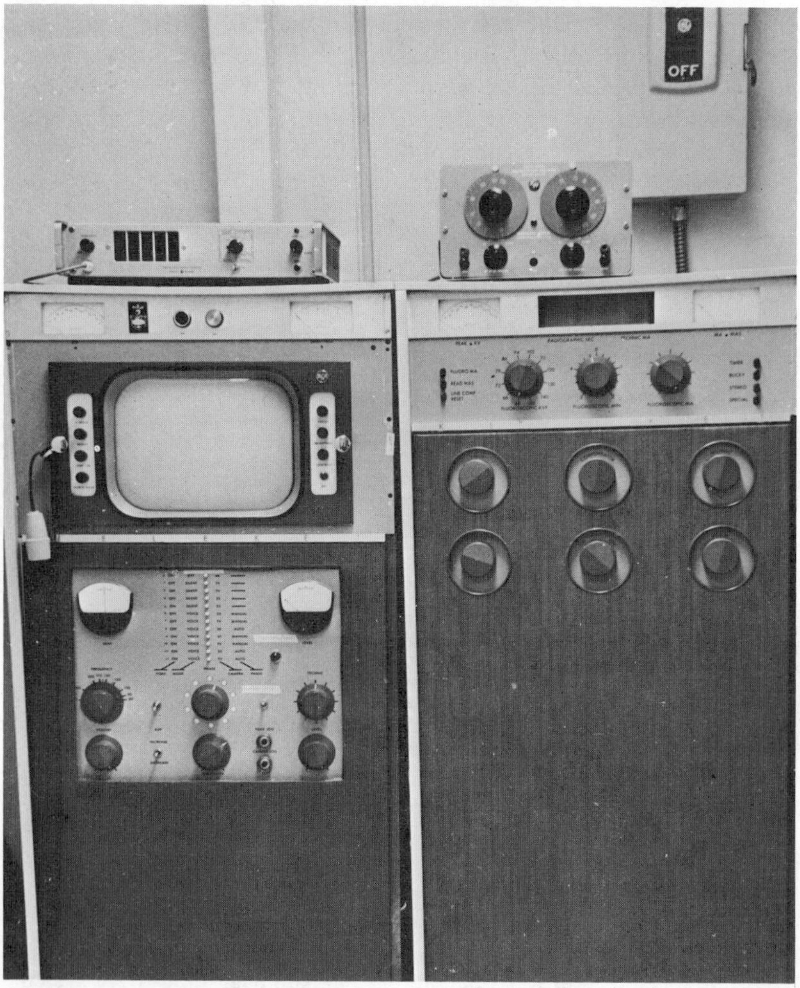

Fig. 5-37. Normal x-ray control console and STROL control console.

The stroboscopic laminagraphic methodology probably offers one of the most accurate methods available for obtaining knowledge about the dynamics of vocal fold vibration and thickness. In addition to the investigations reported, Hollien, Curtis, and Coleman (1968) are continuing studies utilizing this procedure. One of the consistent findings is that there appears to be a systematic trend for the vocal folds to decrease in thickness when increases in the fundamental frequency of phonation occur. Systematic studies treat voice register, vocal intensity, sex of the subject, as well as fundamental frequency of phonation. An excellent description of STROL, current and past studies, and projected investigations, is given in the article by Hollien, Curtis, and Coleman (1968). This article has formed the basis for much of the preceding description.

The second instrument to be described in detail in

this section, because of its considerable potential for investigations into speech phenomena, is the Fundamental Frequency Indicator (FFI), a unit developed for automatically extracting the fundamental period from complex sounds and utilized in a number of studies that have treated fundamental frequency of voice. The accurate description and measurement of fundamental frequency has been a difficult and continuing problem for speech scientists for a number of years.

Within the past 100 years a remarkable series of instruments has been developed by scientists interested in the investigation of the fundamental frequency characteristic of vocal and auditory signals. Fundamental frequency is significant, of course, because it is the component of the complex auditory stimulus which is identified by the listener as the pitch of the sound. The fundamental frequency of the human voice is determined by and is, in fact, identical with the rate of vibration of the vocal cords, measured and reported in Hz.

Two aspects of frequency have contributed to the difficulties encountered in devising instruments for its measurement. First, voice frequency and the frequencies of other stimuli within the auditory range are, compared with other physiological phenomena (respiration, pulse rate), quite high. Hence a fast-acting instrument is required to follow the signal. Second, the fundamental frequency in most acoustic signals is but one component in a complex wave. Therefore, the instrument must be capable of responding only to the fundamental, or of making a response in which the fundamental is clearly to be distinguished from the other components in the sound.

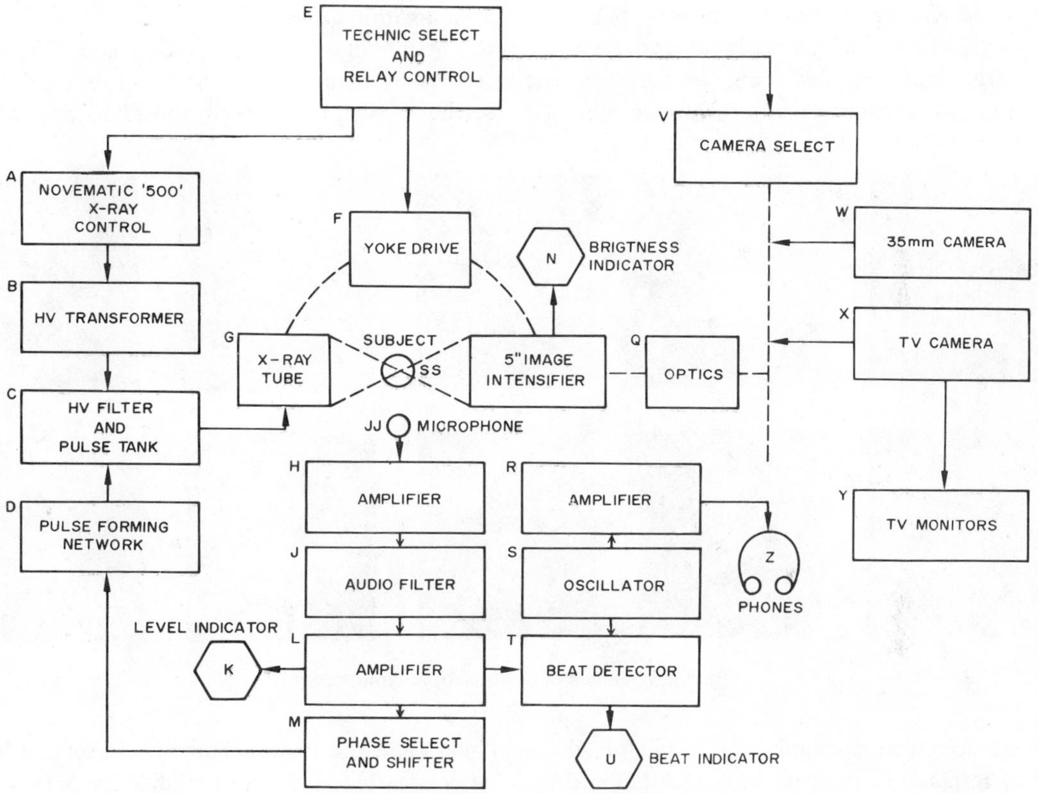

Fig. 5-38. Components of STROL.

Many ingenious devices, dating back to the mid-nineteenth century, have been designed and constructed for frequency measurement. Detailed descriptions of all of these, while of historical interest, would not contribute much to an understanding of the instruments and techniques in use today. Accordingly, brief mention of the major developments in this field of instrumentation will be made in the following paragraphs.

The earliest method of frequency analysis was achieved by comparison of the unknown frequency with a known frequency. The number of beats (rising and falling pulsations of sound) between the known and unknown frequencies was counted within a known time interval, and thus the frequency of the tone in question was determined by adding or subtracting beats per second to the known frequency.

The phonautograph was an early method utilizing the forced vibrations of a diaphragm, mechanically transmitted to recording paper, as a means of measuring frequency. The instrument was developed by Scott and Koenig in 1859 (in Miller, 1916).

Another development by Koenig was the use of the manometric flame in measuring frequency. First described in 1862 (Miller, 1916), the device consisted of a small acetylene gas flame, the height of which varied in response to pressure variations induced by successive sound waves. Major refinements of the technique utilized with the Koenig manometric-flame capsule resulted in the Phono-Projectoscope (Miller, 1937) and Tonoscope (Metfessel, 1926) of Seashore. Metfessel (1928) was successful in applying photography to an instrument which evolved from the tonoscope. He used the glow from a neon lamp, flashing with each major fluctuation in the sound wave, as the visual representation of frequency. Metfessel photographed these flashes of light as they were seen through a stroboscopic disc, containing 66 concentric rows of holes space at precise distances calculated to correspond to specific frequencies of illumination. With speed of disc rotation, number of holes per row, and speed of film movement as known variables, calculation of frequency became possible.

The early tonometer of Scheibler (1834) consisted of a series of tuning forks spread over an exact octave and ascending by equal increments of frequency from lowest to highest. Any source of sound within the range of the tonometer could be determined by counting the beats with the two forks nearest to it in pitch. In the later Koenig tonometer, there were 154 forks ranging from 16 Hz to 21,845 Hz. These forks were provided with adjustable resonators and with sliding weights so that the frequencies could be varied within certain limits.

The Oscillograph of Blondell and Dubbell, described by them in 1893 (Miller, 1916), and Sprachseiche of Scripture (1906), the Phonodeik of Miller (1909), and the Photophonophonelescope, originated by Metfessel (1926) and modified by Simon (1926), by Lewis and Tiffin (1933), and by Cowan (1936), all contributed to the design of the Vibrograph, described by Tiffin and Steer (1939).

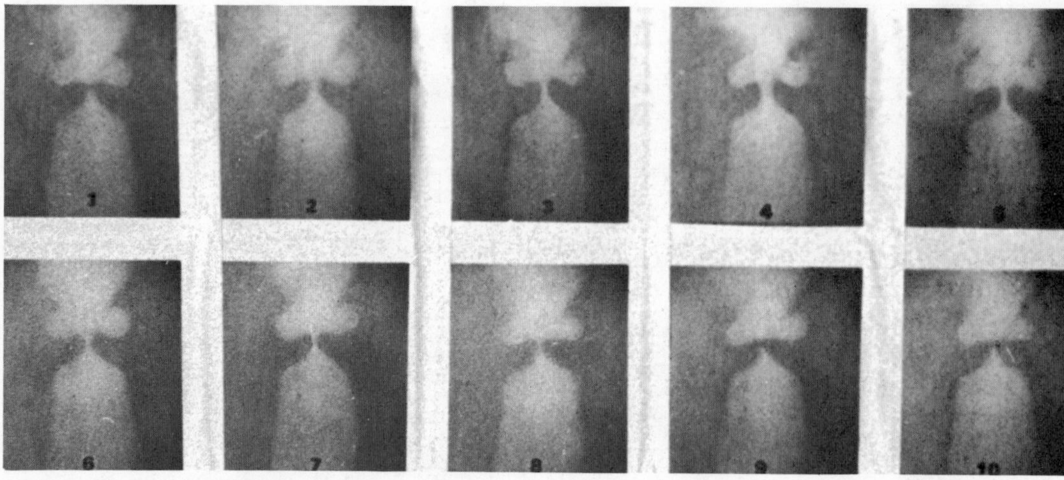

Fig. 5-39 Series of stroboscopic laminagrams.

The vibrograph or its immediate forerunner, the photophonophonelescope, consisted of a combination motor-driven phonograph turntable-film drum, phonograph recording and pick-up heads, amplifier, and a phonelescope optical system on a worm gear for controlled elevation and depression. Standard procedures for making and analyzing phonelegrams, so that pitch measurement is achieved, were described by Tiffin and Steer (1939). Subsequent modifications of the phonellegraph have been made by various investigators. For example, Hollien, Malcik, and

Hollien (1965) describe a modification of the photophoneloscope (Cowan, 1936) that was used for the study of adolescent voice changes in Southern White males. This unit was constructed on the same principles as the photophoneloscope except that it is motor driven and can be constructed from commercially available components.

An instrument capable of direct-reading fundamental-frequency analysis was first reported by Hunt (1935). Second, in point of time, was the recorder reported by Obata and Kobayashi (1937, 1938, 1940). Almost simultaneous publications were achieved by Dempsey (1949) and Gruenz and Schott (1949) with two more versions of pitch-metering devices. Later, Dempsey (1953) described changes in his original apparatus, the Purdue Pitch Meter, and still later he reported the addition of a recording unit (Dempsey, 1955). These devices have several aspects in common, most important of which is the more or less successful attempt to reject higher harmonics in complex sound waves and to meter and/or record the fundamental frequency, either on a linear or a logarithmic scale.

The Fundamental Frequency Indicator (FFI), as described by Hollien (1968), is also based on the principle of isolating the fundamental from other components of the voice signal as were the previous direct-reading fundamental-frequency recorders mentioned above. The FFI utilizes increased sophistication of electronic components, circuitry, and principles including, in addition to filters, logic circuits for isolating the fundamental. A photograph of the instrumental components of the FFI is shown in Fig. 5-40. A system block diagram is given in Fig. 5-41. The system derives the fundamental frequency essentially in the following manner. A tape-recorded sample of speech is played from one channel of a two-channel recorder through an amplifier to a bank of eight low-pass parallel filters arranged with low-frequency cutoffs in half-octave steps. These filter values insure that at least one filter will contain only the fundamental frequency and none of the harmonics of the speech wave. The logic unit passes the output of the filter with the lowest cut-off point that contains a signal in the form of a sine wave to a pulse generator. The pulse generator, in turn, produces a signal for each sine-wave output of the logic unit. These pulses

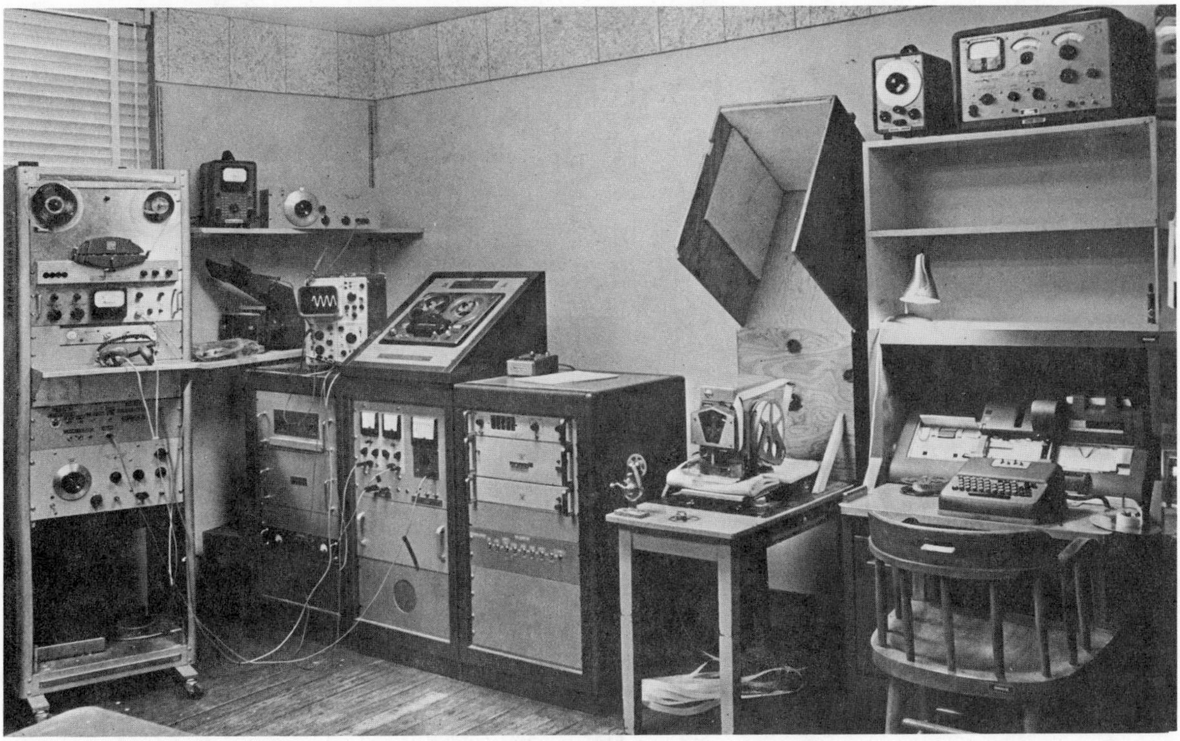

Fig. 5-40. Instrumental components of the FFI.

are recorded on the second channel of the tape recorder that contains the original speech signal. The recorded pulses represent the cycles of fundamental frequency; these pulses are played with the speed reduced by a factor of four, and the intervals between successive pulses are measured by a counter and stored. This information is recorded on punched tape, converted to punched cards, and fed to a computer that changes the information to real time and computes mean speaking fundamental frequency. The FFI also provides variability data, standard deviations in semitones, and melody patterns.

A number of investigations have been completed utilizing the FFI to measure fundamental frequency. Michel, Hollien, and Moore (1966) examined high-school-aged girls to determine the age at which adult patterns are established and concluded that females attain adult speaking fundamental frequencies by 15 years of age. Hollien and Paul (1968) provided additional data on the fundamental frequency of post-adolescent girls. Hollien and Norris (1963), in a report on pitch of adult males, assessed the performance of the FFI. The authors concluded that the fundamental can be accurately derived by this instrument in that the instrument is both reliable and valid in its measurements. For measures of validity, FFI values were compared to those obtained by phonellegraphic methods.

Among the many visitors to the Communication Sciences Laboratory who have made use of FFI in the analysis of tape-recorded speech samples have been Saxman and Burk (1967), who reported on fundamental-frequency characteristics of middle-aged females, and Hanley et al. (1966, 1967, 1968), who examined prosodic features of four different languages in a series of experiments.

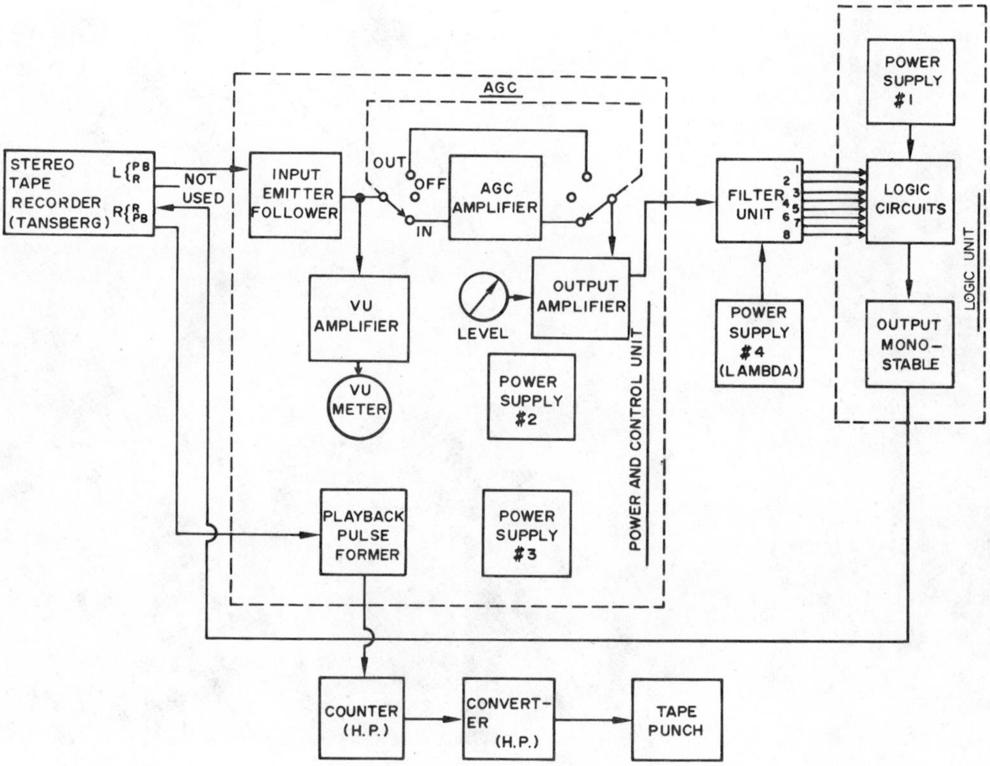

Fig. 5-41. FFI system.

Two major instruments for examining phonatory properties of speech, STROL and FFI, have been described in detail in this section to exemplify the fact that instruments for the measurement of complex phenomena can be developed in a laboratory environment where there are continuous and diligent investigations into specific aspects of speech and hearing.

SPEECH SYNTHESIS LABORATORY

Occupying the ground floor West Wing of a new classroom building on the Santa Barbara campus of the University of California, the Research Laboratory of Experimental Phonetics (Speech Synthesis Project) combines advanced instrumentation for acoustic and physiological analysis with extremely versatile instruments for electronic synthesis of human speech. The general pattern of research performed in this setting and reported in a dozen or more journals and monographs is 1) the meticulous examination of segmental and prosodic features of normal vocal utterances, 2) the reproduction of these features in speech synthesizers, and 3) the validation of the synthesized sequences by crews of trained listeners. Step 2) enables the experimenter to make controlled variations of isolated features and step 3) assesses the effects of the changes upon the ear. Characteristically, the changes introduced involve raising or lowering second- or third-formant transitions or varying the frequency of the burst or frictional noise used for consonant synthesis. Any change is accomplished by varying one cue and neutralizing the others. These variations are interpreted, essentially, as relating to *place* of articulation. In contrast, interpretation of *manner* of articulation is influenced by neutralizing frequency of noise and direction of formant transitions and varying the rate of change in the transitions. Such extreme changes have been accomplished through these techniques as movement from the class of stops, /b, d, g/, through the fricatives /v, z, ð, ʒ/, to the glides /j, w, l, r/, as interpreted by the listening crews.

In recent years emphasis has been placed upon comparisons of prosodic-phonetic features of English and continental European languages. Another comparatively recent venture has been the production of slow-motion, animated picture films with synchronously slowed-down speech produced by synthesis. These films resemble fluoroscopic pictures but permit the filmmakers to show with greater clarity the interactions of the articulators—lips, teeth, tongue, velum, etc.—in the production of normal speech.

A tour through the Speech Synthesis Laboratory starts in the general office area, A in Fig. 5-42, where the visitor is likely to be joined by the Director, Professor Pierre Delattre,* from his office, room B on the plan. Immediately above the general office in room C is a storeroom for office and technical supplies.

* The death of Professor Delattre, July 11, 1969, brought his distinguished career to a close. Professer André Malécot then assumed the directorship of the laboratory. Many of the lines of research described in this section continue under the direction of Dr. Malécot.

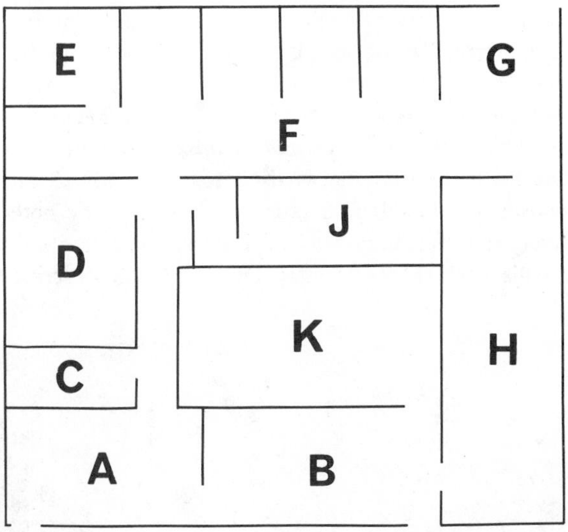

Fig. 5-42. Floor plan, Speech Synthesis Laboratory. See text for legend.

A major data-collection center for the laboratory is in room D, containing high-fidelity tape-recording equipment used in association and ingeniously synchronized with the fluoroscopy instrumentation. The latter consists of a Machlett x-ray tube, a nine-inch Standard-x-ray 3000-gain image intensifier (most effective in reducing radiation), and a 16 mm. Bach-Auricon cine-camera. Linked to this unit is a closed-circuit television system that combines a Fairchild TCS-950 camera and a high-reduction Miratel monitor.

In this equipment assembly the subject sits between the input-phosphor of the image intensifier and the x-ray tube (Fig. 5-43). He is centered correctly in the image-intensifier circle by the operator, who monitors the entire procedure on the closed-circuit TV system. The subject's position is such that he, also, is able to view his performance on the Miratel monitor.

It is noteworthy that in this system there is simultaneous photography of the subject's vocal tract silhouette and the oscillographic image of the sound waves of his voice, ensuring perfect synchronism of picture and sound. The silhouette itself permits a complete lateral view of the phonatory and articulatory mechanism, from below the glottis to above the hard palate, from behind the posterior pharyngeal wall to a space in front of his lips.

Frame-by-frame analyses of photographs taken with this equipment have resulted in a series of research reports, published and in press. Among these is a comparison of vowels and diphthongs in French and American English (Delattre, 1963). A major work is Delattre's *Comparing the Phonetic Features of English, French, German and Spanish* (1965), in which the x-ray technique was used for both vowels and consonants for all four languages. (As will be noted later, acoustic analysis and synthesis also contributed to this work.) Most recently, Delattre (1968) described the instrumentation and its use in "A Dialect Study of American *R*'s."

In the northwest corner of the plan, room E, is a technical library containing books and journals in experimental phonetics, linguistics, and related subjects.

As we mentioned earlier, a fundamental approach of the Speech Synthesis Project is the precise determination of the acoustic composition of the speech elements with which they work. Area F on the floor plan consists of four work spaces in which staff linguists participate in this analytical phase of the research. Although various instruments may be brought into this area, the most common is the Sona-Graph (Fig. 5-34) or sound spectrograph alluded to earlier. Because of the many different uses to which it may be put, a more detailed description of the Sona-Graph than most of the other instruments in this chapter will be provided.

Spectrographic analysis of speech sounds or other acoustic signals consists of recording the signal on a magnetic band within the instrument. The signal is then passed through either a narrow- (45 Hz) or wide- (300 Hz) band-pass filter that is moved progressively upward through the 8,000 Hz range of the Sona-Graph. When energy is detected in the signal, by means of this scanning process, the recording stylus discharges an electric spark and a resulting fine black line appears on the electrostatic recording unit. After the scanning has been completed, the record, a sonagram, is ready for analysis for one or more of the several acoustic parameters revealed.

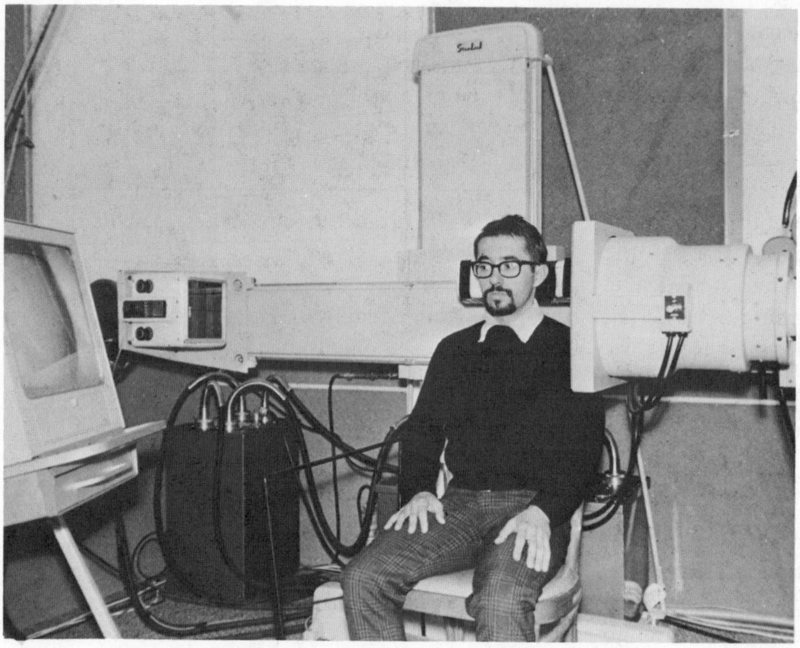

Fig. 5-43. Fluoroscopic examination of articulation.

Since speech sounds are acoustically unique and harmonically individual, though not, as we shall note in a later paragraph, invariant, each is revealed in a unique visual pattern on the sonagram and may be identified by a trained person. Because time is linear on the horizontal axis, the duration of a word, syllable, or phoneme may be measured. Fundamental frequency can be calculated by measurement of the distance between adjacent harmonics, shown as horizontal striations in narrow-band analysis of the signal, again made possible because frequency is linear on the vertical axis. In either narrow- or wide-band analysis, major areas of concentration of acoustic energy, called formants, may be identified. It is these formants, research has demonstrated, that contribute most to the uniqueness and perceptual identifiability of vowel phonemes and, to a certain extent, to consonant phonemes as well.

The power, or relative-intensity aspect, of the recorded signal may be examined in either of two ways. A control within the Sona-Graph, the sectioning circuit, makes it possible to compare the relative intensities of the formants in a given phoneme at a preselected instant in time. When the sectioning switch is thrown, the vertical scanning continues to take place across the frequency spectrum; the horizontal axis now is used for a graphic display of relative intensity. An accessory to the Sona-Graph, the Amplitude Display Unit, retains time on the horizontal axis, but replaces frequency on the vertical with relative amplitude of the whole signal, a summation of the energies contained within the formants. The flexibility of the Sona-Graph makes it possible for the operator to interrupt a standard narrow- or wide-band analysis at any point and shift to a sectioning or amplitude display, thus revealing on the same sonagram two different aspects of the same signal.

So fundamental a role does spectrographic analysis play in the research done in this laboratory that almost any one of its reports may be chosen to exemplify its use. Three, however, are of particular significance, and we shall make note of them. The first, in point of time, is "The Physiological Interpretation of Sound Spectrograms" (Delattre, 1951). In this article the experimental phonetician correlates data from x-ray and spectrographic analyses of vowel production to conclude that the position on the frequency axis of formant one (the lowest) relates to overall mouth opening, of formant two to lengthening of the cavity in front of the most elevated portion of

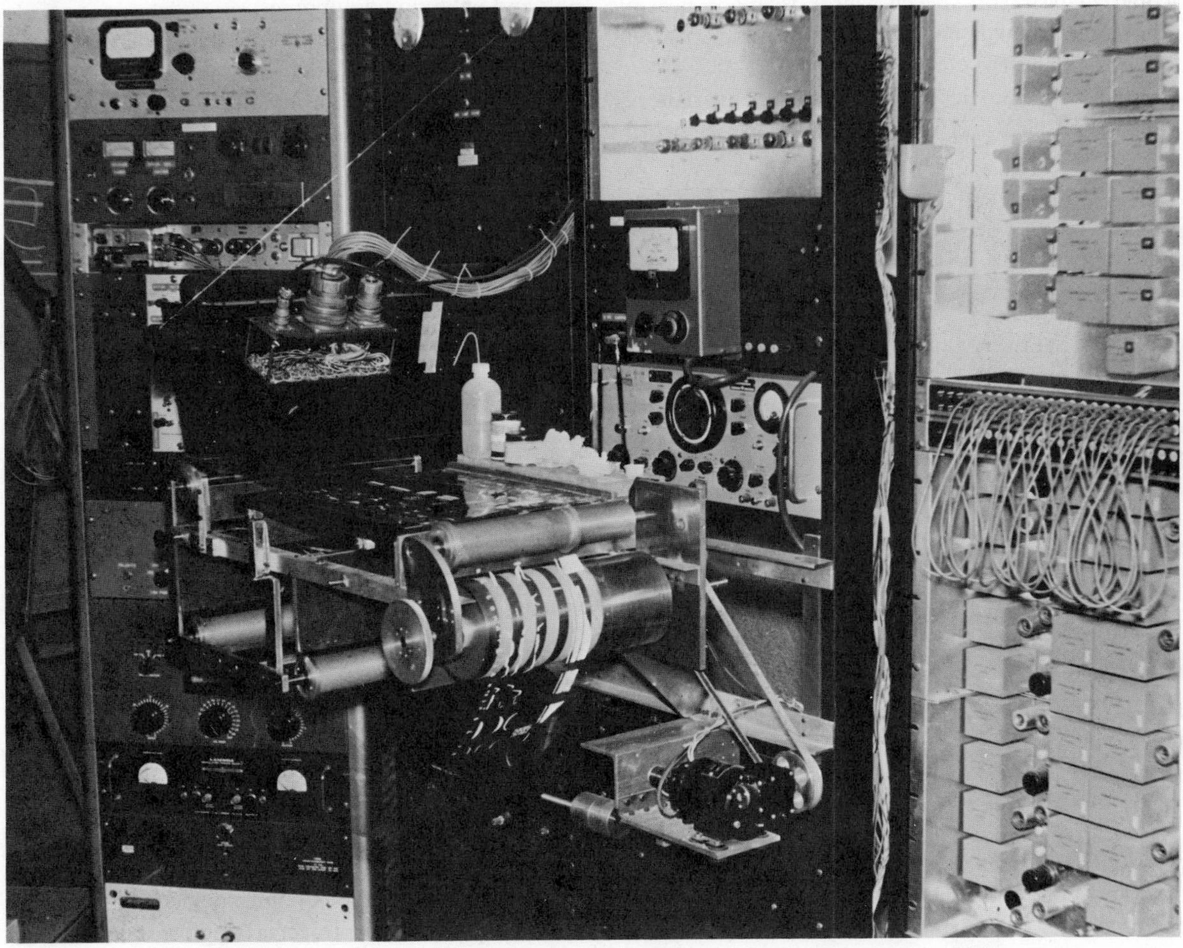

Fig. 5-44. Vocoder.

the tongue, of formant three to tongue-tip or tongue-dorsum raising, as in *r*-coloring.

Mentioned earlier, *Comparing the Phonetic Features of English, French, German and Spanish* (Delattre, 1965) also relies heavily upon spectrographic analysis for its basic data. The conclusions reached in this extensive monograph are too numerous for recapitulation here. Suffice it to say that the spectrographic technique, used in conjunction with fluoroscopic analysis and speech synthesis, made possible numerous comparisons of phonetic and prosodic features among the languages examined.

Finally, "Acoustic or Articulatory Invariance?" (Delattre, 1967) is a close examination of formant positions, particularly transitions, in various combinations of phonemes. The writer shows, for example, that in certain cases two very different *acoustic* patterns are identified as the same phoneme—the /g/ sounds of /ge/ and /go/ are heard as the same consonant in spite of major acoustic distinctions—whereas in other cases two very different *articulatory* gestures are heard as the same phoneme and produce similar spectrograms—the apical-retroflex /r/ and the dorsal-bunched /r/ of American English are identified as the same consonant. From these and other inspections the conclusion was reached that the invariance of phonemes is a perceptual, rather than an acoustical phenomenon. A corollary is that articulatory features of phoneme production also may depart from the invariance sometimes ascribed to them.

On the northeast corner of the wing, room G, is the project engineer's shop area. The standard test and calibration instruments and tools, common to most laboratories, are set up in room G. Several of these instruments will be described briefly in a later section.

Across from the linguists' area in room J is a photographic darkroom, again with standard developing and enlarging equipment.

Below the darkroom, the inner chamber lettered K in the plan is designed for film projection and analysis. The projectors with which the room is equipped are capable of being run, by remote control, at full speed, reduced speed, or frame by frame, forward, or in reverse. Cooling devices within them make it possible to project a single frame, without damage to the film, for protracted periods of time. Thus the precise measurements and observations of transitional movements of the articulators on which many of the significant findings of this laboratory are based can be made with great accuracy.

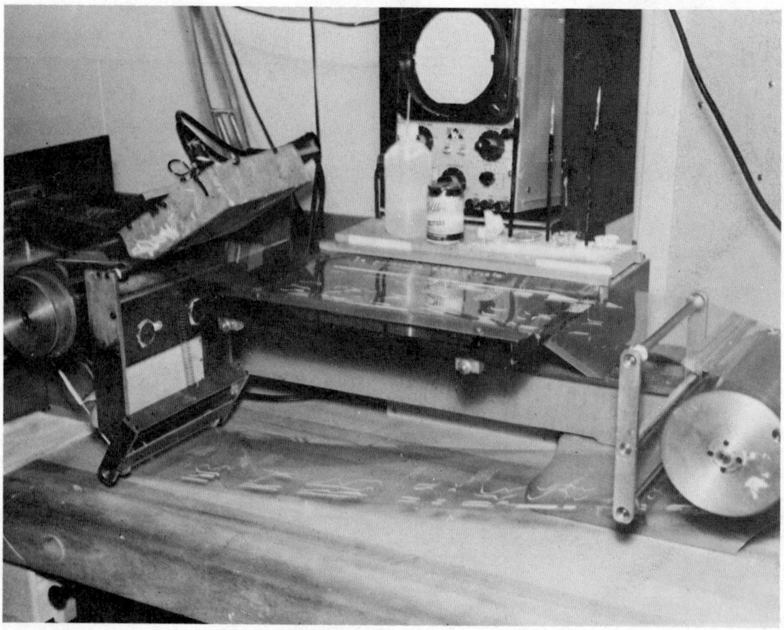

Fig. 5-45. Pattern Playback.

Adjacent to but not communicating directly with the film projection area is the chamber that provides this research facility with its name. Room H is the speech-synthesis room. Of necessity this is the largest of the research areas because both of the synthesizers in use here, the Vocoder (Fig. 5-44) and the Pattern Playback (Fig. 5-45), are large instruments that require extensive electronic and photoelectric circuitry.

Both the Vocoder and Pattern Playback have been described in detail in the journals (see, e.g., Dudley, 1939, and Cooper, 1950). In the Speech Synthesis Project both instruments have undergone extensive modifications in accordance with the particular research goals of the project. The operating principle of the two synthesizers is essentially the same: hand-painted patterns on transparent plastic belts are drawn through a photoelectric scanning system linked to sound-generating electronic sources, linked in turn to speaker systems. The different roles played by the two are a function of the responsiveness of one, the Vocoder, to intonational patterns and the other, the Pattern Playback, to articulatory features of speech, such as are revealed in spectrographic analysis. It is appropriate to refer to the Vocoder as a prosodic synthesizer and the Pattern Playback as a segmental synthesizer.

Representative of prosodic analysis in the synthesizer project is "A Comparative Study of Declarative Intonation in American English and Spanish" (Delattre, Olsen, and Poenack, 1962), in which a principal conclusion was that continuation is generally expressed by a downward inflection in American English, whereas it is typically expressed by a rising inflection in Spanish. Similar analyses have been performed on German intonations (Delattre, Poenack, and Olsen, 1963) and comparisons have been made across four languages in Delattre's (1965) extensive monograph mentioned earlier.

Previous mention has also been made of one representative research report in which pattern playback techniques were used (Delattre, 1967, "Acoustic or Articulatory Invariance?"). Another application was described by Liberman, Delattre, Cooper, and Gerstman (1954), who concluded that in the absence of the typical plosive aspiration, naive listeners were able to make reliable discriminations among synthesized /p-b/, /t-d/, and /k-g/, depending upon direction and extent of the second-formant transitions leading into a sustained vowel. An extension of this experiment was reported by Delattre, Liberman, and Cooper (1955), who discussed probable relationships between acoustic (formant) and physiological (articulatory) loci in consonant production.

This brief description of the Speech Synthesis Project, we believe, is indicative of the thoughtful arrangement of space and instrumentation for most effective processing of the raw data that are the concern of the laboratory. The three-way approach to speech research—spectrography, fluoroscopy, and synthesis—has been a major contribution.

ANALYSIS AND SYNTHESIS OF SPEECH

In the preceding section two instruments for speech synthesis were described. These instruments operate on the principle of reconstruction of spectral data for speech and also upon articulatory and phonetic data of speech. The vocoder was described as portraying prosodic features of speech and the pattern playback was described as a phonetic synthesizer. The interaction and relationship between speech analysis and synthesis is so important for the area of speech and hearing both with respect to instrumentation and speech perception that further discussion of analysis and synthesis is warranted. When speech perception is considered, it is difficult to find aspects that are not related to both analysis and synthesis of speech. Analysis and synthesis are related by the theories of speech perception and also by commonness of their instrumentation. Analysis by synthesis (Stevens and Halle, 1967) is a theory that the perception of speech involves the synthesis of internal patterns and matching these internal ones against incoming speech signals. The abstract rules that govern the generation of the internal patterns are assumed to be largely identical with those utilized for speech production. The motor theory of speech perception (Liberman, Cooper, Harris, and MacNeilage, 1962) makes similar assumptions concerning the role of articulatory features in speech perception. In part, these theories have grown out of investigations of speech synthesis and the resultant realizations that accurate knowledge of perceptual properties of speech is necessary for successful synthesis. There is also an overlap between synthesis and analysis with respect to instrumentation. An instrument that is successful in extracting essential properties of speech for transmission in another form, such as a digital representation, in a reverse mode of operation should also be able to reconstruct speech according to the rules of these properties.

Speech synthesis cannot be, and has not been in actual practice, separated from the problems of analysis because successful synthesis requires that the meaningful properties of speech be isolated and controlled. This has also been true because those laboratories that have been concerned with analysis-synthesis problems have been involved because of their interests, in some cases, in frequency-bandwidth reduction for the transmission of speech. This has required the reduction of the speech signal to narrower bandwidths or the coding of the speech signal in another form. When speech was reduced in either bandwidth or recoded in another form, it was then necessary that a replica of the original speech signal be recovered. In fact, the name vocoder was derived from the words voice and coder (Schroeder, 1966).

There are a number of different methods for analyzing and synthesizing speech. Some methods are based on acoustic properties such as the short-time spectrum of the speech signal or the formant frequencies. Other methods are based on properties of the vocal mechanism such as articulatory features or source and filter characteristics of the vocal tract. In addition, prosodic features of intonation, stress, and duration and abstract rules for the generation of speech such as phonetics and linguistic features may be examined with respect to speech and incorporated into the instrumental instructions for the synthesis of speech. These are the properties and aspects of speech that the speech scientist is interested in for his study of speech processes and the speech pathologist and audiologist are interested in for purposes of diagnosis and therapy. In fact, the instruments, theory, and knowledge of speech analysis and synthesis are all of interest to and potentially useful for workers in the field of speech and hearing.

There are a number of different instruments employed for speech analysis and synthesis. With respect to analysis, the Sona-Graph was described in considerable detail in the preceding section Presti (1966) reported the design of a high-speed sound spectrograph that in addition to providing three basic types of spectrograms, time versus frequency, an amplitude-contour display, and a cross-sectional amplitude display, can automatically advance the tape in order that successive segments of a recording can be analyzed. The instrument also has the ability to record and playback using standard Mylar recording tape and can complete a spectrogram in 80 seconds, thus greatly increasing the possibilities for spectrographic analyses of longer speech samples. Although there have been some studies in speech and hearing that have provided acoustic data in spectrographic form for individuals with either speech or hearing problems, detailed information of this kind is not generally available. These kinds of physical measures, in addition to providing basic knowledge about the disorders, would also be helpful for both diagnosis and therapy.

Although investigators have known for some time that speech could be analyzed into harmonic components, and that speechlike sounds could be produced readily by mixing the proper harmonic spectrum, the first successful electronic analysis was probably represented by the Vocoder (Dudley, 1939). Likewise, the first successful electronic synthesis was represented by the Voder (Dudley, Riesz, and Watkins, 1939). The original vocoder, the type now designated as a spectrum-channel vocoder, measured short-time amplitude spectrum at 10 discrete frequencies each with a bandwidth of 300 Hz. These bandwidths were reduced to 25 Hz, resulting in a transmission bandwidth of less than 300 Hz that included, in addition to the 10 channels, a pitch channel. For the synthesis portion of the device, the speech spectrum was reconstructed from the channel data. In subsequent references to vocoders in this discussion it can be noted that there are many types of vocoders and that the word vocoder has largely become a generic term for this type of analysis-synthesis system where the source or excitation and the filter or transmission systems are separate.

A number of different types of vocoders has been developed in the continuing process of studying speech analysis, transmission, synthesis, and perception. Some of these will be mentioned in this discussion to review some of the possibilities for speech analysis and synthesis and particularly to show some of the potential for workers in the area of speech and hearing. The spectrum-channel vocoder is the oldest method, as was indicated previously, for speech analysis and synthesis. For this kind of vocoder, the speech signal is separated into a number of bands, usually varying in number between 10 and 20. In addition, the channel that carries excitation function, pitch, and voicing, is also included. The original bandpass filters are reduced to narrowband signals so that the total transmission bandwidth is only a fraction of the original channels. The synthesizer section of the vocoder utilizes the narrow-band signals to reconstruct the original speech signal. Other variations of vocoders are formant vocoders, where the analyzer extracts formant frequencies and transmits this information for use by the synthesizer. Again voiced and unvoiced detectors and pitch detectors are part of the analyzer to extract excitation information for the synthesizer. Pattern-matching vocoders are those where a set of stored spectral patterns are matched against incoming short-time speech spectrum to determine the output of the synthesizer.

A vocoder design has been described by Flanagan and Golden (1966) that is called a phase vocoder. This instrument is of interest for at least two reasons: 1) it is designed and modeled on auditory behavior, and 2) it does not require excitation information in terms of fundamental frequency and voicing and unvoicing of the original speech signal. With regard to the modeling of analysis-synthesis devices that correspond to auditory processing by the ear, there is evidence from both psychoacoustic and physiological studies that the human ear makes a type of short-time spectral analysis of acoustic signals (Flanagan, 1967). The auditory system, in this regard, appears to use information that corresponds to smoothed values of short-time amplitude and phase spectra. The phase vocoder attempts to duplicate, to a certain extent, this kind of processing that the ear applies to incoming signals and to retain those features that are perceptually relevant. The phase vocoder encodes the speech signal in terms of smoothed values of the phase derivative spectrum and the short-time amplitude spectrum. An aspect of the phase vocoder is that it is able to expand or compress time and frequency scales. This is a feature that offers possibilities for either individuals who have high-frequency hearing losses or for individuals who require either faster or slower speech-input rates for efficient processing.

Control parameters, other than those based on spectral data, are possible for the synthesis of speech. Coker (1968) has proposed a system for the generation of synthetic speech where the control signals for the synthesizer are derived by rules from phonetic input data through intermediate-step vocal tract area computations. The basic elements of the input data to the synthesizer are phonemes. They are characterized as static context-independent, ideal vocal tract shapes. These phonemes are tabulated in the control programs as sets of parameters of a vocal tract model. These parameters include coordinates of the central part of the tongue, degree of raising of the tongue tip, and degrees of closure and protrusion of the lips. Long-term temporal correlations are incorporated through considering transitions between phonemes and memory that can overlap several phonemes. The control data for this articulatory system model are programmed on a digital computer by means of a typewriter input. Output of the system is through an on-line serial resonance analog synthesizer. In addition to the vocal tract parameter values stored in the system for phonemes, duration and excitation information is also stored. For synthesis, these are also used as acoustic parameters. Although synthesis by rule from articulatory parameters has been presented briefly in this discussion, it is of interest to note that the technique incorporates dynamic vocal tract configurations, coarticulation properties, and the use of instructions from a digital computer for speech synthesis.

Another approach in synthesis is to extract acoustic

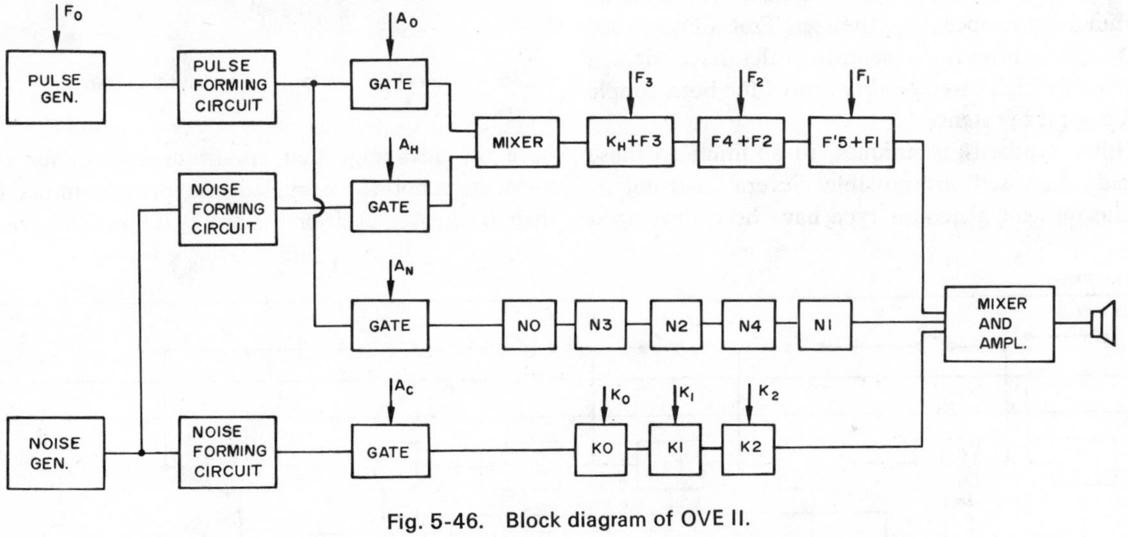

Fig. 5-46. Block diagram of OVE II.

parameters from speech signals and to use these as the rules for synthesis. The use of acoustic parameters has been proposed by Rabiner (1968). In this approach, acoustic information about phonemes is abstracted for use as control parameters. Some of the phoneme characteristics include formant information, source characteristics including voicing or non-voicing, a description of whether the phoneme is nasal or fricative, and a set of frequency values that define the possible variability around target formant positions. Amplitude and durational characteristics are also defined for each phoneme. The input for synthesis is a linguistic description of the utterance including phoneme characteristics, word boundaries, vowel stress marks, pauses, and a terminal marker that indicates an end of an utterance. This input is converted to control signals that in turn drive a serial terminal analog speech synthesizer. Tests of adequacy of speech synthesis by acoustic rules have yielded reasonably high intelligibility scores for both simple and complex sentences.

Other synthesis techniques, in addition to those already discussed, are possible. Several instruments of the formant-generator type have been developed at the Speech Transmission Laboratory of the Royal Institute of Technology in Stockholm. These include the OVE Ib, the OVE II, and the recently developed OVE III. The OVE II (Fant and Martony, 1962) is a formant-generator-type synthesizer that includes three parallel systems to control formants, nasals, fricatives and stops. The block diagram for the OVE II is shown in Fig. 5-46. Series-formant generators have the advantage that amplitude control for the formants is not necessary, because it is determined by their frequency positions. The OVE Ib (Chistovich, Fant, and de Serpa-Leitao, 1966) is a portable vowel synthesizer, shown graphically in Fig. 5-47 and in block diagram in Fig. 5-48. This instrument is a four-formant synthesizer where the voice fundamental and the first two formant frequencies are controlled with

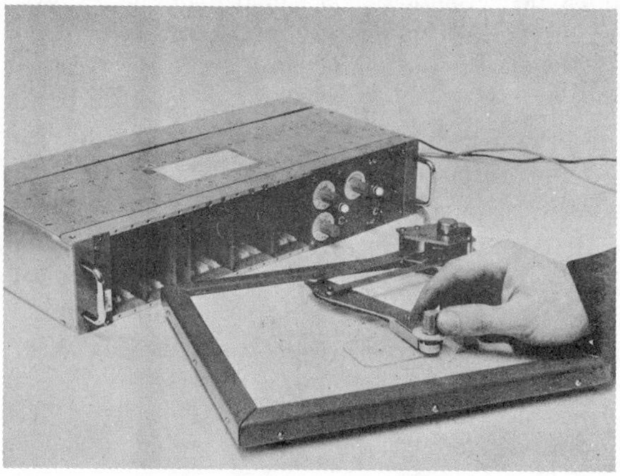

Fig. 5-47. OVE Ib, portable vowel synthesizer.

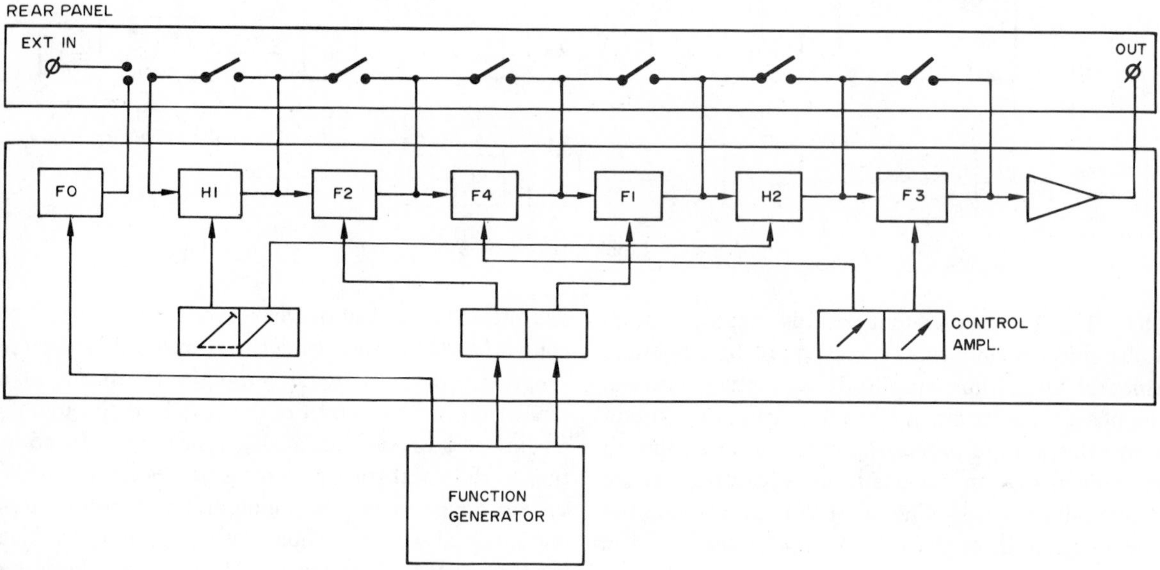

Fig. 5-48. Block diagram of OVE Ib.

a manual function generator. The other formants are separately preset. A unique feature of this instrument is that the function generator consists of a baseplate with a mechanism to which the operator's handle is geared. Movement of the handle over the plate corresponds to movement in formant-one and formant-two space. Voicing is turned on when the handle is pressed downward and the voicing frequency is controlled by turning the handle. An operator, after some practice, can learn to manipulate the device to produce realistic-sounding vowels. The recently developed OVE III, shown in block diagram in Fig. 5-49, is similar to the earlier-developed OVE II. This synthesizer differs in several respects, however. The most outstanding is that synthesis parameters are digitally controlled by a computer. The operator communicates with the synthesizer by use of computer programs. In Fig. 5-49 can be seen the digital computer section and the analog synthesizer section of the OVE III. In this figure can also be seen the three parallel circuits of the synthesizer, formant, nasal, and fricative branches.

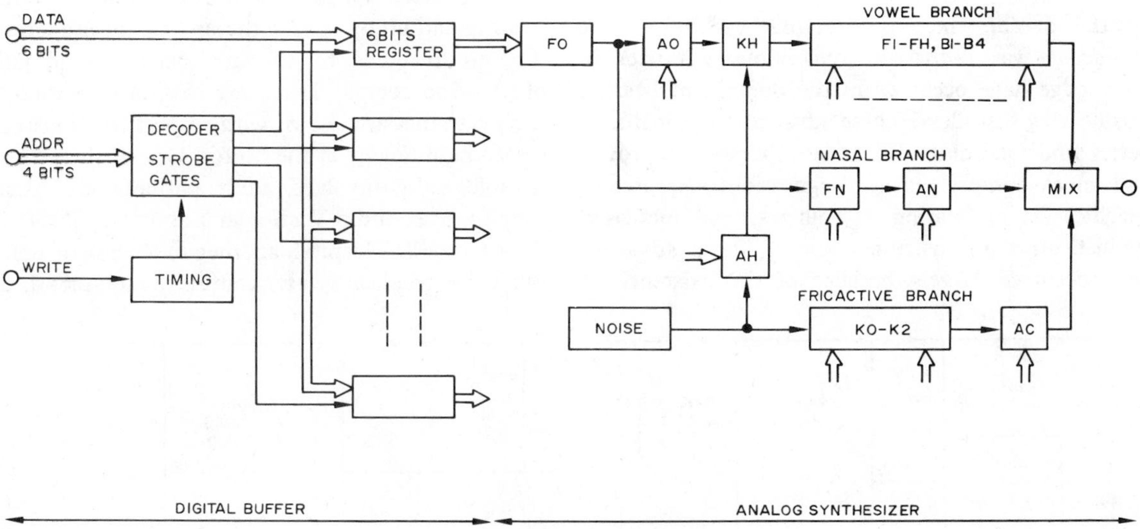

Fig. 5-49 Block diagram of OVE III.

The important and consistent aspect of recently developed synthesizers is that small computers have been utilized as part of the system. Control of synthesis parameters is accomplished by computers that are in some cases instructed in linguistic, phonetic, or acoustic language. Recognition is given to such aspects of speech as coarticulation, variability of formant ranges, and transitional properties of the articulatory system. The fact that basic speech knowledge is employed in synthesis should make these instruments meaningful and useful for workers in speech and hearing. The phase vocoder (Flanagan and Golden, 1966) previously discussed, because of its theoretical implications and its possibilities for multiplying or dividing the frequency spectrum and compression or expansion of the time scale of speech, could be of considerable value for speech and hearing. Computer analysis and synthesis of speech will probably become increasingly commonplace in speech and hearing laboratories and clinical settings,

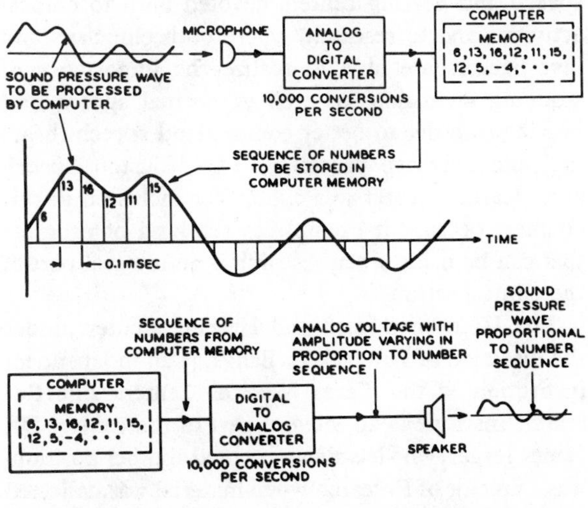

Fig. 5-50. Analog to digital and digital to analog conversion. *Diagram courtesy Bell Telephone Laboratories, Inc.*

particularly with the advent of moderately priced special-purpose computers now available. Fig. 5-50 illustrates analog-to-digital and digital-to-analog conversion for computer processing of sound waves.

HEARING CENTER

In the decade since the original edition of the *Handbook* was prepared, tremendous advances in knowledge have occurred in the domain of hearing and hearing disorders. These advances have included better understanding of hearing processes, improved and more comprehensive diagnostic tests, greater specification of hearing pathologies, and increased sophistication in instrumentation. These advances have occurred largely because of the existence of speech and hearing centers devoted both to clinical activities and to research, where both clinicians and investigators are able to realize the importance of studying anomalous as well as normal speech and hearing in order to better comprehend speech, hearing, and language processes. The Houston Speech and Hearing Center was chosen for inclusion in this chapter, because it exemplifies the kind of progress that can be made when research is an integral part of the clinical setting.

The Houston Speech and Hearing Center, under the direction of Dr. Jack L. Bangs, is an independent institution of the Texas Medical Center. The Research Institute is an integral part of the center. Dr. James Jerger, who has since accepted another position, was Director of Research when material was collected for this chapter. Although the speech and hearing center and the research institute are concerned with a wide range of both normal and anomalous speech and hearing processes, this discussion will only relate to aspects of the center that are devoted to clinical and research audiology. A floor plan is shown in Fig. 5-51 for that part of the center, the basement floor, where most of the audiology activities are concentrated. Not shown is the floor plan for the first floor, where administrative offices, lecture rooms, and group hearing and group speech therapy rooms are located. The group rooms, for the most part, have adjoining observation rooms. There are several exceptions to the plans that are shown with respect to clinical and research audiology at the center. One of these is that neurologically involved adult patients are usually tested in the Audio-Vestibular Laboratory located in the Methodist Hospital, another independent unit of the Texas Medical Center complex, and second, that physical additions to the speech and hearing center that are in progress will result in different locations for particular facilities.

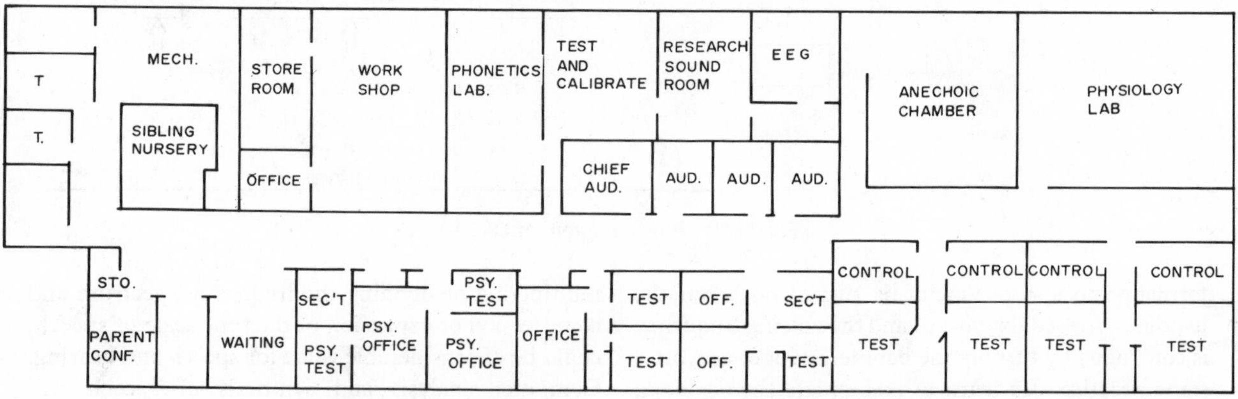

Fig. 5-51. Floor plan, basement section, of the Houston Speech and Hearing Center.

In the plan, lower right corner, are shown two double audiological testing suites. Sound-treatment is incorporated in the structure and complete clinical audiometric equipment is provided for each of the four units. The first room from the right is used for general diagnostic work, the second for child diagnostics, the third for studying auditory evoked responses, and the fourth for adult diagnostic work. The room used for evoked-response audiometry contains equipment specific for this measurement task. The other three rooms can be used somewhat interchangeably for audiological diagnosis. Directly across the hall from these testing rooms is the physiology laboratory, where studies on animals in electrophysiology of hearing are conducted by inducing sensorineural hearing losses through a technique of increasing cerebrospinal fluid pressure. Adjacent to this laboratory is an anechoic (echo-free) chamber, a room in which external noise is reduced to a minimum and ambient sound is broken up and absorbed by acoustic wedges. An illustration of standard anechoic chamber construction is shown in Fig. 5-52. Anechoic chambers are useful for the free-field testing and accurate calibration of such instruments as microphones, loudspeakers, and other audio and audiological devices. To the left, in the diagram, of the anechoic chamber is a room for electroencephalographic study and adjacent to the latter room are two rooms, the testing and control areas, for the Speech Perception Laboratory where work on the identification of synthetic sentences is conducted. On the same side of the hall are a room for calibration of instruments, a phonetics laboratory, and a modern, well-equipped workshop.

In the field of audiology, research, audiometric tests, and instrumentation are closely related. Audiological findings, as they are refined into valid and reliable tests, ultimately become incorporated as part of the capabilities and testing procedures of clinical and research audiometers. Fortunately, electronic components have decreased in size as the number of diagnostic tests have increased. This has resulted in audiometers that are reasonably compact and yet have considerable versatility of signal presentation and control. In general, audiometers can be grouped into three types: clinical and research models; the Békésy type or automatic units; and instruments for pure-tone-threshold and screening usages. The clinical models are the most versatile, providing for a number of special-purpose tests in addition to speech and pure-tone tests. Automatic audiometers are those that allow a patient to test himself and are primarily concerned with responses to pure tones. Pure-tone audiometers are primarily for threshold and screening measures.

The transition from audiological findings to test procedures can be exemplified by reviewing some of the work of the Research Institute of the Houston Speech and Hearing Center. For convenience, this research can be grouped according to the kinds of investigations: those having to do with diagnostic tests for locating the site of a lesion, those concerned with evaluations of auditory measures, studies of hearing-aid performance, the development of synthetic-sentence testing materials, and auditory evoked responses.

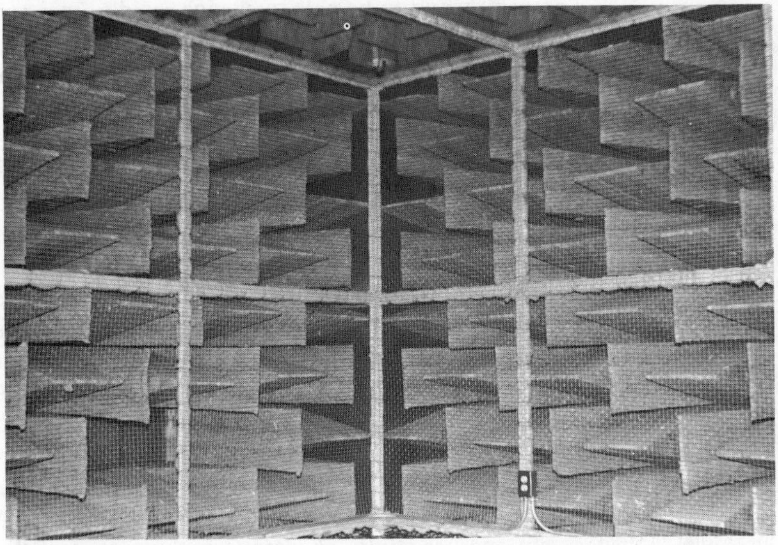

Fig. 5-52. Interior of an anechoic chamber.

One audiological task is that of determining the site of the lesion that produces the hearing loss, assuming that the decision has been made that the loss is sensorineural and not conductive. The problem is that of deciding whether the lesion producing the loss is in the cochlea (cochlear involvement), or in the auditory neural system (retrocochlear involvement), or in both. Retrocochlear lesions may involve the VIIIth Cranial nerve, the brain stem, or the auditory cortex. Tests have been developed that are indicative of either cochlear or retrocochlear involvement.

Several studies conducted at the Houston Speech and Hearing Center pertain to measures that differentiate cochlear and VIIIth Cranial nerve disorders. Jerger and Jerger (1966) reported that subjects with VIIIth Cranial nerve audiometric profiles demonstrate threshold instabilities that are related to critical off-times of periodically interrupted signals. When the off-times were short, thresholds obtained on a Békésy audiometer dropped progressively over time similar to a type III tracing, described below. Jerger (1960) defined four kinds of Békésy audiograms as type I where tracings for continuous and interrupted tones interweave, type II where the tracings for continuous

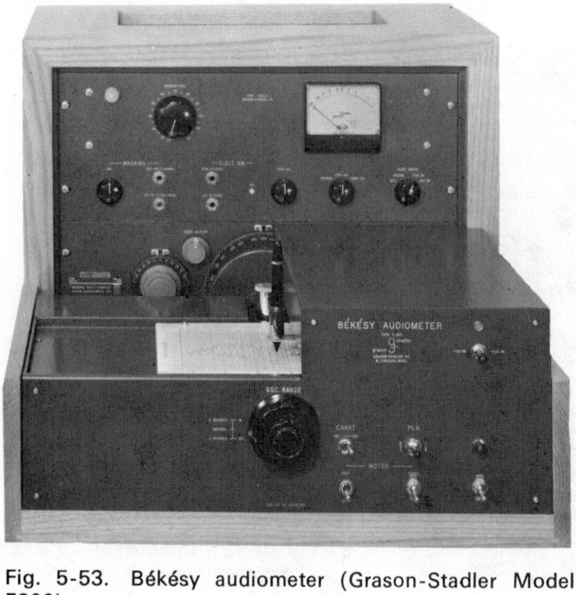

Fig. 5-53. Békésy audiometer (Grason-Stadler Model E800).

tones drop below those for interrupted tones at high frequencies, type III where continuous tracings drop rapidly below interrupted tracings, and type IV where continuous tracings fall consistently below the tracings for interrupted tones. In the study of critical off-time in VIIIth Cranial nerve disorders, Jerger and Jerger (1966) reported that for an on-time of 200 milliseconds critical off-times for six subjects varied from 40 to 200 milliseconds. Although the critical off-times differed for the six subjects, there was a characteristic shape for the function. This was a flat tracing above the critical off-time and a sharply increasing threshold below the critical off-time. The data for this study were collected on a Békésy audiometer, Grason-Stadler, Model E-800 (see Fig. 5-53) that was set to an attenuation rate of two and one-half dB/second and a table speed of one octave/minute. The internal oscillator and electronic switch of the audiometer were replaced by an external oscillator, electronic switch, and interval timer. The external instruments provided control of rise-decay times and of on- and off-times of the signals. The modification of the Békésy audiometer is mentioned because it demonstrates several aspects of audiological research and instrumentation. One aspect is that components of audiometers are basically psychoacoustic instrumentation that include oscillators, amplifiers, attenuators, electronic switches, and similar instruments. Hearing testing could be accomplished using basic laboratory equipment; however, because it is important to be able to test individuals quickly and accurately and to be able to change rapidly from one test to another, the fact that audiometer designs provide this ease and accuracy of testing makes the audiometer much preferred over laboratory instruments for diagnostic testing. Another aspect of audiological instrumentation and research is that investigations into hearing phenomena frequently required capabilities in the presentation and control of signals that are beyond the limits of clinical audiometers. After studies have demonstrated that testing measures and procedures are valid and reliable for the diagnosis of aspects of hearing losses, the facility for the test can then be incorporated into the design of an audiometer. The audiometer does not necessarily need to cover the parameter ranges that were considered in the development of the test, but need only cover crucial values for the test.

In another study, of interest both because of the findings and the instrumentation employed, Jerger and Jerger (1967) administered a variety of psychoacoustic tests to three female subjects, one with normal hearing, one with a cochlear disorder, and one with an VIIIth Cranial nerve hearing disorder. Discrimination measures of loudness, pitch and spectral cut-off, and temporal order were obtained for these three individuals. In addition, critical off-time, the measure discussed in the previous study, and speech intelligibility were measured. Although different configurations of instruments were required for the various measures, oscillators, electronic switches, filters, interval timers, and a programming system were the kinds of devices that were utilized for the study. The programming system, for the most part, was used to control the sequence of signals, tabulate responses, and to provide the subject with information about the accuracy of her responses. A feature of much of the experimentation in hearing at the Houston Speech and Hearing Center is the automation employed in the presentation of signals and in the recovery and tabulation of responses. This is especially true for the studies concerning synthetic sentences and auditory evoked responses.

The findings for the study on a psychoacoustic comparison of cochlear and VIIIth Cranial nerve disorders (Jerger and Jerger, 1967) indicated that the VIIIth Cranial nerve involvement in the area of the discrimination of spectral cut-off was considerably inferior to both normal and cochlear involvement. Jerger, Jerger, Ainsworth, and Caram (1966) report a case study of VIIIth Cranial nerve involvement and audiological responses before and after the surgical removal of a cerebellar tumor. Békésy tracings before and after surgery indicated the reversability of abnormal auditory phenomena after surgery. Jerger (1967) summarizes data and kinds of tests that differentiate cochlear and VIIIth Cranial nerve involvement. These include the short increment sensitivity index (SISI) (Jerger, Shedd, and Harford, 1959; Jerger, 1962) that measures a patient's ability to hear small, short changes in sound intensity and the alternate binaural loudness balance (ABLB), a test for measuring loudness recruitment, Békésy audiograms, and speech intelligibility measures. These kinds of tests, with the exception of the Békésy, are incorporated within the capabilities of most clinical and research audiometers. Several different audiometers are in use at the Houston Speech and Hearing Center. On the Allison model 22, a clinical and research audiometer shown in Fig. 5-54, a number of different tests including the SISI, the ABLB, and speech intelligibility measures can be performed. Patients with cochlear involvement generally show positive SISI, partial or complete recruitment, a type II Békésy, and speech intelligibility that is good to fair (Jerger, 1967). Eighth Cranial-nerve-involved patients show negative SISI, no recruitment, type III or IV Békésy audiograms, and fair to poor speech intelligibility. Reference has been made previously to the Békésy model E800 used in experimentation. Another automatic audiometer is the Rudmose model ARJ-5, shown in Fig. 5-55. It is similar to the Békésy in that the patient has control of the attenuator that charts threshold values.

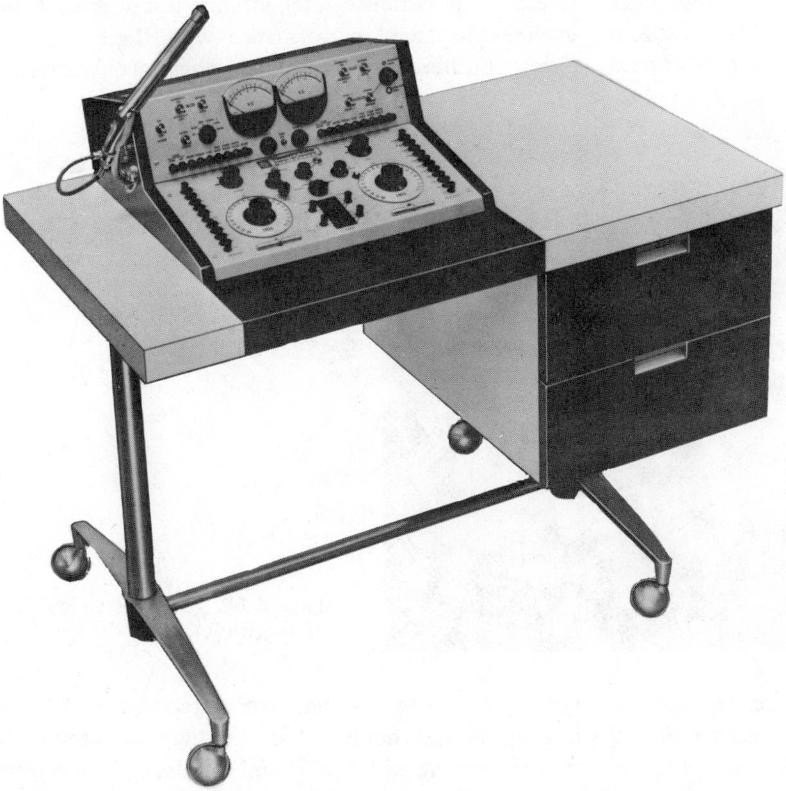

Fig. 5-54. Clinical and research audiometer (Allison Model 22).

Measurements are obtained at discrete rather than continuous frequencies.

Other investigations at the Houston Speech and Hearing Center are those that involve evaluations of audiological tests. One such series of studies treated bone-conduction audiometry in a critical evaluation of sensorineural acuity level (SAL) audiometry (Jerger and Jerger, 1965). In the SAL procedure two thresholds are measured, a threshold in quiet, and a threshold in the presence of white noise presented through an oscillator placed in the center of the forehead. A sensorineural acuity level is computed by comparing the threshold shift that occurs in an impaired ear to that for a normal ear. This difference between normal and impaired threshold shift is taken to be the sensorineural hearing loss in dB. Several variables that relate to bone-conduction audiometry were evaluated in this investigation. Because of the difficulties in both calibration and the coupling of bone vibrators to the skull, specially constructed apparatus was used to couple the bone vibrator to the forehead with known and constant force. The authors concluded that the procedures of SAL audiometry are sound and that factors such as force of application, the acoustic reflex, and the occlusion of the ear canal do not alter the validity of this test.

Another group of instruments useful for audiological purposes is demonstrated by studies done at the speech and hearing center on hearing-aid performance and hearing-aid selection. These instruments are used for evaluating acoustic characteristics of hearing aids and include as a central unit a portable anechoic chamber. A Bruel and Kjaer suggested arrangement of instruments includes, in addition to their hearing-aid test chamber, model 4212, a microphone, amplifier, octave band analyzer, filter, graphic level recorder, and oscillator. A loudspeaker located at the bottom of the test chamber is the signal source. The output of a hearing aid placed in the chamber and under test is analyzed with the instrumental array listed above. The test chamber and some associated equipment were used in two studies at the Houston center to evaluate hearing-aid performance. In one study (Jerger, Speaks, and Malmquist, 1966) that concerned hearing-aid performance and hearing-aid selection, a sentence intelligibility test was used to evaluate listeners' performance with three hearing aids that differed substantially in physical characteristics. The speech materials were prepared by transmitting them through each of the three aids mounted in the hearing aid test chamber, Bruel and Kjaer model 4212. Results of the experiment indicated that speech intelligibility for both normal and hearing-impaired listeners was inversely related to the percent of harmonic distortion that characterized the conditions represented by the three hearing aids. In a companion study, Jerger, Malmquist, and Speaks (1966) utilized similar procedures, including the recording of intelligibility materials through a hearing aid placed in a portable anechoic chamber, for comparing several speech intelligibility tests with respect to both hearing-aid characteristics and type of hearing loss. Again, as in the previous study, sentence intelligibility was inversely related to the percent of

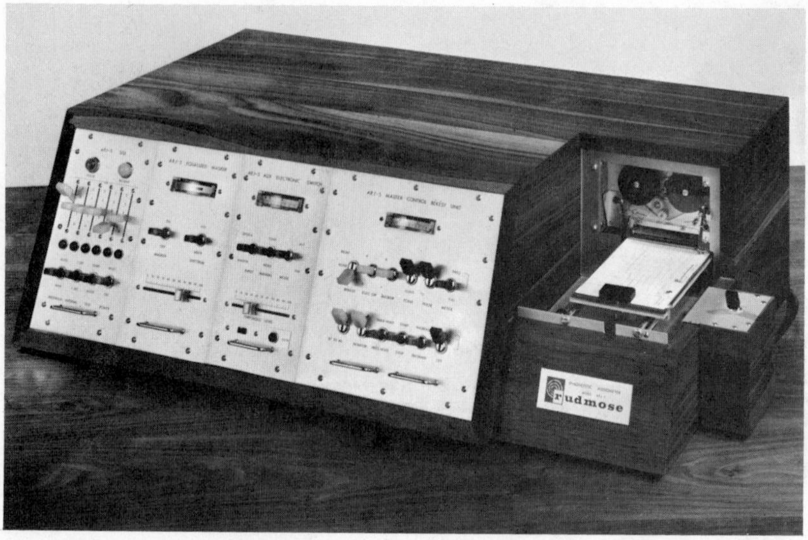

Fig. 5-55. Diagnostic audiometer (Rudmose Model ARJ-5).

harmonic distortion that characterized the hearing aid. Monosyllabic word tests did not systematically reflect performance differences among the aids tested.

A major research effort for several years at the Research Institute, Houston Speech and Hearing Center, has been work on a method for the measurement of speech identification. Several goals are involved in this effort, including the construction and evaluation of methods for the measurement of speech understanding, the relating of acoustic characteristics of hearing aids to speech understanding of hearing-impaired individuals who wear aids, and the identification of auditory impairment that results from damage or disease that affect auditory pathways. Work on these problems has centered around the use of the synthetic-sentence identification test (SSI). The measurement of speech intelligibility has been a difficult problem for a number of years, not only for the audiologist but also for other speech investigators, and has employed a wide variety of verbal materials including nonsense syllables, monosyllabic and dissyllabic words, sentences, and continuous speech. Material that includes words and shorter units has had the disadvantage that it does not sample temporal ongoing properties of speech, while sentences and longer units present the difficult problem of quantification of the listener's responses. A method was developed for the measurement of speech identification that contained sentences constructed as approximations to possible sentences solely on the basis of conditional possibilities of word sequence (Speaks and Jerger, 1965). The message set that was developed contained 10 alternative probabilities as third-order approximations to real English sentences. Advantages of this speech material are that it is a closed message set with controlled length and controlled relative informational content.

The synthetic sentences now have been used in several studies; in particular, this material has been examined for its potential as a diagnostic test of hearing disorders. Temporal interruption and the presentation of sentences in the presence of competing messages appear to make it possible to distinguish VIIIth Cranial-nerve-lesion patients from both normal and cochlear-involved individuals. The performance characteristics of the sentences have been evaluated and studied in several ways. A study of the effect of competing messages on synthetic sentence identification (Speaks, Karmen, and Benitez, 1967) revealed that performance intensity functions were flattened by mixing competing messages with the sentences. Increased flatness of this function improves the capability of the sentences for distinguishing among various individuals tested. In another study, the performance intensity characteristics of the synthetic sentences were compared with other intelligibility testing materials (Speaks, 1967). The potential of the sentences was also evaluated for deriving an unbiased measure of sentence identification. Data were collected to explore the applicability of a statistical-decision-model to performance in sentence identification. Receiver-operating characteristic (ROC) curves were obtained for the sentences that were consistent with the model and suggest that the sentences can be employed to obtain a listener performance score. Apart from the considerable value of the sentences for the measurement of a discrimination function, procedures and instrumentation that have been developed for the synthetic sentence work are of interest. The testing procedure is automated and provides for stimulus presentation and automatic data acquisition and storage. Standard instruments are incorporated into the overall system to provide this automation. A block diagram, Fig. 5-56, shows the arrangement of instrumentation for the synthetic-sentence identification task.

As an example of the utilization of the equipment shown in Fig. 5-56 for a possible synthetic-speech identification study, sentences would be recorded on channel one of the Ampex tape recorder. A series of pure-tone pulses that coded each sentence would be recorded on the second channel, while the third channel could contain continuous speech or similar material as a competing message. If the sentences were to be either temporally interrupted or filtered, the electronic switch or filter could be employed; otherwise the speech signal would be fed to an earphone through the speech audiometer. Channel two of the tape recorder, as was indicated, could provide the pulse code that identifies the sentence presented, signal the listening period, and code the correct answer. Channel three of the recorder, containing a competing message, could be fed directly to an earphone through channel two of the speech audiometer. The response data could be automatically recovered, in that mechanical counters would provide instant readout of such information as the number of messages presented, the number of correct responses, and similar information. The synthetic-speech identification system, as can be observed, provides considerable versatility in signal presentation and recovery of data.

Another research activity at the Houston Speech and Hearing Center involves evoked response audiometry. Although it has been known for some time that electroencephalographic patterns can be altered by auditory stimulation of the subject, the recent advent of special-purpose computers that are able through a process of summation to extract a small evoked potential from background signals has provided a possibility for electrophysiological measurement of auditory sensitivity. McCandless and Best of hearing for infants. The procedures incorporate a telemetry system that avoids connecting scalp electrodes directly to the electroencephalographic instrument (EEG) and thus allows the child to move about during testing. The telemetry system includes a small frequency-modulated (FM) transmitter and an FM receiver. The instrumentation employed in the average-evoked-response studies includes oscillators, an electronic switch with an associated interval timer, and a speech audiometer for delivering signals to a

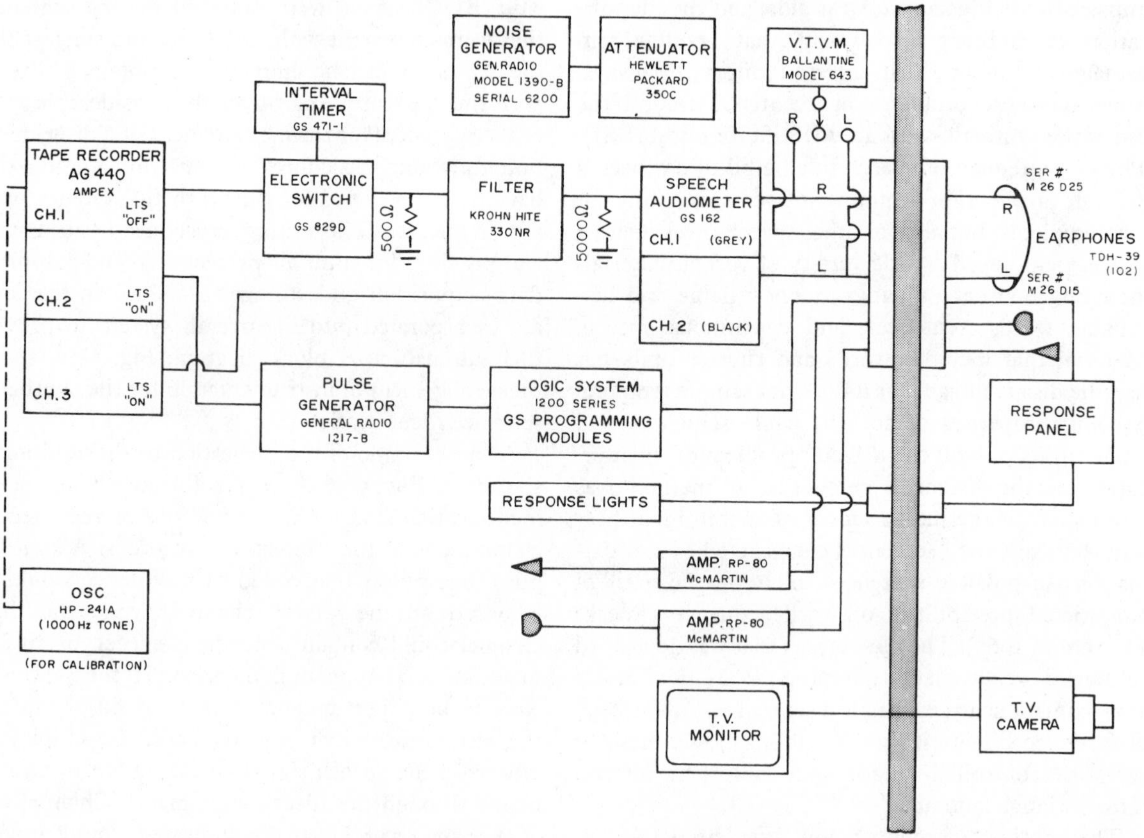

Fig. 5-56. Instrumentation for the synthetic sentence identification task.

(1964) reported on the use of a summing computer for recovery of evoked responses to auditory stimuli for human subjects. McCandless (1967) applied the procedure to the testing of a clinical population of children and adults who were unable or unwilling to respond accurately to conventional audiometric techniques. He concluded that considerable caution is necessary in the interpretation of evoked-response measures. The work in average evoked responses to sound at the speech and hearing center has been directed toward the development of a screening test subject's earphones. Cortical responses are picked up and transmitted from an FM transmitter that is attached to the subject. These signals are received by an FM receiver and fed through a preamplifier to a small special-purpose computer that averages and stores the evoked responses and averages out other random activity of the brain. After a predetermined number of stimulus presentations, the summed and stored data are taken from the computer by means of a graphic X-Y plotter. A normal auditory evoked response will produce a typical waveform with characteristic peaks at time latencies of approximately 135 and 215 milliseconds after the presentation of the stimulus. In order to develop validity and reliability for this procedure, large numbers of children who are in the clinical program of the speech and hearing center are currently being evaluated using the auditory-evoked-response procedure.

Although considerable discussion has been given to research audiology activities at the Houston Speech and Hearing Center in order to demonstrate instrumentation usage and development, the clinical activities that provide diagnostics and treatment for large numbers of children and adults are equally important. The only aspects of this program discussed in the present chapter are the test facilities. The audiometric testing suites were previously indicated in the floor plan, shown in Fig. 5-51. Much of the work concerns the testing of children.

Auditory conditioning techniques have been found to be successful for obtaining threshold measures for children. The testing is usually done by two examiners. One works with the child in the testing chamber, while the other controls the presentation of the auditory stimuli from the audiometric console in the control room.

Audiometric testing of infants and young children is often accomplished by utilizing the illumination of a small, faceted, red light as the reward. The child plays games with the audiological assistant until a stimulus is presented. The child is taught to respond to the presence of the auditory stimulus by turning his head to see the blinking of a red light. Several stimuli are presented simultaneously with the illumination of the light and the child is conditioned to respond by appropriately turning his head to see the light. As the assistant entertains the child visually with toys, the tester presents a variety of signals at different intensity levels. When the signal is perceived by the child, he turns, and the light is lit as a reward.

The light is mounted on the wall at an angle greater than 90 degrees from the child's line of vision and is, consequently, out of sight until the child turns toward it in response to the signal. The tester is capable of controlling the light in such a manner that it is illuminated only when the child turns toward it. Small children appear to think that the signal is generated from the light; however, the audiological examiner is controlling the presentation of the auditory signal as well as the presentation of the light.

Older children, at approximately the age of three years, are conditioned to respond somewhat more directly to the presence of an auditory signal, under test procedures requiring more advanced techniques. The audiological assistant, for example, teaches the child to respond to the presence of a signal by taking a peg. The reward for such a response is for the subject to place the peg in a board or bucket. Several simultaneous presentations of stimuli and peg usually result in the child's reaching for a peg without the help of clues when the signal is perceived.

Another technique involves the use of a pediacometer table. Seven small puppets that are wired electrically are recessed into the top of a table. The audiological assistant teaches the child to respond to the presence of an auditory signal by pushing a button. This response is rewarded by the appearance of a puppet from one of the seven cubicles in the table. Thus, the child is conditioned to respond to the presence of a sound by pushing a button. He is rewarded by the appearance of one of the seven puppets. The assistant can vary the puppet appearances from special controls placed under the table.

Perhaps the success of any conditioning technique resides in the close communication between the audiologist in the control room and the audiological assistant in the test room. A special intercom system is worn by both examiners in order that the assistant receives instructions from the tester without the child and/or parent hearing these instructions. It should also be noted that the intercom circuit allows the assistant to monitor the signals which are being presented to the child's earphones. This type of intercom system eliminates visual clues that often distract children and cause parental anxiety during testing.

The basic instrument for each testing suite is a clinical audiometer that includes a pure-tone circuit that can be fed to earphones, speakers, or a bone oscillator. There is another circuit for speech audiometry. Music stimulation and white-noise masking are also available. The special intercome system described above is a necessary part of the system. The testing chamber is equipped with the jeweled light, the pediacometer table, and other toys. Observation of the testing of children at the Houston Speech and Hearing Center indicates that the success of the procedures depends upon the experience and skill of the audiologists, not only upon the equipment utilized.

As was indicated previously, the audiological testing of adults with neurological problems is usually done at the Audio-Vestibular Laboratory in Methodist Hospital. The audiometric instrumentation utilized in this laboratory includes a two-channel tape recorder, a speech audiometer, a clinical audiometer with a SISI adapter, and a Békésy audiometer. Audiometric procedures include a battery of tests that have been demonstrated to be of diagnostic significance for evaluating hearing disorders. Patients are tested in the audiometric test chamber. In the testing of adults, the procedure that is followed is that first measures are obtained of air- and bone-conduction thresholds. This is followed by both continuous and interrupted Békésy tracings. The particular subsequent tests that are employed will depend upon whether a type I or II tracing or a type III or IV tracing emerges. Subsequent tests include the SISI, PB words, sentence tests, and others having as their goal specification of both the site of the lesion and the degree of auditory impariment. A distinct advantage of the location of the audio-vestibular laboratory in a hospital setting is that audiological diagnoses may be related to medical findings and likewise the medical findings compared with audiological results.

By reviewing some of the work of the Houston Speech and Hearing Center, an attempt has been made to demonstrate various kinds of audiological instrumentation and how instrumentation evolves through the development of meaningful diagnostic tests of hearing disorders.

OTHER AUDIOLOGICAL INSTRUMENTATION

Some instrumentation and associated tests utilized in audiology were not treated in the preceding section where specific features of the Houston Speech and Hearing Center were selected to emphasize certain aspects of audiological instrumentation. Among the instruments and tests that were not included were individual and group screening tests for children and adults, psychogalvanic skin-resistance audiometry, tests for functional hearing loss, auditory training units, and a device for measuring middle-ear impedance.

Screening tests that have as their purpose the identification of those persons with a hearing loss can either be individual tests or tests administered to groups of individuals. Two examples of pure-tone audiometers are shown in Figs. 5-57 and 5-58; both can be used for screening purposes. The second unit is portable and limited to screening uses at three fixed frequencies and three fixed levels. Some group screening tests, of the several that have been developed, used spoken numbers presented at successively decreasing levels. Others have required that the subject signal when he no longer heard tone pulses in a series of pulses presented at diminishing levels, while others have required that the number of tone pulses presented be counted.

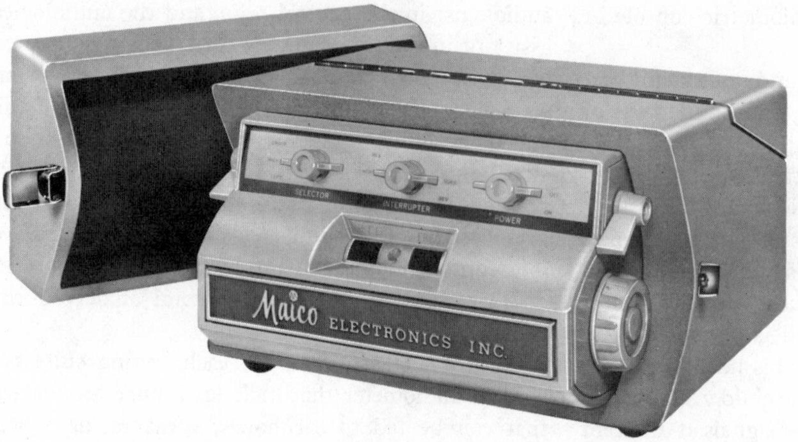

Fig. 5-57. Pure-tone audiometer (Maico Model MA-12).

Hollien and Thompson (1967) report on two forms (A and B) for a group screening test of hearing and subsequently have worked on additional forms for this test. They outline among their criteria that the validity and reliability should be high, that the false-fail rate should be low, that the test should be time-saving, that standard audiometric equipment can be used for testing, and that the test should be a task simple enough for children as young as first- and second-grade pupils. In the most recent work on the test, signals were presented from a Beltone 11-A audiometer through an impedance matching device to 40 Telephonic TDH-39 earphones. In the test procedure for the adult form A, pulse groups of four frequencies at five hearing levels are presented, whereas form B for children involves pulse groups at three frequencies and four hearing levels. Recent forms of the test provide for zero to three pulses at each frequency tested, presented in a descending level from 35 to 20 dB. Evaluation of this test in terms of reliability, validity, and efficiency indicates that the procedure meets the authors' criteria in the screening of large number of children.

Psychogalvanic skin-resistance audiometry is sometimes employed for testing the hearing of young children or individuals with functional hearing loss. The galvanic skin response (GSR), often referred to as the psychogalvanic reflex (PGSR), is an electrodermal response associated with sweating. It is assumed that the response reflects autonomic activity associated with emotional states. In clinical practice, techniques designed to measure the GSR are sometimes employed to explore internal and environmentally oriented factors related to anxiety, apprehension, and depression. In recent years the conditioned galvanic skin response has been used to assist in the determination of auditory thresholds of infants and adults who are difficult subjects when conventional audiometric techniques are employed. The GSR response may also be used as an indicator of a patient's anxiety level in psychotherapy. Current behavioral therapy procedures are based on the identification of anxiety states and subsequent deconditioning of the learned anxiety.

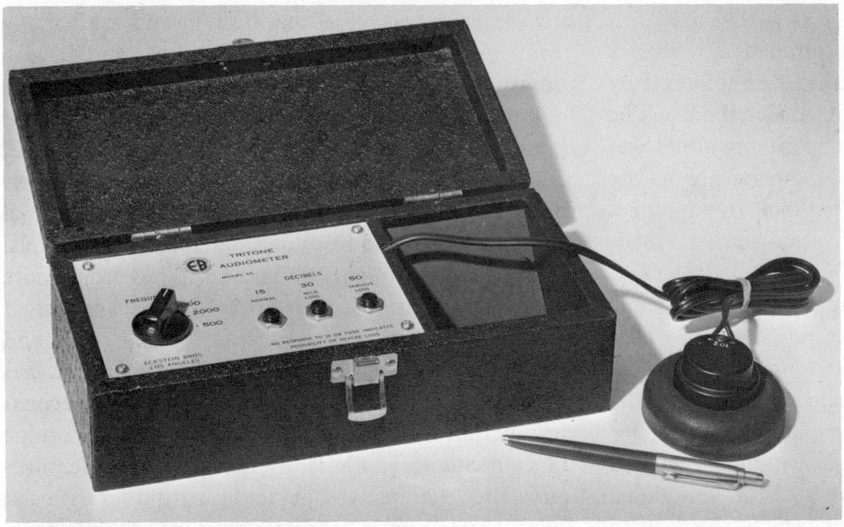

Fig. 5-58. Tritone audiometer (Eckstein Brothers Model 45).

The two basic techniques for investigating the galvanic response related to sweating are the Fere method and the Tarchanoff method. Fere developed the method of measuring skin resistance when an external current is applied; Tarchanoff discovered the skin potential change which arises from currents in the skin. Most investigators employ "resistance" rather than "potential" instrumentation.

In recording galvanic response, skin electrodes are usually fastened to the fingers, palm of the hand, or legs and then coupled to a resistance recorder, often known as a psychogalvanometer. When the indicating meter reveals that a steady-state balance has been achieved between the skin resistance of the subject and the electronic measuring device, the tracing mechanism is then turned on. The resulting trace is a line showing stabilized activity until the individual is subjected to a stimulating or conditioning experience. The GSR is very sensitive to sensory stimuli; factors related to alertness, attention, apprehension, and arousal result in corresponding changes in skin resistance. The magnitude of psychobiological arousal is related, therefore, to the lowering of skin-resistance level and the correlated magnitude of change in the psychogalvanic tracing. Fig. 5-59 illustrates a modern psychogalvanometer. In psychogalvanic skin-resistance audiometry, the conditioning procedure is followed whereby an unconditioned stimulus, electric

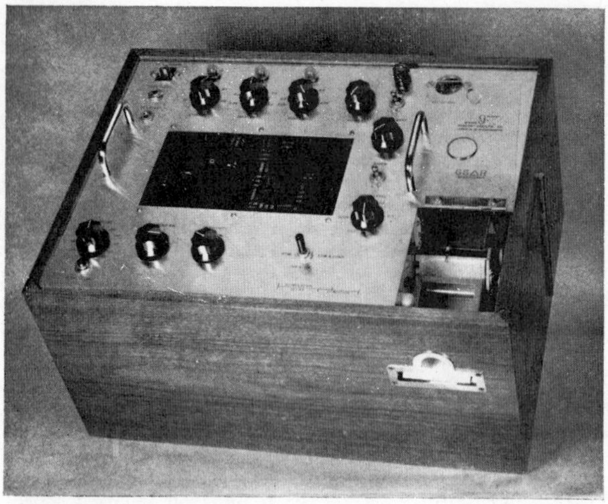

Fig. 5-59. Psychogalvanometer (Grason-Stadler Model E664).

shock, is substituted for a conditioned stimulus, a pure tone. Short tonal presentations are followed by partial reinforcement of the electric shock. The examiner interprets psychogalvanic readings to determine whether or not the responses are to the tones presented. Psychogalvanic audiometry requires an auxiliary unit, such as the Grason-Stadler PGSR shown in Fig. 5-59.

The terms functional hearing loss or nonorganic hearing loss are used to indicate hearing loss where organic involvements cannot be found. The loss is assumed to relate to psychological rather than organic factors. Several testing procedures have evolved for the identification of nonorganic hearing loss (O'Neill and Oyer, 1966). In the diagnosis of functional hearing loss, usually a battery of tests is required to reach a decision. Clinical audiometers include the capability for the administration of tests for functional impairment. The Allison model 22, shown in Fig. 5-54, for example, provides for seven tests which depend upon certain behavioral responses to various types of sensory stimulation, for example lateralization of sound controlled by relative levels at each ear (stenger tests and monaural threshold finding through binaural fusion test), inability of a patient to observe changing levels of speech and noise (Doerfler-Stewart test), the control of voice level by masking noise (Lombard test), conditioned physiologic responses to sound (psychogalvanic skin response test), and cybernetic control of speech (delayed auditory-feedback test). The use of a single clinical audiometer to cover a wide range of tests is an example, as has previously been indicated, of the incorporation of diagnostic test facilities into single audiometric units.

The discussion of audiological instrumentation, so far, has treated devices that are primarily for diagnoses. Less attention has been given to the development of instruments for therapy and rehabilitation, although presumably a number of instruments currently in use could be adapted advantageously for rehabilitative purposes. One class of instruments for the hard-of-hearing is special-purpose instruments for amplifying and controlling the sound level at the patient's ears.

Group hearing aids provide for amplification of speech for a group of listeners and generally control the amplification so that the output level at the earphone is limited. These units contain limitor or compressor circuits that automatically control amplification above a certain level. Auditory trainers also provide compression of amplication and are usually group units that drive several headsets and have a provision for the playing of disc records in addition to speech amplification. Compression amplification is important for use with the hard-of-hearing because, although their hearing thresholds are elevated, their thresholds of pain may not be and, as a result, normal amplification would result in intolerable sound levels.

Another instrument, different in kind from those previously discussed, is a device for the analysis of middle-ear function. In addition to otoscopic and audiometric information for diagnostic purposes, it is sometimes helpful to have an evaluation of the acoustic function of the middle ear. The acoustic bridge (Grason-Stadler model 3, Zwislocki bridge) measures impedance parameters at the eardrum (Zwislocki, 1963). Sound waves are introduced into the ear canal and amplitude and phase relationships of the reflected wave yield a measure of impedance at the eardrum. Values of various frequencies are plotted and an examiner then makes interpretations relative to various middle-ear pathologies. Different patterns, plotting frequency versus impedance, differentiate normal, otosclerotic, and ossicularly discontinuous ears.

TEMPORAL MEASUREMENT AND INSTRUMENTATION

Previous mention has been made in this chapter to digital and analog devices, to small, special-purpose computers, to analog-to-digital and digital-to-analog

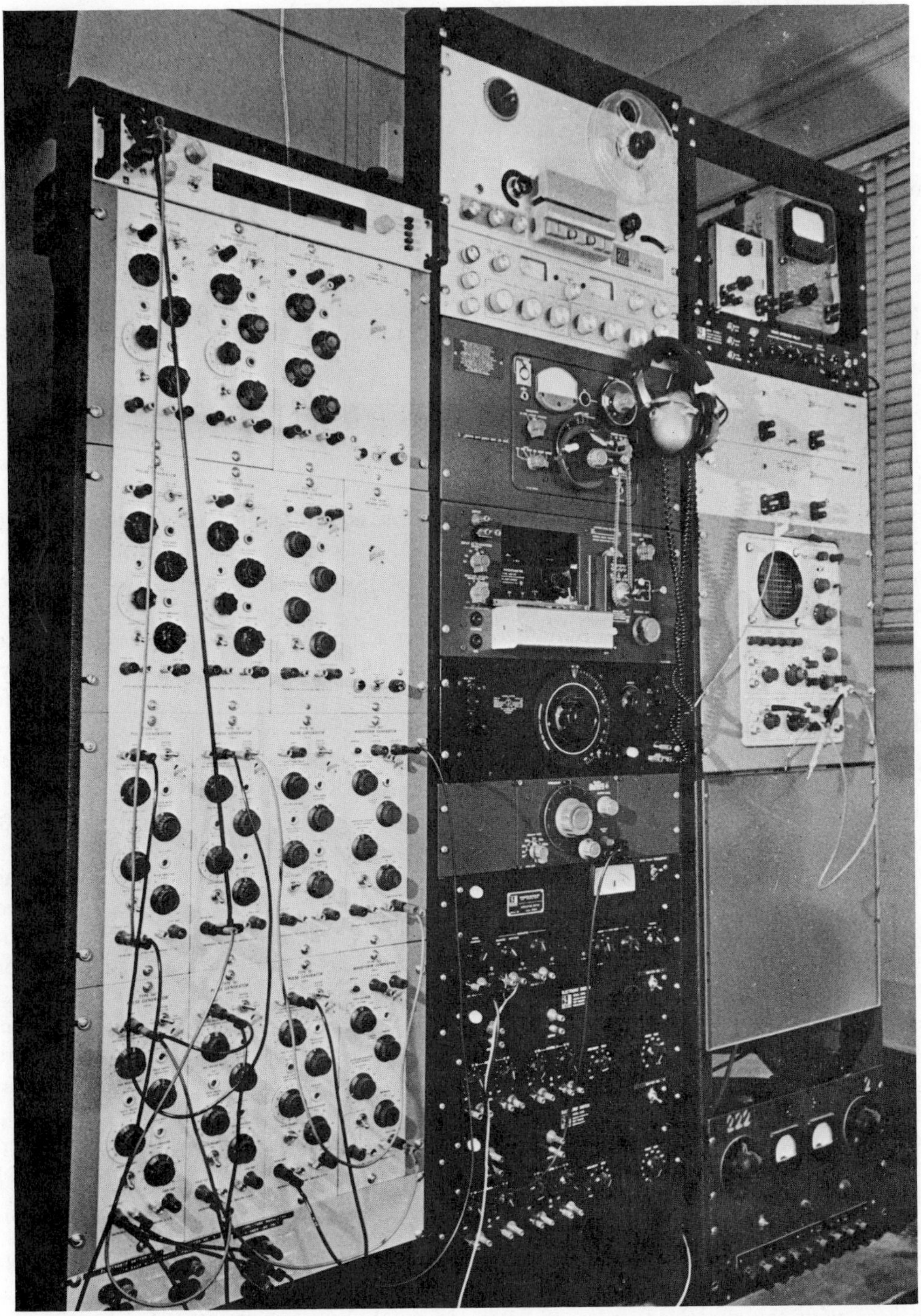

Fig. 5-60. Instruments for the control and measurement of temporal aspects of speech and hearing.

converters, and to automation of experimental procedures. All of these items can be related to measurement and control of temporal aspects of speech and hearing. The most important single parameter for both speech and hearing is time. Speech, a quasi-continuous signal, can be represented acoustically by changing intensity patterns in time. Auditory perception is possible because of these kinds of changes.

Not only can the external speech or hearing signal be viewed in a time dimension, but the internal representation of these signals can also be considered as time based. Auditory perception can be viewed as a discrete time sampling of environmental events by the organism, and speech can be viewed as a series of time-controlled events. Investigators of both normal and anomalous speech and hearing are well aware of the importance of being able to measure temporal aspects of speech and of the hearing signal; they are also aware that temporal aspects are among the most important parameters of speech and hearing. In recent years considerable advancement has been made in the kinds of instrumentation that can make temporal measurements, that can convert an analog signal, such as speech, to a digital form, that can convert digital data, such as a series of numbers, to an analog representation, and that can store and extract information from sizable amounts of data. Actual instruments could include counters, pulse and waveform generators, analog-to-digital and digital-to-analog converters, and special-purpose computers, to mention only a few of those instruments available to workers in the area of speech and hearing. These instruments provide possibilities for analysis and understanding of speech or auditory perception, for the synthesis of speech and speechlike signals to be used in investigations, diagnosis, or therapy, and possibilities for advantageous automation of both experiments and therapy procedures that have not been previously possible except in a few restricted laboratory settings where sizable instrumentation and computation facilities were available.

An instrumental grouping that includes pulse and waveform generators, electronic switches, and counters with associated equipment such as amplifiers, oscilloscopes, and graphic level recorders provides a considerable capability for studies that concern temporal processing by the auditory system or measurement of various time and frequency properties of speech. An instrumental grouping that includes the kinds of instruments listed above is shown in Fig. 5-60. One series of investigations that has been conducted utilizing these instruments has been concerned with the perceived order of tone pulses (Peters, 1967) where the perceptual order of sequential events has been found to be dependent upon other properties of the signal instead of the actual physical order of a series of pulses under certain circumstances. Other work in this laboratory has treated the effect of degree of waveform modulation upon the efficiency of pitch perception (Mahaffey, 1967). Other investigations have been concerned with auditory fusion, judgments of order and successiveness of short temporal events, the effects of uncorrelated and correlated noise upon speech intelligibility, and identification of perceptual units of ongoing speech. Studies like the ones mentioned can be instrumented easily and with precision using equipment of the kind listed above.

An increased capability for controlling and measuring temporal parameters of speech and hearing phenomena, in addition to that provided by the instruments discussed in the preceding paragraph, can be achieved by the acquisition of a special-purpose laboratory digital computer with appropriate input and output facilities. These facilities include analog-to-digital and digital-to-analog converters as well as other computer peripheral equipment for data transformation, control, and display. Analog data can be derived from speech and other sound sources in the form of a varying voltage for conversion to digital information that can be processed by the computer. Digital information, in turn, can be converted to sound by a digital-to-analog process. An illustration was previously shown (Fig. 5-50) that depicted analog-to-digital and digital-to-analog conversion for computer processing of sound waves. The addition of a computer as part of the instrumentation in a laboratory provides capabilities for analysis, measurement, and control of properties of speech and hearing that are beyond those that can be considered to be primarily temporal aspects. The computer and associated equipment provide the potential for various analyses of speech and other signals, for the synthesis of speech and other sounds, for the automation of experimentation that in fact makes the computer part of the experimental process, for modeling or simulating properties of speech or hearing mechanisms, and for data reduction and analysis as well as a number of other possibilities for many aspects of speech and hearing.

INSTRUMENT CALIBRATION

In concluding this chapter, special attention must be directed to the importance of equipment calibration. Electronic instruments and mechanical devices are expected to comply with predetermined specifications. The degree to which such instruments consistently meet established calibration values is of paramount importance in clinical and research application.

Microphones, earphones, amplifiers, filters, speakers, audiometers, galvanometers, recorders, polygraphs, and similar equipment justifiably employed in clinics and laboratories should be checked upon arrival and during scheduled time intervals.

Among the frequent causes of instrument failure are inherent faults in design, laxity in quality control during manufacturing, mishandling during shipment, incorrect assembly and usage, accidental injury, deterioration, improper maintenance, and faulty repair. It is important, therefore, that appropriate calibration procedures should be instituted to reflect instrument stability, reliability, and validity.

Illustrative of calibration techniques are the following descriptions concerning earphones, microphones, amplifiers and associated equipment, speakers, and audiometers. These instruments are component parts of many electronic systems.

Earphone Calibration

Earphones are usually calibrated by checking the frequency response, electromechanical sensitivity, distortion characteristics, and "maximum undistorted" output. In order to accomplish this an artificial ear, consisting of a headset coupler, a calibrated condenser microphone, preamplifier, and power supply, is usually employed. A block diagram of an earphone calibration circuit is given in Fig. 5-61. Subjective loudness-balance tests may be used to supplement objective laboratory measurements. In addition to the artificial ear, one or two vacuum tube voltmeters, a calibrated audio-signal generator, attenuator, cathode-ray oscillograph, and a wave analyzer are necessary for the complete calibration of the earphone.

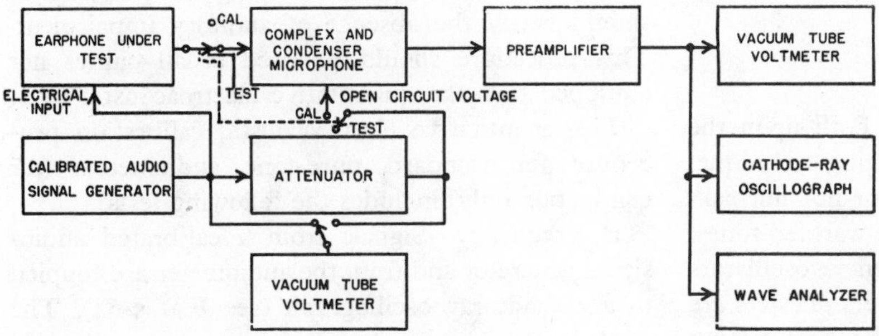

Fig. 5-61. Earphone calibration circuit.

Microphone Calibration

Microphones may be calibrated under either free-field or closed-coupler conditions, depending upon the application of the microphone. The latter method would be employed for a condenser microphone used in an artificial ear. The technique employs a calibrated earphone acting as a standard and the microphone under test as the unknown. The microphone's response would be compared to that of a known or previously calibrated microphone.

For free-field calibration, reciprocity methods may be employed to give absolute measurements of microphone sensitivity and frequency response. Test circuits similar to those employed in testing speakers may be utilized also. The response of the unknown microphone may be obtained by comparing its performance with that of a calibrated standard microphone.

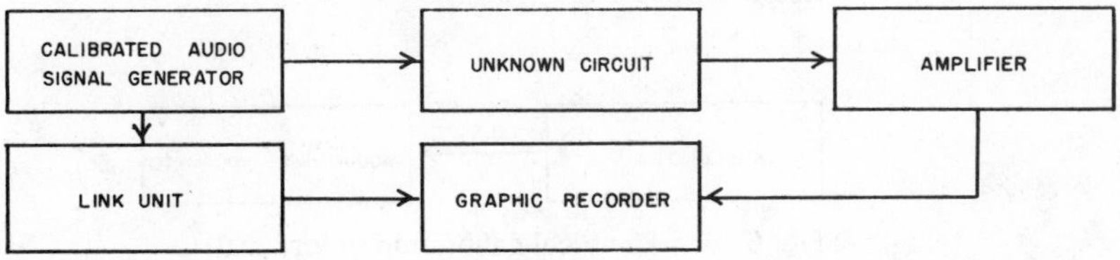

Fig. 5-62. Amplifier filter, equalizer, etc., test circuit.

Amplifier, Filter, Equalizer, etc., Calibration

Tests of amplifier, filter, and equalizer performance will vary with the application and the degree of precision in testing required. Customarily, gain, frequency response, harmonic distortion, intermodulation distortion, and signal-to-noise-ratio tests may be employed in part or in total for the various circuits. Harmonic and intermodulation distortion may be measured by a variety of techniques. Harmonic distortion can be tested using a conventional wave analyzer. Special circuits are available for determining intermodulation distortion.

Frequency-response, gain, and signal-to-noise-ratio measurements may be obtained using a mechanically linked oscillator and graphic recorder test circuit as indicated in Fig. 5-62.

Speaker Testing

The results of speaker tests depend both upon the acoustic test environment and the testing technique. Speakers may be tested in anechoic or in "normal" rooms, using frequency-modulated or warbled tones, band-pass noise, and sweep-frequency oscillators mechanically linked to graphic recorders. Testers are not in complete agreement as to the best testing methods. However, the method selected should give reproducible results. A widely used method of testing speaker frequency response employs a test oscillator whose frequency dial is mechanically linked to the carriage of a graphic recorder (see Fig. 5-63). The

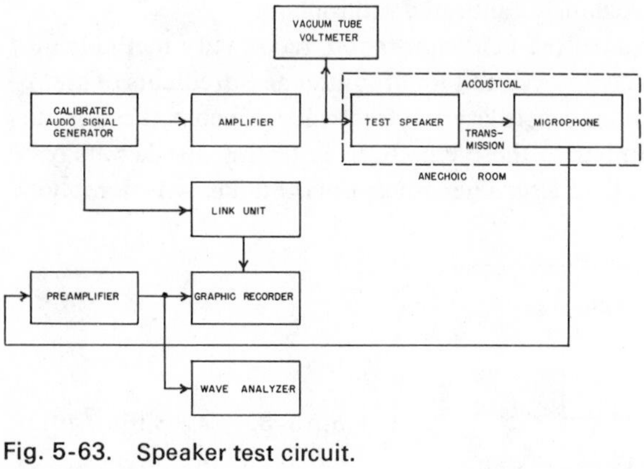

Fig. 5-63. Speaker test circuit.

continuously variable frequency, constant-amplitude output of the oscillator is amplified and coupled to the test speaker. The speaker and a calibrated microphone are placed in an anechoic room. The microphone output is amplified and coupled to the graphic recorder. Thus, a graphic record of the amplitude response versus frequency is obtained. This equipment may be provided with accessory devices for testing speaker directivity. The relative efficiency of speakers may be tested using the above equipment. Wave analyzers may be added to obtain measures of harmonic distortion.

Audiometer Calibration (Pure Tone)

Qualitative calibration of audiometers is conducted by testing the hearing of six to 10 subjects of known hearing acuity. Usually subjects are chosen who have no history of previously known ear disease and who are reported to have normal hearing. The audiometer should verify the absence of auditory impairment. This procedure should be used at all clinics not equipped to make quantitative electroacoustic tests.

The quantitative electroacoustic calibration procedure for standard pure-tone audiometers (air conduction only) includes the following tests:

1. Frequency—Signals from a calibrated audio-signal generator and from the audiometer are coupled to a cathode-ray oscillograph (see Fig. 5-64). The

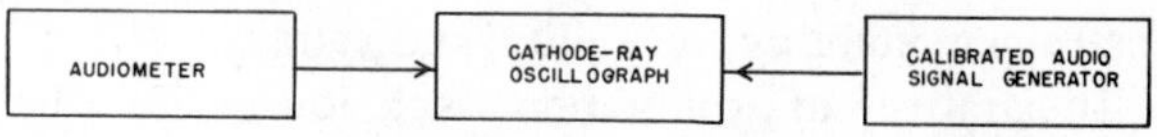

Fig. 5-64. Lissajous frequency calibration of audiometer.

resulting Lissajous patterns indicate the comparison of the known frequency (audio-oscillator) with the frequency produced by the audiometer.

2. Linearity of "Loss Dial"—To check the accuracy of the Hearing Loss Dial (attenuator) readings, the audiometer output is measured at the terminals of the headset with a vacuum tube voltmeter calibrated in decibels (see Fig. 5-65).

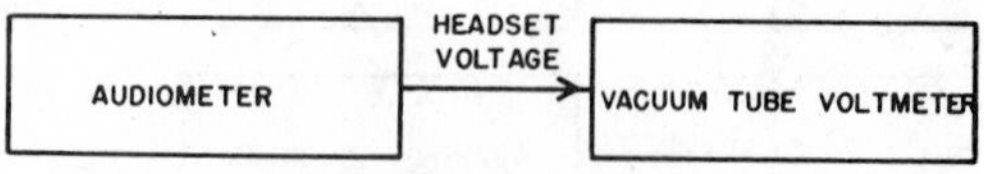

Fig. 5-65. Electrical calibration of loss dial.

3. "Loss Dial"—Accumulative Error—The accumulative error in the readings from the Hearing Loss Dial is calculated from the linearity of "loss dial" measurements.

4. Acoustic Calibration—The acoustic calibration is made by using the maximum permissible output level per frequency of the audiometer and then

expressing the result in terms of the audiometer zero-reference level (see Fig. 5-66). Threshold reference

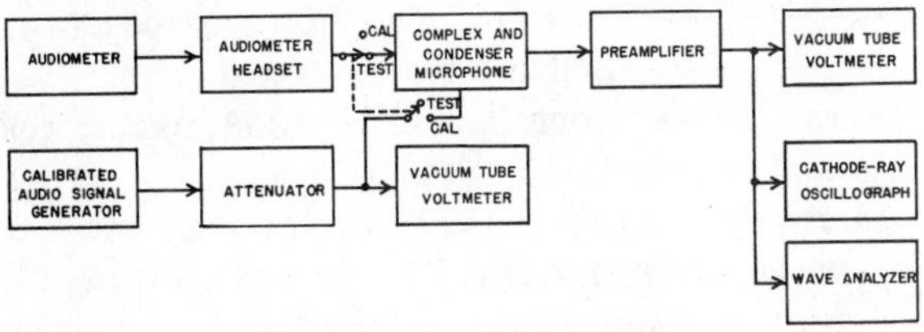

Fig. 5-66. Acoustic calibration of audiometer.

levels for audiometers can be adjusted to correspond to either the 1951 American Standards Association levels or to those recommended by the International Organization for Standardization 1964, using audiometer calibration equipment. The latter (ISO) standards are generally in use today, and sound-pressure levels at various frequencies can be calibrated using, for example, a Bruel and Kjaer model 158 calibration unit. This unit is shown in Fig. 5-67. Components of the calibration equipment include a sound-level meter, an octave filter set, an artificial ear, a pistonphone, and condenser microphone. Calibration is at 60 dB hearing level.

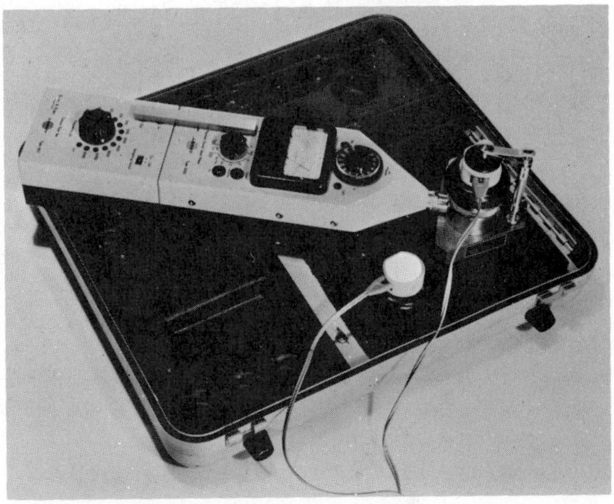

Fig. 5-67. Audiometer calibration unit (Bruel and Kjaer Model 158).

INSTRUMENTS IN USE

As an indication of the wide diversity of instruments in actual use in the present decade, the authors have compiled a listing from the pages of the *Journal of Speech and Hearing Research*, 1960 through June 1967. It is doubtful that we have succeeded in noting all of the instruments named in those pages. Certainly some instrumental arrays that were assembled in individual laboratories could have escaped our notice. However, the tabulation is reasonably complete and should provide some assistance for the laboratory that is just starting or that wishes to add to its armamentarium. The list is presented in alphabetical order, with the generic name, manufacturer, and model number of the instrument followed by the year, volume, and page number of the Journal.

ACOUSTIC BRIDGE. (Zwislocki) Grason-Stadler E8872A. 1965, 8, 214; 1967, 10, 165.

AMMETER, GRAPHIC. Esterline Angus AW. 1964, 7, 57.

AMPLIFIER. Bogen. DB-110. 1962, 5, 145.

———. Bruel and Kjaer 2601. 1962, 5, 238.

———. General Radio Tuned 1232A. 1965, 8, 206.

———. McIntosh. 1960, 3, 306.

———. ———. Type 20W2. 1962, 5, 125.

———. Offner 190. 1964, 7, 154.

———. Presto 900-A4. 1962, 5, 145.

———. Thordarson T30WO3. 1960, 3, 292. Also model T-31W10AX. 1964, 7, 337.

AMPLIFIER, CARRIER. Sanborn 350-1100B. 1964, 7, 234. Also carrier amplifier-recorder system 321. 1967, 10, 134.

AMPLIFIER, MICROPHONE. Bruel and Kjaer 2604. 1965, 8, 254. Also model 2602. 1966, 9, 139. Also model 2603. 1967, 10, 377.

AMPLIFIER, OPERATIONAL. Monroe 203, 1966, 9, 501.

AMPLIFIER-PENWRITER, Offner Dynograph 542. 1963, 6, 5.

AMPLIFIER, POWER. Aerosound Mark II. 1961, 4, 75. Also Ultra Linear Type II. 1966, 9, 279.

———, ———. McIntosh MI-60. 1966, 9, 597.

AMPLIFIER, STRAIN GAGE. Sanborn 64-500B. 1962, 5, 186; 1964, 7, 177.

ANALYZER, OCTAVE BAND. General Radio 1550-A. 1964, 7. 248.

ANECHOIC CHAMBER. Bruel and Kjaer 4212. 1967, 10, 377.

ARTIFICIAL EAR. Audio Instrument Co. 1962, 5, 246.
———. Bruel and Kjaer 4152. 1966, 9, 452; 1966, 9, 501.
ARTIFICIAL HEAD (Custom). 1967, 10, 177.
ARTIFICIAL MASTOID. Beltone M5a. 1965, 8, 255; 1966, 9, 484; 1967, 10, 234.
ATTENUATOR. Daven 2512 and 2514. 1963, 6, 58; 1964, 7, 167. Also T-530F. 1964, 7, 167.
ATTENUATOR, RECORDING. Grason-Stadler E3262A. 1966, 9, 563; 1967, 10, 100.
ATTENUATOR, VARIABLE. Hewlett-Packard 350B. 1960, 3, 250; 1963, 6, 362; also model 350A. 1961, 4, 376; 1962, 5, 104; 1962, 5, 125; 1964, 7, 337; 1966, 9, 182; also model 350AB. 1962, 5, 186; also model 350D. 1966, 9, 598.
AUDIOMETER. Allison Series 21C. 1961, 4, 270; 1967, 10, 142.
———. Ambco Otometer. 1967, 10, 68.
———. Amplivox 61. 1967, 10, 94.
———. Beltone 15A. 1960, 3, 306; 1962, 5, 5; 1962, 5, 246; 1964, 7, 57; 1965, 8, 51; 1965, 8, 151; 1967, 10, 329. Also model 10A. 1962, 5, 114; 1963, 6, 31; 1964, 7, 176. Also model 15C. 1966, 9, 612; 1967, 10, 314. Model 14A. 1963, 6, 102.
———. Purdue Research S-1. 1966, 9, 597.
———. Zenith ZA-100T. 1965, 8, 214; 1967, 10, 165.
AUDIOMETER ACCESSORY KIT. Beltone 15. 1963, 6, 102.
AUDIOMETER, BEKESY TYPE. Grason-Stadler E800. 1962, 5, 5; 1962, 5, 285; 1963, 6, 65; 1964, 7, 80; 1964, 7, 273; 1965, 8, 87; 1965, 8, 105; 1965, 8, 254; 1966, 9, 574; 1967, 10, 105. Also model E800-4. 1967, 10, 234.
AUDIOMETER CALIBRATION UNIT. Allison 3A. 1962, 5, 145. Also model 300. 1961, 4, 271; 1965, 8, 254; 1966, 9, 299.
———. Bruel and Kjaer. 1967, 10, 142.
AUDIOMETER, NOISE. Grason-Stadler 830S1. 1967, 10, 319.
AUDIOMETER, SPEECH. Grason-Stadler 162. 1962, 5, 246; 1963, 6, 266; 1964, 7, 273; 1965, 8, 105; 1966, 9, 139; 1966, 9, 142; 1966, 9, 183; 1966, 9, 228; 1966, 9, 254; 1966, 9, 563; 1967, 10, 112; 1967, 10, 189; 1967, 10, 291; 1967, 10, 391.
AUDIOMETRIC BOOTH OR TESTING ROOM, see SOUND PROOFED ROOM.
BEKESY-TYPE AUDIOMETER, see AUDIOMETER, Békésy-Type.
BONE RECEIVER OR VIBRATOR, see RECEIVER, BONE.
CALIBRATING CUP, MICROPHONE. General Radio 1552-B. 1965, 8, 225.
CAMERA, MAGNETIC SOUND. Cinephonic, 1963, 6, 20.
CAMERA, MOTION PICTURE. Arriflex 16 mm. 1966, 9, 259.
———, ———. Auricon Super-Pro 1200. 1963, 6, 92.
———, ———. Bell and Howell. 1963, 6, 20.
CAMERA, OSCILLOSCOPE. Fairchild F-246A. 1966, 9, 598.
CAMERA, TV. Plumbican. 1966, 9, 259.
CARRIER AMPLIFIER, see AMPLIFIER, CARRIER.
CATHETER, POLYETHYLENE. PE 200. 1967, 10, 134.
CINEFLUOROGRAPHIC UNIT. 1963, 6, 20.
CLICK GENERATOR. Schmitt. 1963, 6, 58.
COMPUTER. Correlogram (Custom). 1966, 9, 492.
———. Enhancetron 1024. 1967, 10, 374.
———. HAVOC (Custom). 1965, 8, 374.
———. IBM 650. 1964, 7, 39. Also model 709. 1964, 7, 84. Also model 1620. 1966, 9, 492.
———. Mnemotron CAT400. 1963, 6, 58; model 400 B. 1966, 9, 361; 1967, 10, 258.
COUNTER, ELECTRONIC. Beckman 7350. 1967, 10, 377.
———, ———. Hewlett-Packard 522B. 1962, 5, 238.
COUNTER, FREQUENCY-PERIOD. Computer Measurements 201C. 1966, 9, 598.
COUNTER, SWEEP. Mnemotron 646. 1967, 10, 258.
DELAYED FEEDBACK UNIT. Echo-Vox Sr. 1966, 9, 597.
DEVELOPER. Eastman D-76, 1960, 3, 320.
EARPHONE. Beyer, DT-48. 1963, 6, 31; 1966, 9, 279.
———. BRUSH. 1964, 7, 37; 1967, 10, 59.
———. Pedersen B-228A. 1965, 8, 105.
———. Permoflux PDR-1. 1960, 3, 71; 1961, 4, 75; 1962, 5, 145. Also PDR-3. 1967, 10, 350. Also PDR-8. 1961, 4, 376; 1962, 5, 125; 1967, 10, 278. Also PDR-10. 1961, 4, 205; 1964, 7, 166. Also PDR-39, 1966, 9, 612. Also PMR 16. 1961, 4, 106.
———. Rudmose Otocup. 1966, 9, 597.
———. Sharpe Type B HA-10. 1966, 9, 373, also type HA-10. 1967, 10, 368.
———. (British) Standard Telephone and Cables 4026. 1961, 4, 3.
———. Telephonic TDH-39. 1960, 3, 328; 1961, 4, 141; 1961, 4, 165; 1961, 4, 270; 1962, 5, 186; 1962, 5, 218; 1962, 5, 238; 1962, 5, 285; 1963, 6, 102; 1964, 7, 83; 1964, 7, 176; 1964, 7, 273; 1964, 7, 326; 1965, 8, 151; 1965, 8, 254; 1966, 9, 142; 1966, 9, 182; 1966, 9, 228; 1966, 9, 254; 1966, 9, 154; 1966, 9, 362; 1966, 9, 463; 1966, 9, 563; 1966, 9, 574; 1967, 10, 95; 1967, 10, 113; 1967, 10, 142; 1967, 10, 234; 1967, 10, 258; 1957, 10, 291; 1967, 10, 315; 1967, 10, 329; 1967, 10, 345; 1967, 10, 391.
———. Western Electric 705-A. 1964, 7, 14.
EARPHONE, CUSHION. Grason-Stadler 001. 1967, 10, 233.
———, ———. MNAF-48490-1. 1967, 10, 278.

BIBLIOGRAPHY

Atkinson, C. 1953. Adaptation to delayed side-tone. *J. Speech Hearing Disorders*, 18, 386–391.

Bilger, R. 1958. Intensive determinants of remote masking. *J. acoust. soc. Amer.*, 30, 817–824.

Black, J. 1951. The effects of delayed side-tone upon vocal rate and intensity. *J. Speech Hearing Disorders*, 16, 56–60.

———. 1957. Multiple-choice intelligibility tests. *J. Speech Hearing Disorders*, 22, 216–217.

Chase, R. 1958. Effect of delayed auditory feedback on the repetition of speech sounds. *J. Speech Hearing Disorders*, 23, 583–590.

Cherry, C. 1961. Two ears—but one world, *In* Sensory communication. Rosenblith, W., ed. New York: M.I.T. and Wiley. Pp. 99–117.

Christovich, L., Fant, G., and deSerpa-Leitao, A. 1966. Mimicking and perception of synthetic vowels. Speech Transmission Lab. Quart. Progress and Status Report. Pp. 1–3 (part 2).

Coker, C. 1968. Synthesis by rule from articulatory parameters. Bell Telephone Lab., Murray Hill. Personal communication received from James L. Flanagan.

Cooper, F. 1950. Spectrum analysis. *J. acoust. soc Amer.*, 22, 761–762.

Cowan, M. 1936. Pitch and intensity characteristics of stage speech. *Arch. Speech*, Supplement.

Darley, F. 1940. A normative study of oral reading rate. Univ. Iowa: Master's thesis.

Delattre, P. 1951. The physiological interpretation of sound spectrograms. *Proc. mod. Lang. Asson.*, 66, 864–875.

———. 1963. Voyelles diphtonguees et voyelles pures. *French Rev.*, 37, 64–76.

———. 1965. Comparing the phonetic features of English, French, German and Spanish. Heidelberg: Verlag.

———. 1967. Acoustic or articulatory invariance? *Glossa*, 1, 3–24.

———, and Freeman, D. 1968. A dialect study of American *r*'s by x-ray motion picture. *Linguistics*, 44, 29–68.

———, Liberman, A., and Cooper, F. 1955. Acoustic loci and transitional cues for consonants. *J. acoust. soc. Amer.*, 27, 769–773.

———, Olsen, C., and Poenack, E. 1962. A comparative study of declarative intonation in American English and Spanish. *Hispania*, 40, 233–241.

Delattre, P., Poenack, E., and Olsen, C. 1965. Some characteristics of German intonation for the expression of continuation and finality. *Phonetica*, 13, 134–161.

Dempsey, M. 1949. The Purdue pitch meter: a direct-reading fundamental frequency analyzer. *J. Speech Hearing Disorders*, 15, 135–141.

———. 1955. Design and evaluation of a fundamental frequency recorder for complex sounds. Purdue Univ.: Ph. D. dissertation.

———, Siskind, R., Hanley, T., and Steer, M. 1953. A fundamental frequency recorder for complex sounds. Technical Report No. SpecDevCen 104-2-34 by the Purdue Univ. Voice Communications Lab. for the Special Devices Center of the Office of Naval Research on SpecDevCen Contract N6 ori-104, T.O. II, Project 20-F-8.

Draegert, G. 1951. Relationships between voice variables and speech intelligibility in high level noise. *Speech Monogr.*, 18, 272–278.

Dudley, H. 1939. Remaking speech. *J. acoust. soc. Amer.*, 11, 169–177.

———, Riesz, R., and Watkins, S. 1939. A synthetic speaker. *J. Franklin Inst.*, 227, 739–764.

Dunn, H. 1930. A new analyzer of speech and music. *Bell Lab. Record.*, 9, 118–123.

Faaborg-Andersen, K., Yanagihara, N., and von Leden, H. 1967. Vocal pitch and intensity regulation. *Arch. Ootolaryng.*, 85, 448–454.

Fairbanks, G. 1954. A theory of the speech mechanism as a servo-system. *J. Speech Hearing Disorders*, 19, 133–139.

———, Everett, W., and Jaeger, R. 1954. Method for time or frequency compression of speech. *Tr. Inst. Radio Engineers*, AU2, 7–12.

———, Guttman, N., and Miron, M. 1957. Auditory comprehension of repeated high-speed messages. *J. Speech Hearing Disorders*, 22, 20–22.

———, and Hoaglin, L. 1941. An experimental study of the durational characteristics of the voice during the expression of emotion. *Speech Monogr.*, 8, 85–90.

Fant, G. 1960. Acoustic theory of speech production. The Hague: Mouton.

———, and Martony, J. 1962. Speech synthesis, *Speech Transmission Lab. quart. Prog. Status Report*, 18–24.

Flanagan, J. 1967. Spectrum analysis in speech coding. *IEEE Tr. Audio and Electroacoustics*, AU-15, 66–69.

———, and Golden, R. M. 1966. Phase vocoder. *Bell System Tech. J.*, 45, 1493–1509.

Fletcher, H. 1953. Speech and hearing in communication. New York: Van Nostrand. Ch. 4.

Franke, P. 1939. A preliminary study validating the measurement of oral reading rate in words per minute. Univ. Iowa: Master's thesis.

Gabor, D., the following references in *J. Inst. Electr. Engineers:* 1946, 93 (Part 3); 427–429; 1947, 94 (Part 3); 369–386; 1948, 95 (Part 3); 39, 411–412.

Griesman, B. 1943. Mechanism of phonation demonstrated by planography of the larynx. *Arch. Otolaryng.*, 38, 117–126.

Gruenz, O., and Schott, L. 1949. Extraction and portrayal of pitch of speech sounds. *J. acoust. soc. Amer.*, 21, 487–495.

Hanley, T. 1951. An analysis of vocal frequency and duration characteristics of selected samples of speech from three American dialect regions. *Speech Monogr.*, 18, 78–93.

———. 1968. Comparative responses to delayed auditory feedback among speakers of four languages. *Phonetica*, 18, 46–54.

———, and Snidecor, J. 1967. Some acoustic similarities among languages. *Phonetica*, 17, 141–148.

———, ———, and Ringel, R. 1966. Some acoustic differences among languages. *Phonetica*, 14, 97–107.

Henrikson, E. 1943. Note on voice recordings. *J. Speech Hearing Disorders*, 8, 133–135.

———, and Irwin, J. 1949. Voice recording—some findings and some problems. *J. Speech Hearing Disorders*, 14, 227–233.

Hirsch, I. 1959. Auditory perception of temporal order. *J. acoust. soc. Amer.*, 31, 759–767.

———, and Sherrick, C., Jr. 1961. Perceived order in different sense modalities. *J. exper. Psychol.*, 62, 423–432.

Hollien, H. 1968. The fundamental frequency indicator (FFI). Personal communication.

———. 1962. Vocal fold thickness and fundamental frequency of phonation. *J. Speech Hearing Res.*, 5, 237–243.

———, and Curtis, J. 1960. A laminagraphic study of vocal pitch. *J. Speech Hearing Res.*, 3, 361–371.

———, ———, and Coleman, R. 1968. Investigation of laryngeal phenomena by stroboscopic laminagraphy. *Med. Res. Engineering*, 7, 24–27.

Hollien, H., Malcik, E., and Hollien, B., 1965. Adolescent voice change in southern white males, *Speech Monogr.*, 32, 87–90.

———, and Moore, P. 1960. Measurements of the vocal folds during changes in pitch. *J. Speech Hearing Res.*, 3, 158–165.

———, and Thompson, C. L. 1967. A group screening test of hearing. *J. auditory Res.*, 7, 85–92.

———, and ———, 1968. Two additional forms of the Hollien-Thompson Group Screening Test. *J. auditory Res.*, 8, 143–150.

Hunt, F. 1935. Direct-reading frequency meter. *Rev. sci. Instrum.*, 6, 43.

Irwin, J., and Becklund, O. 1953. Norms for maximum repetitive rates for certains sounds established with with the sylrater. *J. Speech Hearing Disorders*, 18, 149–160.

Isshiki, N. 1964. Regulatory mechanism of voice intensity variation. *J. Speech Hearing Res.*, 7, 17–29.

———. 1965. Vocal intensity and air flow rate. *Folia Phoniat.*, 17, 92–104.

Jerger, J. 1960. Békésy audiometry in analysis of auditory disorders. *J. Speech Hearing Res.*, 3, 275–287.

———. 1962. Comparative evaluation of some auditory measures. *J. Speech Hearing Res.*, 5, 3–17.

———. 1967. The audiological examination as an aid in diagnosis. *Arch. Otolaryng.*, 85, 552–554.

———, and Jerger, S. 1965. Critical evaluation of SAL audiometry. *J. Speech Hearing Res.*, 8, 103–127.

———, and ———. 1966. Critical off-time in VIIIth nerve disorders. *J. Speech Hearing Res.*, 9, 573–583.

———, and ———. 1967. Psycho-acoustic comparison of cochlear and VIIIth nerve disorders. *J. Speech Hearing Res.*, 10, 659–688.

———, ———, Ainsworth, J., Caram, P. 1966. Recovery of auditory function after surgical removal of cerebellar tumor. *J. Speech Hearing Disorders*, 31, 378–382.

———, Malmquist, C., and Speaks, C. 1966. Comparison of some speech intelligibility tests in the evaluation of hearing aid performance. *J. Speech Hearing Res.*, 9, 253–258.

———, Shedd, J., and Harford, E. 1959. On the detection of extremely small changes in sound intensity. *Arch. Otolaryng.*, 69, 200–211.

———, Speaks, C., and Malmquist, C. 1966. Hearing-aid performance and hearing-aid selection. *J. Speech Hearing Res.*, 9, 136–149.

Kelly, J., and Steer, M. 1949. Revised concept of rate. *J. Speech Hearing Disorders*, 14, 222–226.

LeBel, C. 1951. Fundamentals of magnetic recording. New York: Audio Devices Co.

Lee, B. 1951. Artificial stutter. *J. Speech Hearing Disorders*, 16, 53–55.

Levitt, H., and Bricker, P. 1967. An objective procedure for reading VU meters. Murray Hill: Bell Telephone Lab.

Lewis, D., and Tiffin, J. 1934. A psychophysical study of individual differences in speaking ability. *Arch. Speech*, 1, 43–60.

Liberman, A. 1957. Some results of research on speech perception. *J. acoust. soc. Amer.*, 29, 117–123.

———, Cooper, F., Harris, K., and MacNeilage, P. 1962. A motor theory of speech perception. *Proc. Speech Commun. Seminar*, Vol. 2. Stockholm: Royal Institute of Technology.

———, Delattre, P., Cooper, F., and Gerstman, L. 1954. The role of consonant-vowel transitions in the perception of the stop and nasal consonants. *Psychol. Monogr.*, 68, 1–14.

Licklider, J. 1948. The influence of interaural phase relations upon the masking of speech by white noise. *J. acoust. soc. Amer.*, 20, 150–159.

———, and Miller, G. 1951. The perception of speech, *In* Handbook of experimental psychology. Stevens, S., ed. New York: Wiley. Pp. 1040–1074.

Liljencrants, J. 1967. The OVE III Speech Synthesizer. *Speech Transm. Lab. quart. Prog. Status Report*, 76–81.

Lisker, L. 1957. Closure durations and the intervocalic voiced-voiceless distinction in English. *Language*, 33, 42–49.

McCandless, G. 1967. Clinical application of evoked response audiometry. *J. Speech Hearing Res.*, 10, 468–478.

———, and Best, L. 1964. Evoked response to auditory stimuli in man using a summing computer. *J. Speech Hearing Res.*, 7, 193–201.

Mahaffey, R. 1967(A). Some effects of cosine amplitude modulation on the pitch of tone bursts. *J. acoust. soc. Amer.*, 41, 1591.

Metfessel, M. 1926. Techniques for objective studies of the vocal art. *Psychol. Monogr.*, 36, 1–40.

———. 1928. A photographic method of measuring pitch. *Science*, 68, 430–432.

Michel, J., Hollien, H., and Moore, P. 1966. Speaking fundamental frequency characteristics of 15, 16, and 17 year-old girls. *Language and Speech*, 9, 46–51.

Miller, D. 1937. The science of musical sounds. New York: Macmillan. Pp. 70–91.

———. 1937. Sound waves, their shape and speed. New York: Macmillan. Ch. 2.

Moore, P., and von Leden, H. 1958. Dynamic variations in the vibratory pattern in the normal larynx. *Folia Phoniat.*, 10, 205–238.

———, and ———. 1956. The larynx and voice: the function of the normal larynx. Educational motion picture. Chicago: William and Harriet Gould Foundation.

———, and ———. 1960. The larynx and voice: the function of the pathological larynx. Educational motion picture. Chicago: Institute of Laryngology and Voice Disorders.

———, and ———. 1958. The larynx and voice: physiology of the larynx under daily stress. Educational motion picture. Chicago: William and Harriet Gould Foundation.

Murray, E., and Tiffin, J. 1933. An analysis of some basic aspects of effective speech. *Arch. Speech*, 1, 61–83.

Newby, H. 1964. Audiology (2nd. ed.). New York: Appleton-Century-Crofts. Pp. 246–248.

Obata, J., and Kobayashi, R. 1937. A direct reading pitch recorder and its application to music and speech. *J. acoust. soc. Amer.*, 9, 247–250.

———, and ———. 1938. Apparatus for direct-reading the pitch and intensity of sound. *J. acoust. soc. Amer.*, 10, 147.

———, and ———. 1940. Further applications of our direct-reading pitch and intensity recorder. *J. acoust. soc. Amer.*, 12, 188–192.

O'Neill, J., and Oyer, H. 1966. Applied audiometry. New York: Dodd, Mead.

Peters, R. 1967(A). Perceived order of tone pulses. *J. acoust. soc. Amer.*, 42, 1216.

Peterson, A., and Beranek, L. 1953. Handbook of noise measurement. Cambridge: General Radio Co. P6.

Presti, A. 1966. High-speed sound spectrograph. *J. acoust. soc. Amer.*, 40, 628–634.

Rabiner, L. 1968. Speech synthesis by rule: an acoustic domain approach. Murray Hill: Bell Telephone Lab. Personal communication from James L. Flanagan.

Saxman, J., and Burk, K. 1967. Speaking fundamental frequency characteristics of middle-aged females. *Folia Phoniat.*, 19, 167–172.

Schroeder, M. 1966. Vocoders: analysis and synthesis of speech. *Proc. IEEE*, 54, 720–734.

Scripture, E. 1906. Researches in experimental phonetics. The study of speech curves. Washington, D.C.: Carnegie Foundation.

Simon, C. 1926. The variability of consecutive wave lengths in vocal and instrumental sounds. *Psychol. Monogr.*, 36, 41–83.

Sivian, J., Dunn, H., and White, S. 1931. Absolute amplitudes and spectra of certain musical instruments and orchestras. *J. acoust. soc. Amer.*, 2, 330–371.

Snidecor, J., and Isshiki, N. 1965. Vocal and air use characteristics of a superior male esophageal speaker. *Folia Phoniat.*, 17, 217–232.

Speaks, C. 1967. Intelligibility of filtered synthetic sentences. *J. Speech Hearing Res.*, 10, 289–298.

———. 1967. Performance-intensity characteristics of selected verbal materials. *J. Speech Hearing Res.*, 10, 344–347.

———, and Jerger, J. 1965. Method for measurement of speech identification. *J. Speech Hearing Res.*, 8, 186–194.

———, and ———. 1967. Synthetic-sentence identification and receiver operating characteristic. *J. Speech Hearing Res.*, 10, 110–119.

———, Karmen, J., and Benitez, L. 1967. Effect of a competing message on synthetic sentence identification. *J. Speech Hearing Res.*, 10, 390–395.

Spilka, B. 1952. A study of relationships existing between certain aspects of personality and some vocal effects of delayed speech feedback. Purdue Univ.: Ph. D. dissertation.

Steer, M., and Tiffin, J. 1934. A photographic study of the use of intensity by superior speakers. *Speech Monogr.*, 1, 72–78.

Stevens, K., and Halle, M. 1967. Remarks on analysis by synthesis and distinctive features. *In* Models for the Perception of Speech and Visual Form. Wathen-Dunn, W., ed. Cambridge: M.I.T. Pp. 88–102.

———, and House, A. 1955. Development of a quantitative description of vowel articulation. *J. acoust. soc. Amer.*, 27, 484–493.

Tiffany, W. 1953. Vowel recognition as a function of duration, frequency modulation and phonetic context. *J. Speech Hearing Disorders*, 18, 289–301.

———, and Hanley, C. 1952. Delayed speech feedback as a test for auditory malingering. *Science*, 115, 59–60.

Tiffin, J. 1932. Phonophotographic apparatus. *Univ. Iowa Studies Psychol. Music*, 1, 118–133.

———, and Steer, M. 1937. An experimental analysis of emphasis. *Speech Monogr.*, 4, 69–74.

———, and ———. 1939. The vibrograph: a combination apparatus for the speech laboratory. *Quart. J. Speech*, 25, 272–278.

Van Riper, C., and Irwin, J. 1958. Voice and articulation. Englewood Cliffs, N.J.: Prentice-Hall.

Vennard, W., and von Leden, H. 1967. The importance of intensity modulation in the perception of a trill. *Folia Phoniat.*, 19, 19–26.

von Leden, H. 1961. The electronic synchronstroboscope. *Ann Otol., Rhinol., and Laryngol.*, 70, 881–893.

———, and Isshiki, N. 1965. An analysis of cough at the level of the larynx. *Arch. Otolaryng.*, 81, 616–625.

———, LeCover, M., Ringel, R., and Isshiki, N. 1966. Improvements in laryngeal cinematography. *Arch. Otolaryng.*, 83, 100–105.

———, and Moore, P. 1961. Vibratory patterns of the vocal cords in unilateral laryngeal paralysis. *Acta Otolaryng.*, 53, 493–506.

———, Yanagihara, N., and Werner-Kukuk, E. 1967. Teflon in unilateral vocal cord paralysis. Pre and post operative function studies. *Arch. Otolaryng.*, 85, 666–674.

Werner-Kukuk, E., von Leden, H., and Yanaghihara, N. 1968. The effects of radiation therapy on laryngeal function. *J. Laryngol. Otol.*, 82, 8–15.

Wiener, N. 1950. Cybernetics. New York: Wiley.

Williamson, A. 1935. Two years' experience with recording equipment. *Quart. J. Speech*, 21, 195–224.

Windesheim, K. 1938. The evolution of speech recording machines. *Quart. J. Speech*, 24, 257–264.

Yanagihara, N., and Koike, Y. 1967. The regulation of sustained phonation. *Folia Phoniat.*, 19, 1–18.

———, ———, and von Leden, H. 1966. Phonation and respiration. *Folia Phoniat.*, 18, 323–340.

———, and ———. 1966. The cricothroid muscle during phonation. *Ann. Otol., Rhinol. Laryngol.*, 75, 987–1006.

———, ———, and Werner-Kukuk, E. 1966. The physical parameters of cough. *Acta Otolaryngol.*, 61, 495–510.

Yates, A. J. 1963. Delayed auditory feedback. *Psychol. Bull.*, 60, 213–232.

Yeni-Komshian, G., Chase, R., and Mobley, R. 1968. The development of auditory feedback monitoring: 2 Delayed auditory feedback studies on the speech of children between two and three years of age. *J. Speech Hearing Res.*, 2, 307–315.

Zwislocki, J. 1963. An acoustic method for clinical examination of the ear. *J. Speech Hearing Res.*, 6, 303–314.

6

The Acoustics of Speech

David J. Broad and Gordon E. Peterson

Speech is a form of communication in which one of the essential links is the transmission of information by means of sound waves. An understanding of the manner in which the vocal mechanism sets air into vibration and of the manner in which the resulting sound waves are modified by passage through the vocal tract is thus a fundamental component of a comprehensive view of the human speech communication process. In addition, the sound waves that are emitted from the vocal mechanism are direct results of the physiological processes of speech production, and much can be learned about speech production, particularly about its dynamic properties, by studying the acoustic speech wave. The acoustic waves of speech also stimulate the ear of the listener and a knowledge of the acoustic parameters of the speech sounds which are applied to the sensory mechanism is basic to an understanding of the processes of speech perception. The acoustics of speech thus represents a substantial subdivision of speech science. Here, within the bounds of a single chapter, only a brief review of the subject can be given.[1]

During the past several years, extensive electroacoustical instrumentation has been available for the analysis of speech. One of the most powerful tools of analysis has been the sound spectrograph. More recently, it has become practical to process speech and to measure its parameters with computers. With these devices much has been learned regarding the nature of speech, and it is thus surprising that acoustical analysis techniques are not used more extensively in research in speech pathology and in the diagnosis and assessment of pathological speech.

A wide complement of basic and relatively simple instrumentation is available for speech research. This includes microphones, magnetic-tape recorders, oscilloscopes, volume indicators, sound-level recorders, etc. Accurate circuits for the measurement of fundamental voice frequency are difficult to construct but may be exceedingly useful. The sound spectrograph and the hybrid analog and digital computer are probably the most powerful current tools available for speech research. Instruments which are particularly useful in measuring the acoustical aspect of speech production include devices for measuring low-frequency pressure, which are employed in the measurement of subglottal pressure, and equipment for measuring air flow. All of these tools could provide valuable information about various aspects of speech disorders and, as standard equipment becomes increasingly available, they will probably be used more widely in the study of speech pathology, particularly in experimental research on disorders involving the mechanical aspects of speech production.

While electroacoustical instrumentation and the accurate measurement of sound have been an essential

[1] An excellent discussion of the acoustics of speech is to be found in the book by Fant (1960). Also highly recommended is the book by Flanagan (1965). A lucid discussion of the acoustics of vowel production may be found in the article by Stevens and House (1961). Several of the works cited in this chapter may be found in the book edited by Lehiste (1967).

part of clinical and research audiology since its inception, the use of electroacoustical instrumentation in research on speech pathology has been much less common. That important new empirical information can rarely be obtained without instrumental methods and that the value of the results of experimental research cannot exceed the validity of the instrumental measurements are facts that often seem to be overlooked.

PRELIMINARY CONSIDERATIONS

Some Basic Concepts from Acoustics

Because the study of the acoustics of speech depends upon the general principles of acoustics, it seems, therefore, appropriate to review some elementary concepts from this field. A more complete discussion of these concepts may be found in a textbook on acoustics.[2]

Sound may be considered as a mechanical disturbance of the air which is propagated in the form of a wave. One concept that is fundamental in the study of sound is that of *acoustic pressure* p, which is the short-term deviation of the total pressure P of the air from the equilibrium atmospheric pressure P_{atm}. In other words,

$$p = P - P_{atm}. \tag{1}$$

In speech the magnitude of the acoustic pressure is almost always a very small fraction of the atmospheric pressure so that the acoustic pressure is essentially a small time-varying ripple superimposed on the constant or slowly varying atmospheric pressure. For example, a 100-dB sound has an associated rms acoustic pressure[3] of 20 dynes per square centimeter, while atmospheric pressure is close to a million dynes per square centimeter. Since sound pressure is measured relative to atmospheric pressure, it can assume both positive and negative values. *Condensations* occur at points where the acoustic pressure is positive and *rarefactions* occur at points where it is negative.

Sound also involves a movement or vibration of the air. Movement of the air at a given point is described with the aid of the concept of *particle velocity* v, which is defined as the velocity at which the air is moving past that point. Particle velocity has both a magnitude, called the *particle speed*, and a direction. Thus particle velocity is a vector quantity. The movement of air within a region is described by specifying the particle velocity at every point in the region.

Acoustic pressure and particle velocity are related to one another in a manner whose complexity depends upon the particular situation. One of the simplest examples is that of a piston which is placed in a straight tube of uniform cross section with an area of A square meters as illustrated in Fig. 6-1. The tube is assumed either to be infinite in extent to the right of the piston or else to be sufficiently long that any effects from the distal end of the tube may be neglected. The piston moves within the tube with a velocity v which depends on the time t. This is expressed by saying that the piston has a velocity $v(t)$.

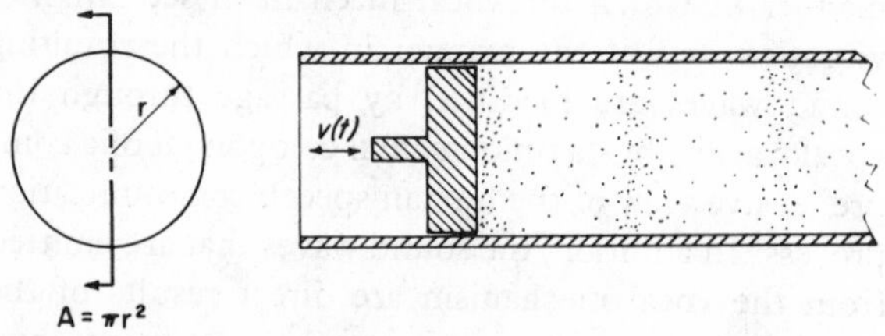

Fig. 6-1. A uniform tube of cross-sectional area A. The piston moves with velocity $v(t)$. The tube is infinite in extent to the right and the velocity pattern of the piston is propagated as a sound wave in the air contained in the tube.

Then the air in the tube, which is in contact with the surface of the piston, will have the same velocity $v(t)$. Assuming that energy losses due to friction or viscosity may be neglected, the particle velocity pattern $v(t)$ will be propagated along the tube away from the piston at a certain speed. We refer to this pattern of propagating particle velocity as a *sound wave* traveling along the tube. The speed at which the pattern is propagated, which is in general different from the particle velocity, is the speed of sound and is usually denoted by c. In air at 20°C and one atmosphere pressure, the speed of sound has been found to be 343 meters per second. In the propagation of the particle velocity pattern along the tube, the air in the tube which is $t_1 c$ meters to the right of the piston will

[2] An excellent text with a basic physical approach is Morse (1948). More advanced and recent material is given in Morse and Ingard (1968). A text which in addition treats a range of topics outside of general acoustics and which is presented largely from the viewpoint of electrical engineering is Kinsler and Frey (1962). The classic work in the field of acoustics which endures as a basic reference is the treatise by J. W. Strutt, Lord Rayleigh (1896) which is available in reprint form (1945). A work which discusses acoustic instrumentation is Beranek (1949).

[3] The abbreviation rms is for *root mean square*. The rms acoustic pressure is the square root of the average value of the square of the acoustic pressure.

have a particle velocity equal to $v(t)$ at time $t+t_1$. For example, the air 343 meters to the right of the piston will have the same particle velocity as the air adjacent to the piston had one second earlier.

If v is chosen to be positive when it is directed from left to right, then the acoustic pressure p at every point in the tube and at every instant in time is related to the particle velocity v in the tube at the same place and time by the equation

$$p(t)=\rho\, c\, v(t). \qquad (2)$$

The quantity ρ is the density of the air and c is the speed of sound. Since ρ and c are physical constants of the air, this means that the acoustic pressure and particle velocity in the tube are directly proportional to one another. That is, except for the constant scale factor ρc, the particle velocity and acoustic pressure have identical waveforms.

At a given point in the air the acoustic pressure may be the result of many sound waves acting simultaneously. Such waves may originate from separate sources, or they may be the result of reflections of a single wave from various obstacles. If the acoustic pressures associated with the individual sound waves are $p_1, p_2, \ldots, p_n$, where n is the number of sound waves present, then the acoustic pressure at the point under consideration will be the sum of the individual pressures.

$$p(t)=p_1(t)+p_2(t)+\ \ldots\ +p_n(t) \qquad (3)$$

Since the pressures combine according to simple addition, Equation 3 is an illustration of the principle of superposition. Particle velocities also combine by superposition, with the understanding that vector addition must be used to add together the particle velocities of the separate sound waves. The use of vector addition in the application of the principle of superposition to the case of particle velocities implies that when more than one sound wave is present the total acoustic particle velocity is in general no longer directly proportional to the total acoustic pressure. This differs from the simple case represented by Equation 2 in which it was assumed that only a single sound wave was present. The principle of superposition often allows the more complex cases to be treated as composites of simpler ones in each of which only a single sound wave must be considered at one time.

When a set of sound waves is propagated through a geometric surface such as a cross section of a tube, then, at any given time, a certain net rate of airflow through that surface results from the acoustic particle velocities at which the air is passing the points of the surface. This rate of flow is the *acoustic volume velocity* $u(t)$ and may be given in units of cubic meters per second. In the case of the tube of uniform cross section of area A, for example, a cross section of the tube for which the acoustic particle velocity is $v(t)$ will have an associated volume velocity $u(t)$ given by

$$u(t)=A\ v(t). \qquad (4)$$

When the particle velocity is not the same at every point on the surface of interest or when the particle velocity is not directed perpendicularly to the surface, the relation between volume velocity and particle velocity becomes more complicated, and an average of the component of the particle velocity which is directed perpendicularly to the surface must be taken. Acoustic volume velocity patterns are propagated at the speed of sound and the acoustic volume velocity waves combine according to the principle of superposition.

A moving body has, by virtue of its mass and its motion, an energy of motion or kinetic energy. When a sound wave is present in the air, then, the air has a kinetic energy that is associated with the acoustic particle velocity of the air. Furthermore, when a body exerts a force or pressure, it can have a potential for doing work, which may be expressed as a potential energy. The acoustic pressure of a sound wave is associated with an acoustic potential energy of the sound. Both kinetic energy and potential energy are thus present in a sound wave. As the wave is propagated, so are the kinetic and potential energies of the wave. The *sound intensity* is the rate at which acoustic energy is transmitted through a surface of unit area. Thus possible units for measuring sound intensity would be watts per square meter. In the example of the uniform tube, the intensity I is related to the root mean square acoustic pressure p_{rms} by the equation

$$I=p^2_{rms}/\rho c. \qquad (5)$$

If more than one sound wave is present, then the relation is again more complicated.

It is often more convenient to use relative logarithmic measures of *sound-pressure level* (*SPL*) and of *intensity level* (*IL*) than it is to use the measures of acoustic pressure or intensity directly. These relative measures are usually expressed in units of *decibels* (*dB*) as follows:

$$SPL=20\log_{10} p/p_o \qquad (6)$$

$$IL=10\log_{10} I/I_o \qquad (7)$$

The quantities p_o and I_o are standard reference values for the acoustic pressure and acoustic intensity, respectively. It is conventional to take $p_o = 0.0002$ dynes per square centimeter. This is approximately the minimum sound pressure that can be heard in the region of maximum auditory sensitivity (1,500–3,000 Hz). It is also conventional to take $I_o = p^2_o/\rho c$ so that, when the situation is as simple as that of the example of the piston in the uniform tube and Equation 5 holds, the two definitions given by Equations 6 and 7 yield numerically equivalent results, i.e., $SPL = IL$. In more complicated situations we usually have $SPL \neq IL$.

When speech is recorded for acoustic study, it is common to assume that the only sound wave which is acting on the recording device is the one that is propagating away from the speaker and that no reflections of this wave are involved. This corresponds to the condition of a *free field*, which can be approximated in an anechoic chamber. Under free-field conditions the acoustic pressure, particle velocity, and volume velocity are related quite simply to one another and have waveforms that are of the same shape. For this reason, it is common to speak of the acoustic speech wave without specifying which of these acoustic quantities is meant. Whether a given recording represents a waveform of acoustic pressure, particle velocity, or volume velocity depends upon the particular recording device used. Also, under free-field conditions the sound-pressure levels and intensity levels of the acoustic speech wave are numerically equal in their decibel expressions.

Some Basic Concepts from Spectral Analysis

One of the main areas of interest in the acoustics of speech is that of the quality of speech waveforms. Quality is commonly studied by means of spectral analysis, and, since this type of analysis is also central to discussions of the acoustics of speech production, it seems appropriate to review a few concepts from the area of spectral analysis. A more complete discussion of these concepts may be found in a textbook dealing with the subject.[4]

PERIODIC WAVEFORMS

A simple type of spectral analysis is the harmonic analysis of periodic waveforms. A waveform is *periodic* if its values repeat themseves in a definite time. The triangular wave illustrated in Fig. 6-2A is an example of a periodic waveform. The *period* T of a periodic waveform is the smallest interval of time such that the values of the waveform repeat every T seconds. Clearly the values will also repeat for every whole-number multiple of T seconds. The number of times a periodic waveform repeats itself in one second (this is not necessarily a whole number) is called its *fundamental frequency* f_o. The period and the fundamental frequency of a periodic waveform are related by the equation

$$f_o = 1/T \tag{8}$$

For periodic acoustic waveforms the *wavelength* λ is defined as the distance traveled by the sound wave during an interval of one period. Thus wavelength is a geometric analog of the temporal concept of period in the sense that a single repetition of a periodic acoustic waveform spans λ meters of space and T seconds of time. Wavelength is an important concept in the consideration of the acoustic properties of the vocal cavities as determined by their geometry. It is interesting, for instance, that the length of the vocal

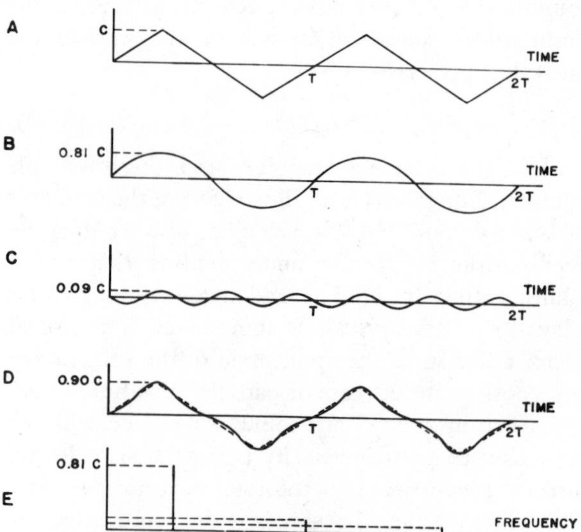

Fig. 6-2. Harmonic analysis of a triangular wave.
A. A triangular waveform of amplitude C and period T.
B. The first harmonic of the triangular wave.
C. The third harmonic of the triangular wave. (The second harmonic has zero amplitude.)
D. The solid curve is the sum of the first and third harmonics. The dashed lines represent the original triangular wave.
E. The harmonic line amplitude spectrum of the triangular wave.

[4] For example, see Chapter 2 of Lee (1960).

tract from the glottis to the lips (about 17 cm) corresponds to the wavelength of a periodic sound of approximately 2,000 Hz, a frequency which is well within one of the most common frequency ranges to be studied in speech (50 to 3,500 Hz). Wavelength, period, fundamental frequency, and the speed of sound are related by the equation

$$c = f_o \lambda = \lambda / T. \tag{9}$$

A periodic waveform can be represented as a *fourier series*, that is, as a sum of sinusoidal waveforms of appropriate amplitudes in which the frequencies are integral multiples of the fundamental frequency of the original periodic waveform. Each component sinusoid is called a *harmonic* of the waveform and is numbered according to which multiple of the fundamental its frequency is. Thus the first harmonic has a frequency equal to the fundamental, and is actually often called "the fundamental." The nth harmonic is the sinusoid whose frequency is equal to nf_o.

As an example of a fourier series representation of a periodic waveform, consider the triangular wave illustrated in Fig. 6-2A. The period of the triangular wave is T seconds and its amplitude is C. In Figs. 6-2B and 6-2C the first and third harmonics of the triangular wave are shown. The even-numbered harmonics of the triangular wave all have zero amplitude and are not shown for this case. In Fig. 6-2D the solid curve is the result of adding together the preceding two curves while the broken line represents the original waveform. The solid curve thus represents the approximation to the triangular wave which is obtained if only the first two nonzero harmonics of the fourier series representation of the wave are taken into account. Inclusion of more terms of the series improves the approximation and if all the harmonics are included, the representation becomes exact.

An expression for a fourier series is

$$\begin{aligned} F(t) = A_o + A_1 \cos(2\pi f_o + \phi_1) + \\ A_2 \cos(4\pi f_o + \phi_2) + \ . \ . \ . \ + \\ A_n \cos(2\pi n f_o + \phi_n) + \ . \ . \ . \end{aligned} \tag{10}$$

Here $F(t)$ denotes the waveform in question, A_n is the amplitude of the nth harmonic, $2\pi n f_o$ is the radian frequency of the nth harmonic, (nf_o is its frequency in Hz), and ϕ_n is the phase angle of the nth harmonic and represents the relative positioning of the nth harmonic along the time axis. Phase has received relatively little attention in speech analysis. The term A_o represents a d-c displacement of the periodic waveform and is actually the time average of the waveform.

The sequence of harmonic amplitudes A_o, A_1, . . . , A_n, . . . is often represented graphically, as shown in Fig. 6-2E for the triangular wave. Vertical lines whose heights correspond to the amplitudes of the harmonics are positioned at the harmonic frequencies. This type of display is called a *line spectrum*. Line spectra are generally associated with periodic waveforms. The graphical representations of line spectra provide a convenient means for appreciating the relative contributions of the different frequency components of periodic waveforms.

NONPERIODIC WAVEFORMS

Although true periodic waveforms are not encountered in speech, the study of such waveforms and their expansions into fourier series provides a useful basis for the development of spectral analysis for other types of waveforms. One way of extending harmonic analysis which leads to the principles underlying spectrographic analysis will now be outlined.

The acoustic speech waveform constantly changes its character as the articulators shift positions and change shape. It is thus desirable to have a spectral representation of the acoustic speech waveform which reflects the dynamic variations of speech. With each time point of the acoustic speech waveform we may associate a *short-term spectrum* which represents the frequency composition of the portion of the waveform which is in the immediate vicinity of the time point in question. The spectral representation of the entire waveform is then given by the continuous sequence of short-term spectra which may be derived from it. There are a number of alternate ways in which the short-term spectrum can be defined, some of which have been discussed by Schroeder and Atal (1962).

To illustrate the concept of short-term spectrum let us consider one way in which it might be derived. Suppose that a short-term spectrum is to be obtained which corresponds to a time point t of a waveform $F(t)$. We may isolate a certain time interval of duration τ from this portion of the waveform by multiplying it by an appropriate "time window" waveform which is zero everywhere outside the interval selected. Let us call the waveform obtained in this manner a τ-waveform. A τ-waveform which has been isolated from the waveform of Fig. 6-3A by multiplication with the time window of Fig. 6-3B is shown in Fig. 6-3C. It is now proposed to analyze the frequency spectrum of the τ-waveform.

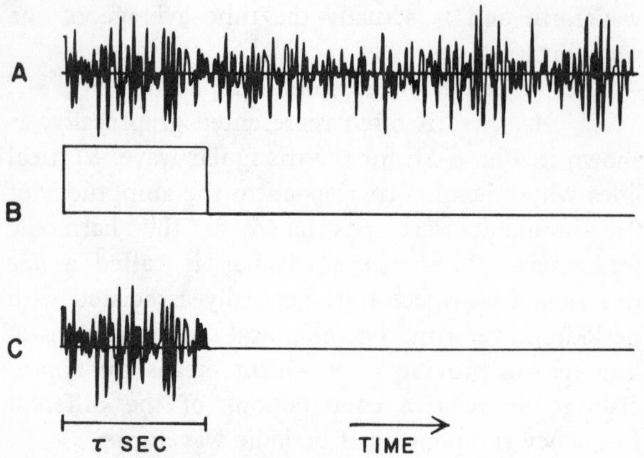

Fig. 6-3. A. A non-periodic waveform.
B. A time-window of duration τ.
C. The product of the original waveform and time window. The result is the isolation of an interval of duration τ from the non-periodic waveform, and the resulting waveform is called a τ-waveform.

An interval of duration T (a T-interval) of the τ-waveform may be considered and treated as if it were a single period of a waveform which actually was periodic with period T. The periodic waveform for which the T-interval is a single period is called the *periodic extension* of the T-interval. The periodic extensions of three different T-intervals of the τ-waveform of Fig. 6-3C are shown in Fig. 6-4A. As the values of T increase, the nonzero portions of the periodic extensions become spaced further apart in time. In the limit, as T tends to infinity, the repetitions of the nonzero interval of the τ-waveform become more widely spaced and the T-interval comes to resemble the τ-waveform itself. This is illustrated by the sequence of T-intervals shown in Fig. 6-4A in which the bottom waveform represents a single infinite T-interval.

Since it is periodic, the periodic extension of any T-interval may be represented in a fourier series for which the fundamental frequency is $1/T$. The spacing between successive harmonics is then also $1/T$. Spectra for the periodic extensions of Fig. 6-4A are shown in Fig. 6-4B. The amplitude scales have been adjusted so that the different spectra can be compared directly with one another. It can be seen that for increasing values of T the spectrum envelope retains the same shape but that the harmonics become more closely spaced in frequency. In the limit, as the T-interval becomes infinite, the harmonics become so closely spaced that for practical purposes they may be thought of as merging with the result that the spectrum becomes a continuous curve, a *continuous spectrum*. As indicated in the preceding paragraph, the infinite T-interval includes the entire τ-waveform, and for this reason the continuous spectrum of the infinite T-interval is identified as the spectrum of the τ-waveform. Thus the continuous spectrum at the bottom of Fig. 6-4B is a short-term spectrum of the interval isolated from the original waveform of Fig. 6-3A. A short-term spectrum, such as the one just described, is generally a continuous spectrum as illustrated.

SPECTROGRAPHIC ANALYSIS

The sound spectrograph is an instrument which implements a type of short-term spectrum analysis to display the varying spectral structures of sounds. Two

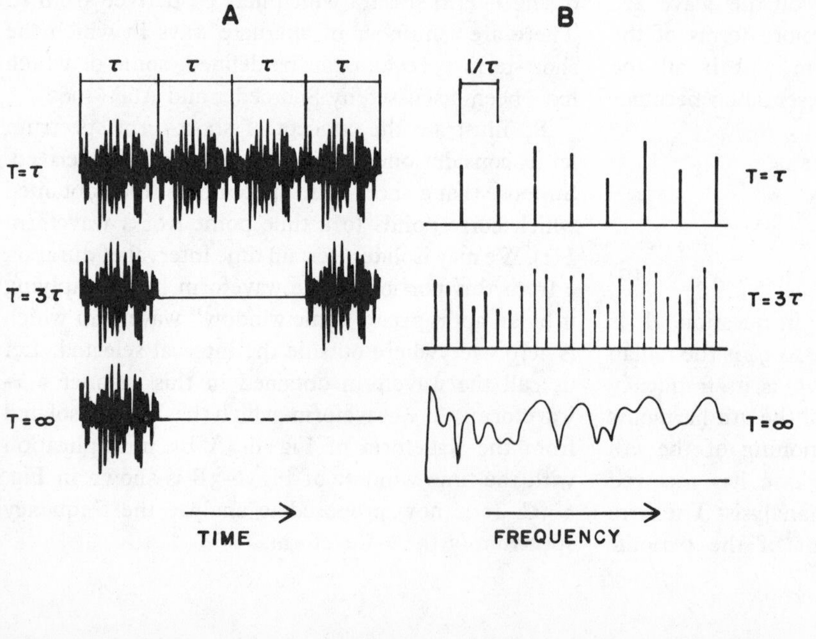

Fig. 6-4. A. Periodic extensions of the τ-waveform of C in Fig. 3, with respective periods of τ, 3τ, and infinity.
B. Frequency spectra of the periodic extensions shown in A.

sound spectrograms of the same vowel sound are shown in Fig. 6-5. On these sound spectrograms time is represented along the horizontal axis and frequency along the vertical axis, while the spectral intensity is indicated by the darkness of the marking. The manner in which a continuous short-term spectrum can be associated with each point along the time axis of the spectrogram is illustrated by the amplitude sections shown below the spectrograms. The particular type of information yielded by spectrographic analysis depends on the duration τ which is selected for the τ-waveforms isolated for analysis. When τ is small, the time resolution of the short-term spectrum is good and events can be specified accurately in time. This is illustrated by the spectrogram of Fig. 6-5A in which each of the vertical striations represents a single vibration of the vocal folds. However, in this case the frequency resolution is poor so that the details of events along the frequency axis become obscured. Increased frequency resolution may be obtained at the sacrifice of time resolution, i.e., by increasing the value of τ. This has been done to obtain the spectrogram shown in Fig. 6-5B in which the separate harmonics of the vowel sound are resolved as solid horizontal bars but the time at which the individual vocal fold vibrations take place are now obscured. The particular choice of a value for τ generally depends on the problem at hand. The *broad-band* spectrogram, as illustrated in Fig. 6-5A, employs a value of the order of a few milliseconds for τ. Broad-band spectrograms are most commonly employed for the acoustic study of articulatory processes. The *narrow-band* spectrogram, as illustrated in Fig. 6-5B, employs a value of approximately 30 msec for τ. Narrow-band spectrograms are most commonly used to study variations in the frequency of the laryngeal source of voicing.

Narrow-band spectrograms of voiced sounds indicate that in these sounds energy tends to be concentrated at nearly discrete frequencies which are multiples of some lowest such frequency. This is the case, for example, in the narrow-band spectrogram shown in Fig. 6-5B. The analogy that this suggests with the discrete line spectra of periodic sounds is one reason for calling these frequencies *harmonics* and for calling the lowest one the *fundamental*. The waveforms of such voiced sounds often display a remarkable approximation to periodicity for a number of periods even though they are never truly periodic. Such sounds are called *quasi-periodic* sounds to indicate their similarity to periodic sounds.

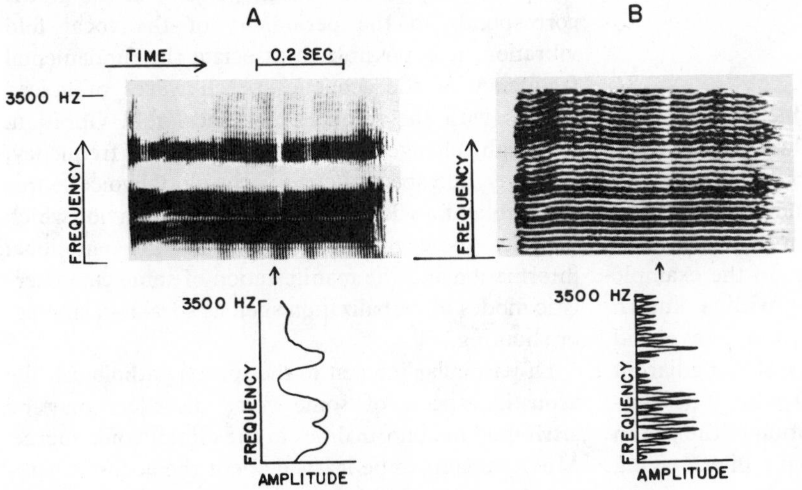

Fig. 6-5. A. Broad-band spectrogram of the vowel [a] and a corresponding short-term spectrum. The broad horizontal bands in the spectrogram show the locations of the resonant frequencies of the vocal tract. B. Narrow-band spectrogram of the vowel [a] and a corresponding short-term spectrum. The narrow horizontal curves in the spectrogram show the locations of the harmonic frequencies of the glottal voice source.

It should be emphasized that a full appreciation of the application of acoustics and spectral analysis to the study of speech requires a more complete and rigorous foundation than that provided in a brief review. While much might be learned without the aid of such a foundation, a sound knowledge of the basic disciplines involved should contribute substantially to an ability to work effectively with concepts in the acoustics of speech.

THE ACOUSTICS OF SPEECH-SOUND PRODUCTION

Of central concern in the acoustics of speech are the processes by which sound is generated and modified by the speech mechanism to produce the acoustic speech wave. Both the manner in which acoustic energy is derived from respiratory work and the manner in which this acoustic energy is modified by transmission through the spaces and openings of the vocal tract are basic to the acoustics of speech-sound production. With a sufficient knowledge of the generation and modification of acoustic energy by the vocal mechanism it should be possible to predict the properties of the acoustic speech waveform on the basis of the physiological actions employed to produce it. Thus the acoustics of speech-sound production involves the study of the physiological-acoustic transformation and provides a basis for the interpretation of the acoustic speech waveform in terms of articulatory processes.

Speech-Sound Sources

A surface or volume throughout which the acoustic pressure, particle velocity, or volume velocity is determined by nonacoustic considerations is known as a *sound source*. Alternatively, a sound source may be thought of as a locus for the conversion of nonacoustic energy into acoustic energy. In the example of the piston moving in the tube with a known velocity $v(t)$, the surface of the piston is a sound source in which the particle velocity of the adjacent air is constrained to be equal to $v(t)$ also. The conversion of a part of the energy of motion of the piston into acoustic energy may be thought of as taking place at this surface.

A common type of sound source studied in acoustics is the vibrating or moving body, such as a tuning fork, which sets the adjacent air into motion. In the acoustics of speech, however, none of the sound sources are actually of this type. Rather, speech-sound sources are almost always associated with the manner in which the kinetic energy of flow and/or the potential energy of pressure buildup of the breath stream is partially converted to acoustic energy as a consequence of the manner in which the vocal mechanism controls the flow of the air stream. In this case it is the air itself which acts as the acoustic sound source.

Three types of breath-stream control which are of particular interest as sources of acoustic energy in speech are 1) the quasi-periodic modulation of the breath stream by the vibrating vocal folds during phonation, 2) the generation of turbulence at a constriction or obstruction in the vocal tract, and 3) the release of a pressure built up against a closure in the vocal tract. These types of control correspond respectively to the quasi-periodic voice source, the quasi-random noise or friction source, and the transient source. The properties of the acoustic sources in speech thus depend directly upon the physiological means of production of the speech sounds.

THE GLOTTAL VOICE SOURCE

As the true vocal folds vibrate during voicing, the area of the glottal opening through which air may pass changes in a quasi-periodic manner. The resulting pattern of volume velocity of airflow through the glottis constitutes the quasi-periodic source of acoustic excitation for the voiced sounds of speech. Since the periodicity in the volume velocity at the glottis corresponds to the periodicity of the vocal fold vibration, it is possible to associate the fundamental frequency of the acoustic speech waves of voiced sounds with the frequency of vocal fold vibration. Through changes in its fundamental frequency, intensity, and spectral quality, the glottal voice source is capable of a wide range of acoustic behavior which includes the signaling of prosodic and emotional information and the manifestation of some characteristic modes of verbalization such as speaking, singing, or shouting.

Of particular interest to the speech pathologist, the acoustic aspects of some voice disorders may be attributed to abnormalities in the glottal voice source. Much remains to be learned about the acoustic parameters of the glottal source which are most relevant for the characterization of the various voice disorders, and the acoustic investigation of voice disorders represents a challenging area for research. Lieberman (1961, 1963) and Smith and Lieberman (1964) have presented some promising results on relations between short-term perturbations in the periodicity of the voice source and pathologies of the larynx. Wendahl (1963, 1966) used synthetic speech to study the influence of this type of perturbation on listener judgments of harsh voice quality. The influence of pathologic voice on the spectrum of the voice source has been investigated by Winkel (1954), Nessel (1960), Yanagihara (1967), and others. These studies indicate that analysis of the acoustic speech wave could provide considerable information about voice disorders.

Owing to the relatively inaccessible location of the larynx, special techniques are usually required for the study of the acoustic volume velocity pattern of the air flowing through the glottis. These include the interpretation of physiological results from high-speed motion pictures of the vibrations of the vocal folds, acoustic analysis of the radiated speech wave by means of inverse filtering, and photoelectric glottography. Theoretical studies of vocal fold vibration and of the nature of the airflow through the glottis serve both to increase the information which can be obtained by experimental methods and to provide a means of formulating knowledge in this area in a precise and unified manner.

Transglottal pressure. The volume velocity of airflow through the glottis depends in part upon the pressure drop across the glottis. This pressure difference, or transglottal pressure, is nearly the same as the subglottic pressure when the air pressure just above the glottis is nearly equal to atmospheric pressure, as is the case when there is no closure or close constriction in the supraglottal part of the vocal tract. This condition is usually satisfied reasonably well during vowel production.

Glottal resistance. The volume velocity of the airflow through the glottis also depends upon the resistance presented by the glottis to the flow of air. The glottal resistance may be defined as the ratio of the transglottal pressure to the volume velocity of glottal airflow for a fixed adjustment of the glottis. By measurements on a model constructed by taking a casting of a cadaver larynx, van den Berg, Zantema, and Doornenbal (1957) determined the resistance of the glottis to various steady-state air flows for different static values of the area of the glottal opening. They found that for a wide range of transglottal pressures and airflows the resistance of the glottis for a constant transglottal pressure was such that for small glottal areas the air flow was proportional to the cube of the area of the glottis while for larger openings the air flow was directly proportional to the area itself. In order to apply this result for flow through a static glottis to the case of a glottis which changes rapidly with vocal fold vibrations, account must be taken of the fact that since the area of the glottis is changing there is no time for the steady-state flow corresponding to a given area to become completely established. Flanagan (1958) estimated the time required for steady flow to be established by a consideration of the inertia of the air in the glottis and showed that for most of the rates of vocal fold vibration of interest, the glottal resistance for the static condition could be used with relatively good accuracy for the dynamic case as well.

Motion picture studies. High-speed motion pictures of the vocal folds were made by Farnsworth (1940) and later by Dunker and Schlosshauer (1958), Timcke, von Leden, and Moore (1958), Hiroto (1966), Soron (1967), and others. In his study of the properties of the glottal voice source, Flanagan made use of the relation between glottal volume velocity and the area of the glottis to derive the glottal volume velocity waveform from measurements of glottal areas obtained from high-speed motion pictures of the vibrations of the vocal folds. His derived volume velocity waveforms closely resemble the area waveforms with the main difference appearing as a slight steepening of the volume velocity waveform with respect to the area waveform for the small glottal openings near closure where the volume velocity is proportional to the cube of the area instead of to the area itself.

In their measurements of the glottic wave, Timcke, von Leden, and Moore determined the excursion of the midpoints of the vocal folds from the midline for different times during the vibratory cycle. Although the lateral excursion of the vocal folds is not precisely linearly related to glottal area, measurements of lateral excursion are generally more easily implemented than area measurements, and the resulting waveforms bear a reasonable resemblance to the area and volume velocity waveforms. Fig. 6-6 shows a period of a

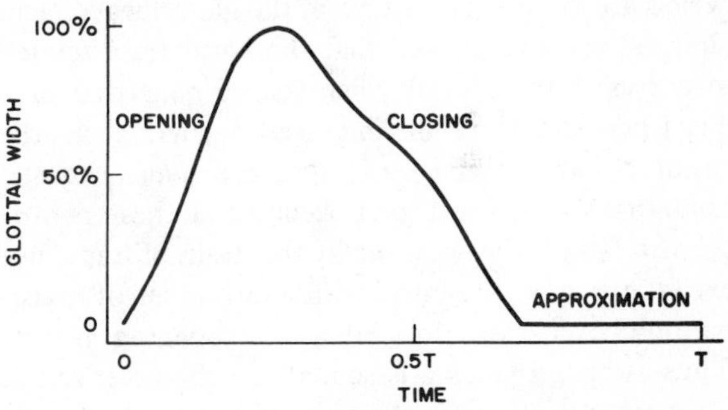

Fig. 6-6 A period of a glottal waveform measured from high-speed motion pictures. *After Timcke, von Leden, and Moore, Copyright 1958 by the American Medical Association.*

glottal waveform as measured by Timcke, von Leden, and Moore. It has an increasing portion corresponding to the opening phase of the glottis, a decreasing portion corresponding to the closing phase, and a section equal to zero corresponding to the interval during which the vocal folds are closed. The relative durations of these intervals were studied by Timcke, von

Leden, and Moore, who defined the *open quotient* as the fraction of time within the entire cycle during which the folds are open and the *speed quotient* as the ratio of the duration of the opening phase to that of the closing phase. They found that the open quotient tends to decrease with increasing intensity and to change slightly with increasing frequency of vibration while the speed quotient increases with increasing intensity and is relatively insensitive to register and frequency of vibration. When there is no complete closure of the folds, as in breathy voice, for example, the open quotient is by definition identically equal to unity. A summary of investigations of the open quotient is given by Sonesson (1960), who cites works on the subject as early as 1935.

Inverse filtering. Miller (1959) obtained records of the glottal volume velocity waveform by the method of inverse filtering in which the acoustic speech waveform is processed by suitable electric filters to remove the effects of the supraglottal cavities from the speech waveform. The volume velocity waveforms to be observed at the output of such a filter correspond quite closely to those obtained from high-speed motion pictures. In his study of glottal waves by inverse filtering, Holmes (1962) demonstrated that the relatively sharp corner to be observed at the end of the closing phase and the one which sometimes occurs at the onset of the opening phase of the glottal period are important features of the glottal waveform. Holmes' records showed that the vocal tract tended to act as if the glottal voice source consisted of a quasi-periodic train of impulses occurring at the closure points in the sense that the main acoustic excitation of the vocal tract occurred at these points. He also found that occasionally this train of impulsive excitations was interlaced with another set of quasi-periodic excitations located at the opening points. Thus although voicing is sometimes characterized as a sequence of air puffs, the end and beginning of each puff and not its maximum point are apparently most important acoustically. A relatively sharp corner in the glottal volume velocity waveform evidently represents a sufficiently rapid change in the slope of the waveform for the second derivative to possess a significant impulselike component at that point in time. This would imply that the glottal source spectrum should possess harmonics whose amplitude tend to decrease at a rate of 12 dB per octave.[5] Of course, a complete representation of the acoustic effect of the glottal voice source would require that the entire source waveform and its shape be taken into account. This would presumably be especially true for the case in which no complete closure occurs at any point during the vibratory cycle with the result that the corners in the volume velocity waveform would be considerably smoothed.

Inverse filtering was employed by Lindqvist (1965), who also noted the sharp corners in the volume velocity waveform at the moments of closure. In addition, he noted that the waveform was in general not identically equal to zero during the interval of vocal fold closure. Lindqvist has suggested that variations in the waveform which occur during closure may be due to vertical movements of the folds which would displace the air in their immediate vicinity.

Glottography. Sonesson (1960, 1963) has reported on glottography, which is a method for observing the glottal area waveform by recording the amount of light transmitted through the glottis from a light source on one side of the glottis to a photocell located on the other side. Since the tissues of the larynx are much less transparent than the air, the amount of light recorded by the photocell is approximately proportional to the area of the glottal opening. This method has the advantage of providing an instantaneous record of glottal area without the necessity of tedious measurements on frames of motion picture film. Coleman and Wendahl (1968) have found some serious discrepancies between glottographic waveforms and waveforms derived from simultaneous high-speed motion pictures of the vocal folds. Although the method is less accurate than the photographic method, it should nevertheless be a source of valuable information if the difficulties of applying it reliably can be overcome. Ohala (1966) has discussed some of the techniques and applications in more detail.

Spectrum of the glottic wave. Spectral analysis of the glottal waveform reveals that the harmonics do tend to decline in amplitude at a rate of approximately 12 dB per octave. From an analysis based on area measurements taken from high-speed motion pictures, Flanagan (1958) reported spectra with amplitudes decreasing at rates between 10 and 12 dB per

[5] Two frequencies differ by one *octave* when one is twice the frequency of the other. For example, a frequency of 1000 Hz is one octave above one of 500 Hz. Thus a decrease in intensity of 12 dB per octave means that every time the frequency is doubled the spectral intensity has been reduced by 12 dB.

octave while Carr and Trill (1964), working with inverse filtering, found spectra decreasing at rates between eight and 16 dB per octave. In addition, there is a tendency for the spectrum to have periodic dips every three to five harmonics (Miller; Carr and Trill), which may be attributed to zeros in the spectrum of a single repetition of the quasi-periodic glottal source waveform. Flanagan (1962) has noted that such a minimum in the glottal source spectrum might influence the perceptual quality of a voiced vowel when the frequency of the minimum corresponds closely to one of the resonant frequencies of the vowel. A typical line spectrum for the quasi-periodic voice source is shown in Fig. 6-7. The power spectrum was derived from the waveform of Fig. 6-6 by means of a fast fourier transform program based on the algorithm introduced by Cooley and Tukey (1965). The envelope represents the continuous spectrum of a single repetition of the wave in Fig. 6-6.

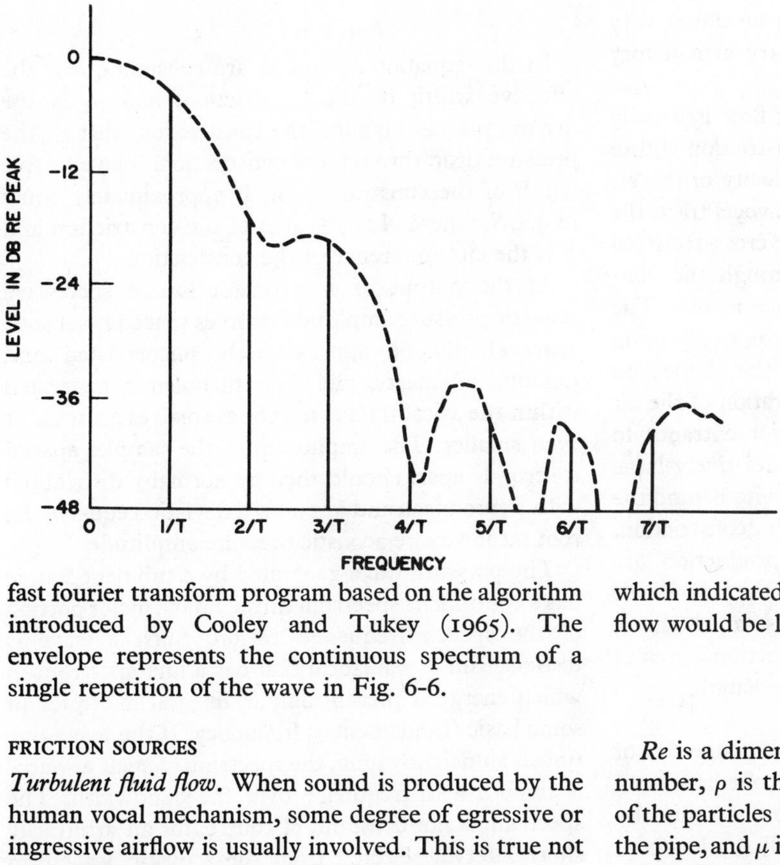

Fig. 6-7. Amplitude spectrum of the glottal wave of Fig. 6-6. The dashed envelope is the continuous spectrum of a single repetition of the wave; the vertical lines show the amplitudes of the harmonics of a source waveform consisting of periodic repetitions of the wave.

FRICTION SOURCES

Turbulent fluid flow. When sound is produced by the human vocal mechanism, some degree of egressive or ingressive airflow is usually involved. This is true not only of normal speech, but also of defective speech. Whenever air flow in the vocal tract is involved in the production of sound there is probably some degree of turbulent flow at certain positions within the vocal tract. Turbulent air flow provides the primary source of excitation for whispering and for the fricatives and sibilants. The opposite extreme of turbulent air flow is laminar air flow, in which the air particles follow paths which are smooth and regular. In turbulent air flow, the air particles follow irregular paths which change direction in a largely random manner. This irregularity in the movement of the air during turbulent flow propagates as a sound wave which has a random or noiselike waveform.

Reynolds number. Whether the fluid flow through a pipe of uniform diameter will be laminar or turbulent is determined by the density of the fluid, the viscosity of the fluid, the inner diameter of the pipe, and the particle velocity of the medium. In the last century Reynolds combined these variables in an equation which indicated whether in a particular case the fluid flow would be laminar or turbulent:

$$Re = \frac{\rho v D}{\mu} \qquad (11)$$

Re is a dimensionless quantity called the Reynolds number, ρ is the density of the fluid, v is the speed of the particles in the fluid, D is the inner diameter of the pipe, and μ is the coefficient of viscosity of the fluid.

The Reynolds number can often be used to predict whether fluid flow under a given condition will be laminar or turbulent. In uniform circular pipes the flow is laminar for Reynolds numbers below 2,100. For higher Reynolds numbers turbulent flow becomes likely. The particular value of the Reynolds number at which turbulence becomes established depends on various conditions, such as the roughness of the inner surface of the pipe.

Different types of boundaries for flows generally have different critical values of the Reynolds numbers at which the transition between laminar and turbulent flow takes place. Flow of a liquid over a flat surface, for example, may be associated with a critical value of 500 for the Reynolds number. In speech the articulatory constrictions probably represent sufficiently great deviations in form from a uniform circular pipe so that the critical values for the Reynolds numbers at such constrictions are likely to be significantly different from the value of 2,100 for a uniform circular pipe. Meyer-Eppler (1953), for example, found a critical value of 1,800 for the Reynolds number in air flow through a model of an articulatory constriction. The critical Reynolds numbers for the different types of flow conditions in speech production no doubt vary according to the shape of the primary articulatory constriction.

In speech production turbulent air flow is usually generated by producing a narrow constriction within the vocal tract. While the volume velocity of the air flow is the same throughout the entire vocal tract, the particle velocity depends upon the cross-sectional area. When the particle velocity through the constriction is sufficiently high, turbulence results. The generation of turbulence is dependent not only upon the particle velocity, but also upon the shape and extent of the constriction. The acceleration of the air particles occurs chiefly at the posterior entrance to the constriction, and there will be a relatively large pressure drop between the air in the cavity behind the constriction and the air flowing in the constriction. Constrictions employed in speech production are relatively short, and the magnitude of the turbulence generated in such a constriction is much more dependent upon the minimum cross-sectional area of the constriction than upon its effective length.

Sound production in turbulent flow. The properties of turbulent air flow through an acoustic tube have been studied extensively, but the generation of sound by turbulent air flow is still not well understood. Turbulence involves an irregular, random fluctuation in the flow of air which is accompanied by a corresponding random distribution of pressures over both space and time. This random pressure field can be viewed as a source of acoustic excitation that is distributed throughout the region of turbulence.

Meyer-Eppler studied the generation of turbulence both in constricted plastic tubes and in the production of fricative consonants. He found that the root mean square sound pressure p_{rms} of the noise measured at a fixed distance in front of the speaker could be expressed as follows:

$$p_{rms} = A(Re^2 - Re^2_{crit}) \quad (12)$$

In Equation 12, A is a constant, Re is the Reynolds number, and Re_{crit} is a critical Reynolds number having a magnitude of about 1,800 below which significant generation of sound does not occur. Fant (1960) has observed that in the study of speech production it is generally more convenient to measure the pressure behind the constriction that is generating turbulence than it is to measure the particle velocity in the constriction. Accordingly, he reformulated the above expression in terms of the driving pressure:

$$p_{rms} = k_1\, h^2 p_d - k_2 \quad (13)$$

In this equation k_1 and k_2 are constants, h is the effective width of the constriction, and p_d is the driving pressure behind the constriction, that is, the pressure drop through the constriction. The effective width of the constriction, h, is approximately equal to $4A/S$, where A is the area of the constriction and S is the circumference of the constriction.

At the output of a turbulent source successive acoustic pressure amplitude samples spaced t_1 seconds apart should be approximately uncorrelated and random in magnitude. For turbulence generated within the vocal tract t_1 may be as small as 0.1 msec or even smaller. The amplitudes of the samples spaced t_1 seconds apart should then be normally distributed with a zero mean and a standard deviation equal to the root mean square acoustic pressure amplitude.

The pressure wave generated by a tubulent source has a continuous spectrum throughout a major portion of the speech frequency region. Such a wave is distinct from a waveform that has a line spectrum in which energy is present only at integral multiples of some basic (fundamental) frequency. If the averaging time is sufficiently long, the spectrum of such a source is smooth with frequency over the bandwidth. The spectrum is not constant, of course, for an arbitrarily short interval selected from the acoustic waveform produced by the source.

Sibilant production. The sibilants apparently employ a more complicated mechanism of generating turbulence. In normal speech production a narrow constriction is formed at the front of the mouth through which the breath stream is directed against the cutting edge of the lower teeth. The teeth divide the air stream so that turbulent eddies are formed. These turbulent eddies normally alternate from one side of the teeth to the other, as in the production of edge tones. This oscillating pattern of turbulent eddies is common in fluid dynamics and may be observed in models employing either gas or liquid. The alternating eddies result in an acoustic wave which has a characteristic frequency pattern so that the spectrum is not uniform. Many variations on the nature of the friction source are found among defective speakers, as in the case of a speaker without the lower incisors.

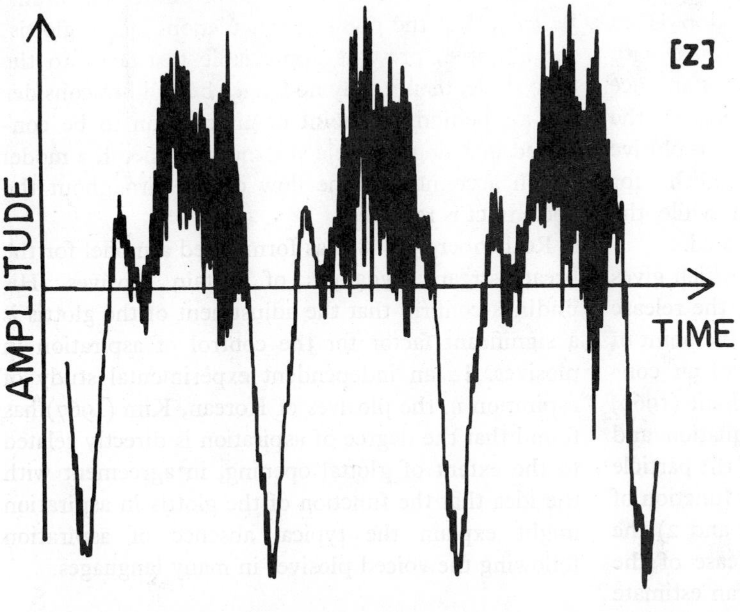

Fig. 6-8. The acoustic speech waveform of 3 periods of a production of the voiced sibilant [z]. The positive portions of the cycles tend to display more friction than the negative portions.

Turbulence concurrent with voicing. In the production of voiced fricatives and sibilants a different source pattern results. During normal phonation the true vocal folds are only open during a part of each laryngeal period. Air flow during the open part of the cycle will normally cause some degree of turbulence to be generated at the constriction for the fricative or at the obstruction for the sibilant. The larynx, of course, introduces considerable resistance into the path of the breath stream. As a result, there is a partial pressure drop at the larynx, and the driving pressure is typically not as great for voiced sibilants and fricative consonants as it is for their voiceless counterparts. The smaller pressure drop across the constriction or the reduced particle velocity against the obstruction results in less turbulence and a lower sound level for the voiced consonants. Since air flows through the larynx during only part of the voiced cycle, the waveforms for voiced fricatives and sibilants may display varying degrees of friction during the different phases of the vibratory cycle of the vocal folds. This is illustrated in Fig. 6-8. This figure shows successive cycles of [z] produced by an adult male. The figure was constructed by band-limiting the fricatives to 14,000 Hz and taking 28,000 12-bit samples per second. The samples were stored in a computer and the waveform was then drawn at a slow rate with a plotter. The smoother portions of the waveform correspond to times at which little turbulence is generated, while the remaining portions of the cycle display considerable friction noise.

The interruption of the turbulence in the formation of voiced fricatives and sibilants might be thought of as a process in which the magnitude of the air flow which produces the turbulence is modulated periodically by the opening and closing of the true vocal folds. Halle and Stevens (1967) have pointed out that the constriction for generating turbulence in the fricatives has substantial resistance, and that the pressure drop across the larynx must be different for voiced fricatives and for vowel production, with the result that the behavior of the voice source is influenced by the friction source. Hence there is a mutual interaction between the voice source and a simultaneously active turbulent source.

The acoustic wave generated by the turbulence at

an obstruction may be substantially greater in amplitude than the acoustic wave generated by the turbulence in a constriction. For example, the sibilants [s] and [ʃ] tend to be more intense than the fricatives [f] and [θ].

Aspiration. In the production of a stop consonant pressure is built up against a closure within the vocal tract. If the pressure is released by opening the closure, then the pressures on either side of the point of articulation tend to equalize quite rapidly. During the brief period of pressure equalization, the air moving past the point of articulation may attain a particle velocity sufficient for the generation of turbulence. Turbulence which results from the movement of air following the release of a stop is an acoustic friction source which is identified with aspiration. In many languages the presence or absence of aspiration is a feature which contributes to the phonological distinction between classes of plosive phonemes. The voiced plosives of English, for example, are predominantly unaspirated while the voiceless plosives are predominantly aspirated.

Stevens (1956) developed an equation which gives the volume velocity of air flow following the release of a stop in terms of the pressure behind the point of articulation and in terms of the volume of air contained behind the point of articulation. Fant (1960) solved a particular form of Stevens' equation and wrote an expression for the time course of the particle velocity past the point of articulation as a function of 1) the volume of air behind the closure and 2) the area of the opening made from the release of the closure. From this relation Fant derived an estimate for the expected duration t_T of turbulent flow following the release of a stop:

$$t_T = \frac{\rho V}{P_{atm} A_o} \sqrt{2p_o/\rho} \qquad (14)$$

ρ is the density of the air, V is the volume of air contained in the cavity behind the closure, P_{atm} is the atmospheric pressure, A_o is the final area of the opening made from the closure, and p_o is the initial value of the pressure difference between the two sides of the closure. Fant's value of 130 msec for one set of assumed conditions is of the same order of magnitude as the durations observed for aspiration in actual speech. One of the major inferences drawn from the equations developed by Stevens and Fant is that an open glottis is essential to the production of prolonged aspiration, since when the glottis is open the volume of the lungs is included in the value of V on the right side of Equation 14. Otherwise the volume is not sufficient to produce prolonged aspiration. This inference agrees with most phonetic observations, for example, that strong aspiration is almost always observed only on voiceless plosives. In some languages, however, voiced plosives are said to be aspirated. The mechanisms by which these sounds are produced must be clarified before it can be determined whether an open glottis is essential for strong aspiration in all cases.

The simple dependency of the duration t_T of the aspiration on the air volume V expressed by Equation 14 requires the assumption that the predominating resistance to the flow of air into or out of the volume be located at the point of articulation. If the glottis, for example, presents appreciable resistance to the flow of air, then it may no longer be valid to consider the air behind the point of articulation to be contained in a single simple volume. In general, a model which accounts for the flow of air throughout the vocal tract is required.

Rothenberg (1968) has formulated a model for the breath-stream dynamics of certain plosives. His findings confirm that the adjustment of the glottis is a significant factor for the control of aspiration in plosives. In an independent experimental study of aspiration in the plosives of Korean, Kim (1967) has found that the degree of aspiration is directly related to the extent of glottal opening, in agreement with the idea that the function of the glottis in aspiration might explain the typical absence of aspiration following the voiced plosives in many languages.

TRANSIENT SOURCES

During the closure for a stop articulation the regions of air behind and in front of the occlusion have different pressures. When the closure is opened these regions come into abrupt contact and a step change in pressure which acts as an acoustic source is applied to the vocal tract. This type of source is called a *transient* source since by its nature it is confined to a brief interval of time. The step change in the pressure within the vocal tract is accompanied by a short period during which the particle velocity can have a considerable magnitude. The particle velocity of the air associated with the transient source thus has the gross appearance of an impulse. The continuous spectrum of a step pressure source should decline with increasing frequency at six dB per octave. Step-pressure sources in speech are nearly always associated with the release of a stop articulation. If a stop is aspirated, then both a transient source and a friction source will be active at the time of release.

The Transmission Characteristic of the Vocal Tract

The acoustic energy generated by a sound source in speech generally undergoes some modification before it is radiated and manifested as a speech waveform. The selective transmission characteristics of the cavities in front and in back of the acoustic source together with the characteristics of sound radiation from the vocal mechanism have significant influences on the character of the acoustic speech wave. The transmission and radiation characteristics depend primarily upon the geometry of the vocal tract as determined by the adjustment of the articulators and depend to some extent upon the location of the sound source in relation to this geometry. For example, the degree of lip opening largely determines the nature of sound radiation from the mouth while the resonant frequencies of the vocal tract are changed largely through changes in the shape and position of the supraglottal articulators.

FREQUENCY DOMAIN DESCRIPTION

Frequency spectra provide a relatively simple description of the effect of the acoustic resonance and radiation characteristics of the vocal mechanism. If $P(f)$ is the spectrum of the acoustic speech waveform and if $S(f)$ is the spectrum of the source waveform, then $P(f)$ and $S(f)$ are related by an equation of the form

$$P(f)=H(f)\,R(f)\,S(f) \qquad (15)$$

The factor $H(f)$ represents the transmission characteristic of the vocal tract and $R(f)$ represents the frequency-dependent characteristic of sound radiation from the vocal mechanism. The transmission and radiation characteristics of the vocal tract may be considered to represent the effect of a sound filter applied to the sound source. The transmission and radiation characteristics emphasize some frequency components of the source (frequencies f for which $R(f)$ H(f) is greater than unity) and attenuate others (frequencies f for which $R(f)\,H(f)$ is less than unity). The product $R(f)\,H(f)$ is sometimes called the frequency response of the vocal tract.

To a first approximation, the behavior of the source and transmission characteristics in speech are independent of one another. This is exemplified by the ability of a speaker to maintain a relatively constant vowel articulation while he changes the fundamental frequency of the voice source or, conversely, to perform a variety of vowel articulations while he maintains a relatively constant adjustment of the laryngeal voice source. The properties of both the source and the transmission characteristics, however, often depend to some extent on the same features of the physiological means of production of the speech sounds, so that, at the physiological level, the source and filter may not be independent in their behavior. For example, the special adjustment of the tongue and teeth necessary for the production of the turbulent noise source of a sibilant sound also helps to determine the filter characteristics for the sound. Similarly, it appears that adjustments of the supraglottal articulators, which determine primarily the transmission characteristic, can also influence the behavior of the laryngeal voice source.

TIME DOMAIN DESCRIPTION

Impulse response. Alternately, the response of the vocal tract to a sound source may be considered in the time domain. If the air contained in the vocal tract is disturbed from its state of equilibrium by a single impulse of acoustic excitation of unit strength, the air will return to its state of equilibrium through vibratory motions which are characteristic of the size and shape of the body of air contained within the vocal tract. The acoustic waveform in the external air which is produced by this characteristic motion is the *impulse response* of the vocal tract. The impulse response characterizes the natural or unforced behavior of the vocal tract in the sense that after the instant of the impulse the behavior of the tract is determined completely by the properties of the system itself. A familiar example of the concept of impulse response is the sound produced by a bell in response to the impulse delivered by the striking clapper.

There is a remarkable relationship between the impulse response of the vocal tract and the frequency response of the vocal tract. If $h(t)$ is the impulse response corresponding to a given vocal tract configuration, then the product $H(f)\,R(f)$ for that configuration will be given by the continuous spectrum of the impulse response $h(t)$. Thus, if the impulse response is known, then the frequency response is also known. This relationship is a basis for using impulse responses to study the transmission and radiation characteristics of the vocal tract.

BEHAVIOR OF A SIMPLE PHYSICAL SYSTEM

Impulse response of a simple physical system. The impulse response of the vocal tract is complex and may be better understood by a preliminary consideration of the impulse response of a simpler physical system. Consider, for example, the motion of a simple pendulum which has been set in motion by an impulsive force, such as a sharp blow from a mallet. If the pendulum is subject to frictional forces, then its oscillations will constantly diminish in amplitude until the pendulum finally comes back to rest. This motion is the impulse response of the pendulum. The actual form of the oscillation will be that of a damped sinusoid. A damped sinusoid is a waveform which has the form of a sinusoid in which the amplitude decays exponentially with time. A damped sinusoid is illustrated in Fig. 6-9. A damped

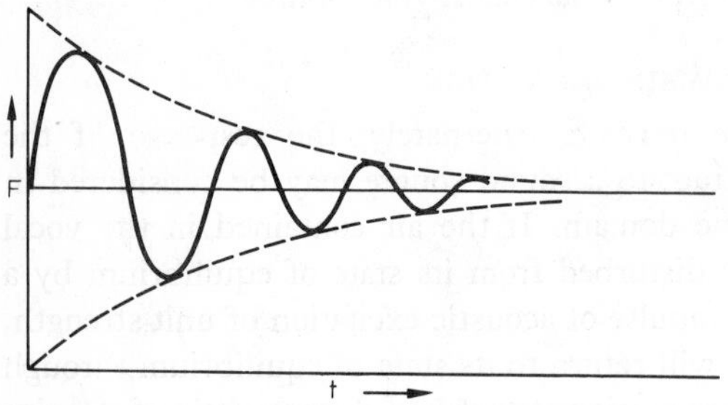

Fig. 6-9. A damped sinusoid.

sinusoid may be specified by the frequency of its oscillation, the rate at which the amplitude decays, and by the initial amplitude. The rate of decay can be given by the *time constant* T_c which is defined as the time interval required for the amplitude of the envelope of the damped sinusoid to decrease by a factor of $1/e$, or about 37 percent. The quantity e is a number which occurs frequently in mathematics and has a value of approximately 2.718. Thus long time constants, for example, correspond to slow rates of decay and indicate a small degree of damping.

Frequency response of a simple physical system. Since the envelope of the damped sinusoid decreases monotonically with time, a damped sinusoid is not a periodic waveform and consequently has a continuous spectrum instead of a line spectrum. The spectra of some damped sinusoids are shown in Fig. 6-10. If the damped sinusoid represents the impulse response of a simple pendulum, then its spectrum represents the frequency response of the pendulum. As might

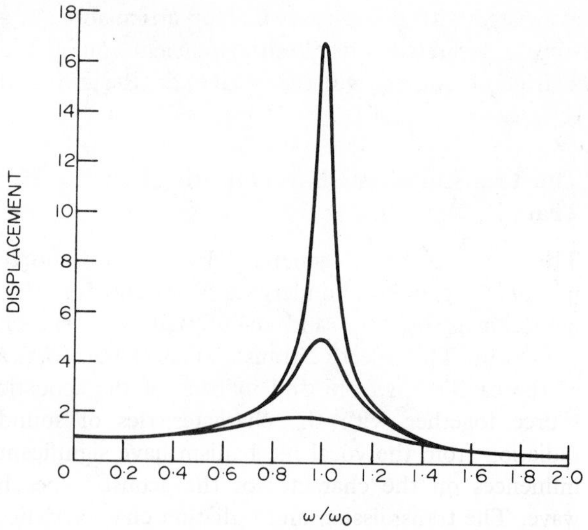

Fig. 6-10. Spectra of 3 damped sinusoids of the same frequency, but with different time constants. The highest curve has the longest time constant, and the lowest one has the shortest time constant.

be expected, the spectrum has its greatest amplitude in the region of the frequency of oscillation of the damped sinusoid. The highest point on the curve of the spectrum, the spectral maximum, is indeed usually close to the frequency of oscillation of the damped sinusoid even though in general the spectral maximum occurs at a frequency slightly below this frequency. In practice the difference between the two frequencies is small enough to be neglected. In addition to the peak in the spectrum, it may also be noted that at low frequencies the curve approaches unity while at high frequencies it approaches zero. Thus a pendulum for which one of these curves is the frequency response will oscillate with only small amplitudes in response to a force which oscillates at a frequency well above the spectral peak.

Relation between time and frequency for a simple physical system. The degree of sharpness of the peak in the spectrum of the damped sinusoid is characterized by the bandwidth Δf, which is defined as the difference between the frequencies of the two points on the curve of the spectrum whose values are $\sqrt{2}/2$ or 0.707 of the value at the spectral maximum. The smaller or narrower the bandwidth, the more the spectrum will tend to be concentrated in a sharp spike centered on the spectral maximum, as illustrated by the upper curve in Fig. 6-10. Thus a narrow bandwidth corresponds to a spectrum which resembles the single vertical line representing the spectrum of a pure sinusoid. The damped sinusoid to which a narrow bandwidth corresponds has a relatively long time constant (slow rate of decay) and hence indeed has more the appearance of a true sinusoid. The relation between the bandwidth Δf and the time constant T_c which this observation suggests proves to be a simple reciprocal relationship:

$$\Delta f = \pi / T_c \qquad (16)$$

Equation 16 resembles Equation 8 for the relation between the fundamental frequency and period of a periodic waveform. When applicable, each of these two equations provides insight into the relation between descriptions of waveforms in the time and frequency domains.

BEHAVIOR OF THE VOCAL TRACT

Formants. For the simple pendulum the impulse response was a damped sinusoid and the frequency response was a curve with a single peak located near the frequency of oscillation of the damped sinusoid. Although the air in the vocal tract is a considerably more complex physical system than a simple pendulum and consequently has an impulse response which is more complex than a single damped sinusoid, the impulse response of the vocal tract can nevertheless be analyzed into simpler components most of which are damped sinusoids. Each damped sinusoidal component of the impulse response of the vocal tract is called a *formant* and represents one of the natural modes of vibration or resonances of the vocal tract. Since a formant has the form of a damped sinusoid, a formant may be specified by a formant frequency, a formant bandwidth, and a formant amplitude.

To see how formants arise, we might consider the relatively simple case for the voiced oral vowels. For these vowels the vocal tract may be considered acoustically as a tube which is open at the lips and nearly closed at the glottis and which has a cross-sectional area which varies along the length of the tube. The transmission characteristic of such a tube depends for the most part upon the manner in which the cross-sectional area changes between the glottis and the lips. The characteristics of the sound radiation through the lips and the effect of the glottal opening on the reflection of sound at the glottis also influence the overall transmission characteristic of the tract. It should be instructive to consider how these effects arise from suitable modifications of the still simpler case of the uniform tube which is open at one end and closed at the other.

Formants in a uniform tube. If sound radiation from the open end of the uniform tube is neglected and if it is assumed that there is perfect sound reflection at the closed end, then the resonant frequencies of the tube are equally spaced along the frequency axis and occur at odd multiples of the first resonance. That is, if f_1 is the frequency of the first resonance, then the sequence of resonant frequencies follows the pattern:

$$f_1, 3f_1, 5f_1, 7f_1, \ldots \qquad \text{(A)}$$

The length l of the tube is just one-fourth of the wavelength λ_1 of the first resonance:

$$l = \lambda_1/4. \qquad (17)$$

The reciprocal relation between frequency and wavelength which was given in Equation 9 then allows Equation 17 to be expressed in the alternate form:

$$f_1 = c/\lambda_1 = c/4l \qquad (18)$$

In Equation 18 c denotes the speed of sound. In terms of the length of the tube, then, Sequence A for the resonances of the uniform tube may be given as:

$$\frac{c}{4l}, \frac{3c}{4l}, \frac{5c}{4l}, \frac{7c}{4l}, \ldots \qquad \text{(B)}$$

Although there are in principle an infinite number of formant frequencies, only a finite number of them fall within the audio frequency range. For example, if the typical value of $l = 17$ cm is taken for the length of the vocal tract between the glottis and the lips, then substitution into Equation 18 yields:

$$f_1 = \frac{343 \text{ m/sec}}{(4)\,(0.17 \text{ m})} = 500 \text{ Hz} \qquad (19)$$

The resonant frequencies of the uniform tube with the same length as the vocal tract are thus spaced approximately 1,000 Hz apart. This suggests that the usual 3,500 Hz telephone channel may be expected to suffice for the transmission of the first three or four formants. Formants higher than the fourth may be important for the naturalness of speech sounds, but it seems unlikely that they are normally important for perceptual discrimination between speech sounds. Experimental studies of the formants have usually been confined to the first four formants, or even to the first two or three.

The above remarks apply to the case of a uniform tube closed at one end and open at the other. It has been assumed that there was no sound radiation from the open end into the external air. To make this simple ideal case more realistic in terms of the human vocal tract, we should consider the effects of 1) sound radiation from the open end of the tube, 2) imperfect sound reflection from the closed end, and 3) deviations from uniform shape along the tube.

Radiation of sound from the open end. In neglecting the radiation of sound from the open end of the tube in this simplified case, it has been assumed that the volume of air outside the open end is so large that the acoustic movement of air within the opening does not significantly compress the external air. Although the actual volume of air outside the open end of the vocal tract is usually of the required size, it must be considered that, as a consequence of the finite speed of sound, not all points within this volume can be acted on simultaneously by the air within the open end of the tube. Thus the effective volume of air outside the mouth opening is limited essentially by the finite propagation time of an acoustic disturbance. This effective confinement of the air at the end of the tube is equivalent to an increase in the effective length of the tube. In view of the relation between the length of the tract and the sequence of resonant frequencies expressed by Sequence B above, this means that the formant frequencies should be decreased to some extent as a result of radiation. A detailed analysis demonstrates this effect more rigorously (Flanagan, 1965).

In an experimental study of acoustic radiation from the lips, Flanagan (1960) found that the radiation causes the higher frequencies of the vocal tract transmission characteristic to be enhanced by an amount which rises at the rate of approximately seven dB per octave. During voiced sounds, this offsets to some extent the 12 dB per octave drop in the level of the spectrum of the speech wave introduced by the glottal source of voice excitation.

In the ideal case of the uniform tube with no radiation and no loss of acoustic energy resulting from imperfect reflection of sound at the ends, the formant bandwidths are equal to zero. That is, if there were no loss of energy from the system the formants would be pure undamped sinusoids. The loss of energy from the system in the form of radiated sound in the real case has the effect of widening the bandwidths. This widening of the formant bandwidths is a common characteristic of all processes which act to dissipate the acoustic energy contained within the tract. Radiation of sound from the vocal tract is of course essential to the use of speech sounds in communication, since it is the acoustic energy which is radiated from the vocal tract that constitutes the acoustic speech waveform.

Effect of the glottis and subglottal system. If the glottis end of the vocal tract is now considered, it is found that the departure from true closure which is implied by the opening of the glottis results in an imperfect reflection of sound waves incident upon this end of the tract. The fact that the soft tissues reflect sound imperfectly may also be expected to have some effect. Part of the acoustic volume velocity of the wave incident upon the glottis end of the tract is dissipated through the resistance of the glottis to the flow of air. As a result, the glottis has the effect of widening the formant bandwidths to some extent.

The mass of the air within the glottis functions as an acoustic element of the vocal tract and acts to raise the frequencies of the formants somewhat (Flanagan, 1965). When the glottis is so widely opened that its area cannot be considered small in comparison with the cross-sectional area of the vocal tract, the manner in which the trachea and lungs are acoustically coupled with the supraglottal cavities must be taken into account and the resonant properties of these subglottal structures must be considered. An electrical analog for the trachea and lungs has been constructed by van den Berg (1960) on the basis of his experiments with the acoustic properties of these structures in cadavers. According to van den Berg, the lungs and trachea possess one rather broad resonance at approximately five to 10 Hz, a minimum at 40–50 Hz, and a series of sharper resonances which begin at 300 Hz and recur at approximately every 600 Hz thereafter. These properties may be of some significance in whispered speech, for example, in which the vocal folds are held apart and allow some degree of coupling between the subglottal and supraglottal parts of the vocal mechanism.

Effect of nonuniform vocal tract shapes. The most significant determinant of the frequencies of the formants is the manner in which the cross-sectional area of the vocal tract varies along its length. It has sometimes been stated that this can be accounted for by supposing the vocal tract to consist of a sequence of cavities separated by constrictions and supposing each of these cavities to determine one formant frequency. Although the first two or three formants can sometimes be accounted for in this manner when there are sufficiently narrow constrictions to provide a clear division of the vocal tract into distinct cavities, such a model cannot account for an infinite number of formants and it cannot account for the values of even the first few formant frequencies when the constrictions within the vocal tract are more open and there is no distinct division of the tract into discrete cavities. In general, even though some portions of the tract may sometimes be more important than others for certain formants, all of the formants depend on the geometry of the entire vocal tract. The dependence of the different formant frequencies upon the overall vocal tract configuration was demonstrated by Dunn (1950), who calculated the formant frequencies corresponding to some simplified tract shapes. In particular, he showed that even for a tract divided into two simple cavities the frequencies of the first three formants depend upon the dimensions of both cavities and upon the manner in which the cavities are coupled together.

More recently, Schroeder (1967) has shown that the vocal tract geometry may be described by a class of features which represent the manner in which the cross-sectional area deviates from uniformity. These features are divided into two subsets of features on the basis of whether or not they influence the formant frequencies. To a good first-order approximation, each feature of the first subset specifies the frequency of exactly one formant by determining the degree to which the corresponding formant frequency for the uniform tube would be perturbed by the introduction of the cross-sectional area change corresponding to that feature. There is a one-to-one correspondence between the formants and the features of this subset. The features of the second subset also describe ways in which the cross-sectional area of the uniform tube can be altered along its length. The features of the second subset, however, have only a minimal perturbation effect on the resonant frequencies of the uniform tube. Thus the features of the second subset characterize the possible compensatory articulations for the production of given acoustical speech sounds in the sense that they describe different vocal tract shapes which give rise to the same formant frequency patterns. This implies that there is not necessarily a one-to-one correspondence between vocal tract configurations and complete sets of formant frequencies. The physiological constraints on the degree to which the articulators can change shape evidently implies, however, that the number of compensatory articulations which are actually possible may in practice be quite limited. Schroeder's analysis has been substantiated and extended by the complementary study of Mermelstein (1967) and generalized in certain respects by the work of Heinz (1967).

THE ACOUSTICAL PROPERTIES OF SPEECH WAVES

We have just reviewed the acoustics of speech production and considered the manner in which acoustic energy is generated and modified within the vocal mechanism to produce the acoustic speech waveform. Attention may now be given to the speech waveform itself, with particular regard for those properties which reflect the mechanisms employed in the production.

The different types of acoustic sources which are employed in speech production give rise to waveforms which can be distinguished from one another by striking general characteristics. When the laryngeal voice source is employed in the production of a sound, for example, a waveform with a strong *quasi-periodic* component usually results. Often voiced sounds may instead have waveforms which are *double-periodic*, in the sense that although the waveform may be recurrent, the alternate periods of the waveform may resemble one another much more closely than the successive periods do. Alternatively, a voiced sound may have an *irregular-periodic* waveform in which there are recurrent "periods" but in which the periods vary irregularly. In contrast to the sounds which employ the laryngeal voice source, the sounds during which a turbulent noise source is active have *quasi-random* waveforms. Closely spaced samples of a quasi-random waveform have randomly distributed values which are nearly uncorrelated with one another. The voiceless fricatives and sibilants and the sounds which employ a whispered laryngeal action characteristically have quasi-random waveforms. If a transient source is employed in the production of a speech sound then the resulting waveform will characteristically have the form of a *burst* in which the waveform typically has a rapid increase to a relatively large amplitude followed by a relatively rapid decrease in amplitude. Speech bursts generally occur in the waveforms of released stop articulations. Naturally, when more than one type of source is active, the acoustic speech waveform can assume a composite form. When no acoustic speech source is active, on the other hand, the acoustic speech waveform is *quiescent* and has an amplitude which approximates zero. The voiceless interval during the occlusion of a voiceless plosive, for example, typically has a quiescent acoustic speech waveform.

The classification of intervals of the acoustic speech waveform according to the acoustic sources which are active during their production leads to the concept of *speech wave types*. In their work on acoustic phonetics, may be present. Acoustical speech parameters such as formant frequencies, formant bandwidths, formant amplitudes, frequencies of antiresonances, fundamental frequency, etc., provide further specification of the acoustic speech wave.

The changes in the frequencies of the first few formants are particularly informative about articulatory events. Broad-band sound spectrograms usually

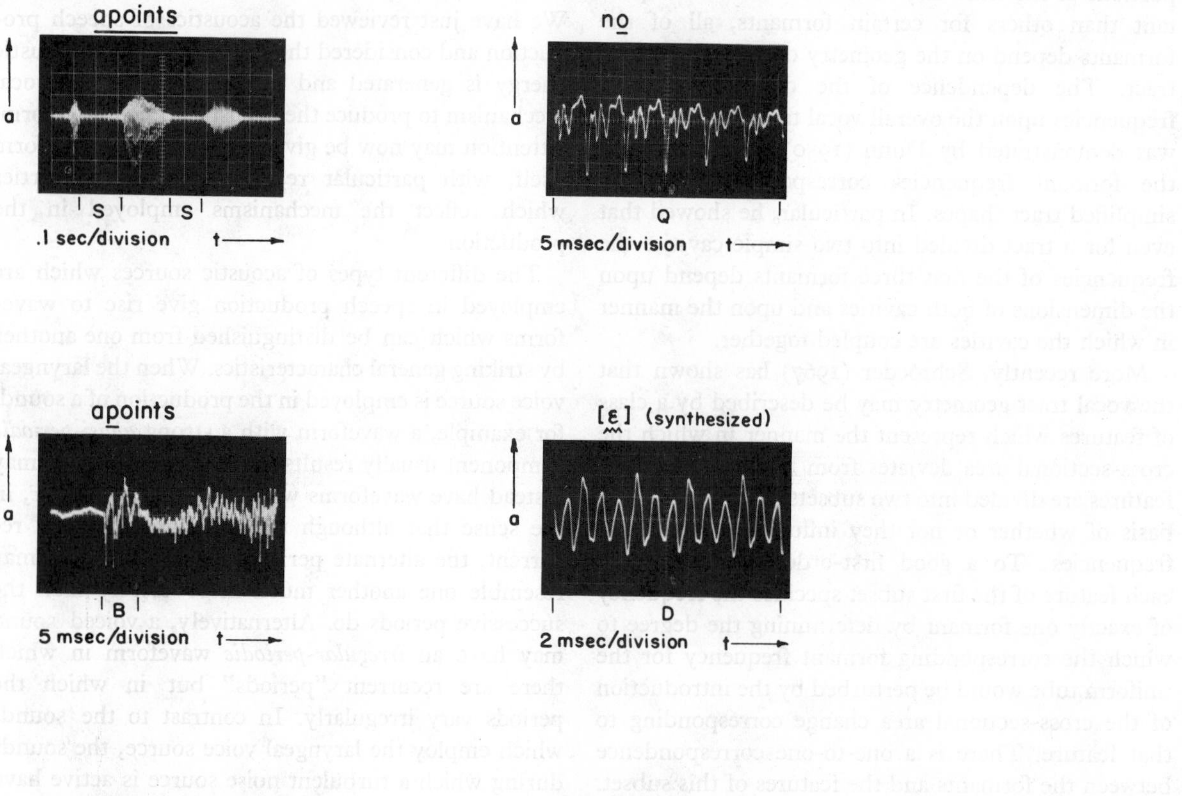

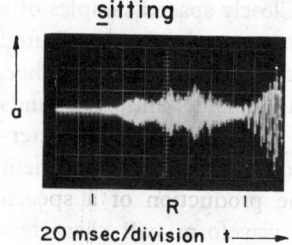

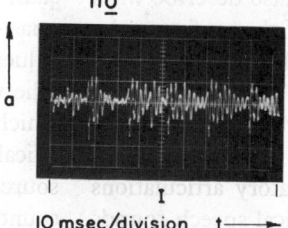

Fig. 6-11. Oscilloscope tracings of the basic speech wave types: S=quiescent; B=burst; R=quasi-random; Q=quasi-periodic; D=double periodic; I=irregular periodic. *Peterson and Shoup.*

Peterson and Shoup (1966) consider the basic speech-wave types to be the quiescent, burst, quasi-random, quasi-periodic, double periodic, and irregular periodic types of waveforms. In Fig. 6-11 an example of each of these basic speech-wave types is shown.

The assignment of a portion of an acoustic speech waveform to a speech-wave type usually accounts for only a part of the significant acoustic detail which provide a good display for observations of changing formant patterns. In Fig. 6-12, for example, is a broad-band spectrogram of the utterance "primed." A good collection of spectrograms of other utterances from American English speech may be found in *Visible Speech*, which is available in a new edition (Potter, Kopp, and Kopp, 1966). The dark bars indicate the positions of the formants. It is also possible to identify the basic speech-wave types on the sound spectrogram. The relatively regular spacing of the vertical striations during the voiced portions indicate quasi-periodic wave types. The blank segment during the initial voiceless plosive indicates a quiescent wave type. The irregularly marked segment corresponding to the aspiration of the plosive represents a quasi-random speech-wave type. To further appreciate the information contained in the spectrographic display, the characteristic acoustic patterns of the different sound formations should be considered. These include the vowel, sonorant, fricative, sibilant, flap, trill, plosive, and nasal manners of articulation as well as the acoustic prosodic parameters of fundamental voice frequency, speech power, and phone duration.

Vowels

FORMANT PATTERNS AND VOWEL QUALITY

The pharynx, mouth, and nose form a complex transmission path for the laryngeal tone. The cross-sectional area along the pharyngeal and oral cavities is variable. A whole series of formant frequencies at which resonance occurs depends upon the specific sizes and shapes of the tract; by adjusting the shapes of the tract, the resonant frequencies are altered.

These resonant frequencies have long been identified with vowel values. They have been specified and described previously by such men as Helmholtz (1895), Stumpf (1926), Paget (1930), and Miller (1926). Much of the early analysis involved men's voices and specific resonant frequency values were usually expressed for the vowels of a particular language. These resonant or formant frequencies are numbered according to their order along the frequency scale from low to high; that is, first formant, second formant, and so on.

Lloyd (1890) was probably the first to recognize that at least certain types of vowels are not well defined by absolute magnitudes of resonant frequency. It is fairly easy to anticipate this fact when it is recognized that men, women, and children do not have vocal tracts of the same size; yet all three types of speakers are capable of producing highly intelligible speech. In general, when such acoustical structures have similar shapes, the resonances of the smaller structures will be higher in frequency. This is illustrated by reference to the equations for uniform tubes in an earlier section of this chapter. An examination of these equations will show that if the length of a tube is divided by some constant k, then the resonant frequencies will all be multiplied by the same constant k.

Lloyd, and more recently Potter and Peterson (1948), developed the hypothesis that vowel sounds are determined in part by the relative values of the formant frequencies, rather than by the absolute

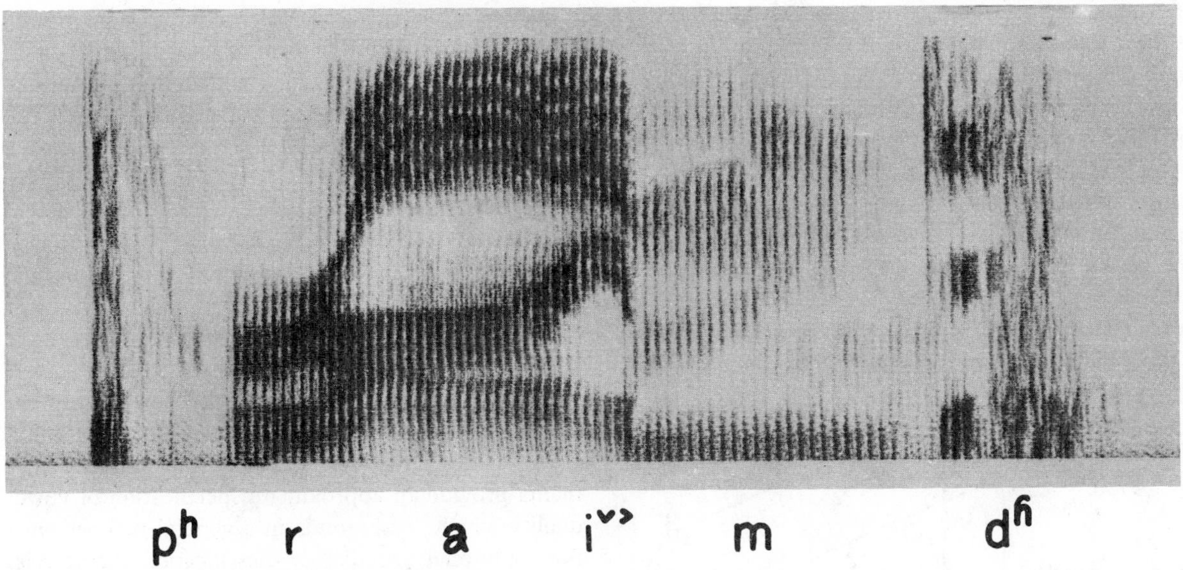

Fig. 6-12. Broad-band sound spectrogram of the word "primed."

magnitudes of these frequencies. Thus the relationships among formant frequencies are considered of significance in determining vowel values. Because of the nature of human perception, however, there is little reason to anticipate that the above principle will hold far beyond the range of normal voice production. These limitations should apply to formant frequency values, damping constants, and fundamental voice frequencies. For example, it is well known that vowel intelligibility degenerates when spectral multiplication or division is obtained by extensive speed change in reproducing recorded speech. As a further limitation on this simple hypothesis, Fant (1967) has pointed out that the relative values of the formant frequencies for men, women, and children do not follow a simple inverse proportionality to the overall size of the vocal tract. He suggests that the significant deviations from simple proportionality may be explained by systematic differences which occur in the shapes of the vocal tracts of men, women, and children. The ratio of the length of the pharyngeal cavity to the length of the oral cavity, for example, tends to be greater in males than in females.

Joos (1948) and Potter and Peterson have noted the relationship of acoustical charts of the formant frequencies to the conventional vowel diagram. Such an acoustical chart is obtained, for example, when the frequency of the second formant is plotted against the frequency of the first formant. The conventional vowel diagram has been employed for many years and has been drawn in several different forms; it is presumed to represent physiological dimensions.

Fig. 6-13 shows the frequency of the second formant plotted against the frequency of the first formant for similar vowels produced by a man, woman, and a child (Peterson, 1951b). The displacement in frequency of these vowel loops is obvious. The frequency scale employed in this plot is that developed by Koenig (1949) as an approximate pitch scale, linear below 1,000 Hz and logarithmic above.

When the origin is placed at the upper right in such a plot, the loop takes the form of the traditional vowel diagram. Separate loops for rounded and unrounded vowels are shown in Fig. 6-14 (Peterson, 1951a). The coordinates on this graph are constructed with a frequency spacing according to the mel or pitch scale of Stevens and Volkman (1940). It is of interest that the unrounded and rounded vowel loops overlap markedly. This indicates the necessity of additional acoustical dimensions for the exact phonetic specification of vowels, even when produced by a single speaker.

Various facts suggest that the lower formant frequencies are of primary importance in determining vowel value. As indicated above, the first two formants provide an approximate specification of vowel quality which corresponds in a general manner with the traditional articulatory classification for vowels. In general, the second formant lies within the most sensitive range of human hearing, and the range of the second formant corresponds roughly to the range of the frequency spectrum which makes the greatest contribution to speech intelligibility. These and other considerations suggest that the higher formants are of somewhat less importance than the first two in determining the phonetic quality of vowel sounds. In general, it appears that the higher formant frequencies primarily contribute to increased definition or exactness of vowel quality.

Peterson and Barney (1952) made measurements of the fundamental voice frequency and the formant frequencies of a series of vowels produced by 76 different speakers; these included 33 men, 28 women, and 15 children. The vowels were located in an *hVd* combination. The speakers represented various dialects throughout the United States, but were predominately General American; a limited number of

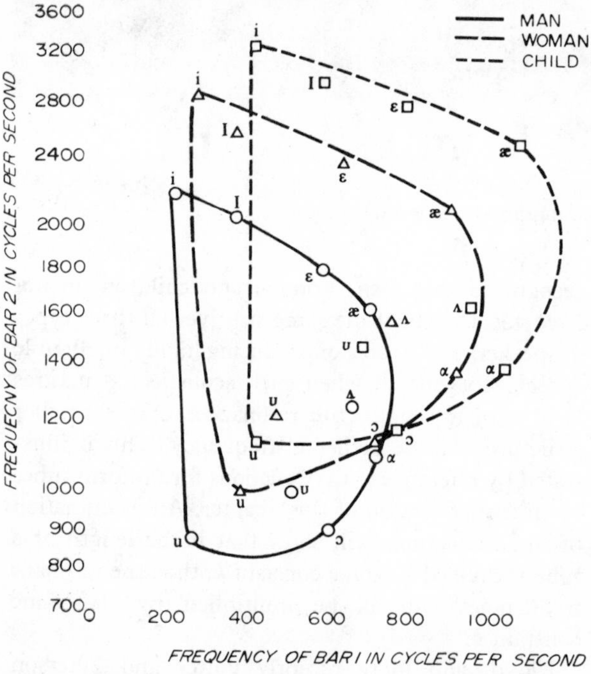

Fig. 6-13. Loops constructed with the frequency of the second formant plotted against the frequency of the first formant for vowels produced by a man, a woman, and a child. *Peterson, 1951b.*

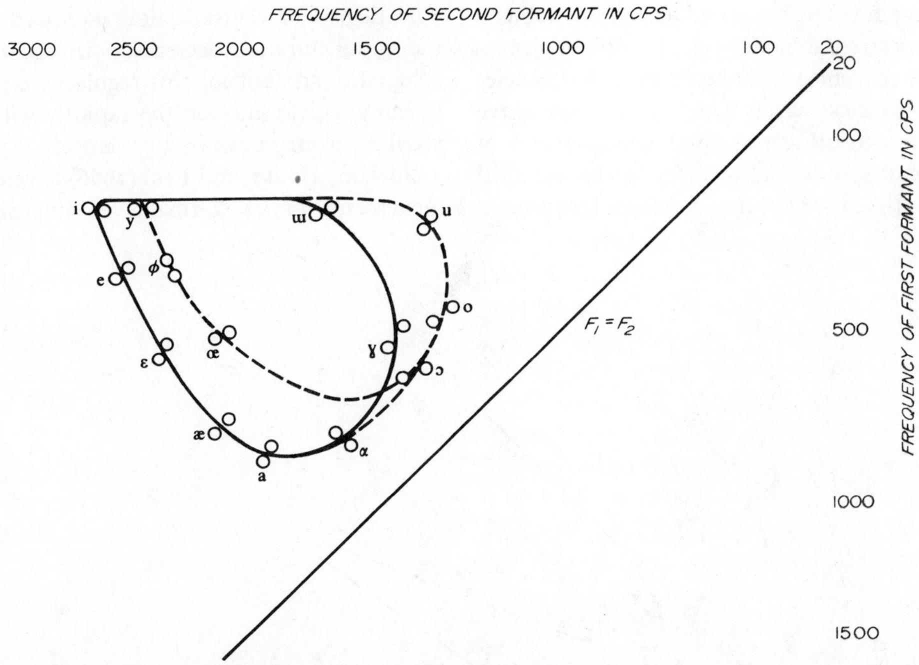

Fig. 6-14. Loops for the frequency of the second formant plotted against the frequency of the first formant for sustained vowels by one speaker. Each vowel was spoken twice, and the points are plotted along a mel scale. The solid line represents unrounded vowels, and the dashed line represents rounded vowels. *Peterson 1951a.*

persons with foreign dialect were included. The individual values for the frequencies of the first two formants are plotted in Fig. 6-15. The coordinates in this chart are linear below 1,000 Hz and logarithmic above. The boundary lines are drawn to provide an optimum discrimination or separation among the vowels. The vowels were also classified by means of a series of listening tests, but the separating lines in Fig. 6-15 are according to speaker classification; that is, the symbol representing each vowel on the chart is determined by the spelling in the *hVd* list which the speaker originally read. From this chart, a table was constructed showing the percentage correct identification for each vowel. The average correct recognition according to speaker classification for the ten vowels is 79 percent. The overlapping points in part illustrate the inadequacy of two formant values for complete vowel specification. Also, considerable formant movement was actually involved in the utterances, since the vowels were formed in a consonant environment.

The formant bandwidths for the vowels in the above set of data were studied by Dunn (1961) in the course of his work on the evaluation of methods for the measurement of vowel formant bandwidths. He found that the formant bandwidths tended to increase with the formant frequencies. For the first two formants the bandwidths widened slowly with increasing formant frequency. Thus for the first two formants the formant Q's[6] actually increased with increasing formant frequency. Dunn found the average widths for formants 1, 2, and 3 for male speakers to be 50, 64, and 115 Hz, respectively. Considerable variation was encountered from vowel to vowel, and appreciable individual variation in formant bandwidths, may also be anticipated.

MOVEMENTS IN VOWEL FORMANT PATTERNS

The patterns produced by the sound spectrograph have emphasized the kinetic nature of speech. The speech organs are in an almost continuous movement as phonemic sequences are produced, and these movements are reflected in the changing acoustical structure of the speech wave. The manner in which the changing formant frequencies determine vowel value is a matter of considerable interest, and there

[6] The *Q*, or quality factor, of a resonator is the ratio of the resonant frequency to the bandwidth. Thus if the frequency of the first formant is 500 Hz and its bandwidth is 50 Hz, then the *Q* of the first formant will be 10.

is much research yet to be carried out on this subject.

In one spectrographic study, Lindblom (1963) observed the movements of the formant frequencies of Swedish vowels which were spoken in three different symmetrical consonantal contexts and at various rates of speech. Between the initial and final portions of the vowels, the formant frequencies followed smooth arcs. The values attained by the formant frequencies in the central portion of a vowel depended in a relatively regular fashion upon the particular vowel intended by the speaker, the consonantal context, and the duration of the vowel. The vowels were characteristically produced with more centralized articulations than would be expected for the same vowel phonemes pronounced in isolation. The degree of centralization increased regularly as the vowel duration decreased. An equation was developed to account for this regularity on the basis of dynamic constraints on the rapidity with which the vocal mechanism can change its state.

Stevens, House, and Paul (1966) have observed the movements of the formants of English vowels in symmetrical consonantal contexts with results which are in basic agreement with those of Lindblom for Swedish vowels. Their work suggests, however, that the regularities of formant movements are complex, and that there is a need for a better understanding of the dynamics of speech at the physiological level.

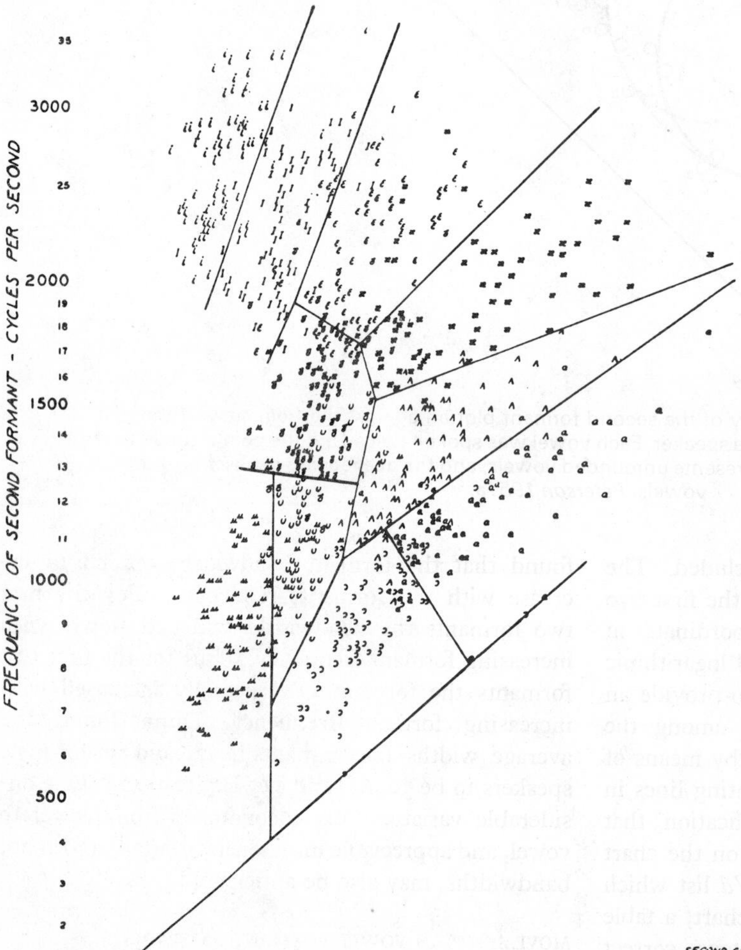

Fig. 6-15. The frequency of the second formant versus the frequency of the first formant for the ten vowels produced in *hVd* series by 76 speakers. The lines have been drawn to provide approximately optimum separation among the vowels according to the two formants, when the vowels are classified according to the lists from which the speakers read. *Peterson and Barney.*

An articulatory model to account for the dynamics of formant movements in VCV utterances has been proposed by Öhman (1966, 1967). He supposes that at any given time the position and shape of an articulator is a composite of the effects of gestures which correspond to both the consonant and the adjacent vowels. In particular, the vocal tract shape during the closure for a plosive is seen as a combination of an ideal shape for the consonant itself and an ideal shape which depends upon the vowel context.

VOWEL NASALIZATION

An interesting problem in the acoustical description of vowels is the effect of nasalization. House and Stevens (1956) have studied some of the acoustic properties of nasalized vowels with the aid of an electrical analog of the vocal tract. Circuits for an analog of the nasal tract were connected to an analog of the pharyngeal and oral portions of the tract. Different degrees of coupling between the oral and nasal tracts were introduced by varying the effective size of the velopharyngeal opening. It was found that increasing the coupling between the oral and nasal tracts had the effect of widening the formant bandwidths and decreasing the formant amplitudes. The formant frequencies were also shifted upward to some extent. Additional resonances introduced into the spectrum were not observed in the analog study. Additional resonances are often found on sound spectrograms of naturally produced nasalized vowels, however, and have often been considered as one of the characteristic properties of nasality. House and Stevens found that in their model extra resonances could be introduced by decreasing the damping which was assumed for the analog nasal tract, but that the values for the damping constants would then be smaller than would be expected for the human nasal cavities. In a perceptual test with the synthesized vowels, House and Stevens found that judgments of nasality corresponded with the degree of coupling between the nasal and oral parts of the analog tract. Thus it appears that additional resonances may not be a necessary cue for the perception of nasality. This conclusion was substantiated and generalized by Dickson (1962), who found that none of the acoustic properties which have traditionally been associated with nasality and nasalization is capable of yielding consistent listener judgments of nasality. Instead, he suggests that combinations of parameters are required for reliable acoustic identification of nasality and nasalization. It would appear that nasality requires more study at both the acoustic and perceptual levels.

Sonorants

The sonorant consonants are normally produced with an airflow that is in an unstable state between laminar and turbulent flow. These sounds, sometimes called semivowels, are usually involved in the production of the English consonant phonemes /j/, /w/, /l/, and /r/. On sound spectrograms the sonorants usually display the quasi-periodic pattern which is typical of vowels, and the sonorants have formant patterns which resemble those of vowels. Some friction is also often evident. A consistent acoustic distinction between sonorants and vowels is in the frequencies of the formants. The most extensive study of the formant frequencies of the sonorants of American English is that of Lehiste (1964). In general, it was found that the first formant of the sonorants was lower in frequency than would be usual for vowels. For /w/ the formant frequencies resembled those of /u/, but both the first and second formants were lower in frequency than for the /u/. The energy in the third formant of /w/ was often not visible on the spectrogram. The formant structure of /j/ was found to resemble that of /i/, but the first and second formants were lower and the third formant was higher than was typical for the /i/.

In her observations of the formants of /l/, Lehiste found many variations, dependent upon the phonetic context of the consonant. These variations were most striking for the second formant, which tended to follow the second formant of the following vowel when the /l/ occurred in initial position. When the /l/ occurred in final position the second formant was displaced less, but in this case the frequency of the second formant of the preceding vowel tended to be lowered. Lehiste observed considerable variations in the formant patterns of the English /r/ phoneme, which depended principally upon the position of occurrence of the /r/ within an utterance and upon the phonetic context. Two properties common to all the variants, however, were the low frequency of the third formant and the consequent relatively narrow separation in frequency between the second and third formants. The position of the first formant varied considerably depending upon whether the /r/ was initial and manifested by the sonorant consonant [r] or whether it was noninitial and manifested by the retroflexed vowel [ɝ]. The consonant form had a consistently lower first-formant frequency in relation to the vowel form.

In a sequence consisting of a sonorant and a vowel, the formant frequencies must naturally undergo transitions between the formant pattern for the sonorant and the one for the vowel. O'Conner, Gerstman, Liberman, Delattre, and Cooper (1957) observed the sonorant-vowel formant transitions in natural speech and manipulated them in listening tests based on synthesized speech. According to their findings, formant transitions gave rise to sonorant judgment if they had durations longer than those associated with stops and nasals, but shorter durations than those of transitions between successive vowels. Transition durations were thus found to influence the perception of sonorants as a consonant class. Variations in the frequencies of the transition onsets were found to influence discrimination between different sonorants. These onset frequencies were in basic correspondence with the steady-state frequencies normally associated with the different sonorants.

Fricatives and Sibilants

Friction sources are active during the production of voiceless fricatives and sibilants and give rise to the quasi-random waveforms of these sounds. For a voiced fricative or sibilant, both a friction source and the laryngeal voice source are active concurrently so that the waveform of voiced fricatives and sibilants characteristically have both quasi-random and quasi-periodic components. Spectrograms indicate that fricatives and sibilants generally have energy distributed continuously across a wide range of frequencies. Formants are often evident, especially when the frequency range of the analysis is extended beyond 3,500 Hz.

The filter characteristics for fricatives and sibilants have been discussed by Heinz and Stevens (1961). As with other formations of the vocal tract, the formant frequencies of fricatives and sibilants are determined chiefly by the vocal tract shape. The effect of the forward placement of the friction source within the vocal tract which is typical for most fricative and sibilant productions is not particularly relevant to the determination of the formant frequencies. The placement of the friction source does, however, account for the existence of antiresonances in the transmission characteristic. An antiresonance corresponds to a frequency region in which the acoustic energy of a source is strongly attenuated by the vocal tract.

Heinz and Stevens constructed an electrical circuit on the basis of their theoretical considerations of the vocal tract transmission characteristic. The circuit had one resonance and one antiresonance and, when driven by an appropriate noise source, produced simulated fricative and sibilant sounds. The parameters of the circuit were adjusted to achieve optimal matches between the spectra of simulated productions and the spectra of natural fricatives and sibilants. The spectra for the naturally produced sounds had been previously obtained by Hughes and Halle (1956). Within the limited assumptions employed in the construction of the circuit, reasonably good agreement between theoretical and measured spectra were obtained.

In addition to the studies by Heinz and Stevens and by Hughes and Halle, the acoustic properties of fricatives and sibilants have been studied by Strevens (1960) and by Jassem (1962, 1965). The results of the different studies have been presented in different ways and it is difficult at present to state with assurance the acoustic parameters and parameter values which are most relevant to the phonetic values of fricatives and sibilants. Hughes and Halle obtained continuous spectra of voiced and voiceless fricative and sibilant productions by four speakers of English. For a given sound there was considerable interspeaker variation in the fine structure of the continuous spectrum. By means of a set of general binary categories, however, it was possible to achieve a fair separation of the sounds on the basis of their spectra. For example, the voiced productions were distinguished from the voiceless productions by the presence or absence of a strong component in the spectrum below 700 Hz.

Jassem measured the formant frequencies of fricative and sibilant productions of three speakers, one each of Swedish, English, and Polish. He proposed a set of three binary categories which accomplished a fairly successful partial categorization of his data. These binary categories were formulated differently from those of Hughes and Halle, however, and it is difficult to compare the results of the two studies.

Strevens recorded sustained voiceless fricatives and sibilants produced by 13 phonetically trained subjects. From the spectrograms of the sounds there appeared to be little regularity in the detailed structure of a given fricative or sibilant and more general categories were employed to organize the results. Strevens grouped the fricatives and sibilants into three categories according to their relative intensity. The least intense sounds were the [ɸ], [f], and [θ], the most intense were the [s], [ʃ], and [ç], while the [h], [x], and [X] were of intermediate intensity. Within these categories further classification was made according to the primary frequency region occupied by the spectrum of a given sound. Within the intermediate intensity category, for example, [x] had the highest lower frequency limit of significant spectral energy, while [h] had the lowest lower limit, and [X] had an intermediate lower limit.

An extensive study of the acoustic properties of fricatives and sibilants has not yet been carried out. As the studies just indicated have shown, however, it is difficult to choose a set of parameters which are both theoretically relevant to the acoustics of fricative and sibilant production and practically relevant to a consistent scheme of descriptive classification.

Harris (1958) carried out a perceptual study to determine the relative significance of the steady-state portions and transition portions of fricatives and sibilants. Tape recordings were spliced so that the fricatives and sibilants could be placed in the contexts of the vowels which had been produced in the context of any other fricative or sibilant. It was found that listeners identified the sibilants /s/ and /ʃ/ primarily by cues present in the sounds themselves and that the transition information contained in the contiguous vowels had relatively little influence. For distinguishing between the fricatives /f/ and /θ/, however, it was found that listeners made identifications according to the transition information contained in the adjacent vowels, and the cues present in the fricatives themselves were less important. Thus the types of cues which are important for a listener's identification of a given fricative or sibilant evidently depend upon the particular fricative or sibilant involved. A better understanding of the perception of fricatives and sibilants probably requires in part a better understanding of the acoustic structures of these sounds.

Stops

The stop consonants involve the buildup of a pressure against a closure in the vocal tract which may be released to produce an acoustic burst. Plosives are stops in which the pressure is built up pulmonically. Other types of stops, such as clicks, ejectives, and implosives, can be formed by nonpulmonic pressures. Plosives, however, are by far the most common type of stop consonants.

During the closure for a stop the laryngeal voice source may be inactive so that the acoustic output of the vocal tract may approximate silence. The acoustic phonetic parameter for an interval of silence is called a gap and on a sound spectrogram a gap is represented by a blank space. On the other hand, the laryngeal voice source may be active during the period of closure so that a quasi-period sound may be produced. Owing to the closure, however, the transmission of the higher resonant frequencies of the vocal tract will be heavily attenuated with the result that usually only one resonance of relatively low frequency can be noted on the sound spectrogram. This low resonance, which occurs when there is voicing during a closure, is called a voice bar. In Fig. 6-12 above, for example, a gap is seen for the closure of the /p/ and a voice bar for the closure of the /d/.

When the pressure buildup for a stop is released by the opening of the closure, the sudden application of the pressure difference to the air in the vocal tract functions as a transient source of acoustic excitation. The acoustic result is a sharp burst which appears on the sound spectrogram as a strong vertical striation at the instant of the release. The properties of acoustic bursts in plosive releases were studied by Halle, Hughes, and Radley (1957). In a perceptual experiment, these authors isolated the burst intervals from plosive productions and found that listeners could identify the plosive from their bursts at a significantly better than random rate. A spectral analysis of the bursts revealed a variety of different types of fine structure in the spectrum, but certain general trends were also observed. For example, the bilabial bursts tended to have relatively strong concentrations of energy in the interval between 500 and 1,500 Hz, the palatal and velar bursts tended to have concentrations of energy between 1,500 and 4,000 Hz, and the alveolar bursts were distinguished either by relatively flat spectra or by concentrations of energy above 4,000 Hz. Bursts were also studied by Fischer-Jørgensen (1954) in an investigation of Danish plosives.

As mentioned previously, the release of a stop can be accompanied by an interval of turbulent airflow which acts as a friction source. As a result, aspiration occurs which acoustically resembles the fricatives and sibilants, which also involve friction sources. Fischer-Jørgensen has observed, for example, that in Danish the aspiration following /t/ has spectral characteristics which resemble those of the Danish /s/.

From these observations, it may be concluded that quite different considerations apply to the separate intervals involved in the production of a plosive consonant: the interval of closure, the instant of pressure release, and the interval of pressure equalization. Another major consideration for the acoustical characteristics of stop consonants is the nature of the transition between the stop and the sounds which are adjacent to it. The behavior of transitions in vowel formants adjacent to plosives has been a particularly active area of study. Cooper, Delattre, Liberman, Borst, and Gerstman (1952) studied the effects of vowel formant transitions on listener judgments of consonant values. This work has been summarized by Liberman (1957). For these investigations a pattern playback machine was employed extensively. The pattern playback is an electro-optical device for the conversion of spectrographic patterns to sound. Sets of simplified spectrograms were prepared in which the formant frequencies and transitions were varied systematically. The spectral characteristics of plosive bursts could also be represented and varied. It was found that the second formant transition could be employed as a particularly effective cue for influencing listener judgments of place of articulation. This was found to be true not only of the synthetic voiced and unvoiced plosives, but for synthetic nasal consonants as well. Harris, Hoffman, Liberman, Delattre, and Cooper (1958) observed that third-formant transitions also have significant influence on the perception of place of articulation. Hoffman (1958) has discussed the relative perceptual influences of burst spectra and transitions in the second and third formants.

Halle, Hughes, and Radley (1957) did a spectrographic study of vowel formant transitions in the plosives of natural speech and concluded that the character of the transitions depended not only on the vowel and consonant involved, but also on whether the vowel followed or preceded the plosive. In addition, it was difficult to determine criteria according to which transitions could be reliably identified in the natural speech. More recently, Öhman (1966, 1967) carried out some elegant empirical studies of vowel formant transitions in VCV contexts. These studies show that both the vowel preceding the consonant and the vowel following the consonant as well as the consonant itself influence both the transition into and the transition away from the consonant.

The so-called voiced plosive phonemes of a language are often realized by plosive phones which are not voiced during their entire duration. Sometimes, for example, the /b/ phoneme of English is realized by the simple nonaspirated voiceless plosive [p]. Thus the voicing may not begin until the following vowel is in progress. The timing of the onset of voicing in relation to the release of a plosive has been investigated by Lisker and Abramson (1964) in a study which included plosives from several different languages. While a considerable variation among individual speakers was observed, a given speaker tended to be fairly consistent in the placement of voicing onset with respect to the burst in a manner which depended upon whether the plosive was to be "voiced" or not. In English, for example, the "voiceless" plosive phonemes typically displayed voicing onset approximately 20 msec later than the corresponding "voiced" plosive phonemes.

Trills and Flaps

Both trills and flaps involve closure of the vocal tract, but, unlike the stops, the closures are so brief that not enough pressure can build up to produce a sharp burst upon release. Trills involve two or more oscillations of an articulator and, although they do not normally occur in English, they are fairly common in other languages. The oscillations for trills involve closures but do not involve bursts. Acoustically, the articulatory oscillations for trills modulate the intensity of the emitted sound waves to produce an alternation between greater intensity and smaller intensity. For each complete oscillation of the articulator, there will be one complete cycle of intensity modulation. On a sound spectrogram this intensity variation is manifested by alternation of intervals of darker and lighter marking.

Flaps, on the other hand, do occur regularly in English. A common example is the "flap t" or "flap r" which can often be found intervocalically in such words as "ladder," "bottom," etc. In these instances the vocal fold vibration is usually not interrupted for the flap and the intervocalic flaps are normally voiced throughout. Flaps may be expected to be associated with transitions in the vowel formants which are similar to those observed in the context of stops and to involve a reduction in the overall sound intensity during the period of closure particularly in the higher frequency components of the waveform.

Nasals

On a sound spectrogram a nasal consonant displays a formant pattern which is in some respects similar to the patterns observed for vowels. Transitions into and out of the nasal formant patterns are often abrupt, and the frequency positions of the nasal formants are often remarkably stable through most of the duration of the consonant. Owing to the greater damping in the nasal passages, the bandwidths of nasal formants tend to be wider than vowel formant bandwidths. This factor together with the relatively small openings provided by the nostrils contributes to an overall attenuation of the intensity level of nasal consonants in comparison to vowels.

House (1957) synthesized steady-state nasals with an electrical analog of the vocal tract which included a cascade of sections for the nasal passages as well as the usual sections for the pharyngeal and oral passages. Perceptual tests indicated that the synthesized nasals were reasonably acceptable and identifiable. Properties of the synthesized nasals which had been noted previously for natural nasal productions included a low-frequency (200–300 Hz) first formant, a strong second formant in the neighborhood of 1,000 Hz, and a lower intensity level than vowels produced with comparable source energy. In addition, an antiresonance was observed whose frequency depended on the place of articulation of the oral closure: for the bilabial articulation the antiresonance was near 1,000 Hz, for the alveolar articulation it was near 3,500 Hz, and for palatal and velar positions its frequency was in excess of 5,000 Hz. These values may be compared to those found by Fujimura (1962) in humanly produced nasals. Fujimura observed antiresonances for /m/ between 750 Hz and 1,250 Hz, for /n/ between 1,450 Hz and 2,200 Hz, and for /ŋ/ in excess of 3,000 Hz.

The nasal antiresonances arise from the closed oral cavity which in the production of a nasal consonant acts as a side branch of the pharyngeal-nasal passage. The length of the side branch is directly related to the wavelength corresponding to the antiresonance frequency. In the ideal case of a uniform side branch closed at the distal end, the length of the branch is one-fourth the wavelength of the antiresonance. Thus the further forward the oral closure is made, the greater the length of the side branch and the lower the frequency of the antiresonance. There is some question about the perceptual importance of the antiresonance, since Nakata (1959) was able to synthesize some intelligible nasals using only resonances and no antiresonances. Hence the antiresonance may not be essential to the perception of nasals, but the extent to which an antiresonance can function as a supplementary cue remains to be determined.

The role of nasal-vowel formant transitions in the perception of nasal consonants has been widely studied. Malécot (1956) recorded some nasal-vowel and vowel-nasal monosyllables and by means of a tape-splicing technique associated the different nasal steady-states with the different nasal-vowel transitions. When the spliced tapes were presented to listeners, it was found that the judgments of the place of articulation of the nasal were significantly more strongly influenced by the transitions than they were by the steady-states. Liberman, Delattre, Cooper, and Gerstman (1954) had previously investigated the perceptual influences of nasal-vowel formant transitions with speech material synthesized on the pattern playback. For their experiments the same steady-state pattern was employed for all the nasals and it was found that judgments of the place of articulation for the nasals were influenced by the vowel formant transitions in a manner very similar to that found for the stop consonants.

Hecker (1961) employed a dynamically controlled vocal tract analog to simulate both the steady-states of the nasals and the nasal-vowel transitions. A particularly appealing feature of the dynamic analog was that its sequential program was based on essentially physiological articulatory information and thus a relatively direct connection between articulatory input and acoustic output could be achieved. In particular, the motions of the velum and the timing of the oral opening and closing movements could then be related to the acoustic properties of the nasal-vowel transitions.

Prosodies

In the above paragraphs the acoustical attributes of the vowels and consonants were discussed. Another aspect of the speech signal which should be recognized is the prosodic variation of the voice. The prosodies are basic to such linguistic concepts as stress and intonation and to nonlinguistic concepts such as individual voice characteristics and emotional characteristics of the voice. Acoustically, the prosodies have sometimes been identified as fundamental voice frequency, voice intensity level, and acoustic phonetic duration. The fundamental voice frequency especially has been studied experimentally in several different contexts.

The acoustic prosodic parameters function in language to signal certain meaningful distinctions between utterances. Syllable stress and sentence intonation in English are manifested primarily by variations in the prosodic parameters. While intensity has often been associated with syllable stress in English, experimental studies indicate that fundamental frequency and vowel duration have greater influence on stress perception than does intensity. In some studies with synthesized speech, Fry (1955, 1958) manipulated the intensity, duration, and fundamental frequency patterns of a set of two-syllable words such as "object" which could be interpreted as either nouns or verbs depending on whether the first or second syllable was stressed. While it was found that all three variables influenced the stress perception in that syllables with higher fundamentals, longer durations, and greater intensities tended to be identified as stressed, the variables differed significantly in influence. Fundamental frequency tended to dominate duration and duration tended to dominate intensity. The differences were sufficiently small, however, that any two of the parameters acting in the same direction could overcome the influence of the third.

The fact that fundamental frequency was found to be a strong cue for stress perception is interesting in view of the theory of Bolinger (1958) to the effect that accent in English is manifested by pitch prominence. According to Bolinger, a sudden change in the fundamental frequency, either upward or downward, can produce a pitch prominence which will be interpreted as accent by a listener.

Fundamental frequency is also basic to intonation which, for example, is sometimes employed by a speaker to change a declarative utterance into an interrogative one. Thus the linguistic function of fundamental frequency is complicated by its simultaneous involvement with both stress and intonation. A good understanding of how variations in the acoustic prosodic parameters are to be interpreted as linguistic signals has yet to be achieved. The analysis of the various acoustic prosodic parameters, including fundamental frequency, is further complicated by dependencies upon the individual vowel sounds and upon phonetic contexts.

House and Fairbanks (1953), Peterson and Barney, and others have found a tendency for the fundamental frequency of the voice to vary systematically from one vowel to another. Thus, ordinarily high vowels such as [i] and [u] tend to have higher fundamentals than a low vowel such as [a]. In addition, vowels following voiceless consonants tend to have higher peak fundamental frequencies and higher average fundamental frequencies than do vowels following voiced consonants. Some physiological mechanisms have been suggested which might explain these trends as consequences of the structure of the vocal mechanism.

The vowels also display significant differences in intensity. A number of authors have observed that more open vowels such as [a] and [ɔ] tend to be more intense than the closer vowels such as [i] and [u]. Lehiste and Peterson (1959) found, for example, that on the average an [a] tended to be approximately five dB more intense than an [i] pronounced under similar conditions. This intensity difference, though significant, is small enough for considerable overlap to exist among the intensities of different vowel tokens, e.g., it should be expected that many tokens of [i] should be more intense than many tokens of [a]. Though contrary trends have been reported by some authors, for example House and Fairbanks, there appears to be a reasonable acoustic explanation for the greater intensity of open vowels. Since the open vowels tend to present larger openings to the external air, they should be more effective in radiating the acoustic energy of the voice source. In addition, the more open vowels have higher first-formant frequencies than do the more close vowels and as a consequence the attenuating effect of the vocal tract transfer characteristic should be reduced. Thus if the source intensity is maintained constant, then the vowel intensities should display the observed trend. It is interesting that when Ladefoged and McKinney (1963) used subglottic pressure as a measure of voice source activity, an /a/ tended to be approximately five dB more intense than an /i/ or /u/ produced with the same subglottic pressure. There are also significant trends for vowel intensity to vary with consonants preceding and following the vowel. Lehiste and Peterson (1959) have reported that vowels tend to be slightly more intense in the context of voiced consonants than in the context of voiceless consonants.

The correspondence between vowel stress and vowel duration was noted by Parmenter and Treviño (1935), who made duration measurements of the acoustic speech waveform from an oscilloscope trace recorded on motion picture film. House and Fairbanks (1953) confirmed earlier observations that the duration of a vowel followed by a voiced consonant in English tends to be significantly longer than the same vowel followed by a voiceless consonant. Denes (1955) showed that this tendency was so pronounced that listener judgments of whether a consonant was voiced or voiceless could be shifted by changing the duration of the preceding vowel.

In languages other than English vowel durations

can be observed to follow quite different patterns. This is evident in languages for which long and short versions of the same vowel belong to different phonemic categories, as the distinction in Finnish between *tuli* ("fire") and *tuuli* ("wind") which is made by changing the duration of the first vowel (Ravila, 1962). Thus it is of some interest to know which predictable features of vowel duration depend on the particular way that the sound system of a language is organized and which features are universal and depend upon more general considerations, such as the physiology of speech production. House (1961), in particular, has suggested that the primary correlates of vowel duration in English are specific to the English language and must be learned by speakers. Another influence on vowel duration which is also probably a part of the language code is the speech tempo. The rhythmic time patterning of speech is at present not well understood and requires further study.

There is in general a need for a better understanding of the acoustic prosodic parameters, their physiological and linguistic correlates, in both normal and pathological speech.

BIBLIOGRAPHY

Beranek, L. 1949. Acoustic measurements. New York: Wiley.

Berg, J. van den. 1960. An electrical analogue of the trachea, lungs, and tissues. *Acta Physiol. Pharmacol. Neerl.*, 9, 361–385.

———, Zantema, J., and Doornenbal, P., Jr. 1957. On the air resistance and the bernoulli effect of the human larynx. *J. acoust. soc. Amer.*, 29, 626–631.

Bolinger, D. 1958. A theory of pitch accent in English. *Word*, 14, 109–149.

Carr, P., and Trill, D. 1964. Long-term larynx-excitation spectra. *J. acoust. soc. Amer.*, 36, 2033-2040.

Coleman, R., and Wendahl, R. 1968. On the validity of laryngeal photosensor monitoring, *J. acoust. soc. Amer.*, 44, 1733–1735.

Cooley, J., and Tukey, J. 1965. An algorithm for the machine calculation of complex fourier series. *Math. Comp.*, 19, 297–301.

Cooper, F., Delattre, P., Liberman, A., Borst, J., and Gerstman, L. 1952. Some experiments on the perception of synthetic speech sounds. *J. acoust. soc. Amer.*, 24, 597–606.

Denes, P. 1955. Effect of duration on the perception of voicing. *J. acoust. soc. Amer.*, 27, 761–764.

Dickson, D. 1956. An acoustic study of nasality. *J. Speech Hearing Research*, 5, 103–111.

Dunker, E., and Schlosshauer, B. 1958. Über Anspannung und Schwingungsform der Stimmlippen. *Arch. Ohr.- Nas.-Kehlk. Heilk.*, 173, 497–500.

Dunn, H. 1950. The calculation of vowel resonances, and an electrical vocal tract. *J. acoust. soc. Amer.*, 22, 740–753.

———. 1961. Methods of measuring vowel formant bandwidths. *J. acoust. soc. Amer.*, 33, 1737–1746.

Fant, G. 1960. Acoustic theory of speech production. The Hague: Mouton.

———. 1967. A note on vocal tract size and non-uniform F-pattern scalings. Royal Institute of Technology, Stockholm, STL-QPSR, January 15, 1967, 22–30.

Farnsworth, D. 1940. High-speed motion pictures of the human vocal cords. *Bell Laboratories Record*, 18, 203–208.

Fischer-Jørgensen, E. 1954. Acoustic analysis of stop consonants. *Miscellanea Phonetica*, 2, 42–59.

Flanagan, J. 1958. Some properties of the glottal sound source. *J. Speech Hearing Research*, 1, 99–116.

———. 1960. Analog measurements of sound radiation from the mouth. *J. acoust. soc. Amer.*, 31, 1613–1620.

———. 1962. Some influences of the glottal wave upon vowel quality. *In* Proc. 4th int. cong. phonetic sciences. Sovijäri, A., and Aalto, P., eds. The Hague: Mouton, 34–49.

———. 1965. Speech analysis, synthesis, and perception. New York: Academic Press.

Fry, D. 1955. Duration and intensity as correlates of linguistic stress. *J. acoust. soc. Amer.*, 27, 765–768.

———. 1958. Experiments in the perception of stress. *Language and Speech*, 1, 126–152.

Fujimura, O. 1962. Analysis of nasal consonants. *J. acoust. soc. Amer.*, 34, 1865–1875.

Halle, M., and Stevens, K. 1967. On the mechanism of glottal vibration for vowels and consonants. M.I.T. RLE-QPR, 85, 267–271.

———, Hughes, G., and Radley, J. 1957. Acoustic properties of stop consonants, *J. acoust. soc. Amer.*, 29, 107–116.

Harris, K. 1958. Cues for the discrimination of American English fricatives in spoken syllables. *Language and Speech*, 1, 1–7.

———, Hoffman, H., Liberman, A., Delattre, P., and Cooper, F. 1958. Effect of third-formant transitions on the perception of the voiced stop consonants. *J. acoust. soc. Amer.*, 30, 122–126.

Hecker, M. 1962. Studies of nasal consonants with an articulatory speech synthesizer. *J. acoust. soc. Amer.*, 34, 179–188.

Heinz, J. 1967. Perturbation functions for the determination of vocal-tract area functions from vocal-tract eigenvalues. Royal Institute of Technology, Stockholm, STL-QPSR, April 15, 1967, 1–14.

Heinz, J. and Stevens, K. 1961. On the properties of voiceless fricative consonants. *J. acoust. soc. Amer.*, 33, 589–596.

Helmholtz, H. 1954. On the sensations of tone, translated by Ellis, A. (reprint ed.) New York: Dover.

Hiroto, I. 1966. Patho-physiology of the larynx from the point of view of vocal mechanism. *Practica Otologica Kyoto*, 59, 229–292 (in Japanese).

Hoffman, H. 1958. Study of some cues in the perception of the voiced stop consonants. *J. acoust. soc. Amer.*, 30, 1035–1041.

Holmes, J. 1962. An investigation of the volume velocity waveform at the larynx during speech by means of an inverse filter. Proceedings of the speech communication seminar. Stockholm: Royal Institute of Technology.

House, A. S. 1957. Analog studies of nasal consonants. *J. Speech Hearing Disorders*, 22, 190–204.

———. 1961. On vowel duration in English. *J. acoust. soc. Amer.*, 33, 1174–1178.

———, and Fairbanks, G. 1953. The influence of consonant environment upon the secondary acoustical characteristics of vowels. *J. acoust. soc. Amer.*, 25, 105–113.

———, and Stevens, K. 1956. Analog studies of the nasalization of vowels. *J. Speech Hearing Disorders*, 21, 218–232.

Hughes, G., and Halle, M. 1956. Spectral properties of fricative consonants. *J. acoust. soc. Amer.*, 28, 303–310.

Jassem, W. 1962. Noise spectra of Swedish, English, and Polish fricatives. Proceedings of the speech communication seminar. Stockholm: Royal Institute of Technology.

———. 1965. The formants of fricative consonants. *Language and Speech*, 8, 1–16.

Joos, M. 1948. Acoustic phonetics. *Language, Monogr. Suppl.* vol 24.

Kim, C. 1967. Cineradiographic study of Korean stops and a note on "aspiration." M.I.T. RLE-QPR, 86, 259–272.

Kinsler, L., and Frey, A. 1962. Fundamentals of acoustics (2nd. ed.). New York: Wiley.

Koenig, W. 1949. A new frequency scale for acoustic measurements. *Bell Laboratories Record*, 27, 299–301.

Ladefoged, P., and McKinney, N. 1963. Loudness, sound pressure, and subglottal pressure in speech. *J. acoust. soc. Amer.*, 35, 454–460.

Lee, Y. 1960. Statistical theory of communication. New York: Wiley.

Lehiste, I. 1964. Acoustical characteristics of selected English consonants. *Int. J. Amer. Ling.*, 30, 3 (part 4).

———. 1967, ed. Readings in acoustic phonetics. Cambridge, Mass.: M.I.T.

———, and Peterson, G. 1959. Vowel amplitude and phonemic stress in English. *J. acoust. soc. Amer.*, 31, 428–435.

Liberman, A. M. 1957. Some results of research on speech perception. *J. acoust. soc. Amer.*, 29, 117–123.

———, Delattre, P., Cooper, F., and Gerstman, L. 1954. The role of consonant-vowel transitions in the perception of stops and nasal consonants. *Psychol. Monogr.*, 68, No. 8, 1–13.

Lieberman, P. 1961. Perturbations in vocal pitch. *J. acoust. soc. Amer.*, 33, 597–603.

———. 1963. Some acoustic measures of the fundamental periodicity of normal and pathologic larynges. *J. acoust. soc. Amer.*, 35, 344–353.

Lindblom, B. 1963. Spectrographic study of vowel reduction. *J. acoust. soc. Amer.*, 35, 1773–1781.

Lindqvist, J. 1965. Studies of the voice source by means of inverse filtering technique. *In* Proc. fifth int. cong. acoust. Commins, D., ed. Liège: 5e Congrès International d'Acoustique.

Lisker, L., and Abramson, A. 1964. A cross-language study of voicing in initial stops: acoustical measurements. *Word*, 20, 384–422.

Lloyd, R. 1890. Vowel-sound. London: Turner and Dunnett.

Malécot, A. 1956. Acoustic cues for nasal consonants. *Language*, 32, 274–284.

Mermelstein, P. 1967. Determination of the vocal-tract shape from measured formant frequencies. *J. acoust. soc. Amer.*, 41, 1283–1294.

Meyer-Eppler, W. 1953. Zum Erzeugungsmechanismus der Geräuschlaute. *Z. Phonetik*, 7, 196–212.

Miller, D. 1926. The science of musical sounds. New York: Macmillan.

Miller, R. 1959. Nature of the vocal cord wave. *J. acoust. soc. Amer.*, 31, 667–677.

Morse, P. 1948. Vibration and sound. New York: McGraw-Hill.

———, and Ingard, U. 1968. Theoretical acoustics. New York: McGraw-Hill.

Nakata, K. 1959. Synthesis and perception of nasal consonants. *J. acoust. soc. Amer.*, 31, 661–666.

Nessel, E. 1960. Über das Tonfrequenzspektrum der pathologisch veränderten Stimme. *Acta Otolaryng.*, Supplementum 157.

O'Connor, J., Gerstman, L., Liberman, A., Delattre, P., and Cooper, F. 1957. Acoustic cues for the perception of initial /w, j, r, l/ in English. *Word*, 13, 24–43.

Ohala, J. 1966. A new photo-electric glottograph. Working papers in phonetics. Univ. Calif., 4, 40–52.

Öhman, S. 1966. Coarticulation in VCV utterances, spectrographic measurements. *J. acoust. soc. Amer.*, 39, 151–168.

———. 1967. Studies of articulatory coordination. Royal Institute of Technology, Stockholm, STL-QPSR April 15, 1967, 15–20.

Paget, R. 1930. Human speech. New York: Harcourt, Brace.

Parmenter, C., and Treviño, S. 1935. The length of the sounds of a Middle Westerner. *Amer. Speech*, 10, 129–133.

Peterson, G. 1951a. The phonetic value of vowels. *Language*, 27, 541–553.

——. 1951b. Vocal gestures. *Bell Laboratories Record*, 29, 500–503.

——, and Barney, H. 1952. Control methods used in a study of the vowels. *J. acoust. soc. Amer.*, 24, 175–185.

——, and Shoup, J. 1966. The elements of an acoustic phonetic theory. *J. Speech Hearing Research*, 9, 68–99.

Potter, R., and Peterson, G. 1948. The representation of vowels and their movements. *J. acoust. soc. Amer.*, 20, 528–535.

——, Kopp, G., and Kopp, H. 1966. Visible speech. (reprint ed.) New York: Dover.

Ravila, P. 1962. Quantity and phonemic analysis. *In* Proc. 4th int. cong. phonetic sciences. Sovijärvi, A., and Aalto, P., eds. The Hague: Mouton, 490–493.

Rothenberg, M. 1968. The breath-stream dynamics of simple-released-plosive production. *Bibliotheca Phonetica*, Number 6.

Schroeder, M. 1967. Determination of the geometry of the human vocal tract by acoustic measurements. *J. acoust. soc. Amer.*, 41, 1002–1010.

——, and Atal, B. 1962. Generalized short-time power spectra and autocorrelation functions. *J. acoust. soc. Amer.*, 34, 1679–1683.

Smith, W., and Lieberman, P. 1964. Studies in pathologic speech production. Final report, AFCRL-64-379, L. G. Hanscom Field, Mass.

Sonesson, B. 1960. On the anatomy and vibratory pattern of the human vocal folds. *Acta Otolaryng.*, Supplementum 156.

——. 1963. Photo-electrical demonstration of the vibratory movements of the human vocal folds. *In* Proc. XIIth int. speech and voice therapy conf. Croatto, L., and Croatto-Martinolli, C., eds. Padua: *Int. Assoc. Logopedics, Phoniat.* 57–61.

Soron, H. 1967. High-speed photography in speech research. *J. Speech Hearing Research*, 10, 768–776.

Stevens, K. 1956. Studies of speech sound production: stop consonants. MIT, Acoustics Lab., Quart. report, Oct.–Dec., 7–8.

——, and House, A. 1961. An acoustical theory of vowel production and some of its implications. *J. Speech Hearing Research*, 4, 303–320.

——, ——, and Paul, A. 1966. Acoustical description of syllabic nuclei: An interpretation in terms of a dynamic model of articulation. *J. acoust. soc. Amer.*, 40, 123–132.

Stevens, S., and Volkman, J. 1940. The relation of pitch to frequency: a revised scale. *Amer. J. Psychol.*, 53, 329–353.

Strevens, P. 1960. Spectra of fricative noise in human speech. *Language and Speech*, 3, 32–49.

Strutt, J. Lord Rayleigh 1945. The theory of sound. (reprint ed.) (2 vol.). New York: Dover.

Stumpf, C. 1926. Die Sprachlaute. Berlin: J. Springer.

Timcke, R., von Leden, H., and Moore, P. 1958. Laryngeal vibrations: measurements of the glottic wave (The normal vibratory cycle). *Arch. Otolaryng.* 68, 1–19. (Part 1.)

Wendahl, R. 1963. Laryngeal analog synthesis of harsh voice quality. *Folia Phoniat.*, 15, 241–250.

——. 1966. Laryngeal analog synthesis of jitter and shimmer. Auditory parameters of harshness. *Folia Phoniat.*, 18, 98–108.

Winckel, F. 1954. Physikalische Kriterien für objektive Stimmbeurteilung. *Folia Phoniat.*, 5, 232–252.

Yanagihara, N. 1967. Significance of harmonic changes and noise components in hoarseness. *J. Speech Hearing Research*, 10, 531–541.

7

Speech and Personality

Bryng Bryngelson

Despite the fact that man exists on paradoxes, inconsistencies, and much that is intransigent, he is compelled by inner forces to keep moving. As long as the basic law of nature is change, our attempts at accommodation to that change will harbor dissension, uncertainty, and sporadic controversy in our daily living. This seems to be inevitably reflected in social, academic, and professional disciplines. It is the nature of our way of life mirrored so baltantly on the political horizons. The price for the risk and daring to participate in the ebb and flow of life's forces seems necessarily costly in terms of the societal disintegrations which each generation must experience. Indeed, it is a task for survival.

From one point of view it might be most satisfying were one able to speak or write with certainty about the subject I am about to discuss. Because I consider truth as a direction rather than an ultimate destination, I am unable to endorse certainty. If finality ever obtains, I would suffer the frustrations of a stifled ego. The myriad problems with which we grapple would all be solved. What then would become of our curiosities, expectations, hopes, and aspirations, which have been so satisfying? From the author's point of view one would experience an end to the joy of creative search. I suggest that, for anyone who deals with the formulated skill of talking and the complicated art involved in the study and understanding of personality—no matter what theoretic or therapeutic approach is employed—his finalized philosophy will always fall short of realistic, scientific insight. Even though I have been involved some 40 years in clinical experiences with the technical and emotional aspects of distraught, talking primates, I find it difficult to speak or write with finality. I am at a loss to find meaningful language with which to relate what I know and feel, regarding such perplexing questions as: "What is speech? What is personality?"

I wish first to discuss "psycho-talk-therapy" for so-called normal speakers. At the outset, let me recall that the clientele for psychotherapy differ from those for psychiatry. Psychiatry is interested primarily in unraveling the behavioral mysteries of pathologic or psychotic organisms, whereas the disciplines employed by psychologists and speech pathologists are programmed for the disturbed people who appear to function tolerably well in our culture. Since the psychotherapist's clients are only partially out of tune with themselves, they do not need drugs, pills, or other so-called medicinal elements in their armamentarium. The two disciplines are also widely differentiated in a clinical population. Psychiatrists treat approximately 600,000 Americans in mental hospitals, a half million in out-patient clinics, and over a million are served by private psychiatrists. Psychotherapists have the rest of the 200 million to process! Needless to say, the accuracy of these figures can be questioned because of insufficient surveys and a paucity of clinicians. In any event, psychologists and speech pathologists do deal specifically with neurotics.

For the sake of interest and clarification it might be appropriate to give a cursory account of the author's involvement in speech pathology, and to a great extent what and who sponsored his professional sojourn.

It is difficult to trace the origin of ideas and how one comes to harbor specific points of view. The events of childhood and experiences in early days of growing up—the people one meets and cataclysmic events one survives—all contribute undoubtedly to one's feelings and thoughts about people. Relative to my own paradigms of change, I shall recite briefly what, how, and where important reference points evolved into a kind of process reality.

A stream of conscious reflections runs something like this: reared in a philosophic environment which was steeped in orthodox concepts relative to the beginnings, milieu, and end of life, I was taught to fear a bewhiskered bookkeeper—a ruler of a heaven and a maker of the earth. It was indeed a literal indoctrination. The first inroad to change occurred in World War I, when during encampment I was forced to witness the hanging of three of my peers. Through this incident I became aware of licensed murder as it was dictated by my government. My response was to seek a course of salvation in the ministry. In this venture I failed to halt the march of sin, corruption, and the ills of society. Studies in biology and zoology while at Yale's Divinity School forced me to make a more realistic appraisal of life and self. Motivated by frustrations that were conditioned into a wholesale smattering of deep-seated fears, guilts, and insecurities, I realized I had to find a discipline other than that of the "cloth."

In addition to the implantation of my personal frustrations to which I have alluded, three persons influenced in large measure my decision to enter a career in clinical speech. While at Yale University I had the good fortune to meet Mrs. William Howard Taft, who entertained her husband's students at Sunday teas. Ex-President Taft was conducting a course in international law and, as was his custom, entertained the class at his home. One of Mrs. Taft's hobbies was to interview hoboes in New Haven Park. What fascinated me was her recital of the personal life stories of the so-called bums from all walks of life. As she listened, she discovered that their lives were in jeopardy due to emotional factors. Mrs. Taft, although not a professional counselor, had great insights into the whys and wherefores of these sordid souls. She ended each recital with a note of the needs and some specific "clinical" help for these people. This experience taught me that talking is more than a mechanically produced phenomenon. At this point in my metamorphosis I began thinking about the symbolic nature of speech.

My second mentor was Dr. Lee Travis, whom I met at the State University of Iowa, forty-seven years ago. I must refer to him as my "professional father." His charismatic spirit and knowledgeable interest in what came to be known as speech pathology solidified my dreams relative to the academic discipline I chose to follow. I am certain I am not alone in this testimony.

Finally, I met Arminda Mowre, who has been my wedded counselor for forty-six years. Not to embarrass her tender and perceptive spirit I shall merely say that she, too, had charisma.

In 1927 I introduced the first speech clinic at the university of Minnesota. Unripened as a beginner usually is—as director, teacher, and clinician—I soon gained full academic support for a program dealing with speech defectives. It was not long, however, before I became aware that deviations in speech could not be managed satisfactorily solely from a mechanical point of view. In dealing with patients, I learned that their defects per se had emotional implications as well. In other words their feelings had been hurt; they were stigmatized because of their difference; their so-called personalities were also in need of reconstruction. It became obvious to me that, when confronted with a person who is in need of aid in communication, one should view him from a twofold consideration. The patient has within him a central nervous system that is integrative in function but may also possess elements of conflict within its boundaries. Because he is a human animal and perforce must operate in a gregarious environment, he faces social competition and possibly conflicts. One ought thus to deal clinically with a client's *neural* and *social* phases as well as his conflicts.

In any consideration of speech one should be aware of the neural heirarchy extant in the central nervous system. One important difference between man and other animals is the evolvement of higher cortical areas that are capable of perceptual, cognitive, and inhibiting functions, which as far as we know operate in the production of talking. Also, the organism with which we deal is still part and parcel of lower levels of neural activity. They too share in the total output of what we call speech. It is also important to be aware of the constant threat to expression by the earlier, lower level patterns which in a sense defy, having been usurped by them, the most recently evolved higher neural centers. The miracle of talking lies in the fact that the newer areas of brain activity are able, in the act of verbalization, to operate control over the older well-established processes most of the time. When lower level interruption does occur, one may have either a cessation of verbal activity or overt misbehaviors that we call defects. I refer to this phase of talking as "*neural* conflict."

Experientially, however, speech clinicians must necessarily concern themselves with a second sort of problem, i.e., social conflict. Clients are living in a dynamic, relating milieu. In this environment they seek to frame their own self-image, craving and hoping for a more comfortable and satisfactory existence among their fellow beings.

It is inevitable that a highly sensitive speech defective becomes involved in problems relating to himself as a person with a handicap. What he is, feels, and thinks may be more important than the specific speech differences he possesses. As most experienced clinicians know, this concern about self-image appears to be more serious in a stutterer. Later in this chapter I shall deal specifically with clinical management relative to the stutterer's need for new experiences.

After having observed what appeared to be a cause and effect relationship between speech differences and personality, I established a group therapy program for people with emotional problems. It was a non-credit course, meeting three hours a week for nine months. The psycho-talk-therapy dealt primarily with clients whose problems lay outside the area of speech defects. Victims of alienation and loneliness in their society, they had been sensitized emotionally because of insecurities in areas of race, nationality, physical habitus, or academic and/or social failures. Their professional and social lives had been stifled by feelings of inadequacy. They felt guilty and fearful and, more importantly, they had been silenced and anonymously imprisoned.

I believe it was a country parson who once said, "Personalities, like fingerprints, are all different—and each leaves its own mark in the world." Despite the basic truth of this statement there are some common speech patterns or modes of expression that are recognizable when one listens interpretatively.

Because of interpersonal needs man talks to:

1. parade his ego
2. grind his axes
3. relieve his guilt
4. avoid being silent
5. keep others from putting him on the spot
6. make himself a good fellow

If speech is basically an emotional act, talking can easily be a vehicle to satisfy one's inner needs. Such needs are usually clustered in a generalized pattern of emotional insecurity. Most of us would admit, if we listen carefully, that our speech reflects symbolically the six needs to which I have alluded.

1. It would be a rare person who had no need to have his sense of personal worth sanctioned. Most of us bid for attention in our own characteristic manner. Indeed, this is such an important factor in our gregarious relationships that it determines our psychologic survival.

2. Our axe-grinding mechanism is conditioned in us by well-meaning parents in our early years. The resulting prejudices are so emotionally charged that, as we mature, we seldom behave in a tolerant and rational manner. This phase of our personality isolates us from insouciant social relationships. A worthwhile goal of therapy, then, is teaching the client to be friendly toward his prejudices. For without the deep-seated feelings which surround them, prejudices become an expression of a delightful, likable, and acceptable human response.

3. The guilt to which most humans are heir is commonly scapegoated through speech. Projecting one's faults onto one's neighbors creates ill feeling and often results in devisive gossip. Our current commentators on radio lend experiential evidence for this mechanism. Most communicasters on 24-hour performances lack insight into this process of guilt assignment. The result is usually a "war of words" which does nothing to facilitate mutual understanding.

4. One does not have to be very perceptive to document our talk due to the dreadful fear of silence. We are in this state of silence self-conscious and not conscious of self. Most of our nonsensical talk is promoted by this fear. As I have often said, "we often talk to see if we are still alive." Speech is a pinching device we use to determine whether or not we are living.

5. Talking can also serve as a front, a ruse, or a mask. In order to avoid being placed on the spot or being asked important personal questions we frequently hide behind our speech mask. As long as we hold forth compulsively with rapid conversation, we avoid the risk of being found out. Thus we constantly get practice as entrepreneurs of "factory noise." As performers in this process we are our own boss, manager, and executioner. We are often termed as people with too much gab. "One can save face by

keeping the lower part of it shut," warns a Chinese proverb.

6. If one listens with an inner ear, whenever one meets an old-time friend, the need to make ourselves good fellows can be documented. What is rehearsed in this situation more often than not falls far short of any sanity. Your desire to have your friend think well of you overshadows your curiosity of finding out what important matters have transpired during each other's absence. You ask questions of no importance to cover up your self-consciousness. Often you could care less that you two met—so you end the tête-à-tête by saying "Good to have seen you!" "Be seein' you, Alice." Thus one can spend a lot of time talking, unmarred by any discovery that "old times" are still old, and about all you have learned really was that your obituary had not yet been written and neither had that of your friend. (I refer the reader to the author's book *Personality Development Through Speech* (1964), Chapter VII, "Put Your Ear to Your Mouth," for a more detailed discussion of why man talks.)

If the above point of view lends any credence to realism, it suggests that talking is couched in symbolic patterns that can be related directly to one's state of security and inner emotional needs. "What you are speaks so loud I can't hear what you say," was said poetically years ago. Speech, when viewed as an emotional act, reveals what goes on inside one. It is also conceivable that these recesses existed long before man discovered he was also endowed with a brain or a thinking apparatus. This alone can be responsible for some of the communicative difficulties our culture has for centuries experienced. The price we pay may be seen in familial quarrels, social unrest, and a war of words which invariably precedes our wars of guns, nuclear weapons, and bombs. The cost is high in human lives. We may be risking individual and social devastation by not keeping our mouths shut. Declaring a permanent moratorium on talking might not be the answer. Altering the talker's personality, via emotional hygiene, would be a more rational approach to our culture's ills.

I have tried to indicate that speech may be used as a diagnostic tool for interpretating the inner needs of patients. In order to collect more reliable data, clinicians must treat talking as a symptom of what may be happening in the deeper recesses of troubled people.

Clinicians conduct the sort of group therapy that is dictated by their professional backgrounds and experiences. To operate effectively a rehabilitation program, each clinician ought to function in his own experiential frame of reference. This doesn't prevent him from experimenting; but the clinician's conviction as to the worth of his approach ought to be made obvious to his clients throughout the clinical process. I say this because I believe that "suggestion" is an important factor in therapy. The theoretical underpinnings of a clinician's approach to therapy are important to him and to his academic colleagues; but his concern with his patients must be with satisfactory results—whether they are proven theoretically or not.

The following patient-oriented goals evolve from my experiences with group therapy. Briefly stated, they are:

1. to overcome devastating inhibitions and guilts
2. to learn to compete with oneself
3. to possess a realistic and honest selfishness
4. to operate with vigorous and healthy feelings
5. to thrive on a continuing, always maturing, adjusting personality
6. to learn to accept oneself for what he is

Inasmuch as I have spelled out in detail the psycho-talk-therapy for normal speakers and for stutterers, I shall not burden the reader of this chapter by repeating what I have written elsewhere (1966).

The remaining portion of this chapter will contain a cursory discussion of some of the main therapeutic principles I have learned from working with emotionally unstable, talking primates. I am of the opinion that whatever personality therapy is to one's liking, he will find a good deal of commonality with the directive approach I have espoused in psycho-talk-therapy.

1. THE SYMBOLIC NATURE OF SPEECH

The general semanticists have outlined this process clearly. They have exposed the irrationality of generalization, allness, trigger reaction, etc., that pervade our language and result in communicative misunderstanding. I look upon this phenomenon primarily as an intellectual process, however. In considering speech as an essentially emotional act, the clinician ought to begin with his patient's feelings, of which his language is only a symptom. If I have a quarrel with general semantics, it is in this context. I suggest that the clinician should prepare his client emotionally before he introduces the intellectual principles of general semantics. This is what I mean when I say "work from within—out." In a sense the "unsane" language patterns described by general semantics are symptoms of maladjustment. A verbal stripping away of this psychologic camouflage is a healthy exercise with which to begin therapy. Too many therapists seem to have lost sight of the fact that emotional catharsis is as important as intellectual adaptation. Both are integral parts of the therapeutic process.

2. THE PERCEPTION OF AN IDEA

By this I mean the holding of an idea in consciousness so long that it wears out its unwholesome quality. When a specific emotional sore spot is verbally acknowledged and continually rehearsed a positive feeling begins to overrule its negative value. A new dimension of acceptance can thus be obtained.

3. EXAGGERATION

Overdoing an act, feeling, or sense of inadequacy gives one a realistic perspective because one learns that whatever one fears is not as unwholesome and as unacceptable as it seems. If one over-limps, over-stutters, or overstates a condition, his problem levels off internally so that it becomes a manageable reality for the patient.

4. NEGATIVE PRACTICE

In brief, this principle of correcting an error by purposefully performing it may be employed for the irradication of almost any deviation in behavior. The essential point to keep in mind is that the patient practises his inappropriate response. The clinician makes him aware of the difference between his inappropriate response and the appropriate one. By consciously practising the inappropriate behavior which he formerly performed unconsciously, the patient gains conscious control of his reflexive behavior. Once he experiences fully the conscious response to his inappropriate behavior, he is free to make the conscious decision to alter it.

5. THE ADJUSTING PERSONALITY

This concept has evolved via my experience in psycho-talk-therapy. I have found that when a client has reached the stage of being "well-adjusted," he tends to live nongregariously. The insights into his behavior that he has acquired in therapy alter his ego drive in the direction of a satisfied complacency. He tends to gloat over his successes in overcoming his former guilts, fears, repressions, and insecurities. In his self-centered, asocial lethargy he is forming a new conceit. This may become so evident to his friends that he is open to criticism. Formerly, as a maladjusted patient he was talked about for being compensatorily social. If he has not learned to interpersonalize with his fellow man, he still must be considered a patient; he is missing the exhilarating joys that can come only from giving of himself in trust to others. If our world were not an everchanging, dynamic, and gregarious process, one would have no legitimate quarrel with his choice of aloneness; but stark reality tells us this is a world of people. Life moves on—each of us has a responsibility to love, respect, and share. Living a life of communicative interaction is an excellent guarantee for warding off the feeling of stultifying futility.

As a patient forms his new self-image, he extends his "self" to others through the communicative act. He consciously attempts to overcome his psychologic aloneless through controlled social experience. Gradually, an awareness of the missing link of human belonging and acceptance evolves. Self-alienation thus becomes self-actualization. This confrontation affords patients the opportunity to appreciate that neglected human needs can be met inviolately via personalized understanding and respect.

In essence I have tried to say that speech clinicians have neglected to stress the importance of verbal and nonverbal communication in enabling man to overcome his social and self-alienation. Talking to oneself, as important as it is for an adjusted personality, may not be sufficient in a world where communicative participation is the core of gregarious living.

In our world today the clamor for understanding of our neighbors of whatever color, creed, or philosophy of life is uppermost in our societal needs. Brotherhood has little or no meaning except through the knowledge one gains from insight into the thoughts and feelings of his fellow man. Mowrer (1964) restates the Delphic Oracle thus: "Make thyself known, and then you will know yourself." His restatement of Shakespeare's utterance, "And this above all, to thine own self be true, and thou can'st not be false to any one," is "and this above all, to other men be true, and thou can'st not then be false to thyself." We have from early childhood been admonished to be our brother's keeper. To me it is also important to be our keeper's brother. I know no better way to acknowledge realistically our inherent, predatory selfishness. We should advertise it verbally, put it into practice instead of enshrining ourselves with an agelong, fictionalized altruism.

In order to obtain a sort of "ultimate" in clinical

group therapy I urge clinicians to introduce what I deem is a broader perspective in helping persons experience a wholeness of self. Here I wish merely to offer one beginning clinical technique. Have two clients stand facing each other in silence, with their eyes closed. Ask them to record or document what they think and feel. Then have them open their eyes and greet each other. Now have them record their feelings toward each other. The first recording will testify to an aloneness which seems somewhat meaningless and stupid. In the second recording the clients discover that as they continue to speak openly, they become conscious of a realistic awareness of an integrated presence, an expression of their higher selves or a holistic charisma. Could this be one aspect of "spirit"? I repeat that what to me at this writing seems to be an important emphasis in dealing with emotionally disturbed persons is that clinicians should awaken them to the need of extending themselves into the communicative act of a "confrontation." Other methods and techniques by which clients can gain experience in this domain I leave to your ingenuity and creative imagination.

Before concluding this discussion on speech and personality, I wish to address myself more specifically to the oncoming group of students in our field. If I appear to be philosophically slanted in my remarks, it is because I believe that speech clinicians and researchers may need a respite from work that can easily become mundane. Those of my colleagues who know me as somewhat of a philosophic sentimentalist will undoubtedly expect me to so wax! So if I espouse you and me as a lauder of our species—a noble hierarchy—I would want you to spell this out to your students and patients. As a matter of fact we are a twofold hierarchy. In your work with the communicative act of talking, you should be aware of the fact that this act is sponsored by neural and physiologic systems not extant in any other organism. Man would not talk did he not possess a cerebral cortex where, according to the latest count, there are 20 billion cells resident and ready for use. I wrote of this earlier in this chapter. The second hierarchy pertains to the fact that because speech is so complicated and so difficult to understand, we must draw on numerous academic disciplines in our work. By such consideration you can obtain and maintain a feeling of security in your profession. Boredom need not haunt you, nor will pleasure of work be wanting if you occasionally ask the philosophic question, "Who, what, and where am I?"

It may not be presumptuous to speculate that when man evolutionally became bipedal, featherless, time-binding, and brain possessed, he experienced self-awareness for the first time and felt that a sense of personal worth was essential to his survival. Self-consciousness may have dawned when he found that his most important needs for psychologic, physical, and emotional security could best be satisfied when he mingled with other men in society. As time went on he accumulated knowledge, whether through revelation or study, about himself and the reality around him. He felt safe and was on his way to becoming a PERSON. This was perhaps the beginning of man's place at the top of the hierarchy in relation to other animals. At the center of his so-called personality was a psychologic force we call the ego. It is well described in the following quotation from Ester and William Menaker when they discuss, *Ego in Evolution* (1966). "The miracle of man is consciousness: but consciousness can only be experienced and implemented by means of the ego (sense of personal worth.) Only when I am aware of "I" can I know that the tree shelters me from the rain, that the sun warms me and all the earth, that another man may help or hurt me, that within limits I can do something to understand and mold my world, and ultimately myself. It is to the ineluctable forces of evolution that I owe my "I-ness" and the very awareness of this is part of the evolutionary process itself."

You will recall in the author's "reflections" in the earlier part of the chapter that due to the fact that speech pathology as a profession did not exist, he was an orphaned man of the holy ministry. Like many other "founding fathers," he wandered into a discipline that was in its swaddling garments. Searching for a professional niche, we were not even neophytes.

Today's oncoming students are entering a vocation that is now well established as a professional discipline. I wish, therefore, to describe two major alternatives which they face, each of which should lead to the satisfaction of their ego-deal.

One is the clinical: this is technology. The other is research: this is science. Let me explain their functional differentiation. The clinician plays the role of one effecting utilitarian results. It is his aim to effect changes in disabled and distraught persons using the knowledge that comes from the laboratory and also from intuitive revelation. In a sense the researcher works with the nature of natures. He has the freedom to establish his own standards of operation, unafraid of results. He generally has no ımpingement from outside authority. On the other hand the clinician perforce is subject in his work to pressures outside of his domain. He is not in this sense as free as the man in the laboratory. Those among us who have served both as scientists and clinicians are well aware of this particular differentiation. The researcher can be his own boss, while the clinician cannot. The latter struggles with not only the patient's needs, but also with social and political interferences within his community. Although he did not sponsor them he has the responsibility of dealing with such problems. The laboratory man is far more alone than the clinician, who is continually exposed to public view.

One cannot conclude, however, that one field has the advantage over the other. The choice, I suggest, should be determined by one's academic background, emotional orientation, and feeling for people. The latter requisite is essential for the clinician. I do not deny the fact that few have both the desire and the ability to work in both areas.

In conclusion I wish to offer some suggestions to those clinicians who work with stutterers. There does not seem to me to be as much emphasis now, as formerly, on the important problem of the personal adjustment of stutterers. I am not speaking here of the early prevention of the development of personality handicaps. The attention now given to parents in the area of sound emotional hygiene seems to be excellent. I am concerned about the experienced stutterer whose real burden of adjustment commences in the schoolroom and on the playground.

We are aware that regardless of etiology a sensitive person with a difference in manner of vocal output runs the risk of developing an overlay of emotional blocks which hinder him from free and easy social adaptations. Our talking world places a high premium on smooth and uninterrupted articulation. (May I here interject an observation for normal speakers, whose speech has recently been cluttered with "you know," "right," and "what not." Its linguistic purpose I know not. Is it related to a fear of silence? Anyway, I must confess my auditory sense would prefer being bombarded with stuttering spasms than by the horrible misplaced "you knows" in the speech of so-called normals.) Back to the stutterer. By societal decree he experiences severe social penalties as he attempts to satisfy his inner emotional needs in being a person. Although a stutterer may be different in his inherent neurologic structure, he may or may not be different from you and me in his feelings. He, too, possesses a spirit and a well-defined personal longing to be accepted by others. Even though his major barrier to social acceptance is his stuttering, he may be maladjusted to a social, academic, physical, race, or nationality sanction. Clinically, he needs more emotional hygiene because of the double strike against him—both as a stutterer and as a person.

A psychologic travesty occurs when we become so concerned with the symptoms of a disorder that we neglect the area of the patient's need to be an acceptable human being. There is no question in my mind about the efficaciousness of reducing the amount of neural overflow inherent in the stutterer's spasms. He can be taught how to vocalize more easily, i.e., to stutter better, via the myriad techniques now available. Be wary, however, of the fact that there is no guarantee your patient will continue as a clear articulator when he leaves you. Relapses are common in the life of stutterers. Unless you have attended to his "hang ups" in his emotional life, you have not prepared him to live happily in spite of his relapses.

There is no utopia in this clinical realm of adjustment for most stutterers. It is too much to hope that your patient will ever learn to enjoy stuttering. My guess is that you will not enjoy his stuttering either. There is no harm, however, in working toward that end. You would have to be considered a genius could you invent a cure for disliking all that takes place peripherally when a stutterer has a block. There are exceptions, of course. Even though I do not know what a "recovered stutterer" is, I am sure there are some who utter that claim; and they certainly have my blessing. Remaining pessimistic and being ignorant on the subject, I prefer to label such people as "professional stutterers." From this point of view there is safety in three respects. One, a stutterer may never reach the goal of removing all his peripheral symptoms. Two, there is no guarantee the symptoms will not return. Three, the stutterer may miss the delightful experience of continuously "doffing his hat" to a past event, which via luck, persistent courage, and the good fortune of fate has brought him from the doldrums of despair to a joyous and exhilarating expression of his ego-ideal. As many of you know, I have not wavered from what I pronounced in the early thirties, "once a stutterer, always a stutterer." During the last decade it has become easier for me to be friendly toward my prejudices in this regard. Recent studies in the medical sciences point more and more in the direction of an organic basis for the aberrant behavior extant in a stutterer. This evidence seems to confirm my statement that structure precedes function. Within the next fifty years speech pathologists may be making neurologic diagnoses of stutterers and of those speech defectives which are now considered functional disorders. If speech pathology is to survive as an entity, it may behoove subsequent students of the subject to include in their training an M.D. degree. Such preparation should more adequately prepare them to understand and clinically manage a stutterer and a maladjusted personality, no matter what label you put on your academic discipline. I feel definitely that the professions of medical and speech pathology should work together.

So to the young in our field who are as knowledgeable as our times allow and as dedicated as the "founding fathers" to their chosen profession, I urge you to be cognizant of the need for emotional hygiene in the treatment of the stutterer. Help him make the most of the potential he possesses. Teach him to live more adequately with his difference. Refurbish his potential toward a new and fresher life. Help him create an acceptance of an indestructible self-image that will withstand the devastating castigations of an uninformed public. Help him unlock the prison that keeps him from self-disclosure, paralyzing not only his hopes, but also his energies. Show him how to simulate and advertise his differences so he can enjoy the role of being off the defensive. Such an approach to therapy focuses on the stutterer as a sensitive human being who needs to learn to deal with a problem, rather than on a patient who is a problem for a speech pathologist.

BIBLIOGRAPHY

Bryngelson, B. 1964. Personality development through speech. Minneapolis: Denison.

———. 1966. Clinical group therapy for problem people: a practical treatise for stutterers and normal speakers. Minneapolis: Denison.

Menaker, E., and Menaker, W. 1966. Ego in evolution. New York: New Grove Press. P. 82.

Mower, O. 1964. The new group therapy. New York: Van Nostrand.

8

Child Therapy

Russell Haney

CONCEPTS

Most therapeutic endeavors made on behalf of children seek either to initiate or to reactivate developmental trends. Such efforts are addressed variously: sometimes toward anatomical or physiological improvement; sometimes toward behavioral or attitudinal change. Although clinicians who are concerned about disorders of verbal communication in children comprehend and respect matters of structure, they vest their therapeutic efforts primarily in modifying function. Their contributions to the general welfare of the child are placed substantially within the broad fields of developmental achievement and learning.

This chapter attempts to identify and explore the use of certain behaviors pertinent to communicative relationships and appropriate to the development or improvement of verbal function in young children. The therapeutic approach to be described is predominantly empirical in origin. Research findings will, of course, be employed wherever they are specifically or appropriately related. This chapter is not an etiological study, but one of therapeutic relationships and processes. No attempt is made to provide a learning theory in detail, or to explore fully the concepts of ego psychology or growth and development phenomena. Such studies are, of necessity, ancillary to our task here and should be viewed as important prerequisites. Information specific to the field of verbal communication and related disorders is assumed to be a part of the reader's knowledge or the subject of his ongoing study.

Child Therapy Defined

In contrast to speech and language therapy as classically practised, child therapy seeks involvement in ways that are more pertinent to the child's own life experiences and ongoing needs. The child's developmental learning of behaviors, attitudes, emotional expressions, and patterns of relating become primary therapeutic properties. Satisfaction of needs, management of anxiety, and efforts at ego achievement are given careful study. Significance is placed on the child's ways of the moment as well as on his developmental efforts. His momentary being is accorded acceptance and respect. His strivings for change are given specific and selective encouragement. Here the child is provided with an unusual opportunity to be a person of influence and consequence. The child is regarded as the central force in the therapeutic relationship. His efforts become both determining and therapeutic. Child therapy is visualized here as a process of dynamic learning and specific growth experiences which are activated in the context of ongoing relationships. It is an arrangement of communicative interaction which involves the introduction of particularly selected people into the child's life. These people will behave in ways that will come to have unique importance to the child, especially in his manner of perceiving them and, most pertinently, himself. Child therapy seeks to discover and offer carefully selected and natural responses to the child's presented behaviors and attitudes. The process is essentially one of careful inquiry rather than one of predetermination. The intent is to provide a climate of communicative interaction which will promote growth. Such a climate will result in the child attaching new kinds of significance to his presence as well as to his many behaviors, including those that assume verbal form. This attachment is accomplished therapeutically as the child, and undoubtedly the therapist, learn increasingly effective forms of relating and therefore of communicating. The term *child therapy* is used to denote the fact that the child is the primary determinant of the various therapeutic acts. This implies that one may anticipate any variety of therapeutic effort. Therapy for the child is as likely to involve instructional activities as it is to require supportive and interpretative responses or to generate life-experience actions. The crucial concept in the approach described here is simple: therapeutic acts must be determined by the child's needs and invited by his ongoing communicative characteristics. Attention is invited to the work of several people (Ginott, 1961; Haworth, 1964; Hejna, 1960; Klein, 1960; Moustakas, 1966). Although differing in theoretical orientation and practical implementation, the concepts and processes described by these authors should provide an excellent basis for initiating a study of the child therapy process.

Therapeutic Questions

The process here termed therapeutic is energized by the child's natural inclination toward exploration and experimentation. To invite such effort, emphasis is placed on the child's capacity for self-determination. Here he is provided with an opportunity to become central, subject, and reciprocal in the therapeutic relationship. Implementation is given when the therapist succeeds in indicating to the child his acceptance of the child's individualized ways of thinking and behaving. Fiedler (1950) described the clinician's capacity for communication and understanding as a basic ingredient for an ideal therapeutic relationship with children. After citing and conceptualizing an impressive amount of data, Barnlund (1968) concluded, "the research suggests that the more genuine, accepting, open, and empathic each person is, and the more each values the experience of the other, the more likely it is that their communication will contribute to the effective functioning and personal growth of each." Barrett-Lennard (1962), as a specific example, was able to demonstrate a positive correlation between certain affective characteristics of a positive sort shown by therapists and congruent therapeutic gain demonstrated by clients. If one views therapist behaviors from the child's perceptual framework, the importance of the conclusions just cited becomes even more apparent. Communicative attempts by the child, whether verbal or more primitive, should be viewed as significant factors in the child's attempts at self-representation. Without regard for the expressive form, the child's acts are important indicators of his being. When the therapist responds positively and accepts these acts of the child, he gives direct and uncontaminated evidence of his regard for the being of that child. Such communication, where successful, contributes to the very matrix in which therapeutic change may occur. By such communication, the child knows that he is free to be as he is or to change. No longer need he search urgently for a way to represent himself to his world. He knows that his presence is recognized and that he is influential. The security thus implied is basic to the therapeutic act. Inherent in such security is the possibility for the use of reciprocal influence of a growth-oriented sort.

The actuation of change occurs not only as a consequence of the child's dynamic nature, but as a function of the clinician's selective responsiveness to the child's various efforts. Church (1961) defined the importance of environmental response when he stated in essence that motivational states have low specificity until courses of action have been given cognitive definition. The importance of environmental help (clinician's responses) in achieving behavioral specificity is another important dimension of the therapeutic act. Particular or selective therapeutic response must be given to those efforts of the child that are deemed to be growth-oriented. By acceptance of his being and his ways, the child is literally invited to reveal his nature and his needs. This is accomplished as he discovers the means by which he can exert particular influence on the course and conduct of therapeutic attempts and, therefore, on the relationship. Such influence provides the child with a growing identity; brings more specificity to the course and content of therapeutic activity; and, finally, indicates to the child that his actions do indeed have an effect on the responses of the therapist. Many therapeutic approaches have already been structured that propose to effect changes in a person's way of thinking or behaving. Some of these approaches contrive to assist the child in the execution of specific and highly circumscribed acts. Other procedures are structured which assist or improve the interplay of sensorimotor, perceptual, and intellectual aspects. Many therapeutic designs offer learning opportunities which are focused on the tolerance of increased anxiety, on improved emotional expression, or on changes in overall ego flexibility or maturity. Some methods assume correction or improvement by virtue of a predetermined procedure. Several approaches appear to provide opportunities for self-correction and, in a sense, may be said to be determined by the child. Although differing in theory and conduct, certain commonalities or issues seem to exist in the preparation of these various approaches. This core of similarity may be conceptualized by answering a single question: in therapeutic efforts that are intended to be growth-promoting, what is to be regarded as significant? The assigning of significance is clearly a vital decision. The question finds comparable application in growth and development studies, in child-rearing practices, and in the discoveries of therapeutic implementation. In practical application, the resolution of this issue prompts inquiry along several dimensions. Who is to decide on the concrete aspects of therapeutic activity? Shall the therapeutic task be procedurally predetermined or shall it develop as a part of therapeutic interchange? What factors are to be used as the impetus for therapeutic change? What is to be changed? Who decides what is to be changed? What factors are to constitute the matrix of a therapeutic relationship? Who is to initiate whatever the activity may be? What, indeed, is meant by the word therapeutic? Answers to these several questions invite comments pertinent to those factors that are thought to initiate change and promote growth. Such is the content of the following concepts and various applications.

The Importance of Play

Behavioral change, whether growth-oriented or regressive, is typically signaled by some kind of arousal. In the developing child, maturational trends are prominently displayed through spontaneous, inquisitive, and exploratory play. Certainly no act is more indicative of his strivings for change or more suggestive of his readiness for new learning. Play provides a natural medium for acquiring and maintaining certain behaviors and discarding others. Commonly visualized in the course of children's play are attitudes, needs, and points of conflict. Play seems to be particularly illuminating of the child's misperceptions. Sources of disturbance and typical adjustment attempts are also available for inspection and study. Of particular value may be opportunities for one to visualize more successful and mature aspects of the child's growth efforts. Play meets the criterion of arousal and is a particularly valuable therapeutic vehicle because of its naturalness and because it originates predominantly with the child.

The nature of play has been given specific study by Friedlander (1966). He described play as stimulus seeking with respect to intent. The differential effects of various stimuli were demonstrated. Of particular interest was Friedlander's impression that the varying effects of stimuli were due primarily to the way each child processed information. This notion places emphasis, therefore, on the individual and unique character of play and seems to illuminate its contribution to the singularity of the child's efforts. Play, as it is described for the purposes of this çhapter, does not imply anything frivolous or light. Observation of children at play will impress one regularly with the force, determination, and purposefulness invested in these efforts. The self-discovery and self-expression purposes of children's play are detailed by Hartley and others (1952) in a particularly useful text. While perhaps having a frolicsome aspect in some instances, the primary character of true play is clearly that of action and persistence. By means of play, children are provided with an unusual opportunity for multidimensional experimentation. And particularly does this seem to be true when the activity has strong elements of self-determination. The primary characteristic of this experimentation is expressive behavior, and the natural link with speech and language development is clear. Play appears to be an important force in growth and development and is certainly not random or capricious in nature. Lieberman (1965) defined play as a unitary factor and hypothesized a relationship between play behaviors and the appearance of certain expressive factors. In a study of 93 kindergarten children he demonstrated a high positive relationship between playfulness and qualities such as ideational fluency, originality, and spontaneity. Play, again defined as a particular force or entity, was studied by Sphere and Kastenbaum (1966). They hypothesized play as growth-giving in nature and, using an interaction research paradigm, studied cerebral-palsied children and their mothers. These authors concluded that parents who did not play with their children, who were excessively anxious, and who emphasized maintaining their children in a dependency role, contributed seriously to the magnitude and generality of their children's problems.

Self-sufficiency, awareness of one's impact, and the requirements for appropriate self-control are realizations available to the child in his playful efforts. The use of play as described here is particularly supportive for children with disorders of verbal communication. It may provide the child with an opportunity for expression and communication where such messages could not be articulated verbally. Play is also an excellent setting in which to exercise certain kinds of learning, particularly that concerning the relationship between the child and the therapist. Communication about this important issue can take place, therefore, whether or not verbal contact is attempted. Relative freedom of activity for the child when combined with carefully selected behaviors on the part of the therapist constitutes an opportunity for child therapy to function. Play is therefore a vehicle. Growth-oriented change is the aim. As the child grows, this exploratory tendency assumes greater complexity. Experimentation is characterized by some reduction of gross motor effort, by improvement in fine motor skills, by stronger cognitive activity, by more accurate perception, and by the appearance of abstract thinking. Time and space orientations take on added dimensions. Both behavior and thinking become more discriminative and impulse control improves. Play assumes greater elements of serious intent and becomes highly channeled and goal-oriented. Verbal function is an inextricable participant in these several developments. The child therapy approach employs exploratory trends from many levels of maturity and consequently may be primitive and concrete, highly symbolic, or pertinently abstract in execution.

Change and Growth

Fundamental to a study of the therapeutic process is the problem of behavioral and attitudinal change. The change phenomenon appears to have two basic properties—change and inertia or resistance to change. These components may be seen in normal growth and development in the form of persistent attempts at behavioral elaboration and increased functional complexity on one hand, and at the stabilization of certain acts and maintaining systems on the other. Inertia is viewed as the maintaining or sustaining component whether one speaks of growth, deterioration, or arousal of tension and its reduction. For example, once a direction that is growth-oriented is assumed, inertia seems to support or maintain the trend until something intervenes. The same kind of inertia is apparently true for states of regression or fixation, or or for conditions of apparent developmental inactivity or failure. Whether change or resistance to change marks the case at hand, the mediating value and purposefulness of both speech and language activities is clear to any knowledgeable observer. Verbal activities both maintain and consolidate present achievement and either support or are responsible for behavioral change.

Although often viewed as a consequence of developmental effort, verbal function may be regarded more dynamically as a critical factor in the implementation of growth. If the "consequence" view is maintained, a restricted therapeutic position may be the result. If the "implementation" view is also employed, a wider spectrum of therapeutic approaches seems possible. The former tends to place the child and his problem, therapeutically, in a respondent role. The latter emphasizes verbal function in the child's general development and seems to implement a need-satisfaction approach in which the child is given a subject role. Child therapy attempts to integrate these views. Here the child's dependency issues as well as his strivings for self-sufficiency may be considered. Whether symptoms of communicative troubles are regarded as consequences (child an object and dependent) or as containing elements of growth implementation (child a subject and only relatively dependent), the therapeutic approach described as "child therapy" may be visualized as child-need-centered. Many therapeutic attempts are centered procedurally and the child seems to be placed in an object role. He is literally acted upon. Few approaches view the child as subject and regard his efforts at verbal communication as implementing factors of general growth.

To say that a human condition is static is fundamentally untrue. The child is always in the process of some change although his distorted efforts at verbal communication are frequently described in static terms and treated in a similar fashion. Important therapeutic problems have to do with how to identify the signs indicative of change, how to link viable change trends to verbal function, how to employ verbal function as a developmental effector, how to give attempts at change appropriate direction, how to induce effort toward change, and, indeed, whether or not to encourage certain tendencies, for example, regressive ones, toward change at all. Another important therapeutic inquiry addresses itself to the problem of interrupting, limiting, or redirecting certain kinds of attempts at change. Many factors seem to contribute relative and dynamic weight to change and inertia-to-change phenomena. Learning is, of course, one of these variables. As an interdependent process of interaction which involves the child and his correspondents, learning is a significant determinant of both change and resistance to change. Growth-oriented change is normally welcomed and consequently supported by the environment. In other instances, attempts at growth are not so perceived by the child's correspondents and are negatively affected. For many children, the inertia component seems to be attached primarily to the maintenance of various immature behavioral or attitudinal systems or even to a readiness for regression. The growing child is continuously in the process of assessing the relative values to be obtained from changing certain behavioral forms, acquiring new behaviors, or maintaining and strengthening old ones. This child is therefore in repeated negotiation with himself and with his various correspondents. The acquisition and use of verbal communication is clearly designed as one of the principle effectors in the conduct of these negotiations. As noted previously, the primary vehicle for child therapy is the child's natural inclinations toward experimentation. Typically, this is an exploratory activity and it frequently contains growth-oriented features. It is clearly oriented to change. Of importance, therapeutically, is its responsiveness to specification and reward. This correspondence feature is often characteristic of child growth and development in general. The factors of specification and reward can be visualized in developmental circumstances where the child achieves self-activated satisfaction as well as in those situations where the child is offered certain kinds of positive responses by other people.

The child's experimentation takes place principally through spontaneous and often self-generated play. This exploratory play is frequently visualized as random or tentative when initiated. If appropriately persistent, however, it comes to acquire greater specificity, complexity, and purposefulness. Such acquisition may be determined by environmental response or demand, or it may be heuristic in nature. Interestingly enough, this concept is apparently true whether the acquired act is inertia-loaded in either the direction of growth or regression. Possibilities for purposefulness and continued efforts at elaboration are significantly greater, however, in those behaviors that are oriented toward change in the direction of maturity. Such efforts by the child require recognition and warrant positive responses. Natural opportunities for the activation of such phenomena will appear regularly in the play of most children.

The potentiality for change is apparently contained in some condition of arousal. Such states are variously termed anxiety, concern, interest, unsatisfied need, activation, motivation, exploration, or deprivation. Milner's (1967) discussion of the crucial relationship between development of the self and indigenous anxiety is of central importance in any discussion of the phenomenon of change. She discusses the normal role of anxiety in human development and specifies both its origins and purposes. Adult responsibility in response to such arousal is also delineated. Although cast in a neurophysiological framework, the implications for growth and development and for child therapy are unavoidable. Arousal of anxiety prompts a seeking for satisfaction or perhaps a relief from anxiety. When applied to child therapy, one may see that anxiety, particularly in the learning of new experiences, seems to have at the point of expression or discharge a searching, restless, often repetitious, and certainly exploratory character. The expressive activity ensuing from this state has channels and purposes that are sometimes discovered or designated by the child, sometimes specified by others, and many times secured by negotiation and mutual concession. On occasion, no expressive channel can be established and the intended expression together with the aroused energies that subserve it must be severely compromised, surrendered, or perhaps rerouted. The consequences may appear in the form of a significant distortion of expression or may be revealed in the form of a deficit in condition or effort. It is not difficult to anticipate the kinds of added distortions or disruptions that might be supplied by the presence of structural pathology. Observation and clinical experience indicate that the likelihood for favorable behavioral change increases when the child's efforts at self-determination or need-satisfaction are not overcompromised. The probability of implementing behavioral change is greater when the challenge to the child falls short of demanding from him such inordinate concessions to his own anxiety that he adopts the form of a pervasive defensiveness. Where the inertia phenomenon supports compromise and finds investment in such defensiveness, the child's normal growth tendency is often contaminated. Inhibition of growth then becomes, for him, an important maintaining function. In other instances, expressive modes adopted experimentally by the child are given indiscriminate reward. Again the inertia component is placed in the service of immature behaviors. These conditions are basic, then, to the state called inertia-to-change (frequently termed resistance) and, of course, will limit seriously the child's inclination to mature. Obviously, changes of certain kinds might occur if the child were to subordinate self-determined intentions, surrender his unique interests or inclinations, and adopt the purposes and release-channels specified by others. If this kind of submissiveness becomes a dominant adjustment, one expects the singularity and thus the identity of the true child to be lost, seriously diminished, or to assume some deviant or substitute form. Child therapy techniques include careful avoidance of such possibilities.

The child therapy approach seeks to complement general growth-oriented change, however it may be initiated and whatever its early directions may be. These directions may not, of course, include changes in speech and language functions, at least not initially. In seeking to implement desired changes, the clinician will typically recognize that they can be effected in a context where the child's ways of being are respected and accepted. When the child's natural inclination toward growth or increased exploratory activity is observed, one can visualize a simultaneous reduction in his need for inordinate defensiveness. Acceptance of the child's nature, of his way of behaving, or of his need to be a particular way at each moment of time will offer him the appropriate opportunity for reduction of his need to maintain compromises previously established. If acceptance is communicated successfully, one can anticipate a resultant increase in experimental or exploratory attempts on the part of the child. In initiating a discussion about human motivation, Cofer and Appley (1966) examine what this writer deems to be a point of view of central importance: "the master motive is anxiety and . . . anxiety underlies other apparent motives." What these authors may be implying is that one should deal with a wide spectrum of behaviors as if they were expressions of anxiety or energy arousal. At any rate, this starting point is exactly that of child therapy—particularly in the instance of new learning or in processes of undoing previously acquired states that seem to be fixed.

One way to describe the acquisition of growth trends that are ongoing is to say that they are accomplished through persistent negotiation between the growing child's ego self, his impulse self, and his structural or physiological self. Dynamic participants in this adaptive effort are the significant people and important conditions of the child's environment or his not-self. These correspondents offer a variety of responses to both ego and impulse aspects. Critical in the changing complexity of the child's growth and his continued learning is this three-way negotation. Many reinforcing responses of external origin assume priority over the child's efforts and become pervasive in the child's attempts at adaptation. Many responses from the environment appear to be given capriciously. Some responses are initiated with minimal regard for the child's needs. Of course, responses of a positive and growth-promoting sort are also seen with great frequency. Considerable contribution to the child's significance (as the child views himself) is also provided by those aspects of himself and his environment to which he may assign perceptual priority. Such priority may be determined by the child's needs but may also be designated by the strength of the demands that are imposed upon him. While such expectations often relate to the true needs of the growing child, they are frequently imposed for the need-satisfaction of others. As such, little impetus may be provided for the child's attempts to grow. Frequently, then, such demands serve only the aims of others, and the child's efforts are unrewarded or fruitless, or value is assigned to the subordination of the child's inclinations. For growth as well as for the therapeutic process to be activated, one must provide not only an interaction situation but an interdependent one in which the child's efforts are accorded importance. The process must be one of mutual and reciprocal influence. Without this condition therapeutic change is likely to be transient, unspecified, negative, or limited with respect to transfer effects. In too many instances in the general course of living, the child is required to invest large amounts of energy in maintaining or defending his way of being; surrendering satisfaction of his many needs is too often required. High priority is thereby given to the acquisition and maintenance of externally designated behaviors or attitudes. Growth efforts and normal synthesizing processes are correspondingly fragmented. Here the child's efforts at achievement are atomized. It is as if the interaction between the child's strivings and the agents of his environment seems to tell the child that growth is of little importance or that change, if it is allowed, is to be substantially a dependent function. Importance is now attached to defensiveness, to the maintenance of immaturity, or to compliance with requirements externally imposed. Demands are thus frequently imposed without regard for their growth-oriented potential. Too frequently the result is that of the child's maintaining behaviors that are below his developmental age or below his potentiality. This child may continue to seek singularity or uniqueness, but that search will now take place through his defensiveness, or perhaps through any variety of immature expressions. Unfortunately, but often unknowingly, the agents of the environment are inclined to participate in this effort, and the child's assumptions that relate to it. Structural deficit or (neuro-) physiological dysfunction appear to intensify the child's tendency toward misassumption or cognitive or perceptual error. When these various things occur, the energies of the child are vested primarily in the maintaining of his fragmented maturity, or, more accurately, in the preserving of his being in its immature state. Available scientific information does not allow one to predict at this point which systems and functions will be accorded freedom to grow and which will be linked with factors of maintained immaturity. The contiguous nature of learning and the pervasiveness of verbal function in serving the aims of growth and development, or the inhibition thereof, offer clear indication of the possibilities for the adoption of pathological speech and language. Bentzen's (1962) study illustrates this general concept. In a study of 40 children, the high incidence of speech and language difficulty in association with emotional disturbance and academic difficulty was noted. One clear inference to be drawn from this study is the importance of treating such children in terms of the interrelatedness of their difficulties in developmental patterning and sequencing. Play or child therapy may be particularly useful in illuminating the interdependent nature of the child's difficulties as well as in facilitating the reactivation of growth trends.

Since the small child does not know (in the sense of logic) but is in the developmental process of knowing, there is a considerable probability that he will tend to link things that are, in reality, only marginally related. In fact, he may tend to link objects, conditions, people, and events that are not related at all. Furthermore, he may (although it is not predictable) link such external factors with many aspects of his own efforts, capacities, or experimentations. When one considers the possibility of the ensuing errors, expressive as well as perceptual, and, if one studies that dynamic in the light of a developing child who is loaded with impulses and possibly damaged structurally, then the child's vulnerability to mistakes in learning becomes obvious. When this anticipated occurrence is focused against a background of cultural demand, parental values, and the child's normal desire for achievement, the potential number and kind of associative links (a large number of them involving verbal function) substantially exceed current comprehension. Observation indicates, however, that if developing but vulnerable speech and language functions find themselves linked with carefully maintained immaturities, then such acts may assume the same burden of inertia. Where this kind of linking has been established, it is not surprising to find certain dimensions of verbal function maintained at the same level of immaturity. The contiguous arrangements between verbal development and the general developments of the child are infinite and undoubtedly reciprocal. When one appreciates the depth and intricacy with which verbal development serves the general needs of the growing child, one can visualize the potential associations that link disorders of verbal communication with the general dimensions and disturbances of growth and development. Typically, the maturing of the normal child is synthesized. The growth of the immature child is still characterized by efforts at synthesis, even at the expense of enormous compromise. Growth of the whole child, of course, invites acquisition of normal development in the various part-functions of the person. Child therapy attempts to make general growth trends dominant. The activation of such trends typically includes the resumption of developmental efforts in verbal communication. The appearance of these attempts, whether specific to speech and language or general in development, warrants the most careful response by the speech clinician.

For the human, the seeking of a singular identity is prominent in his achievement efforts. By reason of his need to live in an organized society, however, efforts toward the establishment of homonymous identities can also be observed. Learning makes a dominant contribution to the child's uniqueness and to the acquisition of necessary identifications with others. It is as if both singularity and similarity are required. Singularity provides the child with self-awareness. Homonymous identities provide the child with awareness and understanding of others. Irrevocably linked with both aims are the various dimensions of verbal function. In no other development does the person display any greater evidence of the acquisition of both singularity and similarity or of failure in those respects. As the child grows, verbal factors become increasingly important in effecting such learning. Verbal function is also affected by such learning. It is as if the reciprocal relation between effect-affect factors are literally activators of the bimodal identities mentioned above. Verbal communication is the primary means by which the child becomes aware of his separateness and singularity. Verbal communication is also the chief means by which the child can identify the presence, purposes, and separateness of others. The child's speech, for example, is unique in some dimensions but is a replica of the speech of others in many ways. His language structure and usage have elements of singularity and elements of similarity with respect to the language of others. Verbal function, containing as it does information about both the person and his environment, is placed in the service of learning and general development as is no other single growth element.

Hertzler (1965) makes the observation that "to speak is to be oneself and to know oneself." He describes language as an environment in itself which functions in a reciprocally orienting way with respect to all other environments. When this concept is applied to the problems of therapeutic conduct it assumes special significance. To this end, one may observe that verbal development is longitudinal in nature, contiguous with other important growth parameters, and prominent in need-satisfaction. Verbal function is literally symbiotic with respect to most of the significant components of the child's growth. It is equally critical in orienting the child to the reality of his surroundings. While specificity is to be provided by research, direct observation finds that verbal communication is associated with a multitude of temporal, spatial, and qualitative features of the child's achievements. It is germinal in his reasoning processes, importantly linked with perceptual and motor developments, and basic to the process of object identification. Speech and language thus come to represent the world to the child and the child to the world. Verbal function also comes to be prominent in the child's growing concept of his communication with himself.

One may examine another dimension of the relation between verbal function and growth. Speech and language behaviors represent that which has occurred and is occurring between the child and his world. His communicative efforts also contain anticipatory elements indicative of his preparation for whatever may be forthcoming. Verbal effort, therefore, may represent the various dimensions of his orientation in time as well as space. Indeed, much of the ongoing speech act contains strong anticipatory elements. It is as if verbal function is an eternal-in-the-present representation of the past and anticipation of the future. The dynamic, synthesizing nature of the verbal act is therefore apparent.

Facilitating Communication

Literature in this field is composed of scientific explanations, descriptions of devices and equipment, anatomical and physiological representations, and data in many forms. Additionally, one will find attempts at etiological accounting, much symptom description, and considerable procedural advice. All of these things are important and necessary. They are descriptive in nature and offer a progressive identification of phenomena which must be understood. Although these components do not yet offer a synthesized understanding of the nature of verbal communication, such aspects become important ingredients in the achievement of clinical goals. The most intangible and perhaps the most elusive factors, however, are those which will bind such ingredients and provide some realization for therapeutic efforts. Useful binding agents seem to be those factors which operate in the context of dynamic communication. Words such as deep regard, personal significance, individuality, personal uniqueness, reciprocal influence, self-determination, and love are seldom seen in scientific literature. A description of the communicative act in a therapeutic arrangement is difficult without an appreciation of these terms. In too many children have their major energies been placed in the service of concealment. Some children identify problems, are properly inquisitive, and find answers. Some children see problems and inquire of others about them only to find no response. Many dream about things and wonder. Still others feel and experience but suffer loss of relatedness. Some children are hungry and search endlessly to fill their loneliness. Too many fear their feelings and consequently seek subtle and often insidious release for them. Others have given up and only hope silently. Structural difficulty has occurred in some and they seek order and purpose or fall prey to the fallacy of assumption. Opportunity for exploration and study appropriate to the needs of each child should be inherent in any child therapy approach. The communicative act in the mutuality of therapeutic search is of vital importance. Bettelheim (1967) says, "It is when language does not make any difference that it loses its value; or if bad events follow in spite of verbal protest."

It is understandable that the word *communication* when used to represent human behavior often implies verbal behavior. In the sense that communication is used here, however, the term is more embracing. Here it is required that all attitudes and all behaviors be viewed as potential communication data. From an interaction point of view the important thing about behavior is probably not the fact that it occurs but the fact that it is communicated. It effects and affects, it influences and specifies. Behavior elicits response and is response. The execution of behavior and the revealing of attitudes begets changes in the behaving organism as well as in its surroundings. Although many communication systems appear to be single-channeled and one-way in their execution, the act in the human is basically designed as an exchange phenomenon. To say it in behavioral and therapeutic terms, communication is dynamic, multidimensional, and interdependent. Each person sends and receives messages. In order to comprehend any particular message each receiver attempts to replicate that message. This apparently consists of some kind of internal reproduction or experiencing of the received message. In the course of comprehension the person may carry out cognitive, perceptual, and even expressive acts. In most instances he must also anticipate or prepare responses. Whether sent or received, each message is distorted to some extent. The nature and accuracy of preparation, transmission, and reception, and the kind and magnitude of distortion may be due to various factors. These factors include anatomical and physiological properties; the medium through which the message passes; the complexity of the message; specificity and applicability of previous learning regarding the message; and the various capacities of the people who are involved. The general history of each person, the needs or current motives of the correspondents, and the conditions of the relationship will also make significant contributions to message sending and message receiving. These several determinants of the communicative act function in a dynamic and integrated way. Their relative weights shift from situation to situation and from need to need. Sometimes appropriate integration is not possible and the resultant effort is termed pathological. Whether pathological or not, however, the ensuing behaviors or attitudes must still be regarded as integrative attempts. In some instances, the child's anatomical or physiological nature may be involved and require improvement or aid. Changes in the transmission medium are sometimes helpful. While little can be done about the constitutional capacities of the person, compensatory education is often effective. Nothing of significance can be done to change the person's history, but it is possible that some supplanting of previously acquired notions or behaviors can be accomplished. The greatest potentiality for change, however, exists in the context of the person's ongoing needs, attitudes, or behavioral expressions. This should be understood to include those events arising out of the conditions of the therapeutic relationship. Such a context also includes, with great frequency, the previously mentioned determinants. The greatest possibility for the accomplishment of change exists within the broad dimensions of new learning or developmental opportunity. This may include the undoing of previous acquisitions, the activation of experimental effort, and the adoption of attitudes or behaviors which are new in the truest sense.

Human messages, regardless of their structure or functional form, typically contain two components. These components are variously described: sometimes as verbal and nonverbal; sometimes as human and more primitive; in other instances as cognitive and noncognitive; or, following Barnlund (1968), as content and intent. These latter terms are more universal in application and suitably embrace all the others. The discussion of these constructs and their operational use is highly pertinent to this general topic, and careful study of Barnlund's material is urged. When messages are viewed in any of the aforementioned two-component ways, it is obvious that some messages and some interaction efforts may be predominantly composed of one component or the other, but careful scrutiny will usually reveal both portions. Some participants in the communicative act assume that the dominant or even exclusive use of one aspect or the other is more effective or at least required. The content portion of messages is the more formal or abstract symbol-sign-system and customarily tends to relate specific information. The intent portion is that part more directly indicative of the person's needs, motives, attitudes, or aims. Intent may be gleaned from semantic variance, from word selection or combination; may be positioned subtly within the abstraction itself; or may be contained within an infinite number of signs which for the most part are nonverbal. This message component is essentially instructional, petitioning, or negotiating in nature. Feldman's (1959) text is an interesting, empirically derived discussion of the intent or nonverbal component. The communicative act in a therapeutic context is one in which both aspects (intent and content) are perceived, both are given careful study, and each is accorded appropriate significance. The interchange which characterizes formal education and much of everyday communication seems to place primary attention on content. The petitioning and nonverbal signs are often given inadequate recognition, sometimes avoided, and too frequently used as a source of conflict. Observation suggests that much disordered communication originates in the matrix of intent. Therapeutic interaction requires purposeful use and careful investigation of this component.

Verbal communication appears to originate in needs and is simultaneously a prime effector with respect to need-satisfaction. Viewed in a therapeutic context it would appear that those needs which subserve messages should be accorded as much significance as their more obvious expressional or behavioral forms. Represented in the child's behaviors and attitudes and thus in his messages are both his ways of being and his ways of attempting to become something else. Many therapeutic efforts are directed at the behavioral and content forms which may appear. Whatever may be the formal or content characteristics, communication is best maintained by a therapeutic speaking to the child's needs or true purposes as well as by therapeutic efforts addressed to behavioral end products. Other approaches will emphasize concern with needs, and little effort may be vested in direct behavioral modification. Child therapy attempts to recognize and give appropriate priority to expressional components, to the needs in which they may originate, and to the several additional determinants which may relate to the child's verbal communication ways. This ability (recognizing and speaking to needs) on the part of the clinician is not only therapeutically maintaining but allows for the implementation of the child's growth capacities. Such an ability also creates a setting in which therapeutic limiting and intervening can be profitably effected. Let us say, then, that the binding, caring, and communicative aspects of a therapeutic attempt are inherent in the significance and respect attributed to the needs of the child. Even those situations where both parties contribute conflict will often be maintained adequately as long as the intent or need portions of messages are accorded recognition. Where content is to be emphasized, contamination of information may be anticipated with some frequency if basic message determinants (often intent) are ignored or disrespected. The execution of this communicative effort is not embodied as much in method and procedure as in the capacity for being deeply, warmly, and distinctly and almost urgently patient in response to the purposes of the child and to his ways of attempting to express and satisfy them. This kind of communication requires the same openness on the part of the therapist that he asks of the child. Therapeutic effort is not implemented by method but by one person's capacity for being thoughtfully and richly involved in the strivings and expressions of another.

The Relationship

Many of the formalities of therapeutic effort would make it appear that the process takes place by activation of a specific method of procedure. Such definition is difficult because of the problem of individual differences and by reason of the present lack of scientific specification. The value of obtaining such definition is obvious and might be questioned only because of the risk involved in the assuming of mechanistic approaches. Perhaps one of the unique values of child therapy is its high emphasis on spontaneity and experimentation. This approach seeks to accomplish change where impetus is provided by the establishment of a particular relationship between two people. Therapeutic possibilities are invited when the child is accorded the right to be subject, relatively self-determined, and appropriately influential in that relationship. The intended effort is implemented when both the child and the therapist become people of unique significance to each other. The relationship assumes therapeutic aspects when the child begins to learn that the therapist is behaving in terms of the child's presented and implied needs. Initiation of the process occurs when the child perceives that the responses of the therapist are usually thoughtful, open, and child-oriented. The relationship, by virtue of the child's position and the therapist's role, allows the child to perceive that the maintenance of previously adopted or overcompromised behaviors is no longer necessary in order to preserve the relationship. In short, the probability for therapeutic change is increased when the child finds himself in an arrangement where certain of his historical protective devices are no longer required and no longer valuable. The appearance of new behaviors, usually exploratory and experimental, or even arousal in the magnitude of anxiety, gives indication of the child's positive response to the relationship and, furthermore, offers evidence of his aims. The conditions just described are not simply methodological in execution. They are accomplished only when the clinician is able to demonstrate a deep regard and, if you will, a considerable amount of thoughtful affection for whatever the child may be or attempts to be. While the theoretical orientation of this chapter is not predominantly existential, the recent publication edited by Moustakas (1966) is pertinent and valuable at this point. Here emphasis was clearly placed on effective communication as a significant part of the relationship.

In many activities that involve learning and caring, and in most situations that are growth-promoting, a particular condition may be observed in the relationship. One finds himself in a position of relative strength and the other in a dependency role thereto. In the former (in this instance the clinician), one presumes to find the existence of motives congruent with his more mature needs and expressive equivalents of those motives which are addressed to the presented needs of the dependent person. In the latter person one may anticipate a variety of signs representing needs at many levels of maturity. It is in the context of this situation that the basic therapeutic relationship must be described. In this communicative experience, both people must make important decisions about self-protection, about new learning, and about the most effective means for handling the problems of wanting and getting. These decisions come to be made by each for himself and, perhaps, for the other. This is a fundamental act involving the whole person. For the therapist, it is essentially the act of perceiving the world of the other in terms of the needs or intentions of the other. Such an act amounts to functioning in the context of another person's psychological realm. Here, indeed, is a transaction in which one person understands or knows the other. The child is free to do this or not. It is therapeutically required that the clinician be able to demonstrate this capacity, however, since it is fundamental to his comprehension of the child. If behaviors and thus communicated acts originate in unsatisfied needs then one is required only to point out that the therapist's needs will be as apparent and well communicated as those of the child. The character, the competence, and the need-satisfying intentions of the clinician will be progressively revealed. Simultaneously, the needs, expectations, and general ways of the child will be progressively expressed. One asks simply whether or not the needs or behaviors demonstrated by the therapist relate primarily to those of the child or ensue from matters of self-concern. It is important that the one in a position of primary accountability be able to identify the needs of others and at the same time maintain cognizance of his own identity and thus his intelligence. Where this is done, therapeutic communication is possible. It is clear that the therapist is to invest his needs and derived energies in the study and appropriate satisfaction of the child's requirements. The identification of such needs, both child's and clinician's, together with the choosing of appropriate responses, is a fundamental therapeutic responsibility. The comments of Goldstein and others (1966) are of particular interest here. He notes that therapist interest in hostility, for example, may produce a person practised in the expression of this emotion. Therapist interest in other and more positive or affiliative affects would lead to the development of "pro-social" attitudes. What Goldstein is implying is clear. The therapeutic relationship must not be used as an arena for the expression of the therapist's needs, and the choosing of the right response is therefore a matter of some importance.

It is seemingly paradoxical that a child who finds himself in the kind of relationship just described would typically demonstrate the activation or intensification of anxiety or at least some condition of excitation. These signs may actually be anticipatory elements which are equivalents of underlying anxiety and which have appeared because of the child's response to the possibility or implied promise of need-satisfaction. An understanding of the change phenomenon would indicate that such an arousal or anxiety state could be expected. The anticipatory aspect of speech production is available to anyone upon inspection and, of course, has been of great interest in speech pathology research. Pertinent to this discussion are the comments of Cofer and Appley (1966). They describe a positive relationship between states of deprivation (need) and arousal (motivation) when anticipation occurs. They identify anticipation as an enhancement of the organism's response to stimuli and suggest, therefore, that the behavior that occurs under these conditions is vigorously augmented—higher in strength than the level that might be expected in the same situation without anticipatory elements. This description corresponds exactly with the arousal and anticipatory nature of so much of one's verbal behavior. Anticipatory elements, therefore, may be viewed as expressive equivalents of some state of deprivation and are, therefore, clear signals by which the child can give an indication of his needs. Moreover, the arousal-anticipatory description parallels much of the activity which can be observed in the general growth efforts of children. The implementation provided for the child's growth by verbal development and by general arousal is pertinent to the study of the therapeutic act. Speech and language functions, particularly in face-to-face communication experiences, are not only consolidating with respect to things such as information and security, but preparatory in nature. As such, verbal effort is clearly both the consequence of and a considerable contributor to the child's growth. At once, then, verbal communication is parametric in the context of human interchange and a major conveyance in its growth movement. Therapeutic action must take place within the dynamic arousal-anticipation context just described. The relationship to be formed between the therapist and child provides the setting in which the child's aroused energies may be profitably employed. This view of anxiety and anticipation appears to be appropriate for those children who must learn ego-control functions as well as those who function by overcompromise and thus seek greater freedom. The importance of a knowing and discriminative therapeutic response is again illustrated clearly. The therapeutic use of arousal is appropriate, furthermore, for those children who demonstrate specific communicative dysfunctions that are contiguous with other and various immaturities. Interestingly enough, clinical observation will also reveal similar ties between anxiety arousal and particular behaviors observed in those children who have anatomical or physiological deficiencies. If anything, the magnitude of arousal in those children tends to be even greater. People often explain this, in speaking of neurologically handicapped children for example, as being the direct consequence of the injury and label it "hyperactivity." Prolonged and varied clinical observation often leads one to suspect, however, that the child's excessive anxiety actually represents the magnitude of need-deficiency. The organic state has made its contribution in that form.

The appearance of some elevated state may be regarded, therefore, as an indication of the child's readiness for change. Certainly, it is to be regarded as an encouraging sign. Naive therapists are inclined to palliate these signals. Therapists who function predominantly in terms of the child's growth needs, however, place significance on the appearance of such anxiety. They realize that the potentiality for change is inherent in the tentative appearance of these historically defended expressions. Read a clinical exemplication of this concept in an account by Moustakas (1964). Here the author describes the relationship between a seizure symptom and anxiety. He illustrates clearly the therapeutic necessity for responding to anxiety elements as potentials for change rather than as pathological end products in themselves. These so-called anxiety expressions are viewed in this child therapy approach as human energy for which new expressive channels must be discovered. From the child's view it is perhaps at this point that the relationship acquires its greatest significance. Here the child has the opportunity to learn that through the use and expression of his historically defended anxiety lies the potentiality for change. Here the child is provided with the unique opportunity to know that those energies which once appeared as anxiety components and were adjusted on a defended or avoidance basis actually contain the potentiality for his becoming a more particular and viable person. The therapist takes the role of an active participant, particularly in a respondent sense. The child is not acted upon as in many instructional arrangements. He is the primary but not sole determinant of his own behavior. He is not subjected to an acceptance of the illusion that his behaviors are determined entirely by forces beyond himself. The therapist is one who is able to give his feelings, his attention, his wisdom, and his selective encouragement without assigning contingencies to them. This is constituted in a paradoxical arrangement, according to typical cultural patterns, where the child is central and relatively independent, influential, and self-determined. The therapist is principally a respondent who is dependent upon the child's giving expression to his basic inclination toward experimentation and, furthermore, dependent upon his ability to perceive accurately the meaning and intent of the child's messages.

PREPARATION

The implementation of therapeutic intent finds the therapist confronted with many questions and issues. This section identifies some of the more common problems. Practical suggestions or solutions are offered. There is little possibility of anticipating all problems, nor can one provide exhaustive directions for each potentially troublesome or questioned area. The basic purpose here is to provide the student with some preparatory or anticipatory opportunities.

Validation

The course of normal relatedness prompts people to perceive, study, and make decisions about each other and themselves. The validity of these attempts is often observable in the quality of the therapeutic result or may be studied while therapy is in process. Verbal communication contains many possibilities for ongoing correction relative to validity maintenance. One of the great advantages in the use of verbal function is its tendency toward change through monitoring and self-correction. This appears to operate in developmental learning; in all thinking-out-loud processes; in most negotiations; and even in verbal pathologies themselves. A unique extension of these processes is found in those situations where one proposes to define and change the behaviors, attitudes, or knowledge of another. Such relatedness is even more critical when the issues are pathogenic. Included in this problem-solving activity is the attempt to understand many variables. Some of these variables may be directly observed and others inferred. If certain safeguards are not employed, some variables may be defined by assumption. The relative validity of decisions ranging from careful, direct, and repeated observation to decision by assumption is obvious. Assessment and consequent therapeutic acts, however, are currently based partly on knowledge and partly on operational constructs. Many of the latter forms are, of course, derived from theory. Operational constructs are used as empirically derived replacements for phenomena which are observable to some extent, but which are not well understood in terms of source. Whether one makes decisions on the basis of fact or by an empirically derived hypothesis, the use of scientific methodology is the validating approach. Clinical judgment is the vehicle. In therapeutic practice many decisions must be made spontaneously and in an ongoing context. Such decisions appear to have improved validity if they are aimed at reflecting the particular uniqueness of the child and if they have been based on directly observable behavioral data. Since this approach is heavily empirical and dynamic in execution, emphasis is placed, furthermore, on the validating of the person who makes the decisions. For example, false deductive approaches are frequently seen in clinical practice. Such an approach is apparent when the clinician, upon visualizing a particular symptom, arrives *post hoc* at certain assumptions about the etiology of the symptom or even about the nature of the person who possesses it. Where data are carefully gathered by direct observation; where one notes whether such behavior appears to originate in the child or in the child's response to the clinician; where one is cognizant of the nature of behavioral change; and finally, if one is adequately self-disciplined with respect to the use of assumption, then the nature and intent of the child will have an optimal chance to be revealed. Individualized clinical observations which can be certified by another observer as characterizing the child is another validating approach. The relativity and clustering of developmental or behavioral signs is still another. For example, it is not uncommon to hear clinicians discuss their clients in terms of behavioral signs from a wide range of maturity levels. The same clinicians constantly shift their notions about the child's maturity or about the meaning to be attached to his behavioral demonstrations. These perceptions by the clinician, while pertinent to his learning about the child, are indicative of unreliability and invalidity in his comprehension of the child. Other clinicians do not speak of behavioral signs or of developmental characteristics, but only of symptom status. This, too, is suggestive of lack of validity in his comprehension of the child. Basic validity occurs when the clinician is willing to make observations and offer responses as if each session were a new experiment, as indeed it is. The foregoing remarks are intended as practical suggestions relative to therapeutic conduct. It is intended that the clinician maintain himself in a perpetual state of new learning relative to his child patient, relative to his own feelings, and to his accumulated observations about the interaction processes that are taking place. If formal research is to be attempted it is hoped that it will address itself to the components of the therapeutic process and not to a study of outcomes alone. The published works of Goldstein and others (1966), Sidman (1960), and Staats and Staats (1966) may be of particular value in design matters and in data programming. The maintenance of therapeutic safeguards through the use of a research design approach would make an excellent contribution to validity in therapeutic conduct.

The Clinician

Preparation of the therapist is a primary consideration. The basic criterion is met if this person possesses the capacity to become openly involved with the intentions and behaviors of others. He should be so involved without any dominating need to impose his expectations, assumptions, or values on the child whom he proposes to help. The academic preparation of such a therapist would, of course, involve the development of a unique curriculum. He should be well grounded in growth and development phenomena. It would be desirable for him to possess a conceptual framework involving learning theory, physiology psychology, ego psychology, and behavioral interaction principles. It is understood, of course, that he will have full academic exposure to the customary subjects in speech, language, and audiology. An extended supervised professional practicum is required. This therapist will possess a clear perception of the management of his own therapeutic attitudes, intentions, and techniques. He will be patiently experimental in his study of the child's needs and in his response to them. Finally, he will be an individual who is himself in the process of seeking change and new knowledge.

The Therapeutic Candidate

The child will, of course, have some kind of speech or language disorder. The typical child candidate will present a pattern of immaturity or developmental difficulty in addition to the verbal communication problem. Many children who may be helped by this approach are those whose development and behavior are maintenance-oriented (immature or fixated) rather than change- (growth-) oriented. Disability in verbal function often produces unreliable results in the evaluation of intelligence. This, together with the fact that speech clinicians work in a wide variety of settings with a full spectrum of handicapped children, makes the specifying of intelligence criteria unwise. It is desirable to have some preliminary diagnostic impression of capacity for improvement in verbal functioning. Many times initial assessment suggests that verbal function has been submerged or partially obscured by other growth and development issues. Selection, therefore, is based primarily on the clinician's judgment that the child is functioning below his capacity and that such an approach as described here could produce successful intervention with respect to the child's resistance to developmental change.

Other Important People

Preparation or involvement of other people who are significant in the child's life must be considered. These people may particularly include immediate family members, relatives, and, in many instances, teachers. It is advised that the therapist maintain close, concurrent, and perhaps simultaneous relationships with these people. This effort may take many forms. Sommers and others (1964), for example, in the course of studying maternal attitudes, provided mothers with direct speech training to employ with their children. Safer (1965) employed conjoint play therapy involving the child and his parents as a means of providing the parents with direct knowledge of their involvement in the child's difficulties. Making the point that the symptomotology of brain-damaged children could not be explained solely on the basis of anatomical impairment, Serrano and Wilson (1963) report the use of family therapy as an intervention attempt. They offer the interesting note that a disturbed or injured child may prove to be a stabilizing influence for the family if his symptoms are used by the family to drain off chronic anxiety. For one interested in techniques of family therapy or in case study approaches, the work of Haley and Hoffman (1967) and Bell and Vogel (1960) will be provocative and instructional. Mottola (1967) has made available an excellent digest of family therapy approaches together with a comprehensive reading list.

Of particular importance is the fact that the therapist should permit no mysteries concerning the nature of the process. This can be done successfully while still respecting the privileged nature of the child's communication. In many instances, it appears to be anxiety-allaying if the parents are given adequate preliminary instruction relative to the therapeutic process. As therapy proceeds with the child, it is often desirable to involve parents and others in a similar therapeutic effort. Webster (1968) describes an interesting and helpful procedure appropriate to this effort. Serious consideration should be given to the possibility of seeing the family (including the child) as a group rather than as individuals. It is common to find that the child-family interaction contains elements which seem to reinforce the child's immaturity. Frequently observed is the fact that the child's efforts at behavioral change meet with family opposition. Increased family understanding and acceptance of the need for change are, therefore, important components of the total therapeutic effort. The successful involvement of the family in this development substantially increases the probability that the child's newly learned attitudes or behaviors will be appropriately transferred and used in his natural setting. Teaching parents how to be concerned with needs as well as with directly observed behaviors is fundamental to this effort. In other words, the same therapeutic concepts used in this child therapy approach are generally applicable for family involvement. The work of Guerney and Stover (1967) is pertinent here. This study involved the training of parents in the processes of child-centered play therapy. In this study, the value of training mothers in the practicalities of conducting play therapy with their children was demonstrated. It is felt that this technique is actually a systematic way of involving the parents in a reeducative process that is something more than training in certain elements of play therapy. The kind of involvement required by the play therapy process seemingly heightened the mother's awareness of the child's needs and improved the sensitivity of her responses to him. Martin (1967) reports the use of family therapy on a current interactional technique. This study demonstrates a practical way of accumulating data and again points to the efficacy of a family approach.

Where interaction problems are severely negative or where the family is strongly threatened by the child's efforts at change, another technique appears to have promise. This requires the use of an observation facility with a one-way mirror. Here one allows the child to be involved with a therapist while other family members are in a therapeutic arrangement with another therapist in the observer's room. Although often producing anxiety in parents, this situation contains striking possibilities for helpful therapeutic intervention and family learning. It also preserves the integrity of the child's efforts which might otherwise be negatively affected by the magnitude of his parent's concern. Many therapists (writer included) would prefer to maintain total family involvement, if at all possible, using conflict issues as simply another source for teaching the child relative to matters of separateness and identity. The decision to employ total family involvement is often related to matters of clinician security. Separation of family and child may be helpful at the outset of the treatment attempt, though, particularly where traumatic anxiety may be anticipated. Actually, every effort should be made to see the child and his family as a unit if all of them are involved in the same treatment goals or are inappropriately entangled in the needs of others. The purpose here is not primarily that of modifying the child's environment. The general aim is to promote a candid and open interchange where the participants are not fearful of their own intent, are respectful of the intent of others, are discriminating but not compromising with their expressions, and hopefully come to be people of reciprocal influence.

Although generally desirable, the conditions and techniques of family involvement relative to the child's therapy are questions of clinical judgment. If preliminary assessment suggests that the parents are enthusiastically oriented to change or characterized by sufficient anxiety so that change is legitimately sought, it would seem perfectly feasible to involve all of these people from the outset. This arrangement might consist of seeing the parents, the child, and siblings in group units of varying composition or as a total unit. Many therapists believe that the child should be reasonably verbal, and often an age of seven or eight is stipulated as requisites for involvement in a family therapy group. It is held by this writer, however, that the purpose of this group work is to effect improvements in general intrafamily communication. Such efforts should be exercised in the very context in which they are going to be used. The general principles of communication, verbal or otherwise, may be learned by all members of the family. Age or verbal facility are not requirements and for that matter actually may represent treatment goals rather than criteria. The therapist becomes a natural member of the group and continues the processes recommended elsewhere in this essay. Many situations present themselves, however, that are neither as positive nor as easily defined. Some parents are rigid, others overprotective, and still others chronically anxious. It is not uncommon to find parents who function primarily by displacement of responsibility. These people apparently expect that all of the efforts and gains are going to be produced by the child and the therapist. Some people appear to be highly indifferent to the therapeutic process. Frequently, one encounters a family with high social consciousness. They are primarily concerned about how the child appears to the world and seem to have little concern about the true child or the therapeutic process. Conditions of this sort tend to inhibit change and are hardly consistent with the developmental needs of the child. It is insufficient and therapeutically inappropriate, however, to pass off parental behaviors with such comments as "they're indifferent, they're rigid, they're rejecting," and so on. These various parental expressions are messages and warrant the same kind of study and response that would be employed had they originated with the child. The decision about whether to involve the child and the parents as a unit, the time of such involvement, and the therapeutic conditions of the involvement must result from this study. In some instances one should consider the possibility of conducting child therapy entirely through the processes of parent-education or parent-counseling. Where this is the approach of choice, it is expected that the clinician will use the same general therapeutic principles set down elsewhere in this chapter. Such concepts may be used in the relationship correspondence with parents or used as guidelines for the promotion of revised parent-child transactions. The criteria for omitting the child from direct involvement are several. One may wish to conduct the treatment effort with parents alone when the communicative disorder is only suspicioned or embryonic. This may occur in instances of non-fluent speech which occur in preschool children, in many situations where speech and language development is questionable and below the child's capacity, or in those instances where, despite normal verbal development, parental anxiety is high and focused on that particular development. Parent involvement of an educational sort is frequently useful in providing developmental guidance for children with anticipated communication difficulties. Those young children with known organic issues are typical examples. The fact of disordered verbal communication is typically not known or specifically felt by young children. Such difficulty with verbal function may not be so identified by the child as long as minimal or immature effort will result in substantial satisfaction for life needs. Recognition of verbal difficulty by the child may also be minimized by the child if he must assign higher priority to other growth or maintaining processes. For that matter, the phenomenological nature of the child's perceptual functions may cause him to assume that his current way of communicating is an adequately effective part of his general achievement effort. Clinicians persistently assign concern to the question of bringing the child's verbal deficiencies or immature communicative efforts to his attention. This is frequently the subject of conversation with the child's parents. The general notion has been that this act might exceed the child's anxiety tolerance and result in symptom fixation. Although this possibility must be respected, the potential importance or value of moderate anxiety arousal cannot be overlooked. Parental involvement is critical where such anxiety is already excessive, or avoidance of child confrontation is desirable, or where the study of these various factors is needed. Certainly it is appropriate to treat many disorders of verbal communication in the context in which they function. The conditions under which such an attempt is activated are unique and individualized and cannot be decided by a preconceived generality. It is thought that the concepts and survey presented by Truax (1968) may prove to be particularly applicable here.

An Approach to Assessment

The extent and kind of preliminary diagnosis or assessment are matters of concern. Careful medical study is a requirement observed by many therapists and should be employed consistently for all child therapy candidates. Other clinicians make "selective" referrals of children for a physician's evaluations. This is a difficult role for the clinician, however, since he places himself in the position of deciding, at least in a preliminary way, which children have symptoms with pathological organic components. By inference, then, the clinician has indicated that the children who are not so referred are free of organic involvement. This kind of assessment approach will probably not meet reliability standards. The word "functional" is often used as an assessment term. This word is as dichotomizing in consequence as the term "organic." Beyond the atomistic aspects just mentioned, however, is the assumption that is implied and the diagnostic responsibility that inures to the clinician who uses the terms.

It is necessary to certify both the symptomatology and the kind and magnitude of any concurrent signs of immaturity or maldevelopment. This writer is not convinced, however, that an extensive and highly detailed history study (as classically used) is a requirement. A careful analysis and an integrated unitary description of current status is perhaps a more judicious approach. Assessment of this kind includes a description of developmental and maturational achievements along multidimensional lines. It would be especially important to carry out studies which might describe not only the child's responses to a variety of situations and stimuli but studies which would indicate the conditions under which the child might demonstrate potentiality, as well as the need, for change. This may well prove to be a part of the therapeutic process itself and should not necessarily be viewed as a "preliminary" study. Experience suggests that in many instances extensive diagnostic effort, particularly that involving a case history study, has provided the therapist with assumptions that may not be at all consistent with the child's needs or capacities. Etiological discoveries, to the extent that they may be unearthed, have a way of determining both therapeutic channels and goals. If done with adequate validity such information, obviously, makes a useful contribution. Too often, however, the ensuing therapeutic effort is procedure-determined and varies little by reason of etiological findings or varies little as the result of direct observation. This is often the consequence of one having preconceived notions about the relationship between symptoms and treatment procedures. In too many instances, assessment findings appear to be derived from an hypothetical construct concerning the nature of the symptom and do not reflect the essential uniqueness of the particular child being considered. In a child therapy approach it seems more desirable for the child to reveal himself in the process of therapeutic change. Free of preconceptions, the clinician may now be more able to maintain a dynamic and ongoing view of the child. Such conceptualization in no way obviates the need for preliminary studies for physical and physiological systems, nor does it preclude the need for careful developmental assessment. Assessment should be implemented in a fashion consistent with the generality of this chapter; namely, to place as much respect as possible on the child's self-determined efforts at change. "The system is then its own best explanation, and the study of its present organization the appropriate methodology" (Watzlawick and others, 1967). The reader's attention is invited to many parts of this text.

Assignment of the Child

Careful consideration should be given to the problem of clinical assignment for the child candidate. The matter of involvement in group or individual situations is a common question. The criteria for assignment of a child on a one-to-one basis appear to be at least three in number. An acting-out child with strong aggression trends or with fragmented attention may be a candidate for individual assignment at least at the outset of therapy. Children with unusual sibling issues may warrant individual care. Sometimes one sees a child with severe isolation trends, and it is apparent that his condition would make any sharing of the therapist actually traumatic. This child is one who should probably be seen individually.

Grouping in terms of symptomatology is a frequently discussed problem. Clinical practice suggests that grouping children according to developmental age is probably more functional and feasible than grouping according to symptom. Such grouping will undoubtedly produce some symptom similarity, but this is not the intent. In the more specifically structured approaches, such as drill therapy, children are often grouped according to similarity of instructional need. The work of Sommers and others (1966) is an example of such grouping and demonstrates, moreover, the comparable value of group work and individual therapy. In the child therapy approach, grouping according to emotional or developmental need or simply by age are more feasible considerations. For further information in this regard Ginott (1961) is helpful, as are the concepts established by Pick and Stewart (1964). Assignment with respect to therapist is a matter for study. When children are seen in groups it may be perfectly reasonable for two therapists to be involved in the activity. It is believed that the classical arrangement which involves the child with a specific therapist is a somewhat rigid or stereotyped approach. Assuming readiness, it is much more natural for a child to have an opportunity to learn the processes of relating with several adults and many children. It is also reasonable to suppose that the wider the child's use of new learning (particularly in a therapeutic setting), the greater the probability of its becoming generalized or transferred into the non-therapeutic parts of his environment.

The initiation of a working relationship is also a matter of concern. Children and therapists sometimes find themselves with each other but with no apparent feeling of mutuality, concern or significant interest. Too often, these situations are allowed to endure and consequently produce only emptiness or perhaps a reinforcement of the child's immaturity and related communicative difficulties. Where possible it seems more therapeutic to allow both parties to seek each other. This is done naturally in many other relationships and may be profitably employed here if the therapist is knowledgeable with respect to his own needs and the opportunity is provided.

The use of groups is generally advised. The situation is more natural and more dynamic. A larger number of people than the customary one-to-one arrangement is far more stimulating and productive of arousal both defensively and in terms of behavioral changes. In this regard, Ginott (1961) says, "however, the usual circumstance is that the group allows the children to experience external reality as satisfying and helpful. To many children reality has become charged with massive negative expectations. They perceive the world as hostile and depriving and expect nothing from it but doom. These children find the conditioned reality of therapy an emotionally moving experience."

Use of Space

Space requirements are best denoted by two words—openness and flexibility. Therapeutic space, therefore, is any area or location which will implement the child-therapist relationship or provide activation possibilities for the child's experimental efforts. Such space may include the use of open grounds or that distance which is required for a walk. Unique intimacy often occurs when people find themselves in the setting of a vista rather than a walled room. The child's home space may also be regarded as a potential therapy area. This particular accommodation may be useful for family study, for establishing contact with extremely insecure and isolated children, or for facilitating application of new learning at a later point in the process.

If one is to describe a particular therapeutic room, several features seem to be desirable. Openness is still the keynote. Flexibility of use is important and, consequently, the area should lend itself to a variety of pursuits. It is not therapeutically helpful if the space contains locked cabinets. Locked storage facilities may be provided in a particular room or in hallway cabinets. This room should not be required to serve as the therapist's office. Clinical practice also suggests that the room need not be specifically assigned. Staff members and children should enjoy flexible and even multiple or simultaneous use of available space.

Equipment and Materials

Equipment need not be particularly unique, exotic, or expensive. Tables and chairs appropriate to the child's age level are necessary. It is desirable to have running water immediately available together with cleanup equipment. Bathroom facilities should be accessible directly from therapeutic areas rather than specifically adjacent to the reception area. Equipment should be acquired which would lend itself to the imaginative interests or experimental tendencies of the child. Too often play equipment specifically determines the child's activities and, consequently, seems to elicit or perhaps reinforce repetitive or stereotyped behavior. Play yard equipment requires cautious evaluation. Many children, particularly those with neurological handicaps, have serious problems with body movement or with space visualization and orientation. Such children do not cope well or safely with many common pieces of play yard equipment.

Therapeutic materials should be restricted in number compared to the large accumulation of objects found in many facilities. Materials which will promote experimentation and exploratory trends are recommended. Many desirable materials are ambiguous or unstructured. Clay, sand, water, painting materials, paper, crayons, and perhaps scissors are examples. Some items which are more specific may serve the same purpose. Human figures, blocks of varying sizes and shapes, and miniature houses are examples. Allowing the child's needs and perceptions to determine the manner in which the materials are used is an important criterion. A paper by Leland and Smith (1962) stressed the use of unstructured material as a means of providing greater patient control of activity and as a means of encouraging the client to see that his efforts can produce effects in reality. Puzzles, intricate games, and many audiovisual devices require high concentration. Experience suggests that such highly structured materials tend to reduce verbalization or to specify the verbal activity within certain limits. Obviously such objects are useful in many educational settings, but their use in a child therapy setting must be carefully evaluated. It is not uncommon to find that certain contrivances are used in the training of specific functions such as visual-motor acts. These approaches and collateral materials are not to be confused with the ambiguously structured materials just described, although their use may be selectively appropriate. When one has decided to use materials that are somewhat structured and which thus tend to determine the nature of the ensuing activity, the selection should be based primarily on the child's developmental status. Many therapists employ a technique where objects representing a variety of developmental ages or developmental interests are available. This approach includes both ambiguous and highly specific devices. Its purpose is to provide the child with a wide spectrum of objects, some of which may be specifically representative of his needs or his maturity level. In terms of assessment, this technique has demonstrable value. It often allows one to visualize any disparities between emotional maturity on one hand and other developmental achievements on the other. As a therapeutic possibility it is equally useful. Presentation of objects from a wide spectrum of maturity levels may be particularly helpful in revealing or revoking any regressive trends which might characterize the child. The use of this multidevelopmental approach should be considered from both the child's and the therapist's standpoint. Frankly, if regressive trends characterize the child, such needs will reveal themselves anyway in the course of therapeutic effort. The use of stimuli from a wide age spectrum, however, seems to be more specifying with respect to the child's needs, particularly those needs which are latent or well defended. The general notion, however, is to provide stimuli which will be more productive with respect to verbal effort. Objects and materials which are ambiguous or which will serve many purposes are seemingly most appropriate. Some objects which are specifically structured to the child's needs may have the same property, but the selection of such stimuli requires careful study. A recent observation also suggested that objects that are unknown may satisfy the same criterion, but this is not so well understood. It was noticed, however, that both pictures and objects that were not within the child's experiences were useful in eliciting heightened verbal activity. Apparently, the newness of the materials was encouraging with respect to exploratory effort. Clinically, it is interesting to note the positive relationship between experimentation and verbal or at least oral activity.

Unless one plans to do some direct speech work in a particular session, it is suggested that no tape recorder be available in the room itself. If a tape-recorded account of the session is needed, the equipment should be remote. For some children the use of such equipment in the therapeutic area often requires the addition of limits which are either difficult in application or inappropriate in terms of the general concept or purpose of limits. If observation facilities are available be prepared to respond honestly if the child questions the area or the window. Appropriately placed windows will double as mirrors, however. The child's spontaneous use of this mirror has been noted with frequency particularly where concern about body image is apparent.

The new therapist would be well advised to promote verbal communication as a function of the relationship. There is some frequent tendency for therapists to evoke speech in response to objects rather than to allow it to develop in relationship to the child's needs or intentions and in a reciprocal human context. Equipment and materials are supportive factors and cannot be viewed as primary therapeutic vehicles.

Time and Schedules

Time, studied therapeutically, is seldom regarded with much interest. Appointments are made for therapeutic sessions. The duration of the session is designated. Frequency of visits is decided upon. The number of sessions is often predetermined, sometimes by such factors as available summer vacation time, occasionally by a designated academic course, often by duration of school semesters, and even by adherence to some stereotyped scheduling pattern. Such decisions are also determined by parents or clinicians according to their personal schedules and general commitments. Length of therapeutic session is often determined by conventional adherence to clock hours. Frequency of session may be determined by schedule limits, by conventionalism, by cost factors, or by "policy." When small children are involved, morning hours are often selected. Such hours are designated, people say, because many children are more calm or "better controlled" early in the day. One must question these as sole determinants, however. Certainly they are reality factors and need to be considered. Of significant importance, though, is that which might be determined by the needs of the child. Perhaps the child should be seen at whatever time of day he is the most anxious. Consider seeing the child for an extended period of time and perhaps with varying frequency. The opportunity to be involved in a variety of settings and experiences may be beneficial. Permit some overlapping of various children's sessions where such meetings might be productive. Whatever the schedule, it needs to be predictable, however. Commitment to a precise and stereotyped schedule does not serve the needs of many children. A highly routinized schedule tends, moreover, to be productive of boredom or repetitive for some clinicians, although this boredom would be suspect as being one of the clinician's defenses. It is indeed difficult to schedule the child's needs, his motivated states, the nature of his anxiety, or his requirements for new learning by conventional clock-hour determinants. It may be added, however, that just such scheduling and careful adherence to time limits may relate pertinently to the presented developmental needs of some children or some families. What is urged here is simply that greater flexibility be considered in the use of therapeutic time and that the needs of the child be given appropriate weight in such decisions. The use of time and the handling of time dimensions, including limits, is a matter of specific importance for the child's developments and for the therapeutic process. Taft (1964) remarks, "the reaction of each individual to limited or unlimited time betrays his deepest and most fundamental life pattern . . . as living things we are geared to movement and growth . . . in terms of this double fear of the static and of the endlessly moving, the individual tries to maintain a balance and frequently fails because of too great a fear of changing or of never being able to change again."

The Milieu

While care is taken with respect to preparation of therapeutic space and management of the therapist's behaviors and cognizance is given to the importance of parental involvement, the nature of the general therapeutic setting is often ignored. Secretaries, volunteer workers and supportive personnel will all benefit from in-service instruction. The attitudes and verbal expressions appropriate to child care and to a therapeutic milieu should be a part of regular discussions in staff meetings. If the general goal is centered on the growth needs of the child then that is the goal for the effort of every person in the environment whether they are called therapist, clerk, custodian, or director. This milieu concept offers the possibility not only for protecting the therapeutic process but for facilitating generalization of the child's learning. It provides a clearly stated purpose for the presence and actions of all adults who are involved.

Record-Keeping

Suggestions relative to record-keeping are explicit. Study of developmental trends, cognizance of factors not immediately recognized, and accumulation of longitudinal data for holistic comprehension of the child are sufficient reasons for the maintenance of careful records. The possibility of reassignment of the child; interprofessional communication concerning the patient; verification of an original assessment; modification of therapeutic planning; information for parental guidance; and gathering of research data are additional purposes.

Of particular importance is the opportunity to record and verify the concurrent or associative nature of behavioral or attitudinal factors. Such longitudinal information may very well identify the presence of developmental needs or issues which function contiguously and which therefore may be significantly linked with respect to the child's verbal difficulties. Such linking, incidentally, is not limited to behavioral phenomena. One may be able to visualize changes in communicative effectiveness in concurrence with changes in physiological condition as may occur in illness, or which might appear in response to medication. Actually, it is common to find the child's verbal behaviors changing in association with a multitude of factors. Shifting of communicative effectiveness may occur in congruence with his manner of emotional expression, relative to his need-satisfying attempts, his defensive modes, environmental demands, the behavior of his correspondents, his functioning in a phenomenological sense, modification of physical attributes or deficits, reactivation of historical issues, changes in physiological variants, or may occur in congruence with a variety of dynamic variables concerned with learning or learning effort. Careful record-keeping increases the accuracy of such observations, or indeed, makes them possible at all. Longitudinally derived information validates the clinician's observation of the links between communication skill and any of the variables just noted.

Records may consist of diagnostic findings, clinicians ongoing notes, or cumulative tape recordings. Although expensive, video-tape records are becoming increasingly feasible. Notes provided by observers, by parents, or by more than one therapist must also be accumulated. Too frequently these notes consist of identification of teaching materials or summaries of the child's responses to the efforts of the clinician.

In some instances, preconceived goals are stated and notes are summaries of the child's responses to those intentions. Data useful for child therapy, however, must be specifically illustrative of the child and accurately reflective of the factors of the relationship. The therapist's statements should describe acts or incidents concretely. The initiator of a given act should be identified. The nature of the response must be described. Where attitudes are labeled, as much verifying information as possible must be offered. Content and intent portions of all correspondents' messages should be summarized. Practicality will place limits on the amount of information that can be accumulated, but the child's need for maximum understanding dictates the necessity of storing all possible data. It should also be stated that persistent collection of clinical information is, in itself, motivating for the therapist. This is particularly true where such data are reviewed consistently by the clinician or shared and discussed with other interested people. Although frequent observations and staff conferences are usually regarded as useful in therapeutic planning and understanding, the motivational value of such interchange is possibly of greater importance. If one is interested in research possibilities, the data-gathering structures required for the studies by Weiland and Legg (1964) and Rousey and Moriarity (1965) will be of interest.

PROCESSES

It was thought feasible to extract and discuss certain major subject areas pertinent to therapeutic conduct. Extensions of these notions can be made to other aspects of the treatment effort with little difficulty. For one thing, it is important to maintain cognizance of the difference between process and method. The former implies something ongoing and changing. The latter seems to define an orderly and prearranged system. Process is somewhat defiant of prediction, resistant to methodological subscription, and inherently promoting of change. Its use is emphasized in this child therapy approach.

Upon First Meeting

When the therapist first meets the child in the reception area it is advised that he speak first and perhaps only to that child. He should express interest in or positive anticipation about the child's presence. He may introduce himself by name. Certainly the therapist is to carry on no significant conversation with the parent unless the intent is to see the child and his parents as a family unit. The purpose here is to tell the child immediately that his position is a central one in the relationship that is being initiated. At this point, if the intent is to separate the child and his parent, the therapist simply takes the child's hand or perhaps puts his hand on the child's shoulder stating to the parent that both the child and the clinician will return presently. If the child appears to be hesitant, speak to him directly and speak in terms of both his feeling and demonstration of doubt or insecurity. At this point, both the parent and the therapist are often inclined to get involved in giving "reassurance" to the child. In many instances parents will want to use admonitions, threats, or bribes. All of this behavior is to be avoided. If this kind of parental communication is initiated, it is the therapist's responsibility to interrupt it. Experience suggests that a quick separation usually reduces anxiety for all parties. It is not uncommon to find therapists offering promises or in some instances stating contingencies. These behaviors are also to be avoided. If the child's anxiety persists, the therapist must speak to the child in terms of respect for that kind of expression. It is unwise to use words that will remind the child of his parent or that will risk intensifying his dependency feelings at this particular point. If crying is encountered, speak respectfully to the crying feelings and proceed to the therapeutic area. If anxiety is high for the child, the therapist becomes the basis for security. This provides an excellent means of establishing the kind of relationship that is intended. When strong conflict is encountered at the point of separation, the most appropriate response would be to study the needs or issues basic to that conflict. This may require the involvement of all parties, but the issue is still that of studying messages and offering a response that is pertinent with respect to the determinants of that message. It is not sufficient, therapeutically speaking, to respond simply to the form of the message in some preconceived or procedural way. The time to cope with conflict is at the point of its arousal, and the coping must include a study of the sources of that conflict.

Separation of the child and his parent immediately upon first meeting is a practice routinely employed by many therapists. Assuming this to be the decision, then follow the axiom that the child must be accepted as he presents himself. This is a first and vital test for all parties. The consequences of this first communication often produce far-reaching effects. In some instances, the child's needs and the therapist's intentions coincide. When they appear to be in opposition it seems appropriate to make the decision in terms of the child. This must not be interpreted to mean that the child's omnipotent or immature adjustments are accorded reward or listed as the only determining factors. The basic issue here is that concerned with the expression of his anxiety and with the impulses or needs which it signals. For the most part, this anxiety can be communicated with and separation continues. It is possible that separation will be traumatic, however. From a therapeutic standpoint, the same communicative principles must be used for all of the people who are involved in this anxiety expression. The very problems which have produced excessive dependency and consequent anxiety at separation may represent a basic therapeutic issue. In many instances this is exactly what is being communicated. The task is to respond to what is being expressed rather than to proceed on the basis of some stereotyped preconception. Of course this may not be the issue at all, and the clinician will simply proceed with his original plans.

If the therapist has planned to involve the parents and the child as a family unit, then this should be initiated immediately. Clinical experience has revealed the fact that many issues arise where the various members of the family are seen individually and then occasionally as a group. While individualized sessions are perhaps required in some instances, therapy as a family unit is desirable and if decided upon would, of course, eliminate any issue concerning separation anxiety.

When the therapist decides on immediate separation and makes that attempt he is committed to carry it through if at all possible. This decision is a matter of clinical judgment. A decision which relates poorly to the child's communicated needs often puts the therapist in a difficult position. This dilemma is one where failure in the attempt is likely to produce only an intensification of the child's original commitment to his own dependency. The therapist is advised to study the basis for his intent to separate the parent and the child. For example, such separation sometimes relieves anxiety for the therapist and consequently may be unrelated to the child's growth needs.

The First Session

The first session finds the child typically engaged in exploratory behaviors. Here is the point at which a crucial concept needs to be observed. The newness of the relationship, the place, the furnishings, and the materials will predictably promote high interest or experimentation on the part of most children. The child's arousal may be above the level of interest and might better be termed anxiety. Whether interest or anxiety, the elevated state will provide an excellent opportunity for the promotion or reinforcement of change. It is perfectly possible that the child may be more highly motivated and more highly susceptible or inclined to change at this time than he may be in many future appointments. This first meeting, then, is one of singular importance. The therapist is often provided with a unique opportunity to select responses that will specify and support change phenomena immediately. The significance of this opportunity cannot be overstated. In the conduct of this situation, the therapist probably says little. He may offer brief comments appropriate to the child's initial curiosity, concern or anxiety. Particular care must be exerted to keep those remarks noninstructional and open-ended. The therapist should not invite the child's attention to any particular object or activity. The opposite view is more appropriate. That is, one should follow the child's interest or inclinations. His behaviour should be treated as an invitation for response. Watching for peaks of interest or high points of anxiety is part of the clinician's task. One should offer encouragement, simple approval, or should comment on the child's intent in response to any reasonably mature effort. The first session is, therefore, commonly one where the child's anxiety or exploratory activity will peak. Or, that session may be one where his most chronic and most secure adjustment will be intensified. If anxiety is the case in point, one is given a rare opportunity to reinforce growth attempts immediately. If immobility occurs, the therapist is given his first challenge with respect to coping with resistance to change. Those children whose adjustments are more strongly characterized by fixed or chronic immaturity may display such issues precipitously. Other children may demonstrate regressive behavior in the face of their anxiety. While one must be cautious with respect to rewarding this trend, the sources of the child's anxiety may be particularly apparent at this time. It is perfectly feasible for the clinician to give illumination of the revealed anxiety source without placing value on the regressive behavior itself. Usually the therapist will have visualized a strongly unsatisfied need or a conflict among needs. The therapist has an immediate obligation to speak to the child's defended or compromised and often concealed need. The nature and intent of this new person, the therapist, is in any case revealed to the child.

Facilitating Exploration

Maintaining exploratory activity is not a particularly difficult task as long as the child is change-oriented or will initiate the activity. Appropriate responses by the clinician are usually rewarding or supportive enough to encourage or maintain the child's efforts. Some children initiate little, offer little, and seem to show minimal effort with respect to change. These are usually children with extraordinary defenses. Their behavior may be characterized, for example, by stereotyped activity, by repetitive play, by considerable isolation, or by obvious denial. When attempting to help such children, one may anticipate the demonstration of conflict signs or defense modes which originated in periods of development much below the child's chronological age. This child is perhaps one in whom inertia has been placed on the side of developmental fixation. By clinical judgment one may determine that if change is to occur some sort of therapeutic intervention will be required. Several factors need to be considered when the need for this particular effort becomes apparent. For one thing, it is possible that the objects or materials available in the therapeutic room are anxiety-producing in some overwhelming way. The therapist also needs to investigate the possibility that the child is being given particular kinds of instructions by his parents before the session commences. If the child has been advised to be "a good child" and, furthermore, has been offered some kind of reward as the consequence of such behavior, he may behave precisely in terms of his understanding of the word "good." Sometimes parents bring siblings to the clinic. The child in question may have some particular sibling issue. His seeming indifference to the therapist is actually an obscure kind of message relative to the other problem. If the therapist has feelings of concern about the child's responses it is important for him to structure and offer a careful expression of this concern. Gendlin (1966) says, "therapy must be experiential . . . change comes through directly felt experiential steps . . . interpersonal relationships carry the experiencing process forward if the therapist expresses his own actual reactions (as clearly his own) and at the same time gives room, attention and reference to the client's felt reactions as the client's own." Frequently, it is helpful to remark on the fact that the child has succeeded in obscuring his feelings. Here again the therapist is to speak to the intent of the child's behavior. Observed with greatest frequency, however, is another factor. In addition to adjustments such as isolation or indifference (these are used only as examples) or interlaced with those behaviors are other, more obscure expressions. Repeated and careful observation reveals the presence of other messages which have gone unnoticed. Wolf and Ruttenberg (1967), in describing an experience with an autistic child remarked that "changes, which in the normal child would be barely noticeable might be of great significance in the autistic child. Fleeting eye contact or the appearance of pitch variations in vocalizations are examples." The clinician's responses to these more subtle expressions will often produce a heightened awareness on the part of the child and a consequent shift in the mode of his expressive attempts. The matter of inducing change is often interpreted by therapists to mean that they are to undertake the directing or initiating of some activity. Related to this inducement is the frequent misinterpretation or misuse of the concept of acceptance. The implementation of acceptance means recognizing, supporting, or reinforcing the presented ways of the child. Strongly isolated children may be offended by direct affectional displays. Motor-oriented children may view puzzles or verbally oriented games as demonstrations of the clinician's failure to comprehend him or appreciate his messages. Reflective approaches may be much more inviting of change than demonstrations of therapeutic initiative by the clinician. Many adults are so strongly intent on change with respect to the child that the initial establishment of conditions which might lead to change are omitted. Initiation of change is often undertaken by the clinician in the guise of "rapport." Good rapport may be highly inviting of arousal and initiative on the part of the child, but it involves initial acceptance of the child's ways, not initiation of change which originates in the notions of the therapist. Examination of the history of the relationship between the therapist and the child will often reveal the fact that the child is not at all indifferent (or whatever may be his message), but simply waiting in perhaps a dependent way for the therapist to initiate the activity. The child may also be attempting to tell the therapist that his (the clinician's) responses do not relate well to the child's messages. A therapeutic behavior which seems to be change-inducing follows something of this course. Identification of the indifference or whatever the message form might be must be made. The therapist speaks of his awareness of the probable importance of that particular behavior to the child. Or he may speak of the child's need for the behavior. Or he may comment on the fact that his behavior is perhaps the only way the child knows of telling an adult about how he feels or what he needs. It is experientially clear that if the therapist successfully gives evidence of the fact that the child does not need to use his typical or immature adjustment techniques, then the child may find his devices to be of less value and may tend to seek their abandonment. In short, here is the purpose of learning to accept the form of the message and learning to speak to the needs which subserve it. Inducing change or creating the conditions in which change might be initiated frequently serves as a precipitant for anxiety expressions. As quickly as such messages appear it is therapeutically critical for the therapist to be supportive, open, and responsive to this changing behavior. Regardless of form or origin, arousal states should be regarded as evidence of change or readiness for change. This concept is axiomatic whether the condition appears in the child or in the therapist. In other words, elevated states literally signal the presence of available energy. The task of the therapist is to give sufficient significance to the heightened state so that its basic source, whether that be a deficient need or inhibited potential, may be expressed. If the therapist uses the attitude that inhibited growth potentials are signaled by this condition then the value of recognizing the signal becomes obvious. Although speaking of infants, Bettleheim's (1967) comments are directly applicable here. He stated, in essence, that when the adult's response to the child is positive, he (the child) may learn that reaching out not only increases his well-being but that it is his own actions that prompted the adult action. Here the value of combined effort is clearly observed. One can visualize the ease with which that potential for change may be again obscured or compromised if the child's anxiety signals are viewed with alarm or treated only as behaviors to be palliated. It is possible, and therapeutically profitable, to be selectively supportive of the child's change signs as a means of inviting the appearance of their sources. Perhaps no other circumstance will be as acutely meaningful to the child as this one. Here he begins to learn that he and another person may be able to do something together that the child was not able to accomplish by himself. He begins to perceive that it is effort—and particularly interrelated and reciprocal effort—that brings about satisfying changes or results in his actually coming to possess more of what he needs. Few circumstances may be as valuable in terms of the child learning about the significance of his impact on others, and, consequently, learning about the significance of himself. Acceptance of (not necessarily reward for) the child's ways of being or his ways of telling others of his being is a basic therapeutic mode. It is clearly an invitation and an inducement to change. Indeed, it may be viewed as a powerful stimulus or a loving and concerned response.

Determinants of the Therapeutic Response

Language is both actuating and integrating in the development and maintenance of social structure. It may be regarded as both germinal and implemental in child development. Child therapy processes require the examination and use of communicative structure in all forms and are not limited to the study of verbal forms alone. An embracing term as used here, language includes expressive forms, meaning (both content and intent), and those many dimensions which constitute the matrix of human feeling and need. Language, then, is the dynamic interface between therapist and child. It is both abstract and concrete; often multidimensional in expression and purpose; assumes verbal or nonverbal forms; and may be explicit or implicit in the communicative context. It is revealing with respect to both formal information and dynamic intention. It is revealing of the person. Furthermore, the clinician must be aware of the impact of his response which, in expression, now becomes a stimulus as far as the child's perceptions are concerned. The clinician's response will not only identify the clinician to the child, but will give motivation, reinforcement, and direction to the child's behavior. Staats (1968) offers some particularly helpful discussion here. He describes some prominent links between motivation and reinforcement. Among them the statement that "many motivational stimuli have their effect before they are applied. That is, they elicit striving behaviors . . . a reinforcing stimulus has its effect when it is applied following behavior." It is apparent by examination of these comments that the therapist is in a situation where he must constantly certify and anticipate the possible effects of his responses. The importance of the adult's response is all the more apparent in further remarks by Staats. "It must be concluded that the organism (child) is never responsible for his behavior. He behaves in accordance with lawful principles. It is the nature of his experiences and the nature of the situation that determine what his behavior will be." The most obvious question is one that asks who is responsible for the experiences and the situations that are provided for the child. Much information is available concerning possible meanings to be ascribed to the child's communicative efforts. Comparatively little discussion is offered appropriate to various purposes and forms of the therapist's communication. Certainly one may discuss matters of interpretation, symbolic inference, response to resistance, and semantic nuance. These are indeed important dimensions of therapeutic interaction and warrant careful study with respect to practical application. In therapeutic communication, however, factors which are more parametric need to be identified and given implementation. Such factors should serve as determinants for selection of the therapist's responses. These factors are empirically derived.

1. The clinician's language should address itself, at appropriate times, to those elements of the child's communication that are beyond (actually "in addition to," of course) the explicit and informational data that are directly observable. The excellent text by Klein (1960) makes the function of this interpretative concept operationally clear. These subsurface elements may be called behavioral or attitudinal determinants and are conveniently described within the general context of needs. This kind of communicative activity provides the clinician with an opportunity to relate to the matrix of the child's ongoingness and reduces the possibility of mechanization of language responses.

2. Where the clinician's language responses are selected in terms of the child's needs, acceptance of that child is as clearly stated as can be conceived. Operationally, this prompts a variety of responses from the therapist, each presumably appropriate to the child's learning or useful in specifying behavioral directions. High chronicity in the themes of the therapist's responses usually implies stereotyped efforts or suggests that the therapist is speaking primarily of his own issues. Communicative behaviors which speak immediately to the child as he is, speak, at least implicitly, of acceptance. Clinically, one can observe an interesting paradox. Where therapists give explicit indication of that which should be changed, the defensiveness of the child is often increased. Perhaps he has interpreted the therapist's urging as criticism or implied threat. When the child feels accepted as he is, his need to be defensive apparently lessens and his readiness for change is increased by his own initiative. This writer believes that children are persistently potentiated as far as change is concerned and that lessening their defensive investment will allow the potentiated energy to become more activate. The forthcoming change attempts may not be readily seen but careful patience will typically produce them.

3. It is interesting to note the frequency with which candid communication is a recommended patient achievement. Seldom does the literature speak of the same behavior on the part of the clinician. True, the clinician must examine his anticipated expressions with respect to their intent and their function with respect to the needs of the child. Beyond this, however, is another concept. Our child is to learn that the expression of his needs is a normal act. These expressions may assume many forms embracing a wide spectrum of maturity levels. He must not work with a therapist whose communicative efforts include such expectations with respect to the child's performance but contain denial or inhibition with respect to the openness of the clinician's behaviors. This child therapy approach urges the expression of feelings or attitudes or the execution of behaviors that are candidly honest as long as the therapist can communicate them within the structure of the child's needs or the child's tolerance. Thus, the child may observe that many feelings, attitudes, or behaviors are normal and that their use is acceptable. The approach described here urges that the therapist speak of his feelings and needs in concert with those which are expressed by the child or expected of him. This therapeutic act must be executed with great care since it requires high selectivity of response. One must guard against the promotion of inappropriate disinhibition; exert care relative to reinforcement of the child's current communicative status; and choose discriminatively with respect to those expressions of the child which are to be given specific encouragement.

4. Most children are subject to some perceptual and cognitive (perhaps the term should be conative) error. This tendency for misperception is probably increased in those arousal states which require regressive adjustments. It is also higher when the child's defensive operations are excessive. The clinician must provide safeguards which might minimize

this kind of error-making particularly as it relates to the child's comprehension of his therapist. One useful measure in this respect can be found in the clinician's willingness to clarify his feelings or anticipated behaviors for the child. This is particularly important when the clinician experiences obvious ambivalence, anxiety, or conflict within his own feelings. Here he must speak of the presence of contradiction, giving voice to as much of its content as is feasible in his clinical judgment. Observation indicates that excessive confusion on the child's part about the feelings or intentions of the therapist has at least two effects. It tends to reactivate previously learned adjustments and it fragments therapeutic interaction. Imminent change trends are thus weakened and often reversed. Siegel (1967) describes an institutional situation where the adults' responses to children appeared to function as dependent variables. It was clear in his study that adult verbal responses were higher with children who themselves were more verbal. Of further interest was the finding that children with low verbal output produced more vocalization during unstructured situations. It is true that there are differences among children with respect to their general activity or energy level. Escalona (1968) makes comments pertinent to several aspects of this discussion. To summarize: inactive babies need more direct response from adults than active ones but, unfortunately, they seem to get less attention because they do not compel it. Further, early ego devlopments are best anticipated during recurring states of arousal of varying intensity, including periods of moderate intensity. Finally, development is implemented when the small child has repeated experiences in which he can effect change and overcome obstacles, this being the foundation for his awareness of reality independent of himself. He must experience, Escalona continues, the fact that his known actions are causal with respect to changes in the environment and changes within himself. It is clear from these remarks that the therapist must consider his responses in the light of the behavior of the child and in terms of the child's centrality in the therapeutic environment. The subtleties of response determination are indeed intricate. The therapeutic purpose is to bring the participants into a position of reciprocal and mutual exchange. The interface between these people must contain as little inappropriate defensiveness as possible. Many therapeutic situations are not reciprocal but characterized by one-way influence attempts. Child therapy concepts do not encourage this over-determined exchange. The language of the clinician then addresses itself to openness, to reciprocal influence attempts, and to an enhancement of the child's accurate understanding of the adult as well as of himself.

5. The needs of the clinician are of equal significance in the therapeutic arrangement. By virtue of his dependency, the child may anticipate being helped with his needs. The therapist is not afforded this opportunity but is required to deal with them on a self-sufficient basis. Candid communication, even here, is a desirable goal. Practically speaking, this means that the therapist must be sufficiently revealing of his needs and particularly of his feelings so that the child is secure with that knowledge and aware of the intent of the therapist's expressions. It would be wise to state at this point, however, that many of the clinician's needs may be satisfied in healthy ways in the execution of his therapeutic task.

Implementation of Therapeutic Response

In the paragraphs just completed, various factors which might act as determinants of the therapeutic response were discussed. Implementation of those factors can be carried out by observing the following precautions:

1. The role of the therapist is predominantly that of a respondent. This requires that the therapist follow the child's expressions with his comments. Wherever the child gives his emphasized attention, and particularly where this represents a point of change in his ongoing behavior, the therapist should consider providing a carefully selected reaction. Therapeutically, one is to watch for those behaviors which represent growth-oriented change and recognize that it is at this point that the response of the therapist is the most helpful.

2. Maintain comments on a noninstructional basis except upon specific request by the child. For the most part, avoid the classical teacher-student relationship in which the teacher is the initiator of most acts and the child becomes primarily a respondent. On occasion, such an instructional arrangement is useful. Caution is advised, however, since many of these teaching relationships seem to increase the child's dependency at least in the therapeutic effort that is being described.

3. Whenever possible, respond to observable behaviors. The child can ordinarily see the direct connection between the therapist's comments and such

behavior. In other words, the child can relate to these experiences more easily and with less defensiveness. This does not contradict the use of interpretation, nor does it restrict talking to things which are beyond immediate observation, but therapists are too often inclined to overlook obvious signals in their search for deeper meaning.

4. When the child is involved in a nonverbal act, stay with him both physically and verbally and regard that behavior as a message. If this is the communicative act the child chooses, then respond to it. The therapist may gently name the behavior. He may comment on its importance to the child or he may relate the behavior to some difficulty the child is having in attempting something new. Direct support or encouragement should be offered predominantly when the child is in a tentative effort position. Offers of specific reinforcement or strong positive responses are appropriate when new behaviors appear and their continuation is desirable. This reinforcing effort should be used with particular specificity when these new expressions are above the child's customary age level performance.

5. The language of the therapist may be used to represent all events or objects in the environment. This usage, of course, is determined by the child's attempts at exploring and relating. It is common to find that therapists are intent upon the promotion of a particular activity and fail to pursue the child's directions. This is done despite clinical observations which suggest that developmental speech seems to originate in the child's needs and not so significantly in his role as a respondent. If the clinician names objects or events or uses a qualifying term it must be offered in response to the child's interests and thus linked with the child's needs.

6. The therapist is advised to avoid the use of contingency, accusative, or critical comments. Rachman (1962) makes the point that undesirable behaviors are more likely to be eliminated if met with no response at all than if met with negative or punishing reaction. Although an obvious and common notion in child therapy approaches, the evaluation of such comments is typically made from an adult view and does not necessarily stem from an appreciation of the child's perception. The attempt to redirect the child's attention or the offering of substitute or avoidance activities is a common limit-setting or anxiety-management technique. The clinician is advised, however, to avoid these approaches if possible and direct his communication toward an understanding of the child's intent and inviting an expression of the issue or impulse which subserves it.

7. When certain of the child's behaviors must be limited the language content needs to be especially clear. Here the clinician must deliver an apparently contradictory message. Part of his expression is directed toward the child's act and is clearly intended to be intervening. The other part of the message places significance and respect on the child's need to behave in that particular way. It becomes possible then to communicate to the child the true extent of the therapist's capacity for being supportive and caring.

8. In those language structures where verbal forms are used, it is advisable to use a high ratio of open-ended questions or simple comments in phrase form. Avoidance of any persistent use of direct inquiry or closed-ended questions is suggested. Children often seem to view such questions as demands or implied criticisms. At best, such a question is limiting with respect to self-determination and certainly requires the child to function in a designated role.

9. Caution must be exerted in the use of assumption statements. These are many times offered in the guise of "interpretations." Too often these are not conceptualizations of data derived from the child, but represent only preconceptions about techniques or are projections of personal issues stemming from the therapist himself. Whether or not the assumption is true, it is not difficult for the child to conclude that the adult can indeed read his mind or at least is attempting to do so. Such assumption also risks increased confusion on the child part, particularly when he can see no tie between his behavior or attitude and the response of the therapist. Such act, then, risk increasing the child's defensiveness rather than reducing it.

10. The verbal activity of the therapist may contribute to fragmentation of the child's attempts at experimentation. This usually occurs when the therapist has assumed the role of subject or initiator and his role-playing represents his uncertainty or insecurity. Many people are inclined to respond to every detail of the child's activity. This undoubtedly dilutes the value or impact of the therapist's responses and in many instances promotes persistent interruption of the child's efforts. While this pedantic behavior may be a popular way for clinicians to maintain their own defensive structure, the act does not function on behalf of the child's needs.

11. The therapist is advised against any direct

palliation of the child's anxiety. As noted previously, anxiety frequently acts as a precursor of attempts at new behaviors or of previously unexpressed aims. Care must also be exerted with respect to the value attributed to the arousal signs. Often, the initial period of anxiety is one of patient waiting and cautious supportive comments as far as the therapist's behaviors are concerned. Specific reward, interpretative remarks, or other reinforcing acts are better employed as responses to growth efforts which appear than as responses to the preliminary signals. The child's arousal frequently exceeds his own adjustment tolerance and results in regressive trends. When these trends assume a release form, controls provided by the therapist are useful and needed. This process of using limits for the child's behavior is another aspect of the therapeutic use of arousal states. The verbal efforts of the therapist, then, must not contain words aimed at diminishing anxiety or discrediting its value; should not attach excess value to the state itself; and may be used to establish controls (within the child) which may promote a more discriminative or purposeful use of the energy involved.

Forms of Therapeutic Response

Specific therapeutic responses take many forms. The selection of an appropriate verbal response is certainly as crucial a decision as its execution. The act of response selection is accomplished by a dual effort on the clinician's part. He must attempt to comprehend the needs, expectations, or intentions indicated by the child. Simultaneously, he must confront himself with what is often a perplexing decision. He must decide on the kind and degree of involvement, commitment, or responsibility to be revealed by his response. Too often does the clinician's response seem to convey a willingness "to take care of things." In many instances the therapeutic relationship simply becomes a situation in which an adult makes most of the decisions, assumes all the responsibility, and fails to accord the child adequate recognition in so doing. This decision is considered to be of vital importance in therapeutic negotiations since it is fundamental to the establishment of an appropriate role for the child. Another problem of importance in working with speech- or language-handicapped children is that of coping with fragmentation. The child's communicative efforts, by definition of pathology, will be fractionated in some fashion. The therapist's response, wherever possible, must not be. In many instances, the clinician's response is a carefully selected completion or complement of the child's message. In other instances, the response amounts to helping the child complete his expression or perhaps give voice to things he has never spoken. Many therapist responses are designed to provide verbal equivalency for certain of the child's behaviors which are communicated in some other form. Some therapist response forms which occur with greatest frequency will now be identified and discussed.

1. The therapist is often called upon to give information responses. These are used where instruction is not the intent. These responses are often requested by the child when he contemplates self-instruction. Children's inquiries often represent interest in phenomena of many kinds. They seek information about objects, events, and themselves or other people. Such seeking is typically representative of moderate arousal and appropriate responses are, therefore, security-giving for the child and reinforcing for his seeking of information. In other instances such requests by the child provide a basis for a testing of the therapist. This testing is usually an act designed by the child to evaluate the therapist with respect to readiness for response and accuracy of response. Most children are sincerely concerned about the clinician's attentiveness with respect to the child's needs. Information is often sought by the child for orienting purposes. He may ask about distances, time, size, color, quality, height, length, the nature of objects, etc. The establishment of self-orientation relative to the factor is the child's usual purpose here.

2. Many responses seem to take an instructional form. These are used primarily to supplement some problem-solving effort demonstrated by the child. Such a response may take an explanatory form aimed at helping the child achieve closure in his comprehension or in improving some motor act. Such responses are probably most effective at the point of demonstrated child readiness. Clinically, one will also note its value in communicating to the child the clinician's interest in growth or new learning. On occasion one will use it as part of a limit-setting act. Instructional responses are often revealing with respect to the therapist's feeling or intentions. Instructions function for purposes of clarification, in many instances. These responses appear to have greatest value when given at the request of the child and if used to supplement some achievement effort which is already activated. In deciding to employ instructional responses the

therapist should be cautioned with respect to responsibility matters. Such responses probably have the effect of maximizing the clinician's responsibility for whatever is achieved or learned. It is not difficult, moreover, to visualize the growth risk involved in reinforcement of the child's dependency position or his role as object in the relationship. These possibilities appear to be lessened when instructional activities are used in association with existing child effort or in response to the child's request.

3. Responses in the form of reflection are employed primarily to illuminate or to give verbal equivalency to the child's behaviors or attitudes. As such, they are particularly useful where the clinician wants to increase the child's awareness of others having received his messages. Identification for the child of the intent portions of his messages appears to be another property of this response form. It seems to be a useful way of telling the child about the nature of the clinician's attention and concentrated interest. It is almost child-identifying particularly with respect to the ongoingness of his communicative efforts. This response is essentially neutral in character. It provides the child with recognition for his efforts without any attempt at interpretation or instruction.

4. Supportive responses are helpful and growth-promoting if used with appropriate discrimination. This response is clearly one which implies a sharing of responsibility. It is useful in giving cautious direction to the child's efforts. Approval-giving and encouraging with respect to its intent, it is particularly useful when new behaviors are tentative. It may be used cautiously to help maintain arousal states where some anxiety is present. Frequently, one may wish to use an intervening effort but wishes to do so with high caution. The selective linking of a supportive statement with a particular behavioral sign may be one of the most subtle approaches available. Supportive statements are essentially reinforcing measures. They appear to bridge the gap between the child's satisfactions being heavily determined by or dependent upon the other person's acts on one hand and the acquisition of self-satisfying achievements on the other. The latter position is not meant to imply neurotic achievements but those which are growth-oriented. Supportive measures, therefore, seem to be particularly useful in the implementation and, to some extent, the maintaining, of behavioral change. A greater amount of separation of child and therapist is involved in the use of this response and thus one sees the development of shared responsibility as a greater possibility than when instructional responses are used.

5. Therapeutic effort often requires the eliciting of additional data. This requires a probing or searching activity and may be known by the word "inquiring." The inquiry technique is implemented by the judicious use of questions or comments. These verbal forms should be open-ended and pertinent to immediately apparent issues whenever possible. This response form is one which seems to place more responsibility on the patient than any previously described approach. It may be used as an intervention device and where employed correctly often produces not only elevated anxiety but resolution of conflict or changes in the child's efforts. The clinician may come to regard this form as an urging but patient method for inducing or initiating effort on the child's part. It may be particularly useful in facilitating further resolution or clarity in the child's messages. This response approach is specifying with respect to conflict issues and with respect to the child's opportunities for and attitudes toward self-determination.

6. Interpretation is a response form designed to give meaning to behaviors or attitudes. It is a cautious accounting process used typically to identify sources for or purposes of various child communicative attempts. Whether offered in response to abstract messages or concrete behaviors, it must be a conclusion derived from repeated observation. To be drawn from a single message or one sign would require high validity in that source. This is essentially an inductive process. While probably used with least frequency of the various forms being discussed, it has the faculty for evoking maximal arousal. When properly or accurately employed, one may anticipate increased illumination of defensive operations or positive changes in expression and affective discharge. It may be aimed at the defense, at that information which is defended or at the link between the two. This response produces increased separation between the communicating agents since it implies responsibility or self-management, and accountability or being answerable to others for both parties. Interpreting comments are to be used judiciously and parsimoniously since they represent significant factors in child growth and in maintenance of therapeutic interaction. This response, when appropriately used, is most pertinent to the naming of the child's need or to a heightened awareness of the intent portion of his communicative efforts.

7. Declarative responses are used most specifically

for the direct expression of affect or for a clear expression of opinion. This kind of verbal operation must contain maximum congruence between the formal content and the affectional components of the message. Such a response may be used as a special kind of supportive or reinforcing statement. It is intended to reveal the therapist's attitudes unequivocally. It may be used in limit-setting operations particularly where emergency action is needed. It appears to have a high impact or influence value when properly timed. This message form undoubtedly contains some risk of misperception by the child, thus its requirement for maximum internal congruence. It is designed to give clear evidence of the clinician's position relative to a given act, achievement, or attitude demonstrated by the child.

The child's behaviors or attitudes, whether verbal or more concrete, or viewed as either symbolic or patently and primitively clear, must be regarded as messages. The therapist is to note those messages with greater prominence or those with greater change potential. His therapeutic task is to identify the message, accept it or the need for it, and answer it. He is to be selective in his decision to respond as well as selective with respect to type of response. The response should be simple, brief, and, wherever possible, linked with observable feelings, behaviors, or identifiable attitudes. Recognition of needs or purposes is dependent on the therapist's perceptiveness with respect to signs. A wide spectrum of sign-clusters will be offered by the child in the course of his communicative efforts. Many messages or signs will be age-related and identifiable on that basis. Major developmental levels have ego-defense signs, ego-achievement properties, conflict signs, and normal developmental characteristics which are unique to each level. Needs for security, belonging, identity, self-determination, self-preservation and the like are represented by expressions which tend to be unique and are thus self-naming. Needs for physiological or anatomical compensation assume many expressive forms—some specific to the pathology inferred and others more complex in their associative mazes and consequent expressive forms. These signs may take any variety of appearance, both release and deficit, symbolic and concrete, and directly appealing or concealed in inferences of perplexing subtlety. The speech clinician finds himself confronted with an abundance of communicative data. Knowing what is being imparted, selecting those messages to which he wishes to respond, and conceiving the response itself are tasks of considerable importance and complexity. The therapist's willingness to offer carefully selected responses indicates to the child the fact that he is important, that his behaviors have impact, and that self-determined intent will be respected.

Many behaviors which appear to be incidental or unimportant to the adult in his own behavior are high in the child's perceptual priority. Such messages, which may operate as incidental behaviors, appear predominantly as intent and consequently enjoy little recognition by the speaker. Apparently, however, many children are concerned about this aspect of the communicative act and tend to respond negatively in too many instances. Anxiety aroused under these conditions is difficult to manage and is often misunderstood as to source. Such message-sending by the therapist occurs of course when his efforts are not child-centered or are not carefully enough conceived. Given child-centered attitudes, one would expect some misperception by the child, but its occurrence can at least be reduced. Instances of this kind of communicative activity may be seen in most therapeutic settings. For example, the therapist and a parent may discuss the child in the reception area while the child waits—and perhaps wonders about the decisions that are being reached by these adults or about the behaviors that the adults are evaluating. Or a therapist may allow the parent to convince the child to demonstrate some newly acquired skill. In another instance, the therapist may decide to carry on a conversation with another staff member on the way to the therapeutic area while the child is in his company. In some situations appointments are too often initiated on a late schedule. In another instance, the therapist promises to remember something for the child until their next meeting but fails to do so. The therapist may be warm and affectionate in one meeting and remote at the next. After being child-centered for a period of time, the therapist decides to change his approach and begins to direct the activity. In all of these instances just named, one may risk a fragmenting or violation of the basic therapeutic relationship. These are behaviors which can be directly identified and for the most part avoided. When avoidance is not feasible then the intent of the act or the mood must be clarified for the child as quickly as the therapist recognizes it. The above occurrences are used only as examples. The number and kind of incidental messages would, of course, be infinite. The deepest understanding of the child and one of the most significant communicative opportunities occurs when the therapist is able to replicate knowingly within himself the child's essential ways of being or of revealing that being. Duplication of verbal expression is relatively simple compared to the requirements for replication of the child's total communicative effort. This is a requirement, however, if the therapist is to treat the whole child. Although carried out automatically in many communicative attempts, the therapist can become a participant in the child's world in a more volitional way than he is customarily inclined to do. To accomplish this, the therapist is required to perceive the child's observed behavior and attitudes as completely as possible. He is to duplicate those messages within himself as purposefully and completely as he is able. Finally, he must carry out a careful introspection. If this replication effort has been at all successful, he has now acquired first-hand knowledge of the child's needs and communicative efforts. In execution, this is perhaps only a momentary act. With practice it yields clearly helpful information. This act is apparently a conscious replica of a portion of the normal communicative act, much of which is carried on automatically. Executed with strong conscious awareness, the therapist has now an opportunity to enter into the world of the child's needs and the child's perceptions. To communicate with the world as the child attempts to do it provides one with a substantial source of new information. Of greater importance, perhaps, is the implementation given to the maintenance of a child-centered relationship. It is interesting to note the frequency with which clinicians give priority to their intentions or techniques and unknowingly allow the child to become subordinate. An important therapeutic language aspect, then, is contained in the ability to communicate within the dimensions of the child's efforts.

Experience Transfer

Although demonstrating general behavior changes or specific speech and language improvements in the clinic setting, children often restrict any wider use of such achievements. The application of these newly learned experiences to the broader aspects of his general life is an issue of considerable importance. Most of the studies which have investigated transfer, or more specifically, transfer application, have addressed themselves to single response learning. These studies, although numerous, are not conclusive, and their results present additional difficulty when studied in dynamic or global behavioral terms. In summarizing the issue of transfer specifically, Brookshire (1967) offers a helpful statement. ". . . if the reinforcing stimulus is not also active in the client's environment, then the reinforcing stimulus will eventually have to be changed to one that is present in the non-clinic environment." Of course, this comment by Brookshire could be extended conversely. One of the purposes of parent counseling, for example, is to place reinforcing stimuli in the nonclinic environment that have been successfully used in the therapeutic relationship. Actually any discussion of transfer is strongly empirical or must be drawn from inference. Earlier periods of therapy may be change-inducing if they are as unlike the other aspects of the child's life as possible. This condition seems to reduce the use or effectiveness of previously learned behaviors or attitudes in the therapeutic situation. It is not uncommon, incidentally, to find that the early hours of the therapeutic relationship produce considerable change in some aspect or another. The care with which therapeutic responses are selected together with the newness of the setting and its people may all contribute to a reduction in the speed or effectiveness of such adaptation. The maximizing of differences between the child's general life and his "clinic life" may simply imply that the child finds less use for previously learned adjustments and is thereby prompted to the seeking of other behaviors. This concept appears to be particularly important for children who are pervasively immature or those whose potentiality for immediate change appears to be limited.

Once specifically desired changes begin to appear it would seem appropriate for the child to exercise those new behaviors in the presence of people from his nonclinic environment. Were he to find such behaviors accepted and rewarded by these people one might anticipate some increase in his tendency to employ those behaviors beyond the specific therapeutic setting. The clinician might therefore want to increase the similarity between the home situation and the therapeutic environment. This could involve the use of the home area as a therapeutic setting. The work of Sommers (1964) could be interpreted as a meaningful effort at transfer and stimulus generalization and could be pursued with potential profit from such a point of view. Transfer may involve sufficient parental participation so that home attitudes or everyone's communicative efforts will assume useful changes. Generalization of newly acquired behaviors may also be encouraged if the child can experience the use of his behaviors with peers. Although anxiety-producing in some instances and questionable in others, the inviting of a playmate to the clinic can have strong positive effects if timed properly. Facilitation of the spread of the child's new behaviors may also be improved by the use of more than one therapist or through involvement of the child client in groups of changing composition. It would seem unwise, once changes have been generated and the direction identified as growth-oriented, to restrict therapeutic activity to a particular place, time, or person.

The clinician involved in this kind of therapeutic approach is well advised to take particular note of the conditions in which desired changes occur. This information may facilitate both parent education and therapeutic planning. Certainly parental acceptance and systematic positive response to new behaviors would seem to carry promise for effecting application of learning. It is also important to note that one may seek transfer applications for specific and finite changes or for implementing the general notion of change. Perhaps one of the difficulties with carryover facilitation has been its high and typical emphasis on the functioning of specific acts or the demonstration of highly specialized skills. Careful encouragement of general change efforts used as a context for the wider application of specific skills would be a more effective approach.

Perhaps many classical therapeutic arrangements are responsible for minimizing transfer applications. Such arrangements simply do not provide for sufficient and widespread use of the new learning under conditions that will specify its value and encourage its being linked with a sufficiently large number of general experiences. Involve peers and family members as systematically and consistently as possible. Produce changes in the therapeutic place in the numbers and variety of people who are involved in those places. When the child begins to demonstrate behaviors or express attitudes that warrant application to his general life, then a critical therapeutic task is to extend the exercise of those behaviors into as many life-experience dimensions as possible. Of equal importance is the therapist's monitoring of those experiences to insure that such behaviors are indeed used and that such use finds acceptance and satisfaction. Goldstein's (1966) discussions are particularly pertinent here and should be thoroughly explored.

The child's awareness with respect to what is being sought, facilitated, or rewarded is a closely correlated problem. The general communicative approach used in child therapy calls for open, candid, and respectfully cautious behavior on the clinician's part. If the child wants to know why he is in this particular setting, he should be told. When he inquires as to the presence of his parents or about his meeting with a new group, he should be answered. Some children rarely inquire and in those instances, the therapist may find it motivating for the child to initiate that inquiry. This is particularly useful if the inquiry can be timed to coincide with changes which the child has already initiated. An increased awareness of the communicative issue or symptom may be productive of some stress for the child but, if that can be tolerated by him, the condition will simply be a motivating one. If increased awareness is desirable, and of course this is a matter of clinical judgment, and the therapist attempts to induce it, that effort should occur as the whole child becomes increasingly change-oriented. It is not uncommon to find that a child will simply develop improved verbal communication incidental to the rest of his maturing. Interestingly enough, transfer applications are less troublesome here. It may be, after all, that speech and language functions are indeed service operations and are better acquired (or reacquired) in association with or even subordinate to other properties or developmental functions of the organism. In order to treat his verbal difficulties the clinician may find himself confronted with the basic needs or purposes of the child. Therapeutic parameters may be defined along lines which include many factors other than verbal function. The speech clinician may find difficulty in deciding whether to address his attention to the specific dimensions of verbal communication or to the attitudinal and behavioral factors with which they may be linked. Both approaches are possible.

Ego Controls and Limits

Although obviously used for safety purposes and certainly prophylactic with respect to the child's reality orientation, the use of limits is not ordinarily viewed as a therapeutic device. In the course of normal growth, children acquire various and effective systems of impulse control. Identifying the boundaries between one's self and others is an important part of reality testing. Not only does the child find it important to learn the values of self-determined action, but he must also come to appreciate the values of identifying the point of tangency between his behavior and rights and the provinces and rights of others. The orientation of himself in his world is given substantial implementation as he discovers ways to satisfy his own needs while being cognizant of and concerned about the needs of others. The use of limits in the therapeutic setting provides the child with guidelines for discovering and constantly evaluating boundaries within which he can learn to function with security, self-approval, and sufficient satisfaction. The appropriate employment of limits also provides the child with directions and channels for the release of the energy that has been aroused in the course of therapeutic confrontation. The implementation of limits, then, is twofold. It protects the child from ego-insult and it provides him with a consistent framework of responses from the environment which will further his self-orienting efforts and will facilitate the selection of appropriate behaviors in negotiations with others.

Limit-setting must observe specific aims. The child's need to behave in a particular way must be given recognition and respect while the behavior itself is limited or actually prevented. If the feelings of the therapist are involved, he is to take responsibility for those emotions without any inference that the child is causative thereto. The setting of a limit is often a declarative act. It is best characterized by clarity, simplicity, and firmness. At this point negotiations, contingencies, and conditions must be specifically avoided. One may be tempted to offer redirection or displacement opportunities for the child. This is usually unwise and customarily not indicated. In other instances silence or lack of response by the therapist proves to be a sufficient limit-setting technique. At the point where the use of limits is required, the child's energy level (motivation or arousal) is typically high. The limiting of its expression in one direction will typically find that energy producing behavioral excursions in other directions. It is of more than passing interest to note that increases in verbal activity are often noted when limits have been imposed on behaviors that were primarily motoric and aggressive in nature. The therapeutic use of limits, then, does involve safety for other people as well as the child, protection of property, preservation of the relationship perhaps, and possible maintenance of social relationships for the child with respect to the group. Of greater importance, however, is the opportunity for ego growth provided for the child. The purpose here is not to limit the child's self-determination but to give it direction and clear purpose. Delay of impulse may originate in the environment as well as in the child. Delay of impulse provides the child with greater opportunity to review alternate plans of action and select one that will be self-satisfying and simultaneously compatible with reality. The critical point is that the child makes the decision. The limit imposed by the therapist simply facilitates that process.

Responses to Conflict

Conflict-oriented behaviors are often seen in intense forms. Pervasive anxiety is the most striking sign, although simple indecision may be indicative of the same phenomenon. This behavior is typically representative of the presence of opposing needs or forces. This kind of demonstration seems to occur with great frequency during initial therapeutic hours. It is felt that such signs may occur early in the relationship because of lack of available adjustments in the new setting, or as an indication of the child's readiness for change. Certainly this is a time when the child is strongly inclined toward shift in behavioral effort. Conflict issues are characteristically impulse-laden on one hand and counterweighted by inhibitory trends on the other. The child's need to express that which is inhibited is often signaled by the appearance of anxiety. The therapeutic task is to view that anxiety as an expression of the child's need for change. This means that the arousal signs are valuable even though they appear in conflict form. They warrant careful consideration and are often worthy of encouragement or supportive response. The therapist is advised to speak to the impulse aspect where possible. Sometimes the impulse is apparent and can be directly labeled. In other instances, some kind of impulse is present but its nature is not apparent. Here recognition, however nonspecific, is still of value. The impulse component is frequently found in that portion of the child's communicative effort which assumes nonverbal forms. While this impulse is not always growth-oriented in aim it must be respected as revealing of the point where the child is growth-inhibited. The weakening of inhibition is often a suitable consequence even though the behaviors which appear are considerably immature. This point, then, at which conflict appears, is a precise invitation for therapeutic intervention. Conflict conditions represent one of the crossroads at which the child is the most vulnerable to specific responses by the therapist.

Regressive behaviors may be anticipated particularly where conflict is strong and expression is difficult. Regression signs need not be viewed as indications of therapeutic failure, nor are they necessarily indicative of further pathology. It is far more probable that such trends occur as the consequences of anxiety that is somewhat overwhelming. Incidents of this kind are typically transient. What is often visualized as regression is likely to be part of the process of undoing or unlearning of certain inhibitory behaviors or attitudes. The actions which ensue simply give evidence of the age-origin of the acquired inhibition. In these instances the child has found it important and possible to weaken his historical compromise. While such trends are regressive momentarily, the clinician should view them as important and required parts of the child's long-range growth efforts. Acceptance of the intent of the regression is important even though its expressive forms may sometimes require limitation and its content an interpretative response. The therapist should make no issue over the regression sign. He is not to give such eager responsiveness to it that it begins to assume unique or inappropriate values of its own. The general axiom is still to be observed. If the child's behaviors are given patient but clear acceptance, at least in terms of need or purpose, his tendency toward behavioral elaboration is frequently implemented. Regression trends also represent valuable points for an intervening response. Behavioral signs which accompany the regressive mode provide particular illumination for the therapist's response selection.

Therapist Self-Management

The general axiom here speaks for open and candid therapist communication or interaction as long as it can be implemented within the structure of the child's needs. The course of action is clear assuming the previous statement to be possible. The therapist is to speak his feelings as long as he is capable of assuming responsibility for their origin. He must also be able to certify that the strength of the expression will not be overwhelming for the child. Observation reveals that for a therapist to be genuinely caring about the child is of importance in the development of that child. It is expected that the therapist will experience normal feelings of warmth, affection, perplexity, anger, or disappointment. If these feelings are offered to the child in genuine and concerned ways they may constitute a kind of teaching where the child is still subject but increasingly aware of the impact and significance of his own feelings and behaviors.

Clinicians frequently discuss the advisability of physical contact with children. The answer to the question appears to be uncomplicated. If the contact represents the affection needs or the anger needs of the therapist then physical contact is contra-indicated. Of course, if this is the situation then the therapeutic effort generally is going to contain questionable values for the child. In many instances, however, reassurance, warmth, and affection for the child can be substantially implemented by some physical contact. These are principally supportive measures. As with all other responses, this one needs to be selected judiciously and used parsimoniously. If used capriciously for the therapist's purposes these responses can prove to be highly fixating for the therapeutic effort and therefore for the child's growth. Setting and maintaining behavioral limits often requires the use of physical contact in the form of restraints. This kind of message can be clear and helpful if the clinician's intent is communicated adequately. If the therapist must prevent the child from striking another child or getting involved in some act that exceeds safety limits, his manner of restraining the child can say clearly, "even here my concern is for your feelings and your needs." The use of physical contact may be helpful in coping with those anxiety situations where the arousal is overwhelming or threatens to traumatize the relationship. Many children may have specific fears attached to certain objects or experiences. The use of mild palliative measures of a physical sort may be supportive here. In addition to being supportive, physical reassurance may be used to separate such fears from the experience or object to which they have been attached. This is a sort of conditioning process and may be helpful if used selectively. Its employment will be particularly pertinent if enlisted at the point at which the child is actually attempting to overcome a specific fear.

Self-management for the therapist also involves some problems relative to self-motivation. For a clinician to be highly interested in the child at the outset of the relationship and then experience some reduction in interest as the interaction proceeds is commonly observed and probably understandable. Just as the child is highly subject to new adaptive efforts at the outset of the relationship, so is the therapist. As these two people carry out adjustment negotiations with respect to each other, the relationship becomes more clearly defined. Once this is accomplished there is some tendency toward reduction in motivation or drive. This kind of deceleration of motivation may be experienced by both parties. Sophisticated clinicians have repeatedly observed the fact that certain kinds of gains are often made initially only to find that the rate of change begins to slow and even the magnitude of change becomes reduced. Regression and loss of previous gains is not unusual. Protection against such an occurrence is maintained to quite an extent as long as the approach is child-centered and as long as reinforcing responses are carefully selected. Such an approach requires that the therapist employ a searching and spontaneous kind of response activity. Probably nothing will produce stereotyped therepeutic activity with any greater rapidity than a decision on the part of the therapist about the mechanics of "what to do." Once this what-to-do decision has been acquired there is a strong possibility that the clinician's behaviors will become technique-determined and contain many elements of redundancy. Child therapy stops at that point. One would need to maintain that few therapists actually know precisely what to do particularly in a child therapy setting. Admittedly it is comforting and security-giving for the therapist to fall into a position of dependency on a method and omnipotence with respect to the relationship. It is relatively simple to offer reinforcing responses capriciously. Frankly, it may be therapeutically healthy for both the child and the clinician to be naive with respect to each other but mutual and reciprocal in their searching and sharing. The child's needs, energies, and messages will serve adequately with respect to therapeutic directions. Motivation for change need not decelerate if the clinician's attention and responses are child-centered. This decline in motivation is also interrupted successfully by the involvement of more than one therapist, by changing group composition, or by frequent opportunities to discuss the child's progress with other people. It also seems particularly helpful to involve therapists in reciprocal observation and subsequent discussion. It is as if therapeutic efforts should be a motivated learning experience for everyone in the milieu—not limited to the child.

It is not always easy to differentiate between that which is therapeutic and that which is simply reciprocal play. The general recommendation here speaks against the therapist playing with the child. The therapist's task is to give structure or meaning to the child's needs and behaviors. Where play is important for the child, ample response will be available from other children in the group. If the clinician is involved with an individual child, play is sometimes indicated, but here the word takes on therapeutic intent. This kind of play occurs primarily with isolated children and particularly with those who have withdrawn energies from motor activity. Play, in this situation, is actually used as a supportive response, and consequently will be employed when the child begins to demonstrate change signs of a particular sort. As the child begins to reinvest energy in these directions, the therapist's involvement in a playful form may be helpful. Intent is critical here. If the therapist is actually playing the consequence is minimally therapeutic. If the clinician can certify that he is using the act for supportive purposes, with instructional aims in response to a child's request, or as a selective kind of reinforcement effort, the response is probably consistent with the word therapeutic. Playing has a way of becoming an activity and an end in itself. It can become subtly defensive for both parties. It seems probable that playing on the part of the therapist risks reinforcing the child's immaturity. It would also seem to remove the therapist somewhat from his specified role.

Fragmentation of the relationship or contamination of the spontaneous aspects of therapeutic interaction can be promoted in many ways. Chief among them is the use of persistent and pedantic verbal responses by the clinician. Interpretative comments, casual supportive statements, and even carefully structured open-ended questions can be fragmenting if used too frequently. Despite the accuracy of such verbal operations, it becomes readily apparent that the clinician is not child-centered but technique-centered. Of course he may be searching aimlessly or illustrating his manner of communicating his own anxiety. This kind of verbal insistence is also fragmenting with respect to the ongoing nature of the child's efforts. One would rather see a response offered which represents a core or thread that has characterized the child's behavior over some period of time. Attention is also invited to the kind of distraction effort employed by many therapists. This is usually the consequence of therapist anxiety and represents a defensive on his part. Anxiety reduction in such instances activity is attempted by directing the child's attention away from certain acts or topics and, of course, this is another effort that is not child-centered. Verbal responses seem to carry far more specific value if they are parsimoniously expressed and bear concept relationship to the child's activity. A study of the therapist's defensive maneuvering is a critical factor. The act just described is only illustrative.

A maximum test in self-management is experienced when the clinician attempts to encounter the child whose defenses prompt him to avoid any such confrontation. Such a situation exemplifies what is probably the most common and difficult therapeutic issue. Resistance to change is that issue. In many instances, it is perfectly apparent that the child's resistance to change is simply a demonstration of the strength and position of the inertia component. In other words, this child has acquired defenses of such magnitude that his natural inclination toward emotional growth has been substantially stopped. The clinician needs to reexamine what messages or what kinds of information the child's behavior is actually imparting. Piercing of this child's protective framework is strongly dependent on the clinician's ability to identify the needs which subserve those behaviors and on his ability to be patiently observing with respect to minimal signs. Reexamining the child in terms of the clinician's concept of acceptance is also required. Acceptance, not reinforcement, not catering, not palliating, but acceptance of the child's condition or behavior of the moment (and this includes his defense) is literally an invitation to change. Careful examination of resistance-to-change circumstances reveals two situations with regularity. In one situation the therapist, in his eagerness to produce change, has become an inquiring, highly verbal, and somewhat pedantic person who has unknowingly slipped into the role of initiator. He has, therefore, simply played into the purposes of the child's defense and has consequently sided with the inertia component of the child's behavior. In the other instance, the clinician has become unnecessarily involved in the content of the child's expressions and has failed with respect to perception of the fundamental determinants of the child's messages. Failure to recognize subtle or low-visibility factors often gives support to the resistance condition. For example, if the therapist talks to the child's parents during the child's therapy time or converses with the parent following the session, it is easy for many children to presume that adults are busy making decisions about him. If the child is motorically inactive, insistence on the part of the therapist that the child be involved in some playground activity infers nonacceptance of the child's chosen way of being. Resistance is also encouraged by the clinician's inertia. The most common example of this phenomenon occurs when the therapist is so preoccupied with "what shall I do next" that he finds his actual attention to the child of the moment substantially diminished.

It is true that the clinician may on occasion find himself appropriately in the role of initiator. This will occur primarily when he is responding to some intent-portion of the child's message and is attempting to relate to the portions of the message that are the determinants of the child's defense. The most powerful intervening act that is available to the clinician, however, is his quiet and concentrated concern with the behavior of the child. Probably nothing is as frankly arousing for the child as a direct and uncomplicated show of acceptance of the very defense which the child has so carefully maintained. It is inevitable that the child's response to this show of concern will be to depart experimentally, even though momentarily, from his chronic way of behaving. It is to these excursions that the therapist should give careful response. It is possible that some children will respond favorably to changes in available activities, objects, or therapeutic conditions. It is also possible that one may see what would appear to be behavioral changes in response to activities that are initiated by the clinician. These changes, unless aimed at sources in the child that are beyond conscious recognition, are suspect and require careful scrutiny since they may represent only compliance or some kind of dependency expression in their execution. This kind of approach, while temporarily reassuring for the therapist, contradicts our general therapeutic notion. Changes thus produced appear to be highly specified and are probably more difficult with respect to transfer applications, and at best are not end products of the child's motivational state.

Duration and Termination

Therapeutic progress may be identified when changes in the child are both directional and growth-oriented. Elaboration of behavior together with an increased variety of adjustment modes may be anticipated. Immature factors which have previously functioned with high chronicity will begin to fragment. Progress can also be identified if the child begins to develop behaviors and attitudes in the clinic setting that are unique when compared to other relationships or adjustments in his general life. The application of these newly acquired capabilities to nonclinic situations would be a most reassuring sign. Since the children discussed here have some pathology in verbal communication, many people would assume that changes in symptomatology would have to be identified as part of a progress picture. Although desirable, such is not a necessity. It is perfectly possible, or perhaps required, that other developmental phases and sequences change prior to growth in verbal function. Despite the fact of the child's difficulties with verbal communication, the status of that development may be among the higher levels in his overall achievement pattern even at the outset of therapy. It follows, then, that if this child therapy approach succeeds at all in activating developmental trends, normal growth sequences would have to be anticipated. The use of verbal function, whether pathological or not, may facilitate other acquisitions, and verbal growth would occur as an integral part of that broader development. The general therapeutic notion is to implement overall development in a normal and unitary way. Such trends would seem to be reflected in similar and concurrent changes in the various specific functions such as speech and language, and this is usually the case. Therapy will continue as long as changes continue or until the child's general performance begins to approximate age-level expectation. Therapy will terminate when verbal communication ability reaches age level or is moving in a growth direction consistent with the individual child's capacities. From the standpoint of the therapist, another factor appears to warrant identification. Clinical experience indicates that progress is more likely if the therapist can certify that he has continued to do new learning about the nature and needs of the child. If an evaluation of recent therapeutic history through the study of clinical notes, for example, suggests that the therapist has done very little new learning, then there is a strong probability that the situation is no longer dynamic but has become a stereotyped and repetitive exercise. It is common to discover that children are maintained in therapeutic arrangements for long periods of time while no visible change occurs. This situation calls for reevaluation, possible termination, or reassignment to another therapist. It is of paramount importance to reassess the therapeutic history with particular attention to the intent and new learning of the clinician.

Speech and Language

The description of a therapeutic context for a child with problems of verbal communication prompts a particular kind of question. What responses or efforts does the therapist offer relative to the specific speech or language symptomatology? Historical and current therapeutic approaches in this field have been predominantly method-centered and have been oriented with respect to focusing attention on the function of specific parts. Etiological thinking has been strongly causal in formation. Treatment planning has been primarily deductive and thus derived from the therapist's concepts about the nature and origin of the symptom. Therapeutic activities defined here emphasize inductive approaches and place significance on associative phenomena rather than on a disease-oriented or causal concept alone. People may ask about the use of particular methods or techniques, the aim of which would be to provide direct improvement in the symptom itself, or they may ask about combining those procedures with a child therapy effort. One may inquire about the use of one sensory channel or another, or about the employment of a structured arrangement for perceptual training, or another may ask about the use of imitative processes. The answer is specific and candid. Of course these processes are going to be used—when the need for them originates with the child or stems from the interaction between the child and the clinician. These are only implementing devices, however, and should be listed among the preparatory effects that have been readied by the clinician. Of course some may question the appropriateness of child therapy as a speech clinician's tool. The answer is unequivocal. It rests in a decision as to whether or not we are going to comprehend the human in his uses of the very core of humanness and learn to function within the realm of his communicated being. These are idealistic and perhaps distant goals. The specialist who works with human, and thus verbal, communication and with the disorders thereof is the most likely candidate for becoming the knowing specialist of man. He does indeed find himself confronted with himself in every communicative effort. To be me as a therapist and identify you or confirm you and come to know you within me and to know, moreover, that I am simultaneously this (whatever I am) within you is distinctly and challengingly human. It defines communicative interaction. This is our field and our task. We have chosen it. The human's capacity for a communicative system called language and his potentiated and anticipatory readiness to give that language a special expressive form called speech allows us to be for each other something that is uniquely human. Such a relationship conceived by this kind of communication is at once terribly concrete in its primitiveness and wonderfully mysterious in its abstraction. Communicative disorders embrace the entire spectrum of maturity and must be so visualized and so treated, and people must be trained in disciplines and behaviors that are appropriate thereto. Weiner (1968), in practical terms, has concluded that to refuse a child who needs this approach would be questionable and perhaps akin to refusing to work with an organically involved child because treatment of the cause is not within the speech clinician's realm.

The kind of communicative attitude recommended in our child therapy approach disallows the therapeutic use of pretense with the child. This means that if the therapist does not understand the child's speech, he does not understand it. If he believes the child's speech to be another immature child way of communicating certain needs, then he must speak to those needs and, if he does so accurately, he will eventually demonstrate the link between the need and the child's particular verbal way of communicating that need. Since this approach minimizes the use of contingencies that originate with the therapist, it follows that all of the child's expressions, whatever their form, will enjoy acceptance or at least acceptance of the need for the expression. Particular value may be placed on some expressions by the clinician's response or by virtue of their usefulness relative to the child's satisfactions. Contingency situations which arise should originate with the child. He may well learn that negotiating in certain verbal ways will produce more effective satisfaction than will the continued use of his historical methods. Here the contingent arrangement originated with the child. Perhaps one will argue that the selective responsiveness of the therapist is a contingency arrangement. It is indeed specifying, but it does not follow the paradigm of the typical conditioning procedure in which the behavior to be changed is decided upon by some person other than the child himself. In the instance of child therapy, each act originates in separate correspondents. The language capabilities of a particular child may be deficient with respect to words for feelings, for objects, for behaviors, or for qualitative descriptions. The therapist may become a teacher if the verbal structuring is a response to the child's communicated request. These requests, not so incidentally, will often appear in the form of deficit behaviors. They may actually occur, or in other words be communicated as blank areas in the child's language, or they may appear in the form of obvious searching for some verbal expression equivalent to that feeling which the child is experiencing internally or equivalent to that which he seeks. A cautious informational response may be helpful in this instance. It is not uncommon to find that the child's level of frustration will prompt him to ask for instruction relative to sounds or words. Even here the therapist is faced with trying to decide whether the child is asking for inappropriate reinforcement of his dependency or for specific instruction that will lead to growth. The latter instance would represent a normal and appropriate use of the child's dependency role, however.

Many therapists who use a play therapy or child therapy approach rarely communicate with the child about the symptom or about factors specifically associated with it. At the same time, however, the clinician is certainly involved in offering responses to many other kinds of behavior. It would seem appropriate for the clinician to include the same responses or offer the same kind of treatment attitude to verbal behaviors as he does to any other kind of performance. Given sufficient data and an adequately strong relationship, the therapist should remark on the conditions under which the child stutters or achieves fluency just as he might comment on conflict behaviors, regression issues, or on the demonstration of any new achievement. A particular child finds the use of reasonably mature articulation possible when involved in an assertive expression, but resumes his partially intelligible speech in accompaniment with passive or dependent attitudes. A cerebral-palsied child with no apparent expressive language demonstrates some verbal capacity under emergency conditions. A child with minimal organic brain syndrome has a measured mean sentence length of two words, but in his aroused response to someone stealing his lunch, for example, produces several sentences of five to seven words in length. Experienced clinicians see great conditional variability in both speech and language factors. These conditions are typically those which occur in response to some sufficiently arousing condition whether that be new effort, stress, fun, or mild fear. Also observed is the frequency with which such expressions are spontaneous and self-determined.

One must be impressed with the value of self-determined effort. It appears to this author that children with disorders of one kind or another are more highly motivated in self-correction attempts than they are in those situations where they function predominantly as respondents. Recently, in response to a child's inquiry or expression of concern about the maturity of his articulation, a particular clinician gave a gentle but candid answer. She described the nature of the child's articulation as she had heard it. The child's next question concerned the possibility of change with respect to the misarticulated sounds. The clinician responded with the notion that although she (the clinician) could produce the sounds in her own speech and could recognize them when made accurately by others it was difficult for her to tell the child precisely how the child was to make the sound. This therapist remarked on the fact that the child seemed to attach a great deal of importance to this desired change and that they should be able to find a way to solve this problem together. Cognizant of the child's potential for self-determination, the therapist asked the child what part he thought each might play. Interestingly enough the child offered a specific suggestion. He proposed to carry out experimentation with respect to the production of sounds if the clinician would show him where the sounds were positioned in the context of words. It was further decided that the therapist would listen as carefully as possible and evaluate the child's experimental attempts. Note here that the therapist gave no auditory stimulation and offered no suggestions relative to phonetic placement. What she did was to place value on the child's willingness to try and, furthermore, she gave specification to the child's attempts as they began to approximate the true sound. In this instance it was noted that the initial acquisition of a reasonable approximation of the sounds in question did not appear as quickly as might have been achieved with the use of a more classical methodology. Once the sound was successfully produced there appeared to be rapid acceleration in the frequency of adequate productions. These efforts, incidentally, occurred in the form of whole words or corrected speech. The application of this acquisition was rapid and uncomplicated. It took place quite spontaneously and, of course, was done by self-direction. Note that this is essentially speech correction, but the process is contrary to the classical one. Here the clinician was the respondent and the child the initiator of the act. The rather rapid generalization of the sound was apparently due not only to the impetus provided by the child but to the fact that the sounds were acquired in clear association with general interests and concerns of the child and were not linked specifically with a procedure, nor were they learned in isolation nor acquired by externally imposed decision.

Many models designed to relate etiology and symptoms have been construed and new ones are being formulated. Some draw data from observation; some from inference. Hopefully, those derived from inference are composed of intervening variables whose functional purposes can be posited and eventually demonstrated even though the functioning of the variable itself may be invisible or unknown. The design of these models is typically causal- or pathology-oriented. Seldom is the symptom viewed as a behavioral component—necessary in formation, purposeful in execution—part of the child's way of knowing himself and presenting himself and being himself—perhaps based in part on perceptual error—and an understandable consequence of the congruence of environmental conditions, reactive experience, and maturational readiness or the lack thereof. The child with disordered verbal communication needs to be studied in terms of the associative ties between that communication form and other maturational acquisitions, developmentally learned behaviors, attitudes, or deficiencies. If one were to study verbal communication as a service function linked in its development and purpose with all major achievements of the child and rooted in the matrix of primitive forms of communication, then a more global understanding of its etiology or its associative links (normal or pathological) would be available. This will require the development of research approaches which will be as dynamic in potential as the human systems to which they will apply. It is almost self-evident that the person's troubles, regardless of origin, will manifest themselves in some form. Some organic states have clear deficit equivalents in verbal communication. Certain emotional issues represent themselves in disturbed verbal behavior. Most disorders of verbal communication do not display this simple equivalency, however, and the two just mentioned probably do not either. Certainly, an absence of soft-palate tissue creates a potential problem with respect to voice quality or articulation. Yes, the human system is apparently capable of displacing or rerouting its feelings and contriving some disguise to allow for discharge of some particular emotion. Incidental learning is a capability and a problem for the human and hypothetically, at least, may account for the origin of certain troubles. There is an observable phenomenon called fixation, and by acquiring this condition the person finds himself stopped developmentally in some dimension or another. Language can be designed to say one thing and intend something else. People are often ambivalent and may display such behaviors in the course of verbal effort; sometimes in self-contradiction with words; sometimes in contradictory and oppositional motor acts. Alterations in effort or in function can be observed in instances where the child finds inordinate compromise to be the only solution. The identity of the person finds itself parametric in his speech and language functions. Many transfer applications are inappropriate although understandable phenomena—foreign dialect speech, for example. Many structural conditions whether peripheral or central in origin or functional site interfere with adequate expression, may fragment cognition, or overdetermine the forms which incoming data may assume. These are rather practical and for the most part observable phenomena. They do not satisfy the requirements for a comprehensive and dynamic view of the child, however. For one thing, symptoms are popularly viewed as consequences and are not regularly studied from the standpoint of their facilitating contributions. Symptoms are too often viewed as deficits and are not visualized as being part of the child's way of maintaining himself or part of his way of attempting to grow. For another thing, one may inquire about the kinds of experiences, maturational levels, needs, satisfactions, neural patterns, and conflict issues with which the child's (disordered) verbal communication may be linked. One should ask this question whether inquiring on behalf of a cleft-palate child, one who stutters, or the child with neurological difficulty. From a maturational and developmental view, one must be as concerned about the growth parameters with which the disorder is linked as he is with the symptom itself. Knowing which to treat in order to help the other is a critical question.

SUMMARY

The clinical approach suggested here is derived from the convergence of three axes. One is composed of information about how people in a particular setting may establish and maintain effective relationships. The second is extracted from child growth and development concepts. The third is supplied by the writer's direct experience with children and adults who have demonstrated difficulties with verbal communication. The attempt, therefore, has been to integrate knowledge with empirically derived data. It would seem appropriate to summarize or restate certain factors. This is done in the following statements:

1. Whether the child's ways (including symptoms of disordered verbal communication) are overdetermined by environmental demand, derived principally from indigenous issues, weighted by lesion, or represented as the consequence of perceptual or cognitive error, the therapeutic concept is the same. Basically, we are to attempt to increase the child's tendency toward exploratory and experimental activity. The therapeutic relationship is a means of giving the child's efforts selective reinforcement, support, direction, and, where needed, specific improvement through instruction.

2. Child development, accomplished by a careful linking of maturational potential and learning, is dependent on several dynamically integrated factors. They may be identified by the following phrases: a) anxiety and obstacle mastery of increasing complexity and strength, b) the child's growing awareness of his particular presence and impact, and c) the characteristics of the child's milieu and especially the nature of the functional interface between the child and that milieu.

3. Anxiety arousal and the processes of therapeutic effort are critically related. The therapist is not only to be involved at the point of arousal as exemplified by exploration and experiment, but may participate in its induction. The therapist is, furthermore, to be carefully and deeply concerned in the expressive acts which represent the discharge of the energy thus accumulated. He is to be an active participant in whatever satisfaction, reward, or behavioral reinforcement may be derived by the child from the expenditure of his efforts. Finally, the therapist is to view the child as subject and with as much viability as the child's status and capacity will allow. This child and this adult, then, are to be reciprocally influential correspondents in the growth-giving acts of anxiety tolerance and mastery, and the development of infinite complexities which inure thereto. This is known as the process of relating.

4. Careful acceptance and exploration of the child's ways of being are acts with a single aim. That aim is to reduce the necessity of the child's maintaining defenses which are or historically have been overdetermined and inhibitory in nature. Conversely, the use of limits is designed to make more effective or purposeful the child's use of his energies if they have historically not been placed under adequate direction.

Both efforts, although antithetical in a sense, propose to promote ego-development and the benefits of self-determination which might thereby accrue.

5. Verbal developments represent a most precise articulation of maturational potentiality and learning. Verbal function is parametric in child development. It is at once facilitating for a wide spectrum of achievements and facilitated by them. Therapeutic approaches must respect both possibilities. The act of linking speech and language developments with general life-needs or interests of the child is a normal course. Increases in exploratory and experimental activity and the accompanying arousal conditions provide a natural context in which such linking may be implemented. The careful use of therapist response is crucial in effecting that linking. Well selected in terms of the child's needs, such responses may be instructional as well as supportive or interpretative. These responses by the clinician, whether emotional, somewhat abstract, or highly concrete in form must be judiciously selected and discriminatively imparted.

6. Growth, or at least its initiation, including appropriate support for maturational effort and adequate satisfaction for achievement, is viewed as a dependent function. It is dependent upon a certain amount of satisfaction being provided for more primitive needs; dependent on a condition where new behaviors are needed to meet new and increasingly complex demands for satisfaction and tension reduction; and dependent, finally, on environmental correspondents and conditions that will allow for or teach, or support, or provide sufficient and safe experimentation. It is understood that this experimentation has a twofold purpose; one is aimed at some immediate tension reduction or satisfaction; the other purpose is to increase the efficiency of achievement of such tension reduction or satisfaction when similar needs again appear. Growth, as a dependent function, is made possible through the child's use of his energies, the arousal of which may be termed interest, concern, or anxiety. Implementation is given to child growth when the child is viewed as central and subject, when his dependency needs are respected, and when his presence is given adequate recognition. While the child is viewed as dependency based, this view is one which originated in the child's correspondents. From the child's view, he (the child) must be strong, important, and particularly unique. Although highly self-centered in their early forms, these notions must be preserved for the child in order to insure the continued growth of his identity and singularity. The achievement of adequate separateness and sufficient security will result in his becoming increasingly interested in the concerns of others and respectful of their needs. Growth, then, is a process in which the child becomes a more and more particular person. Child therapy proposes to support such trends. The uniqueness of the child is perhaps more important than his incidental classification in terms of pathology.

7. Present evidence about neural functioning would suggest that atomistic therapeutic methods, i.e., selection of one variable for control out of a matrix of complex and interrelated variables (many of which are unknown and intervening) will produce many problems. Difficulty in fitting the changed variable back into the child's natural life-experience complex may be anticipated. Attempts at isolating the variable may in themselves be more arousing than the systems choose to tolerate, and the attempt may fail on that basis. If the single variable now takes another form as the consequence of therapeutic effort, then the system may defend against its return or change it back to its original form as it is reincorporated. It is clear, however, that one will have to upset the system, to some extent, if change is going to be feasible. Change is more likely to occur if that effort is associated with the general needs or ongoing purposes of the child. Change appears to be particularly facilitated when the child is a significant and viable participant in the arousal of that effort and is involved in establishing the direction of the achieved change. Finally, the child must derive something of value from that effort whether it be concrete reward, anxiety, reduction, externally offered approval, or personal satisfaction. Selective responses by the therapist may encourage the linking of such values with certain growth factors. Where one is successful in capturing the child's attention or concern, then you do indeed for that moment work with the whole person. The issue probably lies in the fact that our attention to a specific behavior by a particular method does not or may not link that behavior with the stronger needs or concerns of the person. Thus it does not become an integrated or generally used acquisition. One would suspect that where such learning was accomplished the success was due to an intervening occurrence which did allow a linking of the specific behavior and some general or well-motivated factor.

8. Both child-rearing and many therapeutic practices require the child to give significant attention to environmental agents. While a biological necessity in origin, this effort is often overdetermined with respect

to the child's growth needs. Too often the child's attention is drawn away from himself and increased value placed on his giving attention to his correspondents. This may be accomplished at considerable expense with respect to the child's self-knowledge, self-confidence, self-mastery, or self-determination. Verbal function is inextricably linked with this self and not-self issue. It is indeed challenging and fascinating to consider using for therapeutic purposes the very functions which have been labeled pathological.

9. In therapeutic practice one visualizes improvement in children's verbal communication in response to what appears to be a wide variety of therapeutic approaches. In many instances, moreover, improvement seems to take place without any formal treatment whatever. The question exists as to whether the improvement observed is a function of the method or something more fundamental. Empirically, it would appear that only two factors are common to the great variety of clinical methods employed. One factor has to do with the child's tendency toward or readiness for change (self-generated or otherwise). The second factor has to do with the conditions of or the meaning of the therapeutic relationship. While most clinical approaches emphasize methodology, child therapy proposes to implement change in the child as a function of his relationships with others. The many clinical approaches classically employed are viewed as particular ways of implementing the relationship. When visualized in this fashion, the various therapies may be described as authoritative, palliative, instructional, reciprocal, pedagogical, inducing, affective, deeply personal, supportive, directly experiential, highly specific, or broadly actualizing. Critical to this view is one's understanding that these various approaches are relationship conditions. Child therapy seeks to establish and maintain those conditions which will invite growth. Such development is seen as potentiated by the conditions and activities of the relationship—these to be determined primarily by the needs and the ways of the child. Therapeutic subject matter will originate with the child not in schedules of events that are preconceived. Change is invited by minimizing externally imposed demand, by significant acceptance of the child's needs or ways and their consequent expressions, and by carefully conceived therapist responses. The establishment, reinforcement, and growing generality of new behaviors are general therapeutic properties and are made possible by the careful use of a particular relationship between two people.

Relationships which have been established and maintained according to certain criteria and which have as a central purpose that of inviting growth efforts may be termed child therapy. The processes and acts which ensue take many forms. Prominent among the therapeutic negotiations which occur is that concerning the use of initiative, another involving assumption of responsibility, and a third involving influence. When a child is dependent and change trends are obscure the therapist is well tested to invite the child to assume a position oriented toward change. Where the child is relatively mature his readiness for or his seeking of instruction is obviously stronger. It is not difficult to respond to highly resistant or passive children with procedures which have been prestructured and which place great responsibility on the therapist with respect to success. Child therapy seeks to provide a setting where experimentation and self-determined effort are the primary learning modalities. The clinician is an active participant although he functions principally from the standpoint of a respondent. Within the structure of this relationship, the processes may well address themselves to any variety of clinical pursuit. As carefully as possible the activities of the therapist are formed and executed according to information supplied by the child, not by concepts about symptoms, and not by stereotyped adherence to method. Procedural skill, experience, etiological information, general academic knowledge, a concept about the various weights contributed by assorted determinants of the child's communication, and the capacity for comprehending the child's messages, whether verbal or not, are all possible components of the clinician's repertoire. Capacity for appropriate response and a warm belief in the child's potential for growth are also prominent repertoire factors. The person of the child must exercise considerable influence over the activities or conduct of the therapeutic attempt. Change is implemented by acceptance of the child as he presents himself, not by acts initiated by the clinician or others which indicate to the child that his important adult correspondents are dissatisfied with him and seek to change him. Dissatisfaction and other forms of arousal are to originate in the child—and they will—if the conditions for self-generated growth are available.

Conclusion

The unique person of each particular child is composed of many things. Common contributors to the child's being are such elements as his broad genetic-maturational-developmental-learning histories, his anatomical and physiological character, his present needs and present ways, his strivings, and his capabilities. A dynamic view of the whole child must not be limited, however, to these factors. The operational concept of the whole child must also include both his various precincts and the significant correspondents whose persons and precincts are contiguous to the child's.

The continued growth of the human functional hierarchy and its equivalent encephalization processes has apparently prompted behavioral developments which are understandable extensions of those nearly incomprehensible achievements. The human, viewed dispassionately, is an aggregate of specialized cells which function in an intricate and carefully integrated way. Synthesizing of these units together with self-imposed or environmental demands for further development finds application of the cell-specialization concept appropriate to the comprehension as well as the treatment of speech and language functions. To reiterate, the whole person includes the person as one sees him but also includes his many precincts. This view is critical to one's understanding of a whole-dynamic-functioning child. The precincts of the person are parts of the person. Language is viewed here as an abstract, relatively intangible, but demonstrably permeable membrane. It is capable of a relatively high degree of selective reciprocation and is intended to serve as a synthesizing, procuring, and discharging agent for all other cells, both physiological and abstract. Such reciprocation makes possible the maintenance of a continuous surveillance of those points of tangency among the various precincts of various people. Unlike more primitive alerting and orienting systems, however, language also serves to provide a communication structure for the person within himself—about himself. Language is a reciprocal, selective, and highly potentiated membrane. It is listed among the human's critical functions but is simultaneously to be counted among his most important environs (or precincts). Language is an intricately organized structure proving in a reciprocal way a definition of reality to the person and a definition of the person to reality.

At the point at which language needs no longer to be limited to immediate surveillance activities, its functional properties are extended. This development is another high-order response. It is expressive in form, relates significantly to the human's use of his energies, and comes to have a searching and probing aspect. This development is the functional and expressive aspect of language called speech. Speech behaviors have many properties, chief of which is the completion of the person's development in terms of the persistent establishment of extended precincts. Speech, together with its language base, extends the person into his surroundings and in so doing allows him to seek and give information; allows him to probe and intrude; permits him to know and participate in the precincts of others; finds him transcending ordinary time and space limits with respect to his establishing contact with others; provides an accumulation of experiences; is a significant contributor to the person's moment by moment acts and purposes; provides him with an accumulation of knowledge; and offers him a persistent means for probing, rehearsing, and anticipating future events. Structure and function—the person and the development of his precincts—the whole child as he is now and has the potential to become—relationship and process—language and speech. The child in this therapeutic approach is provided with unusual opportunities to know and appreciate his person and to extend his precincts in scope, number, and purpose. Child therapy attempts to visualize the child in the context of his person, his precincts, and his correspondents. The purpose is to provide him with increasing appreciation for the uses of verbal communication in securing his needs, in mediating anxiety, and in identifying the rights, significance, and interdependence of himself and others. Children need to be in a relationship that is warm and deeply believing, with a person who is patiently willing to search and to be open and communicative with respect to his own nature. Children need to be in a therapeutic setting with people who are capable of recognizing growth signs and who are carefully selective in the responses they offer. The process called child therapy is inexact and heavily empirical. The sharing of each one's person within the precincts of another is the process. Reciprocation with respect to influence is sought in the relationship. Child therapy is, indeed, a matter of searching and sharing—a matter of careful receiving and thoughtful giving.

BIBLIOGRAPHY

Barnlund, D. 1968. Interpersonal communication: survey and studies. Boston: Houghton Mifflin. P. 641; pp. 30–68.

Barrett-Lennard, G. 1962. Dimensions of therapist response as causal factors in therapeutic change. *Psychol. Monog.*, 76, 562.

Bell, N., and Vogel, E. 1960, eds. A modern introduction to the family. Glencoe, Ill.: Free Press.

Bentzen, F. 1962. Interdisciplinary research in educational programming for disturbed children. *Amer. J. Orthopsychiat.*, 32, 3, 473–485.

Bettelheim, B. 1967. The empty fortress. New York: Free Press. Pp. 56–57; p. 27.

Brookshire, R. 1967. Speech pathology and an experimental analysis of behavior. *J. Speech Hearing Disorders*, 32, 3, 226.

Church, J. 1961. Language and the discovery of reality. New York: Random House. Pp. 206–207.

Cofer, C., and Appley, M. 1966. Motivation: theory and research. New York: Wiley. Pp. 821–822; pp. 693–797.

Escalona, S. 1968. The roots of individuality. Chicago: Aldine. Pp. 238–247.

Fearing, F. 1968. Toward a psychological theory of human communication. In Interpersonal communication: survey and studies. Barnlund, D., ed. New York: Houghton Mifflin.

Feldman, S. 1959. Mannerisms of speech and gestures in everyday life. New York: International Universities Press.

Fiedler, F. 1950. The concept of the ideal therapeutic relationship. *J. consult. Psychol.*, 14, 239–245.

Friedlander, B. 1966. Effects of stimulus variation, ratio contingency and intermittent extinction on a child's incidental play for perceptual reinforcement. *J. exper. Child Psychol.*, 4, 3, 257–265.

Gendlin, E. 1966. Existentialism and experimential psychotherapy. *In* Existential child therapy. Moustakas, C., ed. New York: Basic Books.

Ginott, H. 1961. Group psychotherapy with children. New York: McGraw-Hill. Pp. 15–36; p. 12.

Goldstein, A., Heller, K., and Sechrest, L. 1966. Psychotherapy and the psychology of behavior change. New York: Wiley. Pp. 237–240; pp. 212–259.

Guerney, B., and Stover, L. 1967. The efficiency of training procedures for mothers in filial therapy. *Psychotherapy: Theory, Res. Prac.*, 4, 3, 110–115.

Haley, J., and Hoffman, L. 1967. Techniques of family therapy. New York: Basic Books.

Hartley, R., Frank, L., and Goldenson, R. 1952. Understanding children's play. New York and London: Columbia.

Haworth, M. 1964. Child psychotherapy. New York: Basic Books.

Hejna, R. 1960. Speech disorders and non-directive therapy. New York: Ronald.

Hertzler, J. 1965. A sociology of language. New York: Random House. P. 396.

Klein, M. 1960. Psychoanalysis with children. New York: Grove Press.

Leland, H., and Smith, D. 1962. Unstructured material in play therapy for emotionally disturbed, brain-damaged, mentally retarded children. *Amer. J. men. Defic.*, 66, 1, 621–628.

Lieberman, J. 1965. Playfulness and divergent thinking: an investigation of their relationship at the kindergarten level. *J. genetic Psychol.*, 107, 2, 219–224.

Martin, B. 1967. Family interaction associated with child disturbances: assessment and modification. *Psychotherapy: Theory, Res. Prac.*, 4, 1, 30–35.

Milner, E. 1967. Human neural and behavioral development. Springfield: Thomas. Pp. 226–239.

Mottola, W. 1967. Family therapy: a review. *Psychotherapy: Theory, Res. Prac.*, 4, 3, 116–124.

Moustakas, C. 1966, ed. Existential child therapy. New York: Basic Books.

———. 1964. The burden of sensitivity and compassion in the onset of a brain seizure. *Psychotherapy: Theory, Res. Prac.*, 1, 2, 67–74.

Peck, M., and Stewart, R. 1964. Current practices in selection criteria for group play-therapy. *J. clin. Psychol.*, 20, 1, 146.

Perkins, W., and Curlee, R. 1969. Causality in speech pathology. *J. Speech and Hearing Disorders*, 34, 3, 231–238.

Rachman, S. 1962. Learning theory and child psychology: therapeutic possibilities. *J. child Psychol. Psychiat.*, 3, 3 and 4, 149–163.

Rousey, C., and Moriarty, A. 1965. Diagnostic implication of speech sounds. Springfield: Thomas.

Safer, D. 1965. Conjoint play therapy for the young child and his parent. *Arch. gen. Psychol.*, 13, 4, 320–326.

Serrano, A., and Wilson, N. 1963. Family therapy in the treatment of the brain-injured child. *Diseases Nerv. Sys.*, 24, 12, 732–735.

Sidman, M. 1960. Tactics of scientific research. New York: Basic Books.

Siegel, G. 1967. Interpersonal approaches to the study of communication disorders. *J. Speech Hearing Disorders*, 32, 2, 112–120.

Sommers, R., Furlong, A., Rhodes, F., Fichter, G., Bowser, D., Copetas, F., and Saunders, S. 1964. Effects of maternal attitudes upon improvement in articulation when mothers are trained to assist in speech correction. *J. Speech Hearing Disorders*, 29, 2, 126–132.

———, Schaeffer, M., Lejss, R., Gerber, A., Bray, M.,

Fundrella, D., Olson, J., and Tomkins, E. 1966. The effectiveness of group and individual therapy. *J. Speech Hearing Res.*, 9, 2, 219–225.

Sphere, E., and Kastenbaum, R. 1966. Mother-child interaction in cerebral palsy: environmental and psychosocial obstacles to cognitive development. *Genetic psychol. Monogr.*, 73, 2, 255–335.

Staats, A. 1968. Learning, language, and cognition. New York: Holt, Rinehart and Winston. Pp. 428–466.

———, and Staats, C. 1966. Complex human behavior. New York: Holt, Rinehart and Winston.

Taft, J. 1964. The time element in therapy. *In* Child psychotherapy. Haworth, M., ed. New York: Basic Books. Pp. 160–163.

Truax, C. 1968. The process of group psychotherapy: relationships between hypothesized therapeutic conditions and interpersonal extrapolation. *In* Interpersonal communication: survey and studies. Barnlund, D., ed. New York: Houghton Mifflin. Pp. 677–719.

Watzlawick, P., Beavin, J., and Jackson, D. 1967. Pragmatics of human communication. New York: Norton. P. 129.

Webster, E. 1968. Procedures for group parent counselling in speech pathology and audiology. *J. Speech Hearing Disorders*, 33, 2, 127–131.

Weiland, J., and Legg, D. 1964. Formal speech characteristics as a diagnostic aid in childhood psychosis. *Amer. J. Orthopsychiat.*, 34, 1, 91–94.

Weiner, P. 1968. The emotionally disturbed child in the speech clinic: some considerations. *J. Speech Hearing Disorders*, 33, 2, 165.

Wolf, E., and Ruttenberg, B. 1967. Communication therapy for the autistic child. *J. Speech Hearing Disorders*, 32, 4, 333.

9

The Psychotherapeutical Process

Lee Edward Travis

Speech pathologists have manifested in both practice and research an ever-quickening interest in psychotherapy. To them have come those suffering from troubles in communication without organic impairment of either the sensory or the motor speech equipment. Voice and speech drills have not always been effective with these cases. The recognition of emotional disturbances as etiological factors in these disorders has forced speech therapists to seek the promising help of psychotherapy as developed by psychiatrists and psychologists. Individual, group, family, play, and activity therapy have all been scouted. Increasing numbers of speech pathologists are familiarizing themselves with the various procedures currently used in psychotherapy. Many of them are undergoing therapy themselves.

In the years to come, it appears reasonable to suppose that speech pathologists will not only apply successfully the principles and practices of psychotherapy to their specialty, but will contribute to the advancement of that from which they now borrow. This supposition would seem to be almost self-evident since speech workers are dealing entirely with problems of communication, and since communication is the matrix of psychotherapy.

COMMUNICATION

Speech as a Stimulus

Speech is a stimulus to both the listener and the speaker. In the listener, speech may arouse feelings, emotions, ideas, action. In listening to another, one may feel lonely and sad, happy and glad; one may hate, become afraid, or love; one may make an induction or a deduction or devise a plan of action; or one may sit down, get up, run, strike, or talk back. One or all or a multiple combination of these responses may be elicited not only by what someone says but also by the way it is said. Words, quality of voice, rhythm and cadence, emphasis, intensity, pitch, all blend in various proportions in their effects.

What the speaker says and the way he says it may frighten, sadden, or excite himself; the content and the style of his utterances may arouse or increase anger or fear or love in him; they may crystallize his thinking; and they may excite him to flee with fear or to attack with anger or to embrace with love. The person's speech has powerful stimulus values to himself as well as to others. In a very significant sense, whenever a person speaks, he speaks only to himself. Others may listen in on his verbal output and constitute themselves as an audience. They may be fooled into thinking that the speaker is talking to them. The speaker may share this illusion as well. But whatever an individual may say and to whomsoever he may think he is speaking, in a deeply telling way, he is communicating fully with himself only. We may say here parenthetically that the "neurotic" is one who does not communicate well with himself, one who does not understand fully what he himself says.

Speech as a Response

Speech is a response. It is an act. In speaking the person moves his lips, tongue and jaw, possibly his whole body. He makes sounds and gestures. He may be both seen and heard in action. Being a response, speech must have a stimulus or stimuli. It must be elicited. Most profitably, speech may be considered as a response to speaker needs and tensions produced by either inner or outer forces, or by both, operating sequentially or simultaneously. Needs and tensions established by forces from within and from without demand action for the satisfaction of the former and the dissolution of the latter. In our culture, individuals of all ages universally resort to verbalization as one means of alleviating, directly or indirectly, needs and tensions. Speech as a response, then, may be considered as serving the following needs:

1. To adventure forth, to reach out, to explore.
2. To control, to probe, to prod, to maneuver, to stimulate, to alter, to influence.
3. To cut, to strike out, to hurt, to destroy.
4. To soothe, to mollify, to love.
5. To receive recognition, status, attention, response.
6. To exhibit, to be found out, to reveal, to expose.

The fate of speech development will depend in a large measure upon the way in which the verbal expression of these needs is managed by the culture.

If speech can be found by the infant or child-speaker to be acceptable as an expression of his pressing needs and mounting tensions, it will develop as a useful and purposeful tool. If he finds he cannot risk an honest, telltale verbal expression, deficiencies and disabilities in speaking may result. To observe him and to listen to him is to acquiesce, and to consider his utterances is to grant identity.

Speaker-Listener Interaction

The speaker-listener interaction is the matrix of society. Speech is the leading character in the drama of interpersonal relationships. The speaker is an actor and the listener is an audience. Regardless of the part the speaker may think he is playing, in a way and to a degree he is always playing himself. And to the act the listener always responds. Sometimes more, sometimes less, sometimes painfully, sometimes joyfully, sometimes feelingly, sometimes intellectually, one's listening and viewing audience invariably responds. And in that response the speaker sees his own reflection. What he sees may not be true of him. It may be distorted by the form and quality of the listener's reflecting surfaces. Unintentionally the speaker may arouse hate or fear or love in another. To his surprise, the speaker may see himself reflected as a hateful creature, or a fearful monster, or a lovable character.

The present intrapsychic structure of the person, which is based predominantly upon his past interpersonal relations, and the present interpersonal relationships determine both his evaluation of himself and others' evaluation of him. And if we may think of inadequacies as being crucially advertised in interpersonal relationships, then maladjustment may be defined in terms of disturbances in communication (Ruesch and Bateson, 1951). If one is considered deluded, withdrawn, mute, feeble-minded, verbally inept, or in one of many other ways abnormal, he is manifesting, rather specifically, disturbances in communication. He is disturbed either in perception (listening) or in transmission (speaking). As shortcomings arise in disturbances of communication, they will be corrected by effective agents found in communication. The primary corrective agent is the communicative interaction between patient and therapist. Psychotherapy may be defined as an effort at improving the communication of the patient within himself and with others. The origin and destination of some messages may be found within the same organism, and we will be dealing with an intrapersonal network. Other messages will originate in one person and terminate in another, and we will be dealing with an interpersonal network. The intrapersonal network will sooner or later be the origin of messages in the interpersonal network, so that the two networks become inextricably linked.

A patient may be defined as a member of our culture who does not speak our language. We do not understand him fully or at all. If the psychiatrist is to converse with the schizophrenic, he will have to decode the symbolic system of the patient. If the speech correctionist is to understand the functional voice or articulatory case or the stutterer, he will have to listen through the speech symptom to hear what is really being said behind the symptom. The therapist tries first to understand the disturbances of communication and then to correct defective processes of communication (Mowrer, 1953).

THE MEDICAL AND EDUCATIONAL MODELS IN PSYCHOTHERAPY

In psychiatry and psychology and now in speech pathology (communicative disorders), students have suffered confusion from such terms as "mental illness" when applied to behavior patterns considered maladaptive by social standards (Albee, 1966). This semantic confusion has existed in psychiatry since 1800; and psychology, when it declared its independence around the latter part of the 19th century, nonchalantly perpetuated the muddle (Adams, 1964; Hirsch, 1968; Sarason and Ganzer, 1968). Now it is being said that there is no such thing as a mental illness in any significantly meaningful sense (Szasz, 1961). Rather, the term is being applied in an indiscriminate way to a motley collection of interpersonal behavior patterns. Consequently, both researchers and clinicians are calling into question the usefulness and value of the medical model from which the concept of mental illness arose.

The Medical or Illness Model

This model is traditionally based upon biological concepts of etiology and pathogenesis of health and disease, of host-pathogen relationship, of disease-specific cure, etc. (Brown and Long, 1968). According to this model, the unhealthy condition is largely beyond the patient's control. He cannot legitimately be blamed or held responsible for it. He is the innocent victim of heredity, or germs, or the unconscious, all of which operate in a deterministic fashion. In psychotherapy the emphasis is upon change in the prebehavioral organization, in underlying attitudes and personality structures. The focus is on diagnostic and causative factors of behavior, on how the patient became what he is.

The Educational Model

This model is traditionally related to learning, habit formation, and conditioning. Its dictum is that behavior, normal or abnormal, is the result of its consequences. A symptom is learned as a means for the manipulation of other people, as a way of controlling the patient's social environment. Symptoms may be thought of as socially deviant behavior but nevertheless learned on the basis of the shaping effects offered by others. Behavior, symptomatic and otherwise, is established and maintained on the basis of its social value. And there are only symptoms, not some neurotic disease behind them. Symptoms alone are the trouble.

Integration of the Two Models

All too often, one of these models, the medical or the educational, is presented as a counterpoint or as an alternative to the other. The polarization of these two approaches in the explanation and management of man's troubles is, in our thinking, faulty (Brown and Long, 1968). They are not mutually exclusive but complementary, both theoretically and practically. In a framework of physiological ecology these two models will fit well as the limits of a short continuum. Man and his culture are reciprocating. Intrapsychic and interpsychic are the two sides of the same proverbial coin. Neither has any meaning without the other. The patient and his symptom are a part of a meaningful whole, part of a system, a culture, or a family, that functions so as to maintain the part he plays. His intrapsychic living is the silent and invisible world of thoughts, feelings and attitudes, while his social life may include overt behavior that can be seen, described, and analyzed. Yet behavior extends from overt actions and movements that a person makes with his hands and his speech organs to what he thinks and perceives and feels and believes. In a significant sense no break occurs in the series of events which encompass both antecedents to overt behavior and movement of the muscles themselves.

In practice, Tate (1967) has brought the two models together in two therapeutic processes that he calls "contrasting and substituting." The aim of contrasting is to improve the patient's understanding of himself which he can then use to improve his behavior. The aim of substituting is to improve his behavior but not his understanding. Therapeutic gains through contrasting are mediated by understanding and through substituting by direct and unmediated behavior change.

Most psychotherapists, regardless of their prejudices, agree in principle that therapy is learning. They agree much less well about just what the maladaptive behavior is and what sort of learning processes therapy sets in motion.

People with disorders of verbal communication may benefit from both the organic and functional approach to their problems. Organic and functional hearing losses, neurological and emotional speech, and language retardation, anatomical, and attitudinal factors in the malformations of sound, all impress the speech pathologist and audiologist with the importance of both medicine and education in their therapeutical consideration. Of all current specialties, the one burdened with the service to those suffering from deficiencies in verbal communication can best apply the concept and tools of its next of kin, medicine and education.

APPROACHES IN PSYCHOTHERAPY

Theories of therapy which have proliferated during the last four decades can be compared and grouped in a relatively large number of ways (Sundberg and Tyler, 1962; Ford and Urban, 1964). Common or popular designations of approaches to the understanding of the troubled person include psychoanalysis (Freud, 1946), Daseinsanalysis or existential psychotherapy (Boss, 1963), client-centered therapy (Rogers, 1951), behavior therapy (Wolpe, 1958), logotherapy (Frankel, 1955), Gestalt therapy (Perls, Heferline, and Goodman, 1965), integrity therapy (Mowrer, 1964), reality therapy (Glasser, 1965), implosive therapy (Stampfl, see London, 1964), "fixed role" therapy (Kelly, 1955), cognitive or rational therapy (Ansbacher and Ansbacher, 1956; Ellis, 1958), will therapy (Rank, 1945), interpersonal therapy (Sullivan, 1953), and individuality-consciousness therapy (Dorsey, 1965).

Depending upon how much and what kind of change he hopes to bring about in his patients, the therapist finds that these many and seemingly different approaches may be grouped into two large, gross kinds of therapeutic operations, the Insight Therapies and the Action Therapies (London, 1964).

Insight Therapies

Practically all of psychotherapy in Western civilization is one or another brand of Insight Therapy subsuming the basic concept of self-increased awareness. Psychoanalysis, the most venerable of Insight Therapies, is popularly taken to be identical with all psychotherapy. Most teaching facilities give training only in the Insight systems, only in man's intrapsychic processes. This situation is changing rapidly, however, as experimental evidence for the efficacy of Action Therapy is mounting at a relatively furious rate. Insight Therapy, however, still prevails in the latter part of the 20th Century.

PSYCHOANALYSIS

In a real sense, the whole structure of modern psychotherapy is Freud's creation. Anyone who wishes to become a therapist soon discovers he must orient himself in some way, positively or negatively, to the classical Freudian position.

The most basic concept in psychoanalysis is that of the unconscious. The unconscious comprises feelings, wishes, and thoughts that have been denied self-reflective consciousness. They are called therefore unconscious processes. Although unknown to the subject, they nevertheless exert a powerful influence over his behavior. What he experiences as symptoms are the disguised outlets of the battle between impulses struggling for realization and repressing forces. Absolutely essential to the theory of psychoanalysis is the concept of conflict between opposing forces. The two main opponents in the struggle are the psychological energies of the id (mainly sexual) and the self-evaluative thoughts of the super-ego. The thoughtful, conscious control of behavior is realized by the ego. All thought and behavior disorders are compromises representing conflicting impulses or wishes. The neurosis may be viewed as a conflict between the id and the ego; the psychoses as a conflict between the ego and situational events. Each symptom satisfies a part of both sides to the conflict, but it is also held in force by them.

The tools of psychoanalytical treatment are primarily free association and the interpretation of dreams. The analysis, as the treatment is called, becomes the center of the patient's life. It looms as an intense and profoundly moving experience. New insights achieved do not transfer automatically to every facet of living. Even after significant unconscious material has been elicited, much working through will be necessary before the patient may be able to carry his responsibilities well and to handle his emotional relationships with others without burdensome anxiety.

Most of the psychotherapy that is practised by both psychiatrists and psychologists is some variation of classical psychoanalysis. A briefer form of psychotherapy that is popular and analytically oriented uses techniques that possess advantages of their own. The patient is asked to talk openly and freely about whatever comes to his mind, but such "free associations" are largely determined by current issues of his anxiety. Small emphasis is placed on the transference neurosis, where the patient defends himself against remembering and discussing his infantile conflicts by reliving them. Attachments to the therapist will occur and the therapist will use them, but he will discourage irrational and overly dependent qualities in the attachments. He will not indulge the patient in the regressive and "neurotic" aspects of a classical transference relationship. Interpretations will not be so classically analytical but more existential. Content and form of utterances by the patient will be used to help him make his own interpretations and to give his own sense of things. Finally in the therapies of modified classical psychoanalysis, the therapist becomes much more active, more disclosing of his own life, more of a participant in the ongoing interactions with his patient. He may become involved with the patient's family and associates, seeking and developing a mutual openness of significant proportions.

NONDIRECTIVE COUNSELING

Carl Rogers (1961) is responsible for the kind of Insight psychotherapy that has as its aim the release of the natural potentiality for growth assumed to be present in every human being. Relief of symptoms may result from the unfolding process, but this is a by-product rather than a primary effect. The real goal is that the client should perceive and accept his unique self so that it becomes free to grow in its own natural way. At the center of the theory is the assumption that man's behavior is innately good and effective in dealing with his environment. Man learns to be hateful, self-centered, ineffective, and antagonistic. Rogers has come to focus on the personal characteristics of the therapist, demanding explicit understanding of his own values and transparent presentation of his true self in relationships to others. The nondirective technique avoids diagnosis, interpretation, advice-giving, and reassurance. The method is mainly to use the reflection-of-feeling responses with the client instead of the usual exploratory questions of the more classical Insight Therapy.

INTERPERSONAL RELATIONSHIP THERAPY

Haley (1963), not a psychiatrist or a psychologist, but a communications analyst, has introduced to psychotherapy a refreshing thought about symptoms and their meaning, and how and why a patient changes his behavior in the psychotherapeutical relationship. His thinking enjoys some success in bridging the chasm between Insight and Action Therapies.

According to the interpersonal theory of Haley, the ills of the individual are not really separable from the ills of his cultural milieu. The emphasis is shifted from the processes within the patient to his relationships with other people. A symptom may be described as some overreaction or some avoidance reaction by the patient which he denies responsibility for doing because he cannot help himself.

Symptoms arise and are perpetuated on the basis of an implicit collaboration with other people. They are the advantages that the patient gains in making his social world more predictable from their use. The crucial aspect of a symptom then is the advantage it gives the patient in gaining control of a relationship with someone else. If the patient suffers distress over his symptom, such distress is preferred to living in an unpredictable world of social relationships over which he might have little or no control. Both the patient and someone else contribute to the perpetuation of the symptom because each has needs satisfied by it. However, generally both parties to the symptom have other needs that are not satisfied by the symptom and the help of a psychotherapist may be sought. The therapy may threaten the patient and possibly his collaborator because of how much control each is going to let the therapist exert over their lives.

It is not abnormal to strive for control of a relationship. When one attempts to control while denying it, however, then such a person is exhibiting symptomatic behavior. By means of dizzy spells, allergies, and stuttering a person may circumscribe another's behavior while denying that he is doing this. After all, he cannot help his trouble. In a sense symptomatic behavior is paradoxical. By it the patient achieves control yet may ask for its removal and thereby lose control. This request for help poses a paradoxical directive, since the other person, possibly a parent or a spouse, has been asked to help in the formation and perpetuation of the symptom, and is now being asked to help in its removal. Really the sought-after helper, be he therapist or some other significant person in the patient's life, is being asked to do contradictory things simultaneously. If a patient asked to be helped not for his sake but for his symptom's sake, then the perpetuation of the symptom is assured. A person who uses a symptom for setting the rules of a relationship cannot be credited or blamed as the one who sets the rules. If one is ever to receive either credit or blame in life, he must take the responsibility for his behavior.

Neurotic and psychotic symptoms occur in relationships where paradoxical directives are common. In his development the patient has had to satisfy conflicting demands by means of symptomatic behavior. Symptoms are the reciprocals to requests made by the patient's culture. If this is true, then all forms of therapy must deal mainly with the problem of control of a relationship, the therapeutic one. And since symptoms arose when the patient continued to receive messages from the culture that were qualified incongruently, they should disappear under the formal pattern of directing while denying direction, which is typical of all forms of psychotherapy.

In both directive and nondirective therapy the attempts by the patient to control his therapist by symptomatic behavior are accepted in such a way that they cannot be continued. Too often the patient finds that he is being directed to direct and he must abandon this type of behavior. A therapist may aim to influence a patient as little as possible within a framework of a relationship whose sole purpose is to influence a patient as much as possible.

Common sense would dictate that if some behavior produces suffering for the patient, sound advice and persuasion to change his way of living would lead to cessation of that behavior. Common observation tells us, however, that certainly many times such help fails. Psychiatry and psychology have taught us that the patient cannot drop his symptom because he is driven by internal forces, mainly unconscious, to persist in it. According to the Insight Therapy theory, the forces behind the distressful symptom are repressed ideas and feelings and, according to the Action Therapy theory, they are past conditionings. Both theories are saying that patients resist change which is in their best interests. But the patients are not saying this. They are saying by the symptom that the distressful behavior is in their best interests, that changes would not be in their best interests, and that they intend to look after these best interests by preserving their so-called symptomatic behavior. These patients are talking to their everyday associates who are free with advice and helpful suggestions. When they talk to a therapist, however, they will not be met with direct requests for change. Rather, they will be met with some other aspect of the interchange between patient and therapist such as gaining self-understanding or realizing fullest potential for growth. In a framework designed to bring about change, the therapist does not ask for change. Instead, he might be encouraging of symptomatic behavior and even ask for an increase in it. Now the patient will resist the suggested change of increase and move in the other direction, a lessening of the symptom. What worked for the change for the better was not an increased self-awareness or self-insight on the part of the patient, but the use on the part of the therapist of a paradoxical strategy to provide a context where the desired change can occur. The therapist not only helps his patient toward increased self-awareness but also traps him in a series of paradoxes which enforce a change in his behavior patterns.

In addition to Haley, whom we have been considering, Corey (1966) proposes a paradoxical concept that is also somewhat difficult to comprehend. He declares that the message of psychotherapy is not normality. "The human problem does not lie at the level of social adjustment or symptomatic behavior." Rather it lies at the level of selfhood. The problem is that the self does not declare and affirm itself. Patients act as though there is something else besides themselves; something in terms of ego-alien factors, such as heredity, early conditioning, unconscious quirks, and so forth. "The problem of therapy is to help the patient to see there is no problem at all, that his situation is just what he wants and is of his own choosing." A patient is one who converts a truly self-made decision into an ego-alien "neurotic disease" that should be cured. The self must embrace itself as it is in the here-and-now, because that is all there is. Therapy must always be restricted to the affirmation of what is. Hard work on problems *is* the problem and is used by the patient to deny the truth that sometimes he will just have to suffer and there is nothing at all he can do about it. Now the paradox enters. The patient can take a step forward. In summary the patient does not have an ego-alien problem such as a reading or speech problem but a selfhood problem. And when he affirms the legitimacy of his "symptom" he may exhibit a new emergent, a new enrichment of his life.

Action Therapies

In Insight Therapy symptoms are significantly not what they seem; they are not the real issue, but rather they are the advertisements of repressed experience and its associated motives and conflicts. This theory at its broadest base holds that all behavior, normal and abnormal, is ground in the psychology of the person as a whole, and it has led the thinking in psychotherapy for over 50 years. As we have already written, Freud has dominated this way of thinking, which may be labeled Insight Therapy.

Action Therapy, on the other hand, holds simply that neurotic manifestations of all kinds are bad habits that are learned. There is no "neurosis" or "complex" as such, which causes the symptoms. There are only symptoms. The so-called symptom is the neurosis, and not symptomatic of anything. There is no disease other than the symptom. Eysenck (1968) has written that it ill becomes those who cannot even cure the symptom to complain that others cure only the symptom.

Behavior or Action Therapy, which is derived from the experiments of Pavlov, is nearly as old as the Insight Therapy of Freud. It has not been nearly so visible or popular until lately when Wolpe (1958) published his theory of the nature of neurosis and the specific techniques for treatment. Wolpe's central idea of therapy is that because neurotic behavior has been learned, it can be unlearned or replaced by more adaptive kinds of behavior.

Uniquely the action therapist is interested predominately in his ability to manipulate behaviors in order to eliminate symptoms; he remains relatively complacent about their origin and what the patient may know about himself. He disregards relatively completely diagnosis and history. Instead, he assumes a strong and direct control over the patient's behavior, both in and out of therapy sessions. Assuming great personal responsibility for the outcome of therapy, he generally does not even discuss the treatment program with the patient. The action therapist thus cannot shift the blame for failure upon any one else, including the patient.

In all of these respects the action therapist stands in contrast to the insight therapist. The latter deals relatively exclusively with the internal states of the person, with self-reflective consciousness, motives, feelings, thoughts, attitudes, beliefs, and intrapsychic conflicts. The former deals relatively exclusively with overt behaviors, with eliminating certain behavioral excesses and/or adding new behaviors. Hyperactivity, phobias, excessive anxiousness, and tantrums would be examples of behavioral excesses. Social withdrawal, underachievement, delayed speech development, autism, and alexia would be examples of behavioral deficits (Clement, 1968). By procedures of extinction and positive reinforcement the patient's behaviors are changed to outcomes that are previously determined as desirable.

Insight therapists feel that the patient's problems are uniquely human, that they are manifestations of his peculiar human condition. In contrast, the actionists say that most human difficulties reflect learnings that are as easily observed in lower animals as in people. The insight therapists are humanistic while the action therapists are mechanistic. Part of being humanistic is to make a great deal of consciousness to think that somehow it inevitably moves behavior. Plainly it does not inevitably determine what a person does. Rather possibly mainly awareness comes after the bit of behavior; it notes the act that has occurred. Also, part of being humanistic is to glorify meaning, to consider the significance of living with its terrible incongruities. In contrast to Insight Therapy, Action Therapy may make too little of the subjective states, especially of thinking as a means of controlling behavior. In contrast with animals human beings can talk about themselves, about their thoughts and behavior, and distinguish between cognitive and affective processes on the one hand and overt behavior on the other. In the response repetoire of human beings is an enormous array of internal behaviors, such as pondering, remembering, and imagining. The humanists say that the behavior of men is signally different from that of animals and that this difference demands a difference between the clinic for the treatment of human beings and the laboratory for the treatment of animals (Bandura, 1967).

In Action Therapy special recognition should be paid Skinner (1953, 1957), Wolpe (1958), and Stampfl (see London, 1964). There are two major kinds of Action Therapy, one focused on changing old maladaptive behavior and the other on shaping new adaptive behavior. In changing old behavior there are two approaches, the counterconditioning of Wolpe and the extinction training of Stampfl. In the shaping of new behavior there are the operant techniques of Skinner.

SKINNER: SHAPING NEW BEHAVIOR

The basis of behavior-shaping is to begin with some form of behavior which the patient has in his current repertoire of acts, and move rigorously and precisely in small steps from this initial performance, differentially reinforcing each step, to progressively closer approximation of the desired final behavior (Holland, 1967). By reinforcement is meant any consequences following an instance of behavior that will increase the likelihood of the behavior reappearing. The timing of reinforcement is critical. It should be presented immediately following the instance of the behavior to be reinforced or else the intervening behavior will be reinforced. Also it is critical that the reinforcer should be a clearly different stimulus from any other stimuli occurring after an inadequate response.

WOLPE: RECIPROCAL INHIBITION

Wolpe believes that all neurotic behaviors are expressions of anxiety. Further he believes that there are numerous psychological states that are inherently antagonistic to anxiety. If the therapist can discover, for any given symptom, precisely which anxiety-inhibiting response would serve to counteract it, and can then teach the patient to produce that response regularly enough, the symptom will gradually disappear and may be replaced altogether by its much more pleasant antagonist. Wolpe's common anxiety-inhibiting behaviors are 1) anxiety-relief responses (avoidance), 2) sexual responses, 3) assertive responses, and 4) deep-muscle relaxation. The aim of psychotherapy is to eliminate an undesired response by reinforcing an incompatible, desired response.

STAMPFL: IMPLOSIVE THERAPY (see London, 1964, pp 95–110)

Briefly stated, Stampfl holds that neurotic behavior is the learned avoidance of conditioned anxiety-provoking stimuli. Symptoms are avoidance responses to unrealistic fears. Every time the individual is confronted with a situation that he thinks will be hurtful, he becomes frightened and in one form or another, even by the symptom, runs away. The wisdom of the street corner says that a person should face squarely the source of his fears and discover through his own experience that they are groundless. Stampfl took his clue from this wisdom and arranged things so that the frightening stimulus would occur in circumstances where the patient could not run away. Then, while preventing his patient from running, he continuously exposed him to the fearsome stimulus until it had lost all power to elicit anxiety. Stampfl's therapeutic technique is to persuade his patients to imagine themselves realistically involved in situations that he describes. He then describes in copious and lurid details the most powerful horrors imaginable in an attempt to frighten his patients most thoroughly. Extinction generalizes from stimuli of greater to stimuli of lesser fear-producing potential. He does not soothe his patients or gradually increase their tolerance for anxiety by first giving them fear in small doses. Rather he tries to terrify them to produce an explosion of panic within them under circumstances where they cannot escape. This treatment by inward explosion has become known as Implosive Therapy.

SUMMARY COMPARISON OF INSIGHT AND ACTION THERAPIES

The points at issue between the two kinds of therapies can be subsumed under three large headings: the role of the therapist, the assessment and treatment of the patient, and training of the therapist.

The Role of the Therapist

THE INSIGHT THERAPIST

He who would serve as an insight therapist must know that to understand another person at the psychological level requires a relationship between the observed and the observer that is distinctive and strikingly different from that between the chemist and his chemicals, the surgeon and his operative field, and the internist and his patient with a heart murmur. Psychological understanding requires as its chief characteristic the highest degree possible of the therapist's identification with his patient, of putting himself into the other person's thoughts, feelings, and emotions. It demands a coexistence of therapist and patient in the therapist's listening and the patient's talking. It demands the therapist's introspection of his own feelings, memories, thoughts, and perceptions as they are aroused by the patient. This is to say, really, that one knows another only through the knowledge of himself, which in turn demands that the therapist must know himself and must be free to be like all others, and yet by great self-knowledge so different from all others. More specifically, when the therapist observes his patient, he must be sufficiently free within himself to know that the patient was expressing hostility, or homosexuality, or guilt, or shame, or patricide, or dependence, or messing interest, or some other condemned feeling or attitude. The therapist, knowing himself, and being free from condemnation of his own feelings and attitudes, will be free to see the condemned ones of those he would help. It might help to say that in a therapeutical relationship the therapist studies himself more than he does his patient. What he really does is to study his own feelings and attitudes aroused by the patient's stimulus value. Realizing his own responses, he can decide the nature of the stimulus that produced them. The therapist studies himself as a responding mechanism to the other person as a stimulus. He is the musical instrument played upon by the patient. If the instrument gives a faithful reproduction of the performer's effort, that effort can then be properly appraised. The therapist must be a relatively perfectly tuned instrument, free from the distorting dissonants produced by the dead and flat strings and reeds of prejudice, compulsion, and defense. What the patient does to the therapist, and the therapist's freedom to see accurately what has been done to him, constitute the basis for assisting in the understanding and development of the patient. The therapist is a unique listener. It is not enough or possibly even beneficial for the patient merely to recite or tell to someone else his misgivings, sins, and mistakes. It is entirely possible that he has been doing this very thing for years and found no real lasting results. We do not find therapeutic effect from mere recital. Telling and revealing are effective if they are followed by no condemnation and no punishment, but rewarded with acceptance, understanding, and forgiveness. The therapist will listen with a permissive and forgiving attitude to the revelation of every little and big personal feeling of his patient. He will receive and understand his patient's every embarrassing, shocking, horrible, cruel, belittling, and shameful disclosure. Truth will be rewarded, especially the most painful truth. Therapy demands the rediscovery or better the recollection of the truth. Mental illness is really the big lie based upon the culture's painful condemnation of the truth. Truth and its painful consequences resulted in illness. Truth and its rewards will result in illness' removal. Emotional disorder is the price man pays for being so lately human. Emotional health will come with the recovery and useful direction of more of man's prehuman qualities.

Clearly the insight therapist orients his practice towards a gentle stance in which his living is an understatement that consists of watching, leading, living, and revealing his own inner core of meaning (Travis, 1966). He offers his patients a life, his own, worthy of emulation and adoption. The patient in turn will have a decisive inner experience of being together with a real human being and in the togetherness sense his own identity and difference.

THE ACTION THERAPIST

The psychologist engaged in behavior modification focuses his attention and efforts upon reliably observed behavior and not upon internal dynamics. He tackles the symptom directly, not as a function of a deeper underlying cause but as though it *is* the trouble, and the only trouble. After assessment the action therapist formulates a program of treatment and assumes full responsibility of selecting behaviors whose emission by the patient are to be changed. He elicits, reinforces, shapes, provides models, changes his own stimulus value, assigns tasks, records changes in the patients' behavior, and finally evaluates the results of the therapy. The action therapist is tough-minded rather than tender-hearted, skeptical rather than credulous, and oriented toward overt behaviors rather than hidden meanings. He is more teacher than doctor and his client is more student than patient. Within this frame of reference of teacher-pupil he does not offer a nonevaluative acceptance of everything the patient says and does, but considers the patient's behavior as having immediate and meaningful consequences, just as it does outside in the community. The action therapist's purpose is to assist the patient to greater independence and responsibility and less dependency on the therapist. From the patient's point of view, therapy changes from a vague and often inexplicable process with an omnipotent therapist, to an understandable learning process between equals.

Assessment and treatment

In assessment, the insight therapist infers the underlying causes of his patient's symptoms, while in treatment he removes those causes. He would rely heavily upon the clinical interview, the case history, and the results of projective tests to understand the deeper significance of his patient's troubles. From the intake interview to the last hour in therapy, the insight therapist is viewing a world of hidden sense. What does the patient actually say, but not know what he has said actually? An adolescent male stutterer gave the five following productions:

December 11. See a whole bunch of clouds and they are forming rings around the moon. A jet black horse with the wings of a bird is there. Then there are a thousand more horses, but they are smaller and a mixture of color; bays, sorrels, roans. There is no other black one. Now a big sorrel appears. He's an outcast and the only stud besides the black. He keeps trying to defeat the black horse but never can.

Down on the earth is a forest of knotted trees without leaves. A whole bunch of little elves, two or three feet tall, are watching this herd of mares and the two stallions fighting. Two of the elves are about six inches bigger than the rest and they're battling it out to see who will be king of this outfit, but neither can win.

Now I see an hour-glass, a very large one, that is sitting out in the desert. It is rolling end over end and instead of sand being in this thing there are snakes. One part has snakes that are hostile to those in the other side so that when the glass is standing up, there is room for only two snakes to go through into the lower part. Slowly the snakes get wiped out as this glass keeps rolling letting snakes through first one way and then the other. Finally there are just two snakes left, one on each side. They are pretty dizzy and pretty battered up by this time and neither one can do a whole lot about killing off the other, although eventually one will have to die. About this time the hour-glass reaches the only tree in the desert and the glass breaks in the middle and each part rolls off in a different direction.

See a waterfall and a river heading out to the ocean. The ocean is calm. There is an ancient sailing ship. Looks like it had been on the bottom of the ocean for several hundred years. It has moss, seaweed, and barnacles all over it. On board are chained the skeletons of the men who worked the oars and on the deck is this huge octopus. A huge black snake is also there. This octopus and snake are having a fight, all wrapped in coils. Snake is wrapped around the octopus and tentacles of the octopus are around the snake trying to crush it. The water gets red and then black and the ship's hold opens up and the ship sinks back down and disappears.

January 19. See a grove of banana and apple trees together. They are intermingled in the same orchard. There is an apple with a worm sticking his head out. He goes back in and starts eating the apple. Slowly he eats the whole inside of the apple out until all that is left is the skin of the apple. It is completely hollow on the inside. What he does with the apple I don't know. The worm gets no fatter and has no discharge. Inside of apple just goes but it has no effect on the worm whatsoever. Pretty soon this apple falls off the tree into a basket which they are putting apples in as they pick them off the tree. This apple doesn't squash or lose its shape for some reason in spite of the fact that all that is left is the skin. All of those apples are put on a sorting table and this one apple is pushed off with the bad ones in a huge dump. The worm is still in this apple. Another worm decides it's a good looking apple too, so he crawls in and they commence to have a fight. As they're fighting they bump around and explode the gases that are in the apple which blows up and throws them out a long way off and they land on the top or side of a mountain. They get pretty hungry and see a mesquite bush which has an apple on it, just one apple. They both make a dive for the apple but when they just about get their hands on it, it explodes. About this time they see a whole bunch of mesquite bushes. Each bush has just one apple. They're running around like mad trying to get these apples. As they just about reach the apples, they explode and disappear. They get underneath an apple and have about given up hope. But as they get under the apple it looks huge. Since they think it will bust they don't pay much attention to it but it falls on them and squashes them. It is solid. As it falls on them it buries them into itself, about one-fourth inch. It starts rolling. It rolls on and on and isn't hurt by the bouncing. Finally it rolls under an apple tree and somebody comes along and picks it up and takes out a knife and sees the two worm holes and cuts that part of the apple off and lets it drop to the ground. The worms' ghosts leave their bodies and go up and up. They have little wings. They see a beautiful apple orchard, the most beautiful one they have ever seen. There are thousands of apples. Instead of each worm picking his own apple they both go for the same one and start fighting. Sparks fly and they fall. They fall down and down. They're on a stick with an apple on each end. The stick is over a fire and the worms are being roasted by all the other apples standing around. They're getting pretty well cooked by this time when the other apples bring out two very beautiful apples which are exactly the same so that one worm may go to one apple and the other worm to the other. But no, both worms go for the same apple and start to fight like hell. The two apples catch them in a squeeze play and bang the two worms together. It so happens one worm is pushed into one apple and the other worm into the other apple. The apples start rolling down hill and the worms have their heads out of their respective apples just cussing the heck out of each other and not bothering to eat. The apples come together every so often to bang the heads of the worms together. The apples decide this isn't going to work as the worms are still mad at each other. So they take them back to the other apples and contemplate what to do with the two worms. They think and think and think and finally two apples which are Siamese twins roll up. They think this is the solution. The Siamese twins are the same apple except they have two stems and two cores and the two worms make a dive for this twin apple and start going around and around eating out the insides. As they're eating out the insides they meet a great big worm which eats both of the smaller worms.

In varying detail and form the same theme is presented five times. In each production, two creatures battle for the possession of something desired by both. By direct statement (stallions) and by implication (size, use of personal pronouns—he and his), the two combatants are male. Also by direct statement and implication the contested things are female. At this point in his therapy, the patient could not clearly admit two men or human males fighting over a woman. Instead he had to use such animals as stallions, worms, and snakes for the human male; and such things as mares, an apple, and an hour-glass for the human female. Still less could he admit his shameful and feared desire to fight his own father for his own mother. Especially at this time was he unable to come to terms with such dreaded desires. At a later time he could and did find peace with these and other practically unbearable feelings.

In Action Therapy assessment starts with questions of what behaviors are disadvantageous, what consequences (reinforcers) maintain current behavior, what new behaviors could replace the maladaptive ones, and what reinforcers can be manipulated in order to increase or maintain socially appropriate behavior. Assessment is based on current observable behavior rather than on invisible internal dynamics. It provides the information by which the treatment program is built.

Treatment is direct, ahistorical, and utilizes any and all appropriate social-influence techniques. For Action Therapy the goal of treatment is to alter maladaptive behavior with other people rather than to give the patient understanding of his feelings and thoughts behind his symptomatic behavior. That changed behavior may precede insight, occur without it, or possibly even produce it, is not of concern to the action therapist.

An example of the use of operant conditioning in behavior or action therapy is given by Clement (1968):

Bruce tried to get the whole group to pay attention only to him, and when they did not do so, he began yelling at them. Since the boys ignored him, the yelling quickly extinguished and Bruce finally sat down and was reinforced.

The boys sat and talked for about 15 minutes. Then they gradually got up and began engaging in cooperative play which lasted throughout the session. They were periodically reinforced for higher levels of cooperation.

During the latter part of the session Bruce began telling Ralph some very bizzarre stories about catching girls and mutilating their bodies. Frequently Bruce's verbal content had become rather loose in the past; therefore, we decided to try to break up the loose talk and fantasies. Before we began to intervene, Ralph had begun to make up some of his own gruesome stories in response to those of Bruce. The following interchange is what took place:

Therapist (T): "Ralph, you didn't really do any of those things you told Bruce."

Ralph (R): "Oh Yes, I did!"

(T): "Oh, come on Ralph. You don't have to kid me. We both know you were just trying to tell stories like Bruce's."

(R): "Well, may be I didn't do all of them." (I reinforced him.)

(T): "What do you mean, 'maybe not *all* of them'?"

(R): "Actually, I didn't do any of them, but I wanted Bruce to think that I had." (I reinforced him.) ....

(T): "But you don't believe any of those phoney stories that Bruce told you."

(R): "Sure I do. He really did them."

Bruce (B): "Sure I did."

(T): "Oh come on Ralph. You don't have to kid me. We know that Bruce was just trying to impress you, but he didn't do any of those things that he was talking about."

(R): "Well, maybe not everything." (I reinforced him.)

(B): "I did too!"

(T): "Let's be honest, Ralph. Bruce didn't do even one of those things."

(R): "I know it. (I reinforced him.) I just wanted to go along with him, but he was making up a bunch of stories."

(B): "They are not stories. They're true."

(R): "No they're not. (I reinforced him.) You made up your stories just like I made up mine. And you know it!"

(B): "Well, some of them were true. Really they were (pleadingly)."

(R): "Not even one was true." (I reinforced him.)

(B): "Okay, you're right. I just like to make up scarey stories like that to get people upset." (I reinforced him.)

For the remainder of the session Bruce and Ralph played together in an appropriate manner.

The Training of the Therapist

A therapist's effectiveness depends upon who he is and what he does. Possibly these two qualifications are saying the same thing; a therapist or anyone else is what he does. Regardless of this possibility, a distinction is made commonly between the person and his behavior. Until relatively recently, specifically until Action Therapy came to the fore, more emphasis was placed upon the person of the therapist than upon his behavior. The important factor in influencing the patient was held to be the personal characteristics of the therapist. He should be an impossibly "good" man. He should be suitable in all treatment settings. He should be able to cross all class, religious, and racial boundaries. Krasner (1963, pp. 16–17) has given us a word picture of this perfect human being who is worthy of being a model for the entire world. But a much less perfect person could still be effective, especially with some patients, and mainly through therapeutic techniques.

The importance of this question is increased when we consider the shift in thinking about the nature and extent of the therapist's participation in the life of his patients. Earlier, but still somewhat even today, the therapist remained quite aloof and impersonal, and unknown. The patient did not have his therapist's unlisted phone number, he did not know his address, his marital status, or his extracurricular activities, and certainly he dared not hope for social intercourse with his therapist now or possibly ever. Dispensing primary rewards (food, candy) is currently not the only activity that a therapist can use to increase his personal and social impact upon the patient. Neither must the therapist be limited to interview and therapy sessions in offering the patient behaviors, values, and styles of thinking that can be modeled. Now therapists may enter the patient's natural habitat and allow him to reciprocate in kind. With younger patients the therapist may participate in basketball games, help obtain valued jobs, or help prepare a progress report for a probation officer. To prepare him to do the things required of a modern psychotherapist the therapist-in-training must have experiences that increase his understanding of himself, of others, and of the community.

In Action Therapy the therapist will be trained in the same manner as a patient, by modeling and selective reinforcement. Only good traits that can be identified in the form of overt behaviors will be taught. Once there is an overt behavior that the supervisor identifies as germane, training then becomes a matter of technique. The action therapist is given techniques that permit him to modify behavior with an everincreasing effectiveness.

In Insight Therapy the meaning of the therapist as channels for producing change in the patient is of more importance than what he actually does. The therapist "does" as he is, and in his selection and preparation as a therapist emphasis is placed upon making him authentic.

Group Psychotherapy

So far we have concerned ourselves with psychotherapy as a somewhat peculiar and unique form of influence upon individuals in what is commonly known today as individual therapy. In this typical relationship we have a trained healer who is socially and professionally sanctioned, a sufferer who seeks relief, and a circumscribed relationship between the two (Frank, 1961). Because pressures for therapeutic services have increased greatly, especially since the end of World War II, group therapy has become a popular context in which to help meet these pressures. It has become a broad and lively area of clinical effort. As yet no particular theory or method has achieved a predominant position.

Some value may be served to consider two viewpoints in group psychotherapy. One may be termed the group-centered viewpoint and the other the therapist-centered position (Goldstein, Heller, and Sechrest, 1966). In the former, psychotherapy is realized through the psychodynamics of the group and in the latter, through those of the individual. The group-centered psychotherapist is less overtly active, serving more as a catalyst in member-to-member or member-to-group interaction. The therapist-centered psychotherapist encourages member-to-therapist interaction and group-wide influences on individual patients. The two positions may be thought of as therapy *by* the group, and therapy *in* the group. Most psychotherapists who work with groups are today somewhere along a continuum between the two extreme positions of group-centered and therapist-centered orientations.

Group experiences permit the individual to explore his acceptance by others and his acceptance of them to see possibly why his impacts on others are as they are, how he can relate more favorably to another one, and how he can behave for better interpersonal relationships such as correcting, replacing, exploring, even creating behaviors of higher social values. Group therapy is a microcosm of the difficulties people have with each other over words, gestures, and facial expressions. Behind these behaviors lie thoughts, attitudes, feelings, and beliefs that can be revealed for appraisal by others, thus acting as determinants of future behavior through feedback effects.

Because an important function of the group is to show its members the effect they have on each other, video-tape equipment is currently in use so that group members can see and hear themselves in interaction. In addition to feeling their impact upon their fellow members, they can literally see and hear it and have objective proof of what others have been telling them and what they have not been able necessarily to believe from the telling. But by seeing and hearing, disbelief in one's reported behavior is practically impossible (Stoller, 1967).

The Marathon Group

Stoller (1967) introduced the concept of the continuous session into group psychotherapy in 1963.

Each session lasts from 24 to 30 hours, often without a break for sleep. The fatigue, and even exhaustion produced by this procedure leads to a lack of interest and energy in being phoney. Adding to fatigue as an induction of honesty, nudity has very recently been explored. This latest innovation awaits further study for its validation as a therapeutic procedure.

Tired and naked people appear to be more truthful and more themselves and undefended by their customary roles. Stoller feels that changes and development are infinitely more rapid than under the conventional "50-minute hour." The marathon has been called a "pressure cooker" because of the tension it builds up. Group members must neither avoid nor dilute their discomforts. They must react to each other immediately and spontaneously at all times and allow feedback to tell them unmistakably what impact they are having on each other. And the marathon gives them time to experiment with this impact upon people and to put it in practice here and now. Anger, fear, and love intermingle in dramatic and moving interchanges as the marathon progresses through its stages.

Stoller makes the group leader's role quite different from that in traditional group therapy. The leader refrains from gathering information for case histories about the members. Instead he builds up his impressions of participants exactly as other members of the group do, and he must share the impact of each of the others. He does not remain the traditional, aloof clinician but becomes a fellow group member, participating in interchanges like anyone else. Every member is a cotherapist and coresponsible for the success or failure of any given marathon meeting. The tendency by some members to depend on the group in a regressive manner is thus counteracted by the demand for everyone to act as a therapist to everyone else.

Family Group Therapy

Since the family is undoubtedly the most important social influence in the development of a person, we naturally look to it in thinking about troubled people. Also, the family is the critical intervening variable between society and the individual. In some way every patient is probably a member of a family, whether parent, spouse, child, or sibling. Generally a patient's symptoms serve a social function, a family function; and generally a family behaves as if it were a unit. Members of a family act to achieve a balance in relationships. They act both overtly and covertly, and their acts may include symptomatic behavior, for example, controlling the behavior of others while denying doing so. In therapy, treatment should thus be oriented to the family as a whole rather than to family members as individuals (Satir, 1967).

CONCLUDING THOUGHT

We are convinced that the therapist is the essential ingredient in psychotherapy. Regardless of his techniques and theoretical stance, he becomes, to an extremely important degree, a model for his patients' subsequent behavior. If this is true, then the existential becoming of the therapist is crucial. He should be fully in charge of himself. He should perceive himself, others, and the culture accurately. He should acknowledge choices and decisions as his and accept full responsibility for their outcome. We might even go to the limit of realizing that nothing in a significant sense exists apart from himself. That everything is his own creation. To change a patient he must change his living of the patient. He must know that his patient is his own mental material, and that his felt need to change his patient is but a preoccupation with himself.

BIBLIOGRAPHY

Adams, H. 1964. Mental illness or interpersonal behavior. *Amer. Psychologist*, 19, 191–197.

Albee, G. 1966. The dark at the top of the agenda. *Clin. Psychologist*, 20 (Spring) 7–9.

Ansbacher, H., and Ansbacher, R. 1956. The individual psychology of Alfred Adler. New York: Basic Books.

Bandura, A. 1967. Behavioral modification through modeling procedures. *In* Research in behavior modification. Kresner, L., and Ullman, L., eds., New York: Holt, Rinehart and Winston. Ch. 15.

Boss, M. 1963. Psychoanalysis and daseinsanalysis. New York: Basic Books.

Brown, B., and Long, S. 1968. Psychology and community mental health. *Amer. Psychologist*, 23, 335-341.

Clement, P. 1968. Operant conditioning in group psychotherapy. *J. school health*, 38, 271–278.

Corey, D. 1966. The use of a reverse format in now psychotherapy. *Psychoanalytic Rev.*, Vol. 53, No. 3.

Dorsey, J. 1965. Illness or allness. Detroit: Wayne State Univ. Press.

Ellis, A. 1958. Rational psychotherapy. *J. gen. Psychol.*, 59, 35–49.

Eysenck, H., 1967. New ways in psychotherapy. *Psychology Today*, Vol. 7, No. 2.

Frank, J. 1961. Persuasion and healing. Baltimore: Johns Hopkins.

Frankl, V. 1955. The doctor and the soul. New York: Knopf.

Freud, S. 1946. Collected papers (five vols., 3rd. ed.). New York: International Psycho-analytical Press.

Ford, D., and Urban, H. 1964. Systems of psychotherapy. New York: Wiley.

Glasser, W. 1965. Reality therapy. New York: Harper & Row.

Goldstein, A., Heller, K., and Sechrest, L. 1966. Psychotherapy and the psychology of behavior change. New York: Wiley.

Haley, J. 1963. Strategies of psychotherapy. New York: Gune & Stratton.

Hirsch, C. 1968. The discontent explosion in mental health. *Amer. Psychologist*, 23, 497–506.

Holland, A. 1967. Some applications of behavioral principles to clinical speech problems. *J. Speech. Hearing Disorders.*, 32, 11–18.

Kelly, G. 1955. The psychology of personal constructs. Vol. 2. New York: Norton.

Krasner, W. 1963. The therapist as a social reinforcer: man or machine. Presented at APA. Philadelphia.

London, P. 1964. The modes and morals of psychotherapy. New York: Holt, Rinehart and Winston.

Mowrer, O. 1953. Psychotherapy, theory and research. New York: Ronald, Ch. 17.

———. 1964. The new group therapy. New York: Van Nostrand.

Perls, F., Hefferline, R., and Goodman, P. 1965. Gestalt therapy. New York: Dell.

Rank, O. 1945. Will therapy and truth and reality. New York: Knopf.

Rogers, C. 1951. Client-centered therapy. Boston: Houghton Mifflin.

———. 1961. On becoming a person. Boston: Houghton Mifflin.

Ruesch, J., and Bateson, G. 1951. Communication. New York: Norton.

Sarason, I., and Ganzer, V. 1968. Concerning the medical model. *Amer. Psychologist*, 23, 507–510.

Satir, V. 1967. Conjoint family therapy (rev. ed.). Palo Alto, Calif.: Science and Behavior Books.

Skinner, B. 1953. Science and human behavior. New York: Macmillan.

———. 1957. Verbal behavior. New York: Appleton-Century-Crofts.

Stoller, F. 1967. The long weekend. *Psychology Today*, 1, 28–33.

Sullivan, H. 1953. The interpersonal theory of psychiatry. New York: Norton.

Sundberg, W., and Tyler, L. 1962. Clinical psychology. New York: Appleton-Century-Crofts.

Szász, T. 1961. The myth of mental illness. *Amer. Psychologist*, 15, 113–118.

Tate, G. 1967. Strategy of therapy. New York: Springer.

Travis, L. 1966. The transparent therapist. *J. scientific Affil.* 18, 127–129.

Wolpe, J. 1958. Psychotherapy by reciprocal inhibition. Palo Alto: Stanford.

PART II

Hearing

10

Mechanics of the Ear

Merle Lawrence[1]

In all sense organs a specialized physiological mechanism has evolved for the purpose of transforming a certain type of physical energy into a nerve impulse. The part of the ear adapted to hearing (instead of linear or radial acceleration) contains unique arrangements for gathering sound and relaying it to specialized cells where a coded neural message is established. This message passes on to the brain, where it gives rise to the auditory experiences that have been quantified by psychoacousticians. The mechanical processes within the ear that enable it to accomplish this have interested auditory theorists for many years.

EARLY THEORIES OF INNER-EAR MECHANICS

At one time it was thought that the nerve fibers were stimulated directly by mechanical vibration. In 1683, Du Verney, who did not know there was fluid in the inner ear, guessed that the nerve fibers were spread out on one side of the spiral osseous lamina, and that stimulation was brought about through the resonant vibration of parts of this bony structure in response to aerial vibrations transmitted into the ear. He felt that this bony shelf not only responded to vibrations but was capable of responding differently to different frequencies. Because the lamina is broader at the base than at the apex of the cochlea, the lower frequencies were supposed to cause the basal end to vibrate while the higher frequencies produced vibrations near the apex. The nerve fibers, presumably spread out over this partition, were thus stimulated selectively by different frequencies and served to analyze the sound. Of course this is the reverse of what we know today. It is the basilar membrane that vibrates, and, where the lamina is broad, the membrane is narrow, which reverses the areas of vibration for different frequencies.

It is probably Aristotle's fault, because of the authority he wielded, that the notion of air in the inner ear persisted. His notion of an "*aer internus*" located in the occiput and separated from the outside world by the tympanic membrane was not refuted for centuries, although the location of this air was moved to the labyrinth during this span of time.

Although it had been suggested earlier, the first author to state clearly that the inner ear is filled with liquid was Domenico Cotugno (1736–1822). He made a precise statement that air is always absent from the labyrinth and cannot penetrate it.

Philippus Fridericus Meckel (1756–1803), in 1777, described observations that provided the final proof. Up to this time dissection of human material employed unpreserved specimens that must have been quite dried out by the time of examination. Meckel

[1] Preparation of this material has been supported, in part, by grant NB-05785 from the National Institute of Neurological Diseases and Blindness, United States Public Health Service.

The considerable assistance of Miss Linda Lawrence in the preparation of this chapter and the one following is gratefully acknowledged.

had managed to obtain some rather fresh heads which he kept outside his window during the freezing winter months. He happened to chop open the petrous region of one of the temporal bones while it was still frozen and noticed ice crystals in the inner ear. Subsequent to this he opened, under water, the inner ears of cats and saw no escaping air bubbles.

Thus, two separate efforts gradually merged as attempts to describe the mechanical action continued. Efforts to explain how the ear responds to different frequencies ran parallel in time with other efforts to learn more about the anatomy and physiology of the system.

The anatomical advances proceeded rapidly with the development of the compound microscope around 1830, and had Huschke (1835) carried his observation a little further the auditory organ might today be known by his name. He noticed the scalloped edge of the spiral limbus as distinct from the spiral osseous lamina and also, possibly, certain characteristics of the sensory area because he called these areas the "teeth of the first order" and "teeth of the second order." It remained for Corti (1851) to describe the complex structure resting on the basilar membrane. Among other things he described the supporting rods, the sensory cells, and the tectorial membrane, but he was the victim of an illusion that led to a misinterpretation of the function of this structure. Looking down from the top he saw the structure as fairly flat, as shown in Fig. 10-1.

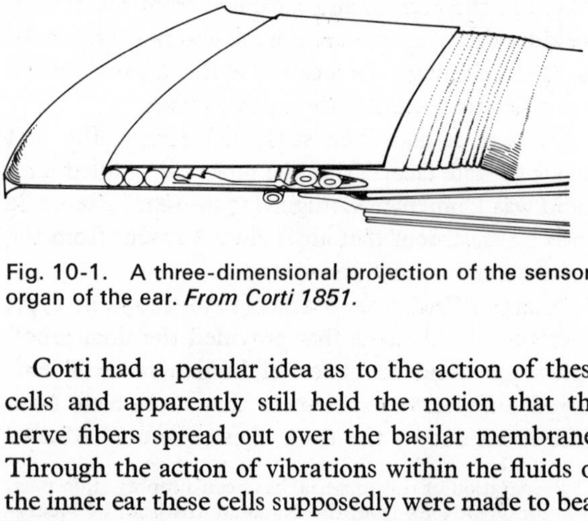

Fig. 10-1. A three-dimensional projection of the sensory organ of the ear. *From Corti 1851.*

Corti had a pecular idea as to the action of these cells and apparently still held the notion that the nerve fibers spread out over the basilar membrane. Through the action of vibrations within the fluids of the inner ear these cells supposedly were made to beat like drumsticks upon the membrane, over which were stretched the nerve fibers. This mechanical beating, presumably, gave rise to the nerve impulse. It is interesting to read what he had to say.

Supported by these observations I do not believe I am making a hypothesis too hazardous in supposing as probable that the oscillations of the air produced following a noise and propagated to the spiral lamina by means of the endolymph of the cochlea are capable of making the processes of the spiral lamina . . . flutter. . . . It is each of the three cylindrical epithelial cells, the anterior branch which supports them and perhaps also the articulating corners [this refers to the articulation of the inner and outer rods] . . . which, during an oscillation, can strike on the narrow dentate band [basilar membrane] almost as the drumstick on a drum. It is natural that the three cells of cylindrical epithelium are not able to strike the membrane of the narrow dentate band except indirectly by means of the anterior branch. This latter, in turn, once beginning to oscillate, should react on the three cells of cylindrical epithelium; and, always following the same oscillation, the membrane of the narrow dentate band will be struck, we suppose, a number of times proportional to the elasticity and suppleness of the various parts. It is possible that the swelling of the posterior extremity of the posterior branch of the [structures] in question [he is referring here to what we now call Hensen's cells] can, by being supported on the membrane of the narrow dentate band, serve to keep up the . . . branches . . . a little distance above the membrane when the lamina spiralis is perfectly quiet. The structures as well as the lamina spiralis on which they are placed, find themselves in this manner in a very favorable position to oscillate at the least vibration of the endolymph. . . . The oscillations produced in the manner we have supposed on the lamina spiralis ought to act immediately on the nervous expansion which is spread out on the tympanic surface of the narrow dentate band.

Other earlier investigators added a great deal to our further understanding of this structure. Reissner (1851), after whom the membrane between the scala vestibuli and scala media is named, Deiters (1860), Claudius (1856), and Hensen (1863), who have cells comprising parts of the organ of Corti named after them, all made immense contributions using relatively low magnifications and crude instruments.

Shortly after this, Helmholtz (1865) proposed a theory incorporating the observations of Corti and, without acknowledgement, the resonance principle already proposed by DuVerney. In this case, however, discrete resonators were designated which supposedly enabled specific nerves to carry messages to the brain. At one time he thought these resonators to be the rods of Corti, but later, after investigations by others had shown that the cochlea of birds has no rods, he reported that probably the transverse fibers of the basilar membrane were more suited to this purpose (Wever, 1949, pp. 25–39). Helmholtz, however, did not identify the hair cells as serving any purpose; although he described these as grouped "like a pad of soft cells on each side of Corti's arches" and directly connected by "fine varicose nerve fibers." Essentially Helmholtz felt the details of the organ of Corti to be a "peculiar auxiliary apparatus" and must have assumed that the nerve fibers were directly stimulated.

We know now that the Helmholtz theory is untenable for at least two important reasons. As we shall see, further careful anatomical observations fail to indicate the presence of structures capable of resonating in any isolated manner, and, mechanically, such characteristics of specific resonance are not compatable with certain psychophysical observations. Any device sharply tuned, when caused to vibrate, will do so for a relatively long period of time. This would indicate that once a tone had been sounded and the resonator activated, the sensation of tone would persist for some time after cessation of the stimulus, but this is not the case. In order for a resonator to cease its activity rapidly after it is no longer driven, the resonator must be highly damped, i.e., the friction must be great—like putting a tuning fork in a vat of oil. A highly damped resonator responds to a broad band of frequencies, however, and thus loses its sharp tuning.

In 1886, Rutherford presented a lecture "On the Sense of Hearing" before the members of the British Association for the Advancement of Science in which he described a theory of mechanical analysis within the inner ear based on principles similar to those which cause vibration to be produced when a sound wave falls on one of the plates of the telephone. Perhaps, for the first time, mention was specifically made that the hair cells transform sound vibrations into "nerve-vibrations" similar in frequency and amplitude to the sound vibrations. His notion of this transformation process is somewhat clouded by his suggestion that the hairs of the auditory cells respond to every tone just as the drum of the ear does. Rutherford believed that there is no analysis of complex vibrations in the cochlea, but that all vibrations, no matter of what frequency or amplitude, or how complex, are relayed directly to the brain. All of the hair cells are supposed to be involved for every tone. The fact that nerve fibers would have to relay impulses for the highest audible frequencies did not seem to bother Rutherford; he felt the auditory nerve might be specially adapted for this kind of activity.

Much evidence exists against this theory as presented by Rutherford; the auditory nerve fibers are not much different, except in their fibrillar termination, than other fibers, and overstimulation by loud pure tones does not destroy the entire length of the organ of Corti but only specific parts of it. Additional anatomical investigations further identified the hair cells as the transducers, and in 1892 Gustav Retzius suggested the proper function of the hair cells, that they are the final receptors for vibration and that the nerve fibers receive their stimulation from these cells.

Because of our concern here, not only with the identification of the transducers, but with the mechanics of their activation, we cannot proceed to modern developments without mentioning a theory of membrane vibration proposed by Ewald. Rejecting Helmholtz's notion of specific resonators, and other modifications of it, Ewald in 1898 proposed a standing-wave pattern for the basilar membrane as it responds to sound. Apparently he thought of waves as starting at the basal end of the basilar membrane, traveling to the apex with little attenuation, and reflecting toward the base. This would establish a series of loops and nodes between the two ends which would be different in number and width for different frequencies. As the frequency rises a greater number of loops, each covering a narrower region, would be produced. Ewald made no mention of how he thought the pattern was transformed into nerve impulses, but the number of standing waves and their width presumably served to provide a neural message adequate for the discrimination of tones of different frequency.

At the turn of the century another class of theories arose purporting to establish some form of peripheral analysis of sounds without resonance or standing waves. These are the so-called traveling-wave theories and are based upon the concept of a displacement wave progressing along the basilar membrane. There have been many of these theories, but since they are adequately covered elsewhere (Wever and Lawrence, 1954) we need only mention their general characteristics before turning to the modern developments.

In all such theories the movement produced by sound in the fluids of the inner ear is communicated to the basal end of the basilar membrane. The wave of displacement proceeds apically along the basilar membrane activating the transducers in ways differing for the various frequencies.

Present-day refinements start with the observations

of Békésy reported in 1928 and have been continued by him to 1960. His work on this subject has been so thorough, accurate, and illuminating that among many other awards he won the 1961 Nobel Prize in Medicine and Physiology.

Before continuing with a discussion of what is now believed to be the true nature of basilar membrane vibration and the exact extent of frequency analysis in the peripheral structures, let us continue the pursuit of experimental evidence that has identified the hair cells with the activation of the nerve impulse. At the same time that Békésy, then in Budapest as a research physicist with the Royal Hungarian Institute for Research in Telegraphy, was observing the action of the basilar membrane in the temporal bones of cadavers and simulating them in models, investigations on the electrical response of the auditory nerve were being carried out in other parts of the world. The history of these experiments is succinctly described in E.G. Wever's book *Theory of Hearing* (1949); suffice it here to summarize the early work pointing out the steps that led to the designation of the hair cells as the transducers.

Because of the limitations of a nerve fiber response, that is, it either conveys an impulse or it does not, with no variation in the size of the impulse, the notion that complex sounds had to be analyzed peripherally dominated the thought on this matter during the early years of this century, and resolving whether this was done in accordance with the frequency theory or place theory became of sizable concern. As E.G. Wever once put it in reviewing the controversy, "one's adherence to a theory of hearing depends upon whether one thinks the 'little man in the brain' is a mathematician or a geographer—either he counted the impulses or he knew where, along the basilar membrane, they came from!"

At about this time high-gain amplifiers using vacuum tubes were being perfected and the time was ripe for someone to place an electrode on the auditory nerve so as to measure directly the impulses to see what the extent of frequency response was. Earlier experiments by Forbes, Miller, and O'Connor in 1927, and by Foà and Peroni in 1930 using the direct-current string galvanometer, had led to confused results, primarily because of the low-frequency response characteristics of the measuring instrument. Subsequently, Wever and Bray (1930a, 1930b) placed electrodes upon the exposed auditory nerve of the cat and electronically amplified responses that were synchronized with the sound waves up to at least 1000 Hz. Eventually two distinct electrical effects resulting from this sound stimulation of the ear were distinguished: the one arising from the nerve response and the other from the cochlea itself.

The responses from the nerve fibers do not show synchronization over frequencies of the entire audible range, a fact which eliminates the frequency theory as a mechanism of peripheral analysis, at least for the high frequencies. Since other lines of evidence rule out a strict resonance-place theory some other explanation must be sought. The traveling waves of Békésy characterize the peripheral action, but only serve to analyze sound in a broad way. We shall return to this shortly.

THE TRANSDUCING ELEMENTS

The response from the cochlea, variously called the cochlear potential or the cochlear microphonic, became the subject of intense investigation and is of importance to us here because of its relation to the action of the hair cells. The source of these electricat effects was unknown for some time, but there were at once several theories, and it is interesting to note thal there really was no concern over the existence of a transducing element until these cochlear effects were observed and the parts responsible for their generation clearly defined.

At first, the fact that vibration in the form of sound gives rise to these potentials suggested some relationship to moving parts and, during the following few years, each structure capable of movement in response to sound was investigated as a possible source of the electrical effects.

A photomicrograph of the scala media, in cross section, is shown in Fig. 10-2. The scala media which contains the organ of Corti is bounded by Reissner's membrane and the basilar membrane. The basilar membrane stretches from the spiral osseous lamina, extending like a shelf out from the midiolus, to an attachment with the spiral ligament. The spiral osseous lamina has already been mentioned in connection with DuVerney's resonance theory (1683). The spiral ligament is interesting to consider because it not only supports one side of the basilar membrane but contains blood vessels and structures that probably have much to do with the chemical makeup of the endolymph.

In 1836 Breschet described the substance which, in a dried specimen, appears as a spiral groove extending around the inner surface of the bony capsule. When dissected, this appears as a gelatinous tissue connected between the bony wall and the basilar membrane. Breschet called this the "yellow band," or "membranous belt."

Some 10 years later Todd and Bowman (1845) described this substance as muscle that could serve the purpose of accommodation similar to that of the eye. They felt, however, that, more than likely, this interesting structure could contract to protect the cochlear nerves from excessive vibrations.

As already mentioned, the following few years were a period of most careful dissection and observation under fairly low magnification, the high point of

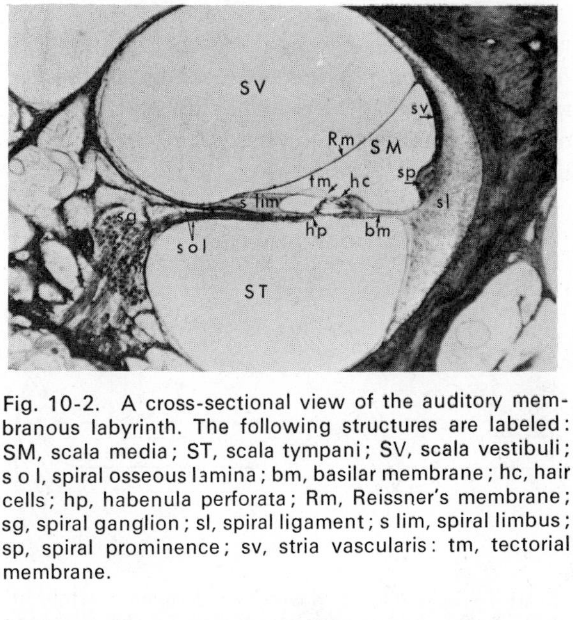

Fig. 10-2. A cross-sectional view of the auditory membranous labyrinth. The following structures are labeled: SM, scala media; ST, scala tympani; SV, scala vestibuli; s o l, spiral osseous lamina; bm, basilar membrane; hc, hair cells; hp, habenula perforata; Rm, Reissner's membrane; sg, spiral ganglion; sl, spiral ligament; s lim, spiral limbus; sp, spiral prominence; sv, stria vascularis: tm, tectorial membrane.

which was the classic description by Corti of the organ which now bears his name. One of these observers was Kolliker (1849), who described in some detail the cells that make up this "cochlearis muscle" of Todd and Bowman. He pointed out that no "Faserzellen" as seen in elements of involuntary muscle could be found. Corti agreed with this, but did not discuss further the question as to whether or not the structure was a muscle, and used Kolliker's name for it, *ligamentum spirale*. Subsequent histological examination has definitely ruled out the existence of muscle fibers in this structure. It is composed of connective tissue cells and many long filamentous extensions from the fibers of the basilar membrane.

Two specialized structures do lie on the endolymph side of the spiral ligament: the *stria vascularis* and the *prominentia spiralis*. These areas are very vascular and have distinct cellular characteristics of their own which, as mentioned, most certainly are related to the regulation of biochemical contents of the endolymph.

Reissner's membrane closes the third side of the scala media triangle. This extends from the upper cells of the *stria vascularis* to the modiolar border of the *limbus laminae spiralis* which juts into the *scala media* to support one end of the tectorial membrane.

The tectorial membrane extends from the spiral limbus to an attachment beyond the hair cells on the supporting cells of Hensen. For some time there has been debated the question of whether the hairs of the hair cells are actually imbedded in the substance of the tectorial membrane, are continuous with its substance, or are merely in contact with it. The latest evidence (Engstrom, Ades, and Hawkins, 1962) from electron microscopic studies has failed to reveal a continuity of the hairs with the membrane or that the hairs are enclosed in it. Rather the evidence is that only the tops of the hairs are in contact and solidly adherent. This must, however, be a strong bond because it is not unusual to find, in normal histological preparations, that the tectorial membrane, in shrinking and pulling free from its end attachment, often has the hairs still stuck to it free of the cell, or even with the cell still attached but released from its normal place atop the Deiters' cell. Whatever the situation, this intimate relationship between membrane and hair cell appears essential for the mechanical action of the hair cell. The hair cells themselves are supported by other cells making up the organ of Corti that rests upon the fibers of the basilar membrane.

Vibrations, in forcing the fluids to move, put the entire scala media into motion so that several sources of electrical potential are possible. The nerve fibers that enter the scala media through small openings, the *habenula perforata*, of the spiral osseous lamina have many fibrils that pass up and down the rows of hair cells giving off numerous smaller branches whose endings are like little buttons around the base of the hair cells. These nerve fibrils also move, along with the other parts, and have been credited with responsibility for the cochlear electrical effects. Thus, there have been three general areas assigned responsibility for the potentials: the membranes (Reissner's and Tectorial) (Bast and Eyster, 1935; Hallpike and Rawdon-Smith, 1934 a); the nerve endings (Adrian,

Bronk, and Phillips, 1931; Hallpike and Rawdon-Smith, 1934 b); and the hair cells (Wever, 1949).

Based on considerable investigation, the weight of evidence indicates the hair cells as the source of these potentials. Three lines of evidence support this conclusion: 1) several species of animals with hereditary deafness show severe abnormality in the structure of the organ of Corti with absence of the hair cells and no electrical response (Wever, 1949); 2) overstimulation of the ear by sufficiently loud sounds destroys the hair cells followed by a loss of electrical response (Wever, 1949); and 3) electrical recording from the interior of the scala media by means of a vibrating microelectrode shows the strongest electrical response from the region of the hair cells (Békésy, 1960). These latter experiments, by Békésy, are particularly ingenious and warrant further consideration.

Because the place of origin of the cochlear microphonic is surrounded by many insulating tissues, measurements made at a distance from the source can be changed considerably. It is, therefore, necessary either to have a thorough understanding of the electrical insulating properties of the surrounding partitions or to explore with an electrode until the strongest electrical effects are found. Békésy did both, but it is not necessary to review the former because the latter are conclusive.

In order to record as closely as possible to the vibrations producing the electrical effects Békésy developed a vibrating electrode, which, after considerable experimentation in order to gain an understanding of the limitations of such a device, he applied to the study of the microphonics of the ear. As Békésy points out, practically ever boundary between two different media produces microphonics when vibrated. In inorganic systems these may be small, but in living tissues they may be 10 to 30 μV[2]. All of the membranes and cells of the inner ear are capable of producing microphonics, but those arising from the cochlea are more than 10 times as great as those arising from other living tissues.

A vibrating electrode in the perilymph produces a smaller electrical effect than when the electrode touches the boundary of the scala media. Therefore the cochlear response must be located within the scala media or at its boundaries.

In order to determine whether the potentials are produced by Reissner's membrane or by the basilar membrane plus the organ of Corti, Békésy built a device capable of pulsating a column of fluid in a small capillary tube. This tube was filled with perilymph and the column set in vibration. A recording electrode was placed in the perilymph and another electrode in an indifferent area.

When this pulsator was placed in the perilymph just above Reissner's membrane, as in (A) of Fig. 10-3, both Reissner's membrane and the basilar membrane moved together; when the tip of the pulsator was placed inside the scala media through a small slit in Reissner's membrane, this membrane would move in a direction opposite to that of the basilar membrane when the fluid was made to pulsate. Consequently, if Reissner's membrane is responsible for the microphonics, the phase of the recorded electrical response should reverse when the pulsator penetrates the scala media. No such phase reversal was observed, indicat- that the microphonics are produced on the basilar membrane. Pushing the pulsator through the basilar membrane immediately reversed the phase, adding further proof.

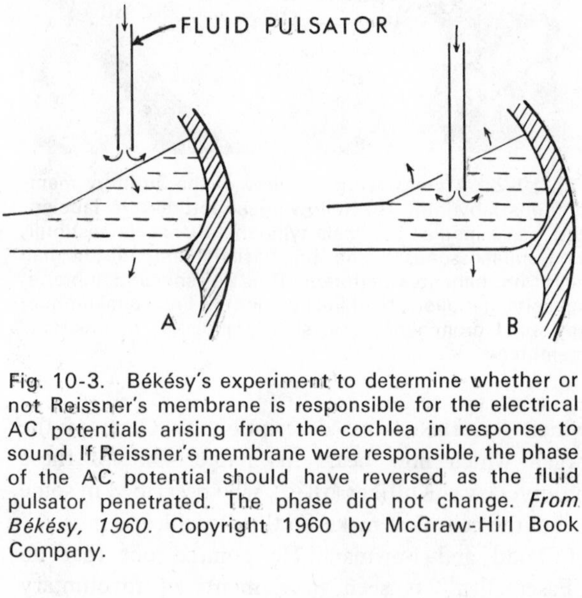

Fig. 10-3. Békésy's experiment to determine whether or not Reissner's membrane is responsible for the electrical AC potentials arising from the cochlea in response to sound. If Reissner's membrane were responsible, the phase of the AC potential should have reversed as the fluid pulsator penetrated. The phase did not change. *From Békésy, 1960.* Copyright 1960 by McGraw-Hill Book Company.

Further experiments with the vibrating electrode lowered into the scala media showed the largest microphonic produced when the electrode touched the outer rim of the tectorial membrane. These were larger than microphonics produced by Hensen or Claudius cells presumably because the stiffer tectorial membrane produces vibration over a larger area of hair cells.

Békésy, rather conservatively, concluded that these

[2] In our laboratory we have obtained more than 100 μV when touching moist cartilage with a vibrating electrode.

experiments indicated that the organ of Corti plays an important role in the production of the microphonics, and that both Reissner's and the basilar membranes protect it electrically.

As an extension of these experiments, Tasaki, Davis, and Eldredge (1954) reported that, while slowly inserting a microelectrode up through the organ of Corti from the *scala tympani* side, there was a sudden reversal of phase in the microphonic at the boundary between the hair cell and the scala media. This, they conclude, is evidence that these potentials are generated exactly at the roots of the hairs of the hair cells, although the presence of the tectorial membrane was not considered in the interpretation of their results. Békésy (1960, pp. 684–703) observed this phase reversal when his electrode touched the scala media surface of the tectorial membrane.

Thus the anatomical observations of Retzius and the evidence presented above combine finally to indicate that the hair cells are the transducers. However they do it, they are responsible for the intermediate step that transforms mechanical vibration into a neural impulse. Without the hair cells there is no cochlear microphonic and there is no hearing.

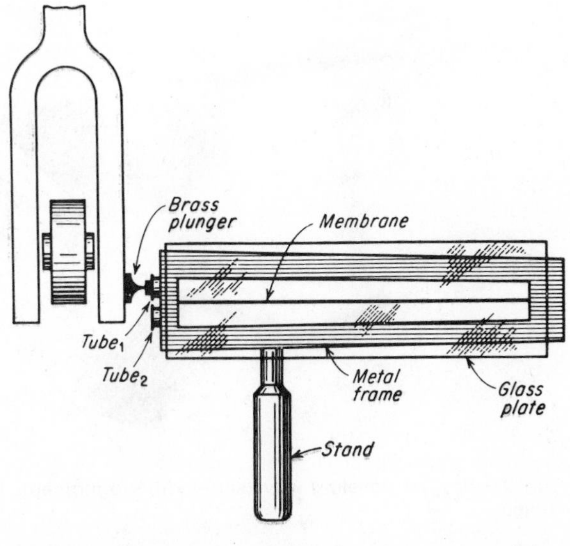

Fig. 10-4. Békésy's model of the cochlea. *From Békésy, 1960.* Copyright 1960 by McGraw-Hill Book Company.

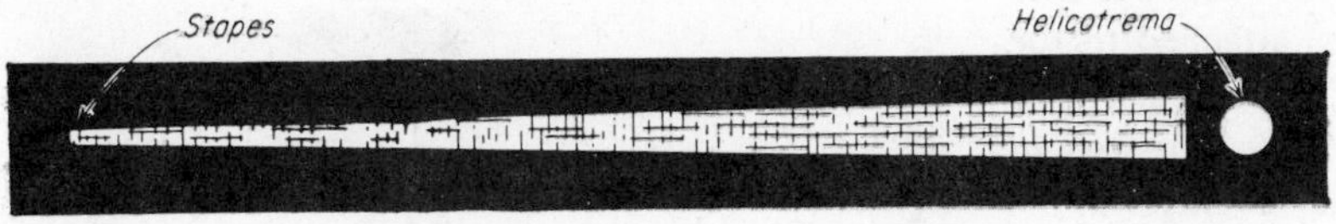

Fig. 10-5. The "basilar membrane" of Békésy's cochlear model. *From Békésy, 1960.* Copyright 1960 by McGraw-Hill Book Company.

It remains now to review the actual mechanical pattern set up along the basilar membrane and within the organ of Corti that initiates this transformation process.

MECHANICAL ACTION OF THE BASILAR MEMBRANE[3]

The various theories (resonance, frequency, and standing wave) proposed to explain how the ear analyzes sound into its different components or discriminates one pitch from another have all run into difficulties for one reason or another. In 1928 Békésy (1960, pp. 404–429) called attention to the fact that the essential difference among the proposed theories lay in the divergent assumptions concerning the magnitude of the elasticity and friction characteristics of the basilar membrane. In order to reproduce the actual conditions as accurately as possible and thus, by observation, make a choice among the different theories, Békésy chose to observe a replica of the ear. So after carefully determining the viscosity of the perilymph, the size of the helicotrema, the varying width and the proper thickness of the basilar membrane, he built a model.

First he fashioned a rectangular metal frame, Fig. 10-4, rather long and narrow, along the middle of which ran a thin metal band so that the cavity of the frame was divided into two long, narrow channels. The middle of the metal band had a long tapering slot, Fig. 10-5, shaped as the basilar membrane would be if stretched out to full length; narrow at the base and wide at the top. Just beyond the wide end of this slot was a hole to represent the helicotrema. The slot was covered by a membrane of rubber cement ingeniously mixed and spread so as to fill completely the slot without wrinkles or other variations. The frame was mounted on a holder, and two glass plates were cemented to the open sides so as to form an

[3] Parts of this discussion (including Figs. 10-4, 10-5, 10-7, and 10-8) are based on material in SENSORY PROCESSES, Alpern, M., Lawrence, M., and Wolsk, D. (pp. 91–96). c 1967 by Wadsworth Pub. and Brooks/Cole Pub., Belmont, Calif. By permission of the publisher.

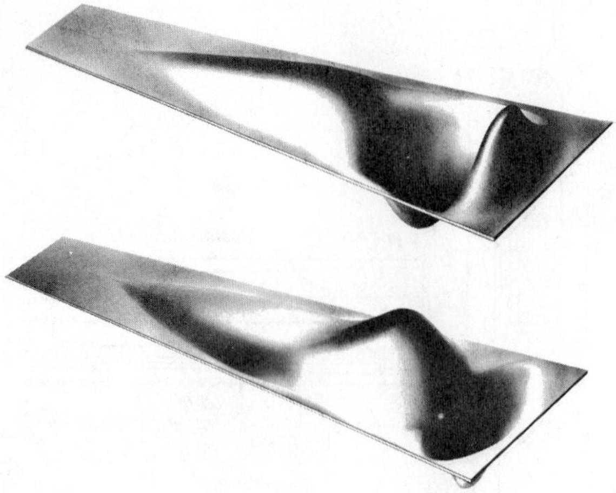

Fig. 10-6. The traveling wave shown at two moments in time.

upper and lower trough above and below the slotted and rubber-membrane-covered dividing plate. The troughs were filled with either a dilute solution of glycerine in water or plain water, depending upon the size of the model.

An opening at the end of each trough was made and each was covered with a rubber membrane. These represented the oval and round windows. Into the "oval window" a brass plunger, attached to the tine of a tuning fork, was inserted. Carbon particles were put into the fluid of the upper trough so as to cover the rubber "basilar membrane" evenly.

When the tuning fork was made to vibrate, the carbon particles were all forced toward the "helicotrema" indicating the presence of a traveling wave going in the direction of the "helicotrema." When a steady state of vibration was reached the pressure variations above the membrane equalized so that there was no longer a movement of the carbon particles over the helicotrema.

Depending upon the frequency used, the portion of membrane extending from the stapes to a certain point along the membrane all moved up and down in phase, increasing in amplitude up to this certain point. Beyond this point, toward the "helicotrema," there was a sudden reversal in phase followed by a series of small waves becoming progressively smaller in wavelength and amplitude, Fig. 10-6. These observations of the traveling wave were later confirmed by experiments on cadaver cochleas.

From the time of that initial observation to the present date Békésy has determined in a precise way many of the actual physical characteristics of the inner ear. The traveling wave and the measurements have been used by many others in proposing mathematical expressions for basilar membrane motion in response to sound, but occasionally the traveling-wave theory itself has been subject to criticism. So, in 1956, Békésy (1960, pp. 539–547) reviewed the theories and showed that by manipulating only two independent physical variables—the absolute stiffness and the coupling of adjacent parts—a continuous series of vibratory patterns could be produced, merging each of the four major theories presented here. Such considerations move directly toward answering the question: what precisely is the pattern of vibration on the basilar membrane and how are the transducers activated in response to vibrations introduced into the fluids of the inner ear? Again Békésy resorted to membrane models, but in this case the elastic properties were varied.

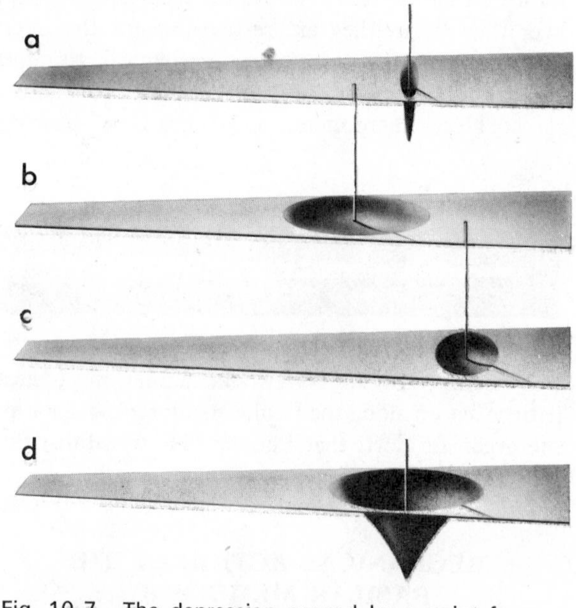

Fig. 10-7. The depression caused by a point force on membranes differing in absolute stiffness and coupling of adjacent parts.
(a) Resonance,
(b) Frequency,
(c) Traveling Wave,
(d) Standing Wave.
From Békésy, 1960.

The displacement resulting from a point force, and the pattern of vibration produced by a continuous tone on different kinds of fluid-immersed membranes, are shown in Figs. 10-7 and 10-8. Békésy had shown earlier that the stiffness of the basilar membrane

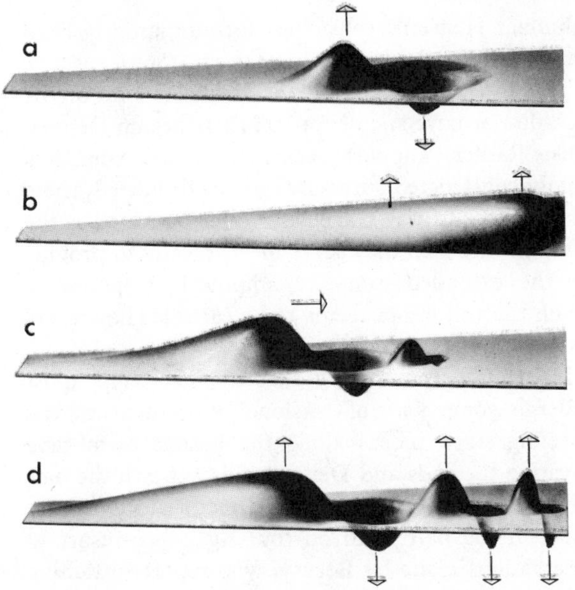

Fig. 10-8. Motion of the model "basilar membrane" produced by a sinusoidal stimulus:
(a) Resonance,
(b) Frequency,
(c) Traveling Wave,
(d) Standing Wave.
From Békésy, 1960.

varies, being about 100 times stiffer near the base than at the apex. This slope of stiffness, therefore, was kept constant, but the absolute stiffness and inherent coupling were varied.

If the membrane were made up of a series of thin elastic fibers stretched across the model frame there would obviously be no coupling between them, and a point force such as a needle would make a sharp localized depression in one fiber only. This condition simulates the Helmholtz resonance theory of freely vibrating resonators, and a limited lateral spread of deformation resulting from a point force is shown in Fig. 10-7, (a). If this membrane is immersed in fluid and a steady sinusoidal vibration introduced, the pattern shown in Fig. 10-8, (a) is produced.

If the relative variation in stiffness of 100-to-1 from base to apex is maintained but the absolute stiffness is increased by coupling the elastic bands tightly together with a plastic sheet, a point force applied to the membrane produces an elongated flat depression as shown in Fig. 10-7, (b). When immersed in fluid and subjected to a sinusoidally varying driving force through the "stapes," the entire membrane moves up and down as described by Rutherford's telephone theory and shown in Fig. 10-8, (b).

When the thickness of the elastic sheet, coupling the transverse fibers together, is decreased, the action of the basilar membrane is that described by the other two classes of theories. As the thickness decreases the deformation produced by a point force increases, as shown in Fig. 10-7, (c). A steady tone presented at the "stapes" of the model under these conditions produces a traveling wave just as was seen in the cadaver specimens and illustrated in Fig. 10-8, (c).

With a still thinner membrane, the same point force sharply displaces the membrane still further, Fig. 10-7, (d). The traveling waves produced by the same steady tone now become shorter and travel farther, so that they are reflected from the far end of the membrane, producing standing waves as Ewald had described, represented in Fig. 10-8, (d).

Thus is it possible to go continuously from one pattern of vibration to another so that an infinite number of intermediate patterns can be produced. What about the myriad of other theories that have been proposed? Békésy says, "Additional vibratory patterns have been proposed, some of which the writer has tried to verify on models, but the conclusion has been reached that they are only drawings and have no physical existence" (1960).

When the actual values of the stiffness and coupling along the basilar membrane are reproduced, a traveling wave results. Further support for the traveling wave comes from Békésy's observation of the traveling-wave pattern along the basilar membrane in various mammals. Also, experiments in which the tip of a needle was pressed perpendicularly on the surface of the basilar membrane of several vertebrates (guinea pig, mouse, cat, pigeon, cow, elephant, and human) produced a deformation of the type shown in Fig. 10-7, (c), almost circular. This indicates that the coupling between adjacent parts of the basilar membrane is too great to permit a resonant type of action, and a side view of the deformation shows that the stiffness of the basilar membrane is too great to permit standing waves.

The organ of Corti, shown in Fig. 10-9, rides upon this undulating basilar membrane. It is necessary to keep in mind that the arch of Corti, with the outer hair cells on the side farthest from the modiolus and the inner cells on the near side, extends for the full length down, more or less, the middle of the basilar membrane. Atop the hair cells, attached to the hairs, is the tectorial membrane (not shown), also running the full length and anchored continuously on the modiolar side to the firmly placed spiral limbus. The entire arrangement appears to be there for the main purpose of supporting the hair cells so that they can be mechanically activated by sound.

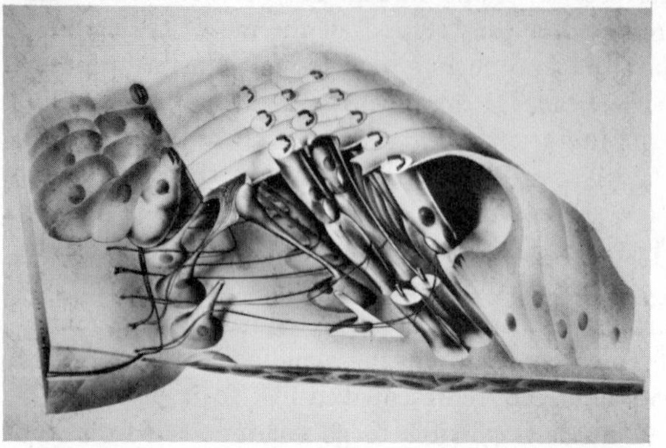

Fig. 10-9. The organ of Corti with the tectorial membrane removed.

The primary elements in this structure are the rods that make up the arch with the feet firmly planted on the basilar membrane. The inner rod may be somewhat weaker than the outer because it invariably seems to be the one most frequently distorted during histological processing, but it gains strength by bending over the top of the outer rod so as to rest upon it. This upper surface of the flat end of the inner rod joins the top plates that terminate the upper ends of the cuticular rods extending as an arm upwards from each Deiters' cell (Deiters, 1860).

The Deiters' cells also have their base firmly placed upon the basilar membrane and their main bodies are of just the right length to support the basal end of the hair cells. Each Deiters' cell contains within its cytoplasm a stiff rod which adds strength in its supporting function, and somewhere near the upper basket holding the hair cell the central rod gives off a cuticular extension which, surrounded by a small amount of cytoplasm, passes up between the hair cells, ending in a flat, oddly shaped plate perhaps three or four hair cells away from the one its main body supports. These flat plates all join together so as to form the reticular membrane continuous with the flat top of the inner rod mentioned above. The odd shape of the plate atop the cuticular rods of the Deiters' cells leaves openings through which the uppermost part of the outer hair cells pass and to which they are attached. The outer border of this reticular membrane attaches to processes from the relatively large columnar Hensen's cells, thus forming a fairly rigid framework for the hair cells (Hensen, 1863).

The inner hair cells on the modiolar side of the arch do not have such support: there are no Deiters' cells. Rather, support seems to come from less rigidly constructed surroundings. And, indeed, these inner hair cells may not be as readily activated as the outer ones, which may serve mechanically to provide for the extended range of amplitude response of which the end organ seems to be capable (Lawrence, 1965).

It can be seen readily that the hair cells must undergo some sort of torsional movement as the traveling wave passes along the basilar membrane elevating the rods and Deiters' cells beneath the hair cells, while the firmly anchored tectorial membrane pulls on the hair from on top. Again we resort to observations made by Békésy, who reports watching the organ of Corti in motion, not only through Reissner's membrane but also from the side through the attachment at the spiral ligament.

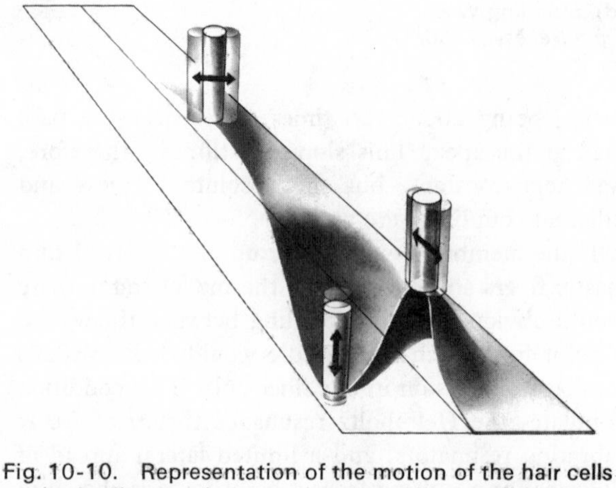

Fig. 10-10. Representation of the motion of the hair cells as the basilar membrane responds to the traveling wave, according to Békésy.

In the initial part of the wave between the stapes and the place of maximum amplitude the hair cells appear to move in a radial direction, that is, back and forth between the spiral osseous lamina and spiral ligament. When seen from the side, the lower ends of the cells appear also to move or rotate slightly in a longitudinal direction. The three characteristic types of movement are shown in Fig. 10-10.

Farther toward the helicotrema, at, or slightly beyond, the region of maximum amplitude, the hair cells were seen to undergo a pure up-and-down movement. And as the undulations become smaller beyond this point, progressing toward the helicotrema, the cells appear to move as a whole longitudinally in the direction of the long axis of the basilar membrane. Further toward the helicotrema all appears quiet.

The significance of these types of movement is not clear; as a matter of fact, no theories have been suggested, nor has any further investigation been carried out since Békésy reported his observations. It seems clear, however, that the vibrations introduced into the fluids of the inner ear induce a traveling wave along the basilar membrane which, through rigid support, causes the hair cells to move in peculiar ways giving rise to a recordable electrical potential. This transduction from the mechanical vibratory motion into the electrically alternating field makes nerve stimulation possible.

Although it is beyond our present scope, it does not seem right, at this point, to leave two important questions as yet unmentioned: if the response of the basilar membrane is broad, what are the processes that enable the ear to analyze sound (Ohm's law; Ohm, 1843); and, is it feasible to stimulate the nerve directly by an alternating current introduced into the inner ear and produce hearing with good discrimination?

We have already mentioned that there is some frequency analysis on the basilar membrane. The region of maximum displacement of the basilar membrane moves toward the basal end and becomes narrower as frequency is increased. This is not sufficient, however, to account for the ear's ability to discriminate frequencies differing by only a few cycles a second. On the other hand, microelectrode studies from single nerve fibers coming from the organ of Corti (first-order neurones) show sharper tuning to particular frequencies than can be accounted for by the broad region of activity of the basilar membrane. This is still not sufficient to account for a listener's actual discrimination ability, so obviously other refinements take place in higher centers, but there is a beginning even in these early neurons. This early process probably is related to the peculiar relationship between the nerve endings and the hair cells. There is no one-to-one relationship between nerve fibers and hair cells; rather the innervation of the organ of Corti is diffuse, one nerve fiber giving off branches to many hair cells and overlapping so that a single hair cell may receive fibrils from several different fibers. There is probably some, as yet unknown, relationship between the peculiar kinds of movement of the hair cells, their electrical field, and and complicated innervation network that initiates the frequency selective process (Lawrence, Wolsk, and Burton, 1959). This "sharpening" mechanism may be the process of lateral inhibition, a subject on which Békésy is continuing to experiment (Békésy, 1967).

Under normal conditions of sound stimulation the organ of Corti demonstrates an extensive dynamic range, i.e., a response to a considerable range of amplitudes. However, when a nerve ending is stimulated directly there is little range of intensity tolerated between the just-noticeable sensation and pain as the upper limit (Stevens, 1958). Whereas, when a stimulus which is adequate for the sense organ is sent in by normal means, this range is quite extensive.

It follows from the above considerations that direct stimulation of the endings of the VIIIth Cranial nerve can never serve to substitute for the peripheral ear. If the fibers are stimulated at all, only noise will be heard, and the range of intensities through direct electrical stimulation is too limited for normal communication.

It is apparent that there must be a healthy organ of Corti in order that normal hearing exist, and it is essential that the vibrations be relayed into the fluids of the inner ear with sufficient magnitude to establish the wave pattern. How this is accomplished is the next consideration.

IMPEDANCE MATCHING OF THE MIDDLE EAR

The vibrating particles of air cannot activate fluids directly without considerable loss, by reflection, of the available energy. To handle mathematically the problem involved in the transfer of energy from the light particles of air to the heavier ones of liquid, physicists have formed a concept of the transmissivity of a surface where two mediums meet. This transmissivity is an expression of the ratio between the energy that gets into the fluid and the energy of airborne sound at the surface.

At the boundary between the two mediums there is a sudden change in density through which the sound must travel. At such an interface there is a considerable amount of acoustic energy that is reflected back and only a little transmitted into the second medium. That which is transmitted into the second medium travels on its way away from the point of entrance, and it would so continue until the energy is dissipated unless the medium were bounded in some way.

The fluids of the inner ear are not boundless, of course, but because of the way the two windows, oval and round, are arranged, the fluid can act, under proper conditions of sound introduction, as if it were boundless. As an initial step in determining the characteristics of the middle ear we must first establish the amount of acoustic energy that could enter the fluid of the inner ear were the middle ear absent.

The two mediums (Fig. 10-11) can be designated by the subscripts 1 and 2 so that in the first medium the pressure of the incident wave is P_1 and that of the reflected wave, P_{1r}. Going out on the other side of the boundary we have a pressure, P_2, and a theoretical pressure, P_{2r}, returning. Under the conditions proposed, for the moment, we are assuming that the wave in the second medium (liquid) travels away to infinity so that P_{2r} is zero.

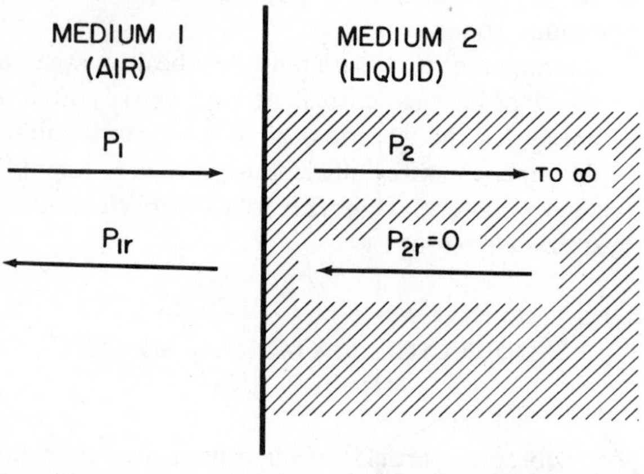

Fig. 10-11. Sound pressure at an interface: P_1, incident sound pressure in air; P_{1r}, reflected pressure in air; P_2, pressure transmitted into liquid; P_{2r}, theoretical nonexistent (in boundless medium) pressure reflected back to source.

There are two boundary conditions that these waves must satisfy: 1) the total pressure must be the same on both sides of the boundary, and 2) the particle velocity into the boundary must equal the particle velocity out on the other side. Considering that $P_{2r}=0$ then $P_1+P_{1r}=P_2$.

When the frequency is held constant, the particle velocity, U, is equal to the pressure, P, divided by the specific acoustic resistance, R, of the medium which in turn is equal to the square root of the product of the modulus of elasticity, ϵ, and the density, ρ: $\sqrt{\epsilon\rho}$. Both of these values can be found in tables describing the fundamental characteristics of various mediums under standard conditions.

If U represents particle velocity and R the acoustic resistance, then

$U_1=\frac{1}{R_1}(P_1-P_{1r})$ because P_1-P_{1r} = pressure into the boundary and

$$U_2=\frac{1}{R_2}(P_2)$$

Equating pressures and particle velocities on the two sides of the boundary gives two equations:

$$P_1+P_{1r}=P_2$$
$$R_2(P_1-P_{1r})=R_1P_2$$

From the first equation: $P_{1r}=P_2-P_1$ which can be substituted in the second equation so that

$$R_2\, P_1-P_2+P_1)=R_1P_2$$

or

$$\frac{R_2}{R_1}(P_1-P_2+P_1)=P_2$$

If we now substitute for the ratio of the acoustic resistances the letter r so that $\frac{R_2}{R_1}=r$ we have

$$rP_1-rP_2+rP_1=P_2$$

transposing gives

$$rP_1+rP_1=rP_2+P_2=P_2(r+1)$$

from which the ratio of pressures can be found

$$\frac{P_2}{P_1}=\frac{2r}{r+1}$$

From this formula for the ratio of pressures the amount of energy transmitted into the second medium expressed as a ratio to that in the first medium can be found.

The power, J, in a sound wave is equal to the square of the pressure divided by the acoustic resistance: $J=\frac{P^2}{R}$

or

$$P_1=\sqrt{J_1R_1}$$

and

$$P_2=\sqrt{J_2R_2}$$

Dividing the above gives

$$\frac{\sqrt{J_2R_2}}{\sqrt{J_1R_1}}=\frac{P_2}{P_1}=\frac{2r}{r+1}$$

Squaring both sides gives

$$\frac{J_2R_2}{J_1R_1}=\frac{4r^2}{(r+1)^2}$$

Again letting $\frac{R_2}{R_1}=r$

reduces the ratio to

$$\frac{J_2}{J_1} = \frac{4r}{(r+1)^2} = \text{Transmissivity (T)}$$

If we now look up the characteristics of different mediums in the appropriate tables we find that for air at 20°C the density (ρ)=0.0012 grams per cubic cm and the bulk modulus of elasticity (ϵ)=1.42×10^6 dynes per sq. cm which gives a specific acoustic resistance ($R=\sqrt{\epsilon\rho}$) of 41.5 mechanical ohms per sq. cm. For sea water (the medium most similar to the inner ear fluids) the density (ρ)=1.024 grams per cubic cm and the bulk modulus of elasticity (ϵ)= 2.53×10^{10} dynes per sq. cm. which result in a specific acoustic resistivity of 161,000 mechanical ohms per sq. cm.

The ratio $r=\frac{R_2}{R_1}$ of the above two resistances is

therefore $\frac{161{,}000}{41.5}=3{,}880.$

Fitting these figures into the formula for transmissivity gives T=0.001, which means that in the case of an air-liquid (sea water) interface only one tenth of one percent of the acoustic energy in air is actually transmitted into the fluids while 99.9 percent is reflected back. This is a loss of 30 dB in the energy as the vibration crosses the boundary.

The fluid-filled inner ear is encased in hard bone, which necessitates the presence of openings through this encasement so the vibrations might have access. Two openings are needed: one exposed to the vibrations, and the other to allow freedom of movement of the fluid as though it were boundless.

Through its special arrangement the middle ear has the property of making the physical properties of air act like those of water, and so prevents the extensive reflection at the interface. There are two mechanisms by means of which the middle ear accomplishes this fact. One is through the difference in area between the tympanic membrane and the footplate of the stapes; the other is through a lever action brought about by the positional relationship of the three ossicular bones (Fig. 10-12).

Measurements which have been made in man of the areal ratio show the tympanic membrane to have, on the average, an area 21 times greater than that of the stapes footplate. Because the membrane is not like a piston, but is more like the cone of a loudspeaker, fastened around its edge, the effective area of movement is somewhat less than its total area. Experimental measurements have shown this effective area to be about two-thirds of the total area, which reduces the ratio to 14 : 1. The pressure per unit area on the drum membrane is transferred to the smaller area of the footplate, decreasing the air-liquid interface disadvantage by 23 dB, thus increasing the effectiveness of the oval window vibrations by this amount.

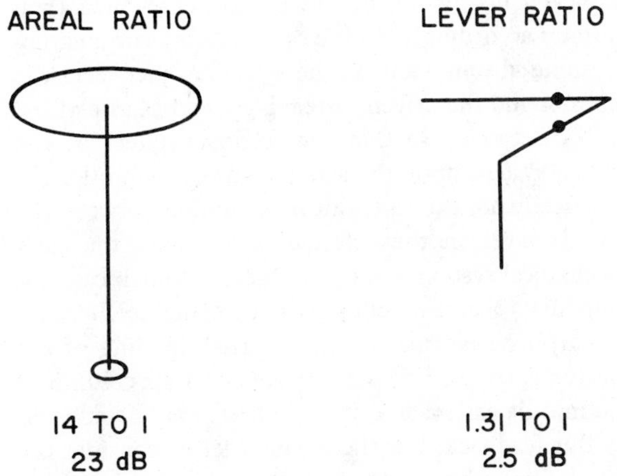

Fig. 10-12. The transformer action of the middle ear.

Some additional advantage is gained through the lever action of the ossicles. Experimental measures of this have indicated a gain in pressure of about 1.31 : 1, which again decreases the air-liquid interface disadvantage, although only by an additional 2.5 dB (Dahmann, 1929, 1930).

This combination of the areal ratio and lever action gives a total increase in effectiveness of vibration transfer of 25.5 dB, which fails by 4.5 dB in making up for the loss of energy at the air-liquid interface. This indicates that the middle ear mechanism is not perfect, but it must be kept in mind that the data on which these figures are based may be somewhat in error because of the difficulties of making the experimental determinations. On the other hand, if the figures are correct, removal of the middle ear system should result in a hearing loss of only 25.5 dB, and not the theoretical 30 dB, providing the round window is protected from vibrations which can cancel the effectiveness of those entering the oval window.

Minute pressure changes at the tympanic membrane associated with the passage of sound produce the movement of the ossicular chain. Thus, the ossicular chain is forced to vibrate, and any object so driven exerts its own characteristics upon the transmitted vibrations and at the same time reflects these characteristics back to the driver.

FORCED VIBRATIONS

The tympanic membrane, with its attached malleus, vibrates because it is linked to sound waves originating in some distant source. Energy from the sound waves is picked up by the middle-ear system which then vibrates accordingly. In the case of sounds originating in some distant source the coupling between the vibrator and the driven system is loose, because of the air in between, so that the feedback effect of the driven system upon the actual source of vibrations is practically nonexistent. But the coupling between the sound waves in the external meatus and the ear's mechanical system is much tighter, in which case the immediate feedback effect is not negligible. Because an earphone closing off the external opening of the meatus is coupled by a relatively short air column to the middle ear system, the earphone may be affected by this feedback. For the moment let us consider the simple case where we need be concerned only with a periodic force supplied by a driving system to a driven, damped system.

In this consideration a mass is maintained in a state of vibration by a vibrating force that may or may not have the same frequency as the natural frequency of the driven mass. We would like to know the characteristics of the forced vibrations just after the force has been applied and after it has been acting for a long period of time. What we have to determine is the resistance to motion that the driven system presents at various driving frequencies.

The damping factor in a driven system is always present, and its effect is to oppose the forcing vibrations. This is called the *mechanical resistance*, R_m, and is proportional to the force applied independent of frequency.

This applied force, in moving the driven mass from its equilibrium position, must overcome the stiffness of the system. This kind of resistance depends upon the frequency, and the greater the stiffness, the higher the natural frequency. In order to distinguish frequency-dependent resistance from the frequency-independent resistance the former is called *reactance*. It is obvious that the stiffer the system the greater this reactance, and the higher the driving frequency the less reactance this stiffness will have. We may say, then, that the stiffness reactance (X_s) varies directly with the stiffness (S) and inversely with the driving frequency: ω or $2\pi f$.

$$X_s = \frac{S}{2\pi f}$$

The inertia of the mass brought into evidence by the change in its position also offers resistance, dependent on the frequency of the applied force. The natural frequency of a system is lowered by an increase in mass. Mass reactance (X_m), then, varies directly with an increase in mass (M) and frequency (ω).

$$X_m = M \cdot 2\pi f$$

Visualize now the tine of a tuning fork being forced to vibrate in simple harmonic motion. As the applied force causes the tine to move away from its equilibrium position the magnitude of the stiffness reactance appears to lag behind the velocity of motion by 90°, whereas the mass reactance appears to lead the velocity by 90°. At the end of an excursion stiffness reactance has reached its maximum, while, by virtue of now being in motion, mass reactance has fallen to zero until the motion is stopped and the tine has started on its return trip. The two reactances oppose each other. The mechanical resistance R_m, on the other hand, is directly proportional to the velocity. The one resistance and two reactances all figure into a total amount of opposition to the applied vibrating force, but, because of the phase differences, they must be added vectorially.

In Fig. 10-13, A shows the way the mechanical resistance, R_m, and mass reactance, X_m, are plotted in magnitude; similarly in Fig. 10-13, B shows the effects of mechanical resistance and stiffness reactance, X_s. Because X_m and X_s oppose each other they must be subtracted, giving the vector, b, as shown in C, Fig. 13.

Applying the Pythagorean theorem the total mechanical impedance, Z_m, can be found.

$$Z_m = \sqrt{R_m^2 + (X_m - X_s)^2}$$

Diagram C, Fig. 10-13 shows us not only the magnitude of the mechanical impedance but also the phase angle of the forced vibration. The tangent of this angle θ is equal to the quotient $\frac{X_m - X_s}{R_m}$ or

$$\theta = \tan - 1 \frac{X_m - X_s}{R_m}$$

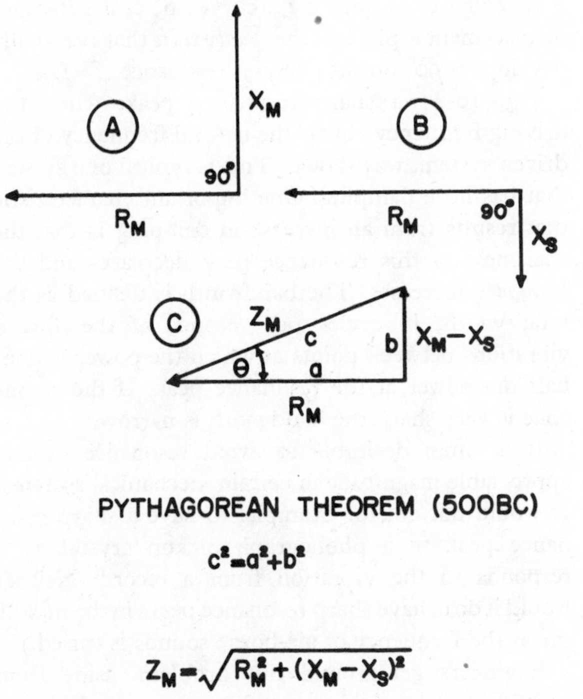

Fig. 10-13. Derivation of the impedance formula : see text.

This diagram also shows that when mass reactance equals stiffness reactance there is resonance of the driven system, because, in this case, the only opposing force is the mechanical resistance of the frictional forces.

At resonance, large amplitudes of vibration may result if the damping is small. A pendulum may be set in motion with large amplitudes if a succession of small forces are each applied at the right moment. A crystal wineglass may be sharply tuned to a certain frequency that causes the glass to vibrate violently and shatter when sound vibrations in the air are of the right frequency. If there is considerable damping in the forced system the vibration produced at resonance will not be as great as with little damping.

It is also possible to force a system to vibrate at frequencies other than its natural frequency, but two things happen. The vibrations are much smaller than those at resonance and the phase is shifted relative to that of the driving system. If the driving frequency is higher than the natural frequency of the driven system the velocity of the forced vibration will lag in phase relative to that of the driver. If the driving frequency is lower than the natural frequency of the driven system, the velocity of the forced vibrations will lead in phase relative to that of the driver. Why this is so can be visualized by reference again to Fig. 10-13.

The size and position of phase angle θ is determined by the relative magnitude of stiffness reactance or mass reactance.

As a driving vibration, which changes frequency from low to high, passes through the resonance point of a driven system there is a rapid phase shift. Recall the illustration of the resonance theory of hearing illustrated in Fig. 10-8, (a) which shows the regions above and below the resonance point in opposite phase. This is shown graphically in Fig. 10-14. At the natural frequency (f_n) of the driven system, the resonance velocity is in phase with the driving vibrations, while displacement lags by 90°. Because in our study of the ear we are primarily interested in the displacement, this has been plotted in the curve of Fig. 10-14. The ordinate shows displacement lagging by 90° at the resonance frequency. When the driving frequency is higher than f_n both the mechanical reactance and phase angle are positive, so that the lag of displacement approaches 180°. When the driving frequency is lower than f_n both the mechanical recatance and phase angle are negative, so that the lag of displacement is reduced.

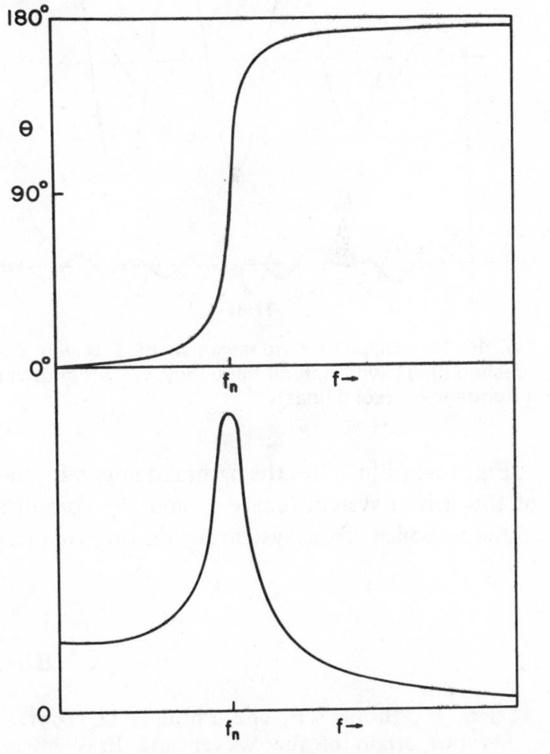

Fig. 10-14. Displacement phase and amplitude of vibrating system with natural frequency, f_n, driven by varying frequency, f.

It is interesting now to see what happens to a driven system when a vibrating force is first applied. At the very beginning of the application the motion is complicated, being a combination of two harmonic motions: that of the driver and that of the natural frequency of the driven system. However, the effect is fleeting and the motion of the driven system soon becomes that of the driver. In the study of hearing, however, this *transient* response may be important because the natural frequency of the conductive system may be in a region of hearing whereas the driving frequency may fall in a frequency region of deafness. Sudden onset of a tone must thus be avoided. An earphone or speaker will, of course, also have these characteristics.

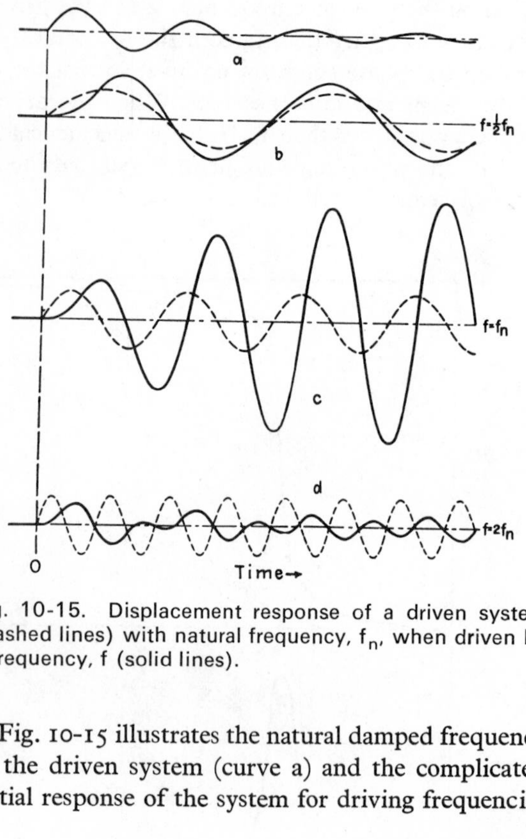

Fig. 10-15. Displacement response of a driven system (dashed lines) with natural frequency, f_n, when driven by a frequency, f (solid lines).

Fig. 10-15 illustrates the natural damped frequency of the driven system (curve a) and the complicated initial response of the system for driving frequencies $\frac{1}{2}$ f_n, equal to f_n, and 2 f_n (curves b, c, d). Because displacement is plotted, the *steady state* that eventually develops is 90° out of phase at resonance ($f=f_n$).

Fig. 10-14 a sharp resonance peak, when the driving frequency equals the natural frequency of the driven system, was shown. This is typical of a system that has little damping. One important characteristic that results from an increase in damping is that the sharpness of this resonance peak decreases and the *bandwith* increases. The bandwidth is defined as the total width, in cycles per second, of the forced vibrations between points at which the power is one-half the power at the resonance peak. If the resonance is very sharp the bandwidth is narrow.

It is often desirable to avoid resonance of any appreciable magnitude in certain mechanical systems. It would not do, for example, to have a sharp resonance peak in a phonograph pickup crystal as it responds to the vibration from a record. Neither would it do to have sharp resonance peaks in the middle ear as the frequency of air-borne sounds is varied.

Engineers get around this problem, aside from building compensating amplifiers (equalizers), in one or any combination of three mechanical methods: 1) by tuning the driven system to a frequency much higher than the frequency range of the driver, called *stiffness controlled*; 2) by tuning the driven system to a frequency much lower than the frequency range of the driver, called *mass controlled*; or 3) by increasing the damping and thereby spreading the bandwidth, called *resistance controlled*. Obviously the ear must incorporate some of these methods in order to avoid resonance.

The frequency-response characteristics of the ear's mechanical system will, of course, be reflected in the threshold sensitivity curve of hearing. Failure of a device to respond equally well to all driving frequencies is called frequency distortion, and the ear certainly demonstrates this. Therefore, because certain diseases of the ear change its mechanical properties, it becomes necessary to analyze how these properties contribute to the sensitivity of the ear.

BIBLIOGRAPHY

Adrian, E., Bronk, D., and Phillips, G. 1931. The nervous origin of the Wever and Bray effect. *J. Physiol.*, 73, 2P-3P.

Bast, I., and Eyster, J. 1935. Tone localization in the cochlea. *Amer. Otol. Rhinol. Laryngol.*, 44, 792–803.

Békésy, G. 1960. Experiments in hearing. New York: McGraw-Hill.

———. 1967. Sensory inhibition. Princeton N.J.: Princeton.

Breschet, G. 1836. Recherches anatomique et physiologiques sur l'organne de l'ouie et sur l'audition. *Mem. Acad. Roy. Med.*, Paris., 5, 229–523.

Claudius, M. 1856. Bemerkungen über den Bau der hautigen Spiralleiste der Schnecke. *Zeits. f. wiss. Zool.*, 7, 154–161.

Corti, A. 1851. Recherches sur l'organe de l'ouie des mammifères. *Zeits. f. wiss. Zool.*, 3, 109–169.

Cotugno, D. 1774. De aquaeductibus auris humanae internae. (1st. ed. Naples, 1760). Viennae.

Dahmann, H. 1929, 1930. Zur physiologie des Hörens; experimentelle Untersuchungen über die Mechanik der Gehörknöchelchenkette, sowie über deren Verhalten auf Ton und Luftdruck. *Zeits. f. Hals-Nasen-Ohrenheilk.*, 24, 462–497, and 27, 329–368.

Deiters, O. 1860. Untersuchungen über die Lamina spiralis membranacea. Bonn.

DuVerney, J. 1683. Traite de l'organe de l'ouie. Paris: E. Michallet.

Engstrom, H., Ades, H., and Hawkins, J., Jr. 1962. Structure and function of the sensory hairs of the inner ear. *J. acoust. soc. Amer.*, 34, 1356–1363.

Ewald, J., 1898. Ueber eine neue Hörtheorie. *Wien. klin. Wochenschr.*, 11, 721.

Foa, C., and Peroni, A. 1930. Primi tentative di registrazione delle correnti d'azione del nervo acustico. *Arch. di. fisiol.*, 28, 237–241, and *Valsalva.*, 6, 105–109.

Forbes, A., Miller, R., and O'Connor, J. 1927. Electric responses to acoustic stimuli in the decerebrate animal. *Amer. J. Physiol.*, 80, 363–380.

Hallpike, C., and Rawdon-Smith, A. 1934a. The "Wever and Bray" phenomenon. A study of the electrical response in the chochlea with special reference to its origin. *J. Physiol.*, 81, 395–408.

———. 1934b. The origin of the Wever and Bray phenomenon. *J. Physiol.*, 83, 243–254.

Helmholtz, H. 1954. On the sesations of tone. Eng. tran. by Ellis, A. (4th. ed.). New York: Dover. P. 576.

Hensen, V. 1863. Zur Morphologie der Schnecke des Menschen und der Saugethiere. *Zeits. f. wiss. Zool.*, 13, 481–512.

Huschke, E. 1835. Ueber die Gehörzahne, einen eigenthümlichen Apparat in der Schencke des Vogelohrs. *Arch. f. Anat. Physiol.*, 335–346.

———. 1844. Lehre von den Eingeweiden und Sinnesorganen des menschlichen Körpers. *In* Vom Bau des menschlichen Körpers. (vol. 5). Von Sommerring, S., ed. Leipzig: L. Voss.

Kolliker, A. 1849. Beiträge zur Kenntniss der glutten Muskeln. *Zeits. f. wiss. Zool.*, 1, 48–87.

Lawrence, M. 1965. Dynamic range of the cochlear transducer. Cold Spring Harbor Symposium on Quantitative Biology. *Sensory Receptors*, 30, 159–167.

———, Wolsk, D., and Burton, R. 1959. Stimulation deafness, cochlear patterns, and significance of electrical recording methods. *Ann. Otol. Rhinol. Laryng.*, 68, 5–33.

Meckel, P. 1777. De labyrinthi auris contentis. Argentorati.

Ohm, G. 1843. Ueber die Definition des Tones, nebst daran geknüpfter Theorie der Sirene und ähnlicher tonbildender Vorrichtungen. *Ann. d. Phys.*, 59, 497, 565.

Reissner, E. 1851. De auris internae formatione. *Dorpat* (Livonia).

Retzius, G. 1892. Die Endigungsweise des Gehörnerven. *Biol. Unters.*, 3, 29–36.

Rutherford, W. 1886. A report of his earlier lecture is reported as A new theory of hearing. *J. anat. physiol.*, 21, 166–168.

Stevens, S. 1958. Measurement and man. *Science*, 127, 383–389.

Tasaki, I., Davis, H., and Eldredge, D. 1954. Exploration of cochlear potentials in guinea pig with microelectrode. *J. acoust. soc. Amer.*, 26, 765–773.

Todd, R., and Bowman, W. 1845. The physiological anatomy and physiology of man. London: Parker.

Wever, E. 1949. Theory of hearing. New York: Wiley.

———, and Bray, C. 1930a. Action currents in the auditory nerve in response to acoustical stimulation. *Proc. Nat. Acad. Sci.*, 16, 344–350.

———. 1930b. Auditory nerve impulses. *Science*, 71, 215.

———, and Lawrence, M. 1954. Physiological acoustics. Princeton, N.J.: Princeton.

11

Sensitivity of the Ear

Merle Lawrence[1]

Before one can analyze the cause of acoustic distortions in the abnormal ear, distortions introduced by the healthy ear must be understood. The first step is a study of the normal threshold sensitivity curve, which reveals that the entire process of hearing, from movement of air particles at the tympanic membrane to conscious registration of sound, demonstrates considerable insensitivity to certain frequency ranges. For threshold sensitivity, the minimum audible sound pressure at 20 Hz is about 10,000 times, and for 15,000 Hz about 100 times, greater than that for 1,000 Hz. This unequal sensitivity constitutes frequency distortion in a physical sense, i.e., all frequencies are not relayed equally for a given driving amplitude, and the immediate question concerns the extent to which the various stages of the hearing process contribute to this distortion.

Because the sound-conduction process of hearing is one of forced vibrations, and because pathological conditions in the ear most often change the characteristics of this process, it is of importance to determine how much the acoustic response of the ear contributes to the threshold sensitivity curve.

DRIVING AMPLITUDES AT THRESHOLD

In a classic investigation reported by Sivian and White (1933), the threshold sensitivity of the human ear was determined for several conditions. The first was a free-field method in which the threshold was established with the observer facing the sound source and listening with both ears. The second was a closed-ear procedure in which the observer listened with earphones, the threshold being determined from the calibration of the earphones or by means of a probe tube whose tip lay within the space enclosed by the earphone and the ear. This latter type of measure was expressed either in terms of binaural threshold or uniaural threshold. Here we are interested in the threshold sensitivity of the single ear at various frequencies, and the curve of this threshold is plotted as the solid line in Fig. 11-1. Whereas binaural free-field listening shows the ears to be maximally sensitive between the frequencies of 2000–4000 Hz, probably because of the sound-reflecting properties of the head and pinnas, the uniaural closed-ear procedure shows maximum sensitivity at 1000 Hz. The sound-pressure

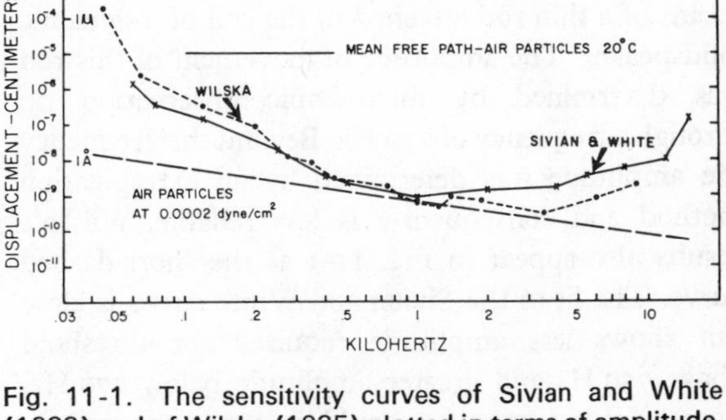

Fig. 11-1. The sensitivity curves of Sivian and White (1933) and of Wilska (1935) plotted in terms of amplitude.

[1] Preparation of this material has been supported, in part, by grant NB-05785 from the National Institute of Neurological Diseases and Blindness, United States Public Health Service.

level as determined by the probe at this point is 0.00035 dyne/cm². The figure 0.0002 dyne/cm², usually used as Sound Pressure Level (SPL) reference, represents an increase in sensitivity of three dB when both ears are used. As shown in Fig. 11-1, the sensitivity of one ear is fairly flat between 1,000 Hz and 4,000 Hz, becoming less sensitive for the higher and lower frequencies.

Because we are interested in the resonance characteristics of the sound-conduction mechanism of the ear this curve has been plotted in terms of the amplitude of vibration at the various pressures needed for different frequencies to reach threshold. The displacement amplitude, A, of air particles in a free sound field can be determined by the formula

$$A = \frac{P}{2\pi f R}$$

where P equals sound pressure in dynes/cm², f equals the frequency, and R equals the specific acoustic resistance. The specific acoustic resistance of sound in air, under standard conditions, is 41.5 mechanical ohms per sq. cm.

Because 0.0002 dyne/cm² is conventionally used as a reference level for sound pressure, the amplitude of displacement of the air particles throughout the audible range of frequencies for this constant pressure is also shown as the long-dashed line in Fig. 11-1. It is immediately obvious that threshold sensitivity as determined by an observer is not linearly related to the amplitude of movement of the air particles at the opening of the ear.

At this point it becomes essential to know the amplitude of movement of the handle of the malleus for the audible frequency range at threshold. Although Békésy and others have had the opportunity to make such determinations by use of the capacitative probe, only one study has been carried out that gives the specific amplitude data.

Wilska (1935) drove the tympanic membrane by means of a thin rod attached to the coil of a dynamic loudspeaker. The amplitude of movement of this rod was determined by microscopic observation up through a frequency of 270 Hz. Beyond this frequency the amplitude was determined by an extrapolation method and consequently is less reliable. Wilska's results also appear in Fig. 11-1 as the short-dashed curve. The fit to the Sivian and White curve is close but shows less amplitude required for threshold above 750 Hz and greater amplitude below 270 Hz. Some of this discrepancy could be due to the calibration in both measurements, but some could also be due to other factors such as the relationship between tympanic-membrane vibration and that of the ossicular chain.

It is obvious that the ear is extremely sensitive to the organized pattern of air-particle vibration. Under normal conditions the air particles move about randomly, traveling over an average distance of 9.29×10^{-6} cm, called the Mean Free Path, before colliding with another particle, and yet the ear is sensitive to movements of 10^{-9} cm, an amplitude of molecular dimensions. Obviously, a sound wave in air organizes the random movements of air particles so as to superimpose the minute movements upon the random ones, effectively moving the tympanic membrane. The random movements are not heard because they are equal on both sides of the tympanic membrane; they must be or one would hear a constant roar. This is similar in principle to a noise-canceling microphone in which the diaphragm is freely exposed to the noise on both sides but the speaker directs his voice to one side only.

In order to achieve this noise-canceling property the temperature on both sides of the tympanic membrane must be equal. The tympanic membrane is recessed in a one-inch hole not only for protection but also so that the external air temperature will be the same as that in the middle ear. Indeed, it is found (Benzinger and Taylor, 1963) that body temperature can be determined by careful measurements made deep in the external meatus.

FREQUENCY RESPONSE OF THE CONDUCTIVE MECHANISM

It must be remembered that the threshold sensitivity curves shown in Fig. 11-1 reflect the entire hearing process, i.e., they include not only the vibration characteristics of the conductive mechanism but those frequency selective properties that might be involved in the transduction process, the nerve-conduction process, cortical and higher-center activities and finally, the response mechanisms by which the listener indicates that he has heard.

In order to determine the role played by the sound-conduction mechanism, methods other than those employing behavioral responses must be sought. There are four different methods that have been used, each of which has certain limitations but they are worth considering.

1. The vibration characteristic of each vibratory part can be studied and then all of these could theoretically be added up to give the total response picture. The trouble is that the vibratory characteristics of any part depend upon the next part and so cannot be considered as an isolated element.

2. A measure of effective vibration such as the cochlear microphonic response can be used with and without the middle ear present, the difference presumably giving vibratory characteristics of the middle ear. Here again the inner ear, driven directly by sound, may not act the same as when driven by the ossicular chain and so the result may be confounded by other factors. Also, the pressure-transformation characteristics are added to the frequency response, confusing the results.

3. The transient response of the system in response to a pulse of energy would give the natural frequency of the entire system, but this would not give an accurate picture of how the system behaves at other frequencies when forced to vibrate.

4. Impedance measures at the tympanic membrane can be used. From these data the transmission characteristics can be determined, but such measures determine only what happens at the tympanic membrane, and if the movement of such parts of the membrane as the *pars flaccida* have little effect in moving the malleus the impedance would not reflect accurately the vibration of the entire system.

Despite the drawbacks of these various methods it is beneficial to review some of the experiments because these represent the only data we have at present from which to gather information on the response to vibrations forced by movement of the air particles.

Method one. The actual vibrating system, as pointed out before, consists of the external meatus, the tympanic membrane, the ossicles, and the fluids of the inner ear from the footplate of the stapes to the membrane covering the round window. In addition to these structures there are certain elements that could influence the vibration in indirect ways. One of these consists of the air cavities of the middle ear, antrum, and mastoid. Another lies in the nature of coupling at the malleoincudal and incudostapedial joints, and a third in the tympanic muscles.

For all practical purposes one must include the external meatus as part of the conductive mechanism. This external ear canal can be considered as a tube closed at one end: about 2.5 cm long and about 0.7 cm in diameter. As everyone who has blown across the mouth of a soda bottle knows, such a tube has a definite resonant frequency and, in the case of the external canal, this is in the vicinity of 3,400–3,900 Hz. Wiener and Ross (1946) have made measurements of this by use of probe tubes, and their results are plotted in Fig. 11-2. This area of resonance is not sharp because the closure of the tube at the membrane end is not rigid but sound-absorbing. This acts as a frictional force broadening the responses with a maximum gain of about 12 dB. Other investigators have made similar determinations using different methods and have come up with slightly different figures, although close enough so as not to be disturbing.

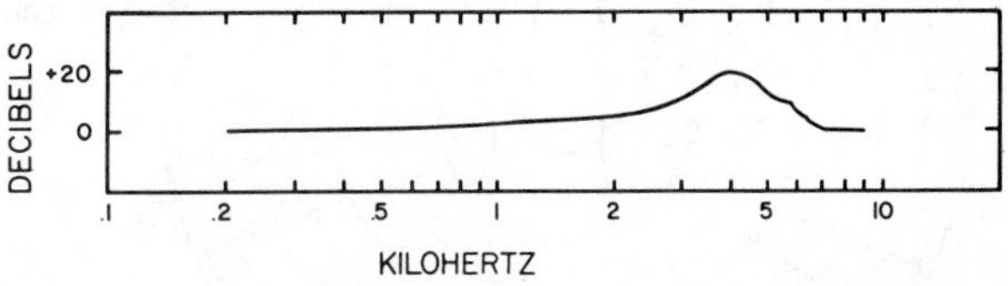

Fig. 11-2. Resonance of the external meatus as determined by Wiener and Ross (1946).

Fleming (1939) established resonance in a broader range: 3,000–4,000 Hz, and Békésy (1960, pp. 270–271), calculating from impedance measures and the cross-sectional dimension of the meatus, arrived at a figure of 2,400 Hz. He states further that because different parts of the tympanic membrane vibrate independently above 800 Hz, there are several areas of resonance. However, in a later paper (1960, p. 101), he says this independent vibration characteristic occurs at a higher frequency (he mentions two figures 2,000 Hz and 2,400 Hz) and hence leaves his several resonances unexplained. Because the Wiener and Ross figure is the most consistent this seems the most acceptable.

As has been described in the preceding chapter, the tympanic membrane plays a most important function in the hearing process. It has many unique anatomical as well as acoustic properties.

A fine description of the arrangement of fibers making up the tympanic membrane is given by Kirikae (1950) and is illustrated in Fig. 11-3. Of particular interest are the groups of "parabolic fibers" and the "transverse fibers." The former presumably transmit vibrations of the tympanic membrane to the "short process of the malleus" (Kirikae), and the latter provide support at the intermediate zone of the inferior quadrant where amplitude is greatest, an observation made by Békésy (1960).

Békésy determined the pattern of tympanic membrane vibration by means of a capacitative probe. This probe is a device that can detect very small displacements by measuring the electrical charge occurring in the space between the vibrating body and a small plate connected to a specialized circuit. The small plate and the tympanic membrane in this case make up a capacitor which gives the probe its name.

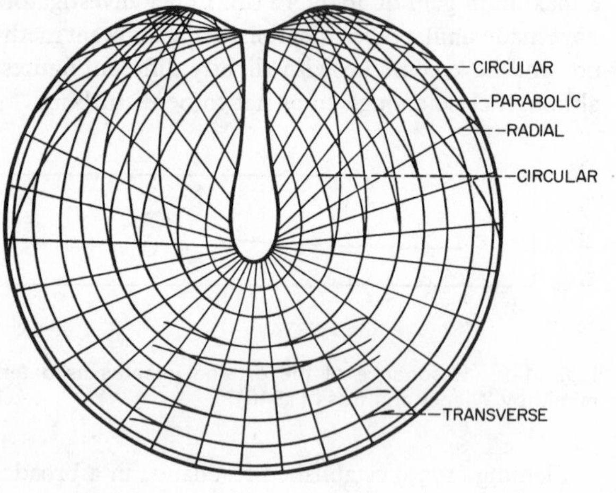

Fig. 11-3. Fibers of the tympanic membrane according to Kirikae (1950).

The entire tympanic membrane behaves as a stiff plate rotating about on axis at the edge of the *pars flaccida*. Because of this stiffness and the nature of the axis, the maximum amplitude is not at the umbo of the malleus but about halfway between it and the annulus. It is possible for the membrane to move in this way because of the presence, at the lower edge, of an elastic fold with a radius of curvature of 0.5 to 0.8 mm. This fold allows the membrane to vibrate as a whole, for frequencies below 2,400 Hz, without any marked deformation except at the edges. Above this frequency the stiffness of the curved portion of the membrane becomes ineffective and the manubrium lags behind the motion of the rest of the membrane as it undergoes rather independent motion, so that all of the acoustic energy is not transmitted to the malleus. In this connection it should be pointed out that the pressure transformation between membrane and stapes is independent of frequency up to 2,400 Hz, indicating that the natural frequency of the tympanic membrane is relatively high.

The motions of the tympanic membrane are not only transmitted to the ossicular chain and fluids but to the air of the middle ear as well. And the acoustic behavior of this entrapped air has an effect upon the movement of the membrane which, in turn, affects the vibratory pattern of the conductive system.

Several factors enter into the determination of the acoustic characteristics of the middle-ear air cavities. Not only is it necessary to consider the total volume but also the nature of the narrow passage between the tympanic cavity and the other spaces, as well as the conversion of energy into heat by the sound-absorbing tissues on the walls of the cavities.

Determining the exact volume of air in the middle ear, antrum, and mastoid is not an easy thing to do, and there are some differences in the published values. By several experimental methods Zwislocki (1962) has determined this volume to be around 8.6 cc whereas Onchi (1961) estimated it to be 3.45 cc. This seems to make little difference, however, as far as Zwislocki is concerned because the impedance of these air cavities is low compared to that of other parts of the middle ear, so the effect upon sound transmission is not critical.

On the other hand, Békésy (1960, pp. 109–110), by an acoustic-bridge method, determined the volume of the middle-ear cavities in cadaver males to be 2.0 cc on the average. These measurements were confirmed on persons lacking an eardrum. He further states that the portion of the middle ear occupied by the ossicles has a volume of 0.5 to 0.8 cc, the rest of the volume being made up of the pneumatic cells of the mastoid. The impedance of an air volume of 2.0 cc is the same as that measured at the eardrum in living persons for low frequencies, so Békésy concludes that the impedance of the eardrum, as measured from the meatus, not only includes the elastic properties of the membrane but those of the cavity air cushion as well. Because of the relatively great compliance of the tympanic membrane compared to the elastic forces of the air cushion, a small perforation in the membrane has little influence on the vibrations.

Békésy (1960, pp. 163–181) has pointed out further that the tympanic membrane could vibrate with the same amplitude as the air particles only by resonance. At the lower frequencies the tympanic membrane, even if weightless, would not have the same amplitude as the air particles because of the presence of the middle-ear air cushion. A cavity of 2.0 cc volume, V, closed with a weightless membrane whose surface area is 0.66 sq. cm., S, would produce a displacement of the membrane equal to:

$$A = \frac{VP}{\rho c^2 S}$$

The vibrations of the tympanic membrane are not determined by its own elasticity but by that of the air cushion. And Békésy points out that this type of vibration is independent of the driving frequency (the driving pressure being held constant). Only at frequencies around 1,000 Hz is the amplitude of the tympanic membrane equal to that of the air particles. Complicated resonances influence the movement of the membrane above this frequency in an irregular manner.

The amplitude of vibration for the tympanic membrane as calculated by Békésy and for the air particles in a free sound field for a uniform pressure of 0.0002 dyne/cm² are plotted in Fig. 11-4. If the volume of the middle ear cavity, influencing the vibration of the tympanic membrane, is 8.6 cc as stated by Zwislocki the amplitude would of course be increased by a factor of 4.3, which would still not be the same as the air particles at low frequencies. The curve for the tympanic membrane in Fig. 11-4 does not take into account the resonance of the external meatus.

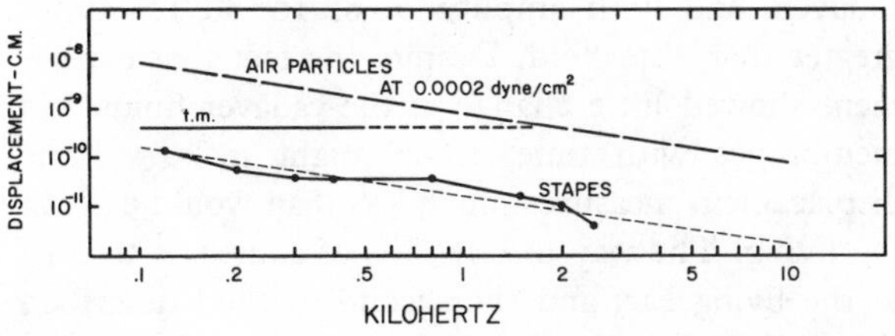

Fig. 11-4. Amplitude displacement of tympanic membrane (t.m.) and stapes according to Békésy (1960). Copyright, 1960, McGraw-Hill Book Company. By permission.

The vibrations of the tympanic membrane are communicated directly to the malleus, then through the incus to the stapes. In between these are two joints, and considerable discussion has been presented concerning the ability of these joints to follow the communicated vibrations.

Anatomically the malleoincudal and the incudostapedial joints differ considerably. The former appears to be a firm attachment through the rather large surface area; the incus fits into the head of the malleus like a rider in a saddle. The latter appears as a flimsy attachment with a small surface area, however, and the incus is capable of some movement even when the stapes is fixed. Some experimenters in the past have even claimed that the malleoincudal joint is ankylosed, but in man it most certainly is not. These are true joints and apparently serve two important functions. They allow for the action of the tympanic muscles in fixing one of the bones with respect to the others, and they allow for some differential movement of one ossicle with respect to the one attached to it as displacement amplitude is lost while pressure is gained through the transformer action. One should be able to measure the amplitude of movement of the handle of the malleus and the footplate of the stapes and obtain an exact measure, not only of the transformer action, but of the frequency-dependent changes caused by the resonance of the three ossicles. Békésy did not give quantitative measures of malleus displacement for a given sound pressure at various frequencies, but he did for the footplate of the stapes (1960, p. 103).

These were determined by the capacitative probe at a constant sound pressure on the tympanic membrane of 1 dyne/cm². Assuming the response to be linear with lesser pressures, the displacement amplitude has been recalculated for uniform pressure of 0.0002 dyne/cm² and plotted in Fig. 11-4. The faintly dotted line through this curve is 26 dB below the 0.0002 dyne/cm² line representing the displacement amplitude of the air particles, and is exactly what the transformer properties of the ossicular chain produce. The curve of displacement amplitude for the ossicular chain varies from this line by no more than five dB, which is well within the experimental error for this type of measure, and, as Békésy points out, the measurements showed considerable variability. The fact that the ossicular displacement follows the movement of the air particles with so little variation with frequency is remarkable. Unfortunately, phase-shift measurements were not made, but the ossicular chain acts like a straight piston without any resonance at all within this frequency range. However, this is not a normal situation, for the stapes is normally backed by the fluids of the middle ear.

A year after the above experiments Békésy (1960, pp. 429–446) reported the determination of the volume displacement of the fluids of the inner ear to uniform sound pressures under various conditions. Rather than using the capacitative probe, a near impossibility because, in the human, the round window lies in a deep bony niche, he used a calibrated sound-canceling earphone in a tube connected to the round window niche by dental cement. By this method he was able to determine the phase-shift and volume displacement of the fluids under conditions in which the stapes and round window membrane were not present, when only the membrane of the round window was present, when the stapes footplate and round window membrane were present, and under normal conditions. It was demonstrated that the membrane of the round window is quite an important structure in controlling the overall frequency response of the entire sound-conduction system.

Some time later Békésy (1960, pp. 163–181) calculated, from the results of earlier experiments, the relative amplitudes of vibration of the tympanic membrane, stapes, and basilar membrane. His plots were on the basis of 134 dB SPL, so we have converted them to 0 dB SPL (0.0002 dyne/cm^2). These are shown in Fig. 11-5.

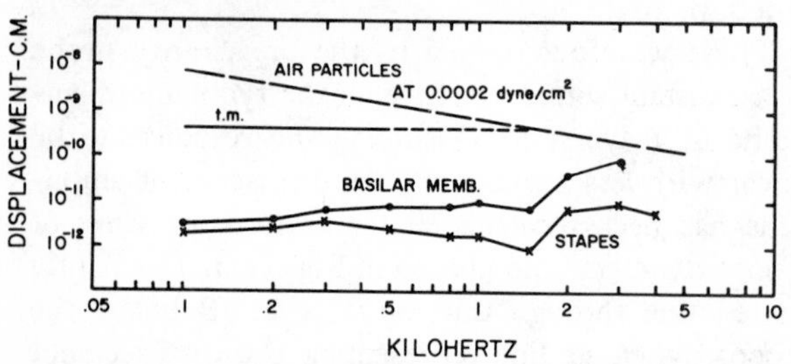

Fig. 11-5. Amplitude displacement of tympanic membrane (t.m.), basilar membrane and stapes according to Békésy (1960). Copyright, 1960, McGraw-Hill Book Company. By permission.

The amplitude of vibration for the tympanic membrane has already been shown in Fig. 11-4, and is repeated here for comparison with the other measurements. According to these calculations only around 1,000 to 2,000 Hz are the membrane vibrations equal to the air particles.

The amplitude of stapes vibration was calculated, first, by determining the pressure transformation caused by the resonance of the external canal, and combining this with figures obtained from the experiments on the volume displacement of the round window, by assuming that this measure is the same as that of the stapes.

From the calculations of the stapes' vibration amplitude Békésy further calculated, by an undescribed method, the vibration amplitude of the basilar membrane, which is greater than that of the stapes "because the surface area set into motion is smaller than the surface of the stapes."

From these curves it is obvious that, except in the external meatus, there are no resonances in the system anywhere, which is odd and certainly in disagreement with results obtained from other methods. It is also odd that the response is linear with sound pressure rather than amplitude but this might well be the result of the sound-canceling method used. As noted in Fig. 11-4, amplitude measures by means of the capacitative probe give different results although the conditions are somewhat different.

One might well be puzzled by the magnitude of these vibrations. As already pointed out, the Mean Free Path of the randomly moving air particles is considerably larger, by a factor of 10^4, than the calculated movement of the particles at threshold. Superimposing a patterned vibration upon a random motion of such relatively large magnitude is amazing and yet this is what Wilska's data show (1935).

The figures given by Békésy for the stapes and basilar membrane are also bewildering, especially when one considers the fact that these are of the order of 10^{-5} times less in amplitude than the thickness of the membrane surrounding a hair cell which is reported to be 60–80 Å based on electron microscopy.

It must be kept in mind that Békésy worked with cadavers and with amplitudes of 10^4 to 10^7 times greater than threshold. Despite the fact that experiment showed little change in the cadaver fluids and membranes with time, these might make volume displacement measures much less than would exist in the living. The way to test this, of course, is to turn to the living ear, and the second method described above has shown that resonances do exist in the middle ear structure.

Method Two. The ossicles do have mass and they are attached to the walls of the middle ear by ligaments, mucosal folds, and two muscles which provide stiffness. And the action of the footplate in the oval window, aside from the stiffness of the annular ligament, encounters frictional forces. The round window, at the other end of the system, also accounts for a stiffness factor, and the mass movement of the fluids contributes a great deal to the frictional or resistive forces.

From the flatness of the vibration curve, based on experiments just described and shown in Fig. 11-5, some sort of resonance control through remote tuning, multiple tuning, or high damping can be expected. That is, the response of the system to the frequencies of interest will not show sharp-resonant peaks because of the presence of control methods discussed earlier: mass control, stiffness control, or friction control. Experiments on the middle ears of animals have been rewarding in furnishing data for analyzing the resonance and phase characteristics.

Wever, Lawrence, and Smith (1948) made measurements of the middle-ear transformer action in cats by use of the cochlear potentials. The amount of sound at the tympanic membrane necessary to give a response of 10 microvolts for various frequencies from 100 to 10,000 Hz was first recorded. This was then compared with the amount of sound needed at the oval window to give the same response after removal of the middle ear. For present purposes the difference in sound pressure required under the two conditions has been plotted to show the resonance of the system. In Fig. 11-6 the abcissa represents the forcing frequency applied to the middle ear, while the ordinate shows the magnitude of response in decibels relative to the cochlear response with no middle ear present. The curve reflects both the transformer advantage of the middle ear and its resonances which, for the most part, determine the shape of the curve.

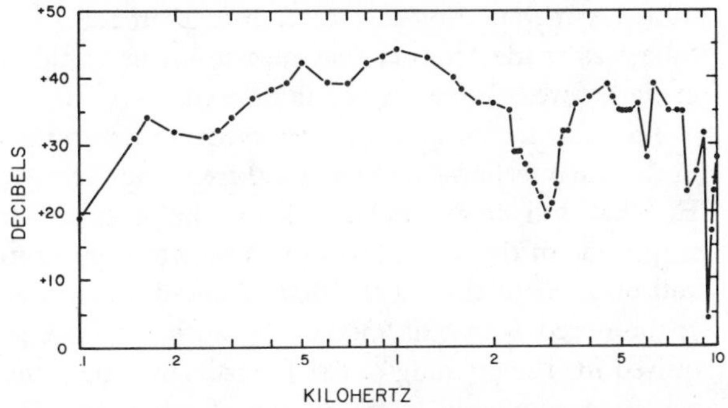

Fig. 11-6. Resonance of the middle ear of the cat as determined by measuring the electrical output of the ear in response to sound before and after removal of the ossicles. The overall gain in decibels also reflects the advantage of the transformer properties of the middle ear.

Several features of this curve are important, keeping in mind that this is the ear of a specific cat. There appear to be two regions of maximum sensitivity, one at 1,000 Hz and another centered in the vicinity of 4,500 to 6,300 Hz. Between these two regions, at 2,900 Hz, there is a point of relative insensitivity. Such a curve is quite common in the cat, and probably represents a double-tuned system having two peaks of resonance and an antiresonance in between. The middle ear obviously does not perform its transformer duties without exerting some of its own characteristics, but even at that the system does a remarkable job considering this is a response to nearly seven octaves. Apparently there is considerable damping present in order for the system to be as sensitive as it is and still be responsive over such a range.

As already mentioned, the phase of the system will also vary as the driving frequency is changed, and these phase changes have a specific relation to the areas of resonance. Where there are several masses and stiffnesses involved the variations of the phase of displacement with that of the force become complicated, but a study of this phase picture throws some light on the characteristics of the resonating system.

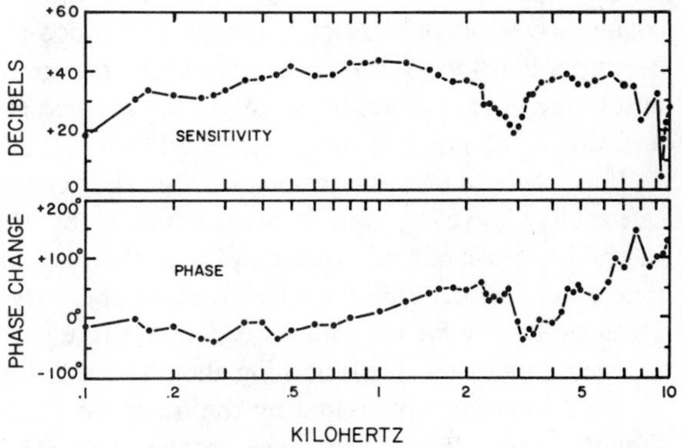

Fig. 11-7. Phase shift produced by the middle ear at indicated frequencies compared with the curve of resonance.

Fig. 11-7 shows the phase changes introduced by the middle ear as the frequency is varied from 100 to 10,000 Hz (Wever and Lawrence, 1954). The curve of Fig. 11-6 is also presented for comparison with the phase changes. Over the lower range, the tympanic membrane and ossicular chain produce a small advancement of phase. At about 1,000 Hz the displacement is in phase, but for frequencies above this, up to about 2,500 Hz, there is an increasing lag behind the driving force. At 3,000 Hz they are again in phase; between 3,000 and 4,000 Hz the middle ear phase is advanced, and at 4,000 Hz they are again in phase.

These measurements are all for the middle ear structures peripheral to the stapes. Similar phase measurements made for the stapes show that it exerts little influence until a driving frequency of 6,000 Hz is reached. Factors determining the response of the stapes are apparently tuned to a high frequency; a fact which should be borne in mind by the otologic surgeons when substitutes for the stapes are improvised.

The significance of these phase findings is that they confirm the triple-tuning characteristic revealed by the sensitivity measurements. In complicated vibrating systems the direction of phase change with frequency indicates the way in which the various masses and stiffnesses are behaving under the vibrations. In general, when, as the driving frequency is raised, a change in the forced phase from an advancement to a lagging takes place, the presence of a resonant point is indicated. At this point there should be a region of maximum amplitude. If the phase changes from a lagging one to an advanced one, a point of antiresonance is indicated, and there should be a region of minimum amplitude. With this in mind it can be seen from Fig. 11-7 that the two regions of resonance are at 1,000 Hz and 4,000 Hz, corresponding with the two points of maximum amplitude. An antiresonance point occurs at 3,000 Hz, and this is the point of minimum amplitude.

The contribution of resonance to the overall sensitivity, however, cannot be ascertained by this method because of the addition of the pressure transformation factor. This was also true of the curves given by Békésy for the cadaver ear. Also this electrical recording method tells nothing about the additions to the resonance contributed by the inner-ear fluids. Only by some method that considers the living ear in entirety can the total resonance of the system be determined.

There are two methods remaining by which this can be done: determination of the transient response and determination of the impedance characteristics. It is of interest to note that by a capacitative probe method Møller (1963) has obtained similar results in the cat to those obtained by the electrical method. He also found that the impedance of the ear as determined at the tympanic membrane is proportional, over almost the entire frequency range investigated, to the velocity (which is proportional to amplitude) of the incus. Unfortunately no quantitative measures were given in this investigation, but the results indicate that impedance measures are fairly good indicators of the vibratory response.

Before turning to impedance measures let us see what has been done in the way of determining the resonance of the sound-conduction mechanism by the transient method.

Method Three. It would seem to be a simple enough matter to displace the malleus and then release it as one would the tine of a tuning fork, or the weight of a pendulum. The resulting vibration would be the natural frequency, and the damping coefficient could be determined by measuring the rapidity with which the vibrations die out. Also revealed would be the frequency of the transient response resulting from sudden onset of a forcing frequency.

Determinations of this sort, however, are not easy to make because of the difficulties encountered in producing a satisfactory initial displacement and of observing the transient response. The sudden application of a direct current to a telephone receiver diaphragm produces transients in the diaphragm which would confuse the picture. Békésy (1960, pp. 314–315) solved this problem by having subjects produce a click by opening their Eustachian tube. When the tensor-veli-palatini muscle attached to the membranous wall of the tube is made to contract it pulls in the direction of the pharynx, expanding this portion of the tube and producing an abrupt change in air volume of the middle ear. The resulting click acts upon the tympanic membrane to produce the desired sudden displacement and subsequent transient response. A condenser microphone recorded the transient response, which was conducted from the tympanic membrane to the microphone through a tube 1.5 meters long and 0.7 cm in diameter. This tube was made long so that measurement could be made before tube resonance interfered.

The transient response of the eardrum determined in this manner indicated a natural frequency of 1,500 Hz that fell to 1,200 Hz during the decay. The amplitude of the second wave was between one-third and one-fourth that of the first. Some difficulty was encountered with this method because the time required for the opening of the Eustachian tube orifice was long compared to the period of vibration. This produced a distortion of the first half-period of the transient.

A few years later Békésy (1960, pp. 104–115) made similar measures on cadaver ears using the sound of an electric spark to serve as the pressure impulse rather than a click from the Eustachian tube. The spark-producing static machine was connected to the external meatus by a tube two meters long so that the ossicular vibrations would die down by the time the sound was reflected back to the source. A small 0.5 sq. mm mirror was attached to the manubrium so that a light beam could be reflected through an airtight glass window made in the side of the meatus.

The natural frequency of the ear's sound-conducting mechanism, as determined by this method, fell between 800 and 1,500 Hz, although some distortion was observed because of the rapid onset of the pulse. Placing cotton in the tube leading to the ear reduced this sharp wave front, and a transient response exactly like that produced in the living ear by a click from the Eustachian tube was obtained. The highly damped natural frequency as recorded from the manubrium is shown in Fig. 11-8.

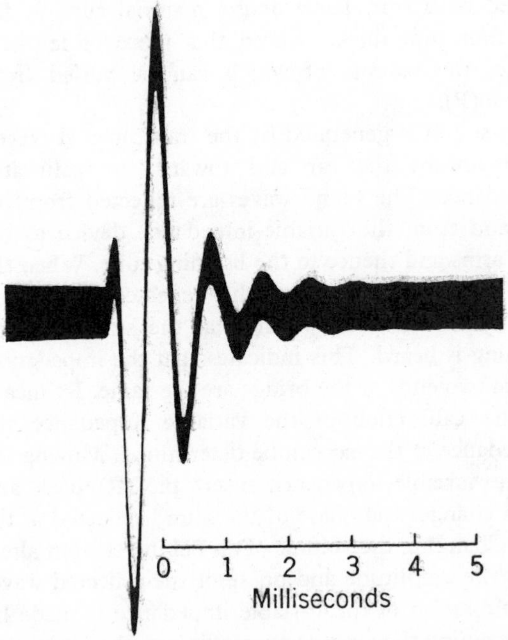

Fig. 11-8. Transient response of the human ear in response to a click as determined by Békésy (1960). Copyright, 1960, by McGraw-Hill Book Company. By permission.

From these observations and others on the vibration of the stapes already reported, Békésy concluded that the middle ear acts as a movable piston with great friction, and that, when loaded with the cochlear fluids, the entire sound-conduction system acts like a strongly damped vibratory mechanism with a natural frequency around 1,400 Hz. Békésy made these measurements both on cadaver ears and on ears of living persons. Because the recorded transient was more clearly portrayed in the cadaver than in the living ear, the cadaver response is the one shown in Fig. 11-8. Actually, for these ears, Békésy said the natural frequency was between 800 and 1,500 Hz, whereas it appears to be somewhat higher for the living ear. However, they are all in the same region and agree fairly well with earlier demonstrations, also on cadavers, by Frank (1923).

Although the damping coefficient was determined as between 0.25 and 0.33, little other information is gained by this transient response method. The frequency range of the ear covers several octaves, and more information is needed before the extent to which the characteristics of the sound-conduction mechanism contribute to the threshold sensitivity curve can be determined.

Impedance measurements can be made at the tympanic membrane and these reflect the resonances of the entire ear over most of the audible frequency range. This is the most satisfactory method to date for finding the answers we seek.

Method Four. In a situation where one listens to sound originating from a distant source there is little direct coupling between the source and the tympanic membrane because of the intermediate air. However, the coupling between the mass of air in the external meatus and the tympanic membrane is more direct, and a condition is encountered whereby the driven system has an influence on the driving system (the air). Sound in air, on meeting an interface, has three things happen to it: some of the energy is transmitted to the second medium, some is reflected, and that which is reflected interacts with the original sound causing diffraction so that a new waveform is produced. We have, in the previous chapter, discussed the relationship between the transmitted energy and the reflected energy.

The nature of the new waveform produced by the process of diffraction is determined by the amplitude and phase of the reflected wave. The feedback of energy from the driven system to the driver depends upon both impedances and the degree of coupling. In the case of a distant vibrator producing sound which reaches the tympanic membrane through the air there is little feedback to the vibrating source: the systems are loosely coupled. If, however, we treat the air in the external meatus as the source, the feedback influence is more direct: the coupling is tighter but not as tight as it would be were a vibrating rod driving the malleus directly.

Actually this is a situation where the diffraction effects in the external meatus are of academic interest only because this column of air is part of the hearing system. However, one can take advantage of the reflected waves in determining the impedance of the ear's conductive mechanism. It has already been pointed out that the mass, stiffness, and damping characteristics of a system determine the phase (with respect to the driver) and amplitude of forced vibrations. The possibility exists, therefore, of using some measure of the phase and amplitude to determine the impedance of the driven system.

Determination of the impedance reveals the extent to which energy is utilized by the system at various frequencies. This is the basis for the interest in determining the impedance of the ear. Such determinations would appear to have considerable clinical use because any lesion that changes the mass, stiffness, or damping of the sound-conducting system will change the impedance.

The acoustic impedance bridges used in determining the impedance of the ear are devices made to measure the amplitude and phase of the sound wave reflected from the tympanic membrane and the system attached to it. The basic design of these bridges was originally devised by Schuster in 1934, and later by Robinson in 1937, for determining the sound-absorbing properties of different materials. The tube used in this bridge was about an inch in diameter, which made it awkward to use in the external meatus for the obvious reason that it would not fit.

In 1938 Waetzmann described a modification of the original Schuster bridge, the essential revision being the use of a six mm diameter pipe tipped with a small olive that could be inserted into the opening of the external meatus. An excellent monograph describing this modified bridge and its use has been published by Otto Metz (1946).

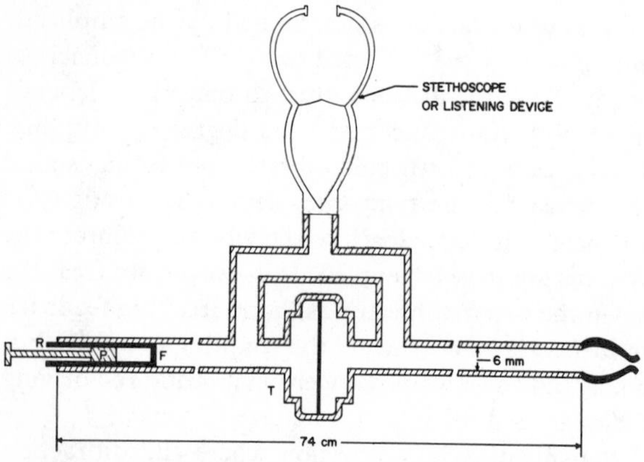

Fig. 11-9. Diagram of the Waetzmann (1938) impedance bridge.

The bridge system is diagrammed in Fig. 11-9. It consists of a sound transducer (T), such as an earphone driven by an electronic oscillator, placed at the center of a 74 cm long, six mm diameter pipe, so that generated sound spreads out within the pipe in both directions. At one end is an olive-shaped insert that can be fitted into the patient's ear while at the other end is a calibrated variable-impedance device. Symmetrically arranged on each side of the transducer are side arms which form a yoke connected to a common tube and a listening device such as a stethoscope.

The calibrated variable impedance consists of a pipe (R) which can slide inside the open end of the longer pipe. The inserted end of this sliding pipe is closed by a soft, fairly dense, material such as felt (F) four mm thick. Behind this piece of felt is a space, the volume of which can be varied by a piston (P).

As sound is generated by the transducer it travels both toward the ear and toward the calibrated impedance. The sound waves are reflected from the ear and from the variable-impedance device to the side arms and thence to the listening tube. When the amplitude and phase of the reflected waves are exactly the same they cancel at the side tube and nothing is heard. This indicates that the impedances at the two ends of the bridge are the same. By means of the calibration of the variable impedance the impedance of the ear can be determined. Moving the entire variable-impedance insert pie (R) back and forth changes the phase of the sound reflected at the felt. Changing the volume of air behind the felt alters both the amplitude and phase of the reflected wave.

Calibration of the variable impedance is made by determining the absorption coefficient, the amplitude reflection coefficient, and the phase change, all in terms of the length of the air column behind the felt pad. There is no need to go into the details here because the method is adequately described by Metz (1946) and in Schuster and Stohr (1939); also, present-day commercially available instruments have their own calibration methods.

Impedance measurements of the ear can be of great clinical value, if they are carefully carried out, because the impedance will be varied by any changes in mass, stiffness, or frictional forces of the middle ear. In order for these measures to have significance, however, the impedance of the normal ear must be established. The impedance of the ear tells us how well the conductive mechanism accepts vibratory energy at various frequencies, and this brings us back to the question raised at the beginning of this section concerning the accuracy with which the ear transfers the patterns of sound presented to it. Any change that the ear introduces represents distortion, but that which is introduced by the normal ear we are stuck with, because this is part of the natural hearing process. Diseases of the ear may introduce further distortions that one is not used to, and these will interfere with the perception of sounds as normally experienced.

By combining the phase and magnitude of the

reflected wave at the various frequencies, the ease of sound transmission into the ear can be determined. The early determinations have been thoroughly discussed (Wever and Lawrence, 1954), and modern refinements have been presented by Zwislocki (1962), Onchi (1961), and Møller (1961). The data from the later methods agree fairly well with the earlier ones, and the methods have now been applied to the pathological ear.

Wever and Lawrence (1954) presented a composite curve, averaged from the early studies, expressed as a transmission loss in decibels for the frequencies with which the studies dealt. This curve showed gradual improvement in transmission to a frequency of about 1,350 Hz. Impedance measures are difficult to make for the higher frequencies because the methods used are limited by the wavelength of the sound wave but the indications are that transmission gets poorer again at the higher frequencies.

These figures represent the transmission characteristics or the resonance of the system and have been plotted as a resonance curve in Fig. 11-10. This is a broad and relatively flat curve. It indicates a highly damped system with a wide resonance peak centering on 1,350 Hz. It is reasonable to have a resistance-controlled system for the ear because in this way changes in stiffness and mass have minimal effect. Normal variation in the size of ossicles or oval and round windows have relatively little effect on the overall resonance. Interference with the pressure transformation or the transduction processes is far more serious.

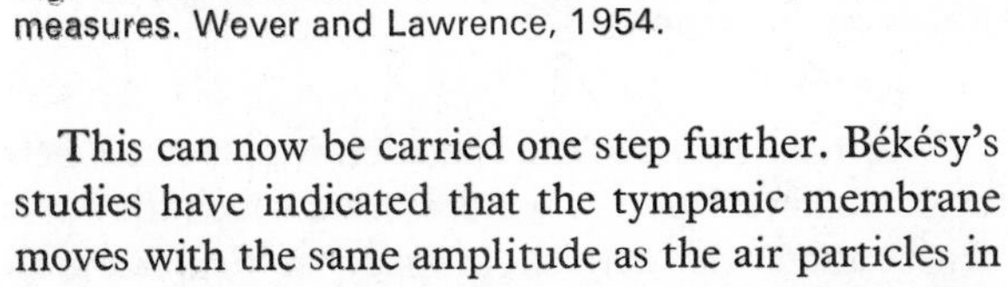

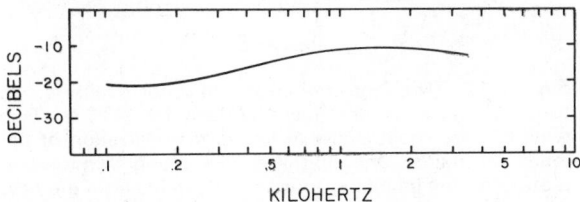

Fig. 11-10. Resonance of ear as determined by impedance measures. Wever and Lawrence, 1954.

This can now be carried one step further. Békésy's studies have indicated that the tympanic membrane moves with the same amplitude as the air particles in the frequency range between 1,000 and 2,000 Hz, and Wilska's data show almost the same thing, although air particle and malleus displacement are more nearly coincident from 300 to 1,000 Hz. It seems reasonable, then, that the resonant frequency for the entire sound-conduction system of 1,350 Hz represents movement of the system with the air particles. The transmission-loss curve as an interpretation of the impedance can be expressed in terms of amplitude displacement with 1,350 Hz coinciding with the amplitude of air-particle vibration at this frequency. This has been done in Fig. 11-11 and is plotted along with the curve representing the amplitude of air-particle movement at the threshold of hearing for the various frequencies over most of the audible range.

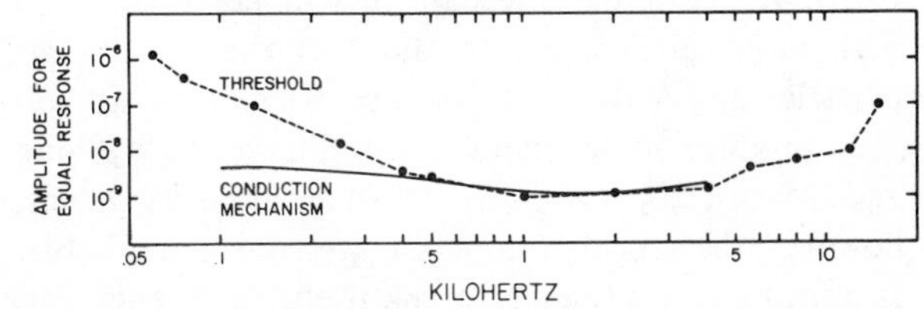

Fig. 11-11. The mechanical resonance curve of the ear superimposed on the threshold curve of Sivian and White (1933).

The rise in the threshold curve at the low and high frequencies indicates that greater vibration amplitude of the air particles is necessary to reach hearing threshold at these frequencies than for the middle range. Similarly, the curve of vibration transmission indicates that it takes a greater amplitude of forcing vibration for equal amplitude of response at the various frequencies. Throughout the middle range, threshold sensitivity is determined by the resonance response of the highly damped sound-conduction system. Although we have superimposed the curves, such a procedure is based on reasonable experimental data.

Below 500 Hz some factors other than remoteness from resonance must account for failing sensitivity, and this is probably equally true for frequencies above 5,000 Hz. For these we must look to processes beyond the mechanical ones: the transduction and neural processes. One might read with profit a discussion of possible contributing factors in Wever's book: Theory of Hearing (1949).

AMPLITUDE DISTORTION

Besides frequency distortion, phase distortion, and transient distortion, another form of distortion of important consideration is that resulting from increased amplitudes of the driving force: amplitude distortion. Any system forced to vibrate beyond its limits of proportional displacement fails to respond with equal amplitudes and produces harmonics of the driving frequency. The ear is no different, and, in the higher intensity regions even below the threshold of feeling, gives rise to aural harmonics. However, it has been shown by extensive experimentation (Wever and Lawrence, 1954) that these harmonics do not first appear as the result of overloading the middle ear structures, but are produced at relatively moderate sound levels in the inner ear. At intense sound levels, levels that would produce damage to the organ of Corti, the ossicular mechanism will fail to respond with amplitudes equal to those of the driving air particles and will itself produce harmonics. It will even produce subharmonics (von Gierke, 1950; Pong and Marcaccio, 1963). At normal intensity levels, however, the sound-conduction system is remarkable. It appears to respond over the useful frequency and dynamic range with little mechanical distortion of any sort.

Conductive Deafness

There are many pathological conditions that can interfere with the sound-conduction mechanism and, generally, when this occurs, a hearing loss results. Fortunately, the otologic surgeon is today equipped with procedures by means of which he can, in the majority of cases, relieve conductive deafnesses. The surgery involves a physiological and mechanical reconstruction of the basic mechanism.

For some operations, for instance those employed in the relief of deafness due to otosclerosis,[2] the procedure to be followed by the surgeon is fairly clear-cut, and he can proceed without any definite knowledge of the acoustic principles involved in his reconstruction. For other operations, however, such as those involving chronic, draining ears, or previous unsuccessful procedures, the surgeon may have to decide on his method of reconstruction as the surgery proceeds, and this requires special knowledge on his part. Interestingly, the first really successful operation for otosclerosis was developed without the acoustic principles being completely understood, but the success of the procedure prompted research that brought to light many aspects of middle-ear acoustics that are now applied in other procedures.

[2] Otosclerosis is a disease of the bone of the otic capsule characterized by an overgrowth of osseous material which, when it invades the stapes, anchors it so as to reduce the acoustic vibrations transmitted to the inner ear.

Fenestration

In 1938 Lempert described a spectacular one-stage operation for the relief of deafness due to otosclerosis. For many years this operation reigned as a masterful success and, although it rarely returned hearing to a normal level, it did return the patient to a level of hearing where he could hear comfortably without the use of a hearing aid, and carry on a normal existence involving communication with his fellow man: listening to concerts, lectures, radio, etc. Fig. 11-12 shows, diagramatically, the anatomical situation within the ear at the completion of this operation. The condition of the ear at the beginning of the operation is one in which the stapes is completely ankylosed so that only one window, the round window, remains as a non-osseous entrance to the fluids of the inner ear.

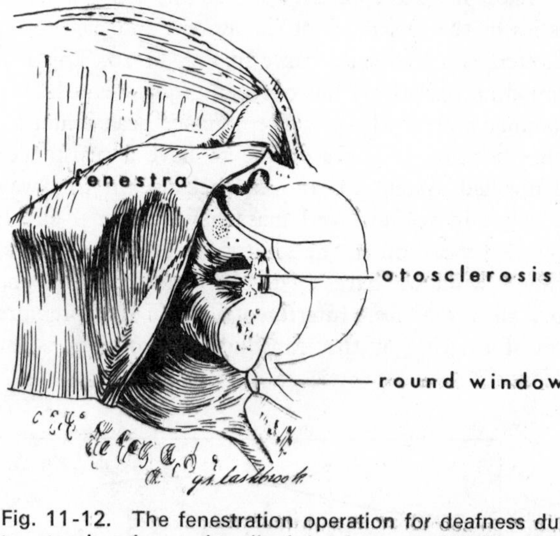

Fig. 11-12. The fenestration operation for deafness due to otosclerosis as described by Lempert (1938). Two windows are again available to allow mobilization of the inner ear fluids. One of these (the round window) is protected from incoming sound so vibrations from the new fenestra will not be cancelled. Hearing, theoretically, returns only to within 26 dB of normal because there is no middle ear transformer.

The main object of the operation is to create a new oval window. This new window from which the name fenestration was derived is made in the "surgical dome" of the horizontal canal. The operation requires extreme skill on the part of the surgeon because it involves sculpturing of the bone to reveal the semicircular canals, at the same time avoiding important nerves and vessels. An additional complication arises from the fact that the membranous labyrinth lies within the hardest bone of the body, the otic capsule.

This new window in the horizontal canal must be made in such a way that the delicate membranous horizontal canal which lies within the bony space is not damaged. Nature has arranged this compact group of vital structures so that the facial nerve lies immediately below and parallel to this horizontal canal, and the surgeon must avoid this nerve in order to prevent facial paralysis, a deformity which causes the complete relaxation of the muscles on the side of the face to which the nerve has been cut.

In preparing to make the new fenestra, the surgeon prepares a flap from the skin tissue of the wall of the external meatus that is connected to the drum membrane. During the course of the operation the incus is removed and, depending upon the surgeon, the head of the malleus may be removed. After preparation of the fenestra and skin flap the portion of the external canal which has been excised is laid down over the new window and the cavity lined with other skin removed from the external canal. As Fig. 11-12 shows, there is an air space over the round window behind the new, displaced tympanic membrane, and this air space is connected to the nasopharynx by the Eustachian tube. The large excavated cavity, through which the fenestra was made, is exposed to the external environment with the fenestration protected by the new skin flap. When this operation is successful, improvement in hearing can be anywhere from normal to 30 dBs below normal with the mean result of the many thousand cases thus operated being around the 26 dB level. Sometimes, for unknown reasons, this operation does not work, and sometimes the new fenestra suffers a bony closure which generally results in a return of the hearing to a preoperative level.

Stapes Mobilization

In 1952 Rosen reintroduced a technique which had previously been tried in the 1890s without too much success. This involves exposing the middle ear by lifting up the drum membrane and attempting to mobilize the anchored stapes. In some instances this procedure has spectacular results. Through the release of the stapes from its otosclerotic anchor, hearing is returned to a normal level, but the results generally do not last long because the active disease process has been disturbed and the otosclerotic bone quickly reunites to anchor the stapes. But this simple maneuver led to a bold gesture involving removal of the stapes, exposure of the labyrinth, and the substitution of the stapes by a prosthesis.

Several attempts were made following the disappointing results of stapes mobilization to get direct mobility from the footplate and avoid the refixation. A, in Fig. 11-13, shows an operation called anterior crurotomy. This is an operation first described by Fowler (1956), the main maneuver of which is to cut free that portion of the stapes which is attached to the otosclerotic growth, thus allowing the rest of the stapes to be moved through the action of the posterior crus. By means of specially devised instruments the anterior crus is cut above the otosclerotic growth and beneath the capitulum; the stapes then is cracked at the point to which the otosclerosis has extended. In the majority of cases, otosclerosis, when involving the stapes, starts from the anterior part of the footplate, making this operation applicable. This is still a

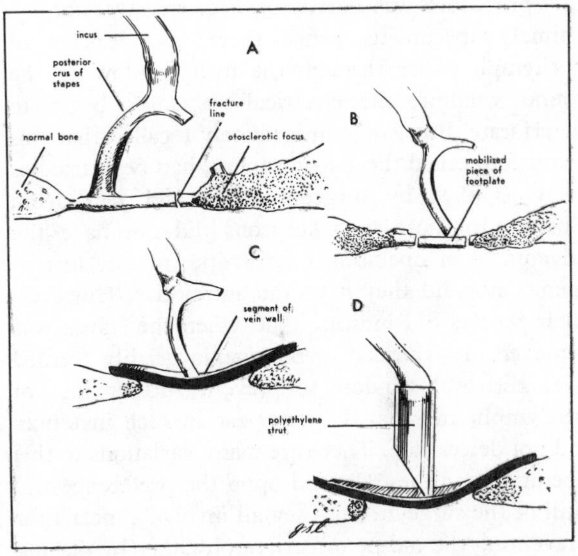

Fig. 11-13. A. The anterior crurotomy operation. The stapes is mobilized by cutting a section out of the anterior crus and breaking free the footplate outside the otosclerotic focus.
B. The crural repositioning operation. In cases of extensive otosclerosis a section in the middle of the stapes is broken free and the posterior crus rotated to rest upon this freed section.
C. This operation is similar to that in B except that the entire footplate is replaced by a vein graft.
D. The stapedectomy operation of Shea (1958) in which the stapes is replaced by a polyethylene strut and the footplate by a vein graft. In present procedures the polyethylene has been abandoned in favor of stainless steel wire. *This illustration reproduced with permission: McCabe, B., and Ritter, F. "The surgery of deafness. IV. The surgery of otoclerosis."* J. Mich. State Med. Soc., *60:1158–1163, 1961.*

successful operation in some cases, but in others runs into difficulty: not only that involved in performing the operation, but the occasional subsequent refixation of the footplate. Other variations have followed.

B, in Fig. 11-13, shows another procedure employed when the otosclerosis is more extensive. Not only is the anterior crus cut and removed, but the posterior crus is also cut near its attachment to the footplate and repositioned to the center portion of the footplate, which has been cracked free from the ankylosing otosclerosis. In general, this operation has the same drawbacks as the anterior crurotomy.

Stapedectomy

In 1958 a bold move was made. Shea introduced an operation in which the entire footplate and its overgrowing otosclerosis were removed, thus exposing the vestibule and perilymph of the inner ear. To the physiologist who had been studying the inner ear, this procedure was horrifying because invariably in animal experiments, when there is a leakage of perilymph either through the oval window or the round window, the electrical responses begin to deteriorate. But it was immediately recalled that this operation, called the stapedectomy, had been tried as early as 1893 by surgeons Blake and Jack from Boston. In those days surgeons did not have the advantages of operating microscopes or fine instruments, nor did they have the antibiotics. However, their reports did indicate that, when the stapes was removed, a cicatricial membrane invariably formed over the oval window to prevent further loss of perilymph, and that the inner ear in such instances did not deteriorate. There are many variations to this operation and these depend upon the preference and skill of the surgeon. But they all involve a means for preventing the escape of perilymph either by placing a vein graft over the oval window or filling it with a plug of vein, fat, or some other tissue and then embedding in it, or on it, a prosthesis (the present favorite is stainless steel wire) which is connected to the long process of the incus if this is feasible in the particular case. (Shea's original operation using polyethylene tubing, is shown in D of Fig. 11-13.) If there are no untoward physiological results it is obvious that the normal mechanism has been restored and, logically, hearing should return to normal.

The drawbacks to this operation are that in rare instances the membranous labyrinth may be damaged with subsequent deterioration of hearing, but this is true of all of the operations which involve working near this portion of the ear. Also in extensive otosclerosis the operation for some reason or other may not return hearing to the expected level. In addition, there are sometimes strange auditory anomalies which follow this operation: there may be peculiar distortions of sound or the patient may experience an inability to withstand the sensation produced by louder sounds.

In order to avoid the use of a prosthesis, Portmann and Claverie (1958) have described a procedure in which a crus of the stapes is repositioned upon a vein graft replacing the footplate of the stapes in the oval window (C in Fig. 11-13). Here again, in many instances, this is a successful operation.

One thing that must be kept in mind is that every case is individual, and the type of surgery involved depends not only upon the state of the art but upon the condition of the patient's ear at the time of operation.

With the many improvements in operative procedures, and with the advent of the use of the microscope, other operations to relieve other kinds of conductive lesions have been developed. New ways of closing perforations of the tympanic membrane and of reconstructing ears that have been riddled with infection over so many years that the ossicles may have been erroded, have been developed and nowadays the surgeon attempts not only to remove the disease and infection, but also to restore hearing.

Myringoplasty

Clinical evidence has shown that, depending upon the size and location of a tympanic perforation, hearing may be more or less impaired. Why this should be so was not always obvious because some perforations seem to have no effect on hearing whereas others may have a profound effect. However, the surgeon has developed many different techniques whereby these perforations can now be closed and in most instances hearing restored to a normal condition. It is true that some of these perforations may not impair hearing to any great extent, but successful surgery not only can return hearing to normal but prevent entrance of disease through the exposed mucosa of the middle ear.

Tympanoplasty

As the surgeons began to understand something of the mechanical principles of the ear's operation they embarked upon a series of procedures designed not only to eradicate the disease in a long-existing draining ear but also to bring hearing back to a serviceable level. These operations have their postsurgery difficulties, but they are of considerable interest because they are based on the acoustic properties of the ear and, if the problems of maintaining skin flaps in their proper position and of maintaining the situation existing at the end of surgery can be solved, these forms of operation may eventually make the surgeon happier about them than he now is. With the successful use of prosthetics and a further understanding of the subtler mechanics of the middle ear, these operations undoubtedly will be replaced, but their basis on the mechanics of the middle ear is of interest.

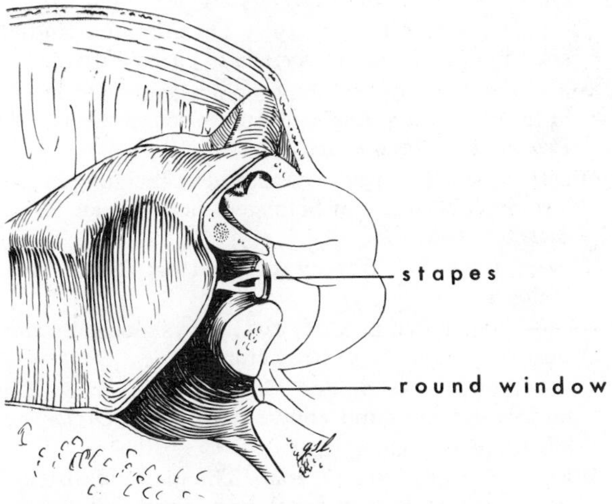

Fig. 11-14. An operation establishing a columella between a large area and the footplate of the stapes; in this instance the stapes is mobile and only the ossicular lever is missing.

Fig. 11-14 shows a postoperative situation in which a skin flap, or the remaining drum membrane, has been attached to the stapes in such a way that a single columella has been formed between the external meatus and the inner ear. This operation, of course, involves a free and mobile stapes. It is performed because of the existence of a chronic draining ear which may have erroded away the incus, possibly part of the malleus, or even the drum membrane. It can also be performed in the event of an injury in which some object has traumatically injured the tympanic membrane and the ossicular chain.

Another form of this operation is shown in Fig. 11-15. This operation is something like the fenestration in its physical characteristics, except that

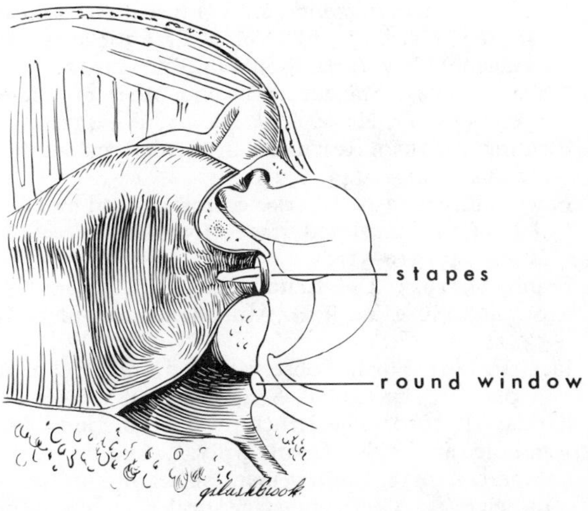

Fig. 11-15. An operation similar in mechanics to the fenestration, except that a mobile stapes serves as an exposed window rather than a new fenestra. The hearing results are no better than the fenestration, but this procedure is employed in cases of chronically infected ears rather than otosclerosis.

no new window is made. Use is made of, again, a mobile stapes on which the crura and capitulum may be present or may have eroded, leaving only the footplate. The object of this operation is to protect the round window from sound by means of a skin flap so that there is no cancellation of vibration by equal amplitudes activating the two windows of the inner ear at the same time. Here again the procedure is based on established acoustic principles, but there are surgical and postoperative difficulties which have led the surgeon to abandon almost completely this procedure.

BIBLIOGRAPHY

Békésy, G.v. 1960. Experiments in hearing. New York: McGraw-Hill.

Benzinger, T., and Taylor, G. 1963. Cranial measurements of internal temperature in man. *In* Temperature: its measurements and control in science and industry. Hardy, J., ed. (Vol. 3, Part 3, Biology and medicine) New York: Reinhold. Pp. 111–120.

Blake, C. 1893. Stapedectomy and other middle-ear operations. *Tr. Amer. Otol. Soc.*, 5, 464–473.

Fleming, N. 1939. Resonance in the external auditory meatus. *Nature*, 143, 642–643.

Fowler, E., Jr. 1956. Anterior crurotomy and mobilization of the ankylosed stapes footplate. *Acta Otolargng.*, 46, 319–322.

Frank, O. 1923. Die Leitung des Schalles im Ohr. *Sitzungsber. Akad. Wiss.*, Munchen, math-phys. Kl. 53, 11–77.

Jack, F. 1893. Further observations on removal of the stapes. *Tr. Amer. Otol. Soc.*, 5, 474–487.

Kirikae, I. 1950. The structure and function of the middle ear. Tokyo, Japan: Univ. Tokyo Press.

Lempert, J. 1938. Improvement of hearing in cases of otosclerosis: A new, one-stage surgical technic. *Arch. Otolaryng.*, 28, 42–97.

Metz, O. 1946. The acoustic impedance measured on normal and pathological ears. *Acta Otolargng.*, Suppl. 63.

Møller, A. 1961. Network model of the middle ear. *J. acoust. soc. Amer.*, 33, 168–176.

———. 1963. Transfer function of the middle ear. *J. acoust. soc. Amer.*, 35, 1526–1534.

Onchi, Y. 1961. Mechanisms of the middle ear. *J. acoust. soc. Amer.*, 33, 794–805.

Pong, W., and Marcaccio, W. 1963. Nonlinearity of the middle ear as possible source of subharmonics. *J. acoust. soc. Amer.*, 35, 679–681.

Portmann, M., and Claverie, G. 1958. Stapediovestibular osteotomy in otosclerosis. *Laryngoscope*, 68, 797–804.

Robinson, N. 1937. An acoustic impedance bridge. *Phil. Mag.*, 23, 665–681.

Rosen, S. 1952. Palpation of the stapes for fixation. *Arch. Otolaryng.*, 56, 610–615.

Schuster, K. 1934. Eine Methode zum Vergleich akustischer Impedanzen. *Physikalische Zeits.*, 35, 408–409.

———, and Stohr, W. 1939. Aufbau und Eigenschaften eines veränderbaren akustischen Vergleichswiderstandes. *Akust. Zeits.*, 4, 253–260.

Shea, J. 1958. Fenestration of the oval window. *Ann. Otol. Rhinol., Laryng.*, 67, 932–951.

Sivian, L., and White, S. 1933. On minimum audible sound fields. *J. acoust. soc. Amer.*, 4, 288–321.

von Gierke, H. 1950. Subharmonics generated in ears of humans and animals at intense sound levels. *Fed. Proc. Amer. Physio. Soc.*, 9, 130.

Waetzmann, E. 1938. Absorptionsmessungen am Trommelfell mit den Schusterschen Brucke. *Akust. Zeits.*, 3, 1–6.

Wever, E. 1949. Theory of hearing. New York: Wiley.

———, and Lawrence, M. 1954. Physiological acoustics. Princeton, N.J.: Princeton.

———, and ———, and Smith, K.R. 1948. The middle ear in sound conduction. *Arch. Otolaryng.*, 48, 19–35.

Wiener, F., and Ross, D. 1946. The pressure distribution in the auditory canal in a progressive sound field. *J. acoust. soc. Amer.*, 18, 401–408.

Wilska, A. 1935. Eine Methode zur Bestimmung der Hörschwellenamplituden der Trommelfells bei verschiedenen Frequenzen. *Skand. Arch. Physiol.*, 72, 161–165.

Zwislocki, J. 1962. Analysis of the middle-ear function. Input impedance. *J. acoust. soc. Amer.*, 34, 1514–1523. (Part I.)

12

Pathology, Diagnosis, and Therapy of Deafness

Victor Goodhill and Paul Guggenheim,[1] *with the collaboration of Gloria Hoversten and Diane MacKay*

BASIC ANATOMY AND PHYSIOLOGY

The auditory system, properly speaking, includes not only the two ears, but their complex central auditory pathways, terminating in the cortex of the temporal lobes of the brain. So conceived, it fulfills its functions by receiving, encoding, transmitting, and decoding sound signals. The central connections include complex afferent and some more recently discovered and as yet poorly understood efferent pathways. The principal neurologic connections are shown in Fig. 12-1.

The temporal bones, major components of the human skull, are by far the most intricate, both functionally and anatomically, of any in the human body (Fig. 12-2). To study and begin to understand them is the work of a lifetime. The temporal bone houses the external, middle, and inner ears, as well as the auditory and vestibular end organs of the VIIIth Cranial nerve, the VIIth Cranial nerve (facial nerve), portions of the internal carotid artery, and the sigmoid venous sinus with its jugular bulb (Fig. 12-3).

The external ear includes the pinna or auricle and the cartilaginous and bony external auditory canal. The latter terminates at the eardrum or tympanic membrane (Fig. 12-4). The auricle collects air-borne sound waves and funnels them through the external auditory canal to the tympanum.

[1] The authors gratefully acknowledge the support of the Hope for Hearing Research Foundation, Los Angeles, California.

Medial to the eardrum lies the middle ear, an air-containing space which is roughly divisible into three portions: the *hypotympanum*, the *mesotympanum*, and the *epitympanum* (Fig. 12-5).

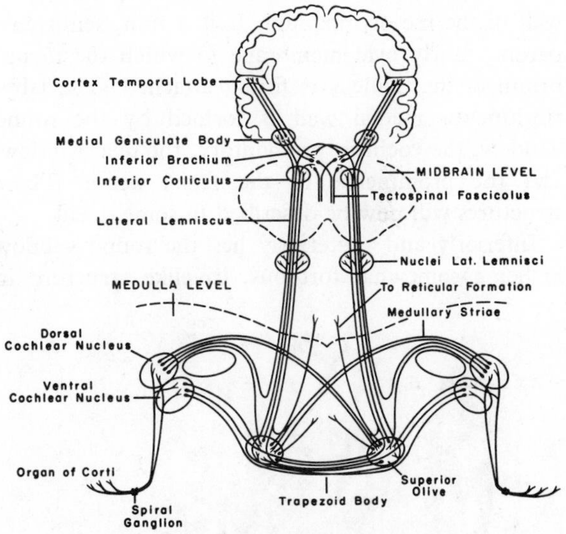

Fig. 12-1. Diagrammatic representation of the neuronal connections of the auditory system.

At the inferior or caudal level is the *hypotympanum.* The jugular bulb lies beneath its floor, rather posteriorly. Near the labyrinthine wall is a small aperture for passage of the tympanic branch of the glossopharyngeal nerve.

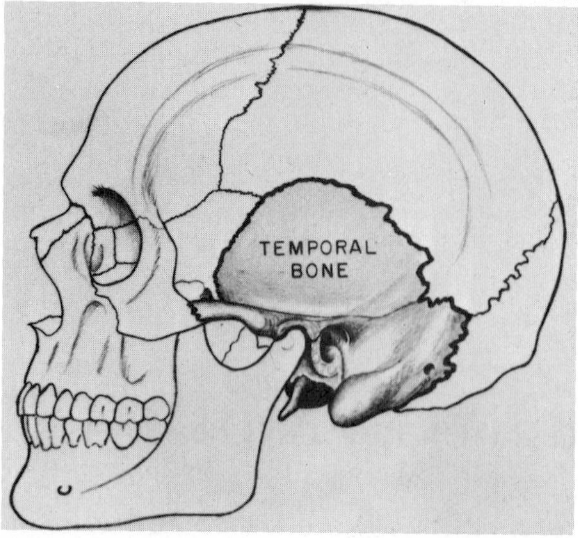

Fig. 12-2. Lateral view of the left temporal bone showing the squamous, tympanic, and mastoid portions. The petrous portion lies more medially and cannot be seen.

Superior to the hypotympanum lies the *mesotympanum*, delimited by the borders of the tympanic membrane. Contained in this area are the stapes and portions of the malleus and incus, and other important structures. The tympanic membrane and the bony ring into which it is inserted form the lateral wall of the mesotympanum. It is a thin, semitransparent, nearly oval membrane to which the manubrium of the malleus is firmly attached. The labyrinthine or medial wall is formed by the round window, the cochlear promontory, the oval window, and the prominence of the facial nerve. These structures will now be described in some detail.

Inferiorly and posteriorly lies the round-window niche, a somewhat tortuous, cavelike structure in which, anterosuperiorly, lies the secondary tympanic membrane or, as it is better known, round-window membrane. This structure is thin like the tympanic membrane but much smaller, and has the shape of an inverted heart. Quite fragile, it is well protected deep within the niche. More will be said presently about its important function.

Above and slightly anterior to the round window, separated from it by a portion of the cochlear promontory, is the oval window. This window, approximately 1.55 mm. vertically by three mm. anteroposteriorly, lies at the bottom of the oval-window niche, which is more shallow and accessible than the round-window niche. The oval window is occluded by the stapes footplate, which articulates with the bony labyrinth in the medial tympanic wall by means of the stapediovestibular joint, consisting of the circumferential annular ligament. This joint permits a modified plunger-type motion of the footplate in response to acoustic energy. It is activated by energy transmitted by the air-borne sound which strikes the tympanic membrane and is transmitted via the malleus (attached to and an integral part of the drum), through the incus to the head (capitulum) of the stapes.

The drum and three ossicles constitute the impedance-matching mechanism or transducer system of the middle ear (Fig. 12-6), which has the task of transmitting air-borne sound waves through its aerial transmission system to the stapediovestibular joint in such a manner that the fluid-containing inner ear receives impulses which set the fluid into vibration without significant loss of energy or change in frequency characteristics. The inner ear is, thus, truly an aquatic organ. Stimulation of the cochlea is

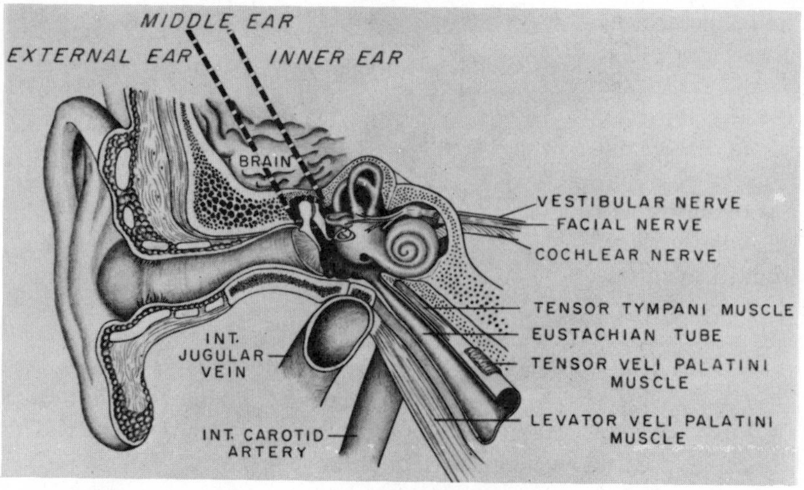

Fig. 12-3. Diagrammatic representation of principal contents of temporal bone.

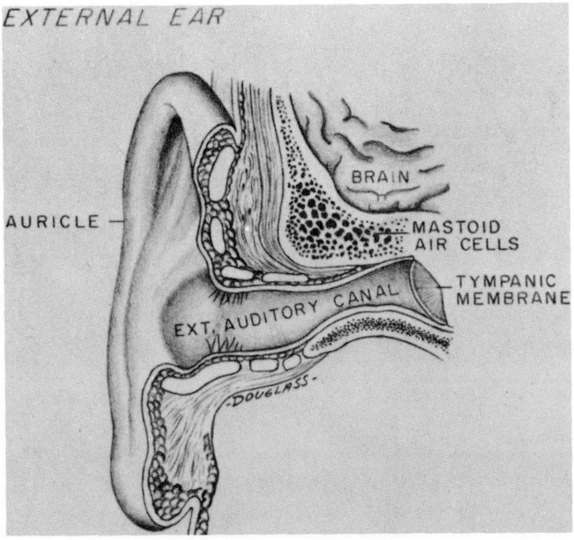

Fig. 12-4. The external ear, showing the auricle or pinna and the cartilaginous and bony portions of the external auditory canal. The external ear terminates at the tympanic membrane (drum).

facilitated by a combination of two mechanical factors: 1) the difference in area between the tympanic membrane and that of the stapes footplate (aerial ratio); and 2) the lever action of the ossicular chain. Of the two, the aerial ratio is the greater factor in the sound-pressure transducer action. In man, this is approximately 22 : 1. The lever action of the ossicular chain is approximately 1.1 : 1. The product of these two ratios yields a result equivalent to approximately 26 dB, which is the essential contribution of the entire middle ear mechanism to the transmission of air-borne sound to the cochlear perilymph. However, it should be borne in mind that loss of the drum and ossicles usually results in a so-called "complete conductive hypacusis," which is considerably more severe than the 26 dB just mentioned. Other factors enter the picture here, and are more fully described in Chapters 10 and 11.

The normal tympanic membrane is partly transparent to acoustic energy, and air-borne sound waves can affect the air contained within the middle-ear cavity independently of the action of the "transmission system." Thus, the round-window membrane is not completely shielded from air-borne sound. One of the functions of the ossicular chain is the production of a significant sound-pressure differential between the two windows and between the two scalae (vestibular and tympanic), allowing basilar membrane motion. Perhaps the position of the round-window membrane, facing as it does, downward and backward, protects it somewhat from direct impingement of air-borne sound waves within the middle ear at a maximally effective angle of 90 degrees. The oval window, by contrast, faces almost directly laterally. If lines drawn perpendicular to the two windows are compared in angular direction in one horizontal plane, they are separated by approximately 67 degrees.

The stapes, the smallest bone in the body, consists of a head, neck, and two crura or legs. The head and neck, like the malleus and incus, consist of ordinary marrow-bone. The crura, however, are extremely fragile and consist of hemi-cylindrical shells of cortical bone from which the marrow has been scooped out, leaving them hollow. The two hollows face one another, forming the boundary of the obturator foramen, and are attached directly to the external aspect of the footplate.

The incus consists of a body, a long process, and a short process. The body articulates with the head of the malleus. The short process projects into the posteroinferior portion of the epitympanic recess; the long process descends behind and parallel to the manubrium and, bending medially, ends in a rounded projection, the lenticular process which articulates with the head of the stapes.

The malleus consists of a head, neck, and three processes—the manubrium, the anterior process (usually vestigial), and the lateral process (Fig. 12-7).

The facial canal, in which the VIIth Cranial nerve is contained, traverses the medial wall above the oval window and then curves vertically downward along the anterior mastoid wall. The two tympanic muscles lie within the mesotympanum. The stapedius muscle, arising from the pyramidal eminence and attached to the neck of the stapes, is responsible for the acoustic reflex to loud sound and sometimes to tactile stimulation. It probably also has some protective function in mitigating the effect of very loud sounds upon the labyrinth. The tensor tympani muscle arises from within a canal in the medial wall of the Eustachian tube, courses posteriorly to a bony eminence known as the processus cochleariformis, overlying the bony canal of the facial nerve in its intratympanic portion, where it makes a right-angle turn to insert laterally upon the base of the manubrium of the malleus. It has the function of tensing or retracting the eardrum.

The Eustachian tube just mentioned is an extremely important structure. Its upper and tympanic orifice lies within the mesotympanum. It is a narrow channel arising high on the anteromedial wall of the

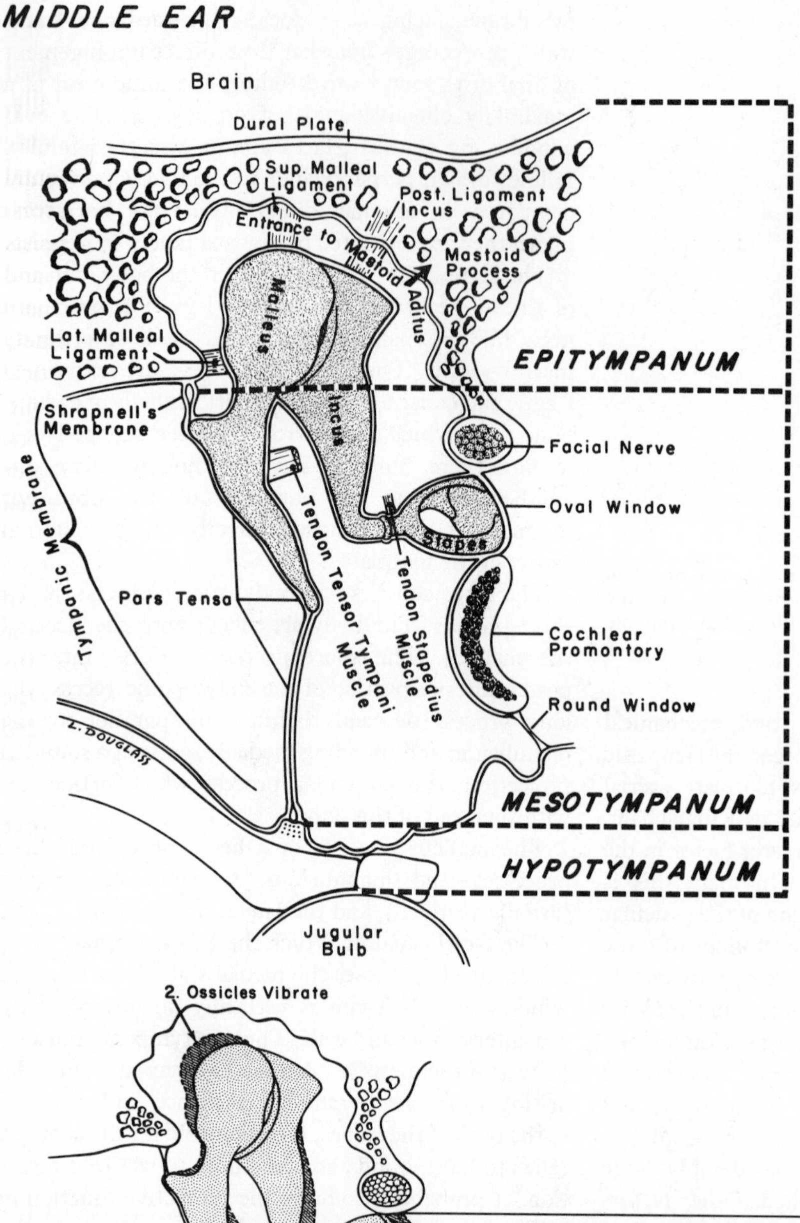

Fig. 12-5. Diagrammatic coronal section through tympanic cavity showing division into three levels: (1) hypotympanum, (2) mesotympanum, and (3) epitympanum or attic.

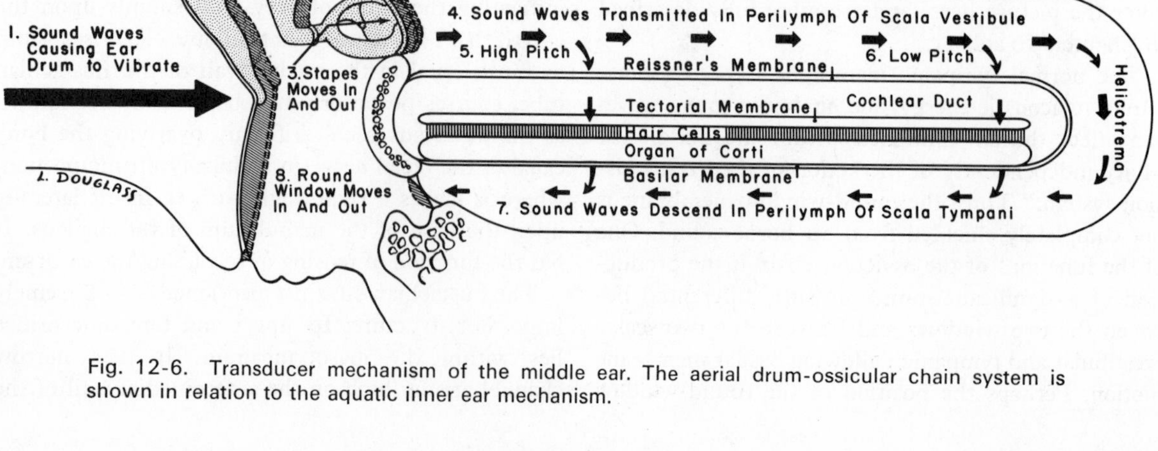

Fig. 12-6. Transducer mechanism of the middle ear. The aerial drum-ossicular chain system is shown in relation to the aquatic inner ear mechanism.

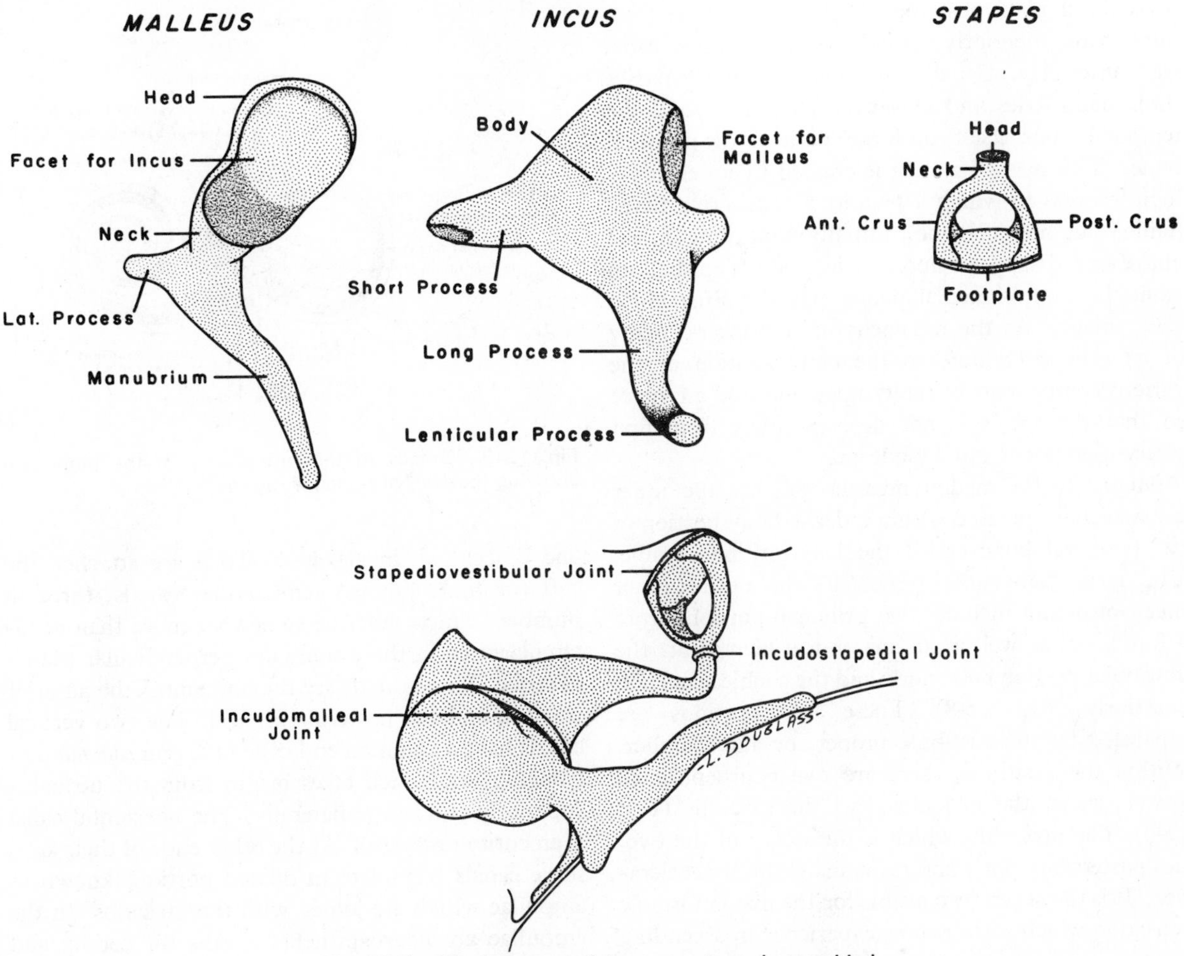

Fig. 12-7. The human ossicles separate and assembled.

tympanic air space. The first portion of the Eustachian tube is bony and rigid, shaped like a thin cone pointing downward, forward, and medially. At the apex of the cone is the isthmus of the Eustachian tube. Below the isthmus, the tube is membranous and cartilaginous in character. Above and on its medial side, it is surrounded with a cartilage to which are attached two important muscles, the tensor palati, laterally, and the levator palati, medially. These muscles are important not only because they play a role in motion of the soft palate but also because they function in regulation of the tubal lumen. The Eustachian tube is normally closed but opens with swallowing, yawning, and palatal elevation. In so doing, it acts to equalize tympanic and external air pressures.

Superior to the mesotympanum lies the attic or *epitympanum*, bounded laterally by Shrapnell's membrane and the external bony attic wall, and superiorly by the tegmen tympani, above which lies the temporal lobe of the brain. The principal structures within the epitympanic space are the head and neck of the malleus, the body and part of the short process of the incus, and the incudomalleal joint (Fig. 12-5). The short process of the incus lies in a groove called the fossa incudis. Just medial to it lies the narrow channel through which the epitympanum communicates with the original and principal air space within the mastoid proper, the mastoid antrum. This passageway is called the aditus (or aditus ad antrum).

The mastoid process is a bony protuberance behind and below the external ear. It begins to develop at two years of age. In ordinary parlance, the term "mastoid" refers not just to this protuberance, but also to the entire interconnected system of air cells with which the temporal bone normally is honeycombed. An area known as the periantral triangle has boundaries defined by the sigmoid sinus and posterior fossa dural plate posteromedially, the middle fossa dural plate superiorly, and the posterior bony canal wall anteriorly. Usually, pneumatization trespasses these boundaries and may even extend beyond the temporal bone itself into the parietal or occipital bones. This air-cell system is created by an embryologic process in which a primitive connective tissue (embryonic mesenchyme), initially ubiquitous in the entire area, disappears upon the invasion of epithelium from the first branchial pouch (via the Eustachian tube anlage). As the mesenchyme disappears, many of its cells contribute to the epithelization of the various components of the tympanomastoid air space so that the lining is not derived solely from first pharyngeal pouch gut endoderm.

Medial to the mediotympanic wall lies the inner ear, which is enclosed within a dense bony portion of the temporal bone called the labyrinthine capsule. The term "labyrinth" refers to the entire inner mechanism and includes two principal portions from a functional as well as an anatomical viewpoint: the vestibular portion posteriorly and the cochlear portion anteriorly (Fig. 12-8). These two portions are separated by the vestibule proper, or antechamber. Within the vestibule, there are two neuroepithelial sense organs, the utriculus and the sacculus (Fig. 12-9). The utriculus, which is the larger of the two, lies posterosuperiorly and responds to linear acceleration. It is the organ responsible for the uncomfortable sensation which some people experience in ascending

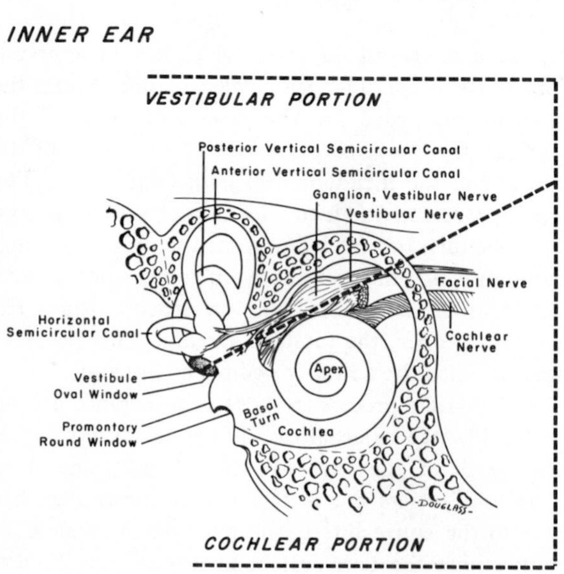

Fig. 12-8. The two divisions of the inner ear shown diagrammatically.

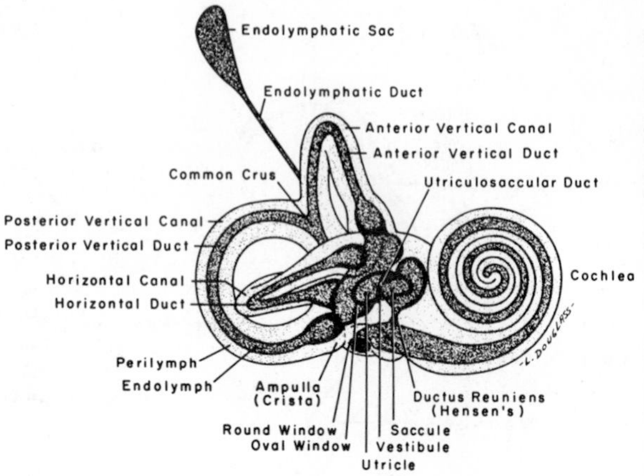

Fig. 12-9. Details of the topography of the inner ear, showing location of principal organs.

and descending in elevators. To it are attached the soft (or membranous) semicircular canals, three in number, which describe somewhat more than semicircular arcs in three mutually perpendicular planes of space. These canals are the horizontal, the anterior vertical, and the posterior vertical. The two vertical canals have a common end called the *crus communis* or common leg, which takes origin from the utriculus superiorly and posterolaterally. The horizontal canal is an entity unto itself. At the other ends of their arcs, these canals terminate in dilated portions known as ampullae which are joined with the utriculus. In the ampullae are neuroepithelial organs for coding and transmitting sensations of rotation. These are called *cristae ampullaris* (singular *crista*). The utriculus is connected anteriorly and inferiorly with the sacculus by a small duct, the utriculosaccular.

From the utriculosaccular duct, an interesting branch is given off, the endolymphatic duct, the entrance to which is protected by the utriculoendolymphatic valve. The endolymphatic duct courses through the depth of the mastoid to a dilated portion, the endolymphatic sac (*saccus endolymphaticus*), which lies immediately adjacent to the posterior fossa dura.

The sacculus may be concerned with sensations of linear acceleration and possibly also with hearing. Its precise function is unknown. It is connected to the basal turn of the cochlea through a small duct called the ductus reuniens, or Hensen's duct. The first portion of the cochlea, known as the hook, begins immediately inferior to the vestibule of the labyrinth and has a long course which traverses most of the anteroposterior width of the cochlear promontory on the medial tympanic wall. At the anteriormost part of the promontory, the cochlear duct bends upward and is then rolled into a three-dimensional, ascending spiral of two and a half turns. Like the threads of a screw, these turns become smaller (tighter) toward the apex. The cochlear spiral points in a generally anterior and lateral direction within the head.

The membranous canals are filled with a clear fluid, *endolymph*, which permeates the entire membranous or soft part of the inner ear, including the utriculus, sacculus, and the cochlear duct. Theoretically, the endolymph is free to circulate through the entire membranous labyrinth, both vestibular and cochlear, including the endolymphatic duct and sac described above. It is questionable whether any gross flow ever occurs from one segment to another. Changes in position of the body and acceleration in any direction, whether linear or angular, cause inertial lag of the endolymph in relation to its containing walls. It is this inertia which causes mechanical stimulation of the *cristae ampullares* and the neuroepithelial sense organs within the utriculus and sacculus. However, pressure changes can be freely transmitted through the entire system since fluid is incompressible, and the entire system is in free intercommunication. The membranous labyrinth is surrounded by perilymph and the whole system is housed within the otic capsule.

Both perilymph and endolymph are clear, but they differ in chemical content. In general, perilymph is virtually identical in composition with the cerebrospinal fluid. It has a relatively high sodium content and low potassium content, like most extracellar fluids. By contrast, the endolymph has a relatively high potassium content and low sodium content, like intracellular fluid. The chemical differences are of the greatest physiologic significance. The perilymph surrounds not only the semicircular canals but the entire membranous labyrinth, including the utriculus and sacculus within the vestibule, and the cochlear duct within the cochlea. Within the perilymph space of the semicircular canal system are small strands of connective tissue (trabeculae) which maintain the membranous canals in position away from their containing, bony walls. To some extent, the same is true of the utriculus and the sacculus lying within the vestibule of the labyrinth. The structure of the cochlea in this respect is quite different.

The cochlear duct, or scala media, is bounded below by the basilar membrane, which stretches across it and gives it firm support so that it is not subject to concussion against its containing bony walls. The basilar membrane is a ribbon of continuously increasing width, suspended laterally (not lengthwise) between the bony spiral lamina centrally and the spiral ligament peripherally. (The bony spiral lamina—*lamina spiralis ossea*—is a thin, ascending bony spiral—a winding ramp—arising from the bony core of the cochlea.) The basilar membrane, in order to cross the approximately constant width of the overall cochlear lumen, is narrower at the base and broader at the apex of the ramp. Since the basilar membrane is the vibratile portion of the cochlea, one would expect that the tones of higher frequency are heard toward the base of the cochlea, and those of lower frequency toward the apex. This is true and constitutes the basis of the famous Helmholtz theory of pitch perception. Fig. 12-10 will illustrate the approximate points on the cochlear partition corresponding to various frequencies in the tonal scale.

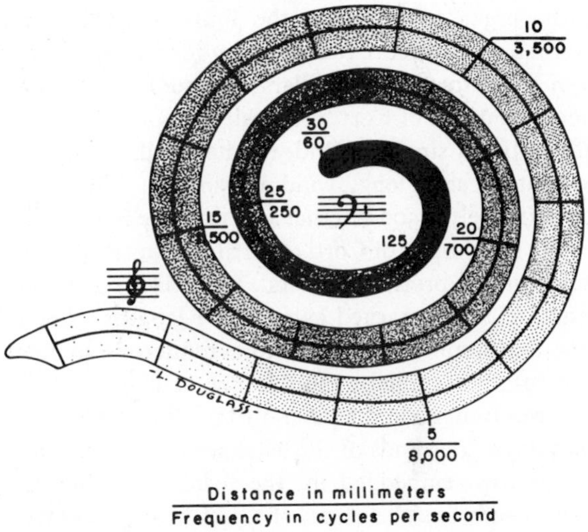

Fig. 12-10. Reconstruction of human cochlea, showing locations of areas of maximum sensitivity to various sound frequencies.

These points are not to be thought of as isolated loci of activity but as critical centers of complex on-going wave disturbances encompassing much wider areas (see Chapters 10 and 11).

The cochlear duct is bounded by the lamina spiralis ossea and basilar membrane below, Reissner's membrane above, and the spiral ligament laterally (Fig. 12-11). Its cross section is roughly triangular in shape. The organ of Corti rests on the basilar membrane within the cochlear duct. It is the essential transducer mechanism by which mechanical waves in the endolymph are converted into impulses in the cochlear

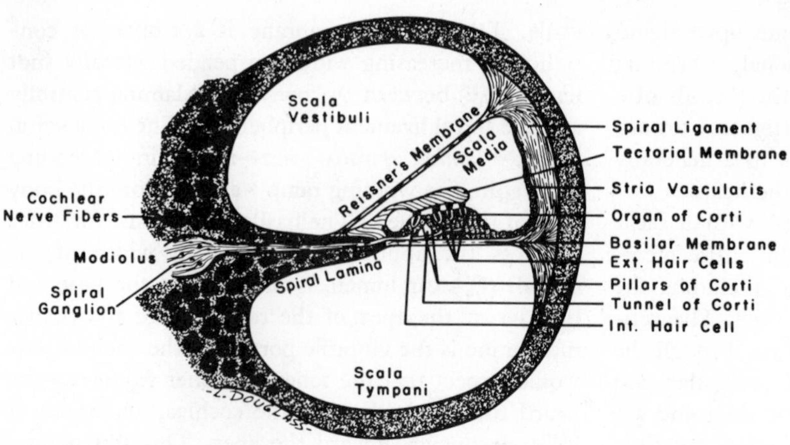

Fig. 12-11. Cross section of the cochlea.

nerve. These impulses are encoded to transmit all the information conveyed by sound energy: loudness, pitch, timbre, etc. Aside from the supporting cells, which are of several types, the *essential* components of the organ of Corti are the four hair cells: one internal, and three external,[2] the former separated from the latter by the pillars and tunnel of Corti. Since the organ of Corti is actually a mountain chain rather than a single mound, the hair cells should be thought of as a long, winding column. There are approximately 3,500 internal and 12,000 external hair cells in each organ of Corti at birth. From the apex of each hair cell protrudes a solid, bristlelike body consisting of closely packed hairs. Their lengths vary, as does the number per cell. More numerous in man than in other animals, the number of hairs per cell increases from 40 in the basal turn to about 100 in the apical turn. The ends of the hairs are in contact with, and perhaps embedded in, the tectorial membrane which overhangs the organ of Corti from its attachment to the vestibular lip of the spiral lamina. Shearing motion between the hairs and the tectorial membrane causes the cell to "fire," resulting in an afferent impulse along a peripheral axon of a spiral ganglion cell. (Limitation of space precludes a fuller discussion of the organ of Corti, which is described in more detail in Chapter 10.)

Above Reissner's membrane is the vestibular duct or *scala vestibuli*, which contains perilymph and which is in direct communication with the perilymph of the labyrinthine vestibule. At the apex of the cochlea is a narrow passage, the *helicotrema*, through which the *scala vestibuli* communicates with the *scala tympani*, also containing perilymph. The *scala tympani* lies beneath the basilar membrane and does not communicate with the vestibule of the labyrinth, as does its companion, but terminates below the labyrinthine vestibule in contact with the round window or secondary tympanic membrane.

[2] Toward the apex, the number of external hair cells increases to four at the middle turn, five in the apical turn.

The function of the round window now becomes clear. If the entire inner ear is filled with fluid, which is by nature incompressible, a wave disturbance could not be propagated by an inward motion of the stapedial footplate unless there were, somewhere within the system, another window allowing for decompression. This is the round window. The motion of the round window has, in fact, a 180-degree phase-difference with respect to that of the footplate. Thus, when the footplate moves inward, the round-window membrane moves outward toward the tympanic air-space (Fig. 12-6). It is interesting that the initial mechanical impulse of sound can be effectively transmitted to the organ of Corti through either of these windows, or, indeed, through an artificial one placed anywhere in the labyrinthine wall, as long as such a window permits "mobilization" of perilymph beneath it.

One might say that the inner ear, taken as a whole, is an organ designed to sense motion. The motion in question covers an enormous spectrum. At one end of this spectrum is the submicroscopic disturbance created by sound waves impinging on the mechanism of the middle ear and cochlea. So sensitive is this mechanism that the amplitude of movement of the tympanic membrane at a sound-pressure level near threshold is of the order of magnitude of the diameter of a single hydrogen atom. We have at least one organ, the utriculus, which senses gross linear acceleration, and the semicircular canals which sense gross motion in the form of rotation in various planes of space. It is possible that the sacculus has something to do with the perception of vibrations in the head.[3] Vibration could well be considered a modality of motion, lying somewhere between the spectrum of frequency represented by sound on the one hand and gross linear or angular accelerations on the other.

HEARING LOSS: TERMINOLOGY AND DEFINITIONS

The term "Deafness"

Because of loose connotation, the term *deafness* creates misunderstandings in otologic literature. As used at the present time, it may describe quantitative speech-threshold shifts of any degree from the relatively minor 15 dB deficit to profound or total loss of hearing in the 80 to 110 dB range. It may also be used to describe specific qualitative communication deficits such as the high-tone, specific-threshold shift in acoustic trauma which is frequently called "high-tone nerve deafness." These quantitatively and qualitatively loose definitions allow confusion that ought to be avoided in order to effect clearer understanding among workers. In the following otologic discussion of hearing losses, more specific terms will be employed.

The term *hypacusis* is used to describe any threshold shift which may be partially or completely corrected by either medical or prosthetic techniques.

The term *anacusis* is used to describe either profound threshold shifts or sensorineural dysfunctions which cannot be helped by medical or prosthetic techniques. (Occasional cases will fit neither the hypacusis nor anacusis category strictly. Such cases will require special descriptions and classifications.)

Dysacusis is a broad term which includes every aspect of disordered hearing—except purely quantitative insufficiency—which causes discomfort or disability. It might include 1. pitch distortion, as in the diplacusis of endolymphatic hydrops; 2. unpleasant timbre—"tinniness"—from the same cause; 3. unpleasant loudness or actual pain from recruitment; and 4. defects in auditory perception on the integrative or interpretive level due to a central lesion. Perhaps one could draw a distinction between *peripheral* dysacuses and *central* dysacuses.

All of the terms mentioned above may be modified by qualitative or anatomic adjectives to designate a large variety of threshold shifts or auditory pathway dysfunctions. They offer further the convenience of being used in adjective form to describe psychophysiologic states heretofore described with difficulty in the English language. The phrase "hard-of-hearing" is used to describe a large variety of mild or moderate hypacuses. Thus, such a patient may be termed *hypacusic*. This will release the word *deaf* to truly describe the person with nonamplifiable major threshold shifts who might then be described as *anacusic* or "deaf" in the educational frame of reference. The term *dysacusis* could then be applied as a general heading for many varieties of central communication defects including aphasia, psychogenic deafness, "mind" deafness, "word" deafness, and so on.

Anatomic-physiologic Types

For purposes of simplicity, all "deafness" in the past was subdivided into two main groups: "conductive" and "nerve."

Conductive. The term *conductive* is still a useful one and will be retained in this discussion. It will be used to describe lesions in the conductive pathway of the hearing organ, namely, the external auditory canal, tympanic membrane, tympanic cavity, ossicular chain, Eustachian tube, otic capsule, and labyrinthine fenestrae (and perhaps cochlear fluids). In other words, any disturbance peripheral to the basilar membrane may be classified within the conductive pathway.

Sensorineural. The term *nerve deafness* has been useful but is ambiguous, and has led to oversimplification of lesions in the neural auditory pathway. In recent years, the term *perceptive* was acquired from psychologic usage and almost displaced the earlier term, *nerve* deafness. This term, *perceptive*, has a useful place, but it is too specific a term for the entire group of lesions in the neural auditory pathway. In the present discussion, we will employ the general term *sensorineural* to describe lesions in the organ of Corti sensory cells and in the neural auditory pathway.

[3] According to two Italian investigators, Bocca and Perani (1960), the sacculus mediates a peculiar kind of hearing which they call "vestibular hearing," and which they believe may be responsible for the low-frequency air-bone gap found in some profoundly deaf individuals. (Such gaps involve frequencies 250, 500, but rarely above this.) Their interesting theory has not been confirmed, and it is probable that such low-frequency gaps represent a confusion of vibration with audition which may affect even a sophisticated subject—possibly because of close physical, physiological, and phylogenetic connections between the two modalities.

These will be further divided into three anatomic subdivisions, namely, *receptive*, *transmissive*, and *perceptive*.

Lesions in the receptor organ (the organ of Corti) may be termed *receptor sensorineural lesions*.

Lesions in the neural auditory pathway, central to the organ of Corti and including the cochlear ganglion, the dorsal and ventral cochlear nuclei, and the ascending tracts, will be grouped under the heading of *transmissive sensorineural lesions*.

Lesions in the subcortical and cortical auditory areas will be termed *auditory perceptive lesions*, inasmuch as true perception of auditory sensation probably does not occur distal to the auditory cortex and associated subcortical integrative areas. It will be difficult to distinguish between *auditory perceptive hypacuses* and *dysacuses* in many cases.

OTOLOGIC DIAGNOSTIC TECHNIQUES

The techniques employed by the otologist in the diagnosis and differential diagnosis of deafness comprise: 1. complete chronological otologic history; 2. pertinent general medical history; 3. physical examination of the ears, nose, and throat; 4. general medical survey; 5. differential audiological studies; 6. laboratory procedures; and 7. roentgenographic studies.

COMPLETE CHRONOLOGICAL OTOLOGIC HISTORY

The otologic history should be complete and should be obtained in chronologic fashion. The patient's own descriptions are important, not only all details pertaining to the hearing loss, but also in regard to tinnitus, vertigo, otorrhea, and otalgia.

PERTINENT MEDICAL HISTORY

Inventories of the respiratory, skeletal, gastrointestinal, neurological, genitourinary, and other systems are mandatory in any medical survey.

PHYSICAL EXAMINATION OF THE EARS, NOSE, AND THROAT

The physical examination should include a complete inspection of the ears, nose, nasopharynx, pharynx, and larynx, as well as the external head and neck. The patency of the Eustachian tubes should be determined by appropriate methods, including not only inflation by Politzerization (mass inflation) or Eustachian catheter, but by visual examination of the Eustachian cushions by one or more of the accepted methods; postnasal (nasopharyngeal mirror), Holmes electric nasopharyngoscope (passed pernasally), or direct peroral inspection employing the Love or Goodhill palate retractor. The last procedure can be carried out in the office—without any anesthesia—upon children. It is uncomfortable but not painful and takes but a moment.

Otoscopic examination should include visualization with magnification and diagnostic compression and rarefaction of auditory canal pressures to determine mobility of tympanic membrane (pneumatic or Siegle otoscopy) (Fig. 12-12). Diagnostic aspiration, either by needle puncture or diagnostic paracentesis, is indicated in questionable middle ear effusions. Disposition of any exudate recovered will be discussed below under *Laboratory procedures*.

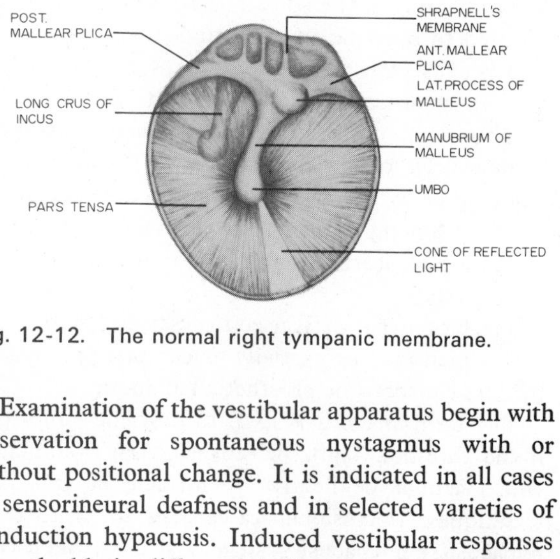

Fig. 12-12. The normal right tympanic membrane.

Examination of the vestibular apparatus begin with observation for spontaneous nystagmus with or without positional change. It is indicated in all cases of sensorineural deafness and in selected varieties of conduction hypacusis. Induced vestibular responses are valuable in differential diagnosis. Such information may be obtained by the Barany rotation technique or torsion swing and from the caloric labyrinthine excitation technique, preferably the Hallpike bithermal method utilizing electronystagmography.

GENERAL MEDICAL SURVEY

The otologist is first a physician and secondly a specialist in ear diseases. His responsibility is to the entire patient, not just to his ears. Accordingly, he will investigate either personally or through a consultant any special medical problems which may coexist. He must remain constantly alert to the otologic manifestations of systemic problems as anemia, hypertension, and other vascular diseases, neurologic problems, endocrinopathies, and all other systemic problems which the true physician will always keep in mind regardless of his speciality.

DIFFERENTIAL AUDIOLOGIC STUDIES

Whereas audiologists, educators of the deaf, speech therapists, and ancillary specialists are all interested in the entire field of audiometry, the otologist is specifically concerned with *differential audiologic diagnosis*. This may be described as audiometric methodology in anatomic localization of auditory pathway lesions. It is concerned with differentiation of conductive from sensorineural lesions, and receptor from transmissive or perceptive lesions (see Chapter 13).

Most otologists feel that no otologic examination is complete without a tuning fork test battery. Of greatest value are the Rinné and Weber tests, using at least the 128, 256, and 512 tuning forks. The Rinné is said to be "negative" (BC > AC) if bone-conducted sound is heard louder than air-conducted sound. This finding bespeaks a conductive loss. The "positive" Rinné (AC > BC) is characteristic of normal ears and sensorineural losses. Because the patient is sometimes unable to appreciate that he may be hearing the sound in the opposite ear when the ear under test is affected by a sensorineural loss, masking is of importance in performing the Rinné test. It is customary to apply the small Bárány noisemaker to the opposite ear for this purpose. The Weber test (butt of fork held at midline of brow and/or at upper central incisor teeth) for lateralization is most sensitive and useful. In normal cases, lateralization does not occur. Lateralization toward a hearing-impaired ear bespeaks a conductive lesion, away from such an ear (to the opposite side) a sensorineural lesion.

LABORATORY PROCEDURES

Exudate may be hidden behind an intact eardrum or manifest in the form of otorrhea through a perforation. In either case, appropriate laboratory studies are indicated on exudate collected either by suction through the canal or by aspiration or paracentesis of the eardrum. Nasal or pharyngeal discharges may also be present and have a bearing on concurrent disease of the ear. In general, exudates, whether from the ear or from the nose and throat, are subjected to the same type of laboratory study. These include smears on glass slides, at least two in number: one stained by the Gram method for the rapid identification of microorganisms; and a second stained by the Hansel method for differential cell count, with particular reference to relative numbers of polymorphonuclear leukocytes, eosinophiles, and lymphocytes. The relative numbers of these cells afford insight into the etiologic roles of allergy and infection and into the relative acuteness or chronicity of the infective component. It is worthy of mention that pathogenic microorganisms in the ears are correlated with those present in the nose and throat in only 60 percent of cases, so that it cannot simply be assumed that identification of pathogenic microorganisms in the nose or throat necessarily give sufficient information for adequate treatment of an ear infection. Exudates are planted in culture media under both aerobic and anaerobic conditions. Sensitivity tests for antibiotics and chemotherapeutic agents are carried out.

Examinations of blood and urine are of paramount importance in all constitutional medical lesions, and the blood count may be of specific importance in the study of ear infections. Serologic examination of the blood to rule out syphilis is frequently required. Leukemia, anemia, and polycythemia, as well as other blood dyscrasias, may produce otologic disturbances and can be revealed by proper hematologic study.

In selected cases where some central nervous system disease may coexist or be suspected, it is necessary to perform a lumbar puncture to measure the cerebrospinal fluid pressure and to withdraw sufficient fluid for chemical, serologic, and cytologic examination.

Recent research indicates that laboratory studies of perilymph obtained through the stapedial footplate may have important diagnostic value in the future.

CONDUCTIVE LESIONS

Audiologic Diagnostic Aspects of Conductive Lesions

Unless otherwise specified in the ensuing descriptions, the term A.C. will be used for air-conduction threshold, and B.C. for bone-conduction threshold. Unless otherwise stated, these thresholds will be described within the speech range (500, 1,000 *and* 2,000 *Hz*). *Calibration is ISO* (1964).

Hearing losses of conduction type are always hypacuses and never anacuses, and are characterized by well-defined criteria. These include the following:

THRESHOLD LOSSES

Threshold losses by pure-tone audiometry do not exceed 60 to 65 dB in the speech range. Any threshold loss in excess of this is undoubtedly due to a coexistent sensorineural loss.

SIGNIFICANT B.C.-A.C. DIFFERENTIAL

The B.C.-A.C. "gap" will give a quantitative measure of the extent of the conduction deficit. This deficit cannot be gauged by A.C. comparison with the zero audiometric reference level for "normal." For example: a patient with coexistent presbycusis and otosclerosis may have an A.C. of 70 dB and a B.C. of 30 dB; his conduction deficit would be roughly 40 dB and not 70 dB. This differential will be confirmed usually by the negative Rinné test when performed with a 128 or 256 cycle tuning fork. Major discrepancy between this test and audiometric B.C. and A.C. tests will call for careful review of B.C. tests with sophisticated appraisal of calibration and masking techniques.

CLOSE CORRELATION BETWEEN PURE-TONE A.C. THRESHOLD AND SRT

The SRT, or speech reception threshold, is the sound level at which 50 percent of spondee words are correctly repeated. Close correlation with pure-tone A.C. threshold is the rule in conduction lesions, but it is not so uniform in sensorineural lesions. Average of the three speech frequencies (500, 1,000, 2,000 Hz) often comes within 10 dB of the SRT in conductive cases.

SPEECH DISCRIMINATION SCORE

Speech discrimination score is the percentage of monosyllabic PB (phonetically balanced) words heard at the most comfortable loudness level, whatever that may be. This is a suprathreshold test. The score is high, approaching 100 percent in conductive cases.

RESPONSE TO AMPLIFICATION

Response to amplification is excellent with little or no recruitment, and there is excellent amplification of whispered voice with the classical speaking tube.

Conduction losses may vary from minor five- to 10-dB losses to the 60- to 65-dB losses mentioned above. In all such threshold estimations, it must be remembered that the zero level used in conventional audiometry is an arbitrary level and may not represent the true predisease threshold of the individual patient.

BÉKÉSY AUDIOMETRY

Conductive lesions characteristically are associated with a Type I Békésy audiogram.

The patient with an uncomplicated conductive hypacusis can never be described as being profoundly deaf. If he has significant difficulty in understanding speech with adequate amplification, it must be assumed, audiometric findings to the contrary, that he has a sensorineural loss in addition to his conductive loss.

Audiologic Evaluation of Surgery in Conductive Hypacusis

Otologic surgeons are always concerned with the efficacy of surgical techniques and, thus, methods for evaluating surgical "success" have been advanced during the past few decades. The principles to be enunciated apply equally to stapedectomy and to tympanoplastic techniques.

The first operation successfully advanced for the treatment of hearing loss was the fenestration procedure for otosclerosis. In this procedure, the physiologic predicted result was fairly constant. Since the operation involves removal of a portion of the ossicular chain and the creation of a new window into the labyrinth, a fixed loss of auditory acuity amounting to 15 to 25 dB could always be subtracted from the ultimate goal of the cochlear reserve as expressed in bone-conduction levels. Thus, the ideal candidate for fenestration surgery, with a bone-conduction level not lower than 10 dB, might well reach approximately a 25 dB level and be rightfully considered a "successful case," since perilymph had been remobilized and basilar membrane excitation increased, even though the impedance-matching mechanism had been partially sacrificed. Thus, a choice of candidates with a 25 to 30 bone-conduction level would almost certainly guarantee a postoperative result no better than 40 to 45 dB regardless of the extent of the preoperative air-conduction level.

Since fenestration surgery involved the use of general anesthesia and major temporal bone removal with creation of a mastoidostomy cavity, an objective of the 30 to 35 dB level was generally adopted as a criterion of "success" with considerable justification. This level was conceded to be that level below which unaided hearing was impractical. With this limitation, prudent surgical opinion dictated the choice of the surgical candidate as one who was likely to achieve this level (30 to 35 dB), the limitation being defined by the preoperative B.C. level.

Since in stapes surgery it is possible to maintain the impedance-matching mechanism and thus eliminate the inherent 15 to 25 dB loss due to its sacrifice, the criteria for selection of candidates for surgery obviously were different from those used in fenestration surgery. Thus, it became possible to consider for surgery patients with significantly poorer B.C. levels than those previously considered essential for successful surgery in the fenestration era. Similarly, in tympanoplastic surgery no arbitrary 30 to 35 dB level could be chosen, since it is possible in certain tympanoplastic procedures to close the air-bone gap completely, although this is less likely than in stapes surgery. Besides, this surgery often is done to alleviate other ravages of disease than impaired hearing, so that other criteria of success must be considered. It thus becomes evident that the magnitude of the air-bone gap and its position on the audiometric "map" as regards superior and inferior limits becomes the crucial indication of the physiologic inefficiency of the impedance-matching mechanism. While other studies such as the SDS, recruitment test, Békésy audiogram, etc., give us valuable information concerning cochlear function, the B.C. measurements, with all respect due to their inherent problems, give us our best quantitative measure of the level of cochlear reserve. The degree of closure of the air-bone gap is the only method available for measuring the efficacy of physiologic reconstruction in surgery for conductive hypacusis. It is obvious that such closure of the air-bone gap must be in an upward direction to be meaningful. If bone conduction drops following a surgical procedure while air conduction remains at the same or at a lower level, the air-bone gap may indeed be "closed" in a downward direction —due to a superimposed sensorineural deficit accruing from the surgery and not to success in removing a conductive block. A consequence of this concept of air-bone gap closure is the necessity for cochlear function studies such as the SDS to be made in addition to B.C. determinations, both pre- and postoperatively, in order to validate the meaningfulness and significance of the air-bone gap. Gap closure is not the sole criterion of successful restoration of hearing, but only of physiologic reconstruction of the middle ear transducer mechanism.

As a result of the need for a mathematical basis for surgical-audiologic evaluation, the percent improvement concept was advocated. The percentage closure is calculated on the basis of comparison between pre- and postoperative A.C. levels with respect to preoperative B.C. level. The formula is:

$$\frac{\text{Preop. A.C. minus Postop. A.C.}}{\text{Preop. A.C. minus Preop. B.C.}} \text{ or } \frac{\text{A.C. Gain}}{\text{Air-bone Gap}} = \% \text{ Improvement}$$

It will be noted that postoperative bone-conduction level does not enter into this equation. It should be understood that, using the above formula, many cases show a postoperative overclosure of the air-bone gap due to mechanical factors that influence preoperative bone conduction adversely, as represented by the Carhart notch concept (Carhart, 1950). The existence of this "notch," and other similar discrepancies recently observed, illustrates the fact that preoperative bone-conduction thresholds cannot be taken as absolute indicators of cochlear reserve and strengthens the case for consideration of postoperative B.C. and SDS measurements in the final evaluation of surgical results. But, again, this consideration is, of necessity, omitted in calculating percent of improvement.

Pathologic Physiology of Conductive Lesions

It is well to recall that it is possible, and in fact common, for conductive lesions to reach decibel loss values far in excess of the 26 dB described previously as the contribution of the drum membrane and ossicular chain to sound-pressure transducer action. In cases with an intact and perhaps thickened drum, behind which an ossicular discontinuity exists, the drum may become worse than useless since it may both reflect and absorb sound energy. Closure of one of the windows by disease may add another 25 to 30 dB of loss, so that a conductive lesion may easily reach a level of 50 to 60 dB in the speech range. In addition, alterations in tympanic physiology may involve the tympanic muscles as well as the suspensory ligaments of the ossicles. Such problems will be reflected in loss of functional efficacy of the ossicular chain lever action and may also produce increased stiffness and frictional resistance resulting in additional deficits in acoustic transmission.

Conductive lesions may be divided into the following groups:

1. *Acoustic reception lesions* involving obstruction of the external auditory canal with or without lesions of the drum membrane involving either a stiffening of the drum or perforations of varying sizes and locations.

2. *Ossicular chain lesions* which may involve any of the three ossicles in the whole or in part. There may be loss of continuity, the most common example of which is the aseptic necrosis of the distal long and lenticular processes of the incus. Arthritic fixation of the ossicular joints may also occur, chiefly from osteoarthritis. Occasionally, atrophic lesions of the

incus or stapes crura may decrease transmission by producing increased elasticity, or softening. Increased brittleness may result in pathologic fracture.

3. *Fixation of the oval window* by ankylosis of the footplate is a common transmission lesion.

4. Blockage of the round window by fibrosis or osteogenic closure may produce a hearing loss.

5. Multiple combinations of any of the foregoing lesions, occasionally combined with some degree of perilymph immobilization by chronic fibrous labyrinthitis.

Basic Surgical Concepts and Operative Procedures

It is necessary at this time to introduce certain basic otosurgical concepts and terms which will be used in describing the management of a number of specific conductive hypacuses in both children and adults.

MYRINGOTOMY

This procedure, involving simple incision of the tympanic membrane, is still the most common ear operation (Fig. 12-13). It is used for the evacuation of fluid under pressure in the middle ear, as during acute infection. Suction may be employed by applying a fine cannula to or through the margins of the incision to effect more complete removal of exudate.

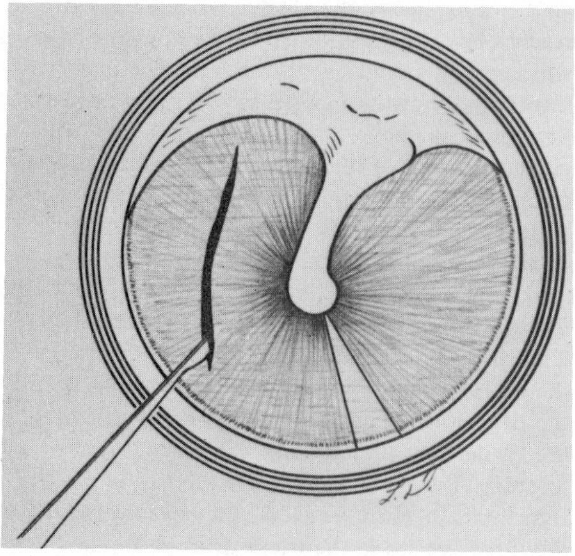

Fig. 12-13. Myringotomy incision in posterior half of drum, as carried out in cases of purulent otitis. Such incisions heal without a visible scar, whereas spontaneous rupture (blowouts) may leave scarring or result in a permanent perforation. A normal drum is shown here for purposes of orientation.

DOUBLE MYRINGOTOMY

This procedure is performed in less acute conditions, usually in cases of subacute or chronic secretory otitis. Instead of one long incision in the posterior quadrant, two short incisions are made, one in each inferior quadrant, anteriorly and posteriorly (Fig. 12-14).

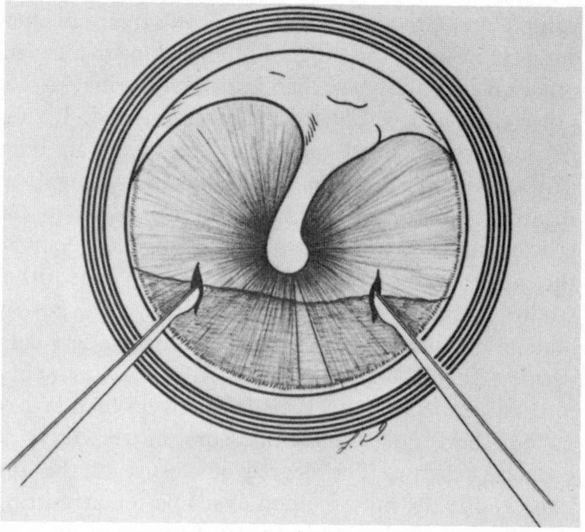

Fig. 12-14. Double myringotomy for secretory otitis. In these cases, the tympanic cavity is usually full, and no fluid level is seen. The tympanic pressure is below normal, and the drum is retracted rather than bulging or full. The condition is usually painless and may go unnoticed in children for long periods of time.

MYRINGOSTOMY

This procedure simply involves the placement of small drainage tubes through the single or double myringotomy incisions described above, with the idea of preventing the usual rapid healing, thus promoting continued drainage and aeration of the tympanic air space when this is required (Fig. 12-15). The principal indication for this procedure is the presence of so-called "glue exudate," a particularly tenacious and stringy substance containing large amounts of D.N.A. It is usually amber in color. Occasionally, such intubation is used when serous or mucous exudate has proved chronic and refractory to treatment. Either prefabricated "collar button" tubes are used or No. 90 polyethylene tubes, with the inner end slightly flanged by holding it in a flame.

EXPLORATORY TYMPANOTOMY

This procedure is exploration of the tympanic air space by anterior reflection of the posterior canal wall

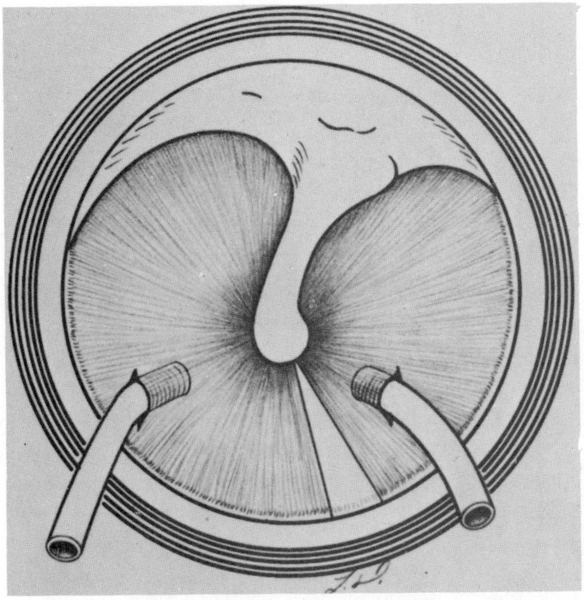

Fig. 12-15. Myringostomy tubes placed through double incisions to maintain patency. Drainage occurs around as well as through tubes. Tubes are left in situ for weeks, sometimes months.

skin and the posterior half of the eardrum, thus exposing the posterior tympanic cavity region and the ossicular chain. This usually involves the use of a posterior omega incision (Fig. 12-16), and frequently curettage of posterior bony canal wall and annulus region in order to get better exposure (Fig. 12-17). With inclusion of canal floor skin by a more generous anterioinferior arm of the incision, it is possible to

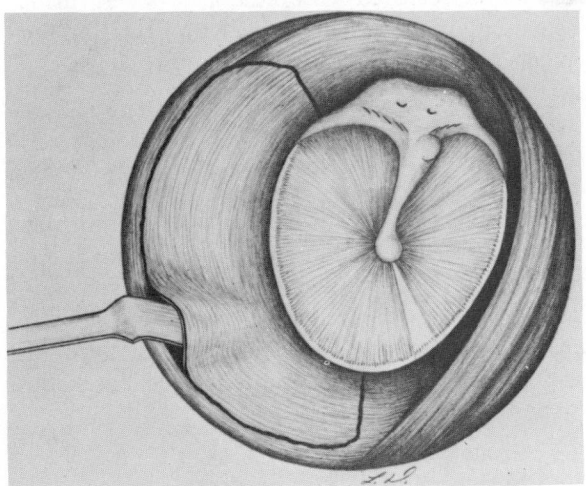

Fig. 12-16. Posterior "omega" incision in skin of bony canal for anterior reflection of tympanomeatal flap for exploration of middle ear space.

expose the tympanic orifice of the Eustachian tube and other structures not available via "posterior tympanotomy."

MASTOIDECTOMY

This is an exposure and removal of mastoid trabeculae and contents of infected air cells. Exenteration of such bony cell walls is seldom anatomically total. The extent of removal is based upon surgical judgment. The incision for any of these following types may be *postauricular* or *endaural.*

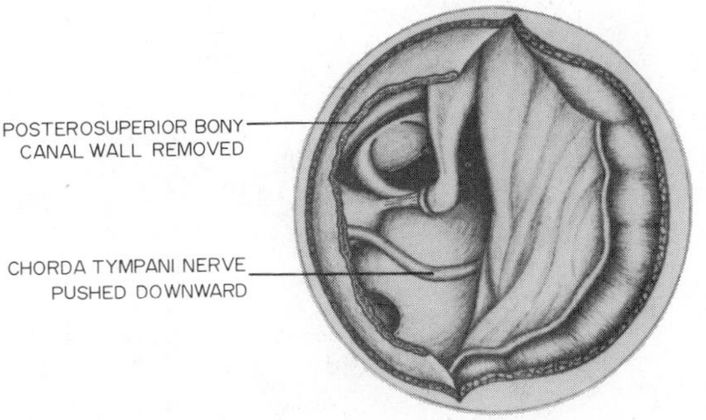

Fig. 12-17. Tympanomeatal flap shown reflected forward and bony annulus resected posterosuperiorly to expose incudostapedial joint and oval window region above, round window below.

SIMPLE MASTOIDECTOMY

This involves an exenteration of the cellular system of the mastoid process and its extensions stopped at the *aditus ad antrum* and omitting exploration of either the tympanic cavity or the attic (epitympanum). This operation is virtually obsolete today.

ATTICOMASTOIDECTOMY

This is the basic mastoid operation which includes exploration of the entire attic or epitympanum, usually through the mastoid approach, permitting visualization and treatment of the head of the malleus, the incudomalleal joint, the body and short process of the incus (Fig. 12-18). This operation usually includes an exploratory tympanotomy which does not require, in all cases, the separate omega incision deep within the external auditory canal described above. It is often sufficient to dissect the skin of the membranous canal away from the bony canal down to the annulus tympanicus, and to disarticulate the latter. It may or may not be necessary to remove annular bone as described previously.

RADICAL MASTOIDECTOMY

This is the classic operation involving removal of the posterior bony canal wall, the drum, the malleus, the incus, and other contents of the tympanic cavity, leaving only the stapes. In the classic operation, no attempt was made to save either the bony or the fibrous annulus. Thus, the middle-ear cavity, the epitympanum, the external auditory canal, and the mastoid were converted into one large space. The modern radical operation attempts to conserve certain structures which may be useful in later reconstruction. Thus, the operation can still be considered a radical mastoidectomy in some instances in which the posterior bony canal wall is left intact. Every effort is made to preserve the fibrous annulus. At the minimum, the modern radical operation would include removal of at least some part of the tympanic membrane, the malleus, and the incus, with or without stapes crura (Fig. 12-19).

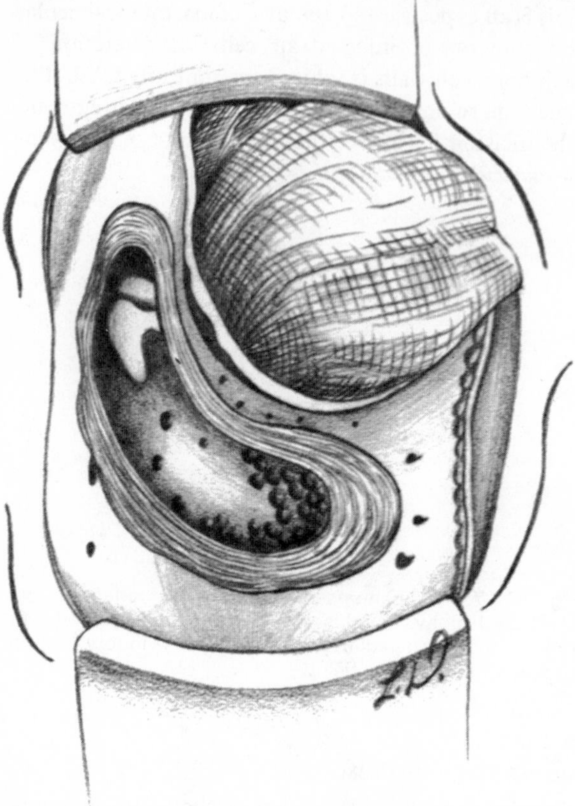

Fig. 12-18. Diagrammatic illustration of an attico-mastoidectomy. The head of the malleus, body of the incus, and short process of the incus are contained in the attic region. Posterior to the short process of the incus lies the mastoid antrum and some mastoid air cells.

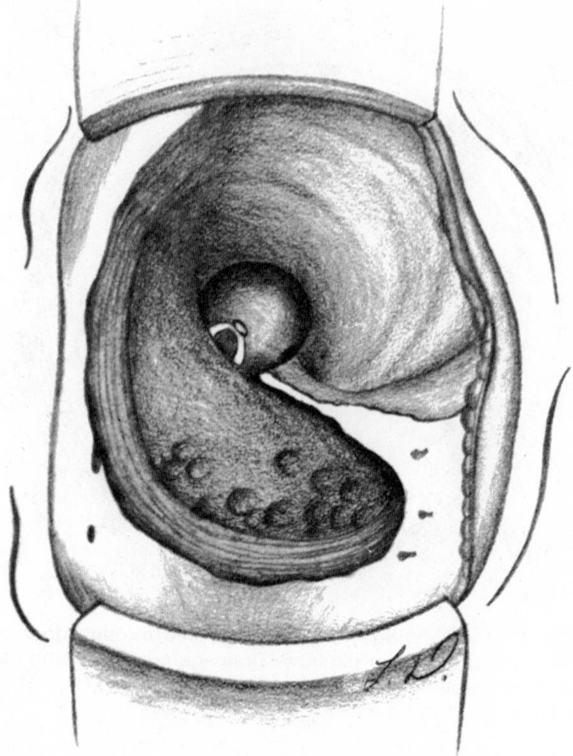

Fig. 12-19. Diagrammatic representation of a radical mastoidectomy showing an intact stapes and complete exteriorization of all the ear spaces, leaving only the stapes intact.

MODIFIED RADICAL MASTOIDECTOMY

This is an operation in which the posterior bony canal wall is removed with creation of a permanent mastoidostomy cavity, but in which the drum and the contents of the tympanic cavity are not too drastically interfered with (Fig. 12-20).

TYMPANOPLASTY

The term tympanoplasty refers to the plastic surgical reconstruction of the tympanic transducer mechanism by means (usually) of autogenous tissues which are used to repair or to bypass existing defects. Tympanoplastic operations are frequently carried out in conjunction with mastoid operations of one type or another. Such procedures are designated "mastoidectomy-tympanoplasty."

The Physiology of Tympanoplasty

The principles of tympanic physiology (Goodhill, 1958, a) are utilized practically in the designing of tympanoplastic operations. Wullstein (1956) has given us a useful classification of five types of tympanoplasty based upon the progression of problems encountered in tympanic defects. With two additions (Extended Type III Tympanoplasty and the Sonoinversion operation) these are:

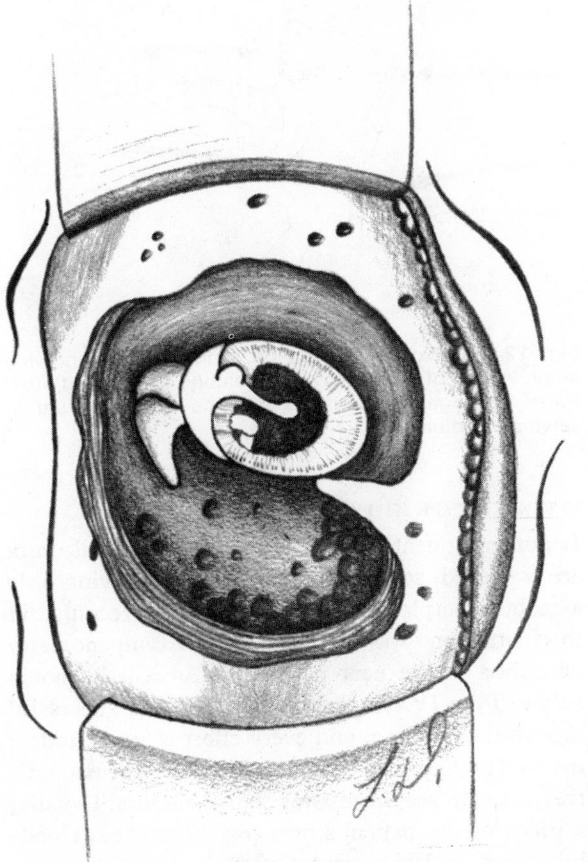

Fig. 12-20. Diagrammatic illustration of a modified radical mastoidectomy (Bondy) showing tympanic membrane remnant, intact ossicular chain, partial removal of posterior bony canal wall with exteriorization of the attic and mastoid.

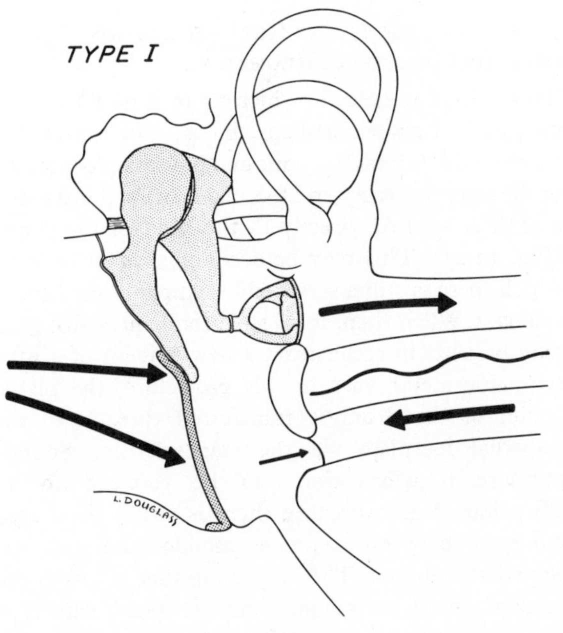

Fig. 12-21. Type I tympanoplasty. A graft is shown closing an inferior marginal perforation. The ossicular chain is intact and mobile.

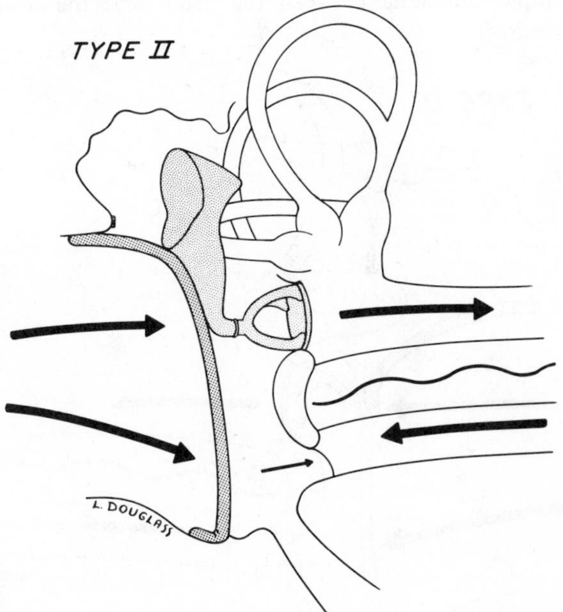

Fig. 12-22. Type II tympanoplasty. A total graft is shown placed against the incus. The malleus has been removed.

TYPE I TYMPANOPLASTY (MYRINGOPLASTY)

This is the simplest problem to solve surgically in tympanoplasty. It describes the closure by an autogenous graft of a perforation in an eardrum in the presence of an intact, normally mobile ossicular chain, and no other significant local pathologic findings (Fig. 12-21).

TYPE II TYMPANOPLASTY

In this situation, it is necessary to sacrifice the malleus. The incus may be partially impaired, but still viable. An autogenous graft is placed upon the incus, producing a reduced ossicular chain (Fig. 12-22). This operation is rarely performed today.

TYPE III TYMPANOPLASTY (COLUMELLIZATION OPERATION OR MYRINGOSTAPEDIOPEXY)

This is used in cases in which there is no longer any continuity between malleus, incus, and stapes, but there is still normal anatomic and physiologic integrity of the stapedial crura and footplate. In such instances, a graft is applied directly to the head of the stapes (Fig. 12-23). This may be accomplished in cases in which there is still a serviceable tympanic membrane remnant. When there is no such remnant, a full graft may be used to reconstruct a new version of a total tympanic membrane. In this procedure, the piston action of the drum is transferred directly to the stapedial footplate via the stapes crura. Sound-pressure transformation can be restored to an efficacious degree because there is still a good *area difference* between the new pseudodrum and the stapedial footplate. The only thing that is lost is the lever action of the malleus and the incus, which, as mentioned previously, is not a great factor in the transducer function of the middle-ear mechanism. Indeed, birds have exquisitely sensitive hearing and lack a malleus and incus altogether, having only a simple columella between the drum and the oval window.

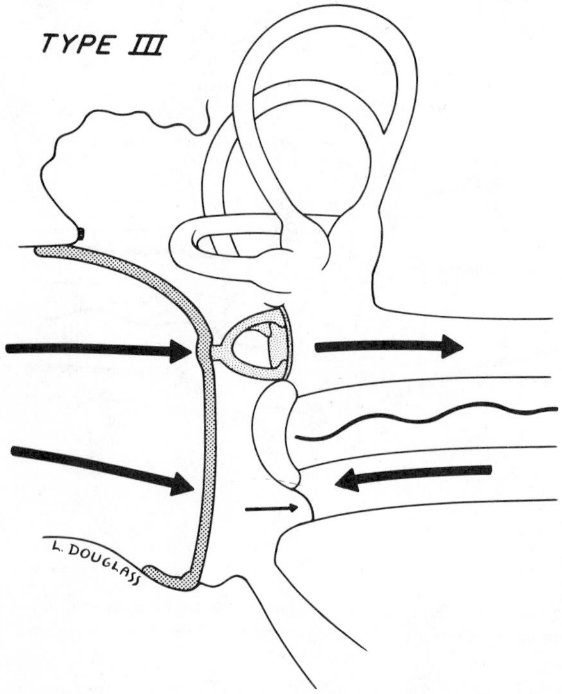

Fig. 12-23. Type III tympanoplasty. Malleus and incus are absent, and a total graft is shown applied to the capitulum of the intact stapes.

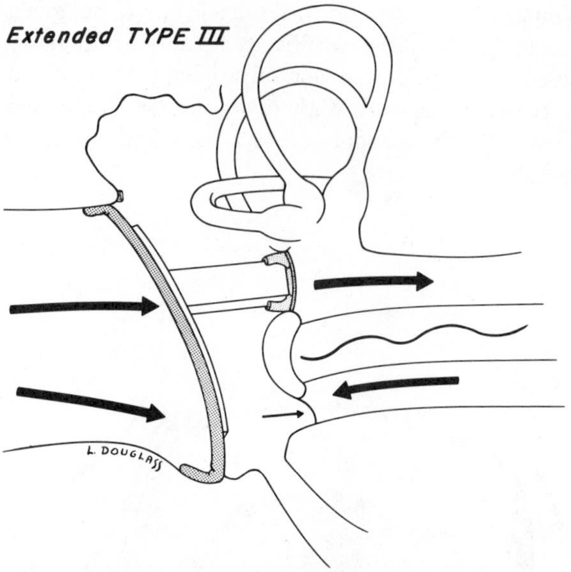

Fig. 12-24. Extended Type III tympanoplasty showing employment of so-called "T-assembly," fashioned from tragal cartilage in continuity with its perichondrium to serve as a columella.

EXTENDED TYPE III TYMPANOPLASTY

It not infrequently happens that the stapedial crura are fractured, sequestrated, or missing, leaving only a mobile footplate. Previously, the only recourse in this situation was the Type IV tympanoplasty described in the next paragraph. As will be noted below, Type IV tympanoplasty is not very successful in restoring hearing, and every effort is made, today, to avoid it. This may be done by utilizing the patient's tissues to replace the missing stapedial crura. Usually, a piece of the patient's own tragal cartilage (Goodhill, 1967, a, Harris and Goodwill, 1967), properly fashioned, is used for this purpose. Often, this piece of cartilage is removed from the tragus in continuity with tragal perichondrium, forming a so-called "T-assembly" (Brockman, 1965) (Fig. 12-24). (It should be explained here that, in general, some sort of connective tissue is used for closing tympanic membrane perforations or for replacing the tympanic membrane altogether. For this purpose, mesodermal tissues such as tragal perichondrium are ideal (Goodhill et al., 1964). Formerly, skin was used, but this led to certain complications and has been abandoned.)

TYPE IV TYMPANOPLASTY (CAVUM MINOR OPERATION OR SOUND-PROTECTION BAFFLE OPERATION)

In instances in which there has been a loss of stapedial capitulum and crura, but in which the footplate is still mobile, a *cavum minor* or small-cavity operation may yield sufficient sound-protection to the round-window membrane so as to restore the sound-pressure difference between the two windows. This "baffle" operation, in which the round window is protected from sound, is usually produced by rotation of a mucosal graft inferiorly from the promontory over the round-window niche and covering of this mucosal graft with a fairly thick, connective tissue graft in continuity with the Eustachian tube orifice. This creates a "small" middle ear which provides continuity of air space between the tympanic Eustachian orifice and round window, but in which the oval-window region and the movable footplate in that window are exteriorized to air-borne sound (Fig. 12-25). The round-window baffle effect will occasionally allow restoration of thresholds from 60 dB to the 30 dB level. The obvious loss of the transducer action of the middle ear still exists, but this improvement in hearing may be significantly helpful in certain cases.

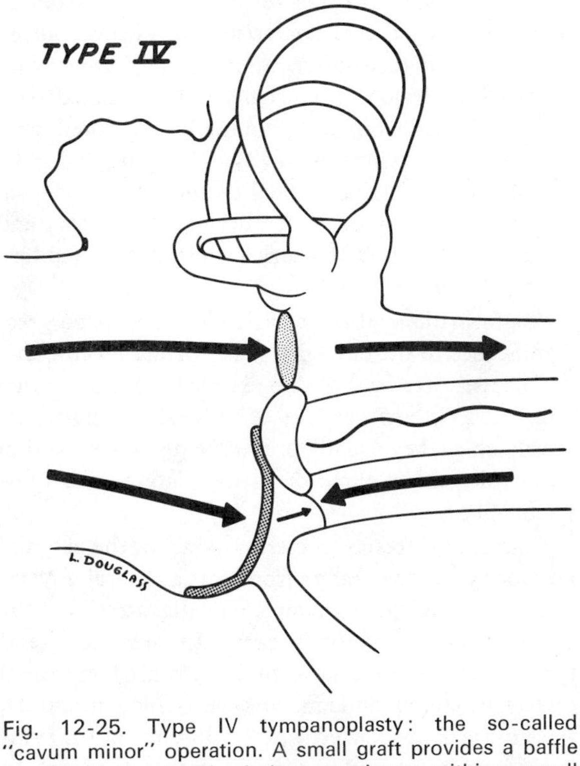

Fig. 12-25. Type IV tympanoplasty: the so-called "cavum minor" operation. A small graft provides a baffle to protect the round window membrane within a small airspace continuous with the tympanic Eustachian orifice. The mobile oval window is left exposed to ambient air. Thus is created a significant phase differential permitting mobilization of the perilymph by air-borne sound waves.

TYPE V TYMPANOPLASTY (FENESTRATION OPERATION COMBINED WITH CAVUM MINOR OPERATION)

In instances in which there is a fixed stapedial footplate, hearing may still be restored by the dual procedure of a round-window baffle and a fenestration of the horizontal semicircular canal (Fig. 12-26). The

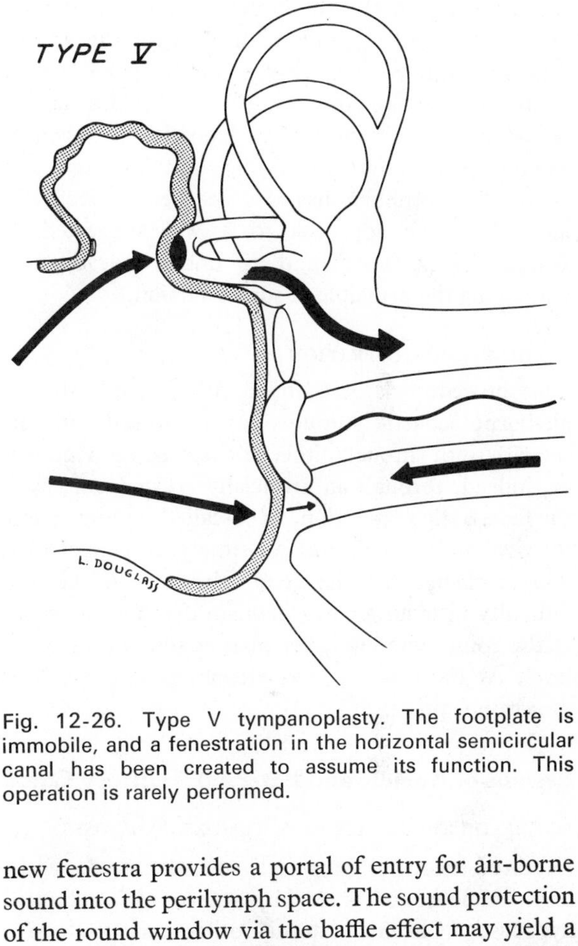

Fig. 12-26. Type V tympanoplasty. The footplate is immobile, and a fenestration in the horizontal semicircular canal has been created to assume its function. This operation is rarely performed.

new fenestra provides a portal of entry for air-borne sound into the perilymph space. The sound protection of the round window via the baffle effect may yield a level of approximately 30 dB in some cases (similar to that of the Type IV tympanoplasty). This operation is rarely performed. One reason is that it is seldom indicated. A second is that fenestration of the labyrinth in an ear which is, or has been, chronically infected is attendant with some added risk to the labyrinth.

The previous classification, according to Wullstein (with, thus far, one American addition, the extended Type III tympanoplasty), represents an oversimplification. Actually, there are many variations of and many deviations from it. Nor are any of these procedures free of problems and difficulties. One of the chief difficulties in tympanoplastic surgery is the avoidance of scar tissue formation (fibrosis) and the maintenance of sufficient depth of the tympanic air space (in a mediolateral direction). This is particularly troublesome in the Type III tympanoplasty in those cases, by no means rare, in which it has been necessary to remove the posterior bony canal wall (radical mastoidectomy). Lacking the buttress which frames the drum superiorly, the graft, resting on the stapes capitulum, tends to involve itself with the mediotympanic wall, particularly the intratympanic portion of the facial canal. This results in a "braking action" which greatly diminishes its acoustic effectiveness. Despite many efforts by skilled and inventive surgeons, this problem has not yet been solved. An altogether new approach to it was suggested by Garcia-Ibanez (1961) and is under investigation, employing the principle of sonoinversion.

SONOINVERSION OPERATION

This procedure is based upon the principle that an air-borne acoustic stimulus can be introduced into the labyrinth through either of the existing windows, or, indeed, through an artificially created one, as in the fenestration operation. In so-called sonoinversion, the oval and round windows simply exchange roles. This exchange has the great advantage of far less difficulty in maintaining adequate depth of air-space at the round-window level than at the oval-window level. At the time of this writing, progress in this direction is promising.

Lesions of Auricle and External Auditory Canal

ACQUIRED LESIONS (ATRESIAS, TUMORS, EXOSTOSES)

Acquired lesions of the auricle and the external auditory canal are of great importance in conductive hypacuses. Chronic external otitis can produce a major conduction loss simply by complete occlusion of the external auditory canal from tissue swelling. No hearing loss will occur as long as even a microscopic opening is present; but, in such instances, conductive hypacuses may occur before such complete closure because of accumulations of cerumen, dead epithelium, or exudate which will close the small remaining opening. Occasionally, such atresias require surgical correction by endaural techniques, which involve resection of edematous skin, subcutaneous tissue, thickened periosteum, and sometimes bone. The surgically widened ear canal is usually covered with a split-thickness skin graft.

Tumors of the external auditory canal may occlude the air-conduction pathway completely and produce a conductive hypacusis. They may be benign or malignant. All common types of tumors may be seen, including those of skin as well as of cartilage and bone. The only safe treatment for such tumors is surgical excision. In some instances, radiation may also be required.

Bony growths due to exostoses and osteomata are not infrequently found in the external auditory canal. They may not only occlude the canal completely as in atresia, but they may extend to the tympanic annulus and into the tympanic cavity. Most of these bony tumors are benign. Exostoses are more commonly found in persons who swim and dive in cold waters, the reason for this being unknown. The proper treatment of exostoses and osteomata is surgical excision by endaural techniques. In most instances, such removal can be accomplished without damage to the tympanic membrane or cavity.

CONGENITAL MALFORMATIONS (ATRESIAS AND APLASIAS)

Congenital malformations of the auricle and external auditory canal are characterized by pleomorphism. They are primarily defects in branchial cleft development. Such lesions are usually not associated with cochlear lesions but are commonly associated with lesions of the tympanic cavity. Thus, normal B.C. thresholds (indicating normal cochlear function) will be found in most cases of microtia (small ear) and congenital defects of the auricle and external auditory canal.

Malformations of the auricle alone are of no great significance to the otologist, being primarily cosmetic problems. Atresias of the external auditory canal (Fig. 12-27), however, are of profound importance, inasmuch as they usually produce a major conduction hypacusis, either alone or in association with tympanic aplasia.

Congenital atresias (imperforations) of the external auditory canal may range from partial lateral atresias (pinpoint openings) to complete medial atresias of the cartilaginous and/or bony canal. In the rare lateral types, it is not unusual to find a normal bony canal and a normal tympanic membrane. In most instances, the atresia is associated with an absence of the tympanic membrane and abnormal tympanic cavity. In these cases, as in the auricular aplasias, the cochlea is usually normal. The tympanic membrane is replaced by the primitive tympanic plate and one, two, or all three ossicles may be absent or deformed in a multiplicity of variations. The surgical treatment of these defects will be discussed below with congenital lesions of the tympanic cavity.

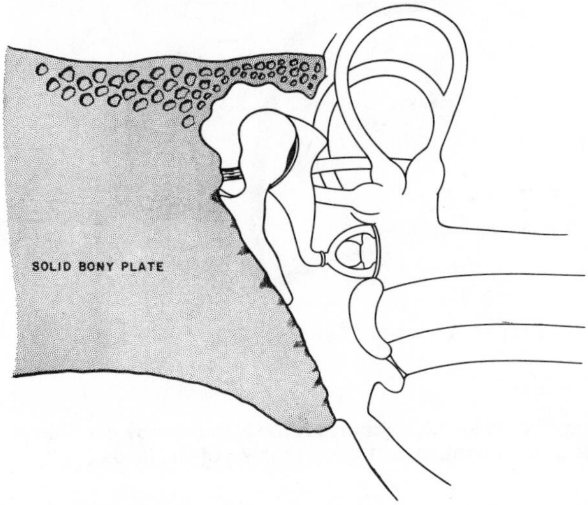

Fig. 12-27. Atresia of the external auditory canal.

Combined External- and Middle-Ear Anomalies

The basic approach to congenital defects of the external- and middle-ears follows the concepts of exploratory mastoidectomy and exploratory tympanotomy. Endaural or postauricular approach to the temporal bone is followed by an exploration of the mastoid, identification of certain fixed surgical landmarks, including the middle and posterior fossa dura plates, and the mastoid antrum. The surgically created external auditory canal is lined with split-thickness skin, but skin is never placed directly over the tympanic air space and its contents, but rather a connective tissue graft, usually perichondrium.

Several definite types of anomalies will be encountered. There is frequently no true canal, nor is there evidence of any functioning tympanic membrane. A thick, bony tympanic plate usually forms the lateral boundary of the deformed tympanic cavity. Most cases share this finding in common, but the following subvarieties of ossicular status will be encountered.

NORMAL MOBILE OSSICULAR CHAIN

Cases with normal mobile ossicular chains show normal formation of all three ossicles and no evidence of discontinuity or fixation anywhere in the chain. In such cases, one creates a new external auditory meatus through the atretic area. A perichondrial or fascial graft (Fig. 12-28) is then placed in direct contact with the denuded manubrium of the malleus, thus providing a tympanic membrane where one had been lacking.

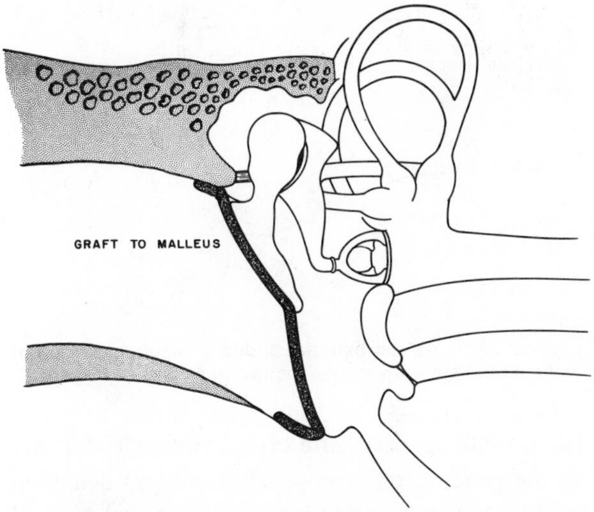

Fig. 12-28. Diagrammatic representation of new external auditory meatus created through atretic area. Graft is placed in contact with denuded malleal manubrium to create a new tympanic membrane.

FUSED MALLEUS, BUT MOBILE INCUS AND STAPES

In this instance, the malleus is fused with the tympanic plate (Fig. 12-29a). However, the incus and the stapes are mobile. A perichondrial or fascial graft placed in contact with the denuded incus after the solid bony plate is drilled out and the malleus remnant is removed produces a myringoincudopexy with transmission of acoustic vibrations from the new tympanic membrane through the incus and stapes to the oval window (Fig. 12-29b).

FUSED INCUS AND MALLEUS, MOBILE STAPES

In this variety, there is fusion of the malleus and incus into one immobile mass, usually attached either completely or partially to the tympanic plate. The stapes, however, is completely formed and mobile (Fig. 12-30a). The procedure of choice is a columellization operation; perichondrial (or fascial) graft applied directly to the head and neck of the stapes after removal of malleus and incus remnants and opening of the atretic external meatus (Fig. 12-30b).

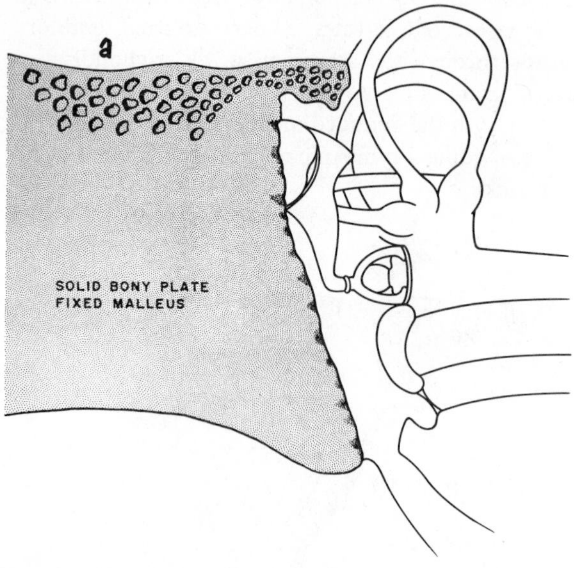

Fig. 12-29a. Atretic external auditory meatus and fused malleal remnant with mobile incus and stapes.

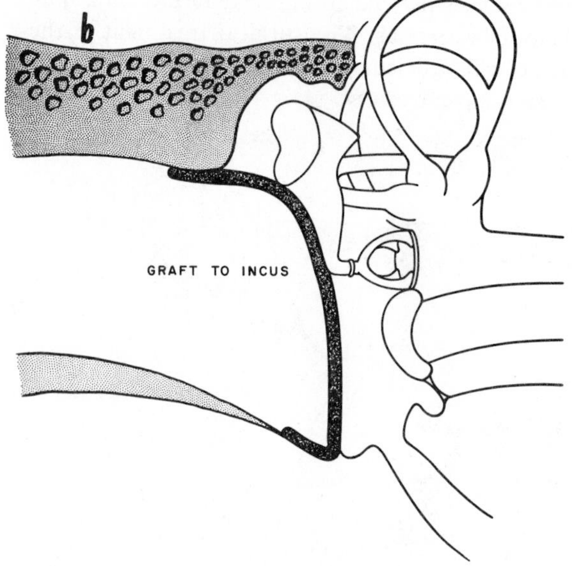

Fig. 12-29b. Myringoincudopexy formed by placement of graft in contact with long process of the incus.

FUSED INCUS, MALLEUS AND CRURA, MOBILE FOOTPLATE

In the presence of a completely fixed and deformed malleus and incus, combined with abnormal crura of the stapes, but with preservation of mobility of the stapedial footplate, an extended Type III tympanoplasty would be done. If this proved impossible, a cavum minor (Type IV) procedure could be tried.

COMPLETE OSSICULAR AND FOOTPLATE IMMOBILIZATION

When there is complete absence or fixation of all ossicular elements with no mobility in the stapedial footplate (Fig. 12-31a), sound can be introduced into the cochlea through a fenestration in the horizontal semicircular canal. A skin graft is placed over the fenestra and in the surgically created external auditory meatus (Fig. 12-31b).

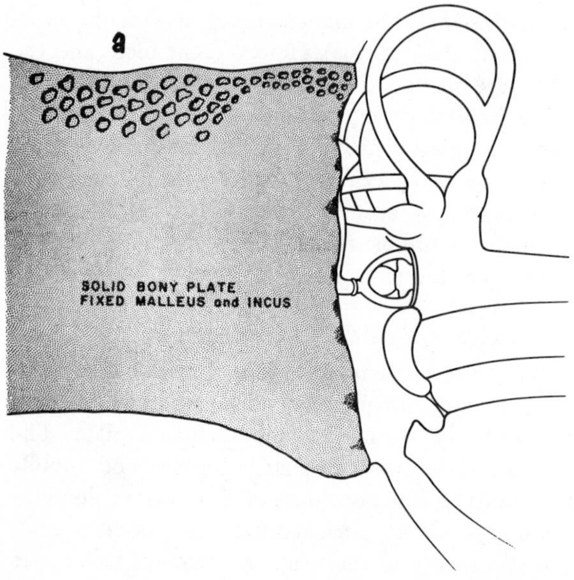

Fig. 12-30a. Atretic external auditory meatus with fixed incus and malleus and normal stapes.

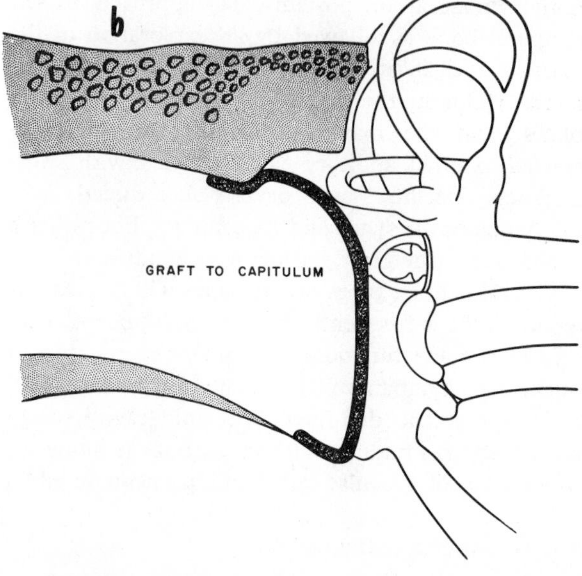

Fig. 12-30b. Surgical excision of bony plate and application of graft to stapedial capitulum.

Thus, by following basic physiologic principles, congenital lesions of the external- and middle-ears can be treated with a high degree of success. However, the problems of tissue grafting must be considered in all tympanoplastic surgery. These procedures may not succeed in one stage, but may require several stages. Only in cases in which there is true deformity of the round window itself with inadequate round window function must fenestration be dropped from ultimate consideration. This is a rare circumstance in congenital lesions.

In dealing with various types of atresia, the technique chosen will depend upon these additional factors: 1) presence or absence of a normal auricle; 2) presence or absence of a skin-lined canal of whatever dimensions or direction; and 3) state of pneumatization of the affected temporal bone.

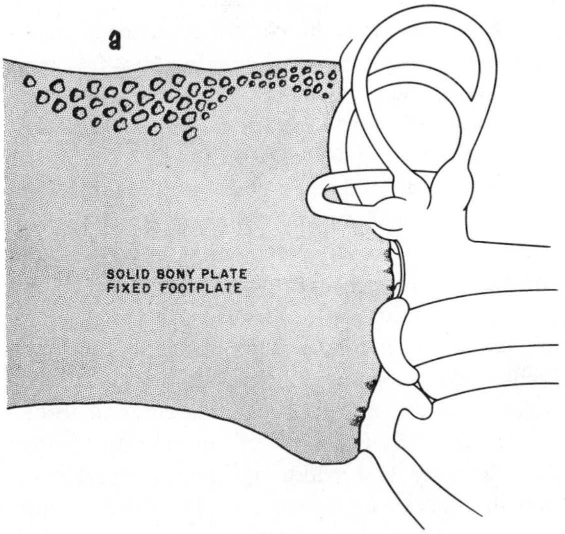

Fig. 12-31a. Atretic external auditory meatus and complete absence of ossicular chain.

Middle Ear Anomalies

Anomalies limited to the middle ear with normal external ear and normal tympanic membrane are more common than hitherto suspected. Exploration of the middle ear under the dissecting microscope in planned stapes mobilization for presumptive otosclerosis has uncovered many such cases. Although exposures during fenestration operations have previously revealed such cases, the extent of middle ear survey in exploratory tympanotomy is more favorable for detailed study of ossicular and fenestral details. Many varieties of such tympanic malformations have been described. Most of these lesions are remediable by combinations of tympanoplasty techniques.

Tympanolabyrinthine Lesions

This is a somewhat theoretical classification, based upon the finding of an apparent air-bone gap in cases of profound sensorineural hypacusis, usually confined to the low frequencies: 250 and 500 Hz, only occasionally at 750 or 1,000 Hz. It is tempting to speculate that this gap may represent a true conductive component in what one might imagine to be a mixed conductive-perceptive deafness. Such cases have been explored surgically. While interesting anomalies of

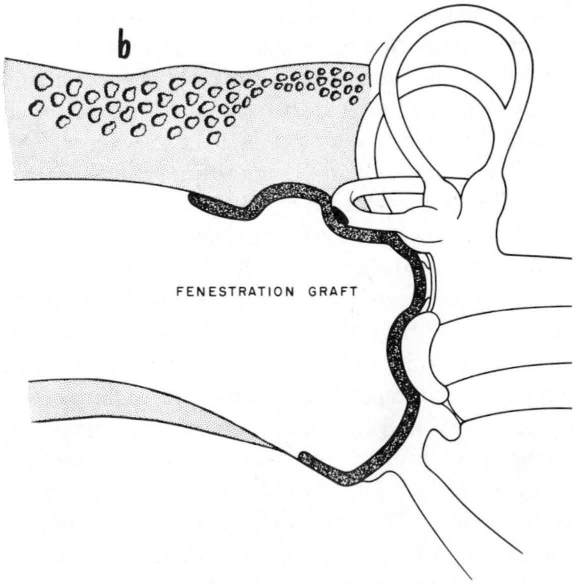

Fig. 12-31b. Fenestration in the horizontal semicircular canal with application of skin graft over the fenestra and surgically created external auditory meatus.

the transmission system of the middle ear have been encountered and some of them repaired, no significant improvement in the hearing results therefrom. It seems likely that these pathological findings are of incidental significance only, and that the apparent air-bone gaps are measurement artifacts based upon a confusion between low-frequency bone-conducted hearing and tactile vibration sense, which is possible even to a sophisticated subject. That such patients may have intralabyrinthine pathologic changes similar to those found in the middle ear (for example, fibrosis) is possible but not yet clearly demonstrated.

Infections

ACUTE OTITIS MEDIA

Acute otitis media is no less common today than it was before the advent of the present antimicrobial era. However, the clinical picture has changed markedly in view of the widespread employment of antibiotics. This use has drastically diminished the incidence of acute mastoiditis. However, it masks symptoms, particularly those of pain, fever, and malaise. It then becomes a difficult problem for the physician to ascertain precisely when the attack is ended and the ear is restored to normal. The only hint that something is amiss may be the persistence of an impairment in hearing, sometimes minimal otoscopic signs. Unless audiometry is employed, the true state of affairs may not be appreciated. The only available alternative to audiometry is the careful performance of live spoken and whispered voice tests under as standard conditions as possible in the physician's office or on a house call. Tuning-fork tests, of course, can be of great assistance here.

The most common mistake in the management of acute otitis media is failure to drain an abscess or collection of seropurulent exudate. Such failure can lead to chronicity of the infection and to numerous complications in the middle ear and its environs. There is a widespread impression in some medical circles that myringotomy (or myringostomy) is virtually an obsolete procedure. This is not at all the case, nor is there any real question of "myringotomy vs. antibiotics." Treatment should always be based on sound surgical principles, and these include the drainage of an abscess or a collection of fluid when an abscess is present. One cannot count on their universal resolution spontaneously. Even when a rhinopharyngeal infection or allergic attack is ended, the mere presence of exudate in the tympanic cavity can cause persistence of "tubotympanitis" with continued tubal blockage and retention of the exudate. The sequelae of such unresolved infection are discussed below. Myringotomy incisions heal without scar.

ACUTE MASTOIDITIS WITH AND WITHOUT COMPLICATIONS

Acute suppurative mastoiditis still occurs and is seen with greater frequency during and following winter epidemics of upper respiratory tract infections. Drug-fast bacteria are often the offending etiologic agents. The pneumococcus, Pseudomonas, and Staphylococcus aureus hemolyticus are the chief offenders causing serious destruction of mastoid trabeculae, frequently with few symptoms.

The treatment of choice for acute mastoiditis which resists antimicrobial therapy is, of course, atticomastoidectomy. The route of approach might be either postauricular or endaural. The extent of removal is entirely dictated by the pathologic findings. Radical mastoidectomy is rarely necessary in acute mastoiditis unless there is concomitant evidence of serious tympanic disease such as cholesteatoma or granulomatous ossicular necrosis or, sometimes, a major intracranial complication. Such conditions are more likely to be encountered in acute exacerbations of chronic otitides which pose the greatest danger of complications of any type of ear disease. Complications in mastoiditis still occur and still require the same vigilance and diagnostic sagacity as in the past. In general, however, the clinical problem is a more serious one, since many of the findings are frequently masked and difficult to elicit. Otitic meningitis (which may occasionally leap from the middle ear directly to the meninges) most usually spreads into the meningeal area via the middle or posterior fossa dura plate within the mastoid portion of the temporal bone. The highest cure rate in otitic meningitis is obtained when appropriate antimicrobial therapy is combined with the removal of the mastoid focus and particularly the removal of osteitic routes for continued thrombophlebitic extension from an infected mastoid process. Lateral sinus thrombosis, otogenous cerebral abscess, and other complications of mastoiditis require mastoidectomy and additional neurosurgical procedures in many cases. Specific details of these complications and their management are too complex for this brief review.

UNRESOLVED OTITIS MEDIA AND MASTOIDITIS

One of the most common problems in recent years has been the latent, silent, or occult otitis media in which a painless effusion occurs in one or both ears, manifested almost entirely by a hearing loss with no other symptoms (Goodhill, 1958, b). The antimicrobial era is certainly the most important cause of the increased incidence of this disease, which is a serious otologic trap for the unwary clinician.

Known by many names and due to many factors, this disease of persistent fluid retention within the middle ear is a major cause of conductive hypacusis in children. It is characterized by variability and confusion in otologic and audiometric findings and is undoubtedly on the increase.

It should be recognized that not infrequently children with unresolved otitis media will be mis takenly diagnosed as having "nerve deafness" because of bone-conduction threshold loss due to the viscosity of thick tympanic fluids which may occlude the round window.

The best treatment for this condition is prophylaxis. Acute otitis media with secretion deserves prompt surgical drainage through myringotomy, along with proper and adequate antibiotic therapy. Even though the acute inflammatory process may subside with antibiotic therapy alone, the persistence of even sterile fluid as a sequel of otitis media not only is a temporary threat to hearing, but also may produce permanent deafness by long-range damage to tympanic structures (fibrosis, necrosis of incudal long process, etc.).

No treatment is satisfactory that does not quickly and thoroughly remove the tympanic fluid. All other modalities which are applied to the Eustachian tube, the nasal and paranasal sinus mucosae, and the pharynx are to no avail if fluid is allowed to remain in the middle ear. This is not to deny the great importance of attention to allergy, to lymphoid tissue, and to chronic infection in the associated nasal, nasopharyngeal, and sinus regions.

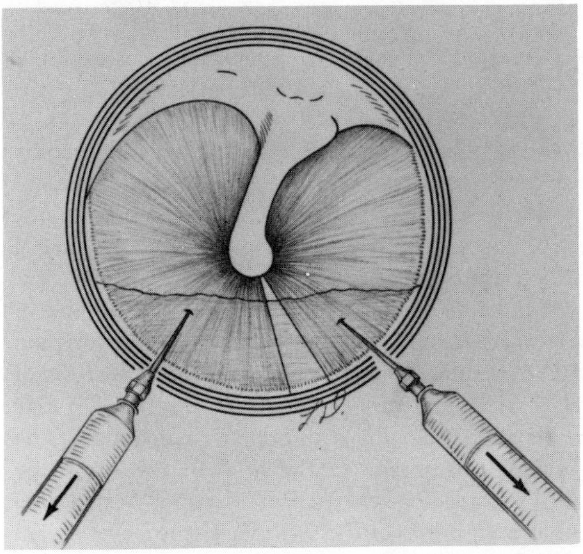

Fig. 12-32. Two needle aspiration of exudate in secretory otitis. Fluid level (meniscus) shown here is not to be expected in the usual case and is not to be depended upon for diagnosis.

Adequate removal of the fluid, then, is the first principle in the proper treatment of this disease and must be accomplished promptly (and repeated if necessary) to ensure an air-filled middle ear, without which restitution of normal mucosa is impossible. Diagnostic aspirations (Fig. 12-32) will be followed in most cases by double myringotomy (Fig. 12-14) and suction to the myringotomy openings (Fig. 12-33). If one encounters fluid of high viscosity, it is usually advisable to insert small polyethylene tubes (Fig. 12-15) immediately for purposes of aeration and drainage. Such tubes may be kept in place for several months, if necessary.

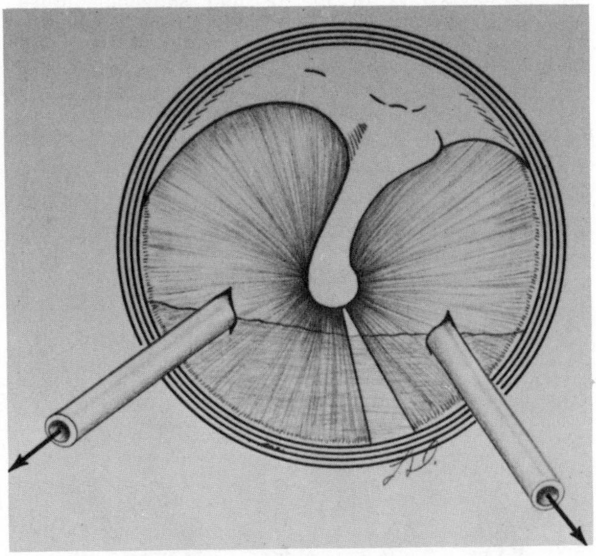

Fig. 12-33. Suction applied through myringostomy incisions using #18 or #15 Rosen suction tubes depending upon viscosity of secretion.

When such measures as described above have been used and there is still no evidence of spontaneous resolution as manifested by recurrent effusion and by continued deformations of the drum and ossicular chain, more thorough exploration is indicated. In most instances of this sort, an exploratory posterior tympanotomy (previously described) is the first step. Such a tympanotomy may be necessary to break up scar tissue bands and drain small pockets of secretion which may not be reached through simple myringotomy and polyethylene intubation. Occasional cystic and polypoid formations may block the tubal orifice. Such a "tympanolysis" may frequently be followed by spontaneous resolution. It is usually advisable to fill the middle ear with hydrocortisone solution to deter recurrence of fibrotic changes.

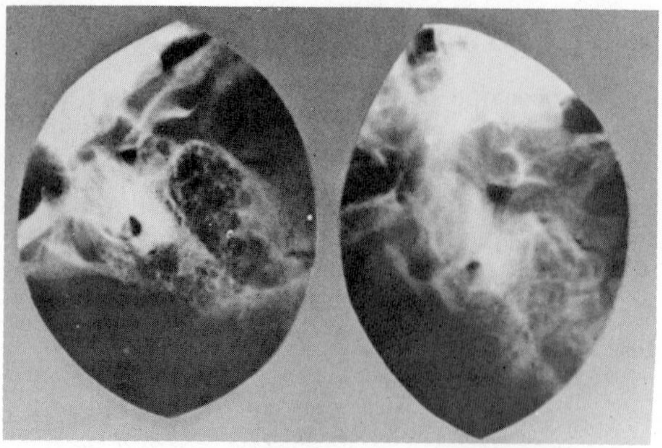

Fig. 12-34. X-rays of the mastoid showing diffuse haziness of the cell structure typical of serous mastoiditis.

In a small number of cases, a chronic unresolved otitis media will be accompanied by a major change in the mastoid cellular mucosa, so that one deals not only with an unresolved otitis media, but also with an unresolved, persistent, nonpurulent mastoiditis. This is clearly diagnosed by x-ray findings (Fig. 12-34).

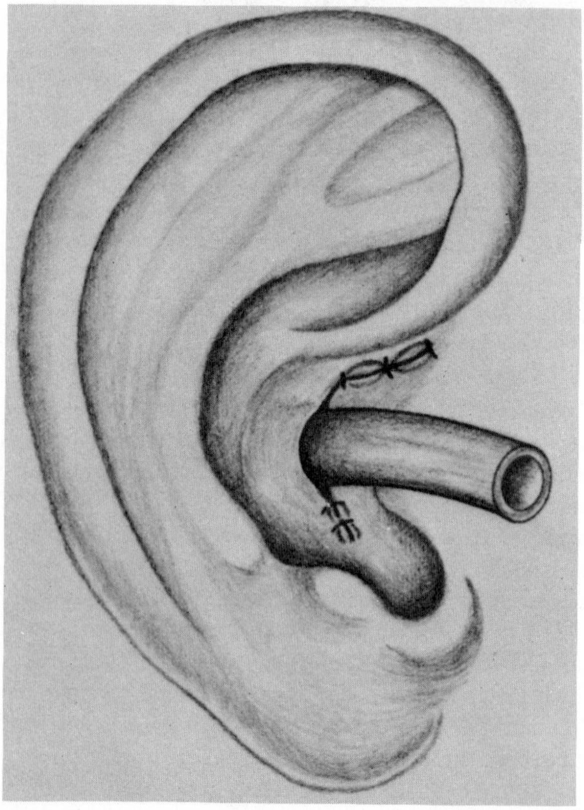

Fig. 12-35. Large polyethylene or rubber catheter drain placed in mastoid antrum and leading out through a portion of the sutured endaural incision.

When this occurs, it is rare to find resolution by simple tympanic therapy. In such cases, exploratory atticomastoidectomy is necessary, followed by prolonged drainage (Fig. 12-35). It is usually advisable to maintain polyethylene ventilation *both* of the *mastoid* and the *middle ear* areas by a large mastoid tube and two small tympanic tubes. During the period of such intubation, it is wise to maintain antibiotic coverage, as indicated by sensitivity tests, along with other necessary therapy to the nasopharynx and the nose.

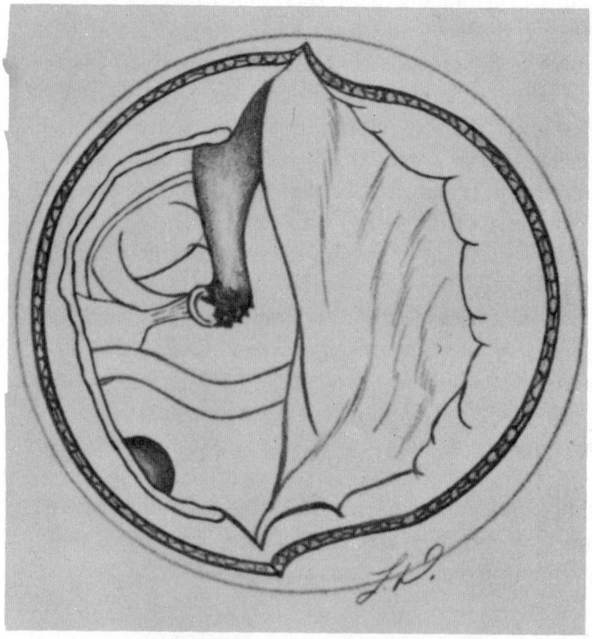

Fig. 12-36. Exploratory tympanotomy exposes aseptic necrosis of the lenticular process of the incus.

In the event that the fibrotic changes disclosed by tympanotomy are accompanied by irreversible mucosal changes and ossicular necrosis, recourse to the reparative procedures may eventually involve one of the various types of tympanoplasty. Fortunately, it is now possible to repair ossicular damage by one of several rerouting operations. Thus, the most common type of acquired ossicular defect, aseptic necrosis of the lenticular process of the incus, (Fig. 12-36) may be repaired by doing a direct approximation of the tympanic membrane to the head of the stapes by myringostapediopexy (columellization) operation. Other deformities of the ossicular chain may respond to other varieties of tympanoplasty.

Pediatricians should also be aware of the lurking, latent cholesteatoma, which may exist behind even an intact eardrum (Fig. 12-37), frequently accompanied by a painless tympanic effusion. Such a cholesteatoma may silently destroy the entire ossicular chain including the stapes, before it is recognised. The early recognition is not difficult if "Siegle otoscopy" (pneumatic otoscopy) and diagnostic Politzerization are a routine part of the otologic examination.

SIMPLE OTITIS PERFORATA (PERSISTENT TYMPANIC PERFORATION)

Perforations of the eardrum are frequently seen in children. They may be due to acute infections which have resulted in pressure-necrosis of the spontaneous perforation margins, or they may be due to trauma.

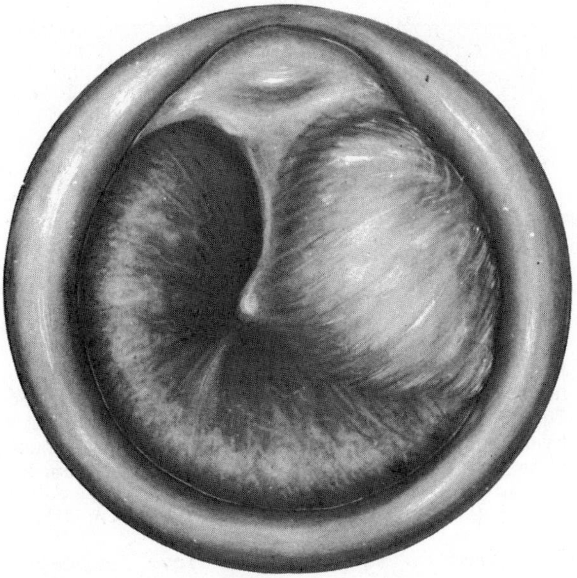

Fig. 12-37. Primary cholesteatoma in a 5-year-old child arising behind an intact drum, now showing a slight bulge. This neoplasm was discovered when a routine screening school audiometry disclosed a one-side conductive loss of 50 dB.

Perforations which are central are usually called simple because they rarely involve bone necrosis. (There are, however, exceptions to this rule, since central perforations may occasionally accompany cholesteatomas.) Marginal perforations are usually not simple because they will involve the bony annulus tympanicus and may involve the ossicular chain.

The problem of the dry central perforations has been virtually solved by the use of tympanoplasty Type I (myringoplasty). This procedure is usually done under general anesthesia in children. It is frequently performed via the ear canal through an

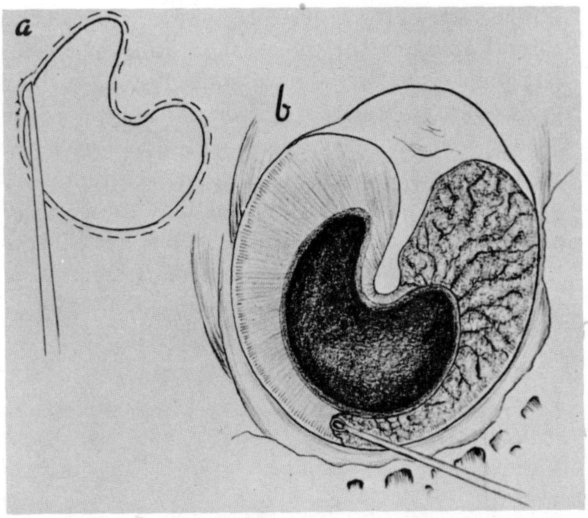

Fig. 12-38. (a) Excision of margin of central perforation to remove epithelized edge which will prevent healing; (b) denudation of the fibrous layer of the drum by systematic removal of the external squamous epithelial layer.

ear speculum with the aid of the dissecting microscope. In narrow or tortuous ear canals, an endaural or postauricular approach may be necessary. The margins of the perforations are excised (Fig. 12-38), and the squamous epithelial layer surrounding the perforation is removed (Fig. 12-38), laying bare the

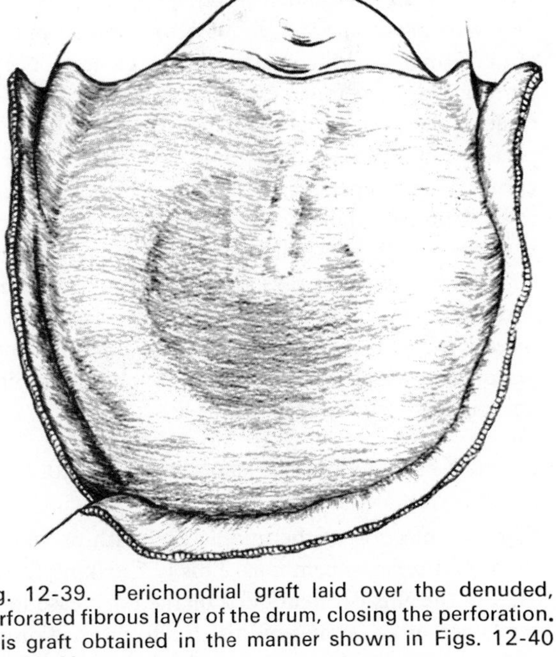

Fig. 12-39. Perichondrial graft laid over the denuded, perforated fibrous layer of the drum, closing the perforation. This graft obtained in the manner shown in Figs. 12-40 and 12-41.

fibrous layer of the drum. This de-epithelialization is carried up along the ear canal in order to create a large supportive area for the graft (Fig. 12-39). The graft is best obtained from one of the connective tissues. Vein wall, fascia, and periosteum have been used, but the best material is perichondrium, easily obtained from the tragus by making a short incision along the lateral edge of that cartilage (Figs. 12-40 and 12-41). As mentioned previously, skin is no longer used for this grafting because the moisture of

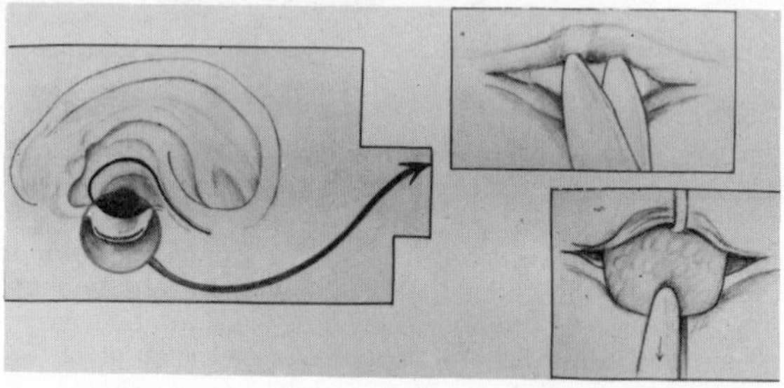

Fig. 12-40. Incision along lateral border of tragus. Endaural incision also shown. The tragal cartilage is dissected free of its surroundings, still covered by its perichondrium, and excised nearly in toto.

the ear canal tends to irritate it and causes it to be inflamed, and, more importantly, because skin can give rise to so-called "flap cholesteatomas." It is particularly tragic when a reparative procedure is vitiated by an iatrogenic complication of this sort.

A warning is in order about a widespread practice of performing myringoplasties in any case of a central perforation, sometimes even one which is draining. Unless one is familiar with the history of such a perforation from its inception, as for example, a clean traumatic perforation due to a blow, it is safer to perform an exploratory tympanotomy concurrently in order to rule out significant intratympanic disease. Of course, mastoid x-rays should always be obtained and the mastoid investigated surgically if evidence of disease is disclosed. In general, the type of central perforation which is safe to close involves a minimal hearing loss, usually of 25 dB or less.

CHRONIC PURULENT OTITIS MEDIA WITH OSSICULAR DESTRUCTION AND MASTOIDITIS

Chronic infection of the middle ear, with or without mastoid disease, is common. This is a striking fact, in view of the already mentioned marked decrease in the incidence of acute mastoiditis. Such chronic disease may rise from inadequately treated acute disease, but, in many instances, the disease may be of a low-grade, chronic nature from the beginning. This is not to say that it cannot assume serious proportions and result in widespread damages and complications. Frequently, a tympanic membrane perforation will be present along with some degree of ossicular destruction. Often, a major discontinuity of the ossicular system will exist. Although there are instances of self-limited chronic otitis in which the damage has been minimized by natural defenses and activity of infection has disappeared, it is, in most instances, difficult to differentiate such relatively benign states from the more serious problems which can continue in a somewhat occult manner.

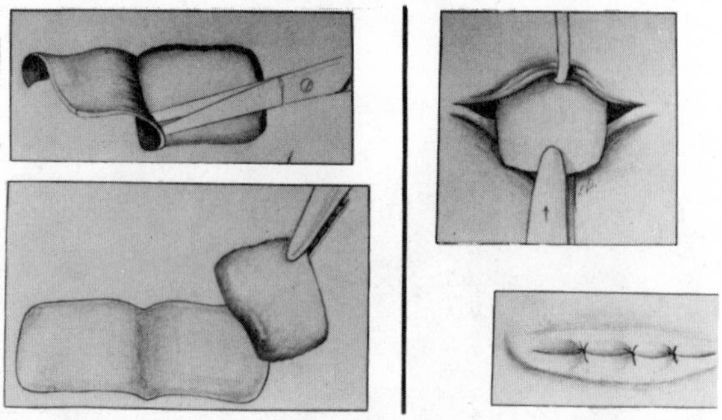

Fig. 12-41. Perichondrium dissected off one face, continuous over lateral edge with perichondrium of other face. The entire removed perichondrial covering is equal to twice the lateral extent of the cartilage itself. Denuded tragal cartilage reinserted into its bed, and incision sutured with 4–0 interrupted silk.

Needless to say, otologists have for decades interested themselves in the medical and surgical treatment of these infections. Mastoidectomy has been the chief approach. The entire attention of the otologist was focused on the removal of infection and the threat to the patient's general welfare. It is only within the past decade that a concerted attack has been made on improvements in middle ear function, along with eradication of disease. The entire concept of functional improvement of the middle-ear mechanism is embodied in the concept of "tympanoplasty," previously described.

The essential ingredients of surgical treatment involve two concepts; 1) tympanomastoid exploration and 2) tympanoplastic reconstruction. Exploratory tympanotomy (previously described) is combined with exploratory mastoidectomy. Pathologic findings and surgical judgment should determine the extent of tissue removal. No predetermined rote operation is ever justified. Decisions should always be based upon observations through the dissecting operating microscope, combined with preoperative information obtained by audiologic, otologic, and roentgen examinations.

Thus, any type of mastoidectomy (simple, modified radical, or radical) may be combined with any one of the tympanoplasty types to suit the specific problem. The goals, however, should always be *safety first* and *hearing second.*

A particular phase of the problem of chronic otitis media has to do with the presence of cholesteatoma or keratoma, in approximately 50 percent of cases (Goodhill, 1960, a). The term cholesteatoma is really a misnomer. These tumors do not contain any appreciable quantity of cholesterol, as their name would imply. They are actually identical with a common skin tumor known popularly as a wen and commonly miscalled "sebaceous cyst." They are not sebaceous (or fatty) but actually composed of concentric layers of squamous epithelium (predominately keratin and hence proteinaceous), surrounded by a thin layer of fibrous connective tissue known as matrix. Keratomas (or cholesteatomas) may occur in widely scattered anatomic sites, but they are most common in the ear. Some are undoubtedly primary, that is, not associated with any infection, and present behind an intact eardrum. Some are caused by invasion of epithelium from the skin of the canal through tympanic membrane perforations, particularly marginal ones. It is likely that many keratomas are mesodermal tumors which may occur, like any other tumor, without apparent provocation, such as the presence of an infection. They may be small and found anywhere within the tympanic cavity. However, they are most frequent in the epitympanum, and the classic site of predilection is said to be Prussak's space, lying between the neck of the malleus and Shrapnell's membrane. Such tumors may be monolocular or multilocular, that is, arising in several places independently. With time, they tend to become diffuse, spreading in various directions and capable of destroying the entire cellular structure of the temporal bone and even invading the cranial cavity. Extensive involvement of the middle ear or its surroundings is described by the term "cholesteatosis." A particular type of this condition is seen in children, who typically have well-pneumatized mastoids. By contrast, keratomas (cholesteatomas) in adults often occur in the presence of sclerotic mastoids, but exceptions certainly exist. A sclerotic mastoid consists of hard eburnated bone with little cellular structure beyond the area of the mastoid antrum, itself, and may be due either to a primary failure of pneumatization or of secondary sclerosis from the filling in of preexisting air cells by bone in response to chronic infection. The sclerotic mastoid, radiologically, appears to be confined to the region of the so-called periantral triangle and does not extend beyond it, as does the well-pneumatized mastoid. The periantral triangle is defined by the middle fossa dura plate or tegmen mastoideum superiorly, the lateral sinus plate posteriorly, and the external auditory canal anteriorly. In sclerotic mastoids, the sigmoid sinus plate is markedly accentuated and stands out in the x-ray picture.

When cholesteatosis of the mastoid occurs, extensive radical mastoidectomy is necessary, and reconstructive surgery in the form of tympanoplasty is contraindicated because of the danger of recurrence beneath a tissue graft. These tumors are particularly prone to recur in children. In adults, in whom they are sometimes less aggressive, a compromise reconstructive procedure is sometimes resorted to, consisting of the placement of a small disc of gelfilm in place of the drum, usually against the head of the stapes. Gelfilm is a proteinaceous material, thin and transparent. It forms a nidus, about which healing may occur with the formation of a membrane replacing the drum which is thin and delicate, but often effective for acoustic purposes. Such is its delicacy, however, that any recurrent cholesteatoma can easily penetrate it so that a dangerous condition is not hidden. Furthermore, the patient has had to make no sacrifice of his own tissue in the form of an autogenous graft.

Cholesteatoma or keratoma is often associated with granulomatous disease. Granulomatous disease, of course, is quite common and often present without keratoma (cholesteatoma). Usually, the granuloma formation is of a nonspecific, pyogenic type. Specific granulomas due to unusual organisms or unusual pathologic processes are sometimes encountered, and their total removal is always necessary. Examples are tuberculous granuloma, which is infectious, and eosinophilic granuloma, which partakes of the nature of tumor.

COMPLICATIONS OF CHRONIC OTITIS MEDIA

Most common is the presence of a tympanic membrane perforation. Some idea of the contribution of the perforation itself to any existing hearing loss may be ascertained by the maneuver of "patching" with plastic material or with cigarette paper. If the perforation is the only lesion, the hearing may be improved to normal. Sometimes, small perforations may be induced to heal by freshening their edges with a knife, painting them with 50 percent trichloracetic acid (in order to destroy the epithelium which has grown around the edges), and then patching the hole as mentioned previously, or, sometimes, placing a small piece of gelfoam within the perforation, followed by a patch. If the perforation is larger, and particularly if the hearing loss is severe, exploration of the middle ear with a small plastic tube or capsule through the perforation may yield a marked improvement in hearing if the "prosthesis" employed happens to touch the stapes or the round window. Gains of 10 to 40 dB may occur with such contact. In the past, many patients were helped by wearing prostheses of this type through their perforations. An example was the formerly well-known Pohlman prosthesis, consisting of a small korojel membrane resembling a small finger cot. It may well be that this type of therapy has been unjustly neglected, and it may have a place even in the present age of tympanoplasty. Its potential usefulness is well worthy of exploration at the present time.

More often, there will be ossicular disease of some degree present. In attic cholesteatosis, it is not at all uncommon for the malleus and incus to be involved in such a way that their sacrifice at surgery becomes mandatory. This may be true whether or not they have undergone atrophy, disruption, or absorption.

One of the most common lesions noted in the middle ear is acquired absence of the long process of the incus which may be due to erosion, infarction (loss of blood supply), or necrosis. The result is an incudostapedial discontinuity which yields a total conductive hypacusis. Formerly, various prosthetic devices of foreign material were used in an effort to reestablish ossicular continuity, such as polyethylene splints and stainless steel or tantalum wires to reunite disconnected components of the ossicular chain. While, as is well known, the use of stainless steel or tantalum wire has become commonplace in stapes surgery for otosclerosis, such foreign materials are poorly tolerated in ears which do, or did, harbor chronic infection. For this reason, it is most desirable to use only autogenous materials derived from the patient himself. The use of homografts (drums and ossicles transplanted from cadavers) is experimental and not generally to be recommended at the present time. There seems, at any rate, little advantage to risking rejection phenomena in transplants to this area, when the patient's own tissues may serve the purpose. This is particularly the case since it appears that some degree of embryonic inductive potency persists in the region of the tympanic annulus, even in adults, so that grafted materials can take on the coloration and texture of the original drum.

A lesion known as tympanosclerosis sometimes complicates the picture of chronic otitis media (Harris, 1961). It consists of a plaquelike, often concentrically laminated, deposition of hyalinized collagen and squamous epithelium which may envelop the ossicular chain and windows, producing varying degrees of conductive hypacusis. It may be either superficial or imbedded. The embedded type tends to be destructive, has osteoclastic tendencies, and may erode the otic capsule, even penetrating the labyrinth. In such cases, tympanoplasty is clearly contraindicated because of the danger of recurrence beneath the graft. Tympanoplasty is only safe when the superficial type of tympanosclerosis can be completely excised.

Tumors

Keratoma (cholesteatoma), described previously, is by far the most common tumor of the tympanic air space. All tumors, including this one, cause hearing losses which are primarily conductive in nature and which only show evidence of superimposed sensorineural involvement if invasion of the cochlear windows or the cochlea itself occurs.

The glomus jugulare tumor is a vascular neoplasm arising from small vascular structures called glomeruli (singular—glomus), usually occurring in the dome of the jugular bulb, but also in other locations within the tympanic cavity, usually near its floor. The most common symptoms are pulsating tinnitus (synchronous with the cardiac pulse) and conductive hearing loss. Otoscopically, the eardrum may show a bluish discoloration. If the tumor has enlarged to such a size as to cause a perforation, a granulomatous-looking mass may be seen protruding into the canal.

Osteoma of the tympanum may accompany osteoma of the external canal. It is a benign lesion but may produce irreversible tympanic destruction and conductive hypacusis.

Carcinoma of the middle ear is a very serious disease with a high mortality rate. Occasionally, tumors will arise from the skin or cerumenous glands of the external auditory canal and invade the middle ear. Rarer still, even tumors of the parotid gland may secondarily involve the external auditory canal, and even the middle ear.

Ossicular Ankylosis

The most common type of ossicular ankylosis is that of the footplate of the stapes in otosclerosis, quite uncommon in children but by no means unheard of. Stapedial ankylosis and ankylosis of other ossicles may occur as the result of adhesive otitis media. Chronic adhesive otitis may be present, strangely enough, in the absence of any history of infection, either acute or chronic. In such cases, the fibrosis is believed to be a result of failure of resorption of embryonal mesenchyme tissue. Whatever the source, the only hope for restoration of middle-ear function is the resection of scar tissue (tympanolysis). This is often difficult and frequently unsuccessful, since such scar tissue tends to re-form.

Arthritis occurs within the ossicular chain and may affect any of the joints. The most common type is osteoarthritis. This is occasionally seen even in children and its etiology is obscure. One might speculate that microtrauma to the ossicular joints as the result of nearly constant bombardment by sound might have some significance.

An interesting condition of obscure etiology is the so-called "fixed malleus syndrome" (Goodhill, 1966, a and 1966, b). In this condition, the head of the malleus is fixed within the attic, usually by calcification of the malleal ligament. The fixation is often massive, and special surgical methods are required to deal with it. These frequently involve amputation of the head of the malleus, and repositioning of the incus in a major attempt at ossicular reconstruction.

It is worthy of mention in this section that a powerful scientific tool for exploration of conductive hypacuses, due to various causes, is afforded by the measurement of acoustic impedance. This is a difficult procedure, best carried out in a research environment. No details will be given here. Suffice it to say that it is possible to obtain a stapedius reflex by sound stimulation which, when confirmed by oscillographic methods, gives reasonably good indication that no conductive lesion exists within the middle ear, although there are some exceptions. It is possible, by means of the "acoustic bridge," to measure such mechanical properties of the middle-ear mechanism as compliance, resistance, reactance, and, finally, overall impedance. In general, impedance is markedly diminished in cases of ossicular discontinuity, somewhat increased by fibrosis, and more increased by stapes ankylosis. The highest figures are obtained in those cases in which the malleus is fixed.

Lesions of the Labyrinth, its Fluids and Windows

Diseases of the bony labyrinth, labyrinthine fluids, and labyrinthine windows are borderline lesions from the point of view of conductive versus sensorineural hearing losses. Since oval and round windows separate the middle from the inner ear, it is difficult to be dogmatic about classification, although from the physical standpoint one must consider the transmission of sound through labyrinthine fluids as a conduction phenomenon. According to this concept, the conduction of sound remains purely mechanical until the displacement of the basilar membrane produces an electrical change in the resting potential in the organ of Corti. Lesions which occur within the organ of Corti itself, or central to it, are lesions in the sensorineural apparatus and might properly be classified as sensorineural losses.

The bony capsule of the labyrinth is composed of dense bone, but nevertheless may be the site of invasion by almost any constitutional bone disease. Some of the invading diseases are rare and will not be discussed in this chapter. There are a few fairly common diseases which invade the otic capsule and produce significant hearing losses by virtue of the invasion. The most common disease in this category is otosclerosis. Less common bone diseases that may mimic otosclerosis include syphilis, Paget's disease, fragilitas ossium, and osteitis fibrosa cystica.

Otosclerosis

The term "otosclerosis" literally means "hardening of the ear." Some confuse it with the sclerotic mastoid, mentioned previously. Otosclerosis is a common cause of deafness in adults. It is primarily a disease of the otic capsule and is represented histologically by a number of pleomorphic forms. The earliest stage of otosclerosis is, actually, a softening, or spongiosis, due to increased vascularity of the affected bone of the otic capsule. This is the form most commonly seen when the disease occurs in children or young adults. The more typical picture, as seen in the mature adult, is one of "sclerosis" which may actually represent healed otospongiosis. Here, one no longer sees the very large vascular marrow spaces, but dense, so-called web bone which has abnormal staining characteristics and which is striking histologically. The disease may occur at any age. It has been described in fetuses and in young children, as well as in adults of all ages. Characteristically, the onset is usually in adolescent or early adult life.

The disease occurs bilaterally in most individuals, and it is present in temporal bones in a large percentage of the population, perhaps as high as eight to 10 percent. In most of these individuals, the otosclerosis is a purely histological curiosity and does not produce hearing losses (Guild, 1944). These are produced only when the otosclerotic lesion involves a critical area within the labyrinth (two percent). Thus, it may well be that instances of unilateral otosclerosis encountered clinically are still bilateral histologically but the lesion has not involved a critical area in one ear.

The bony lesion of otosclerosis is not a tumor, but a change in the consistency of the bony cellular structure. Its growth may be rapid or slow. It is more commonly seen in its growth form during the post-puberty years and in the early twenties. In the thirties and forties, it appears to undergo a quiescent stage. Marked exceptions in activity, however, do occur. The disease is more common in women, perhaps in a ratio of 3 : 1. It frequently becomes worse during pregnancy and during lactation. It is sometimes associated with calcium deficiencies in teeth and, occasionally, in other bones. No systematic pattern of calcium disease, however, is found in all patients. Heredity appears to be a factor. The genetic aspect of otosclerosis is primarily that of a recessive trait.

The disease is limited entirely to the temporal bone and has not yet been discovered in any other part ot the body. It produces no known systemic effects, and its only symptoms are those confined to the auditory and vestibular sensory organs. It more commonly invades the anterior aspect of the oval window (Fig. 12-42) and slowly involves the annular ligament of the stapes footplate and encroaches upon the anterior aspect of the footplate itself as well as upon the anterior crus. When such an encroachment occurs, the stapes footplate becomes progressively fixed.

Although the otosclerotic histologic picture is a classical one, its counterpart has never been found in other parts of the body, and it has been thought by some that the lesion is not a single disease but the histologic sequel of other disease processes affecting the otic capsule. Thus, there may not be just one type of otosclerosis, but several diseases which may have separate etiologic origins. The disease may involve any portion of the vestibular as well as cochlear labyrinth, and in such involvement, vertigo is not at all uncommon. In fact, some instances of otosclerosis closely mimic Ménière's disease, with vertigo, tinnitus, and deafness. It is not unusual to find in a family "riddled" with "classical otosclerosis," an occasional instance of progressive deafness which is entirely sensorineural with no conductive component. This is probably due to otosclerotic invasion of sensorineural components of the labyrinth without involvement of the site of predilection, the oval window. Thus, "nerve deafness" may be otosclerotic in etiology in some patients.

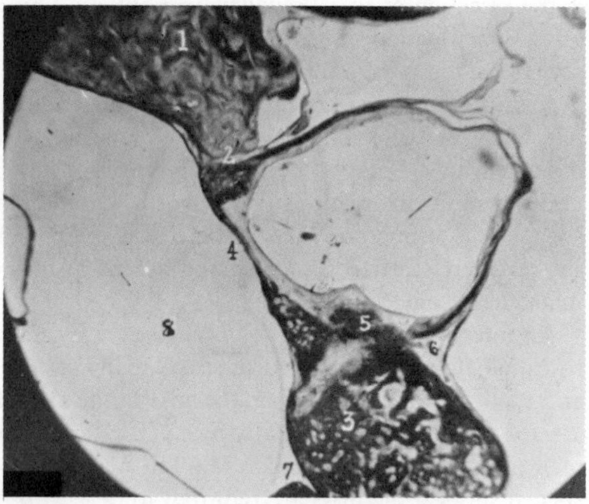

Fig. 12-42. Otosclerosis. (1) Normal capsule. (2) Annular ligament, posteriorly, normal. (3) Focus at site of predilection, obliterating annular ligament and involving anterior half of footplate. Footplate of stapes. (5) Dystrophic bone involving anterior crus of stapes. (6) Fibrous web extending to anterior crus. (7) Fissula ante fenestram almost obliterated by focus. (8) Cisterna periotica. ×20. *From Guggenheim, L. 1935. OTOSCLEROSIS. St. Louis: Zimmerman & Petty.*

SURGICAL PHYSIOLOGIC CONSIDERATIONS

The middle ear is an impedance-matching mechanism, a necessary device to deal with the air-perilymph interface problem. The essential features of this mechanism have been described earlier.

In the pathogenesis of otosclerosis, as a typical anterosuperior lesion increases the stiffness of the stapediovestibular joint, there is a progressive increase in threshold for low frequencies, and a "stiffness tilt" ensues in the pure-tone air-conduction

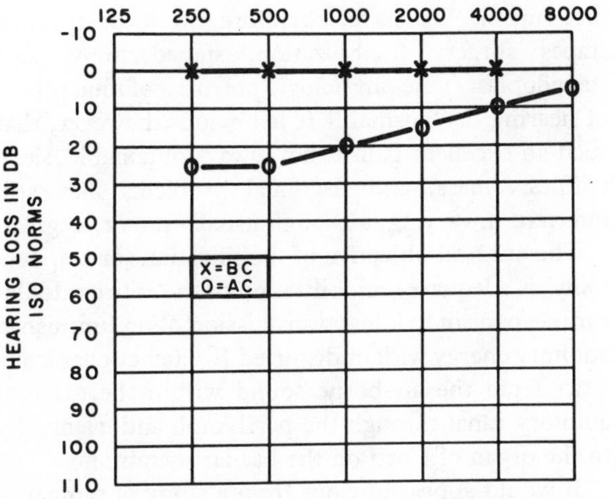

Fig. 12-43. Stiffness tilt in early otosclerosis. Note low-frequency air-conduction tilt with little change elsewhere.

audiogram, exemplified as a drop in the low-frequency hearing level (Fig. 12-43). As the lesion further invades the posterior peribasal region and the footplate becomes completely fixed, there is total loss of the transformer ratio and the plus or minus 26 dB advantage disappears. At this point, the eardrum becomes useless and actually detrimental, since it now blocks the round window as a potential entry of air-conducted sound, being already useless in the normal impedance-matching mechanism to the oval window.

The increased mass of the otosclerotic footplate introduces a "mass tilt" to the air-conduction pure-tone level. A lowering of the high-frequency hearing level causes a straightening out of the total air-conduction level line, as shown in Fig. 12-44.

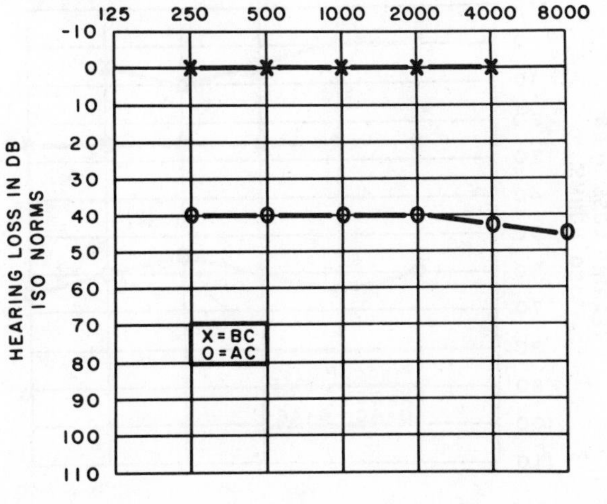

Fig. 12-44. Mass tilt added to stiffness tilt seen in preceding figure.

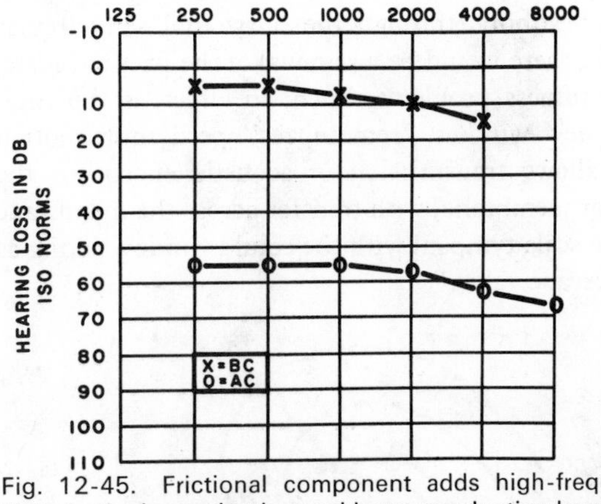

Fig. 12-45. Frictional component adds high-frequency tilt to both air-conduction and bone-conduction levels.

As the disease progresses, frictional elements enter into the picture, and the total air-conduction threshold continues to drop. Fig. 12-45 shows a further drop in the high-frequency air-conduction hearing level and an increasing drop in hearing level throughout the range at all frequencies. In a smaller number of patients, superimposition of a cochlear otosclerotic lesion (most usually at the basal turn of the cochlea) adds a further high-frequency component by both bone conduction and air conduction (Fig. 12-46).

The above sequential story is an oversimplification and omits some known and many unknown acoustic facets, but it does explain the major acoustic sequelae of the progressively ankylosed footplate.

Since the attributes of stiffness, mass, and friction in otosclerosis are all linked to the stapes and oval window, it is logical to expect that, in the fenestration operation, with removal of the incus and malleal head and substitution of a new unimpeded opening into the

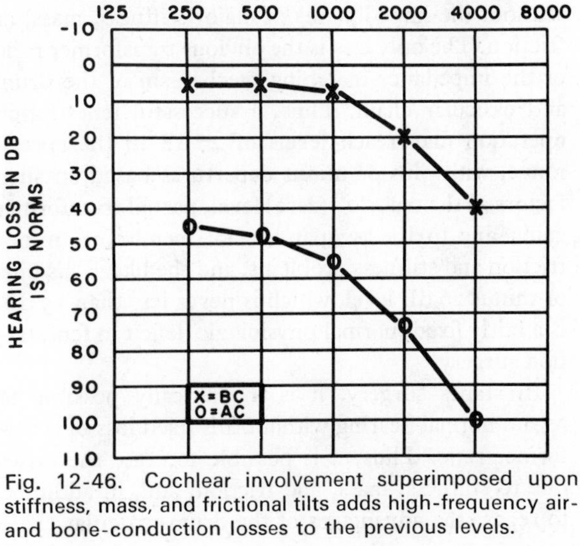

Fig. 12-46. Cochlear involvement superimposed upon stiffness, mass, and frictional tilts adds high-frequency air- and bone-conduction losses to the previous levels.

scala vestibuli (through the horizontal semicircular canal), there would be a removal of the friction, mass, and stiffness problems. Such, in effect, is the case. The new window "remobilizes" perilymph motion and allows transmission of acoustic energy to the basilar membrane, with transfer across the membrane to the scala tympani with the round window acting as an "escape valve."

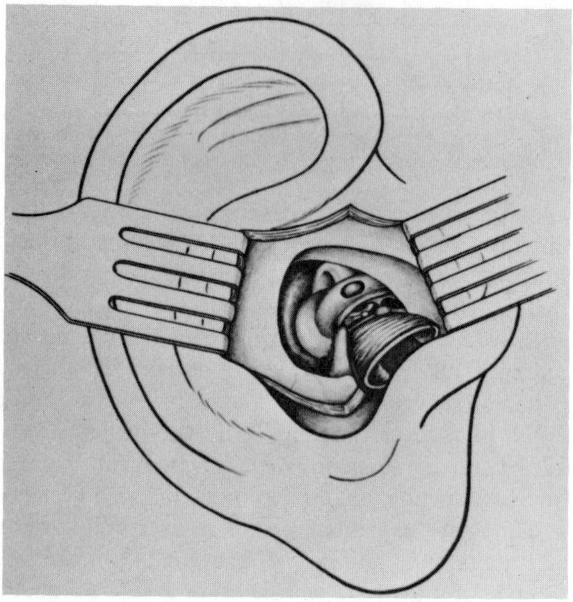

Fig. 12-47. Fenestration of the horizontal semicircular canal. Tympanomeatal flap has not yet been created from the membranous canal, shown here intact.

In the semicircular canal fenestration (Fig. 12-47), the fenestra nov-ovalis functions quite efficiently without the impediments of major stiffness, mass, or friction. The only loss is the obvious transformer ratio of the impedance-matching mechanism of the drum and ossicular chain. Thus, a successful fenestration operation may reach levels of 26 dB in the speech range, with plus or minus departures based on such factors as the true "0" (zero) level, partial transformer gains due to the tympanomeatal membrane, minor friction and stiffness problems, and the like. This plus or minus 26 dB level, which is never less than 15 dB, is a fairly fixed, normal physiologic deficit in fenestration surgery.

In stapes surgery, it is theoretically possible to regain normal hearing without this fixed loss of transformer ratio. Thus, it is possible to erase the losses due to stiffness, mass, and friction, and, in addition, to regain the advantages of the drum-ossicular chain mechanism. We have, therefore, in reconstructive stapes surgery (mobilization, stapedectomy, and stapedoplasty) the physiologic potential of total return of hearing to "normal." It is obvious, however, that such an excellent gain is not always obtainable, since stiffness, mass, and frictional problems may still interfere in varying, although usually minor, degrees.

The surgical objective of mobilization (or stapdectomy) is adequate remobilization of the entire middle-ear mechanism to allow transmission of undiminished auditory energy with undistorted frequency characteristics from the air-borne sound within the external auditory canal through the perilymph and eventually to the organ of Corti on the basilar membrane.

It would appear obvious from a study of tympanocochlear physiology that a direct surgical approach to the obstructed stapes footplate would yield better hearing than a detour surgical approach through fenestration of the horizontal semicircular canal, which dispenses with most of the impedance-matching contribution of the tympanic membrane and ossicular chain. Thus, one would expect, on theoretic grounds alone, to obtain better hearing if the stapediovestibular obstruction could be eliminated and the full force of the middle ear (approximately 26 dB) be brought to bear again upon the sensitive perilymph receptor pathway. That this may actually occur has been demonstrated effectively by a comparison between immediate results following stapedolysis surgery (stapes mobilization) and immediate results following fenestration surgery. Figs. 12-48 and 12-49 show the audiograms of a patient who had a successful

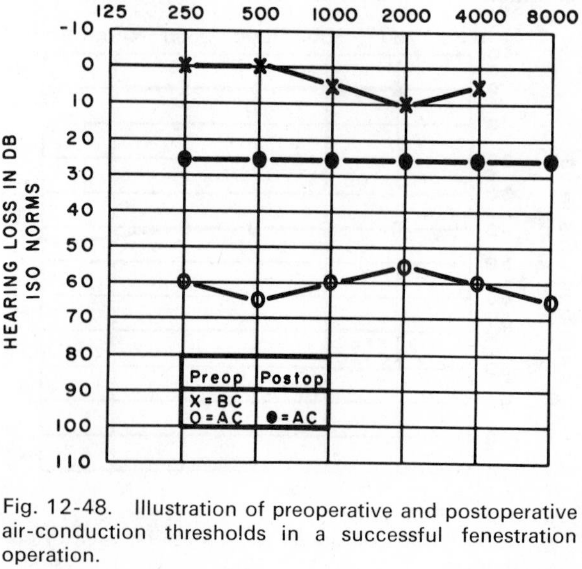

Fig. 12-48. Illustration of preoperative and postoperative air-conduction thresholds in a successful fenestration operation.

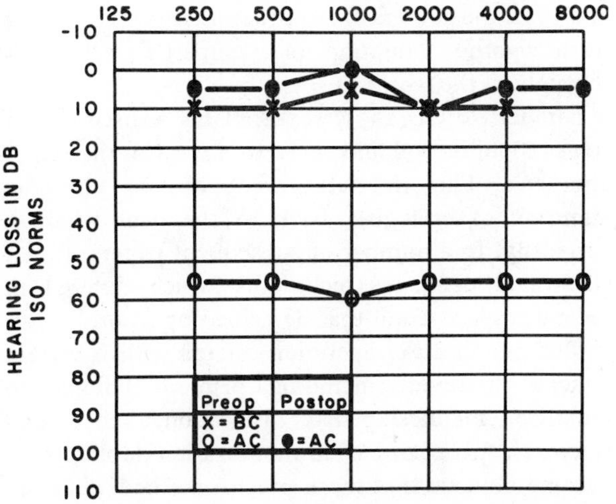

Fig. 12-49. Illustration of preoperative and postoperative air-conduction thresholds in a successful stapedolysis procedure.

fenestration done in one ear and a successful stapes mobilization done in the other ear.

Under ideal conditions, where the fixed stapediovestibular joint can be completely "lysed" or remobilized, it is feasible to expect a return of the air-conduction threshold to the preexisting bone-conduction threshold or, indeed, even to a slightly better level, since it appears that cochlear neural function is at least as good as, and perhaps sometimes better than, bone-conduction measurements may indicate. This should not be interpreted to mean that such results are the rule in all stapes surgery, but that, potentially, such results may be obtained if ideal conditions prevail.

INDICATIONS FOR STAPES SURGERY

The only practical management of otosclerosis at the present time is either through surgery or through amplification with a hearing aid. Medical treatments have been proposed from time to time, but no significant gains in hearing have been reported up to the present.

It may be stated at the outset that surgery in stapes ankylosis may be contemplated if there is evidence of sufficient cochlear reserve so that perilymphatic remobilization will carry with it the probability of effective reception by an active organ of Corti.

The ideal objective of surgery in the treatment of otosclerotic deafness is, of course, the attainment of practical unaided hearing adequate for most social and economic purposes. No one will disagree with this basic concept as a primary objective. It is, nevertheless, true that this ideal objective cannot always be obtained because of a number of modifying factors, the chief of which is the status of cochlear function.

The indications that make patients good candidates for fenestration surgery apply equally for stapes surgery. Thus, the patient with a bone-conduction level from 0 to 20 dB in the speech range, and an air-conduction level of 40 to 70 dB, will qualify well as an ideal choice for stapes surgery as he well might for fenestration surgery. However, this limited group is now greatly expanded so that we may say quite safely that any patient who has a bone-conduction level even as low as 40 to 45 dB and an air-conduction level of 80 to 85 dB may well be considered a standard candidate for stapes surgery since the ultimate aim is restoration of available cochlear function even though this may not carry with it the possibility of unaided hearing. With the lesser severity of stapes procedures and the possibility of completely closing the conductive gap (air-bone), this great benefit should not be denied to any patient unless there is some other serious contraindication to surgery.

It is our present judgment that stapes surgery is indicated for any otosclerotic patient, regardless of age, who has no serious complicating medical problem, who demonstrates an air-bone gap of at least 15 dB (particularly in the lower frequencies), who shows a loss of at least 35–40 dB (ISO) by air conduction, who shows evidence of a speech discrimination score of 60 percent or better, and who demonstrates no anatomic contraindications to exploratory tympanotomy under local anesthesia. For practical purposes, the upper limitation for air-conduction threshold values would be set at approximately 80 to 85 dB. However, it must be emphasized that at the higher levels, one should require a greater air-bone gap than at lower levels. Thus, one should, ideally, require at least 25 dB air-bone gap when the hearing level is 55 dB or lower by air conduction, a 30 dB air-bone gap at 65 dB air conduction, a 35 dB air-bone gap at 75 dB, and a 40 dB level gap at 85 dB.

There are some patients who may not conform to the above requirements but who might well be considered candidates suitable for clinical investigation. These may include patients with lesser air-bone gaps, lower discrimination scores, and patients with tympanic defects involving perforations, fibrosis, and middle-ear anomalies. Exploration is justified in such cases, but only in the hands of an experienced surgeon and only under research circumstances which can be described as ideal for clinical investigation. These patients should not be subjected to routine surgery.

Another category of patient who might not conform to standard criteria but who might merit consideration for surgery would be those with air-conduction levels as low as 95–100 dB and bone-conduction responses at the upper limits of bone-conduction audiometry. If the diagnosis pointing to far-advanced combined stapedial and cochlear otosclerosis is clear-cut, stapes surgery may, indeed, be extremely valuable by allowing the utilization of a hearing aid in an ear which was previously totally useless.

SURGICAL TECHNIQUES—HISTORY AND PRESENT STATUS

For the student of medical history, the development of otologic surgery presents some fascinating chapters. As in all early medical history, clinical discoveries frequently were linked with basic scientific advances with sometimes one and sometimes the other leading the way. Also, tales of dramatic success were frequently followed by sad episodes of failure. Then the phenomenon of rediscovery and reawakening occurred repeatedly. All of these exciting facets were present in early otologic history.

It was Kessel (1876) who first tried to mobilize and then extracted the stapes. In successive decades, a number of European otologists, including Moure (1880), Boucheron (1888), Miot (1890), Passow (1897), Faraci (1899), and others, pursued the stapes surgically. It was Miot, however, who made the most consistent study of the subject. His tympanic approach was based upon a posterior partial myringectomy or myringotomy through which the stapes was mobilized. He reported results in more than 200 cases with many successes. Others at the same time, however, had conflicting experiences. Both poor and good results, both commendations and condemnations, appeared simultaneously in the literature. American observers, including Jack (1891–92), Blake (1892), Burnett (1893), and Alderton (1898) also were involved in these early reports.

It was probably Siebenmann (1900), along with Moure, who closed the door to further stapes surgery at the turn of the century. In their reports, all attempts at stapes surgical intervention were condemned as useless and dangerous.

The dawn of the fenestration era, principally started by Holmgren (1923), modified by Sourdille (1929), and finally climaxed by Lempert's (1938) great contribution, turned the attention of the otologic world back to the surgery of deafness. Between 1938 and 1952, the new era of otologic surgery was launched by a vigorous adoption of Lempert's techniques throughout the world.

Samuel Rosen (1955) reported his rediscovery of stapes mobilization and revived interest in the stapes approach. This dramatic event was to turn the attention of otologists back to the oval window, surgically. In a number of subsequent papers, Rosen elaborated upon his technique, which differed in several respects from that described by Miot.

The mobilization operation carried with it certain deficits, however, including primary failures to mobilize, incudostapedial dislocation, and crural fractures. As experience in mobilization developed, it became obvious that more precise methods directed to the footplate, itself, might increase the number of good primary results.

Stapes surgery evolved from the simple mobilization procedure of Rosen to two major approaches. Both approaches involve subtotal or total footplate removal and substitution of either a tissue graft or a gelfoam pad as a cover for the oval window. 1) Stapedoplasty calls for "interposition" of a portion of the stapedial arch, most commonly the head, neck,

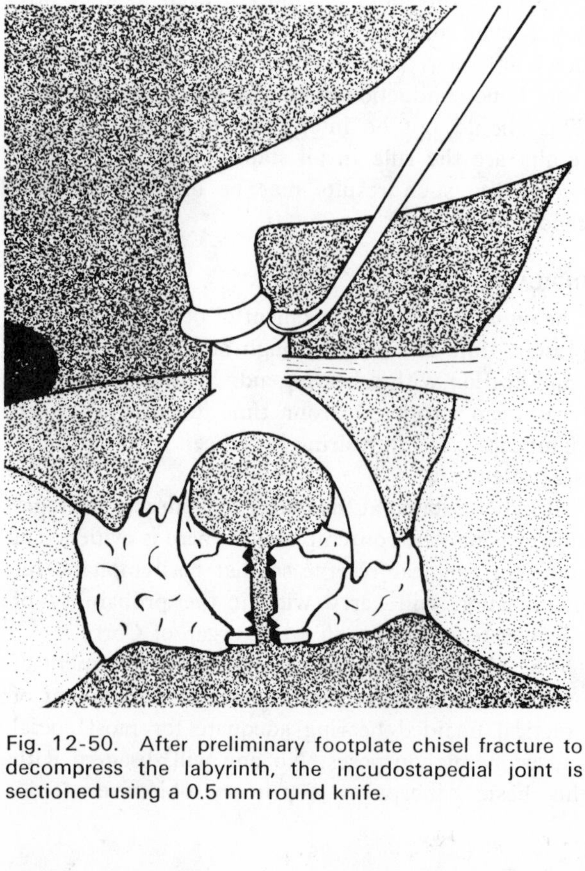

Fig. 12-50. After preliminary footplate chisel fracture to decompress the labyrinth, the incudostapedial joint is sectioned using a 0.5 mm round knife.

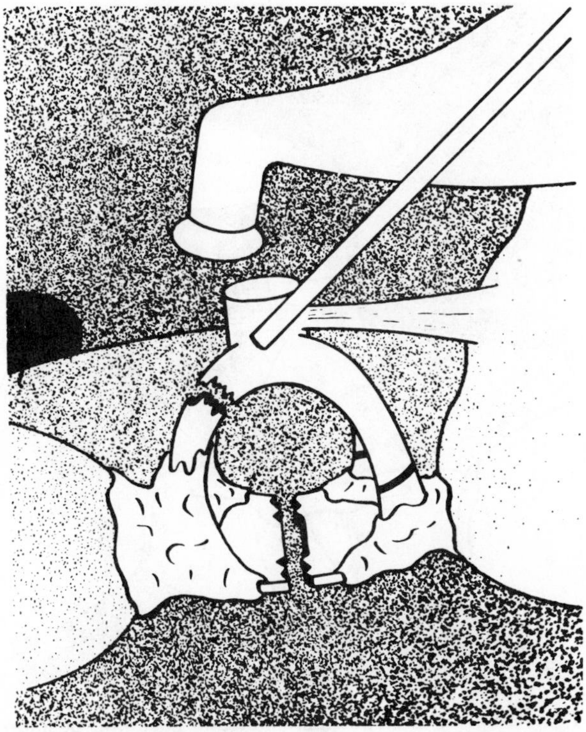

Fig. 12-51. The anterior crus is fractured after partial sectioning of the posterior crus to permit separation of the arch from the footplate. The stapedial tendon is preserved.

and posterior crus. 2) Stapedectomy calls for substitution or "interposition" of a prosthesis. These two major approaches to stapes surgery for otosclerosis are still in common use (1969).

Stapedoplasty technique. Under local anesthesia, an endomeatal microsurgical approach is made through an ear speculum, utilizing the surgical microscope. An incision in the posterosuperior canal wall skin allows exposure through a posterior tympanotomy. Additional exposure, if necessary, is obtained by removal of overhanging annular bone.

After palpation of malleus and incus to rule out lateral ossicular fixation, the incudostapedial joint is sectioned following a preliminary chisel fracture of the footplate to decompress the vestibular perilymph space (Fig. 12-50). The attachment of the posterior crus to the footplate is partially sectioned, and the arch then is separated completely from the footplate by fracturing the anterior crus, preserving the integrity of the posterior crus and the stapedial tendon (Fig. 12-51).

The arch is then rotated temporarily onto the promontory. The footplate is removed in toto or subtotally (Fig. 12-52). The vestibular opening is then covered with either a tragal perichondrium tissue graft or with a pad of gelfoam (Fig. 12-53). The arch then can be swung back into position and the incudostapedial joint rearticulated (Fig. 12-54). Tissues of the joint through surface tension and the normal mesodermal adhesive characteristics cause almost immediate reconstitution of joint integrity. The reconstructed stapedial arch (stapedoplasty) now moves freely on the tissue or gelfoam with immediate subjective hearing improvement. The incision is closed and dressings applied.

Prosthetic Stapedectomy. The incisions and approach are identical to stapedoplasty. The arch, however, is now removed and discarded. This, of course, involves sacrifice of the stapedial tendon.

Following footplate removal and covering of the vestibular opening by either tissue or gelfoam, a prosthesis is now interposed between the incus and the covered oval window (Fig. 12-55). This prosthesis may be made of *plastic* (teflon or polyethylene) or *metal* (stainless steel, tantalum, or platinum) and may be in one of several shapes. Essentially, it is a substitute for the removed stapedial arch.

The choice of procedure is in the hands of the

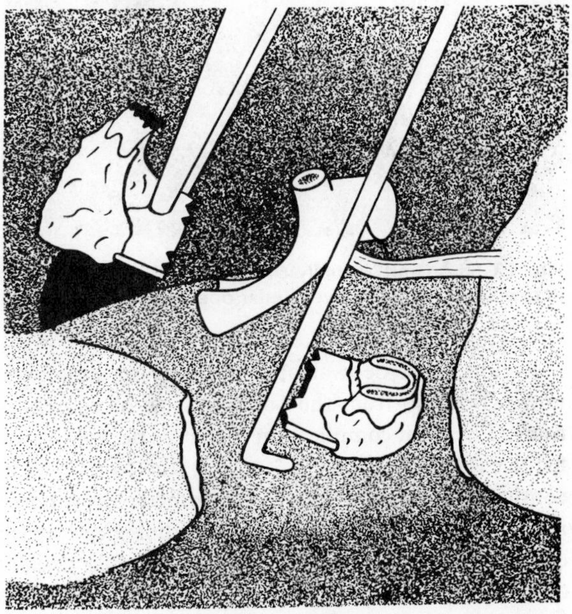

Fig. 12-52. The remaining stapedial arch is rotated onto the cochlear promontory. The anterior half of the footplate is being removed by forceps (left), while the posterior half is shown (lower right) being teased away from the oval window by a microhook.

individual surgeon. Many surgeons will vary the procedure and the prosthesis to suit pathologic conditions. No unanimity exists at the present writing on the merits of various techniques. There are some differences in results, depending upon techniques.

In general, closure or even overclosure of the air-bone gap is obtained in a successful stapedectomy, regardless of technique. However, in a recent unpublished study (Wilber and Goodhill, 1969) of otosclerotic patients, we found some interesting differences between "successful" results comparing interposition stapedoplasty and wire prosthesis techniques. Results are illustrated in Fig. 12–56.

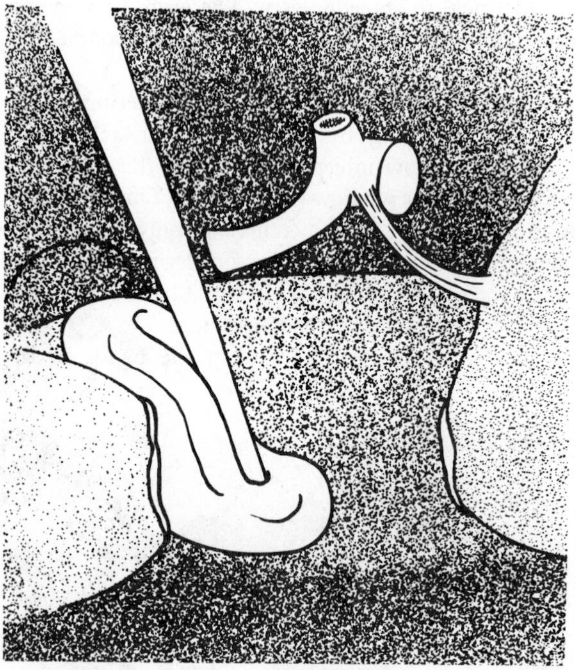

Fig. 12-53. Graft (usually tragal perichondrium) placed in position to cover the vestibular opening (oval window).

Results must be evaluated not only in audiologic terms, but also from the point of view of complications. The chief complication is that of perilymphatic fistulae (Goodhill, 1967, b, 1967, c) due to a break in continuity in the postoperatively formed oval-window membrane. A number of different audiologic sequelae can signal such a complication. The fistula usually carried with it vertigo as well as hearing loss. The hearing loss may range from a minor fluctuating conductive loss to a total sensorineural anacusis.

Further details regarding this complex otosurgical subject should be obtained from the vast literature on

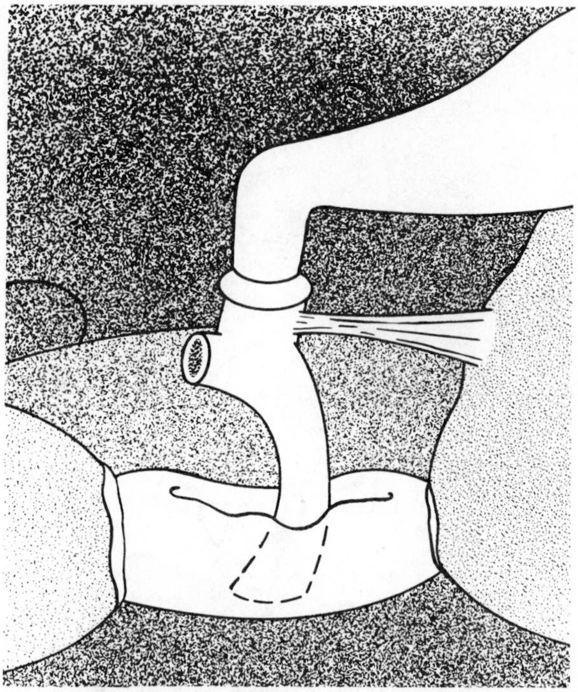

Fig. 12-54. The stapes arch is swung back into position and the incudostapedial joint is rearticulated, accomplishing a stapedoplasty.

the subject (Henry Ford International Symposium on Otosclerosis, 1960; Goodhill, 1961; Shambaugh, 1967).

Diseases Simulating Otosclerosis
(Goodhill, 1960, b)

PAGET'S DISEASE

"Paget's disease of bone" is a systemic disease involving principally the skull, spine, and the shins (tibia). It is manifested by an uncontrolled growth of a dystrophic type of bone strongly resembling the spongiose stage of otosclerosis. They have in common the presence of large vascular marrow spaces. The head becomes progressively enlarged, and the shins become bowed. In the skull, the pathologic process may encroach upon vital structures such as blood vessels, cranial nerves, and even portions of the central nervous system. It can invade the temporal bone and mimic almost any aspect of otosclerosis (Fig. 12-57). It may cause softening of the crura with ossicular discontinuity, or it may produce fixation of the footplate. It may close the round window or may involve the internal auditory canal with pressure upon the auditory nerve. The vestibular portion of the labyrinth may be involved. There is no satisfactory systemic treatment for Paget's disease. If discontinuity occurs between stapes crura and footplate, or if the footplate becomes fixed, surgical intervention is possible, but the prognosis is not favorable inasmuch as growth of dystrophic bone may reclose the oval window. Nevertheless, it may definitely be worth the effort.

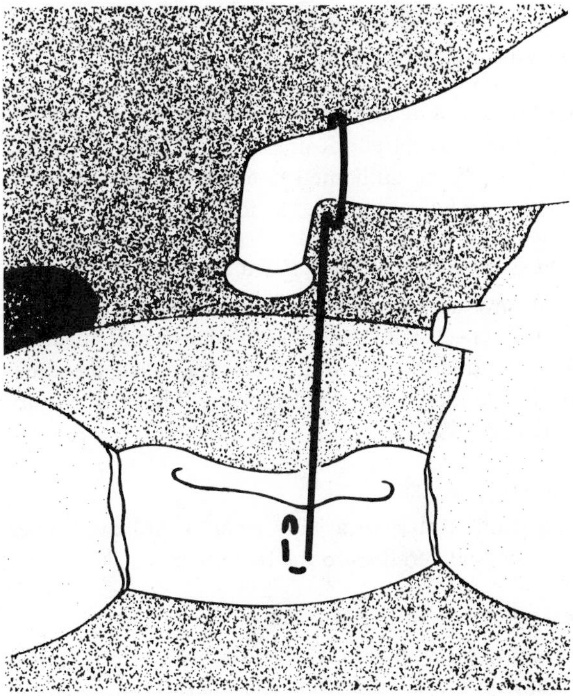

Fig. 12-55. When the procedure requires complete removal of the stapedial arch, a prosthesis is interposed between incus and oval window graft. One end of the wire (upper center) is crimped rather tightly about the long process of the incus, while the tightly curled lower end presses into the perichondrial graft.

FRAGILITAS OSSIUM, OR "BRITTLE BONES"

Fragilitas ossium, or "brittle bones" is a rare disease, usually hereditary in nature, characterized by marked fragility of any of the bones in the body and a peculiarity of the sclerae which robs them of pigment and is described as "blue sclerae." In this disease, multiple fractures occur and it is not unusual for a patient to have as many as 40 to 50 fractures during a 10- or 15-year period, resulting in many deformations. Similar lesions may occur in the ossicular chain, in the tegmen mastoidei, tegmen tympani, and in the otic capsule. Lesions which simulate otosclerosis have occurred in this area, but true otosclerosis can occur in conjunction with fragilitas ossium. With or without

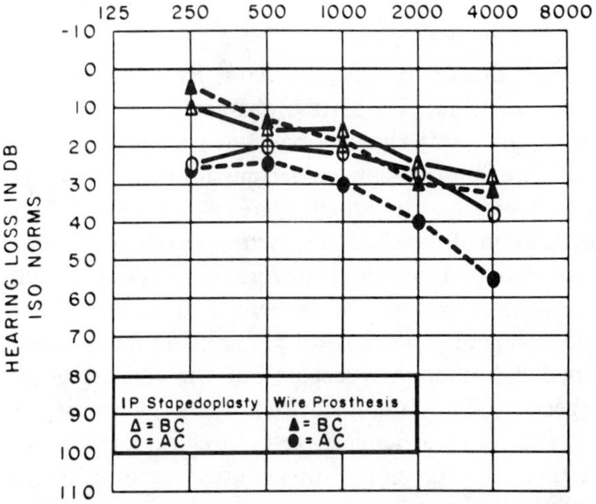

Fig. 12-56. Comparison of postoperative results between interposition stapedoplasty and wire prosthesis techniques on otosclerotic patients.

concurrent otosclerosis, stapedial fixation may occur in this disease. Stapes surgery may be performed, but, as with Paget's disease, the prognosis must be guarded.

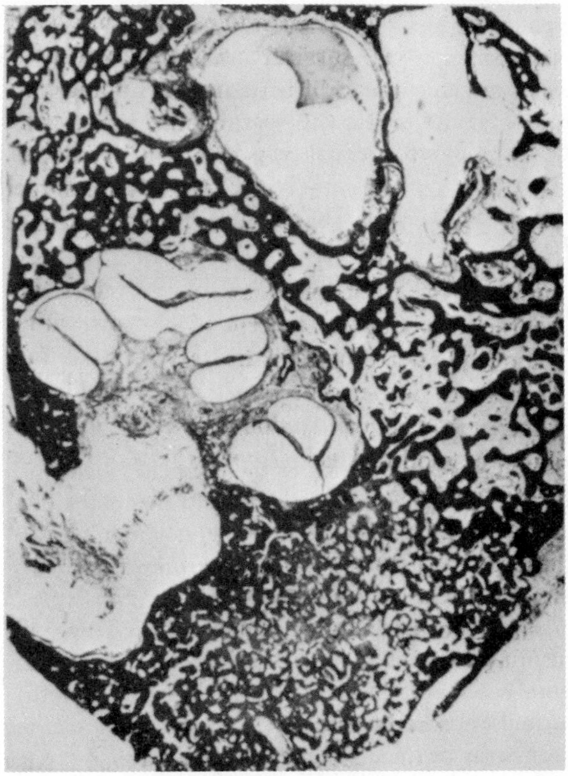

Fig. 12-57. Photomicrograph of case of Paget's disease *From Fischer, J., and Wolfson, L. E. 1943. INNER EAR. New York: Grune and Stratton*

OSTEITIS FIBROSA CYSTICA

Osteitis fibrosa cystica, or von Recklinghausen's disease of bone, is a disease characterized by cystic formations within the long bones as well as within the skull. It is most usually an accompaniment of hyperparathyroidism, in which there is an intense decalcification of the skeletal system. Lesions may occur in the temporal bone and the functional sequelae will depend entirely upon the random occurrence of these lesions. There is no classical picture, and here, again, stapedial fixation may occur, but the treatment by surgery is usually unsatisfactory. Today, when whole batteries of biochemical tests are performed on patients as screening procedures accompanying general physical examination, the presence of hypercalcemia, such as occurs in hyperparathyroidism, is unlikely to escape the internist's attention until so late a sequel as osteitis fibrosa cystica develops. A persistently elevated blood calcium is likely long before to have led to an exploration for parathyroid adenoma.

SYPHILIS

Syphilis, "the great imitator," is fortunately becoming a less common disease in civilized areas since the advent of penicillin and other antibiotics. Nevertheless, its ravages of previous years and the lesions produced through congenital transmission of the disease still make syphilis an important public health problem and a significant etiologic factor in otologic disease.

Syphilis has been known for years to be a serious invader of the temporal bone. It produces a number of lesions (Goodhill, 1939), including periostitis, gumma formation, and sclerosing lesions in various parts of the skull. It may involve any portion of the temporal bone and not infrequently produces sclerosis of the stapes with fixation of the footplate, as well as infiltration of the labyrinth and complete obliteration of the perilymph spaces as well as endolymph spaces. Thus, the syphilitic ear picture may present audiometric evidence of conduction hypacusis at times, with superimposed and fluctuating varieties of sensorineural hypacusis, resulting frequently in neural anacusis as a terminal state. Involvement of the vestibular apparatus is just as common, and Ménière's disease may be imitated by syphilis.

The treatment of early syphilis is quite satisfactory today through the use of penicillin. Late syphilis, however, still remains a problem but can be attacked through combinations of heavy metals and fever therapy. Fortunately, the otologic sequelae of the disease are becoming less frequent and constitute a diminishing problem in deafness. Treatment with steroids such as cortisone is occasionally beneficial.

SENSORINEURAL LESIONS ("NERVE" DEAFNESS)

Diagnostic Aspects of Entire Group

Sensorineural deafness (neural hypacusis, nerve deafness, or perceptive deafness) is characterized by certain typical audiometric and otologic findings. These may be summarized as follows:

PURE-TONE AUDIOMETRIC CHARACTERISTICS

Pure-tone audiometric threshold losses may vary from a mild hypacusis to profound hypacusis and anacusis. Bone-conduction threshold losses are usually equal to air-conduction threshold losses. There is no air-bone gap.

TUNING FORK TESTS

The Rinné test is invariably positive and the Weber test usually lateralizes to the better ear.

SPEECH-RECEPTION THRESHOLD

In contrast with conductive lesions, sensorineural lesions do not always show close agreement between pure-tone air-conduction threshold losses and speech reception thresholds. In some types of sensorineural hypacusis, the agreement may be close, and in other types, the agreement may be poor. If the clarity (discrimination) of speech received is severely impaired (for example, in the abrupt high-frequency loss), the speech-reception threshold may deviate more than plus or minus five dB from the pure-tone average of the speech frequencies (500–2,000 Hz).

SPEECH DISCRIMINATION SCORE

Intelligibility for speech is determined by monosyllabic word lists presented at a sensation level at which the normal ear scores 90–100 percent correct. Speech discrimination may be good in some types of sensorineural lesions but may be poor or even completely absent in other types of sensorineural lesions. Various parameters of speech are affected so that loudness distortion, pitch distortion, asynchronous time relationships may all contribute to the poor perception of speech.

RECRUITMENT OF LOUDNESS

Recruitment of loudness is frequently found in sensorineural hypacuses, particularly in peripheral or organ of Corti lesions.

RESPONSE TO AMPLIFICATION

In sensorineural hypacuses, amplification of speech will yield variable results with frequent examples of poor response to amplification.

Diagnosis of Deafness in Infants

Early diagnosis of hearing impairment in very young infants is a matter of concern to the otologist from the point of view of early *educational* management (Goodhill, 1967, e). Little or no *medical* treatment is available; secretory otitis media does not usually begin to present a problem until after infancy, while surgical attempts to correct malformations of the conductive apparatus certainly should not be undertaken in the newborn. The validity of mass screening programs for neonates has yet to be demonstrated, and, as with any screening program, the primary issue is that of effective follow-up. The process of auditory maturation and the variability from child to child is still largely unknown; therefore, the diagnosis of deafness in the very young infant is difficult, at best, for the experienced pediatric audiologist (who must assume the major responsibility for the auditory testing). Numerous instances have been seen of infants who respond poorly to sound at the age of two to three months, but who, at the age of six to eight months, are quite clearly responding to environmental sounds and the testing stimuli at intensive levels suggestive of normal hearing. Can this be appropriately termed "delayed auditory maturation," and, if so, what are the psychophysical factors involved? If a screening procedure for testing the hearing of infants is elected, what intensity levels are to be used and what stimuli are most effective? If "threshold" determination is desired, the same questions need to be answered, as do the questions concerning the effect of varying activity states, habituation to stimuli, and order of presentation of stimuli. Investigators (Murphy, 1962; Hardy, et al., 1962; Downs, 1967; Suzuki and Sato, 1961; Hoversten and Moncur, 1969; Eisenberg, 1964) utilizing behavioral observations, are beginning to provide answers to some of these questions. It is clear that age is a determining factor affecting the intensity levels at which infants respond, the older infant responding at lower intensity levels than the younger infant, but not at levels standardized as "normal" for adults. Suzuki and Sato (1961), Downs (1967), and Hoversten and Moncur (1969) have demonstrated this in their investigations. It is also clear that infants respond differentially to sound; for example, the voice stimulus secured a considerably higher number of responses than did pulsed-tone stimuli in the Hoversten-Moncur study. Expanding this type of information is absolutely essential for improvement in methods of early auditory diagnosis.

Techniques other than behavioral observation are also employed; the use of computerized-evoked auditory potentials is most promising. H. Davis (1968) summarizes the impressions of a number of investigators that such "physiological audiometry" is useful for infants and young children despite the fact that their responses are slower and more variable. Few investigators are ready to rely solely on the use of evoked auditory potential. Lowell et al. (1968), based on studies of 128 young children, regard the EEG as a helpful confirmatory adjunct to diagnosis but feel that further research is needed.

Classification of Sensorineural Lesions

Sensorineural lesions may be classified by two methods: 1) anatomically (into reception, transmission, and perception lesions), and 2) chronologically.

ANATOMIC CLASSIFICATION

Reception lesions involve the organ of Corti or basilar membrane and represent the majority of cases seen in clinical practice. *Transmission Lesions*—Sensorineural transmissive hypacuses or anacuses involve the auditory nerve and/or the central auditory pathways. Examples of this type of deafness are seen in acoustic neurinoma, in nuclear deafness following erythroblastotic kernicterus, and in other lesions of the neural auditory pathways. *Perception Lesions*—True sensorineural "perceptive" hypacuses or anacuses are rare and involve the auditory cortex and subcortical integrative areas. They are frequently associated with dysacuses.

The accompanying table (Table I) is useful for summarizing basic audiologic features of conduction and sensorineural lesions. It should be remembered that combinations of anatomic lesions (including central neurologic and psychic factors) may result in unusual combinations of findings and a confusing

TABLE I

Conductive and sensorineural "deafness." Basic audiologic differential diagnosis table

	CONDUCTIVE LESIONS	SENSORINEURAL LESIONS Transmission	Reception
Threshold losses	Hypacuses only	Hypacuses or anacuses	Hypacuses or anacuses
B.C./A.C. relationship	Air-bone gap	No air-bone gap	No air-bone gap
Rinné fork test	Negative	Positive	Positive
SRT (speech reception threshold) and pure-tone air-conduction agreement	Excellent	Variable	Variable
SDS (speech discrimination score)	Excellent	Variable	Variable
Recruitment of loudness	None	Variable, often absent	Variable, usually present
Response to amplification	Excellent	Variable, often poor	Variable
SISI (Short increment sensitivity index)	Low score	Low score	High score
Békésy audiometry	Type I	Predominantly Type III (or IV)	Predominantly Type II

diagnostic picture. No one test in and of itself is conclusive, they are best used in combination. A detailed medical history, physical examination, and additional information as provided by vestibular tests and radiographic studies are essential aspects of otologic diagnosis.

CHRONOLOGICAL CLASSIFICATION

The term has been applied to a large number of types of infantile sensorineural deafness. It most properly should be reserved for genetic lesions, or those transmitted by genes, but is frequently used in the sense of "being present at birth" or "with birth." In order to avoid ambiguity, the term *congenital* will be eliminated entirely from this classification and the terms *hereditary* and *acquired* will be used for distinctive purposes. This usage is seen in the context of a chronological classification applying to all age groups, as follows.

HEREDITARY SENSORINEURAL LESIONS

1. Cochlear Aplasia
2. Heredodegenerative Hypacuses
   (a) Infantile heredodegenerative sensorineural hypacusis
   (b) Sensorineural hypacuses of childhood and adult life
3. Otosclerotic Sensorineural Hypacusis
   (a) Infantile variety
   (b) Childhood and adult otosclerotic sensorineural hypacusis

ACQUIRED SENSORINEURAL LESIONS

1. Prenatal
   (a) Toxic factors
   (b) Infections
      (1) Maternal rubella
      (2) Congenital syphilis
2. Natal
   (a) Trauma
   (b) Hypoxia and anoxia
   (c) Rh factor
3. Postnatal and Infantile Hypacuses and Anacuses
4. Childhood Sensorineural Hypacuses
   (a) Viral infections
   (b) Mumps
   (c) Bacterial diseases
5. Adult Sensorineural Hypacuses
   (a) Physical trauma
   (b) Acoustic trauma
   (c) Acquired syphilis
   (d) Presbycusis
   (e) Intracranial tumors
   (f) Toxins—including streptomycin and other drugs
   (g) Acute cochleitis
   (h) Ménière's disease

Hereditary Sensorineural Lesions

COCHLEAR APLASIA

Genetic aplasia, or developmental arrest of the cochlea, spiral-ganglion, and/or neural auditory

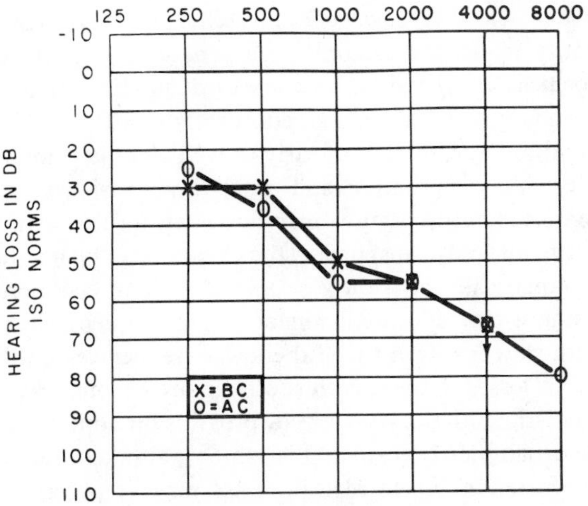

Fig. 12-58. Illustration of a type of advanced sensorineural hypacusis of hereditary etiology.

pathway, has been described histologically and encountered clinically frequently. Microscopic studies have shown in such cases examples where all turns of the cochlea are completely devoid of organ of Corti formation. In contrast to the extreme examples cited, there are innumerable variables with partial aplasias of various elements of the sensorineural auditory system. Thus, both hypacuses and anacuses may be found in this group. The hypacuses may be quite variable in threshold losses and in qualitative differentials within the frequency spectrum (Figs. 12-58 and 12-59). This is undoubtedly a major cause of infantile sensorineural deafness and a major etiologic factor in any survey of the population of schools for the deaf.

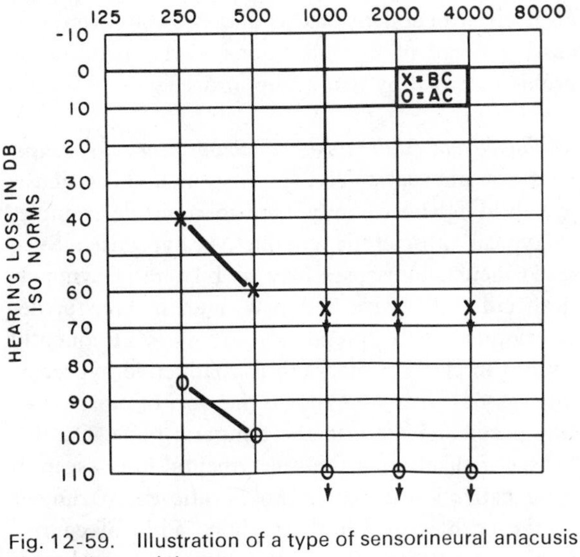

Fig. 12-59. Illustration of a type of sensorineural anacusis of hereditary etiology.

Estimates of this factor in the overall infantile sensorineural deafness picture range from 20 percent to 50 percent of the entire population of profoundly deaf infants. Genetic studies have shown both recessive and dominant trends in this defect. The cochlear aplasias are divided into a number of categories (Schuknecht, 1967).

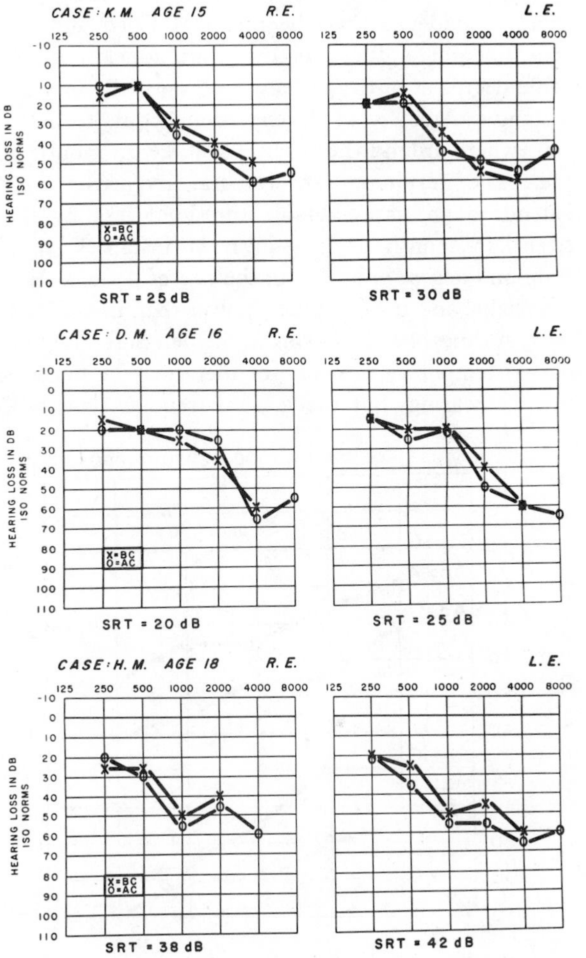

Fig. 12-60. a, b, c – Audiograms of three young brothers with genetic cochlear aplasia. Note the nearly identical bilateral sensorineural hypacuses, present from birth, and not progressive.

For many decades, geneticists have called attention to the prevalence of this defect and have advised against procreation in such families to prevent further dissemination of the genetic trait. Figs. 12-60, 12-60b, and 12-60c illustrate nearly identical hypacuses, bilateral, in three young brothers with genetic cochlear aplasia. There is no satisfactory treatment medically or surgically for this problem.

HEREDODEGENERATIVE HYPACUSES

This variety of hereditary deafness may be grouped as follows.

Infantile heredodegenerative sensorineural hypacusis. There are numerous clinical examples of this peculiar variety of hereditary deafness. In this unusual type there is evidence that the organ of Corti and the sensorineural auditory pathway are functioning to some degree at birth; perhaps even normally in some instances. Atrophy or degeneration begins to occur somewhere around the twelfth or fifteenth month of life. The resultant sensorineural hypacusis may extend to an unpredictable threshold loss by the twentieth month of life—in most instances, to a profound degree of loss—but the rate of deterioration is variable and may be much slower than this. There may, at times, be remissions in the deterioration with partial temporary recovery, or there may be fluctuation in hearing, but the general trend is downhill.

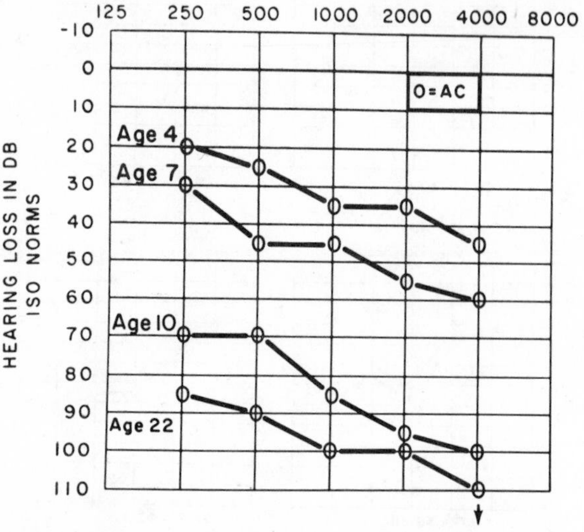

Fig. 12-61. Illustration of a slowly progressive sensorineural hypacusis occurring as a result of a genetic degenerative cochlear lesion.

Onset may, in some cases, be delayed until later childhood or even adolescence. This category of sensorineural hypacusis shades imperceptibly into the type listed below, the sensorineural hypacuses of childhood and adult life, in that pedigrees of one family may show instances of both types. Undoubtedly, they represent different phases of the same disease. There is no medical or surgical treatment of value in this condition.

Sensorineural hypacuses of childhood and adult life. This entity is another example of a genetic degenerative cochlear lesion which may come on at any time in life. Instances have been observed in early and late childhood, in adolescence, in early as well as in late adult life. All quantitative and qualitative varieties of sensorineural hypacuses may occur within this category. In most instances, the losses are bilateral, symmetrical, and slowly progressive. The common lesion is that of a predominantly high-frequency loss with slow involvement of the lower frequencies until major losses in the speech spectrum are encountered. Once the onset is recognized, progression appears to be usually fairly regular (Fig. 12-61), although there are instances where plateau states may be observed followed by precipitous decrements in threshold at unpredictable intervals. There is no satisfactory medical or surgical treatment.

OTOSCLEROTIC SENSORINEURAL HYPACUSIS

Otosclerosis, the major cause of adult conductive hypacusis, may occur in any part of the temporal bone as previously described. In many instances, a strong hereditary tendency has been established for this disease.

Infantile variety. It is theoretically conceivable that some cases of profound infantile neural hypacusis may be due to familial otosclerosis in which the otosclerotic lesion present at birth has involved either the internal auditory meatus region or the ductus cochlearis, per se, with or without stapedial involvement. Such a lesion will present the audiologic picture of a sensorineural hypacusis and possibly even anacusis with all of the educational and rehabilitation problems posed by that group of diseases.

Childhood and adult otosclerotic sensorineural hypacusis. It is not unusual to find a sensorineural hypacusis in a child in whose family there are multiple examples of typical otosclerotic conductive hypacusis. Such sensorineural hypacuses may be bilaterally symmetrical and progressive and may, later in life, further deteriorate with pregnancy—a state frequently noticed in classical otosclerotic conductive hypacusis (Fig. 12-62). It is well known that foci of otosclerosis may occur anywhere in the temporal bone. On this basis, it is likely that the sensorineural losses seen in these patients are due to otosclerotic encroachment on the cochlea or spiral ganglion. This, of course, is in contradistinction to the classical otosclerotic involvement of the stapediovestibular articulation. Furthermore, a well-defined otosclerotic conductive hypacusis may suddenly show evidence (Fig. 12-63) of superimposed sensorineural hypacusis due to this process.

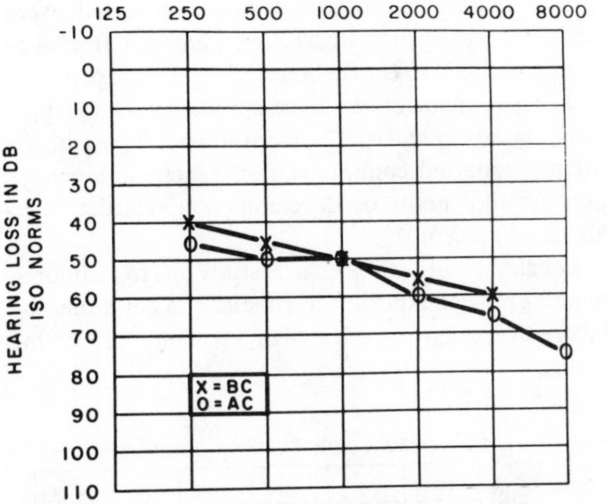

Fig. 12-62. Example of rapidly progressive sensorineural hypacusis in a 25-year-old female in whose family there are multiple examples of typical otosclerosis with conductive hypacusis only. This is probably a case of otosclerotic sensorineural hypacusis, due to cochlear invasion only, without stapes fixation.

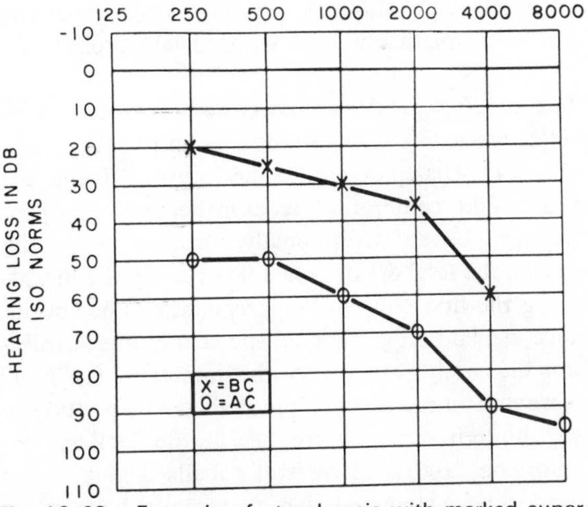

Fig. 12-63. Example of otosclerosis with marked superimposed sensorineural hypacusis, probably due to cochlear otosclerotic invasion.

Since there is no satisfactory medical treatment for otosclerosis, there is no definite therapy for otosclerotic sensorineural hypacusis. Stapedectomy techniques are of no value in these cases, inasmuch as their indication is purely mechanistic and designed to reestablish a functioning acoustic perilymphatic pathway. These surgical procedures have no specific effect upon the basic etiologic nature of the disease itself.

Acquired Sensorineural Lesions

PRENATAL

Under the prenatal acquired category may be included a number of diseases that are due to prenatal factors, traumatic to the development or maturation of the organ of hearing. These may include both toxic and infectious factors.

Toxic factors. A number of toxic factors present during the period of gestation may have an adverse effect on the developing organ of hearing. The toxic effects of certain drugs are considered possible etiologic agents in such developmental trauma. Quinine taken in the early months of pregnancy may have an adverse effect upon the developing cochlea, particularly if there is a specific sensitivity to quinine in the mother. Streptomycin in large doses may similarly produce damage to the developing organ of hearing, again if there is a special susceptibility to streptomycin damage. Even more damaging to hearing is the drug dihydrostreptomycin which has an affinity for the cochlea, whereas, streptomycin tends to be more damaging to the vestibular system. Kanamycin is extremely toxic to the organ of Corti and can result in total and permanent deafness. Neomycin is somewhat less toxic but still dangerous in this respect. These drugs should never be employed, during pregnancy or at any other time, for the treatment of human disease unless there is clear bacteriologic evidence that no other antibiotic will handle the situation and unless the disease, itself, is life-threatening. The threat of total deafness is too great a price to pay for cure of some relatively trivial infection or one that could be handled by less dangerous means.

Alcohol has been cited as a toxic factor, but it exerts its effect, in part, through an associated nutritional deficiency, particularly in relation to the B vitamins. More definitely established is the toxic effect of tobacco. Tobacco has a deleterious effect, both by direct toxic action and also by its effect upon the microcirculation of the cochlea by production of damaging vasospasm. Profound losses with sudden onset have been precipitated by an increase in smoking brought about by nervous stress, which may improve dramatically upon withdrawal of tobacco.

Maternal Rubella. A vaccine is now available which is effective against German measles and which should prevent rubella epidemics in the future. Rubella, one of the mild communicable exanthemata, has been shown to be an exceptionally virulent destructive agent to the fetal organs when it occurs in the mother during the first trimester of pregnancy. The specific effects depend on gestational age at the time of infection. Generally, the earlier the infection, the more severe and numerous are the defects. In a study of 752 children with severe hearing loss (Barr and Lundstrom, 1961), all cases of rubella deafness were found to have stemmed from maternal rubella in the first four months of pregnancy. A more recent study (Bordley et al., 1968) demonstrates that rubella in the second and third trimester may also be teratogenic. In two instances, rubella-deformed babies were born of mothers who contracted rubella in the preconception period.

Past estimates of deafness in postrubella children have varied; Goodhill (1950, a) reported rubella as accounting for at least 20 percent of the population of a school for the deaf.

The 1964 rubella epidemic in the United States was an especially virulent one in respect to production of congenital defects. An estimated 30,000 deformed infants were born to U.S. women who had the disease during pregnancy. Clinical sequelae, found in a group of 100 infants studied at Baylor University (Baylor Rubella Study Group, 1967) were summarized as follows: 29 percent were reported to have a definite hearing loss and 17 percent to have a possible loss. Additional sequelae reported were ocular (65 percent), cardiac (65 percent), thrombocytopenia (30 percent), bone changes (34 percent), and enlargement of the liver and/or spleen (81 percent). Hardy et al. (1969), in a study of 22 postrubella infants, reported communication deficits in about 35 percent and motor or developmental retardation in about 32 percent.

Bordley et al. (1968), in a study of 165 children whose prenatal exposure to rubella was confirmed by laboratory tests, found a high incidence of hearing loss, the children exhibiting live virus at birth having a failure rate for the hearing test of 56.6 percent and the children with positive serology, a failure rate of 41.5 percent. It was also determined that the virus-positive group with hearing loss had a higher percentage of associated defects than those with positive serology and hearing loss. The most commonly associated defects were pulmonary stenosis and cataracts.

Areas of destruction have been found not only in the cochlea but in the central auditory pathway. The picture in the temporal bone, in one autopsy case

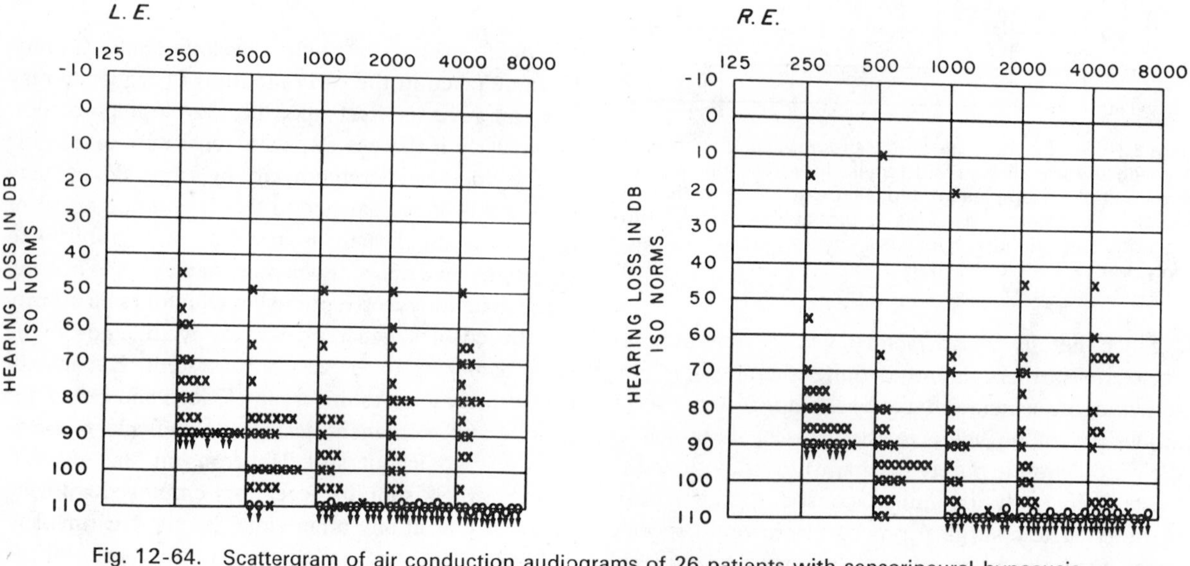

Fig. 12-64. Scattergram of air conduction audiograms of 26 patients with sensorineural hypacusis due to maternal rubella. L.E.=left ear and R.E.=right ear.

showed a cochleosaccular aplasia of the Scheibe type, with changes in the scala media and in the saccule. These included a collapse of Reissner's membrane which was adherent to the stria vascularis and to the organ of Corti. The stria, itself, was small and relatively avascular. The tectorial membrane was compressed into the internal sulcus. The hair cells were not disturbed and the cochlear ganglion seemed intact. The saccule was partially collapsed. The utricle and semicircular canals showed no changes.

The typical audiometric picture in rubella deafness may be described as asymmetrical, flat, and sometimes unilateral (Fig. 12–64, a and b). Vernon (1966), reporting on 8.8 percent of the population of a school for the deaf, found the mean hearing loss to be 82.3 dB, ASA (500–2,000 Hz), and the configuration to be flat. Vernon's psychodiagnostic data corroborates medical research indicating central nervous system dysfunction as one of the sequelae. A greater prevalence of learning disability (including aphasia) and severe emotional disturbance (poor impulse control, excitability, rigidity, emotional instability, distractibility, and emotional shallowness) was reported for the postrubella children.

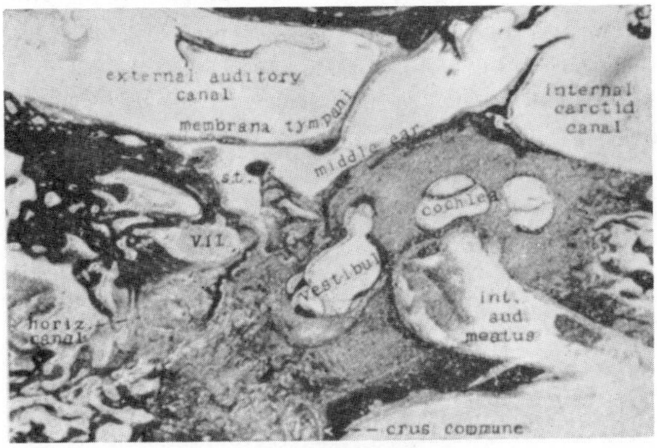

Fig. 12-65. Syphilis. Horizontal section. Note complete cast of new bone filling crus commune, horizontal canal, and part of vestibule; suppurative labyrinthitis; marked deformity of stapes.

In compiling etiologic histories, a history of maternal rubella is often lacking when, in fact, it was the etiologic factor. The infection may have been inapparent, the mother having no clinical symptoms. The virus is recoverable from the young child for some time, and it is believed that it is active in various organs, including the brain, causing a low-grade encephalitis. It can be recovered from blood and various secretions and grown in tissue culture. Antibodies can be demonstrated in the blood. When the child passes the age of two, although viral cultures and antibodies may still be obtained, it becomes increasingly likely that the child may, himself, have suffered rubella of his own, so that the evidence becomes less stringent in favor of an in-utero infection.

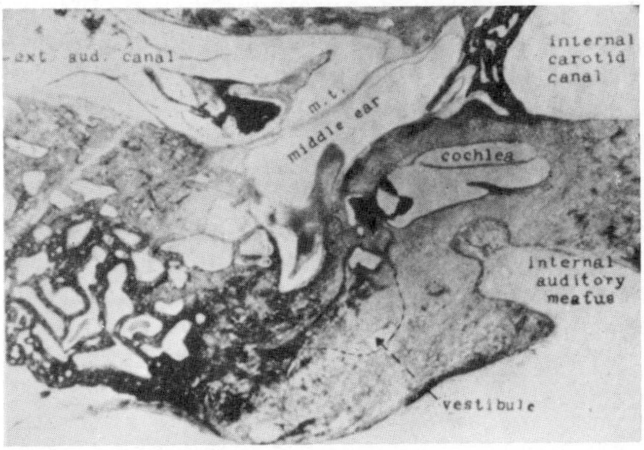

Fig. 12-66. Syphilis. Horizontal section of level of basal turn of cochlea. Purulent invasion of labyrinth occurs via round window. New bone is seen in vestibule here also.

Congenital Syphilis. Syphilis produces many very serious diseases as the result of "congenital" transmission of the disease. Congenital syphilis (Goodhill, 1939) may produce primarily a sensorineural hypacusis (Figs. 12-65, 12-66, 12-67), either unilaterally or bilaterally, which may come on at any time in life. It not infrequently will become manifest during the

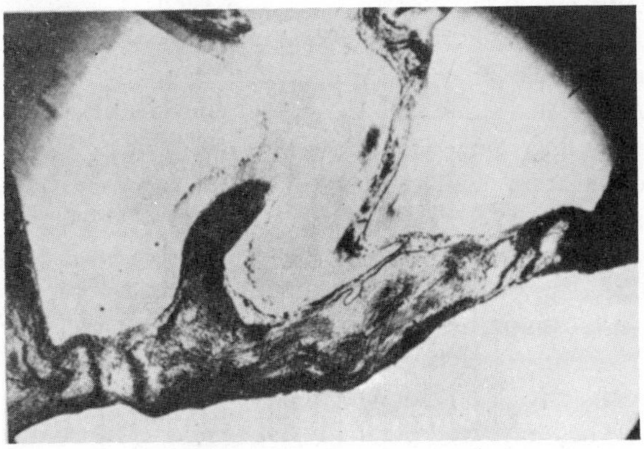

Fig. 12-67. Syphilis. Marked deformity of crura and footplate of stapes.

teenage years, and involvement may be very severe or extremely mild. Variable results are being obtained with antibiotic, heavy metal, and other antiluetic therapy, as well as with steroids. In general, the prognosis today is far better than it was a decade ago. Nevertheless, permanent hypacuses and even anacuses may result and may defy all attempted medical therapy. Frequently, congenital syphilitic deafness is accompanied by other easily recognizable stigmata such as keratitis, Hutchinsonian teeth, and orthopedic defects. The diagnosis is made on the basis of history, physical findings, and serologic evidence in both blood and cerebrospinal fluid.

NATAL

At birth, a number of untoward occurrences may adversely influence the organ of hearing. Trauma, anoxia, and serologic incompatibilities are the chief factors of such natal damage to the cochlea and neural auditory pathways.

Trauma. Physical trauma to the skull during birth occurs infrequently. It may be due to a narrowed pelvic outlet, too close approximation of forceps, or a difficult breech or occiput posterior presentation. In current obstetrical practice, such trauma is becoming increasingly rare; and, unless an intracranial hemorrhage has occurred, it is unlikely that cephalic trauma is at the present time a major cause of natal ear damage.

Hypoxia and anoxia. Probably the most important cause of natal ear injury is prolonged hypoxia or anoxia of the infant. Any disturbance in respiration or circulation will bring with it the possibility of diminished oxygen tension in the circulating blood. Any significant deprivation of oxygen is a severe stress to the delicate neural epithelium of the organ of Corti and produces rapid degeneration and atrophy. Many factors may predispose to hypoxia and anoxia, including long labors, heavy maternal sedation, obstruction of the respiratory passages with mucus, incomplete development of the lungs, and congenital circulatory and cardiac defects. Anoxic sequelae may affect any of the sensory organs and the central nervous system, as well. Thus, cerebral palsy is frequently seen in association with anoxic neural hypacusis.

The only treatment for hypoxia and anoxia is preventative. The sequelae are unfortunately final and irreversible. No medical or surgical therapy can undo the damage; but rehabilitative measures are available and should be offered. Any quantitative or qualitative variety of sensorineural hypacusis may be seen as the sequel of natal hypoxia or anoxia.

Rh factor. Erythroblastosis fetalis is now a preventable disease in most cases. Recently, there became available commercially a gamma globulin concentrate of anti-Rh serum. This material, called RhoGAM, will block or prevent the immunization or sensitization of an Rh-negative woman recently delivered of an Rh-positive infant.

Serologic incompatability between the fetus and the mother is responsible for a variety of hemolytic diseases in which red blood cells are destroyed and the toxic pigment allowed to circulate freely within the fetal circulation. Such circulation of pigment produces a large number of sequelae, principally those due to deposition of pigment in various areas within the central nervous system and in sensory organs as well.

The prime example of serologic incompatability is erythroblastotic kernicterus. The union of an Rh-negative female with an Rh-positive male in which the fetus is Rh-negative produces no unfavorable sequelae. If the fetus, however, is Rh positive in blood type, the possibility of serious incompatibility due to circulating antibodies exists. If such incompatibility assumes major proportions due to high titer of maternal antibody, infantile erythroblastosis will occur, reaching its peak at birth. Circulating pigment would be deposited in the skin, in the liver, in the central nervous system, and in many other vital organs. The deposition of pigment in the pons and medulla will produce the neural pathologic state called "kernicterus" or icterus of the cranial nuclei. Among the sequelae of kernicterus are athetoid cerebral palsy due to involvement of the extrapyramidal tracts and a specific type of central deafness due to involvement of the dorsal and ventral cochlear nuclei which has been termed "nuclear deafness" (Goodhill, 1950, b). There is evidence also that some deposition of pigment may occur in a wide spectrum of possible anatomic sites, namely, the cochlea, the efferent (olivo-cochlear) pathway, the reticular system, as well as geniculate, thalamic, and cortical areas (Goodhill, 1967, d). At any rate, a diffuse type of transmissive and possibly receptive neural hypacusis may occur as the sequel of erythroblastotic kernicterus due to Rh-factor incompatibility.

Hardy (1961) reported somewhat different behavior of children with kernicteric defects than the behavior in children with ordinary peripheral auditory deficits. Not only were language disorders and dysarthria present in 22 percent of the children, but a variety of sensory defects were reported as well.

Hyman et al (1969) studied 405 infants with hemolytic disease of the newborn or hyperbilirubinemia at birth. Of the 405 infants, 396 had hemolytic disease of the newborn (Rh, 348; ABO 48). The children were followed over a four-year period. 85 percent of the children had no evidence of central nervous system dysfunction. 15 percent had one or more of the following: sensorineural hearing loss, athetosis, strabismus, seizures, minimal cerebral dysfunction syndrome, difficulties with auditory rote memory or with visual perception, and other miscellaneous CNC-related problems such as impaired mentality, nystagmus, and psychotic behavior. The authors emphasized that follow-up extending into the school years is needed to clarify the possibility of the incidence of minimal cerebral dysfunction greater than that detected in this study; this would be more apt to be detected under the stress of the school situation.

Keaster, Hyman, and Harris (1969) reported on the 4.2 percent of the children in the above study who had sensorineural hearing losses. High bilirubin exposure was significantly associated with the occurrence of sensorineural hearing loss. However, 16 of the 17 patients had received streptomycin therapy, so it was not possible to separate the influence of streptomycin independent of a high bilirubin level. The hearing losses varied in degree but were most marked in the high frequencies. Fluctuation was not observed. No special speech and language problems (atypical for the degree of loss) were founded except for one child who had a profound loss and aphasia.

A number of investigators have found the usual pure-tone audiogram, in cases of children with kernicteric defects, to be bilaterally symmetrical with a mild to moderate loss in the low frequencies, increasing to a severe loss in the high frequencies. Carhart (1967) compiled group data obtained in major studies and reported the characteristic configuration with ISO 1964 thresholds as follows: about 30 dB for 125 and 250 Hz, about 40 dB for 500 Hz, about 60 dB for 1,000 Hz, about 70 dB for 2,000 Hz, about 75 dB for 4,000 Hz, and about 75 dB for 8,000 Hz. These studies were limited to patients of sufficient maturity to respond consistently. Speech discrimination is variable, and may be good in many instances. Amplification is also of varying benefit. The triad of recruitment, Type II Békésy tracings, and positive SISI scores in the high frequencies is commonly seen.

Matkin (1968) attributed these findings to cochlear lesions but postulated a "dual dysfunction" involving both the cochlear and central auditory system. However, there is considerable postmortem evidence to show that kernicteric foci in the cochlear nuclei are common; cochlear damage has not been shown. Carhart (1967) theorizes that these auditory findings (similar to those found in cochlear disorders), may be produced by central lesions when "normal trains of information from the inner ear suffer disruption in transmission through damaged cochlear nuclei and/or associated basal centers en route to perceptual processing in higher center," and postulates that a normal inner ear and VIIIth Cranial nerve function may be present.

The shape of the audiogram (better hearing for low tones) may be attributed to a differential disruption in acuity located within the cochlear nuclei. Carhart reminds his readers of Wever's (1949) Volley-Place theory and postulates that the place-sensitive mechanism operant for high tones may receive greater damage than the volley-analyzing mechanism (synchronous neural-discharging predominating in low-frequency sensitivity) but at a level within the cochlear nuclei where, he theorizes, the first definitely separate coding may take place.

The evidence of recruitment could have occurred, according to Carhart, if a normal cochlea were present and a gating process were operating within the cochlear nuclei which resulted in tonal stimulation at normal intensities. This could also account for positive SISI scores in that, through action of the gating function, the stimulus level is high enough to evoke a normal response (normal ears usually detect a one-dB intensity increment at levels above 75 dB) despite the kernicteric subject's limited ability to perceive stimuli of less intensity.

Type II Békésy tracings may be attributed to normal peripheral adaptation coupled with a centrally imposed drop in neural activity. Thus, a central auditory disorder (shown by postmortem evidence) may mimic a cochlear lesion and be misdiagnosed as a peripheral sensory impairment. Carhart's hypothesis is as warranted as other and contrary ones and will await further clinical and histologic research.

Erythroblastosis is usually characterized by progressive increase in serologic incompatibility with successive pregnancies. Thus, the first pregnancy with an Rh-positive baby is usually uneventful, but subsequent pregnancies may carry greater concentrations of maternal antibodies and greater risk of icteric deposition with neurologic sequelae. The only treatment available prior to RhoGAM has been prevention, and preventive measures are based upon careful maternal antibody determinations during pregnancy and special measures at birth to prevent kernicterus. These special measures may include blood replacement, transfusions, and the use of some of the newer steroid hormonal drugs. Once the kernicterus lesion has occurred, however, there is no satisfactory medical or surgical therapy at the present time.

Recent studies have shown that incompatibilities within the basic A, B, and O blood classifications may also cause erythroblastotic sequelae with kernicterus. Thus, it is likely that the nuclear deafness previously attributed only to Rh factor incompatibility may conceivably occasionally be due to A, B, and O incompatibility. Further studies along serologic lines may reveal other types of incompatibilities productive of the same sequelae.

Prematurity. While prematurity may be associated with other pathogenic factors such as rubella, Rh incompatibility, or other abnormalities, it can occur as an isolated phenomenon, brought on by physical or psychic trauma or other obscure factors. The fragility of the tissues of the premature infant is such that this factor alone can be responsible for the development of sensorineural hypacusis or even anacusis in the premature infant. Since estimates of the gestation period are sometimes inaccurate, a birth weight of less than five and one-half pounds is usually the criterion for the diagnosis of prematurity.

POSTNATAL AND INFANTILE SENSORINEURAL HYPACUSES AND ANACUSES

A number of the viral exanthemata may occur during the first year of life. Certain bacterial infections of the central nervous system, including encephalitis and meningitis, are also found fairly frequently during this vulnerable period. All major causes of sensorineural hypacusis at this period produce auditory sensory defects which are educationally identical with prenatal and natal lesions. This is the reason for the common, but mistaken, usage of the term "congenital" in categorizing all of these diseases.

Inasmuch as language acquisition during the first year of life is so vitally dependent upon communication input through hearing, any sensorineural hypacusis sufficiently severe to interfere with language input will concomitantly interfere with the development of speech or communication output. The infant who is born with perfectly normal hearing but who, *prior* to the acquisition of speech, loses most of his hearing as the result of meningococcic meningitis, or measles encephalitis, or mumps meningitis, or tuberculous meningitis will pose an educational problem similar to that of a child who has congenital cochlear lesions. Special educational measures (for both parent and child) must begin as early as possible; language input for the hearing-impaired child can be greatly facilitated by early use of amplification, guided enjoyable auditory experiences, and lipreading.

It is imperative that the child who loses his hearing *after* the acquisition of speech receive immediate educational help to assist in conservation of his speech and language and to expedite the learning of new receptive language skills. Thus, a different type of educational approach is needed for the deafened child, and this approach is dependent on the age at which the loss occurs.

CHILDHOOD SENSORINEURAL HYPACUSES

A number of varieties may be classified within this category.

Viral infections. Almost all of the viral exanthemata may produce serious neurological sequelae. These may be limited to one or another of the sense organs, or may involve the central nervous system proper. Thus, sensorineural hypacuses and anacuses may follow measles, mumps, chickenpox, whooping cough, rubella, and members of the so-called virus influenza group. All of these diseases may attack the organ of hearing. Such invasion may be unilateral or bilateral, partial or complete. In general, cochlear involvement by viruses is relatively infrequent except in mumps.

Mumps. Mumps or epidemic parotitis may involve one or both parotid glands and one or both submaxillary salivary glands. It is a highly communicable contagious disease of childhood, and occasionally of adults. Not infrequently, mumps will produce marked otalgia and tinnitus during the acute course of the disease. Examination of the ears at this time will usually reveal no significant changes in the tympanic membranes or middle ears. Nevertheless, the patient may complain of a hearing loss during the actual gland swelling which will become more marked when the swelling disappears. Audiologic examination will reveal no loss due to changes in the middle ears but usually a profound sensorineural hypacusis, usually unilateral, frequently of anacusic degree. Occasionally, such cochlear destruction will be accompanied by vestibular destruction as well, and caloric vestibular studies may reveal total lack of vestibular response on the affected side.

The exact mechanism of invasion of the mumps virus is unknown, as is the percentile incidence of the disease. It is difficult to evaluate auditory sequelae of an epidemic or communicable disease because of the wide disparity of medical care and the fact that most patients are not hospitalized. Nevertheless, it is well recognized that mumps is a major cause of unilateral sensorineural hypacusis and anacusis and, undoubtedly, the major offender among the viral group from the point of view of acquired lesions. Such deafness may occur in adults as well as in children and is usually irreversible.

Bacterial diseases. Bacterial diseases of childhood which invade the central nervous system may also invade the cochlear and central neural auditory pathways with resultant sensorineural hypacuses and anacuses. Meningitis and encephalitis are the two chief examples of this group, with meningitis being the major offender. Any type of meningitis may affect the auditory organ (Fig. 12-68). Epidemic or meningococcic meningitis is just as important a cause of such involvement as the meningitis complicating either streptococcal, pneumococcal, or staphylococcal respiratory infections. Bacterial influenzal meningitis, often of otitic origin, is one of the more common varieties in young children. Tuberculous meningitis may also produce the same type of invasion with the same sequelae.

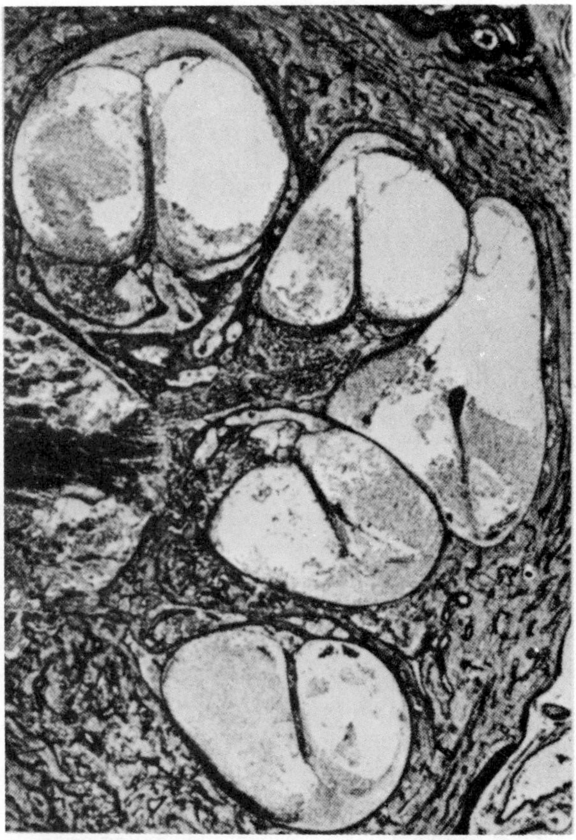

Fig. 12-68. Microphotograph showing the diffuse purulent stage of meningitic labyrinthitis. Pus cells are diffusely distributed throughout the cochlear spaces and the modiolus. Destruction of the cochlear duct has already occurred in the basal coil. *From Jackson, C., and Jackson, C. L., 1945. DISEASE OF THE NOSE, THROAT AND EAR. New York: Saunders.*

Most meningitic sensorineural losses are bilateral, and most of them are profound, primarily in the anacusic category. In some instances, there is also evidence of vestibular disturbance, but this is not a universal finding.

There is no satisfactory treatment for the sequelae of meningitic deafness; but meningitis, per se, can now be treated far more satisfactorily than it was treated one or two decades ago. Consequently, more survivals are reported than ever before. Naturally, many of these survivors will be left with neurologic sequelae, one of which very well may be sensorineural hypacusis. When the meningitis therapy is started very early in the course of the disease, and where the organism is particularly responsive to the antibiotic agent, avoidance of sensory defects may be expected. It is not too much to hope that early thorough treatment of meningitis may result in the virtual elimination of postmeningitic sensorineural hypacusis as a major cause of deafness.

ADULT SENSORINEURAL HYPACUSES

This category contains a wide variety of lesions.

Physical trauma. Physical trauma to the head may produce varying degrees of damage to the auditory organ. A sharp blow on the auricle with resultant compression of air within the external auditory canal may produce a tympanic-membrane rupture and in some instances labyrinthine disturbances. The resultant hearing loss may show evidence of a combined conductive and sensorineural hypacusis, the extent depending upon the degree of damage to each compartment of the auditory organ. Physical trauma to

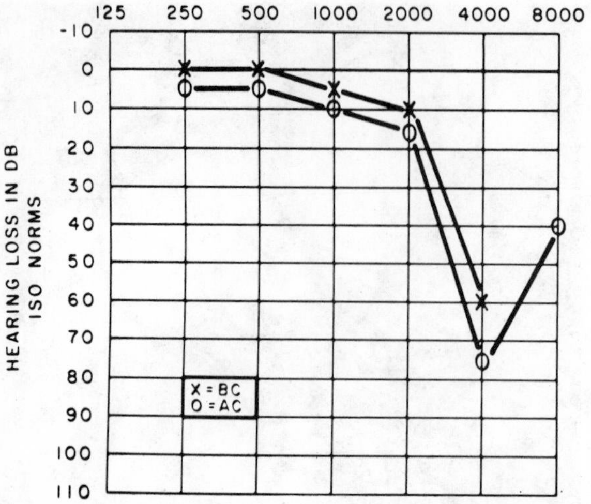

Fig. 12-69. Audiometric example of head injury without fracture of the skull.

the head, itself, may result in concussive damage to the labyrinth (Fig. 12-69) or to an actual fracture of the temporal bone. Concussion of the labyrinth may produce findings similar to those seen in labyrinthine hemorrhage, or in endolymphatic hydrops. Thus, they may include tinnitus, vertigo, and varying degrees of sensorineural hypacusis. Such damage may be temporary or permanent, depending upon the degree of disruption of neural epithelial elements and the degree of disturbance of labyrinthine fluids. Treatment of such conditions is rarely surgical but may include such medical techniques as dehydration therapy and prophylactic antibiotic therapy.

Actual temporal bone fractures may result in variable sequelae, depending upon extent of fracture and location of fracture line. A temporal bone fracture is usually part of a basal skull fracture and sequelae of major importance may occur. If the fracture carries with it a laceration of the dura, there may be an escape of cerebrospinal fluid as well as of blood through the external auditory canal, and this may carry with it the very grave prognosis for life itself. In such instances, there are usually resultant permanent and severe sensorineural hypacuses, along with major vestibular disturbances. Therapy is usually directed along preventive lines and may include antibiotic and other types of supportive therapy.

Acoustic trauma. A subject of major interest to otologists, audiologists, and industrial physicians has been that of increased incident of acoustic injury to the cochlea. It has been known for years that high intensity noise had adverse effects upon the inner-ear. Thus, "boiler makers" deafness was described half a century ago, and its high-tone-loss characteristic was known to otologists of that era. During the past few decades, the increased mechanization of civilized life and the increased part played by noise in military activities have brought with them the inevitable damage to the auditory end organ that one would expect. Thus, sensorineural hypacusis of several varieties is being encountered more and more commonly in clinical practice and is now just as serious a civilian problem as it was a military problem in the last war. The human auditory organ was not created to withstand exposure to high-intensity sounds of the kind encountered in today's mechanization. The jet age has brought with it further instances of such damage, and the entire problem has reached such magnitude that innumerable agencies are devoted to research in this field.

A new phenomenon of considerable interest is that of trauma caused by "Rock and Roll" music. Sound pressure level measurements on the stage occupied by Rock and Roll combos have yielded values in the 90–110 dB range. The amount of attenuation in small bistros or even larger night clubs where these combos play is not great, so that the audiences are exposed to not very much less trauma than the musicians themselves. Temporary threshold shifts, and even sustained losses, are now being observed clinically.

A study by Rosen et al. (1964) among the Mabaans, a primitive African tribe which passes its life in an environment of low psychic stress and extremely low sound-pressure levels, has indicated singular freedom from presbycusis even among the very aged (also significant is the low incidence of coronary arteriosclerotic heart disease in this tribe). Rosen hypothesizes that the presbycusis seen in civilized countries may well be the accumulative result of a lifetime of exposure to sound pressure levels which, in the ordinary sense, we would not consider traumatic. (Reference has been made previously to the possibility of ossicular osteoarthritis as the result of prolonged exposure to sound levels probably not excessive in the ordinary sense. It may, as suggested, be possible that the inner ear is affected by the same noxa.)

Pathologically, selective damage occurs within the epithelial elements of the organ of Corti, the location and extent depending upon the basic intensity and frequency characteristics of the offending noise source (Figs. 12-70 and 12-71). Thus, more and more adult

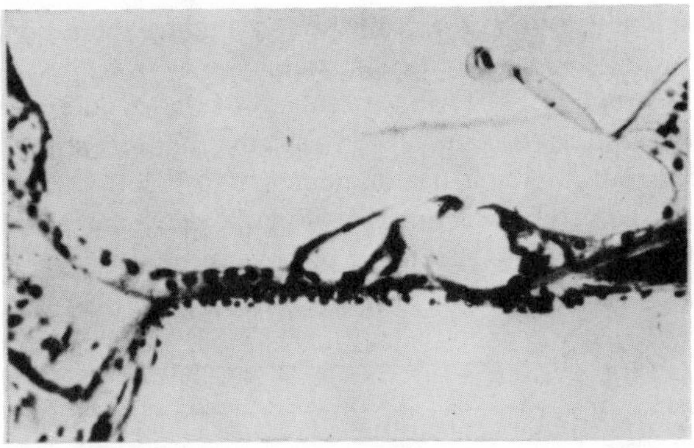

Fig. 12-70. Effect of noise trauma in the guinea pig. The outer hair cells and some of Deiter's supporting cells have disappeared at the beginning of the second cochlear turn. *From Fowler, E. P., 1947. LOOSE-LEAF MEDICINE OF THE EAR. Baltimore; Williams & Wilkins.*

sensorineural hypacusis is being encountered and much of it assumes serious degrees, so that major speech-reception-threshold losses occur. No longer are we concerned about the classical high-tone dip, which was of audiometric interest but which, in itself,

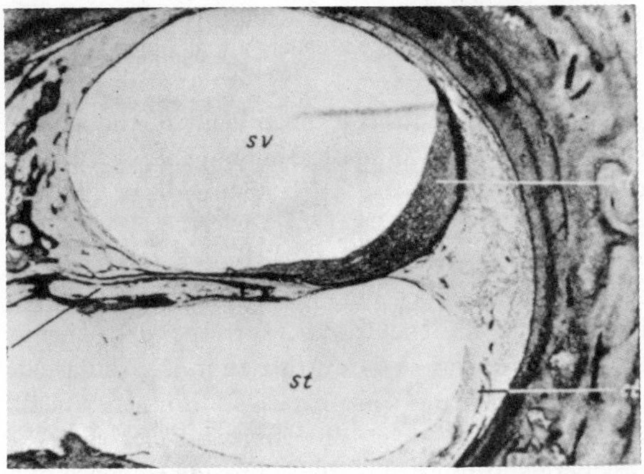

Fig. 12-71. Microphotograph of case of traumatic deafness. Section through basal turn of cochlea, showing organ of Corti destroyed and replaced by connective tissue filling entire scala media, scala tympani, scala vestibuli, as well as complete atrophy of spiral nerve. *From Fischer, J., and Wolfson, L. E., 1943. INNER EAR. New York: Grune and Stratton.*

carried few practical implications for the patient. We now find that prolonged acoustic trauma produces deficits in the entire auditory spectrum, and frequently these deficits assume major degrees in the 1,000 and 12,000 cycle range where they decidedly interfere with the hearing for speech.

Undoubtedly, there is a difference in susceptibility to noise trauma. Many anatomic and physiologic reasons could be offered to explain the reason for such variation in susceptibility. An adequate method for rapid screening techniques to find such susceptible individuals is imperative in an attempt to meet this problem in industry and in military life today.

Individuals who show a characteristic 4,000 cycle dip (Fig. 12-72) bilaterally, by both air and bone conduction, and who have a history of known tinnitus upon exposure to high-intensity noise, should be warned against continued exposure to such noise.

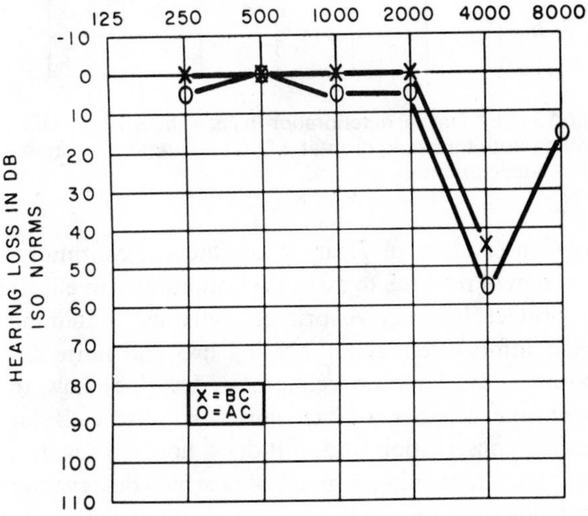

Fig. 12-72. Classic example of dip at 4,000 Hz by both air conduction and bone conduction in traumatic or "stimulation" deafness (high tone sensorineural hypacusis).

Exposure to gunfire in such individuals may possibly cause degenerative changes in the lower parts of the spectrum (Fig. 12-73), particularly at 2,000 and 1,000 cycles, thus rendering that individual a candidate for speech-threshold disturbances as well as speech-discrimination losses.

The treatment of acoustic trauma begins and ends with prevention. There is no treatment for the demonstrable hearing loss which has occurred as the result of such exposure. The efforts of physicians and audiologists must be devoted to 1) prevention of contact of humans with such high-intensity sound areas, 2) selection of adequate sound-protective devices, and 3) screening of individuals to eliminate those who show susceptibility to noise damage in industries where noise is a major problem. In an effort to achieve these goals, the American Academy of Ophthalmology and Otolaryngology's Committee

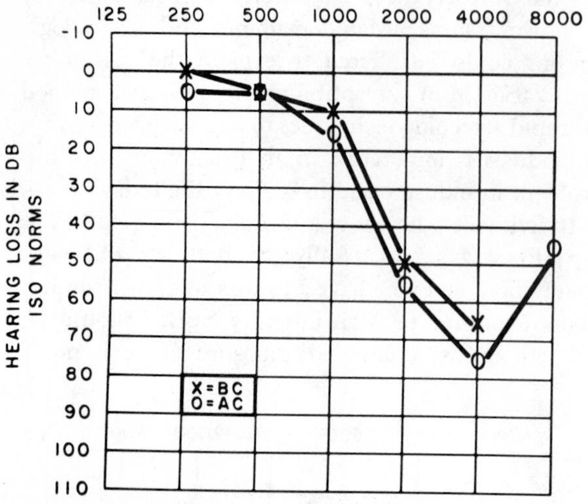

Fig. 12-73. Further deterioration in case shown in previous figure. Note threshold drop at 2,000 Hz due to persistence of acoustic trauma.

on Conservation of Hearing conducts a continuous program of research to assist the community in efforts to protect hearing. A printed syllabus containing basic information about hearing loss and noise exposure is available on request. It describes how to determine whether a given noise exposure calls for hearing conservation, and, if it does, how to organize, conduct, and monitor a practical hearing conservation program.

Acquired syphilis. Syphilis, as a public health problem, is again increasing in importance. Nevertheless, syphilitic deafness, which used to be a major problem otologically, has become a rarity and one requiring little stress from the point of view of therapy. Syphilis has always been known as the "great imitator," and, as such, in the temporal bone (as well as elsewhere in the body), it may imitate any disease, including otosclerosis, Ménière's disease, toxic labyrinthitis, as well as intracranial tumors. By forming large space-occupying gummata and by creating periostitis (Figs. 12-65, 12-66, 12-67), it may produce all varieties of both conductive and sensorineural hypacuses. Treatment must be directed to the basic problem, and syphilis today usually responds to treatment in the majority of cases.

Presbycusis. Presbycusis has been used to designate the deterioration in hearing commonly seen in older age groups. Schuknecht (1964) has shown that aging can affect all the structures of the cochlear duct individually or in combination, including the fluids. Several patterns are demonstrable.

Atrophy of the stria vascularis in the middle and apical turns occurs as an isolated finding and is correlated with a flat audiometric loss pattern and usually good discrimniation (Fig. 12-74). Schuknecht refers to this as "metabolic presbycusis."

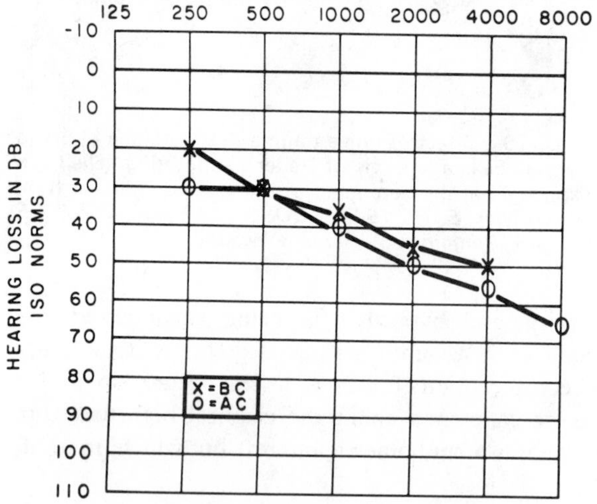

Fig. 12-74. Typical sensorineural hypacusis due to presbycusis, probably of epithelial atrophy type.

Alterations in chemical constituents of endolymph (increased protein content), demonstrable by staining characteristics, can be associated with progressive sensorineural hearing loss.

Atrophic changes in the organ of Corti's with secondary neural degeneration are most severe in the basal end of the cochlea and correspond to abrupt high-tone hearing losses (Fig. 12-75). Schuknecht terms this "neural presbycusis." These patients frequently have poor discrimination for speech. Bredberg and Engstrom (1965) provide evidence of a reduced number of nerve fibers in the basal end of the organ of Corti with increased age. The gradually descending audiometric threshold curve, so characteristic of many cases, has no morphologic correlate and is believed possibly related to basilar membrane stiffening and, thus, to a physical response gradient of this structure. Atrophy of the spiral ligament and basilar membrane may be associated with progressive sensorineural loss and may progress to the point of rupture of the basilar membrane with profound hearing loss.

In general, presbycusis occurs in most adults in civilized countries, but its rate varies considerably. It

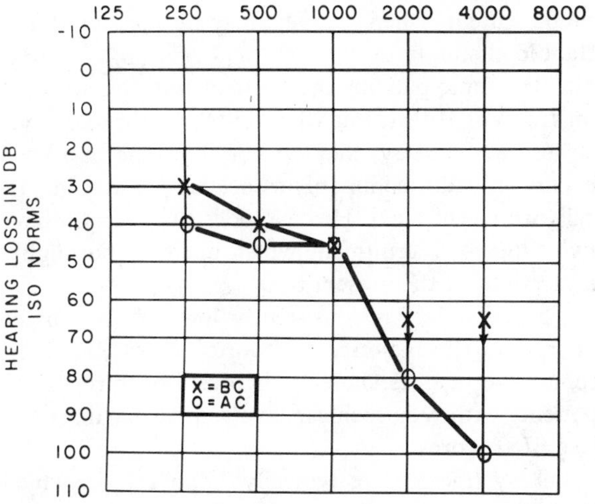

Fig. 12-75. Sensorineural hypacusis due to presbycusis with evidence of neural atrophy and high-frequency damage.

is possible, as mentioned in the section on acoustic trauma, that presbycusis, as we know it, may be the result of chronic exposure to the sounds of our civilization. In our civilization, it rarely becomes manifest until the sixth or seventh decade in the majority of the population. Premature presbycusis, however, may be demonstrated audiometrically in the fourth decade. Recruitment of loudness is not always found in presbycusis, although it may occur in some cases. Premature presbycusis may very well be a concomitant of a familial or hereditary predisposition and, thus, may actually represent a phase of heredo-degenerative sensorineural hypacusis of the adult type.

There is no satifactory treatment for presbycusis at the present time. Its progress continues in spite of all types of medical therapy. Rehabilitation through the use of amplification is not easily accomplished in presbycusis but is of some value in many cases. Liden (1965) suggests that the presence of phonemic regression (in which the hearing for speech is much poorer than the pure-tone audiogram would suggest) may appear as a sign of reduced cerebral function as a result of brain cell degeneration. More refined speech audiometry techniques should be useful in distinguishing cortically-involved hearing loss in presbycusis. Liden suggests that the presbycusic with cortical involvement will have greater difficulty with speech presented in noise, that binaural presentation of speech will not result in an improvement over monaural presentation, and that abnormally large differences in speech understanding will become evident as the difficulty of the speech test material increases.

There is increasing evidence of a conductive component in presbycusis which is presently being explored but about which too little is known to have any practical bearing on treatment at the present time.

Intracranial tumors. Increasingly sophisticated audiologic and vestibular methods of examination have aided the otoaudiologic team in the diagnosis of many central nervous system disorders; however, two intracranial tumors are of particular interest to members of this team.

Cerebellopontine angle tumors may be of any histologic type, either benign or malignant, though usually the former. These tumors compress the VIIIth Cranial nerve secondarily and are capable of producing a variety of symptoms. Eventually, such tumors will cause an increased intracranial pressure, by which time the diagnosis of a brain tumor becomes obvious. Diagnosis as facilitated by appropriate oto-audiological examination.

The acoustic neurinoma represents between one and two percent of all intracranial tumors. These are histologically benign, and may occur in any portion of the auditory nerve, reaching any size (Fig. 12-76 a). Most frequently, they originate within the internal auditory meatus, where they may cause purely cochlear symptoms for a long time. They become intracranial, occupying the cerebellopontine angle, only after a protracted period of growth (Fig. 12-76 b). They may involve either the cochlear or vestibular branches or the entire VIIIth Cranial nerve. With increasing growth, there may be involvement of the facial nerve with ensuing paralysis, and an increasing disequilibrium from involvement of the vestibular nerve. However, due to the slowness of growth, the patient may gradually compensate for the unilaterally diminishing vestibular function, as after unilateral vestibular ablation. For this reason, vertigo is not particularly common in these tumors. Tinnitus and deafness, however, are. Eventually, there may be involvement of other Cranial nerves, notably the fifth, with the production of typical trigeminal pain. Finally, a picture of obstructive hydrocephalus may occur with visual disturbances and other evidences of increased intracranial pressure.

Today, with the help of neurologic, audiologic, and radiographic examination, the diagnosis of these tumors can be suspected much earlier and often established.

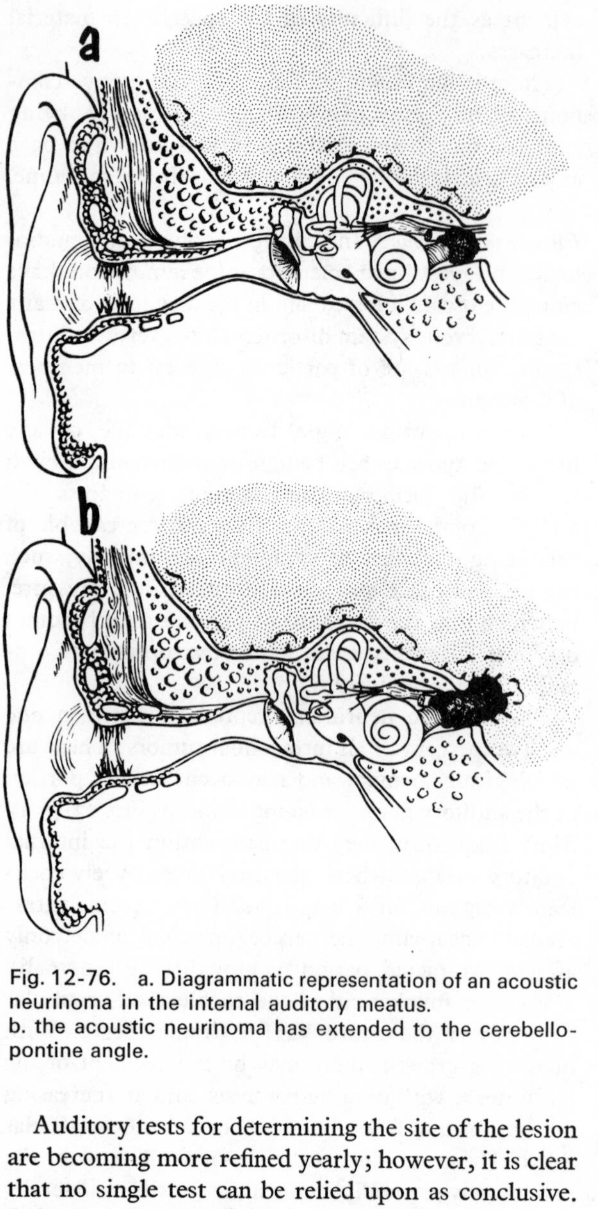

Fig. 12-76. a. Diagrammatic representation of an acoustic neurinoma in the internal auditory meatus.
b. the acoustic neurinoma has extended to the cerebello-pontine angle.

Auditory tests for determining the site of the lesion are becoming more refined yearly; however, it is clear that no single test can be relied upon as conclusive. It is not infrequent to find a contradictory pattern of test results.

A growing body of clinical and research data does, however, permit certain expectations and forms the basis of the diagnostician's determination. A unilateral sensorineural loss is common; speech discrimination frequently is affected beyond the expectations for peripheral pure-tone losses of similar configuration. A mild or moderate loss may yield marked impairment in speech discrimination.

Recruitment is generally absent, but may occur in some cases. Dix and Hallpike (1956) have speculated that the cause of recruitment in the acoustic neurinoma patient, when it exists, may be interference of the blood supply to the cochlea. Reger (1965) points out that some patients may demonstrate recruitment on the ABLB test, but when tested at threshold via Békésy audiometry, they do not show the narrowed excursion width commonly associated but not identical with recruitment. He concludes that we may have two types of recruitment which are not thoroughly understood at the present time.

The SISI test is consistently low (30 percent or poorer) in the majority of reported cases; however, some investigators show as high as one-third of the patients with retrocochlear involvement having positive SISI scores.

Békésy tracings are typically Type III (in which the continuous and interrupted tracings may be superimposed for the low frequencies (100–500 Hz) then the continuous tracing drops below the interrupted to a marked degree, but the width of the continuous excursion remains the same) or Type IV (in which the continuous tracing falls below the interrupted tracing at all frequencies, and the width of the excursions may or may not narrow). A Type I or Type II tracing does not rule out the presence of a neurinoma; 30 percent of the surgically confirmed retrocochlear lesions reported by Johnson (1965) produced Type I and Type II Békésy patterns.

Reger (1965) regards "temporary threshold drift" as one of the most significant audiological responses. Fixed frequency Békésy tracings are uniquely suited to measuring this phenomenon. A steady (continuous) tone presented over a period of time (two to three minutes) may result in rapid deterioration of threshold sensitivity in the retrocochlear loss; threshold drift downward to the maximum output of the audiometer may be seen. Tone decay can also be measured with a conventional pure-tone audiometer (Carhart, 1957) and frequently occurs in VIIIth Cranial nerve lesions at those frequencies showing hearing loss. Stephens and Hinchcliffe (1968) suggest that Dr. Carhart's method of determining tone decay (measured manually with the conventional pure-tone audiometer) is correlated with age, and that a neuronal component of presbycusis may be the determinant. They expressed a preference for the Békésy tracings as being "less age dependent" and as a method of detecting a neuronal lesion other than presbycusis.

The more sophisticated speech audiometry tests (in which the listening task is made more difficult as in filtered speech, time-compressed speech, swinging speech, interrupted speech) are increasingly under investigation for use in differentiating retrocochlear lesions of the brain stem, midbrain, and cortex. Distorted speech may be presented monaurally and the results for each ear compared. In temporal lobe disease, the contralateral ear will yield poorer results; however, normal cochlear function is usually necessary for these tests to be interpreted meaningfully. Binaural presentation of distorted speech is also being utilized, each ear receiving the same or different signals simultaneously or at intervals (Linden, 1964; Matzker, 1959; Bocca and Calearo, 1963). Normal ears (with an intact central auditory pathway) synthesize the sound; pathologic ears do not. Bocca (1965), in his investigations of binaurally presented distorted speech using meaningful sentences (which exclude the coexistent effects of cochlear disturbance), concludes that these tests bring out defects of binaural integration without involving symbolization and memorization. Certain of the tests appear to be more specific to the brain-stem level, others, to the cortical or subcortical level. Currently, research emphasis needs to be placed on selection of those tests most appropriate and on methods of standardization.

Basic research into the psychophysiologic process of temporal auditory summation (Olson and Carhart, 1966; Wright, 1968) should prove a stimulus to designing new auditory tests for differential diagnosis and will also serve an expanding auditory theory. Speaks and Jerger (1965) contributed significantly to the measurement of speech intelligibility by constructing closed-set synthetic sentences which lend themselves more easily to manipulation of temporal parameters than conventional PB-50 word lists or previous sentence lists (uncontrolled as to informational content). Jerger and Jerger (1967) utilized synthetic syntax sentence identification under conditions of temporal compression, temporal interruption, competing message, and filtering and studied the performance of three subjects (normal, cochlear disorder, VIIIth Cranial nerve disorder) as intensity of the speech was increased. Differences in performance were striking, the subject with VIIIth Cranial nerve abnormality demonstrating markedly reduced sentence identification ability as intensity was increased for both the condition of temporal interruption and the condition of temporal compression. The authors also studied the interrelationships of loudness discrimination, pitch discrimination, temporal order, and critical off-time in the three subjects. These areas appear fruitful for investigation. Such mapping of auditory behavior on many listening tasks is essential for progress in the field of human hearing disorders.

Vestibular evaluation is an essential part of the clinical examination for a suspected acoustic neurinoma. Not many years ago, it was thought that vestibular function, as demonstrated by caloric testing, was absent on the affected side and impaired on the opposite side, but now it is known that such a finding is characteristic only of well-developed, advanced tumors. Vestibular testing would show some impairment of function on the affected side but not absence. Involvement of the opposite side (which is a "contrecoup" phenomenon), would not be expected in early cases.

Radiological examination of the skull, with particular reference to the internal auditory canal, is extremely important. While reasonable impressions of the integrity of this structure and comparison of the two sides can be made from the routine Stenvers and Chamberlain-Towne views, laminographic studies are mandatory. Enlargement of the internal auditory canal, erosion of its walls, or loss of the crista which separates it into superior and inferior compartments are considered significant. Exact measurements of the diameter of the canal are important. If a significant abnormality exists in one or both internal auditory canals, it is necessary to obtain information as to possible intracranial extension of the tumor and of the size of such an extension. For this purpose, radiographic dye contrast studies are necessary.

The treatment of these tumors is surgical. The approach consists of a posterior fossa craniotomy in which the neurosurgeon exposes the cerebellopontine angle and removes the tumor which has extended intracranially. The operating microscope is used to facilitate ablation of the posterior face of the petrous bone to open the internal auditory canal for purposes of removing the extracranial portion of the growth. Recent translabyrinthine approaches are under evaluation.

It should never be forgotten that the first symptoms may be limited to unilateral sensorineural hypacusis with mild tinnitus and momentary and not very severe episodes of vertigo. These patients may be in excellent health with little impairment of their ability to carry on their lives. Their symptoms may easily be confused with those of unilateral Ménière's disease or with other conditions. A high index of suspicion is the responsibility of the clinician. Two cases of acoustic neurinoma are illustrated, the first in Fig. 12-77, and the second in Figs. 12-78 and 12-79.

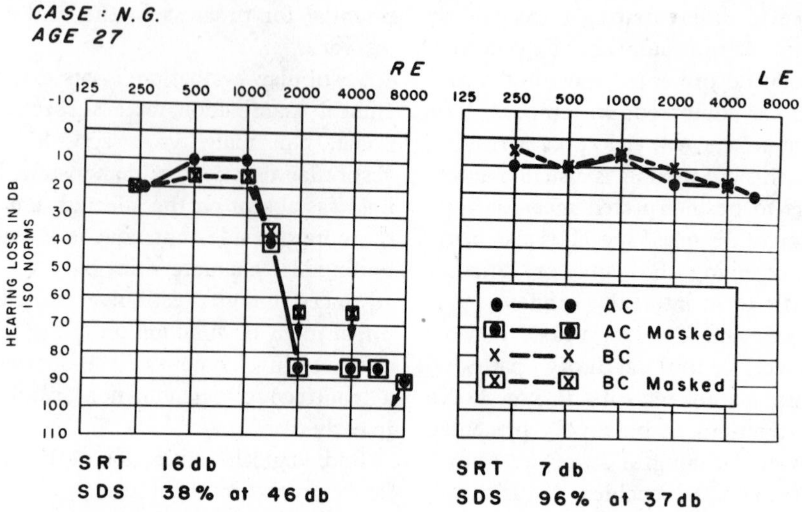

Fig. 12-77. Pure-tone and speech audiometry results obtained on initial examination of a 27-year-old man with a large, right acoustic neurinoma successfully removed 20 days later. The patient gave a history of headaches first noted three months prior to initial otologic examination. One week prior to examination, he began to notice decreased hearing in the right ear, tinnitus, periodic nausea and vomiting, some numbness in the left hand, and some lack of coordination in gait. His fixed-frequency Békésy tests revealed a 30 dB gap between tracings for continuous and interrupted stimuli at 250 Hz. Tracings at the other frequencies did not show a separation of continuous from interrupted of more than 10–15 dB. Of additional significance was the marked drop (60 dB) in sensitivity for the fixed continuous tone at 1,500 Hz. Sweep-frequency Békésy tracings revealed extremely rapid adaptation to continuous tonal stimuli extending to frequencies at least as low as 100 Hz. The gap between continuous and interrupted was as great as 60 dB or more at the low and mid frequencies and then gradually closed at 1,500 Hz. Tracings for both interrupted and continuous tracings then dropped sharply but continuous tracings continued to show a separation of 15–20 dB for frequencies 2,000 Hz and above. This tracing was atypical and could not be clearly classified as a Type IV. Other auditory tests could not be performed, due to the patient's incapacity to tolerate further testing and to his immediate hospitalization.

Cochleo-toxic Drugs. A number of toxic drugs may cause irreversible damage to the organ of hearing. Before the days of antimicrobial therapy, the best known drug in this category was quinine. This drug was given not only for the treatment of malaria, but also for certain other purposes, e.g., hastening labor, treatment of leg aches in women, and in the form of bromo-quinine for the treatment of upper respiratory infections and other ailments. The use to hasten labor has caused the birth of not a few profoundly or totally deafened infants. Taken over considerable periods of time, this drug will cause a tinnitus and a sensorineural hearing loss, beginning in the high-frequency range. It is bilateral and permanent. There is evidence also that such use can make the ears more susceptible to acoustic trauma.

Four antimicrobial drugs deserve special mention: 1. Streptomycin, long the only antibiotic agent useful in the treatment of tuberculosis, was found, after prolonged dosage, to cause an abrupt loss of vestibular function. Despite serial performance of vestibular tests, the onset was unpredictable and based, in part on individual susceptibility. Considering that the drug was unique in its ability to save life in an otherwise potentially lethal disease, the price paid by the patient was not too great. He could still depend upon his visual and kinesthetic senses in order to remain ambulatory, but he had to be sure that his environment was well lighted, as in getting about his bedroom at night. The cochlear effects of streptomycin, while not negligible, were less marked. 2. Dihydrostreptomycin, although possessing little toxicity to the vestibular apparatus, is highly cochleo-toxic and is, therefore, rarely used. 3. Neomycin is sometimes used systemically in life-threatening situations in which no other drug promises a cure, although it is known to be not only cochleo-toxic but nephro-toxic as well. 4. Kanamycin is used in pediatrics for the treatment of Gram-negative septicemias and other infections in very young infants. The dose necessary to produce cochlear damage is unpredictable, and sudden deafness can occur some time after discontinuation of the drug.

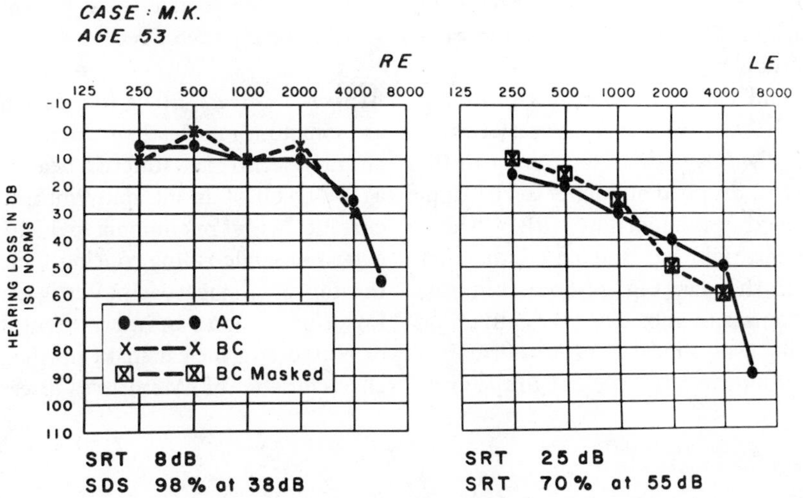

Fig. 12-78. Initial pure-tone and speech audiometry results obtained on a 53-year-old woman with a subsequently confirmed left acoustic neurinoma. A decrease in hearing in the left ear and the onset of tinnitus had been noted four months previous to the initial examination. There were no other complaints. Békésy tracings were Type I for the right ear and Type II for the left ear. SISI scores were low for both ears at 4,000 Hz and were positive for the left ear at 2,000 Hz. Complete recruitment was seen at 1,000 Hz and 2,000 Hz. Caloric studies revealed no directional preponderance. Visual field studies were normal. Radiographic studies revealed enlargement of the internal auditory meatus on the left side. Neurologic examination was negative. Fractional pneumonencephalography revealed no evidence of intracranial masses.

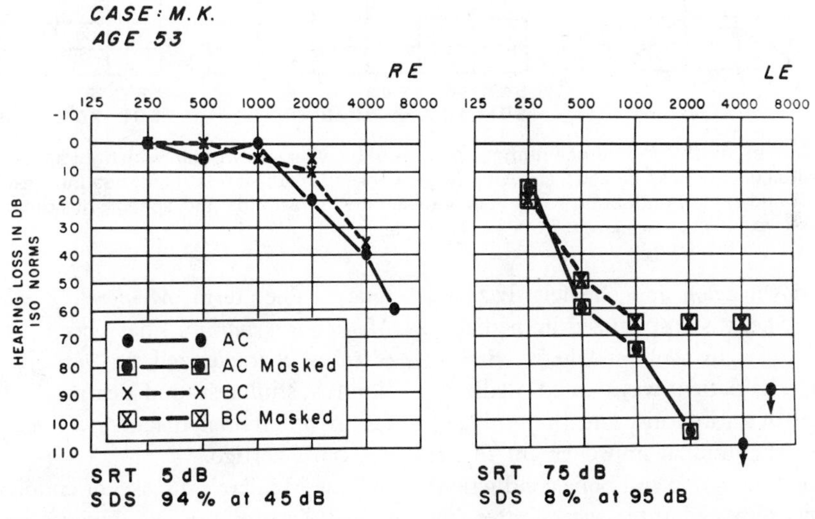

Fig. 12-79. Pure-tone and speech audiometry results obtained three and a half years later on the same patient as in Figure 12-78. Hearing loss in the left ear was progressive over a period of three and a half years. Speech discrimination gradually deteriorated from 70% to 8%. Special auditory tests, initially suggestive of a cochlear lesion' changed gradually to suggest retrocochlear involvement. Nevertheless, Békésy tracings for the left ear remained primarily Type II, but an emerging separation of the continuous from the interrupted tone was seen at frequencies below 1,000 Hz. The SISI score at 500 was negative; no recruitment was seen at 500 Hz. Examination of the cerebrospinal fluid revealed an elevation of the protein. A posterior fossa myelogram did not show an intracranial tumor. The patient complained of transient imbalance, dizzy episodes, and headaches. Eventually, laminography of the internal auditory meatus suggested a tumor mass. Total removal of an acoustic neurinoma with loss of VIIIth nerve function, but preservation of VIIth nerve function was accomplished. Anacusis in the left ear was present, postoperatively.

Acute cochleitis. This is a disease of either viral or microvascular etiology. The following case report is illustrative of the problem.

M.B., a 52-year-old teacher, had had a profound hearing loss in the left ear since having scarlet fever at the age of three. Two days prior to coming to the office, her hearing had dropped suddenly in the right ear. She had awakened in the morning with a "sharp horn blowing" in the right ear and noted that her hearing was down in that ear (Fig. 12-80a). Tinnitus lasted for several hours and subsided gradually. The next day her hearing was almost back to normal in her judgment. The following day, the day of the visit, her hearing was down again and she felt dizzy on getting out of bed. She was hospitalized immediately with the diagnosis of right acute cochleitis, viral or vascular in origin. The patient was treated medically under management of an internist and the otologist. Fig. 12-80b shows the gradual improvement in her hearing for both air conduction and bone conduction; the audiogram was obtained three weeks after her hospital treatment. Four weeks later, her pure-tone thresholds at 1,000 Hz had improved markedly and the speech discrimination score was also improved (Fig. 12-80c). We do not know, of course, if the patient had completely normal hearing in the right ear prior to the onset of the illness. However, we should note that in this case, time was of the essence. If the patient had been treated six weeks later or three months later, treatment would not have been as effective. The sooner these patients are treated, the greater the chance of recovery.

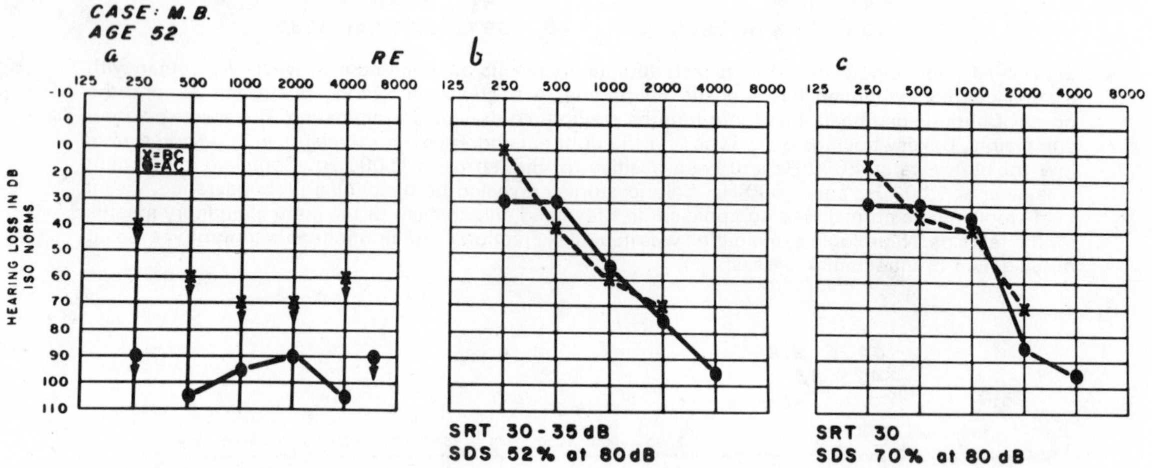

Fig. 12-80. (a) Initial audiometric findings in a case of 52-year-old woman with right acute cochleitis. She was immediately hospitalized; (b) After three weeks of medical treatment, hearing was improved by both air and bone conduction; (c) Four weeks later, thresholds and speech discrimination had further improved.

Ménière's Disease. Eponymic designations in medicine are sometimes misleading. Ménière's original patient, an adolescent girl, suffered hearing loss and vertigo as the result of an intralabyrinthine hemorrhage concurrent with pneumonia which developed from exposure while riding, during inclement weather, on the top of a stagecoach. Vertigo, attacks of hearing loss, tinnitus, and an intermittent feeling of stuffiness or pressure in the ear make up the symptom complex characteristic of Ménière's disease as understood today. The term *Ménière's syndrome*, or *pseudo-Ménière's syndrome*, has been applied to various diseases characterized by vertigo, with or without tinnitus, stuffiness, and deafness. Much care is called for in differential diagnosis, since many conditions can cause vertigo.

True Ménière's disease, or endolymphatic hydrops, is a disease of the endolymphatic labyrinth of unknown etiology. A subtle chemical change in endolymph-perilymph balance results in increased pressure within the endolymph system (hydrops). This causes distention of the membranous labyrinth throughout its extent. Histologically, this is most apparent within the cochlea, where it produces a distention of the scala media, manifested by a bulging of Reissner's membrane away from the basilar membrane, into the scala vestibuli (Fig. 12-81). The

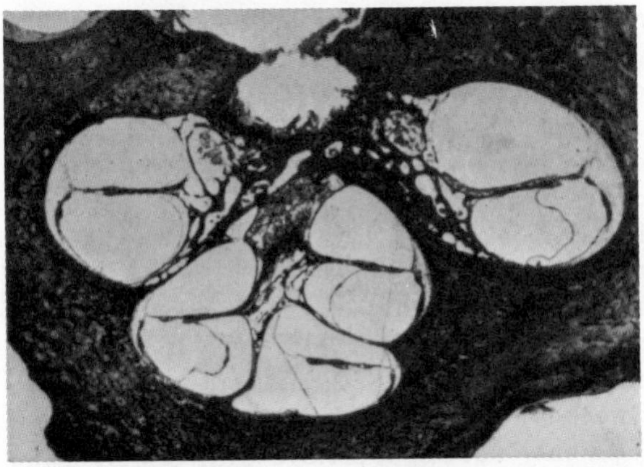

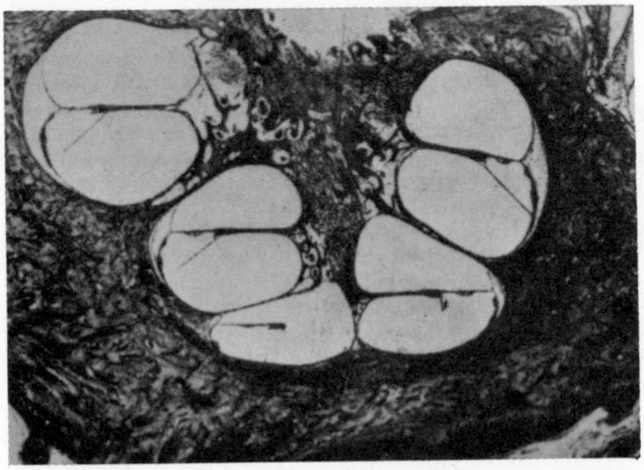

Fig. 12-81. Midmodiolar sections of both cochlea in a case of unilateral Ménière's disease in a man, aged forty-seven. Death from subdural hematoma resulting from a fall during an attack of vertigo. *Top,* horizontal section of right cochlea showing a normal cochlear duct. *Bottom,* vertical section of the left cochlea. The cochlear duct is moderately dilated throughout, almost filling the vestibular scala and extending into the helicotrema. The spiral ganglion of the basal coil shows a reduction from the normal in number of nerve cells and fibers. The organ of Corti shows moderate postmortem degeneration in both ears but is sufficiently well preserved to indicate that the antemortem condition was approximately the same histologically in both ears. Remnants of the hair cells are seen throughout all coils in both ears, and the stria vascularis is similar in both. *From Lindsay, J. R., 1939. MONOGRAPH ON MENIERE'S DISEASE. Chicago: Amer. Acad. Ophthal Otolaryng.*

endolymphatic pressure may be so great that rupture of Reissner's membrane may occur with intermingling of perilymph and endolymph. Such an event causes acute symptoms in the form of violent vertigo, increased tinnitus, and deafness. Partial recovery may ensue, after a time. Prolonged hydrops produces varying degrees of damage to the organ of Corti.

Some comment is necessary in regard to symptoms and their significance. The term *vertigo* refers to a subjective false sensation of rotation, although it is also used to describe a false sensation of linear acceleration. This illusion may involve either the subject or his environment. The clinician should not be mislead by the unfortunate word *dizzness* which is so often used as a synonym. The "dizzy" spell of which a patient complains may, in reality, be a transient visual scotoma, a psychogenic feeling of unreality or depersonalization, a headache, daydream, a feeling of faintness from pooling of blood in the abdomen, even a momentary loss of consciousness—as with petit mal epilepsy. The vertigo of true Ménière's disease is usually of sudden onset and rotatory in character, with an illusion of sufficient severity to produce a noticeable equilibrium disturbance. The patient may feel propelled to one side and will frequently fall down. This sudden attack is frequently accompanied by nausea and vomiting, perspiration, or even mild shock, and may require a day or two of complete bedrest with the use of sedatives before equilibrium returns. It may be followed by a prolonged chronic state of disequilibrium, aptly called "giddiness." The chronic mild "giddy" state may be punctuated by recurrent acute attacks. Great variations exist in the picture of vertigo, and the severity and side effects may vary from one attack to another. It should be stressed, however, that vertigo may be so insignificant that the patient does not voluntarily complain of it. It can be misinterpreted by the patient as a "slightly queasy stomach," or interpreted as an experience of some anxiety provoked by psychological stress.

The deafness of Ménière's disease is characteristically a sensorineural hypacusis. In most cases, the condition is unilateral. The low frequencies are usually involved first, a feature which is distinctive to this condition and found in almost no other. Early in the disease, the increased endolymphatic pressure, transmitted to the perilymph of the labyrinthine vestibule, causes some retrograde pressure upon the stapedial footplate, causing partial fixation and giving rise to a small, low-frequency air-bone gap (Fig. 12-82). This usually disappears at later stages of the disease. Typically, the loss is one of gradual onset and slow progression. Pure-tone configuration may progress from the initial greater loss in the low frequencies to a generally flat and moderate loss (Fig. 12-83), and eventually to a severe loss gradually sloping downward in the higher frequencies (Fig. 12-84). It is not uncommon to find in the early stages of the disease a great fluctuation of the hearing acuity

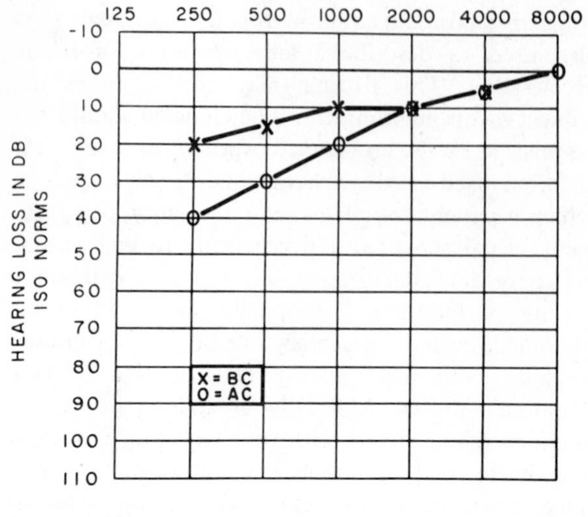

Fig. 12-82. Audiometric threshold in a case of early Ménière's. It is fairly typical of a conductive hypacusis.

occurring over periods varying from hours to days to weeks.

Speech discrimination shows wide variability from patient to patient and in one patient at different times; however, the usual finding is one of poor speech discrimination which varies as the hearing fluctuates.

Special audiologic studies are helpful in diagnosis. The Békésy audiogram is usually of Type II in which the continuous tracing drops below the interrupted tracing above 1,000 Hz, and the excursion width narrows for the continuous tracing in the high

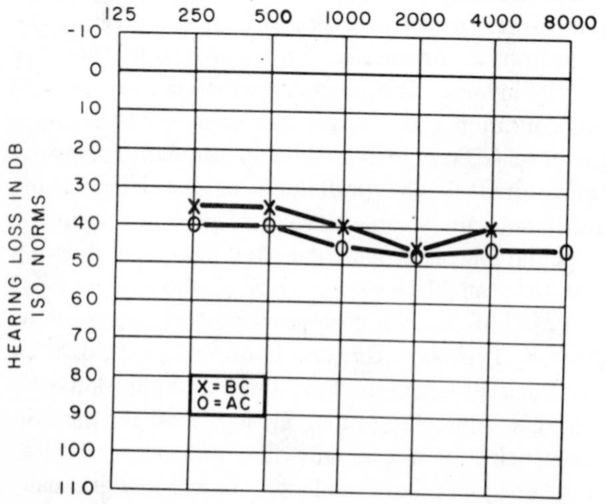

Fig. 12-83. Audiometric thresholds in a case of moderately advanced Ménière's disease. The picture is now typical of a sensorineural hypacusis.

frequencies. Loudness recruitment (measured by the Alternate Binaural Loudness Balance test) is usually complete in the majority of cases. The presence of recruitment is especially helpful in distinguishing cochlear lesions (such as Ménière's) from retrocochlear lesions (such as acoustic neurinoma) which also are frequently unilateral. The SISI test, in which the sensitivity to a one-dB intensity increment is measured, frequently results in a high score (60 percent or greater); however, interpretation of the score must consider the degree of loss at the test frequency (Owens, 1964; Harford, 1965). Mild losses less than 35 dB may not show positive SISI scores; losses

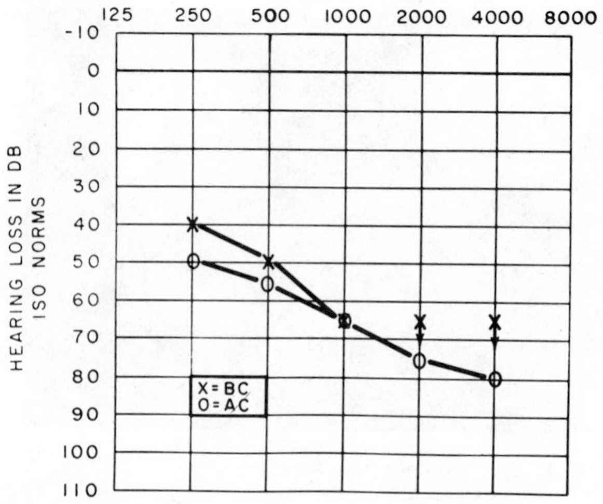

Fig. 12-84. Audiometric threshold in advanced Ménière's disease. This is a severe sensorineural hypacusis and is usually accompanied by marked vestibular hypoactivity, poor speech discrimination, and definite recruitment of loudness.

greater than 80 dB may need to have a lowered sensation level for presentation. Investigations of increment size and sensation level for presentation are continuing. Tone decay (a marked decrease in threshold sensitivity) can be measured by using sustained pure tones and a conventional audiometer or the Békésy audiometer to present continuous discrete frequencies. Results are highly variable depending on various test parameters, although some form of pathologic adaptation is usually evident for frequencies 1,000 Hz and above. Response to amplification is generally poor.

Tinnitus in Ménière's disease is an annoying symptom to some patients. It is usually amorphous and mixed in tonal qualities, usually in a continuous, sustained amplitude. It may be roaring, like an ocean wave, with an occasional bell-like quality. It sometimes varies in intensity, the degree of the annoyance subject to emotional and nervous excitations. A sudden loud environmental sound may accentuate the tinnitus intensity for hours.

The course of disease, untreated and sometimes with treatment, may be progressive, interspersed with plateaus of latency. Usually, there will be some degree of progressive deterioration, at least in the hearing. Treatment of the disease is highly controversial. Because of spontaneous fluctuations in the severity of the disease, the greatest caution must be exercised in attributing virtues to any proposed modality of treatment. No unanimity exists with regard to results with medical therapy. Surgery to the labyrinth involves many approaches to different parts of the labyrinth. The only area of agreement is in the sphere of labyrinthectomy, of one or another type, for patients in whom the vertigo is completely disabling.

TINNITUS

Tinnitus is an otologic symptom. It has many characteristics and can occur as the result of many causes. It is not a disease or syndrome, but a subjective phenomenon common to many diseases and should be viewed in the light of subjective symptomatology in differential otologic diagnosis.

Webster defines tinnitus as a ringing, whistling, or other sensation of noise which is purely subjective. The word is derived from the Latin, *tinnire*, meaning "to jingle."

Basically, two types of tinnitus must be distinguished; tinnitus aurium, and tinnitus cranii (tinnitus cerebri).

Tinnitus cranii is frequently confused with tinnitus aurium and may actually coexist with it. Tinnitus cranii is a nonlocalized subjective sensation of sound which is usually diffuse in the head and has a nonspecific quality. It is frequently described as a roaring or rushing sound not directed to the ear region. Its diffuse character may be confused with somatic sensations of the neck and upper thorax and, indeed, may be due to vascular phenomena in these areas as well as intracranially. Usually, tinnitus cranii is due to organic or functional intracranial vascular disease and is a medical neurological problem, one which does not participate significantly in otologic diagnosis. Tinnitus aurium, on the other hand, is usually localized to one or both ears and is subjectively described with some specificity by the patient.

Tinnitus aurium must be subdivided into two subtypes, each of which has been given a number of names. These two principal subtypes and their synonyms may be described as follows:

1) Subjective tinnitus (static-nonvibratory, true, intrinsic). Subjective tinnitus is the subjective cortical perception of auditory sensations inaudible to anyone but the patient. These sensations are most usually due to auditory paresthesias from any location within the auditory pathway.

2) Objective tinnitus (dynamic, vibratory, false, extrinsic). Objective tinnitus may be defined as the subjective cortical perception of auditory sensations, potentially audible to an examiner as well as to the patient.

Inasmuch as objective tinnitus is a relatively rare phenomenon, its characteristics and significance in otologic diagnosis will be briefly surveyed in order to limit the remainder of the discussion to the principal type of tinnitus encountered in otologic practice, namely, subjective tinnitus.

Objective tinnitus is either vascular or muscular in origin. The vascular type of objective tinnitus is usually due to some type of arteriovenous communication producing an audible bruit or murmur which can be heard with or without amplification. The muscular types of objective tinnitus are due to contractions of tympanic or tubal muscles, usually in bizarre or atypical rhythm. The mechanism for such contractions is exceedingly complex in etiology. Muscle spasms, functional tics, and other neuromuscular phenomena related to metabolic, neurologic, and psychosomatic states play a part in this relatively rare group of cases. An example is a clicking sound emanating from one or both ears in cases of palatal myoclonus. Examination of the pharynx will disclose the fact that each click is accompanied by a spasmodic upward movement of the soft palate. This condition is frequently due to a neurologic lesion of the midbrain and hind brain.

The etiology of subjective tinnitus can be discussed from the standpoints of anatomic location and pathologic change. Subjective tinnitus may arise from any location within the auditory pathway from the external ear to the auditory cortex. The pathologic state responsible for the genesis of the tinnitus may be any histopathologic abnormality in the auditory pathway. Consequently, the potential causes for tinnitus are innumerable and defy simplification.

Tinnitus is a common symptom of many otologic diseases.

In the consideration of subjective tinnitus, it is helpful to differentiate two basic physiologic subdivisions which are quite different anatomically and functionally.

The first subdivision may be described as *unmasked visceral tinnitus*. This tinnitus usually originates in the tympanic region and is usually the sequel of a conduction or impedance lesion. It is caused by the removal of the normal masking effect of surrounding ambient noise and is usually produced by subaudible tympanic and peritympanic vascular and muscular noises. This is the type of tinnitus one meets most commonly in uncomplicated otosclerosis, tympanic fibrosis, and chronic catarrhal otitis with or without perforation. It is also frequently found in glomus jugulare and other tympanic tumors.

The second physiologic type of tinnitus is more common and might be described as *neural discharge tinnitus* of either cochlear or central origin. This is a suprathreshold auditory paresthesia. In this type, there is cerebral recognition of auditory stimuli produced by mechanical cochlear deformation or electrochemical neural hyperirritability in the auditory pathways. This is the type seen in stimulation (traumatic) deafness, some types of presbycusis, Ménière's disease (labyrinthine hydrops), acoustic neurinoma, and in many other lesions involving either the cochlea or any of the neural elements of the auditory pathways.

In addition to the above differentiation, which is important from a localization and management point of view, we must also differentiate tinnitus clinically into *compensated* and *decompensated* forms. *Compensated* tinnitus is present in much of the population. It accompanies the high incidence of minimal cochlear lesions due to various etiologic factors which are productive of neural discharge tinnitus. In most of these instances, the tinnitus is not even noticeable to the patient, except under extremely quiet circumstances. It is not a clinical problem but merely a curiosity.

Decompensated tinnitus may be used as a term to describe tinnitus that is recognized as a problem by the patient. There are two types of otologic problems that will produce decompensated tinnitus. The first is tinnitus of low acoustic intensity accompanied by some type of psychosomatic stress. The second is tinnitus of high acoustic intensity as measured by comparative methods in a tinnitus analysis study. It is the patient with decompensated tinnitus who is really the subject of our discussions. He is the one who comes for help primarily because of the tinnitus. His other etiologic symptoms are frequently subdued and minimized in the history. The tinnitus itself looms as the chief complaint and is the subjective symptom requiring specific otologic management.

As in other medical problems, but especially in cases of subjective phenomena, a double diagnosis must always be considered, designating 1) the actual organic etiologic otologic lesion, and 2) the psychosomatic status of the patient. The latter must take into consideration both the emotional threshold of the patient and the degree of stress impinging upon him. This double diagnostic attack is distinctly the responsibility of the otologist and cannot be shifted to another physician.

The fallacy that tinnitus is a specific otologic disease has been strengthened and amplified by the numerous papers relating to treatment of tinnitus in which the therapy, be it surgical or medical, is directed to the general subject of tinnitus as a pathologic entity. The clinical retention of such a concept will do nothing to advance our knowledge in this field but will deter and retard scientific investigations and logical evaluation of therapeutic techniques. Almost any otologic disease can be accompanied by tinnitus. It is necessary to evaluate the position of tinnitus as a component of that specific disease.

It may be interesting to review briefly some typical organic otologic lesions which may cause tinnitus:

1. *Middle-Ear*

Membrana tympani—perforation, adhesive fibrosis, flaccidity
Fluid collections—hemotympanum, serous effusion, purulent exudate, mucoid exudate
Muscular—spasms, tics
Vascular—anomalies, anemia, polycythemia
Ossicular—joint disturbances, fixation (otosclerosis)
Tumors—glomus jugulare, hemangioma, carcinoma
Cholesteatomas—several types

2. *Inner-Ear*

Bony labyrinth—Paget's disease, otosclerosis, fragilitas ossium
Perilymph diseases—inflammation, chemical alterations, pressure changes
Endolymphatic diseases—hydrops, collapse
Organ of Corti—peripheral neuritis, atrophy, edema, allergy

Cochlear ganglion—ganglionitis, allergy, atrophy
VIIIth Cranial nerve—tumors, inflammation, vascular anomalies

3. *Central Auditory Pathway*

Second order neurons— Third order neurons— Ventral and dorsal cochlear nuclei— Lateral lemniscus tract— Medial geniculate body— Auditory cortex—	Tumors, vascular and circulatory anomalies, focal inflammatory lesions

The Significance of Tinnitus in the Differential Diagnosis of Otologic Disease

In that vast unknown called "nerve deafness," which comprises many diseases occurring in the intricate neural pathway from the endolymphatic labyrinth to and including the auditory cortex, we have few localizing opportunities in differential diagnosis. The pure-tone and speech audiogram, recruitment tests, the SISI test, the Békésy audiogram, and correlated electronystagmographic studies have given us some insight into sensorineural deafness.

Tinnitus is an important symptom in lesions of the neural auditory pathway. The identification, accumulation, and classification of discrete characteristics of tinnitus in these cases, when correlated with other otologic data and later with pathologic findings, may shed much light on the differential diagnosis of sensorineural deafness. Recent studies have shown that much "nerve deafness" originates not only in the organ of Corti and in the cochlear ganglion, but in the nuclei, ascending pathways, and possibly in the thalamus and cortex. Present audiometric techniques do not suffice in the segregation of anatomic locations in patients with "nerve deafness." It is conceivable that correlation of audiometric data with tinnitus analysis data may yield such localizing information.

Methodical Analysis of Tinnitus

A methodical analysis of tinnitus should be an integral part of the otologic examination, particularly in clinical research. The following method of analysis is suggested as an orderly technique in an attempt to obtain useful data.

SUBJECTIVE STATEMENT OF PATIENT

The patient is requested to describe his tinnitus in his own words to the best of his ability without any specific questions.

Subjective analysis. The patient is then questioned for the following specific data:

The general location of the tinnitus. Is the tinnitus *within* the patient or does it seem to be somewhere in the room? Occasionally, the patient will insist that the tinnitus is not in the head, not in the ear, but to the right or to the left of the head and apparently projected several inches or feet away.

The somatic location of the tinnitus. Is it in one or both ears and if so, superficially or deeply; or is it in the head, and if so in what part of the head?

The specificity in regard to loudness. If the somatic location is diffuse and variable, the patient is asked to relate the specificity in regard to loudness. If the tinnitus is stated to be in the head and ear, the predominant intensity is elicited.

Time relations of tinnitus. Is the tinnitus louder during certain times of the day? Is it louder at work or at home? Is it louder at certain times of the week? In women, does it vary with menses?

Positional relations of tinnitus. Does the tinnitus vary with positions of the head or body? Does it increase on stooping? Is it relieved by any specific position of the body or head?

Characteristics of the tinnitus—acoustic analysis. If the tinnitus is a pure tone, it may be identified on the audiometer. For these purposes, the ordinary fixed-frequency audiometer is inadequate. The sweep-frequency audiometer is necessary to accomplish such specific tone localization. By this same technique, the intensity of the tinnitus and intensity of the sound required to mask the tinnitus can be determined.

If the tone is complex, an attempt is made at audiometric analysis, in terms of dominant and accessory tones. Admittedly, in most patients this is a difficult, if not impossible, task, but in musically articulate patients it can frequently be accomplished.

A special type of "tinnitus" is that due to hyperpatency of the Eustachian tube. It consists of audible breath sounds and autophonous reverberation of the patient's own voice, associated with a feeling of stuffiness. It is due to loss of the paratubal fat pad of Rüdiger. It is frequently relieved by lying down because of the induced vascular engorgement of the head, but recurs promptly on arising. Patients often sniff compulsively to relieve the troublesome sensations. While teflon injection about the pharyngeal tubal orifice has lately been a popular treatment method, it seems wise to treat the symptoms like any form of uncompensated tinnitus by reassurance and efforts to gain weight.

Management of Tinnitus

SPECIFIC OTOLOGIC THERAPY

It is important at the present time to reevaluate critically many of the therapeutic techniques previously suggested to avoid therapeutic nihilism as well as mythical tinnitus cures. The organic otologic disease focus in such a case must be approached with the idea of therapy directed specifically to eradication of the tinnitus. In most instances, such therapeutic techniques will also improve the hearing. There are situations, however, when only a slight hearing improvement induced by a particular therapy may be accompanied by a major diminution of tinnitus intensity. It should be the tinnitus that receives the stress of our therapeutic attack, rather than other considerations. For example, the annoying pulsating visceral tinnitus of a tympanic glomus jugulare will usually disappear following surgical removal, yet the hearing may be poorer.

PALLIATIVE MEASURES

Simple reassurance as to the reality of the tinnitus accompanied by encouragement and good prognosis will go far in helping alleviate the anxieties of the patient with decompensated tinnitus.

ACOUSTIC SEDATION

Acoustic sedation is very helpful in many cases of tinnitus, especially in regard to the difficulty in sleep, which is a great problem with many patients. The reason for greater difficulty at that time is, of course, due to the removal of ambient masking noise in the quiet of the night, which allows greater cerebral irritability by the ever-present auditory paresthesia. The use of a pillow-radio or phonograph is helpful in providing an artificial source of ambient noise to mask out the subjective tinnitus.

DRUG SEDATION

Drug sedation is an important palliative measure, not only for daytime use but especially for bedtime tinnitus irritability. In this light, it is valuable to rotate the simple barbiturates, bromides, and other substitutes. No one drug should be used for any long period. It is helpful psychologically to disguise the vehicles and to alternate the medications so that habituation and recognition by the patient are decreased.

SURFACE PSYCHOTHERAPY

In most instances where the decompensation of tinnitus is due to high acoustic intensity acoustically with little or no psychosomatic component, no further measures are necessary. In instances where the decompensated tinnitus is accompanied by major psychologic stresses, a certain degree of surface psychotherapy by the otologist is helpful. Such surface psychotherapy should include a thorough explanation as to the real nature of tinnitus with assurance that it is neither an hallucination nor an illusion.

Patients sometimes have phobias built up around symptoms of tinnitus. This needs careful exploration. A not uncommon phobia is that the tinnitus means that the patient is losing his mind. Usually, an explanation that the symptom has its origin in the ear and has nothing to do, per se, with mental processes, is sufficient. If the phobia persists or if brief inquiry uncovers the existence of major psychological problems, psychiatric referral may be indicated. It is also indicated in those situations in which the tinnitus seems to be organized into either a verbal or musical symbolic communicative process.

Since the treatment is not always satisfactory, the symptoms often being a manifestation of an irremedial degenerative process, one should avoid overoptimistic prognoses in regard to duration and continued severity of the symptom. It is well to explain to the patient that the acoustic characteristics of tinnitus can be evaluated by methods described previously in this section and that observation shows that the amount of distress experienced by various sufferers from this symptom bears very little, if any, direct relation to the loudness or other acoustic characteristics of the tinnitus, as such. Rather, it seems to be a function of individual personality and susceptibility. The patient should be assured that, even if the symptom does not disappear or is not even attenuated, he will find the strength, with help, to adjust or to adapt to it.

BIBLIOGRAPHY

Alderton, H. 1898. Trephining of the stapedial footplate for otitis media sclerosa. *Tr. Amer. Otol. Soc.*, 7, 60.

Barr, B., and Lundstrom, R. 1961. Deafness following maternal rubella; retrospective and prospective studies. *Acta Otolaryng.*, 53, 413–423.

Baylor Rubella Study Group. 1967. Rubella: epidemic in retrospect. *Hospital Practice*, vol. 2, no. 3, 27–35.

Blake, C. 1892. Operation for removal of the stapes. *Boston Med. Surg. J.*, 127, 551–552.

Bocca, E., and Perani, G. 1960. Further contributions to the knowledge of vestibular hearing. *Acta Otolaryng.*, 51, 260–267.

———, and Calearo, C. 1963. Central hearing processes. *In* Modern developments in audiology. Jenger, J., ed. New York: Academic Press. Pp. 337–370.

———. 1965. Distorted speech tests. *In* Henry Ford symposium on sensorineural hearing processes and disorders. Graham, A., ed. Boston: Little, Brown. Pp. 359–370.

Bordley, J., Brookhouser, P., Hardy, J., and Hardy, W. 1968. Prenatal rubella. *Acta Otolaryng.*, 66, 1–9.

Boucheron, E. 1888. La mobilisation de l'étrier. *Bull. Med., Paris*, 2, 1225.

Bredberg, G., and Engstrom, H. 1965. Cellular pattern and nerve supply of the human organ of Corti. *Arch. Otolaryng.*, 82, 462–469.

Brockman, S. J. 1965. Cartilage graft tympanoplasty, type III. *Laryngoscope*, 75, 1452–1461.

Burnett, C. H. 1893. Partial myringectomy and removal of the incus and stapes for the relief of the lesions of chronic catarrhal otitis media. *Med. News*, 62, 509.

Carhart, R. 1950. The clinical application of bone conduction audiometry. *Arch. Otolaryng.*, 51, 798–808.

———. 1957. Clinical determination of abnormal auditory adaptation. *Arch. Otolaryng.*, 65, 32–39.

———. 1967. Audiologic tests: Questions and speculations. *In* Deafness in childhood. McConnell, F., and Ward, P., eds. Nashville: Vanderbilt Univ. Press. Pp. 229–251.

Davis, H., 1968. Averaged-evoked response EEG audiometry in North America. *Acta Otolaryng.*, 65, 79–85.

Dix, M., and Hallpike, C. 1956. Loudness recruitment. *Brit. med. Bull.*, 12, 119.

Downs, M. 1967. Testing hearing in infancy and early childhood. *In* Deafness in childhood. McConnell, F., and Ward, P., eds. Nashville: Vanderbilt Univ. Press, Pp. 25–33.

Eisenberg, R., Hunter, M., Griffin, E., and Coursin, D. 1964. Auditory behavior in the human neonate: a preliminary report. *J. Speech Hearing Res.*, 7, 356–369.

Faraci, G. 1899. Sulla possibilita di riaprire la fenestra ovale in casi di anchilosi ossea del'articolazione stupediovestibolare. *Trans., 6th Int. Otolaryng. Cong.*, London. 240–245.

Garcia-Ibanez, L. 1961. Sonoinversion: a new audiosurgical system. *Arch. Otolaryng.*, 73, 268–272.

Goodhill, V., 1939. Syphilis of the ear: a histopathologic study. *Ann. Otol., Rhinol., Laryng.*, 48, 676–706.

———. 1950a. The nerve-deaf child; significance of Rh, maternal rubella and other etiologic factors. *Ann. Otol., Rhinol., Laryng.*, 59, 1123–1147.

———. 1950b. Nuclear deafness and the nerve-deaf child: the importance of the Rh factor. *Trans. amer. Acad. Ophthal., Otolaryng.*, 54, 671–687.

———. 1958a. The surgical physiology of tympanoplasty. *Laryngoscope.*, 68, 1455–1481.

———. 1958b. Unresolved otitis media. A serious problem. *Texas State J. of Med.*, 54, 579–584.

———. 1960a. The lurking latent cholesteatoma. *Ann. Otol., Rhinol., Laryng.*, 69, 1199–1213.

———. 1960b. Pseudo-otosclerosis. *Laryngoscope.*, 70, 722–757.

———. 1961. Stapes surgery for otosclerosis. New York: Paul Hoeber.

———. 1966a. External conductive hypacusis and the fixed malleus syndrome. *Acta Otolaryng. Supplement* 217.

———. 1966b. The fixed malleus syndrome. *Trans. amer. Acad. Ophthal., Otolaryng.*, 70, 370–380.

———. 1967a. Tragal perichondrium and cartilage in tympanoplasty. *Arch. Otolaryng.*, 85, 480–491.

———. 1967b. The conductive loss phenomenon in post-stapedectomy fistulae. *Laryngoscope.*, 77, 1179–1190.

———. 1967c. Variable oto-audiologic manifestations of perilymphatic fistulae. *Rev. Panamer. Otorhinolaryng.* y *Broncoesofag.*, 1, 100–109.

———. 1967d. Auditory pathway lesions resulting from Rh incompatibility. *In* Deafness in childhood. McConnell, F., and Ward, P., eds. Nashville: Vanderbilt Univ. Press. Pp. 215–228.

———. 1967e. Detection of hearing loss in neonates. Editorial *Arch. Otolaryng.*, 85, 1.

———, Harris, I., and Brockman, S. 1964. Tympanoplasty with perichondrial graft. *Arch. Otolaryng.*, 79, 131–137.

Hardy, W. 1961. Auditory deficits in the kernicterus child. Amer. acad. for cerebral palsy. Springfield, Ill.: Thomas. Pp. 255–266.

Hardy, W., Hardy, J., Brinker, C., Frazier, T., and Dougherty, A. 1962. Auditory screening of infants. *Ann. Otol., Rhinol., Laryng.*, 71, 759–766.

Hardy, J., McCracken, G., Jr., Gilkeson, M., and Sever, J. 1969. Adverse fetal outcome following maternal rubella after the first trimester of pregnancy. JAMA, 207, 2414–2420.

Harford, E. 1965. Clinical application and significance of the SISI test. *In* Henry Ford symposium on sensorineural hearing processes and disorders. Graham, A., ed. Boston: Little, Brown. Pp. 223–233.

Harris, I. 1961. Tympanosclerosis: a revived clinicopathologic entity. *Laryngoscope*, 71, 1488–1533.

———, and Goodhill, V. 1967. Functional viability of tragal cartilage autografts in tympanic surgery. *Laryngoscope*, 77, 1191–1203.

Henry Ford symposium on otosclerosis. 1960. Schuknecht, H., ed. Boston: Little, Brown.

Holmgren, G. 1923. Some experiences in surgery of otosclerosis. *Acta Otolaryng.*, 5, 460.

Hoversten, G., and Moncur, J. 1969. Stimuli and intensity factors in testing infants. *J. Speech Hearing Res.* (In press.)

Hyman, C., Keaster, J., Hanson, V., Harris, I., Sedgwick, R., Wursten, H., and Wright, A. 1969. CNS abnormalities after neonatal hemolytic disease or hyperbilurubinemia. *Amer. J. dis. Child.*, 117, 395–405.

Jack, F. 1891–1892. Remarkable improvement in hearing by removal of stapes. *Tr., Amer. Otolog. Soc.*, 5, 284.

Jerger, J., and Jerger, S. 1967. Psychoacoustic comparison of cochlear and eighth nerve disorders. *J. Speech Hearing Res.*, 10, 659–688.

Johnson, E. 1965. Auditory test results in 110 surgically confirmed retrocochlear lesions. *J. Speech Hearing Disorders*, 30, 307–317.

Keaster, J., Hyman, C., Harris, I. 1969. Hearing problems subsequent to neonatal hemolytic disease or hyperbilurubinemia. *Amer. J. dis. Child.*, 117, 406.

Kessel, J. 1876. Uber das Ausschneiden des Trommelfelles und Mobilisieren des Steigbugels. *Archiv. fur ohrenheilkunde.*, 11, 199.

Lempert, J. 1938. Improvement in hearing in cases of otosclerosis: a new one stage surgical technique. *Arch. Otolaryng.*, 28, 42–97.

Liden, G. 1965. Undistorted speech audiometry. *In* Henry Ford symposium on sensorineural hearing processes and disorders. Graham, A., ed. Boston: Little, Brown. Pp. 339–357.

Linden, A. 1964. Distorted speech and binaural speech resynthesis tests. *Acta Otolaryng.*, 58, 32–48.

Lowell, E., Goodhill, V., and Lowell, M. 1968. Evaluation of averaged evoked auditory response testing of young children. *Presented at ASHA Convention*, Denver, Colorado.

Matkin, N., and Carhort, R. 1968. Hearing acuity and Rh incompatibility. *Arch. Otolaryng.*, 87, 383–388.

Matzker, J. 1959. Two new methods for the assessment of central auditory functions in cases of brain disease. *Ann. Otol., Rhinol., Laryng.*, 68, 1185–1197.

Miot, C. 1890. De la mobilisation de l'étrier. *Rev. de Laryng.*, 10, 49.

Moure, E. 1880. De la mobilisation de l'étrier. *Rev.* de *Laryng.*, 7, 225.

Murphy, K. 1962. Ascertainment of deafness in children. *Panorama*, 3.

Olsen, W., and Carhart, R. 1966. Integration of acoustic power at threshold by normal hearers. *J. acoust. soc. Amer.*, 40, 591–599.

Owens, E. 1964. Tone decay in eighth nerve and cochlear lesions. *J. Speech Hearing Disorders*, 29, 14-22.

Passow, K. A. 1897. Operative Anlegung einer Offnung in die mediale Paukenhohlenwand bei Stapesanklose. *Verhandl. d. Deutsch Otol. Gesellsch*, 6, 141.

Reger, S. 1965. The Békésy audiometer stimulus. *In* Henry Ford symposium on sensorineural hearing processes and disorders. Graham, A., ed. Boston: Little, Brown. Pp. 235–243.

Rosen, S. 1955. Mobilization of the stapes to restore hearing in otosclerosis. *New York J. Med.*, 55, 1.

———. Plester, D., El-Mofty, A., and Rosen, H. 1964. High-frequency audiometry in presbycusis. A comparative study of the Mabaan tribe in the Sudan with urban population. *Arch. Otolaryng.*, 79, 18–32.

Schuknecht, H. 1964. Further observations on the pathology of presbycusis. *Arch. Otolaryng.*, 80, 369–382.

———. 1967. Pathology of sensorineural deafness of genetic origin. *In* Deafness in childhood. McConnell, F., and Ward, P., eds. Nashville: Vanderbilt Univ. Press. Pp. 69–90.

Shambaugh, G. 1967. Surgery of the ear. Philadelphia: Saunders.

Siebenmann, F. 1900. Traitement chirurgical de la sclerose otique. *Cong. Int. de Med. Sect. d'Otol.*, 13, 170.

Sourdille, M. 1929. Techniques chirurgicales nouvelles pour le traitement des surdités de conduction. *Bull. Acad. de Med.*, Paris. Ser. 3, 102, 674–678.

Speaks, C., and Jerger, J. 1965. Method for measurement of speech identification. *J. Speech Hearing Res.*, 8, 185.

Stephens, S., and Hinchcliffe, R. 1968. Studies on temporary threshold drift. *Int. Audiol.* (Leiden) 7, 267–279.

Suzuki, T., and Sato, I. 1961. Free field startle response audiometry; a quantitative method for determining hearing threshold of infant children. *Ann. Otol., Rhinol., Laryng.*, 70, 977–1007.

Vernon, M. 1967. Characteristics associated with postrubella deaf children: psychological, educational, and physical. *Volta Rev.*, 69, 176–185.

Wever, G. 1949. Theory of hearing. New York: Wiley.

Wilber, L., and Goodhill, V. 1969. Auditory rehabilitation aspects stapes surgery for otosclerosis. (Unpublished study.)

Wright, H. 1968. Clinical measurement of temporal auditory summation. *J. Speech Hearing Res.*, 11, 109–127.

Wullstein, H. 1956. Theory and practice of tympanoplasty. *Laryngoscope*, 66, 1076–1093.

13

Clinical Audiology

Hayes A. Newby

RESPONSIBILITIES OF THE CLINICAL AUDIOLOGIST

Audiology has been defined as "the science of hearing" (Davis, 1970, p. 3). This definition encompasses a wide range of professional interests, from microscopy of the cellular structure of normal ears to the teaching of language to a deaf child. The clinical audiologist is concerned with disorders of hearing, or, more properly, with individual children and adults who have disorders of hearing. He is found in various professional environments—hospitals, college and university speech and hearing clinics, rehabilitation centers, community hearing centers, Veterans Administration and other government health facilities—and some audiologists are in private practice with otologists or by themselves.

Wherever the clinical audiologist is found, his primary concerns are with 1. identification of individuals whose hearing is impaired; 2. measurement of the extent of the hearing impairment in terms of loss of sensitivity for pure tones and speech and measurement of the patient's ability to understand what he hears (diagnostic audiometry); 3. description of the patient's hearing behavior on special tests in an effort to specify the site of lesion within the auditory system; and 4. assessment of the patient's needs in learning to live with his impairment, and planning a program of aural rehabilitation.

In performing these tasks, the clinical audiologist works closely with the patient's medical advisers: most frequently with otologists, but also with neurologists, internists, pediatricians, psychiatrists, and specialists in industrial and preventive medicine. In order better to understand the disorders of hearing with which he deals, the clinical audiologist must have some background in such areas as acoustics, phonetics, linguistics, physiology, neurology, and psychoacoustics, to name only a representative sample. The focus of the audiologist's professional existence, however, is the patient, and all of his skill and knowledge are brought to bear on defining the patient's auditory problems and seeking solutions to them.

In this chapter we will discuss the first three responsibilities enumerated above: identification, diagnostic audiometry, and site of lesion specification. Silverman discusses aural rehabilitation of the deaf and the hard of hearing in Chapters 15 and 16.

IDENTIFICATION

The identification of individuals with hearing impairment is accomplished by screening programs in which the object is to separate out for more detailed study those individuals in a population who differ significantly from the norm. With school-age children and adults, screen testing is performed with a pure-tone audiometer. In the case of infants

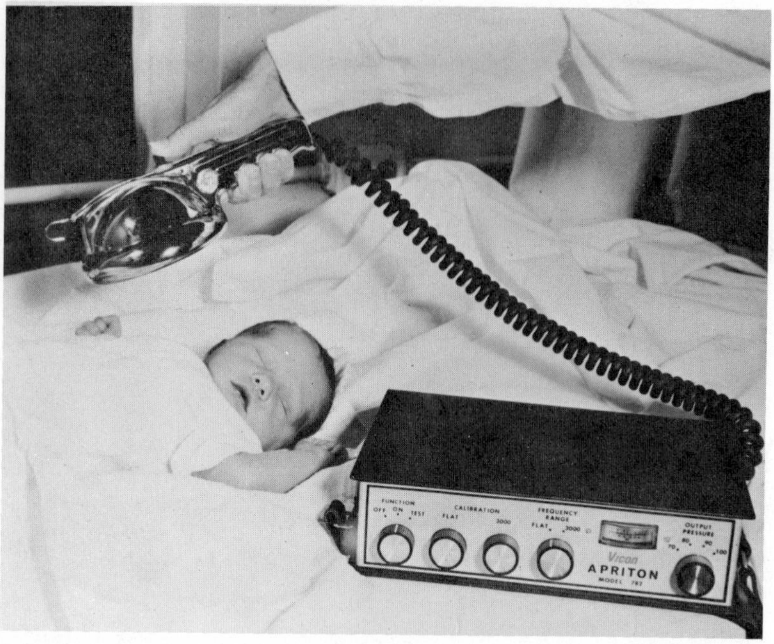

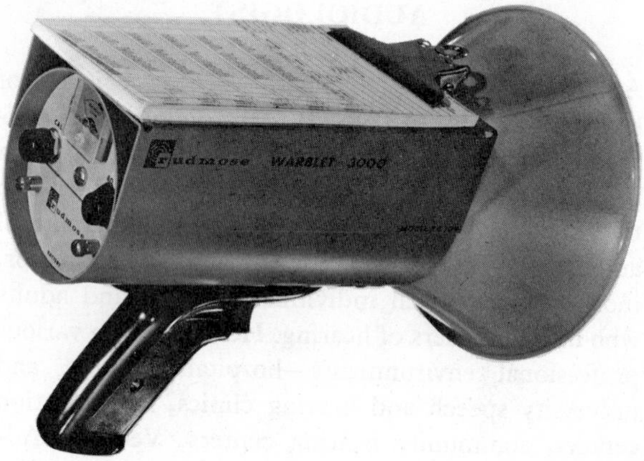

Fig. 13-1 The Vicon Apriton (*left*), manufactured by the Vicon Instrument Co., Colorado Springs, Colo., and the Rudmose Warblet (*below*), manufactured by Tracor, Inc., Austin, Tex.

and very young children, special equipment and procedures are employed.

Infant-Screening Programs

Downs (1967) has pioneered in screening newborn infants in the hospital nursery. The primary purpose of the screening program is to identify those infants who do not give observable responses to fairly intense, electronically generated auditory signals. There are available battery-powered signal generators designed for the screening of newborn infants, of which the Vicon Apriton and the Rudmose Ra-109 Warblet 3000, shown in Fig. 13-1, are representative. The Apriton generates two signals through a hand-held loudspeaker: a narrow band of filtered white noise with peak energy at 3,000 Hz, and a broad-band white noise. Either signal may be presented at sound-pressure levels of 70, 80, 90, or 100 dB measured at a distance of four inches from the speaker. The Rudmose Warblet generates a 3,000 Hz tone that warbles 150 Hz. The warbling tone may be presented at sound-pressure levels of 80, 90, or 100 dB measured at a distance of 10 inches from the speaker.

The frequency of 3,000 Hz was chosen for use in infant screening because generally an inability to respond to this frequency at any of the output levels available would point to the existence of a significant hearing impairment that may be present only for the higher frequencies. Since the typical congenital hearing impairment is sensorineural in origin, and since sensorineural impairments often are characterized by considerably better hearing sensitivity for low frequencies than for high, a screening frequency lower than 3,000 Hz may not succeed in identifying an infant whose hearing is impaired mainly for the high frequencies.

The test is administered by holding the loudspeaker at the prescribed distance from one ear of the infant and presenting a two-second burst of the 3,000 Hz signal. The recommended intensity setting is 90 dB sound-pressure level (Downs, 1967, p. 30). The infant is carefully observed before and during the presentation of the stimulus. Frequently two observers will be employed, especially if the screening is being performed by relatively inexperienced examiners. The observers must note on their charts what response, if any, was observed and the strength or intensity of the response. Typical responses of infants to the presentation of the auditory signal are eye blinking or widening, head turning either toward or away from the sound, sucking activity, movement of limbs or cessation of bodily movements, or perhaps a generalized startle reaction known as a Moro's reflex. Of course any "response" associated in time with the auditory stimulus must be evaluated in terms of observations of the infant's behavior immediately preceding the tonal stimulus. The strength or degree of positiveness of the response is rated on a five-point scale, with one representing no response and five indicating an unequivocal response. Generally the stimulus will be presented at least three times, with a suitable interval separating the trials, and the observers will describe and rate responses for each presentation. If the observers agree that the infant definitely responded to at least one presentation of the stimulus, he is considered to have passed the screening. If responses are absent or equivocal, the state of the infant's hearing is in doubt, and the screening procedure should be repeated at another time. If the infant still does not respond, a note should be made in his chart that he may have an auditory problem and arrangements should be made to have him examined more thoroughly at a later time by the audiologist and appropriate medical specialists.

It should be noted that as of the present writing there is some controversy regarding the usefulness and the validity of the routine testing of infants in the nursery. A joint committee of the American Academy of Ophthalmology and Otolaryngology, the American Academy of Pediatrics, and the American Speech and Hearing Association (1971) refused to recommend the mass screening of neonates pending the results of follow-up studies as to the efficacy of such screening. Goldstein and Tait (1971) urge that at present the emphasis be placed on evaluating only those newborn infants whose family history, or history of pregnancy and birth, suggests that they are in a high-risk category, so far as potential hearing impairment is concerned.

The Ewings (1958) and Hardy, Dougherty, and Hardy (1959) have described methods of screening infants by observing their responses to various stimuli such as whistles, rattles, bells, squeakers, and voiceless and voiced speech sounds. While the Ewings concentrated on screening infants of seven months of age and older, Hardy, Dougherty, and Hardy reported success with selected test items employed with infants as young as three weeks of age. The procedure described by these two sets of workers involves having the infant held in his mother's lap facing one of two examiners. While this examiner attracts the infant's visual attention by manipulating a doll or puppet, the other examiner introduces various acoustic signals behind the mother and child. The examiner in front observes the infant for any evidence of response to the acoustic signal. Younger infants may exhibit "eye responses," body movements, or cessations of activity, head turning toward the source of the sound, or in response to an intense stimulus a Moro's reflex. Older infants (six to eight months old) are not considered to be responding to the signal unless they turn toward the sound source. Since the examiner behind the mother's chair moves from one side to the other, always keeping out of the infant's peripheral vision, any differences in the infant's responses to right- or left-side stimulation can be noted as possible indications of differences between the ears in auditory sensitivity.

Failure of infants to respond either to the nursery screening or to the procedures by these two sets of authors does not necessarily mean that a hearing loss has been identified. It simply means that the infant should be studied more thoroughly to determine if in fact his auditory behavior is deviant from that of most infants of his age. Failure of the screening test may be indicative of a neurological problem, intellectual deficiency, or simply a developmental lag that is not significant of any abnormality, or it may, of course, represent an impairment of hearing due to dysfunction of the middle ear or the cochlea. On the other hand, it can be assumed that the infant who does respond definitely to the test stimuli does not have a profound impairment of his peripheral auditory mechanism.

School Screening Programs

School-age children, particularly in the early grades, are susceptible to upper respiratory ailments and are exposed to a variety of communicable diseases. Because the middle ear is connected with the nasopharynx by means of the Eustachian tube, it is common to have secondary involvement of the middle ear whenever the nasopharynx develops an infection. Thus otitis media is the most common cause of hearing impairment among school children. If otitis media is not discovered early and treated promptly, complications can develop that may lead to permanently impaired hearing. Of course children of school age may also have impaired hearing from other causes, such as congenital defects of the hearing mechanism, or permanent sensorineural losses as the result of the toxic effect of some of the childhood communicable diseases. Children with serious or profound impairments will be easily identifiable because of their obvious difficulties in communication. Those with mild or moderate losses may go undiscovered for years in the absence of any routine check of their hearing sensitivity. Obviously, the longer such children go undetected, the less likely it is they can be helped by medical or surgical treatment, and the more difficult becomes the task of helping them to compensate for their sensory deficiency. Fortunately, the schools have accepted the responsibility of searching out health conditions that may affect their pupils' ability to function in school at optimum efficiency. For some years now, most school systems have conducted regular surveys of their pupils' visual and hearing acuity.

Generally, from five to 10 percent of a school population will be found to have some degree of hearing loss. Many of these children will respond favorably to medical treatment, and some will recover their hearing spontaneously. About one percent of a school population will have permanent, irremediable hearing impairment of sufficient extent to be handicapping. Such children will benefit from special educational procedures such as those described by Silverman in Chapter 15.

Screening tests of hearing in the schools may be individual or group. By far the most common procedure is the individual sweep test performed with an audiometer. We shall confine our discussion of school testing to this procedure. What is required is a portable audiometer, a relatively quiet room in which to test, and an examiner who has been appropriately trained. Mobile testing units—sound-isolated vans or trailers—are ideal for use in school testing programs, because they provide a constant sound-controlled environment.

Since the purpose of a school screening program is to identify children whose hearing differs from "normal," we are interested in determining only whether or not a given child can hear various frequencies at a hearing level representing the limit of normal. If he can respond to each frequency at this level he "passes" the screening test. If he fails to respond to one or more of the test frequencies he "fails" the test, which means only that he is marked for further testing. Generally five frequencies are tested: 500, 1,000, 2,000, 4,000, and 6,000 Hz. If the testing must be performed in environments where background noise is present, the frequency of 500 Hz may be omitted, since noise masks lower frequencies. If many children fail a screening test only at 500 Hz, it is likely that the test environment is unsuited to testing that frequency and it should be eliminated from the screen test.

The recommendation of a group of experts convened at a national conference on identification audiometry in 1960 (Darley, 1961) was that screening levels of 10 dB relative to the ASA 1951 standard for audiometric zero be used for the frequencies of 500, 1,000, 2,000, and 6,000 Hz, and a screening level of 20 dB be used for 4,000 Hz. Since most audiometers today are calibrated to the ISO 1964 standard for audiometric zero (Davis and Kranz, 1964) these recommended screening levels would be translated into ISO-1964 hearing levels of 20 dB at 1,000, 2,000, and 6,000 Hz, and 25 dB at 500 and 4,000 Hz, rounding off the differences between the ASA-1951 and the ISO-1964 standards to the nearest five-dB step. Later in this chapter the calibration standards for pure-tone audiometers will be discussed in more detail.

In performing the pure-tone sweep test the examiner seats the child behind the audiometer so he cannot see the controls and instructs him to raise his index finger whenever he hears a tone, and to lower the finger when the tone disappears. The examiner then places the earphones on the child's head, making sure they are centered over his ears. The test is begun at 500 Hz, assuming the test environment is sufficiently quiet. The examiner first presents a brief spurt of tone at a hearing level of 30 dB, so that the child will have a clear impression of the test signal. Assuming the child responds appropriately, the examiner reduces the hearing level to 20 dB and presents the 500 Hz tone again. If the child raises his finger, the examiner immediately switches to 1,000 Hz without interrupting the signal. If the child hears the tone his finger should stay up. The examiner then interrupts the tone, and the child should lower his finger. The examiner switches to 2,000 Hz and again presents the tone, and the child should raise his finger. Leaving the signal on, the examiner switches to 4,000 Hz, and the child should continue to keep his finger raised. The examiner then interrupts the tone, at which point the child should lower his finger. Switching to 6,000 Hz, the examiner presents the tone, and the child should raise his finger again. Leaving the signal on, the examiner switches the output to the opposite earphone, so the child should now hear 6,000 Hz in his other ear, keeping his finger raised. The examiner interrupts the tone and switches to 4,000 Hz, and the child, of course, should lower his finger. The examiner presents the 4,000 Hz tone, and the child should respond by raising his finger. Without interrupting the tone the examiner switches to 2,000 Hz. If the child continues to keep his finger raised, the examiner cuts off the signal and switches to 1,000 Hz, and the child lowers his finger. Again the examiner presents the tone and the child raises his finger. Without interrupting the signal the examiner switches to 500 Hz. If the child's finger remains raised, the examiner then cuts off the tone. The child lowers his finger and the test has been completed. The child has demonstrated by responding correctly to "tone-on" and "tone-off" conditions that he has heard each test frequency in each ear at a hearing level of 20 dB (re ISO-1964).

Since the recommended screening level at 500 and 4,000 Hz is 25 dB, the examiner will alter the procedure described above and increase the hearing level to 25 dB if the child does not respond correctly to the 20 dB signal at either 500 or 4,000 Hz. But if he responds to all frequencies at the 20 dB level there is no need to take the extra time to change the hearing-level dial settings when changing frequencies. The entire procedure described above should require no more than two minutes to complete. Should a child not respond correctly to the presentation or interruption of the tone at any frequency in either ear (20 dB at 1,000, 2,000, and 6,000 Hz, and if necessary 25 dB at 500 and 4,000 Hz), he is marked for additional testing. No attempt is made at the time of the screening test to determine the threshold hearing levels of a child who fails. Rather, the children who fail the screening test are scheduled for retesting at some later time—preferably on the same day that they were screened. Assuming that the testing program has been planned to keep a steady flow of children proceeding to the test room or mobile test unit, an examiner should have no difficulty in screening from 20 to 30 children an hour.

While ideally every child in a school system should receive a hearing screening test each year, practically it usually is not possible to achieve the ideal. An acceptable compromise is to screen all kindergarteners, first-graders, third-graders, sixth-graders, and tenth-graders every year, plus all new pupils in a school system regardless of their grade. In addition, annual tests should be scheduled for any child who in previous years has been discovered to have a hearing impairment. Any child suspected by his teacher or parents of having a hearing problem should be tested, also, regardless of his grade.

The identification of children who may have hearing impairments is only the first step in a school hearing-conservation program. Those failing the screening procedure must be retested in order to specify their threshold hearing levels at each frequency. In the retesting procedure, some children will demonstrate that their hearing is actually within the acceptable range of normal. They may have failed the screening test because they misunderstood instructions, their attention fluctuated, or for some reason they failed to cooperate with the examiner. Children who on retesting do demonstrate that their hearing is outside the range of normal should have medical and educational follow-up procedures, since the purpose of identifying hearing-impaired children is to provide them with whatever assistance they may need.

While follow-up tests to define a child's threshold hearing levels and to help the otologist arrive at a diagnosis of a hearing impairment should be administered by audiologists, screening tests may be, and often are, given by individuals with a minimum of audiological training. Volunteers may be recruited from the P.T.A. or from various women's service organizations or sorority alumnae groups who are willing to donate several hours a week to screening hearing. Of course any school identification audiometry program dependent on relatively untrained examiners should be supervised by a qualified audiologist, who should also be responsible for training the volunteers and keeping check on the calibration of the equipment. Volunteers are also being utilized successfully in screening infants and preschool children (Downs, 1967; Engh, 1968).

Adult Screening Programs

For the most part adult-hearing-screening programs are found in two contexts: the military induction centers, and industries—or military bases—where noise may be hazardous to the hearing. The purpose of screening in induction centers is to determine if an inductee—or volunteer, for that matter—has a hearing impairment that would disqualify him for military service. Because employers are held financially responsible for noise-induced hearing impairment incurred on the job, they are naturally interested to know of any preexisting hearing loss in the case of a new employee and are concerned with keeping tabs on all their employees who work in noisy locations.

Because of the possible need for proving in court or in a compensation board hearing that an employee had some degree of impaired hearing when he started work, an employer will require a preplacement hearing test, which really is a threshold test instead of a screening procedure. This preplacement audiogram will serve as a reference with which to compare future audiograms in order to determine whether any impairment has occurred since the employee started work.

Once reference audiograms are on file for all employees who work in noisy environments, the employer need only run screening tests periodically to identify individuals whose hearing has shifted outside the range of normal since the last screening test. Employees whose reference audiograms indicated an existing hearing impairment at the time of employment would require more complete periodic reassessment, however, since obviously they would fail a screening test.

Noise-induced hearing impairment is a sensorineural loss of cochlear origin, characterized by a sloping audiogram, i.e., an audiogram that indicates greater losses for the higher frequencies. Usually a noise-induced hearing impairment will manifest itself first by a dip or notch at 4,000 Hz. With increasing exposure to the noxious noise this notch will deepen and widen, but initially the appearance of a slight 4,000 Hz notch in an employee's audiogram will alert an examiner to the fact that the employee is beginning to suffer some noise-induced impairment. Glorig and House (1957) have demonstrated that if an employee's hearing is within normal limits at 4,000 Hz, his hearing at lower frequencies will be normal also. Based on this knowledge, Glorig and House suggested that in monitoring an employee's hearing following a reference audiogram that demonstrated normal hearing, it was sufficient to give him periodic screening tests at only the frequency of 4,000 Hz. They went a step further and suggested that screening tests of school children could also be confined to 4,000 Hz, or to the two frequencies of 4,000 and 2,000 Hz. This latter suggestion stimulated considerable argument among audiologists and resulted in a number of studies of school children that purported to disprove the Glorig and House thesis. At the present writing the adequacy of limited-frequency screen testing in the schools is unresolved, and it is still standard practice to screen school children at four or five frequencies.

In some communities attempts are being made to conduct widespread screening tests of the hearing of adults on a voluntary basis. An individual who fails the screening test is advised to consult his physician, who may refer the patient to an audiology clinic for more definitive testing. It is likely that at some future date screen testing—or even complete audiograms obtained with automatic audiometers—will be as available to the public as chest X-rays and diabetes tests are today. All that is required is an increased awareness on the part of public health officials and the public at large of the prevalence of hearing impairment in the adult population, and an adequate means of financing hearing screening programs.

DIAGNOSTIC AUDIOMETRY

In contrast to screening audiometry, which has as its purpose simply the separation of those with normal hearing from those whose hearing is outside the limit of normal, diagnostic audiometry has as its purpose the measurement of threshold hearing levels and the determination of the category of hearing impairment: conductive, sensorineural, or mixed. Of course the measurement of hearing impairment is but part of the diagnostic process. The patient's history and physical examination findings constitute other important aspects of diagnosis. It is important to note that the physician makes a diagnosis. The audiologist furnishes part of the information on which the physician bases his diagnosis—frequently the most important part—but only the licensed medical practitioner is legally authorized to diagnose physical ailments.

The determination of category of hearing impairment is based primarily on the comparison of a patient's hearing sensitivity for pure tones by air conduction (through earphones) and by bone conduction (through a vibrator placed on the mastoid bone or on the forehead). If a patient hears normally by bone conduction but demonstrates hearing loss by air conduction, he has a "pure" conductive impairment. His problem is in the conduction of sound energy through the outer or middle ear to the end organ of hearing, the cochlea. An audiological finding

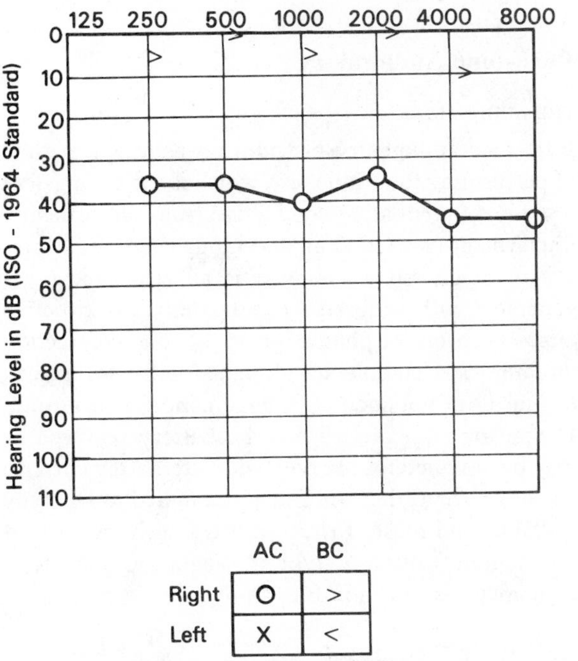

Fig. 13-2. Pure conductive impairment. Results shown for right ear only.

that thresholds by bone conduction are elevated to the same hearing levels as thresholds by air-conduction points to the presence of a "pure" sensorineural impairment, i.e., an involvement of the cochlea or VIIIth Cranial nerve. A mixed impairment occurs when there is some loss by bone conduction but a more extensive loss by air conduction. Typical examples of audiograms indicative of conductive, sensorineural, and mixed impairments are shown in Figs. 13-2, 13-3, 13-4, and 13-5. As can be noted from Figs. 13-4 and 13-5, there are two audiometric patterns that may represent mixed impairment: 1) some losses at all frequencies by bone conduction, but greater losses by air conduction, as shown in Fig. 13-4; and 2) an air-bone gap occurring at lower frequencies but equal losses by air and by bone at higher frequencies, as in Fig. 13-5. The latter pattern is the more typical one.

While pure-tone audiometry yields the information necessary to categorize a hearing impairment, speech audiometry provides valuable information concerning how the patient's hearing for speech is affected. Assumptions as to how the patient hears speech can be made from the pure-tone audiogram, but with speech audiometry the audiologist can obtain direct measures of threshold elevation for speech, and impairment of discrimination for speech sounds. In terms of planning for a patient's rehabilitation, e.g., determining whether or not a hearing aid would be helpful, speech audiometry is superior to pure-tone measurements.

On occasion the audiologist will need to go beyond the usual audiometric procedures that depend on the patient's signaling the examiner or responding in some appropriate way when he hears the test stimulus.

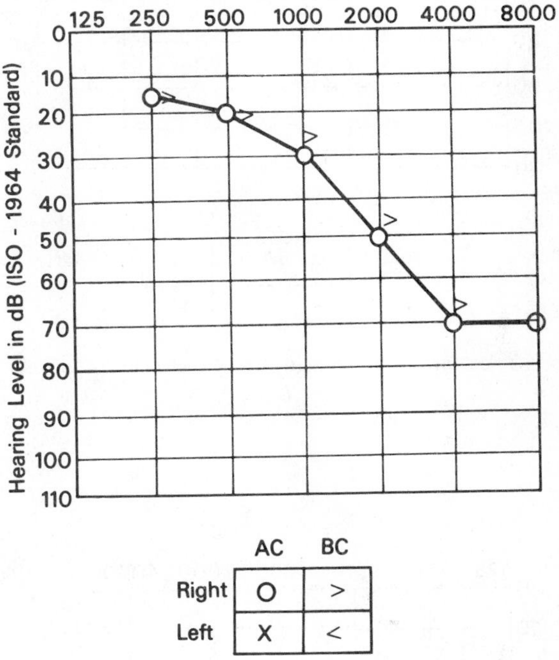

Fig. 13-3. Pure sensorineural impairment. Results shown for right ear only.

While they will not be discussed in this chapter, mention should at least be made of two special diagnostic procedures that are relatively independent of the patient's voluntary responses. Electrodermal or psychogalvanic skin response audiometry is employed in cases of suspected functional or nonorganic hearing problems, or sometimes with very young children who cannot be successfully tested with standard procedures. Electroencephalography, or more properly electroencephalic audiometry, is used primarily with children—again those children who present special problems in testing. Both of these electrophysiologic precedures have been referred to as "objective" methods of hearing testing, because neither requires a voluntary response from the patient.

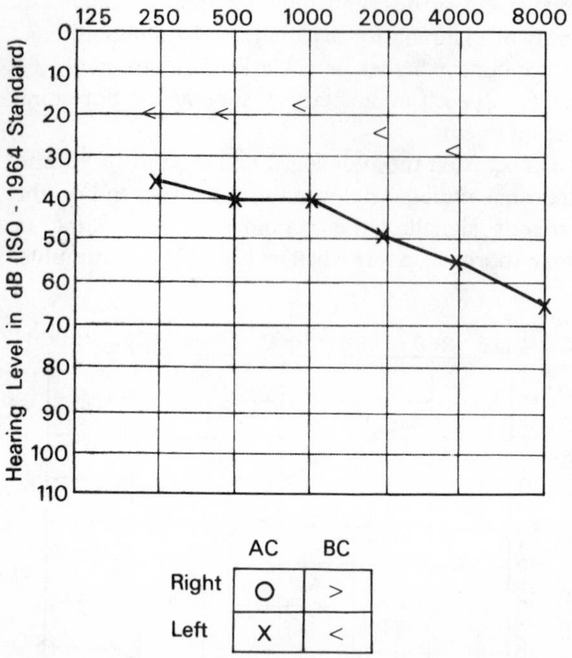

Fig. 13-4. Mixed impairment. Results shown for left ear only.

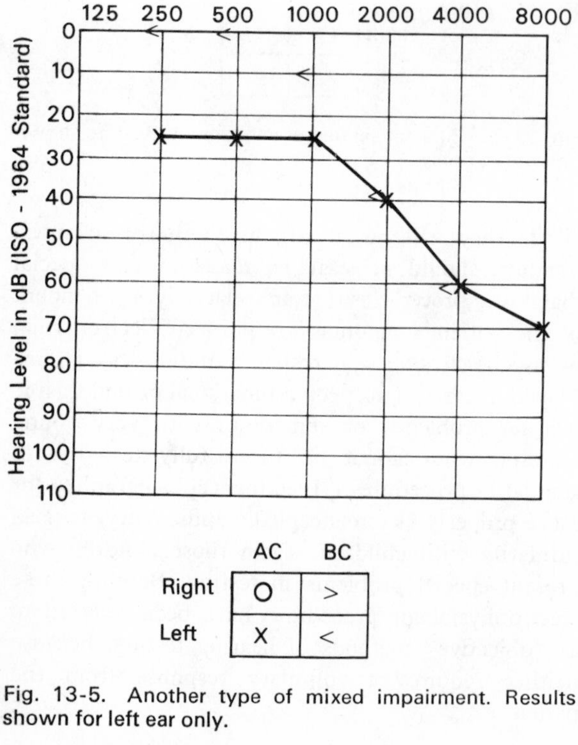

Fig. 13-5. Another type of mixed impairment. Results shown for left ear only.

Pure-tone Audiometry

THE AUDIOMETER

Pure-tone audiometry provides a quantified method of performing the Rinne test, which is the tuning-fork test for differentiating conductive from sensorineural impairment (see Goodhill and Guggenheim, Chapter 12). A diagnostic audiometer is an electronic tone-generator with calibrated output delivered either to air-conduction earphones or to a bone-conduction vibrator. An audiometer designed only for screen testing does not include a bone-conduction output. Diagnostic audiometers may be battery powered or may be designed for use only with alternating current. In either event, they are usually designed to be easily portable, and most of them utilize transistors instead of vacuum tubes. A typical diagnostic pure-tone audiometer is shown in Fig. 13-6.

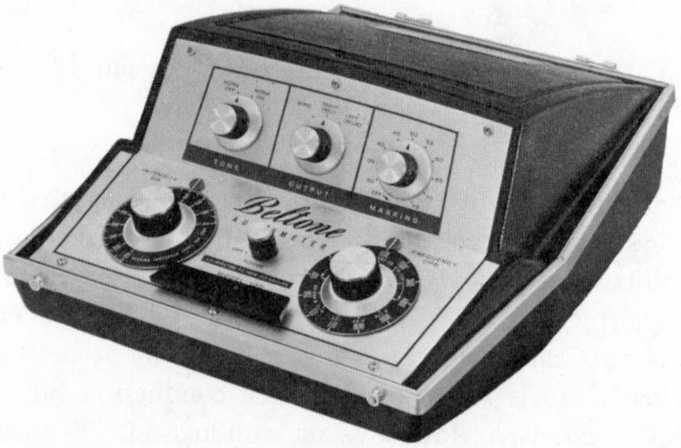

Fig. 13-6. Pure-tone audiometer manufactured by Beltone Electronics Corp., Chicago, Ill.

The frequency selector enables the examiner to choose any of the available frequencies from 125 to 8,000 Hz. Usually testing is performed only at octave intervals, but on occasion it is also useful to test at some of the frequencies midway between the octave limits. The output selector determines whether the acoustic stimulus is directed to the red phone (right ear), the blue phone (left ear), or the bone-conduction vibrator. The intensity of the signal is controlled by the hearing-level control, which on most audiometers is calibrated in five-dB steps over a range of 110 dB. Even where the hearing-level control provides for steps smaller than five dB (as is the case with the instrument in Fig. 13-6), in clinical audiometry threshold hearing levels are measured only to the nearest five-dB step.

CALIBRATION

Earlier in this chapter reference was made to calibration standards for audiometric zero. The so-called American standard—designated ASA-1951, because in that year the American Standards Association (1951) published the sound-pressure level values audiometer manufacturers were to observe for zero-dB hearing level—was based on a widespread national hearing survey conducted in the 1930's. Subsequently it developed that the American standard underestimated hearing levels, especially when compared to standards in effect in various European countries.

TABLE 13-I
Sound-pressure levels in dB re 0.0002 dyne/cm² for audiometric zero (rounded to the nearest one-half dB) according to the ASA-1951 and the ISO-1964 standards

FREQUENCY	ASA-1951	ISO-1964	DIFFERENCE
125 Hz	54.5 dB	45.5 dB	9.0 dB
250	39.5	24.5	15.0
500	25.0	11.0	14.0
1,000	16.5	6.5	10.0
1,500		6.5	
2,000	17.0	8.5	8.5
3,000		7.5	
4,000	15.0	9.0	6.0
6,000		8.0	
8,000	21.0	9.5	11.5

Audiometric zero should represent the average level of normal ears—defined as the average sensitivity of hearing of young adults. When tested with audiometers calibrated to the American standard under conditions of adequate isolation from outside noise, the average hearing levels of young adults was found to be closer to −10 dB than to zero dB. After years of collecting data and exchanging information, the International Standards Organization, composed of representatives from many countries including the United States, recommended a standard for audiometric zero to be used throughout the world. This was termed the ISO-1964 standard, since it was in that year that the international agreement was reached (Davis and Kranz, 1964). The ISO-1964 standard was endorsed by many U.S. scientific and professional societies, and today most audiometric results are expressed in terms of this ISO standard. We are still in a state of transition between standards, however, and it is advisable to indicate on an audiogram which standard was used in obtaining those particular results. Table 13-I compares the two standards.*

The calibration of an audiometer should be checked periodically with an artificial ear, consisting of a sound-level meter and a coupler to which an audiometer earphone is attached. Should the check indicate that output levels in either phone are not accurate to the nearest five-dB step, the audiometer should be recalibrated by a qualified service representative of the manufacturer. Until recalibration is accomplished, a correction chart should be posted on the audiometer indicating what corrections it is necessary to make to obtained hearing-level readings before recording threshold levels on audiograms (Newby, 1964, pp. 87–88). Before giving a test, an examiner should listen to tones through each earphone to assure himself that the equipment is functioning properly, and that the indicated hearing levels are approximately correct.

Other important parts of every audiometer are the interrupter switch, by means of which the examiner is able to present or interrupt a signal immediately and silently, and the masking switch and intensity control, for use when there is danger that one ear may participate in threshold measurements on the other.

AIR-CONDUCTION TESTING

The first step in diagnostic pure-tone audiometry is to obtain threshold hearing levels for each frequency in each ear by air conduction. Threshold is defined as the lowest hearing level to which the patient responds appropriately at least 50 percent of the time. The patient is instructed to signal when he first becomes aware of the presence of a tonal stimulus, and also when he realizes that the stimulus has been discontinued. The most common form of patient signal is to raise a finger to indicate awareness of the tone, and to lower the finger to signify absence of the tone.

If the patient reports any difference in sensitivity

* Since this chapter was written, the American National Standards Institute (ANSI), the present name for what was formerly the American Standards Association (ASA) and for a brief time the United States of America Standards Institute (USASI), has published (1970) "Specifications for Audiometers," ANSI S3.6-1969, incorporating the sound-pressure levels for audiometric zero recommended in the ISO-1964 standard. ANSI S3.6-1969, effective September 1, 1970, replaces the ASA standards Z24.5-1951 and Z.24.13-1953, both of which references appear in the bibliography at the end of this chapter.

between his ears, it is best to test his better ear first. If the examiner is in the test room with the patient, the patient should be seated so that he cannot view the controls of the audiometer, and the examiner must take care that he does not alert the patient to tonal presentation or interruption by visible movements of his arms or hands, or by shifting his eyes toward and away from the audiometer controls in sychronism with the presentation and interruption of the stimulus. Some audiologists prefer to have the patient sit with his back toward the examiner and the audiometer. There is an advantage, however, for the examiner to be able to view the patient's face during the test, as the patient's facial expressions frequently give valuable clues as to whether or not he is hearing the auditory stimulus.

Some audiologists prefer to start a test with the frequency 1,000 Hz, since this frequency has the highest test-retest reliability, and a repeated threshold measurement at 1,000 Hz can serve as an index of the reliability of the entire test. The interrupter switch should be set to produce a tone when depressed and to interrupt the tone when released. Initially at each frequency the threshold can be located approximately by presenting a steady tone and, starting at zero-dB hearing level, increasing the intensity gradually until the patient signals he hears the tone. The tone should be increased to a level 10 to 15 dB higher in intensity to give the patient a clearly audible sample of the test stimulus. Then immediately the examiner should start a gradual decrease in intensity until the patient signals the tone has disappeared. The examiner now knows approximately the patient's threshold hearing level.

At this point the examiner will release the interrupter and from now until the threshold has been determined will present spurts of tone from one to two seconds in duration. The preferred method of determining threshold is to proceed from inaudibility to audibility, that is, from below threshold to above threshold (Carhart and Jerger, 1959). So, after the rough determination of threshold described above, the examiner will present a spurt of tone at the hearing level where he stopped his gradual decrease in intensity. If the patient does not respond, the examiner should increase the hearing level by 10 dB and present a spurt of tone again. He should continue increasing the hearing level by 10 dB until the patient signals he hears the tone. At that point, he should decrease the level by 10 dB and again present the stimulus. If there is no response he should increase the level five dB and present another spurt, continuing in this fashion until he obtains a response. Whenever a response is obtained the examiner should reduce the intensity by 10 dB and then increase in five-dB steps until the patient responds again. The lowest hearing level at which the patient responds consistently to the presence and the absence of the tone will be recorded as his threshold.

Should the patient become confused as to whether or not he hears the tone, it may necessary to increase the tone to a suprathreshold level so that he again has a clear notion of what he is listening for. The examiner should not tire the patient by prolonged attempts to define threshold, which usually occur because the examiner is loath to make a decision as to which of two possible levels is the patient's threshold. In any case of doubt, the examiner should choose the higher (more intense) hearing level, where presumably the patient's response accuracy is well above the 50 percent criterion. The examiner should also vary the length of his tonal spurts and the intervals between spurts, lest the patient respond to his rhythm pattern instead of to the presence or absence of the tone.

Once threshold has been determined for 1,000 Hz, the examiner should shift to another frequency and establish threshold in the same manner. Some audiologists prefer to test lower frequencies next and some higher frequencies. Since a hearing-impaired individual is more likely to respond better to lower frequencies than to higher frequencies because of the preponderance of sloping audiogram patterns, there may be an advantage to testing 500 and then 250 Hz after the initial threshold measurement at 1,000 Hz. In any event, the examiner should return to 1,000 Hz for a second threshold determination before completing the test of the better ear. If the second threshold hearing level at 1,000 Hz agrees within $\pm$ five dB with the first, the examiner can be assured that the test has adequate reliability. On the other hand, if the two tests at 1,000 Hz disagree by 10 dB or more, he should probably start the whole test again—including instructions to the patient—because his test thus far has questionable reliability.

Rarely would threshold be measured at 125 Hz, since there is a high correlation between thresholds at 250 and 125 Hz, and thus the inclusion of 125 Hz adds no useful information. Many audiologists terminate a test at 6,000 Hz instead of including 8,000 Hz, but this is a matter of personal preference. It is true, though, that for several reasons 8,000 Hz tends to be the frequency with greatest variability, and for practical purposes a threshold measurement at 6,000 Hz should suffice as an indication of a patient's hearing for high frequencies. If there should be marked differences in threshold hearing levels at octave intervals, it may be useful to test at the midoctave frequencies. Thus the examiner can observe, for example, whether a slope begins at 1,000 Hz or at 1,500 Hz.

When the patient's first ear has been tested completely the examiner switches the output to the other ear and proceeds to determine thresholds on it. Again it is advisable to begin testing at 1,000 Hz. Should the threshold at any frequency differ by 40 dB or more from the threshold of the better ear, the examiner should be aware of the possibility that he is obtaining a "shadow curve" of the better ear, i.e., that he is actually measuring the hearing of the better ear from the opposite side of the head. The poorer ear's sensitivity may be so decreased that the better ear responds before the signal strength reaches the point that the poorer ear can hear it. Such a "crossover" of the signal occurs in air-conduction testing when the difference in sensitivity between the ears is about 60 dB, and it may occur at somewhat lesser difference. So whenever the examiner notes a difference of at least 40 dB between the ears, he should repeat the test of the poorer ear while introducing a masking noise to the better ear. The masking noise "occupies" the better ear so it cannot participate in the test of the poorer one. For the sake of the record, both unmasked and masked thresholds should be recorded on the audiogram.

Studebaker (1964) suggests that, since a stimulus presented to the test ear presumably reaches the other ear by passing through the bones of the head, masking should be employed whenever the air-conduction threshold of the ear under test exceeds the bone-conduction threshold of the opposite ear by 40 dB. In other words, Studebaker maintains that it is not the difference between air-conduction thresholds of the two ears that is important in determining the need for masking, but the difference between the air-conduction sensitivity of the test ear and the bone-conduction sensitivity of the opposite ear. It may not be possible, then, to determine the need for masking in air-conduction testing until the bone-conduction test has been accomplished.

Most audiometers are equipped with broad-band masking noises. Some are "complex" noises (low-frequency dominated) and some are "white" noises (equal intensity at all frequencies). An attenuator enables the examiner to vary the intensity of the masking noise over a wide range. In air-conduction testing there is practically no danger of making the masking noise so intense that it will interfere through crossover with the measurement of thresholds in the poorer ear, since the "interaural attenuation" of 40 to 60 dB operates for a masking noise as well as for a pure tone. The limitation as to level of masking noise is the patient's comfort. Narrow-band maskers are available as accessory items with some audiometers. These are desirable because an equivalent degree of masking can be achieved with a narrow band centered on the frequency to be masked as with a broad band, and at a lower intensity, thus protecting the patient from discomfort.

BONE-CONDUCTION TESTING

Following the completion of the air-conduction test, the patient should be tested by bone conduction, assuming that the air-conduction results have demonstrated some hearing impairment. Of course there is no need to test by bone if the patient's hearing is normal by air, since obviously in such a case the bone conduction would have to be normal also. Bone-conduction testing evaluates cochlear and VIIIth Cranial nerve function independently of the outer and the middle ear. Since the primary purpose of diagnostic pure-tone audiometry is to categorize an impairment as conductive, sensorineural, or mixed, it is necessary to determine whether or not there are differences in threshold hearing levels as measured by air conduction and by bone conduction. When differences occur, it is said that an air-bone gap exists.

Bone-conduction testing is accomplished by introducing the test tone to a vibrator that is placed usually on the patient's mastoid bone, just behind the pinna, but sometimes on the patient's forehead. The vibrator causes the whole skull to vibrate, producing fluid movement in the cochlea and thus hair-cell stimulation. Regardless of the placement of the vibrator on the head it is virtually impossible to produce fluid movement in only one cochlea, although for certain frequencies mastoid placement results in slightly more intense cochlear stimulation on the side the vibrator is placed. Thus for practical purposes, there is almost zero-dB interaural attenuation for bone conduction. Accordingly, most audiologists believe it is necessary to utilize masking routinely in bone-conduction testing, at least as a check on the validity of thresholds obtained with no masking. The comparison of unmasked and masked bone-conduction hearing levels can often yield important diagnostic information.

Since there is almost no interaural attenuation for bone conduction, there are instances in which it is necessary to test only one ear by bone in order to arrive at a diagnosis. If the unmasked bone-conduction thresholds of one ear agree with the air-conduction thresholds previously obtained on both ears, it is evident that the patient has a bilateral sensorineural impairment. No additional information would be gleaned from testing the other ear by bone conduction, since in the absence of masking the bone-conduction sensitivity of the two ears cannot disagree by more than a few dB. It is obvious, therefore, that both cochleas of the patient are affected.

On the other hand, if an unmasked bone-conduction test of one ear reveals a substantial air-bone gap, it will be necessary to test both ears by bone, using masking of the contralateral ear. In such an instance, the examiner knows only that at least one ear has an air-bone gap. Without masking he cannot be sure which ear has the air-bone gap, or whether both ears might.

The masking noise is introduced through one ot the air-conduction earphones, which, of course, must be placed over the ear to be masked. The ear under test is left unoccluded. Occluding an ear, as by covering it with an earphone, may alter its bone-conduction sensitivity. Even the use of an earphone for masking purposes may cause lateralization of a bone-conducted signal to the covered ear, thus complicating the problem of measurement of the bone-conduction thresholds in the test ear.

The selection of the level of masking to use in bone-conduction testing is critical. Too little masking may not eliminate the participation of the contralateral ear, while too much masking may interfere with the bone-conduction sensitivity of the ear under test. It is probably best to experiment with various masking levels, noting how threshold hearing levels in the test ear are affected by shifts of masking level in the contralateral ear. In the first place, the masking noise must be sufficiently intense to be heard easily before any masking effect occurs. As the level of the masking noise is increased in the contralateral ear, there will come a point at which the threshold in the test ear will shift in proportion to increases in level of the masking noise. When such threshold shifts occur, the question is whether they represent a movement toward the actual thresholds of the test ear, or simply reflect the crossover of the masking noise to the ear under test, i.e., whether they demonstrate the effect of overmasking of the contralateral ear. To determine the answer to this question, it is necessary to continue increasing the level of the masking noise. If a point is reached where the threshold of the test ear remains stable over a range of from 10 to 20 dB in masking level, the examiner can assume that he has now arrived at the actual bone-conduction threshold of the test ear. If, however, the threshold of the test ear continues to shift five dB with every five-dB increase in masking-noise level, then either the hearing level at the point just before the shifts first occurred is the actual threshold of the test ear, or the true threshold lies beyond the limit of the bone-conduction circuit of the audiometer and thus cannot be determined.

Threshold measurement by bone conduction is conducted in the same manner as by air conduction, i.e., using an ascending technique. Because of the limitations of the vibrator, bone-conduction measurements are usually confined to from 250 through 4,000 Hz, and the maximum hearing levels that can be determined range from 50 to 80 dB, depending on the frequency and on the particular audiometer.

To avoid the problems of masking and cross-hearing that occur in bone-conduction testing, a radically different approach has been devised. Rainville (1959) first described the new approach, while Jerger and Tillman (1960) described their modification of the Rainville method which they called SAL, for "sensorineural acuity level." The SAL test revolutionized bone-conduction testing by introducing the masking noise instead of the test signal to the vibrator. The method involves comparing a patient's air-conduction hearing levels in each ear, 1. without masking and 2. with a masking noise of constant intensity applied through the vibrator placed on the patient's forehead. Jerger and Tillman reported that threshold shifts of about 50 dB were produced in normal ears at the frequencies of 1,000, 2,000, and 4,000 Hz by a masking noise that measured 2 volts across the terminals of the vibrator. They found similar shifts in ears with pure conductive impairments, but little or no shift in ears with pure sensorineural losses. The difference between the shift obtained with a normal-hearing subject and that obtained with a patient represents the patient's "sensorineural acuity level," i.e., his bone-conduction threshold hearing level.

Because both ears are occluded during the SAL test, the bone-conduction thresholds determined by that technique may disagree somewhat with those measured by the traditional method of testing. SAL will probably not replace the traditional method, but it is a useful tool for checking on results in cases where crossover and overmasking make bone-conduction testing particularly difficult (Tillman, 1967).

THE AUDIOGRAM

Pure-tone test results are recorded on a form called an audiogram. On an audiogram, air-conduction and bone-conduction thresholds are graphed by frequency and hearing level. Air-conduction thresholds are recorded as O for the right ear and X for the left. When masking was used on the contralateral ear the right-ear thresholds are graphed as △ and the left-ear thresholds as □. The right ear is always graphed in red and the left ear in blue or black for quick differentiation, but when audiograms are reproduced in books or articles the difference in symbols enables the reader to distinguish the right from the left ear, even in black and white.

Unfortunately there is not agreement among audiologists and otologists as to the symbols to use for bone-conduction thresholds. Some prefer arrowheads pointing to the right for the right ear and to the left for the left ear. Others use brackets, but the bracket-users cannot agree among themselves as to which bracket represents which ear. On the logic that the brackets symbolize a patient's pinnas as he faces an examiner, some use [for right ear and] for the left. Unfortunately this logic breaks down if the patient is seated with his back to the examiner! Other examiners reverse the brackets so that [stands for the left ear and] for the right. There is disagreement also as to how to record bone-conduction thresholds when the contralateral ear is masked. Of course if the colors red and blue are used, the ears can be differentiated regardless of the symbols employed. In black and white, however, the reader can easily be confused unless a key to the symbols used is included with every audiogram.

As stated earlier, distinctions among conductive, sensorineural, and mixed impairments are based on comparisons of a patient's air-conduction and bone-conduction threshold hearing levels. While there are characteristic patterns of air-conduction audiogram curves for conductive and sensorineural losses, there are sufficient exceptions that one cannot depend on the air-conduction curve alone in making diagnostic judgments.

For medicolegal purposes it is necessary to translate an audiogram into percentage of disability. The most commonly used procedure for computing percentage of hearing impairment is the AAOO method, so-called because it has the endorsement of the American Academy of Ophthalmology and Otolaryngology (1959). In this method the first step is to average the dB threshold hearing levels for air conduction at 500, 1,000, and 2,000 Hz. These are known as the "speech frequencies," because the average of the threshold hearing levels at these three frequencies usually agrees closely with the speech-reception threshold as measured with a speech audiometer.

The next step is to subtract 26 dB from the average of the hearing levels through the speech frequencies in each ear (assuming measurements are made with an audiometer calibrated to the ISO-1964 standard). The reason for the subtraction is that the limit of normal hearing, so far as compensation is concerned, is considered to be an average loss for speech of 26 dB. In medicolegal parlance this 26 dB is referred to as the "low fence," i.e., the point at which disability begins. The difference between the average dB hearing level through the speech frequencies and the low fence is then multiplied by one and one-half percent, yielding a percentage hearing impairment for each ear.

Finally, it is necessary to combine the percentage of impairment in each ear to arrive at a binaural percentage of impairment—a single percentage that expresses a patient's hearing disability. Based on the assumption that an individual with one good ear is not seriously disabled regardless of the extent of loss in his poor ear, the AAOO method specifies that the

	250	500	1000	2000	4000	6000
Right	25	30	40	50	70	70
Left	50	55	55	65	80	NR

	RIGHT	LEFT
500	30 dB	55 dB
1000	40	55
2000	50	65
	3) 120	3) 175
average	40 dB	58 dB (rounded)
	− 26 (low fence)	− 26 (low fence)
net average	14 dB	32 dB
	X1½%	X1½%
percentage monaural	21%	48%
weighting factor	X5	
	105%	
poorer ear	48%	
	6) 153%	
percentage binaural	26% (rounded)	

Fig. 13-7. Computation of percentage impairment by the AAOO method.

better ear should be weighted five times the poorer ear in computing binaural percentage of impairment. The percentage of impairment in the better ear is thus multiplied by five. This product is then added to the percentage of impairment in the poorer ear. Since six parts have gone into this sum (five for the better ear and one for the poorer ear), it is now divided by six. The quotient is the binaural percentage of hearing impairment. Fig. 13-7 illustrates the method of computing percentage of hearing impairment.

As can be seen by the way in which the air-conduction thresholds are presented in Fig. 13-7, it is not essential to prepare audiograms in graphic form. If the tabular form is used, computations such as percentage hearing loss and air-bone gap are facilitated. When graphs are used, some audiologists prefer to have two audiograms mounted side by side, one for each ear. This procedure eliminates the problem of cluttering that can result when a number of curves are graphed on a single audiogram.

Testing Children

Modifications of audiometric technique are necessary when testing very young children. With patience and ingenuity, an audiologist should be able to obtain at least air-conduction threshold hearing levels on children as young as two to two and one-half years of age. In most cases it will be necessary to schedule the child for more than one appointment. The audiologist must, of course, win the child's confidence and gain his cooperation before he can measure his hearing sensitivity with any degree of precision. Getting the child to accept earphones may be a major battle. It is helpful to have a test assistant available, since there are occasions when the examiner may want to introduce test signals from outside the test room. In such cases, the assistant can be with the child in the test room, keeping him involved in the test procedure and serving as a second observer to evaluate responses. Pure-tone evaluation of a child usually follows some preliminary testing performed with the speech audiometer, about which more will be said later.

In determining a child's pure-tone threshold hearing levels, the examiner must teach the child to attend to signals of weak intensity and to respond positively when he hears the signal. The situation calls for making a game of the test in which the child will be motivated to do his best.

The examiner should have available a number of toys including a set of square blocks and a plastic bucket, and a "Christmas tree" consisting of a peg on which are fitted concentric circular blocks of different sizes. Using one of these toys, say the square blocks and bucket, the examiner teaches the child to drop a block in the bucket when he hears a spurt of tone. It is helpful to teach the child to respond first to tactile stimuli and then make the transfer to acoustic signals. The bone-conduction vibrator is placed in the child's hand, and the audiometer is set at 250 Hz with the output directed to the vibrator at maximum hearing level for that frequency. The examiner places his hand over the child's and then demonstrates that when a vibration is felt in the bone-conduction vibrator a block is dropped in the bucket. For the first few trials the examiner performs the desired response himself. Then he assists the the child to make the response, making sure that the child understands he is not to drop the block until the tactile stimulus is presented. Most children will catch on to this "game" quickly and respond appropriately by holding a block in readiness, and then dropping it in the bucket "on cue." Of course the examiner praises the child when he makes the correct response.

The examiner then puts the earphones on the child. It is usually desirable for the examiner to wear earphones himself, so that the child will be encouraged to imitate the examiner. The examiner then introduces a signal to one of the child's earphones. It is advisable to begin with 500 Hz at a hearing level of 80 to 90 dB. If the child has any hearing ability, he should be able to perceive this frequency, and only rarely should it be necessary to exceed this hearing level. Again the examiner demonstrates to the child that he is to drop a block in the bucket when a signal—this time an acoustic one—is perceived. If a child has learned to respond correctly to the tactile signal, he will usually learn to respond appropriately to the tone in the earphone. When he has responded correctly two or three times, and been praised by the examiner, the examiner lowers the hearing level by 20 dB. If the child responds again, he will lower the level another 20 dB and continue in this fashion until the child does not respond. He assumes, then, that the signal is below the child's threshold. He increases the hearing level 10 dB and presents another spurt of tone. If the child responds again, the examiner records this last hearing level as the threshold and switches to 1,000 Hz. In a similar manner he establishes threshold for 1,000 Hz and then for 2,000 Hz. The examiner then switches the output to the other ear and obtains threshold measurements at the same frequencies—500, 1,000, and 2,000 Hz.

The examiner does not try to pin down the child's threshold any more precisely than to the nearest 10-dB step, and he does not bother with other frequencies until he has information on the child's hearing at the speech frequencies—500, 1,000, and 2,000 Hz—in each ear. In working with a young child there is a premium on haste. At any moment the child may decide to withdraw from the "game," and so the examiner settles for approximate thresholds at a limited number of frequencies. Should the child lose interest, the examiner can switch toys. For example, he can direct the child to put a circular block on the peg of the "Christmas tree" instead of dropping a block in the bucket, and hopefully restore the child's interest and motivation for a long enough time to complete the test.

Should the child demonstrate losses by air conduction, it is desirable to check his hearing by bone conduction. If the examiner has established good rapport with the child and kept his interest at a high level, the bone-conduction check can be accomplished immediately. It may be necessary, though, to postpone the bone-conduction test until another time. Whenever the bone conduction is tested, the examiner will attempt to test with the vibrator on only one mastoid and without the use of masking. He is concerned only to determine if there is an air-bone gap with either ear. If so, he knows that at least one ear has a conductive component and that it is important for an otologist to consider medical or surgical means of eliminating or reducing the air-bone gap.

To reiterate, the examiner is interested first of all in obtaining air-conduction thresholds, or at least approximations of thresholds, for the speech frequencies in each ear, and, assuming the child has losses by air, thresholds at these same frequencies by bone conduction. Only then, if the child is still willing to continue, does the examiner concern himself with determining hearing levels at other frequencies, or make an attempt to define thresholds more precisely. It is the rare child, however, whose interest can be maintained for any period longer than that required to obtain the minimal information about his hearing. Even when a child has appeared to cooperate well, the examiner will usually want him to return at some later time for a retest. If similar results are obtained on a retest, the examiner can place much greater confidence in the audiogram than if he were limited to only one testing session.

Speech Audiometry

Since the primary handicap imposed by a hearing impairment is difficulty with communication, the best way of evaluating the handicap is by the use of speech audiometry. A two-room testing suite is required for speech audiometry: a test room where the patient is situated, and a control room where the audiometer and the examiner are located. Communication between the two rooms is accomplished visually by a window (double or triple pane for acoustic isolation) and acoustically by a talk-back system.

A speech audiometer consists of amplifiers accommodating inputs of live voice through a microphone, tape, disc recordings, and noise generators (for masking). A gain control and VU (for "volume units") meter enable the examiner to monitor inputs to the same level of intensity. Outputs are fed to earphones or to loudspeakers in the test room, and to the examiner's monitoring and talk-back system. Control over the output level is managed by an attenuator, which is calibrated in one- or two-dB steps over a range of 110 to 130 dB. Usually the speech audiometer is built with two channels, so that two inputs may be presented simultaneously and the outputs be directed to the same or different earphones or loudspeakers, each at its own output level. Frequently, manufacturers build pure-tone and speech circuits into the same chassis, so that the one instrument will meet the needs for both pure-tone and speech audiometry. Such a two-channel combination pure-tone

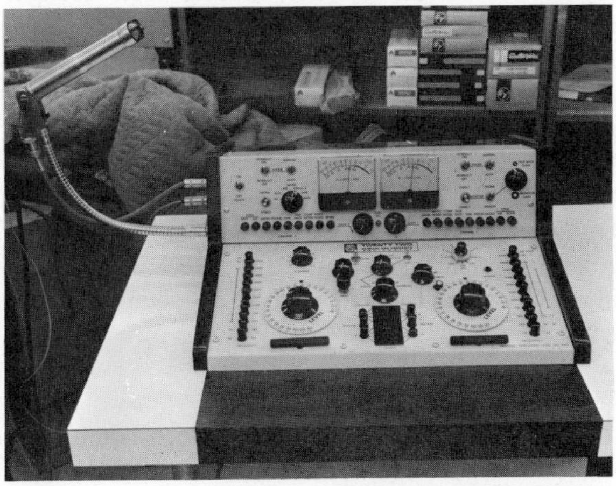

Fig. 13-8. The Allison two-channel combination pure-tone and speech audiometer, manufactured by Tracor, Inc., Austin, Tex.

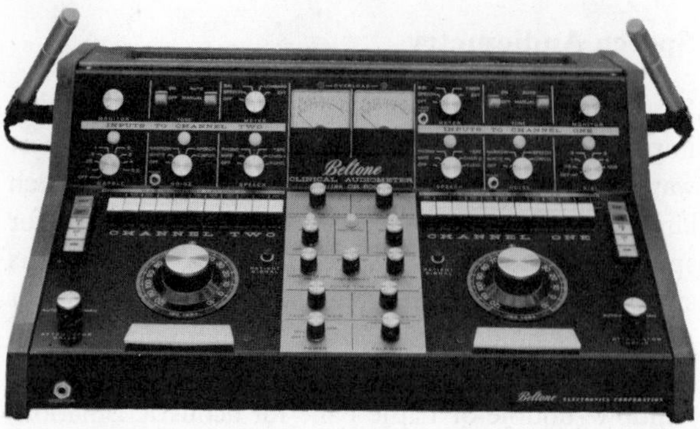

Fig. 13-9. Two-channel combination pure-tone and speech audiometer, manufactured by Beltone Electronics Corp., Chicago, Ill.

and speech audiometer is illustrated in Figs. 13-8 and 13-9.

CALIBRATION

Supposedly zero-dB hearing level for speech represents the minimum average hearing level at which two-syllable words become intelligible for normal ears. The American Standards Association (1953) specified that zero-dB hearing level for speech is a sound-pressure level of 22 dB re 0.0002 dyne/cm^2 with allowable limits for calibration of $\pm$ 4 dB. Hirsh et al. (1952, p. 333) reported that the subjects used in the standardization of the recorded speech tests developed at Central Institute for the Deaf averaged zero-dB hearing level for speech at a sound-pressure level of 18 dB. Extrapolating from the experimental data presented by Jerger et al. (1959) the best agreement between the average hearing level for the frequencies 500, 1,000, and 2,000 Hz and the average hearing level for speech should be obtained when zero-dB hearing level for speech is equal to a sound-pressure level of 20 dB (assuming subjects who are "sophisticated" listeners, and assuming pure-tone thresholds were obtained with an audiometer calibrated to ISO-1964 standards). The Veterans Administration has specified that speech audiometers in its clinics be calibrated to 20 dB sound-pressure level.

PROCEDURES

The measures routinely sought in speech audiometry are 1. hearing level for speech, more commonly called speech-reception threshold (SRT), 2. tolerance level, or uncomfortable level for speech, and 3. speech discrimination ability. Ordinarily these measures would be obtained both monaurally (through earphones) and by sound field (through a loudspeaker).

The speech-reception threshold is defined as the minimum hearing level at which the patient can repeat correctly at least 50 percent of the speech stimuli. In the preceding discussion of calibration, speech-reception threshold has been equated with hearing level for speech. It should be noted that in speech testing we are interested not in the threshold for *detection* of speech but rather in the threshold for the *intelligibility* of speech. At various times in the brief history of speech audiometry two-syllable words, one-syllable words, sentences, and connected discourse have all been used for establishing speech-reception threshold. At the present time, however, two-syllable words—called spondees because they are spoken with nearly equal stress on each syllable—are universally employed for measuring speech-reception threshold. Recorded spondee words are available as CID Auditory Test W-1.[1] The test words may, however, be presented by live voice or in tape-recorded form at the choice of the examiner.

The step-by-step procedures in arriving at the patient's speech-reception threshold will not be detailed here. These procedures have been thoroughly covered elsewhere (Newby, 1964; Chaiklin and Ventry, 1964; Harris, 1965; O'Neill and Oyer, 1966). We may say here only that the spondee words are presented at a hearing level sufficiently above threshold that the patient can repeat them with essentially 100 percent accuracy. The level is then reduced gradually until a point is reached where the patient can repeat only about 50 percent of the words correctly. Usually speech-reception threshold is determined to the nearest two-dB step, but some audiologists present a case for measuring SRT in five-dB steps, as pure-tone thresholds are measured (Chaiklin and Ventry, 1964).

In determining a patient's tolerance level it is advisable to use connected discourse, and it is most convenient to have available a recorded sample of running speech for this purpose. The patient is instructed to signal when the speech becomes so intense that it causes physiological discomfort, and the examiner gradually increases the level of the running speech until either the patient signals, or the maximum output level has been reached. The purpose of obtaining this measurement is twofold:

[1] The records are manufactured and distributed by Technisonic Studios, 1201 South Brentwood Blvd., Richmond Heights, Missouri.

1. to determine the upper limit of hearing level for administering the discrimination test that follows, and
2. to obtain information as to the dynamic range of the patient's hearing within which a hearing aid must function.

It is useful also to obtain information concerning the hearing level at which the patient prefers to hear speech. The recorded sample of running speech can be used for this purpose also. The patient is instructed to signal when the speech is at its most comfortable level as the examiner gradually changes its intensity. Usually it is best to ask the patient to make four judgments of most comfortable level (MCL): two while the speech signal is increased in level above SRT, and two while the speech is decreased in intensity from a level well above MCL. The average of these four judgments is then assumed to be the best estimate of the patient's most comfortable listening level.

Finally, the patient's speech discrimination ability is measured. For this purpose the patient is asked to write down, or to repeat orally, each of a list of 50 monosyllabic words that have been selected for their "phonetic balance" to connected discourse. Each list of 50 words contains the various phonemes of English in the same proportion to their occurrence in running speech, so each list is considered to be phonetically balanced to running speech, and, of course, to every other list. Because of this characteristic the words are called "PB words" (phonetically balanced).

Since normal ears have been determined to achieve maximum scores on the PB word lists when they are presented at a sensation level of at least 40 dB (i.e., 40 dB above threshold hearing level for speech), it is standard practice to administer the discrimination test at a patient's sensation level of 40 dB. While the measure sought is the patient's maximum discrimination ability, referred to as his "PB-MAX" there is little reason to believe that his discrimination score will be enhanced by presenting the word list at any higher level above his threshold. Of course the patient must be protected from discomfort during this test, which is one reason for determining his tolerance level before testing his discrimination. If a reduced tolerance level prohibits the presentation of the PB words at a sensation level of 40 dB, then they will have to be presented at the highest sensation level feasible within his dynamic range, and the examiner will note that the patient's discrimination scores may not, therefore, represent his theoretical maximum discrimination ability.

While it makes little difference in measuring speech-reception threshold whether the spondee words are presented by record or by live voice, it is important to use only recorded test materials for obtaining discrimination scores. The PB words must be spoken with equal effort rather than with equal intensity, because the phonemes of English differ considerably in intensity. Because it has been found that discrimination scores will vary with different speakers, and because it is desirable to maintain the best possible reliability of discrimination test results from patient to patient within a clinic, and from clinic to clinic, it is best to test discrimination only with the CID Auditory Test W-22 records.[2] While there are other tests of speech discrimination that may be more sensitive indicators of a patient's ability to understand what he hears, so much data have been reported on the W-22 recordings—compensation tables have even been based on scores obtained with these particular test materials—that there are practical problems in changing what has become an established clinical procedure.

The discrimination test is scored by allowing two percentage points for each word heard correctly. Preferably, the patient should write his responses, even though each word on the W-22 test record is preceded by the carrier phrase, "You will say. . . ." Assuming that the patient's spelling and writing abilities are reasonably adequate, the test paper is easy to score, and the examiner has a permanent record of any errors the patient made. This record provides interesting information for study and also may shed light on the particular sounds that should be emphasized in speechreading instruction and auditory training. If the patient is unable to write responses with sufficient speed and clarity, the oral response method will have to be used. The problem with oral responses is that the examiner must judge whether or not the patient repeated each test word correctly, so the test challenges the examiner's speech discrimination ability as well as the patient's. Some audiologists have suggested that testing time can be reduced without seriously impairing accuracy of results by using only half a list of words (25) and assigning a value of four percentage points per word. Because the lists were constructed with the notion that each would be administered *in toto*, there was no attempt to balance or equate half a list with the other

[2] The records are manufactured and distributed by Technisonic Studios, 1201 South Brentwood Blvd., Richmond Heights, Missouri.

half. Thus there is no assurance that the patient would score the same on half a list as he would on a whole list.

In testing for speech-reception threshold the same criterion for determining the need for masking applies as in the case of pure-tone air-conduction testing: if the ears differ in sensitivity by 40 dB or more, the SRT test of the poorer ear should be repeated while masking the better ear. Broad-band white noise has been found to be the most effective masker for speech. Because speech-discrimination testing is performed at a suprathreshold level of 40 dB, the examiner may find it necessary to mask the better ear when the threshold difference between the ears is considerably less than 40 dB. Consider the following example:

	RIGHT EAR	LEFT EAR
SRT	10 dB	30 dB
Discrim.	98%	88%

Since the difference in speech-hearing level between the ears is only 20 dB, and we assume an average interaural attenuation of 50 dB, there obviously is no need to mask the right ear while measuring SRT on the left. But the discrimination test on the left ear would be administered at a speech hearing level of 70 dB (i.e., a sensation level of 40 dB). Thus the right ear would be receiving some stimulation at a suprathreshold level (70 dB minus 50 dB for interaural attenuation equals a hearing level of 20 dB, or a sensation level of 10 dB in the right ear). It is conceivable that the limited participation of the right ear with its excellent discrimination could be contributing substantially to the discrimination score obtained in the left ear. When the right ear was suitably masked and another list of PB words was presented to the left ear, the left ear was found to have a discrimination score of only 70 percent. The moral to this example is that whenever there is a possibility that the contralateral ear might be contributing to a discrimination score the test should be repeated with masking.

The primary purpose in performing speech audiometry by sound field is to evaluate a patient's hearing in a way that approximates his everyday listening experiences. When we engage in a conversation with a friend in a quiet room we use both ears, so that what we hear and understand is a function of the interaction of our ears. Naturally, the sound-field test results will usually approximate the monaural results obtained with the better ear. Discrimination in the sound-field test may be better or worse than the better ear alone, however, depending on whether the poorer ear lends enhancement or interference to the better one—or, of course, the discrimination may be the same as the better ear's. Decisions as to whether or not a patient might benefit from a hearing aid are based primarily on sound-field results. When the patient is tested with an aid, the effectiveness of the aid is judged by comparing the patient's aided sound-field test results with his unaided sound-field scores. The decision as to which ear to provide with amplification, however, is made on the basis of a careful analysis of the monaural test results.

INTERPRETATION OF TEST RESULTS

Speech audiometry provides a valuable check on pure-tone test results, contributes some diagnostic information to supplement that conveyed by pure-tone testing, and sheds considerable light on a patient's rehabilitative needs. As stated earlier in this chapter, an average of the threshold hearing levels at 500, 1,000, and 2,000 Hz in most cases should agree well with the speech-reception threshold. There are certain pure-tone configurations, however, with which a better prediction of SRT is obtained by averaging only the threshold hearing levels at 500 and 1,000 Hz and ignoring the frequency of 2,000 Hz. These are the so-called "ski-slope" audiograms that demonstrate sharp increases in hearing loss from frequency to frequency, considering only the span from 500 through 2,000 Hz. If the increase in hearing level from frequency to frequency within this restricted frequency range is less than 20 dB, the three-frequency average will provide the better prediction of SRT. But if the difference between 500 and 1,000 Hz, or between 1,000 and 2,000 Hz should be 20 dB or more, then the two-frequency average will be the better predictor. In either case, if the difference between the predicted SRT and the SRT actually obtained in speech audiometry (referring, of course, to monaural tests) should exceed 10 dB, the examiner should view his test results with suspicion. On the other hand, an agreement between predicted and obtained SRT within ± 10 dB provides reasonable assurance of the validity of both pure-tone and speech-test results. It should be pointed out, however, that agreement between pure-tone and speech-test results is not incontrovertible evidence of the absence of functional or nonorganic factors (see Chapter 14 by Kinstler).

The speech-discrimination ability of a patient as determined by the PB-word tests is usually related to the air-conduction pure-tone configuration through the three speech frequencies. In general, the patient who demonstrates a relatively "flat" pure-tone pattern (nearly equal threshold hearing levels at 500, 1,000 and 2,000 Hz) will obtain close to 100 percent score on a discrimination test, and the more his pure-tone pattern deviates from flatness and approaches a ski-slope configuration, the poorer his discrimination score will be. Thus comparison of a patient's pure-tone audiogram and speech-discrimination results provides another basis for evaluating the validity of a hearing test.

Marked deviations from anticipated and obtained discrimination scores may have diagnostic significance. For example, one of the characteristics of Ménière's syndrome and also of a tumor of the VIIIth Cranial nerve is that a patient's discrimination score is markedly poorer than would be predicted from his pure-tone audiogram. Both of these conditions are also characteristically unilateral impairments. So if a patient with only one affected ear demonstrates extremely poorer discrimination than would be predicted from the pure-tone audiogram, the examiner should suspect that the patient has either Ménière's syndrome or a tumor of the VIIIth Cranial nerve. Other speech-test results can help to differentiate between these two possible diagnoses, as will be brought out later in this chapter.

While generalizations can be made concerning speech audiometric results that are typical of conductive and sensorineural impairments, the only sure way of diagnosing an impairment as conductive or sensorineural is to compare air-conduction and bone conduction results in pure-tone audiometry. Speech audiometry is much more important in determining degree of handicap produced by a hearing impairment and in pointing to a patient's rehabilitative needs than in assisting the audiologist and otologist to a diagnosis. For example, there is little question that a patient with bilateral speech-reception thresholds of 60 dB, no abnormal reduction of tolerance, and discrimination scores of 90 to 100 percent would be an excellent candidate for a hearing aid, or perhaps binaural aids. On the other hand, a patient with speech-reception thresholds of 20 dB, abnormally reduced tolerance level, and discrimination scores in the 60 to 70 percent range is probably not a good candidate for a hearing aid. He may very well benefit, however, from lessons in speechreading and auditory training, as well as from work to prevent his own consonant sounds from becoming blurred or "mushy." Aural rehabilitation is discussed by Silverman (Chapter 16).

While speech-test results may be recorded on a separate form, there is an advantage in using a form that reports both pure-tone and speech-test results. An example of such a form is shown in Fig. 13-10. The boxes to the right of the audiogram are for recording scores obtained on various speech tests for the right ear, the left ear, and by sound field. The tests shown in order are speech-reception threshold (SRT); speech-detection threshold (SDT), for use when for some reason an SRT score cannot be obtained; most comfortable level (MCL); tolerance level (TL); and discrimination score (%PB MAX). Space is provided for recording the sensation level (SL) at which the discrimination test was administered, the identification number of the PB list used, and the level of masking noise in sound-pressure level (SPL) provided masking was used on the contralateral ear. Any scores obtained with masking are marked with an asterisk. Beneath the audiogram are boxes for recording either two-frequency or three-frequency pure-tone averages (PTA) for easy comparison with obtained SRT scores.

TESTING CHILDREN

Earlier in this chapter modifications in pure-tone testing procedures were suggested for testing very young children. It was indicated at that time that attempts to measure pure-tone threshold hearing levels would normally follow some test procedures with a speech audiometer. Because of the flexibility provided by the speech audiometer microphone circuit for the introduction of various stimuli at controlled hearing levels, the examiner can learn a great deal about a child's auditory abilities before attempting to obtain a pure-tone audiogram. Since speech audiometry is performed in a two-room suite, the examiner will require the services of an assistant to be in the test room with the child. Preferably, the assistant and the child should be seated on opposite sides of a child-size table facing each other. The assistant should have available several quiet toys to show the child and with which to engage his attention. The examiner in the control room then introduces a signal by sound field through the microphone circuit. He may say the child's name, he may whisper the child's name, or he may say or whisper isolated sounds, such as individual phonemes or animal sounds. Various noisemakers, such as rattles, bells, and whistles may also be used as well as the masking noise on the audiometer, and if available, warbled

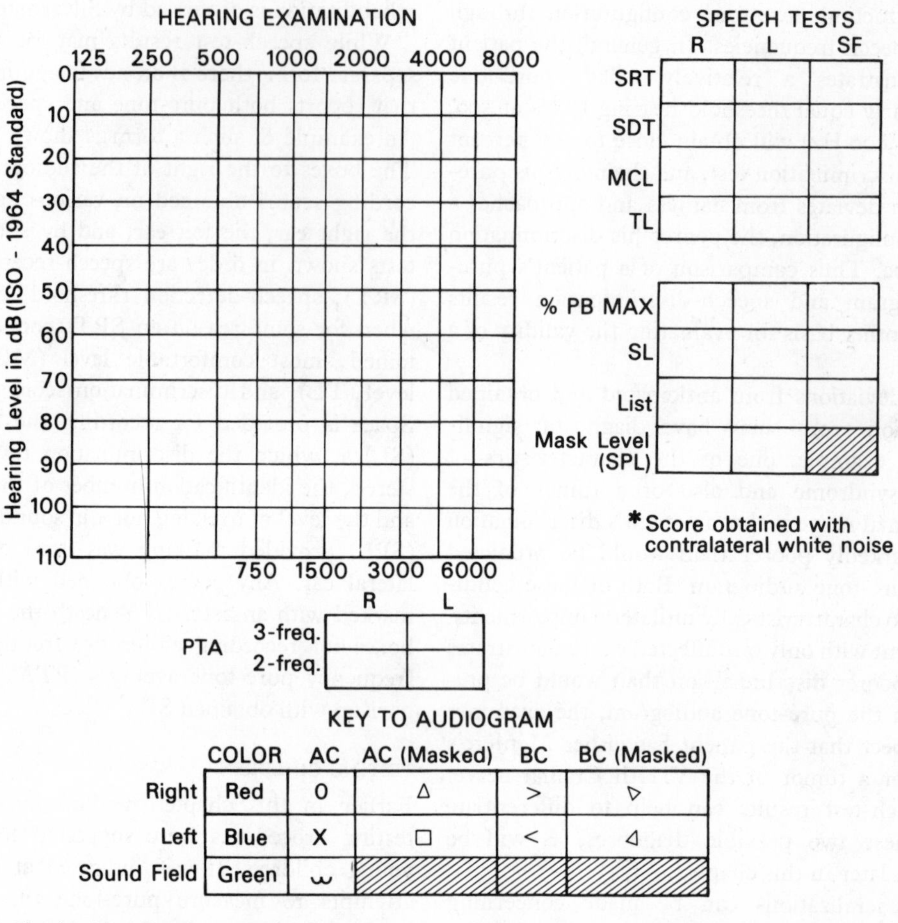

Fig. 13-10. Hearing examination form for recording both pure-tone and speech results.

pure tones. Initially, the examiner is interested in learning which sounds at which hearing levels are successful in distracting the child from the toy in which he is interested. The child may look for the source of the sound (the loudspeaker), or he may give subtler indications of his auditory awareness, such as momentarily stopping his activity with the toy, or looking directly at the assistant as if the assistant had been responsible for making the sound.

The examiner observes the child through the window separating the test room and control room, and the assistant also observes the child closely to detect any indication of his awareness of an acoustic signal from the loudspeaker. Of course the examiner keeps careful notes of the kinds of stimuli and the hearing levels that elicit definite responses from the child. Some audiologists have successfully utilized a reinforcing technique that rewards the child for turning toward the loudspeaker at appropriate times. This consists of a plastic toy, such as a pig or an elephant, in which a lightbulb has been installed, controlled by a switch operated by the examiner. The toy is situated on top of the loudspeaker enclosure, which is located behind the child. When the child, in response to an acoustic stimulus, turns toward the loudspeaker, the examiner causes the plastic animal to be illuminated. The child soon learns to look directly at the animal whenever he perceives an acoustic signal. Should he turn to look at the animal when no signal has been presented, there is, of course, no illumination. By noting the lowest hearing levels to which the child responds in a positive manner, the examiner can determine at least the maximum limit of the child's impairment.

If the child has sufficient language ability to recognize the names of common objects, it may be possible for the examiner to obtain a sound-field SRT —or at least a good approximation of an SRT—by asking the child to manipulate toy objects on the table, e.g., "Show me the cow." "Show me the airplane." "Put the pig in the truck," etc. Each time the child responds correctly, the examiner decreases the hearing level of the sound-field signal, until a point is reached below which no correct responses are made. This would be the child's SRT.

A child with more highly developed language abilities can be tested in ways more closely approximating the testing of adults. Thus pictures can be substituted for toy objects, increasing the range of speech samples to which the child is asked to respond and, therefore, yielding more information concerning the child's auditory behavior. Special lists of spondee words and phonetically balanced words have been devised for use with children who are able to repeat words they hear (Newby, 1964, pp. 377–379). Using these lists, the examiner can obtain SRT and speech discrimination scores not only by sound field, but, the patient willing, also by earphones.

TESTS FOR DETERMINING SITE OF LESION

The comparison of a patient's air-conduction and bone-conduction threshold hearing levels enables the examiner to determine whether the patient's impairment is to be categorized as conductive, sensorineural, or mixed. Frequently it is desirable to obtain more information about a patient's auditory behavior in order to specify more precisely the site of the patient's hearing problem. While there have been reports of the clinical implications of acoustic impedance measurements at the eardrum (Feldman, 1963, 1964; Zwislocki, 1963) and reports describing the auditory behavior of patients with lesions of the central nervous system (Jerger, 1960b; Bocca, 1958, 1967; Bocca and Calearo, 1963), for the most part, site-of-lesion tests have attempted to differentiate between sensorineural impairments of cochlear origin and those resulting from lesions of the VIIIth Cranial nerve. Several such tests will now be described.

Recruitment Tests

Dix, Hallpike, and Hood (1948) pointed out that cochlear and retrocochlear involvements could be differentiated on the basis of recruitment, the abnormally rapid increase in loudness as the intensity of a stimulus is increased above threshold. They reported that patients with cochlear pathology consistently demonstrated recruitment, while those with VIIIth Cranial nerve tumors did not.

The classic test for recruitment is the alternate binaural loudness balance test (ABLB), ascribed to Fowler (1928). In this test, the growth of loudness for pure tones in an impaired ear is compared with that in a normal ear. The test thus is useful only in cases of unilateral impairment. VIIIth Cranial nerve tumors usually produce unilateral impairments, however, so the need is for tests that will differentiate a unilateral retrochlear involvement from a unilateral cochlear impairment, such as Ménière's syndrome.

The patient is instructed to match the loudness of a tone presented to his impaired ear with the loudness of a tone of the same frequency presented to the good ear at a particular hearing level. The examiner varies the hearing level of the tone in the poor ear, presenting brief spurts of the tone alternately to the good and the poor ear, until the patient reports the tones are equally loud. The examiner then increases the hearing level in the good ear usually by 20 dB, and again establishes the hearing level in the poor ear that produces a sensation of equal loudness. Additional points of equal loudness are established until the limit of the audiometer, or the limit of the ear's dynamic range, has been reached. The same procedure is followed for other frequencies. The results of the ABLB test are graphed as a laddergram, illustrated in Fig. 13-11. The laddergram is constructed by connecting the hearing levels that produce equal-loudness judgments in the two ears, beginning at threshold. In Fig. 13-11 are shown four possible laddergrams that might be obtained at a particular frequency. The one labeled A demonstrates the absence of recruitment. Note that the lines connecting points of equal loudness are parallel. The other laddergrams in Fig. 13-11 demonstrate the presence of recruitment, though in varying degrees. Laddergram B shows partial or incomplete recruitment, i.e., the loudness of a given hearing level in the poor ear never does catch up with the loudness of the same hearing level in the good ear. Laddergram C portrays complete recruitment. At the highest hearing levels compared, the loudness of a given hearing level is judged to be the same regardless of which ear is stimulated. In Laddergram D, a result called hyperrecruitment has been obtained. The growth of loudness in the impaired ear has been so rapid that at high suprathreshold levels a given hearing level produces a sensation of greater loudness in the impaired ear than in the good ear. While rare, hyperrecruitment

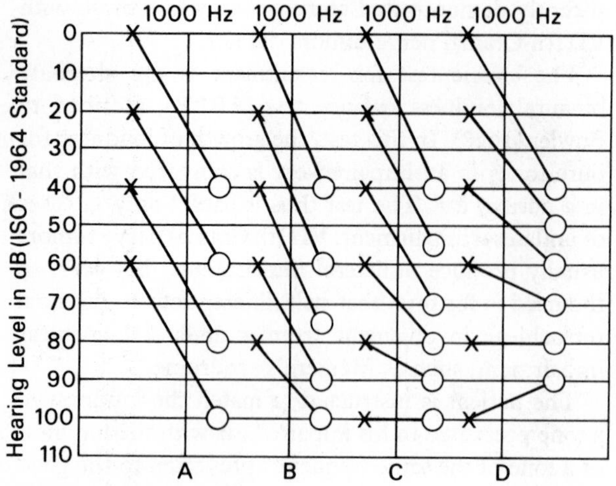

Fig. 13-11. Laddergrams illustrating four possible results in alternate binaural loudness balance test.
A = no recruitment;
B = partial or incomplete recruitment;
C = complete recruitment;
D = hyper recruitment.

does occur clinically at some frequencies with patients who usually have active vestibular and cochlear symptoms of Ménière's syndrome.

There are occasions when it is desirable to check for the presence of recruitment in the case of a bilateral impairment. Another test must be used in such cases, since the ABLB test requires that the patient have one normal ear. The monaural loudness-balance test is suitable for use with bilateral impairments, provided that the patient has at least one frequency in each ear that is normal. Reger (1936) was the first to describe this test. It involves having the patient balance the loudness of two tones of different frequency in the same ear, using the normal frequency as the standard. As in the case of the ABLB test, a laddergram connects the hearing levels at which loudness balance is achieved at each 20 dB step above threshold for the normal frequency. Balancing the loudness of two tones of different frequency is not an easy task even for a trained listener. The farther apart in frequency the tones are, the more difficult is the task. The judgments obtained in the monaural loudness-balance test must therefore be interpreted with caution.

It should be mentioned that some audiologists prefer to increase the intensity by set intervals on the impaired ear or the impaired frequency in the ABLB and monaural loudness-balance tests, respectively, instead of the procedure described here. The results should be comparable regardless of which method is employed. Reger (1965, p. 136) recommends doing both procedures as a check on the reliability of the test results obtained.

The presence of recruitment may also be determined by checking the dynamic range obtained in speech audiometry. The normal ear and the non-recruiting impaired ear should both be able to tolerate running speech at hearing levels close to the maximum output of the audiometer. If the tolerance level for speech is reduced to a hearing level of 90 dB or lower, resulting in a restriction of the dynamic range of the ear, some degree of recruitment is indicated. In cases of Ménière's syndrome it is not unusual to find dynamic ranges as low as 20 to 30 dB.

SISI Test

In the late 1940's and early 1950's there was considerable interest in tests of the difference limen for intensity. Patients with sensorineural impairments of cochlear origin were found to have abnormally small difference limens—i.e., they were able to detect small changes in the intensity of a pure-tone signal—at levels close to threshold. Various methodologies for measuring difference limens were suggested, but none of these tests achieved much clinical popularity. Jerger, Shedd, and Harford (1959), however, developed a difference-limen test that has been widely used. They called their test SISI for "short-increment sensitivity index."

SISI units are available as accessories for pure-tone audiometers, and they are built into some larger audiometers for combined pure-tone and speech testing. What is required is a means for superimposing brief increments of one and five dB of intensity on a steady tone of any given hearing level. The patient is asked to signal whenever he is aware that an intensity increment has been superimposed on the steady tone, which is presented at any frequency desired at a sensation level of 20 dB (20 dB above threshold). The test consists of the presentation of 20 one-dB increments, each having a duration of 0.3 second. The patient receives a score of five percent for each increment heard. Test procedure calls for presenting some five-dB increments for training purposes and to check the patient's responses to increments he should be able to hear, and some zero-dB increments as "control" presentations. If the patient responds positively to control presentations, the test is, of course, invalidated. Only the responses to the one-dB increments are scored.

While the SISI test may be performed at any frequency, the results obtained at 1,000 and 4,000 Hz seem to be the most meaningful in terms of differentiating cochlear from VIIIth Cranial nerve impairments. On the basis of relatively few cases, Jerger, Shedd, and Harford (1959) reported the range of scores for two types of cochlear disorders and for retrocochlear disorders to be as follows:

	1,000 HZ	4,000 HZ
noise-induced	0–40%	95–100%
Ménière's	70–100%	95–100%
retrocochlear	0	0

At a conference in 1965, Harford (1967, p. 232) reported that " . . . the SISI test appears to be withstanding the test of time for the purpose for which it was originally proposed." He did suggest, however, that some modifications in the original test procedure would be indicated in certain circumstances, e.g., altering the sensation level of the steady tone: increasing it to 25 to 30 dB in cases of mild hearing losses, and decreasing it to 10 dB in cases of profound hearing losses.

Owens (1965) reported that the SISI and ABLB tests were duplicative, in that both reflected loudness recruitment. He stated that the SISI test, however, can be utilized in cases of bilateral impairment where the ABLB test would not be usable, and the SISI test provides a more precise measure of cochlear function or dysfunction than does the ABLB test.

Tone Decay

The difficulty experienced by certain patients in maintaining the audibility of a tone at threshold level was reported by Hood (1950, 1955). Designating this phenomenon "per-stimulatory fatigue," Hood reported its presence in patients with Ménière's syndrome. Carhart (1957) described a clinical test procedure called "tone decay," by means of which he demonstrated that patients with Ménière's syndrome and other patients with undefined hearing problems did manifest difficulty in maintaining tones at threshold levels. Carhart's procedure involved determining the lowest hearing level at which a patient could maintain the audibility of a tone for a full 60 seconds. Starting with a tone at the previously determined threshold level, the examiner starts a stop watch. When the patient signals the tone is inaudible, the examiner increases the intensity by five dB and starts the watch again. Successive increments of five dB are added as necessary until a hearing level is reached which the patient can continue to hear for one minute. The difference between his original threshold and the hearing level at the termination of the test is the measure of the tone decay for that particular frequency. The test normally would be performed at several frequencies.

Rosenberg, in a paper read at the 1958 Convention of the American Speech and Hearing Association (Green, 1963), suggested a modification of the Carhart test which reduces the time required for the test to one minute per frequency. The examiner presents a tone at threshold to the patient and starts the watch. When the patient signals he no longer hears the tone, the examiner increases the intensity by five dB but keeps the watch running. He continues to increase the intensity by five-dB intervals as necessary to keep the tone audible until 60 seconds have elapsed. The difference between the starting and ending hearing levels is the amount of tone decay that occurred in one minute.

Yantis (1959) and Sørenson (1962) reported that patients with VIIIth Cranial nerve tumors demonstrated the most extreme levels of tone decay. Owens (1964a) investigated the differential diagnostic capabilities of the tone decay test with Ménière's patients and patients with VIIIth Cranial nerve tumors. Owens started the test at a sensation level of five dB instead of at threshold. Whenever the patient signaled the tone had disappeared, he gave the patient a 20-second recovery period and increased the intensity of the tone by five dB. This procedure was continued until a level was reached at which the patient could maintain the audibility of the tone for one minute, or until four intensity increments had been presented. While Owens found that many of his Ménière's patients demonstrated tone decay at one or more frequencies, all but one of the patients with VIIIth Cranial nerve lesions demonstrated tone decay at two or more frequencies, and there were marked differences between the two groups of patients in the results of the test. In general, the patients with VIIIth Cranial nerve lesions demonstrated decay at all frequencies showing impairment, and the rapidity of tone decay remained the same at each intensity increment, while about 60 percent of the Ménière's patients either showed no decay, or decay at only one or two frequencies, and usually the rate of decay slowed down with increasing intensity above threshold.

Békésy Audiometry

Since Békésy (1947) first described a new audiometer with which a patient could in effect chart his own audiogram, audiologists have been intrigued with the clinical utility of the instrument. In addition to its usefulness as an "automatic" audiometer, the Békésy audiometer yields information of diagnostic importance in differentiating cochlear from VIIIth Cranial nerve lesions, as we shall see. Fig. 13-12 shows the currently popular, commercially available version of the Békésy audiometer.

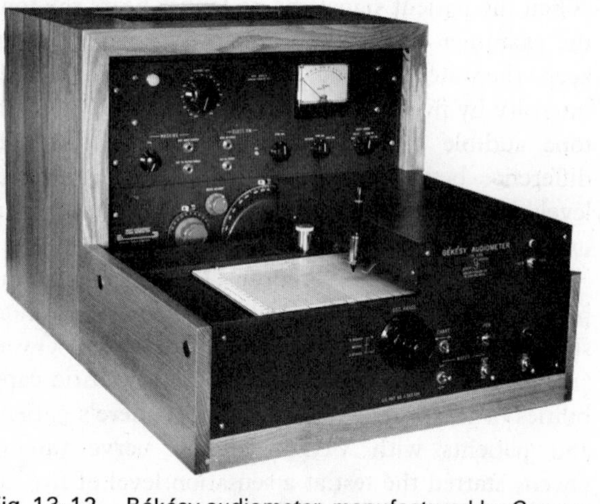

Fig. 13-12. Békésy audiometer, manufactured by Grason-Stadler Co., Inc., West Concord, Mass.

A patient's audiogram is graphed by a pen mounted in a unit that moves vertically in synchronism with a motor-driven attenuator (hearing-level control). The direction of pen movement depends on a push-button control operated by the patient. When the patient depresses the button, signifying he hears a tone in his earphone, the hearing-level control rotates counterclockwise, decreasing the intensity of the tone at a steady rate (usually 2.5 dB per second) and causing the pen unit to move upward. When the patient releases the button, signifying the tone is inaudible, the drive motor instantly reverses, causing the hearing-level control to rotate clockwise and the pen unit to reverse direction, moving downward as the intensity of the tone is increased.

An audiogram form is attached to a plate that moves horizontally under the pen. The plate can be adjusted to move in synchronism with the frequency control of the audiometer, so that a continuous sweep-frequency audiogram can be charted from the lowest frequency available (100 Hz) to the highest (10,000 Hz). Or the plate can be adjusted to move under the pen while the frequency remains constant, thus providing a fixed-frequency chart of hearing level over a period of time. The most commonly used chart speed is one octave per minute. Threshold hearing levels are determined by approximating the midpoint of the up-and-down pen swings that correspond to the patient's depressing or releasing the push-button switch. The audiometer provides either a continuous tone or an interrupted tone (2.5 interruptions per second).

Various investigators (Reger and Kos, 1952; Lierle and Reger, 1955; Jerger, Carhart, and Lassman, 1958; Yantis, 1959) reported that patients with VIIIth Cranial nerve lesions demonstrated marked threshold shifts when tested with a continuous tone on the Békésy audiometer. Jerger, Carhart, and Lassman (1958) noted that threshold shifts did not occur when the Békésy audiometer was set to produce an interrupted tone.

Jerger (1960a) reported on comparisons of continuous-tone (C) versus interrupted-tone (I) Békésy audiogram tracings of more than 400 patients with various kinds of hearing impairments. From his analysis of both sweep-frequency and fixed-frequency Békésy tracings, Jerger described four principal types of audiograms. Type I is characterized by essentially identical tracings obtained with C and with I. Type II demonstrates poorer hearing by C for frequencies above 1,000 Hz, with a separation between I and C usually no greater than 20 dB. In the fixed-frequency tests for frequencies of 1,000 Hz and higher, C drops below I by from five to 20 dB within the first minute but then remains stable over the remainder of a three-minute period.

In Type III, the sweep-frequency tracings show C dropping below I from the beginning of the test, and the gap between C and I widens rapidly as the test progresses until the maximum limit of the audiometer is reached. In the fixed-frequency tracings, C begins to separate from I immediately and plunges to the limit of the audiometer well before the three-minute period ends.

Type IV is similar to the Type II Békésy audiogram, except that C drops below I at the beginning of the test, so that a gap of up to 20 dB between C and I occurs at all frequencies. The fixed-frequency tracings show a constant difference between C and I at all frequencies.

Based on the diagnostic information available on each patient, Jerger (1960a, p. 284) drew the following conclusions:

. . . In lesions of the middle ear (otosclerosis, otitis media) the Type I tracing predominates. In cochlear lesion (Ménière's, noise-induced) the Type II tracing predominates although some fall into the Type I category. No Ménière's case ever showed a Type III tracing. In eighth nerve lesion (acoustic neurinoma) Type III and Type IV tracings predominate. No acoustic neurinoma ever gave a Type II tracing.

It should be noted that the tone-decay test and the Békésy test performed with continuous tone are measuring the same phenomenon: abnormal adaptation or perstimulatory fatigue. As stated in the preceding section, patients with cochlear disorders were observed to demonstrate less severe tone decay than those with VIIIth Cranial nerve lesions. This difference in degree of tone decay is reflected in the difference between C and I in Békésy Type II and Type III audiograms.

Jerger's categories inspired similar studies of clinic populations with known diagnoses, resulting in some disagreements with Jerger's findings. Johnson and House (1964) reported that 12 out of 42 patients with VIIIth Cranial nerve lesions yielded either Type II or Type I tracings. Owens (1964b) studied the Békésy tracings of 92 patients with cochlear lesions and 13 patients with VIIIth Cranial nerve lesions. Twenty-one of the 92 with cochlear pathology had Type I Békésy audiograms. The remainder of this group had variations of Jerger's Types II and IV Békésy audiograms. There were separations between C and I varying from four to 26 dB, and varying also as to the frequencies over which the separation occurred. The patients with VIIIth Cranial nerve lesions all demonstrated varieties of Jerger's Type III Békésy audiogram, although with some of these patients the separation between C and I did not occur until 500 to 2,000 Hz. Owens prefers the fixed-frequency tracings to the sweep-frequency ones, because they provide more precise information, require less time, and are easier for the patients to perform. He believes that the order of importance of the fixed frequencies in most cases is 4,000, 2,000, 1,000, and 500 Hz.

Shapiro and Naunton (1967) reported on Békésy tracings obtained with seven patients with acoustic neurinomas. Six of the seven had Type II Békésy tracings. As a matter of fact, the analysis of various kinds of diagnostic test results with 14 patients having confirmed VIIIth Cranial nerve tumors, including tests for recruitment, SISI, and tone decay in addition to Békésy audiometry, was generally discouraging in terms of the diagnostic value of the test results in Shapiro and Naunton's view. They and Owens (1964b) both suggest that when both cochlear and retrocochlear factors contribute to a patient's impairment the test results will be indicative of only the cochlear involvement. Also they point out that according to Dix and Hallpike (1960) an VIIIth Cranial nerve tumor may produce a cochlear dysfunction by constricting the blood supply to the cochlea. In such cases naturally the audiometric results might be confusing.

Despite the hope of audiologists that test results will be clear-cut and point unequivocally to the site of lesion in sensorineural impairments, they may on occasion, or even frequently, be misleading, as Shapiro and Naunton (1967) have reported. Certainly it is dangerous to make diagnostic conclusions on the basis of one kind of site-of-lesion test. Even when a battery of tests yields consistent information pointing to an impairment as being either cochlear or VIIIth Cranial nerve in origin, the test results are but one part of the diagnostic process. One cannot but agree with the following statement by Reger (1967, p. 242): "It cannot be emphasized too forcibly that the localization implications of all hearing tests must be interpreted in relation to the chronological medical history and physical examination in order to avoid error in otological diagnosis."

BIBLIOGRAPHY

American Academy Opthalmology and Otolaryngology. 1959. Guide for the evaluation of hearing impairment. *Tr. Amer. Acad. Ophthal. Otolaryng.*, March-April, 235–238.

American Standards Association. 1951. Audiometers for general diagnostic purposes. Z 24.5-1951. New York: Amer. Standards Assn.

———. 1953. American standards specifications for speech audiometers. Z 24.13-1953. New York: Amer. Standards Assn.

Békésy, G. von. 1947. A new audiometer. *Acta Otolaryng.*, 35, 411–422.

Bocca, E. 1958. Clinical aspects of cortical deafness. *Laryngoscope*, 68, 301–309.

———. 1967. Distorted speech tests. *In* Sensorineural hearing processes and disorders. Graham, A. B., ed. Boston: Little, Brown. Pp. 359–370.

———, and Calearo, C. 1963. Central hearing processes. *In* Modern developments in audiology. Jerger, J., ed. New York: Academic Press. Pp. 337–370.

Carhart, R. 1957. Clinical determination of abnormal auditory adaptation. *A.M.A. Arch. Otolaryng.*, 65, 32–39.

———, and Jerger, J. 1959. Preferred method for clinical determination of pure-tone thresholds. *J. Speech Hearing Disorders*, 24, 330–345.

Chaiklin, J., and Ventry, I. 1964. Spondee threshold measurement: a comparison of 2- and 5-db methods. *J. Speech Hearing Disorders*, 29, 47–59.

Darley, F. 1961. Identification audiometry. *J. Speech Hearing Disorders, Monograph suppl.* 9.

Davis, H. 1970. Audiology. *In* Hearing and deafness. Davis, H., and Silverman, S. R., eds. New York: Holt, Rinehart and Winston. Pp. 3–6.

———, and Kranz, F. 1964. The international standard reference zero for pure-tone audiometers and its relation to the evaluation of impairment of hearing. *J. Speech Hearing Res.*, 7, 7–16.

Dix, M., and Hallpike, C. 1960. Discussion on acoustic neuroma. *Laryngoscope*, 70, 105–122.

———, ———, and Hood, J. 1948. Observations upon the loudness recruitment phenomenon with especial reference to the differential diagnosis of disorders of the internal ear and VIIIth nerve. *J. Laryng., Otol.*, 62, 671–686.

Downs, M. 1967. Organization and procedures of a newborn infant screening program. *Hearing and Speech News*, 35, 26–36.

Engh, J. 1968. Are you sure your child can hear? *Reader's Digest*, March, 137–140.

Ewing, I., and Ewing, A. 1958. New opportunities for deaf children. London: Univ. London Press.

Feldman, A. 1963. Impedance measurements at the eardrum as an aid to diagnosis. *J. Speech Hearing Research*, 6, 315–327.

———. 1964. Acoustic impedance measurement as a clinical procedure. *J. Int. Aud.*, 3, 1–11.

Fowler, E. 1928. Marked deafened areas in normal ears. *Arch. Otolaryng.*, 8, 151–155.

Glorig, A., and House, H. 1957. A new concept of auditory screening. *A.M.A. Arch. Otolaryng.*, 66, 228–232.

Goldstein, R., and Tait, C. 1971. Critique of neonatal hearing evaluation. *J. Speech Hearing Disorders*, 36, 3–18.

Green, D. 1963. The modified tone decay test (MTDT) as a screening procedure for eighth nerve lesions. *J. Speech Hearing Disorders*, 28, 31–36.

Hardy, J., Dougherty, A., and Hardy, W. 1959. Hearing responses and audiological screening in infants. *J. Pediatrics*, 55, 382–390.

Harford, E. 1967. Clinical application and significance of the SISI test. *In* Sensorineural hearing processes and disorders. Graham, A. B., ed. Boston: Little, Brown. Pp. 223–233.

Harris, J. 1965. Speech audiometry. *In* Audiometry: principles and practices. Glorig, A., ed. Baltimore: Williams & Wilkins. Pp. 151–169.

Hirsh, I., Davis, H., Silverman, S. R., Reynolds, E. Eldert, E., and Benson, R. 1952. Development of materials for speech audiometry. *J. Speech Hearing Disorders*, 17, 321–337.

Hood, J. 1950. Studies in auditory fatigue and adaptation. *Acta Otolaryng.*, *Supplement* 92, 26–56.

———. 1955. Auditory fatigue and adaptation in the differential diagnosis of end-organ disease. *Ann. Otol., Rhinol., Laryng.*, 64, 507–518.

Jerger, J. 1960a. Békésy audiometry in analysis of auditory disorders. *J. Speech Hearing Res.*, 3, 275–287.

———. 1960b. Observations on auditory behavior in lesions of the central auditory pathways. *A.M.A. Arch. Otolaryng.*, 71, 797–806.

———, Carhart, R., and Lassman, J. 1958. Clinical observations on excessive threshold adaptation. *A.M.A. Arch. Otolaryng.*, 68, 617–623.

———, Carhart, R., Tillman, T., and Peterson, J. 1959. Some relations between normal hearing for pure tones and for speech. *J. Speech Hearing Res.*, 2, 126–140.

———, Shedd, J., and Harford, E. 1959. On the detection of extremely small changes in sound intensity. *A.M.A. Arch. Otolaryng.*, 69, 200–211.

———, and Tillman, T. 1960. A new method for the clinical determination of sensorineural acuity level (SAL). *A.M.A. Arch. Otolaryng.*, 71, 948–955.

Johnson, E., and House, W. 1964. Auditory findings in 53 cases of acoustic neuromas. *A.M.A. Arch. Otolaryng.*, 80, 667–677.

Joint committee statement on infant hearing screening. 1971. *Asha*, 13, 79.

Lierle, D., and Reger, S. 1955. Experimentally induced temporary threshold shift in ears with impaired hearing. *Ann. Otol., Rhinol., Laryng.*, 64, 263–277.

Newby, H. 1964. Audiology. New York: Appleton-Century-Crofts.

Owens, E. 1964a. Tone decay in VIIIth nerve and cochlear lesions. *J. Speech Hearing Disorders*, 29, 14–22.

———. 1964b. Békésy tracings and site of lesion. *J. Speech Hearing Disorders*, 29, 456–468.

———. 1965. The SISI test and recruitment of loudness by alternate binaural loudness balance. *J. Speech Hearing Disorders*, 30, 263–268.

O'Neill, J. and Oyer, H. 1966. Applied audiometry. New York: Dodd, Mead.

Rainville, M. 1959. New method of masking for the determination of bone-conduction curves. *Translations Beltone Inst. Hearing Res.* 11.

Reger, S. 1936. Differences in loudness response of the normal and hard-of-hearing ear at intensity levels slightly above the threshold. *Ann. Otol., Rhinol., Laryng.*, 45, 1029–1039.

———. 1965. Pure tone audiometry. *In* Audiometry: principles and practices. Glorig, A., ed. Baltimore: Williams & Wilkins. Pp. 108–150.

———. 1967. The Békésy audiometer stimulus. *In* Sensorineural hearing processes and disorders. Graham, A. B., ed. Boston: Little, Brown. Pp. 235–243.

———, and Kos, C. 1952. Clinical measurements and implications of recruitment. *Ann. Otol., Rhinol., Laryng.*, 61, 810–823.

Shapiro, I., and Naunton, R. 1967. Audiological evaluation of acoustic neurinomas. *J. Speech Hearing Disorders*, 32, 29–35.

Sørensen, H. 1962. Clinical application of continuous threshold recording. *Acta Otolaryng.*, 54, 403–422.

Studebaker, G. 1964. Clinical masking of air- and bone-conducted stimuli. *J. Speech Hearing Disorders*, 29, 23–35.

Tillman, T. 1967. The assessment of sensorineural acuity. *In* Sensorineural hearing processes and disorders, Graham, A. B., ed. Boston: Little, Brown. Pp. 211–221.

Yantis, P. 1959. Clinical application of the temporary threshold shift. *A.M.A. Arch. Otolaryng.*, 70, 779–787.

Zwislocki, J. 1963. An acoustic method for clinical examination of the ear. *J. Speech Hearing Res.*, 6, 303–314.

14

Functional Hearing Loss

Donald B. Kinstler

INTRODUCTION

The subject of functional or nonorganic hearing loss has received considerable attention for many years from the physician and (more recently) the audiologist. Chaiklin and Ventry (1965) list over 400 entries in a bibliography on functional deafness, which is admittedly incomplete and lists relatively few foreign publications.

Although functional hearing loss or functional overlay has long been a recognized clinical entity, only recently have reasonably accurate methods been developed to measure organic thresholds in subjects who are unable or unwilling to respond accurately in the test situation.

As functionality itself becomes more readily identifiable, the problems posed by functional loss—diagnosis, evaluation, establishment of organic threshold, attitude toward the patient, possibility of resolution of functional component or treatment of the patient—are of increasing concern to the clinical audiologist, to the otologist, and to those involved in rehabilitation of the deafened.

This chapter will inquire into the nature of functional loss and its incidence, discuss behavioral clues that may alert the audiologist or physician to nonorganic components, consider the application of conventional and a few of the newer audiometric tests, and add some notes based upon personal clinical experience. Medicolegal aspects of functionality, which should be useful to the student of audiology and to the interested otologist, will be stressed.

DEFINITION OF TERMS

Functional hearing loss, the term used here to designate hearing loss for which no organic basis can be determined or inferred, does not imply that the origin is hysterical or psychogenic, nor does it necessarily imply that the origin is conscious exaggeration of an underlying organic defect, or simply deliberate malingering. A good deal of confusion has resulted from the variety of terms used (and still used) among audiologists and otologists. Brockman and Hoversten (1960) employ the term "pseudo neural hypacusis"; Goldstein (1966) prefers "pseudo-hypacusis"; Doerfler (1951) proposed "psychogenic deafness" to include all nonorganic hearing loss, although the Doerfler-Stewart test is called "a test for malingering"; Dixon and Newby (1959) chose "nonorganic hearing problems"; and several other variants are occasionally encountered. Chaiklin and Ventry (1963, p. 77) have examined the nomenclature problem in some detail and suggest that the term "functional hearing loss" is most meaningful when it is defined " . . . operationally . . . and based on intra-test or inter-test audiometric discrepancies as well as medical examinations that rule out apparent organic conditions that might account for the discrepancies." In an earlier article (Ventry and Chaiklin, 1962, p. 252) they also include " . . . discrepancies between observed behavior and audiometric findings . . . ." They reserve the term "psychogenic hearing loss" for those losses in which the psychological origin is apparent.

Earlier writers carefully distinguish between "malingering," "exaggeration," and "psychogenic deafness." Fournier (1958, p. 3) points out that we have no word for "the deception which consists in an attempt by the traumatized subject to pretend that the very real deficiency by which he is affected is attributable to . . . [a] . . . trauma, when it is, in fact, a deafness due to a different cause and of an earlier origin."

Portmann and Portmann (1961) believed that it was possible to distinguish between psychogenic hearing loss and malingering, and outlined a procedure for making this distinction. However, with the exception of a very few individuals, audiologists today are in agreement that we have no means by which we can distinguish between conscious deception and unconscious or hysterical hearing loss. It is generally agreed that the distinction, if there truly is one, need not be the responsibility of the audiologist. Feldman (1965, p. 107) has stated that . . . "whether or not the patient is aware of hearing better than he admits is of little consequence to the audiologist."

Goldstein (1966, p. 341), however, takes the position that . . . "all [nonorganic] hearing losses in adults and children . . . are feigned and . . . should be designated as pseudo-hypacusis. . . ." He found in an "exhaustive study" of major American journals over the past 10 years " . . . not a single case study in which conscious feigning could be ruled out" (p. 343). In his own extensive clinical practice he found no cases that he could " . . . interpret as anything except simulation or else an organic loss of unusual enough nature to present seemingly conflicting data but which could be resolved into a logical clinical picture. . . ." (p. 344).

Goldstein's two criteria for true psychogenic hearing loss are 1. *consistent* failure to respond at certain hearing levels in behavioral audiometry although there is response to these levels in electrophysiologic audiometry or under hypnosis, and 2. auditory sensitivity to surroundings as good as but no better than that demonstrated in behavioral audiometry. Hopkinson (1967) objects to Goldstein's criteria, pointing out that she sees no basis for expecting psychogenic patients to be any more consistent than patients with organic loss. She supports Feldman's position and states that the question as to whether individuals with nonorganic loss are malingering or are psychogenic is academic.

Whether the patient deliberately or unconsciously fails to respond to certain sound stimuli, he does this because hearing either poses a psychological threat or because he stands to gain in some way from his actions. The gain for a child might be simply attention from his family, friends, or schoolmates. (In screening school children, a high incidence of functional loss is frequently encountered, particularly among children who are members of large families and possibly seek attention in this manner.) With adults, the motivation might be the financial gain to be obtained by an accident victim or an employee who has been exposed to high noise levels. As Feldman (1965, p. 108) has stated, there is ". . . no clear dichotomy between the malingerer and the hysteric. . . ." In all probability the most blatant malingering has some basis in psychological needs. Hopkinson (1967, p. 293) mentions that she has had patients admit malingering ". . . only four or five times" in 17 years of practice. Other audiologists have mentioned small numbers of admissions of malingering in years of clinical work. In his experience with a large number of suspected functional losses, the writer has never had a patient admit or even imply that he was malingering in spite of the fact that, unquestionably, many of them were well aware that their inconsistent slips were showing.

It has been found to be convenient, in written reports, to refer initially to cases of nonorganic loss as "functional or nonorganic hearing loss" and then to rely mainly upon the term "functional." By equating "nonorganic" with "functional," the possibility is reduced that "nonorganic" may be interpreted to mean "psychogenic" or that "functional" may be construed to be simply an impairment of function of unspecified etiology.

The term "malingering" should be avoided entirely. The audiologist may expect to be asked, at a compensation appeals board, for example, if a given patient could ". . . be said to be malingering?" The answer, of course, is "no." It is possible, however, to say that "there are discrepancies in test results" and that, "so far as can be determined, [the patient's] organic threshold of hearing is [at a given level]." Unless the audiologist is fortunate enough to have a patient admit that he is or was lying—and it is difficult to believe that this ever happens—he should refrain from use of the word "malingering" and its synonyms, "simulation," "dissimulation," "exaggeration," " and "faking," and from any implication that the patient's intent is other than completely honest and straightforward.

Apparent functional loss may, in some instances, be due to the fluctuations of undetected middle-ear involvement or even to the presence of an ear canal which collapses under earphone pressure.[1]

INCIDENCE OF FUNCTIONAL HEARING LOSS

The incidence of functional hearing loss is extremely difficult, if not impossible, to determine. The incidence depends upon criteria which may vary enormously. For example, the populations of which functional hearing losses form a part may be entirely dissimilar. The population of a Veterans Administration audiology center, consisting mainly of veterans who are eligible for compensation, would certainly differ from the population of a college outpatient clinic specializing in hearing-aid selection, and both would differ greatly from the population served by an otologist specializing in middle-ear surgery. In addition, in reporting incidence of nonorganicity, some physicians or audiologists may depend solely upon behavioral clues for diagnosis, some may use pure tone-speech threshold inconsistency as a criterion, and some may insist upon confirmation of discrepancies by electrophysiologic audiometry. Some clinics report all cases presenting initial discrepancies and some include only those subjects who persist in presenting discrepant results.

Attempts to obtain relatively current reports of incidence from various governmental agencies, including the Veterans Administration, the Surgeon-General's office, the Department of Defense, and many others, were not successful, although a brief report, which is discussed below, was obtained from the Department of the Army.

There is some information available concerning the incidence of functional hearing loss in World War II, although there is considerable disagreement among authorities. Albrite and Shutts (1955, p. 4), reporting on the activities of the Army Audiology and Speech Center at Walter Reed Hospital, make the following statement: "About 35 percent of the patients tested routinely require additional testing . . . to obtain the true threshold." The population tested was one of army personnel, dependents, and veterans with hearing losses of 30 decibels or more for the better ear in the speech range. In the eight years from 1947 through 1954 nearly 11,000 patients with hearing difficulties were seen at this center.

Bergman (1957), in a report on functional deafness at Hoff General Hospital during World War II, gives a slightly lower incidence among the soldiers admitted to this aural-rehabilitation center between 1943 and 1945. He states that of the 1,375 patients treated during this period for hearing problems, "approximately 84 percent suffered from organic ear disease *or from organic deafness with a functional overlay*"[2] (italics mine). Bergman continues, "A functional basis was suspected in most of the remaining cases but for various reasons could be established in not quite half." Presumably this means that functional loss, entirely apart from organic impairment with functional overlay, *was* established in slightly less than half of the remaining cases, or approximately eight percent.

In an analysis of the 650 patients admitted to the Hoff General Hospital during a nine-month period in 1945, 102 were selected for treatment by narcosynthesis; 17 other patients, who were not investigated, showed greatly improved hearing, and 68 other patients "who were thought to suffer from functional deafness could not be investigated . . . because of inadequate facilities and limited personnel" (p. 479). If these figures are added, we attain an incidence of 29 percent of the patients who were suspected of functional hearing loss.

Truex (1946) reported an eight percent incidence of functional loss among military patients at Deshon Army Hospital; Knapp and Gold (1950) give 10 percent as an estimated incidence of functional hearing loss among military personnel; whereas Martin (1946) estimated that 15 percent of all admissions to aural-rehabilitation centers had nonorganic loss, at least in part.

Johnson and his associates (1956, p. 155) reviewed

[1] Lynn (1967) has described a simple procedure for ruling out this possibility. He suggests the use of a standard MX-41 AR cushion which is alternately pressed against the pinna and released, as a tuning fork or bone-conduction receiver is activated on the midline of the skull. If there is no change in loudness or localization the meatus does not collapse. Coles (1967) reports an extremely low incidence (0.1 percent) of meatus collapse among adults. He suggests that it may occur more frequently only among children and the aged.

[2] This statement is difficult to interpret. Does the author mean that an appreciable portion of the 84 percent have functionality or simply that an unstipulated proportion of the group have some functional component?

the literature available for World War II auditory centers and state that ". . . approximately 10 to 15 percent of the military personnel treated had a hearing loss partly or entirely from nonorganic causes." They declare that there was an increase in the incidence of functional loss in the 10 years following World War II of from 10 percent to ". . . . something approaching 50 percent" among men discharged from military service. These figures were based upon a study of 500 veterans referred to a Veterans Administration Audiology Clinic for service-incurred hearing loss. The authors attribute the enormous increase (from 11 percent in 1951 to 45 percent in 1954) to 1. implementation of a monthly compensation policy rather than the previous lump-sum award, 2. use of the conversational voice test as a basis for award, and 3. inadequate counseling at the onset of the hearing loss. Obviously, increasing efficiency of the audiologic examiners, employing better equipment and more sophisticated techniques would tend, too, to identify many cases of nonorganic deafness which a few years earlier might have remained undiscovered.

Northern (1968) states that 3.1 percent of the total 1967 caseload for The Audiology and Speech Center, Walter Reed Hospital, was diagnosed as nonorganic. He points out that statistics from the center are biased because the center ". . . receives the large percentage of unresolved functional losses from all tri-service hearing evaluation facilities."

It is important to remember that in Army and Veterans Administration centers, incidence of functional or nonorganic loss is reported *after* resolution of cases through the use of advanced audiologic techniques followed by counseling or, in some cases, psychotherapy. These incidence figures, then, represent *unresolved* functional losses. Undoubtedly, the number of cases initially presenting functional loss is considerably greater.

In an effort to sample the incidence of functional loss today, a brief survey was made in one large western city. No reportable figures were obtainable from the Veterans Administration Audiology Center. An otologic group with a large surgical practice and a considerable diagnostic caseload reported an estimated "less than 2 percent" incidence. A group with a similar practice estimated "less than 1 percent," and an otolaryngologist who has a large general and surgical practice, with many patients who are involved in litigation because of traumatic or noise-induced hearing loss, estimates the incidence among his patients as five percent to 10 percent and "probably closer to 10 percent." It is reasonable to expect that the incidence of functional loss will vary in relationship to the proportion of medicolegal cases in the otologist's practice.

Feldman (1965, p. 109) makes the following statement: "The physician may expect 3 percent of his patients with hearing loss to fall in the . . . [functional hearing loss] . . . category. The incidence increases when compensation is a factor." (No source is given for this figure.)

Doerfler (1951, p. 1047) quotes the incidence of "psychogenic" hearing loss as ". . . from 10–20 percent of a series of routine admissions to military hearing centers." (No source is given for this figure.) He states that a University of Pittsburgh survey of 30 audiology centers showed that 53 percent of the centers reported *few cases or only an occasional psychogenic case*, 37 percent reported one to five percent, reported one to five percent, and seven percent and 10 percent reported figures in excess of five percent. Seventy-four percent of the centers reported few or no psychogenic cases for children, 21 percent reported one to five percent, and seven percent over five percent. The incidence at the University of Pittsburgh *was three percent of the caseload.* Doerfler cautions that patient load in audiology centers is highly screened, with the majority of cases referred by otologists, presumably because of difficulties in diagnosis, and therefore these figures may not represent the true incidence of occurrence.

Doerfler adds that those clinics reporting few cases depended for indication of functional loss upon 1. discrepancy of test results with manifest pathology or case history, or with observable behavior; 2. discrepancy of pure-tone and speech-hearing tests; or 3. discrepancy of speech with extent of hearing loss. Those clinics reporting higher incidence used specific tests for functional loss.

With the wide divergence in clinical populations and in the criteria for inclusion of patients in the functional loss category it is probably best to cite incidence figures only for carefully defined populations with carefully specified criteria. It is safe to say, however, that the incidence of functional hearing loss among the civil population is increasing and will continue to increase with the continuing upsurge in compensation claims for hearing impairment due to accidents and to industrial noise exposure. It is suspected that the recent presence at the gates of a California steel plant of a trailer providing free testing of employees' hearing was not a unique phenomenon. The trailer was provided, not by management, but by a firm of attorneys who represent union members in compensation claim cases and were prepared to file suits on the behalf of any employees with hearing impairment. It is reasonable to assume that, in a test situation in which potential financial gain is in inverse proportion to reported sensitivity, some individuals will—consciously or unconsciously—exaggerate impairment.

BEHAVIORAL INDICATIONS OF FUNCTIONAL LOSS

There is a wealth of reports in the literature, especially the earlier literature, listing "clues" which should alert the otologist to the possible presence of functional hearing loss. Indeed, some of the earlier reports detail how distinctions can be made among malingering, psychogenic, and "true" organic loss.

Fournier (1958, p. 3), dismissing malingerers as ". . . young conscripts coming from backward areas for whom the barracks presents a priori fewer attractions than their native hamlets," declares (pp. 7–8) that the malingerer's attitude ". . . fortunately for the expert . . . is quite characteristic." He states that the malingerer pretending unilateral deafness "often mimics the person with bilateral deafness . . . ," asks the audiologist to speak louder and may even cup his hand at his ear. The bilateral malingerer ". . . most often has a stupid expression . . . is afraid of scrutiny and lowers his eyes . . . asks that one write what one expects of him . . . others pretend to know how to read lips," although constant attention to the speaker's face ". . . is not always essential to them."

Inconsistency between pure-tone audiometric responses and conversational ability apart from the test situation is given as a clue to the existence of functional loss by Brockman and Hoversten (1960), Newby (1964), Doerfler (1951), and Feldman (1965). Patients with functional loss often seem to understand conversational or casual speech at levels far lower than their voluntary responses to pure-tone audiometry would suggest.

Johnson, Work, and McCoy (1956, p. 159) list a number of criteria which they believe point toward possible functional loss. They include the presence of serious emotional disorder, exaggerated attempts to hear or understand, excessively loud voice, nervousness, and comments apparently intended to account for discrepancies, such as "the ringing in my ears confuses me."

Doerfler (1951) reports that surprisingly good response to therapy or counseling, in which the hearing quickly recovers or improves disproportionately to expectation, is a sign of possible functionality, as is sudden onset of binaural perceptive hearing loss. (It is rare to find normal or near-normal bone-conduction responses with raised thresholds for air conduction.)

Feldman (1965) counsels that the physician should suspect nonorganicity whenever financial gain is a possibility, when the origin of the loss is vague or uncertain, when the onset is sudden with no obvious etiology, or when the patient has a history of psychosomatic complaints. He adds (p. 108) that hearing screening of children ". . . often acts to suggest a symptom to the child." Feldman lists as clues to possible nonorganicity 1. exaggeration of the impairment's effect upon communication, 2. response of patient wearing earphones to a soft conversational inquiry, 3. exaggeration of the use of the "good" ear and apparent inability with unilateral loss to localize sound, 4. attributing to lipreading skill the ability to sustain communication, and 5. normal loudness, quality, and precision of speech of patients with alleged profound hearing loss.

The use or misuse of a hearing aid has frequently been cited as a clue to the presence of nonorganic hearing loss. Unfamiliarity with the aid, use of insufficient volume, unrealistic statements as to battery life, extraordinary improvement or lack of improvement in hearing with the aid, the successful use of a low-gain aid with a severe loss are typical anachronisms which should warn the audiologist to investigate the possibility of functional loss.

Newby (1964) suggests that the audiologist look for behavior inconsistent with the purported loss. He mentions the patient's apparent difficulty in understanding and suggests that the tester observe how closely the patient is watching him. He also advocates that the examiner occasionally turn his head away from the patient while speaking to him, or drop his voice and speak rapidly. The patient's own speech should be attended to and Newby points out that a well-controlled voice with good articulation is inconsistent with marked hearing loss. Newby and many others have listed the presence of anxiety, especially prior to and during electrodermal response audiometry, as an indicant of nonorganicity.

At this time there has been no published research on the correlation between observed behavior and functional hearing loss. Certainly many of the "clues" mentioned above are useful to the audiologist and suggest possible nonorganicity, but it certainly would be incorrect, at this time, to use these "clues" as a basis for making a diagnosis.

A most serious concern of the clinic director is the effect of behavioral "clues" upon the inexperienced clinician. If the clinician makes a decision that a patient has a functional loss based upon the patient's behavior, the clinician's objectivity (and his usefulness as an examiner) is reduced if not lost. For the clinician already biased toward finding functionality, behavior can easily be misinterpreted. Unquestionably, behavioral clues can be valuable indicants of the need for careful appraisal and further examination, but they should remain just that—clues, not definitive findings.

CLUES IN MEDICAL EXAMINATION

The lack of an apparent physiologic basis (no history of ear disease; normal meatus, tympanic membrane, and middle-ear function; absence of nasopharyngeal pathology or vertigo; negative responses to vascular, electroencephalic, and radiologic laboratory tests) in sudden onset of hearing loss may suggest the possibility of functionality. Lack of agreement between the alleged loss and the results of tuning-fork tests may also point toward the possibility of nonorganic loss. Johnson and his associates (1956) list as discrepancies lack of lateralization to the occluded ear in the Weber test, variations in response to Rinné and Schwabach, momentary response to tone, and inconsistency between tuning-fork and audiometric responses.

Heller and Anderman (1955) describe in detail many "clues" to be found by the physician in the course of history-taking and preliminary examination. However, Chaiklin and Ventry (1965) report, in their NIH multidisciplinary study of functional hearing loss, that few variables in clinical history were significant in distinguishing functional loss. Those variables that were significantly different were tinnitus (higher incidence), subjective loudness of tinnitus (greater), interference with hearing by tinnitus (more), higher incidence of exposure to noise trauma, and more frequent report of history of ear disease. The tuning-fork tests proved not to be very useful in identification, nor did vestibular tests or neurological examinations, including EEG. They found that the combination of medical history, otolaryngolic examination and tuning-fork tests identified 53 percent (N=100) correctly. There were also a few false positive identifications.

CONVENTIONAL AUDIOMETRIC TESTS WITH FUNCTIONAL HEARING LOSS

Pure-Tone Audiometry

Perhaps the most frequently used index of functionality is test-retest reliability of pure-tone audiometry. Lack of consistency in pure-tone response is certainly a strong indicator of the presence of functional loss or overlay (Newby, 1958; Heller and Anderman, 1955; Watson and Tolan, 1949; Chaiklin and Ventry, 1963). Most authorities agree that test-retest differences exceeding 15 dB are suspect (Chaiklin et al., 1961). Differences of 15 dB or more are, barring a known organic basis for fluctuation, certainly sufficient grounds for the initiation of special test procedures. On the other hand, good test-retest reliability should not rule out the possibility of functional loss.

Harris (1958) has described a simple method of screening subjects by requiring responses to alternately ascending and descending tone presentations, which is designed to make maintenance of an artificially raised threshold more difficult. Again, results when negative should not rule out nonorganic loss. It has been demonstrated many times that some subjects have an almost uncanny ability to maintain elevated thresholds consistently.

The flat or "saucer" audiogram has often been mentioned as an indicator of functional loss (Doerfler, 1951; Fournier, 1958). The underlying theory is that the subject is more or less following equal-loudness contours, or is equating loudness for the several frequencies. Doerfler suggests that a subject simulating a hearing loss may take a comfortable loudness level as a reference or criterion for maintaining an elevated threshold. For normal ears this would be an equal-loudness contour at about 60 dB. Chaiklin and Ventry (1965), however, found no significant incidence of the saucer or flat audiogram among their experimental group (N=36) and concluded that presence of this configuration has limited utility in diagnosis. Certainly much care should be exercised in using this "clue", since saucer or flat audiograms often appear in purely organic hearing loss and also an underlying organic deficit may serve to distort the audiometric response pattern.

Lack of lateralization as demonstrated by the absence of a shadow curve, or an unusually high threshold for the poorer ear in cases of unilateral hearing loss, may be a strong indication of functionality. This is especially true with bone conduction audiometry where unilateral loss or losses differing even moderately between ears should produce a shadow curve for the poorer ear when no masking is employed. It simply is not possible to have no response to air-conduction stimuli in the "poorer" ear if the "better" ear is normal or near-normal and no masking is used. You would not normally expect, either, to find differences of 50 or more dB between the two ears especially in the low and middle frequencies when the better ear has not been masked.

There have been many reports as to behavior indicative of nonorganic hearing loss during pure-tone audiometry (Chaiklin and Ventry, 1961; Doerfler, 1951; Johnson et al., (1965). One commonly observed phenomenon is the absence or infrequency of false positive responses. Most patients with organic hearing loss will, on occasion, respond when no stimulus is present or the stimulus is far below threshold. It seems to be true that functional cases rarely have false positive or "false alarm" responses. Chaiklin and Ventry (1965) found that 86 percent of the control group (N=64) in the NIH study gave false alarm responses as contrasted with only 22 percent of the functional group (N=36). They suggest that the absence of false positive responses be used as a criterion of functionality, in conjunction with other criteria.

Behavior accompanying pure-tone audiometry which is considered to be characteristic of functional hearing loss:

1. Attitude implying great strain or painful effort to hear the signal.
2. Frequent adjustment of earphones, ostensibly in effort to hear better.
3. Very slow and tentative response with finger signal; very slight excursion of finger to indicate detection of sound.
4. Slight twitch of finger as signal introduced but no definite response until signal strength has been increased.
5. Inconsistent responses, sometimes followed by improvement in consistency after audiometrist's statement regarding patient's possible misunderstanding of instructions.
6. Patient wearing earphones responds to softly spoken inquiry. (e.g., "In which ear are you hearing the tone?")
7. Flinching or nervousness in subject with alleged total loss when examiner introduces brief burst of very strong intensity. This technique, originally suggested by Fournier (1958), is not recommended.
8. Responses to "booby catchers" (Fournier, 1958) which are sudden unexpected commands or remarks at low intensity (e.g., "Stand up." "Open your mouth." "Your trousers are open.").
9. Response to second or third presentation of tone at an intensity lower than previously determined level.

Speech Audiometry

The relationship between the responses to pure-tone audiometry and speech-audiometry thresholds is perhaps the most widely used tool of the audiologist in the evaluation of functional hearing loss. "In the investigation of medico-legal cases [with this relationship] one can nearly always establish psychogenic overlay" (Lidén, 1967, p. 339). The pure-tone average (PTA) for the three central speech frequencies (500, 1000, 2,000 Hz) should agree within ±5 dB with the speech-reception (spondee) threshold unless unusual conditions are encountered, such as severe sensorineural deficit with consequent elevation of the speech threshold (Lidén, 1960). It is patent that if a subject's spondee threshold is markedly better than his three-frequency pure-tone average, (e.g., ST 14 dB, PTA 40 dB) he has a functional problem. It is highly improbable that any patient can hear and repeat spondee words at levels considerably lower than the levels at which he can just perceive pure-tone signals in the same frequency range. Fortunately for the audiologist attempting to determine organic thresholds in functional hearing loss, many subjects respond to speech signals at considerably lower levels than they respond to pure tones. It is not unusual to observe subjects with allegedly marked or severe hearing loss respond blithely to speech at normal or close-to-normal levels.

Assuming that the speech circuit of the audiometer has been calibrated to approximate pure-tone levels for the central-speech frequencies, it is possible to predict the spondee threshold by averaging the three central speech (500 to 2,000 Hz) frequencies. When there is an interfrequency difference in excess of 10 dB the two lower frequencies are most often used (Graham, 1960). If the audiometer is calibrated differently for speech than for pure tone, allowance must be made for this difference. It is generally agreed that pure-tone average and speech-reception thresholds differing by more than ±10 dB may be suggestive of functional hearing loss with the greater the discrepancy the greater the likelihood of functionality (Brockman and Hoversten, 1960; Feldman, 1965; Chaiklin and Ventry, 1963; Fournier, 1958; Newby, 1958). In the National Institute of Health study reported by Chaiklin and Ventry (1965), the ST-PTA relationship was the most efficient of the five audiometric measures investigated, with 70 percent of the functional subjects identified by this means. (Chaiklin and Ventry used a difference in the same ear of at least 12 dB between PTA and ST as their criterion.)

The PTA-ST difference most often is in the direction of lower spondee thresholds than pure-tone averages, although the opposite condition is occasionally encountered. Subnormal pure-tone response with responses to speech at normal levels are most frequently given by children, but a surprising number of adults give significantly better responses to speech than to pure tones. There have been a number of attempts to explain the reason for the functional subject's admission of lower levels for speech than for pure tones. Juers (1956) attributed this phenomenon in children to regression to an early pattern where the very young infant seems not to respond to pure-tone stimuli although hearing for speech may be normal. Noting wistfully in a later article (1966, p. 1714) that this theory ". . . has not created much of a flurry in audiologic circles," he then hypothesized that, since speech has a broader frequency range than a single pure tone, the total acoustic energy is greater, and more of the patient's sensorineural elements are stimulated with a consequent increase in loudness. He feels, too, that the same condition may account for the Type V Békésy tracing, in which the responses to continuous stimuli are better than those for interrupted stimuli.

In those cases in which the functional loss is a result of conscious design, it may be reasonable to speculate that the patient, unaware of the relationship between pure tone and speech, and pinning his hopes for recompense on "scientific testing" which he would equate with pure-tone audiometry, may relax his guard slightly and respond at lower levels of intensity. If Juers is correct, greater acoustic energy of the speech signals innervates a greater number of neural responses, and since the patient's impression is one of greater loudness, he is willing to acknowledge hearing at lower levels of intensity.

Speech-Reception Thresholds, Speech-Sound-Discrimination Tests

The audiologist who works with functional hearing loss to any extent soon becomes aware of the functional subject's divergent responses to stimulus words in speech-threshold testing. The functional-loss patient may repeat only half of the spondee ("boy" for "cowboy," "ball" for "baseball"), although he has been carefully instructed to guess if he is not certain and has been thoroughly briefed on the test words to be given. Some audiologists (Fournier, 1958; Chaiklin and Ventry, 1963; Johnson et al., 1956) have reported that some patients will repeat only the first half and others only the second half of the stimulus word. Occasionally, a patient will repeat the half-word which is weaker, acoustically, or will fail to respond at all to a word after having easily repeated two or three words at the same or even a lower level. No quantitative analysis was made of these differences until Chaiklin and Ventry (1965) investigated patient errors in the NIH study. They found a greater incidence of total errors and of no-response errors among the experimental group. They also found significant ($P < .001$) differences in 1. errors consisting of the first half or of the second half of the stimulus, 2. errors consisting of one-syllable words which did not contain part of the stimulus, and 3. errors consisting of substitution of other spondee words from the list (e.g., *farewell* for *baseball*). Chaiklin and Ventry's subjects had a disproportionate number of no-responses, half-stimulus word responses, and one-syllable words not containing-part-of-the-stimulus responses. Based upon these findings, a spondee error index (SERI)[3] was constructed and preliminary evaluation with male veterans yielded encouraging results. Eighty-five percent of the functional group ($N=20$) had positive scores and 87 percent of the nonfunctional group ($N=30$) had negative scores. However, it is questionable whether the results obtained, which provide no hint of the organic threshold, merit the time required to analyze

[3] $$\mathrm{SERI} = \frac{\mathrm{NRE} + \mathrm{OS} - \mathrm{SL}}{\mathrm{TE}} \times 100$$

NRE = no response errors; OS = one-syllable response; SL = spondee from list; TE = total errors. Scores of 86 or higher are considered positive; 85 or lower are considered negative.

each patient's responses and apply the formula.

It is important to acquaint the subject with the spondee words before beginning the spondee-threshold test. One technique often used is to read each word aloud as the subject is shown the card upon which the word is typed. In order to avoid giving the patient a loudness reference level amplification should not be used during this preparatory period.

Most clinical audiologists agree that it is better to begin the audiologic examination with speech audiometry in cases of suspected functional loss. Menzel (1960) found that the incidence and degree of non-organic hearing loss is drastically reduced when pure-tone audiometry is deferred until completion of speech audiometry or electrodermal audiometry, or both. The Veterans Administration Audiology Centers' usual procedure for testing veterans where compensation is involved is to begin testing with speech audiometry.

The binaural speech-reception (spondee) threshold test is a logical test with which to begin and you can, if you wish, easily swing into the Doerfler-Stewart and then the monaural spondee thresholds. Monaural speech thresholds obtained with the bone conduction receiver are occasionally useful. If you know the bone conducted speech threshold for normals with your audiometer this level can be subtracted from the patient's acknowledged threshold and his organic speech threshold thereby estimated. Some audiologists proceed from the Spondee Threshold (S.T.) to pure-tone audiometry, but there may be an advantage in going directly from S.T. to speech-discrimination tests. It has been observed that many patients, immediately after having listened for spondaic words at low levels of intensity, respond accurately to the discrimination test words at relatively low intensities, perhaps because these levels then seem, in contrast, to be loud.

Accurate responses to the speech-discrimination test words (C.I.D. Auditory Test W-22s, in most cases) can provide information relevant not merely to the presence or absence of functionality but to the actual organic threshold as well. Regardless of the spondee-threshold level, if a patient achieves a respectable score (let us say 90–100 percent) in sound field at a hearing level of 35–40 dB, it is clear that this patient has binaural hearing for speech which is close to normal. By the same reasoning it is safe to say that a patient achieving a good score binaurally, at, say 55 dB hearing level might be said to have a hearing level for speech which does not exceed 20–25 dB in the important speech frequencies (500–3,000 Hz).

Errors in response to the speech-discrimination test words have been analyzed by Campbell (1965). In an attempt to establish an objective evaluation of "unreasonable" patient response, he developed an index of "pseudo-discrimination loss" (PDL). Errors in patient response are divided into four categories: 1. typical or characteristic errors; 2. uncommon errors; 3. missed easy words; and 4. no response. PDL values are obtained by dividing the sum of the last three categories (2, 3, and 4) by category 1. Values obtained of less than .7 are negative; values from .6 to 1.7 are marginal; and values in excess of 1.7 are considered to be indicative of extra-auditory influence. A validation study (N=80) yielded a Spearman rho correlation of .70 between PDL and the judgment of "three clinical audiologists experienced in discrimination test administration and interpretation."

Although there are numerous advantages in the use of recorded speech tests for normal clinical practice, monitored live voice is frequently preferable in the medicolegal testing of functional loss. It is often necessary to have the greatest flexibility in order to obtain maximal responses, and this can best be attained with live voice. It is surprising how often a subject will give no immediate response to speech stimuli but will respond if the tester simply waits long enough. If a subject fails to respond to a word, repetition of the word with slightly sharper emphasis may elicit a correct response. The radio and television commercial announcer's technique of moving away from the microphone and speaking at a slightly greater intensity produces a sharper tone without increasing the output and often encourages a subject to respond to a lower level of intensity.

Stenger and Speech Stenger

The Stenger test is one of the oldest tests used specifically for the detection of functional hearing loss. It was originally designed for use with a pair of matched tuning forks (Stenger, 1907), but it is now usually performed with a two-channel audiometer. It can be done (Watson and Tolan, 1949) with two perfectly calibrated audiometers or with the use of an accessory box which can be obtained for single-channel audiometers. The Stenger test is based upon the phenomenon that a tone delivered simultaneously to two ears can be perceived only by the ear in which the tone has greater intensity. The Stenger test is effective with unilateral hearing loss or with bilateral loss in which there is a marked difference in hearing levels between the two ears. A minimum of 20 dB admitted difference in threshold between ears is usually considered to be necessary (Newby, 1964).

There is presently no standardized technique for giving the Stenger test although Watson and Tolan (1949), Newby (1958), Fournier (1958), and others have described the test and Altshuler (1970) offers a model procedure for its administration. In essence, a pulsed tone is presented to the "better" ear at threshold level and an identical tone is presented simultaneously to the "poorer" ear at levels below the acknowledged threshold for that ear. As little as 10 dB increased intensity in hearing level will mask out the tone in the better ear. The subject then hears the tone only in his "poorer" ear and is faced with two alternatives: 1. he can signal that he no longer hears the tone which, although inaudible to him, is still present in his better ear, or 2. he can continue to respond to the tone. In the latter case the tester may fade out the tone in the better ear, demonstrating that the patient is responding to a tone in his poorer ear at a level well below his voluntary threshold. The Stenger test is usually considered to be positive if either of these two alternatives occurs. Of course, if the subject does not hear the tone in the poorer ear he will continue to respond to the better-ear stimulus. Chaiklin and Ventry (1965) consider a result positive when the subject indicates an organic threshold 15 dB below his previously admitted voluntary threshold.

The Stenger test is an extremely efficient test for the detection of unilateral impairment. It can be used not only as a measure of functionality but as a means for estimating "true" organic threshold. Obviously, the tone level delivered to the "poor" ear at which the patient ceases to respond to previously acknowledged hearing (in the "better" ear) is a level at which the patient hears, and since at least 10 dB is required to mask the better ear, five dB *less* than this level safely reflects the subject's minimum organic threshold for his "poor" ear. When similar levels are calculated for each frequency, an overall organic threshold for the poorer ear can be estimated.

One limitation in utilizing the Stenger test as a means of determining organic threshold for the poor ear is that this determination depends upon the subject's willingness (or ability) to admit relatively good hearing in the "better" ear. Newby (1964) points out, too, that diplacusis may make this test ineffective, although there is no experimental evidence of this at the present time. Variations of the Stenger test can also be given, such as the Noise Stenger test in which white noise, complex noise, or narrow-band white noise is used as the stimulus. The procedure is the same and problems which occasionally occur with pure-tone stimuli may be avoided.

The efficiency of the Stenger test has been seriously questioned by some writers. Chaiklin and Ventry found in their NIH study that it was the least useful of their five audiometric measures, identifying only 43 percent of the 21 subjects to whom the test was applicable. However, many audiologists have found the Stenger test extremely useful—possibly more useful than any other single test for unilateral hearing loss. For example, Feldman (1965) declares that the Stenger test is the most efficient procedure for validating differences in thresholds between ears. Kinstler, Sheehan, and Lavender (1971) reported excellent results in a study of functional hearing loss patients (N=35) with Speech Stenger tests and found that, contrary to Chaiklin and Ventry's findings, relatively large interaural sensitivity differences were not requisite for obtaining positive results.

The Modified or Speech Stenger test is performed in almost identical fashion to the Stenger test, and the principle is basically the same. The most frequently used procedure is to set the level for the "better" ear at a level slightly higher in intensity than the admitted spondee threshold for that ear, and then deliver speech simultaneously to the "poorer" ear at levels 10 dB or more above the level for the better ear. In a functional loss the patient will either stop repeating the stimulus words as they disappear from the "good" ear, or he may continue to repeat them, in which event the tester may fade out the good ear. It is good practice, in medicolegal audiology, to deliver five or six spondee words to the subject in the good ear and then use the identical words when the speech is introduced simultaneously to the poor ear. A positive Speech Stenger test should produce an approximation of the spondee threshold for the poorer ear and suggest the averaged acuity for the three central (500 to 2,000 Hz) speech frequencies.

There is no standardized procedure for administering the Speech Stenger test, nor is there any commonly accepted criterion for determination of a positive result. Chaiklin and Ventry (1965) consider the test to be positive when it produces a speech threshold which is 15 dB or more below the voluntary speech threshold in the poorer ear. The results of this test were inconclusive in the NIH study; it proved to be only 40 percent (N=15) efficient in identifying functional hearing loss. Chaiklin and Ventry found, however, that subjects with large interaural differences and those with relatively large functional components in the poorer ear were more likely to have positive scores in both of the Stenger tests.

There are audiologists (including this writer) who believe that the Speech Stenger test is an extremely efficient test of functionality in those cases where it can be used. Newby (1958, p. 159) described the test as one which is "practically infallible" when used by an expert, although this statement does not appear in the 1965 edition of his text. Menzel (1960) reported that the Speech Stenger test was 85 percent effective as a "true indicator" of nonorganic hearing loss for applicable cases in his nonorganic group (N=55). Consultation with audiologists employed in two Veterans Administration Centers indicated that they placed strong reliance upon, and confidence in, both the Stenger and the Speech Stenger tests as tests for determination of functional hearing loss.

Lombard

Lombard's test is based upon the observation that a speaker reflexively increases the intensity of his speech as the ambient noise in his environment increases. It is one of the very earliest tests and it was performed originally with mechanical noisemakers, such as the Bárány. The audiometer is now used; a complex or white noise is introduced into one or both ears as the patient reads aloud. He will tend to raise the level of his voice as the noise becomes louder, and it is possible to make a rough estimate of the level at which he hears by careful attention to the intensity levels at which he raises his voice.

The Lombard is a relatively crude test, at best, but since it takes little time and is easy to give, many otologists employ it as a screening device. Unfortunately, some subjects seem to have little difficulty in monitoring the intensity of their voices and there is evidence that sophisticated subjects are able to control their voice levels regardless of the intensity of the noise delivered. The Lombard is considered positive if a patient discernibly raises the level of his voice at an intensity level below his admitted threshold of hearing, and negative if he does not raise his voice below this level. A positive Lombard may suggest the possibility of functionality but a negative Lombard should, by no means, be interpreted to mean that no functional component is present. The test has not been standardized and its usefulness seems to be limited to serving simply as a rough-and-ready device for screening.

Swinging Tone or Speech Test

This test for unilateral hearing loss, which is also known as the shifting tone or voice test, is an old test designed originally to be performed with tuning forks. The procedure is to shift the voice or tone rapidly from one ear to the other in the expectation that the patient with functional loss will become confused and respond to stimuli delivered below the admitted threshold for the poorer ear. Watson and Tolan enthusiastically report (1949, p. 175) that the procedure ". . . will generally confuse and catch all but the cleverest malingerers." They suggest a modification of the test, considered to be "more reliable," in which the patient is asked a question which is delivered to the good ear and then quickly altered in meaning by delivery of a final phrase to the poor ear. The following is an example, given by Watson and Tolan (1949, p. 176): *Delivered to the admittedly good ear:* "Do you hear well in a theatre . . . *To the questionable ear:* . . . if you sit at the back?"

Chaiklin and Ventry dismiss this test on ethical grounds and because of skepticism about the test's utility (1963, p. 108) ". . . we find it difficult to recommend a test which relies on putting pressure on the patient . . . which depends on the patient's confusion. . . ." This writer has long since abandoned its use on the basis that it simply doesn't work very well.

Doerfler-Stewart

The Doerfler-Stewart (D-S) test is based upon the assumption that a patient with a functional loss or overlay establishes and maintains an elevated speech threshold through reference to ambient or environmental noise. The D-S test attempts to disturb this reference level by the superimposition of complex (sawtooth) masking noise at various levels of intensity. Detailed procedures are given by Newby in the 1958 edition of his text. Newby deleted the procedures from the revised edition of his text (1964, p. 161) in saying ". . . there is now some question concerning the efficiency of this test. . . ." Newby was referring to the Chaiklin and Ventry study (1965) in which they found no significant difference between their experimental and control groups on the D-S test. In the NIH study, the D-S test incorrectly identified 50 percent of the Nonfunctional Group as functional and 58 percent of the Functional Group as nonfunctional. It is difficult to account for this finding, as nearly all other available evidence has shown this test to be valid and reliable. Menzel (1960, p. 52) for example, found that 58 percent of the subjects with functional components for whom the test was applicable (N=83) had positive D-S scores, and D-S results were a "true indicator" for the nonorganic component group for 92 percent. The D-S test, of course, should be considered a screening test, and positive results should lead to further investigation of the patient's threshold.

Although there has been little other formal research on the efficiency of the Doerfler-Stewart test, many audiologists (O'Neill and Oyer, 1966; Davis and Goldstein, 1964; Glorig, 1965; and others) have strongly endorsed this test. For example, Glorig (1965, p. 238) states, "This [D-S] is one of the best tests available, for it provides a qualitative and a quantitative estimate of impairment." Consultation with several clinical directors, including two Veterans Administration chief audiologists, supports the impression that the D-S test is held in high esteem and is used routinely in suspected functional hearing loss, and it is always used with hearing losses exceeding 30 dB.

Since adherence to the prescribed procedure for administration of the test is mandatory, a brief outline of the procedure and a form for recording results based upon current practice follows:[4]

Doerfler-Stewart Work Sheet

MEASURE	LEVEL
(*A*) ST[1]	
(*B*) ST[1] +4	
(*C*) NIL	
(*D*) ST[2]	
(*E*) NDT	

DIFFERENCE LIMIT

(*A*)–(*D*)		−4 to +6
(*A*)–(*E*)		−7 to +15
(*B*)–(*C*)		−18 to +3
(*D*)–(*E*)		−18 to +15
(*E*)–(*C*)		−31 to −2

General Instructions: D-S was designed to be administered binaurally, although some audiologists currently perform the test monaurally as well. The norms were established with complex or "sawtooth" masking noise with a 128 Hz base frequency. Doerfler and Epstein recommend performing the test prior to standard speech audiometry.

1. Obtain ST[1] (spondee threshold) by starting at zero dB and ascending in two-dB steps. Record.
2. Add four dB to ST[1] level. Record.
3. Introduce complex noise at zero dB, increase in 10-dB steps initially and then in two-dB steps as patient repeats spondees. When patient no longer repeats any spondees correctly, record as noise interference level (NIL).
4. Increase noise by 20 dB and decrease speech level to 10 dB below ST[1].
5. Decrease noise by five-dB steps with each one or two words given until noise is completely attenuated. (If patient begins to repeat words before noise is completely attenuated, decrease speech intensity by two-dB steps until patient no longer is able to repeat the spondee words. At this point, proceed as previously, reducing the noise until completely attenuated or patient begins repeating spondees again.) Increase speech by two-dB steps to attain ST[2]. Record.
6. Obtain noise detection level (NDT) by having patient signal when he perceives noise. Start at zero dB, use interrupter, and increase in two-dB steps until patient responds. Record.

The test is considered to be positive if any one of the difference scores falls outside the prescribed limits. Doerfler and Epstein (1956) advise that special consideration be given to the NIL and NDT scores, as they believe these to be more sensitive indicators of functional loss. (Ventry and Chaiklin, 1965, found these measures to be the least sensitive and suggest the use of three new norms developed by them.)

It should be stressed once more that, although the D-S test has proved to be extremely useful in the delineation of functionality, it should be considered

[4] The test was described originally by Doerfler and Stewart (1946). The norms, developed by Doerfler and Epstein (1956), have not been published for general distribution. See Newby (1958) for details. A few minor modifications (SRT+4 is now used rather than SRT+5, and, in Step 3, noise is increased until there is *no* response to the stimulus words), in keeping with current procedures have been made here.

a screening test and by no means infallible. Positive results do not necessarily mean that nonorganic hearing loss is present, nor do negative scores necessarily rule out nonorganicity.

Modified Doerfler-Stewart

A modification of the Doerfler-Stewart test is frequently employed for the purpose of obtaining a spondee threshold either binaurally or monaurally when a functional loss is suspected. The procedure entails presenting speech at approximately 5–10 dB below the expected level for ST with the masking noise presented simultaneously at 20 to 30 dB above. The noise is reduced in two-dB steps and, when the patient begins to respond, the speech is gradually reduced until the patient stops responding. The noise is again reduced until the patient begins to respond, and so on. The patient experiences the sensation of the speech emerging from or "arising out of" the noise and may respond to speech at intensities considerably lower than he will admit in routine speech threshold testing.

Electrodermal Audiometry

The principle of the psychogalvanic skin reflex (GSR), or as it is more often called, electrodermal response (EDR), was first described by Feré in 1888 and had been used by experimental psychologists in the measurement of various sensory modalities for many years before its application to the measurement of hearing by Wiersma (1915). More extensive employment of EDR began about 1947 with Bordley, Hardy, and Richter (1948) and Bordley and Hardy (1949) at Johns Hopkins. EDR involves conditioning a subject by presentation of a pure-tone stimulus accompanied by an unpleasant electric shock. Reduction in skin resistance to a low-voltage electric current is effected initially by the conditioned stimulus (shock), and then, after the subject has been conditioned, by the presentation of the unconditioned stimulus (tone), alone. Changes in resistance are amplified and recorded.

EDR is of great value in the determination of the true thresholds of subjects with suspected functional hearing loss. It is not necessary for the patient to cooperate in the testing other than by sitting quietly, and the results have been found to be not significantly different (Burk, 1958, found mean differences of approximately five dB, and Doerfler and McClure, 1954, found only 3.5-dB differences) from voluntary thresholds. Chaiklin et al. (1961) evaluated the reliability of conditioned EDR pure-tone audiometry by a test-retest technique. Their results confirm Doerfler's and McClure's, and Burk's findings, and suggest that reliability is good (95 percent of their 41 subjects had ± five-dB differences between test and retest) ". . . when conducted under well controlled conditions with suitable candidates" (p. 279).

Goldstein raises one of the few dissenting voices as to the efficacy of EDR. He reports (1956) that approximately half of a population of 20 consecutive cases were either difficult or impossible to condition. Commenting on Goldstein's contention, Chaiklin and Ventry (1963, p. 106) state that approximately 80 percent of their clinical subjects are conditioned successfully.

The use of EDR in examination for functional hearing loss provides not only a means for confirming the presence or absence of functionality, but serves also to establish qualitative organic thresholds. Most frequently, testing is done only at 1,000 Hz or at 500 and 2,000 Hz because of time limitations, but if a subject is easily conditioned (and many subjects are), there is no reason why a complete threshold for one or even both ears cannot be obtained. On occasion, application of the electrodes alone has such a salutory effect upon the subject that accurate voluntary thresholds can be obtained before the conditioning procedure is even begun.

Newby (1964) has set down in some detail the procedures utilized at the San Francisco Veterans Administration Hospital, which are fairly representative of current practice. A brief summary of these follows:

1. Pickup electrodes are placed on the index and ring fingers of the left hand; shock electrodes are placed similarly on the right hand and the ground plate is affixed to the right wrist. (The sole of the foot and the calf are also often used.) Set tone for one-second duration, delay .5 second and shock for .5 second.

2. The conditioning schedule is a random one, presenting tone (conditioned stimulus) alone or tone and shock (unconditioned stimulus) at 30, 45, or 60-second intervals, beginning at 10 dB above the best voluntary threshold for each frequency tested. Reinforcement is about 40 percent.

3. "Acceptable" responses are considered to be those with latency of not less than 1.5 seconds nor more than 3.5 seconds. The magnitude of excursion depends upon the sensitivity or gain

setting and should be determined during the sampling period.

4. Threshold "sampling" begins after establishment of conditioning. Again, 40 percent reinforcement is employed. Sampling begins at zero dB and is increased in 10-dB steps with reinforcement as scheduled occurring 40 percent of the time until a response occurs. "The testing is conducted concurrently for the two ears with the examiner switching from one ear when a UCR is obtained, to the other ear, and then back again. Threshold for each ear is based on the results accumulated from at least several 'passes' on both sides" (Barrett, 1969).

There is some disagreement with the concept of alternative presentation of tone to the two ears. Many audiologists prefer to complete one ear before switching to the other. Also, some audiologists, including this writer, do not adhere to a rigid 40 percent schedule but rather reinforce as seems to be required. There are cases where it is unnecessary to reinforce at all and there are cases where frequent reinforcement is required.

The level of shock is important, and an effort should be made to obtain the patient's permission to use enough shock to create at least a modicum of anxiety. It is suggested that, in the ideal situation, the patient is apprehensive and perhaps a bit fearful. Several studies (e.g., Welch, 1953) have indicated that the presence of anxiety is related to success in conditioning. It is best to arouse some apprehension but exercise care not to create overwhelming anxiety. For example, you might say, "This is going to be a bit unpleasant but, I hope, not too painful." Chaiklin, Ventry, and Barrett (1961, p. 272) recommend the use of the strongest tolerable unconditioned stimulus and suggest that the patient be encouraged to permit a gradual increase in intensity until the shock is "distinctly unpleasant but not painful." Gradual increase in the magnitude of the shock as the tone stimulus is reduced is particularly effective.

If the patient coughs, sighs, sneezes, or makes any obvious move, it should be noted on the recording tape. Portmann and Portmann (1961) report that some subjects attempt to disrupt EDR results by surreptitious movement during the test session, and advise patience on the part of the examiner. They cite (p. 252) the case of a subject who wiggled the toes of the foot to which one of the pickup electrodes was attached, each time a tone was presented, and thereby provided the examiner with ". . . perfect voluntary responses of sound perception."

It is useful to indicate the intensity level for each frequency tested by writing directly on the recording tape at the time of presentation. It is recommended that a tabular form be utilized for recording the best conditioned responses obtained at each frequency as they occur. Customary clinical practice is to retest with voluntary response to pure tone after EDR, whether or not good results have been obtained.

Finally, not everyone can be conditioned. Some patients seem to be indifferent even to the strongest UCS and some are so apprehensive that they are impossible to test. Some simply do not condition. Positive results with EDR can be accepted with confidence, but negative results should not necessarily rule out the possibility of functional hearing loss. It is best not to inform the patient if EDR is unsuccessful. On occasion, a patient who has "failed" EDR may respond to voluntary audiometry by giving his organic thresholds if tested immediately after EDR and before the electrodes have been removed. The usual procedure is to ask the patient to say "yes" when he hears a tone. The author is planning to utilize a small light, visible to the patient, which comes on when the tone is presented. The patient will be asked to say "no" when the light comes on if he cannot hear the accompanying tone.

There has been some exploration of the use of speech stimuli in electrodermal audiometry (Ruhm and Carhart, 1958; Ruhm and Menzel, 1959). In speech EDR, as proposed by these authors, electric shock is used to "condition" an electrodermal response to a single speech item which becomes the key stimulus interspersed randomly among other speech stimuli. When the patient is effectively conditioned, a strong electrodermal response occurs whenever the key stimulus is heard, while unconditioned speech items fail to elicit marked electrodermal changes. These tests seem promising, but there has been no great rush by clinical audiologists to employ this technique, and today, clinical use of EDR is still limited almost entirely to pure-tone stimuli.

Békésy

Jerger and Herer (1961) reported that an "unexpected dividend" of Jerger's categorization (1960) of Békésy tracings into discrete diagnostic types was the discovery that a few subjects exhibited distinctly different thresholds from the other several hundred subjects tested. Nearly all of the subjects had Békésy tracings in which the responses to interrupted tones were always equal to, or better than, the responses to continuous tones. However, three subjects, who were strongly suspected of malingering or psychogenic hearing loss, had tracings in which the threshold for interrupted tones was greater than the threshold for continuous tones.

Jerger and Herer point out (1961, p. 390) that the functional-loss patient's discrepancy from tracings given by subjects with organic hearing loss is not extraordinary ". . . if one considers the difficulty such a patient must face in equating the loudness of a continuous tone with that of a relatively rapidly interrupted tone." They suggest that this discrepancy may provide the means for a new instrumentality in the detection of nonorganic hearing loss.

Resnick and Burke support Jerger and Herer's findings and state (1962, p. 40) that in fixed-frequency Békésy audiometry, this inversion of the usual continuous-interrupted response relationship ". . . is almost always present in cases of volitional hearing loss." They found, however, that the Type V tracing, as this pattern has come to be known, does not occur in all nonorganic hearing problems, nor could they find any relationship between the degree of functional hearing loss and the degree of difference between continuous and periodically interrupted stimuli.

Rintelmann and Harford (1963), using Békésy audiometry as one of the tests employed in a test battery, found that nine of 10 pseudohypoacusic children produced Type V Békésy tracings for at least one ear. In two cases, Type I tracings (which are indicative of normal hearing or a conductive loss) were produced. Rintelmann and Harford speculate that if a patient attempts to keep the stimuli from the Békésy audiometer at a relatively high level, a Type V pattern will be produced, but if he attempts to keep the stimuli at a relatively low level (20 dB or less) he will probably produce a Type I tracing. This conclusion is not supported, however, in a study by Hood, Campbell, and Hutton (1969).

Peterson (1963) reports on four cases of children, all of whom showed evidence of functional hearing loss, who exhibited Type V Békésy tracings in which the response to continuous stimuli was better than the response to interrupted stimuli. In a later study Rintelmann and Harford (1967) found that 76 percent of their subjects with functional hearing loss traced Type V Békésy patterns whereas none of the normal subjects and only two percent of the organically impaired patients did so. They defined a Type V pattern as one in which the continuous tracing is found to be at least 10 dB lower for a range of at least two octaves with no overlap in tracings and a maximum separation of at least 15 dB. Hopkinson (1965), however, recommends a 5.5 dB minimal difference between pulsed-tone and continuous tracings.

Békésy audiometry for the evaluation of nonorganic hearing loss is essentially a qualitative test which can be done quickly and with a minimum of supplementary equipment. The Grason-Stadler Model E-800, the Tracor ARJ-5, and the Allison Model 22 audiometers are all widely available in American audiology clinics and can be readily used for this purpose. Production of Type V tracings yields little or no quantitative information as to a patient's organic thresholds, but strongly suggests the presence of nonorganic hearing loss and the need for additional exploration.

Ventry (1971) presents a study of one functional hearing loss subject over a period of two years in which numerous Békésy tests were conducted. He concludes that while Békésy audiometry has "considerable utility in identifying individuals with functional hearing loss" it is not infallible. He emphasizes that the data collected in standard audiometry (ST-PTA discrepancy, SERI analysis, and absence of false-alarm responses) are a powerful tool which does not require a special Békésy audiometer.

Hood, Campbell, and Hutton (1964) have proposed a different approach to the use of Békésy audiometry for detecting functional hearing loss. Based upon the "minimal loudness" principle that the responses of nonorganic patients tend to be influenced by the loudness of the signal initially presented, they developed a test which is somewhat reminiscent of Harris' (1958) proposal, BADGE (Békésy Ascending Descending Gap Evaluation), which compared responses to ascending and to descending stimuli presentations. Subjects in the nonorganic group displayed greater gaps between ascending and descending tracings than did organic subjects. One-minute fixed-frequency pulsed presentations were used. Tracings were compared at presentation, then at 30 seconds and 60 seconds after presentation. Criteria were a minimum of eight dB separation at T_0, four dB at T_{30}, and three dB at T_{60}. Approximately 70 percent of the subjects ($N=54$) were correctly categorized by this means.

Hattler and Schuchman (1970), in another modification of Békésy audiometry, propose lengthening the off time (LOT) of the pulsed Békésy signal from 200 to 800 msec. They correctly identified 99.6 percent of the organically impaired patients and 95.5 percent of the nonorganic patients in a population of 340 with the LOT-Békésy test. If additional studies confirm these results, this test may prove to be one of the most useful methods for identification of functional hearing loss.

Delayed Auditory Feedback (DAF)

Since Lee (1950) wrote his letter to the *Journal of the Acoustical Society of America* describing his discovery of delayed auditory feedback, or delayed side-tone, there has been a voluminous literature (see Chase and others, 1959) dealing with this phenomenon. Azzi (1951) in Italy, and Tiffany and Hanley (1952), apparently independently, proposed using delayed side-tone as a means for detecting nonorganic hearing loss. Speech feedback was most frequently employed (at least, until recently), although Hanley and Tiffany reported (1954b, p. 198) that ". . . to date, no one with normal acuity has been able to 'beat' the test when whistling is included in the measures taken."

The test usually given consists of requiring a subject, wearing earphones, to read aloud a measured passage in simultaneous feedback and then read a matched passage in the delay condition. Since it has been determined that a delay of .175 to 0.2 seconds at an intensity of 20–40 dB above threshold produces marked changes in reading rate, voice quality, intensity, and fluency in many subjects, it is possible to ascertain not only the presence of functional loss but an approximation of the true organic threshold as well (Tiffany and Hanley, 1954a).

There is no universally accepted procedure for delayed speech feedback, but the following technique is often used:

1. Subject reads a measured passage with simultaneous feedback delivered binaurally through earphones at 60-dB sensation level. If a monaural threshold is desired, 60-dB speech feedback is usually delivered to the test ear and 80 dB of complex noise is delivered to the contralateral ear. The subject is instructed to read at his normal rate. A stopwatch is used to time the reading. Three readings are averaged.
2. Subject reads a comparable passage in the delay condition.

The test is considered positive if the subject's reading time varies from the control reading rate by 10 percent or more in the delay condition. (Tiffany and Hanley, 1954a, found that an eight-percent difference in reading time could be expected at hearing levels of 20 to 30 dB above threshold.) The delayed-feedback reading is usually slower than the simultaneous reading, although occasionally a subject will read rapidly, presumably in an effort to offset the effects of the delay. A positive test obtained at a 60-dB sensation level may be interpreted to mean that the patient has a binaural organic hearing threshold, at least in the speech range, which does not exceed the 40 dB level.[5]

Observation of deterioration in voice quality, prolongation or repetition of syllables, slurring, increases in voice intensity, disruption of fluency, etc., may be used to supplement reading time as an index to the presence or absence of delayed side-tone effect.

Unfortunately, many individuals seem to be relatively unaffected by delayed-speech feedback and are capable of maintaining a uniform reading pattern regardless of delay time or signal intensity. Subjects who are experienced choral singers, for example, often seem to have little or no difficulty in preserving their customary reading rates, voice quality, and fluency throughout the delay condition.

The current procedure in many clinics is to avoid telling the subject what he may anticipate during the test. Usually, the subject is instructed to read "in a normal manner regardless of what may happen." However, it has been found that many subjects are more likely to be affected by the delay if they know what to expect. More than one unsophisticated subject has remarked, subsequent to testing, that he "heard someone talking but just ignored it." Apparently, the feedback is more effective if the subject knows in advance that he will hear his voice in a delayed condition.

This test is easy to administer, takes little time, and requires only a modified dual-head tape recorder. It is interesting that some patients, who show no overt effects of delay, freely admit hearing their voices quite clearly in the delay condition, although they have steadfastly adhered to speech-reception thresholds at much higher levels.

An adaptation of delayed-speech feedback for screening unilateral functional loss has been described by Gibbons and Winchester (1957). In this

[5] This value is obtained by subtracting the intensity required to produce the effects of the delay condition (20–40 dB) from the level of the signal delivered (60 dB).

test, a 60-dB delayed-speech signal is delivered to one ear and 80 dB of complex noise to the other. The reading rate is obtained for this condition, the speech and noise signals are then reversed, and a second reading rate is ascertained. A 10 percent or greater difference in the two reading rates is interpreted to mean that there is a real difference in acuity of hearing between the two ears. Also, a Lombard effect when the noise is delivered to the better ear is a good confirmation of the presence of a substantial loss in the poorer ear.

More recently, Ruhm and Cooper (1962, 1963, 1964) have proposed a delayed auditory feedback technique, first described by Chase and others (1959), by Chase and others (1961), and by Chase and Guilfoyle (1962), which uses key-tapping as a motor task. The subject is instructed to tap out a simple rhythmic pattern (e.g., ...) on an electromechanical key which introduces bursts of pure tone to the subject's ear with each tap. The key is modified so as to make no mechanical sound when tapped. The subject practices until he can repeat the prescribed pattern, establishing a clearly defined rhythm. When the pure-tone signal is then switched to the delay condition, the subject's motor performance is disrupted, even at levels close to threshold. The performance is slowed, the rhythm is interrupted or lost, and errors are produced. A strain gauge was originally incorporated into the equipment in order to measure changes in the subject's finger pressure against the key but, since pressure changes proved to be minimal, Ruhm and Cooper (1964) reported that this measurement is not essential for clinical use.

It is possible with DAF (tapping) to obtain a close estimate of the subject's organic threshold in contrast to DAF (speech) in which only a gross approximation of threshold can be obtained. Ruhm and Cooper report also that a measurable disruption of motor performance occurs in nearly every subject tested.

The equipment necessary for this test at the present time must be assembled from various individual components, some of which require extensive modification. However, if the equipment is simplified or made available commercially as a test system the use of pure-tone DAF seems likely to become a useful and reliable tool for the audiologist in the evaluation of nonorganic hearing loss. One drawback to the use of this test, the necessity for the patient to cooperate by active participation in the task, may be at least partially offset by the fact that most subjects probably would not realize the relationship between key-tapping and hearing evaluation, and would be willing to cooperate in performance of the assigned task.

MORE RECENT AUDIOMETRIC TESTS FOR FUNCTIONALITY

Average Evoked Response Audiometry (AERA)

Of all the conventional tests designed to distinguish functional or nonorganic hearing loss from organic loss, only electrodermal audiometry and, most recently, DAF (tapping) yield relatively objective measurement of organic thresholds. Both of these measures have their limitations; some subjects do not condition to EDR, and DAF requires the subject's active participation. Evoked response (electroencephalographic) audiometry offers the possibility of attaining reliable, objectively determined pure-tone or speech thresholds without the necessity for conditioning the subject, nor requiring his overt cooperation.

First reported by Davis (1939), for nearly 30 years researchers (Derbyshire et al., 1956; Lowell et al., 1960; Lowell et al., 1961; Davis et al., 1966) have attempted to measure the minute changes in brainwave potentials produced in the cortex by auditory stimulation. Unfortunately, these small changes are extremely difficult to distinguish from the normal random bioelectric potentials of biologic noise. Recently, the development of small summing computers has made it possible to average out the noise of spontaneous processes and extract the evoked responses to specific sound stimuli. This procedure has been named average evoked response audiometry (AERA). McCandless and Best (1964), and McCandless (1967) have reported that pure tone stimuli at low (less than 20 dB) intensity levels are as satisfactory as the clicks previously used in the eliciting of responses with clinical populations unable or unwilling to respond accurately to conventional test procedures. McCandless and Lentz (1968) studied subjects with nonorganic hearing loss and obtained thresholds which averaged 50 dB better than the results of voluntary pure-tone audiometry.

The procedure usually followed in AERA is to attach an electrode to the scalp at the vertex, fasten the reference electrode to the mastoid process, and the ground electrode to an earlobe, or on the forehead. Pure-tone stimuli are then presented through earphones; each series is summed by the signal-averaging computer and read out on an X-Y plotter oscilloscope or strip chart recorder. When functional loss is suspected, a reference pattern for each frequency is obtained at a suprathreshold level of response and then presentations are made at successively lower (five- or 10-dB) levels until it is no longer possible to visualize the response.

Signal-averaging computers are at present relatively expensive (several companies offer evoked response audiometric systems at prices ranging from $8,300 to approximately $15,000), but it is possible that costs of the comparatively simple averager needed for AERA may be reduced in a few years. Because of the equipment cost, the time required for testing, and difficulties in interpreting results at levels close to threshold, AERA is not currently employed as a standard clinical test, although it is anticipated that, with cost reduction and increasingly simplified test procedure, it may eventually be used more frequently in functional loss test batteries.

AERA at the present time is a relatively crude tool. It is quite time consuming, and it is difficult or impossible, for example, to obtain exact thresholds. Goldstein and Rodman (1967) have been working with the early responses and perhaps these components may offer, eventually, a vehicle for more precise measurement.

Other Audiometric Tests

Numerous other tests have been suggested for use in evaluating functional hearing loss. Galambos and others (1953) proposed the use of cochleopalpebral reflex, or involuntary eyeblink, as a means for measuring response to intense auditory stimuli, and Galloway and Butler (1956) developed a technique in which eyeblink response to a strong light was used to condition subjects to pure tone. Hood (1959) suggested that the inability of the functional subject to maintain the normal relationship between the amount of masking noise and a pure-tone threshold could be used to measure unilateral hearing loss. Menzel and Davidson (1962) found inordinately large pure-tone shifts for subjects with functional loss in Rainville or SAL audiometry. Calearo (1957) used rapid interruption and switching of speech stimuli as the basis for a test of suspected unilateral functional hearing loss. Falconer (1966) described a "lip-reading" test in which homophenous words are presented at various sound levels. The patient reveals the organic level of his impairment by his correct repetition of words which are actually unreadable by lipreading alone.

For various reasons, none of the tests mentioned has as yet attained popularity among otologists or audiologists. The cochleopalpebral reflex operates only at such high intensities (90 dB and above) as to make it useless except for gross measurement; the Galloway and Butler test requires a long period of conditioning. Many audiologic clinics either have abandoned or rarely use Rainville or SAL following Tillman's report (1962) of its limitations, thus reducing the probability of the employment of the Menzel-Davidson proposal. Chaiklin and Ventry (1963) published a brief resumé of Calearo's test and pointed out that supporting data were lacking, and Hood's proposal left many unanswered questions which may have discouraged attempts to use it clinically. Falconer's "lipreading" test is easily given and requires no special equipment. It seems to be a promising test although the possible outcome, an estimated speech-reception threshold, provides relatively limited information which is also attainable through Speech Stenger, Modified Doerfler-Stewart, delayed-speech feedback, and speech-discrimination tests, among others.

In general, it seems to be true that for audiologic tests to become popular, it is necessary to have several reports published including the initial proposal and evaluation, reevaluation studies of test reliability and validity, and, after a reasonable period, publication of a wide-ranging, carefully planned and executed validation study. Tests requiring new and costly equipment, or extensive modification of existing equipment, are less likely to be incorporated into clinical use until their efficacy has been demonstrated in a number of published studies.

FUNCTIONAL LOSS IN CHILDREN

Most of the tests employed with adults can be used with the great majority of children. For the very young, certain tests, such as DAF (tapping) must be modified or eliminated from the test battery. In general, since children are less sophisticated, it is usually not difficult to determine at least a good approximation of organic threshold. The child who consistently adheres to an elevated pure-tone threshold may give normal speech-reception thresholds and respond quite accurately to speech-discrimination tests at normal intensity levels. If the child is too young for speech testing, it may be necessary to rely principally upon EDR or AERA.

The examiner working with children may encourage the child to respond accurately by gently pointing out inconsistencies ("You *did* hear this before, Mary. See if you can hear it again—it will be very soft.").

There seems to be little doubt that functional hearing loss in children is almost always associated with their psychological needs and often takes the form of a simple need to receive, if not love, then at least, attention. Group-screening tests with school children, in this writer's experience, almost invariably produce initial false positive results in one to two percent of the population tested. Nearly all of these pseudo hearing losses are quickly resolved in individual test sessions. Undoubtedly, some of the false positive test results are due to misunderstanding of instructions, intellectual or motoric deficiencies, and even, in a few cases, a simple wish to confuse or "fool" the tester. The child who is one of many children in a large family seems to be peculiarly predisposed to giving false positive indications of hearing loss. The child who manifests functional hearing loss is a child who is in need of counseling or psychotherapy and should be referred for psychological evaluation and, possibly, treatment.

TEST BATTERIES AND ORDER OF TESTING

The more (definitive) tests administered the better seems to be a good rule for the audiologist engaged in medicolegal testing. One of the great difficulties the audiologist engaged in medicolegal activities experiences is in delineating the validity of his tests to the judge or the referee in the court or the compensation appeals board hearing. If he can produce the results of several tests which tend to corroborate each other, his findings are more likely to be accepted, if not understood.

The test battery should include voluntary pure-tone air- and bone-conduction testing, speech (spondee-) reception thresholds, speech sound discrimination tests, Doerfler-Stewart, Modified Doerfler-Stewart, Stenger and Speech Stenger (when applicable), delayed speech feedback, and electrodermal audiometry. Fixed-frequency Békésy, DAF (tapping), SAL, and AERA may be used to supplement the other tests. This writer no longer uses Lombard or Swinging Tone and Speech routinely for the reasons given above, although the Lombard would not be difficult to explain and might be a dramatic test to demonstrate by means of a taped recording of the patient's voice.

In regard to order of presentation, it is recommended that the Doerfler-Stewart test and the monaural speech-reception-threshold tests, followed by speech-sound-discrimination testing, initiate the battery. EDR should be given and if successful, it may eliminate the need for any other special tests. Pure-tone air- and bone-conduction tests should follow and then the remaining tests, in any order, may be given. (Subsequent to EDR and before removal of the electrodes, it is suggested that the pure-tone air-conduction test be given again. Menzel (1960) recommends that pure-tone and speech tests always be repeated at least one time before completion of the test battery. His study suggests that the non-organic component of hearing loss is considerably reduced when either the speech tests or EDR are administered prior to voluntary pure-tone audiometry.)

In accordance with the "minimal loudness principle" the patient should never be exposed to tones or speech stimuli any louder than necessary to evoke a response. Therefore, pure-tone or speech-reception tests should be given in an ascending order of intensity, and tests given at suprathreshold levels should be deferred until the threshold tests have been completed. An exception is the early use of speech-discrimination tests, as noted above. Hood, Campbell, and Hutton (1964) suggest that the loudness of the first stimulus presented may determine the level at which the functional loss patient establishes his reference level for response and, therefore, the louder the first stimulus the higher the level of response thereafter. They observed, too, that the degree of nonorganic hearing loss tends to increase as the test becomes less structured (as in Békésy testing where the subject controls the intensity of the tone presentation), and the examiner less evident. The inference is that highly structured tests should be used where possible, and whenever feasible the examiner should be conspicuously present.

EXAMINER-PATIENT RELATIONSHIP

The audiologist who is frequently called upon to deal with functional hearing loss may find that his attitude toward the patient tends to polarize in the direction of impatience, annoyance, and, ultimately, partial if not outright condemnation of the individual who gives him so much trouble. He may begin to think of the patient as a deliberate malingerer, cunning, irresponsible, and malicious, and think of testing as a game in which he is matching wits with his patient. A real danger in such an attitude, apart from the inevitable loss of good patient-examiner relationship, is the strong probability that the examiner's objectivity will be considerably reduced, if not lost completely, and that his findings will reflect his prejudice.

Ideally, the audiologist will treat his patient as a human being with human fears, needs, confusions, and inconsistencies. Lyman Barrett, Chief of Audiology Services at the San Francisco Veterans Administration Hospital, has summed up his personal philosophy toward the patient-examiner relationship in functional loss (1968):

> Every patient is entitled to the examiner's best job regardless of the symptoms that become apparent. It is the examiner's job to observe and record the symptoms detected, not to prejudge them and thereby limit or color the results . . . Lest we forget . . . more often than not the functional hearing loss case does have an underlying organic deficit. The examiner's responsibility to describe an underlying organic condition accurately is no less great because it is accompanied by a functional component. The job has just been made more difficult. . . . All patients are to be approached as persons entitled to an effective diagnostic work-up and appropriate treatment. . . . The examiner who reacts to the patient . . . as if his aberrant test behavior is a personal affront, or who feels the need to condemn the patient for his "unacceptable" behavior cannot hope to handle functional cases satisfactorily. For that matter, I would suspect that an examiner with this philosophy may fail to handle some purely organic cases satisfactorily. . . .

A patient who has much to gain from establishing a hearing loss may, consciously or unconsciously, fail to respond accurately to tests requiring voluntary admission of hearing at faint levels. This is an understandable reaction and should not be interpreted as evidence of the patient's malevolence toward the examiner.

Possibly the most important element in a good patient-examiner relationship lies in permitting the patient to "save face," to maintain his self-respect. It is vital always to allow the patient to preserve his dignity before the examiner. The patient should not be confronted with his obvious inconsistencies or charged with his failure to respond when it is evident that he is responding inaccurately. Often, a patient with evident functional loss who fears that his responses have not been consistent will attempt to explain ("sometimes my head noises are so bad I can't hear") or will ask, ostensibly out of curiosity but actually due to overwhelming anxiety, "How did I do, Doc?" or "What do you think about my hearing—do I need a hearing aid?" It is best, in this writer's opinion, to make a reassuring but noncommital response. If pressed for a specific answer, and this happens frequently, the audiologist might say, for example, "I want to go over these results and will send in my report in a few days," and if the patient persists, he might say "I think you may be hearing a little better than you think." However, most patients seem anxious to get away as quickly as possible, and refrain from comments or questions.

If at all possible, the audiologist should try to find a way in which the patient may change inaccurate responses without implying that his previous responses (or lack of them) were due to deliberate misrepresentation. One frequently used technique is to repeat the original instructions in great detail with the implication that the original instructions were not made clear (Brockman, 1960; Hoversten, 1960).

Occasionally, a patient with a unilateral loss will admit hearing at normal levels in the "good" ear but will cease to respond at all when the "bad" ear is also stimulated, as in the presentation of sound-field stimuli. Obviously this condition is not possible, physiologically, and the audiologist may be tempted to point this out with annoyance and, possibly, asperity. It is recommended that, in this situation, the audiologist simply say, "You will hear this now, with your *good* ear," prior to reintroducing the stimuli.

In summary, the audiologist must treat the functional or suspected functional loss patient with courtesy and respect. He must, if functional loss is confirmed, refrain from confronting the patient with his inconsistencies, and, above all, he must remain uninvolved emotionally so that he can evaluate the patient's hearing with complete (or almost complete—even audiologists are not quite perfect) objectivity.

MEDICOLEGAL PROBLEMS

The audiologist in private practice, regardless of his background and training, has no official status in the courts and compensation appeal boards other than the nebulous status of "expert witness" which he shares with plumbers, landscape gardeners, bricklayers and practitioners of other skills or crafts. The medical practitioner is paramount and, in evidence relating to the human condition, presumed to be beyond criticism, except by another M.D. This situation creates a problem in introducing evidence and, especially, evidence which may conflict with that presented by a medical doctor. It is hoped that, eventually, the audiologist who possesses a doctorate will be granted equal standing with the M.D. in the measurement of hearing.

Accepting his position, the audiologist should, in submitting written reports concerning functional loss, address and send them directly to the physician who will pass them on to the attorneys, insurance companies, or other interested groups. A copy may be sent directly to the principals, but more often than not the M.D. will prefer to forward the audiologist's report, in whole or in part, with some comments of his own. The audiologist should, if he appears in court or at hearings, appear in conjunction with an M.D. who will endorse and supplement his findings.

One of the greatest difficulties faced by the audiologist is in communicating his results to the court. Some tests (e.g., Stenger, Speech Stenger, Doerfler-Stewart) are difficult to make comprehensible to a judge, referee, or jury who know nothing of audiology. He might try and if he is very skillful he may succeed, at least in part. If he attempts to explain his tests, he should devote considerable attention to how these new and difficult concepts can best be made clear. He may find that it is better simply to state the results of his evaluation in terms of the organic threshold determined, and try to avoid describing the tests employed.

The audiologist occasionally may find that, rather than trying to convince a court that a patient has better hearing than is apparent by voluntary test results, he must establish that a patient truly suffers from the hearing loss he claims. This can be just as difficult as explaining the presence of functional loss or overlay.

PATIENT TREATMENT FOR FUNCTIONAL LOSS

Treatment of functional hearing loss is not really within the province of the clinical audiologist except possibly in his work with children in an aural-rehabilitation setting.

With children, resolution of functional loss occurs quite readily in most cases through counseling, careful explanation of the nature of discrepancies in results, or reiteration of test instructions (Brockman and Hoversten, 1960). With adults, most of the reported efforts to resolve this problem have taken place in military or Veterans Administration settings and have consisted mainly of hypnosis (Rousey, 1961), narcosynthesis (Bergman, 1957), and psychotherapy (Thompson, Hardy, and Pauls, 1947). The audiologist who makes a genuine effort to understand, who is dispassionate and objective yet sympathetic, may provide, through his acceptance of the patient, the first step toward resolution of his problem. It is not an unusual occurrence for a patient, presenting initially a functional hearing loss or overlay, to begin suddenly to respond quite accurately to test stimuli. It might be said that this patient simply wearied of his "pretense" or became discouraged with the difficulty of maintaining elevated thresholds, but we cannot know this; perhaps because he has been accepted, warts and all, his feelings have changed and he need no longer (consciously or unconsciously) dissimulate.

CONCLUSION

A most significant change in the past 20 years of evaluation of functional hearing loss, in addition to the development and/or refinement of the "objective" tests—average evoked response audiometry, electrodermal audiometry, delayed-auditory feedback (tapping)—is in the attitude toward the patient with nonorganic hearing loss. Most of the early audiologists describe tests of functional loss as "malingering" tests and as late as 10 years ago, several audiologists (e.g., Fournier, 1958) attempted to differentiate between malingering and psychogenic loss on the basis of patient behavior. Goldstein (1966) attributed all nonorganic loss to malingering, but he did not rule out the possibility of unconscious motivation. Today, most audiologists agree that we cannot determine the patient's intent through audiologic procedures, and resolutely refuse to define any patient's behavior as deliberate or unconscious on the basis of test results or observation.

The audiologist recognizes that the old labels really are not discrete. Even if we could distinguish clearly between a willful refusal to respond accurately and an hysterical hearing loss, both behaviors are, in essence, an outgrowth of psychological conflict or a breakdown in the individual's adjustment to the mores and values of a most imperfect world.

We are becoming more skillful in the determination of the true extent of hearing loss, whether or not a functional overlay is present, and this is of lasting value. We no longer fear that unveiling of functionality may lead to selection of another symptom by the disturbed patient. We can, by defining his organic threshold of hearing, make it possible for the patient with functional hearing loss to recognize his problem, which may lead him to seek and ultimately find help in his personal battle toward adjustment.

BIBLIOGRAPHY

Albrite, J., and Shutts, R. 1955. Audiology in the Army. *Hearing News*, Nov. 4–5; 16–17.

Altshuler, M. 1971. The Stenger phenomenon—Part II. Maico Audiological Library Series. Vol. 9, Report 5.

Azzi, A. 1951. Le prove per svelare la simulazione di sordita. *Riv. Audiologia Prat.*, 5–6; 23–55.

Bailey, H. Jr., and Martin, F. 1961. Nonorganic hearing loss. *Laryngoscope*, 71, 209–210.

Barrett, L. 1968. Personal communication.

———. 1969. Personal communication.

Bergman, M. 1957. Narcosynthesis in the management of functional deafness. *In* Surgery in World War II—ophthalmology and otolaryngology. Washington, D.C.: Government Printing Office, 474–487.

Bordley, J., and Hardy, W. 1949. A study in objective audiometry with the use of a psychogalvanometric response. *Ann. Otol., Rhinol., Laryng.*, 58, 751–760.

———, and Richter, C. 1948. Audiometry with the use of galvanic skin-resistance response; a preliminary report. *Bull. Johns Hopkins Hospital*, 82, 569.

Brockman, S., and Hoversten, G. 1960. Pseudo neural hypacusis in children. *Laryngoscope*, 70, 825–839.

Burk, K. 1958. Traditional and psychogalvanic skin response audiometry. *J. Speech Hearing Res.*, 1, 275–278.

Calearo, C. 1957. Detection of malingering by periodically switched speech. *Laryngoscope*, 67, 130–136.

Campbell, R. 1965. An index of pseudo-discrimination loss. *J. Speech Hearing Res.*, 8, 77–84.

Chaiklin, J. 1959. The conditioned GSR auditory speech threshold. *J. Speech Hearing Res.*, 2, 229–236.

———, Ventry, I., Barrett, L., and Skalbeck, G. 1959. Pure tone threshold patterns observed in functional hearing loss. *Laryngoscope*, 69, 1165–1179.

———, ———, and ———. 1961. Reliability of conditioned GSR pure tone audiometry with adult males. *J. Speech Hearing Res.*, 4, 269–280.

———, and ———. 1963. Functional hearing loss. *In* Modern developments in audiology. Jerger, J., ed. New York: Academic Press. Pp. 168–190.

Chase, R., Harvey, S., Standfast, S., Rapin, I., and Sutton, S. 1959a. Comparison of the effects of delayed auditory feedback on speech and key tapping. *Science*, 129, 903–904.

———, Sutton, S., and First, D. 1959b. Bibliography: delayed auditory feedback. *J. Speech Hearing Res.*, 2, 193–200.

———, Sutton, S., Fowler, E., Jr., Fay, T., Jr., and Ruhm, H. 1961. Low sensation level delayed clicks and key-tapping. *J. Speech Hearing Res.*, 4, 73–78.

———, and Guilfoyle, G. 1962. Effect of simultaneous delayed and undelayed auditory feedback in speech. *J. Speech Hearing Res.*, 5, 144–151.

Cohen, M., Cohen, S., Levine, M., Maisel, R., Ruhm, H., and Wolfe, R. 1963. Interdisciplinary pilot study of nonorganic hearing loss. *Ann. Otol., Rhinol., Laryng.*, 72, 67–82.

Coles, R. 1967. External meatus closure by audiometer earphone. *J. Speech Hearing Disorders*, 32, 296–297.

Davis, H., and Goldstein, R. 1962. Special auditory tests. *In* Hearing and deafness. Davis, H., and Silverman, S. R., eds. New York: Holt, Rinehart, and Winston. Pp. 225–241.

———, and Silverman, S. R. 1964. Hearing and deafness. New York: Holt, Rinehart and Winston.

Davis, P. 1939. Effects of acoustic stimulation during sleep. *J. Neurophysiol.*, 2, 494.

Derbyshire, A., Fraser, A., McDermott, M., and Bridge, A. 1956. Audiometric measurements by electroencephalography. *EEG Clin. Neurophysiol.*, 8, 467–468.

Dixon, R., and Newby, H. 1959. Children with nonorganic hearing problems. *A.M.A. Arch. Otolaryng.*, 70, 619–623.

Doerfler, L. 1951. Psychogenic deafness and its detection. *Ann. Otol., Rhinol., Laryng.*, 60, 1045–1048.

———, and Epstein, A. 1956. The Doerfler-Stewart (D-S) test for functional hearing loss. Washington, D.C.: Veterans Administration. Unpublished monograph.

———, and McClure, C. 1954. The measurement of hearing loss in adults by galvanic skin response. *J. Speech Hearing Disorders*, 19, 184–189.

———, and Stewart, K. 1946. Malingering and psychogenic deafness. *J. Speech Hearing Disorders*, 11, 181–186.

Escat, E. 1921. Technique oto-rhino-laryngologique. Paris: Maloine et Fils.

Falconer, G. 1966. A "lipreading test" for nonorganic deafness. *J. Speech Hearing Disorders*, 31, 241–247.

Feldman, A. 1965. Functional hearing loss. *Audecibel*, 14, 107–111.

Fournier, J. 1958. The detection of auditory malingering. *Trans. Beltone Inst. Hear. Res.*, 8.

Galambos, R., Rosenberg, P., and Glorig, A. 1953. The eyeblink response as a test of hearing. *J. Speech Hearing Disorders*, 18, 373–378.

Galloway, F., and Butler, R. 1956. Conditioned eyelid response to tone as an objective measure of hearing. *J. Speech Hearing Disorders*, 21, 47–55.

Gibbons, E., and Winchester, R. 1957. A delayed side tone test for detecting uniaural functional deafness. *Arch. Otolaryng.*, 66, 70–78.

Glorig, A. 1965, ed. Evaluation of non-organic hearing loss. *In* Audiometry: principles and practices. Baltimore: Williams & Wilkins.

Goetzinger, C., and Proud, G. 1958. Deafness: examination techniques for evaluating malingering and psychogenic disabilities. *J. Kansas Med. Soc.*, 59, 95–101.

Goldstein, R. 1956. Effectiveness of conditioned electrodermal responses (EDR) in measuring puretone thresholds in cases of non-organic hearing loss. *Laryngoscope*, 66, 119–130.

———. 1966. Pseudo-hypacusis. *J. Speech Hearing Disorders*, 31, 341–352.

Goldstein, R., and Redman, L. 1967. Early components of averaged evoked responses to rapidly repeated auditory stimuli. *J. Speech Hearing Res.*, 10, 697–705.

Graham, J. 1960. Evaluation of methods for predicting speech reception threshold. *Arch. Otolaryng.*, 72, 347–350.

Hanley, C., and Tiffany, W. 1954a. An investigation into the use of electro-mechanically delayed sidetone in auditory testing. *J. Speech Hearing Disorders*, 19, 367–374.

———. 1954b. Auditory malingering and psychogenic deafness. *Arch. Otolaryng.*, 60, 197–201.

Hardy, W., and Pauls, M. 1959. Significance of problems of conditioning in GSR audiometry. *J. Speech Hearing Disorders*, 24, 176–217.

Harris, D. 1958. A rapid and simple technique for the detection of nonorganic hearing loss. *Arch. Otolaryng.*, 68, 758–760.

Hattler, K., and Schuchman, G. 1970. Clinical efficiency of the LOT-Békésy test. *Arch. Otolaryng.*, 92, 348–352.

Heller, M., Anderman, B., and Singer, E. 1955. Functional otology. New York: Springer.

Hood, J. 1959. Modern masking techniques and their application to the diagnosis of functional deafness. *J. Laryng., Otol.*, 73, 536–543.

Hood, W., Campbell, R., and Hutton, C. 1964. An evaluation of the Békésy ascending descending gap. *J. Speech Hearing Res.*, 7, 123–140.

Hopkinson, N. 1965. Type V Békésy audiograms: specification and clinical utility. *J. Speech Hearing Disorders*, 30, 243–257.

———. 1967. Comment on pseudohypacusis. *J. Speech Hearing Disorders*, 32, 293–294.

Jerger, J. 1960. Békésy audiometry in analysis of auditory disorders. *J. Speech Hearing Disorders*, 3, 275–287.

Jerger, J., and Herer, G. 1961. An unexpected dividend in Békésy audiometry. *J. Speech Hearing Disorders*, 26, 390–391.

Johnson, K., Work, W., and McCoy, G. 1956. Functional deafness. *Ann. Otol., Rhinol., Laryng.*, 65, 154–170.

Juers, A. 1956. Puretone threshold and hearing for speech—diagnostic significance of inconsistencies. *Laryngoscope*, 66, 402–409.

———. 1966. Nonorganic hearing problems. *Laryngoscope*, 76, 1714–1723.

Kinstler, D., Phelan, J., and Lavender, R. 1971. Efficiency of the Stenger tests in identification of functional hearing loss. *J. Auditory Res.*, 10, 118–123.

Knapp, P., and Gold, B. 1950. The galvanic skin response and diagnosis of hearing disorders. *Psychosomatic Med.*, 12, 6–22.

Lee, B. 1950. Some effects of side-tone delay. *J. Amer. Speech Assoc.*, 22, 639–640.

Lehrer, N., Hirschenfang, S., Miller, M., and Radpour, S. 1964. Nonorganic hearing problems in adolescents. *Laryngoscope*, 74, 64–69.

Lidén, G. 1960. The assessment of disability caused by being hard of hearing. *J. Laryng.*, 74, 556.

———. 1967. Undistorted speech audiometry. *In* Sensorineural processes and disorders. Graham, A., ed. Boston: Little, Brown. Pp. 339–357.

Lloyd, L., Spradlin, J., and Reid, M. 1968. An operant audiometric procedure for difficult-to-test patients. *J. Speech Hearing Disorders*, 33, 236–245.

Lowell, E., Troffer, C., Warburton, E., and Rushford, G. 1960. Temporal evannation; a new approach in diagnostic audiology. *J. Speech Hearing Disorders*, 25, 340–345.

———, Williams, C., Ballinger, R., and Alvig, D. 1961. Measurements of auditory threshold with a special purpose analogue computer. *J. Speech Hearing Res.*, 4, 105–112.

Lynn, G. 1967. A test to detect collapse of the external ear canal during audiometry. *J. Speech Hearing Disorders*, 32, 273–274.

Martin, N. 1946. Psychogenic deafness. *Ann. Otol., Rhinol., Laryng.*, 55, 81–89.

McCandless, G. 1967. Clinical application of evoked response audiometry. *J. Speech Hearing Res.*, 10, 468–478.

———, and Best, L. 1966. Summed evoked responses using puretone stimuli. *J. Speech Hearing Res.*, 9, 266–272.

———, and Lentz, W. 1968. Evoked response (EEG) audiometry in nonorganic hearing loss. *Arch. Otolaryng.*, 87, 27–32.

Menzel, O. 1960. Clinical efficiency in compensation audiometry. *J. Speech Hearing Disorders*, 25, 49–54.

———, and Davidson, G. 1962. The application of Rainville audiometry to the detection of nonorganic hearing loss. *Asha*, 4, 376.

Molonguet, A. 1933. Manuel d'expertise en otologie. Paris: Masson.

Newby, H. 1958. Audiology: principles and practices. New York: Appleton-Century-Crofts.

———. 1964. Audiology (2nd. ed.). New York: Appleton-Century-Crofts.

Northern, J. 1968. Personal communication.

O'Neill, J., and Oyer, H. 1966. Applied audiometry. New York: Dodd, Mead.

Peterson, J. 1963. Nonorganic hearing loss in children and Békésy audiometry. *J. Speech Hearing Disorders*, 28, 153–158.

Portmann, M., and Portmann, C. 1961. Clinical audiometry. Springfield, Ill.: Thomas.

Resnick, D., and Burke, K. 1962. Békésy audiometry in nonorganic auditory problems. *Arch. Otolaryng.*, 76, 50–53.

Rintelmann, W., and Harford, E. 1963. The detection and assessment of pseudohypacusis among school-age children. *J. Speech Hearing Disorders*, 28, 141–152.

———, and ———. 1967. Type V Békésy pattern: interpretation and clinical utility. *J. Speech Hearing Res.*, 10, 733–744.

Rousey, C. 1961. Hypnosis in speech pathology and audiology. *J. Speech Hearing Disorders*, 26, 258–267.

———. 1963. Some effects influencing pure-tone delayed auditory feedback. *J. Speech Hearing Res.*, 6, 223–237.

———. 1964. Influence on motor performance of simultaneous and syncronous pure-tone auditory feedback. *J. Speech Hearing Res.*, 7, 175–182.

Ruhm, H., and Carhart, R. 1958. Objective speech audiometry: a new method based on electrodermal response. *J. Speech Hearing Res.*, 1, 169–178.

———, and Cooper, W., Jr. 1962. Low sensation level effects of pure-tone delayed auditory feedback. *J. Speech Hearing Res.*, 5, 185–193.

———, and Menzel, O. 1959. Objective speech audiometry in cases of nonorganic hearing loss. *Arch. Otolaryng.*, 69, 212–219.

Stenger, P. 1907. Simulation and dissimulation of ear diseases and their identification. *Deutsch. Med. Wachr.*, 33, 970–973.

Thompson, E., Hardy, W., and Pauls, M. 1947. Hearing disabilities and auditory retraining. *In* Medicine of the ear. Fowler, E., Jr., ed. New York: Nelson.

Tiffany, W., and Hanley, C. 1952. Delayed speech feedback as a test for auditory malingering. *Science*, 115, 59–60.

Tillman, T. 1962. A critical view of the SAL test. *Technical Documentary Report SAM-TDR-62-96*, School of Aerospace Medicine, Brooks Air Force Base, Texas.

Truex, E. 1946. Psychogenic deafness. *Conn. St. med. J.*, 10, 907–915.

Ventry, I. 1971. Békésy audiometry in functional hearing loss. *J. Speech Hearing Disorders*, 36, 125–141.

———, and Chaiklin, J. 1962. Functional hearing loss: a problem in terminology. *Asha*, 4, 251–254.

———. 1965. Multidiscipline study of functional hearing loss. *J. Auditory Res.*, 5, 179–272.

Watson, J., and Voots, R. 1964. A report on the use of the Békésy audiometer in the performance of the Stenger test. *J. Speech Hearing Disorders*, 29, 36–46.

Watson, L., and Tolan, T. 1949. Hearing tests and hearing instruments. Baltimore: Williams & Wilkins.

Welch, L. 1953. Human conditioning and anxiety. *Ann. N.Y. Acad. Sci.*, 56, 266–272.

Wiersma, E. 1915. Over de Waarde van het gelijktijdig registeeren van det Plethysmogram en de psychogalvanische Reactie. *Verslagen Koninklijke Acadamie van Wetenschappen*, 24, 1009–1014.

15

The Education of Deaf Children

S. Richard Silverman

The evolution of Western man's attitudes toward the deaf is perhaps most significantly reflected by his creation of arrangements and systems for their education. The history of our culture is marked by man's slow, faltering, and at times haphazard, frustrating, and irrational struggle toward enlightenment; and the history of the education of the deaf is no exception to this general rule (Silverman, 1960).

The notion that deafness and muteness depend upon a common abnormality and that the deaf were poor if not impossible educational risks persisted through medieval times. The Justinian Code (sixth century) classified the deaf and dumb as mentally incompetent, and the Rabbis of the Talmud classified the deaf with fools and children (second century B.C.). Cardano of Padua in the sixteenth century asserted that the deaf could be taught to comprehend written symbols or combinations of symbols by associating these with the object, or picture of the object, they were intended to represent. Dalgarno, in 1680, suggested the possibility of preschool education, and De l'Epée of France and Heinicke of Germany argued the merits of the language of signs and speech for the intellectual development of the deaf. Edward Miner Gallaudet brought the French (language of signs) system (Garnett, 1968) to the United States, and Alexander Graham Bell applied a science of speech to teaching the deaf. Itard in France, and later Urbantschitsch of Vienna and his student Goldstein of the United States, suggested the values and techniques in training every residuum of hearing.

Universality of educational opportunity for deaf children of school age has now become a reality in our country. The deaf have, although beset by problems of the changes in economic opportunity brought on by the changing technology, by and large, become economically and socially productive men and women. This is an absorbing story that has been set down by many writers and will not be elaborated here (Best, 1943; Farrar, 1923; Hodgson, 1953; Silverman, 1960; Bender, 1960). Rather we shall take up the story in terms of present-day concerns—definition, magnitude of the problem, and the bases of educational procedures—that are likely to determine and shape our approach to deaf children in the future.

DEFINITIONS

The approximately 39,000 deaf children of school age in the United States present a problem somewhat different from that of the more numerous hard-of-hearing children to be discussed in Chapter 16. Most deaf children either are born deaf or lose their hearing before patterns of language and speech have been established. By "deaf" children we here mean those who do not have sufficient residual hearing to enable them to understand speech successfully, even with a hearing aid, without special instruction. And even those children who lose their hearing after patterns of language and speech have been firmly established suffer more deterioration of speech than do hard-of-hearing children. On the other hand, a congenitally deaf child is not dumb. His mechanism for speech is normal, but he has simply never been taught to speak.

In their formative years children learn speech and language, both reception and expression, primarily through the ear. Sectional pronounciations and accents learned as children are likely to be retained throughout life. The New Englander who uses the broad *a* in "park," as distinguished from the Midwesterner who rolls the *r* in the same word, is merely imitating what he has heard as a youth in his section of the country. In the same sense our use and understanding of language naturally depend at first upon hearing. The two-year-old severely deaf child has no useful verbal language, whereas the hearing child of the same age has begun to develop a meaningful spoken and hearing vocabulary. Hence, means of communication with the deaf child must be developed through systematic and, in many instances, laborious procedures.

The detection and diagnosis of deafness and other abnormalities of communication have been discussed in Chapter 13, but it is important to keep clearly in mind the kind of child we are talking about when we refer to the "deaf child." A great deal of unnecessary confusion among the laity and well-intentioned professional workers alike has surrounded the precise classification of hard-of-hearing and deaf children, and unfortunately has frequently obfuscated discussions of their problems. The confusion seems to grow out of the differences in frames of reference to which classification and nomenclature are related. For example, some workers classify the child who develops speech and language prior to the onset of deafness as "hard-of-hearing" even though he may not be able to hear pure tones or speech at any intensity. This child, it is argued, unlike the congenitally, profoundly deaf child who has not acquired speech naturally, behaves as a hard-of-hearing child in that his speech is relatively natural or "normal" and, therefore, he should be classified as "hard-of-hearing." It is obvious that a not too precise educational standard has guided the labeling if not the definition of the child. If, however, we consider the same child from a purely physiological standpoint, it is grossly misleading to term him "hard-of-hearing" when for all practical purposes he hears nothing at all.

The situation is complicated further by the use of terms that suggest not only physiological, communicative and educational factors but also gradations of hearing loss and time of onset. To this category belong such terms as *deaf and dumb*, *mute*, *deaf-mute*, *semideaf*, *semimute*, *deafened*, *partially deaf*, and others. These terms are of little value from the physiological, communicative, or educational points of view, and it would be well to eliminate them from general usage.

For purposes of our chapter we need to define the deaf child in terms of his educational and psychological potential. For some, the significant dimension would be the child's ability to talk. In England, for example, under the School Health Regulations, children have been described as 1. deaf and 2. partially deaf. The former are those who have no "naturally" acquired speech when they are admitted to school, the latter are those who have begun to talk naturally (however imperfectly) before being admitted to school. According to this scheme children with defective hearing are classified in three grades:

Grade I: Children who are found to have defects of hearing (which in most cases are amenable to medical treatment) but who do not need hearing aids or special educational treatment.

Grade II: Children who have some naturally acquired ability to talk but need special educational treatment, on either a part-time or a full-time basis. Many of these children need hearing aids.

Grade III: Deaf children who are without naturally acquired speech when admitted to school. Many of these children are not totally deaf and can be helped by hearing aids in learning to talk and to speak distinctly (Ewing and Ewing, 1954).

For others, the important dimension is the hearing loss expressed by the child's ability to respond to various environmental sounds, speech, and pure tones. Itard, in the early nineteenth century, classified children according to their responses—to bells, drums, and flutes; Urbantschitsch some years later used a harmonica with a six-octave range (E^{-1}—e^4) and an intensity regulator for the same purpose. Both of these workers also used speech stimuli, and Urbantschitsch's classification is fairly representative of the categories that emerge from these approaches: 1. total deafness, 2. tone-hearing, 3. vowel-hearing, 4. word-hearing, and 5. sentence-hearing (Wedenberg, 1951). Huizing's classification (1953a) relates to the loss as expressed by pure-tone audiometry. He suggests the following categories:

Grade I: 0–30 dB = slight loss.

Grade II: 30–60 dB = moderate loss (practical speech span).

Grade III: 60–90 dB = severe loss.

Grade IV: More than 90 dB = deaf (no speech-understanding ability).

We quote Huizing's rationale:

> The principles underlying this scheme have a logical base. An impairment of less than 40 dB means only a remote loss of the whispering world and of the warning element of weak ambient sounds. Under certain circumstances this may be of biological importance. As long as the threshold loss for the middle frequencies (500–2,000 Hz) does not pass the 40 dB level, *grown-ups* encounter no trouble in daily life (Grade I). At the 45 to 50 dB level, however, discommunication troubles arise in auditoria, group conversation, etc.
>
> It is very important to realize that in the case of a *young child* the critical borderline of handicap should be put at a lower level, say at 35 dB. This is explained by a lack of communication experience and language skill. . . . For this reason the 40 dB level appears to be a useful average as the general borderline of a Grade I handicap. The 70 dB level is a more or less critical borderline for the natural development of speech in very young acoustically handicapped children. This is explained by the fact that in life situations the most important part of the speech span is covered by range II. . . .
>
> Finally, the 100 dB line fences off that part of the audibility area in which, notwithstanding the severe loss, speech understanding in most cases is still possible provided that a modern hearing aid is used.
>
> In most cases with more than 100 dB loss there is no speech understanding left, unless it is mainly based on speech reading. Recognition of individual speech sounds has become impossible, although the perception of rhythm, melody and occasionally of some vowels may still provide important clues for understanding.

It is of incidental interest here that Silverman and his coworkers (1948), in relating loss of hearing for speech to the judgment of fenestrated patients as to how they got along in auditory communication, found significant cutting points at losses of 40 dB and 70 dB.

For the National Health Survey of 1935 and 1936, Beasley (1940) classified hearing loss according to the extent to which the individual with impaired hearing performed everyday listening tasks. His classification was based on the following five groups:

1. *Partial deafness, stage 1:* The individual has difficulty in understanding speech in church, at the theatre, or in group conversation, but can hear speech at close range without any artificial assistance.

2. *Partial deafness, stage 2:* The individual has difficulty hearing direct conversation at close range, but can hear satisfactorily over the telephone or can hear loudly spoken speech.

3. *Partial deafness, stage 3:* The individual has difficulty hearing over the telephone at ordinary intensities, but can hear amplified speech by means of hearing aids, trumpets, or other means of amplification.

4. *Total deafness for speech:* The individual cannot hear speech under any circumstances, but acquired the hearing defect after learning to speak language by ordinary means.

5. *Deaf-mute:* The individual was born deaf or acquired severe deafness sufficiently early in life to prevent him from learning speech through the usual means.

Table I shows classes of hearing handicap developed by Davis (1965) and others for the American Academy of Ophthamology and Otolaryngology.

Of course, the time of onset of deafness affects the psychological and educational developmental patterns and should be borne in mind in labeling and classifying a child. In 1937 the Committee on Nomenclature of the Conference of Executives of American Schools for the Deaf recognized the importance of ability to speak, ability to hear (as shown by their use of the word "functional"), and time of onset in proposing the following classification and definitions:

1. *The deaf:* Those in whom the sense of hearing is nonfunctional for the ordinary purposes of life. This general group is made up of two distinct classes based entirely on the time of the loss of hearing. (a) *The congentially deaf:* those who are born deaf. (b) *The adventitiously deaf:* those who were born with normal hearing but in whom the sense of hearing becomes nonfunctional later through illness or accident.

2. *The hard-of-hearing:* those in whom the sense of hearing, although defective, is functional with or without a hearing aid.

Hardy (1952) objects vigorously to the restricting influence of the definitions and classifications of impaired hearing contained in proposals like those of

TABLE 15-I
Classes of Hearing Handicap

dB	CLASS	DEGREE OF HANDICAP	AVERAGE HEARING THRESHOLD LEVEL FOR 500, 1,000 AND 2,000 IN THE BETTER EAR*		ABILITY TO UNDERSTAND SPEECH
			MORE THAN	NOT MORE THAN	
	A	Not significant		25 dB (ISO)	No significant difficulty with faint speech
25	B	Slight Handicap	25 dB (ISO)	40 dB	Difficulty only with faint speech
40	C	Mild Handicap	40 dB	55 dB	Frequent difficulty with normal speech
55	D	Marked Handicap	55 dB	70 dB	Frequent difficulty with loud speech
70	E	Severe Handicap	70 dB	90 dB	Can understand only shouted or amplified speech
90	F	Extreme Handicap	90 dB		Usually cannot understand even amplified speech

* Whenever the average for the poorer ear is 25 dB or more greater than that of the better ear in this frequency range, 5 dB are added to the average for the better ear. This adjusted average determines the degree and class of handicap. For example, if a person's average hearing threshold level for 500, 1000, and 2000 c/s is 37 dB in one ear and 62 dB or more in the other his adjusted average hearing threshold level is 42 dB and his handicap is Class C instead of Class B. (After Davis, 1965.)

the Conference of Executives. He maintains that the continuing increase of fundamental clinical and therapeutic audiological knowledge precludes any "static categorization." For example, study of the thresholds of tolerance for speech and for pure tones has suggested that there is a useful portion of the auditory area even beyond the range of classical audiometry (Silverman, 1947). Some individuals who have heretofore been termed "totally deaf" as a result of audiometric tests may be reached by auditory stimulation using proper amplification. And, it may prove to be more fruitful to classify the person with a physical disability on some psychological scale of behavior that expresses how he lives with his disability.

We are aware that delimiting definitions are hazardous and we recognize that each child's capabilities must be assessed individually by the best methods available to us so that we are not restricted by the tyranny of classification. Nevertheless, we need some orientation as to the kind of child we are writing about and in order that we may discuss him in general terms. This chapter will therefore be concerned with the child who, when we first encounter him, has not developed the expressive and receptive skills of communication before the onset of his deafness. He cannot talk and he cannot understand the speech of others as does a normally hearing child of the same age. We shall also include the child who has acquired some of these skills of communication before the onset of his deafness but whose incompetence in language still calls for special educational techniques. For convenience, we shall refer to both of them as deaf children.

MAGNITUDE OF THE PROBLEM

If we examine the results of mass testing surveys among school children we find a range from two to 21 percent reported as having defective hearing. This great variability in reports of hearing impairment is undoubtedly due to differences in definitions of hearing impairment; in techniques, apparatus, and conditions of testing; and in the socioeconomic status and climate of the communities in which the surveys were carried out.

Our best estimate supported by an extensive detailed study of Pittsburgh school children is that five percent of school-age children have hearing levels in one ear at least outside the range of normal and that from one to two of every 10 in this group require special education attention (Eagles et al., 1963). (These figures do not include children in special schools for the deaf.) The others are likely to respond to medical care or their hearing loss is not apt to reach the handicapping stage. The projections of Educational Statistics of the Office of Education, U.S. Department of Health, Education and Welfare indicate a school-age population of 51,000,000 for 1968–69 resulting in 2,550,000 children with hearing levels outside the range of normal and 255,000 requiring special education services. Table II shows the Pittsburgh findings according to class of handicap developed by Davis (1965). Of course, account should be taken of children below school age. Our judgment is that the statistics would be about the same for them. How most of these hard-of-hearing children are handled we shall discuss in the following chapter.

Of interest is the number of all persons per 1,000 population with binaural hearing loss. Fig. 15-1 shows that there is a striking increase in the incidence of hearing impairments in the older age groups. Of course, the nature of the impairment may vary with age.

As we have described them, how many deaf children are there in the United States? This is

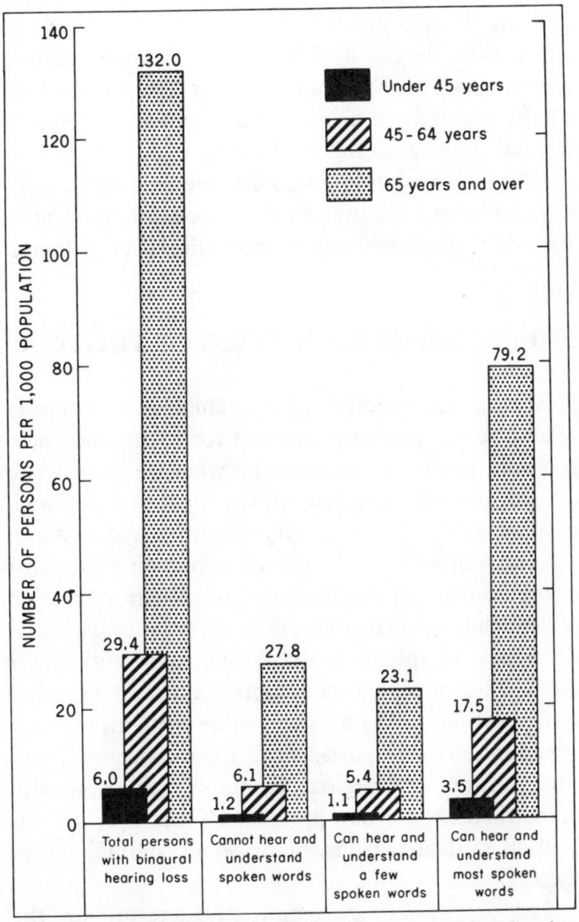

Fig. 15-1. Number of persons with binaural hearing loss per 1,000 population, by age and speech comprehension group. *From CHARACTERISTICS OF PERSONS WITH IMPAIRED HEARING, United States, July, 1962–June, 1963, Washington, D.C., U.S. Department of Health, Education and Welfare, 1967, p. 5.*

TABLE 15-II
Impaired hearing in the Pittsburgh study population
Class of Handicap

	A	B	C	D	E AND F
Ages 5 to 10 years inclusive	Not more than 25 dB*	26–40 dB	41–55 dB	56–70 dB	More than 60 dB
Number 4064	3996	36	19	9	2
Percent 100	98.3	0.9	0.5	0.2	0.05
				← 0.3% →	
		← 1.7% →			

* Impairment refers to the average hearing threshold level for 500, 1,000, and 2,000 Hz. The original ASA-1951 categories have been translated to equivalent ISO categories.

difficult to state precisely because the enrollment in our schools for the deaf is likely to include children who are hard-of-hearing and is not likely to include all the children of preschool age and deaf children who are in schools for the hearing or in other kinds of schools. Our guiding figure is the reported enrollment of 38,391 children in all schools for the deaf in 1967–68, a formidable even if not quite accurate figure.

THE GOALS OF EDUCATION OF THE DEAF

How we go about educating deaf children is obviously related to the goals we have set for them, and these goals are in turn determined by what we consider to be the overall potential of the deaf—educational, psychological, and social. Or, otherwise said, some of the sharp differences of opinion concerning the most desirable arrangements and methods for the education of deaf children really have their roots in fundamental differences of opinion as to the long-range outlook for them. This outlook may be determined among other considerations, by our own value system, by our experience with postschool accommodation and adjustment of deaf persons, by our own education and indoctrination, by our professional training, by our relation to deaf persons, or by some combination of these.

The overwhelming amount of literature on the subject (a bibliography would probably exceed 2,000 titles), ranging from school papers and convention resolutions to lengthy sections of books, reveals an intense polemicism that rests mainly on a nonexperimental empirical foundation. Of course, there are many shades of opinion, but stated views and observed practices suggest what we may term three "schools of thought." We are aware that we may be indulging in caricature and that "it all depends on the individual child," but we believe that a clarification of views is necessary if we are to understand the rationale for particular views on the education of deaf children.

One group appears to stress the limitations, especially the social limitations, of deafness. It is concerned about the exclusion of the deaf from certain types of desirable employment, the effect on the deaf of insurance practices and legislation, the implication of what amounts to minority status in certain educational and social contexts, the impact of isolation from other deaf people, the difficult if not impossible task for some of learning speech and speechreading, and the misunderstandings of the general public concerning the abilities and aspirations of the deaf. This group would suit the method of communication to the child, and its view is best summarized by the following statements (Hardy, 1952):

> The aim of the education of the deaf child should be to make him a well-integrated, happy deaf individual, and not a pale imitation of a hearing person. Let us aim to produce happy, well-adjusted deaf *individuals*, each different from the other, each with his own personality. If a child cannot learn to read lips well or cannot speak well, far better develop other modes of expression and communication, writing and gesturing, than make him feel ashamed and frustrated because he cannot acquire the very difficult art of speech and lip reading. Our aim must be a well-balanced, happy *deaf* person and not an imitation of a hearing one.

The educational program should be geared to the production of contented members of a subculture secure in its sanctions, its modes of communication, and its opportunities for social expression.

A second group emphasizes the great possibilities of the deaf, as yet untapped, particularly for education and for participation in a world of hearing people. It stresses the importance of early education and the great possibilities of auditory training (Ewing and Ewing, 1947; Huizing, 1953; Whetnall and Fry, 1964), and it is apt to emphasize the objective of "normalization." In essence, there is "one world" in which the deaf person must function and that is a world of hearing and speaking people. There is no separate world for the deaf. The adherents of this view reject the validity of the subculture concept for deaf people and strive toward their complete assimilation in the world of the hearing.

A third school of thought points to the record of economic, academic, and social achievement of deaf persons *among the deaf and the hearing* as a strong, tangible justification for the belief that forward-looking, proper, and early fundamental training enables the deaf child to make the fullest use of his capabilities. Yet it is apparent, at least in our present state of knowledge, that there are situations in which the deaf will always be marginal, and our approach to them should be influenced accordingly. Realism urges us to spare parents and the child himself the psychological distress of failure to achieve the "normalcy" that was set up as an attainable goal.

Succinctly put, the first group says there are two distinct worlds, the deaf and the hearing. They communicate little and only when necessary, and the deaf may not be too concerned with devaluation of their group. The second says there is only the world of the hearing and deaf people must adjust to it through integration. For the third group the two worlds overlap. Some deaf people penetrate the majority culture more than others, perhaps because of their education, their native ability, their skill in oral communication, emotional makeup, their families, or for other reasons. These factors require more study in order that the knowledge we gain may enable us to set goals more rationally.

The prevalent attitudes influence not only the means of communication in the classroom and the content and nature of the curriculum, but they have a direct bearing on the organizational and administrative educational arrangements, day or residential, integrated or segregated, that we make for deaf children, and on the important and essential practice of guiding and counseling parents.

A reasonable guiding principle in our present state of knowledge is to reject the notion that deaf persons are an undifferentiated monolithic mass and to avoid the stereotyping to which it gives rise. Deaf persons differ among themselves as do the hearing and therefore there should be a reasonable and carefully thought out range of educational options available to them. After all, this is the essence of our entire culture and we achieve its aspirations to the extent that we increase the opportunities for people to be themselves.

At any rate, until more facts are available to fill the gaps now occupied by opinion, a rational attitude points to the recognition that deafness imposes certain unavoidable limitations that must be accepted. At the same time, proper education in its broadest sense strives to relate the deaf person to the world about him in a psychologically satisfying way.

THE EDUCATION OF THE DEAF

We now turn to consideration of what we judge to be a "proper education." It is both convenient and logical to organize our discussion around the following topics:

1. The Communication Controversy
2. Organization of the Education of the Deaf
3. The Rise of the Preschool Movement
4. Psychological and Educational Assessment of the Deaf Child
   (a) Intelligence
   (b) Educational Achievement
   (c) Personality
   (d) Language Development
5. The Skills of Communication
   (a) Speech
   (b) Auditory Training
   (c) Speechreading
   (d) Language
6. Curriculum Development in Schools for the Deaf.

The Communication Controversy

Because there is universal agreement among educators of the deaf that every deaf child should be given an opportunity to communicate by speech, our attention shall be directed solely to this approach, which is called *oralism*. Some educators also advocate supplementing, or, if indicated, supplanting oral instruction with other forms of communication. One of these other forms is the *manual alphabet*, which is a method of forming the letters from A to Z by certain fixed positions of the fingers of one hand. This is a form of "writing" in the air. A more structured form of the combined approach is known as the Rochester Method after the school in which it was developed (Galloway, 1964). Its aim is to supplement speechreading and it is generally introduced after an oral ground work has been laid. The *language of signs* is another form of communication. This is a system of conventional gestures of the hands and arms that by and large are suggestive of the shape, form, or thought which they represent. A dictionary of signs based on a system of recording them with respect to location, configuration, and movement has been compiled (Stokoe et al., 1965). It is generally agreed that sign language is bound to the concrete and is limited with respect to abstraction, humor, and subleties such as figures of speech which enrich expression. The *combined method*, which attempts to provide speech communication, the manual alphabet, and the language of signs, depends upon the aptitude of the child and the context of the communication. For example, the language of signs and the manual alphabet are frequently employed in public assemblies. The combined method is usually employed in public residential schools.

The "oral-manual" controversy has deep historical roots. In our own country the influence of De l'Epée through Laurent Clerc and Thomas Hopkins Gallaudet established the tradition of manualism early in the nineteenth century, and it was not until well after the middle of that century that oralism began to take hold. At the present time 85 percent of children enrolled in schools for the deaf are reported to be instructed by the oral method of communication at least in their early years. The remainder are taught manually or by some combination of manual and oral methods. Although all organizations of educators of the deaf are on record officially as advocating an opportunity for all deaf children to learn to speak and to speak-read, there is significant (and often heated) difference of opinion as to what properly constitutes a fair opportunity. The criteria for transferring a child from an oral to a manual class, presumably because he shows no aptitude for oralism, are frequently vague and nebulous. Some educators make the transfer during the child's first year in school; others may wait until the child has been in school for three or four years; still others provide oral instruction throughout but permit association in the dormitory with manually taught children. The latter plan obviously makes the oral instruction less effective because the speaking child must adjust himself to the child who cannot talk, and valuable practice in oral communication is lost.

Those who advocate some manualism generally contend that too often the results of exclusively oral teaching are unsatisfactory and that the deaf child cannot make himself understood to an untrained listener. Furthermore, it is argued, many children do not have the aptitude to benefit from oral instruction, and the time spent in this type of instruction could more profitably be used in concentrating on the child's "mental" development rather than on his means of communication. Also, some advocates of manualism feel that the deaf prefer to associate with other deaf and therefore have little or no need for oral communication.

The fundamental assumption of the oralists (advocates of oral instruction for the deaf), on the other hand, is that training in speech and in speechreading gives an easier adjustment to a world in which speech is the chief medium of communication. It does not confine the deaf man or woman to association with those who know the manual alphabet or to those who are willing to resort to pad and pencil. An employer is more inclined to favor a deaf man to whom he can give oral instructions over a man of equal ability with whom he must communicate by gestures or in writing. It is not always possible, especially in smaller communities, for the deaf to find employment or social companionship among other deaf people. Oralists feel that, in the main, orally trained children have done well and are likely to do better as more teachers are adequately trained in the methods of oral instruction.

Recent Trends

Recent (Morkovin, 1968) reports from the Soviet Union's Moscow Institute of Defectology suggest that oral skills may be facilitated by the introduction at the preschool level (unlike the Rochester method which introduces finger spelling somewhat later) of "dactyl speech" or finger spelling which is free of phonetic ambiguity. Preliminary investigations appear to indicate that familiar words could be converted into oral language, speechreading and speech even before the end of the first year of kindergarten. The aim is definitely oral and the gradual elimination of the need for finger spelling except for special difficulties. Signs are excluded. It should be borne in mind that the Russian language is very phonetic. The extent to which control groups using, for example, early and intensive auditory stimulation were employed in these investigations is not known.

There appears to be, too, a significant movement to introduce the language of signs as a major mode of communication with young deaf children on the grounds that the capacity for thinking must be developed early and should not be confused with the capacity for using language. It is argued that we deter the development of thinking in deaf persons by emphasizing at the outset verbal means of communication, be they speech, the manual alphabet, or a combination of the two. In his book on the subject Furth (1966) indicates that by present methods we foster an "experiential deficiency which would be avoidable if non-verbal methods of instruction and communciation were encouraged both at home in the earliest years and in formal school education." This assumption and the belief that this is the only alternative to certain conventional unproductive methods are open to question. For example, we must weigh carefully the accomplishment of parent guidance, the early intensive use of residual hearing, and the impressive academic, vocational, and communicative attainments of many deaf persons.

The idea has been advanced that oral language be taught as a second language preceded by the language of signs and that the latter be used to bring out the advantages of oral language (Kohl, 1966). The sign language, it is suggested, ought to be enriched so that it is less rigidly concrete and situation-bound.

The "oral-manual" controversy is not yet settled. It is encouraging, however, that numerous investigations are under way to study not only the linguistic, conceptual, and intellectual effects of modes of communication for deaf persons but also their influence on such features of personality as emotional maturity and self-identity.

Organization of the Education of the Deaf

Perhaps the most significant fact about the education of the deaf in the United States is that it is universally available to all deaf children of school age. Of course, the quality of education may vary, but it is important that no child need be denied an opportunity for it. Where are these opportunities available

Of 38,391 children enrolled in schools for the deaf in the academic year 1967–68, 18,926 attended public residential schools for the deaf. These schools, open to qualified children without charge, are supported either directly or indirectly by state tax funds. Most funds. Most of the public residential schools are supported by legislative appropriation and hence come under the control of state authorities. The educational services of the remaining schools are purchased by the states on a per diem or per capita basis and are controlled by their own boards. Examples of the first group are the Indiana and Illinois Schools for the Deaf; in the second group we find such schools as the Lexington (New York) and the Clarke (Massachusetts) Schools for the Deaf.

Other tax-supported institutions for the deaf are public day schools and classes. A day school is usually large enough to be a separate entity; for example, Horace Mann School, Roxbury, Massachusetts. Day classes are usually groups within a larger school unit, and there may be as few as one in a school or as many as 10; for example, La Crosse, Wisconsin. In 1967–1968, 2,300 children were being educated in public day schools and 13,070 were in public day classes. The remaining children were being educated in denominational or private schools, such as the Lutheran School (Detroit) and the Central Institute for the Deaf (St. Louis). Such schools may be either day or residential. There were 409 children in schools and classes for the multiple handicapped. The number of children in each class ranges generally from five to 10. Some deaf children have been absorbed into classes for the hearing. Deaf individuals attend high schools and colleges for the hearing (Quigley et al., 1968). Most public residential schools provide education at the secondary level, and higher education exclusively for the deaf is available at Gallaudet College, Washington, D.C. Technical post-secondary education is provided at the National Technical Institute for the Deaf which is an integral part of a larger technical institute for the hearing, the Rochester Institute of Technology, Rochester, New York. Many states are reexamining their arrangements for the management and education of hearing-impaired children. For example, in May 1968 the Illinois Commission on Children published a comprehensive plan for hearing-impaired children in Illinois.

Until we have more evidence to support the point of view of either the day or the residential school, we must study each child's situation thoroughly to determine what educational placement is likely to be most fruitful for him. This points up the crucial need for early identification, diagnosis, and careful assessment. In addition to information about a child's hearing, among the significant points to be considered are the etiology of the deafness, the child's age at its onset, his physical development, his behavioral development, his social maturity, his home environment, and the insight of his parents (Hardy, Pauls, and Bordley, 1951).

The Rise of the Preschool Movement

The encouraging progress in the assessment of hearing of young children has stressed the value of preschool programs for deaf children. The period from birth to the age of five is particularly critical for the learning and overall development of children, whether hearing or deaf. The importance of early auditory experience is now recognized, and hearing aids are being recommended with greater confidence than previously. The extent to which auditory stimulation is combined with discussion is worthy of mention. Indirect evidence from neurophysiology suggests that there is a critical early period of life when the nervous system is still plastic, and sensory experience exerts an important influence on its development (Barnet, 1964). Psycholinguists, too, point to a critical period for the acquisition of language, particularly its syntactic features (McNeill, 1966). Since the young deaf child is denied many of the normal experiences that lead to better socialization, it is all the more essential that he be given help and opportunity for his best development as early in life as possible. This means not just a sensible program for developing the skills of communication which so greatly contribute to socialization, but also a regime that removes wherever possible the barrier which tends to isolate the deaf child from the world about him, from the world of his home, his parents, his sisters and brothers, and from other children. Formal and informal intercommunications (by whatever means) tend to lessen the child's feeling of apartness and hence make him feel wanted and significant.

The child is thus motivated to communicate, and it is the task of the parent and the teacher to show him the usefulness of speech as a tool of communication. "The situations do not happen enough by themselves; they must be anticipated and contrived frequently and deliberately" by all who are in close contact with the child (Ewing and Ewing, 1947).

Although it is not generally mandatory for tax-supported schools to provide preschool classes for deaf children, the need is beginning to be recognized. In the academic year 1967–68, of 18,926 children enrolled in public residential schools for the deaf in the United States 1,028 were under the age of six; of 15,370 children in public day schools and classes 2,453 were of preschool age; and of the 3,686 children in denominational and private schools 1,646 were under the age of six (American Annals of the Deaf, 1968). The proportions reflect the initiative of private groups in promoting programs for preschool deaf children.

It is appropriate, in discussing the young deaf children, to mention the increasing amount of information and guidance for parents of deaf children. Although here and there an effort may be misguided, the proliferation of parent institutes and clinics, and of correspondence courses, reading lists, and literary output is one of the most constructive and forward-looking developments in the education of the deaf. One parent put it succinctly: ". . . the tough thing about deafness is likely to be social isolation, social adjustment. There is no one in the world, and there never can be anyone, as important in determining any child's social adjustment as that child's own parents and his own family at home. For that reason parents are important" (French, 1946).

For the parents of very young deaf children there are now correspondence courses which offer guidance, practical suggestions, and information concerning the home care of the child before the nursery-school years. Probably the first such correspondence course was established by the Wright Oral School in New York City, but the best known at the present time is operated by the John Tracy Clinic in Los Angelos. Intelligent and cooperative parents have found these courses most helpful in giving them specific step-by-step procedures in beginning steps and a good psychological approach to the deaf child. Other procedures include the development of visual discrimination by matching colors and pictures and the comparison of objects varying in size and shape; practice in discriminating odors and tastes; exercise in the imitation of bodily movements; and the use of materials that will aid the child in better muscular coordination. Training of this type is continued in the nursery school on a more extensive and advanced scale. Such a correspondence course is particularly useful for those who are too remote to obtain information and advice in person from one of the well-established schools for the deaf. Children instructed by the parents who have followed a correspondence course of this type are better prepared to benefit immediately from a nursery school.

In general there appear to be no universally accepted specific aims or procedures in guiding parents of very young children. The emphases vary. For some, the primary aim is to create realistic "acceptance" of the child's condition, and counseling is weighted toward psychotherapy. For others, the emphasis is on conveying information in order to create an understanding of sensory deprivation and its effect on the total development of the child in general and of his communication deficit in particular. Wherever possible there is a growing trend toward carrying on parent "training" in homes and homelike settings, sometimes called demonstration homes, where by demonstration and practice parents learn to contrive and take advantage of natural situations in the home to sharpen perceptions and foster communication.

Of great interest to educators of deaf children is the knowledge likely to be gained from the programs of early education, such as Head Start, directed at "culturally disadvantaged" children. Here too, vigorous schools of thought appear to be taking shape. On the one hand there are those who would emphasize "cognitive" approaches that stimulate intellectual functioning. In its extreme form it has been labeled the "pressure cooker" view which aims to compensate for the lack of opportunity for perceptual development. Others would stress the child's social and emotional growth without too much "structured" teaching.

Most of these commendable efforts in orientation and guidance have been directed at parents of children of preschool age. This is natural, since the initial shock of the discovery of deafness must be intelligently cushioned, and crucial and immediate decisions must be made about the child's future. Even though we are here discussing children of preschool age, it should be realized that the placement of a child in a satisfactory educational situation in no way decreases the need for the guidance of parents. This was forcefully driven home to us in a survey made of the parents of present and former pupils at the Central Institute for the Deaf. Parents of teen-agers and young adults wanted an opportunity to share information and experiences about such problems as choices of occupation, marriage with the deaf or hearing, the genetics of deafness, and the choice of companions for the deaf. In short, social adjustment is just as much a problem for the deaf youth as it is for the preschool child, and it is essential that parent institutes and clinics concerned with their problems be fostered also.

Such evidence as exists for the value of particular procedures and programs of parent counseling is meager and is generally anecdotal or based on studies (frequently retroactive) of children's records. It will be helpful, for the programs we undertake, to evaluate all of the following: *genetic counseling* for deaf married couples and parents of deaf children; the use of the *High Risk Register* (Davis, 1964); the *adaptations* necessary because of differences in the intelligence, motivation, and education of parents; the *emotional needs* of parents; the *special training* necessary for those who counsel parents; and the implications of the concept of *critical periods* in development.

Psychological and Educational Assessment of the Deaf Child

INTELLIGENCE

What is intelligence? How we define it determines whether we feel confident in our ability to measure the intelligence of the deaf child. If it is the ability to carry on abstract thinking and to use abstract symbols in the solution of problems as defined by Terman (1916), we are testing an area requiring verbal behavior. In fact, Terman considered the size of vocabulary as the best single indicator of intelligence. Selection of mental tests that satisfy this definition would lead to the conclusions that either deaf children are mentally retarded *or* their ability cannot be measured. However, if intelligence is defined as the aggregate or global capacity of the individual to act purposefully, to think rationally, and to deal effectively with his environment (Wechsler, 1950) then nonverbal tests can yield an estimate of mental ability.

The need for measures of mental ability of the deaf child preceded the development of intelligence scales. In 1889 at the New York School for the Deaf, Greenberger used colored picture books and blocks as a part of the procedure of admission of children to the school. Observation of facial expression and behavior with "test materials" enabled him to weed out the mentally defective child.

Pinter and Paterson (1915) attempted to apply the Binet-Simon Scale to a population of deaf children and concluded that difficulties in the use of the scale occurred due to the lack of comprehension, the lack of environmental experience, and "the peculiar psychology" of the deaf child.

Pinter and his associates were pioneers in the psychological testing of the deaf. They attempted to use and modify existing tests developed for hearing children and finally constructed a performance test, a Non-Language Scale (1921) for group testing, and an Educational Scale for the deaf. The results of a national survey (1928) led to the conclusion that deaf children were mentally retarded (two to three years) and educationally retarded (four to five years or three and one-half grades). These conclusions were accepted by most educators prior to 1930.

With the realization that a child with a hearing impairment must learn to understand language and to communicate came the recognition that a test of mental ability must measure what the child is capable of learning. This required the selection of tests that are nonverbal in administration and response. Pantomine instructions were standardized and gestures substituted for such verbal instructions as: "Watch me carefully and do as I do" or "Put the blocks in the box quickly."

Test batteries such as the Drever-Collins Scale (1928), the Randall's Island Performance Series (1930), the Ontario School Ability Examination (1931), the Grace Arthur Point Scale (1930), and the Hiskey (1941) or Nebraska test of learning aptitude were adapted or constructed for use with the deaf. These tests were administered to hearing populations and their validity determined by comparison with verbal tests. When the performance tests were administered to the deaf, results indicated a normal distribution of intelligence test scores.

The psychometrist using these tests needs to be skilled in obtaining rapport quickly, in stressing the importance of speed in some tests that are timed, in observing carefully the attention of the child, and in recording accurately significant behavior as well as test scores. Many performance-test batteries use the same test items, and the test-retest reliability of some of these items is questionable. Therefore, the psychometrist must be alert to the child's familiarity with a test and be prepared to substitute other test batteries. It is especially important in clinical evaluation to avoid duplication of tests, as many parents take deaf children to clinics throughout the United States to get additional opinions and diagnoses (Lane, 1968).

Recently emphasis has been placed on qualitative differences in the mental ability of the deaf instead of on quantitative measures. There is a tendency to view intelligence on a continuum of concrete-abstract. According to Myklebust (1964), when one type of sensation is missing it alters the integration and function of others. Experience for the child is constituted differently and the world of perception, conception, imagination, and thought has a new configuration. Oléron (1965) feels that conventional tests have not served our purposes and that we need fresh approaches to study difficulties in perceptual analysis and organization, abstract thinking, and concept formation. The Snijders-Ooman Non-Verbal Scale (SONS) (1959) is used in Europe and designed to include nonverbal items requiring conceptual thinking with a minimum of items requiring speed of performance.

Several investigators report the low predictive value of IQ's on performance tests for future academic achievement as evidence that the performance test is inadequate as a measure of the kind of intelligence needed to succeed academically. Otherwise educators have failed to produce academic achievement commensurate with intelligence.

The Hiskey-Nebraska Test of Learning Aptitude has been revised (1966), extending the chronological age limits from three to 18. Tests have been added but are still scored as a learning quotient (LQ), indicating their use to predict learning skills observed in classrooms for the deaf. Birch and Birch (1951) used the Leiter International Performance Scale and the Goodenough Draw-a-Man (1926), together with other test batteries, to predict which children will present serious teaching problems in speechreading, oral speech, and reading. On these tests the children test significantly lower than on the other test batteries.

The performance portion of the Wechsler Intelligence Scales has become one of the widely used tests to measure the intelligence of the deaf. Those used most frequently are Wechsler-Bellevue (W-B) (1946), the Wechsler Intelligence Scale for Children (WISC) (1949), and the Wechsler Adult Intelligence Scale (WAIS) (1955). All of these scales are constructed to have a verbal and a performance section with scores expressed in a Verbal Quotient, a Performance Quotient, and a Full Scale Quotient. It is assumed that in a normal population the mean of differences between the verbal and performance quotients is zero, with a normal distribution of differences. Therefore, psychometrists testing the deaf give only the performance portion and report a score on a test that is meaningful to educators and psychologists. The verbal portion may be significant as an index of the readiness of the deaf child to be integrated into classes for the hearing. When the deaf child achieves a verbal quotient within normal limits, he should be able to cope with the language of the school curriculum for the hearing.

Early identification of deafness and parent-infant programs have created a need for tests from infancy to three years of age. Developmental scales such as the Gesell norms (1949) and the Vineland Social Maturity Scale (1947) serve as guides to which the teacher can supplement her observations of behavior. The Smith Non-Verbal Performance Scale (1960) constructed by Smith at the Tracy Clinic is a behavior scale to be used to estimate levels of development with items graded in difficulty which present a broad clinical picture from two to four years of age.

Testing the multiple handicapped deaf presents additional problems. There are no reliable measures for children with poor motor coordination. Tests of speed are not fair, and tests requiring precision of coordination are frustrating. The psychometrist can estimate ability, and this must be confirmed by a trial period of teaching.

The deaf child with learning difficulties will frequently show a wide range of abilities in the test items. Tests involving memory span are apt to be lower than other tests in the battery. The distribution and pattern of test scores in a battery of tests becomes significant in class placement in order to meet the individual differences of deaf children.

EDUCATIONAL ACHIEVEMENT

Educational progress can be measured by scores on achievement tests, which should be administered at regular intervals, preferably annually, from the time the child reaches the equivalent of second grade until he is prepared to leave the school for the deaf. These tests measure ability in reading, arithmetic, social studies, science, language, spelling, and study skills. There is no need for special tests for the deaf to measure educational attainment in terms of grade and age equivalents. The value of these tests is to compare the educational level of the deaf child with national norms for the hearing. However, Wrightstone, Aranov, and Moskowitz (1963) have developed reading-test norms for the deaf using the revision of the Metropolitan Achievement Test, Elementary Reading Test 2. These norms enable educators to compare groups of deaf children.

There has been great concern about the gap between mental ability and educational level of deaf children from the time of the Educational Survey of Pintner to the present date. Hall (1929) and Fusfeld (1933) reported the educational test level of students entering Gallaudet to be a mean grade equivalent ranging from 9.2 in 1929 to 10.0 in 1932.

The average grade equivalents on the Stanford Achievement Test of deaf children over 16 years of age leaving school programs were tabulated by Boatner (1964) in McClure, 1965) and can be summarized as follows:

	TOTAL N	ACADEMIC DIPLOMAS	VOCATIONAL CERTIFICATES
Residential Schools	1,145	8.2	5.3
Day, Private, Denominational Schools	132	7.3	5.0

These statistics, however, fail to include deaf children leaving special schools before the age of 16.

The Babbidge (1967) report citing the median grade average of 920 students who left residential schools in the 1963–64 school year revealed that at no age was a median seventh-grade achievement attained. Some congenitally deaf children achieve eighth grade, as measured by a battery of standardized tests, and qualify for admission to schools for the hearing at ninth grade. However, they are likely to have spent from 10 to 12 years in a special education program to accomplish this. It is important to emphasize that mean or median scores on a test battery do not give a meaningful measure of the child's achievement. Deaf children do not score equally well on all tests. The poorest scores are found in reading tests (paragraph meaning and word meaning) and in arithmetic reasoning or problem solving. The best scores are recorded in arithmetic computations and spelling.

The deaf child does not learn at the same rate as the hearing child. With the need to master new vocabulary and language, it takes about two or more years to achieve second grade level and an additional one and a half to two years to complete third grade. This plateau in learning is discouraging, but is not the fault of the child or teacher. It can be attributed to the time necessary to build a foundation for future progress.

The gap between mental ability and academic achievement can be reduced but is seldom eliminated. Recommendations to improve the educational level include:

1. Early identification followed by early parent-infant education and a preschool program.
2. Maximum use of residual hearing.
3. Improved reading with the desire to read for recreation.
4. Improved reasoning ability through more opportunities to be placed in problem-solving situations.
5. Higher aspirations of teachers and student teachers for better academic achievement of the deaf.
6. Intelligent use of instructional media like visual aids.
7. Continuous close cooperation of home and school.

PERSONALITY

Results from the administration of personality tests are meager and contradictory and are complicated by language difficulties. Information concerning the personality of deaf children has been obtained from three types of tests: 1. behavior rating scales and questionnaires with the parent, houseparent, or teacher as informant: for example, the Vineland Social Maturity (1947) Scale or the Haggerty-Olson-Wickman Behavior Rating Scale (1930); 2. questionnaires answered by deaf children, for example, the Rogers Test of Personality Adjustment revised for the deaf by Brunschwig (1936) or the California Test of Personality (1953); and 3. projective techniques such as the Rorschach Ink Blot Test (1942), the Draw-a-Person Test (1949) or the Make-a-Picture-Story Test (MAPS) (1952).

All of the questionnaires contain items that are not valid for use with the deaf because they require communication skills and normal hearing. When these items are eliminated, ratings indicate the deaf have more emotional problems and less maturity. When a child fills in the questionnaire the problems of reading comprehension, interpretation of qualifying vocabulary such as "usually," "sometimes," and imagination influence his responses. In a study of the California Test of Personality as a tool for measurement, Vegely and Elliott (1968) found that items that were not understood presented semantic rather than syntactic problems. It was hypothesized that even after revision of items and test norms, deaf children would continue to show poorer adjustment.

Using the Rorschach Test, Levine (1956) found confirmatory evidence of mental "under development" and that personality development is closely linked to language development.

Myklebust (1964) reported emotional immaturity with more emotional stress, conflict, and frustration for deaf children enrolled in day classes and more isolation for those in residential schools. On the Draw-a-Person Test used in his study, the deaf child showed perceptual distortions regarding himself and projected these to others.

Hess (1966) has developed a nonverbal modification of the MAPS test for children eight, nine, and 10 years old. In a preliminary report the deaf differed from the adjusted and emotionally disturbed by showing faster and impulsive reactions to new situations but with indication of adequate involvement. There was evidence of more expansive fantasy life, superficial personal attachment, and depressive emotional tone.

Personality tests are valuable tools in counseling the deaf because they may reveal problems that the school counselor did not suspect existed. They are essential in the vocational counseling program, and tests used for deaf adolescents and adults are described by Vernon (1967). At present there does not seem to be a personality of "the deaf" but rather individual differences that are significant both in teaching and in guidance of deaf children.

LANGUAGE DEVELOPMENT

We know that language is fundamental for hearing-impaired children. Essential for an improved understanding of how it is learned and consequently of how it should be taught is a satisfactory description of language. Investigators and teachers have not been satisfied by vague and frequently misleading assertions about deaf children being "2 to 5 years retarded" or about their having typical "deaf language." They have used such measures as sentence length and complexity, the frequency of occurrence of certain parts of speech and certain orders of words, the extent of vocabulary, so-called "type-token ratios" (the relation between the number of *different* words and *total* words in a sample of language), and subordination and abstractions (Simmons, 1962; Myklebust, 1965). They have used the methods of structural linguistics to analyze the functional and lexical features of the spoken and written language of deaf children. This is one of many possible leads to better description of language and to improved techniques of teaching vocabulary, syntactical patterns, and the semantic rules that relate words or sentences to things or events, not to mention the subtle and little-understood interweaving of the learning of language and the forming of concepts (Rosenstein, 1960). An interesting approach to this problem has been the collection of word-association responses from the deaf (Odom et al., 1965).

Psycholinguists are suggesting descriptive methods that enlighten us on how a child comprehends and manipulates language, particularly syntax. It has been suggested that children have a general capacity to acquire syntax and this may be thought of as an inborn set of predispositions to develop a complex grammar from small amounts of information (McNeill, 1966). Tervoort (1967) studied intensively the relation between "the private, mostly visual, partially esoteric" means of communication of young deaf children and the development in the deaf child of the language of the hearing community. The implications of these views for language instruction for deaf children are being explored.

How and if at all language competence is related to concept formation in deaf children is still an open question. The situation is complicated by generalizing about select groups of deaf children taught by one "method" or another and educated in different environments, day or residential, manual or oral, or combinations of these. In general, the tasks presented to deaf children in studies of their ability to "conceptualize" have been weighted heavily in the direction of categorization (Kohl, 1966). The studies find that deaf children can categorize "concrete"

SOME STEPS OF LANGUAGE DEVELOPMENT

SKILLS
reading, writing,
spelling and composing

MATURE LANGUAGE
involved syntax and inflection
vocabulary of 5000+

CONNECTED LANGUAGE
simple structure – requests
questions

LARGER EXPRESSIVE UNITS
prepositional phrase
participial phrase

LIMITED EXPRESSIVE LANGUAGE
naming – adjectives
few verbs

IMITATIONS
actions including mouthing
sounds including speech

FREE COMPREHENSION
concepts
connected language

SITUATIONAL COMPREHENSION
concrete items
visible actions

AWARENESS
concepts
vocabulary

EXPOSURE

Fig. 15-2. Language development. *After Simmons, 1964.*

material as well as hearing children but do less well in categorizing verbally. The tasks have been quite simple, and higher mental processes seem not to have been investigated. Throughout there is an assumption that verbal performance is equated with linguistic competence, but it may be reasonable to suggest that a sign or gesture, although not verbal, may have linguistic attributes.

In any event, a helpful way for parents and teachers to think of language development is shown in Fig. 15-2.

THE SKILLS OF COMMUNICATION

It is obvious that the skills of *speaking*, of *understanding* speech (speechreading and "hearing"), and of *language* are interrelated in their development. For convenience, however, and without slighting the interrelation, we shall consider separately the following topics: speech, auditory training, speechreading, and language.

Speech

Studies of the speech of deaf children have, by and large, dealt with differences between the speech of the deaf and of normally hearing subjects. By a technique of kymographic recording, Hudgins (1934) found the following abnormalities in the speech of the deaf; slow and labored speech, usually accompanied by high chest pressure with the expenditure of excessive amounts of breath; prolonged vowels with consequent distortion; abnormalities of rhythm; excessive nasality of both vowels and consonants; and imperfect joining of consonants with the consequent addition of superfluous syllables between abutting pairs.

We gain a substantial insight into the speech of the deaf from the investigation of Hudgins and Numbers (1942), who departed from the usual approach of comparing the speech of the deaf and of the hearing and studied the relation between errors of articulation and rhythm and the intelligibility of the speech of deaf school children. Ten sentences spoken by deaf children were recorded and then were analyzed by a group of auditors. They found two general types of error: errors of articulation involving both consonants and vowels, and errors of rhythm.

Consonant errors were classified into seven general types, as follows: failure to distinguish between voice and unvoiced consonants; consonant substitutions; excessive nasality; malarticulation of compound consonants; malarticulation of abutting consonants; omission of arresting consonants; and omission of releasing consonants. The vowel errors were vowel substitutions; malarticulation of diphthongs; diphthongization of vowels; neutralization of vowels; and nasalization of vowels.

In general, our experimental and empirical evidence indicates that the deaf child who lacks an adequate auditory monitor is likely to develop, at least under present methods of instruction, a breathy, nasalized vocal quality, abnormal temporal and intonational patterns, and some surprisingly consistent errors of articulation. These observations do not imply that deaf children cannot be taught to speak intelligibly. Many can. They do, however, show where there is the greatest opportunity to improve our methods of teaching speech to deaf children.

Fundamental attitude

As we have indicated previously, all educators of the deaf endorse the proposition that all deaf children shall have an opportunity to learn to speak. The implementation of this notion in everyday practice, however, reveals fundamental differences in attitudes.

For some educators, speech is a subject to be taught like a foreign language to those who can "benefit" from it. Practice and atmosphere are not aimed at vitalizing speech for the child. Rather, speech is viewed as an eminently desirable but not essential skill to cultivate. For others (including ourselves), a corollary to the proposition of universality of opportunity to learn speech is inescapable: speech is a basic means of communication and hence is a vital mechanism of adjustment to the communicating world about us. Therefore, we set the stage for speech *everywhere*—in the home, on the playground, in the schoolroom—from the moment we learn that a child is deaf, so that speech eventually becomes meaningful, significant, and purposeful for him at all times (Silverman, 1954). We believe that parents, counselors, teachers, and all others who are responsible for the child's development should share this attitude. Only constant practice and actual use of speech will develop fully the deaf child's latent ability to communicate by speech. The absence of a "living speech environment" may account for some of the so-called oral failures in schools for the deaf (Ewing and Ewing, 1954).

The multisensory approach

Obviously the teacher must use all available sensory channels for teaching speech to a deaf child: the visual, the auditory, the tactile, and the kinesthetic.

When we consider the use to which we put *the visual system* in teaching speech we tend to think primarily of speechreading. The child learns to watch with purpose the movements of the lips and the expressions of the faces of those about him and to imitate, however imperfectly, these movements in attempts to express himself. This really is the initial technique with deaf infants. Other well-known uses of vision include systems of orthography, color codes that differentiate the manner of production of phonetic elements, finger-spelling models and diagrams that show position and movement of the mechanisms of speech, and acoustic translators of various sorts that display speech patterns visually and can carry information to the eye about time, frequency, and intensity. A recent symposium at Gallaudet College dealt with a number of electronic possibilities for presenting visual cues to speech (American Annals of the Deaf, March 1968). Now under consideration in some schools is the recently advocated system of "cued speech" which aims to improve the acquisition of speech and its production. It is a system of communication in which phoneme, syllable, or word is identified from lip movements with the aid of 12 cues supplied by the hands (Cornet, 1968).

We know that the literature even of the nineteenth century (Urbantschitsch, 1897) mentions the desirability of using *the auditory system* to aid in teaching speech to the deaf. Today we are better able to exploit this possibility because of the development of modern wearable and group hearing aids designed to deliver speech to the auditory area that the child still possesses. For the kind of child whom we are here discussing the auditory area is greatly restricted, but even a limited perception of stress patterns can help a child achieve better rhythmic and voice quality and better understand speech.

The tactile or vibratory sense is most commonly used by placing the child's fingertips or hands in contact with his own or the teacher's face or head during speech or during phonation (Alcorn, K., 1938; Alcorn, S. K., 1941. Some techniques use sounding boards, including pianos, and diaphragms which are caused to vibrate by speech and music (St. Michiels-Gestel, 1940). Surprisingly good differential sensitivity of the thoracic region of severely deaf children has been demonstrated (Becking, 1953).

Attempts are being made to improve tactile reception by filtering speech electronically and transmitting significant frequencies to each of the fingertips by bone conduction vibrators. The Picketts (1963) described such an instrument called a "tactual vocoder" (VOice CODER) constructed in the Speech Transmission Laboratory, Royal Institute of Technology, Stockholm, Sweden. The Picketts conclude "that the skin offers certain capacities for transmitting speech information which may be used to complement speech communication where only an impoverished speech signal is normally received." Another recently reported instrument is the "Tactus" developed by M. Kringlebotn (1968) of Trondheim, Norway, which transposes frequencies down to the range of maximum tactile sensitivity, 100–400 Hz. Results show that the experimental use of this instrument is helpful when combined with speechreading and as an aid in speech development and improvement. We do know that the capacity for frequency discrimination of the vibrotactile sense is limited and is in the wrong frequency domain for the discrimination of speech. Many past attempts to present speech to the vibrotactile sense have substituted a series of vibrators placed on the hand as representations of different frequencies. Whether the investment in time and money in these refined and sophisticated tactile approaches is justified, compared with conventional methods, is now being studied in a number of laboratories and schools.

The kinesthetic sense is used in "getting the feel" of certain articulatory and vocal movements and in tongue and lip exercises. Some teachers employ rhythmic gross-muscle movements to reinforce kinesthetically the utterance of connected speech and of suitable nonsense syllables.

Many techniques to teach speech to the deaf are in common use. One reason for their variety is the wide difference of opinion concerning the relative emphasis that should be placed on each sensory pathway. Some believe that speech is better learned if attention is concentrated on one sense at a time and the others are deliberately excluded. The opposite view favors mutual reinforcement of the senses and a coordinated sensory input. In support of the latter view, it has been shown that a small fragment of hearing may be trained to supplement vision usefully in a visual-auditory presentation (Sumby and Pollack, 1954). In other words, the eye and the ear together perceive speech better than either one alone. Hence, it is argued, the bisensory approach is likely to produce better speech. The counterargument is that, at least in the early stages, speechreading should be excluded from auditory training because the speechreading is likely to divert the child from full use of his hearing. Shutting the eyes of the child while he is learning to differentiate vibrations has also been suggested.

In developing techniques, it is desirable for the teacher to analyze the speech skill she is trying to cultivate and to select the combination of sensory channels best suited to stimulate the child. For example, the perception of the phonetic element *p* is best accomplished through vision reinforced by feeling, and vowel differentiation is greatly aided by a combination of auditory, visual, and tactile stimulation. We believe that the sum of reinforced multisensory stimulation is greater than any of its parts. It is, in fact, "the nearest approach to the normal that can be made by the deaf child" (Watson, 1951).

Systems of orthography

Students of speech are aware of the irrationality of our symbols for discrete units of speech. The letters of our alphabet bear no consistent relation to the sounds they represent. Furthermore, most of our symbols represent more than one sound and most of our sounds are represented by more than one symbol. This situation has led teachers of the deaf to devise systems of orthography that carry more information about speech units than do the unrelated letters of the alphabet.

The Bells created their system of *visible speech* in 1894. In this system consonants are represented by four fundamental curves that relate to the "articulators," i.e., to the back of the tongue, the top of the tongue, the point of the tongue, and the lips. The insertion of a short "voice" line in the bow of the curve changes a voiceless consonant to a voiced consonant. For example, *a* (which is *k*) becomes *a* (which is *g*). There is also a system for modifying the fundamental symbols to represent the vowels. This system is described in the Bells' book, "*The Mechanism of Speech.*"

The Northampton charts (Yale, 1938), originated at Clarke School for the Deaf and popular with many teachers of the deaf, are arranged to give more phonetic significance to letters of the English alphabet. The charts do this by arranging the symbols in columns and rows according to the method of production of the sounds. Thus the consonants *p*, *b*, and *m* are in the same row because the lips are initially shut in the production of all three. They are in different columns because *p* is voiceless, *b* is voiced, and *m* is nasal. This arrangement shows the differences and similarities among sounds. The multiplicity of letters and combinations of letters that represent the same sound is handled by arranging secondary spellings under the primary symbol, which is the one that occurs most frequently in English usage. Thus *a-e* is the primary symbol for the diphthong in "cake." Here the dash represents any consonant. A secondary spelling under *a-e* is *av*, as in "say."

The diacritical system used in our dictionaries assumes familiarity with the pronounciation of common key words. Where one letter may represent more than one sound, a differentiating symbol is used; thus *e* as in "be" is ē, and *e* as in "bed" is e. Phoneticians and linguists generally use the International Phonetic Alphabet, which has a single standard symbol for each sound and adds new symbols to the Roman alphabet to provide the necessary extra symbols.

Zaliouk (1954) has devised a "*visual-tactile system of phonetic symbolization*" for teaching speech to the deaf. This uses two categories of symbols, static and dynamic. The static symbols represent the hard palate, the tongue, the teeth, and the lips, all of which participate in various "articulatory positions." The dynamic symbols indicate movement.

A recent addition to the pool of orthographic systems that may have value for deaf children is the *Initial Teaching Alphabet* (i.t.a.) of Sir James Pitman (1967). It eliminates ambiguity by having only one symbol for each spoken sound and is arranged alphabetically. It is claimed that it "leads in" easily to reading and writing.

There have been other attempts, too numerous to mention, that have sought through shorthand or other means to convey phonetic information by a logical and consistent system of symbols. An ideal system of orthography would convey information on how to articulate, use the ordinary alphabet, would be within the grasp of children, and would be free of ambiguities. Obviously these criteria are in conflict and some compromises must be made. For example, if we were looking primarily for symbols to convey information on how to articulate, we would probably choose the system of Bell or of Zalicuk. The Northampton charts, with their secondary spellings, represent the letters and combinations of letters used most frequently in the English language, and hence should show how to pronounce the written word. On the other hand, because there are so many secondary spellings and exceptions, the learned combinations may be confusing out of the context of the chart. The diacritical markings of the dictionary are obviously useful, but everyday printed English does not carry these marks. One of the drawbacks of the International Phonetic Alphabet is that some of its symbols are not letters of the alphabet. Some teachers prefer to start children with the Northampton charts and then to teach the diacritical marks when children reach the appropriate academic level. These comments on the various systems are by no means exhaustive, but they may be useful as a guide in choosing a system of phonetic symbolization.

Units of speech

The various approaches to teaching articulation to the deaf may properly be placed on a continuum ranging from an elemental, analytical method to a patterned or "natural" approach. The former would emphasize the development of individual elements out of speech contexts and the latter would begin with words and phrases "as it is natural for hearing children to do." The elementalists argue that in the absence of an appropriate auditory monitor, the kinesthesia of each phonetic element must be fixed before precise articulation can be achieved, lest fluency be attained only at the expense of good articulation. The "naturalists" contend that we must take advantage of the spontaneous articulation, temporal patterns, and voice qualities of young children. These generally are not isolated elements, and the naturalists believe that precision *can* be achieved within the framework of natural spontaneous vocal output without sacrificing fluency.

Most present-day practice lies between these two extremes. It regards the syllable as the basic unit. The syllable is probably the simplest possible utterance in speech. Individual sounds cannot be uttered without somehow making a syllable. As Stetson (1951) expressed it, "when teachers and demonstrators give what they think are 'separate sounds' that are actually uttering syllables; the vowels and on occasion the liquids and nasals constitute separate syllables, as in 'oh, a, rr . . ., ll . . .,' long drawn out fricatives, ss . . . etc., become vowel substitutes, and other consonants are given with a brief vowel, as in "buh, puh, . . ." Of course individual sounds may be corrected, but they should not be considered learned until they are articulated properly in the kinds of syllables in which they are likely to occur. Furthermore, speech rhythm, which contributed to intelligibility, is primarily a matter of grouping, accentuating, and phrasing syllables. The babbled syllable and the building of connected rhythmic speech from syllabic units are used in many methods for the development of speech.

In studies of the development of sounds in young normal-hearing children it has been shown that by the tenth month practically all the different sounds have appeared (Irwin, 1947). Yet it is curious that even though a child may have produced *l* and *r* during his infantile babbling, he frequently cannot at the age of two or three produce these sounds correctly in English words. Apparently he finds it difficult to use the phonetic elements of his babbling as the phonemes of his language (Jakobson, 1941). This relearning comes about by biologic maturation (Lenneberg, 1966), perceptive development, both auditory and kinesthetic, and, in the case of the deaf child, by the use of whatever sensory channels are available.

Evaluation of speech

Frequent critical evaluation of the *intelligibility* of the speech of deaf children is important, both as a guide to modifying existing methods of teaching and, particularly, as an objective assessment of the oral method. Evaluations can be made periodically during the school career of a deaf child, during which he is exposed to formal training in speech by one method or another. Other long-range procedures could be designed to discover how intelligible the speech of deaf pupils continues to be after they have graduated from schools for the deaf.

A child's improvement in speech intelligibility may be evaluated by periodic tests, but the available tests are not as objective or as valid as our corresponding tests of many other skills or of a child's mastery of subject matter. In one popular procedure a child reads a selection and auditors indicate the extent to which the selection has been understood. Or carefully selected word samples are read and scored by the auditors. In a sense, the tests determine the extent to which the deviant talker imposes a loss of discrimination for speech on a normal listener. Although this may yield a limited but fairly reasonable appraisal of the mechanics of the child's speech, it does not simulate the pattern of usual oral intercourse which takes place without benefit of a printed or written visual aid. What is being evaluated is a form of *oral reading* and not speech in broad social terms. The translation of the child's *own* thoughts into intelligible speech is an ability neglected by this type of evaluation.

The use of memorized material without visual aid is subject to similar criticism, since the thoughts expressed usually are not the child's own; or, if they are, they have been memorized. This furnishes the child an advantage which he does not have in a normal social situation. The interview, in which the the child is stimulated to talk freely, may yield a fairly accurate appraisal of speech if it is conducted skillfully. Very often in an interview, however, the child may correctly anticipate the questions; furthermore, the technique fails to appraise the child's ability to initiate speech. The use of speech recordings for periodic evaluation has considerable value. However, the limitations of printed or memorized selections and of the question-and-answer type of sample should be kept in mind. Of course, it would help to capture for study the casual conversation of children. We should be cautious about the inferences we make that relate tests of talker intelligibility to social usefulness of speech. The two are not always linearly related. Attitudes of talker and listener having to do with confidence, encouragement, frustration, motivation—all these play their role in the use a deaf person makes of his speech.

The outcomes of speech-teaching which are most important in the long run are those that reveal the extent to which the benefits of the child's training in speech persist after he has left school. Unfortunately, we have no satisfactory evidence in this area, and the information that comes to us is frequently biased and invariably anecdotal. Good follow-up studies are a task which zeaous oralists might undertake profitably.

Our discussion of teaching speech to the deaf suggests the following guides to practice:

1. An environment must be created or maintained for the child in which speech is experienced as a vitally significant and successful means of communication. Oralism is as much an atmosphere and an attitude as it is a "method" of teaching.

2. Spontaneity of speech should be encouraged, but formal instruction is necessary at the appropriate stage in a child's development. Good speech in deaf children does not come of itself.

3. The proper combination of the visual, auditory, tactile, and kinesthetic pathways should be exploited early, rationally, and vigorously.

4. The syllable is a suitable unit for the development

of articulation and of desirable temporal patterns in speech. Through its use, adequate coordination of parts of the speech mechanism is more likely to be achieved.

5. A functional system of visual phonetic aids is essential.

6. Judicious correction of poor articulation, including individual phonetic elements, and of undesirable rhythm and voice quality is necessary. The acceptance of poor speech encourages its use. The teacher is the only accurate monitor of the child's speech and she must let him know how he can improve it.

7. Periodic and long-range evaluations of the social effectiveness of the speech of the deaf, even though it be informal, is useful both for diagnosis and for educational planning.

Future investigations of the speech of deaf children should be greatly stimulated by the availability of improved tools and methods for the investigation of speech as an acoustic event. Techniques are at hand for analyzing and synthesizing speech, for displaying it visibly and tactually, and for repackaging it by selective filtering, frequency transposition, and temporal expansion and compression. Our understanding of the physiological mechanisms of speech should be enriched by the techniques of high-speed photography of the larynx during phonation and of x-ray views of the articulators in action. Helpful, too, is our study of speech that is deviant because of such structural pathologies as cleft palate, vocal nodules, absent or partially removed larynx, or deficient innervation of speech musculature as in cerebral palsy.

Auditory training

The systematic use of residual hearing potential to improve communication of persons with impaired hearing that has come to be labeled *auditory training*. We have seen previously how, as early as the beginning of the nineteenth century, it was recognized that "very deaf" children may have hearing which if stimulated or "trained" could serve a useful communication purpose. The evolution of this movement has been discussed elsewhere (De Weerd, 1951; Goldstein, 1939; Silverman, 1949; Wedenberg, 1951), but it is interesting to observe that awareness of the possibility of auditory training was spotty and spasmodic during the nineteenth century, perhaps because of wide use of the manual methods of instruction. The great advance in electroacoustic instrumentation of the past three decades, however, both for testing of hearing and for amplifying sound, brought about a revival of interest from many fields in auditory (sometimes in the past referred to as "acoustic" or "auricular") training that has been sustained and substantial.

In discussing hearing "potential," particularly for profoundly deaf children, we need to keep in mind the area available for hearing which we refer to as the auditory area. Silverman (1947c) has likened the auditory area to a building with the foundation represented by the threshold of sensitivity, the in-between stories corresponding to levels of equal loudness, and the roof represented by limits of tolerance. In attempting to determine the maximum desirable acoustic output of hearing aids, he "mapped out" the upper intensity limits of human hearing. If it could be demonstrated that the limits of tolerance were higher than previously supposed, instruments could be designed with a higher level of maximum undistorted acoustic output and thereby the auditory range of usefulness could be improved materially.

In Fig. 15-3 (Davis, 1960) with its accompanying explanation we see the auditory map severely reduced in size because a major portion of it is rendered useless by deafness. In the kind of children we are dealing with in this chapter, the area available for hearing is much less than in Fig. 15-2. Therefore, our task is to "package" sound into the area between the elevated threshold of sensitivity (also greatly restricted in frequency) and the threshold of discomfort. The sound must be intense enough to be perceived in some form and not so intense that the child "can't take it." The surprisingly high level-of-tolerance threshold reached experimentally suggests that in terms of the concept of the auditory area the "hearing" potential is substantial, and it is likely that very few children are "totally" deaf. Instruments directed toward taking advantage of these possibilities have been designed and are available commercially.

We must remind ourselves that in this chapter we are concerned with deaf children as we described them at the outset. They may be in the Grade IV of Huizing (1953a), the "deaf mute" group of Beasley (1940), or the "third group" of Hudgins (1954) with levels above 90 or 100 dB, or groups E and F of Davis. In other words, these are the children whose auditory area is about as restricted as it can be (sometimes as little as 10 dB in the frequencies below 1,000 Hz) with still some residuum of sensitivity. Through this limited sensitivity, however, the central

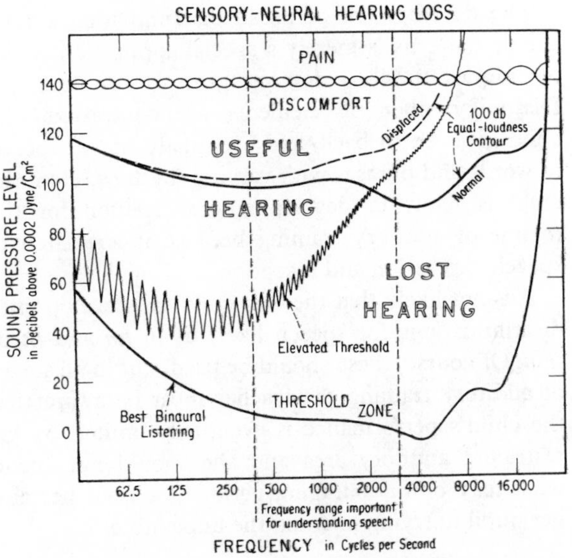

Fig. 15-3. Reduced auditory area in a hypothetical case of sensory-neural hearing loss. The normal free field, binaural threshold zone, and the threshold for pain are shown. The threshold for pain is uncertain above 4,000 Hz. The hearing loss is of the "gradual" high-tone type and is accompanied by strong "recruitment." The 100 dB equal-loudness contour is distorted but is only slightly displaced upward. High-level sounds are nearly as loud as for a normal ear. The threshold of discomfort is unchanged. The zigzag line, representing the elevated threshold as it might be shown by a patient-controlled (Békésy) type of automatic audiometer, covers a wide zone of uncertainty at low frequencies but a very narrow zone where the hearing levels are elevated and recruitment is present. *From Davis, 1960.*

nervous system may get sufficient information and contribute to the attainment of the objectives listed below.

Our understanding of the reception of speech has been aided greatly by the contributions of information theory and by our knowledge of pertinent acoustic properties of speech. Information theory concerns itself with the predictability of elements in communication or, in other words, guessing what comes next based on probabilities of occurrence of a phoneme, a word, or a phrase, according to the particular structure of a language (Fry, 1966). What is important for the hearing-impaired is that it has been shown how much can be "guessed" in the absence of much of a message. The cueing that may be possible with a small amount of residual hearing, properly amplified, may be greater than heretofore supposed.

The presence of low-frequency hearing in many children has stimulated various schemes of signal-processing that re-form the speech signal to improve its perceptibility (Hirsh, 1964). In general speech-compression systems of one sort or another are being tried that reduce the bandwidth much as is done in transmission by radio and telephone. For many children, listening over such systems requires that a new language be learned.

Several objectives of auditory training are within the reach of deaf children:

Improvement in speech perception. Deaf children are not likely to achieve much auditory discrimination for speech, certainly not enough to understand ordinary language through hearing alone. However, they can be taught to appreciate temporal patterns of speech and also to improve their control of the intensity and, in some instances, the pitch of their voices. Refined appreciation of phrasing and stress patterns may be expected to improve the child's ability to attain the "rhythmic grouping" which can contribute greatly to the intelligibility of his own speech. Auditory training improves speech perception, particularly when it is combined with speechreading. Failure of improvement in communication by speech after a regime of auditory training may often be due to the fact that the training was not begun early enough. It should begin in the first year of life.

Improvement in language skills. Although there is no definitive experimental evidence that auditory training improves language skills, it seems likely that the information carried by stressing and phrasing, not easily discerned by speechreading, adds to the meaning and significance of connected language. Vocabulary, particularly words with auditory associations, may be enriched. For example, if a child reads, "The baby cried," the word "cried," which has auditory connotations, has limited meaning for him even though he is able to draw a line between it and the word "baby" in his workbook and he has seen a picture of a baby crying. On the other hand, a recording of the cry of a baby played over an amplifying system, even through not perceived precisely, should enrich the meaning of the word "cry."

Improvement in psychological coupling to the hearing world. Again, convincing experimental evidence is lacking. Nevertheless, consider the deaf child at a ball game. A thrilling play is made on the diamond that evokes a spontaneous outburst of yelling from the crowd. The child sees the hands clap and wave, the spectators rise from their seats, the mouths open, but he has not caught the full emotional impact of the moment because its basic richness lies in the yelling of the crowd and the accompanying noises. This is an auditory experience. If the child could perceive just the presence of these noises, however distorted, through a hearing aid he would share more richly in the group experience. Not to be overlooked are the aesthetic appreciations which may result from auditory exposure to the rhythm of music. Many deaf children who have been trained to appreciate rhythmic cadences seem to enjoy dancing and eurythmics.

Although it is likely that the future will reveal additional and greater values of auditory training, our statements of objectives within reach suggest that we must be cautious of the extravagant claims sometimes made for the use of hearing aids by deaf children, particularly the claim that if they are equipped from infancy with a hearing aid they do not need special education.

With these objectives in mind, we turn now to a consideration of the basis for practices in auditory training for the deaf child. It is important to realize that the child must form the *habit* of listening. Even the very young child under two should be talked and sung to close up to his ear, and he should be encouraged to look at and to listen to sound-producing objects, be it the rattling of a paper bag or the noise of the wind-up toy. Actually, this is the first stage. As the child matures, he needs to develop an awareness for sound and a realization that it can have meaning. Therefore, it is essential that the child be surrounded by sounds that are intense enough to be "sensed." Then, as Carhart (1960) has suggested, the other stages in auditory training are 1) the development of gross discriminations, 2) the development of broad discriminations among simple speech patterns, and 3) the development of finer discrimination for speech.

Gross discriminations can be developed by using objects that produce unique and loud sounds. The child first associates the object with the sound and then is called upon to indicate which object, activated out of his sight, produced the sound. Whistles, drums, borns, bells, cymbals, and chimes are typical of the sound-makers found to be useful with this technique. The same techniques may be applied to identifying dissimilar musical sounds played either live on a piano or produced from recordings. Furthermore, discriminations may arise from association with common sound-generating activities and experience, such as clapping, crying, coughing, and running water. Sounds increasingly alike are used to refine the child's skills of discrimination.

The development of broad discrimination among simple patterns is merely a special application of the techniques used to develop gross discriminations. Dissimilar phonetic elements are contrasted, the child gives them back, and eventually he is exposed to words and phrases with varying rhythms. Here the child is likely to develop an appreciation for the regime of auditory training because it is related to speech expression and reception.

It is not likely that the deaf child can develop finer discriminations for speech like *f* as in *fin* and *th* in *thin*. Of course, these should be tried, but in all stages of auditory training the teacher must be aware that the child's performance is eventually limited by his restricted auditory area and she should not spend what may be discouraging periods for both her and her pupil in trying to attain the impossible.

GUIDES FOR PRACTICE

Despite the unsolved problems that are still with us, there is no longer any question about the usefulness of the auditory system in the education of deaf children. Out of our experience grow the following guides for practice in auditory training:

1. Most deaf children have a small but useful portion of the auditory area that lies above the range of usual audiometry. Consequently, many children who have been termed "totally deaf" as a result of audiometric tests actually can hear properly amplified sound. Audiograms may not tell the whole story of a child's ability to appreciate speech by his hearing. Formal auditory training is essential, however, to teach the deaf child to make use of this remnant of hearing. The hearing aid alone is not enough.

2. Auditory training appears to be more effective, through mutual reinforcement, when hearing is combined with vision and/or touch. There are times when hearing alone is used to teach a child to concentrate on specified information bearing cues.

3. The techniques of auditory training should be geared to a child's auditory capabilities. This requires frequent assessment of his hearing.

4. Auditory training, even without a hearing aid, should be begun as soon as it is determined that a child is deaf.

5. Formal instruction can make hearing aids more acceptable to children by giving them experiences that are meaningful. Such instruction should teach children to discriminate, even though grossly, various environmental sounds, and, within the limits of their hearing, teach them to understand speech by hearing.

Speechreading

Speechreading, sometimes called lipreading because it involves observing more than the lips, is the process through which an individual, regardless of the state of his hearing, understands speech by carefully watching the speaker (Silverman, 1948). It was not until the middle of the seventeenth century that John Bulwer, an English physician, in his *Philocopus* and the *Deafe and Dumbe Man's Friend* suggested the possibility of lipreading as a satisfactory way for the deaf to understand spoken language. However, it may be that the rise of manual methods of instruction in the latter part of the eighteenth century and in the early part of the nineteenth century retarded the development of lipreading despite efforts of German educators like Heinicke to popularize it. The latter half of the nineteenth century saw an increasing acceptance of oralism and with it an enthusiastic interest in lipreading. This writer (1948) has crystallized the latter-day evolution of lipreading.

> Since speech reading (or lip reading) appeared to have value for deaf children, it was inevitable that it should be taught to the deaf child and to the adult whose hearing was so impaired that communication by auditory means was impossible or severely limited. Teachers in schools for the deaf began to instruct adults and in 1902 Martha Bruhn established in Boston a school of speech reading for adults based on the system of Julius Müller-Walle, formerly a teacher in the school for the deaf in Hamburg, Germany. Miss Bruhn emphasized the importance of differentiating the movements of speech through syllable drills as they appeared to the speech reader. Immediately after Edward B. Nitchie founded his school of speech reading in which he stressed the importance of psychological factors in speech reading, primarily the ability to synthesize meaning from contextual clues. Emil Froeschels in Vienna also stressed the need for ability to get meaning of speech movements which were either hidden or ambiguous, teaching first only those with the help of a special phonetical alphabet. In 1917 the Kinzie sisters, Cora, Elsie, and Rose, founded a school in which they attempted to combine the best features of the Müller-Walle and Nitchie systems and they also introduced the idea of speech reading material graded to various levels of difficulty. Later Jacob Reighard of the University of Michigan translated the principles of Brauckmann's Jena method into English and advocated their adoption in America. The Jena method seeks to associate movements of speech with the process of speech reading. . . .

In recent years the emphasis has been on associating lip-reading instruction with hearing, with kinesthesia, and with motion pictures that provide opportunities for learning and practice. Lipreading has come to be accepted as an essential tool of communication for deaf and hard-of-hearing children and adults.

As we have said repeatedly, children with normal hearing learn oral language primarily by hearing, which is reinforced by other sensory experience. The sounds are later associated with the visual symbols, i.e., the movements of the talker's face, that partly represent language. This is speechreading. The deaf child is denied the possibility of learning this by association with auditory language, and is forced to learn his visual speechreading language directly. The extent to which he is able to do this may depend upon a number of factors, some of which are exceedingly complex and difficult to analyze (Simmons, 1959; Frisina, 1967). One group of factors concerns the speaker. These include his distance and position and how well his face is illuminated. They include the character of his speech, his precision of articulation, how fast he talks, the mobility of his face, and the familiarity of the speechreader with the particular speaker. Then there are factors concerning the language material, such as the vocabulary and the language structure. Finally, there is the speechreader himself, his vision, his intelligence, his general information, and his ability to synthesize from contextual clues, his ability to recognize discrete units of speech, his ability to associate his own "feel" for speech with the speech he sees on the face, and the fundamental structure of his personality which may determine his attitude toward speechreading.

Speechreading is further complicated by the ambiguitiest hat result from hidden movements, such as *h* and *k*, from homophenous words (words that look alike on the lips, such as "smell" and "spell"), and from the difficulty of appreciating patterns of stress, intonation, and phrasing.

Numerous attempts have been made to assess the role of these factors in speechreading to diagnose difficulties, to evaluate progress and methods of instruction, and to predict performance (Jeffers, 1967; O'Neill, 1967). Among the possible factors that may be related to skill in speechreading and which have been investigated are intelligence, reading ability, perceptual ability, motivation, and rhythmic skills. These studies have led to no generalizations in which we have confidence. One of the major problems in studying these relations is the adequacy of tests of speechreading. The test constructers are faced with formidable variables that are unique to the population to be tested. Among these are the degree and kind of hearing loss, the time of onset of impaired hearing, the language ability of the subjects, and the standardization of the test material itself and particularly of the manner of its presentation. There is also the difficulty of establishing norms for a heterogeneous population. Furthermore, the validation of the tests appears to rely solely on ratings by teachers. This introduces new problems.

Instruction in speechreading for deaf children is usually not a thing apart. In the beginning, even before the child enters school, he is encouraged to watch the face of the talker. The deaf child is not as aware as the hearing child that he can get information, in its broadest sense, by watching the movements of the face. When formal instruction is begun, the child is taught to associate movements of the lips, jaws, and tongue with objects, feelings, and actions. The objective here is not merely the enlargement of speechreading vocabulary but cultivation of the idea that watching the face of the talker is useful. Finally, speechreading pervades every act of speech perception by the child and becomes an increasingly useful tool of communication as it is practiced in purposeful situations.

The inadequacy of our formal tools for assessment of the ability to speech-read need not deter us from suggesting the following guides to practice in developing this valuable skill in deaf children:

1. An atmosphere of oral communication must be created and maintained. Speechreading must be shown to serve a purpose.

2. Even if the child is not expected to understand every word of a spoken message, he should be talked to and he should be encouraged to take advantage of situational clues.

3. Speechreading should be reinforced by other sensory clues whenever practical.

Language

In our discussion of the skills of communication to this point we have, in a sense, considered the development of the skills of talking and "listening," namely, speech, auditory training, and speechreading. We now turn to the message itself, the stuff of oral communication. This is language. The "ear-to-voice link" is essential for talking and listening (Miller, 1951). It is the basis of a child's attachment of meaning, in speaking, in writing, in listening, and in reading, to words and combinations of words. The absence of hearing is catastrophic for the "natural" but complex development of association of language with experience.

It is the task of the teacher, nevertheless, to develop language in deaf children although they do not have full use of the sensory channel that is considered essential for the growth of language. In the performance of this task the teacher needs to be aware of the unique problems created by the total absence of hearing or by the severe distortions of auditory verbal experience. Among the major problems for the child are vocabulary, multiple meanings of words, the verbalization of abstractions, and the complexity of the structure of language.

Vocabulary

It is difficult to determine when a child really "knows" a word. Does he have it in his spoken, his written, his reading, or his listening vocabulary? The different kinds of vocabulary account for differences in the estimates of the functional vocabulary of children. At any rate, it is interesting that one representative study (Smith, 1926) shows that hearing children "know" 272 words at the age of two, 1,540 at four, and 2,562 at six. Compare this with zero words that the deaf child is likely to know when he enters school, even at the age of three, or more frequently at six.

Multiple meanings

Single words in our language may have many meanings that are eventually clarified for hearing children, chiefly by the repeated auditory experience that is denied the deaf child. An average of almost four meanings per recurring word was found by count in 12 commonly used arithmetic textbooks (Simmons, 1945). For example, the word "over" could mean "above" (the number over five is the quotient); "across" (over the Arctic Ocean); "again" (do your work over); "at an end" (the show is over); "more than" (over half the children); "besides" (left over); "during" (over a period of two years); "present" (turn the meeting over to); "on the other side" (turn the card "over"); or "by means of" (over the radio).

Verbalization of abstractions

Of course, hearing children and, for that matter, adults may experience difficulty in attaching words to abstract concepts, but the deaf child is in particular need of formal and informal but nonetheless deliberate instruction in the meaning of such relatively simple abstractions as *hope* and *want*.

Complexity of structure

Smith (1926) has shown that by the age of five the spoken sentence of the average child has reached five words in length. For the superior child it is about 10 words long. This increase in length is inevitably accompanied by the use of complex syntactical relations that clarify and enrich meaning. These involve such grammatical concepts as pronouns, connectives, tense, person, and word order, as well as relations among clauses and among phrases of various sorts. If the hearing child reaches these levels of complexity at the age of five, we are again struck by the extent of the language gap between the deaf and the hearing. It was found by the Heiders (1940), after their thorough comparison of sentence structure in the written compositions of deaf and hearing children, that the "whole picture indicates a simpler style (for the deaf) involving relatively rigid unrelated language units which follow each other with little overlapping structure or meaning."

In general, the deaf appear to be comparatively deficient in the flexible manipulation of our language to make the best use of it as a tool of communication. This may be due to their educational retardation; it may be due to the methods of teaching language, or, in addition to these, to the idea suggested by the Heiders that "the difference between the deaf and the the hearing cannot be fully expressed in quantitative terms as the degree of retardation and that they represent differences not merely of skill in the use of language forms but in the whole thought structure."

Methods of instruction in language

Methods of instruction of the deaf in language can be divided conveniently into two major approaches: the natural method, sometimes known as the synthetic, informal, or mother method; and the grammatical method, sometimes referred to as the logical, systematic, formal, analytical, or artificial method.

Historically, the *grammatical method* preceded the natural method. It was based on the notion that after memorization of classifications of words and their conjugations and declensions, they could be used as building blocks for connected language. This approach evolved into a multiplicity of "systems" that were created primarily to provide a systematic set of visible symbols to guide deaf children in the use of language. We shall briefly describe three of the more popular ones.

THE BARRY FIVE-SLATE SYSTEM

The assumption underlying this system, developed by Katherine E. Barry (1899) at the Colorado School for the Deaf, is that ability to analyze the relations among parts of sentences is necessary to the "clear thinking" essential to an understanding of language. Five slates or columns are visible on the walls of the schoolroom. The subject of a sentence goes on the first slate, the verb on the second, the object of the verb on the third, the preposition on the fourth, and the object of the proposition on the fifth. Children then learn the rationale of the verbalization of their actions according to the visual aid afforded by the slates. This system, many believe, tends to stultify idiomatic expression and actually may result in ungrammatical, stilted language.

WING'S SYMBOLS

This system, devised in 1883 by George Wing of the Minnesota School for the Deaf, is based on a set of symbols, mostly numbers and letters, representing the functions of different parts of speech in a sentence. These symbols are placed over the word, phrase, or clause in order to demonstrate the form, function, and position of the parts of a sentence, rather than just to illustrate parts of speech. For example, *1* stands for the noun, *2* for a possessive, and *o* for the object. Advocates of the system believe that it is of great value as a corrective tool throughout the child's career and that it encourages correct grammatical usage.

THE FITZGERALD KEY

This system, first published in 1926, was developed by Edith Fitzgerald (1937), a congenitally deaf person, when she was head teacher at the Virginia School. Miss Fitzgerald advocated developing "natural" language but felt that this could be aided by developing the child's power of reasoning, judgment, and discrimination about language. This is accomplished by a set of key words and symbols related to language that was developed as it was needed by the children. There are six symbols, one each for verbs, infinitives, present participles, connectives, pronouns, and adjectives. For example, the symbol for a verb is =. Among the advantages of the method are its comprehensiveness, its flexibility, and the possibilities for self-correction.

The basic feature of the grammatical systems is the emphasis on getting the child to *analyze* functional relations among discrete units of language and, by repetition and visual aids, to impart to him an understanding of language principles or linguistic "rules" including how the arrangement of words affects the meaning of a sentence. Methods that combine an analysis of the structure of language, a Key system, and expanding "kernel" sentences or patterns are also in use.

One of the early advocates of the *natural method* was D. Greenberger, who headed what is now the Lexington School for the Deaf in New York City. He felt that language was best learned by supplying it to children in the situations in which they had need for it. Practice was geared to actual and natural situations. A leading advocate of this approach is Groht (1958), who suggests that prior to the time a language principle is to be introduced formally it should be used in natural situations through speechreading and writing. It is then drilled on in various ways that are interesting and purposeful for the child. In essence, the teacher creates situations which provide many and varied contacts with the principles of language. The method is claimed to be more consistent with the laws of learning of language by hearing children than is a formal, analytical method.

Until we gain more insight into how the deaf child conceptualizes, the teacher of language will need to use all the knowledge and ingenuity at her command to combine the best features of a grammatical method with the obviously excellent possibilities of the natural method. She will use such commonly accepted techniques as general conversation, composition, news items, trips, action work, topical essays, experience stories, letters, and descriptions of places, events, and persons. The child's progress in acquiring language will be governed only by the extent to which the teacher uses her own ingenuity, flexibility, and knowledge of how children grow and develop. Perhaps she may find some help in the following guides to practice:

1. Language teaching should be related to significant and meaningful experiences of children.

2. Language should constantly be made to serve a purpose for the child.

3. All sensory channels should be used to teach language.

4. Teachers need to be alert to the ideas that are developing in children so that they may provide the children with language with which to express them.

5. Children need many varied contacts with the same language in order to make it theirs.

6. Children need formal, systematic aids to the acquisition of language. Many shun language when they feel insecure in its use.

7. Schools and homes should create an atmosphere where language is used and where books are read regularly.

CURRICULUM DEVELOPMENT IN SCHOOLS FOR THE DEAF

In general, curricula of schools for the deaf resemble those in schools for the hearing with appropriate adaptations for difficulties of verbal communication. However, the growing national concern for improving education of all children at all levels has expressed itself primarily in focusing attention, energy, and abundant resources on curricular revision and reform. Stimulated by these efforts, educators of the deaf are seeking ways to improve the performance of their schools. Efforts in curriculum development have centered around considerations of goals, process, and materials, and their dissemination, implementation, and evaluation.

An obvious first question in goal setting is, who sets them? Shall it be school administrators, teachers, parents, deaf adults, mature students, psychologists, social scientists, humanists, employers, psychiatrists, specialists in particular disciplines, funding agencies, or some combination of these? We appear to be a long way from examining on a rational basis the contributions that these and other elements have to make to our formulation of goals. For example, what can students of mental health tell us about the wisdom of such long-range goals as complete integration of the deaf person in the world of the hearing on the one hand, or production of contented members of a subgroup on the other? Certainly the grand design of the educational experience we arrange for our children would be crucially influenced if not fundamentally determined by what we think about this issue.

Another question pertinent to goal setting is: How shall they be stated? Shall they be outlines of "content" like "how a plant grows," shall they be skills like reading, writing, etc., or behavioral objectives like identifying, describing, distinguishing, naming, stating, and applying a rule, etc.? Shall they go beyond the cognitive and apply to total human functioning? What schemes are possible to bring these categories into some reasonable relationship?

Attainability is still another important aspect of goal setting. What is ideal and what are the realistic constraints imposed upon us by the limitations of deafness, by physical facilities, by financial needs, by geography, by the distressing unavailability of enough able and motivated teachers, and by the changing technological and social scene?

Processes and materials

Given a set of goals for a learner it is now the task of the technologists, be they "media specialists," discipline experts, educational psychologists, or just plain teachers in combination or individually, to develop processes and materials to attain the goals. Here we must be careful that the materials do not determine the goals and processes. All too frequently a kind of Parkinsonian principle operates. Goals are developed to use the materials available to attain them, often to the exclusion of more desirable goals.

The impressive array of processes and the increasing abundance of materials underline the growing importance of the educational technologists. The range and kinds of learning and teaching processes that are now or soon likely to be available to us are indeed imposing. They include tutoring, small group discussions, lectures, laboratory demonstrations, individual programmed instruction, textbooks, slides, tapes, films, instructional television, and computer-aided instruction. The contemplation of these possibilities for curriculum improvement is as intriguing as the questions posed by them are formidable.

To assist in the dissemination and implementation of improved materials, the Office of Education of the Department of Health, Education, and Welfare is supporting the development of regional *centers* for instructional materials for special education. In addition courses dealing with curricula in teacher education programs are being updated and elaborated. Yet there are subtle questions related to dissemination and implementation. For example, one of the appealing attributes of outstanding teachers of deaf children has been their spontaneity, their ability to sense an opportunity for learning by a child, and their skill in exploiting the situation. In disseminating and stressing prepared materials are we likely to create a dependence on them that will stultify spontaneity and imagination? The textbook is a classic example of prepared materials (antedating modern technology). There are few among us who do not have grim recollections of teachers who "taught from the book." Nevertheless, we need not face a forced choice. Our deliberations on curriculum improvement point toward the preparation of professional "disseminators" whose performance reflects an understanding of the learning problems of deaf children and how, for better or worse, they are taught.

Evaluation

In his summary of the 1967 National Conference on the Education of the Deaf the chairman said that "a nagging concern was the problem of evaluation whether it be of curriculum, of a method of communication, teaching or guidance, or of a system of organization and administration. Common sense requires that the effectiveness of any procedure, or change therein, be tested by the most objective investigations we can devise, so that substantive grounds are established for eliminating, amending or modifying our arrangements and practices. In education this is devilishly difficult to accomplish. Many of the outcomes we seek resist satisfactory measurement, and some results must await the passage of years before an attempt at evaluation is even appropriate. Nevertheless, the conference time and time again pointed to evaluation as a crucial issue demanding more concentrated attention" (Silverman, 1967).

We may ask what needs to be evaluated? Dyer (1966), in speaking of all schools, suggests a sobering thought; "The extraordinary fact is, however, that in spite of mountains of data that have been piled up from teachers' reports, tests, questionnaires and demographic records of all kinds, we still have only very hazy and superficial notions of what the effects of school experience really are." Of course we have academic achievement tests which, incidentally, may have an undue influence on our goals and which frequently are not pertinent at certain levels to our particular problems in the education of deaf children. Little is done, however, to evaluate the effective and social outcomes of school experience. A teacher may be doing an excellent job of teaching reading as measured by a reading test, but has she also taught some children to despise reading? Do we tend to evaluate only that for which we have tests, and do we accommodate assumptions to requirements of technique rather than to reality? Who should do the evaluating? Should it be members of the closed system we call "the school"—the teachers, the administrators, the school psychologists—all of whom conventionally evaluate their own product? How about parent evaluation? Or extramural individuals or groups? Or employers of deaf persons? Or deaf persons themselves?

Ours is a time of "rising expectations" nurtured by "great advances in technology" with its inevitable idolatry of evangelistic technologists and its comforting faith in equating change with improvement, newness with validity, gimmickry with innovation, and public relations with evaluation. Nevertheless, we must continue to probe for strategies for curriculum improvement with the recognition that it is a complex and demanding task.

Some interesting recent steps in this direction include the symposium on research and utilization of educational media for teaching the hearing-impaired (American Annals of the Deaf, 1965), the special issue of the Volta Review on Curriculum edited by Kopp (1968), and the report of a special study institute on curriculum planning for the deaf sponsored by the California State Department of Education and edited by Lowell (1967).

The need for special provisions for children with handicapping conditions in addition to deafness is being recognized. In the academic year 1967–68 there were, as we have said, 409 children in classes for the multiple handicapped in day and private schools. Data on the number of these children in other schools is not available. Among the more frequently occurring complicating conditions are special learning disability, mental retardation, gross motor incoordination, and abnormalities of vision.

THE NATIONAL CONCERN FOR HEARING IMPAIRMENT

Perhaps the most tangible and significant expression of national concern for the hearing-impaired is the recent enactment of federal legislation aimed at improving and expanding the preparation of professional personnel, stimulating research, and fostering extended services. The major portion of the federal effort is concentrated in the Department of Health, Education, and Welfare, which administers these programs through the Social and Rehabilitation Services Administration, the National Institute of Neurological Diseases and Blindness, and the Office of Education.

A number of specific enactments and projects are worthy of mention to illustrate the growing commitment of the federal government to hearing-impaired children and adults. In October 1965, acting on a recommendation contained in a report to the Department of Health, Education, and Welfare entitled "Education of the Deaf" (1965), Congress established the National Advisory Committee on the Education of the Deaf. NACED was charged:

1. to stimulate the development of a system for periodic gathering of information to make it possible to assess progress and identify problems in the education of the deaf;
2. to identify emerging needs and suggest innovations that promise to improve the educational prospects of deaf individuals;
3. to suggest promising areas of inquiry to guide the federal government's research effort in the education of the deaf;
4. to advise the Secretary on desirable emphasis and priorities among programs.

The Committee is now functioning and has accomplished one of its first tasks, a National Conference on the Education of the Deaf in April 1967. A conference report is available (1968).

The nation is concerned with the increasing number of young people who enter the labor market without any marketable skills or with skills that, at best, are marginal (Silverman, 1964; Williams and Vernon, 1969). The technological revolution that goes on unabated and at a rapidly increasing pace is drastically reducing the employment opportunities for those with marginal or obsolescing skills. Realism compels us to recognize that in any economy persons with severely disordered communication find their economic opportunities limited. Aware that burgeoning technology compounds our problem and underlines our responsibility (Quigley, 1966), Congress enacted legislation establishing a National Technical Institute for the Deaf to provide for a residential postsecondary technical education facility which would prepare young deaf adults for successful employment. In December 1966 the Secretary of H.E.W. entered into an agreement with the Rochester Institute of Technology, Rochester, N.Y., to establish and operate the Institute on its campus, thus making available to deaf students a broad modern range of educational opportunities with hearing students in the technical fields. Of course, the Federal Government continues to sponsor the century-old Gallaudet College, which provides a liberal arts curriculum.

To focus attention on the needs of all handicapped children Congress, in November 1966, amended the monumental Elementary and Secondary Education Act of 1965 to establish a Bureau of Education for the Handicapped within the Office of Education to encourage and support professional training, research, improved demonstrations of services, and the dissemination of information. A measure of the impressive impact of federal support is the increase of badly needed, trained teachers of hearing-impaired children. From 1950 to 1960 existing training centers graduated approximately 125 students annually. At the present time more than 500 graduates enter the profession. Similar relative increases in professional workers in audiology and speech pathology have resulted from training programs in the Social and Rehabilitation Services Administration and the United States Public Health Service.

The National Institute of Neurological Diseases and Blindness is engaged in an extensive collaborative perinatal project that may involve as many as 60,000 pregnancies. A central purpose is to study prenatal and perinatal factors which cause communicative disorders. Subsequent studies and evaluations are made of the children after birth and at various stages of development. Emphasis is thus being placed on the causes of deafness during pregnancy and early childhood and on the development of effective methods for early diagnosis and treatment.

Another encouraging development is the establishment of temporal bone banks in various laboratories to correlate histopathology of cases of deafness with prescribed information obtained during the life of the subject. Perhaps the large number of cases of deafness labeled "cause unknown" will be reduced because of these investigations.

Increased organized activities on the national and international scene by academic, professional, philanthropic, and lay groups is further evidence of the growing interest in the hearing-impaired. This is revealed in the Annual Directory of Services of the American Annals of the Deaf.

Although man has traveled a long, tortuous road from the pre-Christian era in evolving an enlightened understanding of the social problems of deafness, a large portion of society still looks upon the deaf and the hard of hearing as queer, dependent, and, sometimes, ridiculous. We are all familiar with the cheap humor of which they are often the target. Since their handicap is not as visible as that of the blind and the crippled, the deaf often find themselves in embarrassing and humiliating situations because others do not understand their special problems.

The answer of the deaf to such misunderstanding is to continue their social and economic achievements as self-respecting and productive individuals. Our social action for the deaf, therefore, should not aim for special privileges for them but should constantly strive to provide opportunity without discrimination for the deaf to help themselves.

This will happen if we realize that our attainments fall short of what is possible. We can close this gap by improving the quality of professional training, by reducing the shortage of workers in the field, by eliminating a persistent parochialism that is a residue from the days when the education of the deaf was in the hands of a dedicated but professionally inbred few, by communicating information to the public objectively, by increasing and applying scientific knowledge, and by ennobling the legacy of commitment that characterized the early few.

BIBLIOGRAPHY

Alcorn, K. 1938. Speech development through vibration. *Volta. Rev.*, 40, 633–638.

———. 1941. Development of speech by the tadoma method. *In* Report of the proceedings of the 32d meeting of the convention of American instructors of the deaf. Washington, D.C.: U.S. Government Printing Office, 241–243.

American Annals of the Deaf. 1965. Symposium on research and utilization of educational media for teaching the hearing impaired, 110, 508–620.

Amoss, H. 1936. Ontario school ability examination. Toronto: Ryerson Press.

Arthur, G. 1930. A point scale of performance tests. Vol. 1. New York: Commonwealth Fund.

Babbidge, H. 1965. Education of the deaf: a report to the secretary of health, education, and welfare by his advisory committee on the education of the deaf. Washington, D.C.: U.S. Department Health, Education, Welfare.

Barnet, A. 1964. The young deaf child: identification and management. *In* Proceedings of a conference. Toronto, Can., Davis, H., ed. Stockholm: *Acta-Otolaryng.*, Supplementum 206, 210–215.

Barry, K. 1899. The five slate system: a system of objective language teaching. Philadelphia: Sherman.

Beasley, W. 1940. The general problem of deafness in the population. *Laryngoscope*, 50, 856–905.

Best, H. 1943. Deafness and the deaf in the United States. New York: MacMillan.

Becking, A 1953. Perception of airborne sound in the thorax of deaf children. *In* Proceedings of the international course in paedo-audiology. Groningen: Verenigde Drukkerigen Hoitsema N.V., 88–97.

Bell, A. 1894. Sounds and their relations. Washington, D.C.: Volta Bur.

Bender, R. 1960. The conquest of deafness. Cleveland: Western Reserve Univ. Press.

Birch, J. R., and Birch, J. W. 1956. Predicting school achievement in young deaf children. *Amer. Ann. Deaf*, 101, 348–352.

Brunschwig, L. 1936. A study of some personality aspects of deaf children. New York: Teachers College Contrib. to Educ., Columbia Univ. No. 687.

Carhart, R. 1960. Auditory training. *In* Hearing and deafness. Davis, H., and Silverman, S. R., eds. New York: Holt, Rinehart and Winston.

Cornet, R. 1968. Cued speech. *In* Report of proceedings of the 43d meeting of the convention of American instructors of the deaf. Washington, D.C.: U.S. Government Printing Office, 112–113.

Davis, H. 1960. Reduced auditory area in a hypothetical case of sensory-neural hearing loss, Figs. 7–11. *In* Hearing and deafness. Davis, H., and Silverman, S. R., eds. New York: Holt, Rinehart and Winston.

———. 1964. The young deaf child: identification and management. *In* Proceedings of a conference. Toronto, Can. Davis, H., ed. Stockholm: *Acta-Otolaryng.*, Supplementum 206, 13–16.

———. 1965. Guide for the classification and evaluation of hearing handicapped. *Transactions Amer. Acad. Ophthal. Otolaryng.*, July–August, 740–751.

DeWeerd, M. 1951. The development of principles underlying auditory training. St. Louis: Washington Univ. Master's Thesis.

Drever, J., and Collins, M. 1928. Performance tests of intelligence. Edinburgh: Oliver and Boyd.

Doll, E. 1947. Vineland social maturity scale, manual of directions. Minneapolis: Educ. Test Bur.

Dyer, H. 1966. The discovery and development of educational goals. Given at the educational testing service invitational conference on testing problems, New York.

Eagles, E., Wishik, S., Doerfler, L., Melnick, W., and Levine, H. 1963. Hearing sensitivity and related factors in children. *Laryngoscope* Special monog., no number.

Ewing, I., and Ewing, A. 1947. Opportunity and the deaf child. London: Univ. London Press.

———, and ———. 1947. If your child is deaf. London: Deaf Children's Soc.

———, and ———. 1954. Speech and the deaf child. Washington, D.C.: Volta Bur.

Farrar, A. 1923. Arnold on the education of the deaf (2nd. ed.). Derby: Francis Carter.

Fitzgerald, E. 1937. Straight language for the deaf: A system of instruction for deaf children (2nd. ed.). Austin, Tex.: Steck Co.

Frisina, D. 1964. Speechreading. *In* Report of the proceedings of the international congress on education of the deaf and of the 41st meeting of the convention of american instructors of the deaf. Washington, D.C.: U.S. Government Printing Office, Document No. 106, 191–207.

Fry, D. 1966. The development of the phonological system in the normal and the deaf child. *In* The genesis of language. Smith, F., and Miller, G., eds. Cambridge: M.I.T.

French, J. 1946. What can parents do? *Volta Rev.*, 48, 720–726.

Furth, H. 1966. Thinking without language: psychological implications of deafness. New York: Free Press.

Fusfeld, I. 1933. What standard tests have shown at Gallaudet College. *In* Proceedings of the international congress on education of the deaf. West Trenton: New Jersey School for the Deaf. Pp. 197–206.

Galloway, J. 1964. The Rochester method. *In* Report of the proceedings of the international congress on the education of the deaf and of the 41st. meeting of the convention of American instructors of the deaf. Washington: U.S. Government Printing Office, Document No. 106, 440–444.

Garnett, C. 1968. The exchange of letters between Samuel Heinicke and Abbé Charles Michel De L'Épée. New York: Vantage Press.

Gesell, A. 1949. Gesell developmental schedules. New York: Psych. Corp.

Goldstein, M. 1939. The acoustic method for the training of the deaf and hard of hearing child. *Laryngoscope.*

Greenberger, D. 1889. Doubtful cases. *Amer. Ann. Deaf*, 34, 96–102.

Groht, M. 1958. Natural language for deaf children. Washington, D.C.: Volta Bur.

Health, Education and Welfare. 1968. Education of the deaf, the challenge and the charge. Report of a national conference. Altshuler, K., ed. Washington, D.C.: U.S. Government Printing Office.

Haggerty, M., Olson, W., and Wickman, E. 1930. Haggerty-Olson-Wickman Behavior Rating Schedules. New York: World Book.

Hall, P. 1929. Results of recent tests of Gallaudet College. *Amer. Ann. Deaf*, 74, 389–395.

Hardy, W. 1952. Children with impaired hearing. Children's Bur., No. 326. Washington: Government Printing Office.

———, Pauls, M., and Bordley, J. 1951. Modern concepts of rehabilitation of young children with severe hearing impairment. *Acta-Otolaryng.*, 40, 80–86.

Heider, F., and Heider, G. 1940. A comparison of sentence structure in deaf and hearing children. *In* Studies in psychology of the deaf, *Psychol. Monogr.:* Ohio State Univ. No. 232, 42–103.

Hess, D. 1966. The psychology of deafness: understanding deaf persons and their families. *Hearing Speech News*, 34, 20–26.

Hirsch, I. 1964. Communication for the deaf. *In* Report of the international congress on education of the deaf and of the 41st. meeting of the convention of American instructors of the deaf. Washington, D.C.: U.S. Government Printing Office, No. 106, 164–183.

Hiskey, M. 1941. Nebraska test of learning aptitude for young deaf children. Lincoln: Univ. Nebr., Dep't. of Educ. Psychol.

———. 1966. Hiskey Nebraska test of learning aptitude. Lincoln: Union College Press.

Hodgson, K. 1953. The deaf and their problems. New York: Philosophical.

Hidgins, C. 1934. A comparative study of the speech coordinations of deaf and normal subjects. *Jour. genet. Psychol.*, 44, 1–48.

———, and Numbers, F. 1942. An investigation of the intelligibility of the speech of the deaf. *Genet. psychol. Monogr.*, 25, 289–392.

Huizing, H. 1953. Assessment and evaluation of hearing anomalies in young children. *In* Proceedings of the international course in paedo-audiology. Groningen: Verenigde Brukkerijen Hoitsema N.V., 88–97.

———. 1953. Paedo-audiology, its present status and future development. *In* Proceedings of the international course in paedo-audiology. Groningen: Verenigde Drukkerijen Hoitsema N.V., 88–97.

Irwin, O. 1947. Infant speech: Consonantal sounds according to place of articulation. *J. Speech Hearing Disorders*, 12, 397–401.

Jakobson, R. 1941. *Kindersprache, Aphasie und Allgemeine Lautergesetze*, Uppsala, Almquist, and Wiksell. *In* Language and communication. Miller, G. New York: McGraw-Hill.

Jeffers, J. 1967. The process of speechreading viewed with respect to a theoretical construct. *In* Proceedings of international conference on oral education of the deaf. Washington, D.C.: Alexander Graham Bell Ass'n. for the Deaf. 1530–1561.

Kohl, H. R. 1966. Language and education of the deaf. New York: Center for Urban Educ.

Kopp, H. 1968. Curriculum and content. *Volta Rev.*, 70: 6, 359–518.

Kringlebotn, M. 1968. Experiments with some visual and vibrotactile aids for the deaf. *Amer. Ann. Deaf.*, 113, 311–317.

Lane, H. 1968. Personal communication. St. Louis: Central Institute for the Deaf.

Lenneberg, E. 1966. New directions in the study of language. Cambridge: M.I.T.

Levine, E. 1956. Youth in a silent world. New York: New York Univ. Press.

Lowell, E. 1967. Curriculum planning for the deaf. Sacramento, Calif.: State Depart. Educ.

McClure, W. 1966. Current problems and trends in the education of the deaf. *Deaf American*, 8–14.

McNeill, D. 1966. Developmental psycholinguistics. *In* The genesis of language. Smith, F., and Miller, G., eds. Cambridge: M.I.T. 15–84.

Machover, K. 1949. Personality projection in the drawing of the human figure. Springfield, Ill.: Thomas.

Miller, G. 1957. Language and communication. New York: McGraw-Hill.

Morkovin, B. 1968. Language in the general development of the preschool deaf child: a review of research in the soviet union. *Asha*, 10: 195–199.

Myklebust, H. 1964. The psychology of deafness. New York: Grune & Stratton.

———. 1965. Development and disorders of written language. New York: Grune & Stratton.

Odom, P., Blanton, R., Nunnally, J., and Koplin, J. 1965. A collection of word association responses from the deaf. Nashville, Tenn.: Department of Psychol., Vanderbilt Univ.

Oleron, P. 1963. Psychological testing. *In* Report of the proceedings of the international congress on the education of the deaf. Washington, D.C.: Gallaudet College, 140–145.

O'Neill, J. 1967. Frontiers of research in visual communication. *In* Proceedings of international conference on oral education of the deaf. Washington, D.C.: Alexander Graham Bell Association for the Deaf, 1562–1571.

Pickett, J., and Pickett, R., 1963. Communication of speech sounds by a tactual vocoder. *J. Speech Hearing Res.*, 6, 207–222.

Pintner, R. 1927. Psychological survey of schools for the deaf. *Amer. Ann. Deaf.* 72, 377–414.

———, and Paterson, D. 1918. Conclusions from psychological tests of the deaf. *Volta Rev.*, 20, 10–14.

Pitman, J. 1967. Can i.t.a. help the deaf child, his parents and his teacher? *In* Proceedings of the international conference on oral education of the deaf. Washington, D.C.: Alexander Graham Bell Ass'n. for the Deaf. 514–542.

Poull, L. 1931. The Randalls Island performance series. New York: Columbia.

Quigley, S. 1966. The vocational rehabilitation of deaf people. Washington, D.C.: U.S. Dept. Health, Education Welfare, Vocational Rehabilitation Admin.

———, Jenné, W., and Phillips, S. 1968. Deaf students in colleges and universities. Washington, D.C.: Alexander Graham Bell Ass'n. for the Deaf.

Rorschach, R. 1942. Psychodiagnostics. New York: Grune & Stratton.

Rosenstein, J. 1960. Cognitive abilities of deaf children. *J. Speech Hearing Res.*, 3, 108–119.

St. Michiels-gestel Institute. 1949. Perception des vibrations comme bas de enseignement de la musique sensorielle et de enseignement choréographique. The Netherlands: À l'Institut des Sourdsmuets de St. Michiels-gestel.

Shneidman, E. 1952. Make a picture story (MAPS) manual. New York: Psych. Corp.

Silverman, S. R. 1947. Tolerance for pure tones and speech in normal and defective hearing, *Ann. Otol., Rhinol., Laryng.*, 56, 658–678.

———. 1948. Educational therapy for the hard of hearing: speech reading. *In* Twentieth century speech and voice correction. Froeschels, E., ed. New York: Philosophical. Pp. 142–151.

———. 1949. The implications of schools for the deaf of recent research on hearing aids. *Amer. Ann. Deaf*, 94, 325–339.

———. 1954. Teaching speech to the deaf—the issues. *Volta Rev.*, 56, 385–389, 417.

———. 1960. From Aristotle to bell. *In* Hearing and deafness. Davis, H., and Silverman, S. R., eds. New York: Holt, Rinehart and Winston. Pp. 405–412.

———. 1964. Education of deaf children—past and prologue. *In* Report of the proceedings of the international congress on the education of the deaf and of the 41st. meeting of the convention of American instructors of the deaf. Washington, D.C.: U.S. Government Printing Office, No. 106, 113–122.

———. 1968. Some thoughts on curriculum improvement. *Volta Rev.*, 70: 6, 372–375.

———, Thurlow, W., Walsh, T., and Davis, H. 1948. Improvement in the social adequacy of hearing following the fenestration operation. *Laryngoscope*, 58, 607–631.

Simmons, A. 1945. Multiple meanings of words in arithmetic textbooks. St. Louis: Washington Univ. Master's thesis.

———. 1959. Factors related to lip reading. *J. Speech Hearing Res.*, 2, 340–352.

———. 1962. A comparison of the type-token ratio of spoken and written language of deaf and hearing children. *Volta Rev.*, 64, 417–421.

———. 1964. Personal communication. St. Louis: Central Institute for the Deaf.

Smith, A. 1960. Performance of subjects aged 2–4 on non-verbal tasks presented in pantomime. Ohio State Univ.: Ph.D. dissertation. Univ. of Mich.: Univ. Microfilms, Inc., MIC60-6422.

Smith, M. 1926. An investigation of the development of the sentence and the extent of vocabulary of young children. Iowa City: Univ. of Iowa Studies in Child Welfare, 3 No. 5.

Snijders, J., and Snijders-Ooman, N. 1959. Non-verbal intelligence tests for deaf and hearing subjects. Groningen, Neth.: J. B. Wolters.

Stetson, R. 1951. Motor phonetics. Amsterdam: North-Holland Pub. Co.

Stokoe, W., Casterline, D., and Croneberg, C. 1965. A dictionary of American sign language on linguistic principles. Washington, D.C.: Gallaudet College Press.

Sumby, W., and Pollack, I. 1954. Visual contribution to speech intelligibility in noise. *J. acoust. soc. Amer.*, 26, 212–215.

Terman, L. 1916. The measurement of intelligence. Boston: Houghton Mifflin.

Tervoort, B. 1967. Analysis of communicative structure patterns in deaf children. *Report of* Project RD-467-64-65 and Z.W.O. Onderzoek Nr. 585-15. Washington, D.C.: Vocational Rehabilitation Admin., Department Health, Education, Welfare.

Thorpe, L., Clark, W., and Tiegs, E. 1953. Manual for California Test of Personality—1953 Revision, Monterey, Calif.: Calif. Test Bur.

Urbantschitsch, V. 1897. Des exercises acoustiques dans la surdimutité et dans la surdité acquise. *Translated by* Egger, L., Paris: A. Maloine.

Vegeley, A., and Elliott, L. 1968. Applicability of a standardized personality test to a hearing-impaired population. *Amer. Ann. Deaf*, 113, 858–868.

Vernon, M. 1967. A guide to the psychological evaluation of deaf and profoundly hard of hearing adults. *Deaf American*, 19, 15–18.

Watson, T. 1951. Auditory training and the development of speech and language in children with defective hearing. *Acta-Otolaryng.*, 40, 95–103.

Wechsler, D. 1946. The Wechsler intelligence scale for children. New York: Psych. Corp.

———. 1949. The Wechsler intelligence scale for children manual. New York: Psych. Corp.

———. 1950. Cognitive, conative, and non-intellective intelligence. *Amer. Psychol.*, 5, 78–83.

———. 1955. The Wechsler adult intelligence scale. New York: Psych. Corp.

Wedenberg, E. 1951. Auditory training of deaf and hard-of-hearing children. Stockholm: *Acta-Oto-laryng.*, Supplementum 94, 1–129.

Whetnall, E., and Fry, D. 1964. The deaf child. London: Heinemann.

Williams, B., and Vernon, M. 1969. Vocational guidance for the deaf and severely hard of hearing. *In* Hearing and deafness. Davis, H., and Silverman, S. R., eds. New York: Holt, Rinehart and Winston.

Wrightstone, J., Aranow, M., and Moskowitz, S. 1963. Developing, reading test norms for deaf children. *Amer. Ann. Deaf*, 108, 311–317.

Yale, C. 1938. Formation and development of elementary English sounds. Northampton, Mass.: Metcalf.

Zaliouk, A. 1954. A visual-tactile system of phonetical symbolization. *J. Speech Hearing Disorders*, 19, 190–207.

16

Hard-of-Hearing Children

S. Richard Silverman

THE NATURE OF THE PROBLEM

This chapter deals with children whose hearing impairments are mild enough for them to learn without great difficulty to communicate by speech and hearing. The distinction between these hard-of-hearing children and those whom we have called the deaf is not always entirely clear. The reason is that individual children may differ greatly in the use that they are able to make of the remainder of their hearing. It is not simply a matter of hearing level for speech but also of such different factors as the age of onset, of the severity and exact type of hearing loss, the intelligence of the child, the amount of training that the child has had, the age at which the training was begun, and particularly the auditory and language environment of the child. As we have learned from experience with "culturally disadvantaged" children who hear, an impoverished language environment retards development of skills of communication, a condition that is difficult to remedy when the optimum time for acquisition has been passed. It is a matter also of the attitude of parents and their degree of understanding of the significance of the hearing impairment.

Even within the broad group of the hard-of-hearing there is a wide range of the ability to make use of hearing for communication by speech. The relatively mild hearing losses with hearing levels for speech of less than 40 dB cause only a little handicap, except perhaps for faint speech or for hearing at a distance. At the other extreme, with hearing levels for speech of 70 dB or thereabouts and particularly if the hearing loss was congenital or of early onset, the child may require painstaking instruction to learn to hear adequately, even with a hearing aid, and to understand and use language. Furthermore, the impairment of hearing is often not merely a loss of sensitivity that may be overcome by amplification, but may involve also a loss of ability to discriminate between certain sounds. Such a failure of discrimination is common when there is a great loss of sensitivity for the high frequencies.

Just as there are gradations in the usefulness of hearing, so there are gradations in the quality and intelligibility of the speech of hard-of-hearing children. Many hard-of-hearing children speak so well that the lay observer notices no abnormality, whereas the severely impaired may be almost unintelligible to those who are not accustomed to this type of speech.

Many investigators have sought to define the relations of these various factors of hearing impairment: intelligence, personality, emotional stability, social behavior, and the like. Our best generalization from their studies is that it is impossible to draw a *single* composite picture of the hard-of-hearing child. There is too much variation, both in the severity of the hearing impairment and in the many other pertinent factors. The personality structure of a child with hearing impairment is determined by many factors other than his difficulty in hearing.

In this chapter we shall discuss identification of

hearing-impaired children and we shall describe the hard-of-hearing child particularly in terms of his ability to understand speech, his ability to progress in school, and the extent to which these abilities are affected by his hearing loss. In making generalizations about the significance of various degrees of hearing impairment we shall assume that the hearing loss occurred before the child acquired speech and learned to use language. Obviously, if speech and language are acquired before the hearing loss occurs, the handicap imposed by the loss is much less severe. Hence the age of onset of the hearing impairment is an important factor.

Hearing-impaired children may be usefully divided into five classes, depending on their hearing levels for speech. These levels may be estimated quite accurately, by averaging the hearing levels for pure tones at 500, 1,000, and 2,000 Hz.

Class 1: Hearing level for speech 40 dB or better. These children may have difficulty in hearing faint or distant speech but are likely to "get along" in school and to have normal speech.

Class 2: Hearing level for speech between 41 and 55 dB. These children usually understand conversational speech at a distance of three to five feet without great difficulty. They may have some defects in the articulation of their own speech, and they may have difficulty in hearing adequately in school if the talker's voice is faint or if his face is not visible to them.

Class 3: Hearing level for speech between 56 and 70 dB. These children understand conversational speech only if it is loud, and they have considerable difficulty in group and classroom discussions. Their language and, especially, their vocabularies may be limited, and abnormalities of articulation and voice production are obvious.

Class 4: Hearing level for speech between 71 and 90 dB. These children may hear the sound of a loud voice about one foot from the ear and they may identify some environmental noises and distinguish vowels, but, even with hearing aids, they have difficulty with consonants. The quality of their voices is not entirely normal and they must be taught both speech and language. Many, but not all, children in this class should be considered "deaf" for educational purposes until or unless the combination of an adequate hearing aid and sufficient auditory training makes them only "hard-of-hearing."

Class 5: Hearing level for speech 91 dB or worse. These children are deaf, even though they may hear some very loud sounds. They never can rely on the auditory channel as a primary avenue of communication. As we have seen in Chapter 15, their speech and their language must both be developed through careful and extensive training.

The hearing levels that mark the divisions of these classes are substantially the same as those given in Chapter 15 (Davis, 1965). It will be noted that a hearing level of 90 rather than 100 dB is here chosen as the level dividing the fifth from the fourth class. This choice agrees well with a more recent definition of "100 percent hearing impairment" for medicolegal purposes. The scale given by the Committee on Hearing also subdivides what is here the first class into "normal" and "near normal." For the purposes of the present chapter, however, we have grouped all of these children together because they are all likely to "get along" in school and to have normal speech.

IDENTIFICATION OF THE YOUNG HEARING-IMPAIRED CHILD

The following section is taken verbatim from the proceedings of a conference "The Young Deaf Child: Identification and Management" held in Toronto, Canada on 8–9 October 1964. The purpose of the conference was "to bring together a small hand-picked group of 'experts' to exchange information on and to evaluate methods for coping with impairment, whether it be by surgery, hearing aids, special education or the exploitation of other sensory channels" (Davis, 1964).

Auditory Screening of the Neonate

The first opportunity to detect severe auditory impairment in young children is during the neonatal period, within the first few days after birth. Positive evidence of hearing may often be obtained by simple tests based on a startle or arousal response elicited by sudden rather loud sounds. *Methods for routine screening of the newborn infant for auditory impairment have been developed, but before widespread programs are initiated the following points must be considered:*

1. The incidence of deafness or severe impairment of hearing in the newborn is very low. The percentage of children who fail to pass the screening test in the three most extensive studies ranges from 0.1 percent to 2.0 percent. Careful consideration must be given to the value and economy of a screening program whose yield is so low.

2. The validity and the reliability of screening tests of infant hearing are both difficult to establish. Much further research is required. The number of "false positives" and the number of cases missed, which are both rather high, must be considered; the former will cause unfounded anxiety and the latter will give a false sense of security and thus delay later recognition of an auditory impairment. The chance of successful identification of auditory impairment and accurate assessment of its severity becomes progressively greater as the infant grows older.

3. The newborn infant is a very labile organism. He normally sleeps 20 to 22 hours out of each 24-hour period, and on a routine basis it may be difficult to catch him in an optimal state for testing. The best state is asleep, but he may be difficult to arouse sufficiently from deep sleep. He is hyperactive and tense when hungry or cold.

4. Certain conditions which can affect the auditory system, such as anoxic brain damage and particularly hyperbilirubinemia, may not show their effects the first day or two. Hyperbilirubinemia in particular may not cause symptoms before the fourth or fifth day or even later.

5. After they leave the newborn nursery only a small percentage of infants in most communities can be brought together for screening purposes. The maternity hospital thus offers unique opportunity for screening. Against this must be weighed: 1. the economy of a neonatal screening program; 2. the question of whether effective remedial measures, special training or management are available; 3. whether a delay in initiating the remedial measures or the special training and management is of critical importance, and if so 4. how long a delay is critical.

Opinions differ on the matter of how long a delay is allowable in the case of partial auditory impairment. There is no clear evidence that a delay of six months is critical from the point of view of development of language. Most participants in the conference agree that a year is probably critical, and many feel that the sooner auditory experience and training can be provided the better.

6. The possibility of injury to hearing as the result of misplaced and unnecessary use of amplified sound or of other loud and continued noise cannot be overlooked. Certainly the use of amplified sound for infants during the early weeks of life must be instituted with due caution. Indications of pain or discomfort are important guides, and an infant six months old can register them more clearly than a neonate.

A Positive Program

It is not necessary to wait for the methods of routine auditory screening at birth to be perfected and validated or for its economic feasibility to be demonstrated. An effective program for the early identification of children likely to have problems in communication can and should be instituted immediately. Such a program might be developed in two steps.

1. *A high-risk register* should be instituted, containing the names of babies in whom, for one reason or another, the risk of an auditory handicap is substantially higher than it is in the general population. The indications for placing a baby in a high-risk register are given in detail below.

Babies at risk should be followed closely from the point of view of development of normal auditory behavior, and if deviations are suspected definitive testing should be carried out. The children at risk should be seen fairly frequently during the first two years, say at zero, three, six, nine, 12, 18, and 24 months.

2. *All children attending well-baby clinics* or coming to pediatricians' offices might be screened during the latter part of their first year by a simple but well planned test or else by a questionnaire pertaining to auditory behavior. Children who do not yield satisfactory responses on two test occasions or concerning whom doubt is raised by the questionnaire would then be referred for more definitive testing.

The success of such a program will depend on the education of physicians, public health personnel and, above all, parents, with respect to normal expectations for the development of hearing and language and the possibility of auditory impairment. Among physicians it is particularly important to alert both obstetricians and pediatricians.

It would be ideal if impairment were detected and confirmed by six months of age, but a more practical time to try to identify the deaf child and institute appropriate special care and training is during the second half of the first year. This is a compromise between reliable detection of impairment and the earliest possible start on special auditory training. (End of excerpt.)

J. Hardy (1964), has suggested a high-risk register including antenatal factors, complications of labor, neonatal difficulties, early childhood events, and social factors. A useful summary of professional views on identification audiometry is contained in a report of a national conference on the subject (Darley, 1961).

The Significance of the Problem

The problem of the hard-of-hearing child is one of serious social significance.[1] Specifically, the community should feel a concern for the unfortunate financial and social effects of the retardation in school of children whose handicap has been neglected or not recognized. Obviously, the repetition of grades is costly, and, in the long run, it is only a grossly superficial remedy which leaves the root of the problem quite untouched.

To those public school authorities and taxpayers who view with alarm the financial outlay necessary for a really constructive program for the hard-of-hearing child we may point out that the saving from avoiding repetition of grades offsets a large part of the cost of the program. In addition, we must reckon the cost of truancy and various forms of antisocial behavior which characterize the child who becomes bored with the schoolwork in which it is so difficult for him to participate.

The financial aspects of the problem must in no way, however, obscure the solemn moral obligation of every American community to provide for each child the opportunity to develop according to his maximum potentialities. This is the fundamental principle of our system of democratic education, and the community that shirks responsibility for an adequate program for the physically handicapped child stands guilty of its violation.

In the smaller community of the schoolroom itself the teacher is often not aware that the learning or behavior difficulty of a hard-of-hearing child is due to his impaired hearing and not to lack of mental ability or to some fault in her methods of teaching. For example, Goetzinger (1964) and his coworkers in studying children with as low a hearing level as 30–45 dB found the hearing-impaired children to have poorer auditory discrimination and more errors of articulation than normally hearing children. Furthermore, the incidence of comments from teachers stressing poor work habits, poor attitudes, and emotional variability was much higher for the children with even mild hearing loss. Failure to understand the basic cause of the child's difficulties frequently leads to fruitless remedial measures that are time-consuming for both the child and his classmates. And when by good fortune the teacher recognizes the child's hearing impairment, her lack of special training and information and the requirements of other children in the room make quite impossible any adequate solution of the child's particular problem.

In the narrower confines of the family circles, too, the hard-of-hearing child presents a problem that requires wholesome and sympathetic understanding. Apparent inattention to the spoken word is often interpreted as sheer naughtiness. The misdirected punishment often results in tensions within the family which would be avoided if the parents were only aware of their child's handicap. Furthermore, repetition of grades in school delays the day when the child can become a self-supporting individual. In many families the prolonged dependence is a serious problem.

The desirability of identifying hearing losses early by various methods of screening audiometry and individual hearing tests, as well as the possibility of conserving hearing by proper diagnosis and by treatment of the medical conditions that are so disclosed, has been discussed. In detecting hearing losses in children, informal procedures and simple intelligent observation can be of great value. Both teachers and parents should be informed of the clues in a child's behavior that suggest the possibility of a hearing loss. The symptoms include inattention, frequent request for repetition of spoken words, cupping the hand to the ear, cocking the head, difficulty in copying dictation, indifference to music, abnormalities of speech, reluctance to participate in activities that require oral communication, such as dramatics, failure to follow oral directions, daydreaming, and poor scholarship. Not to be overlooked are truancy, lying, stealing, extreme introversion, and other forms of a typical behavior that frequently serve as compensations for the child who feels socially inadequate and wishes to attract attention to himself. Of course, such behavior may also depend on a host of other conditions. We merely note that the possibility of hearing impairment as a cause should not be overlooked by teachers or laymen. Medical indications, such as earache, bad tonsils, frequent colds, and so on, have been discussed in earlier chapters.

EDUCATIONAL NEEDS AND PROCEDURES

The educational needs of the hard-of-hearing child are different from those of the deaf child. The hard-of-hearing child can learn to talk, to understand speech, and to learn language by more nearly natural

[1] Chapter 15 contains statistics about the magnitude of the problem.

means and relying primarily on his sense of hearing. Furthermore, if his difficulties are recognized and if he is given proper assistance, his needs may well be met in a special class for the hard-of-hearing within the public school system, or even in the regular classroom itself. The assignment to a particular class will depend both upon his hearing level and on the availability of special help. The aim should be to educate him with normal-hearing children wherever this is practical.

The particular needs of hard-of-hearing children may be summarized as follows, according to their classification by hearing level for speech:

Class 1: Better than 40 dB. These children should be given the benefit of favorable seating in regular classrooms and may be assisted by special instruction in speechreading.

Class 2: 41 to 55 dB. These children should wear hearing aids and be given training in their use. They should be taught speechreading and also be given the benefit of speech correction and conservation of speech. They should also have the advantage of favorable seating in classrooms.

Class 3: 56 to 70 dB. Hearing aids and auditory training, special training in speech, and special language work are all essential. With such assistance and with favorable seating, some children can continue in regular classes. Others may derive more benefit from special classes.

Class 4: 71 to 90 dB. These children should be taught by means of educational procedures for the deaf child with special emphasis on speech, on auditory training, and on language. After a period of such instruction it is possible that these children may enter classes in regular schools.

Class 5: Worse than 91 dB. These are deaf children who require the special educational procedures described in the preceding chapter. Some of these children, however, eventually enter high schools for the hearing.

AUDITORY TRAINING

As we have seen in the preceding chapter, auditory training, primarily through amplified sound, is aimed at improving speech, speech perception (when combined with lipreading), and at improved psychological well-bearing. For hard-of-hearing children, the potential for auditory training is greater than for deaf children. We may look for development not only of gross discriminations but greater development of discrimination of speech patterns and speech sounds. Actually, lipreading is likely to be the supplementary (to hearing) means of communication for most hard-of-hearing children. Training should be pointed at more extensive discrimination of the kind suggested in the preceding chapter. Most of the techniques for both children and adults reflect the possibility of attaining discriminations sufficient to permit understanding of speech through the ear for all but the severely handicapped (Brentano, 1946; Browd, 1951; Goldstein, 1939; Kelly, 1953; Ronnei, 1951; Utley, 1951; Wedenberg, 1954; Whitehurst, 1947; Oyer, 1966).

In general, hearing aids are useful to hard-of-hearing children and adults who have a loss of 40 dB or more in the speech range and whose hearing loss is such that amplification will not distort speech to the point where the instrument not only does not help but may impair speech perception. Care must be taken not to force hearing aids on children or adults. As long as our culture stigmatizes hearing loss, people will hesitate to display evidence of it. This situation may be aggravated by the tendency of purveyors of instruments to base advertising on ingenious methods of concealing the hearing aid when it is worn on the person. This may be necessary to get people into the shop, but it may also heighten the feeling of stigma and keep the prospective client away. In a study of factors influencing the decision of children to wear hearing aids, Gates and Kushner (1940) found that fear of losing social status and concern over personal appearance caused some children to reject hearing aids. On the other hand, they found that hearing-aid users showed consistent improvement in school achievement and in participation in group activities.

Quantitative information available to us about the effect of auditory training for the hard-of-hearing is fragmentary. We have seen in the preceding chapter that Hudgins (1953) has shown the value of a bisensory approach for the deaf, and Wedenberg (1954) reports encouraging results with selected children, the results varying with the amount of hearing loss. Kelly (1954) claimed some improvement in children for speech perception and social adjustment, and Silverman (1944) reported substantial gains by adults from auditory training in understanding of words and sentences. Siegenthaler and Gunn (1952) questioned some of the results and found in general that previous "acoustic rehabilitation" does not insure more threshold help with a hearing aid. Ling and Druz (1967) found no superiority of a hearing aid featuring transposition of high-frequency sounds to a lower frequency region over a conventional hearing aid. These investigations suffer from the lack of adequate and rigorously valid measuring devices, criteria for gain from auditory training, and control of instruction methods and attitudes.

It is clear that we need more scientifically derived information about the factors that are associated with successful use and acceptance of a hearing aid.

LIPREADING

In the preceding chapter we discussed the evolution of lipreading, its pedagogical basis, and the factors influencing its performance. For the hard-of-hearing child and adult, lipreading instruction may be more flexible and varied because it is not subject to the restriction of limitations in language. As we have said previously, it is the supporting skill for hearing. The skillful teacher of lipreading learns to create situations that stimulate taking advantage of contextual clues and to use material that appeals to the interests of her pupils. Many suggestions of this sort are contained in the recommendations of Bunger (1942), the Kinzies (1931), Nitchie (1950), Hardy (1969), O'Neill and Oyer (1961), and Haspiel (1964).

SPEECH DEVELOPMENT, CORRECTION, AND CONSERVATION

We have already discussed the underlying considerations in the development of speech in the severely deaf. Our major speech problem with the hard-of-hearing is the correction and the conservation of speech. The hard-of-hearing person does not hear speech and speech patterns clearly and therefore has a poor model for imitation. This is particularly applicable to the person with a high-frequency loss. For example, French and Steinberg (1947), using low-pass filtering, found that when only the frequencies below 3,000 were passed, 88 percent of nonsense syllables were heard correctly; but when only the frequencies below 1,000 cps were passed, the score fell to 27 percent. Furthermore, defective hearing prevents adequate monitoring of articulation and phonation.

Characteristic errors of articulation involve the mutilation or omission of sibilants such as *s* and *sh* and of word endings. Deviations in voice that may tax listener effort are the soft voice (with relatively good articulation)—characteristic of conductive deafness; the poorly modulated voice (with incorrect articulations)—characteristic of sensorineural deafness; and various combinations of these, depending, of course, upon the time of onset of hearing impairment and the kind and amount of corrective training. Many hard-of-hearing persons may have no detectable disorders of articulation or voice because of mildness or recency of onset of hearing impairment. Speech may deteriorate, however, with increase in the amount or the length of time of the deafness. It is, therefore, desirable, in order to prevent deterioration, that clinical and educational procedures for such individuals include work in speech conservation.

The procedures in speech correction and conservation for the hard-of-hearing should not differ radically from the measures suggested in other parts of this handbook dealing with disorders of voice and articulation, except that consideration must be given to the difficulties of auditory perception. The techniques should include learning to listen to good models of speech over hearing aids, creating motokinesthetic awareness by feeling vibrations connected with the production of speech, and the encouragement of good speech by the people who live and work with the hard-of-hearing person.

GUIDANCE

Certainly we must not overlook the need for psychological, educational, and vocational guidance which should avert or eliminate the atypical forms of behavior that frequently characterize the hard-of-hearing child. He must be made to understand that speechreading lessons and his hearing aid are as necessary as geography, arithmetic, or any other school activity. In fact, they may be more so. He should be particularly encouraged to join in extracurricular and community activities, such as scouting, athletics, Hi-Y, 4-H, church functions, and other wholesome pastimes of youth. Success in any of these these activities should do much to avert extreme introversion and preoccupation with the impairment of hearing. Of course, extreme cases should be referred for psychiatric study. Vocational plans for the child should take into account the existence of hearing impairment. Obviously we would not suggest preparation for any calling which demands a high degree of accuracy in oral communication. We are too well aware of the psychological distress which inevitably accompanies a trying occupational situation. Bookkeeping, for example, would be preferable to stenography. On the other hand, vocational guidance should stress the child's assets and not his liabilities. There are many occupations at all levels in which hearing impairment is not a barrier to success.

Throughout our discussion we have implied, and it is well now to stress, that, although the welfare of the hard-of-hearing child should be entrusted to specially trained personnel, all remedial measures should be carried out within the framework of the regular school and health system. It is psychologically and educationally desirable that the child should not be prevented from associating with children who hear normally. True, he must be segregated for speechreading lessons and auditory training, but these activities should be considered part of his school program. In fact, we suggest that academic credit be given for participation in such classes, since, for the hard-of-hearing child, they involve the development of communication skills as important as composition or public speaking. They should be so recognized and integrated with the curriculum. When the child is convinced that he is a person with a particular need that has been recognized, he has hurdled the chief obstacle to his eventual adjustment.

In summary, the management of hard-of-hearing children requires:

1. Public information about hearing impairment.

2. Case-finding through appropriate screening and identifying programs in hospitals, in clinics for babies, and in schools.

3. Complete medical diagnosis of hearing difficulties.

4. Appropriate medical and surgical treatment.

5. Thorough assessment of hearing after all indicated medical and surgical procedures have been completed, with particular attention to educational needs.

6. Special educational measures that include auditory training, speechreading, speech correction and conservation of speech, vocational planning, and psychological guidance.

BIBLIOGRAPHY

Brentano, L. 1946. Ways to better hearing. New York: F. Watts.

Browd, V. 1951. The new way to better hearing: through hearing re-education. New York: Crown.

Bunger, A. 1942. Speechreading—Jena method. Danville, Ill.: Interstate Press.

Darley, F. 1961. Identification audiometry. *J. Speech Hearing Disorders., Monogr. Supplement* No. 9.

Davis, H. 1964. The young deaf child: identification and management. *In* Proceedings of a conference. Toronto, Can. Davis, H., ed. Stockholm: *Acta-Otolaryng., Supplementum* 206, 13–15.

———. 1965. Guide for the classification and evaluation of hearing handicapped. *Tr. Amer. Acad. Ophthal. Otolaryng.*, July–August, 740–751.

French, N., and Steinberg, J. 1947. Factors governing the intelligibility of speech sounds. *J. acoust. soc. Amer.*, 19, 90–119.

Gates, A., and Kushner, R. 1940. Learning to use hearing aids. New York: Columbia.

Goetzinger, C., Harrison, C., and Baer, C. 1964. Small perceptive hearing loss: its effect on school-age children. *Volta Rev.*, 66, 124–132.

Goldstein, M. 1939. The acoustic method for the training of the deaf and hard of hearing child. St. Lous: The Laryngoscope Press.

Hardy, M. 1969. Speechreading. *In* Hearing and deafness. Davis, H., and Silverman, S. R., eds. New York: Holt, Rinehart and Winston.

Haspiel, G. 1964. A synthetic approach to lip reading. Magnolia, Mass.: Expression Co.

Kelly, J. 1953. Clinicians' handbook for auditory training. Dubuque: W. C. Brown.

———. 1954. A summer residential program in hearing education. *J. Speech Hearing Disorders*, 19, 17–27.

Kinzie, C., and Kinzie, R. 1931. Lip reading for the deafened adult. Philadelphia: Winston.

Ling, D., and Druz, W. 1967. Transposition of high frequency sounds by partial vocoding of the speech spectrum: its use by deaf children. *J. Auditory Res.*, 7, 133–144.

O'Neill, J., and Oyer, H. 1961. Visual communication for the hard of hearing, history, research, and methods. Englewood Cliffs, N.J.: Prentice-Hall.

Oyer, H. 1966. Auditory communication for the hard of hearing. Englewood Cliffs, N.J.: Prentice-Hall.

Nitchie, E. 1950. New lessons in lip reading. Philadelphia: Lippincott.

Ronnel, E. 1951. Learning to look and listen. New York: Columbia.

Siegenthaler, B., and Gunn, G. 1952. Factors associated with help obtained from individual hearing aids. *J. Speech Hearing Disorders*, 17, 338–347.

Silverman, S. R. 1944. Training for optimum use of hearing aids. *Laryngoscope*, 54, 29–36.

Utley, J. 1951. What's its name. Urbana: Univ. Ill. Press.

Wedenberg, E. 1954. Auditory training of severely hard of hearing school children. Stockholm: *Acta-Otolaryng.*, *Supplementum* 110.

Whitehurst, M. 1947. Train your hearing. Washington: Volta Bur.

PART III

Voice

17

Parameters of Voice Quality

I. P. Brackett

INTRODUCTION

Many textbooks discuss voice disorders under the two general headings of *organic* and *functional*. The professional use of term *organic* relates to conditions affecting structures per se, while the term *functional* applies to the physiology or use of structures in attaining particular objectives. In discussing the nature of speech structures, their conditions, and their use, three concepts must be kept in mind.

1. A normal speech structure may be used in a variety of ways creating the potential for different acoustic stimuli. That is, *a* structure does not necessarily have *a* single function.
2. The way a structure is used may affect the condition of the structure itself. That is, out of the potential use-choices, certain ones may alter the integrity of the structure, such as contact ulcer, vocal nodule, or inflamed edematous vocal folds.
3. The abnormal condition of the structure may restrict its use-potential. That is, the structural aberration such as laryngeal web, papillomas, or insufficient velopharyngeal valving may reciprocally determine its use in the production of acoustic stimuli.

The terms *organic* and *functional*, therefore, are labels which identify the possible antecedents to perceived usage differences. Present understanding does not permit a clear differentiation between the two terms since both the condition and the use of the structures are determinants in the assessment of the disorder.

To assess the nature of a disorder, a number of approaches may be employed. Descriptions of organic conditions rely on visual observation or on technical equipment which aids visual documentation. Terminology often denotes the state of the structure, such as cleft palate or bifid uvula. Visual assessment may also involve the observation of the structure in use. For example, paresis is suspected when one observes that a structure is unable to accomplish an appropriate movement. Visual documentation is basic to understanding of organic factors.

Use of structures often results in acoustic generation; therefore, documentation may rely on auditory sensations. Labeling the disorder then reflects auditory impressions such as "harsh," "strident," "nasal," "breathy," or "denasal." Difficulty often arises when one attempts to correlate visual and auditory information about the disorder because of these differences in labeling. The relationships between the structural aberration and the acoustical output are often assumed since present information does not permit precise comparisons.

Perhaps an example will help. Assume that the client's complaint is that he can't be heard. Specifically, since he is a professor who must teach large sections of a required course, he is distressed about his inability to "project his voice in class." A possible label for the disorder, initially, might be "insufficient loudness." As an aid to more detailed description, his voice may further be labeled as "breathy" or perhaps as having "inadequate breath support" because he exhibits speech samples composed of short phrases with frequent renewal of air supply and gasping. So far, labeling possibilities of the professor's "problem" have been confined to auditory impressions as these relate to his needs in communication. Visual observations of his larynx during phonation by indirect laryngoscopy reveal that the vocal folds do not adduct sufficiently. The disorder, then, may be described as "hypolaryngeal valving." This introduces a physiological label, rather than an acoustic one. Finally, a detailed examination of his vocal folds discloses a partial paralysis and atrophy of the right vocal fold, identified by labels of organic conditions. It may then be assumed that the paralysis and atrophy of the right fold (organic) causes, during speech, laryngeal hypovalving (visual-physiologic) resulting in laryngeal air turbulence which is labeled "breathy" (auditory impression). Lack of laryngeal resistance to air flow accounts for the short phrases, frequent renewal of air supply, and gasping. The minimal laryngeal resistance contributes to reduced amplitude of vocal fold vibration, which is inadequate for the professor's vocal needs in large audience situations. The nature of the disorder remained the same, although different labels may have been used to aid in its description.

Conceptual Delineations of Voice Quality

Within the profession of speech pathology, discussions of *voice* disorders, in contrast to *speech* disorders, demonstrate three general ways the term *voice* may be used. 1. The meaning of the term *voice* may be restricted to laryngeal vibration, or used synonymously with phonation. For example, the term *voiced* consonant indicates the presence of vocal-fold vibration in contrast to *voiceless* where vocal fold vibration is absent. From this point of view, *voice* would be differentiated from *speech* on an anatomical basis, i.e., *speech* being the result of air-stream modulations primarily occurring in the supraglottal cavities, whereas *voice* is the laryngeal modulations or, in the case of esophageal phonation, modulations of a pseudo-larynx. 2. The second meaning of the term *voice* encompasses not only the effects of laryngeal modulations of air flow, but also certain contributions of the resonators. The laryngeal modulations are perceived to initiate certain resonance characteristics within pharyngeal, oral, and nasal cavities which are considered attributes of *voice* rather than *speech*. The differentiation between *speech* and *voice* is now not anatomical, but acoustic, i.e., separating those characteristics required for phoneme identification (speech) from those characteristics not intimately related to verbal coding. For example, one may regard hypernasality on vowels as a *voice* problem, since phonemic identity may remain intact, but view hyponasality as a *speech* problem because the nasal continuants /m/, /n/, /ŋ/ may perceptually become voiced plosives /b/, /d/, /g/ with loss of phoneme identification. 3. Lastly, *voice* is used in an all-inclusive sense, incorporating general impressions which distinguish one person's *voice* from another's. *Voice* is primarily regarded from the viewpoint of the listener, and information is presented about efficient use of *voice*, sensitive response of *voice* to the demands of the speaking situation, *voice* as a revealer of personality, or developing an effective *voice* for speaking. In this context even a whisper is a *voice*. The fundamental interest to persons who hold this point of view is whether *voice* fulfils the requisites of communication.

The delineations discussed above represent valid approaches to voice. The concepts, of course, are academic. For those interested in the phonology of human communication, it is apparent that certain modulations of the air flow from the lungs, produced either laryngeally or in resonating cavities, demonstrate correspondence to meaning within the language code and are therefore phonemic. Other modulations interfere with or detract from meaning and are therefore nonphonemic. The speech clinician, as a decoder, must make decisions as to the appropriateness or inappropriateness of the speaker's code. Generally speaking, the classification of *voice* disorder, in contrast to a *speech* disorder, refers to the nonphonemic attributes which may occur coincidentally with the phonemic coding of the speaker, thereby detracting from the communication process.

The skill of the speech clinician is not only one of differentiating between phonemic and nonphonemic aspects, but, whenever possible, of determining the source of the speaker's encoding difficulty. Nonphonemic attributes coincidental to the verbal code alert the clinician to possible encoding difficulties of:

1. the speech structures themselves, including their use during verbal coding:
2. the central nervous system control or monitoring of neuromuscular impulses to these structures; and
3. the sensorineural feedback (auditory, kinesthetic and tactile) which validates to the speaker the accuracy of his coding.

Nonphonemic characteristics may result from encoding difficulties in any of these, regardless of the traditional category of the disorder, such as cerebral palsy, hearing loss, or cleft palate, and therefore become considerations of *voice*.

The focus of this chapter is directed to the perception of physioacoustic components of the verbal code, with emphasis on the nonphonemic attributes which are not necessarily related to the identification of phonemes themselves.

Basic Elements of Phonology

Success in decoding acoustic speech signals assumes that the speaker will produce 1. acceptable phonemes, variously sequenced or combined, 2. changes in the use of time, 3. changes in fundamental frequency, and 4. changes in intensity or energy. These four comprise the basic elements of verbal communication.

Phonemes

Humans are capable of producing a wide variety of acoustic signals of which only selected ones are recognized as phonemes. Fundamentally, phonemes exist for their linguistic value. Expansion of a statement of Stevens (1964), in which he says that in humans "each source of sound is the consequence of one of several types of modulation of a steady flow of air from the lungs," includes these points:

1. Structures may be placed in apposition in such a manner that air pressure will cause the structure or structures to vibrate. Although the lips or the soft palate may be utilized in this manner, the laryngeal vocal folds are the most frequently used vibrating structures during verbal coding. The vocal folds supply a somewhat regular or periodic sound source. When utilized, the resulting sound generation is amplified or modified by the supraglottal resonators.
2. The vocal tract may be narrowed or constricted at some anatomical area, creating sufficient turbulent fluctuations of the air flow against some obstacle to produce frication. The nature of the turbulence created is the result of a) the extent of narrowing of the tract, b) the rate and volume of air flow, and c) the size of the cavity or cavities through which the turbulence must pass.
3. The vocal tract may be completely occluded with subsequent build-up of air pressure at various anatomical areas producing the acoustic transient, including turbulence, when the pressure is released. The cavity or cavities into or from which the pressure is released also contribute to the acoustic composite.

It is from these three types of air-stream modulation, generated at different anatomical areas, either singly or combined, that man selects some which are designated as phonemes. These three also constitute the types of modulation not directly related to the phoneme. From the standpoint of speech, one might say that the satisfactory frication of a voiceless /s/ is accepted as a phoneme element in the verbal code, but the frication which results from the lateral escape of air for the voiceless /l/ is not.

USE OF TIME

Once a phoneme is identified as significant in a language, it usually must be combined with at least one other significant phoneme before it can be meaningful to the decoder. The sequencing of phoneme events introduces *time* as a variable. All single phoneme elements may be allotted as much time as the volume or pressure of the exhaled air flow will permit. A possible exception might be the plosives, although turbulence following released pressure may be extended similarly in time. During phonation, time, as an element of phonology, is primarily governed by the duration of vocal-fold vibration. Variations in the duration of vibrator oscillation, air turbulence on fricatives or whispered vowels alone or after release of pressure, and varying length of silence within and between words, phrases, or sentences determine gross speech rate. Phoneticians have attempted to set standards for length of time needed to identify phonemes, and writers of *voice* have set arbitrary standards for overall rate of effective speaking (Franke, 1939). However, variations in length of phonemes and gross rate of speech convey to the listener changes in the intellectual and emotional intent of the speaker. According to Fry (1955), the temporal length of the phoneme is one of the determiners of dominance among syllables or words in a phrase. This is true even in whispered speech where the duration of turbulence replaces the duration of vocal fold vibration on vowels and voiced consonants.

Inappropriate use of time, such as in stuttering, disrupts the expected time-use patterns anticipated by the listener. When use of time by the speaker does not match cultural patterns, and therefore detracts from the message, time variables become nonphonemic, and hence are considerations of voice.

USE OF FREQUENCY

Considerations of phonology also encompass the use of a range of frequencies. Variations in fundamental frequency and extent of range use also relate to the intent of the speaker as discussed by Fairbanks and Pronovost (1939). Not only may phonemes be lengthened or shortened for relative dominance of syllables or words, but changes in the frequency of vocal-fold vibration also contribute to dominance. More specifically, the spread of the frequency-change use corresponds to the mood of the speaker, i.e., as Skinner (1935) reports, cheerful, animated speech exhibits greater range-use than serious, thoughtful speech. Changes in duration and fundamental frequency during syllable elements of words are basic to the melody and rhythm patterns unique to English. Unexpected changes in frequency, such as in pitch "breaks," become nonphonemic.

USE OF INTENSITY

Lastly, the study of phonology includes intensity change or variations in energy. Increasing or decreasing total speech power, as discussed by Mol and Uhlenbeck (1956), is another means of achieving dominance of syllables, words, or phrases. Changes of energy signify degrees of emotional involvement, such as shouting when angry. Use of intensity changes also reveals the speaker's perception of physical and psychological distance. Inappropriate use, such as sporadic intensity changes in laryngeal tremor, do not conform to cultural patterns. Speech which is inappropriately soft or loud results in a variety of communication problems which often are a source of irritation to both speakers and listeners.

Phonemes in sequence and changes in duration, frequency, and energy constitute the basic elements of phonology used in verbal coding. To determine when these same variables are nonphonemic requires careful and thoughtful attention on the part of the clinician.

PHONEMIC AND NONPHONEMIC LARYNGEAL VARIABLES

Human acoustic communication results from physiological events which affect, in some manner, a moving column of air. Ordinarily, the air flow is initiated as a result of the processes of exhalation, and proceeds through the bronchial tree, trachea, larynx, supraglottal cavities, and finally to external body space. If no alteration is made in the size of the airway above the trachea, as in quiet breathing, the flow of air proceeds without any marked acoustical effect. Changing the rate of air flow, by increasing pressure, under the same conditions, would create the acoustic signal associated with a sigh. Along the route of exhaled air flow, the larynx (specifically the vocal folds) is the first place at which voluntary valving might be instigated.

Biologically, the larynx functions as a valve to impound air in the lungs or to assist in coughing or the protection of the lungs from the invasion of foreign material. These biolaryngeal actions are achieved by completely closing and opening the laryngeal valve. Should the adjustments of the valve, however, result in vibrating structures, the vocal folds need to be postured between completely open or completely closed. When vibrating, the vocal folds provide a wide spectrum of quasi-periodic modulations of the air stream, accounting for various tonal qualities reflecting different ways the vibrator behaves. When the vocal folds do not vibrate, the larynx may also provide an acoustic output associated with air-flow turbulence. These laryngeal contributions will be discussed under four general headings: 1. the larynx and valving; 2. the larynx and frequency generation; 3. the larynx and energy generation; and 4. the larynx and noise generation.

THE LARYNX AND VALVING

For the vocal folds of the laryngeal structures to function as an acoustic generator, various posturings of the vocal folds between abduction-adduction must be delineated. Abduction (to move away from the midline) and adduction (to bring toward the midline) are means of describing a continuum of laryngeal valving. Along this plane of laryngeal valving, various positions of the vocal folds account for different acoustic outputs.

ABDUCTED APHONIA

Abducted aphonia designates a condition in which the larynx provides no resistance to air flow through the vocal tract, such as in quiet breathing, paralysis of both vocal folds in the abducted position, or after surgical removal of the larynx. If the vocal tract is unable to be constricted in the area of the larynx, acoustic changes resulting from air-flow modulations could only be the product of valvings within the supraglottal resonators. Therefore, modulations are limited to phonemes traditionally labeled as voiceless fricatives, affricates, and plosives. Whispered vowels, nasals, and glides are only minimally possible if air flow is sufficiently increased to cause cavity turbulence.

After laryngectomy, when the airway between the lungs and the supraglottal resonators is interrupted, the effect achieved by buccal speech is similar to that described above. Under this circumstance, however, the voiceless phonemes result from air being impounded in the oral and pharyngeal cavities, since a continuously moving column of air is not available. When a laryngectomized person uses buccal speech, the vowels, glides, and nasals are not perceived as distinct acoustic entities but rather as moments of silence in any connected sequence of sounds. Using buccal speech as an example of abducted aphonia, the word "speech" would be phonetically represented as /sp-tʃ/ with /i/ being orally postured coincidental to the released pressure of the /p/. The turbulence following released pressure is the product of the oral posturing for the /i/. Turbulence characteristics would change should another vowel posture be utilized. A word containing only vowels, glides, or nasals, such as "alone," can only be sequentially postured within the oral cavity, since the phonemes provide no opportunity for turbulence characteristics to be produced.

The absence of any laryngeal behavior subtracts from normal speech signals certain basic components of phonology. Since the signal potential is incomplete, abducted aphonia affects the identification of certain phonemes in addition to other speech-signal elements associated with vibrating structures, such as frequency and energy variations.

WHISPER-APHONIA

Under conditions of partial laryngeal valving, and with vocal folds stabilized, sufficient air flow through the vocal tract on exhalation will produce laryngeal turbulence or frication which is commonly labeled whispering. Whispered speech is the combination of laryngeal turbulence associated with vowels, glides, and nasals, and cavity turbulence associated with the oral production of voiceless fricatives, affricates, and plosives. In soft whisper, laryngeal turbulence is necessary for the identification of vowels where oral cavity size is increased, such as low vowels /ɑ/, /ʌ/, whereas cavity turbulence is more evident on vowels where the oral cavity is reduced in size, such as /i/, /ɪ/, /u/. With loud whisper (stage whisper) laryngeal turbulence is more constant for all vowels, glides, and nasals. Laryngeal and cavity frication provide sufficient core acoustic data for the identification of all phonemes; therefore, whispered speech enables the sophisticated listener to decode the message. Whisper aphonia furnishes additional cues of vowel frication, in contrast to buccal speech, yet still does not possess the advantages of vibrating structures. Phonation provides greater physical dimensions for speech, fundamental frequency change, and additional cues for individual phoneme identification.

Whispering has an appropriateness in our culture by conveying to the listener a spatial intimacy. When whispered speech is the only form of verbal communication, or is inappropriately used for the communication intent, the speaker or listener may perceive it as a vocal fault. Speech pathologists, upon hearing chronic or unexplained sporadic whisper, suspect vocal fold paralysis, an organic condition which prevents sufficient vocal fold approximation for vibration and/or elasticity, or difficulty of the speaker in relating to others.

HYPOVALVULVAR PHONATION

Conditions of hypolaryngeal valving also apply to phonation. By approximating the vocal folds further along the plane of motion between abduction and adduction, vibration may be initiated even though the vocal folds are not optimally positioned. Should vibration of the vocal folds occur during conditions of hypolaryngeal valving, phonation is accompanied by noticeable amounts of laryngeal air turbulence. The combination of quasi-periodic vibration and laryngeal air turbulence has been labeled breathiness.

Vocal fold vibration is difficult to describe concisely, for it is a complex interaction of many variables. For example, the structural properties of the folds themselves, their position in valving, their intrinsic tension, and the amount of subglottal air pressure all contribute to the behavior of the vibrator. High-speed laryngeal photography, which enables observation of the vocal folds by slow motion, shows the vocal folds vibrating in three phases during one cycle:

1. closed (vocal folds touching each other anterior to posterior at the midline),
2. opening (vocal folds moving away from each other),

3. closing (vocal folds moving toward each other).

However, phonation under conditions of breathiness displays the following variations of the closed phase:

1. vocal folds vibrating without a closed phase, i.e., moving away from or toward each other, but never touching along the midline;
2. closed phase involves only a portion of the folds, i.e., the closed phase is confined to the anterior portion of the folds;
3. closed phase is considerably shorter in time than the opening or closing phases.

These variables of the closed phase relate directly to different amounts of laryngeal air turbulence. Assuming constant air flow, absence of the closed phase in the cycle of vibration would result in greater laryngeal air turbulence than when the closed phase time more closely matches the time of the opening or closing phases.

Analysis of high-speed motion pictures of the larynx as reported by Moore and von Leden (1957) demonstrates that change in phase time may be a function of frequency. The closed phase time appears shortened or absent at low frequencies in a person's range, and progressively increased in time as frequency is raised. Consequently, laryngeal air turbulence may be more noticeable at lower frequencies than at higher frequencies. Slight differences in the time devoted to each of the closed, opening, and closing phases are not detected by the listener, but when the closed phase is partially or completely absent, the listener is able to perceive substantial amounts of laryngeal air turbulence as an indication of hypolaryngeal valving.

The observation that lower range frequencies exhibit more laryngeal turbulence is substantiated by Van Riper and Irwin (1958) when they discuss breathiness coincidental with huskiness, i.e., a husky voice is synonymous with breathiness particularly when low-range frequencies are used. Breathiness which does not result from a pathology is expected to reduce as the laryngeal fundamental frequency is raised or subglottal breath pressure is increased, whereas breathiness which is the result of a pathology may not display such an improvement.

Hypolaryngeal valving during phonation has an effect on phrasing during continuous speech. Assuming a constant pressure and air flow provided by the process of exhalation, hypolaryngeal valving would interfere with the "phonemic breath groups" mentioned by Lieberman (1967). Conversely, more optimal laryngeal valving would, in turn, decrease the amount of air flow, increase subglottal pressure, and greater potential phrase length would be available. A possible approach to treatment for breathiness is directed toward altering muscle contractions of exhalation. However, it should be noted that to achieve greater control of exhalation one must also consider the function of the laryngeal valve.

Breathiness is noted for its lack of vocal intensity especially under conditions of increased spatial distance or ambient noise. The degree of turbulence produced by exhaled air passing through partially valved vocal folds results in decreased amplitude of the vocal fold oscillation which is insufficient for certain situational demands. In addition, breathiness is often interpreted by listeners to be an indication of withdrawal, and is assigned personality traits such as quiet, intimate, gentle, shy, timid, insecure, or apprehensive.

To those interested in the sequencing of phonemes, voiceless-vowel frication often accompanies a delay between the release of the position (ergo sound) of a voiceless phoneme when a voiced phoneme follows. Delays in coupling between voiceless and voiced phonemes increase turbulence time during the phrase. An increase in voiceless-phoneme time permits greater amounts of expelled air which may result in a shorter phrase. In identifying isolated phonemes, voicing is necessary, but in the sequencing of phonemes, when other cues to meaning are available, delays of voicing do not appreciably affect meaning. Since breathiness often manifests itself by frequent delays of phonation for the vowel after the release of the voiceless consonant, attention is usually directed toward reduction of this delay time. Phonation delays are more apparent on sentences containing many voiceless phonemes (stop at sister's house) than on sentences containing only voiced phonemes (are you all alone in there?). When delays of phonation occur on initial vowels, it is described as an *aspirate attack* since the movement of the column of air precedes vocal fold vibration.

Breathiness accompanying phoneme sequencing, combined with other attributes described above, affects length of phonation, i.e., phonation time during a phrase will decrease as voiceless-phoneme time increases (Ptacek and Sanders, 1963). A person who speaks rapidly with excessive breathiness often exhibits a short phonation period interspersed by extended moments of whispered speech. Therefore, only certain vowels in the phrase may exhibit phonation.

Breathiness is common as a vocal characteristic. Its use may be appropriate to the intent of the speaker, to certain information content, and during conditions of spatial intimacy. Chronic use, in violation of the above, may result in individuals perceiving breathiness as a vocal disorder.

Breathy voices respond quickly to treatment if the problem is nonorganic and the client is motivated to change. Altering fundamental frequency, achieving more optimal laryngeal valving, increasing total speech energy (Pronovost, 1947), attention to the timing of phonation after the release of a voiceless consonant, all contribute to the reduction of breathiness. When these or other approaches demonstrate reduced laryngeal air turbulence, an organic cause is not suspected. However, should experimental therapy produce no appreciable change in laryngeal air turbulence, breathiness may be the result of an organic condition and further diagnosis should follow.

OPTIMAL LARYNGEAL VALVING

Optimal laryngeal valving is difficult to define precisely, but certain general observations are noted.

1. The vocal folds are postured in such a manner that only marginal variations occur in the amount of time devoted to each of the closed, opening, and closing phases of the vibratory cycle at various frequencies.
2. The degree of laryngeal valving offers sufficient resistance to air flow to accomplish unhampered vibrations of the vocal folds at the desired intensity for speech.
3. The vocal folds vibrate periodically with little noticeable laryngeal air turbulence, so that the laryngeal tone perceived is "clear" or "musical."

Often optimal valvular phonation is expressed in terms of what it is not, i.e., the tone is not "breathy," or "husky," or "strident," or "hoarse." Standards of normalcy vary depending upon the criteria, and obviously there are degrees of valving which are tolerated by listeners as optimal.

HYPERVALVULAR PHONATION

Vocal-fold vibration accompanied by conditions of partial or optimal laryngeal valving logically leads to phonation under circumstances of laryngeal hypervalving. Hypervalvular phonation results when the vocal folds are pressed tightly together during phonation. Time allotment to the closed, opening, and closing phases during the cycle of vibration is then altered toward the opposite of hypovalving. That is, the closed phase would occupy greater time than the opening or closing phases. The vocal folds strike each other vigorously at the beginning of the closed phase and separate violently when the opening phase is initiated. Such changes in the time relationship of the vibratory phases do not alter the frequency generated, but the phonation produced is described as "shrill" or "penetrating."

In hypervalving, the vocal folds offer increased resistance to air flow with subsequent increase in subglottal breath pressure. The laryngeal sound generation has been variously labeled: hypertense, pinched throat, hyperkinetic, laryngeal stridor, strident, or harsh. The vocal folds are nearing the completely adducted state, the phonation is increasingly more difficult to initiate, as reported by Rees (1958). The ventricular folds as an addendum of hypervalving, may also be positioned near the midline, as described by Rethi (1952), Voelker (1942), Jackson and Jackson (1937), and Russell (1936), offering additional resistance to air flow or dampening the vibration of the true vocal folds. For that matter, extremes of laryngeal hypervalving may find the ventricular folds oscillating as well as the true vocal folds, contributing an additional stridor effect.

Hypervalvular phonation is often accompanied by the *coup de glotte* (hard attack, voiced glottal plosive) prior to initial vowel sounds. The vocal folds are vigorously adducted so that subglottal air pressure must be increased before the folds are able to vibrate. A *coup de glotte* is not unlike a cough initiating phonation. Theoretically, phonation could be initiated by the *coup de glotte* for any voiced phoneme, though it is more commonly associated with the initiation of phonation for vowels. When syllables which begin with vowels (VC, VCC) alone or in sequence occur in speech (I ate an apple), the *coup de glotte* is commonly heard interspersed before each word when the larynx is hypervalved.

Hypervalvular phonation often accompanies anger or emotional involvement of the speaker, as in yelling or shouting, and may give the speaker an impression that he is speaking loudly or forcefully. Consistent use of hypervalvular phonation, aspects of which are presented in Moore's and von Leden's film (1958), creates possible use-based laryngeal pathologies, such as inflamed edematous folds, contact ulcers, polyps, and nodules. Reducing excessive hypervalvular phonation is a preventive procedure as well as a therapeutic one. Generally speaking, reduction of hypervalving involves establishing conditions of hypovalving as a contrast to aid the client in the understanding of more optimal valving.

SPORADIC PHONATION

In describing possible laryngeal behaviors, special note must be made of intermittent changes in laryngeal valving during continuous speech. These changes in posturing occur unrelated to phoneme identification and generally do not follow any prescribed pattern. There is an infinite variety of such sporadic changes, but they generally involve the "on and off" phonation unrelated to the phonemes being spoken. Sporadic phonation is that vocal behavior where moments of phonation are interspersed with moments of whispered speech or silence, which results from complete adduction of the vocal folds. An example of the latter would be laryngeal spasms (tonic) associated with stuttering. Intermittent whisper and phonation or phonation and silence considered separately signify essentially normal laryngeal functions. But by occurring inappropriately in connected speech, they alert the speech clinician to potential difficulties the speaker may have in relating to others, such as in hysteria (McCaskey, 1948), or to an organic condition of sufficient size and weight that normal adduction is prevented. Vocal fold vibration then occurs only during moments of increased laryngeal effort. Further diagnosis is usually indicated.

THE LARYNX AND FREQUENCY GENERATION

Whenever a vibrator vibrates, it will oscillate, usually in a complex manner, a certain number of times per second. An integral part of phonation is frequency generation. Frequency, as a physical term, refers to those characteristics of the vibratory motion which provide a fundamental frequency (whole structure oscillating), or segmental frequencies (part structure oscillating). Most vibrators produce a composite of frequencies when they oscillate. The listener is generally not able to perceive discrete frequency components in a composite of frequencies, but rather responds, in some manner, to the total composite effect.

Pitch, as a subjective term, has been used in a number of ways (Flanagan, 1965). One connotation of the term is that *pitch* is a correlate of frequency, i.e., the *pitch* of middle *c* has the fundamental frequency of 256 cycles per second. The word pitch has also been used in a comparative sense, irrespective of fundamental frequency, i.e., voices may differ in pitch, even though the fundamental frequencies are the same. In this sense, the use of the term pitch is not restricted to the fundamental frequency, but includes the contributions of resonators amplifying high or low frequencies. The term *pitch* also has the connotation of vocal intensity, for example, when a voice is referred to as "low pitched," meaning a soft voice. It is often difficult to say what is meant by "the pitch of a person's voice." It cannot be assumed that *pitch* always means *a* fundamental frequency, for it is doubtful that a speaker has one fundamental rate of vocal fold vibration.

The vagueness in the use of the term pitch creates problems of professional intervention. For example, clinicians react to an inappropriate pitch from a comparative frame, and attempt to modify vocal behavior by altering fundamental vocal fold frequency. Manipulations of fundamental frequency are often done without reference to a known standard of comparison, or, for that matter, to the structural characteristics responsible for frequency differences among individuals. *Optimum pitch and habitual or natural pitch* (Pronovost, 1942) are common terms which cannot be clearly defined nor concisely documented. No one phonates without frequency, and rarely without frequency change. Apparent disorders of pitch, then, must be assessed within the framework of the laryngeal structures themselves, their muscle innervations or use in modulations of the air stream which produce fundamental frequency change, and their appropriateness to the intent and circumstances of the communication.

Modes of Laryngeal Oscillation

Normal vocal folds oscillate in a number of ways. Two deserve mention at this time: part-fold (fry or falsetto) and full-fold oscillation.

PART-FOLD

Fry. The fry is produced when the vocal folds are postured to the adducted position before oscillation begins. Using slow-motion photography as an aid to vision, it can be seen that vocal fold vibration is initiated by the appearance of a small glottal chink at the midline near the anterior-posterior center of the adducted folds. The chink spreads and diminishes in size in an anterior-to-posterior, posterior-to-anterior fashion, twice in each cycle, in a somewhat syncopated rhythm. Oscillation is confined to the marginal edges of the folds, which reduces amplitude of vocal fold motion. The sound thus produced is like a "bubbling" or "frying," hence the label *fry* or, according to Cleeland (1948), "the voice quality called X." The rapidity of oscillation may vary so that a range of frequencies can be produced. The restricted amplitude of oscillation and the prolonged adducted state of the folds during the closed phase reduces the amount of air being released in the supraglottal resonators. In addition, there is usually a minimum of subglottal air pressure. The laryngeal valving is offering almost maximum resistance to air flow (McGlone, 1967). Because the acoustic is similar to "rattling," "cracking," or "ticker-like" (Vollker, 1935), some writers describe fry as a type of tonal quality rather than as a frequency range. For example, Moser (1942) discusses fry in conjunction with a "harsh" voice. It is, however, a type of laryngeal adjustment which is capable of producing a relatively low range of frequencies, similar to esophageal phonation. With fry, frequency production and tonal quality become almost synonymous. Differences of opinion exist as to whether fry is a disorder of phonation, as cogently discussed by Hollein, Moore, Wendhal, and Michel (1966).

Professional people occasionally refer to the fry as unsustained phonation, since it is commonly heard as a change in phonation toward the end of phrases or sentences. Fry is also commonly observed when an individual is speaking at frequencies close to the bottom of his range. Listeners variously interpret the fry as an indication of vocal fatigue, lack of physical strength, sophistication, or even indicative of emotional stress. Various causal factors have been cited, such as hypothyroidism and myasthenia laryngis. Assuming no organic cause, fry oscillation can be eliminated by raising the fundamental frequency of phonation, increasing subglottal breath pressure, and by more optimal laryngeal valving which increases amplitude of oscillation with subsequent involvement of the full mass of the vocal folds.

FALSETTO

Falsetto, as discussed by Rubin and Hirt (1960), is another manifestation of part-vocal fold oscillation, sometimes referred to as juvenile, infantile, or eunochoid voice. These terms indicate an artificial frequency range, particularly in the adult male, in contrast to a natural or normal range. The falsetto range is potentially available to most people, children and adults, male and female. However, its appropriate use is often confined to specific circumstances, such as in laughter, singing (Curry, 1940), and possibly screaming. Present understanding does not permit detailed descriptions of subtle changes in vibratory patterns of the vocal folds which produce a falsetto-like range. Two possible oscillation modes are reported. In the first, the vocal fold oscillation is largely restricted to the anterior half of the folds, thereby reducing the length of the vibrator. In order for the oscillation to be restricted in this manner, the cricoid cartilages and the posterior half of the vocal folds are either pressed tightly together, thereby dampening posterior vocal fold vibration, or kept widely separated so that subglottal air pressure is insufficient to activate the posterior portions of the folds. In this latter circumstance, falsetto may be accompanied by noticeable amounts of laryngeal air turbulence. It is also noted that occasionally the whole laryngeal structure is elevated from its "at rest" position during the production of falsetto. This elevation (Weiss, 1950) would tend to reduce the length of the pharynx as a resonator, thereby contributing to resonance changes by amplification of higher frequencies. The second means of achieving a falsettolike range is operative when the vocal folds oscillate along their entire length, but vibration is restricted to the thin, elastic marginal edges of the folds (Judson and Weaver, 1942) rather than the muscle mass portion. The resultant vibration again has limited amplitude, and the production of the higher frequency range is accounted for by the reduced mass of the vibrating structure rather than the limited length of the folds described above. The basic difference between the two modes described is length versus mass as the primary determinant of the frequency range. Regardless of the mode of vibration, falsetto is recognized by its potentially higher frequency range and its limited amplitude.

When the falsetto range is inappropriately or consistently used, particularly by an adult male, professional persons suspect causal factors such as precocious pubescence, glandular disorders, disproportionate growth of the larynx, laryngeal mutations, injuries, growths, or difficulties the speaker may have in relating to others.

FULL-FOLD

Normal laryngeal frequency production as dictated by our usual cultural expectancies involves the full use of the vocal fold mass during vibration. This is especially true at lower frequencies in the range where oscillation appears to involve, in varying degrees, the entire mass of the vocal folds along their entire length. As the frequency is increased, full-fold oscillation diminishes and tends to concentrate more toward the anterior portion of the folds, yet movement is still observable along the full length. Again, a range of fundamental frequencies is available. Full-fold oscillation, which is regarded as normal, provides a *potential range* of frequencies. Customarily, *use-range* is usually less than the individual's *potential range*.

CONCEPTS OF FREQUENCY RANGE

The modes of vocal fold oscillation mentioned above provide three separate means of producing frequency changes. In considering use of these ranges, it must be remembered that voices do not have *a* pitch. Where the phrase "pitch of voice" is used, reference is to an average pitch rather than a discrete frequency which is used to the exclusion of other frequencies. Everyone has a potential range of frequencies as stated by Snidecor (1940), some more extensive than others. Ranges of sampled individuals have been documented by Hollein (1960), Hollein and Curtis (1960), and Hollein and Moore (1960). Comparisons have been made between vocal fold length and range potential with respect to sex and age, and with respect to certain characteristics such as body weight, height, and framework (Jerome, 1937; Wiley, 1942; Lassman, 1942). Yet, there is considerable variation in the range studied depending on subject sample. Potential ranges differ among people, and these differences permit only general observations. If fry and falsetto ranges were included in the estimates of ranges, then the previous estimates would have to be expanded. Hollein's data on ranges, for low and high males and low and high females, reveal a considerable number of discrete frequencies which are common to all individuals sampled. One could conclude that *some* males, females, and children might use essentially the same pitch level. Linke (1953), using a large sample, found a difference of only 3.7 tones between males and females. The listener, however, expects the male voice to be "lower" than the female, or children's "higher" than adults'. It is obvious that "low" and "high" are meaningless terms unless standards of comparisons are known.

The fry, normal, and falsetto modes of vocal fold vibration reflect different laryngeal behaviors during oscillation. Each mode produces a potential range of frequencies. The falsetto range is often presented as a range of frequencies entirely above the normal range. Conversely, the fry consists of frequencies entirely below the normal range. It is important to recognize that certain fundamental laryngeal frequencies can be produced by different modes of vocal fold oscillation. Consequently, these ranges are not mutually exclusive with respect to certain frequencies. Thus, as Curry (1940) reports, singers cultivate transitions from normal range to falsetto with no noticeable "pitch break" or marked frequency-change gap. To the listener, it is often difficult to tell whether a person is speaking in the lower third of his falsetto range or the upper third of his normal range.

In summary, verbal symbols encompass the use of frequency change in communicating with others. The phenomenon of frequency alone is of minor importance to the listener in phoneme recognition, but frequency change is often perceived as important to subtle changes in meaning. However, communication is not seriously affected if frequency change is minimal. Yet some listeners often react, based upon subjective impressions, to the speaker's range use in coding the message, especially if use does not match his expectations. It is curious that the limited use of frequency change by a laryngectomee using esophageal phonation elicits little comment or cultural penalty.

DISORDERS OF PITCH

To assess disorders of pitch is extremely complex. Before labeling pitch as a problem one must determine:

1. the individual's laryngeal or phonatory structure and its capabilities for frequency generation;
2. the individual's use of his potential range under a variety of speaking situations; and
3. the appropriateness of this use to the needs of the speaker in communicating with others.

In most instances, pitch deviations are perceived as disorders because they violate expected patterns of frequency production or change in our culture, and generally are grouped in three ways:

1. disorders which relate to changes in mode of oscillation of the vocal folds, i.e., unexpected frequency differences which result from changes between normal and falsetto (Curry, 1949) or from normal into fry (ordinarily unrelated to meaning, occur sporadically, and evidence

marked differences in fundamental frequency);
2. disorders relating to consistent use of an inappropriate or "artificial" range, i.e., use of falsetto consistently by an adult male, or the use of a falsettolike range by a child with a congenital laryngeal web;
3. disorders of pitch which relate to undesirable use of a range, such as monopitch, limited use of range, average frequency "too high" or "too low," or pitch-change patterns too repetitious in connected speech (Van Riper, 1954).

Each of the above groups requires different approaches in therapy. In the first, therapy is generally oriented to stabilizing a more appropriate range use. In the second, the major goal is to establish normal oscillation either voluntarily or after surgical intervention, and stabilize its use. In the third, the concern is with more appropriate use of fundamental frequency change relative to communication intent and circumstances of the speaker or the expectancy of listeners.

THE LARYNX AND ENERGY GENERATION

Laryngeal modulations of the air stream from the lungs generate energy associated with the acoustic product. Variations in the energy are a function of different types of air-stream modulations which can be produced at the larynx or in the associated resonating cavities. The perception of these energy changes is labeled *loudness*.

The term loudness enjoys a variety of interpretations. It is often used in a gross, relative sense, such as the loudness of one speaker compared with another. Loudness is sometimes equated with physical effort, i.e., the greater the "work" used in speaking, the louder the voice. Loudness is frequently used as a synonym for other terms such as energy, intensity, and amplitude, which leads to confusion. Actually, loudness is the listener's reported evaluation of acoustic energy. For example, certain tonal qualities of phonation, such as breathiness, generate less energy than others. From the listener's evaluation, breathiness may be perceived as a disorder of loudness.

In discussing the laryngeal functions in relation to energy generation, one of the primary attributes of phonation is the extension of man's spatial competency. Phonated speech, in contrast to whispered speech, enlarges man's physical distance of communication. The principle source of increased distance relates to the excursion (amplitude) of the vocal folds' oscillation. Increased amplitude of vibration produces increased energy or intensity of sound which is evaluated by the listener as increased loudness. Amplitude and intensity are physically quantifiable, whereas loudness is a subjective impression. Variations in amplitude are intimately related to laryngeal attributes discussed earlier.

The larynx is responsible for variations of three parameters; tonal quality, frequency production, and amplitude. These three are inseparable in one sense, for any time the vocal folds vibrate they will manifest degrees of laryngeal valving with subsequent changes in modulation, they will oscillate within a range of frequencies, and the amplitude of the oscillation will generate varied amounts of energy. Conceptually, these are independent variables, for altering frequency does not alter amplitude, nor does tonal quality determine frequency or amplitude. However, there is apt to be some correspondence between these three laryngeal variables. During whisper, the sound energy is the result of the amount of air flow through the partially valved larynx. Changes in amount of air flow will produce "soft" or "loud" whispers. During phonation, energy generation is greater with conditions of optimal than with extremes of hypo- or hypervalving of the larynx. There are some areas of the frequency range where energy output is greater or less (Isshiki, 1964), and one expects differences in amplitude as a result of falsetto or fry mode of oscillation when compared with full-fold vibration. The type of laryngeal modulation of the air stream dictates the amplitude potential.

In addition to the effect of laryngeal variants on energy generation, gross speech power must be considered from the requisites of interpersonal communication. Not only does energy change affect syllable or word dominance for meaning, but energy differences result from the speaker's reaction to ambient noise, which makes communication difficult. In the same vein, hearing loss could affect the speaker's use of intensity by disrupting his concepts of physical distance (Black, 1959). Speakers vary in their ability to compensate for or adjust to changes of physical dimensions.

Vocal intensity also reflects the emotional state of the speaker (Moses, 1954). Angry, argumentative, forceful talking is marked by increased energy output. The angry mother or father, sensing that the child is inattentive or resistive, shouts even though the child is only a few feet away. The one who speaks loudly may feel far removed from his listeners, and the one who speaks softly may feel "too close," timid, shy, or withdrawn in his communication with others.

Inadequacies of speech energy which might be regarded as disorders of intensity should never be assessed out of the contexts described above (Benkley, 1949; Steer and Tiffin, 1934). Speech intensity, in and of itself, is rarely a problem. Ordinarily, changes in laryngeal valving toward optimal, changes in the portion of frequency range use, or instruction in speech power needed for particular speaking situations, will demonstrate to the client more appropriate energy output. There are some apparent problems of vocal intensity, such as with a paralyzed vocal fold, where professional speech intervention rarely brings about a change in the speaker's output. The problem then becomes not one of modifying vocal behavior, but of instructing the speaker in voice management under difficult communication circumstances, such as spatial positioning, and the use of amplifying equipment.

THE LARYNX AND NOISE GENERATION

The auditory impressions which have been labeled as "rough," "husky," and "hoarse" defy accurate description. There is a lack of correspondence between the use of such labels and the specific acoustic generation perceived. Consideration was delayed until the three major variables of laryngeal production, tonal quality, frequency, and amplitude were discussed since descriptions of laryngeal noise generation involve all three. There is no doubt that phonation designated as "rough" or "husky" or "hoarse" originates in the larynx (Moore and Thompson, 1965). It is a fallacy to say that these labels delineate *a* particular type of voice, for there are as many "rough," "husky," "hoarse" phonations as there are proportional mixtures of the laryngeal components described earlier (Walford, 1952; Herman, 1942).

Composites of sound previously mentioned are of two general types: *inharmonic* or *harmonic*. *Inharmonic* designates a composite sound made up of a spectrum of frequencies which are unrelated. The sound produced lacks internal consistency, is aperiodic, and reflects a series of unrelated frequency and intensity events. Inharmonic is equated with noise. Laryngeal noise elements may result from irregular vibratory patterns of the vocal folds, or from air turbulence because of incomplete laryngeal valving, or from other acoustic components contributed by laryngeal hypervalving. For example, the adduction and possible oscillation of the ventricular folds may add additional noise elements.

Harmonic denotes the type of sound composite containing frequencies which demonstrate a relationship. The sound produced has internal consistency and periodicity. A laryngeal harmonic is created when the vocal folds vibrate in a regular or efficient manner, and the sound generated is perceived as "clear" or "musical."

It is important to realize, however, that during speech, harmonic and inharmonic sound components may occur at the same moment in time, creating an acoustic composite of both harmonic and inharmonic components. To use phonemes as an example, assume that normal laryngeal vibration of the vocal fold is harmonic and the unphonated frication of /s/ in the oral cavity is inharmonic. The composite acoustic of /z/, therefore, is a combination of harmonic and inharmonic composites occurring from two anatomically separated sound sources. A vibrator may also behave in such a way that harmonic and inharmonic components are produced at the same sound generator source.

The terms "rough," "husky," "hoarse" refer to combinations of harmonic and inharmonic composites of sound resulting from the way the laryngeal valve with its vibrating structures behaves. Phonation could be perceived to be predominantly harmonic or predominantly inharmonic, or any ratio of the two. Breathiness may be cited as an example, for under conditions of hypolaryngeal valving, the vibration of the vocal folds may be harmonic, yet phonation is accompanied by considerable inharmonic air turbulence (Isshiki, 1964).

The terms "husky" and "hoarse," as labels of dysphonia, have been used extensively in the literature. To some, "husky" (Seth and Guthrie, 1935) is that tonal quality produced at a frequency low in the normal range accompanied by considerable turbulence as the air stream proceeds through a partially valved larynx. "Hoarseness," to some, is that tonal quality produced when the vocal folds vibrate in an aperiodic, irregular or haphazard manner. The term "rough" was recently instituted because there was no unified agreement on delineations of the two terms "husky" or "hoarse." "Rough" was introduced as an all-inclusive term of laryngeal noise. Professional people generally agree that regardless of label, laryngeal roughness is an indication of possible laryngeal pathology. Specifically, attention is directed to those pathologies which 1. would prevent the vocal folds from meeting along their entire length at the midline during the closed phase of the vibration cycle, or 2. are of sufficient size and weight to cause the vocal fold(s) to vibrate in an irregular manner. Depending upon the pathology and its location, one would expect different amounts of air turbulence or aperiodic vibration to occur. The speaker, in an effort to initiate or sustain phonation, may also resort to hyperlaryngeal valving, thereby contributing additional inharmonic elements. Considerable investigation has yet to be done with respect to the type, size, and location of the lesion and its relationship to variations in rough tonal quality. Cultural attitudes toward laryngeal roughness need also to be determined since there are evident differences of opinion regarding roughness as a desirable or undesirable vocal characteristic. The relationship of laryngeal noise to the speaker's emotional state or difficulties that he may have in relating to others also needs further study.

When roughness is consistently evident and experimental therapy produces no substantial improvement in tonal quality, medical diagnosis would be strongly indicated. Speech therapy generally consists of manipulating the variables of laryngeal valving, frequency, and intensity toward a more harmonic tonal quality.

PHONEMIC AND NONPHONEMIC CAVITY VARIABLES

Laryngeal vibration excites the supra-glottal cavities which function as resonators. During speech, the processes of phonation and resonation occur in a closed system. The acoustics generated by the laryngeal functions are amplified or modified by the size, shape and openings of the supraglottal cavities. Although phonation and resonation are intimately related, it is helpful to discuss the effects of resonation separately. The acoustic differentiation necessary for the identification of phonemes is largely the result of adjustments within the resonating cavities. To illustrate cavity contributions to phonemes, any voiceless vowel in whispered speech still produces sufficient core acoustic data for vowel identification. The focus of this chapter is not directed to the linguistic phoneme per se, but to those accompanying resonance variables which occur irrespective of phoneme identification. These generally involve centroids of acoustic energy concentrations determined by shaping and coupling of cavities which provide:

1. a preponderance of high or, in contrast, low resonant characteristics; or
2. the effects of coupling or uncoupling of the nasal resonator other than for the nasal phonemes /m/, /n/, /ŋ/.

The Cavities as Resonators of Phonation

Admittedly the laryngeal vibration of the vocal folds may be transmitted both subglottally and supraglottally through the cartilages or bony framework of the trachea, larynx, chest, and head, thereby altering the acoustic signal. However, humans have little direct control over resonance characteristics brought about in this manner. Resonance, though, which results from cavities responding to exitations of the vibrator or the air stream, or these in combination, can be altered, creating innumerable changes in resonance. Changes in the size, shape and openings of the supraglottal resonating cavities, especially the oral cavity, account for changes in resonance for vowels and glides which permit phoneme recognition. Consonants are also produced within cavities which are shaped for vowels either prior to, during, or after the release of the consonant articulation. To describe all of the subtle differences in size, shape, and openings of the supraglottal resonators for a given vowel would be endless. Not only do people differ from one another in vowel resonance, but an individual will vary resonance characteristics for the same vowel presented at different times in contextual speech. Recognition of an individual's "voice" is not only achieved by his laryngeal attributes of tonal quality, use of frequency, time, or intensity, but also by his unique resonant characteristics. It is interesting to note that identification of a speaker is possible by hearing only samples of his whispered speech.

The three supraglottal resonators are the pharynx, the oral cavity, and the nasal cavity. The pharynx, in its "at rest" state, is apt to be the largest of the three resonators. However, during speech, size of the pharynx can be varied in a number of ways. The length of the pharynx can be changed by elevating or lowering the laryngeal structure. Its internal dimensions can be altered by the position of the ventricular folds, or by actions of the soft palate, tongue, or pharyngeal constrictor muscles. The orifice between the pharynx and the oral cavity can be altered by motions of the tongue, such as raising it toward the velum or by retracting it so that the posterior portion invades pharyngeal space. These changes, as well as others, affect resonant characteristics of the pharyngeal cavity.

The oral cavity is even more variable in its size, shape, and openings. Any movement of the tongue, mandible, lips, or soft palate results in changing the dimensions of the oral cavity. The potential variability of the oral space makes it the principal contributor to phonemic characteristics.

Unlike the oral and pharyngeal cavities, the nasal cavity space is fixed in size and cannot be altered significantly by muscle contractions. Rather than changes in the nasal cavity dimension, its effect on verbal signals is determined by the nature of its coupling to the airway system as expressed in degrees of velopharyngeal valving.

Pharyngo-oral Relationships

Perceptually, one must recognize that a linguistic vowel category may have a number of acoustic variants which have been referred to as allophones. Rather than *a* vowel having *a* resonance, there are a number of closely related resonance characteristics brought about by differences in resonators which are perceived by the listener to be within the same linguistic phoneme category. Spectrographic studies (Peterson and Barney, 1952) document differences in centroids of energy within and between vowel parameters.

In considering nonphonemic variants of vowels, one must assume the constant of linguistic identification. That is, although a vowel, as spoken by different persons at different times, may possess different centroids of energy, there is sufficient core acoustic data to permit the listener to identify the phoneme. Therefore, acoustic data which are present coincidental to the core become nonphonemic variables. As mentioned earlier, these nonphonemic variables have been labeled allophones, but the acoustic parameters of vowel allophones have not been delineated with respect to phonemic and nonphonemic components. Generally, pharyngeal-oral cavity attributes to resonance displayed by individuals producing vowel allophones are grouped in three categories:

1. those which manifest amplification of higher frequencies in resonance, although phoneme identification is constant;
2. those which manifest a relative "balance" of high and low frequencies in resonance, while maintaining phoneme identification; and
3. those which manifest amplification of lower frequencies in resonance, with phoneme identification constant.

AMPLIFICATION OF HIGHER FREQUENCIES

The amplification of higher frequencies in resonance relates somewhat directly to those adjustments of resonators which diminish length of the coupled pharyngeal or oral space and increase the size of the posterior and anterior orifices of the mouth. Certain cavity variables are noted:

1. the general posturing of the tongue for all vowels is toward the front of the oral cavity, resulting in a reduction in the length of the oral cavity and an increase in the size of the orifice between the pharynx and the oral cavity;
2. the anterior orifice of the oral cavity is generally larger during the production of vowels because of a more open jaw position, thereby exhibiting increased activity of the jaw and lips and revealing frontal actions of the tongue which under other circumstances are not observed; and
3. the length of the pharynx is reduced during phonation by elevating the thyroid cartilage (larynx) from its rest position, and the circumference of the pharyngeal cavity may be decreased by the adduction of the ventricular folds or by contraction of the pharyngeal constrictor muscles.

The combined effect of the above is an emphasis on higher resonant frequencies concomitant with the acoustic identification core for vowels. The resultant quality has been labeled "oral," "thin," "immature," or "juvenile." The higher frequency amplification has been inappropriately labeled "high pitch," and based on this label, therapy has been directed toward lowering fundamental frequency of vocal fold vibration which achieves little significant change of resonance. With amplification of higher resonant frequencies, the total effect during speech may be "higher," hence the possible confusion with vocal fold frequency. Clinical intervention should be directed toward changing resonator size and openings, rather than altering fundamental frequency of phonation. Such changes would be directed toward increasing the length of the pharynx, for example, by lowering the laryngeal structure itself as in yawning, and assuming a more posterior positioning of the tongue with a reduction of motions of the mandible during vowel production, thereby achieving a more "balanced" use of resonance.

AMPLIFICATION OF A "BALANCED RESONANCE"

For the sake of reference, "balanced resonance" is used to indicate a normal distribution of high and low resonance characteristics as phoneme identification is held constant. In this sense, "balanced resonance" is a "neutral" concept. Within the framework of the present discussion, "balanced resonance" during speech is not perceived to be either a preponderance of high- or low-frequency amplification as determined by pharyngeal and oral cavity contributions, and is therefore considered to be within normal cultural expectations.

AMPLIFICATION OF LOWER FREQUENCIES

In contrast to higher frequency amplification during vowels, amplification of lower frequencies is determined by an increase in size of the resonators and decreasing size of orifices. The following variables are noted:

1. the pharynx may be increased in size either by lowering the laryngeal structures, thereby increasing the length of the pharynx, or by increasing the circumference of the pharyngeal space;
2. the size of the opening between the pharynx and the oral cavity may be reduced by assuming a more posterior and heightened position of the tongue during vowel production; or
3. the size of the orifice at the front of the mouth may be reduced by using a relatively closed jaw position with lips only slightly separated during speech.

The cumulative effect of these resonator changes produces the resonance of lower frequencies which is often associated with speakers who have a severe hearing loss or a neuromuscular impairment. In the writings of professional people, the resultant quality perceived is labeled "muffled," "retracted," "throaty," or "guttural." Since the contributing resonance characteristic is the opposite of the amplification of higher resonance frequencies, therapy would be directed toward altering resonator adjustments toward higher frequency amplification in order to achieve a more "balanced" use of resonators. Suggestions are made to reduce the length of the pharynx by raising the laryngeal structures or to achieve a more forward position of the tongue with increased action of the mandible during speech.

Positive-Negative Nasal Coupling

In the previous section, which discussed the contributions of the pharynx and oral resonators during the production of vowel sounds, the nasal cavity was presented as a resonating system which is coupled to or uncoupled from the pharyngo-oral resonating system. Since speech, at times, requires air flow to pass through the nose, such as for the nasal continuants /m/, /n/, /ŋ/, and at other times through the mouth, the coupling and uncoupling of the nasal resonating system deserves consideration.

NASAL EMISSION

Nasal continuants have traditionally been presented as nasally emitted phonemes, i.e., the oral orifice is closed, the velopharyngeal orifice is open, and air flow is entirely through the nose. The nasal continuants are presented as phonemes requiring laryngeal vibration. Since the nasal chambers are coupled to the other resonators, the resonance derived may exhibit contributions from all the connected resonator spaces. Should phonation not be present, air turbulence, created by the volume of air flow through narrow nasal passages results, and has been described as *nasal emission* or nasal frication.

The individual nasal continuants /m/, /n/, /ŋ/, although each requires nasal resonance, are differentiated by the proportions of coupled cul-de-sac oral resonance. Acoustically, /m/ is differentiated from /n/ not by nasal resonance, which is a constant, but by a greater proportion of cul-de-sac oral resonance. Therefore, /n/, since the oral resonator is closed posteriorly by the tongue touching the velum, depends upon pharyngeal and nasal resonance and not the contributions of a cul-de-sac oral resonator. If phonation is not present, but air-stream turbulence is, no acoustic differentiation is possible between the three nasal continuants because air turbulence is generated in nasal cavity spaces rather than in the cul-de-sac oral space. Phoneme identification of individual nasal continuants requires laryngeal phonation, nasal resonance, proportions of cul-de-sac oral resonance for /m/ and /n/, and any additional contributions of the pharyngeal resonator.

ORAL EMISSION

Isolated phonemes labeled plosives, fricatives, and affricates require oral emission of air flow. If all air flow, regardless of the amount of constriction of the oral passage, is to be through the mouth, the velopharyngeal port must be closed. Uncoupling the nasal chambers may be accomplished either by neuromuscular action of the velopharyngeal sphincter alone or combined with pneumatic pressure coincidental to the impounding of air in the oral and pharyngeal cavities. In normal speech, cavity pressures during the articulation of fricatives, affricates, and plosives may assist the neuromuscular closure of the velopharyngeal port whereas on other phonemes it may not. Cavity pressure for phonemes varies according to the amount of resistance to air flow which is introduced along the vocal tract. In fricatives, for example, oral pressure is less for /ʃ/ than for /s/ or /θ/ (Isshiki and Rengil, 1964). Plosives would logically manifest the greatest pneumatic pressure since during their period of articulation resistance to air flow is maximum. However, plosives in sequence with vowels are often executed more as a "flapping" of structures against each other than as discretely executed oral closures, compression, and release of air. When the plosive is "flapped" there is less cavity pressure than for continuants such as fricatives and affricates.

Vowels and glides possess less cavity pressure than the consonant types listed above. Although oral emission is thought to be a requisite, the closure of the velopharyngeal port need not be complete. McDonald and Koepp-Baker (1951) refer to a critical point in velopharyngeal closure which accounts for the ratio between oral and nasal resonance on vowels. Since oral pressure is not as great for vowels and glides, little pneumatic assistance in articulating the nasal port is available.

Generally speaking, the greater the resistance to oral air flow, the greater the need for complete closure of the nasal port if satisfactory oral emission is to be achieved. That is, /α/ requires less closure than /i/ or /u/ (Moll, 1962), and fricatives, affricates, and possibly plosives require more velopharyngeal valving than vowels.

The identification of vowels and glides depends more upon pharyngeal and oral contributions to resonance than nasal. The presence or absence of moderate amounts of nasal-cavity contributions has little effect on phoneme recognition. In fact, society in general is relatively tolerant of nasal resonance on vowels and glides. Individuals differ as to the degree of velopharyngeal valving while speaking vowels (Sherry, 1954; Nusbaum and Wells, 1935; Kelly, 1934). The presence or absence of nasal resonance on vowels or glides, therefore, is considered nonphonemic. The intent of the next section is to discuss the various effects of nasal-chamber coupling and uncoupling during speech.

Conceptual Model of Positive-Negative Nasal Coupling

If one assumes that complete nasal uncoupling (nose closed at all times) is the opposite of complete nasal coupling (nose open at all times) then the pivotal point between negative and positive nasal coupling assumes an instantaneous change in total air-flow route between the nasal continuant and all other phonemes. Conceptually, then, the nasal continuants are the only phonemes which exhibit sufficient amounts of nasal resonance to deserve the label of nasal. Any contribution of the nasal resonators on all other phonemes would be imperceptible. To achieve instantaneous changes in air-exit routes in contextual speech would require that the oral articulation of the nasal continuant be simultaneous with the disarticulation of the velopharyngeal port and vice versa. Obviously such a statement is ambitious with respect to contextual phoneme production. Variations in the time of oral articulations and disarticulations and valving of the velopharyngeal port are expected to occur, and, in addition, a number of variations in nasal coupling-uncoupling occur with respect to certain impairments. The following parameters are noted.

NEGATIVE NASAL RESONANCE

During speech, negative nasal resonance results when the nasal resonating system cannot be coupled to the pharynx. Other labels have been used to express the inability to couple the nasal resonators, such as negative nasality, rhinolalia clausa (posterior), hyponasality and denasality. These terms refer to the absence of perceived nasal resonance on nasal continuants, resulting from an inadequate free air route through the nose when coupling is attempted. The most apparent perceptual change affects the nasal phonemes, i.e., the nasal continuants /m/, /n/, and /ŋ/ assume the acoustic characteristics of voiced plosives /b/, /d/, /g/. The word "mom" becomes similar to "Bob," "none" to "dud," and "ring" to "rig." When these changes of the nasal phonemes occur, one relates them to such conditions as enlarged adenoids, excessive sinus discharge, nasal congestion, or other similar impairments which block the posterior orifice of the nasal chambers.

A more subtle change occurs on vowels if the entrance to the nasal cavity is blocked. The nasal resonator, which is often partly coupled during vowel production, is thought by some to add "brilliance" to the vowel. Therefore, if the nose is completely closed the vowel will sound "dull," similar to the amplification of lower frequencies discussed earlier. The amplification of lower frequencies could also be the result of excessive mucous secretion on the walls of the pharynx which would dampen high-frequency resonance. The combination of low frequency amplification on vowels, or the change of the nasal continuants to voiced plosives, constitutes the verbal signal change attributed to negative nasal resonance. Speech clinicians regard persistent negative nasal resonance as a problem which deserves medical diagnosis and possible intervention. The speech characteristic rarely occurs without some organic condition.

Visual observation of a person who demonstrates persistent absence of nasal resonance often reveals mouth breathing, i.e., the jaw will be slightly open, the lips parted, and the tongue is apt to be postured forward in the mouth or even resting interdentally in order to provide sufficient airway through the cavity. If such posturing has been maintained over a time, concomitant occlusion abnormalities may result.

MIXED POSITIVE-NEGATIVE COUPLING

It seems contradictory that during production of the verbal signals in a word there may be evidence of both negative and positive coupling of the nasal resonators, yet such a combination may occur with certain impairments. In the foregoing section of negative nasal resonance, the entire nasal resonator was not coupled to the pharyngo-oral resonating system. Assume for a moment that the blockage of the nasal resonating system is anterior to the velopharyngeal port, as with polyps or enlarged turbinate tissue. Assume also that the nasopharyngeal port is only partially valved, as in minimal velopharyngeal incompetencies. There then exists a coupled nasal cavity available for resonance whose exit route is blocked. During the speaking of a word the nasal chamber becomes a cul-de-sac resonator available for resonance, but the nasal continuant, because of the anterior blockage, becomes a voiced plosive. Various labels have been used such as rhinolalia clausa (anterior) or rhinolalia mixta.

Changes in the circumstances described above would produce numerous differences in the perceived mixed effect during spoken words. There are other variations which occur within the allotted time of the nasal continuants and relate more specifically to differences in the timing between the oral articulation of the nasal continuant and the velopharyngeal valving:

1. when the oral articulation occurs prior to the nasal coupling, the result is a voiced plosive release of the nasal continuant, represented by transcribing the word /meɪk/ as /bmeɪk/ (nasal plosion); or
2. when the nasal coupling occurs prior to oral disarticulation, there will be a voiced plosive cancellation of the nasal continuant, represented by transcribing the word /meɪk/ as /mbeɪk/.

The mixed effect on nasal phonemes described above is apparent on speech samples of cleft-palate individuals who have recently been fitted with a prosthetic speech appliance and who are unaccustomed to the velopharyngeal valving associated with the appliance.

By listening to the vowel and then to the nasal continuant for comparison purposes, it is possible to perceive, with certain impairments, negative and positive nasal resonance during the speaking of a given word. Numerous variations and combinations might be expected, and further study is indicated. The occurrence of mixta effects is somewhat uncommon, but they need to be documented as possible perceptual variables of positive-negative nasal resonance.

PERVASIVE EFFECTS OF NASAL COUPLING

The conceptual model stated previously presents the three nasal continuants /m/, /n/, /ŋ/ as the only sounds displaying a preponderance of nasal resonance, whereas all other classifications of phonemes display a predominance of pharyngo-oral resonance or turbulence. The statement is admittedly ambitious because variations might occur in the timing of oral articulation and disarticulation with nasal coupling and uncoupling during normal contextual speech. These expected variations in timing are discussed as pervasive influences of the nasal continuant on adjacent sounds.

The most common influence of the nasal consonant affects adjacent vowels, and as one aspect of similitude, has been labeled 1. anticipatory (regressive) or 2. prolonged (progressive) assimilation.

1. When the nasal resonator is coupled prior to the oral articulation of the nasal continuant, vowels, and occasionally consonants, which precede the nasal phoneme exhibit nasal resonance and/or turbulence, i.e., the /aɪ/ in "time"

contains a proportion of nasal resonance, phonetically represented as /tãĩm/, hence the use of the term anticipatory. One could also say that the nasal continuant has regressively influenced the preceding vowel.

2. When the nasal uncoupling is delayed following the oral disarticulation of the nasal continuant, the effect is to prolong nasal resonance into the following phoneme, i.e., the /eɪ/ in "make" becomes nasalized /mẽĩk/. Hence the use of the terms prolonged or progressive.

Combined, these progressive and regressive influences of the nasal continuant produce hypernasality on vowels as a function of the phonemes of the syllable, word, or phrase. For example, when a sentence contains a number of nasal sounds spaced throughout (many men come home) the speaker may exhibit relatively consistent hypernasality on vowels which, however, would diminish or disappear should the sentence contain no nasal sounds (popsicles are full of spice).

To identify speakers who possess only the similitude effects of nasal resonance on nonnasal sounds, the comparison of vowels in paired words with and without the nasal continuant will display differences in amounts of perceived nasal resonance. Therefore, the vowels in "tide," "road," or "bead" will possess less nasal resonance than the same vowels in "time," "roam," or "mean." Similitude nasal resonance is very common. One would hesitate to describe it as a disorder of speech. However, it should be noted as one of the nonphonemic resonance variables which often accompany normal speech production.

CONSISTENT NASAL RESONANCE ON VOWELS

Clinically, it is important to differentiate adjacency phenomena as a function of sequenced phonemes from consistent hypernasality on vowels during speech. The presence of hypernasality irrespective of the adjacent nasal continuant alerts professional persons to conditions which affect velopharyngeal competency. Under circumstances of consistent hypernasality, it should be noted that there are evident differences in the amount of nasal resonance among vowels (Calnan, 1953; Bloomer, 1953), as a function of the tongue position within the oral cavity. For example, there have been reports of differences in proportions of perceived nasal resonance between high and low vowels, and between front and back vowels. There is evidence which suggests that the trend of these differences may be reversed when comparisons are made between cleft-palate subjects and normally nasal subjects (Spriestersbach and Powers, 1959; Richards, 1966).

During speech, the greatest amount of exhaled air proceeds along the exit route which offers least resistance to its flow. Assume for the moment that the velopharyngeal port is insufficient for neuromuscular closure and is only partially valved during the production of all vowel sounds. Then the oral exit route for the /ɑ/ (father), if the tongue is positioned low in the mouth, could be larger than the orifice from the pharynx into the nasal chambers (McDonald and Koepp-Baker, 1951). This would account for a greater amount of pharyngo-oral resonance than nasal. However, assuming the same valving of the velopharyngeal port, if vowels are produced where the tongue constricts the oral cavity, such as /u/ (boot) or /i/ (beet), then the resonance ratio may be the reverse, thereby displaying greater nasal resonance on the /u/, or /i/ than the /ɑ/ (Hixon, 1949; Johnson et al., 1952). Although the ratio of nasal resonance changes as a function of tongue position in the oral cavity, there is perceived nasal resonance on all vowels which suggests minimal insufficiencies of velopharyngeal valving. The consistent presence of hypernasality on vowels has been labeled by such terms as nasality, rhinolalia aperta, and positive nasality, and the impairments cited include paralysis of the palatal elevators, thickness or heaviness of the velum, or mild congenital insufficiency of the velopharyngeal valve. Under these circumstances, the nasal resonator is partially coupled at all times during speech, but the primary effect is upon the vowels and glides rather than consonants.

An interesting paradox seems to occur when one considers the production of consonant sounds surrounding vowels and glides during the conditions described above. One would assume that if the nasal resonator is partly coupled during vowel production, the acoustics of the plosives, fricatives, and affricates would be similarly affected. However, under conditions of minimal palatal insufficiency, the consonant sound is often produced in an acceptable manner. Evidently, under certain conditions of velopharyngeal incompetency, the speaker is able to create sufficient cavity pressure to produce the consonant with its concomitant oral emission, yet is unable to produce the vowel without noticeable nasal resonance. Present knowledge of velopharyngeal valving during speech does not permit a detailed explanation. Speech, in the manner indicated above, may be attributed to normally nasal speakers or to organic conditions, albeit slight, which permit sufficient cavity pressure, associated with the articulation of the consonant, to compensate for the apparent inadequate neuromuscular valving of the nasal port. Further investigation is indicated.

It should be noted that the perception of nasal resonance on the vowels is influenced by the type of laryngeal phonation (Sherman and Goodwin, 1954; Moll, 1968). According to Curtis (1940) and Potter, Kopp, and Green (1947), the perceived nasal resonance depends upon the reinforcement of frequency bands between 200 and 300 cycles, but there must be sufficient energy generation in the laryngeal phonation to excite the nasal resonators. Therefore, during part-fold laryngeal vibration, such as falsetto or fry, nasal resonance would appear to be less than with full-fold laryngeal vibration. Similar differences exist between hypo- and hypervalvular phonation.

To determine whether an individual has consistent nasal resonance on vowels during speech rather than adjacency effects of the nasal continuant, vowels must be compared with different phoneme environments. As noted earlier, similitude nasal resonance on vowels occurs in conjunction with a nasal sound. Without the presence of the nasal continuant, the vowel will ordinarily not be perceived as being nasal. This is not true if the nasal resonance on vowels is present regardless of the nasal phoneme. For example, the /aɪ/ in "tide" and "time" will both exhibit nasal resonance during speech. When this occurs on a verbal sample, the clinician should suspect that the velopharyngeal closure is not adequate and seek the assistance of other professional personnel. If, after consultation, no medical intervention is recommended, then speech therapy is apt to concentrate on increasing the activity of the soft palate, or lowering the position of the tongue to permit greater oral emission on vowels as reported by Kelly (1934) and Williamson (1944).

CLEFT-PALATE SPEECH

Cleft-palate speech, as a label, distinguishes the speech of those individuals who possess substantial impairments of velopharyngeal incompetence. Impairments, such as inadequate fusion or growth of the oral palate, manifest themselves in the inability to close the velopharyngeal sphincter. All phonemes, except the nasals, may be affected. To be specific, individuals with impairments of the velopharyngeal sphincter are grouped into four categories with respect to their speech characteristics:

1. those who possess essentially normal speech production;
2. those who possess hypernasal resonance accompanying vowels and glides, but demonstrate little adverse effect on consonants (plosives, fricatives, and affricates), discussed previously under consistent nasal resonance on vowels;
3. those where the primary effect is on the consonants, with minimal hypernasality on vowels and glides; and
4. those who demonstrate contributions of the nasal resonator during both vowels and consonants in varying degrees with the exception of the nasal continuants.

These apparent differences have caused professional persons to classify cleft-palate speech as a disorder of voice quality and/or articulation.

Speech which commonly results from marked insufficiencies of the velopharyngeal port exemplifies the opposite characteristics of speech where the nasal resonating system is unavailable for resonance. In negative nasal resonance the nose is unable to be coupled, whereas in certain examples of cleft-palate speech, the nasal chambers are apt to be coupled at all times. Therefore, nasal-cavity attributes accompany all non-nasal phonemes. As a model of the most severe sample of cleft-palate speech, the inability to valve the nasal passage at the sphincter may produce the following changes of phoneme production:

1. all vowels may contain significant amounts of perceived nasal resonance, with high front and high back vowels exhibiting more nasal resonance than low vowels (Kelly, 1934);
2. glide sounds /w/, /l/, /r/, and /j/ may possess amounts of nasal resonance similar to the associated vowels;
3. voiceless plosives, if there is sufficient air flow, will become voiceless nasal fricatives during the oral closure positioning of the plosives (release of the oral articulation may or may not evidence the acoustic of oral pressure release, i.e., voiceless nasal frication may accompany oral pressure release);
4. voiced plosives may become nasal continuants, i.e., /d/ will sound like /n/, /b/ will sound like /m/ and /g/ will sound like /ŋ/;
5. the voiceless fricatives will appear as voiceless nasal fricatives (oral frication and nasal frication could occur simultaneously); and
6. voiced fricatives may appear as the positionally related nasal continuants, and if air flow is

sufficient, voiced nasal frication combined with oral frication could be evident (the expected nasal continuant most commonly perceived would be the /n/, i.e., /z/ and /ʒ/ become /n/, but /v/ may be similar to /m/).

One can conclude from this model that syllables or words containing high vowels surrounded by fricatives and affricates, such as "cheese," may manifest greater effects of nasal coupling than words containing low vowels and glides or plosives, such as "luck."

Compensatory behaviors during speech may bring variations in the above six points. If a person cannot achieve satisfactory production of the sound because of palatal insufficiency, he may seek other means to produce approximately the same acoustical effect. For example, if oral pressure for plosives is difficult, then a similar plosive effect may be achieved at the glottis. Should this choice be made, then oral voiceless plosives appear as voiceless glottal plosives and voiced oral plosives as the *coup de glotte*. Similarly, air can be impounded by placing the root of the tongue against the posterior pharyngeal wall (pharyngeal plosive) with subsequent release of pressure. Voiceless plosives produced at the anterior areas of the oral cavity may be made buccally, especially if the back of the tongue is also postured against the velum. Fricative sounds may be made at different anatomical areas of constriction. Glottal or pharyngeal frication is frequently heard as a substitution for orally produced fricatives. Persons with palatal insufficiency may posture the articulation for a consonant sound without perceived acoustical results, or the sound may be omitted both acoustically and positionally. Samples of cleft-palate speech also reveal sound substitutions which are not necessarily related to the palatal insufficiency.

The speech pathologist can be certain that when the production of consonants and vowels is affected similarly to those described above, the velopharyngeal sphincter is incapable of adequate speech functions. The speech clinician must therefore encourage the assistance of other supportive professional personnel in order to insure a complete habilitation procedure.

COMBINATIONS OF VOICE-QUALITY PARAMETERS AND GENERAL CONSIDERATIONS IN THERAPY

This chapter has documented certain acoustic parameters of voice quality which relate to different laryngeal and cavity adjustments during speech. No two acoustic events requiring different functions of the same structure can occur at the same time during the production of verbal signals. For example, a normal larynx cannot be simultaneously hypovalved and hypervalved, thereby producing both a breathy and a strident phonation. However, such might be the case during sequential speech. The consistency of a particular acoustic event, as well as its inconsistency, provides valuable information for the speech clinician.

Acoustical events resulting from the function of different structures permit the assessment of all parameters of vocal quality. The acoustic variables which occur consecutively and sequentially in time need to be documented so that a profile of vocal characteristics can be determined. For example, breathiness rarely occurs as an isolated entity, but rather accompanies the use of a range of frequencies, degrees of positive or negative nasal coupling, or pharyngo-oral resonance imbalance; all of which contribute to the total impression of the vocal disorder.

Certain clusters of voice quality variants occur commonly in our culture. A few of these deserve mention at this time. The combination of hyperlaryngeal valving with consistent nasal resonance on vowels is often observed. Some clinicians label such a combination as hypertense nasality or nasal twang. The breathy voice is often accompanied by the amplification of higher frequencies on vowels; amplification of low frequencies on vowels is frequently combined with negative nasal resonance. Combinations such as these produce stereotypes of vocal impressions which often are referred to as a vocal personality. The strident, harsh, nasal voice recalls the "shrew," "fishwife," or a "whiner"; breathy, higher frequency amplification suggests a personality which lacks dominance or maturity; the amplification of lower frequencies with denasality gives the impression of a "punch-drunk" prize fighter. Certain vocal qualities are associated with friendliness, alertness, warmth of personality, etc., while other clusters of vocal attributes create a more negative impression. These impressions of a vocal personality develop from associations with people in the past and strongly affect reactions to others in the future. Subjective impressions of this nature should be taken into consideration when assessing vocal disorders.

Therapy for voice disorders relates directly to the manipulation of the resonance and phonatory variables discussed in this chapter as these pertain to specific therapeutic goals. Management of voice disorders must be considered from two points of view: 1. the manipulation of variables which are intrinsic to the client, i.e., the speech clinician assists the client in changing use of his structures to effect a more acceptable acoustic product; 2. the manipulation of those factors which are external to the client, i.e., the guidance in altering the communication milieu within which the individual must speak, in order to permit continued reinforcement of improved vocal use. These viewpoints must both be considered if professional intervention is to be effective. Voice therapy, as it pertains to use of structures, cannot be performed successfully when disassociated from the circumstances of the individual's communication. The significant role of the speech clinician is to institute changes in vocal behavior, and extend their application within cultural and communicative contexts.

It must be assumed that the person with atypical vocal behavior may have no real understanding of more desirable vocal production. He may have the impression that "something is wrong with my voice" from reactions to his speech by others, or he may not. If he feels that his speech is undesirable and he seeks professional help, he expects the speech clinician to "correct the difficulty." The clinician must respond in a positive way to his request for assistance.

Ordinarily, changing vocal behavior will not be successful unless the client is fully informed concerning the processes involved. He will change his vocal behavior with the direct instruction of the speech clinician if the therapeutic process is reasonable, understood, and achieves for him a satisfactory result. The client needs to be informed as much about the "abnormality" of his vocal output as he is about the change he is to achieve, for these provide the basis of comparison and accurate reinforcement. Specifically, the therapeutic process and instruction involve the careful documentation of the boundaries of "normal" as these pertain to the physiological and acoustical parameters which need to be altered.

Modification of vocal behavior becomes a matter of establishing contrasts for reference. Assume for the moment that the client exhibits hyperlaryngeal valving. Not only must he be informed about the use of his larynx in this way, but, more importantly, he must understand the contrast of hypolaryngeal valving as a means of delineating the boundaries of "normal." Therefore, hypovalving and hypervalving become important to the process of achieving optimal laryngeal valving. If a client is unable to demonstrate vocal contrasts of this nature early in therapy, the need for further diagnosis is indicated.

As mentioned earlier, most aberrant vocal behavior exhibits a number of parameters. Evaluation of all parameters, thereby documenting the profile of vocal characteristics, enables the speech clinician to determine the direction and aims of remedial intervention. Once the client understands the parameters of his own vocal profile and demonstrates the ability to change the function of structures toward a more desirable use, therapy is directed toward the stabilization of appropriate vocal characteristics and the application of these to communication within his environment. The speech clinician's role then becomes one of advisor on vocal management.

An advisor-instructor role of the clinician should broaden the sphere of understanding about the professional aims in speech therapy for the client to encompass those persons who could provide continuing reinforcement of improved vocal production. Informed and interested associates remind the client of his own involvement in application, and often provide him with the incentive to continue application over longer periods of time. Wherever possible, the client should be the informer. The clinician also helps by establishing situational cues as a further aid to continued application of improved vocal practices. For example, the bell for recess at school becomes the cue for the child to avoid excessive yelling or talking while on the playground.

Finally, the speech clinician assists the client in the management of communication situations which may have an adverse effect on the improvement of vocal use. If one of the contributing factors to vocal nodules is loud, excited talking accompanied by excessive vocal abuse during sports broadcasts, it is important to return the client to this situation with suggestions for maintaining the improved vocal practices regardless of the situational circumstance. In the final analysis, the speech clinician helps the client solve his problems associated with the verbal signals of communication.

BIBLIOGRAPHY

Benkley, J. 1949. A quantitative measure of loudness. Ohio State Univ.: Master's thesis.

Black, J. 1959. The effect of noise induced temporary deafness upon vocal intensity. *Speech Monogr.*, 18, 74–77.

Bloomer, H. 1953. Observations of palatopharyngeal movements in speech and deglutition. *J. Speech Hearing Disorders*, 18, 230–246.

Calnan, J. 1953. Movements of the soft palate. *British J. Plastic Surgery*, 5, 280–296.

Cleeland, C. 1948. Definitions of a voice quality called x. Univ. Denver: Ph.D. dissertation.

Curry, E. 1949. Hoarseness and voice change in male adolescents. *J. Speech Hearing Disorders*, 14, 23–24.

Curry, R. 1940. The mechanism of the human voice. New York: Longmans.

Curtis, J. 1940. An experimental study of the wave composition of nasal voice quality. Univ. Iowa: Master's thesis.

Fairbanks, G., and Pronovost, W. 1939. An experimental study of the pitch characteristics of the voice during the expression of emotions. *Speech Monogr.*, 6, 87–104.

Flanagan, J. 1965. Speech analysis, synthesis and perception. Berlin-Heidelberg-New York: Springer.

Franke, P. 1939. A preliminary study validating the measurement of oral reading rate in words per minute. Univ. Iowa: Ph.D. dissertation.

Fry, D. 1955. Duration and intensity as physical correlates of linguistic stress. *J. acoust. soc., Amer.*, 27, 765–768.

Herman, D. 1942. An harmonic analysis of hoarse and non-hoarse quality. Univ. Ind.: Master's thesis.

Hixon, E. 1949. An x-ray study comparing oral and pharyngeal structures of individuals with nasal voices and individuals with superior voices. Univ. Iowa: Master's thesis.

Hollein, H. 1960. Some laryngeal correlates of vocal pitch. *J. Speech Hearing Res.*, 3, 52–58.

———, and Curtis J. 1960. A laminagraphic study of vocal pitch. *J. Speech Hearing Res.*, 3, 367–371.

———, and Moore, P. 1960. Measurements of the vocal folds during changes in pitch. *J. Speech Hearing Res.*, 3, 157–165.

———, ———, Wendhal, R., and Michel, J. 1966. On the nature of vocal fry. *J. Speech Hearing Res.*, 9, No. 2, 245–247.

Isshiki, N. 1964. Regulatory mechanism of voice intensity variation. *J. Speech Hearing Res.*, 7, No. 1, 17–29.

———, and Rengil, R. 1964. Airflow during the production of selected consonants. *J. Speech Hearing Res.*, 7, No. 3, 233–244.

———, and von Leden, H. 1964. Hoarseness: aerodynamic studies. *Arch. Otolaryng.*, 80, 206–213.

Jackson, C. and Jackson, C. L. 1937. The larynx and its diseases. Philadelphia: Saunders.

Jerome, E. 1937. Changes in voice in male adolescents. *Quart. J. Speech*, 23, 648–653.

Johnson, W., Darley, F., and Spriestersbach, D. 1952. Diagnostic manual in speech correction: a professional training workbook. New York: Harper.

Judson, L., and Weaver, A. 1942. Voice science. New York: Appleton-Century-Crofts.

Kelly, J. 1934. Studies in nasality. *Arch. Speech*, 1, No. 1, 26–43.

Lassman, F. 1942. An objective study of the pitch characteristics of eight-year-old boys during oral reading. Univ. Iowa: Master's thesis.

Lieberman, P. 1967. Intonation, perception and language. Cambridge, Mass.: M.I.T.

Linke, C. 1953. A study of pitch characteristics of female voices and relationship to vocal effectiveness. Univ. Iowa: Ph.D. dissertation.

McCaskey, C. 1948. Neck surgery as related to otolaryngology. *JAMA*, 137, 1353.

McDonald, E., and Koepp-Baker, H. 1951. Cleft palate speech: an integration of research and clinical observation. *J. Speech Hearing Disorders*, 16, 9–21.

McGlone, R. 1967. Airflow during vocal fry phonation. *J. Speech Hearing Res.*, 10, No. 2, 299–304.

Mol, H., and Uhlenbeck, E. 1956. The linguistic relevance of intensity in stress. *Lingua*, 5, 205–213.

Moll, K. 1962. Velopharyngeal closure on vowels. *J. Speech Hearing Res.*, 5, No. 1, 30–37.

———. 1968. Speech characteristics of individuals with cleft lip and palate. *In* Cleft palate and communication. Spriestersbach, D., and Sherman, D., eds. New York and London: Academic Press.

Moore, P., and Thompson, C. 1965. Comments on physiology of hoarseness. *Arch. Otolaryng.*, 81, 97–102.

———, and Von Leden, H. 1957. Film: The larynx and voice: the function of the normal larynx. Laryngeal Research Lab., W. and Harrison Gould Foundation, Northwestern Univ., Chicago.

———, and ———. 1958. Film: The larynx and voice: physiology of the larynx under daily stress. Laryngeal Research Lab., W. and Harrison Gould Foundation, North western Univ., Chicago.

Moser, H. 1942. Symposium on unique cases of speech disorders: presentation of a case. *J. Speech Disorders*, 7, 173–174.

Moses, P. 1954. The voice of neurosis. New York: Grune & Stratton.

Nusbaum, E., Foley, L. and Wells, C. 1935. Experimental studies of the firmness of velar-pharyngeal occlusion during the production of English vowels. *Speech Monogr.*, 2, 71–80.

Peterson, G., and Barney, H. 1952. Control methods used in the study of the vowels. *J. acoust. soc. Amer.*, 24, 174–184.

Potter, R., Kopp, G., and Green, H. 1947. Visible speech. New York: Van Nostrand.

Pronovost, W. 1942. An experimental study of methods for determining natural and habitual pitch. *Speech Monogr.*, 9, 111–123.

———. 1947. Visual aids in speech improvement. *J. Speech Disorders*, 12, 387–391.

Ptacek, P., and Sanders, E. 1963. Breathiness and phonation length. *J. Speech Hearing Disorders*, 28, No. 3, 267.

Rees, M. 1958. Some variables affecting perceived harshness. *J. Speech Hearing Res.*, 1, 155–168.

Rethi, A. 1952. Rolle des stylopharyngealen Muskelsystems in Krankheitsbild der Taschenbandstimme und der Dysphonia spastica. *Folia Phoniat.* 4, 201–216.

Richards, S. 1966. The establishment of a listener's reliability in judgments of nasality on vowels contained in monosyllable words as spoken by two cleft palate speakers. So. Ill. Univ.: Ph.D. dissertation.

Rubin, H., and Hirt, C. 1960. The falsetto. A high-speed cinematographic study. *Laryngoscope*, 70, 1305–1324.

Russell, G. 1936. Etiology of follicular pharyngitis, catarrhal laryngitis, so-called clergyman's throat, and singer's nodes. *J. Speech Disorders*, 1, 113–122.

Seth, G. and Guthrie, D. 1935. Speech in childhood. London: Oxford.

Sherman, D., and Goodwin, F. 1954. Pitch level and nasality. *J. Speech Hearing Disorders*, 19, No. 4, 432–428.

Sherry, J. 1954. The meatus obturator in cleft palate prosthesis. *J. Oral Surg., Oral Med., Oral Pathol.*, 852–855.

Skinner, E. 1935. A calibrated recording and analysis of pitch, force, and quality of vocal tones expressing happiness and sadness. *Speech Monogr.*, 11, 81–137.

Snidecor, J. 1940. Experimental studies of pitch and duration characteristics of superior speech. Univ. Iowa: Ph.D. dissertation.

Spriestersbach, D., and Powers, G. 1959. Nasality in isolated vowels and connected speech of cleft palate speakers. *J. Speech Hearing Res.*, 2, No. 1, 40–45.

Steer, M., and Tiffin, J. 1934. A photographic study of the use of emphasis by superior speakers. *Speech Monogr.*, 1, 72–78.

Stevens, K. 1964. Acoustical aspects of speech production. *In* Handbook of physiology, Sec. 3, Vol. 1, Respiration. Washington D.C.: Amer. Physiological Soc. P. 347.

Van Riper, C. 1954. Speech correction: principles and methods (rev. ed.). Englewood Cliffs, N.J.: Prentice-Hall.

———, and Irwin, O. 1958. Voice and articulation. Englewood Cliffs, N.J.: Prentice-Hall.

Voelker, C. 1935. Phoniatry in dysphonia ventricularis. *Ann. Otol., Rhinol., Laryng.*, 44, 471–473.

———. 1942. Frequency of hoarseness due to phonation with the thyroartenoid lips. *Arch. Otolaryng.*, 31, 71–78.

Walford, A. 1952. The husky voice. *Practicioner*, 147, 607–614.

Weiss, D. 1950. The pubertal changes of the human voice. *Folia Phoniat.*, 2, 127–158.

Wiley, J. 1942. An objective study of the pitch characteristics of seven-year-old boys during oral reading. Univ. Iowa: Master's thesis.

Williamson, A. 1944. Diagnosis and treatment of 84 cases of nasality. *Quart. J. Speech*, 29, 471–479.

Zimmerman, R. 1938. Stimmlippenlangen bei Sangern und Sangerinnen. (The lengths of the vocal folds in male and female singers.) *Arch. ges. Phonet.*, 103–130.

18

Correlates of Voice Production

John F. Michel and Ronald Wendahl[1]

The *Journal of Speech Disorders*, 10, 1945, p. 153, published the following quote:

> The less a science has advanced, the more its terminology tends to rest upon the uncritical assumption of mutual understanding.
>
> W. Quine, "Truth by Convention," *Philosophical Essays for A. N. Whitehead*, (Longmans, Green), 1936.

If we apply this statement to the study of voice, it is readily apparent that the state of the science is still in an early formative stage. If we ask ourselves "What do we *really know* about voice?" it becomes quickly and disturbingly evident that most of the past, as well as much of the current literature on voice is liberally sprinkled with fiction, mythology, physiological and acoustical misconceptions, and problems of perceptual communication. The terminology consists of an interweaving of fact and fancy within a traditional conceptual framework drawing from the fields of medicine, anatomy, elocution, singing, or any other area that may provide just the "right" words to describe an individual's auditory perception. If we are to be dismayed and confused by this state of the literature, consider for a moment that we do not even have a stable definition of the basic term "voice." It is not unlikely that if we were to ask 10 different people to define the word "voice," we would get 10 different responses.

The Random House Dictionary lists 25 primary and secondary definitions of voice, the first of which is: "the sound or sounds uttered through the mouth of human beings in speaking, shouting, singing, etc." If we expect the "scientific" definitions to be less variable and more precise than the "lay" definitions, we will be disappointed. The authors have, however, included what we consider to be some of the better definitions.

The definition proposed by Travis, Bender, and Buchanan (1934) states:

> . . . the voice producing mechanism is a closed system, the various parts of which have interactive effects. There is a good reason to suspect that the waves or puffs generated by the vocal cords not only affect, but are affected by the resonating system. The vocal cords or generating mechanism and the resonating cavities, or the modifying mechanism, cannot be considered apart from each other.

[1] After being dissatisfied with our attempt to organize and synthesize the literature on voice, we decided to abandon the traditional approach and to step back and take a fresh look at voice from as objective a position as possible. We have tried to develop a framework within which the results of research programs in voice could be compared, interrelated, and ultimately used to provide a clear, accurate, data-supported understanding of voice production. This chapter is by no means a complete product. We have not attempted to present a thorough and detailed review of the literature relating to any single parameter of voice, nor have we tried to include all possible methods of measurement. We hope we have raised more questions than we have answered. It has been our desire to provide neither a tool nor a method or therapy, but rather a philosophical as well as a practical approach to the description and specification of normal and non-normal vocal function.

The glossary of the 1957 edition of this handbook does not consider the interactive effects of the vocal folds and the sub- and supraglottal structures in the definition of voice and simply states: "Sound produced primarily by vibration of the vocal folds." Judson and Weaver (1942) state that "Voice is laryngeal vibration (phonation) plus resonance," and further state that phonation is the "production of tone by the laryngeal generator (vibration vocal folds)." Fant (1960) presents a formula, $P = S \cdot T$ in which the speech sound, P, is the product of the source, S and the transfer function of the vocal tract, T. He states:

> When discussing the production of speech it should be noted that the source S of the formula $P = S \cdot T$ is an acoustic disturbance superimposed upon the flow of respiratory air and is caused . . . by a quasi-periodic modulation of the airflow due to the opening and closing movement of the vocal folds.

Fant goes on to state, however, that "the term voice will be adopted here with reference both to a source category and feature of the speech wave." Thus it seems that the term voice can be used to refer to source characteristics (S) in one case and to a combination of source (S) and tract characteristics (T) in another case.

While commonalities exist among definitions, and each has merit, there still seems to be no precise definition of voice. One person may use the term *voice* to refer only to the laryngeal generation of sound. Another may use the term to mean the product of laryngeal generation of sound plus the transfer function of the vocal tract, while a third person may refer to "a pleasant speaking voice" and mean phonation + resonance + articulation + accent + rate + . . . For our purposes, voice will be defined as the laryngeal modulation of the pulmonary air stream, which is then further modified by the configuration of the vocal tract.

Up to this point we have merely attempted to describe voice as a universal and have made no attempt to describe different types of voices. As we progress toward developing a more complete understanding of various types of voices, our task will become increasingly difficult for many reasons, but mainly because of the existence of a terminology that has been developed without referents. Voices can be discussed under two broad categories—healthy and pathological—with the distinction between these two being arbitrary and negotiable (Michel, 1966). Assuming, however, that this differentiation can be made, the "kinds" or "types" of healthy voices are almost endless. We have all heard the terms, "booming, resonant, pleasant, whiny, rich, full, sexy, timid, weak," etc., when someone tries to describe the voice quality of an acquaintance. The world of music is replete with terms used to convey just the particular shade of meaning desired. Contralto, basso profundo, lyric soprano, and others are all terms to describe the range and quality of singing voices. Within any one voice, the "tone" may be covered or open, the "register" may be falsetto, head, or chest, and the "voice" may be high, mid, low, full, and so on. A plethora of terms has been generated with almost every author and teacher presenting his own terms and his own description of these terms. While there is naturally some overlap in the terminology used by various authors, this overlap should not be construed as agreement, since the explanation of identical terms by different authors is seldom the same.

The origin of this terminology probably lies with the early teachers of elocution and music who, without the advantages of recent developments in electronic and medical technology, were forced, by expediency, to talk about what they heard. Thus, words like "metallic, hoarse, harsh, husky, pectoral, raspy," etc., were used when they related not to what was actually occurring in the vocal mechanism, but rather to the auditory impression of the listener. Brodnitz (1966) wrote that "Much of the terminology conventionally employed . . . is based on incorrect conceptions of vocal function . . ." In a later publication (1967), he further stated ". . . the didactic language that we use habitually in describing voice qualities and forms or faults of voice production mirrors concepts and ideas that have been made obsolete by modern research." While this may be true in many cases, it is probable that individuals who read research literature and who also possess an excellent understanding of the vocal mechanism and its function are still motivated, by convention, to describe voice in subjective, archaic terms. This "tradition" of labeling has persisted in spite of a rapidly growing fund of information currently available on the mechanics of voice. This dilemma was most eloquently expressed by Sarbin (1968). Although he was talking about psychologists and anxiety, the parallel to speech or voice clinicians and voice disorders is disturbingly easy to make. He states:

> Most of my remarks are applicable to many currently used concepts other than anxiety. Historico-linguistic analysis of other concepts would lead to similar conclusions: to wit, we are great mythmakers and myth

users. However, being human and being subject to uncertainty in our efforts to understand the world about us, there are times when we must adopt beliefs so that we are not transfixed for lack of truth (Scheibe and Sarbin, 1965). The psychologist, no different from the man in the street, lacking truth and needing it to provide a course of action, makes it up. In so doing, he runs the risk of locking himself into a conceptual prison from which there is no escape save to explode the myth that he had constructed.

We believe we are indeed locked in such a mythical prison even though there have been suggestions for escape.

In 1959, van den Berg and Vennard proposed three avenues by which objectivity might be introduced into the designations or classifications of voice: 1. the recording of graduated samples (or the arranging of recorded samples in graded sequences); 2. the acoustic analysis of voice samples until the harmonic structure of different recognizable voice productions is understood; and 3. the correlating of changes in tone quality with adjustments of the vocal instrument. Several studies have been reported using the first procedure. The main problem with this approach is that the samples are graded by subjective judgments and little or no information may be available about the aspect of the signal responsible for the judgments. It is possible that different judges could rank a series of samples in the same order, using the same terminology and yet be responding to different parameters of the signal. The second approach is limited to an examination of the harmonic structure of the vocal spectrum. While this may well be one in a series of sources of data, precise measurement and interpretation poses many problems in that important laryngeal functions such as amplitude of laryngeal vibration and laryngeal air flow may not be revealed by spectral analysis. Quantification of the third approach again would appear to be somewhat difficult in that reliance is placed on human evaluation (the reliability of which is tenuous at best) of the signal, and the same change in tone may be accomplished by different adjustments of the vocal mechanism. Moreover, the problems of measurement of changes in the system are a long way from being solved satisfactorily.

Assuming that the two major aims of science are measurement and prediction, the first step in the study of voice must be the determination of pertinent, measurable parameters. Pertinent in that changes in these variables will have a perceptible effect, and measurable in order to quantify and correlate the changes with the effects. What is indicated, therefore, is a thorough, careful study of the mechanism and how it functions. At first glance, the production of voice appears to be dependent upon three primary factors; 1. pulmonic pressure, 2. laryngeal vibration, and 3. the transfer function of the vocal tract with each of these factors having measurable parameters.

It is immediately evident that interactions occur between parameters associated with these factors and that to isolate and study a single parameter is tantamount to introducing considerable error into the results. In an effort to deal with and resolve some of the problems created by the nature of the literature, a program of research will be presented in the following pages which will, hopefully, put the study and evaluation of voice on a more scientific basis. Basically, the approach is to determine the significant parameters of voice production, establish norms for these parameters and, when possible, relate them to perception. This task would appear to be relatively simple as most textbooks present pitch, loudness, duration, and quality as being the primary parameters of voice. Referring to Table 18-I, it is not difficult to see how we can deal confidently with the first three; pitch, loudness and duration. Each parameter can be measured psychophysically and each has a principle physical correlate. We cannot, however, so deal with *quality* as a single entity because there is no single primary physical correlate. While pitch, loudness, and duration can be handled with interval scaling, quality must be treated with nominal scaling due to the existence of many qualities, each with its own underlying parameter(s).

TABLE 18-I

Traditional elements of voice, their principal physical correlates and units of measurement

PERCEPTION	UNITS	PRINCIPLE PHYSICAL CORRELATE	UNITS
pitch	mel	frequency	Hz
loudness	phon, sone	sound pressure level	dB
duration	seconds	time	seconds
quality	?	?	?

We propose, therefore, to present voice as a multidimensional series of measurable events, implying that a single phonation can be assessed in many different ways. We have presented what we feel are the pertinent parameters of voice production, although it is not suggested that because we have listed 12 measurable parameters that there are not 12^2 or 12^3 important parameters of voice. This is merely a tentative list of what we believe to be parameters of voice that have an influence on perception and function. While most can be measured and correlated with specific perceptions, others are more elusive and difficult to talk about in more than ordinal terms. Finally, in no way does the order of presentation of these measures mean to imply order of importance. The major parameters associated with the production of voice include:

1. Vital capacity of the lungs.
2. Maximum duration of controlled sustained blowing.
3. Modal frequency level.
4. Maximum frequency ranges.
5. Maximum duration of sustained phonation.
6. Volume/velocity flow during phonation.
7. Glottal waveform.
8. Sound-pressure level.
9. Jitter of the vocal signal.
10. Shimmer of the vocal signal.
11. Effort level (vocal).
12. Transfer function of the vocal tract.

It would be nice and uncomplicated if the measurable parameters were all physical, all physiological, all acoustic, or all psychophysical. We could then measure one or two parameters and get a relatively accurate estimate of vocal function. Because, however, voice production is an extremely complex event in which auditory, acoustic, and aerodynamic events are produced by the interaction of physiological mechanisms, we need to measure as many vocal facets as possible if we are to get a complete and accurate picture of voice production.

In the following discussion, a definition of each parameter will be presented as needed, together with a brief review of some of the more pertinent literature and methods of measurement. This discussion is not intended to be a complete and definitive review of the literature for all or any of the parameters presented. Its primary purpose is to present a rationale for the study and evaluation of voice and to encourage workers in the field to ask themselves, "What do we *really know* about voice?"

1. *Vital Capacity* is defined as the maximum amount of volume of air which can be exhaled following maximum inhalation. This measure is important only insofar as it provides an estimate of the amount of air potentially available for the production of phonation and is not meant to imply that the entire vital capacity is available or necessary for phonation. Indeed, Yanagihara and Koike (1967) have related vital capacity to phonation volume while Hirano, Koike, and von Leden (1968) have indicated a relationship between vital capacity and maximum phonation time. In the former paper it was reported that the phonation volume and the ratio of phonation volume to vital capacity both decrease as the subject's pitch level decreases. Thus, a correlation between vital capacity and phonation volume was reported with correlation coefficients ranging from .59 to .90. Hirano et al. found that a phonation quotient (vital capacity/maximum phonation time) was correlated with the flow rates from normal subjects, indicating that higher flow rates were generally associated with shorter phonation times or larger vital capacities. Bouhuys et al. (1968) reported singers designated as having "poor quality" also had smaller vital capacities than singers categorized as having average or good quality. One of the criteria for a judgment of "poor quality" was, however, "breaking of phrases in the middle," which may have caused the singers with "reduced" vital capacities not to meet the phrasing criteria, and thus be judged poor.

It is apparent that vital capacity as a single measure will not necessarily be a useful indication of laryngeal function. In conjunction with other measures however, it may be of great value.

2. *Maximum Duration of Sustained Blowing* is defined as the maximum length of time an individual can maintain an oral flow of air. This appears to be a relatively new measure to be introduced into the speech literature (Ptacek and Sander, 1963) and provides an estimate of the amount of control of respiratory mechanics. This estimate may well indicate the capacity of an individual to maintain the subglottal air pressures necessary for phonation. For example, the muscles responsible for the inhalatory preparation to phonation are also active after exhalation (phonation) begins, indicating that they (the inhalatory muscles) exert a "checking" action on the passive forces of exhalation (Draper, Ladefoged, and Whitteridge, 1959) and that variations from the expected durations are probably attributable to laryngeal rather than respiratory function. As with vital capacity, this isolated measure may be of value only to show that the "power" or supportive functions necessary for speech are intact.

The measure of this variable can be coarse or refined. In a coarse measure, one could ask an individual to blow through a common straw, the tip of which was just under the surface of the water. The regularity with which the subject is able to produce the bubbles as well as the time required to complete the task could be noted. Of course, no information concerning rate of air flow or volume of air expended can be obtained from the procedure just described. To obtain this type of data, more refined instrumentation is necessary. A pneumotachograph or some type of flowmeter would be necessary to measure rate of flow while the volume could be determined by integration of the flow. If integration is not possible, a somewhat less accurate but still effective method is simply to multiply flow rate by the duration of the flow.

3. *Modal Frequency Level* is defined as the fundamental frequency most often used by an individual while he is in the act of producing spontaneous speech. The manner in which this measure is obtained may well have an effect on the magnitude of the measure. For example, most of the data that have been reported on fundamental frequency have been obtained from readings of an emotionally neutral passage such as the "Rainbow passage," "My Grandfather," or "Arthur the Young Rat." From these recordings, measures of central tendency (mean, median, and mode) and variability (standard deviation) have been calculated for fundamental frequency. The assumption was that the subjects would read the material with approximately the same frequency level as they would use during spontaneous speech or conversation. However, a study by Tiffany and Hollien (1968) indicates a mean variation of ± five Hz when comparing spontaneous speech with formal reading with some of the differences being as great as 14 Hz. Thus, we propose that this measure should be made during spontaneous speaking, preferably with the subject unaware that he is being recorded. What we then measure is the fundamental frequency most often used, hence the term *modal frequency* level.

The rationale for this measure is that there is a pitch to each person's voice which should be appropriate for his age and sex. Children's voices are generally higher in pitch than adult voices and women's voices are generally higher in pitch than men's voices (Peterson and Barney, 1952). The literature in this area is abundant, with studies by Fairbanks (1942), McGlone (1966b), Fairbanks, Wiley, and Lassman (1949), and Fairbanks, Herbert, and Hammond (1949) providing basic information on frequency levels of children. Curry (1940), Hollien, and Malcik (1962), Hollien, Malcik, and Hollien (1965), and Hollien and Malcik (1967) report data for male adolescent voice change in females. Fundamental frequency has been related to "effective speech" by Murry and Tiffin (1934), to stage speech by Cowan (1936), to superior male speakers by Pronovost (1942), and to superior female speakers by Snidecor (1951). Mysak (1959) and McGlone and Hollien (1963) have published data obtained from aged males and females respectively. Briefly, the results of these studies indicate relatively high and similar modal frequencies for males and females up to the age of puberty. While the voices of both the males and females become lower during this period, the change is much greater for the male. Finally, there is a tendency for modal frequency to rise with advancing age.

This variable may be measured in a number of ways, oscillographic, computer, or by some specially designed pitch-extraction device. The reader is cautioned against confusing "habitual pitch," "natural pitch," or "optimal pitch" with modal frequency level. The former terms are generally undefined or else defined in different ways by different people; the main idea, however, is that every person has a "best" pitch or frequency level at which to speak. At this time, valid, supportive data for this concept are difficult to locate.

4. *Maximum Frequency Range* is defined as the highest and lowest frequencies an individual can phonate in each of three frequency ranges—vocal fry, modal, and falsetto. We have avoided the use of the term "register" and all the terms (head, chest, mid, etc.) associated with the use of the term. Our primary reason for doing this is that we do not know what a register is even though Garcia (1841) gave what is probably the best verbal definition of the term. He stated:

> By the word register we mean a series of succeeding sounds of equal quality on a scale from low to high, produced by the application of the same mechanical principle, the nature of which differs basically from another series of succeeding sounds of equal quality produced by another mechanical principle.

The key phrase in this statement is "equal quality." Because the assessment of the quality of voice is negotiable, we would prefer to deal in terms somewhat less arbitrary and subjective. We are, however, aware that our use of the term "range" is not a great improvement over the use of the term "register." Still, we do feel that the term "range" does not carry the plethora of connotations associated with the term "register."

We recognize the existence of three phonational ranges; modal, falsetto, and vocal fry. To us, all three of these phonational ranges are possible by an individual with a normal vocal mechanism. The modal range is the one most frequently used during conversational speech. We say most frequently because an individual will often drop into vocal fry at the end of a phrase or sentence. For all intents and purposes falsetto is never used during normal speech. The term "range" is used to designate a range of frequencies having the same basic laryngeal waveform. Using this definition, some interesting observations can be made about phonational ranges in humans. In a study by Hollien and Michel (1968) it was reported that while the falsetto and modal ranges occasionally overlapped, phonation in these two ranges could not be produced simultaneously. Thus, the larynx is unable to produce simultaneously the glottal waveforms of falsetto and modal range. The implication is that the perception of modal and falsetto result from the production of two waveforms which are indeed different and not merely two different parts of a continuum. In the case of vocal fry and modal range, however, there was never any overlapping of these two ranges in any individual. There were however frequent examples of phonation which were characterized by the simultaneous production of fry and modal ranges, suggesting that they may be on the same continuum. Supportive evidence for this statement was provided by Coleman (1963), who reported that "when the vocal tract was allowed to decay from 42 to 44 dB of its maximum amplitude for a single pulse, vocal fry was always perceived," and "when the vocal tract wave was allowed to decay only 30 dB between excitation pulses, vocal fry was never perceived." Thus, it seems reasonable to assume that at decay values between 30 and 42 dB, elements of both vocal fry and modal range will be perceived. It has been suggested that this type of phonation has been labeled "creaky" by some authors (John Laver, Edinburgh University, personal communication).

The rationale for obtaining a measure of maximum frequency range is relatively simple. During speech utilizing a normal phonational mechanism, a certain degree of variability in frequency is expected and indeed seemed necessary. The extent to which the mechanism does not or cannot produce a range ot frequencies may be the first indication of non-normal function. It must be mentioned, however, that even though an individual has measured frequency ranges within normal limits, he may still use little inflection during speech.

There are numerous reports in the literature regarding the extent of the "normal" pitch or frequency range of human phonation. Many of these references, however, do not distinguish between the different phonational ranges and report only the lowest and highest frequencies, irrespective of the particular ranges included. For example, Anderson (1942) states that "The total range of the vocal mechanism . . . including the voices of both men and women, extends almost four octaves from a low tone of 70 to 80 d.v. per second in the male voice to upwards of 1,024 d.v. in the female voice." Luchinger and Arnold (1965) state that the "collective human range" from the lowest bass to the highest soprano is from 50 to 2,000 Hz. There are many other references to total pitch range in the literature; Hahn et al. (1957), Fisher (1966), Culver (1956), and Vennard (1967), to name a few, but the most recurring theme is that each person should have a range consisting of a certain number of notes or octaves. Few studies could be found in which an attempt was made to report normative data based on actual measurements of subjects. Hollien and Michel (1968) reported that the mean range for the modal range for males was just over an octave and a half with frequency limits from 71 to 561 Hz. Females had a range of almost two octaves within a frequency range of 122 to 798 Hz. Also reported are data for the vocal fry and falsetto ranges.

It is important also to distinguish between maximum frequency range and the range of frequencies employed during connected speech. As previously mentioned, an individual will almost always go into vocal fry phonation at the end of phrases and sentences. Thus, when we measure fundamental frequency from connected speech, we will undoubtedly be measuring frequencies from both the modal and vocal fry ranges. It is probable, however, that measures of the specific ranges available to an individual can be an indication of the physical condition of the mechanism.

5. *Maximum Duration of Phonation* is defined as the maximum amount of time an individual can sustain phonation after taking a maximum inhalation. While at first this seems to be a relatively simple measure to take, there are a great many variables which can affect the duration. Among these variables are 1. the frequency of the phonation, 2. the sound-pressure level of the phonation, 3. the vowel being

phonated, 4. the general physical condition of the individual, and 5. the amount and kind of training the individual has had, i.e., athletes generally do better than nonathletes and trained singers do better than nonsingers (Lass and Michel, 1969). Ptacek and Sander (1963a) appear to be the first to suggest that the maximum duration of phonation may be influenced by the frequency and sound-pressure level of the phonation. Their results indicated that males could sustain phonation longer than females, especially at lower frequencies and sound-pressure levels. Then, as both frequency and SPL increased, the phonation times between males and females tended to become more similar. However, a considerable degree of variability among subjects was still evident in that significant differences existed for frequency and sound-pressure levels for male phonations, but not for female phonation. Conversely, the frequency-sound pressure level interaction was significant for the females but not for the males. Somewhat different results were found by Lass and Michel (1969). They report that for low-frequency phonations of both males and females and for the moderate frequency phonations of the males there was a general tendency for phonation time to increase as a function of sound-pressure level. However, in the high-frequency phonations for both males and females, there was a decided tendency for phonation time to decrease as sound-pressure level increased.

Van Riper (1954) states that an individual should be able to sustain phonation for at least 15 seconds. Fairbanks (1960) states that 20 to 25 seconds is normal for sustaining a phonation. So far as could be determined, these figures are based on clinical observation. That short phonation times are associated with laryngeal pathology and can be improved by treatment was shown by von Leden et al. (1967), who reported an increase in phonation time from 1.33 to 14.79 seconds in one case and from 3.91 to 8.66 seconds in another case (both of whom had unilateral vocal fold paralysis) after injecting teflon paste into the affected folds. Michel et al. (1968) also demonstrated an increase of from 4 to more than 20 seconds maximum phonation time as a result of teflon treatment of unilateral vocal-fold paralysis.

Ptacek and Sander (1963a) also appear to be the first to try to relate maximum duration of phonation to the perception of "breathiness." Although none of the voices of their subjects were considered to be non-normal, they were able to divide the subjects into two groups; long phonators and short phonators. When these two groups were judged as to the degree of breathiness from least to most on a seven-point scale, they found that the long phonators tended to be judged as less breathy than the short phonators. In addition, perceived breathiness decreased as a function of increased intensity and "high-frequency phonations tended to be rated as more breathy than corresponding low-frequency phonations." In a later study, Ptacek et al. (1966) found that maximum duration of phonation, maximum pitch range, maximum intensity, maximum interoral breath pressure, and vital capacity all decrease as a function of increasing age.

Maximum duration of phonation has been used as a diagnostic tool for some time. Arnold (1959) reports that in cases of paralytic dysphonia, phonation time is always shortened to three to seven seconds. He goes on to state that, "similar findings were made in 1942 by Rieben (5 seconds), in 1937 by Luchsinger (three to 15 seconds) and in 1952 by Brahm (three to 12 seconds)."

The rationale for this measure has been alluded to by Arnold (1959), who wrote that "This simple test gives information of the efficiency of the pheumophonic sound generation in the larynx." He further states that "It also demonstrates the general state of the patient's respiratory coordination." We would modify this statement somewhat to say that this measure *can* demonstrate the general status of the patient's respiratory coordination, but more accurately indicates the relative efficiency of the pneumolaryngeal interaction. If this efficiency proves to be less than expected, then a test of respiratory function per se, such as vital capacity or maximum duration of blowing, is indicated. In the event these measures appear normal, a measure of the amount of air used during phonation as proposed by Hirano, Koike, and von Leden (1968) is indicated.

6. *Volume-Velocity Air Flow.* While the term air flow is self-explanatory, the amount of normative data that we have for flow rates under differing phonatory conditions is small. Flow rates for normal phonation in the modal register appear to be in the vicinity of 100 cc/sec (Kunze, 1962; Isshiki, 1964). Isshiki reported flow rates of around 60 cc/sec to accompany falsetto phonation, and McGlone (1966a, and 1967) observed flow rates of approximately 20 cc/sec during vocal fry phonation.

Isshiki and Ringel (1964) report that flow rates are greater for unvoiced than for voiced consonants; that different flow-rate patterns exist for the various consonant groups; that flow rates for stops, fricatives, and vowellike sounds decrease in that order; and, that consonants in terminal positions are more variable in flow rate than those in initial positions.

Many methods of measuring flow rate are available to the experimenter. Probably the most concise description of a desirable measuring procedure was presented by Isshiki and Ringel in 1964. Their method employed a laminar flow resistor, a differential pressure gauge, and a recording instrument. They state that the principle of measuring flow rate for them was based upon the fact the pressure drop across a resistance (mesh screen) which is caused by an air stream flowing across it varies linearly with flow rate under certain controlled conditions. In their procedure, they heated the screen to prevent moisture condensation during exhalation. They used highly sensitive strain gauges to measure pressure drops across the screen.

Since air flow is quite probably related to fundamental frequency and definitely related to subglottal pressure, it would seem a desirable variable to measure. Normative data should be gathered using the same phonatory ranges suggested for measures of jitter and shimmer. Both shimmer and jitter could be caused by an irregular air flow and could result from irregular subglottal pressures. This measure, then, is necessary as one of the many measures which will allow a differential diagnosis between laryngeal and respiratory dysfunction.

7. *Glottal Wave Form* cannot be as easily defined as some of the other parameters. Basically, however, an index of glottal waveform may be obtained by calculating 1. the opening time of the vocal folds, 2. the closing time of the vocal folds, 3. the time the folds are open, and 4. the time the folds are closed, all during a single vibratory cycle. Of all the laryngeal parameters we have suggested, probably an accurate measurement of the waveform is also one of the more difficult to obtain as the problem is more complex than it appears. To obtain glottal waveform from high-speed photography, one must assume that volume velocity is directly proportional to the area of opening of the folds. This assumption has been shown to be tenuous by Flannagan and Landgraf (1967). A second method of obtaining glottal waveform is through transillumination. Proponents of this technique assume that the output of a photoduo diode is directly proportional to the amount of light passing through the opening folds (Ohala, 1967). The argument might be valid if one were absolutely positive that the folds were completely illuminated (assuming that the photosensor is placed below the glottis) or that (if the light source is introduced below the glottis and the sensor above) the sensor is exactly at the right angle of incidence, and never moves during the portion of the phonation to be analyzed. Coleman and Wendahl (1968) reported the glottal waveforms obtained from simultaneous recordings using high-speed laryngeal photography and transillumination yielded grossly differing waveforms.

A third popular method of obtaining estimates of glottal waveform is through the use of inverse filtering wherein the effect of the transfer function of the vocal tract is theoretically canceled. Although Fant and Sonnesson (1962), using transillumination and inverse filtering on the same subjects, reported similar glottal waveforms, the obvious limitation to inverse filtering is that one encounters the problem of trying to solve the equations involved in individual vocal tracts in which the amplitude of the formants to be cancelled are dependent upon the glottal waveform which is the variable under investigation. In addition, formant frequency cannot be defined as a point of maximum amplitude in the phonated signal. Stevens and House (1955) have stated that:

> Formant frequency is interpreted fundamentally as the frequency of a normal mode of vibration of the human vocal mechanism. As such, formant frequency is a complex number. During the utterance of certain sounds, notably the vowels, the normal modes of vibration of the vocal system are manifested in the acoustic output of the speaker as maxima in the spectra of these sounds. The frequencies of these spectral maxima are closely related to the complex numbers representing the normal modes (or natural frequencies) of the vocal system and to their manifestations in the speaker's acoustic output, i.e., the frequencies of the spectral maxima.

Accepting this definition, even a quasiperiodic signal would cause the peaks in amplitude to change as a function of wave-period. When one attempts to obtain a glottal waveform from a signal having large jitter components, it would seem that inverse filtering would be the poorest choice of techniques. However, inasmuch as formant amplitude and frequency as perceived by the human ear are related to judgments of roughness, even approximations to glottal waveforms may be desirable.

8. *Sound-Pressure Level Range* is defined as the maximum and minimum SPLs an individual can produce at specific points in his frequency range.

This measure is not to be confused with the sound-pressure level most often used by an individual when he is producing phonation. The latter measure is regarded by many as being unnecessary or superfluous, the principal argument being that, "naturally, everyone talks loudly enough to be heard." The assumption is that no matter what the ambient noise levels, no matter what the condition of his speaking mechanism, an individual will monitor his voice production and adjust the loudness to a level appropriate for the situation.

The measure proposed here is not the speaking level, but rather an estimate of what the mechanism is capable of producing. To obtain this measure, it is suggested that after the frequency ranges of an individual have been determined, specific points in those ranges be determined, i.e., the twenty-fifth, fiftieth, and seventy-fifth percentile points of the modal frequency range. Then, at these percentiles sustained phonation be produced as softly as possible and as loudly as possible. Such a procedure is similar to that following by Wolfe, Stanley, and Settee (1935).

9. *Jitter* of the vocal signal is defined as the cycle-to-cycle variation in period that occurs when an individual is attempting to sustain phonation at a constant frequency. That some degree of jitter exists in the laryngeal signal has been accepted for some time and has been accounted for by designating the laryngeal signal as "quasi-periodic." When, however, adjacent periods become so dissimilar that perceptible noise is introduced into the overall spectrum, laryngeal dysfunction is suggested.

Aperiodic laryngeal vibratory patterns have been related to abnormal vocal production over a number of years (Carhart, 1938, 1941; Bowler, 1964). Considerable caution must be taken in interpreting these data, however, because gross changes in wave periods (up to an octave in extent) were reported to be characteristic not only of voices reported to be "harsh," but also of vocal recordings taken from adolescent boys and girls, preadolescent children of both sexes, and from postmenarchal females, Fairbanks et al. (1949); Curry (1940); and Duffy (1958). It seems quite possible that some of the investigators did not recognize the category of vocal fry. The data from human speakers were all obtained from recordings made during continuous speech. A change in range from modal speaking level to vocal fry during conversational speech is not only normal for most speaker, but expected.

An additional problem is the differentiation between changes in adjacent period due to the inherent instability of the oscillator and those due to the inflectional patterns of speech. We take the view that to report measures of aperiodicity or jitter from connected speech without appropriate corrective equations for inflectional changes renders the data extremely difficult to interpret. For example, Lieberman (1961, 1963) and Smith and Lieberman (1964) refer to cycle-to-cycle variations in wave periods in speech as "perturbations" but do not subdivide perturbations into components of jitter and intonation. Thus, to say that an individual has a mean perturbation of 1.0 msec. could mean either that he speaks in a monotone with a pathological larynx or that he speaks with a normal larynx and a great deal of inflection or some combination of the two.

Coleman (1960) and Moore and Thompson (1965) were among the first to report jitter measures obtained from persons producing isolated vowels. They found jitter present in persons with both normal and abnormal larynges. Their data differentiated between the groups, however, showing more jitter in the abnormal group. They reported a great deal less jitter in both populations than previously had been reported. In neither study were octave changes in periods reported. The jitter in the abnormal population was on an average from four Hz to eight Hz with the greatest single cycle-to-cycle shift being around 17 Hz (1.77 semitones).

Wendahl (1961, 1962), used an analog of the larynx to study the effect of aperiodic wave periods on judgments of roughness. He found that very small amounts of aperiodicity, as little as one Hz around a median frequency of 100 Hz, was detectable and that deviations of $\pm$ 10 Hz were reported by listeners to sound extremely rough. Although, as has been stated, some amount of jitter is expected in normal speakers and desirable in speech synthesis to achieve a "natural" sounding tone (Cooper et al., 1967), larger amounts of jitter are probably among the closest correlates of auditory roughness.

10. *Shimmer* of the vocal signal is defined as the cycle-to-cycle variations in amplitude that occur when an individual attempts to sustain phonation at a constant frequency and intensity.

The effect of amplitude modulation on judgments of roughness was first reported by Mathes and Miller (1947). Coleman (1960) later postulated that utterances from human speakers containing large and random amplitude variations were related to listener evaluations of roughness. Laryngeal analog synthesis established a linear relationship between shimmer and listener judgments of roughness with as little as one dB of shimmer between adjacent cycles being sufficient for judges to detect roughness in the signal (Wendahl, 1966).

Sonnesson (1967) reported results of glottograms taken from a patient with a laryngeal hemiparalysis. These glottograms showed a laryngeal wave with amplitude differences between adjacent cycles sufficient to produce considerable shimmer in the voiced signal. Although the period measures from this phonation showed little jitter, the auditory impression of Sonnesson was that this patient had a very rough voice.

It is anticipated that the amount of shimmer in any given voice will be dependent at least upon the modal frequency level, the total frequency range, and the SPL relative to each individual voice. It is suggested, therefore, that shimmer be measured in dB under the same phonatory conditions as jitter is measured, as will be stated in more detail in the measurement section.

It must also be stated that shimmer, like jitter, refers to glottal function and cannot at this time be estimated from signals taken distally from the mouth. Shimmer must then be subdivided into glottal shimmer and oral shimmer.

Inasmuch as the listener's ear attends to oral shimmer, it would seem reasonable to scale this variable under either dimension (glottal or oral) as long as the statement directly defined the point at which the measure had been made.

11. *Effort Level* is defined as the degree of perceived effort in the production of phonation. That this is an important variable was suggested by Curtis (1956), who states that "harsh voice quality . . . is often heard in people for whom voice production seems to be a considerable effort or strain." Later, Lane, Catania, and Stevens (1961) reported that:

> The speaker's numerical estimation of his own vocal level, the *autophonic response*, was found to grow as the 1.1 power of the actual sound pressure produced. When listeners judged the loudness of another speaker's vocalization . . . , the exponent was 0.7. The disparity between these exponents suggests that the speaker does not rely solely upon his perception of loudness in judging his own relative vocal level.

Their main conclusion appears to be that while the listener is responding primarily to the sound pressure level in determining loudness, the speaker or sound producer is probably relying on some physiological dimension as well as sound pressure in his loudness estimation.

In a study of vowel amplitude and stress, Lehiste and Peterson (1959) reported that when a single speaker recorded a series of sustained phonations of 15 different vowels, keeping pitch constant, the absolute sound-pressure levels were not the same. Yet they reported that the vowels appeared to be about equally loud during casual listening. By way of explanation they stated, "This observation doubtless represents a confusion in perceptual judgment, however, for the equivalence is probably in physiological stress, not loudness." The speaker who then recorded sustained vowels at the same frequency level *and* sound-pressure level reported that "some vowels required considerably more effort than others." When tapes of these phonations were presented to listeners, "almost invariably, the listeners identified the vowels that were produced with a greater amount of effort (such as /i/ and /u/ recorded at zero VU) as louder than vowels having greater intrinsic amplitude but produced with normal effort (such as /a/ and /ɔ/)."

Ladefoged and McKinney (1963) measured volume-velocity flow and subglottal pressure during the production of one-syllable words and found that the sound-pressure level of the vowel in *bar* was about five dB greater than *bee* or *boo* produced with the same subglottal pressure. Although they did not measure or estimate "effort" per se, they introduced the concept of "work done" by stating, "To good approximation the rate of work, W, done upon the air in producing a voiced sound is proportional to the product of the subglottal pressure and the volume velocity of air through the glottis; i.e., $W \propto GV$." Applying the results of van den Berg (1956), i.e., the volume velocity is proportional to the subglottal pressure ($V \propto G$) and the results of the first part of their study, i.e., the peak subglottal pressure is proportional to the peak sound pressure level ($Gp \propto Sp^{0.6}$), they derived that the rate of work is proportional to the effective sound pressure ($W \propto S^{1.2}$).

While this finding, $W \propto S^{1.2}$, may be compared with the finding of Lane, Catania, and Stevens (1961) that a speaker's estimation of his own vocal level is proportional to the 1.1 power of the sound-pressure level, any discussion or definitive statement must be tempered by the possibility that the work, W, referred to by Ladefoged and McKinney may not be the *effort* studied by Lane et al. The wide differences in the exponents for the relationship of the loudness of heard speech to sound-pressure level (1.2 in the Ladefoged and McKinney study to 0.6 in the Lane et al. study) may be attributable to the fact that Ladefoged and McKinney did not seek to treat sound-pressure level as an independent variable, i.e., the stimuli to be judged had not been recorded at a constant sound-pressure level and then judged for loudness.

In what is probably the most carefully controlled and executed investigation to date, Brandt, Ruder, and Ship (1968) found they were able to alter the exponents for the relationships of effort and loudness to sound-pressure level by systematically varying the loudness and effort level of the stimuli presented to their judges. One speaker recorded a sentence at eight different sound pressure levels ranging from 60 to 95 dB in five-dB steps. By careful rerecording techniques, they presented the original 80 dB phonation at eight different pressure levels (60 to 95 dB in five-dB steps) and in this way were able to control effort and allow loudness to vary. To control loudness and vary effort, they rerecorded all the original recordings at the same 80 dB level. When these stimuli were presented to judges, exponents for relating loudness and effort to sound-pressure level were 1.12 and 0.89 respectively for normal speech. When loudness was varied and effort held constant, the exponents were 0.92 and 0.38 respectively, and exponents of 0.40 and 0.57 were derived for loudness and effort respectively when loudness was held constant and effort was allowed to vary.

While subglottal pressure may well be a physiological correlate to the perception of effort as well as of loudness, the role of muscular effort also needs to be investigated.

12. *Transfer Function of The Vocal Tract* is defined as the particular modification of the laryngeal signal imposed by the configuration of the supraglottal structures. The authors take the view that the glottis is more closely coupled to the vocal tract than has been indicated by other writers (Curtis, 1968). If the system is closely coupled, it becomes meaningless to describe laryngeal actions in excised larynges unless an artificial impedance or acoustic load is placed above the excised larynges. In addition, the configuration of the vocal tract is related to perceptual evaluations of voice quality (Sherman and Linke, 1952).

The glottal waveform is obviously modified into other waveforms by the supraglottal structures. Among other things, it is this modification that allows us to distinguish one vowel from another, uttered by the same speaker. There are also proponents of the view that the supraglottal structures act in such an unique way as to allow individuals to be distinguished from each other on this basis (Kersta, 1962).

It has been demonstrated in normal speakers that the fundamental frequency of the glottal source is related to the transfer function of the vocal tract. Wendahl and Page (1967) measured fundamental frequency on normal young adult males phonating /ava/ and /ivi/. They found that the production of the constricted /v/ between the two vowels caused the fundamental frequency to be lowered in all subjects. Stevens (1967) had concurrently predicted these results with mathematical theory.

This view, that the vibratory patterns of the vocal folds is partially dependent upon the supraglottal structures, is relatively new. It has been stated by several authors that the vibration of the folds is independent of the supraglottal load into which they work (Curtis, 1968; Farnsworth, 1940). Because previous literature exists which theoretically establishes literally no relationship between the vibratory patterns of the larynx and the supraglottal structures, this point will be discussed in further detail.

Flanagan (1964) showed that the glottal waveform is influenced by the impedance of the supraglottal structures. Since both fundamental frequency and glottal waveform are partially determined by the supraglottal structures, it would seem desirable to specify the vowel phonated by the subjects on which the measures were taken. It would also seem reasonable to assume that the effect of the supraglottal structures upon laryngeal function would be dependent upon SPL and modal-frequency level. Therefore, normative data should be obtained with a typically open oral configuration /æ/ and a typically narrowed configuration /i/ at the same SPL and modal-frequency levels specified in the previous measures. In the abnormal voice, the specification of the conditions of the supraglottal structures seems even more important.

Sherman and Linke (1952) pointed out that high vowels sounded less harsh than low vowels. Subsequently, it was reported by Wendahl (1962) that judgments of roughness were related to the degree of jitter in the signal. In a recent study by Johnson (1969), subjects were instructed to produce sustained phonations of 12 vowels at specified frequency and sound-pressure levels. When analyzed for degree of jitter, the high vowels were found to have less jitter than the low vowels, thus corroborating the results of Sherman and Linke (1952). Cole (1968) and Linklater (1968) also substantiated the conclusions of Sherman and Linke and stated that the effect of the first formant and the formant bandwidths effected listener judgments of roughness, i.e., the lower the first formant, the less rough the vowel sounded. The center frequency of the second formant has also been investigated (Kvols, 1969). Although this study failed to demonstrate that the second formant frequency position was related to judgments of vocal roughness, the results should be considered as only tentative because of the difficulty the judges had in decision making. In general, though, average human formant bandwidths sounded more rough than those either narrower or wider than the listeners were accustomed to hearing.

For the appraisal of a particular voice, it is suggested that jitter and shimmer will most readily be heard and measured with the low vowels, such as /æ/ and least readily on the high vowels such as /u/.

Thus, it is imperative that one states exactly the conditions under which any phonation is obtained. It would be desirable, therefore, to standardize the condition under which voice samples are taken.

AN APPROACH TO MEASUREMENT

The discussion so far has dealt with only the measurable parameters of voice, and no mention has been made with regard to what is normal and what is non-normal phonation. We have concentrated solely on the parameters of production rather than the evaluation of voice. We have suggested that each of these parameters exists on a continuum and that a distribution of each would approximate the normal curve. Yet, while all these measures can be obtained, they are relatively meaningless unless they can be compared against some standard or norm. How do we know that an air-flow rate of 675 cc/sec is not "normal"? How do we know that a mean jitter of 1.34 milli-seconds is not "normal"? How do we know that a pitch range of 7.3 semitones is not "normal"?

To establish such norms, we propose obtaining a body of data from individuals judged to have "normal" voices with "normal" being defined as 1. no past or present history nor reason to suspect pathology and 2. judged as appropriate for the age and sex of the individual. Once these criteria have been established and met, the frequency ranges should be obtained from each individual. After the ranges have been established, which can be diagnostic by themselves, the twenty-fifth, fiftieth, seventy-fifth percentiles of the modal frequency range can be determined. At each of these percentile points, the softest, loudest and median-loud phonation that can be sustained may be determined. Then, at these nine points (three frequencies × three sound pressure levels), measures of jitter, shimmer, volume-velocity flow, and maximum duration of phonation should be made. The purpose of this procedure is to reduce individual differences among speakers by comparing data from the same points in individual ranges rather than by comparing individual performances on the same absolute frequencies and sound-pressure levels. For example, one male speaker may have a modal frequency range of 50 to 150 Hz while another male speaker may have a modal frequency range of 125 to 300 Hz. If we were to compare jitter measurements from these two speakers, we would have common data only between the frequencies of 125 and 150 Hz. A comparison, however, of these two speakers' phonating frequencies common to both will be meaningless due to the fact that one individual was phonating in the upper portion of his frequency range and the other was phonating in the lower portion of his frequency range. And, as we have data indicating that the degree of jitter is dependent upon both frequency and sound-pressure level (Jacob, 1968), any differences we may find may be the result of range rather than of individual differences.

We would expect that once a sufficient body of data has been gathered for each parameter from the "normal" population, measures from non-normal voices would fall at or beyond the extremes of the normal curve. The problem then is to specify how much is too much and how little is too little. For example, we would expect all voices to show some jitter. But while too much jitter may well indicate a laryngeal pathology, too little jitter may cause the voice to sound unnatural (Cooper et al., 1957). We also expect all voices to have a certain amount of unmodulated air flow during phonation, but not enough to cause one to suspect pathology. When the normative data are gathered and tabulated for the pertinent vocal parameters, we would estimate that any measure below the tenth percentile or above the ninetieth percentile would be sufficient to cause one to suspect non-normal function.

CLINICAL IMPLICATIONS

Because this volume has a title which implies there should be some clinical implications as well as theoretical considerations presented, we will attempt to relate our beliefs on how voices should be described for voice therapy. Our basic and most important goal is to see a voice described in terms of a "profile" of measurable parameters. When a medically diagnosed "non-normal" voice is suggested for nonsurgical treatment, the clinician has little to go on until he examines the patient. The medical diagnosis will usually have a complete physical description of the larynx together with some adjectives like "hoarse" or "rough" or "raspy" to describe what the voice sounds like . . . *to the examiner*. The clinician will not really know what to expect until he actually sees the case. Let us suppose, however, that the clinician has received a report which includes measures of frequency ranges, respiratory function, jitter, volume-velocity air flow during sustained phonation, maximum duration of phonation, etc., in the form of a voice profile. The clinician can then compare these values to the norms for each one of the parameters and thus have a relatively good idea as to how to proceed with therapy even before seeing the patient.

If a clinician receives a patient who has not had a voice profile taken, it is not suggested that every parameter will need to be measured for every voice case. The clinician will certainly be able to tell by listening whether or not the pitch level is adequate. In all probability he will also be able to determine whether or not volume-velocity air flow needs to be measured. In any case, it will be up to the discretion of the clinician what parameters should be measured. It should also be noted that periodic measurement of these parameters during the course of therapy may well provide a useful index as to the success of the treatment. Without such objective measures clinicians and patients alike may tend to "perceive" improvement, not because improvement actually has occurred, but rather because they have become accustomed to the voice.

A question that must arise from this discussion is the feasibility of having access to equipment to measure these vocal parameters. In all likelihood, the specialized instrumentation will not be readily available to most clinicians. However, knowing the inventiveness and resourcefulness of most clinicians, we feel that if they have a basic fund of data concerning vocal function, they will devise amazingly simple methods to obtain quite precise information.

BIBLIOGRAPHY

Anderson, V. 1942. Training the speaking voice. New York: Oxford.

Arnold, G. 1959. Vocal rehabilitation of paralytic dysphonia, V. Vocal symptomatology after bilateral loss of abduction. *Arch. Otolaryng.*, 70, 444–453.

Bouhuys, A., Mead, J., Proctor, D., and Stevens, K. 1968. Pressure-flow events during singing, *Sound production in man, Ann. N.Y. acad. sci.*, 155, 165–176.

Bowler, N. 1964. A fundamental frequency analysis of harsh vocal quality, *Speech Monogr.*, 31, 128, 134.

Brahm, K., 1952. Uber den Stimmumfang und die Sprechtonlage bei Kranken mit doppelseitinger Posticuslahmung. *HNO*, 3, 131.

Brandt, J., Ruder, K., and Ship, T. 1968. Listener judgments of vocal loudness and effort. Univ. Fla.: Unpublished manuscript.

Brodnitz, F. 1966. Semantics of voice. Paper presented at 1966 ASHA convention, Chicago, Ill.

———. 1967. Semantics of voice. *J. Speech Hearing Disorders*, 32, 325–330.

Carhart, R. 1938. Infra-glottal resonance and a cushion pipe. *Speech Monogr.*, 5, 65–90.

———. 1941. The spectra of model larynx tones. *Speech Monogr.*, 8, 76–84.

Cole, B. 1968. Judged roughness as a function of formant bandwidth and vowel formant position. Univ. Houston: Master's thesis.

Coleman, R. 1960. Some acoustic correlates of hoarseness. Vanderbilt Univ.: Master's thesis.

———. 1963. Decay characteristics of vocal fry. *Folia Phoniat.*, 15, 256–263.

———, and Wendahl, R. 1968. On the validity of laryngeal photosensor monitoring. *J. acoust. soc. Amer.*, 44, 1733–1735.

Cooper, F., Peterson, E., and Fahringer, G. 1957. Some courses of characteristic vocoder quality. *J. acoust. soc. Amer.*, 29, 183A.

Cowan, J. 1936. Pitch and intensity characteristics of stage speech. *Arch. Speech*, 1, *Suppl.*, 7–85.

Culver, C. 1956. Musical acoustics. New York: McGraw-Hill.

Curry, E. 1940. An objective study of the pitch characteristics of the adolescent male voice. *Speech Monogr.*, 7, 48–62.
Curtis, J. 1956. Disorders of voice. *In* Speech handicapped school children. Johnson, W., ed., New York: Harper.
———. 1968. Acoustics of speech production and nasalization. *In* Cleft palate and communication. Spriestersbach, D., and Sherman, D., eds. New York: Academic Press, Ch. 2.
Draper, M., Ladefoged, P., and Whitterridge, D. 1959. Respiratory muscles in speech. *J. Speech Hearing Res.*, 2, 16–27.
Duffy, R. 1958. The vocal pitch characteristics of eleven, thirteen and fifteen-year-old female speakers. Univ. Iowa: Ph.D. dissertation.
Fairbanks, G. 1942. An acoustical study of the pitch of infant hunger wails. *Child Develop.*, 13, 227, 232.
———, Herbert, E., and Hammond, J. 1949. An acoustical study of vocal pitch in seven- and eight-year-old girls. *Child Develop.*, 20, 71–78.
———, Wiley, J., and Lassman, F. 1949. An acoustical study of vocal pitch in seven- and eight-year-old boys. *Child Develop.*, 20, 63–69.
———. 1960. Voice and articulation drillbook (2nd. ed.). New York: Harper.
Fant, G. 1960. Acoustic theory of speech production. The Hague: Monton.
———, and Sonneson, B. 1962. Indirect study of glottal cycles by synchronous inverse filtering and photoelectric glottography, *Quart. Progress and Status Report*, Speech Transmission Lab, R.I.T., 1-3, Sweden.
Farnsworth, D. 1940. High speed motion pictures of the human vocal cords. *Bell Lab. Record.*, 18, 203–208.
Fisher, H. 1966. Improving voice and articulation. Dallas: Houghton Mifflin.
Flanagan, J. 1964. *Proceedings of the fifth international congress of phonetic sciences*, Munster, Germany.
———, and Landgraf, L. 1967. Self-oscillating source for vocal tract synthesizers. Conference on Speech Communication and Processing, M.I.T.
Garcia, M. 1841. École de Garcia, Traits complete de l'arts du chart. Paris: E. Troupenas.
Hahn, E., Lomas, C., Hargis, D., and Vandraegen, D. 1957. Basic voice training for speech. New York: McGraw-Hill.
Hirano, M., Koike, Y., and von Leden, H. 1968. Maximum phonation time and air usage during phonation. *Folia Phoniat.* 20, 185–201.
Hollien, H., and Malcik, E. 1962. Adolescent voice change in southern negro males. *Speech Monogr.*, 29, 53–58.
———, ———, and Hollien, B. 1965. Adolescent voice change in southern white males. *Speech Monogr.*, 32, 87–90.
———, and ———. 1967. Evaluation of cross-sectional studies of adolescent voice change in males. *Speech Monog.*, 34, 80–84.
———, and Michel, J. 1968. Vocal fry as a phonational register. *J. Speech Hearing Res.*, 11, 600–604.
Isshiki, N. 1964. Regulatory mechanism of voice intensity variation. *J. Speech Hearing Res.*, 7, 17–29.
———, and Ringel, R. 1964. Air flow during the production of selected consonants. *J. Speech Hearing Res.*, 7, 233–244.
Jacob, L. 1968. A normative study of laryngeal jitter. Univ. Kan.: Master's thesis.
Johnson, K. 1969. The effect of selected vowels on laryngeal jitter. Univ. Kan.: Master's thesis.
Judson, L., and Weaver, A. 1942. Voice science. New York: Appleton-Century-Crofts.
Kersta, L. 1962. Voiceprint identification. *Nature*, 196, 1253–1258.
Kunze, L. 1962. An investigation of the changes in sub-glottal air pressure and rate of air flow accompanying changes in fundamental frequency, intensity, vowels, and voice registers in adult male speakers. State University of Iowa. Doctoral dissertation.
Kvols, M. 1969. Perceptual judgments of roughness influenced by second formant frequency. Univ. Houston: Master's thesis.
Ladefoged, P., and McKinney, N. 1963. Loudness, sound pressure, and subglottal pressure in speech. *J. acoust. soc. Amer.*, 35, 454–460.
Lane, H., Catania, A., and Stevens, S. 1961. Voice level: autophonic scale, perceived loudness, and effects of sidetone. *J. acoust. soc. Amer.*, 33, 160–167.
Lass, N., and Michel, J. 1969. The effects of frequency, intensity and vowel-type on the maximum duration of phonation. Univ. Kan.: Unpublished manuscript.
Lehiste, I., and Peterson, G. 1959. Vowel amplitude and phonemic stress in American English. *J. acoust. soc. Amer.*, 31, 428–435.
Liebermann, P. 1961. Perturbations in vocal pitch. *J. acoust. soc. Amer.*, 33, 597–603.
———. 1963. Some acoustical measures of the fundamental periodicity of normal and pathologic larynges. *J. acoust. soc. Amer.*, 35, 344–353.
Linklater, D. 1968. An investigation of vowel formant position and judgments of roughness. Univ. Houston: Master's thesis.
Luchsinger, R. 1937. Zur Behandlung der Kehlkopfstenose bei doppelseitiger Mediansteilung der Stimmlippen. *Schweiz. med. Wchnscnr.*, 67, 1065.
———, and Arnold, G. 1965. Voice-speech-language. Belmont, Calif.: Wadsworth.
Mathes, R., and Miller, R. 1947. Phase effects in monaural perception. *J. acoust. soc. Amer.*, 19, 780–797.
McGlone, R. 1966a. An investigation of air flow and subglottal air pressure related to fundamental frequency of phonation. *Folia Phoniat.*, 18, 313–322.
———. 1966b. Vocal pitch characteristics of children aged one and two years. *Speech Monogr.*, 33, 178–181.
———. 1967. Air flow during vocal fry phonation. *J. Speech Hearing Res.*, 10, 299–304.
———, and Hollien, H. 1963. Vocal pitch characteristics of aged women. *J. Speech Hearing Res.*, 6, 164–170.
Michel, J. 1966. Clinical implications of research in

voice. Paper presented at 1966 ASHA convention in Chicago, Ill.

———, Kirchner, F., Shelton, R., and Hollinger, L. 1968, Acoustic results of teflon procedures. Univ. Kan.: Unpublished manuscript.

Moore, G., and Thompson, C. 1965. Comments on physiology of hoarseness. *Arch. Otolaryng.*, 81, 97–102.

Murry, E., and Tiffin, J. 1934. An analysis of the basic aspects of effective speech. *Arch. Speech*, 1, 61–83.

Mysak, E. 1959. Pitch and duration characteristics of older males. *J. Speech Hearing Res.*, 2, 46–54.

Ohala, J. 1967. Studies of variations in glottal aperature using photoelectric glottography. *J. acoust. soc. Amer.*, 41, 1613A.

Peterson, G., and Barney, H. 1952. Control methods used in a study of the vowels. *J. acoust. soc. Amer.*, 24, 175-184.

Pronovost, W. 1942. Experimental study of the habitual and natural pitch levels of superior male speakers. *Speech Monogr.*, 9, 111–123.

Ptacek, P., and Sander, E. 1963a. Maximum duration of phonation. *J. Speech Hearing Disorders*, 28, 171–182.

———, and ———. 1963b. Breathiness and phonation length. *J. Speech Hearing Disorders*, 28, 267–272.

———, ———, Maloney, W., and Jackson, C. 1966. Phonatory and related changes with advanced age. *J. Speech Hearing Res.*, 9, 353–360.

Rieben, G. 1942. Der Spatverlauf der doppelseiten Stimmbandlamung nach Strumektomie. *Chirurq*, 14, 709.

Sarbin, T. 1968. Ontology recaptulates philology: the mythic nature of anxiety. *Amer. Psychologist*, 23, 411–418.

Scheibe, K., and Sarbin, T. 1965. Towards a theoretical conceptualization of superstition. *Brit. J. Phil. Sci.*, 62, 143–158.

Sherman, D., and Linke, E. 1952. The influence of certain vowel types on the degree of harsh voice quality. *J. Speech Hearing Disorders*, 17, 401–408.

Smith, W., and Liebermann, P. 1964. Studies in pathological speech production. Prepared for Data Sciences Laboratory, Hanscom Field, Mass.

Snidecor, J. 1951. The pitch and duration characteristics of superior female speakers during oral reading. *J. Speech Hearing Disorders*, 16, 44–52.

Sonneson, B. 1967. Photo-glottographical studies of the vibrating larynx. Paper presented at Communication Sciences Short Course on Vocal Function, Univ. Fla., Gainesville, Fla.

Stevens, K. 1967. Discussion of Wendahl and Page, 1967. Presentation at convention of Acoustical Society of America, Miami Beach, Fla.

———, and House, A. 1955. Development of a quantitative description of vowel articulation. *J. acoust. soc. Amer.*, 27, 484–493.

Tiffany, W., and Hollien, H. 1968. Speaking fundamental frequency as a function of type of speech production. Univ. Fla.: Unpublished manuscript.

Travis, L., Bender, W., and Buchanan, A. 1934. Research contribution to vowel theory. *Speech Monogr.*, 1, 65–71.

van den Berg, Jw. 1956. Direct and indirect determination of the mean subglottic pressure. *Folia Phoniat.*, 8, 1–24.

———, and Vennard, W. 1959. Toward an objective vocabulary for voice pedagogy. *Bulletin*, 15, 10–15.

Van Riper, C. 1954. Speech correction; principles and methods. (3rd. ed.). Englewood Cliffs, N.J.: Prentice-Hall.

Vennard, W. 1967. Singing: the mechanism and the technic. Ann Arbor, Mich.: Edwards.

von Leden, H., Yanagihara, N., and Werner-Kukuk, E. 1967. Teflon in unilateral vocal cord paralysis. *Arch. Otolaryng.*, 85, 110–118.

Wendahl, R. 1961. A photophonellegraphic analysis of hoarse voice quality. *Proceedings of the 4th. International Congress of Phonetic Sciences*, Helsinki, 307–310.

———. 1962. The synthesis of harsh voice quality. Paper presented at convention of American Speech and Hearing Association, New York.

———. 1966. Laryngeal analog synthesis of jitter and shimmer, auditory parameters of harshness. *Folia Phoniat.*, 18, 98–108.

———, and Page, L. 1967. Glottal wave periods in VCV environments. *J. acoust. soc. Amer.*, 42, 1208A.

Wolf, S., Stanley, D., and Sette, W. 1935. Quantitative studies on the singing voice. *J. acoust. soc. Amer.*, 6, 255–266.

Yanagihara, N., and Koike, Y. 1967. The regulation of sustained phonation. *Folia Phoniat.*, 19, 1–180.

19

Vocal Function: A Behavioral Analysis

William H. Perkins

INTRODUCTION

Ten years ago this chapter was addressed mainly to the practising clinician concerned with therapy of disordered vocal functioning. He and his problems are still of vital interest. During the intervening years, not only applied but basic studies of voice and its functions have become abundant. Laboratories across this nation, throughout Europe, and in Japan have become heavily committed to unraveling the mysteries of one of the most complex of human mechanisms, the vocal apparatus. This problem has engaged the serious interest of laryngologists and acousticians, linguists and voice teachers, electrical engineers and psychologists, and, of course, phoneticians and speech pathologists. The clinician's applied interests are no longer isolated in the limbo of empiricism. A solid body of information about vocal production is growing. Fortunately, normal functioning is receiving its share of attention, thereby providing a frame of reference from which to assess disordered functioning. The province of this chapter now is to lay a foundation for the scientific study of normal vocal functioning. Practical application of this knowledge to the assessment and therapy of disordered functioning will be the province of other chapters of this book.

Terminology

A pervasive problem in the study of human sound production is confusion about terminology. To avoid compounding this confusion, some definitions are necessary at the outset. Discussion of the topic for this chapter cannot even begin without using such words as: "voice," "vocal production," "speech," and "sound production." These terms, however, do not have the same meanings for all readers. So that it is clear what they mean to this writer, they are defined as follows:

vocal, as used in such phrases as "vocal production," "vocal function," and "vocal apparatus" will refer to the process of phonation, the action of the larynx in the generation of sound.

voice will mean the component of any sound that can be attributed to phonation; it would be applicable to a laugh, a vowel, or a voiced consonant, but not, for instance, to a voiceless fricative.

speech will mean any sound produced that is used within a formal linguistic code; a cough, as an example, would not be considered as speech.

sound, whether used alone or in such a phrase as "sound production" will refer to any sound produced by any process and for any purpose. It is the most inclusive term of this group.

Analysis: The Need and the Price

The test of scientific understanding of vocal functioning is ability to predict and control vocal behavior. This requires exact knowledge. Exact knowledge requires measurement. Measurement requires dimensions that permit quantification. Dimensions require that a complex phenomenon, such as vocal behavior, be analyzed into its component parts, each of which can be measured along a single scale.

Science proceeds by the dissecting operation of analysis. For scientific understanding of vocal functioning, we must first pull the vocal performance apart, measure it piece by piece, specify how the pieces function relative to each other, and then, with much good fortune, we may understand it well enough to reassemble it and control vocal behavior. Indications of our proximity to this goal are apparent in electrical speech synthesizers capable of producing remarkable approximations of human sound.

Although analysis of vocal functioning is essential, it does exact a price. We can easily lose sight of the whole person whose vocal parts we are analyzing. Moreover, an analysis can make what appears to be a simple process seem inordinately complex. If, for example, you were to analyze the structure of something as simple as a kitchen fork, the description could possibly be confined to one page of mathematical symbols that specified the sizes, shapes, angles, and the like of all aspects of the fork—the same description in words would probably take pages. If you were in the business of guiding the production of forks, you would need such a description. Speech pathologists are in the business of guiding the production of voice. They, too, need such descriptions for vocal functions.

Although analysis of voice into its component dimensions appears, at first glance, to make understanding hopelessly complicated, in point of fact, it leads to simplification in two forms. The most obvious form is that dimensions of vocal production are made tangible, hence, measurable, that previously were vague and ill defined. Granted, this form of simplification does not integrate the parts into a simplified whole; it does, however, make explicit what parts need to be integrated.

Integration is the other form of simplification. The conception of vocal functioning that is yielded by detailed analysis is not only more exact, but also simpler, than might be expected: specification of five dimensions of vocal production are necessary and possibly sufficient to account for all of the ways that voice is produced abnormally as well as normally. Furthermore, a rational basis can be established for clinical procedures that, using a few simple operations, permits holistic integration of these dimensions. Before these clinical fruits can be harvested a good deal of analytic cultivating will be needed.

Levels of Analyses of Vocal Functioning

Voice has been analyzed, typically, as an acoustic or physiological phenomenon, but it is just as much a psychological event. Along with determination of the message and of the nuances of vocal expression, the regulation of vocal production is a psychological characteristic. Fig. 19-1 reminds us that the messages we communicate vocally are conceived psychologically, produced physiologically, transmitted acoustically (physically), received physiologically, and interpreted psychologically.

Each level of analysis yields data unique to itself, and each class of data is peculiarly useful for different applications. The acoustic level is characterized by physical data: the various properties of sound waves.

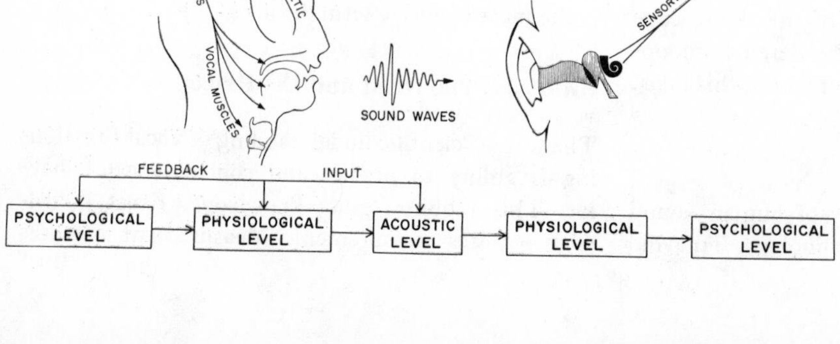

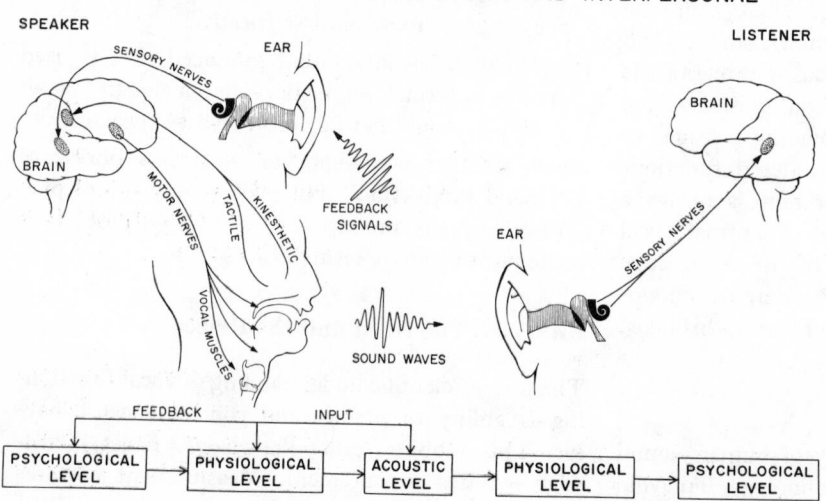

Fig. 19-1. Psychological, physiological, and acoustical levels involved in vocal production for interpersonal and intrapersonal communication. *Adapted from Denes, P., and Pinson, E., THE SPEECH CHAIN, Bell Telephone Laboratories, 1963, Fig. 1.1, p. 4.*

Communication engineers, for example, have special concern for this type of information; it is their primary data. The physiological level yields data of particular value for the physician, who holds exclusive professional responsibility for the somatic integrity of the vocal apparatus. Data of the psychological level, to the extent that they can be objectified, are behavioral—and they are the primary data available to the speech pathologist in his professional responsibility for rehabilitating the vocally handicapped.

Ideally, the voice clinician will understand acoustics of speech. More important, he will understand laryngeal physiology well enough to have a rational basis for his therapy. But these are not the primary phenomena with which he works. He assesses vocal functioning, how the voice is produced; he does not diagnose laryngeal disability (unless asked his private opinion by a physician). He modifies vocal behavior by utilizing the learning process, his only therapeutic tool; he does not modify the organic condition by any form of direct intervention. The speech pathologist's primary data are unequivocally psychological. They encompass perceptual input characteristics of audition, motor output characteristics of vocal production, and the intervening ideational processes in the "black box" of the mind. They also include the various psychological functions of the voice in both interpersonal and intrapersonal communication: the linguistic denotations and the nonlinguistic nuances that link person to person and the sensory feedback information that guides the subjective regulation of vocal production.

Small wonder, then, that a hybrid mixture of concepts and terminology has issued from this melange of physiological, acoustical, and psychological levels of analysis, to say nothing of the multiple communicative functions of vocal production. Obviously, some of the difficulty in understanding vocal functioning stems from mongrel notions, especially with the notoriously difficult term *vocal quality*, whose denotative referents are indistinct and whose conceptual ancestry is undistinguished.

Measurement of Pitch, Loudness, and Quality

Consider, for a moment, how such psychological terms as *pitch* and *loudness* demarcate the perceptual experience from the acoustic, and possibly physiological, stimuli to which they are responses. A simple experiment, first performed years ago, points up the psychophysical problem of pitch as the musician hears it and frequency as the physicist measures it. If a person is asked to sing the pitch heard when a tuning fork is struck, the pitch sung will be relatively accurate if the tuning fork is held a few feet away. If, however, the tuning fork is held a few inches from the ear, the sound will be louder, of course, but the pitch sung to match it will tend to be lower—the sensation of loudness affects the sensation of pitch. Accordingly, psychophysicists have worked out a subjective pitch scale, the *mel* (for melody) scale, in which the pitches of the tones sound as if they are equally spaced. Equal steps on the mel scale do not correspond to equal steps on a physicist's frequency scale, or, for that matter, on a musical scale by which a piano is tuned. Interestingly, they do correspond to equally separated points of stimulation along the basilar membrane in the inner ear. To anchor the psychological scale of pitch perception to the physical scale of frequency, a sound with a frequency of 1,000 Hz and an intensity of 40 dB has, by definition, a pitch of 1,000 mels.

Similarly, loudness is a subjective sensation that, for years, defied accurate measurement. Controversy raged over Fechner's law that clearly did not account for why a sound of 100 dB was heard approximately 30 times as loud as one of 50 dB. It was not until a subjective scale of loudness, the *sone* (from the Latin for "sound") scale, was developed that a straightforward relationship appeared: an increase of 10 dB in intensity of a stimulus sound doubles the sensation of loudness. The two scales have been related to each other by defining a sone as the loudness of a 1,000 Hz tone at an intensity of 40 dB.

Vocal quality has not fared so well. Its problems are unique. On the one hand is the psychophysical problem of relating its subjective perception to its acoustic stimuli. Although this is probably not an insoluble problem, it is a massive one. For one thing, vocal quality has so many perceptual dimensions. Unlike pitch, for which one sound can be judged simply as higher or lower than another, or loudness, for which the judgment is louder or softer, quality cannot be captured within a unidimensional framework. As we will see in the next section, it serves multiple perceptual functions: it has linguistic and nonlinguistic dimensions for interpersonal communication, and it has various perceptual dimensions for intrapersonal feedback of sensory information used for guiding its production. Each of these perceptual dimensions would have to be laid out and quantified as a subjective scale—as has been done for pitch and loudness—if the different aspects of vocal quality were to be clearly related as responses to physical (or physiological) stimuli. Work has been under way for years on phonetic psychophysical problems, but the surfaces of the other dimensions have hardly been scratched (Fairbanks, 1966). This will be a job primarily for experimental phoneticists, psychophysicists, voice scientists, linguists, and, perhaps, audiologists.

The speech pathologist is more likely to have a primary interest in solving the other side of the quality problem—vocal production. The matter of how a speaker regulates his voice to affect all of the different perceptual dimensions is a matter of how voice is produced. The question is, what *behavior* does he regulate? For instance, what does he do vocally to help make linguistic differences between, say, /s/ and /z/, or between /i/ and /ɪ/? What does he do vocally to help differentiate between "yes" spoken in frustrated rage and "yes" spoken in acquiescent pleasure? What does he do differently when his voice sounds harsh and when it sounds pleasant? To the extent that pitch is involved, we can indicate the way he regulates how high or low the tone is, a unidimensional indication. To the extent that loudness is involved, we can indicate the way he regulates how loud or soft the tone is, a unidimensional indication.

To the extent that quality is involved, what do we indicate that he regulates? Throatiness? Pleasantness? Harshness? Hoarseness? Shrillness? Mellowness? The list can be extended beyond three dozen terms used by various authors to describe vocal quality. They all clarify part of the problem, but none provides a clean unidimensional scale along which quality can be quantified and regulated. Moreover, none specifies behavior that can be volitionally managed: what does one *do* to produce a throaty tone, a pleasant tone, a harsh tone, and so on? Terminology for quality has proliferated over the years until we now are mired in a terminological swamp, with terms whose lineage is physiological, anatomical, acoustical, and psychological, all milling around together as referents for what is exclusively a psychological phenomenon: vocal quality.

A major objective of this chapter is to make lucid this problem. This will require that we keep the classes of data straight. The important distinction will be between terms descriptive of psychological dimensions and terms descriptive of correlated physiological processes. The distinctions are tricky, but it is crucial that they be observed.

Functional vs. Organic

A preliminary word is also necessary about the logically incongruous dichotomy of "functional vs. organic." Dorland (1951) defines *functional*, "of, or pertaining to a function," and organic, "pertaining to an organ or the organs." They have come to mean in our literature, however, a dichotomous etiology. Functional disorders are considered a result of how one has learned to use the anatomical structures of speech; organic disorders a result of anatomical or physiological defects. The incongruity of dichotomizing functional and organic disorders becomes apparent if the preceding statement of functional etiology is compared with the organic statement. The latter is presumably concerned with the status of the structures, and the former with how they function. The condition of the structure may limit or alter its function, but the condition certainly does not preclude its function. It is a complementary, not an exclusive, relationship. Vocal production is the behavioral manifestation of the learned patterns of physiological functioning of phonatory and respiratory organs. If the organs are defective, the patterns of voice that are learned may also be defective, but to say that functional disorders are caused by learning while, by implication, organic disorders are not is patently meaningless. This dichotomy with vocal disorders is especially nonsensical. Habitual vocal patterns that are abusive of the voice may produce organic changes, e.g., vocal nodules, that alter the manner of functioning of the vocal mechanism, with possible consequent changes in the manner in which one learns to use the voice.

Vocal Function Emphasis

All human sound production involves resonance as well as phonation. Resonance, however, will not be a major consideration in this analysis. Its effects will be treated in other chapters dealing with such matters as articulation and cleft palate. Its effects will be our concern here, only insofar as they influence vocal behavior. Primary emphasis throughout will be on psychological aspects of vocal functioning, with secondary consideration of physiological and acoustical correlates of psychological dimensions. To establish an analytic framework that permits quantification of the many dimensions of voice, and thereby renders the voice manageable for the clinician and the researcher, receptive and productive functions are delineated. Methods of assessment of the adequacy of vocal functioning and therapeutic tactics, as well as research strategy, derive explicity from this analysis.

PSYCHOLOGICAL DIMENSIONS OF VOICE

A psychological analysis of vocal functioning is plagued with the same problems that haunt psychology as a science. As Stevens (1951) pointed out some years ago, the stature of a science is roughly proportional to its use of mathematics. The more measurable the phenomenon, the more readily can measurement replace description, and calculation replace debate. Little wonder, then, that the science of psychology has had a predilection for psychophysical experiments; the relationship of the perceptual response to the measurable physical stimulus can be quantified. Ostensibly, the methods of psychophysics are applicable mainly to problems of sensation and perception: in other words, to receptive events. Motor responses are, presumably, farther removed from being under the control of environmental stimuli, because how one acts is thought to be dependent on how one perceives his world at the moment, and perception is considered to be a function of the the stimulus condition. Taken literally, this would mean that tactics are more readily available for scientific study of perception than production of speech and voice. And this, of course, is precisely what we have observed as the major thrust of experimental phonetics, in which the acoustic study of perceived sounds of speech has been dominant for years.

The problem is not this simple or straightforward, however; the issue of treating sensation and perception as a psychophysical problem is not altogether on the side of the angels. Speaking strictly, psychophysics is concerned with the relationship between stimulus and response. No prescription holds that the response must be perceptual; it can be behavioral as well. Historically, the response of interest has been perceptual: in audiology, stimulus values that determine thresholds for hearing; in phonetics, stimulus characteristics that distinguish one speech sound from another. The trouble with perceptual responses, in fact with all cognitive responses, arises with the attempt to make them explicit. That the response in question cannot be observed directly, but can only be inferred from behavioral signs, such as raising a finger to signal perception of a tone, places the validity of such internal responses (if, indeed, they are responses) in jeopardy. The problem is basically that of mentalistic psychology, of knowing what goes on in the mind. The most productive solution has come with the advent of the Theory of Signal Detection[1] that questions the concept that a sensory threshold can be established independent of an observable response threshold. Ironically, the salvation for scientific study of receptive processes appears to lie in the production of behavioral events. In fact, Goldiamond (1962) has demonstrated that when perception is considered as a problem in signal detection, perceptual responses can be controlled as operant behavior. So, we have come full circle. The perceptual response can be measured only to the extent that a behavioral response signals detection of a stimulus.

Receptive Dimensions

The receptive functions of voice, as was seen in Fig. 19-1, are twofold: those involved in interpersonal communication, and those utilized in the intrapersonal communication of feedback information for the guidance of vocal production. An extensive analysis of interpersonal communication goes far beyond the province of this chapter, so receptive communicative functions will be considered only to the extent that their clarification can shed light on terminological confusion and provide a basis for quantification of vocal dimensions. More specifically, a purpose of this analysis will be to show how the multiple functions of the vocal property *quality* have contributed to some of the difficulties encountered in dealing with this property. The intrapersonal feedback functions are indigenous to our mission and will be analyzed as an integral part of the discussion of production of voice and its regulation.

Functions of Voice in Interpersonal Communication

The vocal properties, *pitch*, *loudness*, and *quality* function, at least in Western cultures, as shown in

[1] The Theory of Signal Detection requires differentiation among four types of responses: 1) *signal detection* when the stimulus is identified correctly, 2) *signal miss* when the stimulus is present but unidentified, 3) *null detection* when the condition of no stimulus being present is identified correctly, and 4) *false alarm* when an incorrect identification is made of a condition in which no stimulus is present. These responses to perceptual displays can be conditioned by attaching consequences to them.

VOCAL FUNCTIONS IN INTERPERSONAL COMMUNICATION

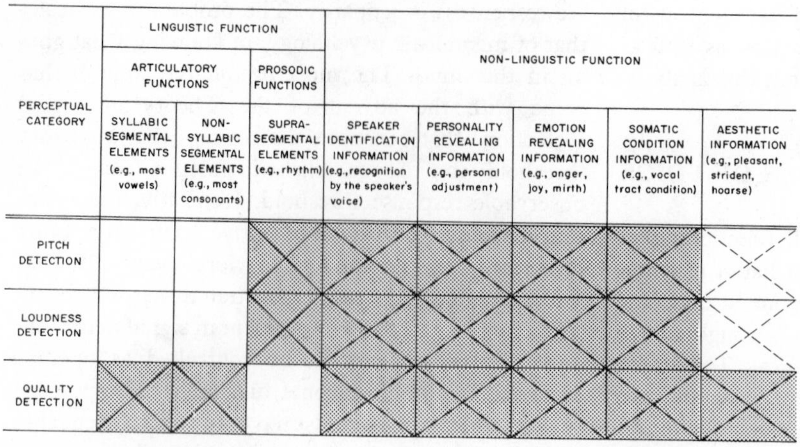

LINGUISTIC FUNCTION
ARTICULATORY FUNCTIONS
PROSODIC FUNCTIONS
NON-LINGUISTIC FUNCTION
PERCEPTUAL CATEGORY
SYLLABIC SEGMENTAL ELEMENTS (e.g., most vowels)
NON-SYLLABIC SEGMENTAL ELEMENTS (e.g., most consonants)
SUPRA-SEGMENTAL ELEMENTS (e.g., rhythm)
SPEAKER IDENTIFICATION INFORMATION (e.g., recognition by the speaker's voice)
PERSONALITY REVEALING INFORMATION (e.g., personal adjustment)
EMOTION REVEALING INFORMATION (e.g., anger, joy, mirth)
SOMATIC CONDITION INFORMATION (e.g., vocal tract condition)
AESTHETIC INFORMATION (e.g., pleasant, strident, hoarse)
PITCH DETECTION
LOUDNESS DETECTION
QUALITY DETECTION

Fig. 19-2. Linguistic and non-linguistic perceptual functions of voice in interpersonal communication that are typical in Western cultures.

Fig. 19-2, in interpersonal communication linguistically and nonlinguistically. Speech pathologists are most familiar with the articulatory linguistic functions that are invariably studied in courses in phonetics. These are the segmental sounds of speech, the phonemes. The suprasegmental or prosodic elements are less often dealt with explicity, but are no less important. These elements also provide empirical raw material for certain of the phonologic aspects of linguistic structures (Peterson and Shoup, 1966). Nonlinguistic functions are omnipresent, but have received scant attention. These involve the myriad ways we communicate connotatively (by tone of voice, by shaded inflection) meanings not necessarily denoted by verbal utterance.

ARTICULATORY LINGUISTIC FUNCTIONS

Of the vocal properties, quality functions predominantly in the differentiation of one segmental phonetic element from another; speech sounds are relatively independent of pitch and loudness for their identity. Of course, all of the changes in quality that distinguish one phone from another are not consequent to laryngeal action alone. The extent, however, that phonation contributes to articulation is by virtue of changes in quality.

For some reason *quality* has been used mainly in reference to nonlinguistic functions for which such words as *harsh*, *hoarse*, *strident*, *resonant*, *pear-shaped*, and the like are variedly descriptive. Why these poorly defined functions are typically thought of as being the primary meanings of *quality* is puzzling.

Curiously, the different sounds of speech rarely come to mind when we think of this term, yet it is precisely with these sounds that a formal system (phonemic symbols for phonemes, phonetic symbols for allophones) for specifying psychological characteristics of quality has been devised. Each phonemic symbol, for example, is at least intended to be descriptive of those qualities considered essential for perceiving a specific phoneme. Moreover, the symbol specifies with minimal ambiguity the perceptual phenomenon for which acoustic and physiologic correlates can be established. For example, /i/ denotes a class of vowel sounds with qualities that should readily distinguish the word *feet* from its nearest phonemic neighbor *fit*. The phonemic symbol, then, denotes a psychological dimension of quality.

PROSODIC LINGUISTIC FUNCTIONS

Speech prosody, the intonation, the stress, the rhythm of language is a function of vocal pitch and loudness as well as of phonetic duration (O'Malley and Peterson, 1966). Although vocal quality is not usually considered a factor in prosody, it probably is affected by stress and intonation. This is to say that prosody is not a function of vocal quality, but quality may well be a function of prosody; the difference lies in which is the independent and which the dependent variable. This comment is based on the observation that vocal stridency is more likely to be associated with strong stress and intonation patterns (prosodic factors) than with relaxed patterns.

NONLINGUISTIC FUNCTIONS

At least five nonlinguistic functions of voice can be delineated: voice can reveal speaker identity, it can reveal personality, it can reveal emotion, it can reveal at least some aspects of the somatic condition, and it can serve an aesthetic function. Recognition of and scientific interest in these problems are in their infancy. The work that has been done, plus causal observation, suggests strongly that all properties of voice contribute to these nonlinguistic functions with quality as a primary contributor. For that matter, the term *quality* is used generally in reference to these functions. In this sense, it has no explicitly specified referents or quantified dimensions.

That human speech can provide simultaneous information about this plethora of nonlinguistic functions, to say nothing of its linguistic load, seems remarkable. Still, that all of us participate regularly in this impressive performance is so commonplace as to hardly need mention. Consider this unremarkable possibility: the telephone rings, you answer it, and within a few seconds of conversation, you manage to recognize the speaker by his voice, understand the words he is speaking, reflect on the generally agressive nature of his personality, note the elation he feels as he talks of his latest administrative coup, observe that he is apparently suffering from a summer cold, and respond with some aversion to the unpleasant harshness of his voice.

That we have the capacity for even more impressive feats is demonstrated by Hockett (1961) in his review of Shannon and Weaver's (1964) classic work that appeared originally in 1948, *The Mathematical Theory of Communication.* He estimates that the linguistic message transmitted at normal conversational speeds utilized only 0.1 percent of the communicative channel space available for speech signals. Viewed in its worst light, if this estimate is valid, speech is 99.9 percent redundant (neglecting noise), which makes it the world's most incredibly inefficient communication system. Viewed positively, however, this astonishing linguistic redundancy means tremendous capacity for the message to resist distortion by acoustic or semantic "noise" (e.g., static in the case of acoustic noise, differences in word meaning for speaker and listener in the case of semantic noise). Observe the considerable difference in the spectrograms of Fig. 19-3 showing the same vowel produced with different vocal qualities, pitches, and loudnesses by the same speaker; yet, it is reliably perceived in American English as /i/. But, more important for this discussion, it means that the human speaking system has vast capability for transmitting nonlinguistic information simultaneously with speech signals.

Whereas phonemes are psychological invariants of linguistic codes, no such invariants for nonlinguistic and metalinguistic codes have been defined explicitly; that they exist implicitly seems apparent. The stability and consistency of response in the areas of most of these nonlinguistic functions suggests strongly that a consensually validated[2] signal system is in operation. A brief look at each of these functions and a bit of speculation about the vocal dimensions that contribute to them should suffice for our purpose.

The accuracy with which the sex and identity of a speaker can be revealed by the sound of his voice is the prime example of a well-perfected implicit code (Voiers, 1964). That the code is on its way to being made explicit is evident from the rapidly increasing interest in voice printing, the telecommunication analogue of fingerprinting. Kersta's (1962) technique utilizes spectographic information as revealed by sonograms. Dreher (1967), on the other hand, has devised ingenious systems for identifying voices. One of these systems involves computer analysis of the distribution of phonated intensities, frequencies, and phonetic durations, and of pauses. Interestingly, the characteristic of duration is the most resistant to distortion by noise. An even more intriguing system of his utilizes a quasi-fourier analysis in which speech power is plotted in a circle, whirled under stroboscopic light, and analyzed in terms of various relationships among standing patterns that can be detected visually with this technique.

Many speech pathologists have received the proposition that voice reveals personality with thunderous disregard. When Moses' pioneering work, *The Voice of Neurosis*, first appeared more than a decade ago, it was generally accorded an unenthusiastic welcome, probably for several reasons; one doubtless being that it was presented as a collection of clinical impressions that, without demonstrable evidence, could be taken as nothing more than one man's speculations. Yet, the notion that voice reflects personality has such vitality that it has prevailed and has been investigated (Starkweather, 1961; Ostwald, 1963; Markel, Meisels, and Houck, 1964). The most convincing evidence to date comes from research by Rousey and Moriarty (1965), who formulated 17 working assumptions about the relationship between personality and speech, three of which specified

[2] The term consensual validation was coined by Harry Stack Sullivan to identify the process by which a child validates the meanings for those symbols that are the consensus of his elders. The term is used here to indicate that a characteristic of a sound has enough identity that the average speaker can recognize it accurately and reliably.

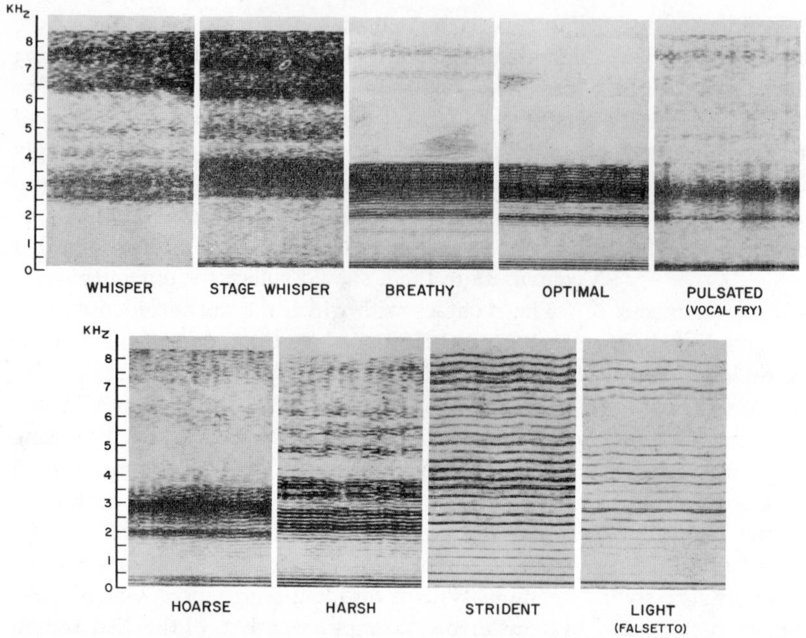

Fig. 19.3 Spectrograms of /i/ produced by the same speaker with different vocal qualities. The terms "pulsated" and "light" are elaborated in the section of this chapter called "Vocal Mode." The term "optimal" is used for reasons presented in the next chapter. Briefly, "optimal" denotes vocal production relatively free of constriction.

features of vocal quality and two of pitch. Based on these working assumptions, 233 "postdictions" (as distinct from *pre*dictions) were made about 24 normal children who had been observed since infancy at the Menninger Foundation for more than a decade. These postdictions were then compared with the psychiatric evaluations and were judged accurate in 83 percent of the instances.

Evidence of the relationship between voice and emotion is available on several fronts. The actor's ability to convey nuances of emotion attests to the existence of consensually validated codes of affect. That his ability involves control of visual and semantic as well as vocal stimuli cannot be argued. But, that the voice can differentiate effectively among the subtle shades of emotion will not be disputed by those who have heard thrilling radio dramas or have been moved by theatrical performances heard, but barely seen, from the last row of the balcony. Scientific attempts to specify these codes have waxed and waned over the years. Fairbanks (1938, 1939, 1941, 1966) conducted studies of prosodic characteristics of pitch and duration almost three decades ago. In one of these studies with Pronovost (1938) listeners demonstrated that they could detect with remarkable accuracy emotions such as anger, grief, and contempt simulated by actors. Recently, Huttar (1967) examined the prosodic features of pitch, loudness, and speed and their acoustic prosodic correlates, fundamental frequency, amplitude, and duration for their relationships with emotion as measured on semantic differential scales. Judgments of emotions often correlated higher with prosodic judgments than with prosodic acoustic parameters. Why research attention has been limited for the most part to prosodic dimensions is perplexing, especially when we usually think of the "tone" of a speaker's voice as the barometer of his emotions. Perhaps it is because prosodic dimensions are easier to quantify. In any event, most of us would probably agree from personal experience that much of the information about affect is communicated by vocal quality. Clearly, the codes of emotion remain virgin territory for adventurous investigators.

The manner in which the voice reveals somatic conditions is of greater clinical significance for the physician than for the speech pathologist. This pronouncement merely reiterates the earlier distinction between the physician's responsibility for the larynx and the speech pathologist's responsibility for the voice. Vocal quality, especially hoarseness, is the auditory clue to a wide range of laryngeal disabilities extending all the way from laryngitis to vocal nodules to benign tumors to cancerous growths. The degree of hoarseness appears to correlate with the extent to which vocal cord vibration "jitters," to which it is perturbed in its periodic vibratory pattern (Cooper, Peterson, and Fahringer, 1957; Lieberman, 1961; Wendahl, 1963; Coleman and Wendahl, 1967). Similarly, a breathy voice may indicate laryngeal paralysis or myasthenia laryngis, an abnormally high pitch may be consequent to a laryngeal web, or an abnormally low pitch to hormonal imbalance. These relationships, though, are far too unreliable to permit anything but the most conservative clinical judgments. For the speech pathologist, the dictum remains: before therapy, refer for laryngeal examination. For now, the point to note is that among the many functions of the voice, one is to reveal, grossly perhaps, some information about the somatic condition of the organism.

The fifth of these nonlinguistic functions to be delineated differs considerably from the others. Whereas the first four reveal an aspect of the speaker, the aesthetic function involves value judgments of the sounds that supply information for these other functions. In other words, the sounds by which we identify a speaker, understand his utterances, reflect on his personality, note his emotional state, and observe his somatic condition are sounds that may appeal to us aesthetically as pleasant, vibrant, strident, harsh, resonant, grating, and on and on throughout the list of terms by which we typically identify vocal quality. As should be apparent, this aesthetic function is the one we invoke almost exclusively when we seek a term descriptive of quality. It is this function, too, by which judgments are made about the desirability of various vocal attributes, that can include pitch and loudness (hence the broken lines for those categories in Fig. 19-2), but probably do not do so normally. Less obvious is the possibility that these judgments also vary with occupational and educational status, at least within our culture. Miller (1957) studied listener evaluation of "good quality" in 133 subjects divided among three educational and three occupational status groups, and found that the more similar the groups in education and occupation the more they agreed in their judgments of good quality. Practically, then, the well-educated speech pathologist who is seeing a laborer for voice therapy would be ill-advised to assume that he and his patient hold identical notions about what constitutes a desirable voice.

By now, a definition of *quality* would doubtless be welcome. Acoustically, this has been attempted: quality is defined, usually, as the distribution of energy among the various frequencies within the acoustic spectrum. This distribution, the spectrum, can be measured at any given instant. It contains so much information that it can serve all of its linguistic and nonlinguistic functions and still have some to spare.

Defining quality physically is not as much of a problem as defining it psychologically. Each interpersonal communicative function of quality offers a basis for its own definition, so a general definition is not too helpful. Anyway, it would have to be cumbersome. Were such a definition attempted, it would be like this: quality, as used for interpersonal communication, is that part of a perceived sound, other than pitch or loudness, that distinguishes among speech sounds, identifies the speaker, the emotion, the somatic condition, and that can be judged aesthetically. If such a definition is useful it is to point up the various perceptual dimensions that must be identified and stabilized if the acoustical stimuli to which they are responses are to be specified. In other words, as with the solution of the psychophysical problems of pitch and loudness, the subjective sensations of the different dimensions of quality must be pinned down before their acoustical correlates can be determined.

Within the interpersonal communicative functions just discussed, quality, is not unalterably more resistant to analysis than pitch or loudness. It may be more intricate in its functions, and an acoustic analysis may be more complex, but it does not pose any problems that are basically more insoluble than those of pitch and loudness—it just poses more of them. Although only its linguistic characteristics are formally denoted by phonetic and phonemic symbols, its nonlinguistic referents could be specified, and implicitly are by virtue of the vocal quality that characteristically identifies the individual, his personality, his feelings, and to some extent his physical condition. Even with aesthetic functions, some agreement can be found among the various descriptive terms and the qualities for which they are intended.

Functions of Voice in Intrapersonal Communication

With the shift of focus to intrapersonal communication of feedback information for the regulation of vocal production, we bog down immediately in the multidimensional terminology of *vocal quality*. Analysis of regulation of any of the dimensions of vocal production—especially those involved in quality—presents quite a different problem than analysis of the sounds produced. For example, regulation of vocal pitch to produce a high note requires a single behavioral adjustment: a pitch change on a unidimensional scale from a low note, let us say, to a high note. Control of this adjustment is based on sensory information that comes in over kinesthetic and tactile as well as auditory channels.

This information is used to guide the behavioral adjustment of pitch. Pitch is but the psychological level at which one manages—directly or indirectly, consciously or unconsciously—what he is doing physiologically. Now, we have not just a psychophysical problem but a psycho-physico-physiological problem. In a psychophysical analysis of perception we can determine all of the different interpersonal communicative functions dependent on acoustic stimuli, so a high pitch may indicate prosodic stress, emotional excitement, aesthetic displeasure, and so on. In a psycho-physico-physiological analysis of pitch regulation, we are concerned with how pitch is controlled to produce these acoustic results. In the case of pitch, the problem is simple: it involves a unidimensional scale of production, so the behavioral adjustment can be made easily along this scale. Similarly, loudness is regulated along a unidimensional scale from soft to loud. To treat the regulation of vocal quality, however, as a unidimensional problem analogous to pitch or loudness regulation is to render its analysis totally impossible.

If the difficulty to which I allude is not immediately apparent, it will become so by attempting to control quality by any of the yardsticks commonly available. Whereas pitch can be regulated from high to low, and loudness from loud to soft, what scale of regulation will fit quality? Good to bad? This would be an evaluative scale of little assistance in quantifying and controlling empirical dimensions, hence, it is no solution. Hoarse to clear? A possible solution, if indeed, increased hoarseness diminishes clearness, and vice versa. Whether or not this scale would provide a continuum for measurement would be less of a problem than would be the difficulty of specifying what must be done to produce some degree of hoarseness or clearness; what behavior is emitted for a hoarse or a clear voice?

Another solution, one which I considered seriously, was to scale quality regulation along a continuum from hypertense to hypotense. This had the merit of providing a behavioral dimension that could be controlled: muscle tension. Two problems scuttled it, however. First, I was unable to specify the laryngeal muscles whose behavior was to be volitionally regulated. Second, the continuum was inadequate. The hypertense end was no problem: it could account for vocal abuse and strident sounds. The hypotense end was the problem: it was ambiguous; it could account for a relaxed hygienic voice capable of adequate loudness, or for a weak breathy voice. This solution was abandoned in favor of more profitable ones to be discussed shortly. Meanwhile, the search for adequate terminology continued, and invariably foundered in the mists of behavioral obscurity. Few, if any, of the terms for quality (e.g., *hoarse*, *harsh*, *resonant*, *husky*, *shrill*) refer to vocal behavior that can be regulated.

Part of this terminological morass stems from differences in background of those who have attempted to describe vocal regulation. Voice teachers and elocutionists, vocal production professionals, have described their subjective experiences with reasonable accuracy. Their terminological problem arises from confusing subjective experiences with physiological reality. Some tones feel as if they are produced in the chest, others in the throat, others in the head. The voice scientist untutored in professional voice usage is inclined to discount these sensations as physiological nonsense; the nonscientific vocalist, on the other hand, experiences and describes his feelings with the certainty of their physiological verity, hence, such terms as *pectoral*, *throaty*, *head*, *chest*, and even *nasal*. In other words, the vocalist describes his subjective sensations, not his behavior, and attributes physiological reality to these psychological data; the nonvocalist scientist, in his quest for objectivity, eschews psychological terminology descriptive of either sensation or behavior in favor of acoustical or physiological accounts.

We see, then, that three albatrosses strangle attempts to analyze vocal quality in terms of regulating its production. Two bear the terminological plumage just discussed, and one the ruffled feathers of a multidimensional bird treated unidimensionally. Let us recapitulate these problems. First, and most basic, existing terminology does not permit explicit delineation of behavior for the regulation of quality. *Pitch*, by contrast, is a term by which we control as well as hear the highness or lowness of a tone. Ask for a higher pitch and a higher pitch is produced; pitch has behavioral significance. Similarly with *loudness*. But not so with that old hulk *quality* with its load of adjectival barnacles. Second, the problem of maintaining clear distinctions among psychological, physiological, and acoustical phenomena is difficult even with pitch and loudness, for which reasonably accurate terminology is available. With quality, the problem is confounded by the miasma of terms that confuse rather than clarify these distinctions. Third, regulation of vocal quality is a multidimensional problem; it cannot be confined to a unidimensional solution. A single scale for its quantification, no matter now precise, will measure only a portion of all of the behavior involved in its control.

Dimensions of Vocal Production

Vocal regulation is a psychological problem; it involves emitting vocal behavior, monitoring it, and guiding it. Although the performance can be analyzed physiologically, and the output acoustically, the performance per se is psychological. It is, however, as much a productive problem as a receptive one, so to split its discussion would be to segment what is essentially a unitary cyclical process that links the guidance of vocal production to the monitoring of its output. Accordingly, we will analyze vocal regulation as an integral aspect of the productive vocal dimensions.

Criteria for Selection of Dimensions

EXPLICIT BEHAVIOR

The dimensions chosen to account for vocal production should meet several criteria. The first is that they involve explicitly defined responses that can be regulated. Many perceptual responses can be identified that are consequent to behavioral responses but do not contribute to their regulation. In fact, the terminology for *quality* is infested with adjectives descriptive of just such perceptual categories. For instance, *harsh* refers to a vocal quality that most of us could recognize, but it in no way makes explicit the vocal behavior that produces it; some behavioral response of the vocal tract would have to be invoked to account for it.

NECESSITY

The second criterion is that the dimensions be necessary to account for the important aspects of performance. The question of sufficiency is, of course, not the same as the question of necessity. A single dimension could be necessary, but whether it would be sufficient would be quite another matter. As for what is an important aspect of performance, analysis of vocal nuances and complexities could continue, conceivably, *ad infinitum*. We must stop somewhere, and we choose to stop with the normal speaking voice produced optimally for vocal hygiene. As will be demonstrated shortly, this criterion will also encompass disordered vocal behavior. Some subtleties of vocal performance important to the professional speaker and singer will doubtless be omitted. Their problems do not exclude them from this analysis, but they do extend beyond it.

QUANTIFICATION

The third criterion is that the dimensions permit quantification on some scale of measurement. Stevens (1951) details these from the most primitive form, the nominal scale, through the ordinal and the interval to the ratio scale that permits the most sophisticated mathematical operations. The important consideration for us at this stage of development of these dimensions is that they permit measurement, regardless of the scale. Future research may perfect techniques that will permit advance from an ordinal to an interval, or from an interval to a ratio scale. For the present, we can be satisfied if any scale will apply.

INDEPENDENCE

The fourth criterion is that the dimensions be independent. Independence of a dimension does not require that it never interact with other dimensions, only that it have the potential for not interacting. It has this potential if it is unidimensional; if it is possible to measure just that dimension alone. This criterion merely accords recognition to the law of parsimony. In the interest of economy, explanatory power is wasted if the properties of one dimension overlap those of another. In other words, if one dimension has not the potential to be altered without altering another, it is not independent and it is not conceived parsimoniously.

CONSENSUAL VALIDATION

The fifth criterion is that the dimensions permit consensual validation (see footnote 2). This, in many respects, is similar to the first criterion. The difference is that the emphasis in the first instance is on explicit delineation of the behavior; the emphasis in this instance is on reliability of the identification. The more easily the behavior can be identified, the more generally useful the dimension. For example, some of the dimensions that could be included if this analysis were extended to the professional vocalist would involve responses of sufficient subtlety that even though the professional could produce and recognize them reliably, the nonprofessional could not. Fortunately, this does not exclude unfamiliar responses that may not be readily recognized because they are rarely, if ever, emitted or noted. Much of the behavior in the regulation of quality falls in this category; many of the responses are so deep in the vocal tract as to be vague or imperceptible, if they occur at all.

Dimensions for Regulation of Vocal Production

Let us now consider the dimensions selected by application of these criteria. Fig. 19-4 presents them in terms, first, of productive characteristics by which the responses are subjectively regulated, second, of the ranges through which they can vary, third, of perceptual categories for their detection and monitoring, and fourth, of the currently most feasible scales for their measurement.

Implied in Fig. 19-4 and specified in Fig. 19-1 are the sensory modalities by which vocal production is monitored. The auditory, tactile, and kinesthetic receptors that Fairbanks (1954) proposed provide guidance in the production of speech, are presumably the crucial channels for vocal regulation. His proposal more than a decade ago that the speech mechanism functions as a servosystem that relies on these senses to monitor output was a germinal concept. It has become almost a canon of speech science, so thoroughly has it been built upon, thought about, discussed, written about, and tested. That auditory and tactile feedback are vital for speech control has been observed time and again (Black, 1950; Fairbanks and Guttman, 1958; Ringel and Steer, 1963; Mysak, 1966). Unfortunately, animals do not speak, and, so far, no human has volunteered himself on the altar of science to demonstrate conclusively that speech (and probably life) is dependent on kinesthetic feedback as well. All in all, we could reasonably assume that subjective regulation of all productive dimensions of voice is guided by feedback information from all three sensory modalities for each of the perceptual dimensions. Accordingly, detection of pitch, loudness, or any of the other dimensions of voice specified in the *Vocal Input* column of Fig. 19-4 implies, for intrapersonal communication, perceptual response to tactile and kinesthetic as well as to auditory stimuli.

PITCH AND LOUDNESS

Turning to the dimensions themselves, we find two familiar dimensions, pitch and loudness, with which the analysis can begin. Both phenomena meet the five criteria for a dimension admirably. Both refer to explicit responses that can be subjectively regulated, which is what the entries in the *Vocal Output* column of Fig. 19-4 are intended to denote. In fact, pitch and loudness can be sufficiently explicit that failure to regulate them according to our intent would likely surprise and distress most of us. Both meet the second criterion in that both are necessary to account for all of the behavior required to regulate fundamental frequency for pitch, and acoustic power for

PSYCHOLOGICAL DIMENSIONS OF VOCAL REGULATION

VOCAL OUTPUT		VOCAL INPUT (FEEDBACK)	
PRODUCTIVE DIMENSION	SCALE	PERCEPTUAL DIMENSION FOR VOCAL MONITORING	CURRENT FEASIBLE SCALE OF MEASUREMENT
PITCH SUBJECTIVE REGULATION	LOW ⟷ HIGH	PITCH SUBJECTIVE DETECTION	RATIO (MEL)
LOUDNESS SUBJECTIVE REGULATION	SOFT ⟷ LOUD	LOUDNESS SUBJECTIVE DETECTION	RATIO (SONE)
VOICING SUBJECTIVE REGULATION	VOICELESS ⟷ VOICED	VOICING SUBJECTIVE DETECTION	ORDINAL
VOCAL MODE SUBJECTIVE REGULATION	PULSATED VOICE (GLOTTAL FRY) — HEAVY VOICE (CHEST) — LIGHT VOICE (FALSETTO)	VOCAL MODE SUBJECTIVE DETECTION	NOMINAL
VOCAL CONSTRICTION SUBJECTIVE REGULATION	OPEN ⟷ CLOSED	VOCAL CONSTRICTION SUBJECTIVE DETECTION	ORDINAL

Fig. 19-4. Unidimensional scales for regulation and measurement of vocal production.

loudness. The third criterion, that they be measurable, is met fully, as the last column of Fig. 19-4 shows. Ratio scales, the ranges of which are also shown in Fig. 19-4, permit quantification of pitch detection in subjective units of *mels*, loudness detection in subjective units of *sones*. The fourth criterion, that requires that pitch and loudness be independent dimensions, is met more fully with trained than untrained voices. Changes in pitch, loudness, or quality typically interact with each other. That these interactions are not necessary, hence revealing potential independence of the dimensions, can be seen in the professional vocalist's ability to vary pitch or loudness while holding other dimensions constant. Finally, both pitch and loudness meet the fifth criterion; they are consensually validated. Most of us can differentiate and detect changes in pitch and changes in loudness.

QUALITY

We are now ready for the more difficult analysis of quality. A preliminary word is necessary about how it was approached and accomplished. The analysis in its present form is a product of evolution. One thing was clear from the beginning: quality is multidimensional. The problem, then, was to determine the minimally necessary and sufficient behavioral dimensions to account for it. At one time, as many as six were specified. While the criteria ultimately used for selection were being formulated, *ad hoc* tests of the adequacy of dimensions under consideration were employed. One was to compile terms descriptive of vocal quality and laryngeal functioning (Peterson and Shoup's (1966) nine distinctive laryngeal actions were especially helpful); the test was to determine the minimal combination of dimensions that would encompass these qualities and functions.

Another test of particular value was undertaken in collaboration with my colleague, William Vennard, a voice scientist and a professional singer. We experimented with the various combinations of dimensions to determine how they would account for important aspects of vocal quality. This proved to be a crucial tactic for answering for the speaking voice the questions of sufficiency, necessity, and independence. This analysis, as it turned out, showed that the three dimensions selected for the regulation of speaking voice quality are also necessary, but not sufficient, for the singing voice nor for the professional speaking voice; at least one additional independent and two dependent dimensions would be required, but the are beyond the scope of this discussion (Perkins, 1971).

VOICING

The three behavioral dimensions proposed as necessary and possibly sufficient for regulation of vocal quality in normal speech are *voicing*, *vocal mode*, and *vocal constriction*. Each will be discussed and tested against our five criteria. Voicing refers to the vocal behavior by which the conversion of continuous air flow into a series of glottal pulses is regulated. An analogy to the concept of alternating current (ac) and direct current (dc) provides a convenient shorthand for referring to a train of glottal pulses, ac, and a continuous current of air, dc. In these short and terms, voicing refers to the behavioral management of the ac/dc balance of air flow.

Voicing meets the second criterion in that it accounts for all aspects of quality that range from voicelessness (dc) to full voicing (ac). Any degree of voicing between these poles represents a balance between ac and dc, so any degree of breathiness or voicing could be located along this scale. Accordingly, the dimension fits normal as well as disordered functioning; phonetically, the degree of voicing for consonants and vowels can be specified; for vocal disorders, aphonic conditions would lie near the dc end of the scale and dysphonias in between the poles.

As far as the third criterion is concerned, no work has been done to develop systematically a scale of measurement for voicing. The fact that so many distinctive differences in phonetics depend on degrees of voicing (Peterson and Shoup indicate four) lends confidence to the speculation that these degrees could be ranked in order along a scale. That voicing meets the fourth criterion, independence, cannot be demonstrated fully until vocal mode and constriction have been discussed. It will have to suffice for the moment to point out that the ac/dc balance can, for practical purposes, be manipulated independent of pitch and loudness. The voicing distinctions made in phonetics are again invoked as evidence that this dimension meets the fifth criterion, consensual validation. If the population at large could not make these distinctions, the phonetic "noise" in our speaking system would be great indeed.

VOCAL MODE

Vocal mode refers to the behavior by which the vibratory modes of vocalization are regulated; it is the basic vocal adjustment that serves as a framework within which the other dimensions are regulated. This dimension corresponds roughly to the concept of vocal register, a term borrowed from the pipe organ and confused beyond usefulness by an opaque mixture of pronouncements and observations of singers, laryngologists, elocutionists, and, of course, speech pathologists. Many of the battles in the register war have been waged over the boundaries between falsetto and head, and between head and chest registers. Fortunately for our primary concern with the untrained speaking voice, these boundary disputes are more vital for the singer than for us. What is vital to this analysis is that vocalization can be regulated among at least three distinct vibratory modes, each of which has a profound affect on vocal quality.

The terms by which these modes are identified were selected to be psychologically descriptive. Therefore, *pulsated voice* is preferred as more accurately descriptive of the feel of the behavior and sound of the voice produced in this mode of vocalization at the low end of the pitch scale than the older terms, *creaky voice*, *dicrotic voice*, and *glottal fry*. The mode is the vocal adjustment that permits emission of the slowest rate of glottal pulses: rates as slow as 10 per second have been measured. Pulse rates below 60 Hz are heard more as a series of popping sounds than as a tone with pitch. These sounds characterize pulsated voice. Those who have experienced this mode are likely to have no question that it is unique. In fact, Hollien and his group (1966) have made a convincing case for vocal fry as a separate register.

For the middle mode, Vennard (1967) prefers the term *heavy voice*, and so do I, to *chest voice* with its anatomical connotation, or, worse yet, to *chest register* which not only mislocates vocal function anatomically but even confuses it with a pipe organ. Heavy voice is the mode used almost exclusively by adult males in our culture, and by many, if not most women and children. It permits wider ranges of pitch, loudness, and quality than any other mode. It is the adjustment that breaks into pulsated voice at low pitches and light voice at high pitches in most untrained voices. In trained voices, adjustments between these modes can be made smoothly.

The mode at the high end of the pitch scale is identified as *light voice* in preference to falsetto, a diminutive of *false* which, when applied to voice means little false voice; the sound produced in this mode may be little, but it is truly vocal. This adjustment permits the highest pitches of which the voice is capable. It is distinguished by the extent to which it limits loudness relative to the loudness that can be achieved with heavy voice. Excessive vocal effort yields increased breathiness more than increased loudness in light voice.

Probably not everyone has produced voice in these three modes, so those who have not been initiated into the behavioral processes of three mode production may remain unconvinced of this analysis. For those who have, the distinctions among the modes need no argument. Let it merely be said that the distinctions are easily made in the untrained voice at the vocal "breaks" or modal transition points (the trained voice blurs these distinctions because one objective of training is to navigate transitions without a break). Proceeding upward in pitch, which, in the pulsated voice will be experienced more as an increase in pulsation rate than as an increase in pitch, a point will be reached at which the voice will "break" into a different mode of vocalization, heavy voice. This mode can be navigated up the pitch scale, with increased effort for the unskilled vocalist, until another transition is reached when heavy voice breaks into light voice.

Vocal mode now can be tested against the remaining criteria. It meets the second by virtue of accounting for all of the behavior that regulates modal adjustments and all of the qualities that characterize these modes. It meets the third in its most primitive form, a nominal scale of measurement. Each mode provides a framework within which the other vocal behaviors are regulated along continuous dimensions, hence, vocal mode meets the fourth criterion of independence. The criterion of consensual validation should pose no problem for any of the modes in the adult male, especially if he is an unskilled vocalist; the qualities peculiar to the modes are unique. If identification were to prove difficult, and no experimental work on this has been done, it would probably be in distinguishing heavy from light voice in the child or in the woman whose heavy voice is relatively light.

VOCAL CONSTRICTION

We come, finally, to the dimension of greatest functional significance for the clinician and probably for anyone interested in nonlinguistic vocal phenomena: subjective vocal constriction.

With this dimension, especially, we must be careful to distinguish psychological from physiological phenomena. It denotes the *feeling* of constriction in the vocal tract, hence, the terms *vocal* constriction and *subjective* constriction. This dimension does not specify the physiology of this feeling. Granted, future research may show that it is dependent on physiological constriction of the vocal tract. But, regardless of what the physiology may be, vocal constriction is the behavior that applies the brakes on the voice. The greater the constriction, the greater the effort to produce a sound, the greater the vocal strain, and the more limited will be the range of pitch and loudness. This is the dimension responsible for most of the qualities for which pejorative adjectives have flourished. Constriction responses, of the various dimensional behaviors, are the most elusive and difficult to identify, probably because they involve pharyngeal and laryngeal functions that are, at best, perceptually obscure. Yet, preliminary experimental work (Beckett, 1967; Joyner, 1967) indicates that these responses can be delineated with reasonable accuracy. The tactic utilized to render them manageable is to define the poles between which they can vary. The pole that is optimal for vocal hygiene involves a behavioral response in which the vocal tract feels maximally open; this response can be elicited universally by yawning. At the other pole, the constriction response is maximal and the feeling of vocal tract closure is greatest; this polar behavioral response is defined reflexively by swallowing.

The term *constriction* was chosen over two close rivals, *tension* and *tightness*, because yawning distends the vocal tract. An open throat, one that the professional vocalist seeks for the hygienic preservation of his voice (Vennard 1967), is not completely characterized by *relaxed* or *loose*—the necessary polar opposites of *tense* or *tight*—these descriptions being more suggestive of a flaccidly collapsed muscular state. This is not to impugn relaxation or looseness. As with athletes, a mark of good condition for the speaker is the ability to relax the muscles for speech when their contraction is not required. Moreover, as Vennard (1967) points out, the feelings of tension in the neck or of the voice being "manufactured" in the throat are signs of poor vocal production; the well-trained vocalist has the feeling of "letting go" in the throat. Yet, a certain feeling of "stretch," as experienced in a yawn, accompanies this letting go of constriction; thus, the decision to choose a behavioral scale primarily descriptive of the degree of openness of the vocal tract.

The second criterion of necessity is especially important for testing the adequacy of this last dimension (vocal constriction) that carries much, if not most, of the load for nonlinguistic functions. The broad issue, though, is whether constriction, in conjunction with the other dimensions, can account for the important aspects of vocal performance in conversational speech. Because this discussion will require extensive consideration of other dimensions, it will be dealt with separately in the next section.

Holding in abeyance the test of vocal constriction against the second criterion, we turn to the third criterion, which constriction appears to meet, namely, that the dimension be measurable. Preliminary experimentation with vocal constriction (Beckett, 1967; Joyner, 1967) indicates that remarkably stable judgments can be obtained regardless of the judge's level of vocal sophistication. So far, only the method of paired comparisons has been used to make relatively gross judgments that permit its measurement on no higher than an ordinal scale. Whether sufficiently refined methods of quantification will ultimately permit use of interval or ratio scales remains to be determined. Be that as it may, the third criterion is satisfied.

The fourth criterion, independence, can also be met. Vocal constriction can vary independently of pitch, loudness, voicing, and vocal mode. It is by virtue of its independence that it contributes in different proportions with the other dimensions to assorted vocal qualities, normal and abnormal. For example, high constriction plus high pitch and loudness is heard by experts frequently as stridency, high constriction plus low pitch as harshness, high constriction plus low pitch and moderate voicing as hoarseness, high constriction plus low voicing as stage whisper. The list could be extended indefinitely with varying proportions of each dimension, but a point to note is that constriction is the key to abnormal quality. With the exception of vocal mode, that must be appropriate to the age and sex of the individual, high constriction is the only dimension that is consistently distinctive in abnormal quality. Low constriction in conjunction with high or low pitch, high or low loudness, high or low voicing will invariably be heard as normal vocal quality.

The studies by Joyner (1967) and Beckett (1967) that demonstrated the feasibility of quantifying vocal constriction, by the same token, have demonstrated that this dimension can be consensually validated. The ability of vocally unsophisticated as well as expert listeners to judge, reliably, differences among numerous voice samples of high, moderate, and low constriction lends confidence that this dimension can be readily recognized, and accordingly, does meet the fifth criterion.

NECESSITY OF DIMENSIONS FOR VOCAL FUNCTIONS

If we consider as important those functions discussed in the section on interpersonal communication and summarized in Fig. 19-2, we have a frame of reference within which to conduct a final assessment of the necessity of all the dimensions, with particular emphasis on vocal constriction.

Taking the important interpersonal functions of voice in the order in which they were presented earlier, the articulatory and prosodic features can be dealt with briefly as far as they are affected by phonation. The prosodic functions can be accounted for by pitch and loudness dimensions (O'Malley and Peterson, 1966). The articulatory functions include syllabic and nonsyllabic elements. Admittedly, syllabic elements (the vowel phones) may be dependent on phonatory action for some distinctions, tense versus lax being a possible candidate. Still, most theories of physiological phonetics invoke supraglottal vocal tract adjustments for differences in syllabic segmental elements. For nonsyllabic elements, the most crucial phonatory distinctions are between voiced and voiceless consonants; Peterson and Shoup (1966) list 46 consonants dependent on one or the other condition, and only eight dependent on other types of vocalization. We saw earlier that they specified in their theory of physiological phonetics nine laryngeal actions; of these, four can be quantified easily along the voicing dimension, one (pulsation) fits the vocal mode class of pulsated voice, and the remainder (e.g., constricted, stopped) can be accommodated on the constriction scale.

The contributions of vocal production to nonlinguistic interpersonal functions are, to a large extent, speculative. That dimensions other than the ones we are considering are involved cannot be argued; no empirical evidence is available to dispute the possibility. The argument is that the dimensions being discussed are *necessary* to account for the important speaking functions. Whether all of them, let alone others, are *sufficient* is not the issue.

For speaker identification, characteristic prosodic patterns of pitch and loudness are doubtless involved along with quality for which voicing and constriction regulation are normally important. *Ad hoc* experimentation with quality dimensions that disguise the voice suggest that all are effective, but some are more so. Probably the most effective is the one least likely to be used normally—vocal mode; aside from Henry Aldrich, whose stock-in-trade was "breaks" across vocal modes, most of us attempt to stay within our habitual mode. Gross changes in voicing and constriction appear necessary before speaker identity is distorted. None of this demonstrates conclusively that these dimensions are sufficient for vocal identification, but that others are required seems improbable. Essentially the same analysis applies to personality- and emotion-revealing functions, so the same points will not be labored and relabored.

This brings us to the most crucial interpersonal functions for the clinician—whose professional responsibility is to keep the voice healthy—the information he derives from vocal production about the somatic condition of the vocal tract, and his aesthetic evaluations of this information. Aesthetic judgments, of course, can be made about any aspect of vocal sound regardless of the functions it serves or the dimensions by which it is regulated. Some dislike high-pitched voices, others loud voices; some think breathy tones are sexy, but only from the throats of lovely lasses; singers generally feel that /æ/ is a flat ugly sound for which /a/ is much preferred. The aesthetic responses that concern us here are those that identify the health condition of the vocal tract and the adequacy of vocal production in the establishment or maintenance of vocal hygiene.

The final test of the necessity of the proposed dimensions, especially constriction, is to assess how well they can account for the various terms descriptive of vocal quality. Many schemes have been offered for classifying quality defects, so classifications were recorded from nine well-known texts in speech pathology and voice improvement (Berry and Eisenson, 1956; Milisen, 1957; Moore, 1957; West, Ansberry, and Carr, 1957; Van Riper and Irwin, 1958, Fairbanks, 1960; Anderson, 1961; Hanley and Thurman, 1963; Van Riper, 1963; Johnson, Brown, Curtis, Edney, and Keaster, 1967). The list included 27 terms, to which were added 16 that appeared elsewhere, and it doubtless could have been continued interminably. Of the 27, only 12 terms are used in more than one text, and of these only two, *nasality* and *hoarseness*, are used by all. The next six contenders for which at least four texts agree, are, in order of preference, *breathy*, *harsh*, *strident*, *denasal*, *husky*, and *metallic*. Of these, *husky* is synonymous with *breathy* in two texts, and with *hoarse* in another; *harsh* means *metallic* or *strident* with one, *strident* and *intense* with another, and *throaty* with still another; *strident* is equivalent to *guttural*, *strained*, *shrill*, *harsh*, or *metallic*. Thurman (1954) found adequate agreement for five of these terms among speech clinicians in experimental situations; Jensen (1965) however, reported poor agreement among six speech pathologists, experienced in work with disorders of voice, who were asked to judge the voices of cheerleaders suffering from vocal strain. They could not agree on the distinctions among hoarseness, breathiness, and harshness. Clearly, we have a Gordian knot of intertwined terminology, which, when unraveled from its overlapping meanings, points to common processes basic to the production of these different qualities.

Using the eight most frequently occurring terms and the qualities to which they refer as a reasonable and final test of the adequacy of our vocal dimensions, two of the terms, *nasality* and *denasality* can, for the most part, be disqualified as outside the province of this analysis. All of the authors agree that these are resonance problems, or, using Fairbanks' (1960) terms, problems of transmission rather than tone generation. To the extent that phonation is involved in them, the dimension of voicing would account for much of the "hooty" sound of hypernasality and constriction for phonatory aspects of "nasal twang." Of the six remaining terms, *hoarse*, *breathy*, and *harsh* are most widely used, yet, these are the ones on which Jensen (1965) reports voice experts could not agree; hoarseness for some was breathiness or harshness for others. This confusion is to be expected if our dimensions are valid. For that matter, several texts (Berry and Eisenson, 1956; Milisen, 1957; Fairbanks, 1960; Van Riper, 1963) described hoarseness as combining the features of harshness and breathiness.

First, then, let us consider harshness, since it is pivotal for strident and metallic as well as hoarse quality. All authors agree that it is characterized by laryngeal strain and tension. Vocal constriction would be the dimension by which we could account for this aspect of its production; after all, if phonation were attempted with constriction approximating a swallow (the closed end of the continuum), the strain and effort to produce a tone would be great indeed. Another feature of harshness included frequently is low pitch, which, of course, would be a function of the pitch dimension. About all that need be said about breathiness is that it obviously fits the voicing dimension.

Now, back to hoarseness, the universally familiar symptom of laryngeal dysfunction whether it be laryngitis or carcinoma. Not surprisingly, it is typically described as a combination of breathiness and harshness. Any laryngeal disability that perturbs the vibratory pattern will tend to reduce the efficiency of the laryngeal generator; the effectiveness of the conversion of air flow from dc to ac is reduced, and breathiness is the consequence. With a loss in glottal efficiency, increased vocal effort is required to maintain adequate loudness, hence the increased vocal constriction and the harsh quality.

This leaves *strident*, *husky*, and *metallic*. Stridency has few characteristics to call its own, having been described as harshness, harshness with high pitch, harshness with high intensity, and hoarseness with high pitch. These correlates have been analyzed, so we come to *husky*. It, too, has had an accounting, being synonymous with *breathy* and *hoarse*. Finally, *metallic* is used as another word for harsh, and as a term for lack of vibrato (a function of rapid periodic pitch and loudness fluctuations); one author has attributed it to oral and pharyngeal tension, and another recommends relaxation of the neck and face for its treatment. Apparently, then, if a metallic voice is a phonatory problem it either resembles harshness, primarily a constriction function, or it involves pitch and loudness regulation. If, however, it is a problem of resonance, constriction is again relevant, although gratuitously so since resonance is not the primary interest here. Vocal constriction is a dimension that probably includes physiological effects in the pharynx as well as the larynx: swallowing, the behavior that anchors the closed end of the scale, not only tightens and constricts laryngeal sphincters, but also narrows and tenses walls of the supraglottal vocal tract; conversely, yawning, the behavioral anchor at the open end of the scale, distends the entire vocal tract with reciprocal relaxation of constrictor muscles.

The closing comment for this section on vocal regulation must reiterate an earlier disclaimer. This five-dimensional model is not intended to account for every characteristic of the vocal sound produced. It was designed with a view to utility. Above all else, it has to be sufficient for the regulation of important aspects of speech, but in the interest of economy, it should not enjoy the luxury of superflous dimensions. Admittedly, one can quarrel with what I selected as an index of importance. In fact, a case is made elsewhere (Perkins, 1971) for a dimension of vocal focus by which one regulates refined and important aspects of vocal performance. The objective here, however, is to provide the minimum number of dimensions necessary for the production of a normal healthy voice.

Strategy for Investigating Vocal Functioning

Psychophysical methods have not yet been, and possibly never will be, developed for the study of motor behavior, the productive aspect of psychology. Granted the problems we considered earlier of classical methods of psychophysics in measuring perception, still, physical stimuli can be quantified and controlled to shed light on sensory and perceptual phenomena. No such stimuli permissible of measurement or independent control are available to aid in the analysis of motor behavior. For those speech pathologists interested in the antecedent events to a behavioral performance, a rough analogue to the audiologist's psychophysical problem in auditory perception, only mediating responses can be inferred. The diabolical "black box" problem of the mind thwarts our scientific study of cognitive processes that regulate motor behavior as it does study of sensation, perception, or even cognition per se.

Perhaps one reason that speech pathology has not advanced more rapidly as a science in the understanding of disordered speech and language is this insoluble problem of being unable to measure and control the stimuli that govern our communicative behavior. The dilemma prevails through all facets of our professional concern. How can we answer definitively why stutterers stutter, or speechless children are without language, or vocal cripples abuse their voices when we cannot specify the independent cognitive variables that control these behaviors? The behaviorist answers that it is an artificial problem, that mentalistic psychology with its cognitive processes does not permit scientific investigation. From this point of view has grown Skinner's solution of the functional analysis of behavior that excludes from consideration those phenomena that cannot be observed and measured (1954). Cognitive theorists argue that this takes the psyche out of psychology, so they continue to work with their hypothetical constructs, intervening variables, and mediating responses.

This is neither the place, nor am I the author to attempt a more successful resolution of this age-old quandary. It is a current reality within which we must work. Having in a sense "begged the question" by analyzing the productive and receptive vocal dimensions as inseparably circular processes, which they undoubtedly are, the imponderables of cognition have been avoided as peripheral to our applied concerns that do permit a behavioral solution. Further discussion of psychological phenomena of vocal production would not be likely to take us much farther. Let us consider, instead, the problems of investigating productive dimensions of voice in terms of the physiological processes correlated with their regulation and the acoustical phenomena that characterize their output effects.

Correlates of Vocal Production: General Issues

A thorough review of physiological and acoustical research is not the province of this chapter. The primary objectives are, first, elucidation of the relationships between the five psychological dimensions of vocal production and the physiological and the acoustic dimensions, and second, clarification of strategy for reducing variance in voice research.

The relationships of the psychological to the physiological dimensions are shown in Fig. 19-5, and to the acoustical dimensions in Fig. 19-6. The scope

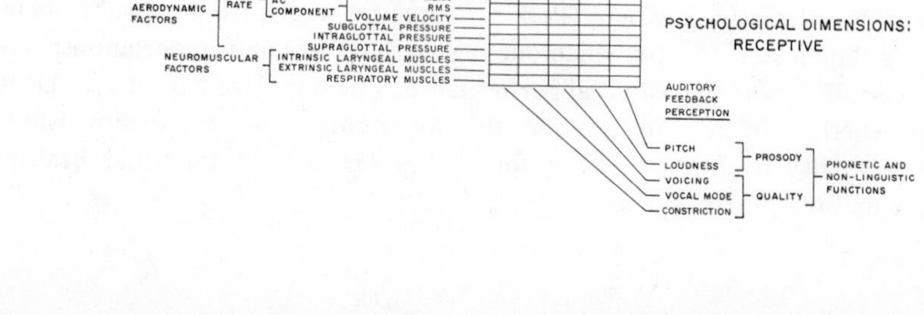

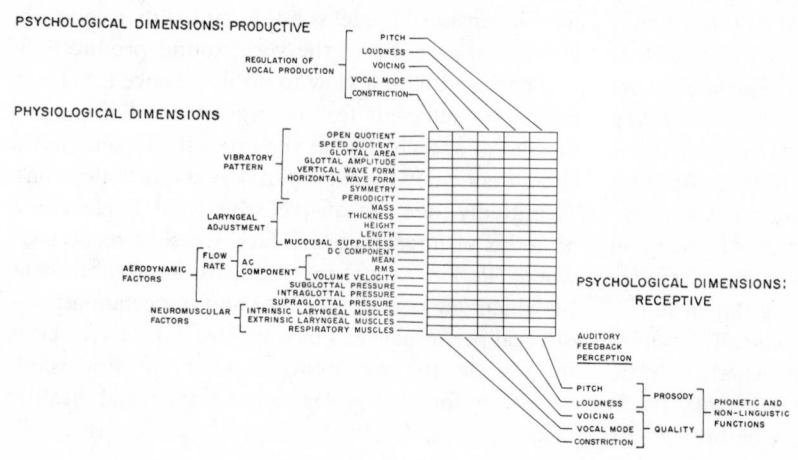

Fig. 19-5. Psycho-physiological model for investigating productive and receptive dimensions of voice. To describe vertical and horizontal vibratory patterns, two terms were coined: "vertical wave form" and "horizontal wave form."

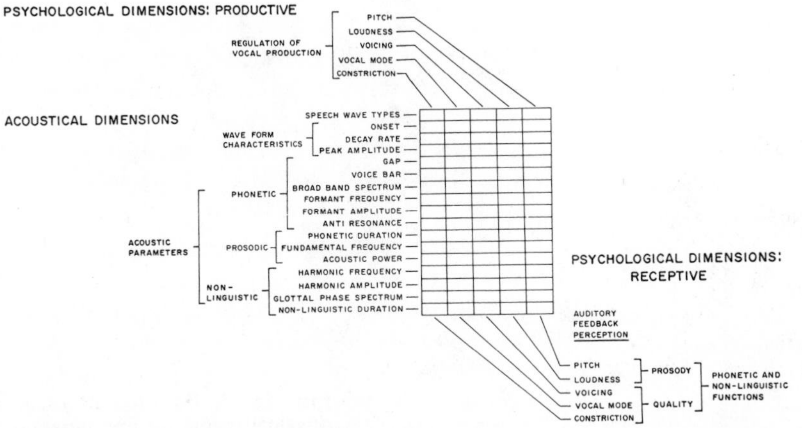

Fig. 19-6. Psycho-physical model for investigating productive and receptive dimensions of voice.

of these relationships, more than their details, is our concern here. These two-dimensional models (discussed in the following chapter under *Assessment of Vocal Functioning*), in a sense, are three dimensional in that the psychological dimension must really be counted twice: productive and receptive psychological dimensions are delineated. The models are not predictive of theoretical relationships, but rather are descriptive of dimensions that can be correlated. They permit relating of each psychological dimension with every physiological and acoustical attribute, a massive prospect for research, to be sure. If only one study were done of the relationship between each dimension of vocal production and each physiological variable, 115 investigations would be required; of the relationships with acoustic dimensions, 85 would be needed.

Admittedly, some studies would appear to be more profitable than others. At the present state of our knowledge, laryngeal adjustment factors seem to be most closely related to pitch regulation, aerodynamic factors to loudness, and vibratory patterns to quality just to mention a few ostensibly good physiological leads. But, the more carefully the problem is scrutinized, the more apparent is the necessity of looking at each productive and each receptive dimension in terms of all physiological and most acoustical correlates.

Consider, for example, pitch regulation. Experience has shown that a change in any aspect of voice tends to be accompanied by changes in all other aspects, e.g., pitch affects quality and loudness. Apparently, the physiology of pitch regulation tends to interact with that of quality and loudness. The question is, then, when pitch is systematically altered as the independent variable and the other four production dimensions are controlled: what are the effects in the dependent variables of vibratory patterns, aerodynamic factors, neuromuscular factors, as well as laryngeal adjustments? If the other dimensions that tend to vary with pitch, when uncontrolled, are held constant during pitch changes, then, it would be instructive to learn whether a variety of intricate compensatory physiological adjustments are necessary to preclude this interaction, or whether the interaction is a consequence of extraneous adjustments unnecessary to the regulation of pitch. Hence the necessity for concern with all of the physiological dimensions.

Numerous other instances could be cited, depending on the question of interest, and the same case could be made for the physiological correlates of receptive psychological dimensions. In fact, the concern in physiological phonetics is with these perceptual characteristics. The point need not be labored, so let us turn to the acoustical dimensions and illustrate the scope of their relevance.

Assume the problem of determining the linguistic and nonlinguistic effects, the perceptual effects, of variations in constriction. If approached from the standpoint of psychophysical methodology, the acoustic properties of the stimulus effects of constriction would be determined and related to the perceptual phenomena of interest, such as perception of vowels under different emotional conditions (a linguistic and nonlinguistic function). Because constriction is a regulatory dimension for the perceptual phenomenon, the relevant acoustic dimensions would include all but the prosodic parameters, and even these would be appropriate if effects of constriction on pitch and loudness were a concern.

The psycho-physio-acoustic problem of vocal production is immensely complex; its scope is made explicit in Fig. 19-7. We have looked only at the possible questions that could be raised about psychological productive dimensions in relation to either

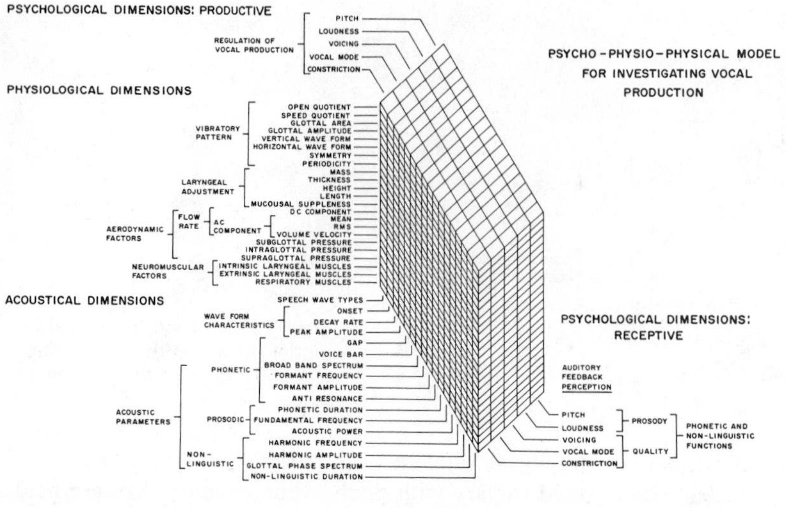

Fig. 19-7. Psycho-physio-physical model for investigating productive and receptive dimensions of voice.

physiological or acoustical factors taken separately. Were the interrelationships among the three classes of phenomena to be studied, a thoroughly legitimate prospect, the number of investigations available in the model would be 1,870—a staggering prospect to contemplate. But, if the psychological receptive dimensions were included, as they would need to be for research in phonetics, this number would be doubled!

These models are not presented to inundate our current work with the immense expanse of the problems awaiting investigation. They are offered, instead, to remind us of the limits of existing knowledge. We can claim, presently, definitive understanding of few, if any, of these relationships. This state of affairs, viewed scientifically, is a challenge; viewed clinically, it is a cause for caution.

The reason for caution is that we are inclined to make judgments about behavioral phenomena on the basis of physiological evidence. Each unit of behavior, say, the utterance of a single phone, subsumes an awesome array of physiological events. To account physiologically for such a simple behavioral task as uttering [i], the neurological phenomena, the respiratory, phonatory, articulatory events, the auditory, tactile, kinesthetic feedback, the metabolic phenomena would all have to be specified, along with the infinitely complex interactions among them. When the difference between hygienic and abusive vocal functioning rests on subtle behavioral adjustments of the vocal constriction dimension, a dimension barely investigated physiologically, we are hardly in a position clinically to make recommendations for hygienic vocal production on the basis of inferences drawn from sketchy physiological data.

Research Strategy

Understanding vocal functioning in human subjects requires, ultimately, that a human produce the vocal samples to be studied physiologically and acoustically. This statement would be trite were not electrical synthesizers[3] and mechanical analogues of the vocal tract available (van den Berg, 1955, 1958; Wendahl, 1963), and if animal research on voice had not been accomplished (Dedo and Dunker, 1967; Dedo and Ogura, 1965; Rubin, 1963). With vocal tract analogues, physiological functions can be simulated and controlled as independent variables, thereby permitting observation of acoustic effects as the dependent variables. Similarly with animal research, selected physiological processes (e.g., electrical stimulation of laryngeal muscles) can be controlled and the vocal output observed. In this type of experimentation, the physiological functions are controlled; they are the independent, not the dependent variables. From such experimentation can come theories of vocal functioning, but these theories must, in the final analysis, be validated by testing them in human subjects.

The significance of the necessary involvement of humans is that, so far at least, no methods have been

[3] Speech synthesizers are of two types; terminal formant and physiological analogue. Terminal formant synthesizers simulate the acoustic speech output, and, thereby, do not attempt to account for the physiological processes that regulate this output. Physiological analogue synthesizers, on the other hand, can simulate the transmission and tone generation characteristics of the vocal tract; their function is analogous to that of the air tube. Because of the immense complexity of the large number of variables, their interrelationships, and the speed with which they interact, these synthesizers are controlled by computers.

developed for controlling their laryngeal physiology; all that current techniques permit is observation of their laryngeal functioning. This means that in research on the human voice, the independent variables are, of necessity, controlled by volitional regulation of vocal production, a psychological function. Not only the independent variables to be manipulated, but also the variables to be held constant must be volitionally controlled.

The point of this discussion of research strategy is that the physiological and acoustical measures of vocal functioning are dependent on the regulation of pitch, loudness, and quality. The measures can be no more valid than control of the vocal production variables will permit. Control of pitch and loudness has not been a serious problem, which is not surprising since both are unidimensional, have subjective units of measure, and can be monitored acoustically. Quality, however, has been another matter. As we saw in the preceding section, it is multidimensional and not subject to direct regulation. Moreover, it tends to vary with pitch and loudness, especially in untrained voices. The consensus in the nine texts mentioned earlier was that quality tends to become harsh at low and strident at high pitches, and that loudness exacerbates both tendencies. In other words, the two dimensions that can be controlled reasonably well are typically accompanied (the poorer the vocal production the more probable the accompaniment) by changes in quality that can be sizable.

The interactions of pitch and loudness with the dimensions of quality can confound the physiological results to such an extent that variations attributed to pitch or to loudness may, in fact, be functions of uncontrolled covarying quality dimensions. We came face to face with this reality in a study of physiological and acoustical correlates of pitch and loudness regulation. At that time, the model of vocal dimensions was in its infancy, but it matured rapidly under the impetus of the results of this study. For this investigation, we manipulated pitch and loudness separately while the other was held constant along with the vowel, the size of mouth opening, and the register (vocal mode), that for this male subject, was chest (heavy voice). The other feature of voice we attempted to control was "style," that varied from "hypertense" to "hypotense" with "optimal" presumably somewhere in between. The subject was a semitrained vocalist who was judged to use his voice optimally during the experiment. As an overall evaluation of the quality of each performance, this judgment was doubtless correct. But, if the judgment were to be made now using vocal constriction on a time segmented basis, brief, but drastic, changes in constriction would probably be observed in some of the samples.

The experiment was to obtain simultaneous recordings of subglottal pressure, mean air-flow rate, electrical potentials of the cricothyroid muscle, and acoustic output. Fortunately, each condition was replicated once and sometimes twice, or we would have been tempted to leap to some drastically erroneous conclusions. After analyzing much of the pitch data, it was found to vary directly with glottal resistance and inversely with mean flow rate. The correlations were so consistently high, often beyond 0.90, that our certainty was soaring that we could account for at least this subject's mechanism for pitch regulation. Our optimism was soon squelched by several records in which the typical pattern was completely reversed for varying periods from brief to long intervals, and the correlations for the reversals were, again, frequently beyond 0.90. Similar reversals occurred in the loudness results. They appeared to occur with variations in constriction, which is probably to be expected because it would appear to be, logically, the psychological correlate of glottal resistance.

This somewhat detailed recital is to stress the necessity of controlling adequately, not just pitch and loudness, but also the regulatory dimensions of quality. That such extreme changes in physiological adjustment could occur with a better than average vocalist who was attempting explicitly to maintain constant quality, and whose performance was being monitored by two experimenters who were listening especially for changes in quality, is a disturbing commentary on voice research.

That such a large enterprise as is delineated in the models of Figs. 19-5, 19-6, and 19-7 for investigating vocal functioning could be jeopardized leads to four strategy recommendations for the control of variance. One is that specific tactics such as proposed here be used to control for the regulatory dimensions of quality. These dimensions can account for so much variance that to leave them uncontrolled in, say, a study of pitch or loudness, would be like trying to detect the effects of a lawn sprinkler during a cloud burst. A second is that judgments of these quality dimensions be made in relatively brief time segments. Vocal mode, voicing, and constriction can fluctuate as quickly as can pitch and loudness. Over all judgments of quality based on a complete performance, even as short as a few seconds, can obscure sizable, but brief, variations. A third recommendation is that subjects capable of controlling vocal production dimensions be utilized for research, at least until the physiological and acoustical correlates for normal vocal functioning are delineated. A fourth, and most basic, recommendation is that quality not be judged or controlled as a unidimensional phenomenon. We were relatively sophisticated judges of quality when we ran the experiment just chronicled. That experience convinced us that behaviorally manageable dimensions of quality would have to be isolated if adequate control of it were to be obtained.

SUMMARY

An analysis of the psychological functions of voice must distinguish receptive from productive dimensions. Receptive dimensions include those involved in interpersonal and intrapersonal communication. For interpersonal communication, the auditory vocal properties, pitch, loudness, and quality, function linguistically in the service of phonetic articulation and prosody; they also function nonlinguistically to reveal speaker identity, personality, emotion, and some somatic conditions, and to provide a basis for aesthetic judgments. For intrapersonal communication, auditory, tactile, and kinesthetic feedback information is utilized to regulate vocal production.

Whereas receptive dimensions are cognitive, productive dimensions are behavioral. The problem in an analysis of vocal production is to delineate the minimal number of parameters that must be controlled to account for the auditory properties of voice that function in interpersonal communication. The criteria that parameters must meet to be adequate are: 1. that they refer to explicitly defined responses that can be regulated; 2. that they be necessary to account for important aspects of vocal performance; 3. that they permit quantification on some scale of measurement; 4. that they be independent; and 5. that they permit consensual validation. The five dimensions that meet these criteria are pitch, loudness, and, for the regulation of quality, voicing, vocal mode, and vocal constriction.

BIBLIOGRAPHY

Anderson, V. 1961. Training the speaking voice (2nd. ed.). New York: Oxford.

Beckett, R. 1968. Pitch perturbation as a function of subjective vocal constriction. Univ. South. Calif.: Ph.D. dissertation.

Berg, J. van den. 1955. Calculations on a model of the vocal tract for vowel /i/ (meat) and on the larynx. *J. acoust. soc. Amer.*, 27, 332–338.

———. 1958. Myoelastic-aerodynamic theory of voice production. *J. Speech Hearing Res.*, 1, 227–244.

Berry, M., and Eisenson, J. 1956. Speech disorders. New York: Appleton-Century-Crofts.

Black, J. 1950. The effect of delayed side-tone upon vocal rate and intensity. *J. Speech Hearing Disorders*, 16, 56–60.

Coleman, R., and Wendahl, R. 1967. Vocal roughness and stimulus duration. *Speech Monogr.*, 34, 85–92.

Cooper, F., Peterson, G., and Fahringer, G. 1957. Some sources of characteristic vocoder quality. abstract. *J. acoust. soc. Amer.*, 29, 183.

Dedo, H., and Dunker, E. 1967. Husson's theory. *Arch. Otolaryng.*, 85, 89–99.

———, and Ogura, I. 1965. Vocal cord electromyography in the dog. *Laryngoscope*, 75, 201–211.

Dorland, W. 1951. The American illustrated medical dictionary (22nd. ed.). Philadelphia: Saunders.

Dreher, J. 1967. Personal communication.

Fairbanks, G., and Pronovost, W. 1938. Vocal pitch during simulated emotion. *Science*, 88, 382–383.

———, and ———. 1939. An experimental study of the pitch characteristics of the voice during the expression of emotions. *Speech Monogr.*, No. 6, 87–104.

———, and Hoaglin, L. 1941. An experimental study of the durational characteristics of the voice during the expression of emotion. *Speech Monogr.*, No. 8, 85–91.

Fairbanks, G. 1954. Systematic research in experimental phonetics. 1. A theory of the speech mechanism as a servosystem. *J. Speech Hearing Disorders*, 19, 133–139.

———, and Guttman, N. 1958. Effects of delayed auditory feedback upon articulation. *J. Speech Hearing Res.*, 1, 12–22.

Fairbanks, G. 1960. Voice and articulation (2nd. ed.). New York: Harper.

———. 1966. Experimental phonetics: selected articles. Urbana: Univ. Ill.

Goldiamond, I. 1962. Perception. *In* Experimental foundations of clinical psychology. Bachrach, A., ed. New York: Basic Books.

Hanley, T., and Thurman, W. 1962. Developing vocal skills. New York: Holt, Rinehart and Winston.

Hollien, H., Moore, P., Wendahl, R., and Michel, J.

1966. On the nature of vocal fry. *J. Speech Hearing Res.*, 9, 245–247.

Hockett, C. 1961. The mathematical theory of communication by Claude L. Shannon and Warren Weaver. *In* Psycholingusitics. Saporta, S., ed. New York: Holt, Rinehart and Winston.

Huttar, G. 1967. Relations between prosodic variables and emotions in normal American English utterances. *J. acoust. soc. Amer.*, 41, 1581.

Jensen, P. 1965. Adequacy of terminology for clinical judgment of voice quality deviation. *Eye, Ear, Nose, Throat Monthly*, 44, 77–82.

Johnson, W., Brown, S., Curtis, J., Edney, C., and Keaster, J. 1967. Speech handicapped school children (3rd. ed.). New York: Harper & Row.

Joyner, J. 1968. Air flow as a function of vocal constriction in normal adult males. Univ. South. Calif.: Ph.D. dissertation.

Kersta, L. 1962. Voiceprint identification. *J. acoust. soc. Amer.*, 34, 725.

Lieberman, P. 1961. Perturbations in vocal pitch. *J. acoust. soc. Amer.*, 33, 597–603.

Markel, N., Meisels, M., and Houck, J. 1964. Judging personality for voice quality. *J. abnorm. soc. Psychol.*, 69, 458–463.

Milisen, R. 1957. Methods of evaluation and diagnosis of speech disorders. *In* Handbook of speech pathology. Travis, L., ed. New York: Appleton-Century-Crofts.

Miller, R. 1957. An experimental study of the evaluations by untrained listeners of efficient and inefficient voice production as to quality. Univ. South. Calif.: Ph.D. dissertation.

Moore, P. 1957. Voice disorders associated with organic abnormalities. *In* Handbook of speech pathology. Travis, L. ed. New York: Appleton-Century-Crofts.

Moses, P. 1954. The voice of neurosis. New York: Grune & Stratton.

Mysak, E., 1966. Speech pathology and feedback theory. Springfield, Ill.: Thomas.

O'Malley, M., and Peterson, G. 1966. An experimental method for prosodic analysis. *Phonetica*, 15, 1–13.

Ostwald, P. 1963. Soundmaking: The acoustic communication of emotion. Springfield Ill.: Thomas.

Perkins, W. 1971. Speech pathology: an applied behavioral science. St. Louis: Mosby.

Peterson, G., and Shoup, J. 1966. A physiological theory of phonetics. *J. Speech Hearing Res.*, 9, 5–67.

Ringel, R., and Steer M. 1963. Some effects of tactile and auditory alterations on speech output. *J. Speech Hearing Res.*, 6, 369–378.

Rousey, C., and Moriarty, A. 1965. Diagnostic implications of speech sounds. Springfield, Ill.: Thomas.

Rubin, H. 1963. Experimental studies in vocal pitch and intensity in phonation. *Laryngoscope*, 73, 973–1015.

Shannon, C., and Weaver, W. 1964. The mathematical theory of communication. Urbana: Univ. Ill.

Skinner, B. 1954. Science and human behavior. New York: Macmillan.

Soron, H. 1967. High-speed photography in speech research. *J. Speech Hearing Res.*, 10, 768–776.

———. 1968. Personal communication.

Starkweather, H. 1961. Vocal communication of personality and human feelings. *J. Communication*, 11, 63–72.

Stevens, S. 1951. Mathematics, measurement, and psychophysics. *In* Handbook of experimental psychology. Stevens, S., ed. New York: Wiley.

Thurman, W. 1954. The construction and acoustic analysis of recorded scales of severity for six voice quality disorders. Purdue Univ.: Ph.D. dissertation.

Van Riper, C. 1963. Speech correction (4th. ed.). Englewood Cliffs: Prentice-Hall.

———, and Irwin, J. 1958. Voice and articulation. Englewood Cliffs: Prentice-Hall.

Vennard, W. 1967. Singing: the mechanism and the technic (4th. ed.). New York: Fischer.

Voiers, W. 1964. Perceptual bases of speaker identity. *J. acoust. soc. Amer.*, 36, 1065–1073.

Wendahl, R. 1963. Laryngeal analog synthesis of harsh voice quality. *Folia Phoniat.*, 15, 241–250.

West, R., Ansberry, M., and Carr, A. 1957. The rehabilitation of speech (3rd. ed.). New York: Harper.

20

Vocal Function: Assessment and Therapy

William H. Perkins

INTRODUCTION

The system of assessment and therapy of defective voice to be developed here is predicated squarely on the behavioral analysis of vocal functioning in Chapter 19. The essence of that analysis is the delineation of measurable behavioral dimensions of vocal production. These are the five dimensions by which normal voice is regulated. Two of them are familiar: pitch and loudness. The remaining three are the minimal number necessary to control the important aspects of vocal quality for hygienic speaking. One of these quality dimensions is *voicing*; voicing behavior is regulated along a continuum from voiceless to full voice. Another is *vocal mode;* the basic vocal adjustment within which the voice functions is, from highest to lowest mode, light voice (falsetto), heavy voice (chest), and pulsated voice (vocal fry). The other dimension is *vocal constriction;* the amount of subjective constriction of the voice is regulated along a continuum from maximal constriction, defined reflexively by swallowing, to minimal constriction, defined by yawning. These dimensions are necessary to account for deviant forms of vocal production and for achievement of a hygienically optimal voice for normal speaking.

When vocal dimensions appear to be indistinguishable from each other in a symbiotic jumble of interrelations, a clinician has no choice but to treat the voice as an undifferentiated unit. When the dimensions by which it is regulated can be delineated, a clinician can recognize and understand each component and how it contributes to the whole, and, if he chooses, he can also join the independent components in a union that permits a holistic conception of their interaction in the rich complexities of the normal speaking voice. That the dimensions of vocal production can be delineated and measured was demonstrated in Chapter 19. That their optimal functioning can be assessed objectively, and that deviations from optimum can be corrected therapeutically, is the subject of this chapter.

ASSESSMENT OF VOCAL FUNCTIONING

Physiological Approach

Assessment of vocal functioning can be approached physiologically and behaviorally. These approaches are not mutually exclusive, but they each have distinctive merits and limits that should be noted. Let us consider, first, a physiological approach. Briess (1957, 1959), for example, has devised an extensive system for identifying and treating specific, intrinsic, laryngeal muscle dysfunction. With selected sounds and phrases, he tests for imbalance among the five sets of intrinsic laryngeal muscles. These imbalances are identified and reported in terms of hyper- or hypofunction of the muscles. He has related the imbalances to subjective symptoms, and, if the abusive conditions persist, to the lesions that result (Brewer, 1964).

The objective to which Briess' system is addressed is commendable. To be able to correlate with confidence the physiological and acoustical phenomena with vocal production would permit both laryngologists and speech pathologists to assess vocal abuse and its consequent symptomatology. But, when this goal is realized, the vast array of psychophysiological problems of voice will be well-defined relationships, not merely proposals for their investigation. We are far from this achievement.

For many speech pathologists, a physiological approach to assessment of vocal functioning is apt to encounter the following difficulties. Brewer, Briess, and Faaborg-Andersen (1960) allude to one major problem when they describe the complexity of Briess' system:

> Clinical voice testing determines the existing ratios only by comparison with expected ratios . . . The expected ratios must be judged from experience. This is gained from testing and working with *thousands of voices* (italics mine) in this manner. Ratios change in a single voice when pitch is changed. However, at the same identical pitch different ratios are expected in voices differing in voice type and degree of voice character.

How to make such a system negotiable for most clinicians might well be an insurmountable problem. Not only would speech pathologists need to be astute laryngeal physiologists (a condition devoutly to be desired), but they would also have to master the complexity of constantly shifting variables; the system, in many respects, is idiosyncratic.

Finally, let us consider the relative merits of an assessment of muscle function as distinct from a behavioral analysis of vocal production. The muscle balance assay is to determine the hypo- or hyperfunction of each set of intrinsic laryngeal muscles. What cannot be determined, at least by the speech pathologist, is whether a hypofunctional muscle is weak and needs strengthening, or whether the vocal response in which a hypofunctional muscle is observed is characterized by a muscle imbalance that would be corrected, or altered, if the response were changed. In other words, is the imbalance a function of weak muscles, or, of normal muscles minimally activated in the vocal response?

If the rationale for a muscle assay is to determine which are too weak and which too strong, then the treatment that should follow, logically, should be a form of physical therapy for laryngeal muscles. These are, of course, not available to direct manipulation, so they could be strengthened only by their involvement in the behavioral patterns of various types of vocal productions (the tactics used by Briess). Thus, we see that treatment of laryngeal muscle imbalance, even if due to weak muscles, cannot be accomplished by direct, or even indirect, physical intervention; it can only be accomplished by control of vocal behavior. The crucial issue is now apparent: what vocal behavior will effect the muscle balance that will afford the most satisfactory use of the voice?

Behavioral Approach

The five dimensions of vocal production delineated in this chapter are intended to account for both normal and abnormal vocal behavior. Such a conception has considerable clinical significance. It means that assessment of the adequacy of *vocal* functioning—as distinct from *laryngeal* functioning—is independent of diagnosis of the anatomical or physiological status of the vocal mechanism. Again, we return to the old theme: the speech pathologist's data are behavioral. Actually, this is not a restrictive conception; quite the contrary: it confronts the clinician with the reality of the patient's potential for realizing his best voice.

This point is illustrated by the man I once saw for therapy who had an almost total glossectomy. The stub of tongue he had remaining was smaller than a little finger. His oral anatomy did not appear to permit intelligible speech, yet the only articulatory defect that he had not been able to correct by himself was a distorted /s/. Probably every clinician can document similar experiences (Brodnitz, 1960). So it is with laryngeal anatomy and physiology. We do not yet know these correlates of vocal behavior well enough to be able to predict accurately what a person with laryngeal disability will or will not be able to do.

Certainly, the clinician must consider the advisability of vocal therapy in terms of the physical condition of the larynx, which can only be determined legally, as well as by training, by a physician. Once the speech pathologist has medical clearance, however, which, of course, often means that laryngeal disability (e.g., vocal nodules) still exists but may improve with therapy, the assessment of the patient's vocal capacity should be based on his performance. Whether the disability is "functional" or "organic," whether it is a nodule or a papilloma, a contact ulcer or a paralysis, is relevant to this behavioral purpose only to the extent that it produces behavioral effects that can be assessed. It is also relevant to the extent that the disability may well set the limits for vocal improvement; again, however, this limiting effect can only be determined accurately by periodic assessment of the behavioral dimensions of vocal performance.

One of the few hallowed concepts in assessment of the voice is determination of what some call "natural pitch" and others call "optimum pitch." Why the concept has not been extended to loudness or quality is a matter for speculation. Probably loudness has been excluded because of the difficulty of measuring it. Optimum pitch can be determined with a piano or a pitch pipe—omnipresent instruments. No comparably convenient measure of loudness is readily available. To conjure up reasons why "optimum quality" has not become a viable notion should require little imagination. Not only has it not been easily measured, but we have not even been able to agree on what it is. Still, the idea of specifying optimal conditions for all aspects of vocal function is important. It would permit definition of the boundary between desirable and undesirable production and, accordingly, a frame of reference for assessing the adequacy of vocal behavior for the individual.

Criteria for Optimal Functioning

The idea of "optimum" implies a standard in terms of which a thing is judged as being best. Selection of that standard can be made in terms of several criteria. Optimal vocal functioning can be defined aesthetically, acoustically, and hygienically. These criteria are not mutually exclusive, except perhaps in rare circumstances. Nonetheless, they can be accorded relative importance.

HYGIENIC CRITERION

The most vital criterion, probably, from the clinician's standpoint, is vocal hygiene. Any form of vocalization abusive to the vocal mechanism would, by any conceivable standard, be undesirable. Moreover, this criterion of hygiene seems to find wide agreement across cultures. The notion that voice is produced most hygienically when it is produced most effortlessly appears to have universal agreement. Admittedly, the observations for this statement are limited, but they cut across a number of different cultures including those of Japan, India, Philippines, Australia, China, Hawaii, Argentina, South Africa, Russia, Iceland, and most of the European countries.

ACOUSTIC CRITERION

Optimum pitch denotes the range of frequencies at which the voice is most efficient for speech. This accords with the concept of glottal efficiency that van den Berg (1956) has defined as the ratio of acoustic power to subglottic power. In fact, both ideas would appear to be acoustic manifestations of the hygienic criterion that specifies that the less the effort for the acoustic output the greater the vocal efficiency (Perkins, 1957). Certainly, achievement of loudness with minimal vocal effort is of paramount concern for the professional vocalist, whose livelihood depends on maintenance of a healthy voice under the most stressful of speaking conditions.

AESTHETIC CRITERION

Although Miller's (1957) results, discussed in Chapter 19, indicate the difficulty in specifying universally acceptable characteristics of an optimally good or pleasing voice, his evidence in no way suggests that vocal strain is any less acceptable to low-status or low-education groups than it appears to be for higher groups. Although I know of no groups or cultures that value aesthetically the sound of a speaking voice produced with strain, it is conceivable that they could exist. If they did, then for them, the aesthetic would conflict with the hygienic and acoustic criteria. My limited cultural sampling has revealed considerable variations in habitual pitch and quality preferences, but no such criterion conflict has appeared. The hygienic voice, that is, the efficient voice, is also, apparently, by virtue of not being excluded, an aesthetically acceptable voice.

Optimal vis à vis Normal Functioning

Specification of optimal functioning is quite different from specification of normal functioning. Designation of optimum is designation of the best. Designation of normal is designation of the average. Perhaps ideally, the norm for vocal functioning would be optimal functioning; certainly, this would tend to be true for the professional vocalist. For the rest of us, we can settle for less, and generally do. The more stressful the conditions for vocal production the closer to optimal will the voice need to function if hygiene is to be maintained. Persons with vocal problems vary widely in their needs for optimal production. Some use their voices so infrequently and in such quiet surroundings as to get by with relatively poor production—

production that might not even qualify as normal, let alone optimal. Others will need to set their standards higher. The clinician should be prepared to offer as much help as a vocally handicapped person needs. By always aiming for optimal functioning, therapy can be terminated at whatever distance from this objective is deemed adequate.

Optimal and Abusive Vocal Functioning

By analyzing vocal quality into the dimensions (delineated in the preceding Chapter) by which it is regulated, the full scope of vocal production can be assessed in terms of optimal functioning. The hygienic criterion, the one of paramount importance, can be applied psychologically and acoustically. In psychological form it can be stated as the ratio of loudness to vocal effort. Although no formal scale of effort has been devised comparable to that for loudness, it seems to involve, nonetheless, a unidimensional evaluation that is easily made by subjects during vocal production and by judges listening to the performance. (Vocal effort is discussed at greater length in a later section on breathing regulation.) In other words, this psychological ratio, crude as it may be, is adequate for clinical assessment and is easily applied. In more exact acoustical form, it is the van den Berg ratio for glottal efficiency: acoustic power compared to subglottic power.[1]

The task now is to assess each of the dimensions for the regulation of vocal production, and to assess breathing regulation (because of its possible clinical importance) against the criterion of vocal hygiene. This criterion will be applied in its most useful clinical form, the ratio of loudness to effort. The criterion in its acoustic form also will be considered, but only for those dimensions to which it has been applied. Throughout this analysis, the objective to remember is that the assessment is to determine for purposes of therapy the behavioral changes needed in each dimension. Implicit in the hygienic criterion is the idea that the farther vocal production is from optimum on any dimension, the more it contributes to vocal abuse. Because optimum often lies toward the middle of a dimension—optimal pitch, for instance, is in between; it is neither too high nor too low—the direction the defective performance must be changed to be improved must also be indicated. The essence of vocal assessment, then, is specification of those dimensions for which production deviates from optimum and, equally important, specification of the direction and extent behavior for that dimension should be altered to achieve satisfactory performance.

What evidence is available of the physiological and acoustical correlates of the dimensions, along with the vocal disorders typically associated with them, will also be considered. Discussion of these correlates may be taxing for those with limited knowledge of laryngeal physiology. The reader whose primary interest is in clinically useful procedures may wish to limit himself to the sections that specify optimal production of the dimensions and the ways that the dimensions can vary from optimum.

Pitch Regulation

SPECIFICATION OF OPTIMUM

Optimal, or natural, pitch has received considerable attention, especially clinically (Pronovost, 1939, 1942; Dreher and Bragg, 1953; Van Riper and Irwin, 1958; Fairbanks, 1960). It has not only been identified as the pitch level or range of pitches at which the voice functions most efficiently (Fairbanks, 1960), but also as the pitches at which optimal quality is observed (Johnson, Darley, and Spriesterbach, 1963). Although research efforts to test the concept of improved efficiency (Thurman, 1958; House, 1959) have not produced verifying evidence of increased intensity at these pitches, these efforts have also not disproved the notion; optimal pitch remains a viable probability that is more likely to be observed by improvement in quality than by increase in loudness. Most authorities agree, though, that the optimal modal point in the range, particularly for males, is somewhere near one-fourth up from the lowest pitch that can be phonated.

The only dispute with determining optimal pitch by a formula such as some propose for measuring this modal point (Fairbanks, 1960) is that it is unnecessarily restrictive. Even though pitch, as a dimension, is independent, its optimal range is not. It is a function, for all practical purposes, of vocal constriction.[2] *Those pitches at which constriction is minimal will be*

[1] The power efficiency of the glottal generator in this ratio is the acoustic power radiated from the mouth during phonation compared to the approximated subglottic power calculated by the product of mean subglottic pressure times mean flow rate (van den Berg, 1956).

[2] Optimal pitch is also a function of vocal mode. The pitches at which the voice functions most efficiently for the modes pulsated, heavy, and light would, obviously, differ. The assumption here is that the voice is functioning consistently in its normal mode, typically, heavy voice.

the pitches that will meet the hygienic criterion for optimum. Granted, constriction is typically minimal near the lowest one-fourth of the vocal range, which accounts for the location of optimal pitch; however, the unskilled vocalist habitually exerts increased effort not only at very high pitches, but also at very low ones. Operationally, this translates into increased constriction at the upper and lower ends of the pitch scale. For those who constrict the voice throughout its range, and this may be a sizable portion of the population judging from the negative research results, no pitches would be discerned at which the voice functions most efficiently. Conversely, for those who do not constrict at high or low pitches (e.g., professional speakers and especially singers), the range would be wide in which their vocal production would meet the hygienic criterion for optimal pitch regulation.

A semitrained subject (in an experiment described in Chapter 19 for whom we gathered simultaneous physiological and acoustical data at varying pitches and loudnesses) afforded a rare opportunity to measure optimal pitch by the acoustic criterion (Perkins and Yanagihara, 1968). We found a low correlation of fundamental frequency with glottal efficiency and the tendency for increases in efficiency to occur in peaklike bursts at a variety of pitches from 135 Hz to 280 Hz, although four-fifths of these peaks were within the middle of the subject's range. Interestingly, the bursts of power occurred despite effort to maintain constant loudness during systematic variation of pitch. At the time, we were aware that these bursts seemed to be associated with reductions in vocal *tension* which we would now classify as decreases in *constriction.*

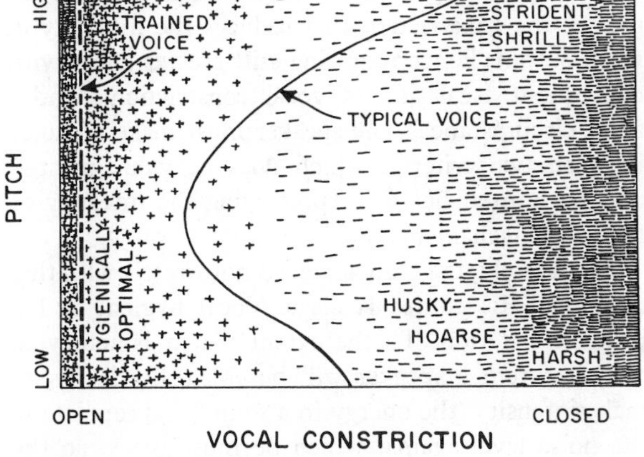

Fig. 20-1. Interaction of pitch with vocal constriction in typical and trained voices.

Assessment of the adequacy of pitch regulation comes down to a judgment of whether pitch is too high or too low. This is not an absolute judgment; it may vary from week to week, day to day, even minute to minute, depending on the status of the constriction dimension. Pitch is too high or too low only insofar as it elicits increased constriction. In other words, pitch, per se, is not the culprit in vocal abuse; it is merely an accomplice for constriction. It works its traumatic effects only insofar as it works in conjunction with constriction. Moreover, these two dimensions interact differently at high than at low pitches, as the pattern for the typical voice shows in Fig. 20-1. The range at which they do not interact, at which constriction is minimal, is optimum. For the well-trained vocalist, as Fig. 20-1 also shows, no interaction occurs, so, for him, the entire pitch range is hygienically optimal.

DEVIATION FROM OPTIMUM

Pitches above optimum are generally associated with strident, shrill, tense voices. Pitches that are deviant in this direction tend to abuse the vocal folds at the point of maximum displacement, the middle of the vibrating glottis. This type of traumatic vocalization will exacerbate existing pathology of the cords, such as neoplasms, will produce laryngitis, and, if prolonged, will lead to the development of nodules—sometimes called "screamer's nodes," "preacher's nodes," "teacher's nodes," or "singer's nodes," depending on the nature of the abusive conditions, all of which are conducive to screechy voices at high pitches (Arnold, 1962; Brodnitz, 1965).

Pitches below optimum interact with vocal constriction in such a way as to produce voice described by terms like *harsh, hoarse, husky,* and *rough.* The physiology of this interaction is uncertain; it might, for example, involve medial compression of the vocal processes of the arytenoid cartilages by hyperfunction of the lateral cricoarytenoid muscles. In any event, the consequence of this form of vocal abuse, in which the anterior tips of the vocal processes grind and pound the mucosal surface in a hammer and anvil effect, is contact ulcer (Jackson, 1928; von Leden and Moore, 1960; Brodnitz, 1961; Brewer, 1963; Luchsinger and Arnold, 1965). Executives seem more inclined to this disorder than, say, truck drivers, suggesting that the laryngeal mechanics for ulceration are more effective in those persons emotionally predisposed to gastric ulcers (Moses, 1959; Brodnitz, 1965).

PHYSIOLOGICAL AND ACOUSTICAL CORRELATES

Vocal pitch is roughly equal to fundamental frequency, a function of the rate of vocal fold vibrations (van den Berg, 1958). This rate, in turn, is a function of myoelastic (muscular) and aerodynamic factors. The myoelastic factors can be summarized in a measure of effective glottal resistance to air flow. It is defined as the complex ratio of effective subglottic pressure (rms) to effective flow rate (rms) (van den Berg, Zantema, and Doornenbal, 1957; Flanagan, 1958).[3] Moore (Brewer, 1964) mentions three physiological adjustments of the larynx that, by affecting glottal resistance, regulate pitch. First is adjustment of the mass of the vocal folds by their elongation. That mass is not entirely a function of length has been clearly demonstrated by Hollien's research (1960a, 1960b, 1962; Hollien and Curtis, 1960; Hollien and Moore, 1960). He and his associates have shown that mass and pitch tend to correlate absolutely, whereas length and pitch correlate only relative to the individual voice, suggesting that mass, more than length, is a crucial determinant of pitch. The second adjustment Moore mentions is of tension in the muscles of the vocal cords that regulate their stiffness or elasticity. The third adjustment involves shortening of the vibrating segment through progressive damping of the posterior portions of the cords.

Van den Berg (1958) includes these three myoelastic adjustments in a conception that integrates them with aerodynamic factors. He accounts for the pulse rate of the glottal generator by five interdependent factors: 1. effective mass of the vibrating folds; 2. effective tension in the vibrating portion; 3. effective glottal area during a cycle, which, in the final analysis, determines effective glottal resistance and the effective value of the Bernoulli effect of "sucking" the folds together; 4. effective value of subglottic pressure; and 5. damping of the vocal folds.

We can now turn to the matter of the physiological pattern of pitch regulation that is optimal, an issue for which only sketchy evidence is available. Van den Berg (1956) has shown that efficiency of voice production is greater at the higher pitches that can be produced easily, a conclusion supported by the work of Perkins and Yanagihara (1968). This evidence specifies the pitches that are optimal, at least by the acoustic criterion, but it does not reveal the necessary physiological adjustments. As will be recalled, both the acoustic and hygienic criteria require minimal constriction for optimal production. Accordingly, *those adjustments that yield greatest acoustic power with the least effort are the most optimal at any pitch.* Rather than cover the same ground twice, these adjustments will be discussed in the next section on loudness.

[3] Instrumentation capacity often limits these measures to mean values of subglottic pressure and flow rate, hence the formula for mean glottal resistance:

$$R = \frac{\text{Mean Subglottic Pressure}}{\text{Mean Flow Rate}}$$

and is reported in dyne sec/cm^5 (Isshiki, 1964; Perkins and Yanagihara, 1968).

Loudness Regulation

SPECIFICATION OF OPTIMUM

Assessment of loudness is more complex than assessment of pitch. For one thing, the criteria for adequacy can be, and sometimes in practice are, mutually exclusive. Hanley and Thurman (1962), for instance, set adequate loudness for comprehension as the primary goal for evaluating loudness, and, of course, they are right insofar as the purpose of speaking is concerned. On the other hand, Fairbanks (1960) posits vocal efficiency, maximum output for minimum effort, as the first objective, and he, too, is right in terms of vocal hygiene.

Ideally, these two criteria are not mutually exclusive; optimally, they complement each other. *The voice that is easiest to hear, even under noisiest conditions, is the one that can be produced effortlessly yet loudly.* The poor vocalist who utilizes considerable constriction will probably, however, have to sacrifice one criterion for the other. The only tone he is likely to be able to produce with minimal effort is soft and breathy. He is trapped in a vicious circle; the louder he attempts to speak, the greater his effort, and the greater the constriction that reduces the intensity of vocal output, hence requiring still greater effort with consequent escalation of vocal constriction. Under these circumstances, the speaker must make a choice between two criteria: which does he value most—making himself heard, or preserving the integrity of his vocal mechanism?

Fortunately, the clinician need not wrestle with this dilemma. His course is clear. Vocal hygiene is his primary criterion. To the extent that it is achieved, to that extent a speaker will be able, effortlessly, to make intensity (the energy in a sound) appropriate to the noise level against which he must speak, so the ultimate goal is to meet both criteria. Were the clinician to reverse priority for the criteria, however, he would reduce the probability of achieving adequate loudness, for constriction breeds constriction, and the achievement of vocal hygiene would be precluded.

DEVIATION FROM OPTIMUM

Loudness, like pitch, interacts with constriction as is shown for the typical voice in Fig. 20-2. Unlike pitch, however, in which the interaction is usually greater at the ends of the scale and lesser in between (an elliptically shaped function), loudness interacts with constriction generally in a straight-line function. Moreover, the interaction is two-way. The louder the voice, the greater the constriction and the greater the vocal effort. Conversely, the greater the constriction, the greater the vocal effort required to maintain a given level of loudness. That this interaction is not necessary can also be seen in Fig. 20-2. For the well-trained vocalist, loudness and constriction do not interact.[4] He can produce the softest to the loudest sound optimally.

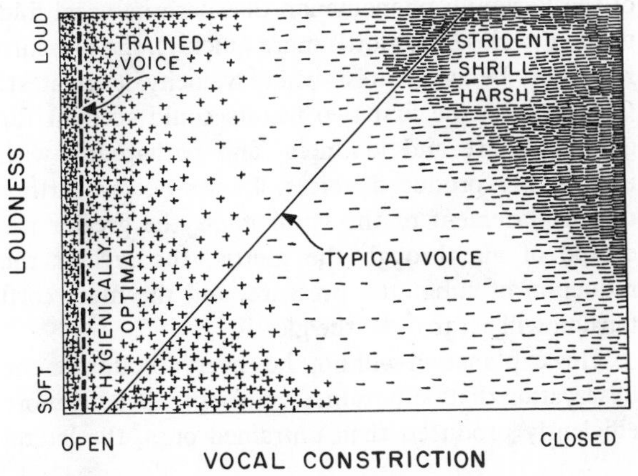

Fig. 20-2. Interaction of loudness with vocal constriction in typical and trained voices.

As the interaction of loudness and constriction spirals upward, the voice becomes increasingly strident, shrill, and even screechy if the pitch is high enough; if the pitch is low, the interaction increases harshness. Either way, this interaction serves to amplify whatever form of vocal abuse is in the making.

[4] Loudness as well as pitch and the other dimensions of vocal production are potentially independent. The trained vocalist capitalizes on this potential and controls constriction volitionally. He is capable of achieving maximal constriction, but avoids it normally for hygienic and aesthetic reasons. Although constriction interacts with pitch and loudness normally in a statistical sense, this interaction is not optimal in a hygienic, acoustic, or aesthetic sense.

Whereas pitch tends to interact with constriction in a manner that selects different forms of vocal trauma (e.g., vocal nodules at high pitches, contact ulcers at low ones), it is the interaction of loudness with constriction that supplies the power to make the selected form of vocal abuse traumatic. This is to say that were the voice to be produced softly, regardless of the interaction of pitch with constriction, no pathology consequent to vocal abuse would be likely to develop. A three-way interaction, then, among loudness, pitch, and constriction is probably necessary to account for physical injury to the vocal cords.

PHYSIOLOGICAL AND ACOUSTICAL CORRELATES

It has been demonstrated mathematically (Flanagan, 1958) and experimentally (van den Berg, Zantema, and Doornenbal, 1957; Timcke, von Leden, and Moore, 1958) that vocal intensity increases, along with efficiency of the glottal generator, as the *Open Quotient* (O.Q.) decreases, that is, as the fraction of the glottal cycle during which the glottis is open becomes smaller. What a small O.Q. describes is a condition in which strong, short glottal pulses excite the vocal tract to resonate high harmonics; the sharper the puff, the richer the glottal wave in these high-frequency components. In other words, high harmonics characterize, acoustically, powerful efficient vocal tones.

We can deduce from the foregoing account, and Ohala (1966) has presented evidence to support the deduction, that the intensity of excitation of the vocal tract is a function of the abruptness of the opening or closing of the glottis. The more abrupt the opening, the greater the differential at any instant between subglottal and supraglottal pressure, the greater the velocity of air escape, and the more explosive the glottal pulse. Conversely, the more abrupt the closure, the greater the negative pressure above the glottis, the greater the velocity of air rushing to fill the partial vacuum, and the more explosive the glottal pulse. Fig. 20-3 summarizes these relationships. It was constructed as a schematic composite of the 21 graphs of the performances of six subjects reported by Timcke, von Leden, and Moore (1958). An important feature of Fig. 20-3 is the stability of the opening phase, which, apparently, is not related to loudness; the small variations that did occur in this phase showed no consistent relationship to loudness. Conversely, loudness was clearly a function of the closing phase. The ratio of the time of lateral excursion of the cords during the opening phase to their medial excursion during the closing phase has been termed *Speed Quotient* (S.Q.); it has been found to vary consistently with the intensity of the sound produced (Timcke, von Leden, and Moore, 1958). We can see, then, that the rate at which the cords close is a primary determinant of the percentage of the vibratory cycle during which they will be approximated (hence, it affects both O.Q. and S.Q.) as well as of intensity of the voice.

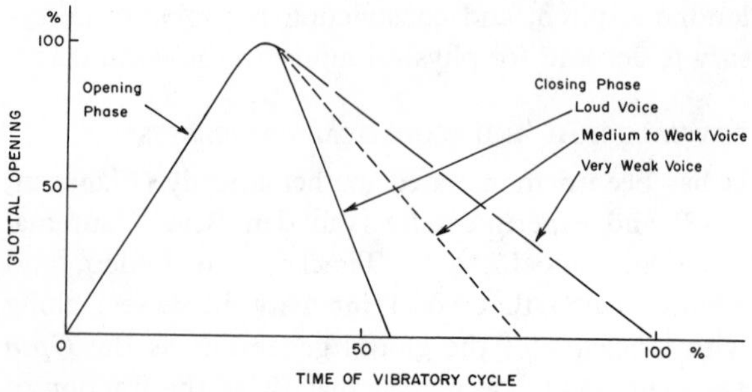

Fig. 20-3. Schematic composite of opening and closing phases of glottal cycles of six subjects at different levels of loudness. *Based on work reported by Timcke, von Leden, and Moore.*

One more point of evidence must be considered. Investigators frequently have found, as might be expected, that, as loudness increases, so does the lateral displacement of the vocal folds as they are blown open more vigorously (Timcke, von Leden, and Moore, 1958). For trained voices, however, some have observed less lateral excursion and a longer period of closure during a vibratory cycle than for untrained voices (Bell Labs, 1937; Fletcher, 1954). This suggests that loudness and vocal efficiency are more dependent on the abruptness with which the cords close than on the distance they are driven apart.

The physiological adjustments to account for the optimal production of loudness have not been described definitively. We have, though, in the foregoing analysis, enough reasonably firm points to predict with some confidence what the myoelastic-aerodynamic mechanisms will prove to be. As we have seen, the key to vocal efficiency is an adjustment that permits a short closing phase for each cycle. The fact that the closing phase, not the opening phase, varies with intensity points to some condition operating during closure that does not operate during opening.

With the demise of the Neurochronaxic (neuromuscular) Theory (von Leden, 1961)—it proposed that neural impulses controlled glottal opening, with air pressure only assisting the process—little argument exists for this alternating condition being increased vocal cord tension during the closing phase of each vibratory cycle. On the other hand, van den Berg, Zantema, and Doornenbal (1957) have made a strong case for this alternating condition being the Bernoulli effect, first mentioned by Tonndorf in 1925 as a factor in laryngeal functioning. This is the phenomenon that accounts for why, when two pieces of paper are together, they cannot be separated by blowing between them. It also accounts for the lift of an airplane wing. Practically, what the Bernoulli principle explains is why the density and pressure of a gas or liquid, in our case, air, decreases as its velocity increases.[5]

Van den Berg (1958) proposes that glottal closure is accomplished by three basic factors: 1. decrease of subglottic pressure as air escapes through the glottis, 2. tension of the vocal folds, and 3. the "sucking" effect of the escaping air (the pressure-reducing effect of the Bernoulli phenomenon that permits vocal fold tension to close the glottis more quickly), the pressure reduction being greatest where velocity is greatest. Conceivably, the first two factors could account for glottal closure and loudness, and perhaps do with inefficiently produced voices. Logically, the farther the displacement of the vocal folds, the greater the escape of air through the glottis, the greater the reduction of subglottic pressure, and the more cord tension will act to close the glottis.

This explanation will not, however, account for the observation that with trained voices, presumably more efficiently produced than untrained ones, the lateral

[5] The formula for the Bernoulli effect is: $p + \frac{1}{2}dv^2 =$ constancy in which d is density, v is velocity, and p is pressure (van den Berg, Zantema, and Doornenbal, 1957). This relationship between pressure and velocity can be demonstrated with a garden hose. If pressure within the hose is constant, then, the force of the water from the hose would be the same (barring friction) whether the nozzle is large or small. If the nozzle is large, a relatively large volume will flow slowly; if the nozzle is small, a small volume will flow rapidly. Because the same number of water molecules pass through the nozzle each second, when they go through quickly fewer are in the small nozzle at any one time than are in the large nozzle. Now, consider the glottis as analogous to the nozzle. The smaller the glottal opening, the faster the air will flow through it, so, the fewer will be the molecules exerting pressure against the vocal folds at any given instant. This reduced pressure, often loosely labeled as *suction*, permits the forces within the vocal folds that resist displacement to close the glottis more quickly when velocity of the volume of air flowing through is high than when it is low.

excursion of the cords tends to be relatively small. This means that in the trained voice, the size of the glottal opening through which air can escape tends to impede, rather than enhance, pressure reduction. We should recall, though, from the discussion of the physiology of pitch, that the smaller the glottal area in a cycle, the greater will be the velocity of air escape, and, consequently, the greater the tendency for the cords to be "sucked" together; this is the Bernoulli effect. Not only does it accord with experimental evidence from the laboratory, but it also accords with what Vennard (1967), from the professional singer's point of view, considers best for singing, and with what Luchsinger and Arnold (1965) from the laryngologists' point of view, observe as the laryngeal functioning of trained voices.

At low pitches in good voices, the laryngologist observes a glottis that remains slightly open with the vocal cords appearing relaxed and vibrating over their full length. As pitch rises, the cords appear increasingly elongated, tensed, and closed. When they have become maximally elongated and tensed, further increases in pitch are accomplished by an apparent damping or shortening of the vibrating glottis. Increased loudness at high pitches extends the vibrations into the damped sections (Luchsinger and Arnold, 1965). This account agrees with the factors specified for pitch regulation by Moore (Brewer, 1964) and by van den Berg (1958).

It also agrees with Vennard's (1967) conception. He points out that both pitch and loudness can be regulated by the Bernoulli effect. "Singing on the breath," a time-honored objective in singing, is accomplished by a laryngeal adjustment in which the glottis is almost, but not quite, closed. By regulating the velocity of air flow, a function of size of glottal opening and subglottal pressure, the Bernoulli effect can be controlled. As its "suction" (reduced intraglottal pressure) is increased, the cords will close more quickly, thereby increasing intensity, and, presumably, by virtue of shortening the cycle, also increasing pitch. The mechanism by which "suction" affects intensity is reasonably clear, but how it controls pitch is little more than speculation. Subjective observation suggests that it is possible, but beyond that, we have no evidence bearing directly on the physiology of pitch regulation by the Bernoulli phenomenon.

In the final analysis, the physiology of vocal functioning hinges on the regulation of the mechanisms of glottal resistance as they interact with subglottal pressure. Too much resistance applied in a pattern that compresses the tips of the vocal processes apparently predisposes development of a contact ulcer; resistance applied in a pattern that slams the muscular glottal edges together at the site of maximal displacement predisposes development of a vocal nodule. Too little resistance to effective subglottal pressure results in turbulence and a breathy tone. The optimal balance of resistance and pressure yields maximum velocity of air flow in each glottal pulse, and, relative to pitch, thick, relaxed glottal edges and supple mucosal surfaces.

Yet, our knowledge about the physiology of pitch and loudness control is, in many respects, still meager. Exactly how the larynx contributes to the generation of a train of acoustic pulses remains puzzling. Soron (1967) has developed sound-synchronized high-speed cinematography equipment with which he has produced data relevant to this problem. He has found from preliminary evidence (1968) that the position of the positive air-pressure peak within the glottal cycle varies with the proportion of time that the cords are closed (O.Q.). With the cords closed about 50 percent of a glottal period, the acoustic peak appears during early opening time of the glottis. As the proportion of closure time decreases, the position of the acoustic peak moves to a later point in the glottal cycle: when the cords barely close, the acoustic peak and glottal area peak coincide; when the glottis does not close, the acoustic peak occurs during the closing phase.

Ohala (1966), on the other hand, has used a glottograph with which he has found peaks of pressure during the closing phase of glottal cycles in which cord-closure time was relatively long. This evidence appears to be in opposition to that of Soron's, yet there is no reason to question the accuracy of the work of either investigator. What these divergent results point to, probably more than to anything else, is the complexity of the relationship among a large number of variables that affect vocal production. Much work remains, especially to determine how all of these variables interact as pitch and loudness are regulated.

Voicing Regulation

SPECIFICATION OF OPTIMUM

The assessment of voicing involves many of the same issues as are involved in loudness, largely because loudness is, to a considerable extent, a function of voicing; obviously, a whispered or even a breathy voice will not be potentially as loud as one fully voiced. Voicing and loudness are similar in that the same two criteria are available for assessing them: is voicing sufficient to produce a loud enough voice for communication, and, is the degree of voicing hygienically optimal? As with loudness, these criteria can, and, ideally, should, complement each other, but they can also be mutually exclusive. Fig. 20-4 shows that voicing and constriction do not interact in the well-trained vocalist, but that they do interact in the typical speaker; an accelerated curve describes this relationship.

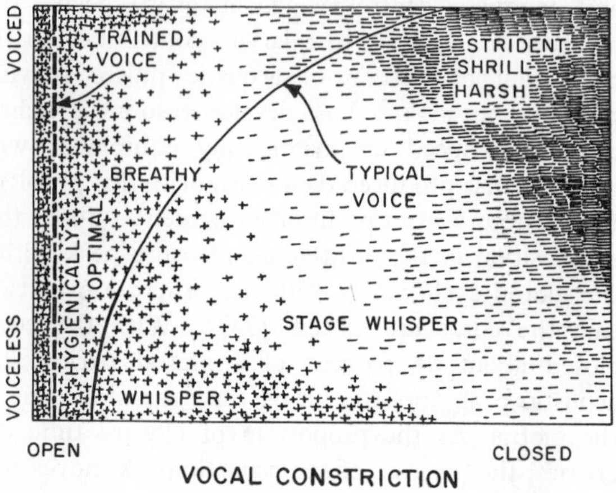

Fig. 20-4. Interaction of voicing with vocal constriction in typical and trained voices.

The interaction between voicing and constriction is not surprising when one remembers that the glottis ranges for the voicing dimension from open (voiceless), through any number of stages of closure, to fully closed, while vocal constriction involves physiological constriction of the laryngeal sphincters, as well as of the supraglottal vocal tract. Clearly, maximal laryngeal constriction (a physiological correlate of behavioral constriction) precludes breathy or whispered degrees of voicing, and *vice versa*. That is, if the vocal tract is highly constricted, as in a swallow or in lifting a heavy object or in vocalizing with much strain, production of a soft breathy voice or an easy whisper would be all but impossible. Conversely, *a condition in which effortless partial voicing is possible would be one in which constriction would be reduced.*

DEVIATION FROM OPTIMUM

We have just seen how voicing can be a function of constriction; now let us consider the reverse relationship. Constriction can be a function of voicing because of the problem of achieving adequate loudness. This problem is manifested in conjunction with emotional conflict and with organic disability. Functional (hysterical) aphonia, spastic dysphonia, and ventricular dysphonia have been widely discussed as symptoms of emotional conflict (Bloch, 1965; Kiml, 1965). Whether they are or not need not concern us at the moment; evidence has been presented that suggests that spastic dysphonia may have a neurological basis (Robe, Brumlick, and Moore, 1960; Aronson, Brown, Litin, and Pearson, 1968). Be that as it may, the behavior that distinguishes these symptoms is of interest. Brodnitz (1965) makes the point that the person with functional aphonia has given up his will to communicate, so he produces a breathy whisper; voicing and constriction do not interact appreciably because this person is apparently unconcerned with making himself heard. The person with ventricular phonation, on the other hand, seems to be concerned with loudness. For whatever reason, he is thought to have ceased to use his true vocal cords for phonation. Instead, he constricts the ventricular folds sufficiently to produce a rough, high-pitched voice. Brodnitz goes on to describe the person with spastic dysphonia as one who speaks with violent contraction of the vocal cords, who exerts great pressure to overcome laryngeal cramps in much the same way a stutterer exerts pressure to overcome blocked speech. My experience with more than a dozen persons with spastic dysphonia has been that none were able volitionally to produce a fully voiced sound. Either they produced a barely audible whisper or they overcame it with the type of voice Brodnitz describes; this would appear to be an example of constriction and vocal effort being compensatory functions of inability to control the voicing dimension adequately.

Organic disability also can prevent complete voicing and can, accordingly, impair the achievement of adequate loudness with consequent increase in vocal effort and constriction. Any laryngeal condition that interferes with complete closure of the glottis, or perturbs the vibratory pattern of the vocal cords, would, logically, limit the extent of voicing; breathiness should, presumably, be proportional to the interference or perturbation. Support for this conclusion comes from several sources. Von Leden, Moore, and Timcke (1960) and later Iwata and von Leden (1970) showed the irregularity of vibratory patterns in laryngeal pathology; Isshiki and von Leder (1964) showed the increased turbulent air flow with hoarseness and pathology; Wendahl (1963) demonstrated with an electrical laryngeal analog that listener judgment of rough harsh voice is a function of aperiodic vibratory pattern; Koike and Hirano (to be published) have developed a *vocal velocity index*, the ratio of mean air-flow rate to vital capacity, with which they have shown the index to be above normal for paralyses and neoplasms, but below for contact ulcer, which is not too surprising considering the medial compression of the cords typically associated with this problem; and Koike (1967) has also found remarkable differences in periodicity of the vibratory pattern for normal and pathologic larynges.

Since practically all forms of vocal cord disability, whether myasthenia laryngis or carcinoma, paralysis or papilloma, prevent full voicing, a characteristic consequence of organic involvement is hoarseness and impaired loudness (a possible exception may be contact ulcer). In an effort to achieve adequate loudness, persons with laryngeal disability typically exert greater vocal effort with a consequent increase in constriction. They then become trapped in the additional problem of the vicious circle of loudness and constriction: the harder they strain, the more they constrict, and the more they have to strain. Needless to say, this spiral not only holds little reward by way of achieving adequate loudness, but also exacerbates the existing laryngeal disability.

PHYSIOLOGICAL AND ACOUSTICAL CORRELATES

The physiological difference between the production of voiced and voiceless sound is described by Luchsinger and Arnold (1965). Voiceless, or whispered, production is characterized by: 1. incomplete closure of the vocal cords, the glottis resembling an inverted Y; 2. relaxed vocal cords[6] whose margins do not vibrate, at least visibly; 3. increased air flow; and 4. because of low glottal resistance, decreased subglottic pressure. The acoustic characteristic of voiceless performance is the noise of escaping air set into nonperiodic frictional turbulence.

If, as is proposed here, constriction accounts for the strain of a stage whisper, then its affect on whispering can be seen in Pressman's (1942) photographs of the laryngeal adjustment for a harsh effortful whisper (stage whisper) and its relaxed counterpart. Both show the typical "whisper triangle" formed by the incompletely closed cartilaginous glottis. Although the transverse arytenoid muscle does not approximate the arytenoid cartilages posteriorly in either case, the lateral cricoarytenoid muscles obviously do perform differently. For a harsh whisper, the tips of the vocal processes appear to be tightly compressed, whereas in a relaxed whisper, they approximate but do not touch. The latter adjustment would permit positioning of the vocal folds along a continuum that would account for the ability to achieve various degrees of voicing. An optimal whisper would be a function of sufficiently incomplete approximation of the vocal processes that the cords would not be "sucked" into vibration by the Bernoulli effect. That this distance could be as much as three mm. in relaxed vocal folds is suggested by von Leden's (1961) report that he has induced vibration with this much separation of the flaccid folds of freshly excised larynges. Apparently, by regulating subglottic pressure, as well as extent of approximation, the Bernoulli effect could produce any degree of voicing.

That optimal regulation of voicing is a function, physiologically, of the Bernoulli phenomenon is pointed up by Vennard's (1967) judgment of proper vocal attack. He maintains that initiating a tone with a glottal plosive, in which the cords are compressed and the glottis is closed tightly, is akin to producing a cough. The adjustment is tight, the larynx is tense. Instead of initiating phonation by closing the glottis and then applying pressure to force the cords open, he recommends an aspirate approach to tonal attack. By "sucking" the cords into the initial vibration, the larynx is adjusted properly for optimal vocal production.

Vennard's position is based on Moore and von Leden's (1958) physiological analysis of the laugh. As most who have laughed can attest, this can be one of the most vigorous forms of vocalization used. Yet, it seems to be remarkably free of vocally traumatic consequences. When we consider the traditional form of laughter, "ha-ha-ha," we again encounter that panacea for vocal abuse, the Bernoulli effect. Moore and von Leden document the aspirated initiation of the laugh-pulse. Their description of its physiology captures the essence of what is proposed as hygienic phonation:

> During adduction the vocal cords are relatively flaccid, and their medial borders, from the ends of the vocal processes to the anterior commissure, bulge into the glottal area. . . . The initial swing of the flaccid cords is into the air stream toward each other. . . . This movement occurs relatively slowly, and . . .

[6] Moore (1967) makes the point that to prevent the vocal folds from vibrating in a whisper, they must be stiff and tense.

gives the impression of relaxed cords being disturbed gently by the air stream. As soon as they reach the limit of their medial excursion, they are tossed upward and laterally in the opening phase of the first complete cycle.

Finally, Koike (1967) has delineated three distinct types of vocal attack: hard, breathy, and soft. Typical hard attacks corresponding to glottal plosives, are distinguished, aerodynamically, by no air leakage prior to attack, but considerable air usage following initiation of sound; electromyographically, by conspicuous preparatory electrical activity of intrinsic laryngeal muscles; cine-radiographically, by rapid closure of the glottis, but, a lengthy period of adjustment (possibly for tense powerful closure of the glottis) prior to initiating sound; and acoustically, by rapid rise time with corresponding rapid increase in amplitude. The breathy attack is characterized by air leakage prior to vocalization, and only somewhat more air usage following it than in hard attack; by minimal preparatory electrical activity in the vocalis muscle; by prolonged closure of the glottis, but a brief period of adjustment prior to phonation; and by a moderately long rise time. The soft attack is distinctly different from breathy as well as hard attack. Like hard attack, it shows no air leakage prior to phonation, but, it utilizes less air, once sound begins, than either hard or breathy attack. Like breathy attack, it shows inconspicuous preparatory electrical activity, especially in the cricothyroid muscle. Also, like breathy attack, the glottis closes slowly and, once closed, adjusts quickly for vocalization. Acoustically, soft attack shows the longest rise time.

By integrating Vennard's conception of proper vocal attack with Moore and von Leden's analysis of the laugh-pulse, and, particularly, with Koike's study of vocal attack, *we can specify the hygienically optimal, acoustically efficient vocal attack: soft attack.* Hard attack wastes air after the sound begins, breathy attack before and after it begins. That soft attack is uniquely different from hard or breathy is attested by Koike's (1967) finding that persons with pathologic larynges were rarely able to produce soft attacks; what they did produce resembled either hard or breathy attack.

Vocal Mode Regulation

SPECIFICATION OF OPTIMUM

The hygienic criterion is less appropriate for the assessment of vocal mode than for any other dimension of vocal functioning. This is because the voice can be produced hygienically in the pulsated, heavy, or light mode. Conversely, it can probably also be abused in any of these modes. Ironically, the one used most habitually, heavy voice, is the one in which greatest trauma occurs, not only because of its high frequency of usage, but also because it doubtless permits the greatest abuse; greater loudness can be achieved with greater vocal effort and constriction. By contrast, light voice can also be constricted and produced with effort, but the extent to which it can be pushed is limited. With much constriction, the sound shuts off altogether. With vocal effort that does not constrict the larynx and shut the sound off, the voice becomes breathy; the greater the effort the greater the breathiness, thus limiting loudness. Similarly with pulsated voice, the extent to which this mode can be produced loudly with constriction, or with vocal effort, is sharply limited. It is least likely to permit vocal abuse.

Pulsated voice, in fact, is so limited in the amount of constriction and vocal effort that it can tolerate, and still be produced, that I have used it clinically as a model for optimum production. In fact, Vennard (1967, 1968) reports that it is the most efficient vocal adjustment of any for sustained phonation on a single breath. To achieve maximum loudness with it requires minimal constriction and an optimal balance of vocal effort and voicing. The sound that is then achieved resembles a series of discrete explosive pulses, the rate of which can be controlled.[7]

Were selection of vocal mode to be made in terms of the hygienic criterion, we would all be speaking in pulsated voice, and if we could not achieve that, in light voice. Obviously, other criteria predominate in our selection of a mode to use for daily living, and, equally obviously, a major one is that we have a voice loud enough for communicative purposes. Although some women and children manage with light voice, the mode preferred by most, at least in this culture (and that is exclusively acceptable for adult males) is heavy voice. As Fig. 20-5 demonstrates, heavy voice provides a greater pitch and loudness range for the typical speaker than either other mode. Discussion of the trained voice is omitted because it presents complexities that will rarely concern the speech

[7] The dimension of pitch is not altogether appropriate for pulsated voice. The pulses occur at 10 to 50 Hz (McGlone, 1967), too slow a rate to be perceived as a tone having pitch. Instead, each pulse can be distinguished, so the equivalent of pitch is perceived pulse rate.

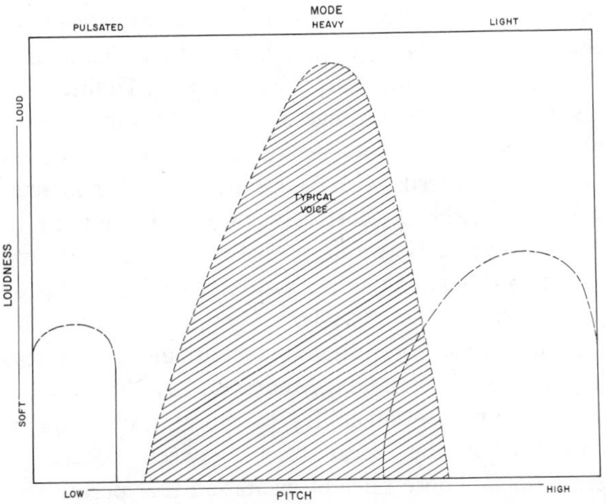

Fig. 20-5. Interactions among vocal mode, pitch, and loudness in typical voices.

pathologist. Singers and some professional speakers use a blending of heavy and light modes (often called *head voice*), especially for high pitches. Speaking broadly, the optimal mode is not exemplified much more clearly in the trained than in the typical voice, so we will not need to concern ourselves with distinctions among more than pulsated, heavy, and light modes.

DEVIATION FROM OPTIMUM

A vocal mode is optimal by virtue of the loudness it permits and by cultural standards. The only deviation from optimal mode that is a relatively serious problem in our culture is mutational voice. This condition is restricted for the most part to adolescent boys, and occasionally adult males, who, usually for psychological reasons, resist the voice change forced on them at puberty by a growing vocal mechanism. Light voice permits them to continue producing sounds similar to those they produced as children. Their preference for this voice, and the problems it may pose for them, has far more to do with mental than vocal hygiene.

Another culturally based problem superficially similar to mutational voice is virilization of the female voice by hormonal imbalance. Damsté (1967) states that an early sign of the condition is the patient's feeling that her voice is out of control, that she cannot prevent its becoming heavier and more masculine. He assigns virilization to endogenous or exogenous factors: endogenous being tumors of the ovary or the adrenal gland that produce androgenic hormones, exogenous being administration of androgens for medical reasons. The masculinized female voice is usually produced at abnormally low pitches in the heavy vocal mode. It is not as likely to pose a hygienic as an aesthetic problem. Unlike light voice, that is unacceptable in the adult male, heavy voice is frequently, if not typically, used by females. The virilized voice is not faulty because of its mode, but, rather, because of the low pitch range in which it functions within the heavy mode.

The reverse of this difficulty is seen occasionally in the adult male whose voice sounds as if it is being produced in the light mode. To assess whether or not it is a modal problem requires testing for a "break" in the voice as pitch is systematically raised. If it breaks into a higher light voice, then it is being produced in the heavy mode even though it may have the characteristic sound of light voice.

PHYSIOLOGICAL AND ACOUSTICAL CORRELATES

Because pulsated voice is the key to the system of therapy to be presented shortly, let us save its discussion until last; we will work from the top mode to the bottom. Light voice is characterized acoustically by weak harmonics, and by a range of fundamental frequencies that overlap but are predominantly above the range for heavy voice. Physiologically, this mode is distinguished by a thin glottal edge that, according to van den Berg (1958), provides resistance to the air stream by virtue of tension in the vocal ligament. That the major longitudinal bundle of the vocalis muscle is not a primary contributor to glottal resistance in light voice is supported by two types of evidence. First, if it did contract, it would thicken the glottal edge—this does not seem to be the case. Second, if it did contract, it would oppose the cricothyroid muscle and require its increased contraction as it elongates the vocal folds—this, too, does not seem to be the case. Faaborg-Andersen (1957) has shown that, with pitch increases, considerably less electrical activity is seen in the cricothyroid muscle when the increase is accomplished by shifting to falsetto (light voice) than when it is accomplished in chest (heavy) voice. More conclusively, he has also shown little or no electrical activity in the vocalis muscle in falsetto. Another distinguishing feature of light voice is a large O.Q. (Open Quotient); it is never small, and frequently, the glottis does not completely close.

Heavy voice is characterized, acoustically, by a wide range of fundamental frequencies that overlap the ranges for light and pulsated voice; it is also characterized by relatively strong harmonics and a much wider range of intensities than either light or pulsated voice. Physiologically, heavy voice is distinguished by varying degrees of contraction of the vocalis muscle. The glottis is typically deep, but thickness of the cords can be regulated; they may be relatively relaxed or tense, but the vocal muscle provides resistance to the air stream by its mass, its tension, or both (van den Berg, 1958). As for the O.Q., it, too, can vary over a wide range from a condition of incomplete closure, in breathy production, to an optimal condition in full voice in which the closing phase is abrupt, thereby productive of intense sound with high harmonics. Overall, the feature that best typifies heavy voice is its flexibility in all dimensions.

Now we turn to pulsated voice. It has been considered, traditionally, as a clinical form of harshness. Hollien, Moore, Wendahl, and Michel (1966) first proposed formally that it may be a normal, rather than a pathological, mode of laryngeal operation. Although it is not used much, and would probably pose a cultural problem if it were, it can be heard often at the bottom of downward inflections, especially in well-produced low-pitch male voices. The fact that everyone cannot produce it with ease probably attests as much, if not more, to unfamiliarity with it than to innate lack of capacity. My own experience with it began about a decade ago when I stumbled onto it as a therapeutic tool quite by accident. I found that it could only be produced at slow pulse rates, roughly below 50 Hz, if the feeling of tension in the throat (identified now as constriction) was minimal; the greater the capacity to reduce the rate to as low as 10 Hz (McGlone, 1967), the less the subjective tension (constriction). More important for therapeutic purposes I found, to my surprise, that when those who produced very slow pulse rates shifted to heavy voice, they invariably produced their normal voice optimally, at least briefly, without apparent volitional effort. I have yet to find an exception to this observation; it appears to apply irrespective of sex, age, or habitual patterns of constriction. The limitation on this conclusion is that pulsated voice can be produced with some constriction at rates above 50 Hz. At these higher frequencies, it is not likely to be a stable series of pulsations; the voice tends to fluctuate erratically between heavy and pulsated modes in much the fashion described by Moore and von Leden (1958). Moreover, heavy voice in these fluctuations is typically produced with moderate constriction.

Having argued that pulsated voice is hygienic, not harsh or pathologic, let us consider its acoustical and physiological characteristics. Two features distinguish it acoustically: pulse rate and damping. Hollien and his group (1966) estimated 20–90 Hz would be a reasonable fundamental frequency range, but 10–60 Hz, which accords with McGlone's (1967) evidence, would be closer to what I have observed; a pulse rate much above 60 Hz would probably be heard as heavy voice. Although Coleman (1963) found that faster pulse rates (up to 85.1 Hz) were less likely to be judged as vocal fry (pulsated voice) than slower rates, he, along with Wendahl, Moore, and Hollien (1963), attributes perception of fry to the almost complete damping of the vocal tract between successive excitations. Those rates of excitation that permit the energy in each wave to decay from 42 to 44 dB of its maximum amplitude will, apparently, always be heard as pulsated voice; conversely, this mode is not heard when the decay between excitation pulses is 30 dB or less.

Physiologically, pulsated voice is of interest, not only to understand the basis for its therapeutic value, but also to account for the mechanism that permits women and children, as well as adult males, to produce pulses in the same frequency range. McGlone (1967) has demonstrated this curious ability of women experimentally, and many of us have doubtless witnessed children playing "motor boat" with these slow glottal pulse rates. The puzzlement is why the pulse generator, the larynx, produces such a different range of pulse rates for men, women, and children in the heavy mode, yet, in the pulsated mode, they all function at the same rate. Obviously, much remains to be understood about pitch and vocal mode regulation.

We are somewhat closer to a glimmer of understanding of the physiological basis of the hygienic value of pulsated voice. The most singular feature apparently necessary for its production is abrupt glottal closure. Moore and von Leden (1958), in their early account, describe a double glottal opening for each cycle in which the second opening differs markedly from the first by virtue of abrupt closure of the glottis almost simultaneously throughout its length. Their subsequent report also shows this rapid closure (Timcke, von Leden, and Moore, 1959). Ohala (1966), using glottography that permits equating of glottographic pulse to glottal volume velocity waveform, reports, similarly, what can be interpreted as double and sometimes triple glottal openings per cycle. He found, though, that only the closing phase is generally sufficiently abrupt to excite the vocal tract and produce an acoustic pulse. His finding agrees with that of Wendahl, Moore, and Hollien (1963), who reported perception of vocal fry with or without dicrotic excitation of the vocal tract.

Perhaps the most persuasive argument for abrupt glottal closure as the distinctive physiological feature of vocal fry can be inferred from the necessary acoustic condition for pulsated voice. Assuming its perception to be a function of almost complete decay of energy in each glottal pulse, then, to achieve such a highly damped sound requires a pulse that will excite a response in the vocal tract rich in high harmonics. We have already seen, from our earlier discussion of loudness, that the shorter the closing phase of the glottis, the more intense the sound and the more high frequency components it will have. Hence, the conclusion that abrupt closure of the glottis is a requisite of pulsated voice.

Theoretically, this vocal mode is produced with low subglottal pressure and air flow through thick, but not necessarily tense, vocal folds (Hollien, Moore, Wendahl, and Michel, 1966). McGlone (1967) has confirmed the prediction of low air flow. From this evidence, and from Ohala's (1966) report that glottal openings are roughly one-tenth those for normal voice, we can infer the probability of low subglottal pressure. If the remainder of the prediction is accurate, that the cords are thick and relaxed, their rapid closure, then, can only be explained by the Bernoulli principle. If this analysis is essentially accurate, we can understand why the pulsated mode establishes hygienically optimal vocal production in heavy mode: pulsated voice can only be produced with the Bernoulli effect; it can only be produced with relatively intense excitation of the vocal tract considering the minimal effort involved; and this adjustment that relies heavily on "sucking" the cords closed apparently persists, involuntarily, when vocal mode is shifted back to heavy voice.

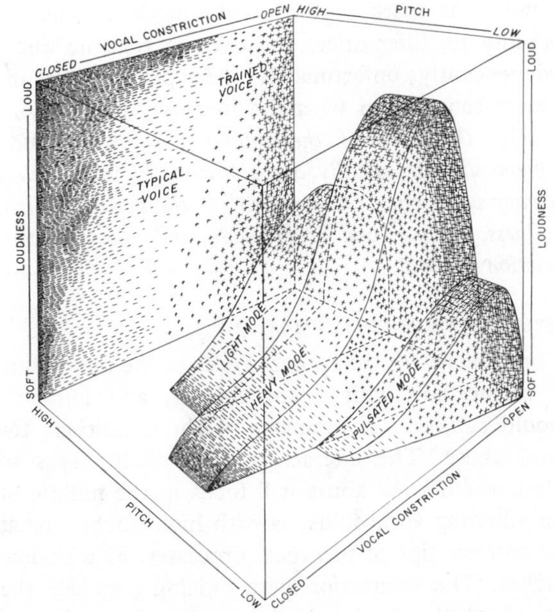

Fig. 20-6. Interactions among vocal mode, pitch, loudness, and vocal constriction. This figure summarizes the interrealtionships shown in Figs. 20-1, 20-2, and 20-5. The effects of constriction in typical and trained voices are shown on the back wall and in each "shoe-shaped" vocal mode.

Vocal Constriction Regulation

SPECIFICATION OF OPTIMUM

That the regulation of vocal constriction holds the key to vocal hygiene has been iterated and reiterated. The ways in which it interacts with each dimension have already been discussed, so all that remains to be stressed is that optimal constriction is minimal constriction. Like weeds in a garden, constriction has no useful place in the cultivated voice (or the uncultivated one for that matter), and, like weeds, it tends to spread. The effect it imposes on the other vocal dimensions, except voicing, is to limit them. Fig. 20-6 shows three-dimensionally the extent to which constriction restricts pitch, even vocal mode, and, most vividly, loudness. The "+" and "−" marks along the side of the vocal constriction dimension in this Fig. remind us that constriction increases as the vocal tract feels closed and decreases as it feels open. These marks are projected to the "shoe-shaped" areas (each show is for a vocal mode) to show how constriction interacts with the various other dimensions shown. Vocal constriction spreads because it thrives on its accomplice, vocal effort, with which it is directly proportional, and which must be increased to overcome the limiting effects of constriction on pitch and, especially, on loudness.

The relationship between constriction and vocal effort needs a word of clarification. Typically, vocal effort and constriction interact, but, ideally, they would not. In other words, constricted vocal production cannot exist without vocal effort, but effort can, and should, be exerted without constriction. Some degree of effort is required for any form of vocalization, so effort is necessarily ubiquitous, but constriction is not. The mark of the poorly produced voice is inability to differentiate the two, to regulate effort independently; unfortunately, the typical speaker increases constriction when he increases effort. Conversely, *the mark of the optimally produced voice, hygienically, acoustically, and aesthetically, is the ability to vary vocal effort proportional to the needs of pitch, loudness, voicing, and vocal mode while keeping constriction minimal.*

DEVIATION FROM OPTIMUM

A brief review of the consequences of the interaction of constriction with pitch, voicing, and loudness should suffice as a summary of the conditions for vocal abuse. The interaction with pitch serves to select whether the abuse will focus in the middle of the vibrating vocal folds, as with high pitches, or at the anterior tips of the vocal processes, as with low pitches. The interaction with voicing provides the framework that limits the traumatic effects of vocal abuse; the less the voicing, the less the potential for tissue damage. The interaction with loudness provides the force with which abusive patterns of vocalization can injure the vocal cords.

Combine these interactions with constriction into the four-way interaction among the component dimensions and we can account for a wide variety of vocal abuses. Proceeding with the effects of constriction along the voicing dimension, at the voiceless pole is functional aphonia, with little effort, little constriction, and little loudness. A stage whisper requires more effort, more constriction, and more loudness; ventricular dysphonia considerably more; and spastic dysphonia even more. Neither of these latter dysphonias involves full voicing in terms of true vocal fold vibration—the false folds may vibrate in ventricular dysphonia, and in spastic dysphonia, the larynx is so cramped and constricted that it produces more noisy turbulence than strident tone, which probably accounts for why these two dysphonias, with all of their constriction and strain, do not seem to damage the cords appreciably.

With full voicing comes the potential for application of the damaging force of loudness interacting with constriction. When this force is applied at high pitches, the voice sounds strident, shrill, even screechy. If this application is prolonged, especially if the cords are not healthy (e.g., inflamed following a cold), laryngitis and eventually nodules can be expected. If this combination occurs at low pitches, the voice will sound harsh, husky, hoarse, or rough, and the pathology that may ensue will be laryngitis and contact ulcer.

PHYSIOLOGICAL AND ACOUSTICAL CORRELATES

The acoustic characteristics of constriction as an independent phenomenon have not been studied systematically, so little can be said about them with authority. Yanagihara (1967) has shown that, as hoarseness becomes more severe, three abnormal acoustic patterns become more apparent: 1. noise components in the main formant of each vowel; 2. high frequency noise components above 3,000 Hz; and 3. loss of high-frequency harmonic components. Although these findings are applicable to perceived hoarseness, for which constriction is a major component, they are based on data from patients with laryngeal problems for whom inability to achieve full voicing may have contributed as much to the noise as constriction. That Yanagihara's evidence for hoarseness may also be applicable to harshness and stridency, constriction being the common characteristic for all three, can be seen by inspecting Fig. 19-3 in Chapter 19. These three samples, as well as the others, were produced by a normal male voice simulating the conditions that were perceived as identified.

Koike (1967) has also produced some acoustic evidence relative to constriction during vocal attack. Hard attack in normal voices (an attack with constriction) was found to show large pitch perturbations of considerably greater magnitude than were seen during steady phonation. These perturbations, as well as amplitude fluctuations, were even more apparent in pathologic cases.

Because the dimension of constriction is of recent vintage, little work has been done on it physiologically. Still, Joyner (1967) has manipulated it as an independent variable to determine its effects on air flow in normal voices ranging from professional to average caliber, and Beckett (1967) has done a companion study with the same population to determine its effects on pitch perturbation. Although Beckett's results are what might be expected, greater perturbation with greater constriction, Joyner's are more difficult to interpret. As a group, his subjects showed significantly more air flow with minimal than maximal or moderate constriction, yet a few of his best-trained vocalists showed just the opposite pattern. Although air flow may be typically related to constriction, clearly, it is not related invariantly. Again, our knowledge of the dynamics of glottal resistance as a regulator of air flow is incomplete.

Much of the evidence presented for the other dimensions bears tangentially on constriction. Let us synthesize what we know about it and speculate a bit on how it may contribute physiologically to laryngeal abuse. The condition specified for optimal phonation is freedom from constriction. Physiologically, this condition is characterized by closure of the cords being accomplished mainly by the "sucking" action of the Bernoulli effect. This phenomenon accounts for the abrupt closure of relaxed vocal folds, an aerodynamically economical and acoustically productive adjustment. We may, then, *define the physiology of constriction as any vocal tract adjustment, given a positioning of the cords for vibration, that weakens the Bernoulli effect.*

Physiological evidence of vocal constriction would be such as just mentioned from Joyner, Beckett, and Koike, all of their findings pointing to inefficiency with constriction. Having participated in two of these studies, I can report that, when a moderately soft tone was produced optimally and the intensity level was noted, then, to produce the same intensity with constriction required considerably more vocal effort.

Speculations are always risky, but, they are also sometimes profitable. This speculation has to do with the mechanism by which vocal abuse can injure the cords. Arnold (1962) has accounted for the predilection of nodules for the junction of the anterior and middle thirds of the cord, the point of widest vibratory amplitude and mechanical impact, and of contact ulcers for the medial surface of the cartilaginous vocal processes, the point at which the processes grind and hammer together when forcefully adducted. This account cannot be faulted, but it leaves open some puzzling paradoxes. Why, for example, do speakers of Germanic languages full of glottal stops, presumably conducive to excessive adduction, not show high incidence of contact ulcer? How can many professional singers, whose vibratory patterns are characterized by abrupt glottal closure that slams the cords together, perform for a lifetime vocal feats that would reduce most of us after a few minutes to laryngitis and eventually nodules—yet, never suffer vocal abuse?

Probably, a portion of the answer, at least for contact ulcer, is that it is a psychosomatic disorder (Arnold, 1962). But, may we not speculate that another portion, for all vocal abuse, is a function of constriction? Curiously, constriction, if anything, probably reduces the force with which the vibrating cords slam together, but this force cannot, by itself, be the mechanical basis of abuse. If it were, those voices that function by virtue of the Bernoulli effect would suffer the greatest damage—we have seen that it is probably this "sucking" effect that produces the most abrupt closure, *ergo*, the greatest force on impact, and the longest, and, probably most compressed, glottal closure—but, these are the voices that function most hygienically. In fact, if the Germans produce a glottal stop utilizing the Bernoulli phenomenon in the manner described by Vennard and Isshiki (1964), then we can even explain why they are not all afflicted with vocal trauma.

Vocal constriction tightens the sphincters of the vocal tract. Two especially relevant manifestations are tension in the vocalis muscle and medial compression of the vocal processes by contraction of the lateral cricoarytenoid muscles. At low pitches (with which contact ulcer is generally associated) for optimal production utilizing the Bernoulli effect, the vocal processes are approximated, but not compressed, and may not even touch. This would be the adjustment for soft attack. The relaxed cords are set into vibration by "suction." The adjustment for hard attack, however, involves vigorous compression of the glottis in which the cords must be driven apart. Presumably, medial compression of the vocal processes in this adjustment is considerable, hence, the grinding action at low pitches with constriction.

We can account for the shifted locus of trauma in high-pitch constriction responses by the increased longitudinal force with increased pitch that tends to keep the vocal processes parallel and offsets their medial compression. As pitch increases, so does elongation of the vocal folds. The stronger the anterior pull on the vocal processes the less likely they are to grind together and ulcerate the mucosa. But, as the vocal folds are elongated with increased pitch, tension in the vocal muscle tends to increase. The greater the tension the firmer the surfaces the cords present to each other when they slam together; the mucosal lining is pounded between two hard muscles—little wonder that nodules develop at high pitches. Obviously, hygienic production of high pitches, if this formulation is valid, would involve minimal possible tension in the vocalis muscle for that pitch.

Breathing Regulation

The regulation of breathing is of importance to this behavioral analysis of vocal production only insofar as it is related to the regulation of the other vocal dimensions. The concern here is not with how long the voice can be sustained, rather, it is with how well it can be produced. Accordingly, vital capacity is not a primary issue, but management of subglottal pressure is. Assessment of the adequacy of breathing, then, is in terms of which pattern provides optimal support for the optimal regulation of pitch, loudness, voicing, vocal mode, and, above all else, constriction. Although work has been done to establish normal relationships among vital capacity, air flow, pitch, and loudness, this is not a focus of major interest here (Yanagihara, Koike, and von Leden, 1966; Yanagihara and Koike, 1967).

VOCAL EFFORT

Phonation is powered, physiologically, by subglottal pressure. That it is manifested psychologically as vocal effort has been demonstrated by Ladefoged (1963) and by Ladefoged and Mckinney (1963). They have also demonstrated that word stress is regulated more physiologically, with kinesthetic feedback from the control of subglottal pressure, than acoustically. They, along with others (Isshiki, 1964; Perkins and Yanagihara, 1968), have even shown that pitch, as well as loudness, is a function of subglottal pressure. Similar correlations could, in all probability, be demonstrated empirically for the other dimensions of voice if they were to be investigated. They have not been, so we must content ourselves with subjective observations of these dimensions as they relate to vocal effort, a reasonably well-established psychological correlate of subglottal pressure.

For our purpose, we should consider the vocal dimensions as independent variables and vocal effort as dependent on them. The importance of considering the relationship this way is because the vocal dimensions are the behavioral phenomena that are regulated volitionally; vocal effort depends on the extent to which these dimensions need effort for their support. Stated in this frame of reference, optimal vocal effort is that which is necessary for the regulation of the productive dimensions of voice. Conversely, vocal effort deviates from optimum to the extent that it becomes an independent variable, i.e., to the extent that any dimension of voice, especially constriction, becomes its dependent function.

What this means in practice is that the effort necessary to produce a given pitch, for example, should be discretely limited to the regulation of that pitch; it should not spill over into other dimensions and produce unintended changes in loudness and constriction. Even voicing is, in all likelihood, functionally related to vocal effort; the subglottal pressure necessary to displace vocal folds approximated for phonation is probably a bit more than that required for a whsiper. Certainly, differences can be discerned in the range of vocal effort that can be utilized for the different vocal modes, and as for constriction, it is all but synonymous with strain and stress.

Although vocal effort typically functions as an independent variable in its interactions with pitch and loudness, this deviation from optimum is a problem only for the singer who must maintain discrete control of these two variables; the fact that the effort involved in changing loudness tends, inadvertently, also to change pitch is not of much consequence as far as vocal hygiene is concerned. What is consequential is that this same vocal effort tends to function independently to elicit unwanted vocally abusive constriction responses.

Optimal regulation of breathing, then, permits any respiratory pattern that does not increase the tendency toward a constriction response. Granted, the clavicular or pectoral pattern is inefficient as far as vital capacity is concerned, and this limitation alone could disqualify it; still, the more severe indictment is that it tends to spread tension to the throat and elicit constriction. As for so-called diaphragmatic control of breathing that, in the layman's mind, is the style devoutly to be desired, it is one of the purer forms of physiological claptrap that has been perpetrated on the public. The only time the diaphragm is active in normal phonation is when it is needed to resist relaxation pressure that would otherwise produce too much subglottal pressure (Draper, Ladefoged and Whitteredge, 1959). The abdominal muscles compress the viscera and push up the diaphragm during speech, so it is control of abdominal as well as thoracic muscles that is vital to the regulation of breathing.

THERAPY OF DISORDERED VOCAL FUNCTIONING

A Rational Basis for Therapy

All that has been said so far has been by way of preparing a rational basis for the therapy of disordered vocal functioning. What will be proposed in this section is deduced from the foregoing analysis, it follows logically as a necessary consequence. But, it is more than a theory of vocal therapy. The analysis derives from 20 years of experience with problems of voice. These ideas have been molded in the crucible of clinical practice in which the search has been for a conception that will simplify the immense complexity of vocal disorders, yet will preserve the rich detail of the normal as well as the disordered voice; the search has also been for therapeutic procedures that permit delineation of disabled vocal behavior that can then be modified effectively. Finally, and most important, the search has been for simple explicit techniques that will synthesize all of the vocal dimensions into an optimal balance. Not only were techniques selected that effectively integrate the dimensions holistically, they were also selected as being easily grasped and applied by patients as well as by clinicians.

The system of therapy in its present form has been tested clinically during the last five years. It was designed for the explicit purpose of modifying vocal-production behavior; for this purpose, it has been gratifyingly successful. It was not intended to ameliorate emotional distress, except as it may be a function of defective vocal performance; it has also lived up to this intent: it has not been very effective with problems such as spastic dysphonia in which gains in vocal functioning are quickly lost to what are apparently overriding symptom-serving needs.

Conditions for Vocal Abuse

The conditions under which the voice may be traumatized are external to this system of therapy for reducing vocal abuse. The system itself involves the assessment of behavior, discussed in the preceding section, the specification of desired objectives to be achieved, and the description of a set of procedures for achieving them. The therapy is based on a functional analysis of vocal behavior; as such, etiological issues are relatively immaterial. The crucial questions are, what is the behavior, and, how does it function in the person's overall performance? How the behavior came to be is of more historical than practical value, unless the conditions that produced it are still operating and would limit or prevent its amelioration. Because conditions that preserve abusive vocalization often prevail and disrupt the effects of therapy, they will be considered briefly for both children and adults.

ABUSE IN CHILDREN

Hoarseness is the danger signal of the larynx, and it occurs in children far more frequently than most of us are inclined to suspect (unless we hover on the brink of acoustic trauma from having children of our own). The figures range from 40 percent in a European report in 1907 (Luchsinger and Arnold, 1965) to a recent one of seven percent of elementary school children who were chronically hoarse (Wilson, 1966). The same triad of conditions found in adults are also present in children to account for these startling figures: organic disability, emotional stress, and situational stress. We will examine them in that order.

The laryngeal disabilities that afflct children are not as varied or as plentiful as are usual among adults. Von Leden (1967) has said that acute laryngitis is, by far, the most frequent condition he has observed, followed by vocal nodules, occasionally benign tumors (congenital or traumatic), and, rarely, a laryngeal web. Others have reported, additionally, hyperkeratotic plaques, polyps, structural anomalies, and endocrine disturbances (Luchsinger and Arnold, 1965; Wilson, 1966). It is the province of another chapter to present the details of these organic disabilities. The purpose here is to indicate that optimal vocal functioning is limited to varying degrees, determinable only by behavioral assessment, as long as any of these conditions prevail. Moreover, because they reduce the acoustic efficiency of the voice, excessive vocal effort is exerted to achieve loudness, and the tendency toward abusive vocal functioning is heightened.

Emotional stress, situational stress, and vocal performance interact so quickly with each other as to make them a functional unit. Fortunately, the child's habitual vocalization may be close to optimum. His use of abusive vocal production is often a reaction to a combination of situational factors, and it invariably involves screaming and yelling; it is such a characteristic reaction that the typical pathological consequence has been named for it: screamer's nodes. Consider a typical playground situation. An aggressive, insecure child is attempting to make his presence felt, so he yells. The other children like him even less when he is loud, which frustrates him all the more, so he yells louder and longer, and now the children exclude him. The interaction spirals out of control until he is screaming himself hoarse—obviously, not an uncommon occurrence.

Children are engrossed with gut-level issues of living. They are not much interested in the minute-to-minute, day-to-day attention required to change patterns of vocal production, even if it is for their own good (so very many parental and teacher admonitions are for their "own good"). The value of vocal hygiene is just not likely to loom as large for the child as for the clinician, the physician, the teacher, or the parent. To ignore this reality in attempts to effect therapeutic change is to try to empty the ocean with a teaspoon—both will be about equally effective.

This prelude is to the point that the clinician will be well advised to assess situational and emotional stress as well as vocal production before undertaking therapy. Unless vocalization is habitually traumatic, attention would be more profitably directed to control of circumstances that elicit abusive vocal patterns. Control is considerably more certain of the conditions in which the child performs than of the child's performance once he is in those conditions; a frustrated child is a loud-voiced child, vocal hygiene or no vocal hygiene. Control of such situations is doubly important if the child is in poor health, especially if he has upper respiratory infection or a laryngeal disability; these conditions make him vulnerable to tissue damage of the vocal cords. Not only should attention be directed, particularly during these health circumstances, to minimizing use of loud voice, but also to eliminating, if possible, vigorous throat-clearing, singing at extremes of pitch or loudness, and vocalization during inhalation. This is not an exhaustive catalog of "don'ts," but it is suggestive of conditions to be avoided.

ABUSE IN ADULTS

As with children, so with adults, the conditions conducive to vocal abuse include organic disability, emotional stress, and situational stress. Organic disabilities range from lesions of laryngeal tissues including inflammations, benign and malignant tumors, functional disabilities, to paralyses and manifestations of systemic disease. These disabilities are detailed elsewhere. They are discussed here for the same reason they were with children: they tend to limit, or preclude, optimal vocal functioning, and because they reduce acoustic output, they increase the probability of excessive vocal effort and strain. These effects are realities that should be recognized in undertaking therapy.

Emotional stress and its treatment is also, for the most part, beyond the scope of this chapter. The aphonias and dysphonias that are symptomatic of personality conflict and that function, albeit maladaptively, to alleviate personal distress, require management of behavior beyond that for which the system of therapy proposed here is intended. This system is particularly effective with those adults with whom voice and emotion interact, one with the other. Men frequently report, for example, that a thin, weak voice makes them feel socially impotent; strengthen the voice and they feel stronger.

The dimension of voice that could almost be called the *emotional* dimension is *constriction*. Emotional stress and vocal constriction typically go hand in glove. As with children, again, so with adults: emotional stress, situational stress, and constriction are an interacting functional unit. Increase any one and all tend to rise; decrease any one and all tend to diminish. The clinician, before undertaking modification of habitual vocal performance, would have time well spent if he were to investigate this interaction carefully. It may well hold conditions that would limit or undo therapeutic gains.

The important issues to consider in vocal abuse are twofold. On one hand, they include such questions as: Do you clear your throat vigorously? Do you speak loudly or yell? Do you sing too high, too loud, or too long? On the other hand, they include: Where do you do it? When? With whom? For instance, a retired business executive of my acquaintance uses a relatively pleasant soft voice with his wife, but when he serves on a panel that ajudicates business differences, he reverts to his executive's voice; it is loud, harsh, and vocally abusive. An analysis of the daily conditions in which speaking is done is vital for planning tactics to extend vocal improvement in the clinical laboratory to everyday situations.

Behavior Therapy

Behavior therapy comes in several forms these days, the number of which seems to be proliferating rapidly. The popularity of this therapy is not surprising in a field that values empirical phenomena, yet, has had an inflated diet of subjective impressions. We have for many years seen speech disorders as intertangled with emotional problems, but many have eschewed the nebulous uncertainties of personality conflicts for the behavioral tangibilities of defective patterns of speech and voice. Some have agreed with the definition of psychotherapy as "an unidentified technique applied to unspecified problems with unpredictable outcomes." Therapies, designed to modify anxiety as well as behavioral responses, that provide the clinician with the equivalent of a procedural blueprint have been welcomed, especially by those uneasy about the wisdom of therapy by intuition and feeling.

OPERANT THERAPY

The choice of operant therapy over other behavior therapies is made with recognition of its limitations. For one thing, the effects it can produce with certainty are limited to the behavior that can be controlled. It would not, for example, be expected to alter anxiety (whatever it may be behaviorally) if the behavior at which it is aimed is vocal. In this respect, it is diametrically opposite to reciprocal inhibition therapy, one of the earliest forms of behavior therapy, with which Gray, England, and Mohoney (1965) report successful remission of vocal nodules in a 29-year-old woman. Their therapy is intended to relieve anxiety and tension, the presumed underlying subsoil from which vocal difficulties grow. This is not to disagree with their conception, but rather to identify anxiety in relation to voice for subsequent discussion.

Operant therapy was chosen because it permits greater prediction and control of behavior that can be identified than any other existing approach. It was not chosen because it is based on the best theory of learning. It is, in fact, an application of experimental analysis of behavior that yields a functional account of behavior, but in no way attempts a theoretical explanation of what transpires in the "mind" between stimulus and response. The analysis of vocal production in the foregoing sections is what makes this a feasible therapy of choice. If crucial vocal behavior could not be specified, an operant analysis would be severely hampered.

Two additional considerations made this the therapy of choice over those intended to reduce anxiety. The first is that anxiety is a hypothetical construct; it is not explicit behavior. Accordingly, it is not subject to direct control. True, it can be observed subjectively, and its observance can be signaled, but an observer has no way of verifying the truth of that signal. Normally, any reinforcement or punishment is made contingent on the signal; if it is false, therapy proceeds in the opposite direction from that intended. Even if anxiety could be managed directly, however, the second consideration would weaken any preference for this approach. It presumes that vocal disorders are functions of anxiety. Although this presumption may be true in many instances, it probably is not in many others. Unless means were available for differentiating the two groups, considerable time and effort could be wasted by clinician and patient alike. Operant therapy, by contrast, can be applied with reasonable certainty of the effects it will produce.

Not all persons with voice problems may be candidates for these effects, but that can be determined by careful assessment before embarking on an extensive therapeutic venture. If evidence of the desired improvement is not seen after two or three sessions utilizing this operant system of therapy, to be described next, it would probably not be the therapy of choice; its effects are quickly apparent. Emotional resistance to vocal change has been, in my experience, the only consistent basis for failure—especially if the emotional problem is manifested in spastic dysphonia.

On the other hand, we must consider the possibility that "the cure may be worse than the disease." If the vocal disorder is serving an anxiety-binding function, removal of the vocal symptom would, presumably, expose the patient to problems and anxiety with which he might be unable to cope. To deal with this possible consequence, a clinician has at least two alternatives. He can assume an underlying emotional problem and attempt to resolve it before or during direct attention to the voice; a lengthy alternative to be sure, especially when pursued without certainty that the vocal complaint is emotionally based. Moreover, if the speech clinician is not prepared to treat underlying conflict that might exist, then he must refer the patient to a competent psychotherapist. The route for a person seeking vocal therapy would then be from the laryngologist via the psychiatrist or psychologist to the speech pathologist.

An alternative to this circuitous course is for the clinician to perform a differential diagnosis with his vocal therapy procedures. Three possibilities will be apparent within a few sessions. First, the patient may fail to improve or to carry over improvements into daily living, a possibility suggestive of emotional conflict and resistance. Second, he may improve vocally but become increasingly anxious, a possibility that points to a symptomatic function of the vocal disorder. Third, he may improve without undesired side effects, a possibility that indicates the independence of vocal difficulty from whatever emotional problems he may face. If the first possibility is encountered, vocal therapy is likely to be neither helpful nor hurtful. If the second, it can be hurtful, helpful, or both; the emotional conflict is exposed and must be dealt with either by reinstating vocal symptoms, or preferably, by finding more successful methods of coping with life—psychotherapy may be needed to help find these methods. Finally, if the third possibility occurs, vocal therapy is helpful; it is the treatment of choice.

A System of Operant Therapy of Disordered Vocal Functioning

We will now examine the system of therapy by which the various dimensions of voice can be brought toward their most optimal condition of functioning. Discussion of details of the system may tend to obscure the relative simplicity of it as applied in practice. It is no more complex than articulation therapy, which in many ways it resembles. By making explicit the vocal performance to be achieved in each dimension, a tangible goal is available towards which to work: optimal production of each dimension is the target that corresponds to the center of a phoneme in articulation therapy. The farther off target, the more defective the articulation or the vocalization. Therapy, of course, is aimed at bringing the performance as close to the bull's eye as the patient's capacity permits.

This approach would be immensely complex if optimal production of each dimension had to be worked out separately and then be integrated into an optimal balance for normal speech. Both patient and clinician would be as busy as ataxic centipedes trying to coordinate everything. Fortunately, procedures are available for integrating these dimensions holistically into a unified optimal vocal performance. Underlying this approach is the conception that deviation from optimum in one dimension signifies deviation in others. Ability to analyze each dimension separately increases ability to detect not only that the voice is out of balance, but also, how it is out. The following system of therapy has been designed to put it back in balance, often within four or five half-hour sessions.

A system of operant therapy requires of the clinician four distinct operations. First, the behavior to be managed must be identified, and the desired, or terminal, performance specified. Second, the existing behavior must be selected to be shaped to the ultimately desired form. Third, the selected behavior must be successively approximated to the desired form by managing schedules of reinforcement that are made contingent on acceptable performance. Fourth, stimulus control of the terminal behavior must be extended to normal living conditions. Let us, now, consider each operation.

Goal of Therapy

An assumption basic to this system of therapy is that any behavior that can be identified, and for which reinforcement can be made contingent, can be modified. The relevance of defining dimensions is best illustrated with an analogy. We speak often of "simple articulation disorders." Nothing about them is simple, of course, if one tries to understand why, for example, /s/ is more frequently deviant than /t/. I would venture that the illusion of simplicity is a function of the relative ease with which articulatory behavior can be modified, and this ease, in turn, is a function of how explicitly the behavior to be modified can be identified. Not only can it be readily identified in its defective form, but the form it should take to be normal is equally clear. As a facet of phonetic behavior, articulation and its disorders have been made abundantly explicit. Its linguistic functions have been defined phonemically; the behavior that must be emitted to produce an acceptable allophone in each phoneme is clearly delineated; in fact, its physiological and acoustical correlates are well on the way to being specified. The obvious point of this analogy is that if the dimensions of voice were as well defined as those of articulation, we might, then, be able to speak of "simple voice disorders."

Therapy of voice has been notoriously difficult because the vocal behavior to be managed, except for pitch and loudness, has not been made explicit. The purpose of the preceding sections of this chapter has been to rectify this difficulty. Five dimensions by which the important aspects of the speaking voice are regulated have been identified. Optimal behavior for each dimension has been specified; this behavior is optimal regardless of organic or emotional conditions that may have contributed to habitual deviations from it, or limit therapeutic approximations of it. In other words, the desired phonatory ability is constant; it is not different for the child or the adult, for the person with myasthenia laryngis, vocal nodules, or laryngitis. *Hygienically optimal vocal behavior for one is hygienically optimal for all.*

OPTIMAL REGULATION OF VOICE

The goal of this therapy is to delineate the regulation of each vocal dimension so that it can function independently and in optimal balance with the others. Because vocal effort is required for all five dimensions, it should be the only dependent function during vocal production, and it should be responsive only to the dimension being regulated; it should not elicit responses in any other dimension. This means, most importantly, that vocal effort required for any dimension, especially loudness and pitch, should not elicit constriction responses. To reiterate, the hygienically optimal voice is produced without constriction.

A consequence of this analysis that may be a bit startling for some is that *any pitch or loudness level that can be produced without constriction is hygienically optimal.* This does not deny that the voice will tend to operate around a modal pitch and loudness that, typically, will involve the least constriction of which the person is capable at the moment. Nonetheless, the closer to optimal (minimal constriction) the voice is produced, the wider the range of acceptable pitches and loudnesses.

Implicit in the preceding statement is a word of caution. Any tactic utilized to approximate "optimal" pitch, loudness, voicing, or vocal mode that results in increased constriction has missed the mark. If, for instance, the voice is analyzed a few days following recovery from a chest cold, it will function, typically, at a lower pitch level than usual. If "optimum" pitch is calculated by measuring one-fourth of the way up from the bottom of the range, a pitch too low for the voice under normal health conditions would be established as a goal to achieve. Following recovery, attempts to approximate this "optimal" pitch would probably require increased vocal effort and constriction. The test of optimal production that should be made continuously, is whether the pattern of regulation of any dimension at any instant is eliciting constriction.

Selection of Behavior to Shape

The purpose of assessment of vocal behavior is to ascertain the segment of each dimension in which the voice functions closest to optimal. Therapy should begin with the emission of those behaviors that most closely approximate their ultimately desired form. A test of whether or not these behaviors have been clearly delineated is to obtain a reliable baseline, or base rate, on them. This is done by measuring the rate at which the response occurs during a given set of conditions. When the response rate becomes stable, it can be taken as a base against which to compare future performances. More specifically, a base rate provides a frame of reference for determining therapeutic effects.

Although merit can be found in the strategy of beginning therapy with the classical procedures of speech therapy, ear training (Van Riper, 1963), this is probably not the most efficient point of departure practically or theoretically. Perceptual responses are functionally related to motor responses, but are nonetheless distinct from them. The rationale for ear training is based on the assumption that the production of a desired response is a function of the perception of the form that response should take. Yet, a case has been made for the opposite of this assumption. Lieberman and the Haskins group (1963) have proposed that speech perception involves a decoding process in terms of equivalent motor speech patterns. This suggests that we perceive in terms of what we can produce.

It can be argued, of course, that we can perceive a wide range of sounds, yet our utterances are so narrowly limited by the consistency of production that our identity is easily revealed by our patterns of speech. This argument attests to two points. First, it suggests strongly that production and perception are independent phenomena. They may well be linked by a common cognitive guidance system for coding and decoding, but one is not a direct function of the other. As Goldiamond (1962) has demonstrated, perception can be conceived as an operant class of behavior. As such, perceptual responses are determined by their consequences. Perceptions that are differentially reinforced become differentiated perceptions. Similarly, motor responses that are differentially reinforced also become differentiated. But, differential motor responses are not established by manipulating perception, nor *vice versa*.

The second point to which the argument attests is that the sensory modalities by which we monitor and guide speech output are not identical to those by which we perceive the speech of others. Teleceptors (i.e., audition and vision) are the channels for interpersonal communication. Of these channels, audition alone functions in speech production, but also functioning, of course, are the tactual and kinesthetic senses. These latter senses, being proprioceptive, respond to private stimuli, whereas teleceptive senses respond to public phenomena. The speculation proposed is that the breadth of the sounds we can perceive is a function of the public teleceptive sense, audition; auditory perceptual responses are reinforced on a broad phonemic basis permitting perceptual recognition of any phone that makes a distinctive difference. Conversely, the consistency of the sounds we produce could be explained as primarily a function, not of public auditory stimuli, but of private tactual and kinesthetic feedback information. Since the only conditions under which these private stimuli occur require a motor response, little merit is apparent in initiating modification of speaking behavior with ear training.

If the foregoing analysis is valid, then we have a theoretical basis, as well as evidence from successful clinical experience, for beginning therapy with production of the vocal dimensions as close to their optimal form as possible. Of course, this assumes that the desired response is motor production of optimal vocal behavior; if the terminal response sought is perceptual discrimination of various vocal dimensions, therapy should emphasize differential listening, i.e., ear training. Naturally, the closer the behavior selected initially for shaping is to the terminal form, the less differential reinforcement required, and the shorter the course of therapy.

Success in the selection of behavior to shape is, in the final analysis, dependent on the success of tactics for eliciting or obtaining emission of desired behavior. Techniques for eliciting that behavior reflexively would, of course, provide greatest certainty of success. Such respondents as are elicited in a yawn, a laugh, or in the chewing activities utilized in the method of therapy devised by Froeschels (1952; Wyatt, 1951) are among the few reflexive responses that inhibit constriction. Yet, as respondent behavior, they require considerable shaping to transform them into useful operants for optimal vocalization. In other words, although the yawn defines the optimal pole on the constriction dimension, and the vegetative action of chewing (but not swallowing) partially inhibits constriction responses, reflexive responses such as these, and also laughing, are valuable mainly as devices for providing the "feel" of a low-constriction condition. The problem of extending this "feel" to constriction-free vocal production is the problem of bringing a respondent under operant control, and then shaping it as an integral part of the vocal response, no mean trick. Still, one must start somewhere, and these respondents are universally available. If, after careful assessment of vocal operants, none approaches optimal as a starting point for therapy, yawning, laughing, and chewing can be utilized as a certain foundation on which to build.

A few techniques have proven sufficiently useful in reducing constriction during vocal production that I utilize them in a system, and rarely have to deviate from them. These techniques for initiating therapy capitalize on the typically most optimal portion of each vocal dimension: *pitch extremes are avoided, soft rather than loud tones are used, soft and breathy vocal attacks are sought, partially voiced sustained tones are preferred to full voicing, and the modes in order of constriction reducing capacity are pulsated, light, and heavy.* Although conceivably, other portions of the dimensions could be found by assessment to function more optimally than those just cited, and would, to that extent, alter the behaviors selected with which to begin therapy, nonetheless, I have not encountered deviations from these typical conditions for optimal. If exceptions do appear to prevail, they should be acted on cautiously lest the initial assessment be determined later to be in error.

FIRST ALTERNATIVE SEQUENCE

The system that has worked well involves a set of alternatives arranged to accomplish different purposes. The first alternative, if it can be achieved, is somewhat superior to the others insofar as it requires minimal shaping for optimal vocal responses. It is built around the pulsated vocal mode. This mode is sharply limited in the amount of constriction it can tolerate; that is, if it can be achieved at all, it is reasonably close to optimal. The slower the rate of pulsations, the more discrete, and the more explosive each pulse can be made, the freer of constriction is the production and the more effective it will be for establishing spontaneously optimal vocal production.

The sequence of procedures for this first alternative is as follows: swallow, yawn, pulsated vocal-mode production of /a/ and /eɪ/, breathy, heavy vocal-mode production of /hmeɪ/, /hmaɪ/, and /hmɔɪ/, counting, reading, and speaking. The rationale for this sequence is that it permits extension of a constriction-free condition from a reflexively elicited activity through a series of increasingly more complex and difficult vocalization tasks to its ultimately desired form in conversational speech; in other words, the rationale, to state it in terms of operant conditioning, is that of behavior shaping. As in all operant shaping, successive approximations of the finally desired behavior must meet criterian at each stage before the next, more complex, approximation is attempted. This means for voice therapy that if freedom from constriction is lost at any stage, the progression should immediately stop; the patient should be encouraged to relax during a few minutes of silence, deep breathing, and yawning; then, the entire sequence should be recycled. During the first session, one can proceed as far through the sequence as the patient demonstrates consistent success and easy mastery of the techniques: only one or two new skills requiring concentration should be assigned for practice between sessions.

A word about the efficacy of the procedures per se. A swallow followed by a yawn (preferably a genuine full-blown yawn) provides proprioceptive contrast of high and low constriction. Clear perception of this contrast should be established before undertaking the next approximation, the most difficult step in the sequence; this is the crucial point of transition from reflexive elicitation of constriction-free respondent behavior to volitional emission of constriction-free operant vocalization. The purpose of the yawn is to provide the "feel" of the vocal tract for an optimally produced /a/ and /eɪ/ in pulsated vocal mode. When ready for the transition, follow the yawn, without changing vocal "posture" (the feel of the vocal tract condition), with an easy inhalation, and then attempt pulsated phonation of /a/ or /eɪ/. The success of obtaining, initially, emission of pulsated vocal mode depends, in large measure, on the ability of the clinician to demonstrate the phonation desired. It is not used frequently in speech, except at the ends of falling inflections in optimally produced male voices, so it is often difficult to discover. Once the pulsated mode is emitted, even with constriction, reinforce it; removal of constriction is easier to achieve than the first emission of pulsated phonation. By obtaining control of the pulse rate, by slowing it and making each pulse as discrete a "pop" as possible, constriction will be removed spontaneously.

For the first alternative, mastery of pulsated voice is vital. If it cannot be achieved, this alternative must be abandoned. Not uncommonly, however, it can be obtained later following the use of other alternatives. The prospect of its achievement will dwindle as frustration from futile attempts mounts, so pressing for it should be avoided; periodic returns to it are more profitable. When, and if, pulsated voice can be obtained, as much time and effort as are necessary to shape it to its most optimal form will be well worth the investment. It will provide a therapeutic "home base" to which the patient can return to check "alignment" of his voice for all other forms of optimal vocal production.

The shaping procedures utilized following establishment of a home base are the same for all of the alternatives. Production of /hmeɪ/, /hmaɪ/, /hmɔɪ/ is used because the /h/ provides a soft, breathy tonal attack, /m/ provides a vocal posture that has a feel of balance about it, and /eɪ/, /aɪ/, /ɔɪ/ sample high, low, front, and back vowels and end with a sound that adds "brilliance" and carrying power to the voice. When these diphthongs are produced optimally, the voice feels and sounds big, effortless, and vibrant. Again, this stage should be thoroughly mastered before attempting to extend it. Counting is the next step, and is used because it requires little attention to the content of what is being spoken, yet provides a varied phonetic sequence through which vocal alignment must be maintained before success could be expected with reading. To begin this stage, reading material that requires minimal attention to content should be selected. The remainder of therapy is devoted to extending optimal vocal alignment into increasingly distracting and stressful speaking situations.

SECOND ALTERNATIVE SEQUENCE

The second alternative emphasizes the hygienic value of soft, breathy phonation. It differs from the first alternative only in the omission of pulsated voice. It is the alternative of choice under two conditions: when minimal voice usage is indicated, and when pulsated phonation cannot be achieved. The first condition provides the most compelling justification for this alternative. Some laryngologists recommend complete vocal rest from a few days to a few weeks following laryngeal surgery, and also as a means for permitting spontaneous remission of such functional pathologies as vocal nodules and contact ulcers. Complete silence, however, poses problems. For one thing, it is difficult to maintain. Ours is a verbal world. Even with the best of intentions we can hardly exist in it silently. But even if we could, prolonged silence has the undesired side effect of weakening muscle tone. A partial solution to these problems is to have the patient use an electrolarynx during the period of enforced silence. This does not lessen the tendency to weakened muscle tone, but it does relieve vocal abuse during the period of laryngeal recovery.

Many laryngologists prefer, instead of silence, minimal use of the voice under conditions that minimize vocal abuse. Soft, breathy phonation accomplishes this objective admirably. Fortunately, it can be obtained easily in its most desirable form by asking for the use of a "confidential voice." This guards against the constriction and force that frequently creep in to convert an easy whisper to a "stage whisper." The conditions under which the confidential voice should be utilized must be carefully restricted. Talking at cocktail parties, in an open car, in group conversations all preclude soft, breathy phonation. Under such conditions, vocal usage that starts out as "confidential" can soon become consequential in exacerbated laryngeal distress. When minimal speaking has been recommended, no attempt to progress to a full voice should be made without medical clearance.

Confidential voice can also be used as an alternative when pulsated voice cannot be achieved as a means of acquiring full-voiced optimal phonation. The second alternative follows the same sequence as the first, except that for the unavailable pulsated vocal mode, a sigh to terminate the yawn followed by confidential voice are substituted. They can, then, be followed by a laugh to help shift vocal initiation from breathy attack (hygienic but aerodynamically and acoustically inefficient) to soft attack (hygienic and efficient). By bringing the laugh under operant control, it provides an optimal soft attack that can be extended through the other procedural steps. This alternative can yield a voice minimally optimal for ordinary purposes. If, at any time during this alternative, pulsated voice can be achieved, reversion to the first alternative will normally yield a wider optimal range for the dimensions of vocal production.

THIRD ALTERNATIVE SEQUENCE

The third alternative is built around chewing functions. This approach has the advantage of providing a condition for operant vocalization simultaneous with the constriction-reducing effects of the vegetative function of chewing. Chewing sounds and words offer some good from both worlds; reduced constriction from the world of respondents combined with vocalization from the world of operants. If chewing speech freed the voice as effectively of constriction, and provided as balanced a vocal posture as does pulsated voice, it would offer the *best* of both worlds. But, in my experience, it does not. Others may find more success with it, and for them, it might be the therapy of choice. For me, it is a useful adjunct to the second alternative. When it is incorporated, the sequence is altered as followed: swallow, yawn-sigh, laugh, chewing sounds, confidential voice, and so on through the procedures as described for the first alternative.

A final word to stress what many clinicians already know: it is more important to master well each step in the successive approximations of optimal vocal functioning than to cover many steps rapidly or to provide the patient with an abundant variety of exercises. The gate to an optimally produced voice is strait. A plethora of techniques may bespeak therapeutic ingenuity, but it is no substitute for a few incisive procedures designed to accomplish specific purposes.

Contingencies of Reinforcement

The behaviors to be elicited or emitted have been specified, and the forms towards which these vocal responses are to be shaped have been defined. They are applicable for children as well as adults, for women as well as men, for the vocally gifted as well as the vocally handicapped. We will now turn to some tactics by which the frequency of occurrence of these performances can be managed by contingencies of reinforcement. This problem can be resolved into two basic issues: types of reinforcement available, and schedules by which reinforcement can be applied.

TYPES OF REINFORCEMENT

Types of reinforcement are determined by their consequences. Those conditions contingent on behavior that increase its frequency of occurrence are reinforcing; those that decrease its frequency are punishing. Reinforcement comes in two forms, as does punishment (Brookshire, 1967). Those stimuli that are rewarding, that a person will approach, characterize the condition for positive reinforcement. Those behaviors that offer escape from or avoidance of noxious aversive stimuli are negatively reinforced. Both forms of reinforcement increase frequency of response, one of approach behavior, the other of avoidance. Curiously, even in this business of behavioral management, two negatives can make a positive: by making aversive stimuli contingent on avoidance behavior, a condition is established in which avoiding avoidance is negatively reinforced; the result equals emission of approach responses. As for the two forms of punishment, one decreases frequency of response because positive reinforcement for it is withheld, the other decreases response rate because the contingent stimuli are aversive.

The system of operant vocal therapy presented here is not designed to extinguish responses, but rather to increase the frequency of occurrence of constriction-free responses. Accordingly, positive reinforcement is the most relevant. True, negative reinforcement increases the frequency of responses, but of avoidance responses. Moreover, it relies on aversive conditions, and the possibility of negative side effects from the use of noxious consequences still hovers ominously around this type of stimulus. The safest course currently available to the clinician is to utilize positive reinforcers.

The problem of managing positive reinforcement,

is, in one sense, easier with children than adults, and in another, more difficult. Children present an easier problem in that they want so many things. Pennies, candy, intriguing toys can all be rewarding, especially if their availability can be linked to what the child wants at the moment. This idea has been systematized by Addison and Homme (1966) in what they call the reinforcing event (RE) menu. It consists of a "menu" of stick drawings of the reinforcing events available to the child. Before the desired task is performed, the child selects the event he would prefer; he then completes the task, and if it is satisfactory, receives his reinforcement immediately.

Adults, on the other hand, are not likely to exert themselves mightily for extrinsically rewarding trinkets and tidbits. In fact, extraneous positive reinforcers for adults are hard to find: one man's meat is another's poison. Still, unlike children, adults who are good candidates for therapy are good candidates by virtue of their desire to improve their vocal production; improved performance for them has its own intrinsic rewards.

An approach to reinforcement, applicable to children and adults, is based on work by Premack (1959, 1961, 1963a, 1963b, 1963c) and has been elaborated by Homme (1965, 1966). The basic conception, sometimes called the Premack principle, is that given a pair of responses, the less probable one will be reinforced if the more probable one is made contingent on it. This notion takes cognizance of the tendency for motivations to fluctuate; what is reinforcing one minute may be neutral or aversive the next, or restated, what is high-probability behavior one minute may be low in probability the next. Practically, what is required of the clinician, in this approach, is a continual alertness for high-probability behavior that can be made contingent on the desired vocal performance. For instance, suppose a clinician notices that a child is pulling at a button on his coat instead of attending to the therapeutic task: button pulling at this moment is high-probability behavior and desired vocal production is low in probability. Following the Premack principle, if button pulling is made contingent on vocal performance, the vocal response will be reinforced. The principle is so simple that one is reluctant to credit its effectiveness, but effective it seems to be.

Two general points remain to be stressed in this brief discussion of types of reinforcement. First, an absolutely essential condition that must be observed continuously is that reinforcement follow the desired behavior immediately. Behavior does not occur in isolation; each instant of it occurs in a temporal stream of responses that flows within the larger context of a constantly changing stimulus environment. Delayed reinforcement, then, has the consequence of reinforcing the wrong behavior, occurring later in the sequence and in the wrong stimulus setting.

The second point to stress is that the reinforcing stimuli or events that are used in the clinic be available in the person's daily environment. Unless careful consideration is given to the conditions for reinforcement outside of the clinical setting, no permanent change in behavior is apt to be forthcoming.

SCHEDULES OF REINFORCEMENT

The schedules of reinforcement available are plentiful, and their differential effects could be discussed at length. Fortunately, for clinical purposes, we can content ourselves with two major considerations: schedules of reinforcement to initiate and to terminate therapy (Brookshire, 1967). Generally, a continuous reinforcement (crf) schedule should be used early in treatment when the rate of emission of desired behavior is low. Although reinforcement of each occurrence of a response is the most effective procedure for increasing its frequency of occurrence, this schedule is not especially effective for making a response resistant to extinction. Therefore, the schedule of preference, once an adequate response rate is achieved, is one of large variable ratios (VR) and intervals (VI). This schedule makes the sequence of reinforcements and the interval of time between reinforcements unpredictable, and produces steady emission of the desired response in expectation of its eventual reinforcement. Moreover, a variable schedule is more typical of reinforcement conditions encountered in everyday living.

Stimulus Control

Finally, we come to what, for many speech clinicians, is their nemesis: carry-over. This is, essentially, a problem of stimulus control of desired responses. All learned behavior is acquired in environmental contexts. We not only learn what to do, but equally as important, when to do it. Discrimination among various stimulus patterns is our basis for appropriate behavior. Conversely, the stimulus patterns under which responses are acquired, in turn, control emission of those responses whether we like it or not. I have often had the experience of obtaining constriction-free vocal responses from a patient anywhere in our clinic, but, upon leaving the building where all of the therapeutic modifications have been obtained, of then having the new responses deteriorate progressively with each step toward the street. Systematic manipulation of stimuli is as crucial to a permanent new response as is control of the behavior itself. Again, the conditions for initiating and for terminating therapy are of particular importance. The beginning of treatment will be facilitated if it bears little resemblance to daily conditions in which the undesired responses are emitted. The less the similarity between the stimulus conditions under which, let's say, abusive vocalization occurs and the clinic conditions, the less probable the emission of vocally abusive behavior in the clinic. This consideration offers an additional advantage to starting therapy with responses that bear little resemblance to normal speech, e.g., pulsated voice, chewing, laughing, yawning, sighing, confidential voice.

The opposite arrangement is sought toward the end of treatment; the stimulus conditions in the clinic should be modified systematically until they resemble, as closely as possible, those that the patient will encounter outside of the clinic. Naturally the modifications should be gradual enough not to imperil the adequacy of the new response. Several approaches to carry-over are possible. All involve analysis of the patient's typical speaking activities for the most predominant and the most troublesome conditions (these conditions are not necessarily identical). Those deemed most important are selected for simulation in the clinic. Some, such as telephoning, can be simulated easily. Others will require different tactics. One of the most effective is to bring a crucial person in the patient's life, a spouse, a friend, a parent, into the treatment sessions at the clinic; their presence then exerts stimulus control over the desired behavior at home, at school, at work. If this arrangement is impossible, as it will often be for professional colleagues, the alternative is to extend stimulus control by sending some part of the clinical setting, possibly the clinician, into the patient's environment.

The Whole Person

Implicit throughout this system of therapy is the idea of its application with a view to the needs of the whole person. To the extent that these needs include improvement of vocal performance, the procedures described will facilitate management of this part of his life. The presumption is that desire for accomplishment, alone, is not enough. Without knowledge of exactly what to do, uncertainty and frustration more than progress will result. This system is intended to provide the necessary knowledge.

The procedures have been designed for holistic application. The key to optimal vocal functioning is freedom from vocal constriction, so the techniques are intended to establish this freedom in all dimensions simultaneously. Alertness for signs of constriction in other dimensions must accompany work focused on a single dimension: constriction shifted from one dimension to another does not represent therapeutic progress.

A favorite site for emotional tension is the voice; it is easily pulled out of optimal balance by various forms of stress. The objective of this therapeutic system is to give a person the tools with which to rebalance the voice, usually in a few minutes, when it has become constricted. Once the voice is in optimal balance, the techniques described here are unnecessary to maintain it. Even during the period of work in the clinic when optimal vocal functioning is being established, the procedures being used do not require prolonged practice. Throughout, they need be used for only a few minutes at a time; but, they should be used as frequently as is necessary to maintain optimal vocal alignment as constantly as possible.

SUMMARY

The aim in this Chapter has been to objectify vocal functioning, and thereby to make its disorders manageable for the clinician. First, criteria have been established by which optimal performance can be assessed. Second, the criteria have been applied to the five dimensions of vocal production—pitch, loudness, voicing, vocal mode, and vocal constriction—to establish a tangible goal for voice therapy: an integrated balance of optimally hygienic vocal functions. Third, a group of simple objective procedures for altering vocal production holistically toward an optimal balance have been organized into a system of alternative sequences. Key techniques for each sequence are sufficiently varied and universally available that any patient seriously interested in vocal therapy can easily, quickly, and closely approach the most hygienic voice of which he is capable. Finally, these alternative sequences have been organized with-in the framework of operant behavior therapy to establish and strengthen optimal vocal functioning in the clinic, and to insure its carry-over into normal daily life.

BIBLIOGRAPHY

Addison, R., and Homme, L. 1966. The reinforcing event (RE) menu. *NSPI J.*, 4, 8–9.

Arnold, G. 1962. Vocal nodules and polyps: laryngeal tissue reaction to habitual hyperkinetic dysphonia. *J. Speech Hearing Disorders*, 27, 205–217.

Aronson, A., Brown, J., Litin, E., and Pearson, J. 1968. Spastic dysphonia. II. Comparison with essential (voice) tremor and other neurologic and psychogenic dysphonias. *J. Speech Hearing Disorders*, 33, 219–231.

Beckett, R. 1968. Pitch perturbation as a function of vocal constriction. Univ. South Calif.: Ph.D. dissertation.

Bell Telephone Laboratories. 1937. High speed motion pictures of the vocal cords. New York: Bur. of Publication.

Berg, J. van den. 1956. Direct and indirect determination of the mean subglottic pressure. *Folia Phoniat.*, 8, 1–24.

———. 1958. Myoelastic-aerodynamic theory of voice production. *J. Speech Hearing Res.*, 1, 227–244.

———, Zantema, J., and Doornenbal, P. 1957. On the air resistance and the Bernoulli effect of the human larynx. *J. acoust. soc. Amer.*, 29, 621–631.

Bloch, P. 1965. Neuro-psychiatric aspects of spastic dysphonia. *Folia Phoniat.*, 17, 301–364.

Brewer, D. 1963. Contact ulcer of the larynx. *N.Y. State J. Med.*, 63, 3100.

———, Briess, F., and Faaborg-Andersen, K. 1960. Phonation: clinical testing versus electromyography. *Ann. Otol. Rhinol. Laryng.*, 69, 781–804.

Briess, F. 1957. Voice therapy: identification of specific laryngeal muscle dysfunction by voice testing. *Arch. Otolaryng.*, 66, 375–382 (Part 1).

———. 1959. Voice therapy: essential treatment phases of specific laryngeal muscle dysfunction. *Arch. Otolaryng.*, 69, 61–69 (Part 2).

Brodnitz, F. 1960. Speech after glossectomy. *In* Current problems, phoniatrics and logopedics. Trojan, F., ed. Basel, N.Y.: Kerger. Pp. 68–71.

———. 1961. Contact ulcer of the larynx. *Arch. Otolaryng.*, 74, 70–80.

———. 1965. Vocal rehabilitation. Rochester, Minn.: Amer. Acad. Opthal. Otolaryng.

Brookshire, R. 1967. Speech pathology and the experimental analysis of behavior. *J. Speech Hearing Disorders*, 32, 215–227.

Coleman, R. 1963. Decay characteristics of vocal fry. *Folia Phoniat.*, 15, 256–263.

Damsté, P. 1967. Voice change in adult women caused by virilizing agents. *J. Speech Hearing Disorders*, 32, 126–132.

Draper, M., Ladefoged, P., and Whitteredge, D. 1959. Respiratory muscles in speech. *J. Speech Hearing Res.*, 2, 16–27.

Dreher, J., and Bragg, V. 1953. Evaluation of voice normality. *Speech Monogr.*, 20, 74–78.

Faaborg-Andersen, K. 1957. Electromyographic investigation of intrinsic laryngeal muscles in humans. *Acta Physiologica Scandinavia, Suppl. 41.*

Fairbanks, G. 1960. Voice and articulation (2nd. ed.). New York: Harper.

Flanagan, J. 1958. Some properties of the glottal sound source. *J. Speech Hearing Res.*, 1, 99–116.

Fletcher, W. 1954. Vocal fold activity and subglottic air pressure in relation to vocal intensity: A brief historical review. *Speech Monogr.*, 21, 73–78.

Froeschels, E. 1952. Chewing method as therapy. *Arch. Otolaryng.*, 56, 427–434.

Goldiamond, I. 1962. Perception. *In* Experimental foundations of clinical psychology. Bachrach, A., ed. New York: Basic Books.

Gray, B., England, G., and Mohoney, J. 1965. Treatment of benign vocal nodules by reciprocal inhibition. *Behavior Res. Therapy*, 3, 187–193.

Hanley, T., and Thurman, W. 1962. Developing vocal skills. New York: Holt, Rinehart and Winston.

Hollien, H. 1960a. Some laryngeal correlates of vocal pitch. *J. Speech Hearing Res.*, 3, 52–58.

———. 1960b. Vocal pitch variation related to changes in vocal fold length. *J. Speech Hearing Res.*, 3, 150–156.

———. 1962. Vocal fold thickness and fundamental frequency of phonation. *J. Speech Hearing Res.*, 5, 237–243.

———, and Curtis, J. 1960. A laminagraphic study of vocal pitch. *J. Speech Hearing Res.*, 3, 361–371.

———, and Moore, P. 1960. Measurements of the vocal folds during changes in pitch. *J. Speech Hearing Res.*, 3, 157–165.

———, Moore, P., Wendahl, R., and Michel, J. 1966. On the nature of vocal fry. *J. Speech Hearing Res.*, 9, 245–247.

Homme, L. 1965. Perspectives in psychology—XXIV: control of coverants, the operants of the mind. *Psychol. Record*, 15, 501–511.

———. 1966. Contiguity theory and contingency management. *Psychol. Record*, 16, 233–241.

House, A. 1959. A note on optimal vocal frequency. *J. Speech Hearing Res.*, 2, 55–60.

Isshiki, N. 1964. Regulatory mechanisms of voice intensity variation. *J. Speech Hearing Res.*, 7, 17–29.

———, and von Leden, H. 1964. Hoarseness-aerodynamic studies. *Arch. Otolaryng.*, 80, 206–213.

Iwata, S., and von Leden, H. 1970. Pitch pertubations in normal and pathologic voices. *Folia Phoniat.*, 22, 413–424.

Jackson, C. 1928. Contact ulcer of the larynx. *Ann. Otol., Rhinol., Laryng.*, 37, 227–230.

Johnson, W., Darley, F., and Spriestersbach, D. 1963. Diagnostic methods in speech pathology. New York: Harper & Row.

Joyner, J. 1968. Air flow as a function of vocal constriction. Univ. South. Calif.: Ph.D. dissertation.

Kiml, P. 1965. Reserches expérimentales de la dysphonic spastique. *Folia Phoniat.*, 17, 241–300.

Koike, Y. 1967. Experimental studies on vocal attack. *Practica Otologica Kyoto*, 60, 663–688.

———, 1967. Personal communication.

———, and Hirano, M. Significance of vocal velocity index: Laryngeal pathology (to be published).

Ladefoged, P. 1963. Some physiological parameters in speech. *Language and Speech*, 6, 109–119.

———, and McKinney, N. 1963. Loudness, sound pressure, and subglottal pressure in speech. *J. acoust. soc. Amer.*, 35, 454–460.

Lieberman, A., Cooper, F., Harris, K., and MacHeilage, P. 1963. Motor theory of speech perception. Abstract. *J. acoust. soc. Amer.*, 35, 1114.

Luchsinger, R., and Arnold, G. 1965. Voice-speech-language. Belmont, Calif.: Wadsworth.

McGlone, R. 1967. Air flow during vocal fry phonation. *J. Speech Hearing Res.*, 10, 299–304.

Miller, R. 1957. An experimental study of the evaluations by untrained listeners of efficient and inefficient voice production as to quality. Univ. South. Calif.: Ph.D. dissertation.

Moore, P. 1967. Laryngeal physiology. Short Course. ASHA convention.

———, and von Leden, H. 1958. Dynamic variations of the vibratory pattern in the normal larynx. *Folia Phoniat.*, 10, 205–238.

Moses, P. 1959. Emotional causes of vocal pathology. *In* Psychological aspects of speech and hearing disorders. Barbara, D., ed. Springfield, Ill.: Thomas.

Ohala, J. 1966. A new photo-electric glottograph. *Working papers in phonetics*, 4, 40–52.

Perkins, W. 1957. The challenge of functional disorders of voice. *In* Handbook of speech pathology. Travis, L., ed. New York: Appleton-Century-Crofts.

———, and Yanagihara, N. 1968. Parameters of vocal production: 1. some mechanisms for the regulation of pitch. *J. Speech Hearing Res.*, 11, 246–267. 2. Some mechanisms for the regulation of loudness (to be published).

Premack, D. 1959. Toward empirical behavior laws: 1. positive reinforcement. *Psychol. Rev.*, 66, 219–233.

———. 1961. Predicting instrumental performance from the independent rate of contingent response. *J. exper. Psychol.*, 61, 163–171.

———. 1963a. Rate differential reinforcement in monkey manipulation. *J. exper. Analysis Behavior*, 6, 81–89.

———. 1963b. Prediction of the comparative reinforcement values of running and drinking. *Science*, 139, 1062–1063.

———. 1963c. Running as both a positive and negative reinforcer. *Science*, 142, 1087–1088.

Pressman, J. 1942. Physiology of the vocal cords in phonation and respiration. *Arch. Otolaryng.*, 35, 355–398.

Pronovost, W. 1939. An experimental study of habitual and natural pitch levels of superior speakers. Univ. Iowa: Ph.D. dissertation.

———. 1942. An experimental study of methods for determining natural and habitual pitch. *Speech Monogr.*, No. 9.

Robe, E., Brumlik, J., and Moore, P. 1960. A study of spastic dysphonia neurologic and electroencephalographic abnormalities. *Laryngoscope*, 70, 219–245.

Soron, H. 1967. High-speed photography in speech research. *J. Speech Hearing Res.*, 10, 768–776.

———. 1968. Personal communication.

Thurman, W. 1954. The construction and acoustic analysis of recorded scales of severity for six voice quality disorders. Purdue Univ.: Ph.D. dissertation.

———. 1958. Frequency-intensity relationships and optimum pitch level. *J. Speech Hearing Res.*, 1, 117–123.

Timcke, R., von Leden, H., and Moore, P. 1958. Laryngeal vibrations: measurements of the glottic wave. *Arch. Otolaryng.*, 68, 1–19.

———, ———, and ———. 1958. Laryngeal vibrations: measurements of the glottic wave: physiologic variations. *Arch. Otolaryng.*, 69, 438–444 (Part 2).

Tonndort, W. 1925. Die Mechanik bei der Stimmlippenschwingung und beim Schnarchen. *Hals-, Nasen-, u. Ohrenheilk*, 12, 241–245.

Van Riper, C. 1963. Speech correction (4th. ed.). Englewood Cliffs, N.J.: Prentice-Hall.

———, and Irwin, J. 1958. Voice and articulation. Englewood Cliffs, N.J.: Prentice-Hall.

Vennard, W. 1967. Singing: the mechanism and the technic (4th. ed.). New York: Fischer.

———. 1968. Personal communication.

———, and Isshiki, N. 1964. Coupe de glotte, a misunderstood expression. *N.A.T.S. Bulletin*, 20, 15–18.

von Leden, H. 1961. The mechanism of phonation. *Arch. Otolaryng.*, 74, 660–676.

———. 1967. Personal communication.

———, and Moore, P. 1960. Contact ulcer of the larynx. *Arch. Otolaryng.*, 72, 746–752.

———, ———, and Timcke, R. 1960. Laryngeal vibrations: measurements of the glottic wave.—The pathologic larynx. *Arch. Otolaryng.*, 71, 16–35 (Part 3).

Wendahl, R. 1963. Laryngeal analog synthesis of harsh voice quality. *Folia Phoniat.*, 15, 241–250.

———, Moore, P., and Hollien, H. 1963. Comments on vocal fry. *Folia Phoniat.*, 15, 251–255.

Wilson, K. 1966. Laryngeal voice problems of children. Paper presented ASHA convention.

Wyatt, G. 1951. The application of Froeschels' chewing method in the treatment of disorders of the speaking voice. *In* The chewing approach in speech and voice therapy. Weiss, D., and Beebe, H., eds. New York: Kerger.

Yanagihara, N. 1967. Significance of harmonic changes and noise components in hoarseness. *J. Speech Hearing Res.*, 10, 531–541.

———, Koike, Y., and von Leden, H. 1966. Phonation and respiration. *Folia Phonat.*, 18, 323–340.

21

Voice Disorders Organically Based

G. Paul Moore

When an individual speaks habitually with a voice that differs in pitch, loudness, or quality from the voices of others of the same age and sex within his cultural group, he is considered to have a voice disorder. This traditional definition recognizes that there are children's voices, adult voices, male voices, and female voices, and that these may vary normally among cultural groups. The definition also presumes that there is a normal pitch, loudness, and quality for each population group and that differences between normal and abnormal vocal sound can be readily and uniformly identified. Recognition and differentiation are accomplished by the auditor; it is he, as the definition indicates, who identifies the voice disorder. It follows that the perceived defectiveness of any one voice will vary among listeners without change in the actual voice. It is apparent that a voice is abnormal for a particular individual when he judges it to be so. Judgment implies a set of standards that are learned through experience and that are related to the judge's own aesthetic and cultural criteria. Judgment also implies that standards are not fixed, that there is opportunity for more than one conclusion. This flexibility in determining the defectiveness of voices does not alter the validity of the basic definition of voice disorders, but it does underscore the observation that vocal standards are culturally based and environmentally determined. The child, the parent, the adult, the employer, and the speech pathologist may have markedly different concepts of voice, and this possibility must temper the approach of the latter to voice evaluation, diagnosis, and therapy.

Since the focus of this chapter is on voice disorders that are related to organic abnormalities in contrast to functional problems, the discussion will center on those defects of pitch, loudness, and quality that are associated with deviations in size, shape, tonicity, surface conditions, and muscular control of the phonating and resonating mechanisms. These differences result from such causes as heredity, disease, injury, abuse, and surgery.

The foregoing statement identifies three kinds of information that are essential in a consideration of voice defects and their management. The first is the symptom, the acoustic element, that which is heard and labeled as the voice defect. The second is the abnormal function of the mechanism, that which is the immediate cause of the acoustic deviation. The third is the pathology, the basic organic condition that alters the function and is of primary concern in diagnosis and treatment. These three levels are intertwined, but for systematic presentation each requires separate consideration.

The problems that are heard as abnormal pitch, loudness, or quality are directly related to the mechanisms of the respiratory tract and to their associated structures. When voice defects are present, it means that the vocal folds or the resonators are not operating normally. These abnormal functions may result from the way the individual learned to produce voice, or they may stem directly from such organic disorders as tumors, infections, loss of tissue, debilitating disease, systemic conditions, structural anomalies, or paralysis. Differentiating between so-called functional and organic disorders is a division of logical convenience, but in reality there is often no clear distinction between these types of voice problems. Malfunction may cause structural change; and conversely, structural anomalies or disease may produce malfunctions that remain after alleviation of the organic problem.

PHONATORY THEORY

Phonation is the process of producing vocal sound. It normally occurs when the breath in the course of exhalation sets the vocal folds into vibration. This action generates a series of pressure pulses that travel as sound waves through the respiratory tract, where they are modified by the process of resonance.

The pitch of the vocal sound is directly related to the frequency of vibration which is determined by the mass, elasticity, length, and compliance of the folds. The heavier and more massive the vibrators, other factors constant, the slower is their movement and the lower the pitch. Conversely, the greater the elasticity, the quicker is the recoil of the vibrators after displacement, the faster the vibratory excursion, the greater the frequency of vibration, and the higher the pitch. The longer the vibrators, other factors constant, the slower the frequency and the lower the pitch. However, if the vocal folds are elongated, or stretched, their elasticity is increased and the unit mass decreased, which in combination counteract the greater length and thereby cause a higher frequency. Compliance refers to relative ease of displacement and compression at various regions of the glottis. This factor is determined by the shape of the vocal folds, the texture of the mucosa, and the degree of firmness of the underlying tissues. The most compliant areas of the glottal border are displaced first by subglottal pressure and are compressed most completely during the closed phases of the vibratory cycle. When massive compression of compliant areas occurs, the time of the vibratory closure is lengthened and frequency is reduced.

The loudness of vocal sound is determined by the pressures that are generated in the released pulsations by the combination of volume and velocity of air flowing through the glottis at any instant. Increased pulsatile pressure causes greater amplitude of movement of air molecules, which, in turn, extend the excursions of the ear mechanism and thereby generate the sensation of a louder sound.

The quality of voice is determined by both vocal fold vibration and resonance. The phonatory aspect includes the manner of air-pulse formation and the sequencing of vibratory cycles, both of which are regulated by the movements of the vocal folds. Resonance is related to the adjustments of the size and shape of the several regions of the respiratory tract and of the diameter and length of the spaces connecting them.

Textbooks typically describe phonation as occurring when the vocal folds are adducted to close the glottis, after which the breath pressure increases subglottally until it becomes great enough to force the folds apart. At that moment a pulse of air escapes which reduces the subglottal pressure sufficiently to allow the vocal folds to restore the glottal closure. This occlusion results from the elasticity of the folds and the Bernoulli effect created by the flow of air through the glottal space. When the folds close the airway, the activating pressure again increases to the breakthrough point and the vibratory process is repeated. This repetitive starting and stopping of the air flow will continue regularly so long as the alternating relationship between vocal fold resistance and air pressure continues. When this type of sequence is maintained, the voice is classified as normal.

The preceding traditional description of phonation is not inaccurate; it is incomplete. It presents one form of vocal fold vibration, but it neglects other types that are important in the consideration of both normal and abnormal voice production. The vocal folds often are set into vibration when they are not completely adducted. With this adjustment the air flows through the glottis, alternately in greater and lesser amounts, thereby creating a chain of pressure variations that are heard as tone. Concurrently, the more or less continuous flow of breath also creates turbulence in the air stream that generates other pressure changes which are heard as noise superimposed upon or combined with the vocal tone. Together these two sound sources produce a breathy type of sound that may be heard in aspirate initiation of vowel sounds, in pseudo whispering, and in chronically breathy voices.

The paired vocal folds are customarily pictured as a functional vibratory unit. In the normal larynx both folds have the same length, contain similar muscle masses, maintain comparable tension, have about the same compliance, adduct symmetrically, and are activated uniformly by a common air pressure. As a result of these features, both vocal folds normally vibrate synchronously and simultaneously. However, this normal function should not obscure the fact that each fold is a distinct unit capable of vibrating independently. The significance of this observation becomes evident through an analysis of the vocal cord vibration that causes hoarseness characterized by vocal roughness.

Study of sound-wave patterns of vocal roughness reveals a random variability in the lengths or amplitudes of consecutive vibratory cycles. Parallel analysis of ultra high-speed motion pictures of vocal fold vibration occurring during the production of vocal roughness demonstrates random variations of vibration that are comparable to the acoustic patterns. Each vocal fold may move as a semiindependent vibrator having a frequency that differs from that of the other fold and having vibratory movements that are often aperiodic. Furthermore, when two somewhat asynchronous vibrators act concurrently upon the glottal closure, and consequently upon the pressure variations of the sound wave, they create irregularly spaced glottal openings and thereby form an aperiodic sound source. The differences between the frequencies of the vocal folds, the number and length of glottal closures, and the manner of pulse release combine to influence the character of the sound produced. Vibrational differences between the vocal folds can be caused by such factors as increase of the mass of one fold, by change in elasticity, or by modification of effective length. Details of these and other factors affecting vocal fold vibration will be considered in some detail in succeeding sections.

DESCRIPTION OF VOICE DISORDERS

Phonatory Voice Deviations

PITCH

There are three types of vocal-pitch deviations: 1. those that are consistently higher (in relation to the musical scale) than are customarily found among persons of the same age and sex in a particular cultural group; 2. those that are lower (in reference to the same circumstances as indicated under point 1); and 3. those that do not fit the meaning being expressed, including such deviations as bizarre melody patterns, monotone, and tremulousness.

LOUDNESS

Disorders of vocal loudness may be classified as follows: 1. voices that are too loud in relation to the place and circumstances; 2. voices that are not loud enough to meet communication needs; and 3. vocal variations that do not convey the intended meaning of the speaker.

QUALITY

Quality deviations are the most frequent and the most complex of the voice problems. They are commonly classified as phonatory, those disorders associated with sound generation at the vocal folds; and resonance, those problems related to sound modification in the spaces of the respiratory tract. The phonatory defects, often listed as dysphonias, are determined by the complexity of vocal fold movement and can be placed along a continuous scale extending from aphonia through intermittent phonation, breathiness, hoarseness, and rough hoarseness. The resonance disorders are related most commonly to the patency of the nasal passages and vary from extreme hypernasality to extreme denasality. Voice qualities rarely exist as isolated entities; instead they tend to combine and thereby to create extremely complex vocal disorders. However, it is essential that the features of each be recognized, so that they can be identified even in combination.

The aphonic voice is a whisper. In complete aphonia the whispered speech flows smoothly; the vocal folds do not interfere with the outgoing breath and they do not vibrate. However, in some so-called aphonias, the air flow is interrupted by momentary spasmodic closure of the glottis, which causes the speech to be halting and arhythmic. This type of disorder is sometimes designated as spastic dysphonia or hysterical aphonia. Occasionally, as the spasmodic closure is released, there will be a moment of voiced sound. When this occurs frequently, it produces one type of intermittent phonation. Another form of intermittency may occur in direct relation to the force of the exhaled air stream. In this instance, the voice breaks suddenly from a whisper to phonated sound and back again at frequent intervals, often several times within a word. Almost always the phonated portions are of defective quality, either breathy or hoarse.

Breathy voice, as described previously, is composed of a combination of vocal fold sound and whisper noise produced by turbulent air. Usually pitch variation is present, and frequently the overall intensity is diminished. The quality of the breathy voice varies over a wide range that is determined by the ratio of breath noise to phonatory sound. At one end of this spectrum the phonatory aspect predominates; at the other extreme the turbulence noise is relatively prominent and is usually caused by increased air flow, related either to an effort to force more sound from an impaired larynx or to a laryngeal condition that requires high air-flow rates and pressure to initiate and maintain vibration.

Hoarseness has been experienced at some time by most persons during an attack of laryngitis. The complex acoustical structure of this voice quality is characterized by the combination of a low-pitched phonatory sound from the vocal folds and a noise that is similar to the relatively constant static noises from a radio. These vocal noises probably result from many concurrent high-frequency oscillations and transient disturbances of the mucosa, mucus, tumors, or other flaccid, soft, moist surfaces on the vocal folds. An extreme example of hoarseness resulting from the vibration of flaccid structures and secretions is often heard in esophageal speech.

Hoarseness has many varieties and degrees of severity. It may be similar to breathiness, and in fact some voices vary between that quality and hoarseness in relation to sudden extra vocal effort or following a period of vocal abuse or during a "cold." In contrast, hoarseness may contain very little audible phonatory sound and be composed instead almost entirely of noise accompanied by evidence of vocal effort.

The term "rough hoarseness" indicates a common phonatory defect that is associated with hoarseness but also contains an impression of auditory roughness. Occasionally the element of roughness gives the impression of a second sound superimposed at a lower pitch. As indicated in the preceding discussion of phonatory theory, the rough quality comes from a randomly variable series of sound pulsations caused by different vibratory frequencies and patterns in the two vocal folds. The degree of roughness varies among voices and is related to the amount of variation in time or intensity from one vibratory episode to the next in a phonatory sequence.

Harshness is a term that is often used to describe an extremely low-pitched vocal sound that falls well below the lowest part of the ordinary phonatory range. It is recognized by a popping or ticking component that is determined by the glottal pulse release. The vibratory pattern is distinguished by a relatively brief glottal opening followed by an extremely long closed phase in the vibratory episode. Irregularity of the length of successive vibratory periods often occurs and adds a roughness factor to the sound. Harshness is very complex acoustically, containing a large number of high-frequency partials. This complexity probably accounts for its classification as an unusual quality rather than as an abnormally low pitch. The quality is almost always voluntarily or functionally produced, but it is also possible for marked increase in the mass of the vocal folds to contribute to its production, which accounts for its inclusion in this discussion.

Resonance Voice Problems

There are many subtle variations in voice quality that are related to resonance phenomena, but the two problems that are associated most frequently with organic conditions and which therefore deserve mention here are excessive nasality and its physiological opposite, denasality.

NASALITY

Nasality is a general symptom classification that includes all those voices that have an excessive nasal component. Acoustically, nasal speech is composed of the customary sounds of language with a simultaneous overlay of nasal sound. That is, the vowels are recognizable, yet they are distorted by the additional nasal element. The intensity of the audible portion of the nasal component determines the severity of the voice defect. This variation seems to be directly related physiologically to the size of the velopharyngeal opening and the degree of closure of the mouth cavity. It may be related acoustically also to the formants of the vowels in such a way as to emphasize the characteristic nasal-frequency components with some vowels and to suppress the nasal component with others.

Nasal voices of organic origin vary considerably in quality and severity. Some speakers are almost unintelligible, while others differ only slightly from normal. The quality may be openly resonant (rhinolalia aperta), as found typically with such disorders as cleft palate, paralysis of the velar muscles, congenitally short palate, or perforated palate; or the quality may be "twangy," the type of voice that anyone can produce by pinching the nostrils and "talking into the nose." Frequently the open nasality is accompanied by superfluous noises caused by the uncontrolled rush of air through the nose during the production of plosive and fricative consonants. The "twangy" voice referred to is caused either by the combination of an anterior blockage in the nose and an open velopharyngeal channel or by a small velopharyngeal oriface and normal nasal passages. The anterior obstruction allows the nose to serve as a resonator as far forward as the region of blockage, which causes the nasal formants to be emphasized and the "twang" sound to be heard. The constricted velopharyngeal opening creates a resonating system that emphasizes nasal components while maintaining relatively normal resonance and articulatory function in the pharynx and oral cavities. The nasal twang is a piercing sound often used intentionally by news vendors and others who hawk their wares. Under these circumstances the problem has a functional rather than an organic cause.

DENASALITY

Denasality, rhinolalia clausa posterior, is acoustically different from excessive nasality, but because both nasality and denasality are associated with abnormalities of the nasal passages, they are usually discussed together. Denasality results from the reduction in, or absence of, the normally expected nasal sounds and consequently is most obvious in the production of the nasal consonants, m, n, and ng. This vocal characteristic has been experienced by most persons during a severe "head cold," when the nasal passages were blocked. If the voice defect is chronic, there is a relatively constant obstruction in the nasopharynx or posterior part of the nasal passages which eliminates use of the nose as a resonator. Denasality often interferes seriously with the intelligibility of speech and consequently deserves careful remedial attention.

Rhinolalia becomes complicated further in those instances where there is a partial posterior obstruction associated with inadequate velopharyngeal closure. This voice may be illustrated by the person with a head cold who purposely tries to nasalize his speech. The sounds that are normally non-nasal become somewhat nasal, and the nasal consonants are more or less denasal. Both qualities are audible in the same voice.

THE PHYSIOLOGY OF ORGANIC VOICE DISORDERS

In the foregoing section, an attempt was made to describe the acoustic aspects of voice defects, which are the symptoms of abnormal behavior or function of the voicing mechanism. In the present section, the acoustic phenomena will be linked with the organic deviations that cause the atypical behavior. Somewhat later in this discussion, the underlying pathologies that produce the organic changes will be introduced.

Pitch Defects

CHRONICALLY HIGH PITCH

A consistently high-pitched voice in the late adolescent and adult male is one of the most distressing of voice defects. The resemblance to the female voice suggests a lack of masculinity. It is this implication, with its psychosocial sequelae, that creates the seriousness of the disorder, since the voice proper does not interfere with communication; nor would it be unpleasant if it were produced by a female.

Most "juvenile voices" are functional and psychogenic, but there are three organic causes that are found occasionally. The first of these is the failure of the larynx to develop to the necessary size to produce a masculine pitch. In this instance the vocal cords are small, as in the female larynx, and consequently vibrate more rapidly, producing a higher pitch than is normally expected. Sometimes this small larynx accompanies a general structural retardation or is part of a characteristic familial body size. The larynx may fail to develop, also, as a result of insufficient gonadal influence. This glandular lack is usually demonstrated simultaneously in the retardation of hair growth on the face, masculine physique, and other secondary sex characteristics.

The second organic cause of high-pitched voice is laryngeal web, a defect that is usually congenital but which may also be cicatricial. Webs vary considerably in size, and when large will interfere with breathing, thereby demanding early medical attention. However, those that are small often go undetected until the voice is observed as being abnormal. The speech pathologist is obligated to be alert for this problem since he is often the first professional worker to become aware of its possible presence.

A web is a shelf-like membrane that is usually located in the anterior portion of the larynx and ordinarily extends from one vocal fold to the other, but webs are also found both subglottally and supraglottally. When a web is attached to the vocal folds, it shortens their vibrating portions and consequently produces a faster oscillation and a resultant higher pitch. It may also be wedged into the anterior commissure when the vocal folds are adducted, thereby effectively shortening the vibrators and contributing to a high pitch. This obstruction may also impair the regularity of the vibratory pattern and consequently cause a hoarseness or roughness. Frequently, the high pitch and roughness are accompanied by the audible evidence of vocal strain or effort, particularly in adult males who have attempted to force a vocal pitch that is below the capability of their larynges.

The third organic cause for a chronically high pitch is an abnormal approximation of the vocal cords. In this condition a structural asymmetry causes one vocal process of an arytenoid to slide under or over the other so that the posterior segments of the vocal folds are pressed together, thereby damping the movement in these areas and effectively limiting the vibration to the anterior portions of the folds, which increases the vibrating rate and raises the pitch.

ABNORMALLY LOW PITCH

A masculine voice in a female is as distressing to the one possessing it as is the high-pitched voice in the male, and for the same psychosocial reasons. The persistent low pitch is almost always caused by an increase of the mass of the vocal folds through such organic lesions as edema, tumors, or the changes of virilization. The three most common etiologic factors in abnormally low pitch of women's voices are hormonal therapy, tumors, and nerve damage.

Masculine voices have developed in adult females following periods of male hormone therapy. The defect persists after the cessation of the therapy and there is no known method of reversing the process. Mirror views of the virilized larynx reveal what appears to be slight bulging of the vocal folds into the glottal area anteriorly from the vocal processes. However, this observation is subject to question since the larynges involved are usually seen only after the vocal changes have occurred and, consequently, the size and shape of the vocal folds prior to the change were not known. An assumption of psychogenic involvement is not justified by the data.

Weighting of the vocal folds by tumors, edema, hyperplasia, and other enlargements produces low pitch and hoarseness by slowing the vibration rate and causing irregular vibrations. Usually, a swelling or tumor that is extensive enough to cause a defectively low pitch will also produce hoarseness, and the voice is apt to be classified under the latter heading.

Damage to the nerve supply of the larynx may cause a flaccid paralysis in one or both vocal cords, and consequently a low pitch. With both folds involved, there may be an aphonia unless the arytenoids can be approximated. In the latter instance, and also where only one fold is paralyzed, this elasticity is reduced, which causes the folds to vibrate more slowly. The low pitch of paralysis is often accompanied by hoarseness, which is usually more prominent than the low pitch and therefore represents the customary classification of the defect.

In the preceding description of pitch defects, a reference was made to tremulousness, monotone, and similar pitch disorders. Most of these are functional rather than organic and consequently are discussed in the appropriate chapter of this book. However, there is an occasional tremulous voice or a voice without pitch changes that is caused by deterioration or injury to the central nervous system. In these cases, in which Parkinsonism is probably the most common disease, the other physical symptoms are so pronounced that the voice is of relatively minor importance and deserves no more than simple recognition here.

Loudness Defects

Voices that are too loud or not loud enough to satisfy the immediate communication needs are almost always functional in origin. The most evident partial exception to the general statement is in those loudness differences that are associated with hearing loss. In this situation the symptom is corrected by improving the hearing rather than by attention to the voice.

Weak voices are often caused by paresis, or paralysis, in the larynx or in some of the muscles of respiration. When the cords cannot interrupt the flow of breath enough to allow subglottal pressure to develop or when the muscles of exhalation are unable to provide sufficient air pressure in the trachea for vigorous activation of the cords, a weak voice will result. This weakness is almost always accompanied by breathiness which becomes increasingly prominent as the patient attempts to speak louder.

Quality Defects

APHONIA

The absence of vocal sound indicates that the vocal folds are not vibrating. There are two general organic conditions under which this circumstance may occur: when the vocal folds cannot be approximated sufficiently to be set in motion by the air stream; and when they are not capable of vibrating, regardless of their relation to the breath flow. The former condition may occur under three circumstances: 1. adductor paralysis; 2. ankylosis of the cricoarytenoid joints; or 3. the presence of an interarytenoid mass large enough to prevent approximation.

The second general condition exists, or tends to be present, under three circumstances also: 1. when the vocal folds have been surgically removed; 2. when there is a tumor on or adjacent to the folds in such a position that it prohibits their vibration; or 3. when they are too stiff with scar tissue, thickened tissue, or edema to oscillate in the air stream. These concepts may be restated for diagnostic application by saying that when there is an organic aphonia, there is either a paralysis, a fixation of the cricoarytenoid joints, a massive growth, the absence of one or both cords, a destructive disease, or a systemic condition producing extensive edema.

Occasionally there are persons who are intermittently aphonic. Their voices represent a wide range of vocal inadequacy. Some are aphonic most of the time; others are so only occasionally. The underlying conditions in these patients are similar to those in persons with chronic aphonia, but there is a smaller degree of impairment in those factors that influence vocal cord vibration.

Breath pressure may also be an important factor in intermittent aphonia. Sometimes stiff or relatively inactive folds can be vibrated by sharply increasing the flow of air in exhalation. It should be observed also that a swelling along the glottal margins that improves approximation without stiffening the folds can contribute to vibration and sound generation. This factor accounts for the occasional improvement of breathiness or intermittent aphonia despite increased swelling.

Some persons exhibit an intermittency in which the whispered and phonated sounds change from one to the other rapidly and repeatedly, often several times within a word. The condition frequently accompanies large vocal nodules or edematous cords. The phonated portions of this speech are always defective, and may be so breathy, hoarse, or rough that the casual listener does not notice the intermittency.

BREATHINESS

Vocal folds vibrate in the production of a breathy voice, but they are unable to impede the air stream long enough for much increase in infraglottal pressure. There is either a very short closed phase in the vibratory cycle, or, as is more commonly present when breathiness results from organic disorders, the glottis cannot close completely. The air flows in alternately greater and lesser amounts, thereby producing audible turbulence with a weak phonated component.

The organic conditions related to breathy voice are similar to those associated with aphonia, but there are some differences. The most prominent are: 1. the involvement of one vocal fold rather than two; and 2. smaller tumors, other enlargements, or more limited areas of pathology. Each of the organic conditions deserves brief mention.

Unilateral laryngeal paralysis usually results from impairment of the recurrent nerve on the affected side and may cause the involved fold to be located anywhere between complete abduction and a median position. The degree of approximation achieved by the abduction of the healthy fold is inversely related to the amount of breathiness in the voice. As a general rule, the width of the glottal opening during the vibratory cycle is directly related to the prominence of the breathy component. However, in most of the glottal conditions if the breath flow is increased, breathiness will also increase. The exception occurs when the glottal width is small and the increased flow draws the folds together in the Bernoulli effect. Impairment of glottal closure and breathiness may also be increased by involvement of the external branch of the superior laryngeal nerve that supplies the cricothyroid muscle. When this muscle is paralyzed unilaterally, the muscle on the healthy side tends to draw the thyroid and cricoid cartilages horizontally toward each other, thereby shifting the anterior part of the glottis toward the nonparalyzed side. This action may increase the glottal opening to reduce both pitch range and control.

An incomplete glottal closure and breathiness usually accompany the fixation of an arytenoid cartilage resulting from ankylosis of the cricoarytenoid joint. The glottal condition and vocal symptoms are similar to those accompanying unilateral paralysis.

Breathiness is also one of the symptoms of myasthenia laryngis. This disease produces muscle weakness and rapid fatigue that contribute to a relatively poor glottal closure which becomes less competent with continued phonation. As vibratory closure deteriorates the voice becomes increasingly breathy, but unlike paralysis, there is considerable temporary restoration of function with rest.

The common factor responsible for breathiness in the conditions just discussed is the inability of the vocal folds to approximate properly. Other organic disorders that can prevent the approximation of the arytenoid cartilages and thereby produce breathy quality include structural enlargements and other modifications that occur on the medial surfaces of the arytenoid cartilages or in the posterior commissure. They include contact ulcer, thickened tissues, and both benign and malignant tumors. It should be noted that these conditions do not invariably cause breathiness. The amount of relaxation, the degree of approximation permitted by the obstruction, and the urgency of the vocal effort, as reflected in both the flow of air and the muscle tension in the larynx, will determine whether the voice is aphonic, breathy, or hoarse at any particular time.

Circumscribed enlargements on the glottal edges of the membraneous portions of the vocal folds provide another mechanical interference with vibratory closure that may cause a breathy voice. During the vibratory cycle, any protrusion on the cord edge will meet its opposite member and prevent an adequate closure. Infraglottal air pressure is reduced, and the constantly escaping air creates turbulence which is the source of the defective sound.

The size, location, and degree of hardness, or compliance, of the enlarged areas influence the voice quality. Usually, a large mass produces more breathiness than a smaller one, but an equally faulty voice may be caused by a smaller mass that is hard and not compressible. Furthermore, a small protruberance located in or near the anterior commissure interferes more with glottal closure than the same size mass located more posteriorly. The proximity of the vocal folds at their anterior attachments and their angles of convergence cause the protruding masses to be squeezed into the commissure when the folds are adducted. The same size protrusion located posteriorly will not affect closure until the folds are more nearly adducted. As indicated previously, vocal quality will vary with the amount of vocal effort; a tumor or other mass that causes a breathy voice in quiet conversation may produce hoarseness when the individual attempts to speak loudly.

The common tumors on the vocal cords that are responsible for breathiness and other voice deviations include, in the benign group, papilloma, pedunculated and sessile polyps (the latter including vocal nodules), hematoma, keratosis, and the malignant tumors commonly called cancer. The speech pathologist does not diagnose such disorders, but he is obligated to understand their causes when they can be known, as well as their implications related to voice therapy.

When part of one vocal fold has been removed, three conditions remain that affect phonation. 1. The missing tissue, usually in the anterior section, creates a concavity that the unaffected cord cannot close and through which air escapes, causing turbulence. The excision of the whole cord produces a larger opening, and, from the phonation standpoint, approaches the situation that is present in adductor paralysis or ankylosis of the cricoarytenoid joint, when the arytenoid is fixed in a lateral position. 2. Scar tissue forms at the site of the surgery, thereby presenting a relatively stiff shelf that has little or no vibration but which may assist the mobile cord toward a vibratory closure. At best, the function is inefficient and there is considerable air wastage. 3. The removal of some or all of the thyroarytenoid muscle tissue limits the adducting movement of the aryntenoid cartilage, with the result that any portion of the cord remaining after surgery can be made only incidentally effective in the vibratory movement.

Edema may be associated with such factors as trauma, systemic conditions, and a variety of diseases, but the important consideration is that the swelling can interfere mechanically with a normal vibratory pattern and may cause a breathy voice. Clinical observations suggest that edema, either inflammatory or noninflammatory, causes a nonuniform swelling and stiffening of the flexible edges of the folds. The effect of these changes is somewhat analogous to the inflation of a balloon: the extent of inflation determines the size and degree of stiffness. The stiffness reduces the flexibility of the folds so that the undulating movements that begin at the most compliant area of the glottis, which is usually just anterior to the midpoint of the cords, are reduced or eliminated. The swollen, stiffened areas are noncompliant; they interfere with closure and allow air to escape in a turbulent stream.

A variable factor that can modify the influence of edema on vibration is the constantly changing muscle tension in the vocal folds. That is, a relatively small amount of swelling might produce breathiness at high pitches, when the folds are stretched and their muscles are tensed; in this adjustment, the swelling becomes effective by adding to the stiffness of the glottal border. However, at the lowest pitches, when the vocal folds are shortened and relatively flaccid, edema may serve only to increase both their mass and compliance, slow their rate of movement, and cause a lower pitch.

Discussions of breathy voice usually imply some association with the adequacy of breath supply, which may be expressed in two ways: the amount of air available, and the force with which it is delivered to the glottis. Clinical observation reveals that a reduced air supply, such as that resulting from the collapse or removal of one lung, is not in itself a cause of breathiness. The condition may result in shorter phrases and "shortness of breath," particularly under stress, but this is not a true breathiness. There are many persons with a low vital capacity who have normal voices.

There is also substantial clinical evidence that reduced breath pressure alone is not a cause of breathiness. If low pressure produced the defect, a person with a normal voice would necessarily have a breathy voice whenever he uttered a tone of low intensity. It is obvious that trained singers can intone a clear non-breathy voice which is scarcely audible. The critical element is the adjustment of the vocal folds in relation to the breath pressure.

In view of the foregoing observations recognition should be made of the fact that persons who are fatigued or ill or who have a paralysis involving the muscles of breathing, often have a breathy voice. Under most circumstances, the factor of breath is only part of the involvement. In these cases, the basic condition is usually not limited to the muscles of respiration but includes also the muscles of the larynx. The laryngeal component is responsible for the voice defect, but the combination of reduced breath pressure and weakened vibratory control in the larynx tends to exaggerate the vocal defect that would have resulted from the laryngeal weakness alone. The heightened effect comes, at least in part, from the person's lessened ability to compensate in some measure for the reduced muscular control. That is, patients with only the laryngeal involvement probably learn to regulate the breath stream for maximum possible efficiency of voice production. Those with paralysis limited to the breathing musculature, probably learn compensatory laryngeal adjustments.

HOARSENESS

The vocal defect called hoarseness has many variations; it differs from one person to another and it changes within each individual. At one extreme it is scarcely distinguishable from breathiness, and in fact some persons will exhibit hoarseness at one moment and breathiness at another. At the other extreme, hoarseness may contain so much noise that there is little evidence of vocal sound as such. It is probable that the primary or common factor in hoarseness is noise of a relatively high frequency that is produced by transient or highly unstable vibrations. These sounds are combined with other phonatory sounds that are frequently at low pitch as the result of laryngeal disease or other condition that would lower the frequency of vocal fold vibration. The transient disturbances seem to occur on the surfaces of the vocal folds, particularly along the glottis, but other laryngeal structures may also contribute to the total effect.

Transient vibrations are relatively brief disturbances that occur in structures, electrical circuits, resonators, and so on, as the result of a sudden change of conditions (Baranek, 1949). Transient waves are created in a vibrating sound source, such as a string, when it is touched, struck, or shortened suddenly. Similar transients can be created on the vocal cords by any condition that would interfere momentarily with the normal cycle of vibration. Transient vibrations may also be caused by multiple random disturbances of the type created by air bubbles through water. Sources of laryngeal transients can be grouped into four categories for this discussion: 1. accumulations of sticky mucus secretion in the larynx; 2. relative flaccidity of one or both of the vocal folds; 3. additions to the mass of the folds; and 4. the destruction of all or part of a fold. Each of these sources deserves brief consideration as a basis for diagnosis and investigation.

When there is too much mucus on the vocal folds from any cause, hoarseness will be present. The characteristic sounds of this voice defect seem to be produced by any one or a combination of three factors. First, excessive mucus tends to interfere with the normal undulating movements of the cords by weighting them unevenly and by damping their excursion through causing them to adhere to each other. Accumulations of sticky mucus, particularly at the anterior and posterior commissures, appear to cling to the cords and to act as elastic bands or membranes between the cords. These accumulations probably add a vibratory factor of their own and concurrently slow the rate of vibration of the cords, thereby producing a lower pitch. Mucous sounds are also probably produced when the vocal folds pull away from each other during the opening phase of the vibratory cycle. The elastic mucous particles stretch and break, creating many transient disturbances. It is possible that this action is somewhat similar to separating pieces of adherent adhesive tape. The adhesive action will be more pronounced when larger areas of mucous membrane are brought into contact, a condition that is present, for example, when the person with a normal larynx purposely produces a hoarse voice. The vocal folds are pressed together forcibly so that they are flattened against each other during the closed phases of the vibration. This provides larger areas of contact between mucosal surfaces and increased amounts of mucus to stretch and break as the cords separate in the opening phase of each vibratory cycle.

The second way in which mucus may contribute to hoarseness is through the vibration of mucous globules. These accumulations on the surfaces of the vocal folds become secondary vibrators that are agitated by the folds and thereby probably produce many transients. This disturbance of the mucus is commonly visable in high-speed motion pictures of the vocal cords.

The third influence of mucus on hoarseness is its somewhat independent vibration in the glottis. When secretions accumulate on the vocal folds, this material is moved into and out of the glottis by inhalation and exhalation. When adduction occurs the glottal area may be more or less filled with mucus which is set into complex random vibratory motion by the air stream. The liquid may be dislodged toward the laryngeal ventricles and the hoarseness lessened momentarily, but where there is excessive accumulation, its effect will be persistant in the vocal sound. Most persons have experienced this type of hoarseness during respiratory infections involving the larynx. The vocal problem is usually relieved temporarily by coughing or clearing the throat.

Flaccidity of the vocal folds can exist with adductor paralysis, with the lateral fixation of an arytenoid cartilage, or with looseness of the mucous membrane that covers the folds. The first two conditions were associated with breathiness in preceding comments, but it is obvious to the clinician that these conditions may also cause hoarseness. The affected fold may interfere with the motion of its unaffected partner, or the flaccid fold may be set into somewhat independent vibration. Either of these situations can create transient disturbances. It should be observed, also, that excessive mucus is usually present in these conditions and that it also contributes to the vocal disorder.

When there is difficulty in approximating the vocal folds, a compensatory sphincterlike contraction of the superior parts of the larynx frequently occurs. The ventricular folds have been observed in motion pictures to approximate for vibration, and the epiglottis may swing downward to meet the upper anterior surfaces of the arytenoid cartilages. In this adjustment the epiglottis often vibrates toward and away from the arytenoids, and the mucosa over the latter structures is displaced in progressive waves by the flow of air. These complex movements probably contain many transient vibrations that contribute to the hoarseness.

Loose mucous membrane has been observed in high-speed motion pictures of the vocal folds to slide over the firmer underlying structures. This membrane is sometimes free enough to swing over the glottal rim to meet the opposite member following the impact of the folds against each other during vibration. When the muscle masses of the folds reach their maximum lateral excursions and start their medial motions, the mucosa can be seen to continue its lateral movement momentarily, after which it is drawn medially, trailing the leading edge of the glottal border. These disturbances of the surfaces of the folds probably create many high-frequency transients.

It was pointed out previously that a mass on a vocal fold may cause a pitch change, breathiness, or hoarseness by weighting it, by stiffening it, by influencing its compliance, or by keeping the glottis from closing completely. A tumor, such as a papilloma or a polyp, may rest on one or both folds in such a way that it is vibrated with the cord, thereby becoming a secondary sound source; or it may be jiggled if it rests more or less loosely on a cord. In the latter case, it interferes with the vibration of the folds and causes additional semi-independent vibrations that create noise. Furthermore, a tumor is usually accompanied by excess mucus which contributes to the generation of hoarseness, as described in the preceding paragraph.

Hypertrophic conditions in areas adjacent to the cords may also cause hoarseness. An example of the kind of structural modification indicated has been observed in larynges where an enlarged ventricular fold rests on the opposite vocal fold. The impinging member interferes with the motions of the true folds and, in addition, is jostled into movements of its own. Flaccid, moist surfaces contribute to the complex vibratory disturbances and the hoarse sounds.

The surgical removal of all or part of a vocal fold

often causes hoarseness. Following this type of structural modification, vocal sound may be produced by the remaining normal fold and the residual fold or scar on the opposite side, or by vibration of the ventricular folds and other structures in the superior part of the larynx. Under these circumstances many random vibrations and transients occur that cause hoarseness. Frequently, surgical removal of one vocal fold will create a permanent glottal opening that causes a breathy component in the hoarseness.

ROUGH HOARSENESS

The voice quality called "rough hoarseness" is often associated with the types of hoarseness that have just been described, but it contains additional low-pitched sounds that produce the "rough" characteristic. As indicated in the dicussion of phonatory theory earlier, auditory roughness is perceived when successive sound waves in a sequence vary randomly in time or amplitude. Variation in patterns of movement result from asymmetrical elasticity, mass, compliance, or position of the vocal folds. The organic problems that determine these physical elements in vibration are the same as those causing the other phonatory disorders described above.

The differences in audible vocal characteristics result from the location, size, extent, shape, and firmness of the disabling condition and not the condition independently. Usually the sound of the voice does not reveal the specific disease or type of tumor.

Resonance Defects

NASALITY

Any condition that prevents a velopharyngeal closure between the oral pharynx and the nasal pharynx will produce excessive nasality. The organic conditions responsible for this voice defect may be classified under two categories: 1. the absence of sufficient structure to make the closure; and 2. the inability to manipulate the structure. The absence of tissue may be congenital, as with the cleft palate and short palate; or it may be the result of destructive disease, such as tumors or syphillis; or it may follow surgery, either on the palate or for the removal of adenoids. In the latter instance, excessive nasality that occasionally results from the removal of adenoid tissue usually does not indicate damage to the velum; instead it demonstrates that this tissue sometimes contributes to the velopharyngeal closure and that upon removal the velar structures are unable to compensate.

The inability to manipulate the velopharyngeal valve is associated primarily with paralyses. Unilateral or bilateral involvement of either velar or pharyngeal muscles will interfere with the proper closure. It should be noted that the opening into the nasopharynx need not be very large. This means that relatively little organic involvement may cause a marked nasalization of speech. It also means that vocal recovery may occur more slowly than functional restoration in cases of paralysis or surgical repair. It is not unusual to observe a patient with satisfactory velopharyngeal control for swallowing and for the production of isolated vowel sounds but who has inadequate closure in the rapid movements required for speaking.

DENASALITY

This voice deviation is almost always an organic problem, resulting from obstruction in the posterior portion of the nasal passages or nasopharynx. The organic conditions are varied and include: 1. tumors of many types; 2. hypertrophy associated with chronic disease in the nose and nasopharynx; 3. allergies that cause swelling of the nasal membranes; and 4. trauma, with its sequel of deviated septum, nasal spurs, and congestion.

Denasality is most evident on the normally nasal sounds, but it gives the whole speech pattern a characteristic dullness, similar to that observed in persons having a "head cold."

Obstruction of the nasal passages produces other problems also, that are potentially significant in evaluating vocal reeducation for the patient. The obstruction causes mouth breathing that results in drying of the pharyngeal and laryngeal mucosa which may adversely affect phonation. Obstruction in the anterior part of the nose interferes with breathing as does posterior blockage, but the anterior closure may also create excessive nasal resonance if the velopharyngeal closure is incomplete. That is, the location of a nasal obstruction can cause characteristically different acoustic results.

Summary: Voice Disorders Related to Organic Impairment

The normal physiology of sound generation and resonation may be altered by tumors, paralyses, malformations, swelling, or loss of tissue. From the physioacoustic standpoint, the importance of these anomalies in causing voice defects is in the way they modify the basic functional pattern of voice production. These modifications can be grouped into six categories: 1. those that distort the customary resonances, either by occluding the upper parts of the respiratory channel or by impairing the capacity to control the size of the orifices that connect the sections of the resonators (tumors, velopharyngeal paralysis, congenitally inadequate palate, cleft palate, and nasal disease); 2. those that impair the movements of the arytenoid cartilages and the adduction of the cords (adductor paralysis, ankylosis of the cricoarytenoid joints, interarytenoid tumors, and other tissue masses); 3. those that interfere mechanically with the vibrations of the vocal folds (tumors, edema, engorgement, scars, hyperplasia, asymmetrical arytenoid approximation, and excessive mucus); 4. those that alter the contractile ability and tonicity of the cords (paralysis, anemia, and myasthenia laryngis); 5. those that change the character of mucosal surfaces of the vocal folds and cause extraneous noises (excessive sticky mucus, loose mucous membrane, dry mucosa, and scars); and 6. those in which essential tissue is absent (surgical removal, injury, destructive diseases).

ETIOLOGIES OF ORGANIC CONDITIONS THAT CAUSE VOICE DEFECTS

In the earlier parts of this presentation, an attempt was made, first, to describe the sound characteristics, the audible symptoms, of the various voice disorders that have an organic basis; and, second, to describe the physiology of these problems, with particular attention to the organic deviations causing the vocal defects. The purpose of the present section is to present the underlying organic pathologies, insofar as that can be accomplished in this type of discussion. This review of organic pathology does not imply that the voice therapist should attempt any type of medical diagnosis or therapy; rather, it is intended to provide some insight into the basic causes that are the foci of therapy for voice disorders. An understanding of the organic problems increases the effectiveness of professional relationships between the medical profession and speech pathology and lessens the chance of professional encroachment.

Almost any disease or disorder that affects the vocal folds can influence their vibration and consequently the voice. An extensive catalog of specific diseases and structural modifications could be compiled, but for the current discussion the most important factors can be grouped into four classifications that have significance in diagnosis and therapy of voice disorders: 1. injury; 2. tumors and other diseases; 3. loss of laryngeal tissue; and 4. congenital factors. These categories are not completely distinct, but they represent discrete types of etiology that can be managed in this brief review. The first classification includes trauma from vocal abuse and other irritants; the second refers to tumors of all types and to both infection and neural diseases; the third encompasses the removal or destruction of tissue by surgery or disease; and the fourth indicates disorders that are present at birth.

Autogenous Trauma and Its Sequelae

Ballenger (1969, p. 318) lists four types of trauma to the larynx: mechanical, both external and internal (automobile and other accidents); burns from hot liquids, foods, or chemicals (lye, ammonia, bleach); irradiation; and autogenous trauma, by which he means vocal abuse. The first three may cause chronic laryngeal changes with attendant vocal problems that require rehabilitative procedures, but the vocal disorders are so rare and so individually unique that they require only incidental attention. However, the fourth classification, vocal abuse, is of central concern and requires detailed consideration.

VOCAL ABUSE

Excessive vocal use, whether of continuity or loudness, is the most common cause of voice disorders. Vocal abuse initially is a behavioral or functional problem, but as it persists, changes occur in the mucosa and other structures that are true organic problems. Most textbooks of laryngology describe the deleterious effects of excessive speaking and singing, but one of the statements that has almost become a classic was published by Jackson and Jackson in 1942 (1942, pp. 39–40) and is just as pertinent today as when it was first written.

> Unquestionably the greatest of all causes of laryngeal disease (and hence phonatory problems—*author*) is the excessive use of one of its normal functions, phonation. . . . The patient with chronic laryngeal disease is almost always a person who either talks constantly or uses his voice professionally, or often, both. There is little use asking the patient if he talks much. For some curious reason a patient who talks all the time he is awake will insist he talks little. It is not only the singer,

the lecturer, and the huckster who suffer from occupational abuse of the larynx. Teachers are especially frequent sufferers and persons who talk in noisy places such as factories where machinery is running often develop chronic hoarseness . . . There is a great variation in the amount of abuse the larynx of different individuals will stand; but every larynx has its limit. To go beyond this limit means thickening of the cords, and a thickened cord means a hoarse voice. Not only is a thickened cord a poor vibrator but it throws great additional work upon the thyroarytenoidei. These muscles instead of growing stronger grow more and more feeble, less and less able to cope with the increased requirements. A vicious circle is established and this renders cure a long tedious process.

FUNCTIONAL VOCAL FATIGUE (myasthenia laryngis)

Weakness of the vocal muscles, primarily the thyroarytenoids, produces the condition known as *myasthenia laryngis*. It is very common but often overlooked. Ballenger (1969, p. 389–390) refers to this condition as hyperkinetic phonasthenia and says,

Phonasthenia or functional vocal fatigue is due to vocal abuse. The amount of abuse necessary to produce the condition is quite variable. Persons using their voices professionally and the elderly are more prone to develop intermittent vocal fatigue.

The underlying disorder is weakness or fatigue of the vocalis or thyroarytenoid muscle. As a result, the tension and form of the vocal folds cannot be maintained. This occurs most often in singers and public speakers as a result of overuse of the voice. With senility, the thyroarytenoid muscle is subject to atrophy and loss of tone which may precipitate phonasthenia with normal voice use.

Clinical Manifestations. The patient complains of the voice "breaking" so that there is a drop in pitch and increased roughness or frank hoarseness. Elderly people will complain of increasing hoarseness towards the end of the day and frequently after telephone conversations. In an effort to compensate and avoid pitch alteration, professionals tend to carry the voice at an abnormally high pitch by increased activity of the cricothyroid muscle.

Vocal trauma often leads, also, to other types of laryngeal disorder. Vigorous shouting and cheering may cause vascular engorgement, injury to the joints or musculature, resulting in arthritis, myositis or, more often, hematoma. These subepithelial hematoma "do not always become absorbed; often they become organized into fibrous tumors that increase in size as the result of irritation and inflammation." (Jackson and Jackson, 1942, p. 378). They are often on the vocal fold edges, where they cause breathiness or hoarseness according to associated conditions.

VOCAL NODULES

Prolonged vigorous use of the voice frequently causes vocal nodules. These lesions are by definition a type of polyp, but their unique relationship to vocal trauma causes them to be treated in the literature as an entity. In referring to the etiology of nodules Ballenger (1969, p. 351) states:

The factors important in the causation of chronic laryngitis are influential here. However, it is probable the persistent vocal abuse of hyperkinetic phonation is the single most important precipitating factor. As a result, the lesions are seen most commonly in professional voice users and in nervous, hyperkinetic individuals. The lesions occur at the center of the membranous cord because this area is the center of vibratory motion of the cord. . . .

The genesis of vocal nodules is related to the peculiar anatomy of the true vocal cords. At the free margin of the membranous vocal cord is a subepithelial potential space (*Rienke's space*). . . . This potential space is easily infiltrated by edema fluid or blood and this is what probably occurs at the onset of the condition due to the trauma of vocal abuse. Since nodules are an inflammatory response to mechanical trauma they would be expected to exhibit progressive inflammatory changes. Young or early nodules tend to be soft and reddish. . . . More mature nodules will be more firm and contain areas undergoing fibrosis and hylinization. Mature nodules, as seen in professional singers, are fibrous and pale.

VOCAL POLYPS

A lesion that is similar to vocal nodules in its effect on phonation and its origin in vocal abuse is the vocal polyp. It is usually located near the middle of one membranous vocal fold and is not paired. It may be sessile or pedunculated and can vary in color from dark red to pale buff. Unlike vocal nodules the trauma producing a polyp

. . . need not be of long duration and frequently the onset of the lesion can be related to a single episode of vocal strain. Polyps may also develop acutely following an upper respiratory infection. . . . The pathology is localized to the area of Rienke's layer of the true vocal cord. The lesion consists of varying amounts of edematous stroma, dilated blood vessels, fibrous tissue and hemorrhage. The early polyp represents an exaggeration of the early polypoid stage of vocal nodule and tends to be more vascular. As the lesion matures, fibrosis and fibrinoid and hyaline degeneration become apparent in the stroma, old hemorrhages and vessel walls.

The lesion that is generated by glottal trauma has a vocal disorder as its initial symptom. The size and location of the polyp will determine the quality of the voice, which may encompass such disorders as aphonia, breathiness, and many varieties of hoarseness.

CONTACT ULCER

Another disease that is caused chiefly by vocal abuse is contact ulcer. This entity is an ulceration that occurs on the medial surface of one or both arytenoid cartilages where they meet each other. It is related in the literature to a "throaty" method of phonation (Jackson and Jackson, 1942, p. 163; Peacher, 1947). The term "throaty" probably means that the person speaks habitually with a vocal pitch at the lowest part of his range and that there is audible evidence of muscular effort to keep it there. These patients, who are almost always adult males, do not speak loudly, but they talk more or less continuously. They give the impression, and some have admitted this, that they use the low, effortful pitch in an attempt to sound more masculine.

Jackson and Jackson attribute the formation of the ulcer and its typical location on the arytenoid cartilage to the "trauma of the hammer and anvil." They suggest that the constant hammering of the arytenoids against each other is the chief mechanical cause of the ulceration. Ballenger (1969, p. 332) states that it

> . . . develops on the medial surface of the arytenoid in response to excessively forceful apposition of the two arytenoid cartilages during phonation. The ulceration may be unilateral or bilateral. . . . Vocal abuse is undoubtedly the most important etiologic fctor. The disease is usually seen in preachers, salesmen, managers, and lawyers who use forceful speech. Smoking and persistent coughing may also be etiologic factors. Frequently, the onset of symptoms is related to an acute upper respiratory infection.

The implication in the literature is that contact ulcers develop over a period of time. This is probably true, but there is evidence in this author's experience of one case in which the initial trauma that developed into an ulcer occurred within a period of about two minutes, although it did not become apparent with granulation tissue in the ulcer until approximately two weeks later.

VOCAL ABUSE AND CHRONIC LARYNGITIS

Vocal abuse is one of the causes of chronic laryngitis, and chronic laryngitis almost always causes hoarseness. Furthermore, chronic inflammation of the larynx is extremely common, which suggests that much of the hoarseness that is heard is caused by chronic laryngitis.

The term chronic laryngitis includes many different conditions and implies long standing inflammatory changes in the laryngeal mucosa. These conditions often blend into one another so that exact diagnoses are not always possible by either the clinician or the pathologist.

Often the exact cause is not apparent. Probably chronic laryngitis most often results from repeated episodes of acute laryngitis. Constant use (or misuse) of the voice such as may occur in singers and public speakers aggravates the condition or may produce it in a person with an otherwise normal larynx.

In addition to vocal abuse, other causes of chronic inflammation in the larynx that are regularly observed include infections in the respiratory tract, such as the sinuses, from which purulent material may flow to the laryngeal area; smoking; mouth breathing, particularly of dry, hot air; and alcohol. "Alcohol contributes to chronic laryngitis probably not because of a toxic effect of the alcohol itself, but because a drunk usually abuses his voice." (DeWeese and Saunders, 1964, p. 134.)

The mechanism by which these laryngeal irritants generate the mucosal changes that cause the hoarseness is the production of ". . . vasodilatation and hyperemia. This may in turn precipitate submucosal hemorrhages, interstitial edema and production of an inflammatory exudate consisting mainly of mononuclear cells. Eventually, the injured area is invaded by fibroblasts, causing fibrosis and hyalinization with thickening and deforming of structure. The pathophysiologic cycle may be arrested at any point with a resulting clinical entity." (Ballenger, 1969, p. 348.)

The vocal folds appear pink, the small vessels on their surfaces are dilated, and their glottal margins are rounded when they are approximated for phonation. The thickening of the mucosa and alteration of the shape modifies the mass of the vocal fold, its compliance, and the manner of glottal closure. The result is atypical vibration that can produce breathiness, hoarseness, or even roughness if the changes are sufficiently advanced.

Chronic inflammation often exists in localized areas

of the larynx in contrast to the diffuse chronic laryngitis discussed previously. There are several of these conditions that occur occasionally, but two that are frequent enough to have significance for the speech pathologist are hypertrophic laryngitis and hyperplastic laryngitis.

The first of these diseases is referred to as "diffuse vocal polyposis" by Ballenger (1969, p. 353) and as "polypoid corditis" by DeWeese and Saunders (1964, p. 141). Both references report the causes to be vocal abuse and smoking. The appearance of the polypoid lesion is described by Ballenger (1969, p. 354) as follows: "Symmetrical pale, sausage like masses will be seen hanging from each membranous cord. They frequently are in approximation and obliterate the interior glottis so that the only airway is between the arytenoids. The masses are usually a translucent grayish-pink color but inflammation may produce bright redness." As might be expected with this type of lesion, hoarseness and low pitch are present continuously, with variation in severity depending upon the size and location of the offending masses.

Hyperplasia refers to the development of excess tissue. Hyperplastic laryngitis indicates a thickening of the mucosa or the presence of keratosis. The symptom of both is hoarseness. The etiologies that have been reported include the usual types of irritants such as smoking, vocal abuse, chronic laryngitis, and so on, but the basic cause is not known (Ballenger, 1969).

"The usual location of hyperplastic growths is on or under a portion of the vocal cords or in the interarytenoid space . . . (This tissue) may interfere with the movements of the cords so that approximation is often incomplete. . . . The color of the hyperplastic tissues varies from a pale pink to a deep red. In some cases edema is present." (Ballenger and Ballenger, 1954, p. 173.)

Tumors and Other Diseases

TUMORS

The word tumor means a swelling or enlargement, but it refers more specifically in the medical literature to a tissue mass that has no function and that develops from structures normally present. Some tumors remain at their original sites and while they may displace or crowd adjacent structures they do not infiltrate neighboring tissue and they do not migrate to other locations. For these reasons they are classified as benign. In contrast, some tumors do invade and destroy adjacent structures, and these tumors may also metastasize. That is, tumor cells migrate by way of the blood or lymph circulation systems and establish themselves at new sites where they continue their destructive course. The evil character of these tumors causes them to be classified as malignant. They are commonly called cancers.

Both benign and malignant tumors may develop in the larynx and other parts of the respiratory system. When they are located where they can interfere with the normal adjustment and vibration of the vocal folds or with the function of the resonators, they cause voice disorders. The type of vocal sound produced does not reveal the kind of tumor or other conditions that cause it. As indicated in earlier comments, it is the size and location of an offending mass in combination with the pitch and loudness of the voice that determine its effect upon the vocal product.

A common benign tumor and consequently one of great importance in voice disorders is papilloma, a wartlike growth that may appear on the vocal folds or adjacent parts of the larynx. It occurs often in children, it is not directly associated with vocal abuse, and it tends to regrow after removal. Papilloma usually reveal their presence by causing hoarseness that will disappear following surgical excision, but, since these tumors often recur, repeated excision causes scar tissue that may interfere with phonation and cause a chronic voice problem.

Malignant tumors are critically important in voice therapy because hoarseness is often their first symptom, and voice disorders usually remain as evidence of their eradication. The initial observation emphasizes the necessity for medical referral of phonatory problems. The second stresses the need to understand the structural conditions that follow medical therapy so that rational vocal reeducation can be devised.

The physician has two major therapeutic means for the treatment of laryngeal cancer, irradiation and surgery. When the first is selected, it is with the presumption that the tumor can be destroyed by X ray or other means without major modification of the structures that surround it. When surgery is employed, there is recognition that the tumor and its adjacent structures must be removed. This means in some instances that only a part of one vocal fold will be excised; under other circumstances the entire larynx and sometimes additional structures must be taken. Following treatment by irradiation, hoarseness usually persists because the mucous glands and some of the normal muscle tissue have been destroyed. The absence of mucus leaves the membranes dry; the loss of muscle fibers reduces the size and probably the flexibility of the involved vocal fold. These circumstances often cause irregular vibration and rough hoarseness.

When part or all of one vocal fold is removed, a glottal closure is not possible; consequently the voice is breathy and weak. Sometimes a cicatricial protrusion will develop at the site of the diseased fold that reduces the glottal space and thereby improves the vocal sound. Occasionally also the ventricular or aryepiglottic folds can be vibrated to contribute sound. This latter voice is usually quite rough and hoarse.

With the excision of the entire larynx, breathing occurs through a stoma in the neck to which the trachea is attached. The patient is aphonic until he introduces into his mouth and adjacent spaces a sound that substitutes for that previously made by the vocal folds. The usual procedure is to develop esophageal speech, which is described later in the discussion.

INFECTIONS

In the earlier discussion of the misuse of the voice, particular reference was made to causal relationships between vocal abuse, certain diseases, and chronic changes in the larynx that produce voice disorders. Other diseases, particularly infections, may also cause organic voice defects but without the association of vocal abuse. These infections are of four general kinds: 1. airborne; 2. contactual (kissing, silverware, cups, etc.); 3. focal; and 4. specific (tuberculosis, mycoses, syphilis, measles). The common routes of invasion are: a) flotation (from some area on the mucosa to the larynx); b) the air current; c) the lymph channels; and d) blood vessels (Jackson and Jackson, 1937, p. 53).

Infections influence the voice through the modifications that they produce in the vocal folds. The changes take many possible forms, including scars, tumors, thickening of the membranes, atrophy, fixation of the cricoarytenoid joint, edema, and paralysis. The influences of these conditions on the action of the vocal folds have been discussed in other parts of the chapter and therefore need not be reviewed here. The reason for including this general reference to infections is to stress, for the voice therapist, that there are many kinds of damaging infections and that their detrimental effects may last a long time.

NONINFLAMMATORY EDEMA

One of the causes of hoarseness that has been mentioned several times in a variety of ways is edema. The presence of this extra vascular fluid in the areolar, submucosal space causes changes in the mass, compliance, and sometimes the elasticity of the vocal cords. In the preceding discussion, most of the edematous conditions have been associated with inflammation. However, it is evident that edema may occur also without inflammation and be just as detrimental vocally.

Internal medicaments, such as iodides and acetylsalicylic acid, frequently produce edema (Ballenger and Ballenger, 1954, p. 166). ". . . of the internal medicaments potassium iodide is the commonest as a cause of hoarseness. Its selective effect on the larynx may go so far as to produce acute edema of the larynx or a chronic engorgement; . . ." (Jackson and Jackson, 1937, pp. 54–55).

Noninflammatory edema may be caused also by mechanical compression of the venous return flow or by lymphatic obstruction. This mechanical compression may be a tumor pressing on a vein, or any condition that reduces the flow of blood or lymph (Ballenger, 1969, p. 343).

The majority of books that are concerned with diseases of the ear, nose, and throat state that noninflammatory edema may be caused by glandular imbalance, autonomic dysfunction, and allergy. The mechanisms of these relationships are extremely complex and are not completely understood, but there is general agreement that each of these anomalies is capable of producing edema.

Clinical observation and systematic research also suggests a very close relationship between hypothyroidism and voice problems. This form of endocrine imbalance frequently produces edema. There is evidence that the amount of hypothyroidism need not be great to cause hoarseness, and it is apparent that many borderline hypothyroid persons are not aware of their condition. It follows that some of the unsatisfactorily diagnosed cases of hoarseness may be caused by a hypothyroid condition. (Luse, 1948).

ENGORGEMENT

The effect of vasodilation and engorgement on the function of the vocal cords is similar to that of edema. In both instances the mass and contractility are affected. According to Jackson and Jackson (1937, p. 51), ". . . alcohol is a potent cause of laryngeal disease. . . . Observation in thousands of patients justifies our opinion that it is the prolonged, peripheral, vasodialator effect of alcohol that is so injurious to the laryngeal mucosa. . . . The mucosa of the larynx of the victim of alcohol . . . was always engorged. It was evidently the chronic engorgement of the cords that was responsible for the hoarseness. . . . It is the constant repetition of alcohol that results in the vasomotor condition resembling paralysis and the chronic engorgement."

PARALYSIS

In the earlier parts of this presentation, several references were made to relationships between paralysis and voice problems. The various paralyses and their causes are not uncommon and deserve considerable emphasis in vocal rehabilitation.

Sensory impairment in the pharynx or larynx produces an anaesthesia in these regions that can affect swallowing and aspiration of foreign material into the trachea and lungs. The problem is rare and vocal deficits are not regularly associated with the disorder.

Motor paralysis of the larynx may be classified into five types according to the location of the lesion. The four neural origins are ". . . cortical, corticobulbar, bulbar and peripheral" (Ballenger 1969, p. 395). The fifth cause is myopathic disease. The first three causes referred to are in the brain and, according to location, may cause the laryngeal musculature to be either spastic or flaccid, but the associated motor problems that usually are present produce such extensive incoordinations that voice is a relatively minor factor. The fourth, or peripheral, origin of neural lesions accounts for almost all of the laryngeal paralyses affecting voice. These lesions occur in the vagus nerves and their branches and may be located anywhere along their courses from emergence at the medulla to their attachments in the laryngeal musculature. When a vagus nerve is damaged above the origin of the superior laryngeal nerve, both the sensory and motor functions on the involved side are affected. If injury occurs to the vagus below the superior nerve or to the recurrent laryngeal nerve, paralysis of the laryngeal musculature will result in all muscles on the same side except the cricothyroid muscle, which is activated by the external branch of the superior laryngeal nerve. Damage to the recurrent nerve may result from ". . . enlarged cervical lymph nodes, traumatisms, goiters (before and following operations), aneurysms, mediastinal tumors, tumors of the esophagus and the pharynx, pleurisy, scoliosis of the cervical vertebrae, tuberculosis of the apices of the lungs, and even paricarditis or mitral stenosis." (Ballenger and Ballenger, 1954, p. 180.) The result of lesions along the recurrent laryngeal nerve can be either an abductor or adductor paralysis or both. The form depends upon the extent of the damage and the part or branch of the nerve affected.

The fifth cause of laryngeal paralysis is disease of the muscles. Myopathic paralysis "is characterized by some form of pathologic process in one or more of the intrinsic laryngeal muscles. It may be of toxic origin such as typhoid fever or tetanus, or it may follow trichinosis, tuberculosis, local infections, and tumors of the vocal cords." (Ballenger and Ballenger, 1954, p. 181.)

A vital concern about voice therapy and laryngeal paralysis is the possibility of recovery of motion of an affected vocal fold. Various writers indicate that vocal folds that have remained relatively fixed for a period of six months or more will not recover their motion. The immobility to which reference is made is adduction and abduction, not vibration. Paralyzed vocal folds vibrate readily when located where the air stream can activate them. The vocal sound produced by paralyzed vocal folds is usually breathy and often rough, particularly at lower pitches.

Loss of Laryngeal Tissue

The removal, destruction, or modification of vocal fold tissue almost always produces a voice defect. There are three primary causes for this loss: surgery, trauma, and disease. Surgical procedures may affect the vocal folds, and hence the voice, either directly through the removal of part or all of the larynx, or indirectly through injury to the nerve supply. In the former, the absence of vocal fold tissue precludes the normal vibratory closure and results in an abnormal voice. In the latter, except in abductor paralysis, there is an incomplete closure of the glottis and sometimes an atrophy of the involved cord tissue. This problem was discussed earlier along with paralysis and other neurological conditions.

The removal of part of the larynx is made necessary usually by some form of tumor. The location and the amount of material excised varies from patient to patient, but the size of the involved area is not a positive indicator of the severity of the vocal disorder. The absence of even a small amount of the glottal border may cause a marked hoarseness, while, in contrast, a voice may not be appreciably worse when one complete cord has been removed.

When a malignant tumor extends beyond certain limits within the larynx, the laryngeal surgeon usually performs a laryngectomy. The total absence of the larynx produces complete aphonia and necessitates the development of a substitute type of phonation. This is not difficult for most patients to accomplish, and some suggested procedures are available in the section on therapy.

Another, but relatively uncommon, cause of tissue destruction in the larynx is external trauma. Automobile accidents in which the passenger is thrown against the dashboard, steering wheel, or other protrusions are common sources of laryngeal injury. Blows on the larynx that fracture the cartilages may result in the deterioration of the thyroid cartilage and the loss of tissue support. Such injuries also produce scar tissue and both laryngeal and vocal distortions of various kinds. The voice is almost always defective and can vary from aphonia to mild hoarseness.

There are some diseases that cause tissue destruction and which, when present in the larynx, can result in voice problems. The two that are referred to most commonly are tuberculosis and syphilis. Fortunately, these diseases are under reasonably good medical control and rarely involve the larynx. When they do, the detrimental effect upon the voice usually results from cicatricial tissue.

Congenital Factors

An infant may be born with a laryngeal paralysis, a cyst, syphilis, papilloma, abnormally large laryngeal structures, a laryngeal web, and so on. If any one of these disorders is marked enough to receive medical attention, it may be remedied. On the other hand, those diseases and structural abnormalities that go unnoticed or are recognized as relatively insignificant anomalies, may become important later as causes for voice defects. Since these minor difficulties are apt to be observed only after some years and since they may develop subsequent to the time of birth, it would be difficult or impossible to determine whether or not they were congenital in any particular case.

CONGENITAL WEB

One of the exceptions to the preceeding statement is the congenital web, which is not too uncommon. "The causes of congenital web are unknown, but are possibly atavistic.

"The most frequent location for congenital web is the level of the glottis, usually in the anterior portion where it attaches the two cords together for more or less of their anterioposterior extent" (Jackson and Jackson, 1942, p. 60).

The web is apt to cause a high-pitched voice, accompanied by effortful phonation and hoarseness. Therefore, wherever pitch problems are present, the possibility of a web should always be considered.

Resonance Voice Defects

The organic etiologies of the resonance voice defects could have been discussed along with the organic etiologies of laryngeal problems, since many of the causative conditions are common to both. However, for simplicity of treatment, they have been considered separately.

EXCESSIVE NASALITY

It was pointed out earlier that the two principal resonance defects associated with organic etiologies are too much nasal resonance and insufficient nasal resonance. The former defect is caused by incomplete nasopharyngeal closure and results from four possible organic causes: 1. congenital deformity; 2. paralysis; 3. destructive disease; and 4. surgery.

The congenital deformity takes two forms: cleft palate and short palate. In both conditions the nasopharyngeal closure cannot be made, thereby allowing sound from the larynx to pass into the nasopharynx and nose.

Paralysis of one or both sides of the pharyngeal constrictor muscle groups or of the velum will prevent a velopharyngeal closure and will therefore provide a condition similar, in effect, to a cleft or short palate. Such diseases as poliomyelitis and measles can cause the lesions in the nerves to the muscles of the pharynx and velum.

The destructive diseases that can produce excessive nasality include malignant tumors on the hard or soft palates and syphilis with a gumma extending through the hard palate. The voice quality is similar to that accompanying paralysis or cleft palate.

Surgical removal of adenoid tissue sometimes results in excessive nasality. If the mass of the pharyngeal tonsil contributed to the velopharyngeal closure prior to surgery, thereby reducing the amount of velar movement necessary, and this gland is then removed, excessive nasality often results and remains until the habits are modified and the closure is again established. When the palate and the other velopharyngeal structures are not adequate to make a closure without the adenoid tissue, the voice will remain hypernasal.

DENASALITY

Occlusion of the nasal passages posteriorly causes the vocal disorder known as denasality. The chronic obstructions that may produce the problem include enlarged adenoid, polyps, papilloma, nasal spurs, edema, and mucosal congestion from chronic and allergic rhinitis and sinusitis. Traumatic occurrences, such as a broken nose, also produce swelling which may become chronic.

In all these conditions the acoustic results are essentially the same. The exception exists when a growth or spur is located well forward in the nose, thereby allowing the posterior part of the nose to act as a resonator. In these instances, hypernasality, rather than denasality, may be associated with a stoppage of air in the nasal passage. The vocal disorder is referred to sometimes as rhinolalia clausa anterior.

Summary

The pathologies of the organic phonatory defects are extremely complex and often interrelated. The discussion just presented has arbitrarily grouped the various pathologies into the following four categories to simplify presentation:

1. Autogenous trauma and its sequelae, including such conditions as myasthenia laryngis, vascular engorgement, vocal nodules, and contact ulcer. This section also touched on vocal abuse and chronic laryngitis, chronic hypertrophic and hyperplastic laryngitis, and chronic atrophic laryngitis.
2. Tumors of various kinds and other diseases not related to vocal abuse, encompassing infections, paralysis, engorgement, and non-inflammatory edema caused by internal medicaments, mechanical compression of lymph channels and venous blood flow, glandular imbalance, and allergy.
3. Loss of laryngeal tissue by surgery, trauma, or disease.
4. Congenital factors, in which most of the emphasis was placed on congenital web.

The organic causes for the more common resonance problems were discussed separately under two headings: those that cause excessive nasality; and those that produce insufficient nasal resonance. The former included such conditions as cleft palate, congenitally short palate, paralyses of the velopharyngeal constrictors, and surgery. Denasality was related to nasal growths, trauma, and allergies.

The successful management of organically caused voice defects requires an extensive understanding of the pathologies involved. It is imperative that the voice therapist be aware of, and informed about, the various anomalies of the larynx and other parts of the respiratory tract. This does not imply any encroachment upon the field of medicine; it simply recognizes the fact that the laryngologist, the rhinologist, and the voice pathologist must work together and understand one another.

MANAGEMENT OF ORGANIC VOICE DISORDERS

The management of organic voice disorders encompasses two distinct stages, diagnosis and therapy. Yet the former may continue after the latter has begun. Diagnosis, which is the process of determining the cause or causes of symptoms, may be accomplished in four well-defined steps: 1. analysis of the voice in terms of pitch, quality, and loudness; 2. investigation of the history of the voice problem; 3. examination of those structures potentially related to the voice defect, such as nose, mouth, pharynx, and larynx; and 4. evaluation of nonspeech skills and abilities, including intelligence, emotional stability, motor skills, general health, and hearing. Briefly and for practical purposes, these four phases of the diagnostic process may be identified by the terms listen, question, look, and test. The data from these steps determine recommendations and the specific therapeutic procedures.

Diagnosis

Diagnosis should be done systematically. However, the order of items in the suggested four-part evaluation is not fixed; the setting, immediate situation, and characteristics of the persons involved will determine both the sequence and the specific items included in each part. Furthermore, the experienced diagnostician collects data for several parts of the evaluation simultaneously; for example, the history interview provides an excellent opportunity to assess the voice of the patient in conversational use. To gather information in an orderly manner and at the same time to maintain a flexibility of approach, requires the examiner to have a carefully prepared outline with which he is thoroughly familiar. In most situations this outline should be used as the data-collecting form, and it should be standardized to fit the needs of each school system or clinic.

To systematize the immediate discussion of the diagnosis of organic voice defects, the four aspects of the process have been elaborated briefly in the following presentation. An effort has been made through specific suggestions and wordings to provide practical information without being prescriptive. The intention is to suggest a progression through a diagnostic procedure.

EVALUATION OF THE VOICE

Since the voice is the focus of interest, its analysis begins with the first words spoken at the initial meeting and continues throughout the time the patient or student is present. The examiner may wish to put the patient at ease by conversing casually about some local event, or he may prefer to introduce direct questions to gather identification data that usually occupy the first part of an information questionnaire. These identification items include name, address, telephone number, date of interview, birth date, school and grade or occupation, parent or guardian, number of siblings and the patient's position in the series, the name of the informant (if different from the subject), the referral source, and the interviewer.

During this interview, the examiner should note the habitual pitch level and its normalcy in relation to contemporaries of the same age and sex. He should also observe the loudness and its suitability to the situation, and he should be aware of the quality of the voice. This informal voice evaluation supplements the more formal testing to be reviewed later.

By the time the identification data have been recorded, the examiner should have a fair estimate of the patient's ordinary vocal usage. The subject usually has some concept of his difficulty and is willing to supply his own evaluation of this voice problem. It is important to know what he thinks is wrong with his voice and why he wants to improve it. He should be asked to report the comments that have been made by teachers, friends, or employers. His report should also contain his reason for seeking help with his voice at this particular time. If the voice defect that the examiner has observed is not mentioned by the subject, leading questions should be asked to learn the true extent of his information and comprehension.

The next logical item under the analysis of the voice is the examiner's description and evaluation of the voice. This should contain comments on pitch, quality, intensity, rate, and other communication problems such as articulatory disorders, language problems, and stuttering. Sometimes the interviewer will wish to complete the case history before carrying out the formal steps of the voice evaluation. Under these conditions, he would explore next the questions pertaining to the development and history of the voice problem. However, where the examiner uses one office space for interviewing and voice evaluation, and where the same person makes the analysis and takes the history, the vocal analysis can be carried out with some advantage at this point in the procedure. As an aid to the examiner in the analysis, the voice should be recorded whenever possible for use in subsequent checking of the initial impressions of the voice.

Voice testing should concentrate on one vocal element at a time, even though the experienced clinician will simultaneously note quality differences while testing the pitch or loudness of the voice. However, even those who are thoroughly familiar with voice problems should establish a routine that includes tests for pitch, loudness, and quality. Unintentional variations in procedure are apt to produce incomplete data and faulty evaluation. Careful, systematic, routinized operation is essential in diagnosis.

The tests of pitch should discover the total pitch range and the voluntary control of pitch. The subject should be asked to sing or hum a tone near the middle of his range (the examiner may need to supply a starting tone for imitation), and then to proceed by scale steps to the lowest note possible and to the highest, including falsetto. If the clinician does not have a pitch pipe or piano with which he can determine the pitch range, an estimate of "adequate" or "inadequate" range should be noted. Concurrently, the control of pitch can be assessed by observing the ease and accuracy with which the subject changes from one musical tone to the next. A "speaking" test should also be given in which the subject is asked to repeat a few questions with rising inflection, such as, "Oh?" "Are you going *home*?" or "Do you have the *book*?" Some persons cannot voluntarily change from one note to another on a musical scale, yet they use normal inflectional patterns in speaking. The primary concern in diagnosis is whether or not the activity can be performed; it is secondary to discover how well it can be accomplished.

If the voice is completely monotonous in both sung and spoken sounds and is also somewhat hoarse, the superior laryngeal nerve, or its central attachments, or the muscles supplied by it, are suspect. However, it must be remembered that monotonous pitch can be habitual or related to emotional problems. If the pitch is regularly very low, combined with rough hoarseness, some asymmetrical weighting of the vocal folds from a tumor or edema is to be suspected.

When vocal pitch is abnormally high, particularly in the adult male, the most probable cause is functional, but the basis may also be a failure of laryngeal development or the presence of a laryngeal web. The delay in laryngeal development is usually paralleled by the absence of secondary sex characteristics, such as beard growth and masculine physique and by the presence of effeminate behavior patterns. Two factors in loudness should be evaluated: 1. its suitability in the conversational situation and 2. the maximum loudness that the individual can produce. The latter may be gauged by turning down the volume control on the recorder and asking the person to speak as loudly as he can. Many people are more willing to try to speak loudly into a microphone than to a person only a few feet away. If the patient is unable to produce a loud voice, it is because the glottal closure is incomplete, the breath pressure is insufficient, or the individual is embarrassed. Questions about the patient's ability to call to someone at some distance or to cheer at a sporting event may help to differentiate the causes. If the quality is breathy or hoarse, particularly when a loud voice is attempted, an organic involvement may be present.

Analyzing the quality of the voice means systematically listening for five qualities under different conditions of pitch and loudness. These qualities include breathiness, hoarseness, rough hoarseness, excessive nasality, and denasality. Usually the interview conversation and the vocal use during the checks of pitch and loudness will provide adequate material for classifying the quality, but it may be desirable to use a standard test passage, such as those to be found in speech pathology textbooks. In this instance, the patient should read and record the test paragraph in the habitual manner, then repeat it loudly. He should also produce sustained tones softly and loudly at several pitches. If the voice becomes increasingly breathy at higher pitches, it suggests a protruberance, such as a nodule, or polyp, on the glottal border; or perhaps inadequate arytenoid approximation as in unilateral paralysis. If the voice is hoarse at low pitches and becomes clearer at higher pitches, it creates suspicion of some inflammatory condition producing excess mucus or edema or some general swelling.

Resonance problems may exist independently or they may accompany the phonatory deviations just listed. They are vocally important, sometimes they are organically critical, and they always deserve careful evaluation.

Listening for nasal sound deviation is carried out easily and simply. If the test passage selected previously for reading is one without nasal sounds, the presence of excessive nasal resonance will be markedly evident. Resonance of the aperta type immediately suggests an organic pathology in the velopharyngeal area. The presence of nasal twang indicates either an occlusion anteriorally in the nose or a functional narrowing of the velopharyngeal oriface.

If the opposite condition of denasality is present, there is almost certainly a partial or complete obstruction in the nasopharynx or posterior nasal passages. The most common cause is a hyperplastic adenoid.

Recording the voice during the several tests provides material for objective post-test listening. It is advisable to rehear the voice from a recording in order to separate the voice from the person producing it, for the appearance of the patient often influences the auditory judgment of the examiner. It is always advisable to listen to the recorded voice from a good recorder before making a final evaluation of the patient's voice.

The terminology of voice defects is notoriously inexact. There are several reasons for this lack of precision, but a discussion of them does not properly belong in this presentation. However, it is possible, and desirable, to indicate the relative severity of each type of deviation noted, and it is advised that at least three modifiers be used, such as *mild*, *moderate*, and *severe*. These terms will be useful to the therapist as a device for noting progress, or the lack of it, in therapy.

DEVELOPMENT AND HISTORY OF THE VOICE PROBLEM

The collection of identification data at the beginning of the information form gives the interviewer some idea of the patient's background, family size, type of work, and so on. The description and evaluation of the voice by the patient and the examiner identify the problem and focus the attention of the patient upon it. Ordinarily, at this stage questions about the voice difficulty will be answered readily and as completely as memory will allow.

To simplify the discussion of the development and history of the voice problem, a series of key questions are presented here and are used to outline the steps in gathering pertinent information. These questions have been thoroughly tested in clinical situations. (The student is advised to relate the previous discussions of organic pathology to the questionnaire items if the purposes and significance of the questions are not evident.)

What were the circumstances under which the voice problem was first noticed? The informant frequently gives this information when he is describing his voice difficulty. However, some elaboration is usually necessary and may be accomplished through such questions as these: Was the voice problem noticed suddenly? Did it develop slowly? Have you been aware of it for some time? How long has it existed? Who first noticed it? Had you done any shouting, singing, extensive speaking, or heavy lifting before the problem was noticed? Had you been ill, in an accident, or had any surgery about this time?

It is important to distinguish the problems of sudden onset from those of long or indefinite development. The former may indicate a condition that is a threat to life, and although all patients with phonatory problems should be examined by a laryngologist, the acute problems demand immediate referral.

What do you think caused the voice difficulty? If a specific statement has not been made previously to answer this question, the direct question should be asked. The answer may provide insight into the individual's concept of his problem.

Does it vary in severity? Has it become better or worse recently? Does it vary during the course of a day? Do seasons or daily weather changes seem to affect it? Does it vary with your feelings of happiness or discouragement? Does it vary significantly with the degree of fatigue? The long-term trend and the daily or short-term variations can suggest a variety of potential causes, such as developing tumors, allergies, glandular imbalance, anemia, and chronic disease.

Is your voice similar to that of anyone else in your family? It is often necessary to ask the patient if his voice is confused with anyone else's on the telephone. Where the voice is similar to that of another member of the family, it usually indicates an imitation factor. However, in a large family, there is often vigorous vocal competition which may cause thickening of the vocal cord tissue, edema, nodules, or other vocal-cord damage. It is not unusual to find several in a family who demonstrate this vocal similarity as the result of vocal trauma rather than some hereditary or learned factor.

Are there any speech defects or other voice problems in your family? (Include aunts, uncles and grandparents.) Sometimes the answer to this question reveals other speech problems and gives insight into family attitudes regarding speech deviations generally. Occasionally, also, when nasality is the voice defect, the patient may reveal cleft palate or other structural anomalies that have potential significance and necessitate further questioning.

What remedial attempts have been made? Frequently, the answer to this question is given in the individual's comments about his first awareness of the disorder. The information is important and should include the names and addresses of physicians and clinicians who have worked with the patient on his problem. It is also helpful to discover what therapy was administered, what its effects were, and why the work was stopped.

It may be desirable to get additional information from previous therapists, and it is always wise to learn all one can about previous therapeutic experiences. Successful voice therapy requires careful, serious work. There is no magic. It is helpful to be able to recognize the person who "shops around" looking for a ready-made "cure."

Do you have any information about your early vocal usage? As an infant, was there excessive crying, screaming, or yelling? Excessive vocal use in young children often produces vocal nodules which are sometimes called screamers' nodes. Was there any abnormality in respiration, such as noisy breathing? Stridorous breathing may mean a laryngeal abnormality, with obvious potential relationship to the voice defect.

In childhood were you talkative and vocally noisy? Did you ever lose your voice? Was there anything unusual about the change of voice? When did it occur? Have you ever been a cheer leader? A singer? Did you ever work in a noisy place, where it was necessary to speak loudly? It is obvious that these questions are intended to probe into areas of vocal misuse. Occasionally the answers to them are insightful and lead to more specific search.

The previous questions have concentrated on the origin and development of the voice problem itself.

The following enquiry focuses on the individual's general development and health history. These questions are particularly important in chronic voice cases of indefinite origin.

HEALTH HISTORY

What diseases have you had, and at what ages? (Note particularly measles, scarlet fever, diphtheria, poliomyelitis, mumps, ear trouble, and any high-fever diseases diagnosed or undiagnosed.) Special attention should be given to the so-called childhood diseases named, to their aftereffects, and to their time relationship to the origin of the voice problem. Peripheral or central nerve damage may be associated with any of them.

What injuries have you had? The nature, extent, and date of injuries, particularly in the head and neck area, should be investigated thoroughly. If one of these is related in time to the start of the voice problem, a report should be obtained from the attending physician if possible.

What operations have you had? Usually, when an operation is related to a voice defect the patient is aware of the association. The voice therapist is interested in knowing the nature of the surgery and whether the resultant voice defect is caused by tissue removal or nerve lesions and paralysis. A report from the surgeon is particularly advisable when the surgery is of recent date.

Do you have any allergies? What is your "blood count"? Do you know what your metabolic rate is? The conditions of allergy, anemia, or glandular imbalance should be suspected, particularly where a voice defect exists without a visible pathology. When a laryngologist refers a patient for speech therapy and reports no visible laryngeal pathology, a metabolism rating and a red-cell determination are desirable. The person who has sufficient allergic reaction to produce a voice problem usually knows that he has an allergy, although he may not have associated the voice problem with it. The mechanism of the voice deviation in these conditions is usually noninflammatory edema.

When the voice therapist must carry out his diagnostic procedure without the immediate assistance of a physician, he seeks evidence of need for referral before asking an individual to see a medical doctor for metabolic tests or general physical evaluation. The following questions are not diagnostic and no question is significant alone, but if there are a number of positive answers, the therapist can feel justified in suggesting a medical examination: 1. Have you ever had a metabolism test? What were the results? 2. How long ago was this determined? Who suggested that you have it, and what was the circumstance? Did you take any medication? How long did you continue with it? 3. Is your pulse rate a little slower than the average? 4. Is your temperature usually a little lower than 98.6°? 5. Do you often feel tired without real cause? 6. Do you often have bodily aches and pains without specific cause? 7. Do you have an abnormal dryness in your nose and throat? 8. Do you have sinus infection? 9. Do you have dry skin and hair? 10. Do you perspire less than the average person? 11. Do you perspire more than the average person? (Either of these last two symptoms may be present with hypothyroid imbalance.) 12. Do you often feel chilly when others are comfortable or warm? 13. Do you have any eye trouble? 14. Do you have any ear trouble? 15. Do you have any dizziness? 16. Do you have any pain or sensation of pressure in the region of the larynx? (Luse, 1948).

Where there has been a previous history of thyroid imbalance or other metabolic disturbance, the physical condition is suspect as a cause of the voice problem, and the patient should be urged to report regularly to his physician if he is not already doing so. If a recent metabolic rating is not available, the voice therapist should be reluctant to accept a "functional" diagnosis and should insist upon a reliable medical opinion.

Do you smoke? How much? How long have you been smoking? The amount of smoking and the length of time the subject has been smoking may have etiological importance. Heavy smoking associated with hoarseness, particularly if the hoarseness has developed recently, deserves careful and immediate laryngological attention.

Has swallowing ever been difficult? Has food often become lodged in the throat, causing coughing and discomfort? Have foods or liquids ever gone into the nasopharynx during swallowing? Has water ever escaped from the nose while drinking from a fountain? When either nasality or denasality has been noted in the patient's voice, these questions may be diagnostically revealing. If he answers affirmatively to one or more, it can be assumed that there is, or has been, a structural inadequacy or a paralysis in the velopharyngeal area.

Observation of the facial structures may be as diagnostically revealing as careful listening when considering nasal stoppage. Interference with the flow of air through the nose causes mouth breathing, which, after a time, is usually accompanied by a shortened upper lip and a large, pendant lower lip.

Questions about difficulty of breathing through the nose and whether or not the stoppage occurs at certain seasons, in particular geographic locations, or under other allergenic circumstances, will usually reveal the general nature of the problem.

By the time the examiner has progressed this far in the diagnostic procedure, he should have formed a detailed description of the voice defect and should also have acquired a substantial understanding of the patient, along with a concept of the origin and development of the voice problem. At this point it is appropriate that a careful study of the structure and function of the voice-producing mechanism be conducted. The tentative assumptions that have been made need to be confirmed or rejected.

EXAMINATION OF THE VOCAL MECHANISM

There is a tendency to think of the examination of the vocal mechanism as being identical to the examination of the larynx. The latter is very important and persons specializing in voice therapy should become skillful examiners of the larynx, but the careful observer can learn much without instruments and without attempting to see into the larynx. It is necessary to recognize also that in most school systems the examination of the larynx may be done only by a physician, which undoubtedly is a wise practice.

Observation requires a bright light that can be directed easily onto any desired area, and two chairs placed to allow the examiner to face the patient. The simplest light source is a flashlight, which is completely adequate for everything except examination with instruments. In the latter case, a concave mirror with a hole in the center is supported over one eye by a headband in such a position that light from a light bulb can be directed and focused onto a specific spot. The hole in the mirror allows shadow-free observation.

The examination should start with a scanning of the face and neck areas for scars or asymmetries. Usually this is done unobtrusively during the interview, but, where any abnormalities have been observed, further questioning at this time is indicated. These items may be clues to structural anomalies, injuries, surgical procedures, or neural lesions that were not revealed previously.

The functioning and control of the facial muscles should also be checked, not because they are directly related to voice defects, but because a deviation may signal a neurological disorder that involves the velopharyngeal area or the larynx. This examination is accomplished by observing asymmetry when the patient is asked to pucker his lips and to smile, alternately.

A similar type of interest motivates the observation of the tongue. The patient should be asked, first, to protrude the tongue beyond the lips. If it deviates definitely to the right or left, there may be a unilateral paralysis on the side toward which the turning occurs. Next, he should be asked to pass his tongue completely around his lips. Failure in any part of the movement again suggests neurological involvement. The third test of tongue movement is done by asking the patient to speak a word, such as "kitty" or "Tucker," slowly at first, and then to accelerate to the highest rate possible. Persons with a coordination problem in the tongue will reveal it in a quick failure of the diadochokinesis.

Light directed into the oropharynx will reveal the position of the soft palate, the contours of the faucial pillars, the presence of scars, the size and color of the tonsils, and the relative dryness of the posterior pharyngeal wall. Of greatest importance, however, is the observation of the movement of the velum and the related pharyngeal walls. A simple procedure is to ask the patient to open his mouth, to protrude his tongue, curl it down toward the chin, and to voice a prolonged "eh," as in *end*. The normally active soft palate will lift vigorously against the forward displacement of the tongue. At this time it is easy to see any irregularities in palatal elevator and tensor action. A further test of the velopharyngeal closure is to ask the patient to produce a loud, prolonged "th" sound, as in *thin*. If he can accomplish this without nasal escape, the closure is potentially adequate.

The openness of the nasal passages can be determined if the examiner will press the nostrils closed, alternately, while the patient is humming a long "m" sound. Partial, or even complete, blockage of one side may not affect the voice noticeably, but it should be investigated further through questions about allergy or the presence of a cold, or through medical referral unless the patient reports adequate medical care.

If a phonatory problem exists, the diagnosis cannot be considered complete until the larynx has been carefully observed. The examination of this structure with a mirror is relatively simple in principle. However, in practice it is apt to be difficult because most people have sensitive pharyngeal reflexes that interfere with the proper placement of the mirror in relation to the vocal folds and the light source. The examination technique can and should be learned by the voice pathologist, since it is a help to be able to observe laryngeal conditions and to follow the changes that occur in the course of therapy. It should be emphasized, however, that the diagnosing of laryngeal diseases and disorders is the province and responsibility of the laryngologist. This implies at once that the laryngologist is a necessary and extremely important person in the management of voice defects.

It is obvious that a complete diagnosis of a phonatory problem cannot be made until a laryngologist has examined the patient and reported his findings. This means that one of three procedures can be followed: 1. have a laryngologist as a regular member of the diagnosing team; 2. ask all persons requesting assistance to be examined by a laryngologist before they come for the initial interview; and 3. refer all patients who have phonatory problems to a laryngologist after their voices have been evaluated and other data collected. The last is the least desirable, since it delays the completion of the diagnosis, but it is the most common.

Where a close working arrangement can be made with laryngologists and they can be informed of the types of information that the voice therapist needs, it often helps to use a prepared form for acquiring data. Some public school speech correctionists have developed such forms, with the assistance of the local laryngologists. These forms should be clear to everyone using them, and it is important that they be brief.

Those speech pathologists who plan to concentrate on voice disorders and who should learn, therefore, to examine the larynx skillfully, are advised to follow three steps: 1. study the examination procedures for indirect laryngoscopy set forth in at least two books on laryngology; 2. become skillful with self-examination procedures; and 3. practise on some friends. It is emphasized that two or more descriptions of laryngeal examination technique should be studied because the various authors follow somewhat different procedures.

The self-examination can be worked out in several simple steps, as follows: first, buy a No. 3 or No. 4 laryngeal mirror from a surgical supply house; second, place a flashlight or a slide projector so it will shine into your mouth when you are seated; third, attach a small mirror of the type found in a woman's purse to the side of the flashlight or projector lens, and adjust the mirror to permit a view into your own mouth when you are seated in the proper position and the lamp is turned on; fourth, protrude your tongue, and hold it down toward your chin; and, fifth, with the other hand, place a warm laryngeal mirror back in the pharynx. By adjusting the laryngeal mirror properly, the interior of the larynx will come into view by reflection in the external mirror. The development of the technique is substantial reward for the necessary patience and practice.

When the time comes for practice on friends, the examination equipment must be changed to conform with that described in the laryngology texts. Practice in the manipulation of the head mirror and laryngeal mirror should be accomplished before an examination is attempted, even on friends. The examiner should approach all of these practice examinations seriously and with a sincerity of purpose. There is certainly no place for levity in such situations, but the examiner should not be surprised if associates feel self-conscious and laugh in the initial phases of practice.

EVALUATION OF NONSPEECH SKILLS AND ABILITIES

The fourth step in the diagnostic procedure is the evaluation of certain nonspeech skills and abilities. These include intellectual ability and emotional stability, motor skills, general health, systemic conditions, and hearing. If the patient's general level of skill and abilities are not included within the diagnostic evaluation, the stated causes of the voice defect may be inaccurate; and the plan for therapy is almost certain to be incomplete.

There is no implication here that organic voice disorders result from low intellectual ability or emotional instability. However, these factors influence learning ability, and they need to be evaluated as part of the plan of therapy. Furthermore, the intimate association of intelligence and emotional problems with psychogenic voice disorders causes these factors to be importantly present in the diagnostician's thinking.

Ideally, a clinical psychologist should be a part of the diagnostic team, but where this is not feasible, a qualified person should be available for referral. It is not necessary for all, or even a majority, of the persons having organically caused voice disorders to be examined by a psychologist. Usually the patient's reactions to the interview and the testing procedure, plus the school and employment records, provide sufficient evidence to determine the advisability of referral.

Occasionally an individual who seeks assistance for

a voice disorder will also exhibit an incoordination of the face or tongue, peculiarities of gait, or random movements. It may be obvious that there is a neurological disorder, but it may not be possible to determine immediately whether that problem has any influence on the voice. Observation and questioning will usually indicate whether the patient should be referred to a neurologist, a laryngologist, a psychiatrist, or kept for voice therapy.

During the case history interview, it is usually possible to conclude whether or not further information on general health and the systemic conditions, such as glandular imbalance, are indicated. If they are, the referral should be made, with specific questions to the physician.

The hearing acuity of a person rarely contributes significantly to his voice defect. The exception is where it causes him to speak very loudly and thereby creates social problems or produces vocal abuse. Such a hearing loss would be evident and would require immediate referral to an otologist or audiologist. A milder hearing loss should be known to the voice therapist if it exists because it may make certain phases of the therapy more difficult. It follows that an audiometric evaluation should be a routine part of each voice diagnosis, and a qualified audiometrist should be a member of the diagnostic group.

The processes of listening, questioning, looking, and testing that have been described provide basic information about voice problems and the persons having them. The study of the relationships among these data, the elimination of nonapplicable items, and the final synthesis of the pertinent factors provide the diagnosis. Usually, it can be set forth briefly in two parts: first, a classification, or descriptive statement, of the vocal symptoms; and second, a summary of the factors that seem to have caused them.

Such a diagnostic statement constitutes a hypothesis on which to base recommendations. These ordinarily follow one of three directions. When voice therapy is indicated, the patient is either scheduled for remedial work with the diagnosing clinic or he is referred to another voice therapist, if one happens to be located more conveniently. When voice therapy is not recommended, the decision is explained to the patient in terms most beneficial to his welfare, and when it will be helpful, he is referred to another type of service.

The preceding diagnostic routine has implied a need for a complete effect-to-cause investigation. This is not always necessary, however, since some surgical conditions are immediately evident and do not need a detailed diagnostic procedure. The primary example of this situation is the laryngectomized person. Ordinarily the laryngeal surgeon's report is available, which, in combination with a few basic questions, will establish the advisability of vocal reeducation.

In the case of the laryngectomee, the therapist needs to know something about him as a person, and about his pre- and postsurgical history. The following questions have been found to be helpful in a clinical situation as items on a brief questionnaire: When and where was the surgery performed? Who was the surgeon? Were there any complications? Before the operation, was there hoarseness or aphonia? When, and under what conditions? Was speech important to the patient's occupation? Did he sing? Did he smoke? How much? How long? Since the operation, what is the patient's attitude toward his condition? (Upset and disturbed; unconcerned acceptance; eager to develop speech.) Has there been any attempt to learn to speak? When? Where? What procedures were used? Were they successful? Have artificial devices been tried? What types? What is the reason for the present interest in voice therapy?

What is the laryngectomee's present level of speech ability as indicated by the following scale:

1. no sounds.
2. occasional sound, uncertain control.
3. single sounds and short words under voluntary control.
4. words and short phrases used in communication.
5. sentences used frequently, occasional sound failure.
6. fluent speech.

Therapy

The diagnostic procedures outlined above stressed the close affiliation of voice therapy with laryngology and other medical specialities. When an organic anomaly is present, the condition of the patient must be improved as much as circumstances will allow before active voice therapy starts. The following discussions are based on the assumption that all such treatment has been done or is being done.

Voice therapy is an art and the therapist is an artist in the same way that medicine is an art and the physician an artist. Each of these practitioners, as a painter with a palette full of colors, chooses from a variety of procedures based on scientific investigation and clinical observation. Each therapist must use his best judgment in the selection of techniques that form a rational therapy specifically for an individual who has a unique personal problem. Fortunately, there are basic principles of therapy that apply to voice disorders and that offer an opportunity for generalizations about treatment.

Vocal therapy for organic voice disorders may be focused toward either the restoration of normal voice or the development of a compensatory voice. The therapeutic approach that is chosen for a particular remedial program will depend upon the extent to which the vocal structures can be restored to normal. That is, if the vocal condition can be alleviated by vocal therapy alone or if surgical and medicinal procedures can provide a normal structure, the goal of vocal therapy is the reestablishment of normal phonation. On the other hand, if the mechanism and voice are permanently altered, the voice therapy has three compensatory objectives: 1. to establish the greatest possible efficiency in the use of the remaining structures; 2. to develop physiological compensations; and 3. to help the patient accept his "different" voice.

RESTORATIVE THERAPY

Therapeutic procedures that aim to restore a normal voice are applied to the following three kinds of disorders: first, voice problems resulting from vocal abuse that has produced the intermediate mechanisms of thickened vocal fold tissue, myasthenia laryngis, vocal nodules, contact ulcer, or chronic laryngitis; second, vocal deviations that follow surgical intervention that provides an essentially normal larynx; and, third, voice problems resulting from endocrine imbalance or anemia that persist despite medical treatment.

The procedures that the speech pathologist can use in restorative therapy are psychological, environmental, and physiological. Their combined aim is to establish a method of voice production in which the natural rejuvenating processes can occur, since normal structures tend to reestablish themselves when given the opportunity; and to develop vocal habits that can be used effectively to meet the ordinary demands of living.

The psychological factors that are applicable in restorative therapy include informing each patient, as completely as his ability will permit, that continued misuse of the voice will create serious vocal problems in the future, that vocal recovery is a long process, that it will occur in relation to the completeness with which he follows the therapeutic program, and that he must learn to eliminate his vocal noisiness and to talk less. Throughout his therapy he should be encouraged to maintain the best vocal usage possible at all times, in order to avoid the recurrence of the anomaly. Vocal improvement in these cases occurs slowly, and the therapist must be sensitive to those forms of encouragement and motivation that apply to the individual patient and that can provide a favorable atmosphere for progress.

Perhaps the most important single psychological ingredient in successful therapy is the attitude of the patient. Admonition, encouragement, and motivation from the clinician have little effect unless the individual with the problem wants to modify his voice. An effective means of establishing a contributing attitude is through the process of problem solving in which the patient arrives at a clear understanding of his problem and recognizes realistic goals toward its solution. Therapeutic maneuvers can have little effect unless the patient understands their purpose and willingly agrees to apply them effectively.

Environmental therapy refers to the recognition and alteration of factors in the work, home, or recreational situations that are detrimental to normal vocal usage. If the patient must speak in a noisy environment or if he competes vocally with members of his family or others, vocal abuse and its sequellae are present. There is little value in efforts to retrain a voice if vocally harmful practices are regularly present. Parents, employers, and the patient himself can often modify the environment or change the requirements within the environment to accomplish less detrimental vocal use. Vocal reeducation is an all-day, every-day process that involves almost every aspect of the patient's pattern of living, and careful attention must be focused on his total environment if therapy is to be successful.

The physiological aspects of therapy must be concrete and positive. In some instances, where healing must occur or inflammation allowed to subside, the first step in direct therapy is the prescription of complete silence. This means that all communication must be by pencil and paper for a period of from a few days to a week or two. However, silence alone is not enough to produce the required change in voice production. Silence will not improve the *habits* of voice any more than absence from a piano will give the pianist a new pattern of finger movements. The period of silence provides the environment for recovery of the structures, but the patient will use the only habits he knows, which are the abusive ones, when he resumes talking unless he has been taught a new and nondamaging method of phonation.

The second specific step in the reeducative process is to train the patient to phonate in a relaxed, easy manner. This instruction can proceed during the period of communicative silence, and its importance should be vigorously emphasized. Training in relaxed phonation provides a bridge from the previous type of vocal abuse to the recommended way of phonating.

Relaxed voice production can be acquired through a combination of at least the following five types of training: 1. learning general physical relaxation; 2. development of emotional control; 3. training in the recognition of adequate and inadequate voice production; 4. development of the awareness of tense and relaxed phonation; and 5. learning to produce voice without excessive effort.

General physical relaxation can be achieved by systematic training. Relaxation, as discussed here, encompasses two concepts: first, that relaxation is a general reduction in muscular activity, causing the individual to be motionless and flaccid; and second, that relaxation is a dynamic balance, in which the opposing groups of muscles exert just enough reciprocal tension upon each other to accomplish the desired movement with perfect control. It is this second concept that applies in efficient phonation. Training in generalized relaxation is desirable as an aid to achieving dynamic relaxation, since management of the voluntary skeletal muscle groups can be accomplished more readily than relaxation of the involuntary muscles, many of which are active in phonation. Dynamic relaxation as presented here is the basis for muscular coordination, and good coordination of the phonatory musculature is essential for efficient voice production.

Several methods and techniques have been advocated for general and differential, or localized, relaxation, and each has claimed success. The three ingredients that seem to be necessary for general relaxation are: 1. a comfortable position for the patient; 2. skill in the recognition and localization of muscle tension; and 3. the ability to release excessive tension either directly by voluntary attention to it, or indirectly by substituting another sensation, such as "heaviness" or "lightness." The amount of training required to achieve relaxation will vary widely with the attitude of the patient toward the process and toward his voice problem. Unless he is able to practice frequently each day and unless there is real motivation, relaxation will probably not be achieved. It hardly needs to be added that the voice therapist should be thoroughly familiar with the various relaxation techniques and should be able to apply them to himself.

The mechanical procedure of general physical relaxation is relatively ineffective if the individual who is trying to relax is chronically worried or easily upset emotionally. It follows that learning to relax requires personal insight and control of emotional responses, as well as the physical ability to release muscular tension. This discussion cannot deal with the psychological and counseling techniques that are useful in this phase of relaxation, but it can stress the fact that the voice therapist should be thoroughly familiar with such procedures. It can point out, also, that the counselor, the psychologist, and the psychiatrist can be helpful in dealing with muscular tension in vocal defects.

The principles of general relaxation that have been mentioned establish the environment for relaxed phonation. Next it is desirable to direct the patient's attention to the phonatory process proper, in order to help him gain control over it. As indicated earlier, the aspects of phonation to which he must attend before starting direct vocal training are the acoustic and the kinesthetic. The patient must learn to hear the characteristics of other voices, as well as his own; and he must develop the ability to recognize the sensations of tension and relaxation that are present when he voluntarily produces various kinds of voice quality.

Learning to hear one's own voice, and particularly learning to recognize vocal faults in one's self and others, requires training in listening. The most direct approach to this ability is through the combination of a skillful clinician and a good recording machine. The clinician's role is to help the patient record many samples of his voice, and, as they listen to the recordings, to identify the good and poor characteristics of the various qualities. This often requires a number of training periods and may be facilitated by critically listening to samples of other voices.

After the patient has learned to hear vocal differences, he can be taught to associate various kinds of vocal sound with the kinesthetic sensations of their production. Specifically, he can learn to recognize hypertension both by hearing the sound and by the concurrent kinesthetic sensation. At this stage the individual begins to gain a positive control of phonation, and he is ready to start direct vocal training.

Direct training in voice production is the last part of the reeducative program for a defective voice produced by a relatively normal larynx. The general aim of the program is to teach the patient to produce a pleasant and servicable voice that will allow the larynx to function in a normal manner. This type of phonation helps the natural healing and rejuvenating processes to occur and prevents the recurrence of vocal abuse and its sequelae. The reeducative program is composed of five well-defined types of exercise and instruction. Each deserves a brief review:

1. The voice must be used quietly. The patient should realize that he must speak in a subdued way, without any exceptions, for perhaps as long as a year or two. The therapist will need to remind the patient frequently to speak at a low-loudness level, particularly at the beginning of corrective work, but it is a necessary part of the therapy.

2. Phonation should be started with a breathy quality. To establish this concept, one helpful exercise is to instruct the patient to produce a phonated sigh on a downward inflection. He is asked to inhale deeply, to let the air out as in a sigh, and, at the same time, to produce a vowel sound on a downward pitch glide. This exercise can be modified rather quickly to a gently phonated downward pitch glide which is breathy but without the extreme air escape of the sigh.

As work progresses, another exercise that can be used is the quiet production of words and sentences containing initial aspirate sounds, such as *home*, *hurry*, *He hit Henry's hat*, and *Hold hope high* (Moser, 1969). When the patient can manage these materials, he should be encouraged to read ordinary prose and poetry in a slightly breathy voice.

Breathiness, purposely produced, keeps the vocal cords from striking each other as vigorously as in other types of phonation, and the closed phase of the vibratory cycle is shortened, thereby reducing the time in which the cords are in contact. The relaxed breathy-voice production also reduces the pressure between the arytenoid cartilages, which is particularly advantageous with contact ulcers.

3. The patient must be instructed and helped to use a middle-pitch range. Quiet, breathy phonation can be of maximum benefit only if the individual uses a pitch that averages at least four or five tones above the lowest note of his range. In contrast, when the vocal pitch is held within one or two notes of the bottom of the range, there is excessive muscle tension evident in the larynx. This type of voice production is often associated with contact ulcer.

Exercises for learning to raise the average pitch level begin with listening to recorded pitch changes and comparing them with the patient's habitual pattern. The individual should listen to recordings of his own voice and that of his clinician, in which the two have alternately produced sounds with rising and falling inflections. Such vowels as "ah" and "oh," spoken as though asking questions, and the speaking of actual questions are useful drill materials. A successful ear-training technique for pitch discernment is the "saying" of a sentence with the lips closed. This effectively eliminates the words but leaves the tune of the sentence. Variations in meaning produce different melody patterns. The preceding exercise can be extended easily into phrases and sentences, spoken with several melodies to express different meanings: for example, "*I* am going downtown." "I *am* going downtown." "I am going *down*town." Eventually the patient can learn to read prose quietly and with meaningful pitch changes, which is an excellent pitch exercise. This step must be delayed, however, until he can both hear and control the pitch of his own voice. Many good exercises for varying the pitch and for using the most advantageous average pitch can be found in textbooks for voice and diction classes. The pitch exercises mentioned in this section have been included to stress the need for attention to pitch when working for effortless phonation.

Variation in pitch at once eliminates monotony and raises the average level of those voices that are too low. The attempt to raise the average pitch level by direct instruction to "Raise the pitch," or through chanting and singing exercises is usually unsatisfactory. Ordinarily the patient is unable to comply with the first request, and he is apt to feel silly trying to carry out the second. Furthermore, it is difficult to make a transition from the sung tones to normal speech. On the other hand, an emphasis on meaningful expression of ideas through pitch variation accomplishes the change of pitch level in a normal way and generally improves the expressiveness of the speech.

4. The patient must be taught to use his breath efficiently. To learn to hear one's own voice defects and to develop the ability to phonate easily at a comfortable pitch are fundamental to vocal rehabilitation. However, the ability to sustain single sounds and otherwise to use the breath stream efficiently must be learned and practised if the habits of easy phonation are to be made permanent.

There can be little doubt that many persons with

harmful vocal habits expend more effort on breathing than is necessary. Most patients have an adequate vital capacity but have poor vocal control. Some persons, particularly those who do sedentary work, develop breathing habits in which the expansion and contraction of the thoracic and abdominal regions are asynchronous. That is, when they depress the rib cage, they not only move air through the trachea and larynx as they intended, but the intrathoracic pressure also forces the diaphragm downward and hence distends the abdominal wall. This breathing pattern seems to contribute to undesirable, compensatory muscle tensions in the neck and larynx, particularly when additional vocal effort is necessary.

Usually it is possible to improve the efficiency of breath use without specific attention to the respiratory movements. This can be done most simply by improvement of posture, combined with the sustaining of tones and the uttering of progressively longer sentences on one breath. The latter, of course, does not imply that in ordinary conversation the patient should say as many words as possible on one breath. The prolongation is a drill and should be so explained.

A breathy type of phonation was recommended earlier to avoid hypertension in the laryngeal musculature and to foster a subdued type of voice production. This voice quality, however, is not desirable if it can be improved. One of the simplest and best methods of reducing breathiness without increasing harmful tensions is to sustain tones as suggested above. This is another aspect of efficiency in the use of the breath in vocalization.

5. Frequent, short practice sessions are necessary in restorative voice therapy. Overuse of the voice is always detrimental and must be avoided. Furthermore, the rest periods have a positive benefit, for they provide the opportunity for recovery if misuse happens to occur. The frequency of the practice sessions will be determined by many circumstances, but an ideal schedule, one found to be practical in many cases, is to practise the last few minutes of each hour, six or eight times per day. During the initial one to two weeks of therapy, three minutes of active practice at each session are enough. If that period of activity is tolerated, the practice time can be increased to five minutes and then to 10 in each session. At this point, an occasional practice session of 30 minutes should be tried. When this period can be handled with ease, more responsibility for the vocal usage should be given to the patient. Regular instructional sessions should be continued at weekly intervals for several months, and if the patient demonstrates sufficient progress, he should be started on a series of lessons in which the time interval between sessions is gradually increased. This gives the voice therapist an opportunity to guide the patient into a sound program of self-directed vocal hygiene that he can manage alone.

Restorative therapy for organic voice problems usually is a long reeducative process. It requires the patient to understand the goals of therapy and to cooperate willingly in the therapeutic process. The reeducative procedures that have been employed successfully include relaxation and the use of quiet phonation, a breathy type of voice production, attention to the pitch level and the speech melody, the sustaining of tones and the production of progressively longer sentences for phonatory control and breathing efficiency, and the use of frequent, short practice periods. The specific exercises and their use must be determined by the therapist as he arranges the therapeutic program to fit the needs of the patient.

COMPENSATORY VOICE THERAPY

At the beginning of the discussion of therapy, a differentiation was made between treatment for persons with essentially normal structures and those who have had structural modifications that are permanent and that preclude the likelihood of normal voice production. The pathologies that illustrate the latter situation include the surgical removal of all or part of the larynx, destructive diseases, ankylosis of the cricoarytenoid joints, and paralysis. The purpose of voice therapy, where these structural changes exist, is to help the patient acquire as effective voice production as possible without developing harmful vocal habits or unpleasant associated behavior. This therapy, therefore, has been labeled "compensatory."

The discussion of compensatory therapy has been divided into two parts: first, procedures for patients who have a larynx; and, second, procedures for the laryngectomized. Again, it should be stressed that each person requires careful planning of therapy to fit his particular case. However, there are some suggestions which can be generally applied in compensatory therapy.

The voice program for a person who has a modified larynx ordinarily does not require a period of silence beyond that necessary for the proper healing of the surgically treated areas. When the patient is released by his physician for voice therapy, it may begin immediately with a systematic and careful sampling of what the patient can do vocally. The patient should be asked to attempt tones over his complete pitch range to discover whether or not certain parts of his range are less hoarse, louder, or produced with less effort than others. These pitch changes should be tried with many vowels and with variations in intensity. Frequently, particularly in cases having one vocal fold removed, there will be a significantly better quality with one vowel sound at a particular pitch.

There are several other evaluative procedures that should be employed. One is to ask the patient to cough and thus demonstrate the presence or absence of complete laryngeal closure. He should be instructed, also, to turn his head first toward one shoulder then the other, and to produce selected sounds and words. When the head is in a rotated position, the vocal folds sometimes are approximated to a greater degree, thereby producing a louder, less breathy voice. A similar assistance may result from asking the patient to press lightly on the sides of the thyroid cartilage while attempting to phonate. The effect of this manipulation is to improve approximation of the vocal folds. Turning the head and pressing the thyroid cartilage are devices only and do not represent any real advancement in vocal recovery. They are valuable in therapy in two ways: they sometimes encourage the patient to greater effort; and they may be useful "crutches" in difficult communicating situations, such as telephone conversations or talking in noisy places.

These exploratory procedures are both diagnostic and therapeutic. Ordinarily they extend over a period of weeks, and often a favorable response does not come until after a prolonged period of exploration and training. Discovering what the patient is capable of doing is the real beginning point in direct therapy. Exercises to help him improve and extend what he can do constitute the second step in therapy, and they require all the imagination and ingenuity the clinician posesses. Adaptations of the types of vocal drills suggested in the discussion of restorative therapy are very useful.

The patient with a permanently modified larynx requires careful management and supervision to avoid excessive practice and vocal abuse. Short practice periods are imperative. Some of these individuals need much encouragement, since their progress is apt to be slow and therefore frustrating. On the other hand, so long as the therapist believes some additional progress can be made, the patient should not be allowed to become satisfied with his results. The patient who loses his desire to improve has lost his ability to improve.

The second type of compensatory therapy applies to persons without a larynx. It is commonly known that any complex sound put into the upper respiratory tract can be formed into audible speech by the adjustments of the articulating and resonating mechanisms. It follows that a laryngectomized person can learn to speak again if he can introduce or create a sound in his pharynx or mouth. Consequently, the primary focus of therapy is the generation of the necessary sound (see Chapter 22).

There are three common substitute sound producing mechanisms used by laryngectomees. One is the reed type of artificial larynx in which the reed element is activated by the exhaled air which passes through a tube from the tracheal stoma. The sound that is generated by the reed travels by way of a second tube into the mouth, where it is articulated into speech. The reed instrument has several disadvantages and has been almost entirely replaced by a battery-operated buzzer that is placed against the neck in such a position that its vibrations activate the tissues of the neck and consequently the air in the pharynx. The resulting sound in the respiratory tract is articulated in the customary manner. There are several brands of electrical artificial larynges, some of which are available through local telephone companies and hearing aid dealers. The third mechanism that can produce sound for speech is a body structure that is trained to function as a pseudoglottis. This sound generator is a constriction capable of vibrating and is usually located at the junction of the esophagus and pharynx. However, it may occur higher in the pharynx or in the mouth. The air is customarily taken into the esophagus and expelled as in eructation, which causes the voice to be called "esophageal speech." The skillful esophageal speaker presents an entirely normal appearance, his speaking is fluent, he can often change the pitch of his voice, and, although there is always some hoarseness present, the quality of his voice is relatively normal. Laryngectomized persons usually prefer esophageal speech to one of the artificial devices. It approximates the speaking process, it causes fewer aesthetic problems, it is more reliable, and it is always available.

It is desirable to begin speech therapy as soon as possible after it is known that a laryngectomy is necessary. In some situations, training may be started before surgery, but ordinarily the voice therapist does not see the patient until after the operation. Usually vocal restoration with esophageal speech occurs more quickly when therapy is started as soon after surgery as healing permits. However, many laryngectomees have learned esophageal speech after years of voicelessness or use of an artificial device. Therefore, both the patient and the therapist have reason to expect success, providing there is proper motivation and adequate physical structure following the surgical procedures.

The first step in speech retraining with a laryngectomee is to ask him to belch voluntarily. If he cannot or if he is not sure, ask him to imitate either you or a good laryngectomized speaker who can be present at the lessons. The teacher should produce a sound and ask the patient to follow immediately with his own effort. It is helpful if the instructor demonstrates with a word, such as "yes" or "no," rather than an ordinary eructation. The formation of a word is esthetically more pleasant and also indicates specifically what the patient is expected to do.

If the individual cannot imitate, ask him if he has produced a belch noise at any time since his laryngectomy. If he has, and almost everyone is able to do so, it indicates that he probably can learn esophageal speech. However, if he has not done so, the voice therapist should talk with the surgeon, if this is possible, to learn of the presence of any structural reasons why the patient cannot be expected to develop esophageal speech. If there are reasons to doubt successful speech, it might be wise to consider the immediate acquisition of an artificial larynx. The patient needs to have a means of communication as soon as possible, and decisions about the use of an instrument should not be delayed unnecessarily. However, esophageal speech should be taught and used wherever possible.

When imitation does not produce sounds in three or four lessons, it is wise to add description and explanation in the teaching of esophageal speech. The first step is to inform the patient, if he does not already know, that his larynx was only a sound-producer, and that the tongue, soft palate, lips, and related structures formed the sound into speech. He should be told that any other sound that can be put into the mouth can also be used for speech and that the best one is the natural belch sound made by the escape of air from the esophagus. Through descriptions and diagrams, he can be told about the surgical changes that have occurred and why he needs to learn to take air into the esophagus. This instruction reduces the patient's reluctance to try, and prepares him to follow the therapeutic program.

Another phase of the preparatory motivation is the presentation of a good esophageal speaker to the new patient. This is often the most important single step in therapy. It should be pointed out, however, that if a speaker is not available, the therapist should not substitute recordings of other laryngectomized speakers at this stage of therapy. It is usually very difficult to obtain a faithful recording of esophageal speech; consequently, since the new patient is familiar only with normal rather than esophageal speech, his comparison with the recording may be more disturbing than helpful. Later, after the patient has some skill, he can appreciate a recording of a fluent speaker and will profit from hearing it.

There are several methods used to teach laryngectomized persons to take in the air for speech. The therapist should be familiar with all of them, since a particular approach may be successful with one patient but fail with another.

Perhaps the most normal-appearing way of taking air is called the "inhalation" technique, and for this reason it should be tried first. In this approach the therapist simply asks the patient to open his mouth, to relax the mouth and throat areas, and to inhale suddenly. Often the reduction of pressure within the the thorax causes the air in the pharynx to be drawn into the esophagus. It will help if the patient places his finger over his tracheostomy momentarily at the start of inhalation, so that the inhalation movement will inflate the esophagus. If he is successful, he should be encouraged to expel the air immediately with as much noise as possible. It should be emphasized that the momentary obstruction of the tracheostomy is a device for helping the patient in his first attempts at speaking. It should not, and need not, be continued.

Another temporary assisting device used with the "inhalation" technique is a forward and upward projection of the chin. This pulls the anterior structures of the neck forward, thereby helping to open the entrance to the esophagus. The head movement should be stopped after the patient learns to inhale the esophageal air, since it is not necessary for speaking and calls attention to itself as an abnormality.

If the patient is not successful with the "inhalation" technique, he should be taught the "injection" method of obtaining air. The critical element in this procedure is pressure on air held in the mouth and pharynx of such nature that the air is squeezed, or "injected," into the esophagus. When the velopharyngeal closure has been made and the mouth passage occluded at the lips, alveolar ridge, or velum, as in the formation of plosive sounds, there is a certain amount of air enclosed within the mouth and pharynx. When pressure is exerted on this air, it will move if an opening is available. In this instance, the only place the air can possibly go is through the esophageal sphincter into the esophagus. The air in the esophagus is then expelled by an increase in intrathoracic pressure, as in respiration. The sound is made by vibratory interruptions of this air movement at one of several places in the pharynx or mouth.

The patient may be taught to "inject" the air in either of two ways. The first starts from the "b" position, the second from the "d" position. In either instance, the patient is asked to place his lips or tongue in the position for one of these sounds and then to "squeeze" the air in the mouth. The tongue and cheeks compress the air and force or pump it into the esophagus. The patient should be instructed to expel the air immediately in an attempt to produce sound.

A variation of this procedure has been described by Moolenaar-Bijl (1953), who believes that some of the articulatory movements of speech, particularly the plosives, produce pressure pulses that recharge the air in the esophagus during the utterance of a phrase or sentence. This replenishing of the esophageal air probably accounts for the long sentences that some speakers can produce.

The first purposeful sound is usually a great encouragement to the patient. Often, however, he will be unable to repeat it immediately, since his excitement and desire to speak create excessive tensions that he cannot control. This may disturb him unless the therapist explains what has happened. This situation offers an excellent opportunity to point out the need for regular and frequent practice periods in a calm, quiet atmosphere. The ability to produce controlled sounds varies widely. A few patients speak words in the first lesson, but most require from several weeks to several months to achieve control of single words. Those who believe they cannot learn require a little longer!

The controlled production of sound is of greatest importance, but it is only part of the development of esophageal speech. In addition, the patient must learn to increase the number of words spoken on one "breath," and he must eliminate the individual eccentricities that sometimes develop.

The speech rehabilitation process usually advances rapidly after the patient knows how to produce esophageal sounds voluntarily. For a short time, while he is concentrating his attention on the control of sound, he should be allowed to produce single vowels, but it is advisable to substitute real words soon. Single syllable words that begin with a vowel or voiced consonant (particularly "b" and "d") and end with an unvoiced sound are particularly valuable, for example, boat, bat, bait, ate, date, dot, eat, it, but, boot, and so on. In these words, the final unvoiced sound is added after the phonation has ceased, and no more esophageal sound is required to complete the word. The patient recognizes that he is actually speaking, and thus is motivated more than with the linguistically meaningless repetition of vowels.

Two and three syllables in words and phrases should be introduced as soon as there is a reasonably consistent production of monosyllabic words. Usually, the patient is so anxious to talk that he will indicate what he is able to do and consequently will determine his own progress. Talking in conversation is perhaps the best possible practice as long as the patient makes a consistent effort to speak well.

Environmental factors can also contribute to the success of the reeducative program. The therapist should explain to the patient that the ease of speaking will vary with fatigue, excitement, the speaking situation, and other conditions. Learning will often be accelerated by the cooperation of the family. The speech clinician should confer with members of the patient's family to explain what is being done and to point out the need for patience with him and respect for his attempts to learn to speak again.

From the very beginning of therapy, the patient should be instructed regarding the esthetic aspects of his problem. He must be encouraged to keep the neck area and the tracheostomy tube clean. Men should keep their shirt collars closed and should wear a tie when in the presence of others. This not only protects the patient by shielding the opening; it also keeps the exhaled air from striking persons standing in front of the patient. Women can be shown how to wear neckerchiefs, collars, and brooches on special neck bands to cover and protect the tracheal opening. Such esthetic care will help the patient to be more socially acceptable and will, in consequence, add to his opportunities for conversional practice.

THERAPY FOR RESONANCE PROBLEMS

The resonance problems of organic origin that have been discussed in this chapter have included excessively nasal and denasal voices. The causes of the former were described as cleft palate, congenitally short palate, surgical procedures, and paralyses of the velar and pharyngeal muscles. The organic causes of the latter are stoppages of various kinds in the nasal passes or nasopharynx.

The voice defects associated with a cleft palate deserve every consideration; but since they are only part of the total problem, they should be discussed in their proper perspective in an integrated therapy. For this reason the reader is referred to Chapters 29 and 30.

The congenitally short palate is, first of all, a medical and surgical problem. After repair has been accomplished, the voice therapist can contribute by providing appropriate palatal and pharyngeal exercises and by supervising their use. These are identical with those used in postsurgery speech training for cleft palate. Therefore, to avoid needless duplication the reader is referred again to the section on cleft palate.

Surgical procedures, primarily tonsilectomy and adenoidectomy, sometimes leave scar tissue in the faucial area that reduces the mobility of the velum. If the disability is extreme, additional surgical procedures can reduce the scar tissue and improve the mobility. Following corrective surgery, velopharyngeal exercises, of the type recommended for paralyses in the paragraphs below, are helpful.

When the removal of adenoids produces hypernasality, it means that this tissue had been used in the formation of the velopharyngeal closure. If the velum and other structures are normal, the ordinary swallowing and articulatory movements will modify the habits, and normal action will be developed. Sometimes voice exercises to stimulate velar activity are indicated to accelerate the speech improvement. These exercises are the same as those suggested in the following section on paralysis.

Paralysis in the velopharyngeal area may be slight, or it may be extensive. Where it affects many muscles, the prognosis for speech is unfavorable. Ordinarily, however, therapy should be tried even in severe cases on the chance that there may be some beneficial development. The less extensive the involvement, of course, the greater the expected response.

Exercises can begin with the passive lifting of the velum with a tongue blade or the handle of a spoon. In addition, the eliciting of a gag reflex is also beneficial. When some constrictive motion or lift of the palate is present, the patient should be shown how to observe his own structures with a mirror so he can develop his voluntary control to the fullest extent. This can be facilitated by having the patient protrude the tongue and say such vowels as "ah," "uh," "eh," and so on. Thrusting the tongue out pulls actively against the palatal elevators and tensors, thereby stretching and stimulating them. It should be pointed out to the patient that one of the best exercises is swallowing, which he should practice regularly and frequently. Liquids should be taken with many small sips and the swallowing act carried through as completely as possible each time.

The types of speech exercises that are applicable to paralysis include: 1. teaching as wide-mouth opening on all sounds as is both possible and consistent with sound production; 2. alternating open vowels with nasal sounds; 3. blowing exercises, in which the air is directed through the mouth as completely as possible and in which the blowing is frequently changed into "oo" and "oh" sounds without altering the positions of the articulators; 4. developing gentle plosives to reduce the apparent nasality and air noises; and 5. the development of the patient's ability to listen carefully to his own voice and speech in an effort to produce the most intelligible communication possible.

Organically caused denasality always represents a complete or nearly complete occlusion of the airway above the soft or hard palate. The obstructions are not amenable to voice therapy; they can be remedied only by surgery or medical treatment, depending upon the nature of the obstruction. The voice therapist is often the first person consulted professionally by the patient with denasality. Proper referral to a rhinologist or a rhinolaryngologist constitutes a service to the patient and usually alleviates the voice problem. However, in those instances where chronically swollen nasal membranes caused by allergy or some other condition that does not respond to medical treatment exists, speech therapy can help the patient compensate for this problem. Careful attention to the production of nasal sounds, training in listening, and slowing of the speaking rate are helpful procedures.

SUMMARY

This discussion of organic disorders of voice has been developed through six main divisions that included: 1. introductory perspective; 2. phonatory theory; 3. description of voice disorders; 4. physiology of organic voice disorders; 5. etiologies of organic conditions that cause voice defects; and 6. management of organic voice disorders, in which both diagnosis and therapy were sketched.

The presentation attempted to be practical, to relate practice to theory, and to stimulate a research interest in this extremely complex field. The author is aware that there is much yet to be learned before voice problems can be managed adequately. Careful observation, systematic research, and detailed reporting should eventually provide answers to most of the problems.

BIBLIOGRAPHY

Arnold, G. 1962. Vocal nodules and polyps: laryngeal tissue reaction to habitual hyperkinetic dysphonia. *J. Speech Hearing Disorders*, 27, 205–217.

———. 1963. Vocal rehabilitation of paralytic dysphonia. X. functional results of intrachordal injection. *Arch. Otolaryng.*, 78, 179–186.

Ballenger, H., and Ballenger, J. 1954. A manual of otology, rhinology and laryngology (4th. ed.). Philadelphia: Lee & Febiger.

Ballenger, J., and contributors. 1969. Diseases of the nose, throat and ear (11th. ed.). Philadelphia: Lea & Febiger.

Beranek, L. 1949. Acoustic measurements. New York: Wiley.

Brodnitz, F. 1959. Vocal rehabilitation. *Amer. Acad. Ophthal. Otolaryng.* (Section on instruction-home study courses).

———. 1961. Contact ulcer of the larynx. *Arch. Otolaryng.*, 74, 70–80.

———. 1963. Goals, results and limitations of vocal rehabilitation. *Arch. Otolaryng.*, 77, 148–156.

Cooper, M., and Nahum, A. 1967. Vocal rehabilitation for contact ulcer. *Arch. Otolaryng.*, 85, 41–46.

Daly, J. 1963. The hoarse patient. *Postgrad. Med.*, 34, 488–492.

Damsté, P. 1967. Voice change in adult women caused by virilizing agents. *J. Speech Hearing Disorders*, 32, 126–132.

Darley, F. 1964. Diagnosis and appraisal of communication disorders. Englewood Cliffs, N.J.: Prentice-Hall.

DeWeese, D., and Saunders, W. 1964. Textbook of otolaryngology (2nd. ed.). St. Louis: Masby.

Diedrich, W., and Youngstrom, K. 1966. Alaryngeal speech. Springfield, Ill.: Thomas.

Dolowitz, D. 1964. Basic otolaryngology. New York: Blakiston Division, McGraw-Hill.

Holinger, P., Johnston, K., and McMahon, R. 1952. Hoarseness in infants and children. *Eye, Ear, Nose and Throat Monthly*, 31, 247–251.

Jackson, C., and Jackson, C. L. 1937. The larynx and its diseases. Philadelphia: Saunders.

———. 1942. Diseases and injuries of the larynx. New York: Macmillan.

Levin, N. 1962, ed. Voice and speech disorders: medical aspects. Springfield, Ill.: Thomas.

Luchsinger, R., and Arnold, G. 1965. Voice-speech-language. Belmont, Calif.: Wadsworth.

Luse, E. 1948. A study of vocal structures and speech in relation to metabolic rate. Northwestern Univ.: Ph.D. dissertation.

Moolenaar-Bijl, A. 1953. The importance of certain consonants in esophageal voice after laryngectomy. *Ann. Otol., Rhinol., Laryng.*, 62, No. 4, 979–989.

Moore, G. P. 1971. Organic voice disorders. Englewood Cliffs, N.J.: Prentice-Hall.

———, and Abbott, T. 1969. Defects of speech. *In* Diseases of the nose, throat and ear (11th. ed.). Ballenger, J., ed. Philadelphia: Lea & Febiger.

———, and von Leden, H. 1958. Dynamic variations of the vibratory pattern in the normal larynx. *Folia Phoniat.*, 10, 205–238.

Moser, H. 1969. One-syllable words. Columbus, Ohio: Merrill.

Myerson, V. 1964. The human larynx. Springfield, Ill.: Thomas.

Robe, E., Brumlik, F., and Moore, P. 1960. A study of spastic dysphonia: neurologic and electroencephalographic abnormalities. *Laryngoscope*, 70, 219–245.

———, Moore, P., Andrews, A., Jr., and Holinger, P. 1956. A study of the role of certain factors in the development of speech after laryngectomy: 1. type of operation; 2. site of pseudoglottis; 3. coordination of speech with respiration. *Laryngoscope*, 66, 173–186; 382–401; 481–499.

Rubin, H., and Lehroff, I. 1962. Pathogenesis and treatment of vocal nodules. *J. Speech Hearing Disorders*, 27, 150–161.

Senturia, B., and Wilson, F. 1968. Otorhinolaryngic findings in children with voice deviations. *Ann. Otol., Rhinol., Laryng.*, 77, 1027–1042.

Snidecor, J. 1962. Speech rehabilitation of the laryngectomized. Springfield, Ill.: Thomas.

Sound Production in Man. 1968. (Collection of papers presented in a conference under the same title.) Krause, M., Editor-in-Chief and Bouhuys, A., Consulting Editor and Conference Chairman. *Ann. N.Y. Acad. Sci.*, 155, 1–381.

Van Riper, C. 1963. Speech correction: principles and methods (4th. ed.). Englewood Cliffs, N.J.: Prentice-Hall.

———, and Irwin, J. 1958. Voice and articulation. Englewood Cliffs, N.J.: Prentice-Hall.

von Leden, H., and Moore, P. 1960. Contact ulcer of the larynx: experimental observations. *Arch. Otolaryng.*, 72, 746–752.

Wilson, K. 1961. Children with vocal nodules. *J. Speech Hearing Disorders*, 26, 19–26.

———. 1962. Voice reeducation of adolescents with vocal nodules. *Arch. Otolaryng.*, 76, 68–73.

22

Speech Without a Larynx

John C. Snidecor

HISTORICAL PERSPECTIVES

Man has suffered from cancer of the larynx and other laryngeal disorders and injuries since ancient times. Only until recently has there been real hope of surgical or medical palliation and cure. Tracheotomy, the first step towards laryngectomy, was performed by Antyllus (Wright, 1914) as early as 120 A.D., and thus the results of stoppage of the larynx could be at least temporarily relieved. However, the tracheal tube was not invented until our revolutionary war, and thus we must assume that even this relatively simple life-saving operation was not routinely performed until the third quarter of the eighteenth century.

The first great step in the knowledge of the living larynx was deferred until 1855, when Manuel Garcia published on the laryngoscope. Although only one of the independent discoverers of the laryngoscope, Garcia exploited and publicized the instrument and added much to our knowledge during his long and productive life. He died in 1906 at 102 years of age honored by laryngologists throughout the world.

Billroth (MacKensie, 1880) performed what was probably the first laryngectomy for cancer in 1872, although Watson had performed one a few years earlier for a syphilitic infection. Within six years of Billroth's operation, 19 laryngectomies had been performed, all but one or two only temporarily successful. By 1900 at least 200 laryngectomies had been performed and the rate of success had substantially increased.

Today, according to Ranney (1968), there are 3,000 surviving laryngectomees added each year to approximately 23,000 total laryngectomees alive in the United States. That cancer of the larynx is largely a male disease is supported by the fact that approximately 18,600 of these cases are men. Within the last 10 years, according to the National Cancer Institute, there has been a 75 percent increase in cancer of the larynx with, however, only a 42 percent increase in mortality. Currently, the total incidence is approximately four in 100,000 of the general population.

The result of increases in numbers of survivors plus the general increase in longevity of the population is obvious to those concerned with various aspects of rehabilitation following laryngectomy. More and more laryngectomees present themselves for speech therapy, and it is essential that improved procedures be developed so that the present success rate of 60–70 percent for esophageal speech learning be raised to a significantly higher figure. It is equally desirable to improve attitudes towards the artificial larynx so that those who cannot learn esophageal speech will learn to use and be accepted as users of this reasonable mode of communication.

SURGERY FOR TOTAL LARYNGECTOMY: THE STANDARD OPERATION AND THE ASAI LARYNGOPLASTY

What is the nature of modern total laryngectomy? In standard total laryngectomy the larynx is removed and, at times, the hyoid bone as well. When neck glands are involved, drastic resections may be performed on one or both sides of the neck. The primary and appropriate goal is preservation of life, while all other considerations must remain secondary.

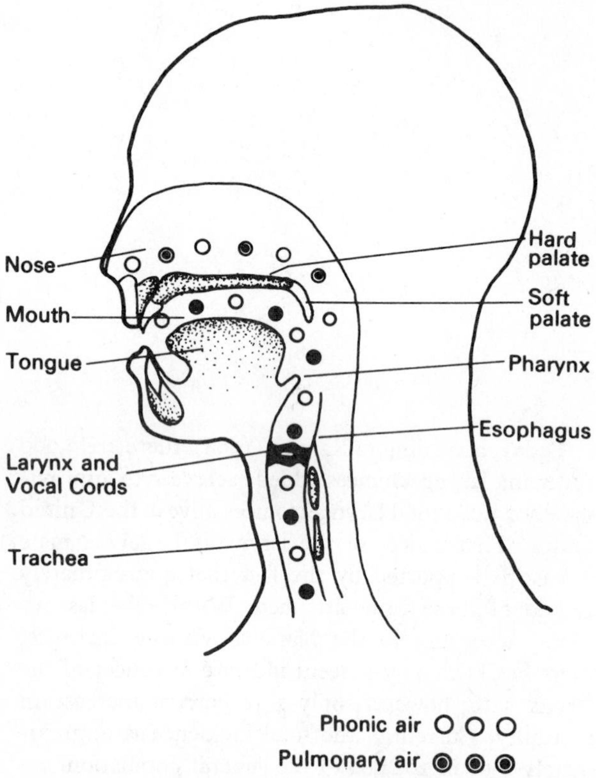

Fig. 22-1. Head and neck of a normal speaker. Pulmonary and phonic air follow the same path.

The general nature of the normal speech mechanism and the mechanism for esophageal speech is shown in Figs. 22-1 and 22-2. In normal speech, pulmonary and phonic air pass through the larynx with the vocal chords vibrating in a complex manner subject to the finest of physiological and neurological controls. In esophageal speech, pulmonary air must move in and out of the tracheal stoma, for there no longer remains an airpath between the mouth and the lungs. Phonic air for esophageal speech is physiologically sucked, pumped, or injected into the top of the esophagus, and when this air is forced upward the top of the esophagus vibrates and the resonators and articulators form this acoustic energy into speech. The vibrator, as might be expected, is relatively crude and not subject to the delicate control systems common to normal speech. Fig. 22-3 illustrates the simple sphincterlike vibrator under consideration. The above description suffers from oversimplification, a fact which will be corrected in part by further discussion.

Because of the great variety in operations necessitated by the location and extent of cancer, one might assume that the nature of the operation would condition substantially the effectiveness of esophageal speech. Robe et al. (1956) have shown that, within broad limits, the nature of the standard operation has little influence on the effectiveness of speech. One of this writer's most effective speakers has had two operations and, *in toto* has lost his larynx, a small portion of the esophagus, and has a neck resection on each side. He lost his esophageal voice after the second and most involved operation and had to learn speech all over again. He now speaks effectively and serves as an adjunct interviewing patients in the hospital, lecturing to students, and assisting in speech instruction for other laryngectomees.

A special and new type of total laryngectomy is

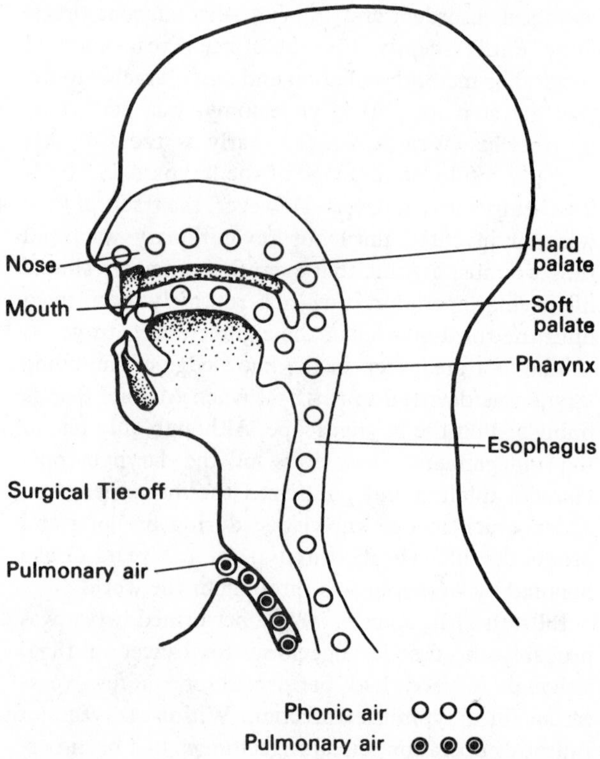

Fig. 22-2. Head and neck after standard laryngectomy. Pulmonary air passes in and out of the tracheal stoma. Phonic air passes from the esophagus into the hypopharynx, mouth, and nose.

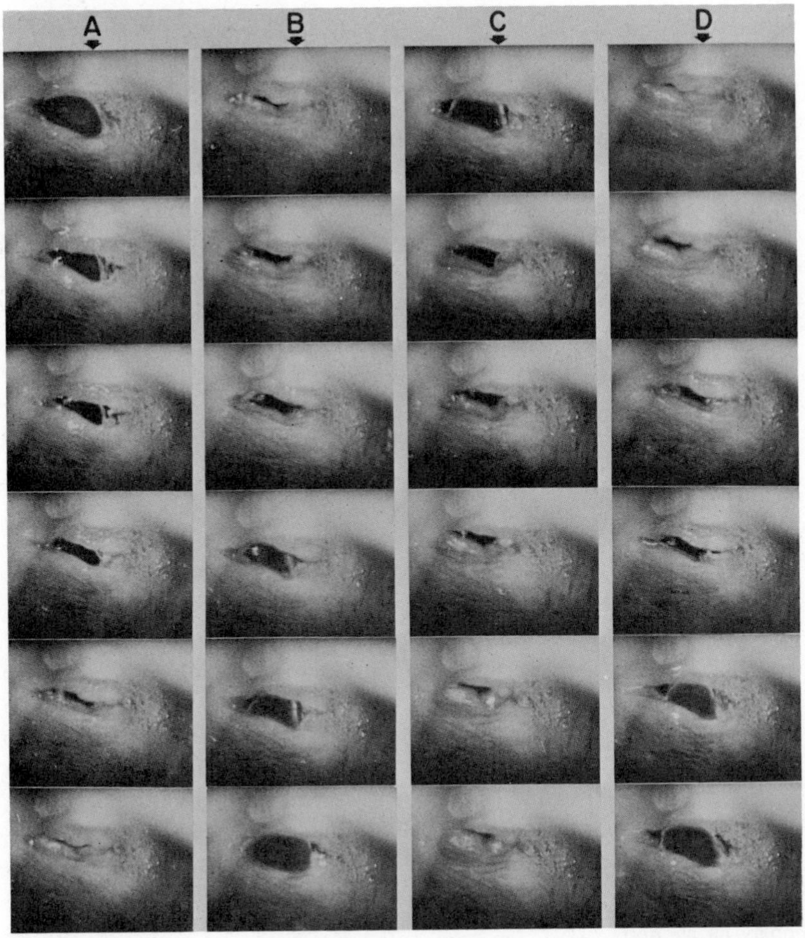

Fig. 22-3. Ultra-high-speed motion pictures of the top of the esophagus during esophageal speech. Note bubbles of mucus at the top of the pseudoglottis. The tone is "burbly" and rough. *Courtesy of Henry J. Rubin, M.D.*

pictured in Fig. 22-4 with considerable exaggeration of the size of the air passages so that they may be seen easily in the sketch. The laryngoplasty operation is usually called the Asai operation after Dr. Ryoso Asai of Kobe University Medical School (Japan) who originated the operation. In this three-stage operation, a dermal tube is formed which leads into the top of the tracheal stoma. Extending from this point upward the tube follows the midline of the neck and turns inward directly below the base of the tongue and ends in the hypopharynx. At either the point of turning or opening into the pharynx, the tube vibrates much as does the top of the esophagus in esophageal speech. To generate a power source, a finger or thumb is placed over the tracheal stoma and air is forced upward to vibrate the neoglottis. Special metal valves have been devised so that quiet normal breathing is possible, and then with greater force, the valve closes and speech is possible without use of fingers or thumb. Such valves pose problems that are not yet altogether solved. The great advantage of the Asai operation is that speech can be initiated once the third stage of the operation is completed. This writer has observed phonation when the patient was still on the operating table. A study by Snidecor, Isshiki, and Kimura (1968) indicates that speech after laryngoplasty can be rapid, well phrased, and loud with a hoarse-breathy quality present. The major advantage of "Asai speech" is that it is supported by pulmonary air which has already been thoroughly conditioned to the speech act rather than by any special superiority of the vibrator itself. A certain clumsiness in swallowing liquids, especially for those who salivate copiously, is an inherent aftermath of the operation, for liquids can move down the tube just as air moves up the tube. If the edge of the hand is held under the chin, difficulty in the act of swallowing is minimized. If the surgeon turns the tube downward as it enters the hypopharynx, infiltration of liquids is minimized. The writer has observed speakers who used the index

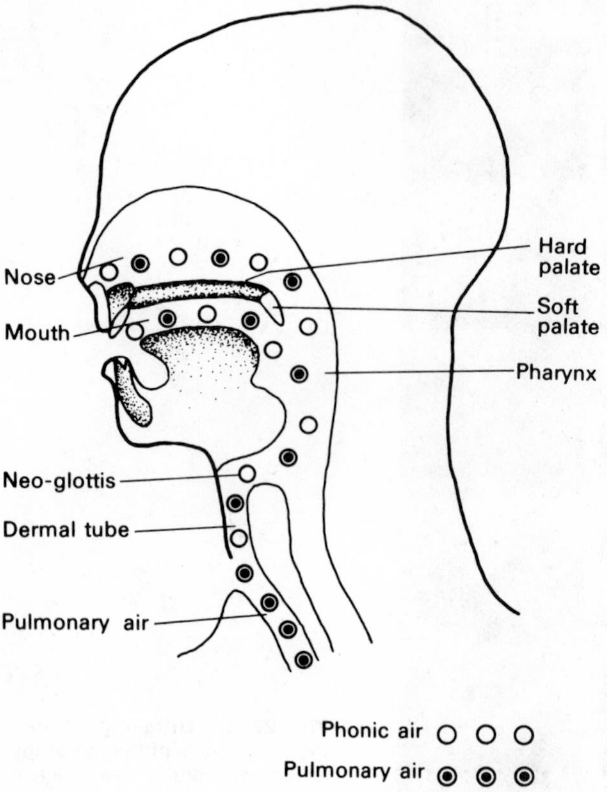

Fig. 22-4. Head and neck after the Asai laryngectomy and laryngoplasty operation. In normal breathing, pulmonary air flows in and out of the tracheal stoma. In speech, the stoma is closed, and pulmonary air supports phonation. The size of the dermal tube and the vibrating passage under the tongue is exaggerated.

finger and thumb to manipulate the flesh surrounding the vibrator, thus controlling both pitch and loudness.

Perhaps the most dramatic example of the Asai operation performed in the United States was the operation on Cpl. Walter Lopata which was reported in *Newsweek* magazine, January 23, 1967. Lopata had lost his larynx as a result of grenade fragments which tore the larynx away and had fractured his left leg. Dr. William W. Montgomery of the Massachusetts Eye and Ear Infirmary in Boston and Lt. Comdr. Robert Toohill operated on Lopata with a basic Asai operation.

This writer has a recording of Lopata's voice shortly after the operation and again several weeks later. In the first recording the voice is intelligible but not well modulated. In the second recording a rate of 211 words per minute can be maintained, and the voice is well modulated. Because Lopata's rate of speech is too rapid, it should be reduced, but he is obviously and technically an efficient speaker. The pitch level is somewhat above that of the average male. The voice is breathy but requires no more breaths for a 55-word reading passage than does the normal speaker.

Several practitioners are performing the Asai operation in the United States, but no one contacted by the writer believes that laryngoplasty will completely supersede standard laryngectomy. Nearly 100 Asai operations have been performed in Japan, 70 of these by Professor Asai himself. Compulsory health insurance in Japan minimizes the relative out-of-pocket costs for the series of three operations and resultant extended hospitalization.

DANGER SIGNALS

Speech pathologists are aware, and should make their clients aware, of the danger signals of laryngeal cancer which the American Cancer Society states should be heeded and for which medical attention should be sought if one or more signals persist for more than two weeks. Among these danger signs are: hoarseness, difficulty in swallowing, bleeding, coughing, and soreness. These signals *need not be accompanied by pain.* A famous surgeon recently stated, "all laryngectomies would be subtotals if the cancer could always be detected early enough."

There is no single cause of laryngeal cancer, but heavy smoking is the most important contributing factor according to the American Cancer Society. Excessive talking and drinking may well be additional causes.

HOW EFFECTIVE CAN ESOPHAGEAL SPEECH BE?

Because esophageal speech is and will be the usual means of communication for laryngectomees, it will be profitable to look at the performance of superior and average speakers.

One of the most effective speakers ever subjected to detailed study is M.W., who performed many detailed vocal tasks for a study by Snidecor and Isshiki (1965). In terms of age, physique, and personality, M.W. presented high potentials for esophageal speech. At 52 years of age he was slim and wiry, a successful businessman, and an aviator by hobby. M.W. was generous and outgoing, giving unlimited time to the experiment.

In brief summary: 1. M.W. speaks rapidly for an esophageal speaker. He can sustain speech at 153 words per minute which is in the lower limits of satisfactory rate as defined by Franke (1939). 2. This speaker both "inhales" and injects and can count to 14 (19 syllables) without any reversal of air flow, using as much as 615 cc of air at a rate of 98 cc/sec. This is an "athletic" performance utilizing air volume over seven times the capacity of the esophagus. Normally, M.W. uses short, yet effective phrases. 3. Intensity levels of /ɑ/ were 85 dB contrasted with 95 dB for a normal speaker under identical conditions. Although loudness is satisfactory, the nature of the vibrator limits dynamic range and the intensity profile is "rough." Generally speaking, pitch and intensity are related, as in normal speech. 4. Pitch level was low (70 Hz) and almost one full octave in range. 5. In terms of quality (waveform), harmonic elements were clear and distinguishable from each other even though the voice contained a noise component up to 6,000 Hz. 6. M.W.'s mean flow rate of esophageal air during sustained phonation of the vowel /ɑ/ ranged from 20 to 100 cc/sec, depending on the intensity of the voice. The mean flow rate for easy phonation was 72 cc/sec, a figure substantially lower than that for normal speakers. 7. During the period of reading the "Rainbow Passage," he produced voice almost entirely (97 percent of the time) synchronously with exhalation. 8. Most of the air (76 percent) was insufflated into the esophagus synchronously with the inhalatory movement of the thorax. Fig. 22-5, from Robe, illustrates full air intake for a superior speaker.

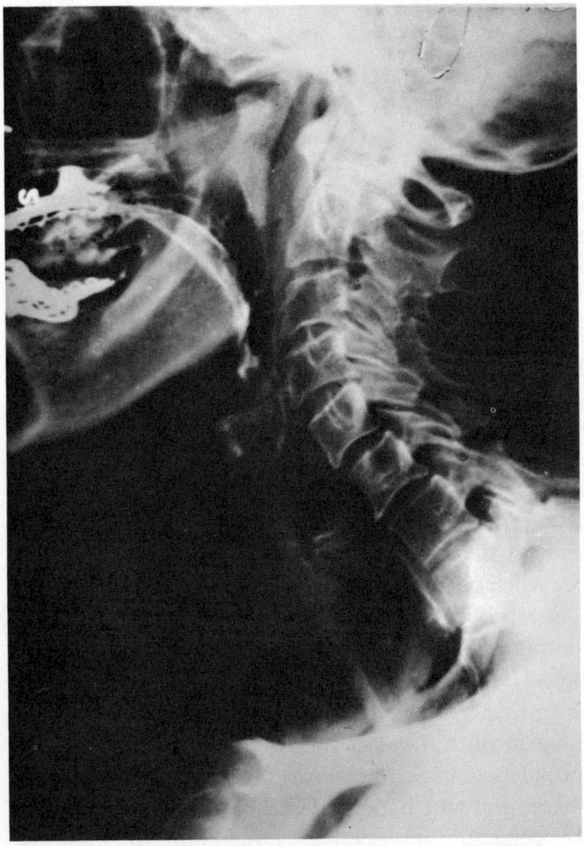

Fig. 22-5. X-ray photograph of a superior speaker following maximum intake of air. The vibrator is probably at the level of the fifth and sixth cervical vertebra. *From Robe.*

M.W. has been seen regularly for four years. Once dominantly an "inhaler," he now uses injection as much as inhalation. The only difference in vocal efficiency noted is increased loudness, and this has resulted in part by the need to communicate from an airplane to the ground, and to pilots who are in the plane and under instruction. For loud, brief bursts of speech, M.W. either "inhales" or uses three rapid injections prior to phonation.

Few can obtain M.W.'s performance levels, but his generally effective performance may serve as a goal for speech therapists when individuals of high potential present themselves for therapy.

The average esophageal speaker who can use his speech in day-to-day situations differs from M.W. as follows: 1. He can speak from 85–120 words per minute, which will be judged as very slow. 2. He will also use a combination of methods for air intake but will encompass only three to four syllables, which is a sufficient number providing air intake is rapid. Average flow rate will be about one-third that of the normal speaker and substantially less than M.W.'s, and it will be broken into smaller units. 3. Intensity levels will be lower but sufficient for an audience of 25 people under quiet conditions. In general, public address systems should be used for larger audiences or where ambient noise prevails. M.W. was able to use a microphone to talk from his airplane to the ground, a task beyond the limits of most esophageal speakers. 4. Pitch level will be comparable to M.W.'s i.e., 70 Hz or slightly lower. 5. In terms of voice quality the average speaker will have more noise components than M.W. Vowels will not be as clear, perhaps a result of less effective air support.

THE PROBLEMS OF MOST LARYNGECTOMEES ARE COMPLEX

The nature of the laryngectomy operation, the usual age of the patient, and other physiological and psychological factors present problems which are diverse and complex.

The laryngectomee first of all brings to the speech pathologist a difficult, yet essential task of speech rehabilitation. Speech completely lost, when once relearned, bridges again the gap between the person and the spouse, other family members, the employer, and the general social and economic world of which he had been a part. In other words, *the skill of speech is adjustive*. Effective speech alone will do much to readjust the laryngectomee to the complex world he lost when he lost his voice.

Second, few if any speech problems are so complicated by concomitant physical and psychological factors as is the acquisition of effective esophageal speech. Speech with the artificial larynx and subsequent to the Asai operation are, to some extent, special cases in point and will be discussed separately. Pharyngeal and buccal speech are rarely heard, and are generally undesirable. Discussion of these is purposefully excluded.

Diedrich and Youngstrom (1966) have pointed out that there are physical factors which, though under the supervision of the surgeon or other physician, must nevertheless be taken into account by the speech pathologist. Some of these are: postoperative complications such as innervation problems; limitations in the esophagus resulting from extensive surgery; upper respiratory problems; and spasms of the hypopharynx. Unrelated to the operation but of importance are such factors as: general senility; hearing loss; lack of teeth or dentures that are unsatisfactory; arthritis; colostomy; aerophagia; edema of the hypopharynx; and asthma.

Directly within the province of the speech pathologist are those environmental and psychological factors which impinge upon the man or woman who has lost a larynx as a result of cancer, an automobile accident, shotgun wound, or war injury.

Travis, in lectures given as early as 1937, made the point that psychological illnesses are generally accompanied by physical correlatives, and, conversely, physiological problems have their psychological concomitants. Two questions then arise: 1. Are there psychological patterns that were present before the operation; and 2. are there feelings and attitudes which limit or accelerate learning esophageal speech subsequent to excision of the larynx?

In answer to the first question, Webb and Irving (1964) in a lengthy study of 77 male laryngectomees using, in the main, Szondian procedures, concluded that: 1. Most of the laryngectomees manifested the oral triad of excessive speaking, drinking, and smoking; and 2. there were other signs of instability and adjustmental difficulty leading in the direction of asociality (Woltisbuel Index) rather than in the direction of neuroticism. Research in progress by Blake (1968), utilizing methods more precise than Szondian, supports in general the view of Webb and Irving. Webb and Irving (1964) believe that if there is postoperative shock, it is no greater than that which occurs after any other major operation.

Snidecor (1962) and others take a contrary position and believe that psychological and environmental factors are very important indeed. Although seldom do all the factors stated below apply to any one person, nevertheless, multiple psychological limiters are usually present. 1. Diedrich and Youngstrom (1966) state that because of the operation the patient has suffered amputation and resultant deformation. The deformation is far more subtle than, for example, the loss of a leg or arm. 2. The patient suffers shock and subsequent depression not only because of his amputation but also because of fears which include a) fear of recurring cancer; b) fear of permanent loss of voice; c) fear of old age; d) fear that he cannot reestablish previously valued social and sexual relationships; and e) fear of loss of job or of being unable to find a new job. It should be noted that fear tightens and closes the esophagus as confidence and relaxation open it. Heaver (1962) has indicated the presence of a generalized sense of futility for the above and other reasons. 3. Auxiliary functions of the larynx, and of mouth and nose breathing, are lost or substantially changed. It is no longer possible to laugh or cry audibly, and this proves a severe secondary handicap to those who had reputations for gaiety and those who need the catharsis of tears. The men seem more affected in the first instance, and the women in the second. Smell and perceptually related taste are limited, and this has proven to have important impact on professional cooks and housewives who enjoy cooking. Glossopharyngeal press and release can be learned, which will bring back partial stimulation of olfaction.

The tracheal stoma itself may limit previous behavior. For example, cosmetic liabilities apply to both men and women and must be adjusted to; these include special devices to cover the stoma such as high collars, bibs, scarves, and special jewelry (see Fig. 22-6). Coughing and wheezing often occur as a result of taking cold, dry, and contaminated air directly into the trachea. Under conditions of dust and noxious fumes, special filters must be used. Gardner (1964) has presented information on special filters in detail. Hobbies such as swimming, fishing, and very strenuous sports are lost or limited. However, one client remarked that his golf game had improved because he could no longer lift his head quickly and thus had to keep his eye on the ball.

More important, as a rule, are problems of general adjustment that often represent areas of special sensitivity that become out of proportion subsequent to laryngectomy. Some patients, even when relatively successful in learning a new voice, refuse to use it. Many of these individuals were marginal communicators prior to the operation and find limitations of rate, pitch, and quality more than they can adjust to. Individuals who have been independent shift to dependency and slowly or never traverse the road back to their former position in their family and social group. In this category of the maladjusted, one finds especially the woman whose children have grown and left home, and the man who has recently retired and no longer feels the need to be competitive. One who has lived alone prior to laryngectomy will be even more likely to live alone subsequent to the operation. To all of these individuals essential activities must be planned and carried out. Visits with friends, participation in social clubs, Lost Chord Clubs, and other organizations are examples of activities that bring the individual "back to life."

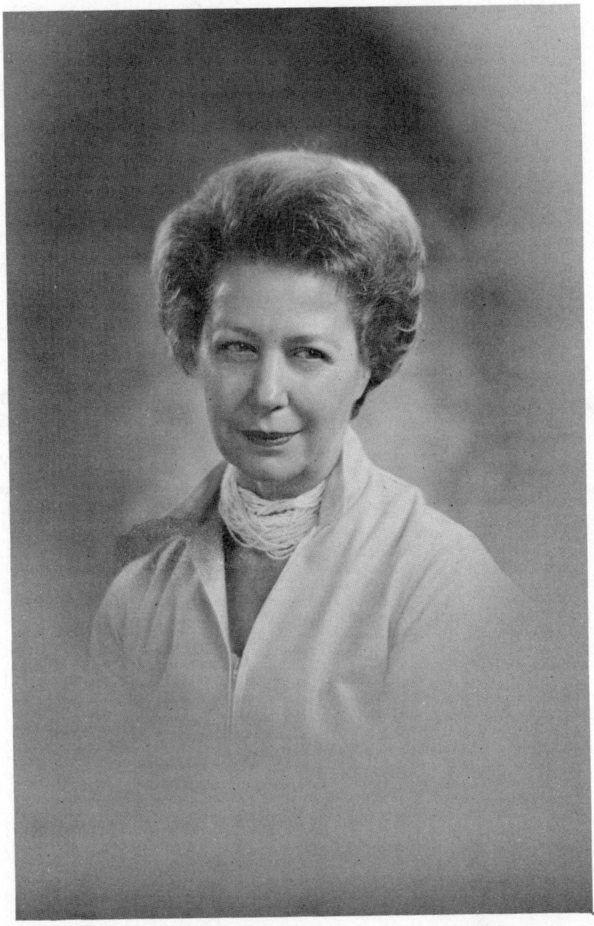

Fig. 22-6. A well-chosen necklace covers the tracheal stoma in addition to accenting the costume. *Photo by Brooks, Bethesda, Md.*

Fear of job loss or downgrading of economic position become obsessions with feelings of inadequacy prevailing even when professional and vocational efficiency remain high. Thoughtful counseling will often make the difference between vocational adequacy and utter failure. One client of the writer's held a position in which he found it necessary to take orders over the telephone, but he could no longer be understood by those who called. Practice in the use of the telephone enabled him to continue work in the same job he had held for 15 years.

SPECIAL PROBLEMS OF WOMEN

In addition to the problems encountered by both sexes, are those special problems of women (Gardner, 1966). The special problems of 240 women laryngectomees were given definitive study in 1966 by Gardner with certain differences obtained between men and women. First, women react with more despondency than do men when threatened with removal of the larynx. Three-fourths of the women were married at the time of surgery, and more than three-fourths of these married women were bolstered by the presence of their husbands when the report of cancer was given. The picture is not completely pleasant because two husbands asked for a divorce; one said his business relations would be jeopardized. The total picture, however, favors the married women in regard to support, sympathy, and the ability to face the operation. Directly before the operation, women wished to be counseled by female laryngectomees and, when they were not available, they preferred to write to a female laryngectomee rather than to talk with a male laryngectomee. Of course, counsel from the surgeon is necessary and desirable. Sixty percent of the women were shocked at their appearance and several fainted.

Upon returning home, 46 percent of reporting wives stated their husbands avoided them, pitied them, or babied them too much. Fifty-four percent wrote about the loyalty of their husbands and their display of optimism and confidence.

Specific to speech, the subjects were somewhat embarrassed at the low pitch and rather coarse quality of esophageal speech. More married women accepted esophageal speech than did unmarried women. Eighty-two percent of those with a favorable reaction to speech succeeded whereas only 64 percent of those with unfavorable reactions succeeded. Two-thirds of the wives were assisted in speech by their husbands, by such acts as taking them to speech classes and bringing visitors to the home. It proved a common complaint that esophageal speech was not easily understood. This, in some cases, was due to the fact that spouses were at an age where hearing had been lost.

Women insisted that laryngectomees should be taught by trained teachers. They noted that determination was essential in learning, and affection and confidence important. The importance of motivation and self-discipline was stressed. One woman worked hard to give her sons and grandchildren her new voice as a Christmas present. One woman wisely identified herself over the telephone so that she would not be called "Sir." Effective speakers emphasized that women should return to work as soon as possible and speech would improve thereby. More than half of the women returned to work after surgery. Successful job holders advised others to: "1. dress neatly; 2. cover the stoma with an attractive scarf, bib, or lacy material; 3. return to work as soon as possible; 4. with good speech there should be no employment problem." Gardner goes on to emphasize, as we do, the desirability of attending Lost Chord Clubs, and he further emphasizes the need for sympathy and realistic attitudes.

WHO IS YOUR TEACHER?

There has been considerable discussion in regard to who should be the teacher of the laryngectomized individual. The opinion of this writer is that the individual should be initially instructed by a speech pathologist. *Members of the American Speech and Hearing Association Available for Referral of Laryngectomees* is the title of a publication issued by the American Cancer Society in 1967. It may be obtained either from the IAL or the American Speech and Hearing Association. Speech pathologists will normally enter into the teaching situation without prejudice concerning the way in which the individual should inject and use air. It is also to be noted that the speech pathologist will, in all probability, have psychological training so that he may counsel with both the laryngectomized individual and family members. He also may be in a favorable position of going "to bat" for the laryngectomee with his employer. The nature of the operation can be explained to the employer and it can be noted that speech, if once established, will gradually become more fluent and intelligible. Emphasis can be given to the fact that the individual remains physically and intellectually capable, and that he may even be more motivated than he had been in the past. The assistance of laryngectomees is essential to effective instruction. A surgeon with whom this writer works desires that a laryngectomized individual who is a good speaker, visit an individual prior to his operation. On occasion he has asked that I do the same thing. Once speech is even partially established, association and communication with other laryngectomees is essential to the training program. However, it is important to initiate phonation and develop a pattern of speech prior to the client's close and continuous contact with another esophageal speaker. With good luck this may only take a week or two. When at least a temporary speech pattern is established, the new esophageal speaker should contact individuals who will be compatible with him or her for reasons aside from their mutual problem. A New Voice Club or Lost Chord Club may be just what the individual needs if such a club is available. However, it must be remembered that outside of metropolitan areas there may be too few esophageal speakers to make practical the organization of group instruction, whether formal or informal.

THE FIRST CONTACT IS IMPORTANT

In the first formal contact with the new laryngectomee, it is good to set up three appointments on one day. These appointments are usually set up at a morning hour, say 9:00, 11:00, and 3:00 or 4:00 in the afternoon. The establishment of three appointments in one day is of substantial importance in our local situation because a number of our clients must travel a considerable distance. Perhaps even more important than this convenience factor is the advantage that comes from initiating phonation in the first day of contact with the teacher. If the client initiates phonation during the first meeting, he is dismissed with practice exercises, and the same holds true for the second meeting. Usually, but not always, some phonation is generated by the end of the third meeting on the first day. It would be unwise to overemphasize the desirability of phonation on the first day, but to gain phonation constitutes a satisfying experience on the part of both the client and the teacher. This morale in turn is transferred to members of the family if the laryngectomee can go home and say even a simple word or two. Daily or triweekly appointments are deemed essential until basic speech habits are established. This period may last from a few days to several weeks.

Preferably before, or, if necessary, during the first meeting, background materials are gathered. The brief but usable case study outline (Table 22-I) developed by Knepflar (Snidecor, 1962) is stated below. It will be noted that the digits in each line represent the number of lines needed for filling in information.

TABLE 22-I

Speech Therapy Evaluation Form for Laryngectomized Patients

K. J. Knepflar

Name...................... Age.... Date ......
Address........................... Phone .....
Source of Referral ....

1. Operative Factors
   - Date(s) of surgery (1)
   - Extent of surgery (3)
   - Post operative complications (2)
   - Irradiation (2)
2. Physical Factors
   - General physical condition (2)
   - Spread of cancer (2)
   - Upper respiratory conditions (2)
   - Other physical factors (3)
3. Geriatric Factors (4)
4. Auditory Factors
   - Audiometric results (3)
   - Comments (3)
5. Emotional Factors
   - Depression (1)
   - Motivation (2)
   - Degree of dependency (1)
   - Acceptance of esophageal speech (2)
   - Other personality traits or problems (2)
6. Social Factors
   - Educational background (1)
   - Cultural background (1)
   - Patient's sociability (2)
   - Family attitudes (3)
   - Vocational aspects (1)
7. Intellectual Factors (3)
8. Articulation Factors
   - Motor factors (1)
   - Dental factors (1)
   - Accuracy of articulation (2)
   - Foreign accent (2)
9. Language Factors
   - Language comprehension (3)
   - Language usage (3)

Summary of pertinent factors (3)
Apparent prognosis (2)
Recommendations (4)

METHODOLOGY

There are many procedures for teaching the client to get air as quickly as possible. Of course, the first effort is limited simply to the process of getting some air into the esophagus and then releasing it. Gardner (1962) has the patient whistle and follow with a /t/. It is this writer's interpretation that this may help to inject air by the so-called plosive method. Berlin at times uses an inflated balloon, the contents of which are injected into the esophagus provided, of course, the patient can relax the top of the esophagus sufficiently to let the air go in. Diedrich and Youngstrom (1966) have recommended the sniff-inject-pah method: air is brought in through the nose and is then injected by tongue-pumping action facilitated by the previous plosive. Snidecor (1962) uses a method which is especially useful with the extroverted male. The individual is asked to imagine that he has finished a full meal and that he has some gas on his stomach. One can go into detail here and have the meal finished perhaps with mince pie, etc. It is explained to him that when a person desires to burp or belch that air is taken rather forcibly into the top of the esophagus and then injected with whatever gas or air that may be in the stomach. This will sometimes bring vocalization on the first or second trial. It should be immediately noted that there is no assumption that the individual will continue to talk by this method, or at least not by this method alone; it is simply to demonstrate to him that he can insufflate air into the top of the esophagus and use it for the purpose of phonation. It is most encouraging to get phonation by any method whatsoever as soon as possible. At a later time other methods may be used, and obviously refinements will develop gradually. One speaker, who was a client of the writer, went home and used his son's bicycle pump for the purpose of injecting air into the top of the esophagus. He held his nose and pumped a good-size bubble of air into the top of the esophagus which gave him the "feel" of the process. Before long he was not dependent upon the bicycle pump. For several reasons this method is not recommended for general use, nor is the use of a catheter for air injection.

Where to begin and how? The writer favors, as a starter, the Diedrich and Youngstrom sniff-inject-pah concept. "Sniff" gets air in the mouth, "inject" makes use of the tongue as an injector pump (see Fig. 22-7), and /p/ takes advantage of possible use of plosive "backfire" for air injection. Sniff-inject-pah may and should become one continuous movement.

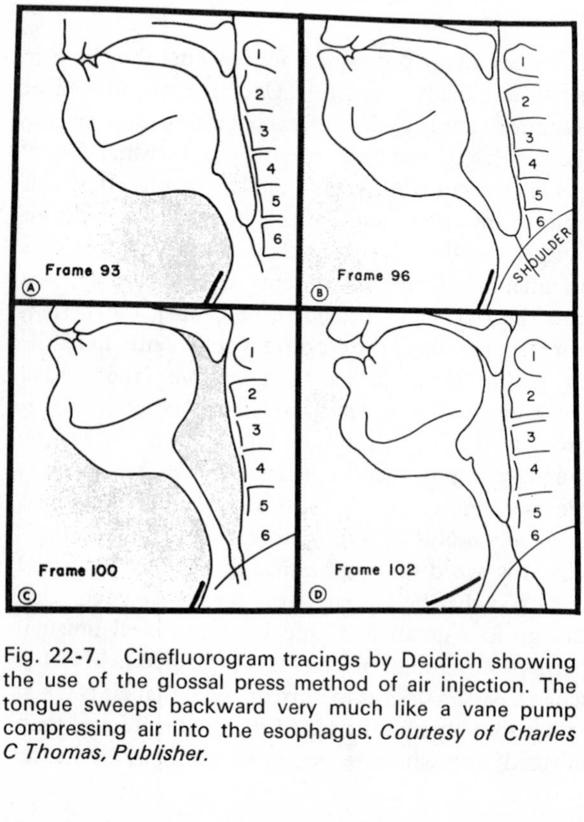

Fig. 22-7. Cinefluorogram tracings by Deidrich showing the use of the glossal press method of air injection. The tongue sweeps backward very much like a vane pump compressing air into the esophagus. *Courtesy of Charles C Thomas, Publisher.*

If this method fails, air injection can sometimes be started by having the client take a small amount of liquid on the front of the tongue and inject it down into the esophagus. The liquid need not be carbonated and should not be sweet. The client will be inclined to use the term "swallow" but it is desirable to use the word "inject" from the first. Shipp et al. (1967), have shown by electromyographic techniques that the acts of swallowing and injecting are not analogous. As we have mentioned, for the strong extroverted male the "forced belch" method is often a good starter. A 52-year-old operator of heavy road machinery was able to speak in short bursts of crude speech within one hour of initiating therapy. He later developed smooth inhalation, always with the mouth open, sure proof that he was an "inhaler" (see Fig. 22-8). Later this client added injection to his repertoire. Plosive injection, by itself, may be tried and may be useful for those who are old or weak. The

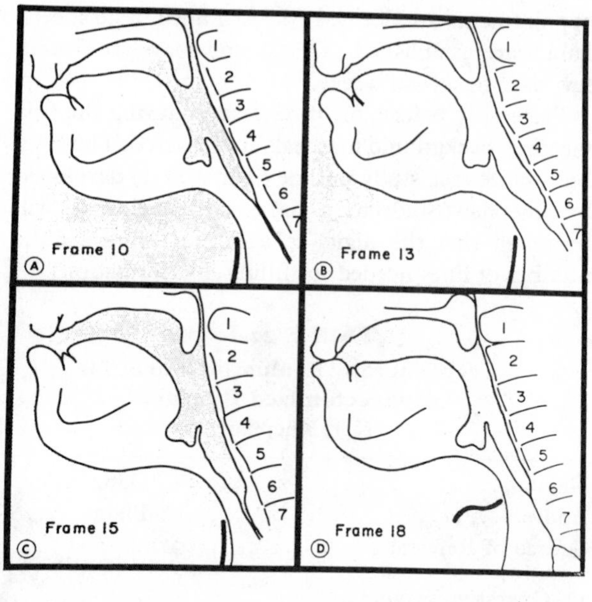

Fig. 22-8. Cinefluorogram tracings by Deidrich showing the use of the inhalation method. Note that during the insufflation of air the subject's mouth remains open, sure proof that injection was *not* utilized. *Courtesy of Charles C Thomas, Publisher.*

taking of air by mouth compression, which is the essence of the plosive method, is simple to learn but seldom supplies sufficient air for easy speech. In this method the tongue is relaxed in the floor of the mouth, the neck muscles are relaxed, the cheeks are puffed out as if for a loud /p/ and the air pushed down into the esophagus. At the beginning it may be necessary to hold the nose. A microphone placed just below the locus of the thyroid cartilage will pick up the noise of air moving down into the esophagus as it will for taking air by other methods. Most normal speakers can easily inflate the esophagus and stomach with this method. Unless released at once, much of the air will soon go out through the intestinal tract often accompanied by stomach rumble. This suggests that one abstain from practice before formal dinner parties. Of course, all clients should be counseled concerning flatulence, which is to be expected in early practice. It is some relief to know that swallowed air does not have the noxious qualities of intestinal gas.

From the very first, quick air intake should be taught. Damsté (1958), Snidecor and Curry (1959), Diedrich (1966), and others have shown that air injection can occur in less than half a second with that figure as an approximate average for good speakers. The act of insufflation on demand must be taught in a relaxed yet motivated situation.

Phonation must follow immediately upon intake. To teach a quick, easy, yet even brief phonation, is better than to demand initially loud and long phonations which will often be accompanied by struggle. Cooper (1967) has pointed out the desirability of stressing good quality from the very first. His concern for quality is supported by Nichols (1968), who has carefully pointed out the acoustic rationale for practice of clear vowel articulation. It is obvious that good consonant articulation also adds to intelligibility. If and when phonation extends to one and a half to two and a half seconds, as Berlin (1963) has pointed out, the prognosis for success can be made, assuming, of course, that intake has been relatively quick. If extended phonation has been achieved and diminishes in length, the client should be sent at once to his surgeon, for there is the possibility that cancerous growth is again present (Berlin and ZoBell, 1963).

It is important that the laryngectomee not whisper as his first method of speech communication, for to do so may develop bad habits of communication that are difficult to cancel. It is preferable, in our opinion, that the individual write rather than whisper until usable esophageal speech is learned or until an artificial larynx is used.

If the client can take air but it "poofs" out of the top of the esophagus without vibration, it may be possible to use the handkerchief trick to compress the throat and thus help to initiate vibration. The corners of the handkerchief are firmly pulled in opposite directions and as the throat is compressed, phonation may result (see Fig. 22-9). As speech progresses, it may be necessary to continue permanent neck pressure by fingers pressed against the front of the throat or by tight collars or elastic bands (Spandex). Throat compression retrieves a significant number of failures and should be tried when appropriate.

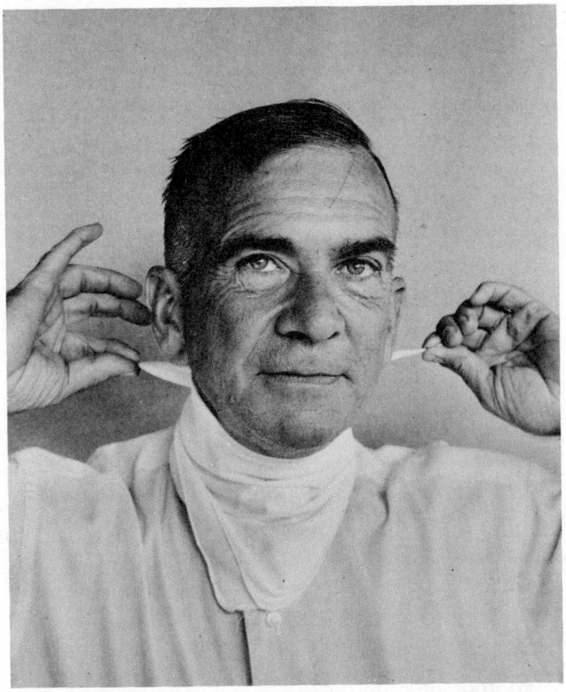

Fig. 22-9. The handkerchief test. Varying degrees of throat compression can be tried by the client to ascertain if speech can be initiated or improved with pressure.

The specific exercises given below do not imply that we take the "cookbook" approach to speech therapy. It will be noted, however, that principles stated above are incorporated in the drills. After speech is established one moves from one level to the other for practice. It is impossible to predict how long an individual will work at each level. In a motion picture, Diedrich has demonstrated a young woman who uses words and phrases in the first session of therapy. Snidecor elicited "Carpenteria," the man's home town, in the first meeting. On the other hand, we have a client who is, after three months, still working at levels three and four. There is no hard-and-fast line between levels.

Examples of exercises:

First Level: Stress speed of intake and relatively relaxed phonation. Good vowel quality should be taught from the beginning.

Sniff-inject-pah (one movement) sniff-inject-pah, etc.
/i/ /ɪ/ /e/ /ɛ/ /æ/ /ʌ/ /a/ /ɔ/ /o/ /ʊ/ /u/ /aɪ/ /aʊ/ /ɔi/

Each vowel and diphthong is linked with each plosive sound. Example s (niff) ɪ (inject) ba, ta, da, ka, ga. Then (s ɪ) bi, bɪ, beɪ, etc.

Later fricatives are linked with vowels and diphthong, e.g. (s ɪ) ʃi, ʃɪ, ʃeɪ, ʃɛ, etc.

If liquid is necessary, then liquid . . . inject . . . pah, etc.

Second Level: Prolong each vowel in the plosive vowel combination as long as possible. Time and record results. One and one-half to two seconds is very satisfactory. Three seconds is longer than necessary.

1. pah ....
2. bee ....
3. too ....
4. deh ....
5. kuh ....
6. go ....

Third Level: Repeat each syllable as many times as possible on one air charge. Record results and improve them. Three at a time is a good start. Ten to twelve is not impossible.

1. pay pay pay pay pay pay (etc.) ....
2. toot/toot/toot/toot/toot/ ....
   tootootootootootootootoot ....
3. calm calm calm calm calm ....
4. boy boy boy boy boy boy ....
5. gag/gag/gag/gag/gag/gag ....
   deedeedeedeedeedeedeedeed ....

Fourth Level: Strive to increase the number of syllables you can deal with on one air charge.

1. Put the paper plumes on the carpet.
2. Grab the bear cub and put him in the cab.
3. The teacher saw ten kittens today.
4. To dine on bread is better than to dine on candy.
5. The cook baked a cake and biscuits for the Christmas party.
6. My great big gray goose lays golden eggs.

Fifth Level: Increase the clarity of vowels and consonants with practice. Vowel quality is inherently difficult in esophageal speech, so shape the mouth precisely.

1. Bee keepers teach bees.
2. Big Bill caught the kingfish.
3. Ben put the keg on the deck.
4. (diphthong) Pay day is a great day.
5. Jack gave Dan the crabapple.
6. The pup and the duck loved the cook.
7. Bob and Tom caught John.
8. Crows cawed and caught hawks.
9. (diphthong) Joseph rode the polo pony.
10. The cook put the cookies on the book.
11. Bluegoose flew to school.

Sixth Level: This level calls for practice on articulation, stress, pitch, quality, loudness, and time in a conversational situation at first with guidance from the therapist. Note: In using the telephone the lower edge of the mouthpiece should touch the lower lip with the mouthpiece pointed upward, thus increasing intensity and shielding from stoma noise. Because of low pitch level, women should identify themselves on the phone, i.e., "This is Miss Jones calling Mr. Smith."

There is almost no end to gradual improvement. Experienced clinicians note improvement over a period of from two to four years.

During the whole process of therapy it should be remembered that most esophageal speakers will eventually combine two or more methods of speaking (Isshiki and Snidecor, 1964). Further, N. M. Bork (1967), in a recent cinefluorographic study of esophageal speakers, found sufficient differences in morphology from speaker to speaker to preclude any highly consistent use of the new speaking mechanism from speaker to speaker.

Within the program of teaching esophageal speech, emphasis on vowel and consonant articulation is appropriate. The crude vibrator in esophageal speech gives a low-pitched fundamental, low loudness level, considerable noise, and energies that shift into the higher partials. It follows that vowels must be articulated carefully. The unvoiced aspect of the consonants can be made with buccal air alone. For example, the final (t) in "bat" need not be supported by esophageal air.

THE ARTIFICIAL LARYNX

Inevitably, some individuals find it impossible to learn esophageal speech. For them the artificial larynx provides functional communication (see Fig. 22-10). Acceptance of this instrument must be increased in both the social and occupational milieu, otherwise 20–30 percent of laryngectomees must remain speechless. Further, we know of no evidence which proves that the availability of the artificial larynx limits the learning of esophageal speech. As a matter of fact, the reverse may be true. It is our current practice to have an artificial larynx on the table when the individual comes in for his first lesson.

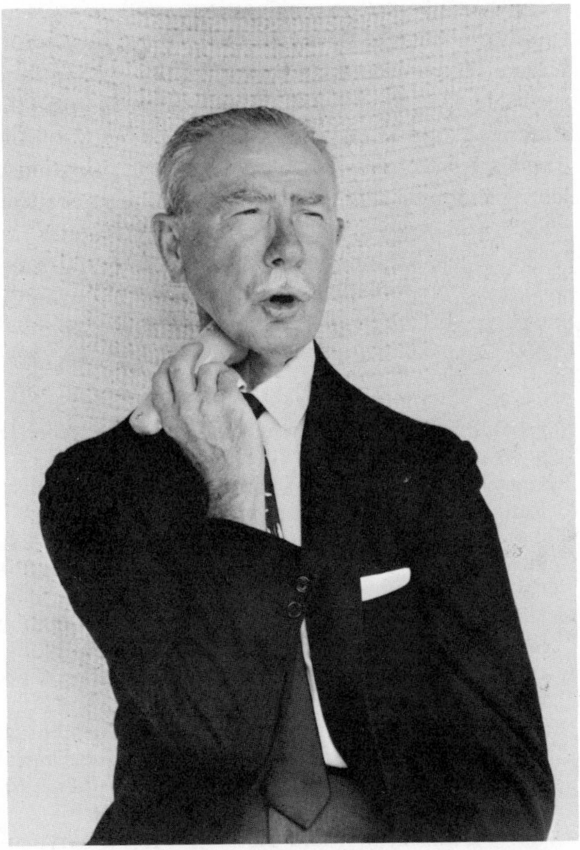

Fig. 22-10. A modern artificial larynx in use.

Sometime during the first lesson the instrument is discussed and demonstrated. It is pointed out that many people are carrying on relatively normal lives with the use of the instrument. It must be recalled that fear tightens the esophagus whereas relaxation opens it, and thus the presence of a speech aid may be conducive to a relaxed atmosphere, and may even assist in developing esophageal phonation. The artificial larynx is, all factors considered, a less effective and desirable vibrator than is the top of the esophagus, so here too instruction is essential in vowel and consonant articulation. Because of monotony in all of the parameters of tone, phrasing and other temporal factors become important for emphasis and intelligibility.

ASAI SPEECH

Speech therapy for Asai speech is yet to be evaluated. Speech after the third stage of the operation develops at once, then gradually improves for several weeks or months. This writer is of the opinion that the period of spontaneous improvement might be speeded by speech therapy. In those cases where manipulation of the dermal tube improves speech, the speech therapist can probably speed up the trial and error process.

AMPLIFIERS AND HEARING AIDS

Esophageal speakers, with very few exceptions, experience certain business, professional, or social social situations where they cannot be heard. For example, a sales manager must make reports to those at a large conference table; a college professor must lecture to a class of 30 or 40. There are several transistor-speaking-aid amplifiers on the market that can be carried in the pocket, placed on the desk (see Fig. 22-11), and utilized in such situations. For large audiences, it is of course more realistic to use a standard public address system. A client of the author's wired a good transistor radio in such a way that the radio was cut out of the system and the amplifier reacted only to the speaker's voice. It is a satisfactory and inexpensive aid to speech.

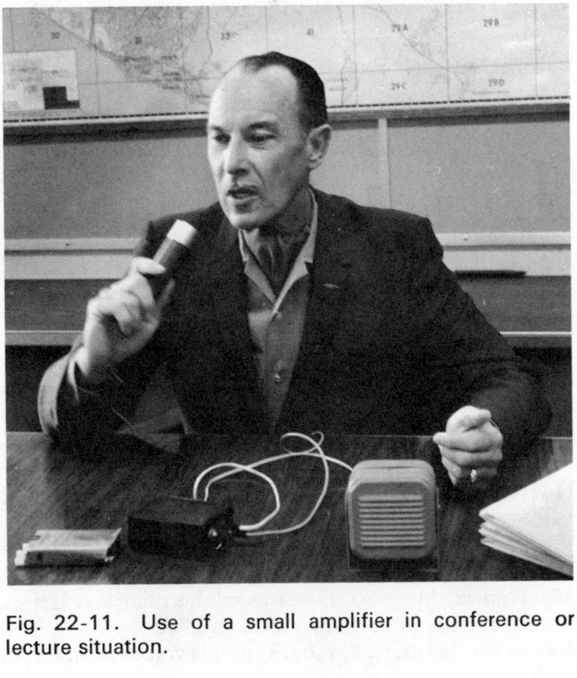

Fig. 22-11. Use of a small amplifier in conference or lecture situation.

THE INTERNATIONAL ASSOCIATION OF LARYNGECTOMEES

The cause of those with laryngeal cancer, which can be mentioned here only briefly, has been helped by many agencies and individuals. The social and educational sides of the problem have been attacked by IAL (International Association of Laryngectomees), an autonomous agency supported by the American Cancer Society since 1953. IAL was conceived by Warren H. Gardner, Ph.D., of the Cleveland Hearing and Speech Clinic in 1951, and was first made truly international in scope through the travels and efforts of Edmond C. Johnson, Lawrance Phelps, and others. The *IAL News* is a bimonthly periodical distributed without charge to over 18,000 persons in 55 countries. IAL, located at 219 East 42nd Street, New York, New York, 10017, keeps a directory up to date which includes clubs and their locations, and sources of supply for such aids as tracheal tubes, bibs, stoma screens, and amplifiers. Training manuals, films, and recordings are also listed. The local branch of the American Cancer Society will have a copy of the directory, which is a valuable source of information to laryngectomees and the professionals who serve them.

BIBLIOGRAPHY

American Speech and Hearing Association. 1964. Members of the American Speech and Hearing Association available for referral of laryngectomes.

Berlin, C. 1963. Clinical measurement of esophageal speech: I. methodology and curves of skill acquisition. *J. Speech Hearing Disorders*, 28, 42–51.

———, and ZoBell, D. 1963. Clinical measurements during the acquisition of esophageal speech: II. an unexpected dividend. *J. Speech Hearing Disorders*, 28, 389–392.

Blake, I. 1968. Personal communication.

Bork, N. 1967. A cinefluorographic study of four alaryngeal speakers. UCLA: Ph.D. dissertation.

Cooper, M. 1967. Personal communication.

Damsté, P. 1958. Oesophageal speech after laryngectomy. Groningen: Boekdrukkerij Vorheen Gebroeders Hoitsema.

Deidrich, W., and Youngstrom, K. 1966. Alaryngeal speech. Springfield, Ill.: Thomas.

Directory. 1967. The International Association of Laryngectomees, 219 East 42nd Street, New York, N.Y., 10017.

Franke, P. 1939. A preliminary study validating the measurement of oral reading rate in words per minute. Univ. Iowa: Master's thesis.

Gardner, W. 1962. The whistle technique in esophageal speech. *J. Speech Hearing Disorders*, 27, 187–188.

———. 1964. Laryngectomees (neck breathers) in industry. *Arch. Environmental Health*, 9, 777–789.

———. 1966. Adjustment problems of laryngectomized women. *Arch. Otolaryng.*, 83, 31–42.

Heaver, L., and Arnold, G. 1962. Rehabilitation of alaryngeal aphonia. *Post-grad. Med.*, 32, 11–17.

Isshiki, N., and Snidecor, J. 1964. Air intake and usage in esophageal speech. *Acta Otolaryng.*, 59, 559–574.

MacKensie, M. 1880. Diseases of the pharynx, larynx and trachea. New York: William Wood.

Newsweek, January 27, 1967. Find his voice again. P. 86.

Nichols, A. 1969. Quality and loudness. *In* Speech rehabilitation of the laryngectomized. Snidecor, J., and others. Springfield, Ill.: Thomas.

Ranney, J. 1968. Personal communication from Jack Ranney, Executive Secretary, IAL.

Robe, E., Moore, P., Andrews, A., and Hollinger, P. 1956. A study of the role of certain factors in the development of speech after laryngectomy: 1. type of operation. 2. site of pseudoglottis. 3. co-ordination of speech with respiration. *Laryngoscope*, 66, No. 3, 173–186 (Part 1); 66, No. 4, 382–401 (Part 2); 66, No. 5, 481–499 (Part 3).

Shipp, T. 1967. Frequency, duration, and perceptual measures in relation to judgments of alaryngeal speech acceptability. *J. Speech Hearing Res.*, 10, No. 3, 417–427.

———, Deatsch, W., and Ross, J. 1967. Pharyngoesophageal activity in laryngectomees. Nat'l Institute Neurological Disease and Blindness progress report.

Snidecor, J., and Curry, E. 1959. Temporal and pitch aspects of superior esophageal speech. *Ann. Otol., Rhinol., Laryng.*, 68, 1–14.

———, and others. 1962. Speech rehabilitation of the laryngectomized. Springfield, Ill.: Thomas.

———, and Isshiki, N. 1965. Vocal and air use characteristics of a superior male esophageal speaker. *Folia Phoniat.*, 17, 3, 217–232.

———, Isshiki, N., and Kimura, T. 1968. Speech after laryngoplasty (The Asai operation). Proceedings des Séances du. XIV Congrès de L.I.A.P. Paris.

Travis, L. 1937. Class Lectures in Clinical Psychology. Univ. Iowa.

Webb, M., and Irving, R. 1964. Psychologic and anamnestic patterns characteristic of laryngectomees; relation to speech rehabilitation. *J. Amer. Ger. Soc.*, 12, 303–322.

Wright, J. 1941. A history of laryngology and rhinogology. Philadelphia: Lea & Febiger.

23

Modern Techniques of Vocal Rehabilitation for Functional and Organic Dysphonias

Morton Cooper

INTRODUCTION

Vocal rehabilitation is the process of retraining a misused voice to alleviate or eliminate a dysphonia. Dysphonias may be generally classified as functional or organic. Functional dysphonia denotes the absence of an organic involvement of the vocal folds and indicates a misuse or abuse of the vocal folds within a normal laryngeal structure. The broad category of functional dysphonia includes hysterical aphonia and dysphonia, spastic dysphonia, falsetto, ventricular phonation, nasality, and a major grouping of functional vocal disorders (excluding the specific types mentioned above), generally known as functional dysphonia. Other terms for this last specific classification are hyperfunctional and hypofunctional dysphonia (Froeschels), executive dysphonia (Gardner), aggravated voice (Tarneaud), phonasthenia (Flateau), hyperkinesia and hypokinesia (Bloch), chronic, nonspecific laryngitis (Baker), and myasthenia laryngis (Jackson). The term used by this author is functional "misphonia," which literally means functional "wrong voice." This voice may also be alluded to as a "tired voice," a "hoarse voice," a "weak voice," with or without laryngeal and/or pharyngeal tensions.

Organic dysphonia indicates an organic or neurological origin for the dysphonia, such as growths on the vocal folds (nodules, polyps, contact ulcer, papillomata, and leukoplakia), laryngeal nerve paralysis or paresis, and partial excision of the vocal folds (partial or complete unilateral cordectomy).

Vocal rehabilitation as discussed in this chapter is directed primarily to the most frequent type of functional dysphonia—functional misphonia—and the most prevalent type of organic dysphonia—growths on the vocal folds (nodes, polyps, polypoid degeneration, and contact ulcer). Adaptations of vocal therapy for the less frequent types of functional dysphonias (falsetto, ventricular phonation, spastic dysphonia, nasality, and hysterical aphonia and dysphonia) and of organic dysphonias (papillomata, vocal fold paralysis, Parkinsonian, partial excision of the vocal folds, leukoplakia, and keratosis) will be included.

To define the three most common lesions producing organic dysphonia in terms of anatomical and physiological considerations, contact ulcer of the larynx is a unilateral or bilateral lesion, occurring at the posterior third of the vocal folds on the medial surfaces overlying the arytenoid cartilages and/or the vocal processes, resulting in a granuloma, an ulceration, or both. Nodes or polyps, which may be unilateral or bilateral, are usually located at the junction of the anterior and middle third of the vocal folds. Nodes are generally sessile; polyps may be either sessile or pedunculated. An early form of node may be referred to as a nodule; however, the terms node and nodule are often used interchangeably. Polypoid degeneration may vary from mild edema and thickening to extensive polypoid growths involving one or both vocal folds.

Over the past ten years, 1261 nonselective patients have been seen for vocal rehabilitation. This group includes 660 patients with functional dysphonia (486 functional misphonia, 33 falsetto, 11 ventricular phonation, 63 spastic dysphonia and incipient spastic dysphonia, 44 nasality, and 23 hysterical aphonia and dysphonia) and 601 with organic dysphonia (254 nodes, 68 polyps, 63 polypoid degeneration, 85 contact ulcer, 24 papillomata, 59 vocal fold paralysis, 14 Parkinsonian, 11 partial vocal-fold excisions, and 23 leukoplakia and keratosis). Where applicable throughout this chapter, appropriate findings from this group will be cited, using the results from functional misphonic patients (486) and organic dysphonic patients—nodes (254), polyps (68), polypoid degeneration (63), and contact ulcer (85). The results for this group of 956 patients, plus the remaining 305 patients discussed briefly at the end of the chapter, definitely justify direct vocal rehabilitation with vocal psychotherapy for the treatment of functional and organic dysphonias.

VOCAL MISUSE AND ABUSE

Direct vocal rehabilitation relieves and eliminates the causes and symptoms of vocal misuse and abuse. Vocal misuse is the use of an inappropriate pitch level and pitch range, tone focus, quality, volume, breath support, and possibly rate, either singly or in combinations. Vocal misuse is generally due to vocal confusion, poor vocal dynamics and usage, and a lack of correct vocal knowledge (Cooper, 1968). Vocal abuse occurs during, and as the result of, vocal misuse. As Loughlin (1920, p. 15) states: "Very few people speak correctly." Clerf (1952, p. 6) concludes: "I know of no organ or structure in the whole body that is more abused than the larynx."

Many individuals are totally unaware of good vocal dynamics, and once such good vocal production is brought to their attention, with practice, patience, and good meaningful vocal direction, they cooperate and improve. Most people do not use the vocal instrument as it can and should be utilized. Insofar as the professional voice user is concerned, Brodnitz (1962, p. 455) writes: "Technically, the lack of proper instruction during professional training in the use of the speaking voice is responsible for many voice disorders." McClosky (1959, p. 73) concurs: "The vast majority of patients who have come to me for voice therapy have been suffering from vocal abuse, that is to say, misuse."

Effect of Vocal Misuse and Abuse

Vocal misuse and abuse are essentially responsible for the onset and continuation of functional misphonia which is a known prelude to the occurrence and maintenance of benign organic lesions of the vocal folds, including contact ulcer, nodes, and polyps. Jackson (1928), Jackson and Jackson (1935), Jervey (1946), Peacher (1947a, 1947b, 1947c, and 1961), Peacher and Holinger (1947), New and Devine (1949), Baker (1954), Wright (1954), Wolcott (1956), Holinger and Johnson (1960), von Leden and Moore (1960), Levin (1962), Brodnitz (1963), and Myerson (1964) all consider vocal misuse and/or abuse the essential factor in the creation of a contact ulcer or a contact ulcer granuloma.

Vocal misuse and abuse are also major considerations in the creation of nodes and polyps according to Cunning (1934) (nodules), New and Erick (1938) (nodes and polyps), Delph (1940) (nodes and polyps), Moses (1940) (nodes), Friedberg and Segall (1941) (polyps), Ash and Schwartz (1944) (nodes and polyps), Harris (1948) (nodes and polyps), Holinger and Johnston (1951) (nodes and polyps), Kelly and Craik (1952) (nodes), Brodnitz (1958) (nodules), Fitz-Hugh, Smith, and Chiong (1958) (nodules and polyps), Withers and Dawson (1960) (nodules), DeQuiros, Sisatzky, and Tormakh (1960) (nodules), Wilson (1962a and 1962b) (nodules), Baker (1962) (nodules), O'Neil and McGee (1962) (polyps), Arnold (1962c and 1963c) (nodules and polyps), and Baker (1963) (polypoid degeneration).

Vocal abuse may be a factor in other types of lesions, as Jackson and Jackson (1939, p. 210) state: "The location of 85 percent of cancers on the most abused part of the larynx, the middle third of the cord, renders it logical, even if not probable, that vocal abuse is one cause of cancer of the larynx." Other authors who hold a similar view include Cavanaugh (1923), Waugh (1929), Tucker (1935 and 1937), Mitchell (1943), and Froeschels (1943). Vocal misuse and/or abuse may also create acute and/or chronic laryngitis (Clerf, 1937, and Murphy, 1967). According to Greene (1964, p. 91): "Chronic laryngitis and sore throats are frequently the result of bad habits of voice production." Froeschels (1943, p. 129) writes that:

> Hygiene of the voice may even prevent organic disorders of the respiratory tract. The epithelium of the vocal cords, as well as that of the mucous linings of

the throat, is injured by the continuous attack due to a hyperfunctional state and therefore may be more susceptible to infection.

Gabriel and Jones (1960) stress that in 10 percent of 101 patients, chronic laryngitis progressed to cancer; they report that vocal abuse is a chronic irritant (among others) which causes chronic laryngitis (Cooper, 1970a).

Voice strain may lead to hematoma and then papilloma (Kerman, 1937, and Briess, 1957). Vocal abuse may also be a causal factor in keratosis and leukoplakia (Cracovaner, 1965, and Brewer and Briess, 1960a).

Contributing Factors to Vocal Misuse

Constitutional factors (Wendler, 1966, and Meano, 1967) and altered body activity or functions may lead to a laryngeal effect that may contribute to a functional misphonia, which in turn may result in an organic dysphonia. Colds (Brodnitz, 1967, and Jackson and Jackson, 1935), hormonal changes, observed during pregnancy (Voorhees, 1914; van Thal, 1961), during medical treatment (testosterone) (Goldman and Salmon, 1942; Bauer, 1963; Calvet and Coll, 1964; Grimaud and Bonneville, 1964; Damste, 1964; Imre, 1965; Van Deinse, Dieleman, and Drost, 1966), and during the premenstrual period (Frable, 1962), postnasal drip, allergies (Maximov, 1965), and sinusitis may result in inflammation or edema of the vocal folds. This condition of the vocal folds may result in a slower vibratory pattern, thereby creating a lowered pitch. Unfortunately, this temporary vocal disability may become permanent.

Body fatigue, during or after a cold or illness, depressed emotional states, and medications (tranquilizers) may cause reduced volume and a subsequent drop in pitch.

The untrained speaker may well have his speaking voice shadow his feeling states. Brodnitz (1962, p. 456) explains: "But there can be no doubt that the lack of technical training makes the voice even more vulnerable to the effects of emotional tensions and anxieties."

Connecting emotional state and cold, Goldman (1967, p. 34) writes: "Some pneumonias of uncertain etiology ('non-specific,' or 'virus' pneumonias) and prolonged course, are often associated with severe emotional change, particularly depression, to the degree that a kind of vicious cycle is set up."

One major condition contributing to a functional misphonia is the cold, or upper respiratory infection. The altered vocal pattern that began during the cold, or infection, and which creates vocal misuse, continues long after the cold or infection has disappeared. This vocal pattern may also be continued because the patient likes the subsequent low voice. A number of patients have dated the onset of a functional misphonia (20 percent) and organic dysphonia (17 percent) from a recent or long past cold.

Other external factors, such as smoking, may set up a spiraling effect in that the smoking creates laryngeal irritation which in turn may lead to vocal misuse which results in further irritation. Wallner (1954, p. 260) reports: "Speaking with chronically inflamed vocal cords may lead to voice strain that results in the formation of polyps or of polypoid degeneration. The prolonged irritation of the mucosa may cause keratosis or even malignancy." Myerson (1950) states that smoking may cause irritation, inflammation, and edema, which can eventuate into a neoplasm.

Thus, although colds, allergies, sinusitis, postnasal drip, and smoking are not the direct causes of the dysphonia, they may be contributory factors by creating vocal misuse which leads to functional misphonia or organic dysphonia. Inflammation of the vocal folds can be created primarily from vocal misuse and secondarily from these conditions. These conditions may also be responsible for the alteration in resonance, volume, or breath support. However, despite the possible inflammation of the vocal folds, the excessive mucus, and the affected quality of voice from postnasal drip, allergies, sinusitis, and smoking, these patients have generally responded to direct vocal rehabilitation. Lack of vocal rehabilitation may result in a continued inflammation even during medical treatment or after a temporary disabling condition has been resolved. Brodnitz (1953) has pointed out that postnasal drip is entirely normal for healthy individuals. Other factors that may influence the pitch level and range, tone focus, volume, and quality include food intake and sexual orgasm (both may tend to lower the pitch), hearing defect, alcohol, smoking, drugs (tranquilizers), and chlorinated water (Manser, 1939).

One basic concept that should be noted is that vocal disorders do not occur because of overuse or excessive use, but rather are created by misuse and abuse of the voice. Knight (1901) made that very point almost 70 years ago. The human speaking voice when well used does not fatigue and does not afford any negative symptoms. Overuse of the speaking voice does not usually incline toward or result in a dysphonia, except in specific critically adverse circumstances, such as during a cold, protracted depressed feelings, and bodily illness. Anderson (1961, pp. 18–19) writes: ". . . nor should the vocal organs become fatigued or irritated even after prolonged, steady use under normal conditions. Ordinarily there should be no feeling of strain or tension in the throat during vocalization." In agreement are West, Ansberry, and Carr (1957, p. 76), who state: "No amount of vigorous vocalization can damage the edges of the vocal folds if the voice is properly used."

Pitch and Vocal Misuse

The primary cause of misphonia and dysphonia has been found to be the use of too low a pitch level by many, including Cunning (1934) and Cooper and Nahum (1967). Peacher (1963) states that most laryngeal pathological conditions are due to too low a speaking pitch.

Peacher (1966, p. 19) also explains: "Most people who have vocal problems will have to raise their pitch from two to five notes. This is contrary to the popular conception that a beautiful speaking voice is always low-pitched." Hanley and Thurman (1963, p. 144) write: "But far too many persons, in our experience, self-diagnose 'too high' (rarely 'too low' for either sex) pitch levels, set about lowering pitch, and by so doing perhaps lay the groundwork for future serious vocal disturbances." Boland (1953, p. 110) has found: "The obviously hoarse patient is usually speaking at the bottom of his pitch range, his pitch is a monotone, and he uses too much energy in speaking." Gardner (1958, p. 180) concludes: "Practically all of the executives spoke below their respective normal levels of pitch." Williamson (1945) reports that nearly all of his 72 hoarse patients had too low a pitch for the speaking voice, while Flower (1959) finds patients utilizing usually only three or four tones at the lower end of the pitch range. Moses (1954, p. 40) also says: "Actually many people insist on talking in a range not intended for them."

By raising the pitch to the optimal pitch level and range, this author found that reports from laryngologists indicated that the redness and edema of a misphonia had disappeared; the node or polyp was usually reduced during and eliminated following vocal rehabilitation. The same holds true for contact ulcer of the larynx (Cooper and Nahum, 1967; Peacher, 1961; and Gardner, 1958).

The pitch range may be too limited. However, some individuals with wide pitch ranges present voice problems because they use a limited vocal range, usually the lower notes, almost exclusively.

Another type of vocal misuse of pitch is singing solo or in a group or chorus using the wrong pitch range with poor tone focus, and inadequate breath support.

Organic lesions on the vocal folds, by reason of increased mass, may have the effect of slowing the vibratory pattern, thus resulting in a possible lowering of the pitch. The size or extent of the lesion also may influence the degree of the pitch variation. However, a growth on the vocal folds may not affect the pitch per se; the factors which do influence the pitch change in an organic dysphonia may be the same factors—vocal image, morning voice, and other influences—which affect the pitch level in functional misphonia. One organic lesion which does affect the pitch level markedly is polypoid degeneration (an extended form of polyps). This lesion restricts and lowers the pitch level and range.

Basal Pitch

The basal pitch is defined by Van Riper and Irwin (1958, p. 300) as: "The lowest note on which . . . (one) . . . can sustain utterance." A prominent factor which may create a voice problem is the use of the basal pitch or near basal pitch, which may be referred to as the basal pitch range. This author found that 91 percent of functional misphonic patients and 92 percent of organic dysphonic patients were using pitch levels much lower than their estimated optimal pitch levels; the habitual pitch levels were at or near the basal pitch levels.

A study by Cooper and Yanagihara (1971) indicates that the basal pitch is not stationary throughout the day. In nearly all individuals, the basal pitch is lowest in the morning. It rises one to three semitones during the day, with the rise being greater in some individuals than in others. In some subjects the basal pitch continues to rise in the evening, and in other subjects the basal pitch drops in the evening. The time of day appears to influence the basal pitch level.

One of the most common types of vocal misuse is the continued use of the basal pitch level and range. Two types of voices in which the basal pitch level and/or range is used are the "morning voice" (Perkins, 1957, p. 867) or "post-sleep voice" (Ladefoged, 1964, personal communication) and the vocal image voice (Cooper, 1968).

MORNING VOICE

The morning or postsleep voice occurs following sleep and is due to a relaxed laryngeal musculature which produces a lowered pitch. Russell (1936, p. 114) writes that there was a hoarseness or "heavy quality" to the voice upon awaking. Perkins (1957) has stated the morning voice is the voice to emulate by the patient. He maintains that the morning voice is the most relaxed voice, the most effortless voice. This author agrees that the morning voice is physiologically the most relaxed level and range in the voice. However, it is not the most physiologically oriented to proper usage for functional or artistic longevity.

This low pitch level or range, if used exclusively or to the exclusion of the optimal pitch level and range, is conducive and productive of pharyngeal and laryngeal tensions; this voice thus predisposes to laryngeal pathologies, since it tends to remain static and contained within a very few notes. The pitch level of the morning voice is but one segment or part of the speaking voice. The morning voice utilizes a pitch level too low and too constricted to afford the flexibility and melody, comfort, and carrying power necessary for daily conversational activities. The tone focus of this voice is almost always located within the laryngopharyngeal area rather than a balanced placement within the oro-, naso-, and laryngo-pharynx, thus necessitating the use of excessive volume for carrying power since the laryngopharynx does not allow for a great deal of carrying power or intelligibility. The morning voice is not operational; it is not functional; it is not utilitarian. This voice stresses a a tone which is heavy and throaty. This author has found that the use of the morning voice throughout the day is detrimental to the pharyngeal and laryngeal musculature, producing an inefficient voice. Clinical experience with 956 patients revealed that 71 percent of functional misphonic and 71 percent of organic dysphonic patients had a low morning or postsleep voice that was at the basal pitch level or range of the speaking voice.

In regard to the morning voice, patients have said, "I dread the first utterance in the morning—it's always a strain, that first conversation." "I can barely talk in the morning." "People can always tell when I've just gotten up."

The patient who experiences the morning voice and hitherto has employed that voice is instructed to raise the pitch immediately upon arising in the morning to the optimal pitch level. Simple exercises to accomplish this include: "Me-me" or "Ahem" counting one to ten, such as "Me-me one, me-me two," etc. utilizing the higher optimal pitch range and running up and down the scale, gently, for a few minutes, as will be more fully explained later.

VOCAL IMAGE VOICE

The vocal image is that aspect of voice whereby the individual either pursues or rejects a given sound because it either appeals or does not appeal to his esthetic sense or to his needs. In this group, 76 percent of functional misphonic and 78 percent of organic dysphonic patients had a vocal image.

Voice culture constricts the voice, according to Kallen (1959). This condition begins in childhood and continues into adulthood. Emotional and/or psychological considerations may contribute to the onset and development of voice troubles. Kallen further explains that the optimal pitch is distorted by the voice culture which identifies habitual pitch with natural pitch and thereby creates functional vocal inefficiency and voice problems. Moses (1954, pp. 42–43) writes: "But though the potential range of a person's voice is constitutionally given, his speaking range is a matter of training, custom, and personal preference."

The vocal image voice is usually at a pitch level that is basal or near basal in nature. The quality, volume, and focus of voice usually also are affected.

The positive vocal image voice is that which the patient identifies with and thereby seeks to emulate throughout the daily routine or for special circumstances of speaking. The vocal image may be purposeful (conscious) or nonpurposeful (unconscious) in nature. Although he makes no mention of a vocal image, Holmes (1931, p. 244) writes: "The cases which present a below the normal pitch level, are, generally, those who have made a conscious effort to lower their voices." Rousey, Moriarty, and Ostwald (1965, pp. 31–32) state: "Our assumption is that hoarseness of any degree results from an attempt to phonate at a level below the individual's optimal or expectable pitch. It will be immediately recognized that the crucial point in this discussion is the motivation for phonating at such a low level." The individual may lower his pitch, seek a certain tone, and/or foster a certain volume in order to consciously identify with another individual or type of individual. On the other hand, there may be an identification with a family member, friend, associate, or famous personality which results in an unconscious attempted imitation.

An additional point to note is that during a cold or upper respiratory infection, some patients have a tendency to pamper or overprotect their voices. They use subdued voices during the cold and continue this practice long after the cold has disappeared. The temporary vocal identity which was created to meet an immediate need, namely the difficulty of talking through a cold, results in a permanent vocal image and vocal identity. Harris (1960) finds the low voice beginning during an acute infection.

The negative vocal image voice is that aspect of voice where an attempt is made to avoid a given pitch level, quality, volume, or tone focus. An individual may feel negative toward the voice of a family member, a friend, an associate, or a personality, and thereby consciously or unconsciously seeks to avoid one or more aspects of that voice. Patients who have a sinus condition and want to avoid a nasal tone may force the pitch lower and find that this low pitch avoids a nasal twang or quality. Representative comments by patients include: "I don't like a squeaky voice," "A nasal voice offends me," "That voice is too high," "I can't stand a shrill voice," and "It is an uncultured and uncultivated tone."

The voice patient may be influenced or guided in his choice or direction of a vocal image, either positive or negative, by the vocal likes and dislikes of someone meaningful to him, such as a spouse, a parent, or a friend. Typical comments depicting this circumstance were: "My husband thinks my voice is too high," "My wife likes a low voice," and "My son sounds like a girl."

The vocal image voice, both positive and negative, is often contributory to the onset and development of functional misphonia and organic dysphonia. A few studies mention the vocal image as an entity, but fewer explore this phenomenon as one of the basic causes of vocal misuse and abuse. This author has found that most adults and children have a vocal image; in the adults, the vocal image is of long duration. The vocal image is a basic and overriding factor in the continuation of voice disorders.

Many patients whose vocal identities have long been established due to a vocal image are responsive to a more realistic and natural voice after a thorough review and analysis of the vocal image. The change of pitch, quality, tone focus, or volume within the first session may result in patient comments that the new voice is artificial, phony, different, funny, superficial, not representative, strange, contrived, strained, or unnatural.

Van Riper and Irwin (1958) explain that the habitual pitch is tied up with the self-concept. Establishing a new pitch makes the patient feel strange and uncomfortable, resulting in varying defensive behavior. Weiss (1955) writes that the patient does not hear himself as he really sounds and violently resists changing to a new voice.

A large number of patients experiencing the changeover from the old pitch to the new optimal pitch level and range react sharply and immediately. The essential complaint of male patients is that the voice is too high, too thin, too weak, and effeminate. Female patients express the view that the new voice is shrill, squeaky, strident, nagging in tone, lacking in grace and charm, monotone, unnatural, and uncultured.

Assurance that the new voice is natural and that it will affect listeners in a positive, not a negative, fashion needs to be underscored. Mention may be made of the negative listener reaction that the old voice may have invoked with its grating quality and basal pitch. Without the exploration and quick resolution of the vocal image (in cases where it exists) at the outset of therapy by the voice therapist, the rehabilitation of the misphonia or dysphonia cannot be readily achieved.

The types of vocal image voices which could possibly create a functional misphonia and organic dysphonia include the authoritarian voice, the intimate or confidential voice, and the siren voice. The authoritarian voice or the voice of authority utilizes a pitch that is low (Moses, 1965) or basal in level or range. Professional speakers (lawyers, doctors, and teachers) and people involved in entertainment (actors, radio and television announcers) reveal a marked tendency to pursue this type of voice. Moses (1954), p. 43) writes: "Authority speaks low. The male teacher, lawyer, judge, the preacher often use a low voice to express authority, utilizing the deepest part of their potential range." This voice is restrictive of pitch, and quality, predisposing to inadequate tone focus. Inherent in this voice is an effortful and forced increased volume. The basal pitch range and relatively loud volume of this voice appear to be associated in the patient's mind with a strong, masculine, knowledgeable person with confidence, assurance, and authority, and therefore the patient seeks to acquire this vocal identity. Many people are trying to push their voices down seeking to add status or stature through this lower pitch level. The basis for this vocal identity rests upon the long-term vocal image which has shaped and formed the patient's voice.

The intimate or confidential voice is often used under special circumstances, such as on the telephone, in restaurants, and in offices. Many patients habitually use the intimate voice. This type of voice results in a drop in pitch level to the basal pitch range, is breathy, with little carrying power, and may lose its natural tone focus, resulting in spasm or prolonged contraction of the laryngeal and pharyngeal muscles.

The siren voice is utilized by women who desire to sound "sexy." The basal pitch level and range is once again utilized for this type of voice. The same type of problems which accrue to the voice of authority and the intimate voice also accrue to this type of voice. Moses (1954, p. 42) states: "If we scan our preferences today, it becomes evident that deep female voices are admired. Most of the ranking actresses in the legitimate theatre have deep voices." The siren voice is a long-term vocal image that has created a vocal identity for both the speaker and the auditor. Some women, however, place the voice at such a low pitch level that they create the impression of being a man and are called "mister" and "sir" on the telephone. This male designation activates some of these women to seek vocal assistance.

A special type of vocal imitation is the vocal cue. A vocal cue is the pursuit by the patient of the pitch, quality, volume, or rate of the immediate speaker in a conversation. This may occur on the telephone, at parties, or in face-to-face conversation.

All of these types of voices may be used as a general mode of speech or may be utilized for special circumstances and conditions. The progressive and continued use of these voices may eventually result in mild to severe functional misphonia and organic dysphonia, depending upon the extent of vocal usage and duration of vocal images.

Regarding the misused pitch level of the voice, the patient must be trained to use the optimal pitch level and range. Optimal pitch range is that area within the total extended pitch of the voice where a maximum amount of voice is produced with a minimum amount of effort. Optimal pitch level is the best level and should be the most frequently used pitch level within the optimal pitch range. Habitual pitch level and range is that portion of the pitch range utilized by an individual for normal and routine speaking situations. The habitual pitch level and range may be too high or too low. The habitual pitch level and range should be the same as the optimal pitch level and range. When these two differ, the individual is misusing his voice. Habitual pitch level and range have been investigated by Snidecor (1943 and 1951), Lynch (1934), Tiffin (1934), Pronovost (1942), Mysak and Hanley (1958), Mysak (1959), and McGlone and Hollien (1963), among others.

Tone Focus and Vocal Misuse

Tone focus is the placement or emphasis of resonance in one or more portions of the naso-, oro-, and/or laryngopharynx. The tone focus may be basically within the lower portion of the pharynx (laryngopharynx), which results in a throaty, effortful voice. Tone focus primarily in the upper pharynx (nasopharynx) may create a nasal voice. Good tone focus is produced by balancing oral and nasal resonance (with some laryngeal resonance) and by focusing or directing the tone to the "mask" (an area embracing a point at about the bridge of the nose, down to and including the lips).

Volume and Vocal Misuse

The volume may be excessive (which places a strain on the musculature) or inadequate (which affects intelligibility). There is a tendency to increase intensity when the distracting noise level is increased (Hanley and Steer, 1949). Competition with industrial noise leads to voice problems (Brewer and Briess, 1960b). Even noise at cocktail parties reaches levels of 80–85 dB (Legget and Northwood, 1960).

The use of excessive volume for audibility or listenibility often results in an inappropriate pitch level (too high or too low) and a placement of tone within the laryngopharynx. Therefore, misuse and abuse of voice, such as yelling at a baseball game, may result in a sore throat, hoarseness, and a lowered pitch level; this pitch level may be continued after the sore throat has passed.

Patients who need to supervise within a noisy situation, such as construction work and in factories, or who need to conduct business at cocktail parties, can be taught to comfortably increase the volume markedly without adverse effect to the voice. Most important, they must learn to use the optimal level of pitch combined with a greater nasopharyngeal resonance.

Quality and Vocal Misuse

The quality of voice may be forced and unnatural, presenting a deviant tone, which may sound breathy, hoarse, husky, raspy, squeaky, or foggy. Hoarseness is the most prevalent quality. The vocal image may play a role in hoarseness also. Boland (1953, p. 109) reports that

> . . . *the number of persons who are being treated for hoarseness is infinitesimal compared to the number of people who need treatment.*
>
> . . . .
>
> An individual's opinion about his own voice may not be reliable. People who are hoarse often think of their own voices as being "mellow" or "deep and resonant."

Most individuals who are seen in voice therapy, though they present a hoarse voice, are unaware of the extent of the hoarseness, its duration, or its communicative impairment. They fail to hear themselves as hoarse, to identify themselves as hoarse, and to define hoarseness in others both in and outside of the therapeutic situation. Of the patients in this group, 91 percent of those with functional misphonia and 94 percent of those with organic dysphonia were hoarse.

Breath Support and Vocal Misuse

Breath support may depend upon an incorrect type of breathing, such as clavicular or upper chest breathing, rather than a relevant and comfortable medial or midsection (central, abdominal, or diaphragmatic) breathing for good support of tone. Sustained interpersonal conversation must rely on active midsection breath support in order to avoid laryngeal, pharyngeal, and bodily tensions. Hundreds of patients have indicated that the lack of midsection breath control has added and contributed to the onset and development of voice disorders. Of these patients seen, 86 percent of the functional misphonic patients and 89 percent of the organic dysphonic patients had upper chest breathing.

Abnormality or irregularity in breath control for speech related to voice problems is noted by Brodnitz (1962, p. 466), who states: "The prevalence of chest breathing is very frequent in disturbed voices." He also believes (p. 475): "The treatment of almost any voice disorder requires correction of the breathing habits of the patient." Among those who advocate breath control for speech are Holmes (1930), Drake (1937), and Anderson (1961). Moore (1957, p. 694) adds: "There can be little doubt that many persons with harmful vocal habits expend more effort on breathing than is necessary."

Lindsley (1929) notes that women tend toward upper chest breathing. The prevalence of abnormality or the acceptance of irregular breath control need not be cause to accede to such a state, especially when a voice disorder prevails. The continued use of upper chest breathing for males or for females becomes a matter of concern in vocal rehabilitation when a voice is impaired, and inadequate breath control exists and contributes to the ongoing vocal impairment.

Studies under the editorship of Gray (1936) compositely find that specific types of breath control are irrelevant to audibility (Sallee, 1936) and to loudness (Wiksell, 1936). Huyck and Allen (1937) in a fluoroscopic study of good and poor speakers explain that regular diaphragmatic movement prevails in good voices. Drake (1937) strongly favors abdominal breath support because such breathing allows the greatest amount of control and best affords an absence of laryngeal and pharyngeal tensions.

Rate and Vocal Misuse

The rate of speech, a minor consideration, is involved only if a fast rate creates hyperventilation or a labored voice. Most patients undergoing vocal rehabilitation find it necessary to slow the rate of speech so as to allow them time and effort to concentrate upon the elements of concern, such as pitch, quality, tone focus, and breath support.

Therefore, the most basic causes of vocal misuse are one or more of these factors: inappropriate pitch level, pitch range, tone focus, volume, breath support, and quality. Tone focus and pitch level are the two most vital elements in creating and continuing vocal misuse.

Allied Areas and Vocal Misuse

General areas in which vocal abuse tends to occur are parties, meetings, sports events, in and about transportation facilities, around machinery, television, radios, and record players—any area in which environmental noise or sound is excessive or abnormal for normal conversation, thereby demanding an altered vocal pattern. This vocal pattern usually emphasizes an abnormally lowered or raised pitch level, excessive volume, and laryngopharyngeal tone focus. Usually vocal misuse and abuse are insidious and are not identified as such by the speaker who is experiencing the resultant symptoms and subsequent functional misphonia or organic dysphonia.

Summary

Functional misphonia is a basic and overriding step which leads to organic dysphonia, such as nodes, polyps, and contact ulcer. These organic dysphonias are not usually discrete entities which occur full-blown by vocal misuse or abuse. An exception is sudden and immediate vocal trauma, which may be caused by abusive yelling, leading to a vocal fold hemorrhage and which in turn may create an organic lesion. Normally, functional misphonia is an ever-present, ongoing continuum which eventually creates the vocal pathology known as nodes, polyps, or contact ulcer. The circumstances and conditions, both external and internal, define the duration of the misphonia and predicate the development of the organic dysphonia. Defining the treatment of functional misphonia essentially specifies the treatment of organic dysphonia.

SYMPTOMS OF FUNCTIONAL MISPHONIA AND ORGANIC DYSPHONIA

The various attributes indicating the existence of functional misphonia and growths on the vocal folds may be: 1. visual, as seen during a direct or indirect laryngoscopic examination; 2. sensory, as experienced by the patient; and 3. auditory, as noted in the sound of the voice by the patient and/or the listener. These attributes may exist singly or in combination.

Visual Symptoms

In the visual sense, functional misphonia refers to an impairment of the vocal folds which may be evidenced by an inflammation, a redness, or an edema of the vocal folds; no visible organic lesion per se exists. Functional misphonia may also exist when no visible signs of vocal fold irritation appear, but when the sensory and/or auditory symptoms of vocal misuse and/or abuse are present. In organic dysphonia, such as nodes, polyps, and contact ulcer, the lesion is self-evident to the laryngologist.

Sensory Symptoms

The sensory symptoms are: nonproductive throat clearing; coughing; progressive vocal fatigue following brief or limited vocal use; acute or chronic irritation or pain in or about the larynx or the pharynx; sternum pressure and/or pain; neck muscle cording; swelling of veins and/or arteries in the neck; throat stiffness (Glassburg, 1925); rapid fatigue and voice breaks (Hunt, 1906); a feeling of a foreign substance or "lump" in the throat; ear irritation or tickling; repeated sore throats; a tickling, a tearing, soreness, or a burning sensation in the throat; scratchy or dry throat; tenderness of anterior and/or posterior strap muscles; rumble in the chest; stinging sensation in the soft palate; a feeling that talking is an effort; a choking feeling; tension and/or tightness in the throat; earache; back neck tension; headache; and mucus formation (Russell, 1936, and Mithoefer, 1940). Other symptoms may include arytenoid tenderness, trachael pressure, anterior or posterior cervical pain, and pain at the base of the tongue (Brewer and Briess, 1960a).

Almost all patients complained of one or more of the above symptoms. The most common symptoms were vocal fatigue (functional misphonia, 92 percent; organic dysphonia, 94 percent); throat clearing (functional misphonia, 61 percent; organic dysphonia, 65 percent); and coughing (functional misphonia, 16 percent; organic dysphonia, 15 percent). According to Hunt (1906), the great majority of voice problems due to poor use of the speaking voice remain at the stage of vocal fatigue. It has been our experience that vocal fatigue prevails in many speaking voices unrecognized as a symptom of vocal misuse, and is seldom, if ever, considered abnormal, irregular, or treatable. In general, vocal fatigue remains a routine, if not standard, aspect of many speaking voices. Throat clearing and coughing may be contributory to the initial and continued irritation of the vocal folds, which may influence the extent or duration of a misphonia or dysphonia.

Auditory Symptoms

The auditory aspect may be noted in: acute or chronic hoarseness; reduced vocal range; inability to talk at will and at length in variable situations, such as direct conversation or on the phone without vocal fatigue; tone change from a clear voice to a breathy, raspy, squeaky, foggy, or rough voice; repeated loss of voice; laryngitis; voice breaks; voice skips; voice comes and goes during the day or over a period of months; clear voice in the morning with tired or foggy voice in the afternoon or evening; and missed speech sounds.

The most typical auditory symptom is hoarseness;

the hoarse voice that does not present a pathological cause is frequently seen by the laryngologist. However, hoarseness is the basic symptom which brings the patient to the physician (Levin, 1962).

When the quality of voice is markedly hoarse or rough, and there is a lack of throat irritation (acute or chronic), this may be indicative of long-term extended vocal misuse and abuse. The patient no longer exhibits sensory symptoms.

Functional misphonia can be seen, felt, and/or heard in variable combinations. It can sometimes be seen; it can usually be felt; it can almost always be heard. Organic dysphonia (growth) can essentially be seen, felt, and heard.

VOCAL REHABILITATION

Vocal rehabilitation is the retraining of the patient's voice in a single parameter or in all parameters of the voice; pitch, volume, quality, tone focus, breath support, and rate. Vocal rehabilitation generally requires vocal education or vocal reeducation. Almost invariably a patient must learn vocal techniques for the speaking voice.

It is imperative that all voice patients be seen for an initial laryngeal examination by a laryngologist prior to vocal rehabilitation. A medical report on the visual aspects of the vocal folds is essential to exclude pathology and/or to establish the state of the vocal folds. Periodic laryngeal checkups are necessary to complement the vocal rehabilitation and to determine the extent of improvement visually. No voice patient should be seen by a voice pathologist if a laryngoscopic examination is declined by the patient.

Approaches to Vocal Rehabilitation

The literature has long been divided concerning the types of approach for treatment of vocal disorders. Each group respectively supports its own view of the causation of vocal disorders, and thus presents its own method of treatment for a given disorder. Two groups believe the problem is medical and prescribe surgical or palliative measures. Another group indicates that the disorder is psychological and advocates psychotherapy as the main, if not total, approach. These two types are indirect in their approach.

A fourth group believes the voice disorder is due to functional misuse and utilizes direct vocal rehabilitation. Still a fifth group, also indicating the functional causation, recommends essentially direct vocal rehabilitation with requisite *vocal* psychotherapy. Our experience reveals that the large majority of voice patients require this fifth or combined approach.

These five methods of treatment, except surgery, apply to both functional misphonia and organic dysphonia. Organic dysphonia can and often does involve surgical intervention. Organic dysphonia may be treated by surgery alone, by surgery followed by any of the other methods above, or by any of the other methods without prior surgery.

SURGERY

Surgical intervention alone for the treatment of nodes, polyps, and contact ulcer has been pursued by some laryngologists. A review of the author's patients referred following surgery indicates that surgery alone may not be sufficient, since the patient is frequently left with a functional misphonia following surgery.

Brodnitz (1958, p. 113) describes the need for vocal rehabilitation for contact ulcer, nodes, and polyps, as well as definining his point of view concerning the relationship between surgery and vocal therapy.

> Surgical removal is necessary in the majority of benign lesions of the cords. But in small lesions of relatively recent standing, such as small nodules, thickenings of the cords, small contact ulcers without pronounced granulation, vocal therapy alone may effect a disappearance of tissue changes together with the restoration of a normal voice.
>
> On the other hand, larger and solidfied nodules, well-defined polyps, general polypoid thickenings of the cords, and contact ulcers with extensive granulation require surgical intervention, to be followed by vocal rehabilitation. Without such vocal retraining recurrences are frequent since the underlying cause of the lesion continues to be effective.

From clinical experience this author recommends either surgery followed by the fifth method (direct vocal rehabilitation with *vocal* psychotherapy) or the fifth method alone, depending upon the discretion of the laryngologist who determines the feasibility for surgery. A surgical procedure apparently activates the patient to enter vocal rehabilitation. Of 246 patients seen who had undergone a surgical procedure to remove a vocal fold growth(s), 75 percent entered therapy and 91 percent of this group completed therapy. Of the 224 non-surgical patients seen, 71 percent entered therapy but 94 percent of these completed therapy. In comparing patients who completed vocal rehabilitation, of those who had had surgery, 69 percent received excellent ratings, while 74 percent were rated excellent in the group who had not had surgery prior to vocal rehabilitation. These statistics indicate slightly better results for non-surgical patients.

Peacher (1961), in a follow-up of 70 contact ulcer patients, states that surgery prolonged the vocal rehabilitation process. Regarding contact ulcer of the larynx, Cooper and Nahum (1967, p. 64) explain:

> The surgeon must always keep in mind that any surgical procedure for this disease has only temporal value and does not alter the basic etiologic factors which are operating and which will continue to operate. Without concomitant vocal therapy, surgery alone will usually fail to correct the problem and may aggravate and accelerate the disease process.

PALLIATIVE MEASURES

The two indirect types of treatment are palliative measures and psychotherapy. Palliative measures include vocal rest, bed rest, vacation, suggestion, hypnosis, relaxation, diathermy, steam, and medications (lozenges, syrups, sprays, pills, gargles, and intravenous injections). These measures can and do reduce the inflammation of the vocal folds temporarily, but do not affect the basic causation—vocal misuse and abuse. Lozenges merely tend to mask the laryngeal and/or pharyngeal irritation or fatigue. Vocal rest is not a relevant treatment for functional misphonia or organic dysphonia (Brodnitz, Myerson, West). Following vocal rest or limited vocal usage as the voice is used again, the misuse and abuse reoccur, thereby recreating the functional misphonia or organic dysphonia. Vocal rest is seldom observed because of personality demands and communication needs. Vocal silence pursuant to vocal rest creates negative reactions from listeners as well. Therefore, vocal rest is seldom fulfilled by or fulfilling to the patient.

Hypnosis has been suggested by some as a means or a method of meeting the vocal problem. This point of view is without foundation and based upon opinion. Brodnitz (1963) indicates hypnosis has disappointing results. For most patients, the power of autosuggestion or hypnosis cannot alter a mechanical vocal problem and habit.

Vacation, relaxation, and/or bed rest are often prescribed by some physicians, since they consider functional misphonia to be a problem of "nerves." "Nerves" may be a contributory factor, since tension affects the voice, and feeling states do influence it. However, the term "nerves" is misleading, since tension or "nerves" is only one aspect to be considered for some patients with functional misphonia. Also, a certain amount of tension is normal and must be utilized for active living. If a patient is using his voice well, tension or "nerves" basically do not cause misuse; if misuse is already present, tension adds to the misuse. Vacations and relaxation are of little, if any, help. Once poor vocal habits have been established, temporary relaxation may attenuate and not resolve the misphonia or dysphonia.

Some of the patients seen had been given numerous medications by physicians other than the referring laryngologists in an attempt to relieve and resolve the hoarseness. One patient with functional misphonia was given ultrasonic medcolator treatments as well as 25 different medications, including Librium, Sulfa, Polycillin, Tetracycline, Atropine, and ACTH for hoarseness and laryngitis over a period of years. Vocal rehabilitation resolved this misphonia. As Douglas (1950, p. 383) notes:

> The patient is alarmingly frequent who has been treated for hoarseness supposedly due to sinusitis, deviated nasal septum, enlarged palatine tonsils, infected or noninfected, for one or two years prior to seeking other medical advice, when his symptoms have either failed to have been alleviated or have progressed. Not infrequently the patient is seen to have had a uvulectomy or wholesale dental extractions performed in an attempt to treat the hoarseness or laryngeal sensations.

Tarneaud (1947, p. 14) agrees: "The patients often receive wrongly and unsuccessfully treatment for chronic laryngitis, whereas only phoniatric treatment —considering the somatic and psychological etiology —is promising."

The palliative measures, alone or in combination, afford some comfort and ease to the patient; however, these measures do not afford a permanent or realistic confrontation, dissolution, and resolution of the essential components of a misphonia or a dysphonia. Hoarseness has been known to disappear for short periods of time, but this condition persists despite palliative treatment. Palliative measures are useful if and when they are utilized for immediate symptom containment and relief only as a prologue in the context of a total program of vocal rehabilitation.

PSYCHOTHERAPY

The psychotherapy or psychodynamic position holds that voice disorders are psychosomatic in nature, and that with a resolution of the external and internal stresses upon the patient, the vocal disorder will terminate. The group of authors viewing vocal disorders from a psychodynamic position include Duncan (1947), Thorn (1947), Moses (1954), Wyatt (1950), Heaver (1958), Bloch (1959), and Nemec (1961). Under this presentation vocal therapy apparently is to be pursued under the guise of psychotherapy. However, despite the etiological viewpoint of some of these authors, they utilize modified or direct vocal rehabilitation techniques.

Few psychotherapists, be they psychologists or psychiatrists, are trained or knowledgeable in the dynamics of voice production. Psychotherapy may afford the patient a modicum or marked degree of relaxation, but easing the psyche is really not resolving the voice problem. Verbalization regarding the feeling states and their effect upon voice may clarify the voice problem and offer catharsis, but this does not alter the pattern of vocal misuse or abuse. Psychotherapy cannot direct a poor voice into a good voice. Two psychiatrists, Weiss (1955) and Schick (1966), representing some of the psychiatric overviews of voice disorders, maintain that voice needs to be dealt with by a direct functional voice training approach rather than by a psychiatric approach. Schick (1966, p. 140) states: "From our long and varied experience we have learned that vocal disturbances are treated far more efficaciously by functional therapy than by psychotherapeutic measures alone." Weiss (1955, p. 215) concludes:

> The voice and the psychological make-up of an individual mutually influence each other. If a person is psychologically disturbed, the voice suffers, and in turn the deterioration of the voice exerts a negative influence upon the psyche. We can approach this vicious circle from either the psychological or the vocal angle. Psychotherapy is often a hazardous and always a lengthy procedure and, as mentioned above, the voice would have to be treated in any case. On the other hand, in the treatment of the voice we feel on pretty firm ground. Attacking the formerly vicious circle from this point, we arrive, by improving the phonation, at influencing the psyche in a favorable manner. This, in turn, creates more favorable conditions for the voice itself. Thus the vicious circle has been converted into a "virtuous" one.

The patients we have seen with voice problems fell into these three categories: 1. Patients with voice defects and no psychological involvement. These patients responded to vocal rehabilitation and vocal psychotherapy, if needed. Most patients were in this category. 2. Patients with voice defects unaffected by accompanying emotional or psychological problems. These patients improved their voices with vocal rehabilitation without changing the psychological problems. It is seldom essential or appropriate to pursue this concern or consideration, since it does not interfere with the voice. Thus, an individual may be emotionally disturbed, may have psychological involvement, and still have a clear voice, if the voice is properly used. 3. Patients with voice defects affected by psychological problems. In these patients the psychological problems were too involved for the voice to be helped by vocal rehabilitation. The personality problem needed to be resolved before the voice could be treated. Only a very few patients in this study fell into this third category—those needing psychotherapy alone prior to vocal rehabilitation.

From a review of these 956 patients, the direct approach, namely, educating the patient to use the voice properly, is the basic approach. As Anderson (1961, p. 10) writes: "It is much easier to effect changes in the voice than in the personality." Murphy (1964, p. 107) explains: "A large number of functional voice disorders are cases of faulty vocal behavior in individuals who do have major personal stresses affecting vocal functioning, but who are essentially normal in terms of general emotional stability." Thus, psychotherapy may be essential as an adjunct to vocal rehabilitation when the patient is made aware of the vocal dynamics by the voice therapist, understands the process, but elects to ignore or thwart purposefully and consistently vocal direction and rehabilitation assistance.

TRADITIONAL APPROACH

The traditional or direct school does not ignore psychological causation as a contributory factor, but maintains that voice disorders are overcome by concentrating on the basic elements of voice production itself.

Some therapists, including Froeschels and Brodnitz, follow a basically nondirective approach. They demand that the patient, through a given set of exercises, develop the proper pitch level. One of these exercises is vocalization while chewing. Specific breathing exercises are afforded the patient to prevent laryngeal and pharyngeal construction of the tone.

This chewing method, so named and developed by Froeschels, has been advocated by Froeschels and associates as the essential approach to vocal rehabilitation and as a singular method to use in order to locate the correct pitch level. This method is an attempt to remove hyper- and hypofunctional voice disorders (Froeschels, 1943; Weiss and Beebe, 1950).

The method appears to be effective basically in the hands of those who are familiar with its purposes and its limitations, and who are also knowledgeable in vocal rehabilitation. However, the recommendation that the chewing method is *the* method is without foundation. This method affords many limitations in actual practice aside from all theoretical considerations. The optimal pitch level and range are neither given by the therapist nor requested of the patient. The new pitch that is afforded the patient via the chewing method may well create extended or extensive hyper- and/or hypofunction of the voice. The chewing method is indirect or nondirect and places the responsibility on the patient who must determine which pitch range or level feels comfortable. (The traditional approach is directive in that the optimal pitch level and range are afforded the patient.) Nondirective vocal rehabilitation is highly dangerous in that it allows a patient to become his own therapist and thereby presumes that vocal assistance can be rendered by a basically nonassistant therapist. In actuality, experience has shown that the optimal pitch level and range are uncomfortable for many at first since the vocal muscles are being realigned. The discomfort quickly disappears as the optimal pitch level is utilized. However, the patient would not originally choose this range as comfortable, functional, satisfactory, or aesthetically appealing. In addition, the chewing approach is concerned with neither a development or extension of range nor with the aesthetic element of voice—namely, the tone. Although not having had intensive training in the chewing technique, Van Riper and Irwin (1958, pp. 293–294) find that many patients resist the method, that improvement is often temporary, that the method is distracting to the patient, and that "the transition from overt chewing to 'mental chewing' is not accomplished easily."

Direct vocal rehabilitation emphasizes specific parameters of voice: pitch level, pitch range, tone focus, quality, intensity, breath support, and rate. Those pursuing direct vocal rehabilitation include Anderson, Van Riper and Irwin, Wilson, Williamson, Flower, Gardner, Peacher, West, and Holmes. This type of therapy is utilized for functional misphonia and organic dysphonia (nodes, polyps, and contact ulcer).

MODERN VOCAL REHABILITATION

This approach is similar to the direct traditional approach except that it incorporates vocal psychotherapy and differs in the sequential order and emphasis in treating the vocal variables.

In our experience *vocal* psychotherapy, not psychotherapy per se, is involved in the vocal rehabilitation program, such as the discussion of the formation of the vocal image and the subsequent vocal identity that the patient pursues. According to Van Riper and Irwin (1958), all therapy, including voice therapy, has some psychotherapy in it. Moses (in Bloch, 1959, p. 116) "affirms that well-planned vocal psychotherapy is capable of replacing a more extensive type of routine psychotherapy." Greene (1964) says that commonsense exploration of human problems suffices for most voice therapy. Brodnitz (1958) suggests limited psychotherapy, a quiet hour with the patient. Thus, essentially the voice disorder is viewed as a bad habit based upon poor vocal production, poor vocal culture and image, and poor vocal hygiene.

Tone Focus

Most therapists advocate determination of the optimal pitch level and range as the basic step in vocal rehabilitation. Direct methods for this location are found in Pronovost (1942) and Fairbanks (1960). However, an inherent concomitant and essential part of the location of the optimal pitch level is the establishment of the correct tone focus or resonance.

The pharynx is composed of the laryngo-, the oro-, and the nasopharynx. To the patient, these areas are described in terms of resonance: the lower resonance (laryngopharynx); the middle resonance (oropharynx); and the upper resonance (nasopharynx). The lower resonance alone is guttural and throaty; the middle resonance alone is flat, colorless, and possibly denasal; the upper resonance alone is too sharp, nasal, and aesthetically unacceptable to speaker and listener alike.

The expression "Don't speak in the throat" is a meaningless and highly confusing statement. Since the larynx is located with the laryngopharyngeal area, one must speak "in the throat" in the sense that the basic sound emanates from the laryngopharynx. However, this sound should be focused or placed in the proper balanced tone focus within the oro-, naso-, and laryngopharynx.

The lower resonance is quite easy and natural in

vocalization, since sound initiates from this area. However, emphasis upon this type of resonance places undue stress and strain upon the laryngeal and/or pharyngeal muscles and concomitantly affords limited projection to the voice. The result of such lower resonance stress is both sensory and auditory. The patient complains of throat throbbing or pain in the throat, tautness in the neck, and a tired voice after speaking, and says that he seems to have trouble being heard.

Since the lower resonance will naturally occur, the emphasis must be placed on the acquisition of upper and middle resonance which may be lost due to vocal misuse and abuse. To a knowledgeable and experienced voice therapist, this balance of middle and upper resonance in combination with lower resonance, if naturally produced and not forced, has a "ring." This "ring" refers to a clarity of tone which is easily projected, effortless, and buoyant, making the voice melodious and appealing. Tarneaud (1958) refers to this "ring" as a "sonorous" quality.

West, Ansberry, and Carr (1957) state that many outstanding voices have a marked degree of upper resonance. This nasal resonance is not detected as such; nasal resonance does not mean nasality. Weiss, a discussant in Vennard (1962, p. 419) notes Reszke as saying: "The sound should be in the nose but the nose should not be in the sound." The correct oro-naso-laryngo-pharyngeal resonance as discussed here may well be noted in such voices as Peter Ustinov, Edward G. Robinson, Lawrence Olivier, Julie Andrews, Joan Crawford, Franchot Tone, and Richard Burton.

A balanced oral and nasal tone or resonance must be identified, discriminated, and established by the patient as afforded through the therapist's highly positive and definite vocal direction. A motorkinesthetic approach is utilized as part of the methodology to make the patient aware of the different types of resonance.

The therapist produces first lower resonance and then upper resonance while the patient is asked to place his hands on the laryngeal area and the nasal area in order to contrast these types of resonance. Next the patient is directed to produce tone in exercises (counting, etc.) and in speaking to determine which resonance he is using. Almost inevitably the patient produces lower resonance.

With the demonstration followed by a discussion of resonance, the patient is made aware of the emphasis he is placing on lower resonance and made cognizant of the need to balance the resonance of tone. Mechanical exercises to establish the approximate tone focus are initiated after the location of the optimal pitch level, since the same exercises are used to afford the patient his own guideline to experience optimal pitch and the proper tone focus. The need is to balance the middle and upper resonance so that nasal resonance is inherent yet not outstanding in the new tonal quality. This tone focus is often referred to as "mask" placement, which means balanced oral and nasal resonance. This type of focus can be felt internally and externally by the patient through vibration at the anterior portion of the hard palate and lips (Anderson and Holmes) and in or about the nasal area or "mask" (Zaliouk, 1963). Some others report that this tone focus can also be experienced within the forehead and the crown of the skull.

Holmes (1931, p. 236) writes: "Efficient voice production cannot be achieved unless 'frontal' placement is established." Regarding the relationship between pitch and placement of tone, Holmes (1931, p. 244) has found: "All of the cases which have incorrect 'placement' present pitch levels which are either above or below the normal pitch."

Optimal Pitch Level and Range

In order to ascertain the optimal pitch level and range, we utilize the following steps.

1. The patient is directed: a) to sustain the vowels [ɑ] and [o] at the lowest comfortable pitch (basal pitch), and b) to speak at the normal speaking level (habitual pitch). These two pitch levels, the basal and the habitual pitch levels, are compared. They are usually quite similar, if not identical.

2. The patient is directed: a) to vocalize a natural spontaneous "uh-hum" or "ahem"; b) to laugh naturally, (a person's natural spontaneous laugh is often representative of the optimal pitch level.); c) to vocalize "me-me" or "nim-nim"; d) to vocalize while chewing (occasionally used); e) to vary these vocalizations in pitch, four or five notes or tones above the basal pitch level, as the therapist directs; and finally, f) to vocalize on a pitch level which has the most "ring" or "mask" focus to the therapist. The competent voice therapist is able to hear the ring of this optimal pitch level immediately.

The therapist must direct the patient to this new pitch level, since the patient is unable to monitor himself in relation to the basal, habitual, and optimal pitch levels. One important point must be noted. Our experience has shown that almost all patients have a tendency to drop the optimal pitch level to a lower level which results in a loss of both optimal pitch and tone focus. The resurgence of old symptoms of vocal misuse are then immediate. For this reason, the patient is usually directed to a higher pitch level referred to as the elevated or supraoptimal pitch level within the optimal pitch range. Thus when the usual pitch drop occurs, the patient is at the optimal pitch level. Also, this supraoptimal pitch level has enabled us to locate the tone focus more easily and quickly and has enabled the patient to hear and maintain the tone focus better.

For illustrative purposes, let us take the case of a bass-baritone. First the supraoptimal pitch level is developed in the baritone portion of the range, and a balanced oral-nasal or mask focus is attained. Once the tone focus and pitch level are established, the pitch is dropped to the optimal pitch level. Following this, development of the total bass-baritone range is sought.

3. The patient is directed to vocalize at the basal, the habitual and the supraoptimal pitch levels in order to compare these pitch levels and to begin ear training.

4. The patient firmly establishes the supraoptimal pitch level and tone focus in the mask, both of which require varying amounts of time and training, with the following procedure: a) He vocalizes *gently* using the nasal exercises "um-hum" and "ahem" at the supraoptimal pitch level, attempting to feel the mask focus. This is done for variable periods of time as required to locate the focus. b) He vocalizes *gently* using the nasal exercises "um-hum one, um-hum two," or "me-me one, me-me two," or "nim-nim one, nim-nim two," on the supraoptimal level, again feeling the mask focus. He stays on one pitch level. There is a marked preference among patients as to which of these exercises best serves to define and to determine the mask focus and the supraoptimal level. Either a) or b) or both are repeated at the beginning of each therapy session as a warm-up after the pitch level and focus have been mastered. c) The patient talks on the supraoptimal pitch level, feeling the mask focus. This is compared directly with the pre-recorded "um-hum" and "me-me one" to be certain that the patient is speaking on approximately the same level he used for the nasal exercises. This speaking is practiced first in therapy and then used outside the therapy situation. In speaking, the tone focus should be within the mask area, but not as much vibration is felt as compared to the nasal exercises.

The use of "ahem" is extremely important outside of therapy, since it can be used during conversations in order to attain the mask focus, or to assure the patient he is using the correct focus. The word "ahem" is socially acceptable and does not create any negative connotations; thus, the patient is able to practice guidelines for the new voice in public. Gentle humming at the optimal pitch level is very effective in securing tone focus for outside practice.

5. After the supraoptimal pitch level and mask focus are definite, the patient is directed to drop the pitch level to the optimal pitch level. Conversation is to be maintained at this optimal pitch level which is well focused and comfortable.

6. The patient then practises on developing the optimal pitch range. This range is a variation of tones above and below the optimal pitch level and prevents the voice from being monotonous, lifeless, colorless, or flat. The tone focus must always be maintained in the anterior oro-naso-pharynx or mask area. This practice is as follows: a) The patient starts on the highest comfortable pitch level in the optimal pitch range and continues down the pitch range, using one of the nasal exercises "me-me one" or "um-hum one" (personal choice). This exercise is repeated 10 times on each pitch level, such as "me-me one, me-me two, me-me three," etc. b) The patient prolongs the sound "me" and vocalizes from the top to the bottom of the range, smoothly and easily, and then reverses the procedure, going from the bottom to the top. c) The patient reads aloud using the optimal pitch range. d) The patient speaks in spontaneous, unprepared conversation utilizing this pitch range first in therapy and then outside of therapy. This carry-over to normal routine situations is challenging and a vital step in the creation of a new voice.

During the first therapy session, the optimal pitch level may appear but briefly and then flicker out. The patient is generally unable to maintain the new pitch level once the session is over. In fact, within a few moments following the first session, the new pitch level is lost. During the next few sessions, the pitch level may be held for longer and longer periods of time. Generally the pitch pattern can be maintained during mechanical exercises in the office, carried over into conversation in the office, and then transferred into outside situations involving spontaneous speech. Regressions and plateaus often occur in maintaining the optimal pitch level in mechanical exercises or conversational speech, in the office and outside the office.

EAR TRAINING

Ear training is one of the most essential elements in vocal rehabilitation (Van Riper and Irwin, 1958). Anderson (1961, p. 71) believes: "In general, ear training should precede voice training." Since the vocal cords cannot be touched or viewed by the patient, he must rely basically upon auditory monitoring of vocal cord function. Intensive ear training is carried on until the optimal pitch is isolated, identified, discriminated, and established. For this training the patient uses recording devices which provide an instantaneous comparative playback (Bell and Howell Language Master). Thus, automation has been instrumental in expanding the field of vocal rehabilitation. It enables the patient to instantaneously compare and monitor the habitual and optimal pitch levels. We employ intensive and extensive use of automation with highly directed positive vocal guidance that adheres closely to the needs of each patient's voice.

Automated equipment is appropriate and advisable as a helpful device for home use. The Language Master allows precise carry-over from the therapy situation to the patient's practice sessions at home. Home practice is more frequent of necessity than office sessions, and is therefore extremely pertinent to the carry-over of the very elements of voice presented and practised under guidance in the office. The optimal pitch level and tone focus is recorded on an automated card in the office by the patient and is used as an example for comparative purposes by the patient during practice at home.

Moses, in a discussion (Flower, 1959), opposes tape replay. Moses believes that voice playback has a critically adverse effect upon the patient and should not be used. Henrikson (1943) reports variable reactions to tape replays. Henrikson and Irwin (1949) believe that voice recording is a legitimate and valuable aspect of voice training.

Tape replays have always been employed in our therapy and have been of great use and assistance in altering the individual's inadequate voice production. If the patient does not hear the inadequate voice, he is not cognizant of a need or a desire to alter the voice. Nearly all patients were unable to idenitfy their own voice from a replay of the original recording. Comments such as "Whose voice is that?" "That's not my voice," "It sounds awful," were representative. Of the 1261 patients seen, only a minuscule number initially objected to the tape replay of their voices, but this negative reaction was minimal and temporary. It is surprising to realize that little mention is made in the literature of the effectiveness of automated tape replay in vocal rehabilitation.

PHYSICAL CHANGES

Certain physical and/or mental factors may occur as the result of pitch change. The therapist must prepare the patient for these natural reactions. The attempt to alter the pitch level and range almost always results in one or more of the following: vocal-chinning (raising the chin), furrowing of the forehead, body posturing while sitting or standing, and posturing of the tongue or jaws. Mental sets such as imagery of tone placed against the teeth, lips, or hard palate, placed in the nose, or a combination of these areas are common. These vocal reactions are normal and transient. As the new pitch range is established, a feeling of irritation or burning in the soft palate, a tug or pressure within this area, tension under the mandible, and possibly tension extending to the ears and dryness of the mouth may occur. These are also entirely normal and transitory.

Quality

Closely related to the change in pitch level is the resulting change in quality. With the elevation of the pitch and the use of nasalized exercises for mask-tone focus, hoarseness and its related symptoms disappear. The use of nasalized vowels is noted by Pahn (1964), who explains that functional dysphonia patients are unable to produce their habitual distorted quality while vocalizing nasalized vowels.

Following the establishment of the optimal pitch level and range, if the tone focus has too much nasal or upper resonance, a more balanced oro-, naso-, laryngopharynx resonance is sought at this time. Again, a highly positive, direct approach by the therapist is accorded the patient.

Volume

Voices that are too low in pitch level and range have little carrying power. In order to gain intelligibility and required volume for various situations and people, effortful vocal production may ensue, resulting in vocal misuse.

In the initial stages of vocal rehabilitation, limited volume is produced. More often than not, patients find that it is essential to increase the volume in order to maintain the new pitch level and firm focus. This increased volume at the higher pitch level is non-injurious to the vocal folds as long as the tone focus is correct. As soon as the optimal pitch level and mask focus are reached, a marked increase in volume occurs. When this pitch level and focus are firmly controlled, it is often necessary to reduce the volume since the new voice now has too much carrying power. The effortful volume needed for the old voice is no longer required for the new voice.

Breath Support

With the correct tone focus, pitch, and midsection breath support, the patient who needs volume uses projection, not shouting. Shouting is effortful and creates vocal abuse. Projection of the voice requires little effort and is not injurious to the vocal folds but facilitates a great amount of carrying power and intelligibility.

Most patients seen have had clavicular or extreme upper chest breathing. We have found that this type of breathing may lead to pharyngeal and laryngeal tensions and may interfere with voice production.

Concentration on midsection breath support is begun only when the tone focus and optimal pitch level have been firmly established, since good midsection breath support with an inadequate pitch level and a poor tone focus is highly punitive to the voice and accelerates the destruction of the voice. Also, the additional variable of midsection breath support is disconcerting and distracting to the patient. Even at this time, the new voice often does regress, and the tone focus and optimal pitch level become uncertain, but within a short period of time the voice will respond and be supported by midsection breathing.

After ascertaining that the patient has upper chest or clavicular breathing, the therapist demonstrates this type of breathing and midsection breathing for the patient. The patient, in a standing position, is asked to count from one to ten with one hand on his chest and the other hand on his abdomen, in order to realize that he is using upper chest breathing. When the patient accepts the fact that he is breathing incorrectly for speech, he is ready for the following steps. Each step must be mastered before going to the next step.

1. Lying in a supine position, the patient places one hand flat on his abdomen and the other hand at his side at the waist and breathes normally through the nasal cavity. The patient is instructed not to take a deep breath or an irregular breath.

2. When the patient feels the midsection moving up and down, or in and out, and the waist slightly expanding on the side, he is directed to follow the same procedure in a standing position.

3. The patient does the same in a sitting position. This position is the most difficult; the supine position is the easiest.

4. The patient repeats the first three steps, attempting to monitor his breathing without feeling the process with his hands.

5. The patient again repeats the first three steps, this time breathing through the oral cavity instead of through the nasal cavity, first monitoring with his hands, and then removing his hands.

6. The patient, in a sitting position, begins to combine breathing and speech by using mechanical exercises. The patient is directed to continue this activity in as many circumstances outside the office as possible, using spontaneous speech during interpersonal conversations. For this latter portion, the patient attempts to monitor his breathing without direct manual contact with the midsection. If this is not possible, the patient is instructed to place one hand on the waist.

Because of the pressure of circumstances, the commitment of time and expense, the lack of patience, and the satisfaction with the results already acquired, vocal rehabilitation may be terminated before midsection breathing is attempted. Though nearly all patients are in need of midsection breath support for the production of voice, it is sometimes appropriate to settle for a clear easy tone which allows for a basically effortless, durable voice for routine speaking.

We have found with most patients that lack of midsection support affords little projection of voice and makes a difference in ease of production, quality, and longevity of voice for the professional speaker. For those who use their voices as a livelihood for artistic purposes, and have need of a comfortable voice, midsection breath support becomes essential.

Rate of Speech

The rate of speech often needs to be slowed during the initial stages of vocal rehabilitation. The need to concentrate upon the process rather than on the content—the concern of the "how" instead of the "what"—may be emphasized. During the practice on mechanical exercises and until the completion of correct tone focus, optimal pitch level and range, and midsection breathing, rate may be a dominant factor.

The suggestion that the patient slow down his rate is of no consequence without direction; the patient does not comprehend or understand the relationship between rate and voice.

Frequency and Duration of Therapy

The frequency and duration of vocal rehabilitation may be posited upon the following factors: the extent and severity of the vocal problem (chronic or acute, long term or short term); the extent of the lesion; the factor of surgery; how quickly the patient wants to overcome the problem; the cooperation of the patient; the amount of time that can be alloted to therapy sessions and outside practice; the patient's ability to pursue or follow vocal directions (ability to monitor the pitch, tone focus, and breath control); and the financial situation of the patient.

Functional misphonias can usually be resolved within one to six months, which should be considered short term therapy. The majority require three to six months. A small percentage requires only a month or two, and some need only a few sessions. In contrast, another small group requires a protracted period of vocal rehabilitation, ranging in time from six to 12 months, which is considered long-term therapy. We found that about 84 percent of patients required short-term therapy and 16 percent required long-term therapy.

For organic dysphonia, the percentage requiring long-term therapy was slightly higher. Approximately 28 percent required long-term therapy, while 72 percent achieved a resolution with short-term therapy.

The majority of voice cases may appear to be short term, because the vocal diagnosis is simple. However, alteration of the vocal image and of the habitual vocal pattern is not simple.

At the outset of therapy, it has been found most appropriate to begin with basically two and sometimes three sessions per week, in order to inculcate and establish new vocal patterns and practices. This intensive therapy is necessary in the beginning; infrequent meetings find the patient forgetting or ignoring the therapy and possibly dropping out of therapy due to lack of comprehension or lack of results. As the patient is able to master the various elements of voice, and the initial vocal symptoms begin to disappear, the patient is given more responsibility to handle his vocal progress. Frequency of meeting is diminished in this order: weekly, semimonthly, monthly, six-weeks, and a follow-up three months later. After this the patient is requested to call if any difficulty occurs.

Sessions may be long or short, depending on the above factors. If the sessions are long in the beginning, as the frequency of meetings is diminished, the length of the session is also reduced.

Patients vary in their ability to understand and master a new voice. Some progress more quickly than others at the beginning; of this former group, a few may regress following a fast start. A difference also occurs in ability to grasp various elements of vocal rehabilitation, such as mastery of breath support, pitch level, and tone focus.

Assurances of any kind regarding the time required for vocal rehabilitation cannot be given to the patient prior to therapy. The prognosis can be given during the initial evaluation and an approximate length of time and frequency of sessions outlined. The patient per se will determine how intensive and extensive the therapy need be.

Although therapy is not an overnight affair, the therapist has an obligation to direct and assist the patient to overcome the functional misphonia or the organic dysphonia within the shortest possible period of time. However, the solution to a voice problem is not as simple as it may appear. The number of failures in vocal rehabilitation has borne out that fact. Although pitch change was a basic factor for most patients in the alleviation of the hoarseness, fatigue, or irritation of the throat, there is much more to vocal rehabilitation than altering the pitch range, tone focus, and breath support.

Group Therapy

Vocal rehabilitation has been attempted in groups. Group therapy appears to be effective when used on a limited basis to ventilate feeling states and vocal concepts. The best groups are those composed of patients in varying stages of vocal rehabilitation. Patients who have completed therapy are persuasive in explaining and convincing current patients to respond positively toward vocal training. Group therapy alone or as a mainstay has been found to be totally ineffective. Group therapy as an adjunct has been found to be helpful.

Science and Art

Some people think that vocal rehabilitation is an art, a mystic given to those few who can master its elements. Others of us believe that vocal rehabilitation is an art and a science. It is a science in that it can be duplicated, repeated on any level anywhere, by anyone who has the background, qualification, and ability to pursue the given points of view. Within the science, the practice of vocal rehabilitation becomes an art. This occurs in the therapist-patient relationship and the ability of the therapist to direct the patient to the correct pitch level, tone focus, and other elements, to explain the vocal image and other vocal concepts, and to guide the patient from one element to another in therapy at the right time.

Problems of Vocal Rehabilitation

Two problems are apparent in the area of vocal rehabilitation. One is that the vocal retraining should be done by someone who is qualified in that area—a voice therapist—not a speech therapist. Voice therapy is a specialty, which requires additional training and interest in this aspect of rehabilitation (Williamson, 1946; Froeschels, 1948). The other problem is that few voice therapists, although trained in vocal analysis, are themselves able to produce a good voice, the type of voice which they are supposedly directing their patients to produce. In combination, many of those practising speech therapy have, as part of their caseload, taken on voice cases when they themselves have voice problems and little vocal knowledge.

The question of leadership in the program of vocal rehabilitation is often academic and of little pertinence to the therapy. Leadership is determined by the situation and circumstances, not by any invariable pattern. Some medical authorities believe that the laryngologist should always direct the program (Moses, 1948; Ferguson, 1955; Tarneaud, 1958; Garde, 1961; Brodnitz, 1962; Zaliouk, 1964). The difficulty in this is that the laryngologist usually does not have the time, the training, the patience, the interest, or the ability to do vocal therapy. Moses (1948), Brodnitz (1954), Ferguson (1955), Tarneaud (1958), and others who espouse the point of view that the laryngologist control and supervise vocal retraining emphasize the fact that the field of laryngology is currently unprepared, unsuited, and unaware of the relationship between vocal misuse and dysphonia and the treatment for dysphonia. These authors agree that vocal misuse needs to be treated by vocal retraining. Although Tarneaud (1958, p. 10) believes in physician-directed programs, he admits: "If they have not learned to appreciate the sonorousness, physicians are obviously not in a position to control vocal manifestations." (Sonorousness is defined by Tarneaud to refer to pitch, intensity, ring, cadence, and melodic characteristics of voice.)

In this author's experience, the voice therapist has directed the vocal rehabilitation, after the laryngologist has done the initial laryngeal examination and reported his diagnosis. Throughout the therapy program, the voice therapist has sent periodic progress reports to the laryngologist for an up-to-date medical file. The patient is periodically reexamined by the laryngologist so that he may visually determine the progress of vocal rehabilitation.

Thus, combined efforts by the laryngologist and the voice therapist, each contributing as much as possible from diverse abilities and training, has afforded the most success. Brodnitz (1966, p. 270) states: "More and more laryngologists have begun to realize that voice therapy by a well-trained clinician should form an integral part of the over-all plan of treatment of these patients."

The ear of the voice therapist is like the eye of the laryngologist—both vital in the examination of the patient. It has been estimated that it takes ten years to develop a good ear for vocal evaluation. Brodnitz (1963) writes that the trained ear of the therapist is the best means of determining results of vocal rehabilitation.

Progress in Vocal Rehabilitation

Progress in vocal rehabilitation is highly individual. Some patients are able to bring patience and insight to therapy along with a desire to practise and to rehearse a new voice pattern and quickly overcome self-consciousness. These patients are adept at reforming their vocal problem. Other voice patients are slow to change their defective vocal patterns. They are lethargic about altering the voice, lacking in insight and ability to modify their usual routine, and not willing to listen to the therapist. Although no definite means of prognosticating the rate of progress exist, generally, progress depends on the following factors: 1. acceptability of the problem, 2. understanding of the variables influencing the problem, 3. motivation, and 4. special needs of the patient.

ACCEPTABILITY OF PROBLEM

Acceptability of the problem begins with the reason the patient comes in for a vocal evaluation and vocal rehabilitation. Strong physician referral may activate a patient to seek vocal rehabilitation, whereas anything less than a whole-hearted endorsement of the program by the physician may result in an abbreviated and all too brief program that leaves the vocal problem basically unresolved. Unfortunately, many physicians are unaware of vocal rehabilitation or have misunderstandings of the process. Ferguson (1955) states that laryngologists are not knowledgeable about voice problems. Many are not cognizant of the symptoms of vocal misuse or that vocal rehabilitation will alleviate and eliminate the symptoms their patients describe. Many believe that vocal rehabilitation is a long-term, expensive procedure that seeks to alter the personality structure of the individual. Therefore, many voice problems are not referred and treated by vocal rehabilitation. Tarneaud (1958, p. 8) writes:

> All laryngological consultation rooms are crammed with people suffering only from functional dysphonias or dysodias, wrongfully considered as chronic laryngitis and treated as such, without ever succeeding in suppressing the hoarseness and in fully restoring the voice.

Basically, most voice patients come in because of physician referral, but only a small number of laryngologists refer. Often the physician utilizes many other means of treatment and uses vocal rehabilitation only as a last resort. Occasionally, the patient himself will request a different type of treatment that will eliminate the symptoms on a permanent basis. Family and friends may suggest that something be done about the voice; word of mouth by former patients may initiate a patient to seek a vocal consultation.

Many cases of functional misphonia go unrecognized for a period of years because of their gradual onset. Some are postpubertal problems in that the natural voice was never utilized following the voice change. Sensory and/or auditory symptoms may become severe before the patient seeks medical attention. Some fear cancer. The existence of a voice problem often comes as a surprise. The patient does not relate the symptoms to the misuse of voice. The use of the voice is thought to be a natural function, one that does not require direction or training. They are unaware of how they sound, of the extent of their impaired tone, of the fact that the voice can be easily and comfortably used. Impairment of the voice is attributed to smog, allergy, postnasal drip, smoking, tensions, and nerves. They view laryngitis as a commonplace occurrence. Despite strong physician referral many wait in the hopes that the problem will disappear until the functional misphonia is severe or until an organic dysphonia has developed.

Patients with voice problems react quizzically to the findings they are in need of voice therapy. "But I have always used my voice this way." "Why doesn't —— need voice therapy? He does the same as I do . . ." "I sounded like this as far back as I can recall," or "If anyone would have told me I would have to learn to talk all over again at my age, I'd have said he was crazy, but now . . ."

Some of the patients with a most severe functional misphonia or organic dysphonia may resist vocal therapy because of their subjective overview regarding what is a good or bad tone. They equate a hoarse, husky, or gruff voice as being attractive, charming, masculine, or feminine. A tape replay of the patient's voice is often instrumental in alerting the patient to his vocal deterioration. An explanation of the difference in hearing oneself through the bones of the head as compared to air conduction is in order.

Before production of voice can be altered the patient must be aware of the reasons for change. Therefore, a basic grounding in what is the problem and what is producing the voice problem must be understood by the patient. To gain acceptance of the voice problem, the patient must accept the therapist as able and knowledgeable and feel confidence from the therapist that the problem can be solved.

Securing the understanding, if not the assistance, of a patient's spouse, parent, or other close relative or friend for vocal rehabilitation is done in the initial or early stages of therapy when possible. One such meeting is usually sufficient. Acceptance of vocal rehabilitation by any of these individuals makes for a more cooperative patient and for an easier and better carry-over to home and other outside situations.

In summary, the patient must accept the fact that he has a functional misphonia or organic dysphonia, that the symptoms are caused by the voice problem, and that vocal rehabilitation will eliminate the symptoms and the problem.

VARIABLES OF VOCAL PROBLEM

The many variables influencing the progress of vocal rehabilitation must be understood by the patient. Most of these revolve around the use, control, and acceptance of the new voice. The new voice is often felt to be a physical strain as the musculature of the laryngeal and pharyngeal area, as well as the midsection, is being realigned. The patient must understand this is a temporary condition. Mental vocal discipline stress is inherently involved in the acceptance and the maintenance of the new voice. The patient must internally accept the new voice. He must understand the factors of the vocal image and its influence upon the utilization of the new voice. At times he may find it necessary to explain to his family and close friends the need and use of the new voice; only the closest of associates or friends may be aware of the patient's new voice. Most colleagues, acquaintances, and the general public are totally unaware of any change in voice. The one exception is the recognition by some of the new voice when heard on the telephone. The patient, himself, is quite cognizant of a new vocal pitch level and range, new tone, and new tone focus. The patient is quite incredulous that the new voice creates little reaction from others. The essential reaction to the new voice is by the patient to his own new voice.

The patient must understand that many factors can episodically affect and influence the voice. These include air-conditioning, chlorinated water, and a gym workout, all of which may contribute to hoarseness; certain foods or beverages which may change the vocal quality; sexual orgasm, body and/or mental fatigue, feeling states, and the morning voice which may result in a lowered pitch. Regardless of the understanding of correct vocal production, the patient must observe good vocal hygiene, avoiding vocal abuse. As one patient commented, "I shouted him down. I won the argument, but I lost my voice." To summarize, the patient must understand the multifarious variables influencing progress, which include effects on the voice, vocal image, vocal hygiene, and acceptance of the new voice.

MOTIVATION

Motivation may be categorized into several aspects, such as need to change, desire to change, willingness to change, and ability to change. The need to change is often based upon the immediate concrete need for a durable comfortable voice which is necessary to fulfill business or professional needs. The desire to change may be based on aesthetic demands from within the individual or from society. The realization of his vocal disorder as exemplified through hoarseness or breathiness or other tonal impairments may motivate the patient to seek a new voice. If the culture in which the individual resides sponsors or approves a given tone, though it be a symptom of dysphonia, this aspect of motivation is negated. If the symptoms of misphonia are progressively cumulative, the individual may either desire or need to change, depending upon the severity of the symptomatology and the condition of the vocal folds. When an organic dysphonia prevails, the patient may be activated to attempt reduction of the growth through vocal rehabilitation in order to avoid surgery. If and when surgery does occur, the patient is actuated to retrain the voice so that a recurrence of the original growth does not develop. Brodnitz and Froeschels (1954) stated that surgery traumatizes; we have found that surgery traumatizes and then motivates.

Willingness to change may be based upon multiple factors. The patient must be willing to devote time for therapy sessions and for outside practice, must be willing to change his vocal patterns, and must be willing to follow the directions of the therapist. The involvement of the patient with problems other than voice will hinder progress. Distraction is a basic factor in slowing down the vocal rehabilitation progress.

Patient effort varies considerably in the vocal rehabilitation program. Some patients afford little effort and secure little results; some patients afford little effort and secure fine results. Some patients afford much effort and achieve only limited results at first; continued effort by these patients often affords excellent results.

The patient must have the ability to change, to alter the habitual vocal patterns. One of the key demands is that of "vocal awareness." The patient often characterizes himself as having a "tin ear" and as being unable to carry a tune or hum a melody, having been vocally traumatized from childhood. The patient is afraid that his "tin ear" will prevent him from benefiting from vocal rehabilitation. Assurance and early therapeutic proof should dispel the patient's fear and anxiety. It is a myth that a good musical ear is needed to improve the voice. Training and specific direction, together with tape replays and consistent practice, are necessary to create an awareness of the proper pitch level and tone focus.

Too often the patient is not afforded essential, specific, and direct vocal training, and, therefore, blames the failure of vocal rehabilitation upon his poor musical ability. Eisenson, Kastein, and Schneiderman (1958) note that voice defectives appear to be inferior in pitch discrimination, yet fifteen of their patients receiving therapy showed significant gain in pitch discrimination. Riker (1946) notes that the ability to judge pitch is not confined to specially trained or musically talented individuals. A recent study by Davis and Boone (1967, p. 814) concludes that: "Voice patients are probably similar to the normal population in their ability to discriminate pitches and remember tonal sequences." This study presents a much needed review of the topic of pitch discrimination among normal and dysphonic patients.

SPECIAL NEEDS

Some patients undergoing vocal rehabilitation have special needs which must be considered. Sometimes a patient is available for a limited period of time. That period may be so short that it is imperative to have intensive therapy so that an extensive revision of the voice can transpire. Some patients who are singers must perform regardless of the state of their voice. If these individuals are misusing their speaking voices, an improvement in the speaking voice will improve the singing voice. A fair number of singers have poor speaking voices. Need to correct the singing voice (tone focus, pitch range, and breathing), as well as the speaking voice is imperative for some of these individuals (Cooper, 1970b).

Some professional speakers, including radio and television announcers, actors and actresses, desire and need a highly polished and versatile voice (Cooper, 1969). The artistic voice is far more demanding in practice, in control, and in essence (Cooper, 1970e).

A few patients have need of a loud, carrying voice. These include factory supervisors, referees at ball games, and others who must be heard above noise. Other patients, such as teachers, telephone operators, trial lawyers, ministers, and executives, must have an extremely durable voice. In the vocal rehabilitation program, emphasis is placed on providing the type of voice which will meet the special needs of each patient.

The extent of voice disorders among the geriatric population from clinical experience indicates an extensive problem. These patients generally are not referred for treatment until they demand symptom relief other than palliative and temporary measures (Cooper, 1970d). This segment of the population will be more often referred as the awareness of vocal rehabilitation and its resolution of functional misphonia and organic dysphonia becomes recognized by the laryngologists and other physicians.

The incidence of voice problems in elementary school children is estimated to be seven to 10 percent by Baynes (1966), five percent by Frick (1960), and six percent by Senturia and Wilson (1968). Curry (1949) reports that 55 percent of 10-year-olds and 80 percent of 14-year-olds have husky voices; hoarseness is common in elementary and high school children, according to White (1946). Froeschels (1943, p. 130) states: "Many children, especially school children, show symptoms of hyperfunction, and a smaller number exhibit symptoms of hypofunction." Lore (1950, p. 825) adds: "Hoarseness in children is far more widespread than is usually supposed."

The etiology of voice disorders in children is vocal abuse (Murphy, 1967), choral singing (Moses, 1940), poor reading, speaking, and singing (Froeschels, 1943), functional misuse (Manser, 1939), and aggressive behavior (Nemec, 1961). The misuse and abuse of the speaking and singing voice in childhood leads to adult misuse and abuse, according to Pahn (1966).

Cornut and Venet (1966) report that of 50 dysphonic children, 19 mothers and five fathers were dysphonic, also. Our clinical experience with children affirms the existence of some parental voice problems as influencing or initiating the voice disorder in their respective dysphonic children (Cooper, 1970c).

Wilson (1962a and 1962b) outlines the routine orthophonic method of treatment for children and adolescents. O'Neil and McGee (1962) believe that vocal rehabilitation techniques adapted from adults to children are not meaningful. Our experience with dysphonic children indicates that direct vocal rehabilitation is dependent upon the needs and abilities of the child. Parental assistance is often sought as a means of carryover of voice therapy from the office to the home.

The Art of the Therapist

One of the most important aspects in vocal rehabilitation is the personality of the therapist and his relationship with the patient. These factors contribute heavily to the motivation of the patient and to the success or failure of the program. Rapport must exist between therapist and patient. The therapist develops this by being aware of the fears and anxieties of the patient regarding his vocal recovery. The therapist must give constant reassurance that the patient is not unique with his voice problem, that many others have recovered from a similar problem; the patient is given the opportunity to meet or talk with by phone, if he so desires, others who are in therapy, or who have completed vocal therapy. The patient must also be assured that all of his questions concerning his voice and vocal rehabilitation are pertinent and meaningful. The willingness of the patient to expose his vocal confusion must never be slighted. The therapist must attempt to answer all questions posed concerning the vocal problem as clearly and definitively as possible.

The therapist must also be extremely sensitive to

the patient's feelings and total personality. At one extreme, the therapist can push too hard or too far and make the patient a vocal hypchondriac, afraid to use his voice and overly conscious of every vocal nuance or sensory discomfort from the change in voice. On the other hand, the therapist can push minimally causing vocal progress to be limited, and the patient becomes discouraged and discontinues therapy. The therapist must be able to determine the amount of pressure to apply to each patient in order that vocal progress continues as smoothly, as easily, and yet as quickly as possible.

Unless it is enjoyable and satisfying, vocal rehabilitation becomes and is a monotonous and boring affair. The therapist must possess authentic enthusiasm, must be fresh in feeling, must have insight, and must have patience. Transference may occur in vocal rehabilitation, but it is seldom necessary to discuss it.

Rapport and empathy are vital, but without real vocal direction for the patient, vocal progress is merely verbalized and not realized. The personality of the therapist can be a decisive factor in affecting the program of vocal rehabilitation, but the therapist must also be knowledgeable and able in vocal retraining. Wolberg (1967a and 1967b) discusses qualifications of the therapist, such as warmth, empathy, sensitivity, and flexibility.

The voice therapist must also be able to predict the progressive stages in the process of vocal rehabilitation and the symptoms of progress, which again affords reassurance to the patient. There appear definitely to be stages within the patient's own vocal rehabilitation recovery. Initially the patient is unable to grasp the variables for the new voice and a control of the new voice. Realization occurs in that the patient needs mechanical exercises, a great deal of ear training, and a new vocal concept. In the second stage, vocal rehabilitation becomes a laborious and demanding process which involves constant awareness and vocal activity within the therapeutic situation and outside the office. The third stage is the acquisition of a new voice, acceptance of it, use of it, and control of it under all circumstances. The patient now generally understands the process and is at the point of making the new voice automatic.

Reasons for Failures in Vocal Rehabilitation

One of the most vital aspects of vocal rehabilitation is a topic seldom reviewed and less considered; the failures we confront in our practice of vocal rehabilitation. We cite our successes and discuss the reasons for them. We deplore our failures, but we do not explore the multiple factors contributing to the "cancellation" or the straightforward dropout of a patient.

Most patients drop out of therapy during the first stage of vocal rehabilitation. They are not able, willing, or concerned enough to undergo the *process* of vocal rehabilitation. They find the exercises do not meet their preconceived idea of vocal rehabilitation, are not intellectually stimulating, and do not provide an immediate resolution of the problem. Their philosophy seems to be "Tomorrow is too late and today is not soon enough." Some discontinue because malignancy is not present. Others feel that vocal retraining is for a professional person who needs an artistic voice and not for the average person who uses his voice routinely. Vocal retraining is considered a luxury item and basically irrelevant to their norm of living. Some also believe that they are unpleasantly unique if they begin or continue vocal retraining. Some have cited the cost as the reason for terminating or not beginning therapy. Personality conflict has been an inconsequential factor.

Partial vocal success can be disastrous. In functional misphonia, the laryngologist's favorable report on the improved condition of the cords, or in organic dysphonias, the report of a reduced lesion, may be a motivating factor in the continuation of vocal rehabilitation. In other patients, the improvement noted by the laryngologist results in a discontinuation of therapy. The patient's fears and anxieties about the condition of the vocal folds and his desire to improve this condition seem to disappear. The laryngologist must be strongly supportive regarding continued therapy or else only a partial resolution of the vocal problem is achieved.

Criteria for Success in Vocal Rehabilitation

Vocal rehabilitation is complete when the following occurs: 1. the patient is free of the visual, auditory, and/or sensory symptoms of functional misphonia or organic dysphonia, 2. the patient is able to produce an efficient voice, and 3. the patient is able to handle regression and thus prevent recurrence of the problem.

SYMPTOMS

The symptoms originally presented by the patient, or those inherent in his voice problem, should be resolved. In the visual aspect, the laryngologist should see smoothly approximating vocal folds, free of redness or edema, or free of the original benign lesion in organic dysphonias.

In the auditory aspect, the patient should have a clear tone with no hoarseness or other deviant quality. In the sensory area, the patient should experience no pain, tension, discomfort, or fatigue during or after speaking.

EFFICIENT VOICE

Vocal therapy is complete when the patient is able to produce the best, most efficient voice possible for him. This voice is one that the patient can control, that is comfortable, durable, easily produced, usually clear, and that can be used under special circumstances if special training were afforded.

ACCEPTANCE OF REGRESSION

Regression occurs during the vocal rehabilitation process and is a normal, natural, and inherent part of all vocal therapy. It is essentially impossible to overcome a voice problem without a vocal regression or a series of such regressions. Combining the elements of voice, such as pitch, tone focus, volume, and breath support, and making this vocal approach natural and automatic (both in the therapy situation and in spontaneous conversation in outside situations) is a difficult task to achieve without periodic or sporadic failures. As therapy nears its final stage, the patient understands the circumstances and conditions of vocal regression, and learns to handle the regressions and overcome them.

If the patient cannot deal with regressions, then a recurrence of the problem is likely. Recurrence is not a matter of purposeful design on the part of the patient. It is a temporary disability to control the recently learned elements of vocal training. Recurrence will also occur if vocal therapy is incomplete; the new voice must be stable and natural, requiring no conscious effort for production.

Occasionally, a patient may experience a recurrence of functional misphonia or organic dysphonia after a period of time following the completion of vocal therapy. Prominent causes of this are upper respiratory infection, severe body fatigue, mental stress, or demanding and unusual speaking situations. Usually only brief vocal therapy is required for these patients.

DIRECT VOCAL REHABILITATION FOR OTHER TYPES OF DYSPHONIAS

Direct vocal rehabilitation as outlined in this chapter can be modified to meet the needs and demands of patients experiencing other types of dysphonias. This list includes functional dysphonias such as nasality, ventricular phonation, falsetto, spastic dysphonia, and hysterical aphonia, and organic dysphonias such as papillomata, vocal fold paralysis, Parkinsonian, partial vocal fold excisions, leukoplakia, and keratosis.

Nasality

Nasality is amenable to direct vocal rehabilitation. It has been pointed out by Williamson (1944) that increased oral resonance, tongue control, and adequate breath control are important factors in the elimination of nasality. Although Sherman and Goodwin (1954) maintain that a lowered pitch level should not be a routine technique for limiting hypernasality, in the cases we have seen, hypernasality has been modifiable by pitch consideration, by using lowered pitch levels as well as Williamson's techniques. We have had success with about 78 percent of patients with nasality. As with all voice training, ear training is a vital aspect. Acceptance of a new vocal image is an important part of the program. Non-nasal vowels [o] [u], [ɑ] should be used to establish an oral sound.

Ventricular Phonation

Ventricular phonation is infrequently seen in a voice practice. Hoarseness is sometimes misdiagnosed as ventricular phonation. The essence of therapy for this type of lesion is location of the optimal pitch level, maintainance of good midsection support, and extensive ear training.

Falsetto

The falsetto voice is more often than not responsive to direct vocal rehabilitation. Bryngelson (1954) reports outstanding success in the retraining of the falsetto voice by direct vocal rehabilitation. Our experience is that the falsetto voice should be first contained to the basal or near-basal range (van Thal, 1967), and then with the acquisition of a new low voice, a changeover to the optimal pitch range must be sought. Vocal psychotherapy is vital. The patient hears the clear natural tones as hoarse or husky and at first is negative to the new voice (Satou and Cooper, 1968). Weiss (1955, p. 214), in a case history, explains: "It took some time and much persuasion to make the patient accept his new and impressive voice." Ferenczi (1926) presents two psychoanalytically oriented falsetto voice cases. Most falsetto cases are resolvable within three to six months; we have had about 79 percent success with falsetto voice.

Spastic Dysphonia and Incipient Spastic Dysphonia

Spastic dysphonia is by far the most trying and difficult of all voice problems. Elimination of spastic dysphonia remains a mystery. Bloch (1965), Heaver (1959), and Arnold (1959) posit a psychiatric basis for this disorder and advise psychiatric treatment plus vocal rehabilitation. Aronson, et al. (1968a and 1968b) indicate that once the condition takes hold it is seldom relinquished. Our experience is similar to Aronson's in that patients with an established pattern of spastic dysphonia are at best subject to containment of some of the symptoms. The percentage of even partial success in eliminating the symptoms remains poor. A much more rewarding outcome in therapy has been afforded those experiencing incipient spastic dysphonia. A review of the patients with incipient spastic dysphonia reveals excellent results with those completing therapy. Our case histories indicate that this condition may be actuated by psychological trauma, physical trauma, and vocal misuse. Ferguson (1955) indicates that spastic dysphonia may have a gradual insidious onset, and that a practised ear is necessary to detect it in the early stages.

This type of syndrome lacks a correct tone focus in the mask and an optimal pitch level and range as well. Easy, relaxed initiation of voice is essential. Breath support is often erratic and forced. Supacek and Lacina (1961) have discussed the effect of spastic dysphonia on the respiratory system. Unless this condition is diagnosed and treated in its early, incipient stages, the chances for recovery are minimized. Considerations that this problem may be in some part neurologically or organically created have been presented by Robe, Brumlik, and Moore (1960) and Aronson, et al. (1968a and 1968b).

Hysterical Aphonia and Dysphonia; Functional Aphonia

Hysterical aphonia was the diagnosis in 23 patients seen by this author. However, it appears more appropriate to define this condition in terms of onset and symptoms into three categories: functional aphonia due to vocal misuse or abuse, a cold, or laryngeal surgery (no psychological reaction); hysterical aphonia and dysphonia due to psychological or physiological trauma, vocal misuse or a cold (followed by psychological reaction). Aphonia is the absence of voice; a whisper is used. Dysphonia is an impaired voice. Psychological trauma may include accidents, divorce, family conflicts, religious conflicts, death, and personal problems. Physiological trauma may include injuries from accidents or surgical procedures. A primary or secondary gain may exist in the loss or impairment of voice.

Hysterical aphonia is a condition infrequently seen. Of nine patients seen, three were treated in therapy; a resolution was effected in two cases. Clerf and Braceland (1942), Jackson (1949), Wolski and Wiley (1965), and Boone (1966) indicate a psychological means of treatment in addition to voice therapy. Sodolowsky and Junkermann (1944) note loss of voice due to cold in the majority of cases. Aronson *et al.* (1964) report cold or flu symptoms preceeding the onset of the voice disorder. Psychiatric attention alone for aphonia is recommended by Barton (1960).

Of 14 patients seen experiencing functional aphonia (six) and hysterical dysphonia (eight), 10 entered therapy. All of these cases were resolved by direct vocal rehabilitation. The treatment of true hysterical aphonia remains a challenging problem for the knowledgeable voice therapist.

The treatment of hysterical aphonia, hysterical dysphonia and functional aphonia is essentially dealt with by direct vocal rehabilitation. The patient is given the assurance and knowledge that the speaking voice does exist as experienced by a series of vocal exercises, such as the "um-hum" or sonorous cough. Discrete exercises emphasizing vowel formation, such as "o, one," "o, two," etc., allows the patient to produce some voice and gain confidence that the voice still exists. Step-by-step recovery programs in vocal rehabilitation are outlined by Bangs and Freidinger (1949 and 1950).

Papillomata

A papilloma may be classified as a peudomalignant lesion, the causation of which remains unknown or the subject of speculation. Papillomata appear to form at the same site on the vocal folds as do nodules and polyps, mainly the anterior third. Cooper (1964) studied the pitch level, intensity, quality, and air-flow rate of patients with papillomata (under the direction of Isshiki). The findings of these subjects were compared to normal subjects in frequency, intensity, quality, and air-flow rate (Isshiki and von Leden, 1964). A review of the methods of treatment for papillomata has been presented by Cooper (1964, 1971). Vocal rehabilitation has been found helpful by Brodnitz (1963) and by this author. Vocal rehabilitation for this lesion is the same as for nodes, polyps, and functional misphonia.

Vocal Fold Paralysis

The treatment of paralytic dysphonia has been reviewed by Moses (1940), Arnold (1962a, 1962b, 1963a, and 1963b), Rubin (1965 and 1967), Lewy (1966), Toomey and Brown (1967), and Boedts, Roels, and Kluyskens (1967). Laryngeal nerve lesions following thyroidectomy result in approximately three percent of voice problems (Moses, 1940). Vocal rehabilitation as a method of treatment for vocal cord paralysis is presented by Froeschels (1944), Froeschels, Kastein, and Weiss (1955), and Cooper (1970f). Arnold (1962b) indicates that a period of six months should be afforded for vocal rehabilitation; Arnold (1963a, p. 386) also states: "Intrachordal injection should not be considered before all possible attempts at vocal rehabilitation by voice therapy have been made." Arnold (1963a, and 1963b) and Rubin (1965a, 1965b, and 1967) have written on intrachordal injection.

Effortful emphasis upon vowels, such as [i], [aɪ], [o], and [u], beginning at the top of the vocal range and descending step-by-step in pitch until the basal range is reached, is a basic method of compelling the vocal folds to close. Forced sustained vocalization of these vowels alternating with staccato production of vowels is essential before normal speech is attempted. Optimal range and level is nearly always lacking in these patients. Definition of the optimal pitch level for the patient must be made and repeatedly used in all speaking situations. Periodic practice sessions throughout the day on the vowelization must be continued until the vocal folds approximate without effortful vocalization. Volume is necessary to approximate the cords and loud vocalization should be encouraged during the early stages of recovery. Normalization of the volume, the tone, and breath support occurs when the voice is obtainable by easy, effortless endeavor. Patients using effortful speech normally object to the loud volume and to the forced effort involved in this technique. The patients are assured that this heightened laryngeal, pharyngeal, and midsection breath support effort is temporary and essential. The length of time for vocal rehabilitation with excellent results lies between six and 12 months. Vocal rehabilitation and intrachordal injection afford good voice results.

Parkinsonian

Parkinsonian speech is seldom referred for vocal rehabilitation. The voice inherent in this condition is often considered secondary if not inconsequential to the affliction itself. Parkinsonian voice problems are difficult to deal with because of the body fatigue and depressed feeling state associated with this condition. The vocal image remains that of the old preaffliction period, and the patient is unable or unresponsive to alter readily or easily that vocal concept now outdated by general body deterioration. Few patients seek vocal assistance and still fewer are able to abide by vocal rehabilitation demands. The prognosis is often poor, although the ability to phonate clearly and easily has been found to remain intact.

Greene and Watson (1968) outline the value of speech amplification in Parkinsonian cases and indicate the variable need for voice training. Canter (1963) reports that the pitch of Parkinsonian patients is not basically deviant; Parkinsonian patients utilized a median fundamental vocal frequency of 129 cps, while normal subjects in the control group were at 106 cps. He also indicates that vocal intensity levels were comparable for the two groups, and the two groups did not differ in speaking rate. Delaini, as reported by Luchsinger and Arnold (1965), found marked monotony of voice in six out of 10 cases. Our experience indicates that the voice is often markedly impaired as regards pitch, tone focus, quality, volume breath support, and rate.

A basal or near basal range occurs, and inaudibility due to an established vocal rate now outmoded is present. The patient is mentally traumatized by the inability to be heard or understood and soon turns to selective communication. The patient attempts to be understood, using normal phonation technique, such as sustained sentences in and about noisy situations. Even within normal context the voice does not carry and is not sustainable. The patient requires a new vocal technique and a new vocal image. Short phrases, frequent breath intake with midsection support, louder volume, and the use of an optimal pitch level and range are essential for audibility and intelligibility.

Partial Vocal Fold Excision

Excision of any lesion, benign or malignant, may well require vocal rehabilitation assistance. Removal of a malignant lesion on the vocal folds can well lead to a dysphonia. Treatment of this type of excision by voice training is appropriate in that the training will prevent irritation or trauma. The same type of vocal rehabilitation technique as utilized for misphonia, or for nodes or polyps, is pertinent.

Leukoplakia and Keratosis

Leukoplakia and keratosis are pseudomalignant lesions that have as their possible causation smoking, alcohol, and vocal abuse (Cracovaner, 1965). Jackson and Jackson (1939, p. 180) also write: "Alcohol, tobacco smoke, vocal abuse, residue of acute infections, chronic laryngitis, dust and syphilis have seemed in many cases to be the cause of precancerous conditions." Brewer and Briess (1960a, p. 462) state:

> Screamers, speakers, or singers nodes have long been reckoned as the wages of voice strain, yet many swollen vocal cords without other evidences of inflammation, polyps, papillomas in the adult, contact ulcers, hyperkeratoses, and leukoplakia, as well as localized edemas and inflammatory areas, can now be traced to specific intrinsic laryngeal muscle dysfunction for their etiology.

Vocal rehabilitation as practised with benign organic lesions, such as nodes and polyps, is essentially the same for leukoplakia and keratosis. Moderate volume is always suggested to patients with these lesions. Brodnitz (1963) and Briess (1957) find that vocal rehabilitation is helpful. Good to excellent results were achieved in our group of 13 leukoplakia and keratosis patients completing therapy.

VOCAL REHABILITATION: SUMMARY AND CONCLUSIONS

Vocal rehabilitation has been in need of a new and definite approach to functional misphonia and organic dysphonia. Brief vocal rehabilitation plus vocal psychotherapy is the essence of this modern and meaningful way to view voice disorders. In order to overcome a functional misphonia or organic dysphonia, it is posited that direct vocal rehabilitation regarding pitch level and range, volume, tone focus, quality, rate, and breath support be considered in isolated elements and then combined into a normal voice after being mastered separately. Automation is extremely useful and meaningful in gaining new vocal acceptance and new vocal patterns and abilities through repetitive directed practice on a consistent basis.

Generally speaking, the onset and development of functional misphonia and organic dysphonias are due to poor vocal knowledge and habits actuated by multiple factors. Understanding of personality needs, cultural demands, and emotional involvements should be considered to whatever degree that is necessary and pertinent for the individual patient.

Direct vocal rehabilitation must be buttressed by

TABLE 23-I
Standards for those Completing Voice Therapy

	EXCELLENT	GOOD	FAIR
VISUAL	No inflammation; cords normal in appearance; no lesion.	Cords basically normal; perhaps slight inflammation.	Some inflammation; reduced lesion.
AUDITORY	Optimal pitch and clear tone 90–100% of the time.	Optimal pitch and clear tone 80–90% of the time.	Optimal pitch and clear tone 70–80% of the time.
SENSORY	No laryngeal or pharyngeal irritation or discomfort during or after speaking.	Slight irritation or discomfort, occasionally.	Some irritation or discomfort either during or after speaking.

TABLE 23-II
Results of those Completing Voice Therapy

	EXCELLENT		GOOD		FAIR		TOTAL
Functional misphonia	233	74.4%	54	72.2%	26	8.3%	313
Contact ulcer	49	88.0%	5	8.0%	2	4.0%	56
Polyps	27	58.7%	9	19.5%	10	21.7%	46
Polypoid Degeneration	23	66.0%	8	23.0%	4	11.0%	35
Nodes	125	70.0%	29	16.0%	24	14.0%	178
	475	72.8%	105	16.7%	66	10.5%	628

many allied areas of learning, and the approach to the problem of misphonia or dysphonia must be patterned upon the patient's needs and problems in conjunction with the therapist's insights and abilities. Direct vocal rehabilitation is requisite for a large number of patients with functional misphonia or organic dysphonia. Vocal therapy plus vocal psychotherapy is the approach. The goal of vocal rehabilitation is to afford the patient a natural voice, one that is comfortable in continued sustained usage, that affords clarity and grace, and fulfills all communicative situations.

Concerning the outcome of direct vocal rehabilitation for those patients completing therapy, the vocal results were judged as excellent, good, or fair. These judgments were based on the three previously discussed attributes representing functional misphonia and organic dysphonia—visual, auditory, and sensory. These criteria are relative and do not apply fully to all patients, since some patients may have experienced a single impaired parameter rather than two or all of these aspects. The final determination of excellent, good, or fair was made in regard to the original parameter of the misphonia or dysphonia that was impaired or disturbed subsequent to its partial or complete resolution. The visual judgment was rendered by a laryngologist; the auditory judgment was made by the therapist and the patient; the sensory judgment was evaluated by the patient alone.

Out of 956 patients seen originally (functional misphonia, nodes, polyps, polypoid degeneration, and contact ulcer only), 273 were seen for an evaluation only (did not elect to enter therapy), 55 entered but did not complete therapy, and 628 completed therapy. The results for these 628 patients are shown in Table 23-II.

Of all patients completing therapy, 83.7 percent of functional misphonia, 73 percent of nodes, 80.4 percent of polyps, 77 percent of polypoid degeneration, and 55.4 percent of contact ulcer were seen for short-term therapy (six months or less). Of functional misphonic patients, 19.2 percent were seen for less than one month of therapy, with 11 percent being rated excellent with less than one month of therapy. Long-term therapy (over six months) for functional misphonia, nodes, polyps, polypoid degeneration, and contact ulcer was quite often successfully concluded with excellent results; 125 out of 141 patients in the long-term therapy group were rated excellent.

Direct vocal rehabilitation with vocal psychotherapy speaks for itself.

BIBLIOGRAPHY

Anderson, V. 1961. Training the speaking voice (2nd. ed.). New York: Oxford.

Arnold, G. 1959. Spastic dysphonia I. *Logos*, 2, 3–14.

———. 1962a. Vocal rehabilitation of paralytic dysphonia. VII: paralysis of the superior laryngeal nerve. *Arch. Otolaryng.*, 75, 549–570.

———. 1962b. Vocal rehabilitation of paralytic dysphonia. VIII: phoniatric methods of vocal compensation. *Arch. Otolaryng.*, 76, 76–83.

———. 1962c. Vocal nodules and polyps: laryngeal tissue reaction to habitual hyperkinetic dysphonia. *J. Speech Hearing Disorders*, 27, 205–217.

———. 1963a. Alleviation of aphonia or dysphonia through intrachordal injection of teflon paste. *Ann. Otol., Rhinol., Laryng.*, 72, 384–395.

———. 1963b. Vocal rehabilitation of paralytic dysphonia. X: functional results of intrachordal injection. *Arch. Otolaryng.*, 78, 179–186.

———. 1963c. Vocal nodules. *N.Y. State J. Med.*, 63, 3093–3098.

Aronson, A., Brown, J., Litin, E., and Pearson, J. 1968a. Spastic dysphonia. I: voice, neurologic, and psychiatric aspects. *J. Speech Hearing Disorders*, 33, 203–218.

———, Peterson, H., and Litin, E. 1964. Voice symptomatology in functional dysphonia and aphonia. *J. Speech Hearing Disorders*, 29, 367–380.

———, ———, ———, and ———. 1968b. Spastic

dysphonia. II: comparison with essential (voice) tremor and other neurologic and psychogenic dysphonias. *J. Speech Hearing Disorders*, 33, 219–231.

Ash, J., and Schwartz, L. 1944. The laryngeal (vocal cord) node. *Tr. Amer. Acad. Ophthal. Otolaryng.*, 48, 323–332.

Baker, D. 1954. Contact ulcers of the larynx. *Laryngoscope*, 64, 73–78.

———. 1962. Laryngeal problems in singers. *Laryngoscope*, 72, 902–908.

———. 1963. Polypoid vocal cord. *N.Y. State J. Med.*, 63, 3098–3099.

Bangs, J., and Freidinger, A. 1949. Diagnosis and treatment of a case of hysterical aphonia in a thirteen-year-old girl. *J. Speech Hearing Disorders*, 14, 312–317.

———, and ———. 1950. A case of hysterical dysphonia in an adult. *J. Speech Hearing Disorders*, 15, 316–323.

Barton, R. 1960. The whispering syndrome of hysterical dysphonia. *Ann. Otol., Rhinol., Laryng.*, 69, 156–164.

Bauer, H. 1963. Die Beeinflussung der Weiblichen Stimme durch androgene Hormone. *Folia Phoniat.*, 15, 264–268.

Baynes, R. 1966. An incidence study of chronic hoarseness. *J. Speech Hearing Disorders*, 31, 172–175.

Bloch, P. 1959. Goals and limits of vocal analysis. *Logos*, 2, 111–118.

———. 1965. Neuro-psychiatric aspects of spastic dysphonia. *Folia Phoniat.*, 17, 301–364.

Boedts, D., Roels, H., and Kluyskens, P. 1967. Laryngeal tissue responses to teflon. *Arch. Otolaryng.*, 86, 562–567.

Boland, J. 1953. Voice therapy for hoarse voice. *J. Okla. State Med.*, 46, 109–113.

Boone, D. 1966. Treatment of functional aphonia in a child and an adult. *J. Speech Hearing Disorders*, 31, 69–74.

Brewer, D., and Briess, F. 1960a. Voice problems. *Med. Times*, 88, 461–464.

———, and ———. 1960b. Industrial noise: laryngeal considerations. *N.Y. State J. Med.*, 60, 1737–1740.

Briess, F. 1957. Voice therapy; part I: identification of specific laryngeal muscle dysfunction by voice testing. *Arch. Otolaryng.*, 66, 375–381.

Brodnitz, F. 1953. Keep your voice healthy. New York: Harper.

———. 1958. Vocal rehabilitation in benign lesions of the vocal cords. *J. Speech Hearing Disorders*, 23, 112–117.

———. 1962. Functional disorders of the voice. *In* Voice and speech disorders. Levin, N., ed. Springfield, Ill.: Thomas.

———. 1963. Goals, results, and limitations of vocal rehabilitation. *Arch. Otolaryng.*, 77, 148–156.

———. 1966. Training of students in the management of disorders of voice. *Asha*, 8, 270–273.

———. 1967. Semantics of the voice. *J. Speech Hearing Disorders*, 32, 325–330.

———, and Froeschels, E. 1954. Treatment of nodules of vocal cords by chewing method. *Arch. Otolaryng.*, 59, 560–565.

Bryngelson, B. 1954. The functional falsetto voice. *Speech Teacher*, 3, 127–128.

Calvet, J., and Coll, J. 1964. Trois cas de masculinisation de la voix par pellets de testosterone. *J. Franc. ORL*, 13, 287–290.

Canter, G. 1963. Speech characteristics of patients with Parkinson's disease: I. Intensity, pitch, and duration. *J. Speech Hearing Disorders*, 28, 221–229.

Cavanaugh, J. 1923. Benign neoplasms of larynx. *Ill. Med., J.*, 43, 59–64.

Clerf, L. 1937. Treatment of chronic laryngitis simplex. *Amer. Acad. Ophthal. Otolaryng.*, 42, 384–391.

———. 1952. Laryngeal disease. *Proc. First Institute Voice Pathology*, Cleveland Hearing and Speech Center, Cleveland, Ohio, 3–7, 15–18.

———, and Braceland, F. 1942. Functional aphonia. *Tr. Amer. Laryng., Rhinol., Otol. Soc.*, 48, 69–82.

Cooper, M. 1964. Vocal manifestations of laryngeal papillomatosis. UCLA: Ph.D. dissertation.

———. 1968. Vocal suicide in the legal profession. *Los Angeles Bar Bull.*, 43, 453–456.

———. 1969. Vocal suicide in the theatrical profession. *Screen Actor*, 11, 8–9.

———. 1970a. Vocal rehabilitation—Current opinion. *Med. Trib.*, 11, 11.

———. 1970b. Vocal suicide in singers, *Bull. Nat. Assn. Teachers Singing*, 26, 7–10, 31.

———. 1970c. Speech disorders and problems—III. *Ped. News*, 4, 27, 48.

———. 1970d. Voice problems of the geriatric patient. *Geriatrics*, 107–110.

———. 1970e. A broadcaster's artistic voice. *Quill*, 58, 19.

———. 1970f. Rehabilitation of paralytic dysphonia. *Eye, Ear, Nose, Throat Monthly*, 49, 532–535.

———. 1971. Papillomata of the vocal folds: a review. *J. Speech Hearing Disorders*, 36, 51–60.

———, and Yanagihara, N. 1971. A study of the basal pitch level variations found in the normal speaking voice of males and females. *J. Communication Disorders*, 3, 261–266.

———, and Nahum, A. 1967. Vocal rehabilitation for contact ulcer of the larynx. *Arch. Otolaryng.*, 85, 41–46.

Cornut, G., and Venet, C. 1966. Les dysphonies chroniques de l'enfant d'âge scolaire. *J. Franc. ORL*, 15, 837–852.

Cracovaner, A. 1965. Premalignant diseases of the larynx. *Pacific Med. Surg.*, 73, 176–180.

Cunning, D. 1934. Benign neoplasms of the larynx. *N.Y. State J. Med.*, 34, 56–58.

Curry, E. 1949. Hoarseness and voice change in male adolescents. *J. Speech Hearing Disorders*, 14, 23–25.

Damsté, P. 1964. Virilization of the voice due to anabolic steroids. *Folia Phoniat.*, 16, 10–18.

Davis, D., and Boone, D. 1967. Pitch discrimination and tonal memory abilities in adult voice patients. *J. Speech Hearing Res.*, 10, 811–815.

Delph, J. 1940. Benign tumors of the larynx. *Quart. Bull. Northwestern Univ. Med. Sch.*, 14, 26–30.

DeQuiros, J., Sisatzky, D., and Tormakh, E. 1960. Consideraciones sobre la evolución y la terapéutica de los nodulos de las cuerdas vocales. *Fono Audiol.*, 6, 39–47.

Douglas, T. 1950. Hoarseness. *Northwest Med.*, 49, 383–385.

Drake, O. 1937. Toward an improved vocal quality. *Quart. J. Speech*, 23, 620–626.

Duncan, M. 1947. Personality adjustment techniques in voice therapy. *J. Speech Disorders*, 12, 161–167.

Eisenson, J., Kastein, S., and Schneiderman, N. 1958. An investigation into the ability of voice defectives to discriminate among differences in pitch and loudness. *J. Speech Hearing Disorders*, 23, 577–582.

Fairbanks, G. 1960. Voice and articulation drillbook (2nd. ed.). New York: Harper.

Ferenczi, S. 1926. Psychogenic anomalies of voice production. *In* Further contributions to the theory and technique of psychoanalysis. London: Hogarth.

Ferguson, G. 1955. Organic lesions of the larynx produced by mis-use of the voice. *Laryngoscope*, 65, 327–336.

Fitz-Hugh, G., Smith, D., and Chiong, A. 1958. Pathology of three hundred clinically benign lesions of the vocal cords. *Tr. Amer. Laryng., Rhinol., Otol. Soc.*, 61, 476–496.

Flower, R. 1959. Voice training in the management of dysphonia. *Laryngoscope*, 69, 940–946.

Frable, M. 1962. Hoarseness, a symptom of premenstrual tension. *Arch. Otolaryng.*, 75, 66–68.

Frick, J. 1960. Incidence of voice defects among school-age speech defective children. *Penn. Speech Ann.*, 17, 61–62.

Friedberg, S., and Segall, W. 1941. The pathologic anatomy of polyps of the larynx. *Ann. Otol., Rhinol., Laryng.*, 50, 783–789.

Froeschels, E. 1943. Hygiene of the voice. *Arch. Otolaryng.*, 38, 122–130.

———. 1944. Experiences of a bloodless treatment for recurrens-paralysis. *J. Laryng. Otol.*, 59, 347–358.

———. 1948. Should the speech therapist be a voice therapist? *J. Speech Hearing Disorders*, 13, 346–350.

———. 1960. Remarks on some pathologic and physiologic conditions of the human voice. *Arch. Otolaryng.*, 71, 787–788.

———, Kastein, S., and Weiss, D. 1955. A method of therapy for paralytic conditions of the mechanisms of phonation, respiration, and glutination. *J. Speech Hearing Disorders*, 20, 365–370.

Gabriel, C., and Jones, D. 1960. The importance of chronic laryngitis. *J. Laryng. Otol.*, 74, 349–357.

Garde, E. 1961. Nodules et polypes des cordes vocales. Considérations nouvelles. *Ann. d'Oto-Laryngol.*, 78, 378–398.

Gardner, W. 1958. Executive's dysphonia: a study of 49 patients. *Cleveland Clin. Quart.*, 25, 177–186.

Glassburg, J. 1925. Throat stiffness and the voice. *Laryngoscope*, 35, 469–472.

Goldman, D. 1967. Management of psychosomatic problems in young adults. *Psychiatry Digest*, 28, 33–37; 39; 42–43; 46.

Goldman, J., and Salmon, U. 1942. The effect of androgen therapy on the voice and vocal cords of adult women. *Ann. Otol., Rhinol., Laryng.*, 51, 961–968.

Gray, G. 1936. Studies in experimental phonetics. Baton Rouge: *State Univ. Louisiana Studies*, 27.

Greene, M. 1964. The voice and its disorders (2nd. ed.). London: Jittman.

———, and Watson, B. 1968. The value of speech amplification in Parkinson's disease patients. *Folia Phoniat.*, 20, 250–257

Grimaud, R., and Bonneville, J. 1964. Anabolisants de synthèse et voix. *Rev. Laryngol. Otol.-Rhinol.*, 85, 734–742.

Hanley, T., and Steer, M. 1949. Effect of level of distracting noise upon speaking rate, duration, and intensity. *J. Speech Hearing Disorders*, 14, 363–368.

———, and Thurman, W. 1963. Developing vocal skills. New York: Holt, Rinehart and Winston.

Harris, H. 1948. Benign lesions of the true vocal cords. *Ann. Otol., Rhinol., Laryng.*, 58, 189–196.

Harris, R. 1960. Comments on a particular type of hoarseness. *Tr. Amer. Laryng., Rhinol., Otol. Soc.*, 63, 182–183.

Heaver, L. 1958. Psychiatric observations on the personality structure of patients with habitual dysphonia. *Logos*, 1, 21–26.

———. 1959. Spastic dysphonia II. *Logos*, 2, 15–24.

Henrikson, E. 1943. A note on voice recordings. *J. Speech Disorders*, 8, 133–136.

———, and Irwin, J. 1949. Voice recording—some findings and some problems. *J. Speech Hearing Disorders*, 14, 227–233.

Holinger, P., and Johnston, K. 1951. Benign tumors of the larynx. *Ann. Otol., Rhinol., Laryng.*, 60, 496–508.

———, and ———. 1960. Contact ulcer of the larynx. JAMA, 172, 511–515.

Holmes, F. 1930. An experimental study of individual vocal quality. *Quart. J. Speech*, 16, 344–351.

———. 1931. The problem of voice placement. *Quart. J. Speech*, 17, 236–245.

Hunt, M. 1906. A discussion on laryngeal disturbances produced by voice use. *J. Laryng., Rhinol., Otol.*, 21, 519–528.

Huyck, M., and Allen, K. 1937. Diaphragmatic action of good and poor speaking voices. *Speech Monogr.*, 4, 101–109.

Imre, V. 1965. Hormondebingte stimmstörungen und ihre behandlung. *International Assn. Logopedics Phoniatrics*, 13, 139–142.

Isshiki, N. 1964. Personal communication. Kyoto Univ., Kyoto, Japan.

———, and von Leden, H. 1964. Hoarseness: aerodynamic studies. *Arch. Otolaryng.*, 80, 206–213.

Jackson, C. 1928. Contact ulcer of the larynx. *Ann. Otol., Rhinol., Laryng.*, 37, 227–230.

———. 1949. Psychosomatic aphonia and ephemeral adductor paralysis. *Laryngoscope*, 59, 1287–1298.

———, and Jackson, C. 1935. Contact ulcer of the larynx. *Tr. Sect. Laryng., Otol., Rhinol., AMA*, 86, 69–88.

———, and ———. 1939. Cancer of the larynx. Philadelphia: Saunders.

Jervey, J. 1946. Contact ulcer of the larynx: a personal experience. *Ann. Otol., Rhinol., Laryng.*, 55, 431–433.

Kallen, L. 1959. What is "optimal" for the human voice? *Logos*, 2, 40–48.

Kelly, H., and Craik, J. 1952. Laryngeal nodes and the so-called amyloid tumour of the cords. *J. Laryng. Otol.*, 66, 339–358.

Kernan, J. 1937. Fundamental pathology of the larynx. *Laryngoscope*, 47, 77–91.

Knight, C. 1901. Vocal nodules. *Tr. Amer. Laryng. Assn.*, 23, 165–173.

Ladefoged, P. 1964. Personal communication. UCLA.

Legget, R., and Northwood, T. 1960. Noise surveys of cocktail parties. *J. acoust. soc. Amer.*, 32, 16-18.

Levin, N. 1962, ed. Benign and malignant lesions of the larynx. *In* Voice and speech disorders. Springfield, Ill.: Thomas.

Lewy, R. 1966. Responses of laryngeal tissue to granular teflon in situ. *Arch. Otolaryng.*, 83, 355–359.

Lindsley, C. 1929. An objective study of the respiration accompanying speech. *Quart. J. Speech*, 25, 45–48.

Lore, J. 1950. Hoarseness in children. *Arch. Otolaryng.*, 51, 814–825.

Loughlin, A. 1920. The voice in speaking and singing. *Quart. J. Speech Educ.*, 6, 8–23; 11–27.

Luchsinger, R., and Arnold, G. 1965. Voice-speech-language. Belmont, Calif.: Wadsworth.

Lynch, G. 1934. A phonophotographic study of trained and untrained voices reading factual and emotional material. *Arch. Speech*, 1, 9–25.

McClosky, D. 1959. Your voice at its best. Boston: Little, Brown.

McGlone, R., and Hollien, H. 1963. Vocal pitch characteristics of aged women. *J. Speech Hearing Res.*, 6, 164–170.

Manser, R. 1939. Voice problems of university students. *Proceedings Amer. Speech Correction Assn.*, 9, 90–102.

Maximov, I. 1965. Les monocordites allergiques circonscrites. *International Assn. Logopedics Phoniatrics*, 13, 143–146.

Meano, C. 1967. The human voice in speech and song (rev. ed.). *Trans.* by Khoury, A. Springfield, Ill.: Thomas.

Mitchell, H. 1943. Tumors of the larynx: a review of 105 cases. *Tr. Amer. Laryng., Rhinol., Otol. Soc.*, 46, 249–268.

Mithoefer, W. 1940. A simple treatment for defects of the singing and of the speaking voice. *Arch. Otolaryng.*, 31, 16–22.

Moore, P. 1957. Voice disorders associated with organic abnormalities. *In* Handbook of speech pathology. Travis, L., ed. New York: Appleton-Century-Crofts.

———. 1971. Organic voice disorders. Englewood Cliffs, N.J.: Prentice-Hall.

Moses, P. 1940. Is medical phonetics an essential part of otorhinolaryngology? *Arch. Otolaryng.*, 31, 444–450.

———. 1948. Vocal analysis. *Arch. Otolaryng.*, 48, 171–186.

———. 1954. The voice of neurosis. New York: Grune & Stratton.

———. 1965. Auditory versus visual diagnosis in laryngology. *Eye, Ear, Nose, Throat Monthly*, 44, 55–56, 58.

Murphy, A. 1964. Functional voice disorders. Englewood Cliffs, N.J.: Prentice-Hall.

Murphy, R. 1967. Hoarseness. *Nova Scotia Med. Bull.*, 56, 177–179.

Myerson, M. 1950. Smoker's larynx: a clinical pathological entity. *Ann. Otol., Rhinol., Laryng.*, 59, 841–846.

———. 1964. The human Larynx. Springfield, Ill.: Thomas.

Mysak, E. 1959. Pitch and duration characteristics of older males. *J. Speech Hearing Res.*, 2, 46–54.

———, and Hanley, T. 1958. Aging processes in speech: pitch and duration characteristics. *J. Gerontol.*, 13, 309–313.

Nemec, J. 1961. The motivation background of hyperkinetic dysphonia in children: a contribution to psychologic research in phoniatry. *Logos*, 4, 28–31.

New, G., and Devine, K. 1949. Contact ulcer granuloma. *Ann. Otol., Rhinol., Laryng.*, 58, 548–558.

———, and Erich, J. 1938. Benign tumors of the larynx: a study of seven hundred and twenty-two cases. *Arch. Otolaryng.*, 28, 841–910.

O'Neil, J., and McGee, J. 1962. Management of benign laryngeal tumors in children: preoperative, operative, and postoperative. *Ann. Otol., Rhinol., Laryng.*, 71, 480–488.

Pahn, J. 1964. Der therapeutische Wert nasalierter Vokalklänge in der Behandlung funktioneller Stimmerkrankungen. *Folia Phoniat.*, 16, 249–263.

———. 1966. Zur Entwicklung und Behandlung funktioneller Singstimmerkrankungen. *Folia Phoniat.*, 18, 117–130.

Peacher, G. 1947a. Contact ulcer of the larynx; I: history. *J. Speech Disorders*, 12, 67–76.

———. 1947b. Contact ulcer of the larynx; III: etiological factors. *J. Speech Disorders*, 12, 177–178.

———. 1947c. Contact ulcer of the larynx; IV: a clinical study of vocal re-education. *J. Speech Disorders*, 12, 179–190.

———. 1961. Contact ulcer of the larynx; a follow-up of seventy patients. *Laryngoscope*, 71, 37–47.

———. 1963. Voice therapy. *N.Y. State J. Med.*, 63, 3104–3107.

———. 1966. How to improve your speaking voice. New York: Frederick Fell.

———, and Holinger, P. 1947. Contact ulcer of the larynx; II: the role of vocal re-education. *Arch. Otolaryng.*, 46, 617–623.

Perkins, W. 1957. The challenge of functional disorders of voice. *In* Handbook of speech pathology. Travis, L., ed. New York: Appleton-Century-Crofts.

Pronovost, W. 1942. An experimental study of methods for determining natural and habitual pitch. *Speech Monogr.*, 9, 111–123.

Riker, B. 1946. The ability to judge pitch. *J. exper. Psychol.*, 36, 331–346.

Robe, E., Brumlik, J., and Moore, P. 1960. A study of spastic dysphonia: neurologic and electroencephalographic abnormalities. *Laryngoscope*, 70, 219–245.

Rousey, C., Moriarty, A., and Ostwald, P. 1965. Diagnostic implications of speech sounds. Springfield, Ill.: Thomas.

Rubin, H. 1965a. Intracordal injection of silicone in selected dysphonias. *Arch. Otolaryng.*, 81, 604–607.

———. 1965b. Pitfalls in treatment of dysphonias by intracordal injection of synthetics. *Laryngoscope*, 75, 1381–1397.

Rubin, H. 1967. Histologic and high-speed photographic observations on the intracordal injection of synthetics. *Tr. Amer. Acad. Ophthal. Otolaryng.*, 70, 909–921.

Russell, G. 1936. Etiology of follicular pharyngitis, catarrhal laryngitis, so-called clergyman's throat; and singer's nodes. *J. Speech Disorders*, 1, 113–122.

Sallee, W. H. 1936. An objective study of respiration in relation to audibility in connected speech. *State Univ. La. Studies*, 27, 52–58.

Satou, A., and Cooper, M. 1968. Psychiatric observation of falsetto voice. *Voice*, 17, 31–33; 35–37; 39; 41.

Schick, A. 1966. Functional therapy in vocal disabilities. *Folia Phoniat.*, 18, 138–143.

Senturia, B., and Wilson, F. 1968. Otorhinolaryngic findings in children with voice deviations. *Ann. Otol., Rhinol., Laryng.*, 77, 1027–1041.

Sherman, D., and Goodwin, F. 1954. Pitch level and nasality. *J. Speech Hearing Disorders*, 19, 423–428.

Snidecor, J. 1943. A comparative study of the pitch and duration characteristics of impromptu speaking and oral reading. *Speech Monogr.*, 10, 50–56.

———. 1951. The pitch and duration characteristics of superior female speakers during oral reading. *J. Speech Hearing Disorders*, 16, 44–52.

Sokolowsky, R., and Junkermann, E. 1944. War aphonia. *J. Speech Disorders*, 9, 193–208.

Supacek, I., and Lacina, O. 1961. Pneumographic findings in cases of hyperkinetic and spastic dysphonia. *Logos*, 4, 19–27.

Tarneaud, J. 1947. Une laryngopathie fonctionnelle: la voix aggravée. *Folia Phoniat.*, 1, 7–14.

———. 1958. The fundamental principles of vocal cultivation and therapeutics of the voice. *Logos*, 1, 7–10.

Thorn, K. 1947. 'Client-centered' therapy for voice and personality cases. *J. Speech Disorders*, 12, 314–318.

Tiffin, J. 1934. Applications of pitch and intensity measurements of connected speech. *J. acoust. soc. Amer.*, 5, 225–234.

Toomey, J., and Brown, B. 1967. The histological response to intracordal injection of teflon paste. *Laryngoscope*, 77, 110–120.

Tucker, G. 1935. Observations on chronic inflammatory lesions of the true vocal cords. *Tr. Amer. Acad. Ophthal. Otolaryng.*, 40, 390–402.

———. 1937. Tumors of the true vocal cords: malignant, benign. *Tr. Sect. Laryng., Otol., Rhinol. AMA*, 88, 171–177.

Van Deinse, J., Dieleman, F., and Drost, H. 1966. La révalidation des troubles de la voix virilisée par des médicaments. *Practica Oto-Rhino-Laryngologica*, 28, 288–293.

Van Riper, C., and Irwin, J. 1958. Voice and articulation. Englewood Cliffs, N.J.: Prentice-Hall.

van Thal, J. 1961. Dysphonia. *Speech Pathology Therapy*, 4, 11–21.

———. 1967. Vocal rehabilitation. *British J. Disorders Communication*, 2, 23–29.

Vennard, W. 1962. An experiment to evaluate the importance of nasal resonance in singing. *International Assn. Logopedics Phoniatrics*, 12, 418–419.

von Leden, H., and Moore, P. 1960. Contact ulcer of the larynx: experimental observations. *Arch. Otolaryng.*, 72, 746–752.

Voorhees, I. 1914. Vocal fatigue in singers and speakers. *Tr. Amer. Acad. Ophthal. Otolaryng.*, 19, 340–348.

Wallner, L. 1954. Smoker's larynx. *Laryngoscope*, 64, 259–270.

Waugh, J. 1929. The significance of chronic hoarseness in adults. *International Clinics*, 3, 60–67.

Weiss, D. 1955. The psychological relations to one's own voice. *Folia Phoniat.*, 7, 209–217.

———, and Beebe, H., eds. 1950. The chewing approach in speech and voice therapy. Basel, Switzerland: S. Karger.

Wendler, H. 1966. Behandlungsergebnisse bei funktionellen Dysphonien. *Folia Phoniat.*, 18, 401–416.

West, R., Ansberry, M., and Carr, A. 1957. The rehabilitation of speech (3rd. ed.). New York: Harper.

Wiksell, W. 1936. An experimental analysis of respiration in relation to the intensity of vocal tones in speech. *State Univ. La. Studies*, 27, 37–51; 99–164.

Williamson, A. 1944. Diagnosis and treatment of eighty-four cases of nasality. *Quart. J. Speech*, 30, 471–479.

———. 1945. Diagnosis and treatment of seventy-two cases of hoarse voice. *Quart. J. Speech*, 31, 189–202.

———. 1946. Symposium on adequacy of training of voice specialists. *Quart. J. Speech*, 31, 145–160.

Wilson, D. 1962a. Voice reeducation of children with vocal nodules. *Laryngoscope*, 72, 45–53.

———. 1962b. Voice reeducation of adolescents with vocal nodules. *Arch. Otolaryng.*, 76, 68–73.

Withers, B., and Dawson, M. 1960. Psychological aspects . . . treatment of vocal nodule cases. *Tex. State J. Med.*, 56, 43–46.

Wolberg, L. 1967a. The psychological management of individuals with speech and hearing problems. Part I/Introduction. *J. Communication Disorders*, 1, 66–74.

———. 1967b. The psychological management of individuals with speech and hearing problems. Part II/Conclusions. *J. Communication Disorders*, 1, 75–84.

Wolcott, C. 1956. Contact ulcer of the larynx. *Ann. Otol., Rhinol., Laryng.*, 65, 816–819.

Wolski, W., and Wiley, J. 1965. Functional aphonia in a fourteen-year-old boy: a case report. *J. Speech Hearing Disorders*, 30, 71–74.

Wright, E. 1954. Contact ulcer of the larynx. *So. Med. J.*, 47, 148–154.

Wyatt, G. 1950. The application of Froeschels' chewing method in the treatment of disorders of the speaking voice. *In* The chewing approach in speech and voice therapy. Weiss, D., and Beebe, H., eds. Basel, Switzerland: S. Karger.

Zaliouk, A. 1963. The tactile approach in voice placement. *Folia Phoniat.*, 15, 147–154.

———. 1964. La restauration de la voix dans les dysphonies hyperkinétiques. *J. Franc. ORL*, 13, 247–265.

PART IV

Speech

24

The Incidence of Speech Disorders

Robert Milisen

Knowledge of incidence of speech disorders is of importance to clinicians as well as to experimenters, but it can serve different purposes today than it did three decades ago. Early workers had to demonstrate the number of people who had disabling speech handicaps before superintendents would hire clinicials and before college presidents would allow courses in speech pathology to be listed in their curricula.

Now that the need for speech rehabilitation has been demonstrated and accepted in most areas, the study of incidence can be directed toward the solution of other problems. Of course, the student clinician should have up-to-date information about the frequency of occurrence of each disorder. Unfortunately, most of our sources do not reflect changes that may have been produced by thousands of members of our profession over the past 30 years. Surely the impact of modern methods of communication that have distributed quantities of information to every village will have created a change in incidence as well as in the mean severity of disorders. Some informal observations of this phenomena have been made. For example, one school system in Indiana found so few stutterers that group therapy sessions were no longer feasible. Another observation made by the author relates to the severity of stuttering among college students at Indiana University. In the past 10 years, few of the university students enrolled in the clinic demonstrated as severe symptoms of stuttering as were seen so frequently 20 and 30 years ago. However, during the summer of 1968 while off campus the author did see some teenagers whose stuttering was very severe. They came from a sparsely populated state where clinical services are not so readily available since many of the towns are small and are separated by many miles.

Regardless of whether or not these observations are indicative of changes in incidence of disorders in the general population, a new need is developing which requires more accurate information. This need grows out of the maturation of the profession. We must be able to measure the impact of speech pathology on the communication skills of the population as a whole. Although we do have emperical evidence relevant to changes that occur in our clients, we do not know whether changes are also taking place in speech of people who are not receiving therapy. Successful prevention is the true basis for measuring our achievement, especially since speech disorders have learning components which can be manipulated.

Assessment of these changes will be dependent on long-term longitudinal studies. Speech samples representative of each type of disorder must be kinescoped and preserved for posterity. More objective measurements of severity such as was demonstrated by Sherman and Cullinan (1960) must be used so a sample of speech evaluated today can be compared objectively to speech 20 years hence.

These studies will require a sizeable investment of money and time since results are so difficult to analyze and compare. Unfortunately, speech behavior can not be represented by such finite numbers as the number of TB patients or the number of cavities in the patient's mouth, since the learning component always effects etiology as well as management. This component imposes its characteristics on speech behavior so that measures will always be represented by areas on a continuum (involving interactions between a speaker and an audience) rather than by finite numbers.

Determining the incidence of speech disorders is not, therefore, a simple matter of counting those who are defective. Speech may be defective in many and complex ways. Nevertheless, speech disorders must be classified if the data are to be presented meaningfully. No system of classification has proved completely satisfactory since the nature and severity of speech deviations are distributed on continua and are, therefore, hard to separate into distinct classes. Each class is really an area on a continuum and therefore is composed of the numerous variations found within the area on the continuum. Unfortunately, many responses fall between classes and are not easily represented. Some of the variables complicating speech disorder classification are as follows:

1. Speech is a dynamic process which makes impossible the establishment of any standard of speech. No sound is made exactly the same way twice even by the same person. The variability increases as the speech pattern becomes more complex and as the situation becomes more difficult. The speech pattern of each individual goes through a constant change from birth to death.

2. Speech may be defective because of the overemphasis or underemphasis of any element of the speech act. Any effort to analyze the speech act into its component elements is bound to lead to a number of artificial divisions which do not really represent the whole of speech. Because the behavior is really on a continuum, the discrete classes provided by a system force the examiner to make arbitrary judgments regarding responses which fall between two classes. The more widely the classes are separated on the continuum, the less descriptive will any class be of the response assigned to it.

3. Speech is a medium of communication and as such involves both a speaker and an audience. In order for speech to be defective, either the audience, the speaker, or both must be reacting to the process of speech in such a way as to interfere with the communication of the content. This interference is frequently unintended and unpleasant.

The amount of attention directed by either the speaker or the listener to speech deviations, which are an aspect of the process of speech, changes constantly. The total changes in listener or speaker responses may take place gradually. Each speech act at any moment is likely to present an either/or condition for each person involved in the act. That is, at any moment each person is reacting either to how one speaks or to what is said. The person is speaking "defectively" at the moment when attention is directed to process (how he is speaking), whereas he is speaking "normally" when attention is directed to content (what he is saying). This complete switch may occur many times during a short conversation. The listener's or speaker's reactions range on a continuum from complete acceptance to complete rejection. Either or both may be disturbed by speech deviations at the beginning of a speaking situation and then become adjusted to them later on, or *vice versa*. Thus, a type of deviating speech may be considered defective at one time by the listener and/or the speaker; however, if adaptation has taken place the deviation may not be reacted to at all. These changes in reaction may occur even though the nature and extent of the deviations may remain relatively constant. Thus a measurement of the extent of a deviation (even if this could be done with mathematical accuracy) would not necessarily indicate the extent of the speech defect, because the deviation is important only as it interferes with communication and is reacted to by the speaker or the listener.

4. The judgments used in determining the incidence of speech disorders have a low reliability and validity. Frequently the judgments have been made by persons who have no training in the scientific method and, what is worse, have little interest in the accuracy of the judgments they are making. This is especially true of questionnaire studies. The investigator is faced with the dilemma of whether to use trained or untrained examiners in determining which deviations may be classified as speech disorders. If only trained examiners are used, the reliability of the judgments will be greater but the validity will be more questionable. If untrained observers are used, just the opposite may be true. This is because the trained observer may report accurately many minor deviations which would seldom attract anyone else's attention and therefore should not be classified as speech defects, whereas the untrained observer may not identify many deviations, but for the most part those he does report will either be severe or will have some particular quality which disturbs him. Pronovost (1951) has

pointed to wide variations in percentages, according to the type of person making the survey, such as nurse or speech teacher.

No experimental work on the incidence of speech defects has been done which has successfully controlled all of the above variables, simply because the task is impossible. One cannot analyze a dynamic whole into a series of parts and then synthesize those parts back into a whole. In spite of these limitations, the incidence of speech disorders can be reported if the reader will use his own common sense and experiential background to modify reports which do not fit his situation precisely. The only alternative is for each person to satisfy his own professional needs by using his own definitions, classifications, and testing methods when studying incidence.

All good clinicians will, to some extent, investigate speech conditions in their own communities, but few will have the time to carry on extensive investigations. Furthermore, if they did, they would be confronted with the same difficult problems which have confronted all previous investigators.

Definition of terms may eliminate at least one source of error. As much as possible, the discussion by the writer will be couched in the terms which follow. A speech deviation refers to any demarcation from the assumed "normal or standard speech pattern." Defective speech refers to a segment of speech behavior which is sufficiently deviant to attract attention to the process of speech, or to interfere with communication or affect adversely either the speaker or listener. A speech defective is one who frequently demonstrates defective speech.

Deviations in speech may involve: 1. articulation—the way a sound is formed; 2. rhythm—the time relationship between sounds in a word and words in a sentence; 3. voice—the sounds produced by the vibrating vocal folds and modified by the resonators and articulators; and 4. language usage—difficulty in comprehending speech of others or in projecting one's own ideas through the medium of speech.

INCIDENCE OF SPEECH DEFECTS IN GENERAL

Estimates of the incidence of speech defects in the general population are few and probably inaccurate. Estimates of the incidence in the school population are more readily available. The White House Conference (1931) reported that seven percent of 10,033 school children in Madison, Wisconsin, who were carefully examined by speech pathologists had defective speech, compared to a median percentage of 6.9 in their questionnaire survey which covered 48 cities. However, the results reported from these cities varied from 21.4 percent (Fresno, California) to 1.0 percent (Philadelphia). Hawk (1945) reported that individual diagnosis of elementary school children in Ohio showed 9.5 percent with defects. Johnson (1942) stated that 10 percent of 30,000 individually tested Iowa school children were judged to have defective speech. Irwin (1948) reported that 10 percent of Cleveland children between kindergarten and grade six were defective in speech. Only 7.7 percent of the children above kindergarten were defective. Mills and Streit (1942) reported 33.4 percent of 1,196 individually tested children in the first three grades of Holyoke, Massachusetts, had speech defects, 12.6 percent of them serious. In the first six grades, 10.1 percent of 4,685 children had speech defects, 4.5 percent of them serious. Blanton (1916) in a personal survey of 4,862 school children in Madison, Wisconsin, and including only those serious enough to be evident to the casual observer, reported that 5.7 percent had speech defects with a gradual decrease from lower to higher grades. He reported a pronounced leveling off at the fourth grade and a sharp decline between the seventh and eighth grades, ascribed to large numbers of children with defective speech leaving school at that time.

The relative number of males and females with speech disorders varies according to the age of the subjects and too often from one study to another. The White House Conference (1931) reported 1.9 speech-defective males to each speech-defective female for the entire school population. Mills and Streit (1942) found 1.8 boys to one girl in the first three grades and 3.3 boys to one girl above the third grade. In an early study, Blanton (1916) found 1.7 males to one female for an entire school population. All workers report more males than females for all age levels, and more speech defectives, both male and female, in the first three grades of school.

Surveys of speech defects in high school and college populations show wider discrepancies, probably because of more varying standards of what constitutes a speech defect at these ages. Carhart (1939), in a questionnaire survey of 405 Illinois high schools, listed as speech defective 23.3 percent of freshmen, 21.0 percent of sophomores, 20.0 percent of juniors, and 17.8 percent of seniors, with a sex ratio of 1.3 to 1.

Evans (1938) found three students or 1.3 percent of 224 grade 9A students defective in speech, with 92 students or 43 percent showing slovenly and inaccurate pronunciation and enunciation. Morris (1939) reported speech defects in 16.8 percent of a random sample of 178 high school sophomores in Kansas City.

Blanton (1921) reported that personal examination showed that 18.0 percent of 2,240 members of the freshman class of the University of Wisconsin "were found to be unable to meet the necessities of English Speech." Six percent of these stuttered, while the remainder exhibited foreign accent, oral inactivity, mispronunciation of "s" and "z," abnormally rapid or slow speech, or severe vocal defects. In contrast to this, Morley (1952) reported an incidence over a 10 year period at the University of Michigan of 3.9 percent with speech disorders. The number of students with defective speech decreased over the years. Half the cases had articulation defects and one-fourth stuttering defects. There was a sex ratio of 2.1 to 1. Partridge (1945) described 47 percent of students at Ohio University as having speech defects, but localisms in pronunciation apparently accounted for the bulk of the cases.

It is certain that a college population is highly selected and not representative of the population as a whole, and since the definition of a speech defect in these studies obviously is as individual as the examiner, it would seem desirable to attempt to study speech defects in a more random sample of the adult population. Carhart (1943) reported that 0.1 percent of draftees in World War I were reported as having defective speech. This varied from 0.23 percent in the longer settled states to 0.02 percent in the recently settled western states. Of the 0.1 percent, well over half were rejected for military service. In World War II, Peacher (1945) has reported that 0.04 percent of men examined between November 1940 and February 1941 were rejected for speech defects. Johnson (1943) estimated there were five to eight stutterers alone per thousand of the draft-age population, so the percentage of draft rejections cannot be considered indicative of speech defects in the general population.

It is obvious that reports of speech disorders in the general population vary so much that it is necessary to attempt a summary statement which may estimate a median incidence. From kindergarten through fourth-grade level, roughly 12 to 15 percent of the children have seriously defective speech. In the next four grades, between four and five percent are seriously defective. General estimates above the eighth grade are based on highly selected samples and therefore the best guess as to the incidence of speech disorders in persons over 14 years of age would be about the same as for the upper elementary grades—four to five percent. This statement is justified by studies of specific disorders which show that little or no change takes place in the speech condition after the child has reached 10 to 14 years of age, unless special therapy is offered.

INCIDENCE OF SPEECH-SOUND DEVIATIONS IN INFANTS

Before presenting information about speech defects and speech defectives, one should study deviations in the child who does not talk or who is in the early stages of developing speech. These deviations are important because they may be the precursors of speech defects to follow. Many deviations—voice quality, pitch, loudness, duration, body movement, and others—have been studied. However, the ones most extensively studied and the ones probably most highly correlated with speech development are the frequency and variety of production of speech sounds, particularly as they are reported by Irwin and his co-workers.

Deviations of this sort can be measured in infants by counting the number of times sounds are made during any unit of time and also counting the number of different sounds or phonemes produced during the same period. These results can be placed in distributions; the results farthest from the mean being the significant deviations.

Irwin (1946), in studying the oral behavior of infants, has shown that the frequency of production of sounds increased until 30 months of age. Irwin and Chen (1946) found that the variety of phoneme types produced also increased until 30 months of age, at which time the average child presented a speech-sound behavior pattern similar to that of an adult. In both studies, at each month the frequency of production as well as the variety of phonemes differed considerably from one child to another.

The variations in infant speech sounds indicate that retardation in frequency of production of speech sounds as well as a reduction in the variety probably are related to retarded speech development and perhaps to the emergence of defective speech. Boys are slower to develop speech and have a greater percentage of speech defects than girls. Irwin and

TABLE 24-I
Deviant Speech-Sound Development Showing Inferior and Median Responses up to 30 Months of Age[1]

BI-MONTHLY AGE GROUP	PHONEME TYPE VARIABILITY AMONG INFANTS		PHONEME FREQUENCY VARIABILITY AMONG INFANTS	
	10TH PERCENTILE	50TH PERCENTILE	10TH PERCENTILE	50TH PERCENTILE
1–2	4.8	6.9	49.9	57.7
3–4	6.9	10.7	53.7	66.4
5–6	7.4	12.4	60.6	72.5
7–8	10.9	14.4	60.4	75.1
9–10	10.6	15.5	65.0	76.0
11–12	11.2	18.5	68.0	90.2
13–14	11.9	17.8	62.9	85.9
15–16	14.3	19.4	68.0	91.3
17–18	15.2	21.2	76.0	97.4
19–20	15.9	23.0	76.3	94.1
21–22	16.2	23.3	77.4	102.6
23–24	20.1	24.6	84.8	110.8
25–26	20.6	26.6	94.8	129.5
27–28	18.9	26.9	103.0	132.0
29–30	23.5	27.0	107.7	148.3

[1] Extracted from O. C. Irwin (1947). Any child who performs in the region of the 10th percentile may be retarded in speech sound development.

Chen (1946) reported that boys tended to be inferior to girls after the second year in the variety of speech sounds produced. Spiker (1951) found girls to be significantly superior to boys from the twentieth to the thirtieth month in the variety of speech sounds produced. Mentally defective children also develop speech more slowly and have more speech defects than do normal children. Irwin (1942) found mental defectives to be inferior in the frequency of production and the variety of speech sounds produced.

Cerebral-palsied children also learn to speak more slowly and have more speech deficiencies. They too were found by Irwin (1952) to be retarded in infancy.

Orphaned children who received a reduced amount of speech stimulation and reinforcement were definitely inferior in both frequency and type of phoneme produced to the infants living in their own homes. Thus the developmental age of speech-sound responses as well as the frequency of usage and the adequacy of production may be closely related to a variety of environmental and organic conditions. It is necessary to observe that none of the conditions can be measured in isolation. The behavior studied is always an interbehavior between a speaker and an audience in which case the speech behavior is always the product of environmental and organic influences.

Speech pathologists, ever alert to materials of use in making an early diagnosis, may find Table 24-I helpful. Only the score results of children functioning in the tenth and fiftieth percentiles are presented here. The data, reported by Irwin and Chen (1946), were gathered in the following manner: A total of 1,622 records was transcribed in the International Phonetic Alphabet from the spontaneous speech of 95 infants throughout a period of 2.5 years. Each record consisted of the sounds uttered on 30 breaths.

To use these for diagnostic purposes (see Irwin, 1947), sounds transcribed from each of 30 breaths should constitute the sample at a given visit and at least two such samples should be at hand before a diagnosis is made.

The developmental pattern presented in Table 24-I can be extended into the upper age levels, at least for articulation skills, by using the Templin (1953 and 1957) and Roe and Milisen (1942) studies.

INCIDENCE OF ARTICULATION DISORDERS

It is difficult to assess the incidence of articulation disorders. Marked differences are not only found between persons, but also within each person. The quality of the individual's speech production will vary with age and situation. Evaluations may vary from day to day and from examiner to examiner. Errors in articulation may vary from complete omission to substitutions to distortions. Reports on incidence, even when they are the result of carefully planned studies, must be recognized as being subject to considerable error.

All children who learn to speak will produce some sounds defectively at the beginning. Speech sounds have not been "learned" when the first word or sentence is forthcoming. This is just a midpoint in a long process. Templin and Steer (1939), reporting on nursery school children, said that none of the 51 children tested made all sounds correctly in all positions. Roe and Milisen (1942), in a study of the articulation of elementary school children found that all of 772 first- and second-grade children tested made at least one error. Not until the third grade were children tested who did not make a single error. The developmental study by Templin (1957) reported age of maturation for all American speech sounds. The age of maturation of a sound was defined as being that age when 75 percent of her subjects could produce the sound correctly. All sounds did not satisfy this criterion until her subjects reached the age of eight. These studies show the tendency of most experimenters to ignore some speech-sound errors in young children, since none of them have reported 80 to 90 percent of all first- and second-grade children to have defective speech.

In the first grade, from 15 to 20 percent of the children are likely to be described as having defective articulation. There is a marked decrease (Mills and Streit, 1942; Reid, 1947) in the percentages reported through the first three or four grades, after which the decline is likely to become small or nonexistent. Table 24-II illustrates this trend in the columns in which the incidence is given in percentages.

Apparently, articulation is likely to improve until the age of 9 or 10; but after that age, for the most part, misarticulated sounds remain defective unless therapy is provided. The defect is not only likely to remain, but it is also likely to appear to be a more serious handicap as the child becomes older, since most people of the same age with whom he will be compared will have achieved normal articulation. Thus the high school student or the adult who has defective articulation has an entirely different type of problem of adjustment from that faced by the first-grader.

The decrease in the percentage of children who are reported as having defective articulation with increase in grade level is strikingly paralleled by the decrease in the number of defective sounds per child. According to Roe and Milisen (1942), the mean number of defective sounds per child (all children in the grades, not just "defective speakers") decreased from 13.30 percent in grade one to 9.99 percent in grade two, 8.85 percent in grade three, 7.62 percent in grade four, 7.61 percent in grade five, and 8.01 percent in grade six. A similar study by Sayler (1949)

TABLE 24-II
Articulation Defects by Grade in School

GRADE	ROOT (1925)* QUESTIONNAIRE %	REID (1947) (FRANCIS) PERSONAL SURVEY %	MILLS AND STREIT (1942) PERSONAL SURVEY %	WHITE HOUSE CONFERENCE (1931) QUESTIONNAIRE NO. OF CASES
K		27.8		
1	5.70	19.3	28.9	10,217
2	3.60	11.5	22.2	7,745
3	2.50	9.0	22.1	5,745
4	1.04	3.1	2.1**	4,375
5	2.70	3.6	2.1**	3,364
6	1.01	2.1	2.1**	2,612
7	.60	2.6		1,241
8	1.00	4.7		839
9		2.6		
10		6.7		
11		2.1		
12		4.7		

* Lispers and lallers.
** Average for the three grades combined

showed only a small and inconsistent decrease in the mean number of errors per child in grades seven through twelve. In short, there is significant improvement in articulatory skills up to and through the fourth grade, at which time the average child has achieved much of his adult articulatory skill. In the absence of speech therapy as such, there is likely to be little improvement in articulation after the fourth grade.

Age, as indicated by grade in school, is only one of many factors which must be taken into consideration in the study of defective articulation. Boys tend to develop articulatory skill more slowly than girls. The White House Conference report (1931) covering 31 cities showed a sex ratio of 1.58 to 1 in county schools and 1.44 to one percent in city schools. Mills and Streit (1942) gave figures which showed a sex ratio for the first six grades of 1.9 to one percent. Root (1925) gave figures for various types of articulation defects which average 1.7 to one percent. Young (1940) gave figures which showed a sex ratio of 1.4 to one percent. Studies by Roe and Milisen (1942) and Saylor (1949) showed a slight but not statistically significant difference in the mean number of errors per child, the boys making more errors.

Other factors, such as intelligence, influence the incidence of articulation defects; Loutitt and Halls (1936) found 2.5 times as many children in classes for subnormals with articulation defects as in the total school populations. Wallin (1926) stated that defects of articulation were "distinctly more prevalent among mental defectives." However, as Van Riper (1954) pointed out, the speech problems may contribute to the apparent subnormality. Lima (1927) reported that Binet tests of 402 children with speech defects (type not specified) in the St. Paul, Minnesota, schools showed a median I.Q. of 97.7 percent, well within the normal range. This sample, however, must not be considered random, since it was a school population from which the "uneducable" would be excluded.

Weaver, Furbee, and Everhart (1960) investigated the relationship between parental occupational class and articulatory defectiveness in 594 first-grade children. On the basis of their data, they reported that parental occupational status is significantly related to early speech maturation; that more children without defective articulation come from homes in the upper occupational groups, and more children with defective articulation come from homes in the lower occupational groups; and that only the two lowest occupational classes affect significantly the number of articulatory defects exhibited by children.

A study of Schlitt (1961) conducted in the Norfolk, Virginia, public schools indicated that 49 percent of the Negro sample evidenced phonatory and articulatory defects as compared with 16 percent of the white sample.

Certain organic disorders, particularly cleft palate and cerebral palsy, are frequently associated with articulation disorders. Shover (1945) reported that in 1,000 cleft-palate, cleft-lip cases, surgery was in 90 percent only a partial rehabilitation and speech therapy was necessary. With the improved surgical techniques, it would be expected that this figure would be significantly reduced today.

In the report of the White House Conference (1931) articulatory defects, associated with structural anomalies, many of which can probably be ascribed to cleft palate, constituted 8.6 percent of the total speech defects. Pronovost (1951) said that 1.2 percent of total speech defects were due to cleft palate while Johnson and Gardner (1944) estimated that 5,000 school children in the United States had defective speech caused by cleft palate. Loretz, Westmoreland and Richards (1961) reported a ratio of one case of cleft lip and/or palate per 851 live births or 1.18 cases per 1,000 live births in California in 1955.

Fraser and Calman (1961) studied a number of factors in relation to cleft lip and palate at the Churchill Hospital (England). Among their findings were: 1. for the combined groups the incidence is slightly greater for males than females; and 2. there are substantially more left clefts than either right or bilateral clefts.

Tretsvn (1963) reported a collection of seven years of data that showed incidence of cleft palate in Montana Indians was one in 276 births as compared with the non-Indian occurrence of one in 583 births. Another incidence study of a minority group conducted by Millard and McNeill (1965) indicated that the cleft-lip and -palate incidence of a group of Negro or Negro-mixed individuals in Jamaica was one cleft to 1,887 births. This incidence rate is particularly low as compared to other incidence figures.

Serious difficulties in accurate determination of incidence figures have been observed by Milham (1963). He reported that of a total of 143 patients with cleft lip and/or palate ascertained in 79,536 births at three upstate New York Hospitals from 1950 through 1960, 18.2 percent would have been missed if ascertained through hospital records alone while 27.2 percent would have been missed if vital records alone had been consulted. From these data he concluded that underreporting may have been responsible for variations in reported incidence of cleft lip and palate.

The other organic disorder responsible for many articulation disorders is cerebral palsy. Wolfe (1950) reported that 30 percent of 50 cases (a random sample from 746 cases between ages five and 30) of cerebral palsy had normal articulation and that of the 70 percent with inadequate articulation, 40 percent were due to the cerebral palsy, four percent to other organic causes, and 26 percent were functional. Shover (1945) reported that 50 percent of 3,000 cerebral-palsied children were in need of speech therapy.

The 1931 White House Conference report showed that the largest group of the paralytic articulatory cases can probably be ascribed to cerebral palsy. They constituted less than one percent of the population of speech defectives. However, Pronovost (1951) said that 11 percent of total speech defects were due to cerebral palsy. Johnson and Gardner (1944) estimated that 65,000 school children in the United States had defective speech caused by cerebral palsy. Wallace, Meinert, Dieter, and Bearman (1961) reported a prevalence of 1.3 percent cerebral-palsied individuals per 1,000 total population in Minnesota. Of the cerebral-palsied population, Mecham, Berko, and Berko (1960) reported 70 to 80 percent to have speech and/or hearing problems with the incidence of hearing loss varying from five to 40 percent.

Other organic conditions may cause or complicate speech defects, but they are present in much smaller percentages. Fletcher, Casteel, and Bradley (1961) collected data which indicated that the subject with a tongue-thrust swallow was much more likely to have associated sibilant distortion than was the subject without this pattern of swallowing. A study by Miner (1963) of the incidence of speech deviations among visually handicapped children found an incidence rate of 33.8 percent, a rate four or five times higher than that among public school pupils. A similar study conducted by LeZak and Starbuck (1964) revealed an incidence of speech disorders of almost 50 percent among the residents of the New York State School for the Blind. Of this group, approximately 37 percent had articulatory problems and about 10 percent demonstrated voice problems.

INCIDENCE OF STUTTERING

Definitions of stuttering vary widely, and figures on incidence will vary with the definition used and the method of survey. The question of differentiating between 1. speech deviations involving rhythm and 2. the speech defect of stuttering is beyond the scope of this chapter. However, it is interesting to note that Davis (1939) in a study of repetitions in the speech of 62 young (24 to 62 months) children, found that 16 did not present any syllable repetitions, and one boy who was judged a "stutterer" by parents and teachers alike was 12.4 standard deviations beyond the mean of four-syllable repetitions per thousand words, with 66 syllable repetitions per thousand words. The child (a boy) with next most frequent repetitions of syllables, 3.6 percent standard deviation from the

TABLE 24-III
Incidence of Stuttering for the First Eight Grades

GRADE	MILLS AND STREIT (1942) PERSONAL SURVEY	BURDIN (1940) QUESTION-NAIRE	ROOT (1916) QUESTION-NAIRE	BLANTON (1916) PERSONAL SURVEY CASES			WHITE HOUSE CONFERENCE (1931) QUESTIONNAIRE CASES		
	%	%	%	BOYS	GIRLS	TOTAL	BOYS	GIRLS	TOTAL
K				1	0	1			
I	1.5	.48	1.10	2	0	2	623	203	826
II	4.3	1.66	.70	4	0	4	829	244	1073
III	2.5	1.13	.60	1	1	2	966	265	1231
IV	1.1*	1.59	1.80	3	1	4	1052	253	1305
V	1.1*		2.10	5	2	7	1172	271	1443
VI	1.1*		1.60	5	1	6	1095	255	1350
VII			1.30	3	2	5	842	178	1020
VIII			.60	2	1	3	678	177	855

* Average for the three grades combined.

mean, was considered a "stutterer" by one teacher and was later voluntary taken to a speech clinic as a stutterer by the mother. Templin and Steer (1939), in a study of growth of speech in preschool children, described two boys out of a group of 27 the first semester and two boys out of a group of 24 the second semester as having severe disturbances of rhythm. However, they emphasized that most of the children repeated sounds, syllables, or words, but the frequency and severity of repetitions and blocks varied greatly.

According to Van Riper (1954), the vast majority of cases of stuttering begin in early childhood, usually between the ages of two and four years.

As shown in Table 24-III, there seems to be a marked tendency for stuttering to increase between the second and fifth grades and then to decrease again. Note that the columns headed Mills and Streit, Burdin, and Root are percentages of the total enrollment, whereas those headed Blanton and White House Conference are numbers of cases reported. There is an interesting parallelism in the small group studied personally by Blanton in 1916 and the large number studied by questionnaire by the White House Conference in 1930. The marked increase in cases of stuttering in the middle elementary grades in both reports was largely due to the great increase in incidence of stuttering among boys. The incidence among girls remained relatively constant.

Statistics on the incidence of stuttering among high-school students are inadequate. Morris (1939) reported five boys and one girl in a random sample of 178 sophomores. This would be an incidence of three percent and a sex ratio of five to one. Louttit and Halls (1936) show an incidence in grade nine of .69 percent, in grade 10 of .66 percent, in grade 11 of .39 percent, and in grade 12 of .41 percent, with a sex ratio for these grades of 3.3 to one.

In college students, Blanton (1921) found that six percent of members of the freshman class at the University of Wisconsin stuttered, while Morley (1952) reported figures indicating that approximately one percent of 33,339 students examined at the University of Michigan were stutterers and that boys outnumbered girls 4.3 to one.

Peacher (1946) reported seeing 77 preinduction and 37 postinduction stutterers at Brooke and McGuire General Hospitals but gave no figures on actual incidence in the army in World War II. However, Johnson (1943) estimated that there are five to eight stutterers per thousand draft-age men.

Although the ratio of boys to girls always points to more speech defects in boys, this is nowhere more apparent than in stuttering. While the ratio for articulation defects is something less than two to one, for stuttering it varies from 2.2 to one (Root, 1925) through 3.9 to one (White House Conference, 1931) to 5.3 to one (Mills and Streit, 1942). Travis (1931) has reported a range of from two to one to 10 to one. In considering these figures, it must be kept in mind that there is a possibility of various factors influencing these ratios. Perhaps girls with defective speech are more likely to drop out of school, perhaps they make themselves less conspicuous, perhaps a speech defect in a girl is considered less important. At least until the sex ratios can be more carefully studied, we should consider the possibility of other factors affecting or exaggerating the ratios as reported.

Another factor possibly influencing the incidence of stuttering is intelligence. Lima (1927) reported on the results of Binet testing of 402 children with speech defects. A median I.Q. of 97.7 was found for this group, 122 of whom were stutterers, but no separate figures were given for stutterers. Wallin (1926) reported that "stuttering is more prevalent among normal, retarded and backward children than among mental defectives . . . only one of our morons stuttered, while none of the imbeciles stuttered." Travis (1931) gave the following I.Q. distribution of 73 public school stutterers in Madison, Wisconsin:

I.Q.	60–69	70–79	80–89	90–99
Percent:	1.4	2.7	12.0	19.0

I.Q.	100–109	110–119	120–129	130–139
Percent:	37.0	16.4	8.2	1.4

However, Louttit (1936) described 3.22 percent of subnormals as stuttering compared to 0.77 percent of stutterers in the total school population. Williams (1954) reported at a meeting at Indiana University on the results of tests thus far completed on mentally defective persons at the State School for the Retarded at Butlerville, Indiana. Twenty-seven of 1,700 tested who ranged in age from 14 to 64 years presented severe rhythm problems. Seventeen of the 27 persons were definitely diagnosed as stutterers. Root (1925) found a retardation in school progress of 20.65 months for children with thick speech compared with 8.55 months for stutterers. The average for all speech defects was a retardation of 10.49 months. Whether the retardation was caused by the stuttering, by lower intelligence, or whether there was some other relationship is impossible to say on the basis of the available data.

Fruewald (1936) reported that the incoming stutterers at Ohio State University ranked definitely higher than the general freshman college population. Travis (1931) said that "stutterers in the University of Iowa have been distinctly superior to the average college student in intelligence," but attributed this to a selective factor which may keep the less intelligent stutterer from attempting college.

Numerous other factors have been related to the incidence of stuttering. Laterality, especially handedness and change of handedness, has been considered (Bryngelson, 1939; Milisen and Johnson, 1936; Orton, 1937; Travis, 1931; Van Riper, 1954) to have an important relationship to at least some cases of stuttering. However, emphasis on this area has decreased with reports (Daniels, 1940; Heltman, 1940; Van Dusen, 1939; Williams, 1952) which presented contrary evidence.

Birth conditions (Milisen and Johnson, 1936), allergy (Card, 1939), bilingualism and race (Travis, Johnson, and Shover, 1937), position in family (Rotter, 1939), familial incidence (Wepman, 1939), blindness (Weinberg, 1964), and many other physical and environmental conditions can be related to the incidence of stuttering, but in most cases the relationships are not entirely clear or have limited application. The annotated bibliography can be used by the reader who wishes to explore further the relationships of these factors with the incidence of stuttering.

INCIDENCE OF VOICE DISORDERS

Defects of voice were reported in 1.5 percent of the total group of 4,685 elementary school children studied by Mills and Streit (1942). In the Madison, Wisconsin, personal survey (White House Conference, 1931), out of a total of 10,033 children examined, 69 or 0.7 percent were classified as functional voice cases, 30 or 0.3 percent as structural voice cases, and one or .01 percent as paralytic voice cases, giving a total of 1.0 percent of voice defects in the population studied. Pronovost (1951) reported speech defects in 7.8 percent of the 87,288 individuals tested. Of those having speech defects, 6.6 percent were defective in voice; thus about 0.5 percent of the population tested had voice defects.

Evans (1938) found no cases of defective phonation in 224 students in grade 9A. Morris (1939) reported four boys and one girl with voice defects, an incidence of 2.8 percent, in a random sample of 178 high school sophomores.

Morley (1952) in an examination of 33,339 university students found that 15.04 percent of the speech defects were in voice, which is an incidence in the total number of students of .58 percent. However, Blanton (1921) found an incidence of voice defects of 4.5 percent of 2,240 members of a freshman university class.

Voice disorders presented after laryngectomy (usually due to carcinoma of the larynx) have been studied. Of course, the incidence rate would be 100 percent after operation; however, other conditions such as age may also be contributing factors. Glass and Fraser (1965) reported that about 25 percent of persons with laryngeal malignancy are over 70 years old. A study conducted in Prague by Konecny (1960) showed the average age of the patients studied to be 52 years with the condition requiring treatment being most frequent between the ages of 51–60 years. Of the 117 patients studied, 113 were men and four were women.

A summary of incidence of voice disorders is difficult to make not only because of the great variety of types of voice disorders but also because results of studies vary considerably. However, studies would seem to indicate that approximately one percent of the total population of this country is hampered by defects of voice and that they constitute between five and 15 percent of the defective-speech population.

INCIDENCE OF LANGUAGE DISTURBANCE INVOLVING COMPREHENSION AND EXPRESSION

Speech as a means of communication is used insufficiently or not at all by people who have delayed speech. In addition to the paucity of expression some persons, such as the deaf, aphasic, mentally defective, and many others may also have difficulty in comprehending speech. Before the incidence of delayed speech can be studied and reported reliably, it would be necessary to establish norms of language development for children up to eight years of age. Language retardation could then be determined by comparing a child's language development with the norm. The establishment of such a norm would involve many complications which would be most difficult to control, such as 1. obtaining a random sample of children; and 2. obtaining a random sample of speech behavior of each child which would be representative of his overall language behavior. This would involve creating a natural situation involving parents and other members of an audience in a strictly laboratory type of experiment. As of the present time, no such study has been reported. However, a few studies have been made relating delayed speech to various organic and environmental factors.

Beckey (1942) found retardation in speech to be more common in children with histories of abnormal conditions during pregnancy and birth, in children with poor motor control, in children who had had two or more severe infectious diseases, especially measles, and in children who were in poor physical condition. Boys tended to outnumber girls. From an environmental standpoint, retardation in speech was more common among more isolated children, in children from lower socioeconomic levels, in children who had had severe frights, in children who had had their wants anticipated, and in children with inferior ratings in intelligence. Children with retarded speech tended to substitute gestures for speech. It should be noted that the incidence of delayed speech is 100 percent among preschool deaf children. Furthermore, it should be noted that large numbers of mentally defective children have delayed speech, although no reliable data can be cited.

Persons studying incidence of aphasia in young children are subject to even more problems than those who are studying delayed speech. A major stumbling block is the establishment of a criterion which will separate aphasic from nonaphasic language behavior. Without such a criterion, data on incidence of the disorder are quite meaningless. The examiner of these children receives little language behavior upon which to make judgments and little opportunity to compare the child's speech at the time of examination with his speech at other times. A study by DiCarlo (1960) illustrates this difficulty in diagnosis. A group of 67 children previously diagnosed as congenitally aphasic were reeaxmined at the Syracuse Hearing and Speech Center by him. It was found that only four of the group had aphasoid characteristics as defined by DiCarlo. Of the remainder, 17 had I.Q.'s below 58, 11 had I.Q.'s from 60 to 75, 20 were emotionally disturbed with normal intelligence, and 15 had defective hearing.

Reports of incidence of aphasia in adults might be more meaningful, since most adults had adequate speech and comprehension before the brain damage which usually preceded their aphasic behavior. However, most groups available for study are not randomly selected. They are usually hospitalized patients. Many aphasics may not have had brain damage and may not, therefore, have needed hospitalization. Furthermore, the individual symptoms which are seemingly so clear-cut in the textbooks can be duplicated thousands of times in the speech of the so-called normal speaker.

With all these reservations, the following data are presented: The enormity of the uncharted field may explain in part the wide variation in the results reported by various experimenters. Young (1942) reported 18 cases of aphasia in a total grade- and high-school enrollment of 9,448, or an incidence of 0.2 percent. Morris (1939) reported one case of aphasia in a random sample of 178 high school sophomores, or an incidence of 0.6 percent. Mills and Streit (1942) in their breakdown into type of defect did not mention aphasia. Blanton (1916) included aphasia in the 1.71 percent of miscellaneous defects. Pronovost (1951) recorded 0.5 percent incidence of aphasia in a group of speech-defective subjects he studied. When this percentage is projected to a total population it would indicate an incidence of aphasia of about 0.04 percent. Childhood aphasia, then, may be found in between zero percent and 0.6 percent of a school population. Since, by its very nature, aphasia is likely to make success in school very difficult, it is probable that a sizable proportion of "child aphasics" are not included in the school population.

At upper age limits, there are few figures available on incidence of aphasia. Surveys of speech defects on the college level rarely if ever mention aphasia, probably due to the difficulty the aphasic would have with college work. Since brain tumors and cerebral hemorrhages may be more common in older people and aphasia is not often completely "cured," there are almost certainly more aphasics among older people.

Cerebral trauma as a cause of aphasia has received the most attention, since such trauma was often caused by injuries in war. Frazier and Ingham (1927) reported that of 200 head-injury cases at a general hospital in World War I, language involvement lasting six months or more was seen in 16 cases.

Peacher (1945) described patients seen at Brooke General Hospital from May 7, 1943, to September 1, 1944. Admission was not on the basis of language difficulties alone, but for medical or surgical reasons.

Of 120 patients with speech problems, 32 were dysphasic: 18 from craniocerebral traumata, seven from cerebrovascular disease, six in association with brain tumor, and one following acute meningo-encephalitis.

A summary statement of the incidence of language disturbances, especially involving delayed speech and aphasia, would be meaningless. This area of defective communication must be more carefully described and studied before incidence reports will be more than "best guesses."

The incidence of defective hearing is a particularly difficult figure to arrive at with any degree of accuracy. One reason for this is pointed out by a survey by the Federal Office of Vocational Rehabilitation as reported by Ogles (1961). According to this survey of 2,992 hard-of-hearing adults, 68.9 percent were having communication problems a minimum of 10 years prior to referral, and 47.2 percent were having problems 24 years prior to referral. These data would seem to indicate that a great number of hearing problems go officially unrecognized for several years, making the establishment of an accurate incidence figure particularly difficult.

Since this chapter deals specifically with the incidence of speech and language disorders, it would be most applicable to be able to cite figures for the number of speech disorders associated with impaired hearing. However, data dealing with this area of incidence seem to be particularly scarce at least as reported in the literature. Angelocci (1962) conducted a study involving 10 vowels spoken by 18 deaf and 18 normal-hearing boys. When these vowel sounds were judged by college students for intelligibility, the vowels spoken by the deaf revealed an overall intelligibility of 32 percent in contrast with 81 percent for the normal hearing.

The incidence of communication problems involving speech deviations, defects, and defectives needs to be more carefully studied. At present, better testing methods are available, more people are well trained, and therapy programs are well established, all of which should permit the establishment of long-term studies which could control more of the variables. Until these studies are completed, we must continue to quote incidence data as "approximations."

BIBLIOGRAPHY

Angelocci, A. 1962. Some observations on the speech of the deaf. *Volta Rev.*, 64, 403–404.

Backus, O. 1938. Incidence of stuttering among the deaf. *Ann. Otol., Rhinol., Laryng.*, 47, 632–635.

Beckey, R. 1942. A study of certain factors related to retardation of speech. *J. Speech Disorders*, 7, 223–249.

Bender, J. 1939. The organization and guiding principles of the New York City survey of the speech handicapped child conducted Oct., 1939–June, 1940. *J. Speech Disorders*, 5, 357–362.

Berry, M. 1939. A study of the medical histories of stuttering children. *Speech Monogr.*, 5, 97–114.

———. 1949. Lingual anomalies associated with palatal clefts. *J. Speech Hearing Disorders*, 14, 359–362.

———. 1956. Speech disorders. New York: Appleton-Century-Crofts.

———, and Eisenson, J. 1942. The defective in speech. New York: Crofts.

Bilto, E. 1941. A comparative study of certain physical abilities of children with speech defects and children with normal speech. *J. Speech Disorders*, 6, 187–203.

Blanton, S. 1916. A survey of speech defects. *J. educ. Psychol.*, 7, 581–592.

———. 1921. Speech defects in school children. *Ment. Hyg.*, 5, 820–827.

Bryngelson, B. 1939. A study of laterality of stutterers and normal speakers. *J. Speech Disorders*, 4, 231–234.

Bullen, A. 1945. A cross-cultural approach to the problem of stuttering. *Child Develop.*, 16, 1–88.

Burdin, L. 1940. A survey of speech defectives in the Indianapolis primary grades. *J. Speech Disorders*, 5, 247–258.

Camp, P. 1923. Survey of speech defects. *J. Speech Educ.*, 11, 280–283.

Card, R. 1939. A study of allergy in relation to stuttering. *J. Speech Disorders*, 4, 223–230.

Carhart, R. 1939. A survey of speech defects in Illinois high schools. *J. Speech Disorders*, 4, 61–70.

———. 1943. Some notes on official statistics of speech disorders encountered during world war 1. *J. Speech Disorders*, 8, 97–107.

Carrell, J. 1936. A comparative study of speech defective children. *Arch. Speech*, 1 (3), 179–203.

Chen, H., and Irwin, O. 1946. Infant speech vowel and consonant types. *J. Speech Disorders*, 11, 27–29.

Daniels, E. 1940. An analysis of the relation between handedness and stuttering with special reference to the Orton-Travis theory of cerebral dominance. *J. Speech Disorders*, 5, 309–326.

Davis, D. 1939. The relation of repetitions in the speech of young children to certain measures of language maturity and situational factors. *J. Speech Disorders*, 4, 303–318.

Davis, I. 1937. A survey of speech defects in Akron public schools. (Unpublished report to Board Educ., Akron, Ohio).

DiCarlo, L. 1960. Differential diagnosis of congenital aphasia. *Volta Rev.*, 62, 361–364.

Evans, D. 1938. Report of a survey in grade 9a. *Quart. J. Speech*, 24, 83–90.

Evans, M. 1947. Problems in cerebral palsy. *J. Speech Disorders*, 12, 87–103.

Fletcher, S., Casteel, R., and Bradley, D. 1961. Tongue-thrust swallow, speech articulation and age. *J. Speech Hearing Dis.*, 26, 201–208.

Fraser, G., and Calman, J. 1961. Cleft lip and palate: seasonal incidence, birth weight, birth rank, sex, site, associated malformations and parental age: a statistical survey. *Arch. Dis. Childh.*, 36, 420–425.

Frazier, C., and Ingham, S. 1927. Neurological aspects of gunshot wounds of the head. Medical department of the U.S. army in world war 1. Washington, D.C., Gov't. Printing Office. 11, 795–803.

Fruewald, E. 1936. Intelligence rating of severe college stutterers compared with that of others entering universities. *J. Speech Disorders*, 1, 47–52.

Glass, E., and Fraser, W. 1965. Malignant disease involving the larynx in the elderly patient. *Geriatrics*, 20, 228–235.

Gratke, J. 1947. Speech problems of the cerebral-palsied. *J. Speech Disorders*, 12, 129–134.

Hawk, E. 1945. A survey and critical analysis of speech needs in the elementary schools of an Ohio city of 15,000 population with a suggested remedial program in speech. Ohio State Univ.: Ph.D. dissertation.

Hawk, S. 1936. Speech defects in handicapped children. *J. Speech Disorders*, 1, 101–106.

Heltman, H. 1940. Contradictory evidence in handedness and stuttering. *J. Speech Disorders*, 5, 327–331.

Henderson, F. 1940. The incidence of cleft palate in Hawaii. *J. Speech Disorders*, 5, 285–287.

Henderson, P. 1947. The incidence of stammering and speech defects in school children. *Monogr. Bull., Minn. Hlth, and Emerg. Publ. Hlth. Lab. Serv.*, 6, 102–105.

Henrikson, E. 1945. A semantic study of identification of speech defects. *J. Speech Disorders*, 10, 169–172.

Hill, H. 1944a. Stuttering: I: a critical review and evaluation of biochemical investigation. *J. Speech Disorders*, 9, 245–261.

———. 1944b. Stuttering: II: a review and integration of physiological data, *J. Speech Disorders*, 9, 289–324.

Hood, P., Shank, K., and Williamson, D. 1948. Environmental factors in relation to the speech of cerebral-palsied children. *J. Speech Hearing Disorders*, 13, 325–331.

Ingram, C., Pintner, R., and Stinchfield-Hawk, S. 1941. The auditorially and the speech handicapped. *Rev. Educ. Res.*, 11, 297–314.

Irwin, O. 1942. Developmental status of speech sounds in ten feebleminded children. *Child Develop.*, 13, 22–29.

———. 1946. Development of speech during infancy: curve of phonemic frequencies. *J. exp. Psychol.*, 37, 187–193.

———. 1947. Infant speech variability and the problem of diagnosis. *J. Speech Disorders*, 12, 287–289.

———. 1952. Speech development in the young child: 2: some factors related to the speech development of the infant and young child. *J. Speech Disorders*, 17, 269–279.

———, and Chen, H. 1946. Development of speech during infancy: curve of phonemic types. *J. exper. Psychol.*, 36, 431–436.

Irwin, R. 1948. Ohio looks ahead in speech and hearing therapy. *J. Speech Hearing Disorders*, 13, 55–60.

———. 1949. Speech and hearing therapy in the public schools of Ohio. *J. Speech Hearing Disorders*, 14, 63–68.

Johnson, W. 1942. The Iowa remedial education program: summary report. Iowa City: Child Welfare Res. Station.

———. 1943. The status of speech defectives in military service. *Quart. J. Speech*, 29, 131–136.

———, Brown, S., Curtis, J., Edney, C., and Keaster, J. 1948. Speech handicapped school children. New York: Harper.

———, and Gardner, W. 1944. The auditorially and speech handicapped. *Rev. Educ. Res.*, 14, 241–248.

Konecny, L. 1960. Partial operations of the larynx for carcinoma. *Cesko. Otolaringol.*, 9, 367–374.

Krantz, H., and Henderson, F. 1947. Relationship between maternal ancestry and incidence of cleft palate. *J. Speech Disorders*, 12, 267–278.

Krebiel, T. 1941. Speech sounds of infants in the fourth, fifth and sixth months. Univ. Iowa: Master's thesis.

Larr, A. 1944. A county speech and hearing conservation program. *J. Speech Disorders*, 9, 147–151.

LeZak, R., and Starbuck, H. 1964. Identification of children with speech disorder in a residential school for the blind. *Inter. J. Educ. Blind*, 14, 8–12.

Lima, M. 1927. Speech defects in school children. *Ment. Hyg.*, 795–803.

Loretz, W., Westmoreland, W., and Richards, L. 1961. A study of cleft lip and cleft palate births in California, 1955. *Amer. J. Public Hlth.*, 51, 873–877.

Louttit, C. 1936. Clinical psychology. New York: Harper.

———, and Halls, E. 1936. Survey of speech defects among public school children of Indiana. *J. Speech Disorders*, 1, 73–80.

McCurry, W., and Irwin, O. 1953. A study of word approximations in the spontaneous speech of infants. *J. Speech Hearing Disorders*, 18, 133–139.

McDowell, E. 1928. Educational and emotional adjustments of stuttering children. *Teach. Coll. Contr. Educ.*, No. 314. New York: Teachers College, Columbia.

Mecham, M., Berko, M., and Berko, F. 1960. Speech therapy in cerebral palsy. Springfield, Ill.: Thomas.

Metraux, R. 1950. Speech profiles of the preschool child 18 to 54 months. *J. Speech Hearing Disorders*, 15, 37–53.

Midcentury White House Conference. 1952. Speech disorders and speech correction. *J. Speech Hearing Disorders*, 17, 129–137.

Milham, S. 1963. Underreporting of incidence of cleft lip and palate. *Amer. J. Dis. Child.*, 106, 185–188.

Milisen, R., and Johnson, W. 1936. A comparative study of stutterers, former stutterers and normal speakers whose handedness has been changed. *Arch. Speech*, 1, 61–86.

Millard, D. and McNeill, K. 1965. The incidence of cleft lip and palate in Jamaica. *Cleft Palate J.*, 2, 384–388.

Mills, A., and Streit, H. 1942. Report of a speech survey, Holyoke, Massachusetts, *J. Speech Disorders*, 7, 161–167.

Miner, L. 1963. A study of the incidence of speech deviations among visually handicapped children. *New Outlook for the Blind*, 57, 10–14.

Moncur, J. 1950. Environmental factors differentiating stuttering children from nonstuttering children. *Speech Monogr.*, 18, 131–132.

Morley, D. 1952. A ten-year survey of speech disorders among university students. *J. Speech Hearing Disorders*, 17, 25–31.

Morris, D. 1939a. A survey of speech defects in central high school, Kansas City, Mo. *Quart. J. Speech*, 25, 262–269.

———. 1939b. The speech survey. *J. Speech Disorders*, 4, 195–198.

Morrison, C. 1914. Speech defects in young children. *Psychol. Clinic*, 8, 138–142.

Ogles, C. 1961. Procedures in discovering persons with communication problems. *Hearing News*, 29, 9–12.

Orton, S. 1937. Reading, writing and speech problems in children. New York: Norton.

Palmer, M., and Gillett, A. 1938. Sex differences in the cardiac rhythm of stutterers. *J. Speech Disorders*, 3, 3–12.

Partridge, L. 1945. Dyslalias of southern ohio. *J. Speech Disorders*, 10, 249–250.

Peacher, W. 1945a. Speech disorders in world war II. *J. Speech Disorders*, 10, 155–161.

———. 1945b. Speech disorders in world war II: III. Dysarthria. *J. Speech Disorders*, 10, 287–291.

———. 1945c. Speech disorders in world war II: II. *J. nerv. ment. Dis.*, 102, 165–171.

———. 1946. Speech disorders in world war II: VIII. Stuttering. *J. Speech Disorders*, 11, 303–308.

Phair, G. 1947. The Wisconsin cleft palate program. *J. Speech Disorders*, 21, 410–414.

Pintner, R., Eisenson, J., and Stanton, M. 1941. Psychology of the physically handicapped. New York: Appleton-Century-Crofts.

Poole, I. 1934. Genetic development of consonant sounds in speech. *Elem. Eng. Rev.*, 2, 159–161.

Pronovost, W. 1951. A survey of services for the speech and hearing handicapped in New England, *J. Speech Hearing Disorders*, 16, 148–156.

Reid, G. 1947. The efficacy of speech re-education of functional articulatory defectives in the elementary school. *J. Speech Disorders*, 12, 301–313.

Roe, V., and Milisen, R. 1942. The effect of maturation upon defective articulation in the elementary grades. *J. Speech Disorders*, 7, 37–56.

Rogers, J. 1931. The speech-defective school child. Bull. No. 7. Office of Educ., Washington, D.C.

Root, A. 1925. A survey of speech defectives in the public elementary schools of South Dakota. *Elem. Sch. J.*, 26, 531–541.

Rotter, J. 1939. Studies in the psychology of stuttering. XI: stuttering in relation to position in the family. *J. Speech Disorders*, 4, 143–148.

Rutherford, B. 1938. Speech re-education for the birth injured. *J. Speech Disorders*, 3, 199–206.

———. 1944. A comparative study of loudness, pitch, rate, rhythm, and quality of the speech of children handicapped by cerebral palsy. *J. Speech Disorders*, 9, 263–271.

Sayler, H. 1949. The effect of maturation upon defective articulation in grades seven through twelve. *J. Speech Hearing Disorders*, 14, 202–207.

Schlitt, R. 1961. Socioeconomic status as a correlate of speech defects: A study of the white and negro children in the Norfolk, Virginia, public schools. *J. Speech Hear. Assn. Va.*, 2, 11–15.

Schuell, H. 1946. Sex differences in relation to stuttering: Part I. *J. Speech Disorders*, 11, 277–298.

———. 1947. Sex differences in relation to stuttering: Part II. *J. Speech Disorders*, 12, 23–38.

Sherman, D. and Cullinan, W. 1960. Several procedures for scaling articulation. *J. Speech Hearing Res.*, 3, 191–198.

Shover, J. 1945. Illinois program for speech and hearing. *J. Speech Disorders*, 10, 117–122.

Snidecor, J. 1948. The speech correctionist on the cerebral-palsy team. *J. Speech Hearing Disorders*, 13, 67–70.

Spadino, E. 1941. Writing and laterality characteristics of stuttering children. *Teach. Coll. Contr. Educ.*, No. 837. New York: Teachers College, Columbia.

Spiker, C. 1951. An empirical study of factors associated with certain indices of speech sounds of young children. Univ. Iowa: Ph.D. dissertation.

Stinchfield, S. 1925. The speech of 500 freshman college women. *J. appl. Psychol.*, 9, 109–121.

Sullivan, E. 1944. Auditory acuity and its relation to defective speech. *J. Speech Disorders*, 9, 127–130.

Suydam, V. 1948. Speech survey methods in public schools. *J. Speech Disorders*, 13, 51–54.

Templin, M. 1947. Spontaneous versus imitated verbalization in testing articulation in preschool children. *J. Speech Disorders*, 12, 293–300.

———. 1953. Norms on a screening test of articulation for ages three through eight. *J. Speech Hearing Disorders*, 18, 323–331.

Templin, M. 1957. Certain language skills in children. Minneapolis: Univ. Minn. Press.

———, and Steer, M. 1939. Studies of growth of speech in pre-school children. *J. Speech Disorders*, 4, 71–77.

Travis, L. 1931. Speech pathology. New York: D. Appleton.

———, Johnson, W., and Shover, J. 1937. The relation of bilingualism to stuttering. *J. Speech Disorders*, 2, 185–189.

Tretsvn, V. 1963. Incidence of cleft lip and palate in Montana indians. *J. Speech Hearing Disorders*, 28, 52–57.

Van Dusen, C. 1939. A laterality study of non-stutterers and stutterers, *J. Speech Disorders*, 4, 261–265.

Van Riper, C. 1954. Speech correction: principles and methods (3rd. ed.). Englewood Cliffs, N.J.: Prentice-Hall.

Voelker, C. 1944. A preliminary investigation for a normative study of fluency; a clinical index to the severity of stuttering. *Amer. J. Orthopsychiat.*, 14, 285–294.

Wallace, H., Meinert, C., Dieter, R., and Bearman, J. 1961. Cerebral palsy in Minnesota: method of study, prevalence and distribution, Part I. *Amer. J. Publ. Hlth.*, 51, 417–426.

Wallin, J. 1916. A census of speech defectives among 89,057 public school pupils. *Sch. and Soc.*, 3, 213–216.

———. 1926. Speech defective children in a large school. *Bull.* XXV, No. 4, Miami Univ., Oxford, Ohio.

Weaver, C., Furbee, C., and Everhart, R. 1960. Paternal occupational class and articulatory defects in children. *J. Speech Hearing Disorders*, 25, 171–175.

Weinberg, B. 1964. Stuttering among blind and partially sighted children. *J. Speech Hearing Disorders*, 29, 322–326.

Weiss, D. 1948. Organic lesions leading to speech disorders. *Nerv. Child*, 7, 29–37.

Wells, C. 1945. Expanding state speech correction services. *J. Speech Disorders*, 10, 123–128.

Wepman, J. 1939. Familial incidence in stammering. *J. Speech Disorders*, 4, 199–204.

West, N. 1939. The heredity of stuttering. *Quart. J. Speech*, 25, 23–30.

West, R., Kennedy, L., and Carr, A. 1947. The rehabilitation of speech (rev. ed.) New York: Harper.

White House Conference on Child Health and Protection. Special education. 1931. New York: Century.

Williams, D. 1952. An evaluation of masseter muscle action potentials in stuttering and non-stuttered speech. Univ. Iowa: Ph.D. dissertation.

Wolfe, W. 1950. A comprehensive evaluation of fifty cases of cerebral palsy. *J. Speech Hearing Disorders*, 15, 234–251.

Young, J. 1940. Speech rehabilitation in rural schools of Waukesha County, Wis. *J. Speech Disorders*, 5, 25–28.

———. 1942. A city and county speech reeducation program. *J. Speech Disorders*, 7, 51–56.

25

Methods of Evaluation and Diagnosis of Speech Disorders

Robert Milisen

TRADITIONAL CONCEPTS OF DIAGNOSIS

In the traditional concept of diagnosis, the examiner should be able to identify and describe the speaker's disorder, its etiology, and the symptoms that developed after the onset. The format for the diagnostic report should facilitate forecasting of the kind of clinical program to be used in eliminating or compensating for the conditions that stand in the way of normal speech.

To be successful, a diagnosis based on this concept depends on the accuracy of the following assumptions: 1. that each disorder can be described definitively; 2. that etiologies are known; 3. that changes in speech behavior (symptoms) occurring after the onset are caused by conditions that are independent of those involved in etiology; and 4. that therapies, specific to each individual's disorder, are known and can be predicted from the diagnostic report. Unfortunately, our testing methods at present do not provide definitive information which will permit precise separation of many disorders, nor are speech pathologists in agreement on the nature of etiology and therapy.

Fallacies in traditional concepts of diagnosis

Before a chapter dealing with diagnosis can be written meaningfully, since opinions vary on matters relevant to diagnosis, assumptions made in the traditional concept of diagnosis should be reexamined with an intention of modifying them. Perhaps the assumptions that are most disruptive to diagnosis are those involving the relationship between etiology and developmental symptoms of speech disorders. If the causes of a disorder are not understood, how can tests be constructed so they will provide information that will be helpful in treatment? It is possible that a fallacy of considerable importance to the diagnostician occurs because traditionally only those conditions occurring prior to and during the onset of the disorder can be considered etiologic but not those which emerge later on. This traditional pattern is an extension of our heritage from medicine which is concerned primarily with biological malfunctioning. Since physiological equilibrium is maintained by a process called homeostasis, the physician can determine whether or not health is impaired by comparing body balance at the time of examination with predetermined standards of physiological processes such as body temperature, blood pressure, pulse rate, etc. The processes evaluated by the physician resemble, to a degree, the all-or-none function of the nerves—the body is either healthy or unhealthy. The key issue is that developmental events occurring after the onset of imbalance do not alter etilogy of the illness. These events may, however, provide symptoms that are helpful in diagnosing some diseases such as scarlet fever and measles since the spots develop on the skin after the period of onset and are specific symptoms of the diseases. However, these spots do not change the etiology. Of course, various conditions occurring after the onset of some diseases may alter the effectiveness of treatment. For instance, a pneumonia patient whose lungs are filling with fluid will be more difficult to treat than one whose lungs have not reached this state.

The physician's diagnostic pattern does not fit the needs of the speech diagnostician. Whereas the physician is dealing, for the most part, with physiological processes, the speech pathologist is dealing with learning processes superimposed on the more fundamental physiological ones. Furthermore, the overt evidence of basic physiological processes of the body, such as body temperature, remain essentially the same throughout life. This is not true of learned behavior since it changes considerably as a person gets older and as changes in environment and physical conditions occur.

The learning component involved in speech production is dynamic and progressive. The nature of speech production at any moment is affected by all relevant experience up to the moment when the speech response is made. For example, the etiology of the speech behavior of a child of five will be determined by all relevant influences (environment, physical conditions, and situation stresses during the testing period) occurring up to and during the period of examination. If this is true, the speech diagnostician must abandon the traditional concept of separating etiology and symptoms. He must recognize that all developmental events relevant to the production of speech at any moment play an important role in determining its nature. As such, they are a part of the etiology of behavior which occurs at any time. Hence (for the speech pathologist) etiologies of the disorder at its onset may be identified, but all of those affecting subsequent speech cannot because they are always changing as long as the person lives and speaks. Therefore, it can be hypothesized that developmental events which modify speech behavior play an important etiological role in those disorders and should be considered as an integral part of all diagnosis and therapies. This hypothesis not only affects the conceptualization of diagnosis, it also raises questions about the propriety of criticism of certain procedures which are directed toward management of so-called "symptoms" emerging after onset. (Most articulation and stuttering therapy falls into this category.) If the nature of the speech production is affected by all relevant speech experience up to the moment when the response is made, then those responses and the conditions that precipitated them contribute to learning. They become a part of the experience relevant to all subsequent speech behavior and thereby become etiologic of it. Therefore, by treating these "symptoms" one may be dealing with one aspect of the etiology of the speech disorder.

In this chapter etiology of the various speech disorders and their diagnoses will be treated as a dynamic process starting on or before the first observation of the disorder and continuing to the time of examination.

ACQUISITION OF SPEECH

Speech—a form of learned behavior

Until recently, speech pathologists have had little reason to doubt that speech behavior was learned. In the early thirties Travis (1931) reported speech to be a form of acquired or learned behavior superimposed on the primary physiological processes. Recently some psycholinguists have questioned whether learning plays so omnipotent a role. They have suggested that many of the characteristics used in speech encoding are wired in and therefore do not need to be learned. Occasionally some students read into this concept much more than was intended when they hypothesize that language is wired in genetically and therefore learning is not necessarily a component of its acquisition.

There is little question that the nature of the characteristics used in encoding and decoding speech will be restricted to the physiological capacity of the organism. For instance, man cannot hear sounds above 20,000 Hz while some other animals can. By the same token, human infants from all cultures tend to produce similar preverbal sounds, but other animals do not simulate our preverbal sounds because they have a different physiological capacity. The physiological capacity to produce many distinctive phonemic features is demonstrated by infants in many nonlinguistic acts such as breathing and vocalization and their modification during eating, crying, vocal play, etc. These features are essential parts of the speech act. Clearly, they do not have to be learned by the child, but whether he will convert them into a code and use them as a part of a communication system does.

Lenneberg (1967) has presented a scholarly treatment of this subject, and he concluded that the human is restricted by his biological processes to a certain type of form for language and that all languages are within this form. However, there are an infinite number of possibilities that may fall within the large-form category. He also contends that the human organism, through a genetic process, develops to a state called "language readiness" and is then able to take the language used by those around him and turn this "latent structure" into "realized structure." This process "gives the underlying cognitively determined type a concrete form."

For the purposes of this chapter it will be assumed that speech development is dependent on the child's learning to adapt various physiological processes so they will serve as a medium of communication. Many of these processes will not have to be learned because they are genetically wired into the child, who uses them during the prelinguistic period as a part of vital functioning of his body. Obviously, these processes are available for the development of language if the proper interaction takes place between the child and his environment.

The inverse process of self-evaluation and regulation as it affects the speech-learning process.

This inverse process must also be reckoned with by the diagnostician since it is pertinent to the development and maintenance of many of our speech patterns (Milisen, 1967). In essence, this concept is based on the assumption that a person does not perceive his speech productions as do other people nor as he perceives many of his other motor skills, such as shooting arrows at a target. In shooting he can see easily how close he comes to the center of the target and in turn can tell what his error was and try to correct it. However, he can never determine precisely how close his speech production comes to the model. There are many reasons why it is impossible to make this evaluation with precision, but one of the more important reasons is that a person's speech response feeds back to him over a different set of sense organs than he uses in receiving model sounds from his environment. Since he cannot tell precisely the difference between speech models he receives and those he produces, he must depend on some other source to make up for his deficiency. This source is environmental reinforcement. If the environment inadvertently gives positive reinforcement to his error responses, he will be conditioned to reproduce them habitually. If error responses are rejected and correct ones positively rewarded, he is likely to learn to articulate in a standard manner.

This inverse process of self-evaluation and -regulation described by Milisen (1966) is important in diagnosis since it not only effects the etiology of some speech disorders but their management as well. It is significant to the speech pathologist that he must learn that he cannot deal with the learning of speech as he does the learning of many other skills. Special methods must be introduced into the therapy process if the client is to become efficient in learning to identify his errors and replace them with standard responses. The inverse process used in learning phonemes should be considered when making a diagnosis and designing a therapy.

COMPILATION OF DIAGNOSTIC DATA

The next problem confronting the speech pathologist is how to arrange the enormous quantity of information gathered during diagnosis. First a rationale must be developed which will facilitate the separation of the relevant from the irrelevant data. This rationale must also bring into focus the especially pertinent information and provide a way of constricting the remainder. It is difficult to plan a rationale that will fit all disorders and all people who have those disorders, but failure to do so causes the diagnostician to perform in an incoherent and often unprofessional manner. Unfortunately, attempts to conceptualize the matter may lead to oversimplification, in which case important bits of data are omitted or other bits are assigned a faulty role in the etiological process. In spite of these dangers, the diagnostician must have rational goals and methods to use in achieving them.

A rationale for diagnosis of speech disorders

Communication must be looked upon as a whole process. In practice, quite often, the whole must be separated into parts for convenience in testing. Some dangers are inherent in this practice. The diagnostician may not isolate for study all of the important parts. He may also fail to reconstitute the bits of information into a whole that accurately represents the behavior of the person being studied.

The parts to be studied may be referred to as determiners, i.e., those conditions which determine the nature of the speech act. This speech act is one form of interaction between a speaker and his environment. It is necessary, therefore, that both be represented in the diagnosis since each will have influenced the nature of the speech pattern produced by the client.

There are three determiners of the nature of speech: 1. the *physical* characteristics of the speaker, 2. his *environment*, and 3. the *situational stresses* affecting him at the moment of speech. The physical determiners consist of all organic conditions of the client occurring prior to the onset of the disorder and up to the time of examination. Environmental determiners consist of all stimulation and reinforcement (relevant to the speech condition being examined) of the client by the environment. Situation determiners consist of all stresses influencing the interactions between the speaker and his environment which will in turn influence the nature of the speech act during the period while the speech is being assessed.

Although these determiners function as independent variables in their influence on speech behavior, the influence of each one is always being inhibited or facilitated by the other two interacting variables. For example, a physical determiner such as a cleft palate will usually have an inhibiting effect on the environmental determiners involved in development of some speech sounds, especially those dependent on high oral breath pressure. However, the cleft palate might actually have a facilitating effect on the environmental determiner if it motivates the parents to put forth extensive efforts to train the child to compensate for the faulty palate. Under this interaction of the variables the child may acquire good articulation as soon or sooner than other children who have normal palates. This type of interaction between the determiners makes the task of diagnosis a difficult one. It demonstrates why it is unwise to use a single determiner as the cause of a speech disorder as is done by many clinicians who refer to speech disorders as functional or organic. Therapy which is really based on such a diagnosis will usually be inappropriate.

Since each speech act is affected by different values of the three determiners, it is logical that the role of each be assessed when diagnosing the problems of the defective speaker. A successful diagnosis should report the manner in which each determiner interacted with the others in precipitating and maintaining the disorder. Information received by the clinician about the relative importance of each determiner will guide him in planning his management of the disorder.

CLASSIFICATION OF COMMUNICATION DISORDERS

In order for a classification system to be developed, the speech behavior of many people must be observed and compared. Additional information from tests and historical background will contribute to the refinement of the system. It is necessary to keep in mind that communication disorders will tend to be related to the processes of decoding and/or encoding. Although both processes may be defective in any person, usually only one is faulty in the majority of defective speakers.

The diagnostician must be prepared to compare the abnormal behavior with that which is standard in the patient's environment, but he must also be able to compare it to other types of anomalous speech behavior. The following classification of speech disorders is designed for this purpose.

Classification of communication disorders of which speech is a part

1. Failure to develop a skill of meaningfully decoding and encoding language. Examples of this class are frequently found in sensory-impaired persons such as the profoundly deaf who have received no compensatory assistance in developing language. Also many severe mental retardates who have likewise been neglected will fit this category. Some patients with severe physical disabilities such as cerebral palsy (which usually affects encoding) who have not received compensatory assistance may also be found to have a complete failure of language usage as a medium of communication. Some persons without linguistic skills may also be found who have no observable physical or intellectual impairment but have had no opportunity to develop language as a medium of communication.

2. Failure to develop the skill of encoding language even though ability of decoding is adequate. Examples of this class are most likely to be children with delayed language. Many of these children have no obvious physical anomaly, but marked anomalies involving environmental determiners are common.

3. A nonstandard encoding process is found in many people who are able to decode with complete adequacy. Their encoding is meaningful if the imperfection of the end product (speech behavior) is

ignored or adjusted to. Examples of this type of disorder are found among people most frequently referred to as defective in speech, i.e., defects of articulation, voice, and fluency.

4. Deterioration of decoding and/or encoding skills which occurs after the talent of language has been learned. The most obvious example is that of aphasia, which is usually associated with brain damage, but it may also accompany many other physical and environmental aberrations.

Once the examiner has determined the nature of the disorder, he should seek to describe its etiology with reference to conditions occurring both prior to and after the onset.

Many factors may interfere with linguistic processes. A defect of one part of the linguistic process is not due to one determiner acting independently of the others. It is instead the product of all determiners acting in concert. This is important in diagnosis, since to oversimplify the condition and to see it in too narrow a perspective can only result in defective therapy.

ETIOLOGY OF DISORDERS

The determiners of behavior can be divided into three groups: environmental influences on the speaker, his physical condition having long-term cumulative effects, and situational stresses affecting the client at the time of examination having less lasting ones. Many persons who have communication disorders demonstrate no gross physical abnormality, but one seldom if ever finds a language disorder associated with a gross physical anomaly persisting over a period of time which has not also been complicated by environmental conditions.

The situational stress determiner is of special importance to the diagnostician since it may markedly increase or decrease the severity of the disorder at time of examination. Speech behavior observed at this time may not be representative of that which is habitual, regardless of the cumulative strength of physical and environmental determiners. Thus, while the physical and environmental determiners have a continuing effect on the speaker, the situational stresses may cause him to change his habitual speech behavior temporarily.

In order to study the effect of environmental behavior on linguistic disorders, one must begin with an assumption that language is a form of learned behavior superimposed on nonlinguistic experiences and capacities. As such, it is obviously necessary that the child have the cooperation of the environment if he is to become capable of comprehending speech as well as using it. Environment can also affect adversely the development of linguistic skills or disrupt them after they have been established.

Although systems of classifying human behavior may be designed for a variety of purposes they usually are dependent on a process which consolidates various relevant events under various umbrellas and excludes all irrelevant ones. A good classification system may aid the diagnostician in identifying and describing speech disorders. It may also facilitate diagnosis by focusing attention on etiology. A poor classification system may misdirect the diagnostician. For the most part no attempt should be made to serve both as a description of the disorder and its etiology, as is true of the term "dysarthria," unless there is no question of etiology of the disorder being described.

The terms "physical" and "environmental" determiners of etiology of speech behavior should not be used to imply that either one functions with complete independence, since speech is dynamic and one event leads to modification of subsequent events. The conjoining of all conditions that determine the nature of speech disorders under the terms "environmental" and "physical" gives the diagnostician some direction. Further assistance will come from more definitive subdivisions of these two determiners. This is possible if one realizes that both will have a different effect on speech behavior during the periods when speech is developing and when it is deteriorating. For example, the environmental influence on behavior will be quite different during infancy than during the geriatric stage. In like manner, the physical capacity of the person changes considerably during the same periods. In addition to the "normal" changes that come gradually and can be predicted, are those bizzare, precipitous ones that seem to be correlated with sudden changes in determiners. A few of these conditions involve various psychological disturbances and injury or disease of bodily tissues.

The reader is likely to say that such classifications are the same as the age-old ones used by medicine, i.e., functional and organic. However, real differences do exist. Since speech is learned and all speech disorders are dynamic because of their continued use in communication, it can be demonstrated that all disorders have a functional component which is the outgrowth of the interaction between environmental influences and the physical organism of the person during the speech act. The debilitating effect on speech behavior may be affected more by the environment in one instance or by the physical condition in another, but both are involved at all times. So the use of either functional or organic as definitive of a "single cause" is evidence that the diagnostician has not recognized that the disorder involves learned behavior. Such thinking is likely to cause him to ignore interaction between the determiners in his programming of therapy.

Besides the division of determiners into physical and environmental, each of these categories lends itself to further subdivision relating to the development and deterioration of speech. The *developmental* conditions are those that occur prior to the time when an individual attains comparatively stable speech patterns. Most children achieve this level between six and 10 years of age whether the pattern that is stabilized is normal or defective. The developmental conditions overlap the prelinguistic (infancy) period and early linguistic experiences of children. Both environmental and physical determiners may significantly affect the child's speech during this period. The *deteriorative* factors are those which occur after a constancy of speech pattern has been attained. During this period both environmental and physical conditions may contribute to the deterioration of habitual speech patterns.

Environmental determiners occurring during the developmental stages of speech in the prelinguistic (infancy) period:

1. Failure to associate noises made by the infant with a need he may be expressing. For instance, adherence to a rigorous feeding time schedule may cause the mother to overlook the infant's cries as being associated with a desire for food. This may slow down the development of a communication attitude.

2. Failure to reinforce the infant's vocal play sounds. This may result in a reduction in the number and skill of oral movements developed by the infant.

3. Failure of the mother to accompany care of the infant with verbal output. This failure to talk to the infant reduces his attention to speech, since comprehension will come only through the association of speech with meaningful behavior.

4. Failure to provide for imitation model sounds which are relatively new to the infant. Thus, a skill in producing new sounds is not stimulated and practice in these sounds is reduced.

5. Failure to provide reinforcement when relatively new sounds are produced by the infant. Failure of operant conditioning may result in the extinguishing of further attempts to produce the sound.

Environmental determiners occurring during the developmental stages of speech in the linguistic (childhood) period:

1. Failure to comprehend, accept, and positively reinforce the early speech attempts. This is likely to result in a regression to nonlinguistic patterns and a slowing of the development of speech as a medium of communication.

2. Overacceptance and encouragement of pantomime as a tool of expression. This encourages the continued use of gestures as a means of communication since in the beginning they are easier to use than speech.

3. Acceptance and reinforcement of infantile speech behavior, which will result in the maintenance of this type of behavior.

4. Undue positive reinforcement of irrelevant conditions, such as extraneous lip, tongue, jaw, and breathing movements associated by chance with the speech act. This results in the maintenance of this undesirable behavior.

5. Undue penalty, such as hitting, shouting, etc., directed toward faulty speech patterns. This may cause the individual to withdraw from oral communication even though the speech as a medium is well established. It may also produce an exaggeration of the abnormality when speech is produced.

6. In some cases there may be a generalized dearth of reinforcement of communication and other learned behavior. There may be so little motivation to learn and so little reinforcement of success that the child, in addition to being seriously deficient in language, is also seriously deficient in so many other skills that he, in fact, has a "learned mental deficiency."

Environmental determiners relating to the deterioration of established speech:

1. Undue penalty associated with the speech act. This may cause the individual to withdraw from oral

communication even though the medium is well established.

2. Placement of the individual in an atmosphere which is emotionally upsetting and therefore not conducive to speech. This too may cause the individual to withdraw from speaking even though the medium is well established.

Physical determiners occurring during the developmental stages of speech in the prelinguistic (infancy) period:

1. Sensory disabilities, such as audition and vision, are likely to limit the infant's interaction with his environment. This limitation will slow down subsequent language acquisition that is an outgrowth of preverbal experiences. Sensory disturbances of hearing, touch, and proprioception may reduce the effectiveness of the infant's self-evaluation, self-regulation, and self-reinforcement. Inability to control his behavior will affect him adversely when he needs this skill while trying to talk.

2. Motor disabilities limiting the coordination of movement will also limit the ability to achieve precise postures of the speech mechanism. Usually the effect will limit speech and language acquisition.

3. Damage to the brain may be an important deterrent to meaningful nonlinguistic communication between the infant and his environment. However, the relationship, insofar as infants are concerned, has not been well established and therefore its effect can only be hypothesized.

4. Ill-health during infancy and childhood may not only reduce the child's physical ability to perform nonverbal communication acts but may also have an adverse effect on the environmental reactions so that the infant is neither stimulated to interact nor reinforced when he does. Another effect it may have is to cause the environment to anticipate all of the infant's needs so he does not have to learn to initiate any nonverbal communication act.

Physical determiners occurring during the developmental stages of speech in the linguistic (childhood) period:

The extension of conditions as listed above under the preverbal period may also be present in the verbal period and may likewise be determiners in dysfunctions of oral language.

Physical determiners relating to the deterioration of established language and speech:

1. Injury, disease, or age as it effects the *sensory mechanism* may influence the speech pattern if it interferes with the speaker's ability to evaluate his own speech adequacy. This will be especially relevant to disorders of hearing, touch, and proprioception. Sensory deficiencies may also interfere with the effectiveness with which the person can recharge his storehouse of information about how standard speech sounds as related to how he "sounds" to himself.

2. Injury, disease, or age as it affects the *central nervous system.* This anomaly does not lend itself to precise predictions. It can unquestionably disturb habitual language patterns. It can also affect articulation, fluency, and voice.

3. Injury, disease, and age may affect *body structure and muscle coordination.* They in turn may affect articulation, fluency, and voice.

THE EXAMINATION

Preinterview investigation

When a person is admitted for examination, the first problem is to identify the type of disorder so that appropriate diagnostic tests can be chosen. As a rule, observations of speech behavior enable a skilled examiner to identify the type of disorder, especially if the case history verifies his evaluation.

Most adult clients are not accompanied by any other member of the family at the time of examination; and most children are accompanied by only one parent, usually the mother. This is likely to limit the extent of information that can be obtained during the first interview. It is essential, therefore, that additional sources of information be tapped prior to the first interview. A simple way of obtaining this information is by sending brief questionnaires to appropriate sources such as the family, physician, school, or employer to be returned before the first interview. Reports can be requested from hospitals, social agencies, and other speech and hearing agencies that have provided services to the client. Other individuals and organizations may be contacted informally by mail or telephone. Sample forms such as those shown at the end of this chapter may be useful.

The histories received through correspondence and information from other sources obtained prior to the examination should be reviewed before the client is observed. This will acquaint the examiner with the problem that is alleged to exist as well as the type of people with whom he must deal. It may save time by eliminating redundant examinations. It may also result in a more thorough and accurate case review since much of the information that is needed will not be known or easily recalled by persons participating in personal interviews. Information received through correspondence also gives the examiner a referent with which to compare information received in the personal interview. However, it should be kept in mind that the history obtained by personal interview is in most respects far superior. An example of such a psychodiagnostic blank is reported by Louttit (1947).

Personal interview

The personal interview allows the examiner to: 1. evaluate testimony for important clues about the client that can be followed up immediately, 2. help ease the pain when unpleasant personal matters are discussed, 3. check answers which are unclear, incomplete, or of doubtful accuracy, 4. relieve the parents of some anxiety or guilt feelings about some of their past behavior toward the child. At the same time the examiner is able to observe and record the nature of the parental reactions, 5. establish a friendly rapport with the family, school, or agency, and 6. above all, follow up the leads which come from observations of the client. In a sense, the case history should be considered an extension of the observation period as far back as the birth of the child. (Many of these "observations," however, will not have been made by a clinically trained person, hence they must be accepted with caution.)

Autobiography

Another valuable source of information is the autobiography, which can be used as a supplement to the case history when dealing with teenagers and adults, especially those whose disorders will persist long enough that the client will have to learn to adjust to them. Usually, the examiner must give some supervision, but he must be careful that the supervision is suggestive in a way that stimulates the person to write expansively rather than restricting him to a set pattern. Such suggestions as the following may create a permissive situation which will enable the person to write his thoughts without fear of penalty.

> We need to know as much about you as possible because the better we know you the better we can help you. If you will just think of your life as a story and begin to write about it, you will find it interesting and so will we. Don't feel that you must tell us what caused your disorder; simply tell us what you know about yourself. No detail in your life is too small or uninteresting for us. You have lived a number of years and had a lot of experiences and thought a lot of thoughts; so you will probably find that fifty pages is not too much. Don't worry about your writing, grammar, or spelling; we are interested in you, not how well you write.

Occasionally the autobiography will be written in a brief outline form and must be filled in; however, most people enjoy writing about their lives if they believe the examiner is really interested and friendly. Once the autobiography has been finished, the examiner can always ask for additional information if some period of the person's life has been excluded.

Establishing rapport

When the client being examined is a child, one may observe him first as he interacts with family members and other people who are present. The tester should direct attention briefly to the adults but should not talk about the child. Some friendly reference should then be directed toward the child, by reacting to his clothes or a new toy, or mentioning what a strong boy he is. An effort must be made to direct his attention to real-life activities which the child is happy about. Under no circumstances should attention be directed to his speech, mouth, or ears, or any other structure or bodily action which the child may associate with punishment, shame, or anxiety.

If, after a reasonable period of time, the child does not interact with the examiner, it may be wise to turn from the child to others in the room so as to give the child little or no overt attention. Presently, the child may insert himself into the situation and demand some attention, and this should be given him only after he shows some willingness to cooperate. However, if the child persists in withdrawing from the examiner and from the situation, it may be necessary to transfer him to another examiner in another room (playroom if available) and, if possible, without the presence of the parents.

Assessments of client's behavior

Observation made of the child in his home would, of course, be most desirable but is often impossible to achieve. Observation on a playground or in a room with other children will often be helpful.

During these first observations, information should be gained about the following: 1. general behavior and level of maturity; 2. physical appearance and parental reaction to it; 3. adjustment of child while speaking and during nonlinguistic situations, and parental reactions during these situations; and 4. parental reactions while child is being examined and at times when parent is unaware he is being observed, and methods of discipline and child's reaction to them.

Observations of this sort should provide a descriptive picture of the child and his behavior which is far superior to one gained from either the preexamination sources or the personal interview history since the examiner has an opportunity to assess at first-hand the child's behavior rather than to depend on second-hand testimony. Actually, the personal interview should describe the bases of some behavior. It will often focus attention on behavior that might have been overlooked. For this reason the period for personal interviewing and for observations should overlap.

General information examinations

Physical examinations are routinely required by many clinics. Whether one accepts this position depends partly on where he performs his service and partly on the types of disorders his clients present. The observations of another professional person can be helpful and the health of a client is always important. However, in many cases the health information is known and the value of further investigation is questionable for many clients, especially if their problems are not ordinarily associated with chronic or acute illness or physical disorders. Many speech disorders fall into such a grouping.

The physical examination is a must if the speech disorder is associated with an illness or physical anomaly. The physician might be expected to give information about the nature of the disorder, kinds of treatment, and the limitations the condition imposes on the clinical process.

Psychological tests should be routinely given. They give the diagnostician another way of comparing the behavior of the client with that of controlled samples of people under standardized conditions. They point out strengths and weaknesses of many psychological processes. They also assist in prognosis in that they suggest the complexity of tasks that can be performed.

Mental testing of the speech-handicapped is complicated by faulty communication. Some clients are unable to understand what the examiner says or to make the examiner understand them. In spite of these difficulties, a communication barrier must not be allowed to depress the intelligence quotient. We are measuring intelligence, not language performance. In order to attempt to avoid this hazard the diagnostician must choose his tests carefully and on occasion vary the standard test procedures to fit the capacity of the client.

For those who can neither decode language or encode it, the examination must be strictly nonlinguistic insofar as both instruction and responses are concerned. The following test meets this criteria. The Hiskey-Nebraska Test of Learning Aptitude (1966) is one of the few intelligence tests particularly applicable to deaf children. This test not only has norms for deaf subjects, but it has also been administered to and has norms for a normal hearing population.

For those who can decode language but cannot encode it, the instructions can be linguistic in nature but the responses expected of the client must not be. Several tests have been developed which give some indication of the individual's intellectual ability by requiring a strictly performance task. One such test is the Goodenough-Harris Drawing Test (1963). The individual is asked to draw three pictures—man, woman, and self. These pictures are scored according to stringent criteria. The score yields a high correlation with an individual intelligence test for children between the ages of five and 10. However, the instrument is used primarily as a supplemental procedure.

Another performance test is the Point Scale of Performance Tests developed by Grace A. Arthur (1925, 1947). This test may be administered to subjects ranging in ages from four and one-half to adult and has been standardized on the same sample.

Several picture tests have been developed to use in assessing the individual's intellectual level. One of the more recent of these is the Pictorial Test of Intelligence (1964) developed by Joseph French. In this test, questions are presented orally by the examiner while he shows the subject some large picture cards on which are represented four possible choices or answers to the questions. The results are used in assessing general intellectual level of both normal and handicapped children.

Other tests have been developed which attempt to assess the individual's intellectual ability by sampling his behavior. Sources and descriptions of these tests as well as their experimental applications can be found in Buros' 1970 edition of Personality Tests and Reviews published by Gryphon, Highland Park, New Jersey. The Peabody Picture Vocabulary Test (1965) is one such attempt. The test has norms for ages three to 18. Several plates of four pictures are shown and the subject is asked to indicate which picture best depicts the word said by the examiner. Results have been standardized to give some indication of intelligence quotients and mental age.

In the Van Alstyne Picture Vocabulary Test (1960) 60 cards each with four pictures are presented and the child is asked to respond to each of the cards by indicating the picture which illustrates a stimulus word or phrase presented orally by the examiner. The results provide an estimate of the mental ability of children in the mental age range from two to seven years.

For those who can decode as well as encode language but have a disability in the final process of encoding, the instructions can always be linguistic. The responses expected of the client can also be verbal provided the examiner can understand them and provided the client is not penalized because of slow responses as might occur with stutterers.

A test particularly applicable to young children below the age of six is the Stanford-Binet, Form L-M (1960). Above the six-year level the test becomes primarily verbal and may not be suitable for children with communication problems.

The Wechsler Intelligence Scale for Children (1949) is divided into verbal and performance sections and thus may give a better idea of a child's ability when a communication problem impairs his verbal performance. The Wechsler Preschool and Primary Scale of Intelligence (1967) has recently been developed to extend the Wechsler series downward to younger children.

The Wechsler Adult Intelligence Scale (1955) is particularly adaptable for adult intelligence testing. It too is divided into verbal and performance sections. The division into verbal and performance sections affords the examiner an opportunity to compare verbal performance abilities within an individual subject.

The performance items from the Stanford-Binet, the Wechsler Intelligence Scale for Children, and the Wechsler Adult Intelligence Scale may also be used separately with those who can decode language but cannot encode it to give some indication of the intellectual functioning of these individuals when encoding is not required.

In addition to mental tests, a number of other psychological tests can be used for specific purposes. An exemplary offering in the area of testing is the Illinois Test of Psycholinguistic Abilities (Kirk, McCarthy, and Kirk, 1968). This test is not an intelligence test but is an attempt to study a child's ability to use language both in the decoding and encoding processes.

One of the few available tests to compare the social maturity of a child with others of his age is the Vineland Social Maturity Scale (1947). Questions are asked of the parent regarding eating habits, skills in dressing, playing, etc.

There are several personality tests which can be administered to children and adults and interpreted by a competent examiner. The Minnesota Multiphasic Personality Inventory (1951) is a self-administered personality questionnaire composed of 550 items. It was designed for the purpose of screening deviant personalities though some of the scales have been found to be particularly weak in predicting the defect they purport to predict.

The Children's Apperception Test (1949) is applicable to ages three to 10 and is made up of pictures of animals aimed to elicit information on feeding conflicts, sibling rivalry, and other childhood problems.

The Thematic Apperception Test (1938) requires the subject to interpret 20 pictures by telling a story about each—what is happening, what led up to the scene, and what will be the outcome. The trained interpreter derives an hypothesis from each story and checks it with subsequent stories. The interpreter must integrate the information on intellectual powers, emotional conflicts, and defense mechanisms indicated by the test protocol.

In the Rorschach Inkblot Test the subject is asked to tell what he sees in 10 inkblots. The interpretation begins with a systematic scoring according to fairly objective rules. Simultaneously, however, the examiner collects impressionistic interpretations.

There is also a group of tests designed to investigate the perceptual motor abilities of individuals. One such test is the Bender Visual Motor Gestalt Test (1946). The subject is asked to copy eight separate figures. Scoring rules have been developed, but the examiner generally attempts a qualitative integration.

A large variety of school achievement tests are available which give an indication of the individual's performance in various subject areas. The Stanford Achievement Test (1953) is applicable to grades one through nine; the Metropolitan Achievement Test (1959) may also be administered to grades one through nine; and the Iowa Tests of Basic Skills may be administered to grades three through nine. The Durrell Analysis of Reading Difficulty and the Gates tests provide information specifically about reading ability.

Identifying disorders of speech or language

The diagnostician is usually able to "label" the client's problem by the time the history, general observation, and physical and psychological tests have been finished. As a matter of fact, he will have progressed further in his diagnosis than identification with most clients. For the few whose disorder is still obscure, more definitive interviewing and observation will be needed.

Identification should involve data relevant to the nature of the faulty speech behavior, not its etiology. All clients should be assigned to one of the following four groups:

1. Those who neither decode speech or encode it as a means of communication.
2. Those who do decode speech but do not encode it as a means of communication.
3. Those who do decode speech and do encode it in expressing themselves but have a defective encoding process.
4. Those who have lost some of their ability to decode speech and/or encode it as a means of expression.

Once this assignment is made, the diagnostician is ready to focus on the next stage of diagnosis—etiology.

DIFFERENTIAL DIAGNOSIS

Many speech disorders with essentially the same overt symptoms have different sets of determiners. Both the nature of the disorder and the conditions that bring it about must be determined if a scientifically planned therapy is to be designed.

Persons who neither decode speech nor encode it as a means of communication

The language dysfunction of those who neither understand speech nor use it as a medium of communication is a good illustration. Failure to use language is easily identified, but this fact is not too helpful to the clinician unless he also knows something about the determiners that brought about the disorder.

The primary determiner of this disorder may be either physical or environmental. Deafness, brain injury, and structural disabilities represent the first, and psychological disturbance and cultural deprivation represent the second. Mentally retarded children often are found in either group.

Differentiation between these etiologies will be revealed by nonverbal behavior. The deaf child shows little or no response to verbal and nonverbal sounds while the others, with the exception of autistic children, will respond to nonverbal stimulation. Pantomime is often effective, provided it is meaningful, with all except the autistic child. Usually a stranger will have to spend some time conditioning these children to their pantomimes. However, samples of this form of the child's communication are readily available by observing him and his parents in real situations in lunchrooms, playrooms, etc.

Differentiation between the etiologies can also be obtained by physical examinations since they will locate children with physical anomalies. Furthermore, thorough examinations will also reveal the nature of the organic problems.

Investigation of major environmental determiners depends largely on good interviews and careful observations of interactions between the child and family or others.

Prognoses for these clients are difficult to make. Certainly the more serious the anomalous behavior the less hopeful is the prognosis. However, no anomaly functions independently as a predictor since other determiners which are also present may completely change the picture. (A child with marked mental retardation is likely to develop better language if he has good environmental assistance than a mildly retarded one with poor environmental help.)

Children who decode language but do not encode it

These children are not so difficult to deal with as those who are unable to understand and express. The diagnostician has a medium for communicating with these children and by careful planning can enable the child to give meaningful nonverbal responses. Although profound deafness as a determiner can be ruled out, less severe hearing losses might be present.

These losses are more likely to interfere with some of the phases of the encoding process, i.e., articulation and voice rather than to disrupt the whole process.

Personality disorders leading to such conditions as autism will usually affect both the decoding and encoding processes. However, less severe disturbances may have caused the child to withdraw from oral verbal expression. Careful case history related to the early development of speech may be helpful. Information that the child did say words or phrases at one time and then stopped is common. It shows that a serious breakdown of environmental behavior occurred and is a major determiner of the disorder.

Severe physical anomalies are more likely to interfere with the encoding than the decoding process. Since these children may have a difficult task in formulating sounds and words well enough to be understood, they may receive poor feedback from their environment. They may find it easier to withdraw into gestural language. (Fortunately, most children do muddle through and learn to speak anyway.) The relevance of these physical disorders to the speech condition is a matter for the clinician to decide, but the nature of the physical condition and the method of its treatment is up to medical specialists.

Intellectual retardation is one of the more common etiologies of language retardation. In a cooperative child, it is usually possible to measure the level of intelligence. For the most part, the level of language will not exceed the mental age of the child, and the diagnostician must remember that expressive language of the average three- or four-year-old child is complex.

Unfortunately, the calculation of the level of intelligence will not determine the cause of retardation. Two and three decades ago it was almost universally thought to be caused by some kind of organic anomaly. Currently, it is believed that many children with "normal bodies" have literally learned to act retarded until the behavior pattern became fixed. The reason for mentioning this theoretical explanation of some cases of mental retardation is that the very conditions that interfere with mental growth in children may also interfere with their language development.

DEPRIVATION OF ENVIRONMENTAL FACILITATION

The development of language skills in any child requires numerous meaningful stimulations of the child by his environment and reinforcements of his responses during interpersonal interactions.

A child will not develop language if for any reason he is unable to receive stimuli from his environment or to produce responses that are meaningful enough to warrant reinforcement. In a sense all children who have delayed language may be said to have been deprived, to some degree, of environmental facilitation. Of course, the greater the physical limitations the greater the likelihood the child will be deprived even though his environment makes a real effort to develop compensations.

Many rejected or ignored children do not learn to encode language even though they were born with the physical components needed for language acquisition. Children reared in their natural homes and orphans may be rejected in such a way as to keep them from receiving environmental stimulation and reinforcement. Cries and other noises produced by these children are ignored and no effort is made to talk to them while they are being fed and cared for. Not only will these children fail to develop language, they may also fail to acquire other skills needed in eating, walking, dressing, toilet training, etc. As environmental horizons for these children are expanded, the greater the likelihood that they will begin encoding language, but the longer they depend on nonverbal media the poorer their prognosis will be.

Children smothered with love and attention may also fail to acquire encoding skills—there is no need for speech since their pantomimes are willingly interpreted by overly solicitous parents.

Excessive attention given to some children may have grown out of great love for the child, insecurity of parent, or illness of child. As one mother said whose 10-year-old daughter had a language level of a five-year-old, "We waited for ten years before she was born and we just wanted her to have everything she wanted." This mother was on her feet to serve the child before the child knew she needed something.

Insecure parents may hover over their child in order to ward off criticism from relatives and neighbors. One very intelligent war bride had a beautiful five-year-old daughter who did not speak. Her husband was sure the child's defect was due to the foreign accent of the mother. The mother overcompensated for her own defective speech by overprotecting the child.

Perfectionistic parents may also force their unreasonable expectations on their child. They expect such excellent performance of their child that they refuse to reward him for speech that is not normal and may even punish him. A child whose best efforts are rejected may withdraw to an easier mode of communication than speech.

Resentment felt by perfectionistic parents may be revealed in such statements as, "he is so stubborn," "he won't do anything I tell him to do," or "he used to say words when he was little but he just stopped talking."

DISORDERS OF PROCESS OF ENCODING IN PERSONS WHOSE LANGUAGE USAGE IS OTHERWISE ADEQUATE

Disorders of articulation

In this disorder, phonemes used in encoding speech deviate markedly from standard. The deviation may be due to acoustic or to physiological variations so that speech either sounds or looks defective to the audience.

It may also attract the attention of the speaker himself through a direct feedback circuit which is activated when he hears his own speech and feels the movement of the speech mechanism. It is more likely to be brought to his attention, however, when the indirect (interpersonal) circuit between himself and his audience feeds back a rejection of his speech pattern. These feedback circuits were described by Milisen (1966).

Deviant phonemes are not evidence of articulation disorders unless they affect communication. Those that interfere with intelligibility of speech are likely to be severely deviant or the listener is not well trained in the decoding process.

The act of articulation changes in a multitude of ways from one situation to another. Its variance may affect some people in a situation and not others. The great variance of the act itself and the manner in which it affects participants make this type of speech behavior difficult to evaluate.

A rationale for the disorder of articulation was given by the author in 1954. An attempt was made to correlate the description, development, diagnosis, and rehabilitation of the disorder. The basic concept proposed that the disorder of disarticulation is learned as a result of disruption of the developmental process growing out of interactions between the child and his environment. This disruption may grow out of limitations of the physical make-up of the child interacting with inadequacies of his environment. It also proposed that the disorder need not be maintained by any child if he receives suitable help that begins early enough and continues long enough.

In addition to the developmental articulation disorders, the defect may result from a deterioration of stable articulation patterns of older children and adults. The principles used in diagnosing disorders of articulation are much the same whether the etiology relates to developmental arrest or to deteriorated learning. Materials and methods used in testing do differ not only because of age of the clients but also because of the different physical and environmental determiners.

The articulation test

Essential to a description of this disorder is a careful phonetic analysis of habitual articulation used in conversational speech. This analysis includes the faulty acoustic and visual characteristics of each defective sound in all positions in words. Reports should also be made on the variance of articulation produced as the phonetic environment of the sound is changed. The effects of phonemic environment on speech-sound production have been described in detail by MacDonald (1964). He has also published the Deep Articulation Test that is admirably designed for this type of assessment. Another articulation test often used by clinicians was published by Templin and Darley (1960). This is an excellent test for research purposes but tends to be too rigid in its procedure to meet many clinical needs.

Anomalous physiological behavior that is used in producing misarticulations must be reported. These anomalous conditions represent the pattern the client has learned to use. They often point directly to the conditions that must be changed if better articulation is to be achieved. The best information is provided by the acoustic characteristics of the phonemes and the way the physiological process looks. However, many features cannot be heard or seen, so the examiner must turn to other measures such as nasal olives and candle flames for measuring nasal air emission and tubes held against the teeth to measure air flow of lateral lispers. (Some of these methods were described by the author in 1966.)

Tests of speech-sound discrimination are recommended by many people. For the most part, the child who is efficient in decoding oral language has demonstrated efficiency in speech-sound discrimination. Discrimination ear-training of the traditional type for these children is of doubtful value. However, for those children whose discrimination reduces efficiency of decoding language, traditional types of discrimination tests are available. Travis and Rasmus (1931) describe a test of speech-sound discrimination. Their pattern has been followed by Templin (1957) and by Van Riper (1954).

Discrimination involving self-evaluation is always of value and should be used by diagnosticians. It assesses the speaker's ability to identify his own errors and the manner in which he deviates from a standard. This can be done informally by asking the person if he has trouble making some sounds. If the answer is yes, follow-up questions would be "which ones?" and "how?" Negative answers may not represent the client's self-evaluative capacity. They should be followed up by concrete speech experience in which the client says a word or sentence. The accuracy of his articulation should be evaluated by him. Results from this test will indicate his self-evaluative efficiency level while attention is directed to his process of encoding. (His ability to self-evaluate will change when attention is directed to content of speech, rather than to its process.) Of course, the examiner must pay close attention to the physical mechanisms used in speech, especially those parts that are closely involved in the production of misarticulated sounds.

After the habitually misarticulated sounds have been identified and described, the examiner is ready to administer additional articulation tests for the purpose of determining the level of difficulty at which various misarticulated sounds can be improved or corrected by the client. In order to achieve this goal, a series of tests should be used which are arranged on a continuum from easy to difficult. The easy tests should facilitate good articulation and the difficult ones should not. The judgment of improvement can be made on the degree of approximation to normal that is achieved by the client and the difficulty of the test on which the achievement occurred.

A test program was published in 1968 by the author that is patterened after the one reported in 1954. It provides for brief reports of the physical condition and extensive analysis of habitual (phonetic) behavior, of anomalous behavior used in producing sounds, and of the level of skill achieved by the client for each of his misarticulated sounds.

This test, referred to as the BASIC DATA SHEET, requires a comparatively short time to administer (20 to 30 minutes for most clients) but it gives the diagnostician an opportunity to make many comparisons of the client in order to separate relevant from irrelevant information. These data also help the clinician in planning his therapy, whereas most articulation tests do not since they identify the misarticulated sounds and the nature of articulation responses under only one testing condition.

INSTRUCTIONS FOR ADMINISTERING BASIC DATA SHEET

This form provides a quick over view of various communication and organic disabilities and was published by Milisen (1968). In addition, special attention is devoted to articulation since this disorder is present in such a large percentage of people who have speech and hearing handicaps. The goal of the data sheet is to provide maximum visibility of the various disorders of communication with a minimum of time devoted to recording. Multiple-handicapped individuals with articulation difficulty as well as patients with other types of disorders of communication should be examined further and the results recorded on data sheets specifically designed for those specific disorders.

Identification of communication disorders

The purpose is to bring into focus all types of language, speech and hearing disorders. A patient is marked defective if his performance is below that of other people of the same age. Hence the examiner always compares *test performance* with *developmental expectancy*. The examiner must, therefore, develop standards for judging behavior of individuals of different age levels for the various skills being measured.

Organic conditions

Various anatomical and physiological processes are to be judged as normal or defective. Since no absolute criteria exists for separating normal from defective, the examiner must make a subjective judgment as to whether the organic deviation from "hypothetical perfect" is sufficient to warrant further testing. In other words, does the organic condition deviate enough to interfere with communication? If the answer is *yes*, the item should be checked in the defective column; if not, it should be marked in the "normal" one.

Articulation behavior

This disorder should be measured in depth only if the examiner observes defective articulation during conversational speech, or if the patient is specifically referred for an appraisal of his articulation skill.

Items in the data sheet which deal specifically with articulation

1. The column labeled *Sound* lists the consonants in a specified order to facilitate testing and diagnosis. The order is determined by the probability that a sound will be misarticulated, its frequency of occurrence in the language, and similarity of distinctive features. The phonemes which are misarticulated by more people and occur more frequently in the language are placed toward the top. Cognates are paired with the unvoiced phoneme listed first.

Vowels, diphthongs and consonant clusters are given less attention than single consonants. Vowels and diphthongs are listed in the order of their production. Only a sample of consonant clusters are listed.

2. *WAT* represents the word articulation test. Speech responses are elicited spontaneously, by pictures, without giving the client cues as to how the phonemes should be articulated. (The chief weakness of this test is that patients often use better than their habitual articulation. When this occurs, it may be due to the fact that the test is composed of single words making it possible to attend to the process of articulation rather than to the content of speech.)

3. *CAT* represents the conversational articulation test. Speech responses are elicited by engaging in conversation with the patient. Conversation may take place between the client and the examiner or some lay person such as the mother. The recording is, of course, performed by the examiner. Usually, it is accomplished by writing on a scratch pad a sample of words which are misarticulated. The nature of the error is recorded above that letter in the word which was misarticulated. Results of this informal testing are transferred to the data sheet.

4. *Anomalous behavior* provides space for a brief description of the feature of the speech process which is defective. Generally, a description is not necessary since the speech characteristic can be identified by studying the nature of the response on the WAT or CAT. For instance, a substitution of /*θ*/ for /*s*/ describes satisfactorily the nature of the faulty response if the examiner knows how those sounds are normally produced. If, however, the response is in the form of a lateral lisp, no phonetic symbol will suffice since the air may be emitted between the teeth on the right side, the left, side, or both. Hence the nature of the anomalous behavior should be described.

5. *SST* represents the (isolated) sound stimulation test with the sound elicited by imitation of the model sound presented orally by the clinician.

6. *SYST* represents the syllable stimulation test with the syllable elicited by imitation of the model syllable presented orally by the clinician.

7. *WST* represents the word stimulation test with the word elicited by imitation of a model word presented orally by the clinician.

8. *WCT* represents the word control test with single-word responses uttered *carefully* by the client as he attempts to articulate the word correctly. Models are not provided for the client to imitate, nor are other cues provided that may enable him to articulate better. (This test is not administered if the client is very sensitive about his speech.)

9. *SORT* represents the oral reading articulation test composed of sentences. Speech responses are elicited by having the client read paragraphs containing words within the level of the patient's reading ability. (This test is not administered if the client has insufficient reading skill.)

10. *Frequency* refers to the rank order of frequency of usage of speech sounds in the written language (Dewey, 1923). It indicates how often a defective phoneme will occur in conversation; and, therefore, how often the phoneme may disrupt communication if it is defective.

11. *Developmental age* refers to the developmental age at which approximately 75 percent of the children demonstrate an ability to produce the phoneme correctly. The age norm listed in this column is an extrapolation from the study by Templin (1945).

12. Separate cells are provided for recording responses in the initial, medial, and final positions of words or syllables for all tests except the SST. (This test is composed of isolated sounds and can only be administered in isolation.) Cells that are blocked out indicate that the phoneme does not occur in that position. For example, all voiced plosives are blocked out in the SST since they cannot be produced in isolation but can be produced in syllables.

13. The WAT and CAT constitute the *Descriptive Articulation Tests* and are administered during assessment of the habitual articulation of the client. When results of these two tests differ markedly, responses from the CAT should be retained and those from the WAT should be rejected since the CAT is likely to be more valid.

14. The *Prognostic Series* of tests begins with the SST (the easiest of the tests for most clients) and

progresses through the SYST, WST, WCT, and SORT, and ends with the CAT (the most difficult of the tests). This prognostic series provides the diagnostician with a systematic measurement of the client's speech behavior to be used in predicting the defective phonemes which may be more easily corrected. It also provides evidence as to how much learning has been achieved for each sound. This information is helpful in planning the client's therapy program.

HOW TO RECORD ARTICULATION RESPONSES

Although each production of a phoneme differs, all deviations can be assigned to one of five classifications to facilitate diagnosis, prognosis, and management. These classifications are: normal, mildly distorted, severely distorted, substituted, and omitted. The following system is to be utilized in evaluating articulation skill: the numeral "1" is recorded in the cell for each normal response, "2" for each mild distortion, "3" for each severe distortion, a phonetic symbol for each substitution, and "om" for each omission.

Each time the examiner elicits a response from a patient, it is recorded in the appropriate cell. No cell should be left blank if a response has been obtained. A blank space would mean that no response was obtained.

After all testing has been completed, it is possible for the examiner to *see at a glance* those phonemes which are misarticulated, the nature of the errors, the consistency of the errors, and the misarticulated phonemes which may be more easily corrected.

HOW TO ADMINISTER THE DESCRIPTIVE ARTICULATION TEST

Beginning with the establishment of rapport, the examiner should write on a scratch pad a sample of words misarticulated while engaged in conversation with the client. The nature of the misarticulation should be transcribed phonetically immediately above the misarticulated "letter." This process should be continued until at least six speech-sound positions (i.e., six responses in I, M, or F positions of two or more phonemes) have been recorded. This same process should be continued during the remainder of the diagnostic period. The evaluations should be transferred to the cells of the CAT as soon as is practical.

Following a general assessment of the client's articulation and the appropriate number of samples of habitual articulation obtained during conversational speech, the examiner should administer the WAT. Pictures for eliciting responses from children can be obtained from magazines and children's books. The pictures should be arranged in a booklet with three pictures to a page. The picture used to elicit the phoneme in the intial position should be placed at the top of the page, the picture used to elicit the phoneme in the medial position should be placed in the middle of the page, and the picture used to elicit the phoneme in the final position should be placed at the bottom of the page. Words representing each picture *should not* be written on the test. When possible, each phoneme should be represented by two different pictures of two different words placed on adjacent pages. (The advantages of having two pictures for each phoneme in each position are: a) when one picture does not elicit a response, the other can be used; b) when an examiner suspects that a misarticulation was primarily a mispronounciation, the alternative picture can be used to reevaluate the phoneme questioned; and c) when the examiner is not sure of the nature of the articulation rather than asking the child to repeat the word, another response may be obtained by pointing to the alternate picture.)

Materials for testing adults are more difficult to develop if the goal is to assess habitual articulation. Pictures tend to be insulting to the older person, although pictures from magazines may be less objectionable. Reading of lists of words, sentences, and paragraphs cannot be used in assessing habitual articulation because the printed letter will facilitate articulation (Wolfe, 1959) and, therefore, reduce not only the number of errors that occur habitually but also the severity of misarticulations. For example, few omissions will occur in oral reading even though the phoneme may be omitted in conversational speech. When a habitually omitted phoneme is changed in response to cues from reading, the change is usually to a less severe form of misarticulation rather than to "normal."

Fortunately, most adults do not misarticulate as many phonemes as children. It is usually possible to obtain longer samples of conversational speech from adults than from children. Therefore, it is wise to depend on conversation as a source for eliciting speech samples to be used in evaluating articulation of adults. The results of the conversational speech sample should be transferred to the cells in the CAT.

When the examiner is satisfied that he has obtained a valid sample of the client's habitual articulation, he is ready to begin the prognostic test series. The purposes of this series of tests are to enable him to:

1. predict the phonemes which may be more easily corrected.

2. determine, in an objective manner, the phonemes which should be emphasized in therapy, the level at which training should be initiated, and to some degree the kind of management to recommend.

HOW TO ADMINISTER TESTS IN THE PROGNOSTIC SERIES

The Prognostic Test Series is an in-depth assessment of articulation skill. Most Articulation Tests are not. The Prognostic Test Series evaluates the relationship between the adequacy of articulation responses and the:

1. complexity of the speech pattern.
2. method of eliciting the response.

These tests are arranged on a continuum, the SST representing the lowest level and the CAT representing the highest level on the continuum.

Since the Prognostic Test Series is arranged on a continuum, administration should begin with the easiest and continue with each succeeding test until one of the two following conditions has been obtained: 1. either the client's articulation has regressed to a level of defectiveness comparable to that of his habitual speech pattern, shown on CAT or WAT tests, or 2. the client has completed all of the tests up to the most difficult (the CAT) without regressing completely to his habitual level of articulation.

When to administer the Prognostic Test Series

These tests should not be initiated until the examiner is finished with the Descriptive Articulation Tests.

Phonemes to be tested in the Prognostic Series

The examiner must remember that the only phonemes to be tested in depth are those misarticulated habitually as shown by data from WAT and CAT. Furthermore, only those *speech-sound positions* misarticulated habitually should be reexamined in the Prognostic Series.

The administration of the SST involves vigorous integral stimulation and reinforcement of the client by the examiner. The goal is to determine how well the client can articulate the phoneme in isolation after receiving maximal stimulation and reinforcement from the examiner. The client should be afforded an opportunity to imitate the phoneme two or three times. The best response should be recorded. Instructions should be "watch me and listen and try to say the sound as I do."

The SYST should be administered in much the same manner as the SST. A syllable is presented orally as a model to be imitated and the phoneme is evaluated in the initial, medial, and final positions. Generally, the examiner should combine the consonant with the neutral vowel /ɑ/. Instructions should be "watch me and listen and try to say the syllable as I do."

The WST is administered in much the same way as the previous two tests. Words are presented orally as the model to be imitated. The same words as those used in the Descriptive Articulation Test should be presented with stimulation.

The WCT test is a valuable diagnostic tool since it demonstrates how well the patient can articulate a phoneme in a word when he is specifically trying to say the phoneme correctly. On the other hand, it may damage the client's self-confidence and the rapport between the client and the examiner if not presented in a thoughtful manner. The WCT should be administered only if the client appears to be aware of his misarticulations and is willing to accept his disorder with objectivity. (According to a study by Hadjian, 1961, phonemes produced in WAT have more errors and on WST fewer than on the WCT.)

The test words should be the same as those used in the WAT or CAT. The instructions should be as follows: "when I showed you this picture you had some trouble saying the sound at the beginning (or middle or end) of that word. Think about it and see if you can say it better." Good responses are reinforced.

The SORT test is a valuable diagnostic tool. It provides an opportunity to evaluate the client's articulation in speech samples comparable to those of conversation. Further advantages over CAT are: a) the speech sample can be predetermined, thus making certain that all sounds are produced quickly and easily, and b) evaluation of phonemes can be made more accurately than in conversational speech since the examiner is aware of the phonemes which are to be evaluated.

Fewer phonemes may be defective since the printed symbol often facilitates articulation of phonemes which are habitually misarticulated in conversation. When this result is observed it gives valuable therapeutic clues.

Administration of this test requires duplicate sets of reading materials. The testing material should be printed and double-spaced. The type should be large enough to be easily read. The examiner's copy should be the same as that read by the client; however, the test words in the examiner's copy should be underlined.

Instructions should be "Read this material out loud and be prepared to answer questions about it after you finish." (This latter instruction reduces the chances that the patient will be attending only to the processes of speech.) The examiner should record misarticulations immediately above the letters in the underlined words. These misarticulations should be transferred to the cells in the SORT as soon as the test is completed. Occasionally, the examiner may have to ask the client to reread a portion of the passage due to the client's rapid reading rate, cluttered speech, or weak volume.

Consonant clusters

The procedure used in testing articulation of consonants clustered with other consonants in words is quite different from that used in testing consonants produced adjacent to vowels. The objective of the consonant cluster test is to assess the assimilation effect on the articulation of commonly misarticulated sounds by other adjacent consonants. (Sometimes the effect facilitates and sometimes it disrupts production.)

In this test, careful selection of the phoneme that is adjacent to the test sound is important, not the position of the test sound in the word. In order to meet this criteria, a representative sample of phoneme clusters was chosen for each of 13 frequently misarticulated consonants. These clusters are composed of two or three phonemes each. Test words (in which these clusters are located) should be elementary enough to be found in the vocabulary of children and at the same time of such nature that they can be elicited by pictures.

The test words are listed on the articulation data form with the key sound underlined. The examiner elicits the key word from the client and records the articulation response in the proper cell as in the preceding tests. Most sounds can be tested three times, twice in double clusters and once in a triplet cluster. Each can also be examined in WAT and WST. Decision as to which sounds to examine in the WAT will depend on observations made during the Descriptive Articulation Series, especially during conversation. (Any sound produced defectively in a single element would be reexamined in a cluster.) Decision as to which sounds to reexamine on the WST is easily made since any sound misarticulated in a WAT cluster should be reexamined in a WST cluster.

Vowels and diphthongs

The procedure for evaluating these phonemes is essentially the same as that used for consonants with the exception of the Prognostic Test Series, which has been reduced to one test—the WST. The other prognostic tests are not included in this form because vowels are infrequently misarticulated and interfere with intelligibility less than do consonants. They are, therefore, less likely to require therapy and hence less attention.

Identification of all communication disorders is essential before a diagnosis can be completed and therapy planned. When multiple disorders are present, examination in depth should be conducted for each one. At the completion of diagnosis for the multiple handicapped, two decisions must be made: 1. which disorder is more severe, and 2. which disorder should be given the major role at the onset of the therapy program. (It is not always wise to place greatest stress on the client's most severe problem at the onset of therapy.) Subsequent to this decision all other disorders must play a minor role. For instance, one might initially completely exclude from the therapy design some aspect of behavior in need of improvement if it is felt it might interfere with rehabilitation of the major area.

Organic conditions provide cues as to whether further investigation is needed before a diagnosis can be made.

Descriptive tests provide the chief source of information included in the written report of the client's habitual articulation at the time of examination. These tests also identify the phonemes that must be studied further in the Prognostic Test Series. The descriptive test data also reflect the client's speech behavior at the most difficult level of the speech continuum represented by the Prognostic Test Series.

Prognostic Test Series provide a sequence of tests

ranked according to difficulty. They are useful to the diagnostician in predicting which phonemes may be more easily corrected. These tests also indicate which level of behavioral therapy should be initiated for each phoneme. An additional value produced by these tests is the guidance they give in choosing the type of learning processes to use for each misarticulated sound in each position. The types of learning processes which might be selected are: 1. raw learning, 2. transfer learning, and 3. extinction learning.

USES OF BASIC DATA SHEET

The data for diagnosis of articulation found in the Basic Data Sheet enable the clinician to describe with some accuracy the nature of the habitual articulation as well as the anomalous behavior which is present when misarticulations are produced.

When these test results are followed by analysis of data from the prognostic series the diagnostician has a basis for predicting ease of correction of sounds. Essentially, two factors are used in making this decision: the level of the prognostic continuum, and the degree of approximation of speech responses.

The level on the continuum at which a sound more nearly approximates normal than its habitual production provides vital data for forecasting improvement. For example, if two sounds are omitted habitually but in the prognostic series it is demonstrated that one is produced correctly in the SST and the other can be produced correctly as far along the prognostic series as the SORT, it is clear that the latter will be more easily corrected by therapy since it is already produced correctly in sentences that are read orally. The other sound will be more difficult to correct because it is produced correctly only in isolation, and considerable training will have to be given before the client will be able to produce it correctly at the SORT level. The same conclusions might be drawn for production of sounds on the prognostic series that do show improvement in degree of approximation but not enough to reach normal. For example, if the same two sounds were omitted habitually and if one were improved to the level of distortion in the SST and the other to the same level of approximation on the SORT, the latter sound would be more easily corrected than the first because the client more nearly approximated normal speech at a higher level of the prognostic series.

Change in degree of approximation in producing of sounds with the level of test held constant is also vital to prediction of prognosis of various sounds misarticulated by the same client. For example, if a child habitually makes substitution errors but changes one more than the other in the prognostic series, this change may be used in predicting the ease of correction of the two sounds. If one sound is still produced as a substitution at a given test level while the other is changed to a mild distortion, it is clear that the second sound more nearly approximates normal speech and should require less training.

These two measures (level on continuum and degree of approximation) of the client's skill in articulation provide the diagnostician with an objective basis for predicting which sounds misarticulated by his client will be more easily corrected. These measures also provide, in part, the answer to the question why are they more easily corrected. The reason is that the prognostic test series samples the etiological factors that are present and functioning at the time of the examination. The articulation responses made to the tests are a summation of all communication experience of the client as he has interacted with his environment. This summation provides information about achievement levels for each sound and also the kinds of deficiencies that are still present and interfering with articulation. These deficiencies may be consolidated into three speech variables: nature of speech pattern, method of elicitation of speech, and the audience effect.

The nature of the articulation therapy can also be predicted to a degree from the prognostic series since each response samples the skill of the client in producing sounds at specific levels of each of the three therapy variables. For example, if one sound is produced correctly on the SST and another on the WST it is clear that therapy for each should differ. The first should not begin with the stimulation of the sound in isolation since the client has already demonstrated skill at this level. The level of either the speech pattern or the elicitation variable should be advanced. Thus speech level might be advanced from the sound in isolation to syllable, or the elicitation variable might be advanced from stimulation to the control level. *One of these changes or the other should be made but never the two simultaneously*. The same principles of therapy can be applied to the sound that was produced correctly at the WCT level. Therapy would not begin at the stimulus level of the word since skill has already been demonstrated. The level of either the speech pattern or elicitation variable might be advanced, but not both. The level of the speech pattern variable might be advanced from the word to the sentence or elicitation variable might be manipulated by advancing from the stimulation to control level.

NONFLUENCY AND STUTTERING

Methods used in diagnosing the disorder of stuttering range from the measurement of blood chemistry to the evaluation of emotional stability. The methods of therapy range over an equally wide territory. It is obvious that no specific diagnostic approach will meet the needs of all clinicians. Nevertheless all clinicians, whether of one school of stuttering or another, must observe the client's speech behavior to relate it to the development of the disorder and environmental influences on it. The primary goal for observation should be to obtain qualitative assessments of the overt speech behavior and attitudes rather than quantitative ones. Frequency and severity of interruptions and attitudes change so markedly from one situation to another that enumeration of symptoms will have little meaning unless they are related to other situations where conditions are controlled. In spite of the fact that no so-called standardized tests are available, the diagnostician must seek special kinds of information. Attitudes of the client toward his disorder are of paramount importance because to a large degree they guide his behavior. The Iowa Scale of Attitude toward stuttering and stutterer's self-rating of reaction to speech situations scales are reported by Johnson, Darley, and Spriestersbach (1963). For the most part one must depend on lengthy interviews for the assessment of attitudes, and these will be successful only if good rapport has been established. Often a written autobiography is helpful since it saves much of the clinician's time and will also give the client time to think through his life's story. This time factor is often important when dealing with stutterers. The autobiography also has definite therapeutic catharsis that is not available in interviews because the client has a direct feedback of his statements about himself without contamination of the biases of his examiner. Another advantage comes from the fact that writing is often easier for the stutterer than speech.

Behavior and attitudes of people in the client's environment are also essential to the understanding of stuttering behavior. Although the case-history interview is a valuable source, careful observation of interactive behavior between the stutterer and other people provides a more vivid picture as well as a more accurate one. Every effort should be made to bring the mother, wife, or other members of the family into the clinic so they can be unobtrusively observed by the clinician while he is talking to the client.

Overt stuttering behavior observed in a variety of situations is the most instructive information for the diagnostician. In order to make use of these observations he must be able to distinguish between interruptions which are relevant to stuttering and those that are symptomatic of "normal speech." Stuttering interruptions are composed of speech processes to which the client reacts either overtly or covertly. Other interruptions, which are typical of the normal speaker, are those to which the stutterer reacts neither consciously nor unconsciously. They do not interfere with his train of thought even though the forward movement of speech may be interrupted.

Nonfluencies of the normal speaker tend to cluster around filled and unfilled pauses plus a few syllable, phrase word repetitions, and prolongation of sounds. Pauses are likely to be filled with meaningless sounds, words, and phrases. They are used in filibustering until the person can clarify his thoughts before encoding them.

Development of nonfluencies and other stuttering behavior are definitely correlated with interactions between the stutterer and his environment in which reinforcement is directed to the speech process, not to its content. The symptoms of this abnormal behavior begin to emerge from a welter of "normal speaker" nonfluencies. Although some of the interruptions must be sufficiently bizzare to upset the communication process, the child or his family will not necessarily be aware of the interruptions or of the fact that either is reacting "consciously" to them. Nevertheless their subliminal sensitivity to the interruptions will cause them to react differently to some types of interruptions than to others. Once these changes begin to take place, Pandora's box has been opened and all manner of speech interruptions will begin to emerge. Each one is designed to stop or avoid or cover up the stuttering. The wider the lid of the box is opened, the further will the client's speech behavior deviate from standard communication patterns.

A developmental pattern followed by many stutterers is as follows: *Primary stuttering* interruptions are usually composed of repetitions or prolongations. The individual usually shows no overt awareness of the interruptions and the audience may or may not be overtly aware of them. Regardless of the presence or absence of overt awareness on the part of the individual or his audience to the interruptions, the fact remains that changes begin to occur which will ultimately erupt into an obvious stutter and distress will be felt by both the speaker and audience. As soon as the distress associated with any type of interruption becomes greater than the speaker can live with, he tries to make an adjustment. *Release mechanisms* emerge when the speaker tries to stop the interruptions so he can go forward with his speech. He is not aware of an interruption until it emerges. From that time on he is very much aware until it stops and his speech behavior returns to that of the normal speaker. The release mechanism may involve tensing up, trying to "push out the word," speeding up speech, or the use of a limitless number of body movements not ordinarily associated with speech. As soon as the release mechanism fails to accomplish its purpose of stopping the interruption, it becomes so unpleasant for the speaker that he changes his speech process. *Avoidance mechanism* is the procedure the individual introduces in an attempt to prevent the interruption from emerging. The speech process no longer follows the spontaneous one of the normal speaker because the speaker attends directly to the process as well as to the content of speech. He is so afraid he will stutter that he tries to forecast the words on which interruptions will occur so he can do something to avoid the anticipated stuttering. These avoidances may follow many forms. *Postponements* may be used in an effort to put off saying the word until he thinks he can say it without stuttering. Usually the putting-off period is filled with meaningless sounds or movements that will serve as filibusterisms. *Starters* are another type of avoidance mechanism. They occur when the person introduces some sound or movement designed to speed him into the feared word so the interruption will not "have time" to erupt. After a while these postponements and starters fail to serve their purpose of helping the person repress his interruptions. In fact, they now become the stutterer's bogeyman and come to be identified by him as "his" stuttering. The feeling develops that certain sounds and words cannot be spoken without stuttering. When this attitude emerges, the person is ready to retreat further from normal spontaneous speech, and he begins to omit certain feared sounds and words. *Complete avoidance* is the practice of omitting feared words and/or situations. This type of behavior may provide some relief from fear of stuttering but sooner or later the need for speech becomes so great that the stutterer has to talk. Usually at this time stuttering is so bad that the client feels a compulsion to keep from stuttering which leads him to make a new change. He believes that if he could just keep from anticipating his stuttering (rehearsing the encoding process before speaking) he would not stutter. *Antianticipation* processes are introduced to mask out the feared sound, word, sentence, or situation so they will fade into a facade of nonfeared speech. Any sound, movement, or concept that can be superimposed over every word as it is spoken may serve as a device which distracts the stutterer's attention from the feared condition.

If this description of stuttering development is representative of most stutterers, it is obvious that evaluations of stuttering speech will tell much about the person's feelings about his stuttering. It will also reveal the attitudes of many people who lived with him and the way they influenced his speech behavior.

In the text by Johnson, Darley and Spriestersbach (1963) five methods of quantifying disfluency were described. These were: 1. Total Disfluency Index; 2. Disfluency Type Index; 3. Repetition Index; 4. Sander's Disfluent Word Index (1961); and 5. Young's Disfluent Word Index (1961). This text also contains normative data that gives frequency of nonfluencies for speaking and reading.

Since the amount of speaking an individual does is also important in the evaluation of stuttering, there are two ways in which the clinician can measure the amount of speaking a person does. Either the speaker can be required to keep a concise and accurate account of his speaking situations over a period of time, or the clinician may observe and record the individual's verbal output in specific situations.

VOICE

Voice disorders are difficult to identify since no clear-cut border separates the normal from the abnormal voice. Effectiveness of voice testing depends to a large extent on two conditions; the representativeness of the voice sample and the training of the examiner. A sample should contain voice that is produced during conversation while the client is unaware of the examination and also under other conditions when he is conscious that a test is in progress. There is evidence of psychogenic determinants if marked differences are obtained between these samples. The sample obtained during conversation represents a model of habitual voice pattern used by the client. All subsequent decisions about voice must be related to this habitual pattern.

Voice disorders that are consistent from one situation to another and from spontaneous to controlled speaking are less likely to respond to therapy than those that are more variable. Organic correlates often are present in the stable voice disorders.

A qualified examiner must have a well-established concept of voice deviations. He should use a classification system that will facilitate identification of type of voice disorder as well as its etiology. He must recognize that all vocal behavior is the product of an interaction between the organism and the environment, and therefore both determiners must be allowed for when making a diagnosis and in planning therapy.

Voice deviations may be classified according to the attributes of pitch, loudness, and quality. A voice with defective pitch may deviate toward high, low, monotonous, and double pitches. Loudness may deviate toward excessive loudness, softness, and monotonous loudness patterns, intermittent moments of voice, and voicelessness. Some people have prolonged periods of aphonia or voicelessness.

Deviations in voice quality are more complicated and more difficult to classify. Voice disorders associated primarily with faulty functioning of resonating chambers are nasal, denasal, metallic, and muffled. Those associated primarily with malfunctioning of the vocal folds are the harsh, hoarse, and breathy.

Pitch examination

Pitch range can best be measured in the singing voice. A note near the middle of the client's range can be used as a reference point. He can sing the scale up and down. The examiner can count the notes toward the high range and those toward the low range and by combining the results determine the full range of voice. During this test the voice quality should also be evaluated for each note since the quality varies with pitch changes. Usually voice at the extremes of the range are of poorer quality and often can be produced only with much strain. These two bits of information can be most useful in planning therapy. It enables the diagnostician to determine the pitch levels that represent good voice quality and those that do not as well as the usable pitch range.

Median pitch for conversational speech is often important when the speaker is vocalizing too high or too low. Evaluation of this level depends on subjective evaluations of the examiner; however, the examiner objectifies this evaluation by either recording the speech on a tape recorder or imitating aloud the client's speech and voice pattern. Playing back the tape or repeating the imitation will provide more opportunity of rechecking the client's voice pattern.

Pitch inflection may vary greatly from one conversational situation to another and certainly from one type of oral presentation to another (oral reading, memorized material, or spontaneous speech). The purpose of evaluating pitch inflection must be determined before the method of testing is chosen.

All measurements of pitch should be rechecked by the examiner in an effort to determine how much change can be obtained after a sample of therapy has been administered.

Loudness examination

This attribute of voice is sensitive to situational pressures. For this reason it is expedient that the examiner be sensitive to the client's feelings of insecurity before reporting loudness disorders or predicting outcome of therapy. (It is not uncommon to have great reduction of loudness even to a point of aphonia while the speaker is under stress.)

Habitual loudness level can be determined only by observing the speaker in a friendly conversational situation. Potential loudness range can be assessed only if the client is aware of the goal and is cooperative enough to try to produce a very loud voice in nonconversational situations. Even in this situation the results may not represent his capacity, but may instead demonstrate the loudest voice he could make while feeling embarrassed and inhibited.

Test of voice quality

Habitual voice quality, like the other attributes, can be assessed only in a truly conversational situation; however, stress may not change quality as readily as they will loudness and pitch. The interactive influence of pitch and loudness on some voice qualities must be kept in mind while testing. Metallic voice qualities will almost always increase as the pitch is raised, and pitch tends to rise as loudness increases. Muffled voices will become more extreme in the lower ranges. Harsh and hoarse voices become exaggerated as voice loudness increases.

The qualities of voices are often the replication of speaking voices of the family or region. This is especially true for nasal-metallic voices which are so common in parts of America adjacent to the Ohio, Mississippi, and Missouri Rivers.

Voice quality deficiencies are often associated with organic anomalies and malformations of the resonating chambers and larynx. Nasal obstructions, both temporary and permanent, may interfere. Temporary conditions often involve pathology of adenoids, sinuses, and various virus infections and asthma. Permanent ones involve the deviations of the medial septum, excessively high palate, and various nasal growths. Anomalies of the oral cavity may also be temporary or permanent. Enlarged tonsils, infections of mouth and throat that cause swelling, and injuries represent some temporary disorders. The more permanent ones are clefts of the palate and lip, and tumors.

Organic disorders of the larynx may also be temporary or permanent. The transient ones come mostly from infection originating in the nose and oral cavity, allergic reactions, and some tumors. The more permanent type on the vocal folds are growths, both malignant and benign, scar tissue, paralysis, webs between the folds, and nodes on the folds that are essentially a form of callous that has developed as a defense against too much contact. Whereas anomalies of the resonation cavities interfere with the moulding of the voice after it leaves the larynx, those affecting the vocal folds interfere with the initial production of voice.

The speech diagnostician should rely on physical examinations by a physician in determining the nature, causes, and treatment to be used for various organic disorders. The limits to be imposed on voice therapy as well as the probability that medicine, surgery, or prostheses can reduce the effects of the organic disability upon voice are to be decided by the physician in consultation with the speech pathologist.

Two good sources of information about voice disorders are Van Riper and Irwin (1964) and West, Ansberry, and Carr (1957). Both books have good reviews of organic conditions related to voice.

Personality maladjustments often carry a vocal trademark. A diagnosis of clients with this etiological involvement requires considerable psychological background and training. Voice symptoms of these people may reach into all attributes of voice. Often the psychological withdrawal is demonstrated vocally by excessively soft infantile voices. Patterns of aggression often lead to very loud voices. Other patients use voice quality that is flat, nonresonant, and lackluster. Although these voice patterns and many others may be found in maladjusted patients, it is important that the diagnostician not use them to diagnose personality problems. All of these voice disorders can be found in well-adjusted clients.

DISORDERS THAT DEVELOP AS A RESULT OF DETERIORATION OF STABLE LANGUAGE AND SPEECH PATTERNS

Disorders with this etiology (except aphasia and laryngectomy) have not received as much attention from either the researcher or the clinician as have those which originate during the developmental period. One large area that is open for investigation involves the geriatric patient whose speech behavior has gone through a long, slow period of deterioration. Another group of patients whose speech disorders have received little attention are those who might be called "medical" patients. They have a wide range of acute and chronic illnesses and diseases as well as tissue deterioration. West and Ansberry (1968) have set forth a description of some of these conditions as they affect speech, language, and voice. Two groups that have been studied extensively by speech pathologists are the voice and articulation client with laryngectomy and the language handicapped aphasic with brain damage.

Laryngectomy

An individual who has undergone a laryngectomy due to carcinoma or some other trauma will, without question, present a complete aphonia. Identification is not a problem for the diagnostician because the fact is made clear by the surgeon's report. The diagnostic goal is to describe the behavior of the patient that will be relevant to speech rehabilitation and the attitudes that may facilitate or interfere with it.

Often these people are so depressed that they completely withdraw and well they might, because their world has been shattered. Life without speech seems to be no life at all. The first goal for the diagnostician is to restore confidence and hope for the future. Even a skilled clinician may meet resistance because the patient cannot help thinking, "What does he know about my feelings and future? He has never lived through such an ordeal." With these people rapport is established more effectively by other patients who have recovered from the "ordeal" and look forward to a long and well-adjusted life. Once the client begins to plan for the future, the clinician may expect to conduct an examination that will provide useful data.

The clinician must determine the attitudes of the family so he will know the kind of support the patient will receive during rehabilitation. He must also assess the client's attitudes because they will determine, to a large degree, the extent and direction of support the client will give during rehabilitation.

Another area of investigation involves the nature of the speech mechanism that is still available after surgery. Most of this information can be obtained from the surgeon. However, studies showing the ability of the client to inhale air into the esophagus and make a noise as it is exhaled will indicate whether it will be difficult to develop an esophageal voice. The age and vitality of the person will also predict the direction rehabilitation will take. Younger or vigorous clients will probably aim at developing esophageal speech. Older people of low vitality and especially those who have little or no success in expelling air for esophageal voice will probably use a prosthetic device to produce a substitute voice.

Some patients, by the time they see a speech clinician, have already established some means of oral communication of their own. If this is the case, the clinician should note the methods of voice production, the number of sounds that can be emitted, and the length of time the patient can sustain a sound. Special attention should be given to methods of production that have a poor prognosis such as ducking of the head as a means of swallowing air, trapping air in the mouth in an effort to make a noise in an unnatural manner, and excessive lip movements that are not accompanied by voice.

From this information, the diagnostician should be able to recommend procedures to be followed by a clinician and the family, procedures that are adapted to the interests and capacities of the patient and his family.

Some sources available which relate to the area of laryngectomy are the publications by Snidecor (1960), Brodnitz (1961), Murphy (1964), and Gardner (1971). There are also several publications written specifically to introduce the laryngectomized patient to a new manner of voice production (Doehler, 1953; Waldrop and Gould, 1956; Nelson, 1949; Marland, 1949; and Moorlenaar-Bijl, 1953). The American Cancer Society also makes available certain pamphlets to aid the laryngectomee ("Helping Words for the Laryngectomee"; "Rehabilitating Laryngectomees"; "First Aid for Laryngectomees").

Aphasia

The loss of language is also a shattering experience and aphasia represents one of the most devastating of language disorders. It distresses the patient, his family, and most of the professional people dedicated to his care.

The etiology of this disorder has been assigned to some form of brain damage for nearly a century. It was not until recently that clinicians have recognized that the language deficit was due to a number of determiners in addition to the cerebral anomalies; and it was not until this concept became accepted that examinations were aimed at data that were more relevant to languages rehabilitation and the plight of the aphasic became less dismal. We still have a long road to travel before the diagnostician will be able to exploit fully information about this patient's behavior that is clinically manipulable. Fortunately, we are moving in that direction as evidenced by the fact that more diagnostic time is spent in studying the patient's behavior and less with the cerebral mechanism. Certainly the role of the speech and language pathologist involves manipulation of the client's attitudes and language behavior, and most recovery, except for that which is spontaneous, depends upon it.

Diagnosis must be shared by two professions—medicine and speech pathology—if the patient is to be rehabilitated. The task of the physician is of major importance during the acute stage of the cerebral disease or injury. During this period the speech pathologist assumes a consultative role with all persons who will be communicating with the patient. Later on the role will be reversed after the patient's physical condition is stabilized and as soon as he is well enough to talk and interact in other ways with people around him.

Examinations begin with the case history of the patient with special reference to his language background. Attention is directed to the family attitudes: extreme reactions of pity or rejection, or feelings of hopelessness that will interfere with rehabilitation. These conditions must be investigated so the clinician can be prepared for them when formal therapy begins. Early communication attempts must be observed and the patient's behavior recorded as well as descriptions of the situations in which they occurred.

When examining for aphasia it is important that the examiner always be aware of two processes involved in the act of communication—decoding and encoding. The decoding process involves the reception (visually and auditorally) and comprehension of incoming information.

The act of encoding is concerned with the formulation and expression (orally and graphically) of ideas that the individual wishes to express. The wise and organized examiner will be careful to construct tests so that he knows whether he is examining the decoding or encoding process and, further, which modality of reception or expression (auditory, visual, oral, or graphic) is being tested.

Test construction is difficult because the patient's interactions usually involve a number of modalities in each communication circuit. If the test does not isolate the modalities when the aphasic patient fails, it is difficult to determine what aspect of the loop is responsible for the failure. The following examples represent communication behavior where a single variable of verbal behavior is represented in a whole communication circuit. If a breakdown occurs, it is easy to isolate that aspect of language which caused it.

Single linguistic variable involving the decoding process:

Test item—Patient is asked to point to an object.
Instructions by examiner are linguistic (speech).
Sensory modalities used by patient are visual and auditory.
Response modalities used by patient are nonlinguistic and should be performed easily if he understands instruction.
Failure to perform successfully indicates patient has faulty decoding of speech.

Test item—A number of objects are placed on the table and a card is given to the patient on which is written a single word that represents one of the objects. By pantomime, the tester can instruct the patient to place the card next to the appropriate object.
Instructions by examiner are linguistic (graphic-written).
Sensory modality used by patient is visual.
Response modality used by patient is nonlinguistic.
Failure to perform successfully indicates patient has faulty decoding of written language.

Single linguistic variable involving the encoding process:

Test item—An object is presented to the patient and in pantomime the examiner asks what it is and the patient is encouraged to give the name.
Instructions by examiner are nonlinguistic (pantomime).
Sensory modality used by patient was visual.
Response modality used by patient was speech.
Failure to perform successfully indicates patient has faulty encoding for speech.

Test item—A piece of paper and pencil are placed in front of the patient.
An object is held in front of him by the tester who, by pantomime, indicates that the patient should write the name on the paper.
Instructions by examiner are nonlinguistic (pantomime).
Sensory modality used by patient was visual.
Response modality used by patient in encoding was graphic.
Failure to perform successfully indicates patient has faulty encoding for writing.

The foregoing examples demonstrate one form that tests should follow if the diagnostician is to identify that aspect of the communication feedback circuit which is defective in the patient. By manipulating only one linguistic unit at a time it is possible to judge more accurately which aspect of communication was defective. Unfortunately, many test items that are presently available have not met this criteria as well as would be desired. However, a number of the tests, developed recently, have made giant strides toward a better diagnosis of aphasia:

1. Language Modalities Test for Aphasia (LMTA) (1961). This test is composed of a series of filmstrips to which the subject is asked to respond. The test is made up of a screening section and a standardized section. Failure to comprehend the screening item may indicate that further testing would be of minimal value. This test calls for auditory, visual, oral, and

graphic responses. Scoring of these responses is done on a six-point scale according to: 1. correct responses; 2. phonemic or orthographic errors; 3. grammatical and syntactic errors; 4. semantic errors; 5. jargon errors; and 6. no response. The authors define five different aphasias: pragmatic aphasia, semantic aphasia, syntactic aphasia, jargon aphasia, and global aphasia.

2. Minnesota Test for Differential Diagnosis of Aphasia (MTDDA) (1955). This diagnostic test presents items which are designed to investigate the following areas: auditory disturbances; visual and reading disturbances; speech and language disturbances; visual motor and writing disturbances; and disturbances of numerical relations and arithmetic processes. Administration time is approximately two to three hours.

3. Examining for Aphasia (Eisenson, 1954). Section I is composed of items to investigate primarily evaluative and receptive disturbances. Under this section are agnosias (visual, auditory, and tactile) and aphasias (auditory verbal comprehension and silent reading comprehension). Section II deals with predominantly productive and expressive disturbances, i.e., apraxias (nonverbal apraxia and verbal apraxia) and aphasias (automatic speech, writing numbers and letters, spelling, writing from dictation, naming, word finding, arithmetic processes, clock setting, and oral reading).

4. The Sklar Aphasia Scale (1966). This diagnostic test is a short screening device with eight to 10 items to test each of the four modalities. The test attempts to examine only one modality at a time. This instrument examines at a fairly basic level and, therefore, does not test very well for subtle language problems. The test covers a range from the phoneme level to paragraphs. It yields a classification of mild, moderate and severe for each modality according to the number of errors. It also allows for an average of the errors to give a total score with a prognosis given for each particular classification. Administration time is approximately 20–45 minutes.

5. The Porch Index of Communicative Ability (1967). This examination procedure separates modalities. The test is built on a set of words for common objects, each subtest using these same items regardless of the modality or complexity of the task. The examination procedure begins with the most difficult subtest and proceeds to the simplest. There is a rating scale of 1–16 for each response. The scale is well defined as to what rating a particular response would receive. There are explicit instructions which accompany this test and an examinee is supposed to take a course in order to learn how to administer it. Administration time is approximately two hours.

Other tests used in the diagnosis of aphasia though not primarily designed for that purpose include the following: Peabody Picture Vocabularly Test (1959); Bender Gestalt (1938); Raven Progressive Matrices (1938); Ammons Full Range Picture Vocabulary (1948); Columbia Mental Maturity Scale (1953); Goldstein-Scheerer Object Sorting Test (1951); Illinois Test of Psycholinguistic Abilities (1968); and the performance section of the Wechsler Adult Intelligence Scale (1955).

CONCLUSION

The therapy for most speech disorders varies so much from clinician to clinician that no set of examination methods will be completely suitable. Perhaps as determinants of disorders become better known and universally accepted, more standardized testing procedure can be recommended. In the meantime, the greatest tool of the examiner is *observation.* He must never sacrifice this tool in favor of the standardized testing procedure.

INDIANA UNIVERSITY

Speech and Hearing Center

BLOOMINGTON, INDIANA 47401

MEDICAL EXAMINATION

NAME: ______________________ AGE: __________ BIRTHDATE: ______________

ADDRESS: ____
(street and number)

____
(city) (state) (zip)

DATE OF EXAMINATION: ____________________

I. GENERAL HEALTH: Poor ________ Fair ________ Good ________

A. HEARING: Normal ________ Other (explain): ________

Tests: ________

B. VISION: Normal ________ Other (explain): ________

Tests: ________

C. SPEECH & LANGUAGE: Normal ________ Other (explain) ________

D. MOTOR COORDINATION: Normal ________ Other (explain): ________

II. SIGNIFICANT DISEASES:

german measles	___	diphteria	___	encephalitis	___	whooping cough	___
measles	___	influenza	___	poliomyelitis	___	asthma	___
chicken pox	___	scarlet fever	___	otitis media	___	heart disease	___
mumps	___	meningitis	___	diabetes	___	allergies	___

Please give dates and other pertinent information such as treatment, severity, accompanying fever, outcome, etc. for items checked above.

III. SIGNIFICANT INJURIES AND OPERATIONS: (give dates and describe)

IV. EARS: normal ________ other (explain): ________

Is there any contraindication to using earmold? ________ R L

NOSE: normal ______ other (explain): ________

THROAT: normal______ other (explain):____________________
tonsils: yes _____ no _______ explain ____________________
adenoids: yes _____ no _______ explain ____________________

LARYNX: normal _______ other (explain) ____________________

Is there any medical reason to limit amount or kind of voice therapy for this patient? ______ If yes, please specify:____________________

V. PHYSICAL DEFORMITIES: (list and describe)

VI. NEUROLOGICAL & PSYCHOLOGICAL:

retardation	_______	depression	_______
CNS dysfunction	_______	anxiety	_______
cerebral palsy	_______	spatial disorientation	_______
hyperactivity	_______	bizarre behavior	_______
distractibility	_______	other	_______

Please explain any items checked above.

VII. Is the patient presently being treated by you for a medical problem which may be related to the speech and/or hearing problem?________ Explain:

VIII. Is the patient presently taking prescribed medication? ________ Explain:

IMPORTANT: If special examinations (otological, neurological, psychological, etc.) have been done, please send copies of reports or send information in detail.

PLEASE PRINT OR TYPE NAME AND ADDRESS OF EXAMINING PHYSICIAN:

NAME:____________________ ADDRESS: ____________________

SIGNATURE: ____________________

DATE: ____________________

INDIANA UNIVERSITY

Speech and Hearing Center

BLOOMINGTON, INDIANA 47401

TO THE PRINCIPAL AND TEACHER: In order that we may have complete information about this child, we are asking you to fill out this form and send it directly to the Coordinator of Clinical Services at the above address. Thank you. (If there is not enough room for comments, please attach a separate sheet.)

Name of child ______________________ Birthdate: ________

Address ____
(street & number) (city) (state) (zip)

Parents (guardians) ______________________________

Name of school ______________ N ow in __________ grade

Address ____
(street & number) (city) (state) (zip)

At what grade did child enter your school __________ Age ____ What grades, if any, were repeated? ______________________

I. Achievement in current school subjects (if possible we would appreciate having a transcript of the child's record):

A. Elementary

	Poor	Average	Good
Reading	____	____	____
Spelling	____	____	____
Arithmetic	____	____	____
Writing	____	____	____
Language	____	____	____
Art	____	____	____
Citizenship	____	____	____

B. High School

	Grades
English	____
Mathematics	____
Science	____
Social Studies	____
Foreign Language	____
Industrial Arts	____
Citizenship	____
Other	____

What is your estimate of the child's current academic functioning in relation to his classmates?

II. Has any remedial work been done in academic subjects? ______________

If so, what? ______________ For how long? ______________

Success of remedial work? ______________________________

Would you recommend any remedial work for the child? ______________

III. Tests that have been administered at school:

Date of test	Name of test	Results
____________	______________________________	______________
____________	______________________________	______________
____________	______________________________	______________

IV. Communication Skills:

Does the child have normal speech? ________ If not, describe ____________

____

____

To your knowledge does he have a hearing loss? __________ Has remedial work been done? __________ For how long? ____________ If so, please describe.

____

____

Name of speech clinician or other person doing this remedial work: ______

________________________ Please have a report sent to us by this person.

V. Attitude of child toward school:

How does child relate to other children in school? ____________________

____

Does the child seem to like to come to school? ____________________

How does the child cooperate with teachers? ______________________

Is attendance regular? ______________ If irregular, why? ____________

____

Please describe any special behavior problems:

____
(Date of report)

____
(Child's teacher)

____
(Approved by: Principal)

(Child form)

Date Sent ____________________
Date received ________________

HISTORY QUESTIONNAIRE

C O N F I D E N T I A L

Indiana University Speech and Hearing Center

Bloomington, Indiana 47401

1. Name of person for whom appointment is requested:	Age	Sex	Date of Birth

2. Address:	Phone Number
______________________________ (Street and Number)	

____
(City) (State) (Zip)

3. Name of person completing this form:	Relationship to client

4. Address:	Phone Number
______________________________ (Street and Number)	

____
(City) (State((Zip)

5. Name and address of person who referred you to this clinic:

____

____

6. Why has appointment been requested?

____

____

FAMILY HISTORY

7. Mother's Name:	Age:	Occupation
8. Father's Name:	Age:	Occupation

9. If other than natural parents are guardians, please give name and relationship:

Name: Relationship:

10. Names of brothers and sisters	Age	Sex	Grade in school	Speech problem?

11. Relatives or others living in home:	Relationship:

BIRTH HISTORY

12. Birthdate: Born at:

(Hospital) (City) (County) (State)

13. Pregnancy (mos.)	Labor (hrs.)	Birth weight	Was mother given drugs: ___ During pregnancy? ___ At birth? ___

14. Any previous miscarriages?
No _____
Yes _____ How many _____

Mother's health during pregnancy
Excellent _____ Good _____ Fair _____
Poor _____

15. Describe any complications at birth:

16. Describe any past or present feeding or sleeping problems:

DEVELOPMENTAL HISTORY

17. Give approximate dates for the following:

sat alone . . . . . _____

crawled . . . . . . _____

stood alone . . . . _____

walked alone . . . _____

climbed stairs with alternating feet . _____

weaned . . . . . . _____

fed self with spoon _____

toilet trained:

bladder . . . . . _____

bowel . . . . . . _____

night . . . . . . _____

first three words . _____

sentences . . . . . _____

MEDICAL HISTORY

18. Name and address of regular family physician or pediatrician:

19. List illnesses, injuries, childhood diseases and operations. Give dates and length of disability. Include any physical handicaps, prolonged fever, convulsions, etc.

Illness, injury or operation	Date	Hospital

20. Does child have any hearing problem?

No ______ Yes ______ Explain: ______

21. Is there a history of hearing loss, ear infections, etc.?

No ______ Yes ______ Explain: ______

22. Does the child wear a hearing aid?

No ______ Yes ______ Where and when was it fitted? ______

23. Has child been examined by an otologist?

No ______ Yes ______ Date of last examination: ______

Name and address of otologist: ______

SCHOOL HISTORY

24. Name of school presently attending	Address

25. Name of teacher	Grade	Name of Principal

26. Schools previously attended	Address	Grade

27. List any special classes attended:

SPEECH AND HEARING

28. Describe the speech and/or hearing problem:

29. In what way has any member of the family tried to help the child with his speech problem?

30. What situations at home do you feel have influenced the child's speech hearing problem?

31. List any psychological, speech or hearing testing and/or therapy that has been done and the name(s) of the therapist(s). (Please sign attached release form if you answer this question.)

Testing or Therapy	Institution	Name	Date

32. Write down any additional information you feel will help us in understanding the child and his speech/hearing problem.

SIGNED:

RELATION: DATE

BIBLIOGRAPHY

Ammons, R., and Ammens, H. 1948. Full-range picture vocabulary test. Missoula, Mont. Psychological Test Specialists.

Arthur, G. 1925, 1947. Point scale of performance tests. Chicago: Stoelting.

Bellak, L., and Bellak, S. 1949. Children's apperception test. New York: C. P.S. Co.

Bender, L. 1938. A visual motor gestalt test and its clinical use. *Res. Monogr. Amer. Orthopsychiat. Assn.*, No. 3.

Brodnitz, F. 1961. Vocal rehabilitation. Rochester, Minn.: Whiting Press.

Burgomeister, B., Blum, L., and Lorge, I. 1953. Columbia mental maturity scale. Yonkers-on-Hudson, New York: World.

Doehler, M. 1953. Esophageal speech. Boston: American Cancer Society.

Doll, E. 1947. Vineland social maturity scale. Minneapolis: Educational Test Bureau.

Dunn, L. 1965. Peabody picture vocabulary test. Minneapolis: Amer. Guidance Service.

Eisenson, J. 1954. Examining for aphasia. New York: Psychological Corp.

First aid for laryngectomees. 1962. American Cancer Society, 219 E. 42nd. St., New York, N.Y., 10017.

French, J. 1964. Pictorial test of intelligence, Boston: Houghton Mifflin.

Gardner, W. 1971. Laryngectomee speech and rehabilitation. Springfield, Ill.: Thomas.

Goldstein, K., and Scheerer, M. 1951. Goldstein-Sheerer object sorting test. New York: Psychological Corp.

Hadjian, S. 1961. Comparisons of sound productions in word articulation test, word stimulation test, and word control test. Ind. Univ.: Master's thesis.

Harris, D. 1963. Goodenough-Harris drawing test. New York: Harcourt, Brace & World.

Hathaway, S., and McKinley, J. 1951. Minnesota multiphasic personality inventory. New York: Psychological Corp.

Helping words for the laryngectomee. 1965. American Cancer Society, 219 E. 42nd St., New York, N.Y., 10017.

Hiskey-Nebraska test of learning aptitude. 1966. Lincoln, Nebr.: Union College Press.

Iowa tests of basic skills, 1956. Boston: Houghton Mifflin.

Johnson, W. 1961. Measurements of oral reading and speaking rate and disfluency of adult male and female stutterers and nonstutterers. *J. Speech Hearing Disorders, Monogr. Suppl.*, No. 7.

———, Darley, F., and Sprietstersbach, D. 1963. Diagnostic methods in speech pathology. New York: Harper & Row.

Kirk, S., McCarthy, J., and Kirk, W. 1968. Illinois test of psycholinguistic abilities. Champaign, Ill.: Univ. of Ill. Press.

Lenneberg, E. 1967. Biological foundations of language. New York: Wiley.

Louttit, C. 1947. Clinical pyschology of child's behavior problems. New York and London: Harpers Bros.

Marland, P. 1949. A direct method of teaching voice after total laryngectomy. *J. College Speech Therapists.*

McDonald, E. 1964. Articulation testing and treatment: a sensory-motor approach. Pittsburgh: Stanwix House.

Metropolitan achievement test. 1959. Yonkers-on-Hudson, New York: World.

Milisen, R. 1954. Rationale on articulation. *J. Speech Hearing Disorders, Monogr. Suppl.*, No. 4.

———. 1966. In Speech pathology. Reeber, R., and Brubaker, R., ed. Ch. 13. Amsterdam: North-Holland Pub. Co.

———. 1967. Programmed therapy for misarticulations resulting from inverse processes of self-evaluation. *Brit. J. Disorders Communication.*

———. 1968. Basic data sheet. Bloomington, Ind.: Ind. Univ.

———. 1968. Instructions for speech pathologists in the use of basic data sheet. Bloomington, Ind.: Ind. Univ.

Moolenaar-Bijl, A. 1953. The importance of certain consonants in esophageal voice after laryngectomy. *Ann. Otol., Rhinol., Laryng.*

Murphy, A. 1964. Functional voice disorders. Englewood Cliffs, N.J. Prentice-Hall.

Nelson, C. 1949. You can speak again. New York: Funk and Wagnalls.

Porch, B. 1967. Porch index of communicative ability. Palo Alto, Calif.: Consulting Psychologists Press.

Raven, J. 1949. Raven's progressive matrice test. London: H. K. Lewis.

Rehabilitating laryngectomees. 1960. American Cancer Society, 219 E. 42nd. St., New York, N.Y., 10017.

Rorschach test. Chicago: Stoelting Co.

Sander, E. 1961. Reliability of the Iowa speech disfluency test. *J. Speech Hearing Disorders, Monogr. Suppl.*, No. 7.

Schuell, H. 1955. Minnesota test for differential diagnosis of aphasia. Minn.: Univ. Minn. Print. Dept.

Sklar, M. 1966. Sklar aphasia scale. Beverly Hills, Calif.: Western Psychological Services.

Snidecor, J. 1960. How effectively can the laryngectomee expect to speak? *Laryngoscope*, 70, 62–67.

Stanford achievement test. 1953. Yonkers-on-Hudson, New York: World.

Stanford-Binet, form L-M. 1960. Boston: Houghton Mifflin.

Templin, M. 1943. A study of sound discrimination ability of elementary school pupils. *J. Speech Disorders*, 8, 127–132.

———. 1957. Certain language skills in children. Institute Child Welfare, *Monogr. Series*, No. 26. Minneapolis: Univ. Minn. Press.

———, and Darley, F. 1960. The Templin-Darley tests of articulation. Univ. Iowa: Bur. Educ. Res. and Service, Ext. Div.

Travis, L. 1931. Speech pathology. New York: Appleton.

———, and Rasmus, B. J. 1931. The speech sound discrimination ability of cases with functional disorders of articulation. *Quart. J. Speech Educ.*, 17, 217–226.

Van Alstyne, D. 1960. Van Alstyne picture vocabulary test. New York: Harcourt, Brace & World.

Van Riper, C. 1965. Speech correction. Englewood Cliffs, N.J.: Prentice-Hall.

———, and Irwin, J. 1958. Voice and articulation. Englewood Cliffs, N.J.: Prentice-Hall.

Waldrop, W., and Gould, M. 1956. Your new voice. American Cancer Society, Ill. Division, Chicago, Ill.

Wechsler adult intelligence scale. 1955. New York: Psychological Corp.

Wechsler intelligence scale for children (WISC). 1949. New York: Psychological Corp.

Wepman, J., and Jones, L. 1961. Studies in aphasia: an approach to testing. Chicago: Education–Industry Service.

West, R., and Ansberry, M. 1968. The rehabilitation of speech. New York: Harper & Row.

Wolfe, D. 1959. The nature and frequency of misarticulation relating to the method of eliciting speech. Ind. Univ.: Master's thesis.

Young, M. 1961. Predicting ratings of severity of stuttering. *J. Speech Hearing Disorders. Monogr. Suppl.*, No. 7.

26

Cerebral Palsy Speech Syndromes

Edward D. Mysak

This chapter is concerned specifically with a description of the possible speech syndromes that may accompany the various neurological conditions known as cerebral palsy. The next chapter is devoted to a discussion of habilitation procedures designed to treat these syndromes. For more inclusive discussions of the multifaceted problems in cerebral palsy, the reader is referred to general texts by Cardwell (1956) and Cruickshank (1966).

Cerebral palsy as used in this chapter refers to the full range of chronic, childhood brain syndromes—from the minimal, where the major symptoms may be primarily behavioral in nature, to the severe sensorimotor involvements. More specifically, the cerebral palsies will be viewed here as disease complexes which have their inception during the period of infancy, reflect nonprogressive damage of multiple causation to cortical and subcortical areas of the brain, and which may appear in various forms and combinations of sensorimotor, perceptual, and behavioral disorders.

Admittedly, the definition is broad. The only limitations are that the lesion should have been incurred during the period from conception to about two or three years of age and that the lesion be nonprogressive. In short, it includes all those CNS disturbed children that are usually seen by speech clinicians who work with the cerebral-palsied: that is, those children who are "born with it" and are most frequently referred to as either "spastic," "athetotic," "ataxic," or mixed.

The discussion of cerebral palsy speech syndromes will focus on those problems which are relatively specific to the speech system. No attempt will be made to discuss in any detail the special oral communicative problems of the cerebral-palsied who have major emotional, intellectual, or hearing problems. Further information on how these conditions contribute to oral communicative disorders will be found in appropriate chapters in the Handbook.

In short then, the central purpose of this chapter is to describe the frequently encountered problems in the development and production of oral linguistic symbols which accompany the more common forms of childhood cerebral palsy. Pertinent normative data, clinical and clinical-research findings, diagnostic implications, as well as research needs will be included in each major area of discussion.

CEREBRAL PALSY AND CENTRAL AND PERIPHERAL NEURAL MECHANISMS FOR SPEECH

It might be obvious to the reader that to attempt to describe the full range of speech symptoms that may accompany the various conditions known as cerebral palsy means not only the possibility of describing all of the presently known speech pathologies but also implies the need to speculate on relatively unknown speech pathologies.

More specifically, lesions of the central nervous system which cause cerebral palsy are also lesions which may directly or indirectly affect central neural mechanisms supporting the central speech system (e.g., areas including the midbrain, basal nuclei, thalamus, and speech cortex). Such lesions may also have direct or indirect repercussions on the peripheral neural mechanism (i.e., Cranial, cervical, and thoracic nerves) serving the interrelated and interdependent peripheral speech subsystems of respiration, phonation, and articulation. In addition, there may also be lesions in the peripheral auditory system and secondary malocclusions due to irregular oroneuromaturation. Further, there may be adverse environmental reactions to the organism and its involved speech system. Hence, because of the possible involvements of central and peripheral speech systems, a discussion of speech disorder in cerebral palsy must include reports on varieties and combinations of disorders of respiration, hearing, articulation, phonation, resonation, rhythm, and oral language.

Before beginning the discussion of the possible components to cerebral palsy speech disorders, a series of comments from various authorities should contribute to an appreciation of the completeness of the range of speech disorder reflected by the cerebral-palsied. No other clinical population will show such a variety of conditions which can delay the use of oral language (Westlake and Rutherford, 1961); there is no speech and language disorder that is uniquely characteristic of the cerebral-palsied, with problems ranging from mild to severe (Lencione, 1966, p. 221); a high proportion of children with cerebral palsy and defective speech fall into the category of mixed cases (Ingram and Barn, 1961); wide variations exist in all areas of cerebral palsy involvement including speech (Rutherford, 1956); and the speech output of the cerebral-palsied may range from complete lack to slight or no differences from the normal (Mecham, 1966, p. 24). With respect to the average incidence of oral communicative disorder among the cerebral-palsied, the following figures have been offered: about 75 percent (Hopkins, Bice, and Colton, 1954); 86 percent (Achilles, 1955); 70 percent (Wolfe, 1950); and 79 percent (Lorenze, 1962).

DISORDERS OF THE SPEECH SYSTEM AND ITS SUBSYSTEMS IN CEREBRAL PALSY

As previously indicated, the production of oral symbols among the cerebral-palsied may be affected by involvement in any or all of the central and peripheral speech systems and subsystems. Problems in the respiratory, auditory, phonatory, articulatory, rhythm, and linguistic systems will be described here.

Respiratory System

There are many dimensions of breathing which should be of interest to the speech pathologist; for example, comparisons between normal and cerebral-palsied children in respiratory maturation—specifically in the characteristics of inspiratory and expiratory phases during vegetative and speech functioning. Since speech clinicians are frequently not too familiar with developmental sequences in vegetative and speech-breathing functioning, and since the description of breathing anomalies among the cerebral-palsied will include references to symptoms of breathing immaturity, a short discussion of these sequences follows.

MATURATION OF VEGETATIVE BREATHING

Peiper (1963, pp. 310–312), in his review of the neurology of respiration, provided the following information with respect to respiratory maturation.

An infant at rest indulges in nasal respiration. Lung expansion takes place principally by the lowering of the diaphragm causing abdominal-wall respiratory activity to be extensive and thoracic respiratory activity to be minimal. Further, respiratory cycles are comparatively shallow and their frequency is high. After the sixth month of life, the predominantly diaphragmatic pattern is replaced by a mixed pattern in which both diaphragm and thorax participate. By the sixth month, breathing has also become deeper and slower. Finally, thoracic breathing is predominant at about the seventh year of life.

With respect to changes in the frequency of respiration, or breaths per minute (bpm), Peiper has reviewed the findings of various investigators. Ranges of reported bpm's include: 22 to 72 bpm (mean of 35·0) for the first to the seventh day of life; 21 to 58 bpm (mean 33·3) for the first to the sixth month of life; 19·5 to 45 bpm (mean of 27·8) for the first half to the second year of life; 15 to 31 bpm (mean of 20·4) for the fifth to the tenth year of life; and, finally, 14 to 31 bpm (mean 19·1) for the tenth through the fifteenth year.

DEVELOPMENT OF SPEECH BREATHING

Breathing for speech purposes requires that vegetative breathing patterns undergo certain modifications. These include higher center control of central breathing mechanisms, transition from nasal to oral respiration, and a transition from rather regular inspiratory-expiratory phases to a rapid inspiratory phase, approximately one-sixth of the complete respiratory cycle, followed by a prolonged expiratory phase (Perlstein and McDonald, 1953). One investigator (Heffner, 1949) has reported that in normal conversation the ratio of the length of inspiration to the length of expiration varies from 1 : 3 to 1 : 10.

Respiratory Disorders Among the Cerebral-Palsied

Breathing anomalies of almost every type have been reported among the cerebral-palsied by clinicians and investigators. Shallow or irregular cycles, high frequency of cycles, predominantly diaphragmatic or abdominal patterns, "oppositional" or "reverse" breathing patterns, and the use of vegetative patterns during speech are among the conditions reported. Various figures have been presented concerning the frequency of breathing anomalies among the different types of cerebral-palsied children. Investigators report that 70 percent of the breathing anomalies are found among athetotics. Wolfe (1950) stated that 80 percent of his ataxics showed respiratory involvement, while Achilles (1955) reported that 40 percent of his ataxics showed such involvement. Sixty percent of the spastic group in Achilles' (1955) study had breathing problems.

It should be of theoretical as well as clinical value to discuss breathing symptoms which result from the persistence of infantile patterns and those which are caused by paralytic involvement. By infantile-pattern symptoms, or arrest or retarded development symptoms, is meant those symptoms characterized by patterns which may be considered appropriate for earlier periods of life; and by paralytic symptoms, or pathological movement or lack of movement symptoms, is meant those symptoms resulting from the defective innervation of muscles directly or indirectly associated with respiratory activity. An attempt to describe cerebral palsy speech manifestations in terms of duplex symptomatology, that is, in terms of persistence of infantile patterns vs. paralytic or specific patholgic patterns, will be made in each of the major disorder areas.

INFANTILE-PATTERN SYMPTOMS

Persistence of infantile breathing symptoms in cerebral palsy are associated with those effects of the original lesion reflected by general arrest or retardation of the neuroevolution of the child. Such symptoms include infantile bpm rates accompanied by shallow breathing cycles; predominance of diaphragmatic-abdominal patterns; periodic, simultaneous activity of inspiratory and expiratory musculature; predominance of nasal respiratory patterns; and difficulty or inability to shift easily from a vegetative to a speech-breathing pattern.

There have been numerous descriptions of breathing anomalies among the cerebral-palsied which are suggestive of infantile-pattern symptoms. For example, high and irregular bpm's have been reported by Berry and Eisenson (1956, pp. 364–365), Westlake (1952), Achilles (1955), and Palmer (1952); simultaneous inspiratory and expiratory movements, or so-called "reverse" or "oppositional" breathing has been reported by Hull (1940), Morley (1965, pp. 208–209), Westlake (1952), Achilles (1955), and Perlstein and Shere (1946); shallow breathing and reduced vital capacity have been reported by Palmer (1952), Achilles (1955), and Blumberg (1955); and predominance of the diaphragmatic-abdominal pattern has been reported by Achilles (1955).

PARALYTIC SYMPTOMS

Paralytic breathing symptoms are those related to a lack of, or to irregular innervation of, those muscles directly or indirectly involved with respiration. Such symptoms could include paretic thoracic and abdominal muscles, involuntary or uncoordinated movements of the diaphragm and other muscles of respiration, irregular air flow due to associated movements of the trunk, asynchrony of respiratory and laryngeal movements, and deficits in sensory feedback from respiratory muscles.

Reports of breathing anomalies suggestive of paralytic symptoms include: air-stream obstruction due to irregular movements of the vocal folds, posterior tongue, or oropharynx (Berry and Eisenson, 1956, pp. 364–365); irregular air flow due to trunk dystonia (Crothers and Paine, 1959, p. 45); and respiration accompanied by retracted abdominal muscles and little movement of the diaphragm (Morley, 1965, pp. 208–209).

Breathing anomalies associated with secondary bony problems have also been reported; for example, thoracic-cage anomalies which, in turn, are related to a lack of or inefficient sitting and standing postures and prolonged use of chest and stomach bands.

DIAGNOSTIC IMPLICATIONS

On the basis of the information presented on respiratory involvements among the cerebral-palsied, it is clear that the speech pathologist who is conducting a differential diagnosis of a cerebral palsy speech syndrome must examine carefully for various breathing anomalies and their possible speech repercussions. Certainly the following relationships betweeen speech involvement and differences in breathing patterns deserve attention: 1. inability or delay in voluntary phonation, and the child's difficulty in initiating a smooth transition from a nasal-symmetrical phase vegetative pattern to an oral-asymmetrical phase speech-breathing pattern; 2. ability to produce only one or two syllables per expiration, slow and irregular rate, and difficulty in modifying vegetative into speech-breathing patterns; 3. inspiratory voice, forced voice, sudden arrest of phonation, uncontrolled loudness, and asynchrony of respiratory and laryngeal movements; and 4. asthenic voice, and shallow breathing patterns.

Numerous investigators have reported on certain respiratory anomalies and associated speech problems among the cerebral-palsied. Blumberg (1955) studied the respiration and speech of spastic, athetotic, and ataxic children and concluded that respiratory function and control in these children were important to speech. Poorer speech among the athetotic children was attributed to poorer respiratory control caused by damage to hypothalamic respiratory regulating centers. During the speech of a group of spastics, Hull (1940) found an unusual amount of thoracic expansion and asynchrony between thoracic and abdominal muscle activity. Morley (1965, pp. 208–209) found relationships between asthenic and inspiratory voice and asynchrony of thoracic and abdominal muscle activity; and between "forced" voice and fixation of respiratory muscles during speech. Finally, McDonald and Chance (1964, p. 89) present a list of speech-breathing anomalies and associated speech symptoms which includes the following: rapid respiratory rate and reduction in infant vocalization; rapid respiratory rate (above 30 bpm's) in older children and poor speech; asynchrony of thoracic and abdominal movements and difficulty in sustaining vocalization and interruption of vocalization; and involuntary respiratory movements and uncontrolled loudness variation.

RESEARCH NEEDS

Much in the way of basic and clinical research in breathing and speech among the cerebral-palsied needs to be done. It would be well if more data were available on the normal sequential development of vegetative and speech-breathing patterns among normal and cerebral-palsied children from the period of prelingual vocalization through the first six or seven years. Details on the relationships between prolonged supine-lying, supported sitting with thoracic bands, crutch-walking, and thoracic-cage and associated breathing anomalies are also needed. More information on the presence and proportion of infantile-pattern breathing and paralytic breathing symptoms and their respective relationships to voice and speech symptoms is also needed.

Auditory System

General discussions of auditory functioning, hearing disorders, hearing measurement, and aural rehabilitation will be found in appropriate chapters in the Handbook. However, it is in order to discuss here those aspects of hearing and its disorders which are related, more or less specifically, to cerebral palsy, and which may affect the cerebral-palsied child's speech perception and production. As in the case of respiratory functioning, it is believed that speech clinicians are often not too well aware of normal sequences in the maturation of auditory behavior, and since the discussion of auditory problems among the cerebral-palsied will include references to symptoms of immaturity of auditory behavior, and since the clinician may want to gain an impression of the auditory maturation of a particular cerebral-palsied child, a short discussion of these sequences follows.

The maturation of auditory behavior in children may be described from various standpoints. For example, data may be provided in terms of general body reactions to various sound stimuli, or in terms of progressively more specific localizing reactions to sound stimuli, or in terms of specific body reactions to changing stimuli (i.e., changing distances and intensity and frequency characteristics of the stimuli)—all as a function of age. Increasing ability in the auditory perception of speech signals with respect to span, discrimination, analysis, and synthesis of signals is still another way of describing auditory maturation.

AUDITORY MATURATION AS A FUNCTION OF GENERAL BODY REACTIONS TO SOUND

In Peiper's (1963, pp. 83–92) discussion of the development of hearing in the human infant the following kinds of reaction to sound are mentioned;

cochleopalpebral reflex, fright reaction, change of respiratory rhythm, motor restlessness, facial grimacing, cessation of crying and cessation of movements including suckling movements, opening of the eyes, startle reaction, wrinkling of the forehead, mouth opening, arm extension and finger spreading, initiation of suckling movements, noisy crying, smiling, and tongue protrusion.

In particular, Peiper has observed a change in respiratory tracing in response to sound stimuli in four out of six infants during the first hour of life. Peiper cites investigators who found blinking in reaction to noisemakers and high-pitched tuning forks in newborns and premature infants; who elicited conditioned suckling movements in newborns in response to sound stimuli on the twenty-seventh day; who have observed suckling movements and smiles in response to human voice during the third week and second month, respectively; and who observed cessation of crying in infants by words or musical sounds. Reactions to auditory stimuli of fetuses in utero have also been reported. Peiper elicited "kick" and "restlessness" reactions in fetuses by the sounding of a loud and shrill automobile horn near the position of the head. Sound stimuli have also been said to increase temporarily the heart rate in the fetus. It has been reported that fetal auditory reactions do not begin until the seventh month and are strongest by the ninth month. Murphy (1964) found that the peripheral auditory mechanism is stimulable by the twentieth to twenty-fifth weeks of pregnancy.

AUDITORY MATURATION AS A FUNCTION OF SELECTIVE INHIBITION OF STARTLE

Murphy (1964) stated that the "first sign of cortical function in relation to auditory stimuli is the development of selective inhibition of startle"; that is, the ability of the infant to ignore familiar sounds, while less familiar and even softer sounds may cause startle. Murphy suggests that "rudimentary cortical function precedes selective inhibition and at this stage hearing can be distinguished from auditory reflex."

AUDITORY MATURATION AS A FUNCTION OF LOCALIZING BEHAVIOR

There are at least two forms of "localizing" behavior in response to sound—the orientation of the head toward the source of sound, and the orientation of the head and eyes, or just the eyes, toward the source of sound. Again, Peiper cites investigators who report inital head and eye orientation to the source of sound by about the third month with eye orientation lagging behind somewhat.

Murphy (1964) indicates that normally the eight- to 10-week-old infant in supine will quickly orient his head in the direction of a 50 dB sound source, a movement which is frequently preceded by "stilling" and often accompanied by a "batting" of the hand or a "kicking" of the leg on the side stimulated. Eye turn toward sound often accompanied by appropriate head roll may be noted at nine to 12 weeks. Murphy states that from the age of 12 weeks on, head control in the normal infant is sufficient to allow for testing in the seated position. He has found that localization downwards occurs before localization upwards and that in 60 percent of cases maturation toward the right precedes maturation toward the left. Finally, Murphy states that mature localization is indicative of binaural hearing and that consistent turning to one side irrespective of location of sound indicates monaural defect, while consistent turning toward only one source of sound with no reaction toward the other is usually a function of maturation with respect to being able to turn the head in either direction, and not monaural defect.

The author (Mysak, 1966, p. 35) recently attempted to describe the maturation of auditory behavior in the infant as a function of general and specific body-part reactions to acoustic stimuli. It appears that first, startlelike reactions and "auditory staring" (immobilization of eyes) may be observed in response to certain acoustic stimuli; then, at about three months, in addition to the startle and stare behaviors, "searching" (side-to-side head movements in response to sound) and incipient localizing behaviors may be observed. By about six months, localizing behavior is well developed. This evolvement from startle-staring, to searching-localizing, and finally to localizing is in keeping with the developmental principle of progression from gross, undifferentiated behavior to fine, differentiated behavior.

AUDITORY MATURATION AS A FUNCTION OF SPEECH PERCEPTION

Auditory maturation with respect to speech perception may be judged by observation of the infant's reaction to speech sounds made by others, as well as by the infant's ability to reproduce these sounds. The author (Mysak, 1966, pp. 35–37), in his effort at describing stages of speech development, referred to these behaviors. It has been observed that even during the first weeks of life "whimpering" may cease in response to a nearby soft voice; later, at about three months, the infant may stare or smile in response to his mother's voice; at about six months, the infant is usually able to immediately localize his mother's voice and may respond differently depending on the tone of the mother's voice; at about nine months, he may show meaningful reactions to the calling of his name, he may respond appropriately to "no" and "bye-bye", attempt to imitate sounds made by adults such as lip-smacking, brr, and so on, and he may repeat self-produced sounds. Finally, at about 12 months, the infant recognizes and quickly responds to his name, usually responds to simple "give me" requests, and can imitate speech sounds made by others.

The sequence of behavior with reference to speech stimuli appears to be: first, immobilization or an infantile listening attitude, then smile or recognition of maternal voice behavior, then differential response depending on the tone of the mother's voice, then appropriate response to the calling of his name and repetition of self-produced speech sounds, and, finally, increased ability to respond to requests and to imitate the speech sounds made by others.

Hearing Disorders Among the Cerebral-Palsied

Hearing disorders of every variety and degree have been found among the cerebral-palsied population; typically high-frequency sensorineural losses, conductive losses, and central and intermittent hearing losses. Figures of incidence and types of hearing loss have been provided by various investigators. McDonald and Chance (1964, p. 46) stated that reports of hearing losses among the cerebral-palsied have ranged from 10 percent to over 30 percent. In Nober's (1966, p. 277) review of reports of hearing losses among the cerebral-palsied, he found a range of from six percent to 41 percent. He adds that it is easy to accept high-incidence figures since 22 possible etiologies of cerebral palsy can also cause central auditory disorders, while 73 percent of them might also be responsible for peripheral disorders of hearing. Various investigators have indicated that these children characteristically show high-frequency hearing losses (e.g., Hardy, 1953; Perlstein, 1952; Crabtree and Gerrard, 1950; Rutherford, 1945). It has also been reported that the highest incidence of hearing loss is found among the athetotic groups (Hardy, 1953; Illingworth, 1958; Phelps, 1950). Hopkins et al (1954, p. 11) reported incidence figures in terms of type of cerebral palsy as follows: athetotic, 22·6 percent; ataxic, 18·4 percent; rigidity, 13·7 percent; and spastics, 7·2 percent.

Variations in incidence figures have been attributed to factors such as differences in definition of hearing loss, differences in methods and types of testing, actual differences in hearing among the different groups of cerebral-palsied, age at which testing was done, and so on.

As with the section on respiratory problems, the discussion of hearing disorders among the cerebral-palsied will be divided into descriptions of symptoms of auditory immaturity and of symptoms of hearing pathology.

SYMPTOMS OF AUDITORY IMMATURITY

Symptoms of infantile auditory behavior in cerebral-palsied children could include the persistence of "startle" behavior, and of crying, facial grimacing, motor restlessness, and released suckle and smile behavior in response to auditory stimulation. A delay or retardation in the development of localization behavior, for example, retention of startle-staring rather than searching-localizing behavior, and a delay in the ability to discriminate between familiar and unfamiliar sounds may also be viewed as symptoms of auditory immaturity. Also included would be the persistence of infantile head and neck and thoracic activity which, in turn, would disturb the development of auditory localization behavior. The author is unaware of any substantial research or clinical data specifically concerned with symptoms of infantile auditory behavior among the cerebral-palsied.

OTOPATHIC SYMPTOMS

Otopathic symptoms include those auditory involvements related to specific lesions in the external, middle, and inner ears and to lesions of the auditory tracts and cortices.

One investigator (Lassman, 1951) has indicated that the cerebral-palsied can present all kinds of hearing losses. He reported that they showed a susceptibility to middle-ear diseases and that all of his spastic subjects showed such impairments. He also found that most unilateral losses were due to middle-ear involvement.

The most frequently cited otopathic condition is that associated with cerebral palsy resulting from Rh incompatability between mother and child. Blakely

(1959) found evidence of cochlea damage in the Rh athetotic, hearing-involved child. According to McDonald and Chance (1964, p. 46), "Central deafness may also be found among athetoids with a history of kernicterus." Other investigators who have reported on hearing loss and kernicterus include Hardy (1953), Crothers and Paine (1959, p. 148), Perlstein (1950), and Gerrard (1952).

Clinical reports of variable auditory acuity, or intermittent hearing loss, may also be found (e.g., McDonald and Chance, 1964, p. 46). Crickmay (1966, p. 89) states, "It is interesting to note that sometimes there is a marked connection between a cerebral palsied child's ability to hear at a certain moment and the degree of his spasticity at that particular moment." She believes that when a child is experiencing severe spasms accompanied by abnormal reflex activity he will not hear as well.

The author (Mysak, 1968b, p. 31), in a review of 15 cases of children with minimal cerebral dysfunctioning, found deficits in auditory acuity, memory span, and discrimination. Inconsistent responses and rapid accommodation to auditory stimuli were also observed. In this regard, Wepman (1941) found that his group of children with cerebral palsy fell far below the norms in the auditory discrimination of speech sounds.

Various types of secondary auditory problems have also been reported by the author. "For example, when actual auditory problems exist and these are not detected or properly treated, the child may eventually find it unrewarding to attend auditorially, and he may begin to use less of his auditory capacity. Consequently, a type of 'auditory atrophy' may manifest itself." Or, "because of his problems, the involved child may be exposed to many unpleasant auditory experiences such as verbal criticism, punishment, and so forth, and he may eventually begin to reject auditory events." (Mysak, 1968b, p. 24.)

Finally, Fisch (1964) includes cerebral-palsied children in the category of children who may suffer from a pathology of listening. According to him there are three basic physiological processes involved in listening; neuromuscular, neurosensory, and automatic involuntary processes. The neuromuscular process is concerned primarily with "improvement of acoustic conditions" or the adoption of a listening attitude. This involves keeping still to eliminate body movement noises, and proper orientation of the head and body toward the sound source. The neurosensory process involves "the ability to eliminate or inhibit, in varying degrees, the other channels of communication of information from the environment, in order to be able to process as many items as possible by auditory communication." In other words, Fisch is referring to the process of selective inhibition and enhancement, or the ability to make the auditory channel "figure" and the other sensory channels "ground." The automatic involuntary processes include momentary cessation of respiration, change in respiratory rate, or shift in breathing pattern from thoracic to abdominal or vice versa, and possibly a change in heartbeat and the production of adrenalin.

In view of what is known about cerebral palsy, such children may possibly suffer listening pathology from the standpoint of all three basic physiological processes mentioned by Fisch. For example, with respect to the neuromuscular process, such children may be unable to orient the head toward the sound source and show inability to keep still. The latter difficulty is especially true in the case of the athetotic child whose involuntary body movements may generate as much as 30 to 40 dB of noise.

DIAGNOSTIC IMPLICATIONS

The information presented in this section on hearing has numerous implications for the diagnosis of auditory and speech disorders among the cerebral-palsied.

In the area of hearing evaluation, the clinician should be prepared to test for conductive losses, for neural receptive, transmissive, and perceptive losses, for intermittent hearing losses, and for auditory "atrophy" and "rejection" problems. Specifically, the clinician must keep in mind the high correlation among athetosis, kernicterus, and hearing loss. Numerous investigators (Crabtree and Gerrard, 1950; Hardy, 1953; Perlstein, 1952) have reported that the audiometric configuration in the athetotic child is characterized by a gradually sloping, bilateral, symmetrical high-frequency loss. Further, the clinician must also keep in mind the higher incidence of hearing loss among all types of cerebral-palsied. The implications of Fisch's discussion of listening pathology in the auditory assessment of cerebral-palsied children should also be remembered. The clinician must also cope with the great difficulty in using conventional pure-tone and speech audiometry testing with this population, and with the questionable use of electrodermal and evoked potential audiometry.

The diagnostic implications of substantial hearing disorder to speech-sound development, speech perception, and speech monitoring in the noncerebrally handicapped are well known to the speech pathologist. In the cerebral-palsied, it represents still another component of the speech complex. Fisch and Beck (1961) reported that 19 of 76 cerebral-palsied examined had hearing loss sufficient to produce difficulties with speech and language. Byers, Paine, and Crothers (1955) stated that hearing loss is present in the majority of cases of extrapyramidal cerebral palsy due to erythroblastosis and that the loss is severe enough to interfere with speech development and language acquisition.

With respect to the effects of persistence of infantile auditory behavior on speech development, it might be appreciated that persistence of auditory startle behavior, the inability to inhibit body movements in order to listen to speech sounds, difficulty in localizing speech sounds, and so on, may all affect speech sound and oral language development to various degrees. In terms of auditory perceptual functioning, the author (Mysak, 1968b), in reviewing the literature on the minimally brain-damaged, reported difficulties among these children in organizing and perceiving auditory stimuli; in confusing similar speech sounds, and in reversing or omitting syllables within words.

RESEARCH NEEDS

With reference to improving the hearing evaluation of cerebral-palsied children, it would be important to accumulate more comparative data on the maturation of auditory behavior in these children and normals. Because of the frequent involvement of head and neck and thoracic balance among the cerebral-palsied, it would not be unexpected to find deficits in the development of auditory localizing behavior, or problems in Fisch's neuromuscular aspect of listening. More information on this population relative to auditory memory span, discrimination, analysis, and synthesis of speech sounds and their relationships to speech-sound production should also prove useful.

Other areas of research interest include studies of better and earlier assessment of auditory acuity, investigations of the relationship of spasms and abnormal reflex activity to hearing, and of the phenomena of variable auditory acuity and rapid accommodation to sound.

Articulatory System

Articulatory disorders among the cerebral-palsied are frequently the most obvious aspect of the possible speech syndromes. Such disorders may stem from numerous sources; for example, hearing involvement, mental retardation, and various neurological deficits of the articulatory system. Again, since we will discuss here not only the articulatory problems associated with CNS impairment, but those associated specifically with CNS impairment in children, that is, associated with developing organisms, the discussion will be divided into two sections: those articulatory problems which reflect interference with speech-sound maturation, and those which reflect various types of irregularity in the innervation of the articulatory musculature. It should be apparent that the latter condition may also contribute to the former.

SPEECH-SOUND IMMATURITY IN CEREBRAL PALSY

According to various investigators (e.g., Wellman et al., 1931; Davis, 1938; Templin, 1957), speech-sound maturational processes among normal children may continue through the sixth, seventh, and eighth years of life. It is easy to understand how speech sound maturational processes may be disturbed among cerebral-palsied children, who in association with their CNS impairment may present respiratory, hearing, convulsive, intellectual, and perceptual complications during this same period.

With respect to speech-sound maturation in cerebral palsy, Irwin (1955) studied the speech of 128 spastics, 86 athetotics, and 52 tension athetotics, who ranged in age from one through 12 years, in an attempt to discover whether there were significant differences among these groups in consonant and vowel production, and in the frequencies of their production. No strong statistical evidence for differences in mastery of speech-sound elements among the groups studied was shown. However, a significant increase in the mastery of speech sounds as a function of age was noted.

Information on some specific backgrounds for speech-sound immaturity in cerebral palsy follows.

Speech-sound immaturity related to arrested or retarded oroneuromotor maturation. The author (Mysak, 1963) has reported on the persistence among the cerebral-palsied of infantile oroneuromotor patterns such as mouth opening, rooting, biting, suckling, and chewing reflexes, and how these may interfere with the development of speech sounds. It was indicated that ". . . when attempted articulatory movements also elicit infantile reflexes which, for example, cause involuntary jaw deviation, lip movement, mouth opening, and tongue protusion, it may be appreciated how these extraneous movements may make adequate articulation more difficult." Further, ". . . most of the reflexes associated with infantile feeding behavior are certainly inhibited by the time the normal child utters two- or three-word sentences. In other words, articulatory movements, which require higher integrated motor activity, are more adequately performed when infantile oral reflex behavior has been inhibited." In addition, abnormal facial-masticatory muscle activity, including persistence of infantile suckle-swallow patterns, may contribute to malocclusion (Lyons, 1956) and malocclusion, in turn, may also interfere with speech-sound maturation.

Sheppard (1964), in response to the author's observations, studied 51 children with cerebral palsy for the incidence of infantile cranio-oropharyngeal motor patterns and their relationship to age, feeding competence, speech intelligibility, and progress in speech therapy. She found that 1. infantile patterns were frequently found in the subjects, and 2. an inverse relationship existed between the number of patterns elicited in a subject and speech and feeding proficiency, progress in speech therapy, and age.

Speech-sound immaturity related to problems in developing adequate intraoral breath pressure. Hardy (1961) tested the hypothesis that some of the problems of children with cerebral palsy may be related to their inability to produce sufficient intra-oral breath pressure for speech-sound production. Sixteen of 41 children with speech ditheutics were found to have problems in velopharyngeal closure. He reported that problems in attaining sufficient intraoral breath pressure may be related to malfunctions of at least three musculatures—the palate, the respiratory mechanism, and the articulators—and that the ability to develop sufficient intraoral breath pressure may be considered one indicator of an individual's physiological readiness for speech.

Speech-sound immaturity secondary to mental retardation or hypacusis. Ingram and Barn (1961) have stated that there is a tendency to regard all children with cerebral palsy and speech disorder to be suffering from dysarthria; however, they believe that simple retardation of speech development, usually associated with mental retardation or defective hearing, is a more frequent cause of unintelligible speech.

Speech-sound immaturity viewed as a specific developmental speech disorder. According to Ingram and Barn (1961), specific developmental speech disorder is the commonest cause of abnormal speech in the general population of children. Such disorders include misarticulation not attributable to abnormal articulators or to other diseases and, except for slow development of intelligible speech, children with such disorders are usually normal in all other respects. It is expected, therefore, that a certain number of children with cerebral palsy may also evidence such speech symptoms.

CEREBRAL-PALSY DYSARTHRIAS

Various types of dysarthria have been identified in children with brain damage. Morley (1964, p. 179), in reporting on the variability of developmental dysarthrias, has observed near-normal articulation in the severely handicapped child, severe dysarthria in children with minimal brain symptoms, and dysarthria in the absence of any other neurological symptoms, or isolated dysarthria. With respect to incidence figures and types, Wolfe (1950) reported that 31 to 59 percent of cerebral-palsied cases studied showed some degree of dysarthria; Mecham (1966) reported that 70 to 80 percent of the cerebral-palsied have some type of articulation problem ranging from adequate to no ability; Achilles (1955) found that 43 percent had poor articulation, 45 percent had fair articulation, and 12 percent had adequate articulation; and Paine (1962) in a study of 41 minimally brain-damaged children found normal speech in about half of the group and nine who showed varying degrees of dysarthria, slowing, slurring, or dysarticulation.

It is clear from these reports that the incidence of articulatory disorder among the cerebral-palsied is high and may vary in severity from near normal to very severe.

To be discussed next are the speech characteristics of the various types of dysarthria which have been reported among the cerebral-palsied, such as spastic dysarthria, athetotic dysarthria, ataxic dysarthria, apraxic dysarthria, and somesthetic dysarthria.

Speech characteristics of spastic dysarthria. The following speech characteristics have been identified in spastics by various investigators: difficulty with linguadental, lingua-alveolar sounds, and frictives (Clement and Twitchell, 1959); ". . . grave articulatory problems which reflect the inability to secure graded, synchronous movements of the tongue, lips, and jaw" (Berry and Eisenson, 1956, p. 357); and ". . . articulation is slow, clumsy, and particularly defective in those vocables that require delicate movements of the intrinsic muscles of the tongue." (West et al, 1957, p. 122.)

Speech characteristics of athetotic dysarthria. The speech of the athetotic has been described in the following ways: ". . . articulatory problems varying from the extremes of complete mutism or extreme dysarthria to a slight awkwardness in lingual movement" (Berry and Eisenson, 1956, p. 358); and "In athetosis all sounds are articulated poorly, if at all, except at those rare moments when the patient is quiet, and is free from surges of convulsion that sweep over his neuromuscular system, from the labial muscles of articulation to the abdominal muscles of exhalation. In such moments the articulation of the purely athetotic patient is startlingly normal." (West et al, 1957, p. 122.)

Speech characteristics of ataxic dysarthria. Ataxic speech has been described as ". . . characterized by slurring of articulation which lapses into unintelligibility if speech is continued beyond phrases or short sentences" (Berry and Eisenson, 1956, p. 360). West et al (1957, p. 122) state that ataxic dysarthria is characterized by a lack of consistency in incoordinations. "Ataxic clumsiness alone may be thought of as a sensory, or afferent, deficiency; when labored scansion appears, it should be regarded as an associative failure."

In an analysis of the articulation problems of the major types of cerebral palsy, Rutherford (1944) stated that athetotics are generally able to make movements for speech but few movements are under constant control, that spastics may be limited in the direction and extent of movement but control is consistent, and that the ataxic, who shows mainly defective feedback, does not know whether he has made appropriate movements and is not always certain the movements have taken place.

Speech characteristics of apraxic dysarthria. Apraxic dysarthria (or articulatory apraxia, or oral dyspraxia) is contrasted with dysarthria by Morley (1965, p. 175) in this way: there are those ". . . who apparently have no difficulty in moving the tongue, lips, or palate for spontaneous movements but have difficulty in directing them for voluntary imitation of movements or for reproduction of the correct articulatory sounds when hearing is normal." Morley associates such articulatory dysfunctioning with higher level involvements of the nervous system. Affected children may acquire only a limited number of consonant sounds and usually have insufficient audiokinesthetic control to reproduce such sounds when they appear in conversational patterns.

Referring to children with cerebral palsy, Morley (1965, p. 182) states, "Developmental articulatory apraxia of severe degree may also occur in these children, whether in isolation or in association with dysarthria or dysphasia." According to Morley, such apraxic dysarthria may be further complicated by the acquisition of abnormal, sensory model patterns for articulation arising as a consequence of experiencing abnormal, dysarthria-associated movements.

Speech characteristics of somesthetic dysarthria. Recent studies (McCroskey, 1958; Ringel and Steer, 1963) have reported on induced disturbance of articulation as a result of tactile alterations in the oral region. McCall (1964), in a study of tactile sensibility and kinesthetic function, primarily of the tongue, found the cerebral-palsied to be inferior to the normal in most of the tasks.

With respect to lack of progress in speech therapy among certain cerebral-palsied individuals, Wilson (1965, p. 56) has reported that "It has been our clinical experience that a limited number of cerebral palsied have reasonable motor functioning and yet do not respond to the usual therapeutic techniques. Upon more careful evaluation we found these children to have measurable breakdown in sensory feedback."

Dysarthria as related to cerebral palsy classification. Ingram and Barn (1961) related speech examination data of 258 cerebral-palsied children to the types of cerebral palsy manifested. Some of their findings appear below.

Among those with *hemiplegia,* they reported that dysarthria as an isolated problem is uncommon and that it is more often associated with retardation of speech development or with dysrhythmia; that dysarthria was no more frequent among those with acquired than among those with congenital hemiplegia; that dysarthria among the hemiplegia group was characterized by a slowing of rate and misarticulation, most frequently, of the plosives, labiodentals, and interdentals; and that hypernasality due to palatal involvement was not common.

Among those with *bilateral hemiplegia* (involvement of all four limbs, upper limbs more affected), they reported that dysarthria was almost inevitable since the bulbar musculature is involved; that most have more or less severe feeding difficulties in infancy which may involve both suckling and swallowing, or swallowing only, and associated drooling; that most are severely mentally defective and hence the associated retardation of speech development usually conceals the extent of articulatory organ paresis; and that these children usually acquire no more than a few single words and rudimentary phrases and show gross misarticulation and usually marked nasal escape.

Among those with *diplegia* (lower limbs more involved than the upper limbs), they reported that dysarthria was commoner than among hemiplegics, occurred more often in tetraplegic than in triplegic or paraplegic children, and was usually accompanied by impairment of voluntary movements of the lips, tongue, or palate; that a high proportion of those with severe dysarthria or no speech presented histories of feeding difficulty in infancy or drooling and many showed a positive suckling reflex; that there is a characteristic dysarthria among diplegics marked by slowing of utterance and intonation, unchanging and monotonous stress patterns, frequent slight or moderate nasal escape, and labored production of speech sounds with better production of vowels than of consonants.

Among those with *ataxic diplegia* (more severe paresis in lower limbs and ataxia of cerebellar type) and *ataxia* (incoordination of movement and impaired balance), they reported that most of these children showed speech retardation usually proportional to the degree of mental impairment and which might occur alone but more frequently was associated with dysarthria and other abnormalities, including a characteristic type of dysrhythmia; that the slowness and ataxia of movements of the articulatory organs in ataxic disorders causes articulatory problems which may be very similar to those resulting from the slowness and weakness of their movements in children with extensive diplegia, but that in ataxic disorders the articulatory differences tend to be less consistent; and that it was not unusual to observe excessive nasal escape during conversational patterns, even though palatal movements appeared intact upon examination.

Finally, among those with *dyskinesia* (disorder of involuntary movements which may be of the choreoid, athetoid, tremulous, or dystonic varieties), they reported only a small proportion of these children spoke normally and that a majority have complex speech problems; that about 70 percent of their children showed dysarthria with practically all the patients showing involuntary movements of the face, tongue, palate, and often other parts of the body whenever the child attempted to move his articulators; and that the speech sounds which were defective varied widely but that θ, r, l, ʃ, and p were of particular difficulty.

DIAGNOSTIC IMPLICATIONS

The discussion of articulation disorders among the cerebral-palsied is replete with implications with respect to the differential diagnosis of possible articulatory complexes in any one case.

The discussion suggests that a thorough evaluation of speech-sound immaturity should include an investigation of the possible contribution to the problem of oroneuromotor maturation, of adequacy of intraoral breath pressure, and of mental retardation and hypacusis. The factor of specific developmental articulatory disorder must also be considered.

Further, the diagnostician needs to distinguish among the spastic, athetotic, ataxic, apraxic, somesthetic, and mixed features of cerebral palsy dysarthria. However, it should be pointed out here that there is some question about the extent of the value and validity of such groupings. Twitchell (1965) has indicated that from a neurophysiological view the separation of cerebral-palsied children into various categories is artificial and that, regardless of classification, the physiological substrata for, as examples, spasticity and athetosis can be demonstrated in all patients. He urges "... that more attention be paid to the physiological basis for the motor deficit in each individual patient so that treatment could be oriented to that individual patient rather than to some arbitrary grouping." This expresses well the long-standing beliefs of neurophysiologically oriented treatment specialists in cerebral palsy.

In line with a more individualized, physiologic approach to the dysarthria under scrutiny, the diagnostician should remember that adequate speech articulation is based on controlled movements in appropriate directions, and of appropriate range, speed, accuracy, and coordination. Hence, he must determine whether the phonetic lapse under consideration is related to consistent limitations to direction and range of movements of the articulators; to inconsistency in moving in appropriate directions with appropriate range; to problems in intra-articulatory system coordination (e.g., lack of coordination between labial and velopharyngeal closure activities for production of [b]); to difficulty in voluntarily reproducing certain movements which can be effected spontaneously; to difficulty in moving separately various articulators within the articulatory system (e.g., moving the tongue tip separately from the lips); to problems in the adequate and accurate reception of sensory feedback from the articulatory system; and, finally, to various combinations of the above.

After identifying the various possible movement deficits in a particular articulatory complex, the diagnostician should then attempt to determine whether the problems are caused by disturbances in oroneuromaturation, such as reflected in retained infantile feeding reflexes, or in lack of differentiation among articulators, or to active stretch reflexes, or to higher order involvement of the neuromotor system, and so on.

A discussion of additional areas of interest for diagnosis of articulatory problems in cerebral palsy follows.

Implications of a clinical study of children with minimal chronic brain syndromes to diagnosis of articulation problems in cerebral palsy. The author (Mysak, 1968b), in a review of the speech findings of 15 children (boys and girls with age range of three to 13 years) with minimal brain damage, found that: three showed abnormal velar activity, four showed normal nonspeech but abnormal speech movements, three showed excessive involuntary movements of the tongue in the rest position, two showed abnormal nonspeech and speech movements of the articulators, and six showed excessive nasality. Of the total group, only two children reflected near-normal speech-sound development.

Implications of certain research data to diagnosis of articulation problems in cerebral palsy. Pertinent to the area of speech-mechanism examination is a study by Hixon and Hardy (1964). They studied 50 cerebral-palsied children for possible relationships between speech defectiveness and repetition rates of certain nonspeech and speech movements of the articulators. They found that, in general, speech movements were faster than nonspeech movements, and that speech-movement capacity predicted with fair accuracy speech defectiveness while nonspeech activities were not highly related to speech activities. These findings led to the conclusions that the neurophysiological mechanisms which evoke speech activities may be dissimilar from those which evoke nonspeech movements of the same structures, and that an adequate evaluation of the restricted motility of the speech articulators cannot be determined by testing capacity for nonspeech movements.

In a discussion of neuromuscular involvements of the speech mechanism in cerebral palsy, Mecham (1966, pp. 30–33) indicated that among spastics may be found hypertonicity, pathologic stretch reflex, and flaccidity; among athetotics may be found involuntary movements, or a series of involuntary movements; and among ataxics may be found disordered feedback mechanisms for positional and directional orientations. Such a disordered feedback mechanism may exist in other cases, too, but represents a primary disorder in ataxia.

A series of reports by Irwin should also be of interest here. Irwin (1956) studied the articulation of 96 cerebral-palsied children aged four to 16 years and found that, unlike normals, omissions occurred significantly more often than substitutions. In another report of a study of 147 children, aged three to 16 years, Irwin (1961) indicated that factors of chronological age, mental age, and I.Q. did not appear to have a significant influence on articulatory ability. He also stated that final consonants in words were most difficult and that spastics made higher scores on an integrated articulation test than did athetotics. There were no significant differences between hemiplegics, quadriplegis, and paraplegics, although the third group tended to make higher scores than the other two. No differences were found between the performances of right and left hemiplegics. Categories of mild, moderate, and severe involvement had a significant influence upon articulation within the hemiplegia, quadriplegia, and paraplegia subgroups.

Also of diagnostic importance are statements by Berry and Eisenson (1956, pp. 366–369). Among the cerebral-palsied they have identified problems in velopharyngeal closure, and failure of tongue tip and blade to rise to the alveolar ridge without the approximation of the mandible. They reported that ". . . 75 percent of athetoids have great difficulty in elevating the tongue." (Berry and Eisenson, 1956, p. 358.)

Many findings by Lencione (1966) also have diagnostic implications. Lencione studied the speech-sound ability of 129 spastics and athetotics aged eight to 14 years. With reference to rank order of correct production of sounds, in terms of the position of the sounds in words, she found a progression from the initial, to the medial, to the final position. She found that her subjects showed highest proficiency for tongue tip simple, lip, and back-of-tongue sounds. Tongue tip complex sounds were significantly more difficult than the other three, and voiceless sounds were more difficult than voiced sounds. Lencione also found a marked relationship between age and consonantal proficiency. Byrne (1959), who studied 74 children aged two to seven years, also found that the greatest accuracy in speech-sound production was on sounds in the initial position followed by sounds in the medial position of words. Highest proficiency was found for production of bilabials followed by tongue tip simple, back-of-tongue, lip complex, and tongue tip complex sounds. Byrne also found that voiced sounds were less difficult than voiceless. Both Byrne and Lencione found that, in general, spastics were better than athetotics in speech-sound production.

Finally, Clement and Twitchell (1959) studied the speech of children with infantile spastic quadriparesis and congenital bilateral athetosis. In the cases of spastic dysarthria, they found that the tongue at rest was flattened and pulled slightly back from the teeth; that there was a thin lip line with corners retracted, and there was difficulty in raising the velum. In cases of athetotic dysarthria, they found that, except for some movement, the tongue at rest was similar to that of the spastics; that lip movement was also similar to the spastics although lips were more rounded with frequent alternation between pursing and parting of the lips; and that there was difficulty raising the velum, which was less than in the spastics. It was believed that athetotics learned speech sounds slightly better than spastics.

Implications of certain neurological considerations in the diagnosis of articulation problems. Clement and Twitchell (1959) have attempted to differentiate between spastic and athetotic dysarthria in terms of disequilibrium between grasping and avoiding responses.

It is believed that different cortical regions subserve positive exploratory reactions while others subserve negative withdrawal reactions. Normally, positive and negative reactions are in equilibrium with each other; however, a lesion abolishing one type of reaction will release its opposite.

They believe that disturbed grasping and avoiding responses in cerebral palsy, for example, the unstable equilibrium of responses shown in athetosis, and the overactive avoiding responses shown in spasticity, are also reflected in the speech mechanism. They view lip pursing, tongue protrusion, and velar elevation as positive or grasping responses; and lip parting, tongue retraction, and velar depression as negative or avoiding responses.

In spastic dysarthria, then, the primary problem is one of a depression of positive responses and exaggeration of negative responses rather than spasticity of the speech musculature. In athetotic dysarthria, the primary problem is overactive negative responses plus occasional alternation with positive responses rather than involuntary movements of the speech musculature; positive, grasping responses are not depressed in athetosis but are in unstable equilibrium with negative, avoiding responses.

RESEARCH NEEDS

It should be clear from the incomplete and contradictory findings in the discussion of articulation disorders in cerebral palsy that a great deal of research remains to be done. For example, much more work must be done in attempting to identify all of the factors possibly responsible for speech-sound immaturity. The roles of persisting infantile oroneuromotor activity and reduced intraoral breath pressure must be explored further. The value of the concept of specific, developmental articulation disorder in misarticulation in cerebral palsy also needs to be appraised.

The value as well as the means of better differentiating among spastic, athetotic, ataxic, apraxic, somesthetic and mixed forms of cerebral palsy dysarthria must be considered. Related to the problem of improving methods of evaluating the articulatory system, Shelton et al (1967) have reported on the development of a test for oral stereognosis ability. Much more needs to be done in studying oral sensation and perception and their significance to articulatory disorders among the cerebral-palsied. The clinical implications of viewing cerebral palsy dysarthrias from the standpoint of disturbed oral grasping and avoiding responses should also be examined.

Phonatory System

Efficient phonatory behaviour depends on coordination between inspiratory and expiratory muscles which, in turn, must be coordinated with laryngeal, velopharyngeal, and articulatory muscle valving activity. The vocal product of this complex coordination must then be monitored primarily by the auditory system. In light of the already discussed respiratory, auditory, velopharyngeal, and articulatory system anomalies among the cerebral-palsied, it is apparent that many of these children will manifest various types of dysphonias. Further, in a review of the concept of normal voicing, the author (Mysak, 1966b) has stated that of the two possible theories of voice production, the myoelastic-aerodynamic theory, which indicates that the vocal folds are activated by the air stream from the lungs and trachea, is the most supportable. Again, in terms of what has been stated with respect to respiratory anomalies and coordination problems, dysphonias among the cerebral-palsied should certainly not be unexpected.

CEREBRAL PALSY DYSPHONIAS

Because of the interdependence of respiratory and laryngeal muscle functioning in voice production, frequent reference will be made to material previously presented in the section on respiration. And, as usual there will be an attempt to separate voicing problems in terms of whether they reflect predominately infantile or paralytic patterns.

Symptoms of infantile laryngeal functioning. The author (Mysak, 1968a) recently discussed the nature of the glottic-closing reflex in infants. For air-breathing creatures, reflexive laryngeal closure is important during swallowing and during periods of immersion. Excessive rehearsal of this reflex during fetal life has been cited by one author as a possible cause of congenital laryngeal stridor. Irregular persistence of this primitive laryngeal behavior in the child with cerebral palsy could result in voice disorders associated with involuntary, open-close or over-close activity of the glottis; that is, voice disorders characterized by interruption of voicing, intermittent and forced voicing, and inspiratory voicing.

Other anomalies possibly reflective of infantile respiratory-laryngeal behavior are: delay in initiation of voicing due to slowness in shifting from vegetative to speech-breathing patterns; short duration of phonation due to use of vegetative breathing patterns during speech attempts; paucity of phonation due to a high bpm rate, and weak phonation due to shallow breathing cycles.

Symptoms of laryngeal paralysis. Mecham (1966, pp. 38–40), in his discussion of problems of voice production among the cerebral-palsied, reported that aspirate and breathy voices have been attributed to flaccid paralysis of the cords. Mecham also reported on the following conditions which affect voice production: spasms of intrinsic and extrinsic laryngeal muscles and of the ventricular folds, asynchrony between expiratory and laryngeal muscles, irregular and arrhythmic laryngeal activity, and hoarseness usually resulting from tension in the vocal folds.

McDonald and Chance (1964, pp. 90–91) have indicated that adductor spasm of laryngeal muscles in cerebral palsy may prevent the initiation of voicing, or, if the spasm takes place during speech, may result in interrupting phonation. On the other hand, abductor spasm may prevent phonation by not allowing for the approximation of the vocal folds or may pull them apart during voicing. Irregular shifts in pitch, intensity, or quality may reflect uncontrollable variations in laryngeal muscle tension. It is not possible to determine how many of the vocal conditions described by Mecham and McDonald and Chance are really reflections of infantile laryngeal functioning rather than of laryngeal paralyses.

Numerous investigators have reported on perceived differences in the dysphonias reflected by the major groups of cerebral palsy. The voice of the athetotic has been described in the following ways: 1. pitch basically low, intensity weak and forced, quality throaty and forced, duration broken and wavering (Clement and Twitchell, 1959); 2. whispered, hoarse, or ventricular phonation (Berry and Eisenson, 1959, p. 358); 3. weak in volume, irregular episodes of intense volume associated with involuntary spasms of the diaphragram, fluctuations in pitch and intensity (Mecham et al, 1966, pp. 38–40); and 4. inspiratory voice, periodic, involuntary abduction of the vocal folds or intermittent dysphonia (Ingram and Barn, 1961). As is apparent, the various clinical descriptions of athetotic dysphonia show consistency in various respects.

The voice of the spastic has been described in the following ways: 1. pitch generally high, intensity weak and forced, quality breathy and forced and hypernasal, duration broken with short vowel duration (Clement and Twitchell, 1959); 2. lack of inflection, gutteral or breathy quality, uncontrolled volume (Berry and Eisenson, 1959, pp. 356–360); and 3. marked nasal escape in cases of bilateral hemiplegia, and moderate nasal escape because of palatal paresis in cases of diplegia (Ingram and Barn, 1961). Again, there is some consistency among reports on the voice of the spastic; however, it is also apparent that there is overlap in the reported characteristics of athetotic and spastic dysphonias.

The voice of the ataxic has been described in the following ways: 1. ". . . vocal pitch, loudness, and quality tend either to be monotonal or to vary spasmodically and without respect to meaning" (Berry and Eisenson, 1959, p. 360); and 2. excessive nasal escape, abnormalities of intonation and stress, and pitch rise during speech acceleration and pitch fall during speech deceleration (Ingram and Barn, 1961).

Brown (1967, pp. 382–383), in speaking of the voice of the cerebral-palsied, indicated that it is often ". . . of poor quality, with breathiness, harshness, and nasality being the undesirable qualities most often encountered." He also cites weakness, reduced pitch, and loudness variability as additional factors. One writer (Wilson, 1965, p. 53) has indicated that "In all likelihood, the structure [larynx] will be adequate, but functionally incapable of the rapid transitional movements necessary for phonation." Wilson indicated that "The ability to start and stop phonation is most closely related to the speaking act." He believes that five alternations in five seconds is a minimal requirement. Finally, it has also been reported (DiCarlo and Amster, 1955, p. 219) that the child with cerebral palsy may show symptoms of vocal abuse because of his difficulty with voice production.

DIAGNOSTIC IMPLICATIONS

The discussion of infantile as opposed to paralytic voicing symptoms suggests that whenever possible such symptoms should be differentiated by the diagnostician. For example, examination for the irregular persistence of the infantile glottic-closing reflex and its possible relationship to interrupted, forced, or inspiratory voicing is in order.

Also, it would be useful to differentiate voice disorders at the laryngeal level from those stemming from respiratory disorders, or from problems of coordination between laryngeal and respiratory activities.

RESEARCH NEEDS

For purposes of better identification of all the possible components of dysphonias in cerebral palsy, it would be well if the question of symptoms related to infantile laryngeal functioning vs. symptoms related to laryngeal paralysis is explored further. The role of respiratory involvement alone, and the role of lack of coordination between respiration and laryngeal functioning in cerebral palsy dysphonia also need further investigation. The validity of the concept of the "spastic voice," or the "athetotic" or "ataxic voice," needs further study. Studies of voicing in cerebral palsy involving the use of cineradiographic, electromyographic, and air-flow instrumentation should also prove useful.

Speech-Rhythm System

Manifestations of irregularities in the flow of speech have been described in various ways. Interjections of sounds or syllables; repetitions of sounds, syllables, words, or phrases; prolongations of sounds or syllables; and revisions either in pronunciation or grammar are disruptors of speech fluency commonly observed in normal speakers. When speech flow is increased in an irregular fashion in conjunction with articulatory deterioration, or when speech flow is interrupted by abnormal repetitions and prolongations of sounds or syllables, the conditions may be referred to as cluttering or stuttering, respectively. This discussion will be confined to those speech rhythm problems which are associated with CNS involvements and which, therefore, may be found in children with cerebral palsy. For more general discussions of stuttering, the reader is referred to appropriate chapters in the Handbook.

Since there will be an attempt to discuss cerebral palsy speech dysrhythmia in terms of manifestations of immaturity of central neural mechanisms for control of speech rhythm, as well as neuropathology of these centers, a short discussion of speech-flow maturation is appropriate.

The author (Mysak, 1966a, p. 86) described the developmental sequence of speech flow approximately in the following way: 1. the regularizing of speech flow depends first, on the maturation of associational cortex in and around neuronal arrangements representing percept, heard-word, and spoken-word patterns, and second, on control over external factors which may contribute to speech-flow disturbance such as inability to gain, or the fear of losing a listener's attention, or the fear of interruption by the listener; and 2. speech-flow automaticity proceeds from syllabic, to word, to phrasal, to full articulatory cycle levels. It should be apparent that children with CNS involvement may reflect speech dysrhythmia because of problems in, for example, establishing intact neuronal patterns representing percepts, heard-words, or spoken-words, or in developing automatic and reciprocal relationships among these nervous arrangements; or in development of sensorimotor integration capacity which allows for speech automaticity on phrasal and full cycle levels rather than on only phonemic or syllabic levels.

Various neurological bases for dysrhythmia have been presented by numerous investigators. Travis

(1931, p. 95) stated, "The stutterer . . . reflects a certain lack of maturation of the central nervous system which either does not afford integration of the highest neurophysiological levels involved in speech or predisposes these levels to disintegration by various types of exogenous or endogenous stimuli." West (1958, Ch. 4) postulated that the fundamental disorder of stuttering may well be related to pyknolepsy and hence may be described as speech epilepsy; Zentay (1937) identified similarities between disorders due to lesions in the striopalidum or mesencephalon and stuttering; and Weiss (1964, pp. 65–66), in a discussion of the differential diagnosis of cluttering, states, "The first step . . . is exclusion of cases of symptomatic cluttering, i.e., the cluttering-like symptoms that result from neurological disease." According to Weiss, any kind of brain lesions such as those caused by trauma, infection, or tumor can upset language function and produce clutteringlike symptoms. Finally, palilalia, or the repetition of a phrase which is reiterated with increasing rapidity, is most frequently found as a symptom of postencephalitic parkonsonism and in pseudobular palsy due to vascular lesions (Brain, 1961, p. 106).

A related finding concerns the statement by Dinnerstein et al (1966) that stuttering could be explained on the basis of an anxiety-induced delay in audition and proprioception. The concept grew out of their work on explaining tremor and hypokinesis in parkinsonism on the basis of delay in proprioception.

Reports on the effects on speech of electrical stimulation of certain parts of the brains of patients undergoing brain surgery contribute further to the concept of central, speech rhythm control centers. Penfield and Roberts (1959, p. 133) described hesitation, slurring, distortion, and repetition of words resulting from electrical stimulation of various areas of the brain, while Guiot et al (1961) reported that electrical stimulation of the thalamic area, prior to a surgical ablation procedure for the relief of parkinsonism, in some instances caused an arrest or hesitation followed by a slowing of speech, and in other instances caused an acceleration of speech. With respect to irregularities in speech rhythm in parkinsonism, problems such as speech festination, inability to initiate speech, or speech "freezing," drawling, clonic blocks, and increased amount and frequency of pause time have all been reported.

It would appear that there is sufficient evidence to support the concept of a speech rhythm control center existing in the central speech system and that such a center could easily be affected in those cases of neuropathology identified as cerebral palsy.

CEREBRAL PALSY SPEECH DYSRHYTHMIAS

Speech dysrhythmia among the cerebral-palsied has been reported by many investigators (e.g., Rutherford, 1944; Palmer, 1949; Ingram and Barn, 1961).

Specifically, Ingram and Barn (1961) state, "The proportion of children who stammer or hesitate because of organic disease of the nervous system is small, but it includes a relatively high proportion of the children whose speech disorder is due to cerebral palsy." They believe that "Speech dysrhythmia is common in children suffering from dyskinesia, but it also occurs, less commonly, in those with hemiplegia, ataxic diplegia and ataxia." In their study of speech disorders among 258 cerebral-palsied children, they reported the following with respect to the characteristics of speech dysrhythmia among the various forms of the disease.

Among the *hemiplegics*, dysrhythmia occurred in 14 percent of the cases and was manifested as a combination of arrest or hesitation with stammer; among *ataxics*, dysrhythmia and associated abnormalities of intonation and stress occurred in a high number and were manifested by irregular division of phrases and irregular speech acceleration and deceleration; and, among those with *dyskinesia*, irregularities of speech rhythm were present in more than half of the children and were manifested by irregular, involuntary action of the respiratory muscles which moved out-of-phase with muscles of articulation. Under these circumstances, speech might be suddenly arrested, or unexpected inspiratory activity would cause inspiratory speech episodes. Periodic speech arrest also appeared to be related to obstruction of the speech air stream at the glottic level.

With respect to differentiating between those symptoms of speech dysrhythmia that may be associated with retarded or arrested development of central neural mechanisms for speech rhythm control, and those associated with direct or indirect neuropathology of such mechanisms, it should be understood that such symptom differentiation among children with cerebral palsy will be mostly conjectural since this writer is unaware of the existence of actual data in this area.

Symptoms of speech dysrhythmia associated with immaturity might include those disfluencies apparently related to slowness in developing oral symbols and in using them automatically, and those disfluencies marked by childish whole-word and phrasal repetitions. Symptoms of pathology of central neural mechanisms for speech-rhythm control might include irregular speech acceleration and deceleration, episodic inability to initiate speech and arrest of speech, disfluency accompanied by articulatory and phonatory irregularities, disfluency associated with physiologic delays in transmission of auditory and proprioceptive feedback, and disfluency associated with out-of-phase respiratory, laryngeal, and articulatory muscle activity.

DIAGNOSTIC IMPLICATIONS

Numerous diagnostic implications arise from this discussion of cerebral palsy and speech rhythm. For example, the value of attempting to differentiate between speech dysrhythmia due to maturational factors in certain central neural mechanisms and that dysrhythmia due to neuropathology of these mechanisms. In this regard, consideration would need to be given of the integrity of the neuronal arrangements representing percept, heard-word, and spoken-word patterns, of the influence of external or listener reaction factors on speech flow, and of whether speech-flow automaticity had reached the word or phrasal levels.

It would also be necessary to determine whether the disruption of speech rhythm was due to problems in auditory and proprioceptive feedback systems, to respiratory or laryngeal spasms, or to dyssynergies between respiratory, laryngeal, and articulator muscle systems.

RESEARCH NEEDS

It would be useful if further electrical stimulation of the brain studies were done to provide additional information on the role of central neural mechanisms in speech rhythm control. Additional study also needs to be done of the roles of central mechanisms and respiratory and laryngeal functioning in cerebral palsy speech dysrhythmia.

Finally, studies of the concept of duplex symptomatology in speech dysrhythmia, (i.e., symptoms associated with immaturity of central neural mechanisms devoted to speech rhythm control and those associated with damage to these mechanisms) and of ways of discriminating between symptoms also need to be done.

Oral Language System

The author (Mysak, 1961) has described the organismic development of oral language as ". . . the result of the simultaneous maturation of the perceptorium, the vocalization mechanism, and the general motorium." The perceptorium important for oral language development includes the eye-ear-hand unit (i.e., basically a visual-auditory-tactile receiver) and central mechanisms, the vocalization system including the respiratory-phonatory-articulatory subsystems and central mechanisms, and the general motorium (locomotor system) for transporting the perceptorium and vocalization mechanism about the environment.

In terms of an organismic nature of the development of oral language, it is apparent that the cerebral-palsied child, who may show involvements of the perceptorium, the vocalization mechanism, and the general motorium, may potentially display any and all varieties of oral language dysfunctioning.

As is the case in the description of all the other possible components of cerebral palsy speech syndomes, oral language problems will be discussed in two ways: first, those problems which may be identified as symptomatic of oral language immaturity, and second, those which may be identified as symptomatic of direct or indirect involvement of brain centers which subserve oral language functioning.

ORAL LANGUAGE IMMATURITY

Factors which contribute to oral language immaturity may include substantial hearing loss, mental retardation, perceptual dysfunctioning, psychosocial problems, and limited stimulation and experience. In this vein, Brown (1967, p. 381) stated, "In addition to neuromuscular problems, the child with cerebral palsy may have visual, hearing, perceptual, intellectual and behavioral difficulties interfering with normal speech development."

That oral language retardation is a frequent symptom in cerebral palsy has been reported by numerous investigators. A sampling of these reports follows: 1. in a study of athetotic and spastic quadriplegic children between two and seven years, all children were found language-retarded with respect to the appearance of first words and two-word and three-word sentences, and further, it was stated that their language maturation reflected that of normals but at a reduced rate (Byrne, 1959); 2. in a study of 334 spastic hemiplegics, it was found that there was a delay of nine months in uttering first words and a delay of six months in the use of sentences, and further, those considered mentally defective spoke their first words 14 months later (Hood et al, 1956); 3. in a study of 200 cerebral-palsied individuals, there was found an average retardation of from three to four years in vocabulary and verbal recall (Dunsdon, 1952); 4. in an analysis of the communicative disorders of 151 cases of cerebral palsy, it was found that 66 percent either had no speech or no more than one year of oral language development (Achilles, 1955); and 5. in a study of 67 spastic hemiplegics under 13 years, it was found that the development of language depended on mental potential rather than on degree of impairment, or preferred hand, or presence or absence of convulsive disorder (Kastein, 1951).

Ingram and Barn (1961), in their discussion of speech disorder among various forms of cerebral palsy, indicated that "The most frequently observed abnormality is simple retardation of speech development, usually associated with mental retardation or defective hearing." In terms of associating symptoms of speech retardation with various forms of cerebral palsy, they offered the following: in *hemiplegia, bilateral hemiplegia*, and in *diplegia*, the commonest disorder was simple retardation of speech development associated with mental impairment; in *ataxia and ataxic diplegia*, the commonest problem is again retardation of speech development in proportion to the degree of mental impairment and, like diplegic children, those ataxic diplegics with tetraplegia show greater degrees of speech retardation than those with triplegia or paraplegia; and in *dyskinesia*, because of the smaller proportion of mental retardation among those with dyskinesias, speech retardation due to mental retardation is less frequent, but speech retardation due to hearing impairment is higher in this group than in the others.

The discussion of oral language immaturity has been limited to the report that it is frequently observed in all forms of cerebral palsy and that it is most commonly associated with the problem referred to as mental retardation. There is, of course, the large question of identifying those factors which contribute to intellectual impairment in cerebral palsy.

ORAL LANGUAGE PATHOLOGY

An attempt will be made in this section to identify those symptoms of oral language disorder apparently related to involvement of those particular brain centers that subserve oral language functioning. Obviously, separating symptoms of oral language immaturity from symptoms of oral language pathology in the cerebral-palsied is difficult even under ideal circumstances. Of course, in those rare instances where intellectual, hearing, articulatory, and psychosocial factors are relatively within normal limits in any one cerebral-palsied child, it may be possible to identify language symptoms suggestive of direct involvement of CNS language centers. It should be expected that some of the symptoms may be similar to those found in children and adults with normal language who suffer loss of language due to brain trauma.

In line with the latter statement, there have been numerous reports of oral language dysfunctioning among the minimally brain-damaged child (e.g., Strauss and Kephart, 1955; Ingram, 1960; Lewis et al, 1960; Hagberg, 1962; Mysak, 1968b). Because many of these children are considered to have normal or near-normal intellectual potential, and because some of their other symptoms may also be minimal, language evaluations of many of these children may help clarify the concept of a relatively specific language disturbance in childhood due to CNS impairment.

Language symptoms reported among this "minimally" involved population include: definite retardation or marked reduction in language behaviour, confusion among similar sounding words, syllable reversals within words, neologisms, grammatical confusions, omitted or mistakenly used functional or "little" words in sentences, lack of meaning associated with verbalization, irregular verbal associations, word-finding problems, circumlocutionary verbalization, near-normal comprehension with substantial lag in expression, excessive use of gesture, verbal perseveration, and pathologic echolalia. Many of these symptoms appear similar to the auditory perceptual problems and irregular language behavior frequently found in normal language users following trauma to language centers in the CNS. Aphasiclike symptoms have also been reported among children who present frank diagnoses of cerebral palsy.

Cohen and Hannigan (1956) studied 22 cerebral-palsied, 19 of which were athetotic (16 of these due to kernicterus), for speech problems which could not be accounted for solely on the basis of dysarthria, mental deficiency, or hearing loss. They found that a significant number had language difficulties resembling aphasia in adults; in addition, they showed symptoms such as inconsistent response to speech stimuli, perseveration, disinhibition, and disturbances of auditory and visual perception. Greene (1964, p. 81) indicated that among brain-injured children may be found auditory agnosia and lip and tongue dyspraxia, and hence inability to imitate speech not due to paralysis.

She stated further that both agnosia and apraxia are accompanied by profound language learning disorders. Palmer (1949) also reported on the presence of aphasic symptoms and lingual apraxias among the cerebral-palsied. Ingram and Barn (1961), in discussing speech symptoms among hemiplegics, state that it is important to distinguish between temporary arrests of speech due to dysrhythmia or to dysphasia. They reported that an inability to use previously acquired words correctly in order and at will, or "true acquired aphasia," was found in three congenital and five acquired hemiplegics in their group. In two of the congenital cases, the verbal symptoms were observed following severe epileptic attacks. In contrast to the reports above are findings by Love (1964), who indicated that when he studied 27 cerebral-palsied individuals with a matched control group of physically handicapped, the finding of deviant language among the cerebral palsied was, in general, not supported.

Finally, Mecham (1964) has discussed clues for differentiating between psychogenic and organic backgrounds for language involvement in cerebral palsy. Symptoms which may be indicative of organic influences include varying combinations and degrees of deviate propositionality, perseveration, catastrophic behavior, fluctuations in perceptual functions, and deviate forms of abstraction and categorization; symptoms which may be indicative of mild psychogenic influences include fearfulness, unwillingness to interact with peers and adults, phobic reactions, and excessive habit spasms; and, finally, symptoms which may be indicative of severe psychogenic influences include lack of interpersonal contacts, autistic behavior, failure to distinguish between persons and things, and no attempt to communicate in any form, even through gesture.

DIAGNOSTIC IMPLICATIONS

The diagnostician in attempting to analyse the oral language of a language-involved cerebral-palsied child may be challenged indeed. First, the large question of whether the disorder represents simple slowness in language learning or irregular language learning, or a combination of both. Second, in the case of simple retardation, it will be necessary to identify and ascertain the relative influence of factors such as general intelligence, hearing loss, speech system paralysis, reduced mobility and range of the organism and hence reduced sensory-perceptual stimulation, and the tendency for infantilization of the child.

Then, it will be necessary to attempt to identify those language symptoms which appear related to involvement of central language centers and those language symptoms which appear to arise from more serious psychological problems. As is apparent, to discriminate among all the possible components of a cerebral palsy language complex would be difficult indeed.

RESEARCH NEEDS

In the way of research in the oral language area, it would be good to know of the relative effects on language learning in the cerebral-palsied of visual perceptual dysfunctioning, of reduced organism mobility and range of experience, and of the home environment engendered by the presence of a child with cerebral palsy. It would also be valuable to collect additional data to help distinguish among simple, specific oral language retardation, oral language retardation secondary to intellectual, hearing, and paralytic factors, and oral language pathology due to involvement of brain centers subserving language functioning in the cerebral-palsied.

SUMMARY

This discussion of the various possible speech involvements in cerebral palsy emphasizes the polycausal, polymorphous nature of cerebral palsy speech syndromes. It should also be apparent that the speech pathologist should expect to find some form of speech syndrome when examining the cerebral-palsied child, and must be prepared to examine for speech pathologies of every known variety. He must remind himself that all of the central neural mechanisms serving the central speech system (i.e., centers for linguistic, respiratory, phonatory, articulatory, and speech rhythm functioning) are vulnerable to the CNS lesions which may be responsible for cerebral palsy, and that involvement of the central neural mechanisms for speech will usually be reflected in involvement of the peripheral neural mechanisms serving the peripheral speech system (i.e., subsystems involved in the innervation and coordination of respiratory, laryngeal, velopharyngeal, and articulatory musculatures). It is obvious that to become an expert diagnostician in this area is an accomplishment indeed.

This chapter also forms the basis for the discussion of speech habilitation procedures which is the central subject of the next chapter. It should be obvious that the degree of effectiveness of such procedures will depend largely on how well all of the components of any particular cerebral palsy speech syndome have been identified, and on how well the speech clinician is able to generate and apply individualized therapy regimens designed to counteract the particular syndrome.

BIBLIOGRAPHY

Achilles, R. 1955. Communicative anomalies of individuals with cerebral palsy: I: analysis of communicative processes in 151 cases of cerebral palsy. *Cerebral Palsy Rev.*, 16, 15–24.

Berry, M., and Eisenson, J. 1956. Speech disorders. New York: Appleton-Century-Crofts.

Blakeley, R. 1959. Erythroblastosis and perceptive hearing loss; responses of athetoids to tests of cochlear function. *J. Speech Hearing Disorders*, 2, 5–15.

Blumberg, M. 1955. Respiration and speech in the cerebral palsied child. *Amer. J. dis. child.*, 89, 48-53.

Brown, S. 1967. Cleft palate; cerebral palsy. *In* Speech handicapped school children. Johnson, W., Brown, S., Curtis, J., Edney, C., and Keaster, J. New York: Harper & Row.

Byers, R., Paine, R., and Crothers, B. 1955. Extrapyramidal cerebral palsy with hearing loss following erythroblastosis. *Pediatrics*, 15, 248–254.

Byrne, M. 1959. Speech and language development of athetoid and spastic children. *J. Speech Hearing Disorders*, 24, 231–240.

Cardwell, V. 1956. Cerebral palsy. New York: Assn. for the Aid of Crippled Children.

Clement, M., and Twitchell, T. 1959. Dysarthria in cerebral palsy. *J. Speech Hearing Disorders*, 24, 118–122.

Cohen, P., and Hannigan, H. 1956. Aphasia in cerebral palsy. *Amer. J. phys. Med.*, 35, 218–222.

Crabtree, N., and Gerrard, J. 1950. Perceptive deafness associated with severe neonatal jaundice. *J. Laryng. otol.*, 64, 482–506.

Crickmay, M. 1966. Speech therapy and the Bobath approach to cerebral palsy. Springfield, Ill.: Thomas.

Crothers, B., and Paine, R. 1959. The natural history of cerebral palsy. Cambridge: Harvard.

Cruickshank, W., ed., 1966. Cerebral palsy. Syracuse, New York: Syracuse Univ. Press.

Davis, I. 1938. The speech aspects of reading readiness. *17th Yearbook Depart. Elem. School Principals*, NEA, 17, 282–289.

Denhoff, E. 1955. Cerebral palsy: medical aspects. *In* Cerebral palsy. Cruickshank, W., and Raus, G., eds. Syracuse, New York: Syracuse Univ. Press.

———, and Robinault, I. 1960. Cerebral palsy and related disorders. New York: McGraw-Hill.

Di Carlo, L., and Amster, W. 1955. Hearing and speech behavior among children with cerebral palsy. *In* Cerebral palsy. Cruickshank, W., and Raus, G., eds. Syracuse, New York: Syracuse Univ. Press.

Dinnerstein, A., and Lowenthal, M. 1966. Anxiety, perceptual latency and behavioral disability. *J. nerv. ment. Disorders*, 142, 562–567.

Duncan, M. 1955. Emotional aspects of the communication problem in cerebral palsy. *Cerebral palsy rev.*, 16, 19–23.

———. 1953. Anxiety as a speech deterrent among cerebral palsied children. *West. Speech*, 17, 155–162.

Dunsdon, M. 1952. The educability of cerebral palsied children. London: Newnes Educ. Pub.

Fisch, L. 1955. Deafness in cerebral palsied school children. *Lancet*, 269, 370–371.

Fisch, L. 1964. The functions of listening and its disorders. *In* Learning problems of the cerebrally palsied. Loring, J., ed. London: Spastics Soc.

———, and Beck, D. 1961. The assessment of hearing in young cerebral palsied children. *Cerebral Palsy Bull.*, 3, 145–155.

Gerrard, J. 1952. Kernicterus. *Brain*, 75, 526–570.

Guiot, G., Hertzog, E., Rondot, P., and Molina, P. 1961. Arrest or acceleration of speech evoked by thalamic stimulation in the course of stereotaxic procedures for parkinsonism. *Brain*. 8, 363–369.

Greene, M. 1964. Speech and reading disorders in cerebral palsy. *In* Learning problems of the cerebral palsied. Loring, J., ed. London: Spastics Soc.

Hagberg, B. 1962. The sequelae of spontaneously arrested infantile hydrocephalus. *Develop. med. Child Neurol.*, 4, 583–587.

Hardy, J. 1961. Intraoral breath pressure in cerebral palsy. *J. Speech Hearing Disorders*, 26, 310–319.

———. 1966. A physiological approach to the study of speech disorders associated with neuromuscular problems. A paper presented at the annual convention of the Amer. Speech and Hearing Assn., Washington, D.C.

Hardy, W. 1953. Hearing impairment in cerebral palsied children. *Cerebral Palsy Rev.*, 14, 3–7.

Heffner, R. 1949. General phonetics. Madison: Univ. Wis. Press.

Hixon, T., and Hardy, J. 1964. Restricted motility of the speech articulators in cerebral palsy. *J. Speech Hearing Disorders*, 29, 293–305.

Hood, P., and Perlstein, M. 1956. Infantile spastic hemiplegia: V. oral language and motor development. *Pediatrics*, 17, 58–63.

Hopkins, T., Bice, H., and Colton, K. 1954. Evaluation and education of the cerebral palsied child—New Jersey study. Washington, D.C.: Inter. Council Except. Child.

Hull, H. 1940. A study of the respiration of fourteen spastic paralysis cases during silence and speech. *J. Speech Disorders*, 5, 275–276.

Illingworth, R. 1958. Recent advances in cerebral palsy. Boston: Little, Brown.

Ingram, T. 1960. Pediatric aspects of specific developmental dysphasia, dyslexia, and dysgraphia. *Cerebral Palsy bull.*, 2, 254–277.

———, and Barn, J. 1961. A description and classification of common speech disorders associated with cerebral palsy. *Cerebral Palsy Bull.*, 3, 57–69.

Irwin, O. 1955. Phonetic equipment of spastic and athetoid children. *J. Speech Hearing Disorders*, 20, 54–57.

———. 1956. Substitution and omission errors in the speech of children who have cerebral palsy. *Cerebral Palsy Rev.*, 17, 75.

———. 1961. Correct status of vowels and consonants in the speech of children with cerebral palsy as measured by an integrated test. *Cerebral Palsy Rev.*, 22, 21–24.

Kastein, S., and Hendin, J. 1951. Language development in a group of children with spastic hemiplegia. *J. Pediatrics*, 39, 476–480.

Lassman, F. I. 1951. Clinical investigation of some hearing deficiencies and possible etiological factors in a group of cerebral palsied individuals. *Speech Mongr.*, 18, 130–131.

Lencione, R. 1954. A study of the speech sound ability and intelligibility status of a group of educable cerebral palsied children. *Speech Monogr.*, 21, 213–214.

———. 1966. Speech and language problems in cerebral palsy. *In* Cerebral palsy. Cruickshank, W., ed. Syracuse, New York: Syracuse Univ. Press.

Lewis, R., Strauss, A., and Lehtinen, L. 1960. The other child. New York: Grune & Stratton.

Lorenze, E., Sokoloff, M., and Cruz, R. 1962. Prognosis for deficiencies in speech accompanying cerebral palsy. *Arch. phys. med. Rehab.*, 43, 621–626.

Love, R. 1964. Oral language behavior of cerebral palsied children. *J. Speech Hearing Res.*, 7, 349–359.

Lyons, D. 1956. An evaluation of the effects of cerebral palsy on dentofacial development, especially occlusion of the teeth. *J. Pediatrics*, 49, 432–436.

Manning, J. 1953. A descriptive study of some interrelationships between speech, laterality, and other aspects of behavior in the cerebral palsied. *Speech Monogr.*, 20, 189–190.

McCall, G. 1964. Study of certain somesthetic sensibilities in a selected group of athetoid and spastic quadriplegic persons. Northwestern Univ.: Ph.D. dissertation.

McCroskey, R. 1958. The relative contribution of auditory and tactile clues to certain aspects of speech. *So. Speech J.*, 24, 84–90.

McDonald, E., and Chance, B. 1964. Cerebral palsy. Englewood Cliffs, N.J.: Prentice-Hall.

Mecham, M. 1964. Differential identification of factors related to language delay in young cerebral palsied children. *Cerebral Palsy Rev.*, 25, 8–9.

———, Berko, M., and Berko, F. 1960. Speech therapy in cerebral palsy. Springfield, Ill.: Thomas.

———, ———, and ———, 1966. Communication training in childhood brain damage. Springfield, Ill.: Thomas.

Milisen, R. 1966. Articulatory problems. *In* Speech pathology. Rieber, R., and Brubaker, R., eds. Amsterdam: North-Holland.

Morley, M. 1965. The development and disorders of speech in childhood. Baltimore: Williams & Wilkins.

Murphy, K. 1964. Development of articulation and hearing. *In* Learning problems of the cerebrally palsied. Loring, J., ed. London: Spastics Soc.

Murphy, M., and Hardy, J. 1966. Speech physiology problems in athetoid and spastic quadriplegic children. A paper presented at the annual convention of the Amer. Speech Hearing Assn., Washington, D.C.

Mysak, E. 1961. Organismic development of oral language. *J. Speech Hearing Disorders*, 26, 377–384.

———. 1963. Dysarthria and oropharyngeal reflexology: a review. *J. Speech Hearing Disorders*, 28, 252–260.

———. 1966a. Speech pathology and feedback theory. Springfield, Ill.: Thomas.

———. 1966b. Phonatory and resonatory problems. *In* Speech pathology. Rieber, R., and Brubaker, R., eds. Amsterdam: North-Holland.

———. 1968a. Neuroevolutional approach to cerebral palsy and speech. New York: Columbia Univ., Teachers College Press.

———. 1968b. Disorders of oral communication. *In* Evaluation and education of children with brain damage. Bortner, M., ed. Springfield, Ill.: Thomas.

Nober, E. 1966. Hearing problems associated with cerebral palsy. *In* Cerebral palsy. Cruickshank, W., and Raus, G., eds. Syracuse, New York: Syracuse Univ. Press.

Paine, R. 1962. Minimal chronic brain syndromes in children. *Develop. med. child Neurol.*, 4, 21–27.

Palmer, M. 1949. Speech disorders in cerebral palsy. *Nerv. Child*, 8, 193–202.

———. 1952. Speech therapy in cerebral palsy. *Pediatrics*, 40, 514–524.

Peiper, A. 1963. Cerebral function in infancy and childhood. New York: Consultants Bur.

Penfield, W., and Roberts L. 1959. Speech and brain mechanisms. Princeton, N.J.: Princeton.

Perlstein, M. 1950. Neurologic sequelae of erythroblastosis fetalis. *Amer. J. Dis. Child.*, 79, 605–606.

———. 1952. Infantile cerebral palsy, classification and clinical correlations. *JAMA*, 149, 30–34.

———, and McDonald, E. 1953. Nature, recognition, and management of neuromuscular disabilities in children. *Pediatrics*, 11, 166–173.

———, and Shere, M. 1946. Speech therapy for children with cerebral palsy. *Amer. J. dis. Child.*, 72, 389-398.

Phelps, W. 1959. The cerebral palsied. *In* Textbook of pediatrics. Mitchell, M., ed. Philadelphia: Saunders.

Ringel, R., and Steer, M. 1963. Some effects of tactile and auditory alterations on speech output. *J. Speech Hearing Res.*, 6, 369–378.

Rutherford, B. 1944. A comparative study of loudness, pitch, rate, rhythm, and quality of the speech of children handicapped by cerebral palsy. *J. Speech Hearing Disorders*, 9, 263–271.

———. 1945. Hearing loss in cerebral palsied children. *J. Speech Hearing Disorders*, 10, 237–240.

———. 1956. Give them a chance to talk. Minneapolis: Burgess.

Shelton, R., Arndt, W., and Heatherington, J. 1963. Testing oral stereognosis. *In* Symposium on oral sensation and perception. Bosma, J., ed. Springfield, Ill.: Thomas.

Sheppard, J. 1964. Cranio-oropharyngeal motor patterns in dysarthria associated with cerebral palsy. *J. Speech Hearing Res.*, 7, 373–380.

Strauss, A., and Kephart, N. 1955. Psychopathology and education of the brain-injured child. Vol. 2. New York: Grune & Stratton.

Templin, M. 1957. Certain language skills in children. *Institute of Child Welfare Monogr.* Series No. 26. Minneapolis: Univ. Minn. Press.

Travis, L. 1931. Speech pathology. New York Appleton-Century.

Twitchell, T. 1965. Variation and abnormalities of motor development. *J. Amer. phys. ther. Assn.*, 45, 424–430.

Weiss, D. 1964. Cluttering. Englewood Cliffs, N.J., Prentice-Hall.

Wellman, B., Case, I., Mengert, I., and Bradbury, D. 1931. Speech sounds of young children. *Univ. Iowa Studies in Child Welfare*, 5.

Wepman, J. 1941. Speech therapy for cerebral palsy patients. *Physiotherapy Rev.*, 21, 82–87.

West, R., Ansberry, M., and Carr, A. 1957. The rehabilitation of speech. New York: Harper.

———. 1958. An agnostic's speculations about stuttering. *In* Stuttering a symposium. Eisenson, J., ed. New York Harper. p.60.

Westlake, H. 1952. A system for developing speech with cerebral palsied children. Chicago: Nat. Soc. Crippled Child. and Adults.

———, and Rutherford, D. 1961. Speech therapy for the cerebral palsied. Chicago. Nat. Soc. Crippled Child. and Adults.

Wilson, F. 1965. Differential diagnosis in speech and hearing with the cerebral palsied child. *In* Speech and language therapy with the cerebral palsied child. Daley, W., ed. Washington, D.C.. Catholic Univ. Amer. Press.

Wolfe, W. 1950. A comprehensive evaluation of fifty cases of cerebral palsy. *J. Speech Hearing Disorders*, 15, 234–251.

Wood, N. 1953. A study of the speech and language development of right spastic hemiplegics as compared with left spastic hemiplegics, with reference to motor, intellectual, and visual perceptual findings. *Speech Monogr.*, 20, 191–192.

Zentay, P. 1937. Motor disorders of the central nervous system and their significance for speech. Cerebral and cerebellar dysarthrias. *J. Speech Disorders*, 2, 131–138 (Part I).

27

Cerebral Palsy Speech Habilitation

Edward D. Mysak

In the previous chapter, cerebral-palsy speech complexes were described as having various forms and backgrounds and as appearing in organisms experiencing various degrees of anomalous overall development. In short, these speech syndromes were viewed as polycausal, polymorphous, and polyphasal.

Because of the nature of these syndromes, wide-spectrum treatment approaches to speech habilitation should be considered in order to ensure that each child actualizes his maximum potential for spoken communication. By wide-spectrum speech treatment is implied 1. a total speech system rather than a speech organ approach, and 2. a treatment which begins at the time the child is identified as having cerebral palsy instead of when the child has reached the "cooperative age." Amplifications of these two points follow.

SPEECH SYSTEM vs. SPEECH ORGAN APPROACH

Emphasis on a speech system rather than on a speech organ approach means that the speech and hearing clinician should consider more than just the child's respiratory, auditory, phonatory, and articulatory mechanisms. He must remind himself that speech and hearing systems are located within the total system—the organism—and further, within the total system and its mode of interaction with the environment. This concept, which is important when planning speech therapy in general, is especially important in the area of cerebral palsy because of the frequency of primary and secondary problems in the organism as a whole as well as in various parts of the speech and hearing system.

Hence, the speech clinician working with the child with cerebral palsy must know about his general developmental patterns—for example, his perceptual, motor, emotional, social, and intellectual developments—and the interrelatedness and interdependence of these developments with each other and with the development of the speech system.

INFANT SPEECH vs. SPEECH AGE TREATMENT

Speech clinicians should realize that their contribution to the habilitation of the child's speech system could begin at the moment the child is identified as cerebral-palsied and not at some arbitrarily selected age, for example, at three or four years when he may be more "cooperative." And, because of the nature of the problem, the clinician should have suggestions and ideas to offer to physician and parents alike, as well as direct assistance to offer, even when the child is identified as early as at the moment of birth. One obvious purpose of such an orientation is to attempt to counter the frequently found "immaturity" as well as "pathology" symptomatologies of the speech system as discussed in the previous chapter.

In accordance with a total speech system approach

begun as early as possible, the discussion of habilitation procedures will be divided into three major sections: speech prophylactic, speech etiologic, and speech symptomatic procedures; and two subsections: speech compensatory and speech palliative procedures. In view of the nature of the cerebral-palsy speech syndromes, and the personal and individual nature of the therapy encounter, the chapter will be devoted basically to a presentation of a philosophy of therapy and some principles and methods based on that philosophy. Further, those readers who have a special interest in this area are encouraged to familiarize themselves with the many sources of additional information that exist, for example: Berry and Eisenson (1956, Ch. 15), Crickmay (1966, Ch. 6–8), Di Carlo and Amster (1955, Ch. 5), Lencione (1966, Ch. 5), McDonald and Chance (1964, Ch. 7), Mecham et al (1966, Ch. 4–7), and Westlake and Rutherford (1961).

SPEECH PROPHYLACTIC PROCEDURES

Speech prophylactic procedures describe all those activities the clinician may employ or stimulate which may contribute to the child's reaching the highest possible level of speech maturation. Hopefully, they should also reduce to a minimum the emergence of possible secondary problems. Reference will be made to how such procedures may contribute to respiratory, auditory, articulatory, phonatory, and linguistic aspects of spoken communication. Further, it should be understood that these procedures are designed primarily for the prespeech period or period of infancy; however, it may be found that many of the techniques described could also be used to good advantage during the speech period.

Parents' Role

The parents' role in the habilitation of any congenitally handicapped child is important; this is especially true in the case of the child with cerebral palsy, who is usually more generally handicapped. Parents must be guided to understand the contribution to the speech development of the child of positive interpersonal relationships, a positive speech environment, appropriate feeding experiences, and adequate sensory, sensorimotor, and perceptual experiences.

PARENTS AS EARLY WARNING SYSTEMS

Parents must be instructed to bring to the attention of their child's habilitation team any previously undetected problems so that these problems may receive early attention. In terms of the speech system, symptoms to which parents must especially be alert are those which may herald hearing loss, visual and emotional disorders, and incipient malocclusion. For example, it is hoped that identification of hearing involvement within the first months of life of the child would reduce the adverse repercussions of such an involvement in the already vulnerable and usually affected speech system. It is too frequently the case that hearing problems among the cerebral-palsied go relatively unattended until well past the first year of life, and hence serve to compound the speech syndromes. This unnecessary compounding of speech problems may be reduced or eliminated if speech specialists instruct parents properly as to their roles as early warning systems.

FEEDING

For the sake of facilitating the best possible development of the child's speech articulatory system and his dental occlusion, parents should be encouraged to nurse their children whenever possible and to use foods that require increasingly greater degrees of oral manipulation. The general rule to be followed here is that the oral vegetative system should be required to work at maximum potential at each stage of development even though this may mean that feeding time is substantially extended. It is believed that such a procedure will make a positive contribution to the child's oroneuromotor maturation and hence to his speech-sound development.

SOCIOEMOTIONAL DEVELOPMENT

Parents should be informed of the positive effects on the development of their child's speech and hearing system which may derive from their efforts to create an environment which will encourage maximum socioemotional maturation. The clinician could indicate that, in general, parents should allow the child to do as much for himself as is possible at every stage of his development. In other words, parents must assess continually whether each additional day, week, or month has made it possible for their child to do something else for himself, no matter how small. The goal is for parents to move the child as quickly as possible from the "what can you do for me" stage to the "what can I do for myself" stage and, hopefully, whenever and wherever possible, to the "what can I do for you" stage. Parents should be reminded that not only does this kind of effort on their part contribute to the overall socioemotional development of their child, but that it should make a contribution to his speech development as well.

POSITIVE SPEECH ENVIRONMENT

With respect to the child's speech environment, parents of the cerebral-palsied should make special efforts to create and to keep active a "communisphere" (Mysak, 1968a, p. 81). This means having speakers come within at least the 12-foot range, as well as the arms' length range of the child as often as possible during each day. It also means providing the child with extensive speech stimulation at those times which are associated with pleasant happenings, for example, feeding, rocking, bathing, and play activities.

Development of Bipedal Head and Thoracic Balance

In keeping with the total speech system approach, clinicians should remember that speech respiration, phonation, and articulation are more efficient when produced by an organism which is able to support its own head and thorax in the normal upright position. Hence, the speech clinician should view the accomplishment of head and thoracic self-support, at least in the sitting position, not only as an important goal in general motor development, but also as an important goal in speech system development. Such an orientation requires that the speech clinician learn how to stimulate such development and to incorporate appropriate techniques into his overall speech habilitation program. The author has already described techniques designed to stimulate head and thoracic balance in his discussion of principles of neurospeech therapy (Mysak, 1968a, pp. 93–102); for example, such balance may be facilitated by inhibiting infantile tonic neck and tonic labyrinthine reflexes, if present, and stimulating righting reflexes of the head and body and equilibrium reactions in supine, prone, crawling, and sitting positions. Details on the application of neurospeech therapy techniques may be found in the source cited. Of course, physicians, parents, and therapists also contribute to the child's development of bipedal head and thoracic balance.

Respiratory Functioning

In the preceding chapter it was indicated that breathing anomalies of almost every type have been reported among the cerebral-palsied. The symptoms were divided into two categories: infantile or immature-pattern symptoms and paralytic symptoms. It may be recalled that symptoms of immaturity include: infantile rates of breaths per minute (bpm); shallow breathing cycles; predominance of diaphragmatic-abdominal patterns; periodic, simultaneous activity of inspiratory and expiratory musculature; predominance of nasal respiration; and difficulty in shifting from a vegetative to a speech-breathing pattern. During the first months of the child's life, the speech clinician should concentrate his efforts on facilitating the transition of these infantile breathing patterns into patterns more appropriate for later speech behavior.

In general, the clinician should encourage the transition from 1. the predominant diaphragmatic-abdominal pattern observed during the first six months to a mixed pattern in which both diaphragm and thorax participate after the sixth month; and 2. the rather rapid range of 21 to 58 bpm observed during the first six months to the more appropriate range of 19 to 45 bpm observed during the first half to the second year of life (and steadily less after this). The clinician must also help the child to shift voluntarily from nasal to oral respiration and to change rather regular inspiratory-expiratory phases to rapid inspiratory followed by extended expiratory phases (an inspiratory-expiratory ratio of about 1 : 3 to 1 : 10). There are at least two ways of helping the child to achieve these respiratory goals and hence to contribute to his phonatory and articulatory development. The first is via special handling and stimulation techniques and the second is via the use of respiratory-assist devices.

SPECIAL HANDLING AND STIMULATION

Techniques for developing deeper and more regular vegetative breathing patterns have been discussed by the author (Mysak, 1968a, pp. 98–99). For example, in a supine position, the child's legs may be flexed and the knees brought toward the axillae and then returned to the starting position. Depending on the age of the child, the rate of cycles of such activity should be in accordance with the appropriate bpm rate. In a seated position, simulating the movements of the yawning reflex should also prove useful. Here, the child is seated with knees abducted with his hands clasped behind his head. First, the head and elbows are brought to extreme dorsiflexion-abduction positions, respectively; then there is a slow and steady head-thorax ventroflexion and elbow adduction movement pattern imposed with the ventroflexed head and adducted elbows finally brought between the abducted knees. Again, the rate of cycles of such activity is in accordance with the appropriate bpm rate for the child. The clinician is able to guide the activity by appropriate handling of elbows, head, and thorax.

After appropriate guidance and supervision by the clinician, these procedures may be done several times a day by the parent and should prove beneficial to the child in general, as well as in regard to his breathing and voicing ability.

SPECIAL DEVICES

There have been numerous reports of the use of various electronic devices in assisting cerebral-palsied children with respiration. For example, Jones (1963) used an electro-muscle stimulator on two athetotic children and reported some positive results including reduced rate of rest breathing and some increase in tidal volume.

Auditory Functioning

Prophylactic procedures in the area of audition include early detection of hearing loss, early use of amplification, and facilitation of the maturation of auditory behavior.

Since discussions of the use of amplification with infants and infant auditory training programs will be found in appropriate chapters in the Handbook, no attempt will be made here to discuss these procedures, except to indicate that the author is in favor of the earliest use of amplification in established or suspect cases. Amplification might be in the form of reducing the speaker-listener distance, or in using a microphone and speaker, or a personal hearing aid, or all three.

More will be said with respect to the facilitation of normal sequences in the maturation of auditory behavior, since it is believed that efforts in this area are not frequently made by either clinician or parent.

In the previous chapter, a number of sections were devoted to the various ways of describing the maturation of auditory behavior. For purposes of the present discussion, the reader is reminded of the following sequence: headroll and eyeturn toward the source of sound by about three months; after three months and in a seated position, downward localization before upward, and usually localization toward the right before the left; progression from auditory startle-staring behavior in the early weeks to auditory searching-localizing by about three months; and infant stare or smile in response to maternal voice at about three months and localization of maternal voice at about six months. Meaningful reactions to the calling of the child's name, attempts by the child to imitate sounds made by others (echolalia) and a tendency for him to repeat self-produced sounds (lalling) may be seen to occur by about nine months. Finally, the child usually recognizes and quickly responds to his name and can imitate the speech sounds made by others by about 12 months. It should also be recalled that in the previous chapter symptoms of auditory immaturity were identified as: persistence of infantile startle, crying, restlessness, and suckle behavior in response to auditory stimulation; retardation of auditory localizing behavior; and a delay in the ability to discriminate between familiar and unfamiliar sounds.

Some techniques designed to facilitate normal sequences in the maturation of auditory behavior will now be described.

SELECTIVE INHIBITION OF STARTLE BEHAVIOR

Weakening of infantile startle behavior in response to sound, the persistence of which does not easily allow higher center processing of auditory stimuli, may be accomplished by "overpresentation" of auditory stimuli in the child's environment. This may be done by presenting auditory stimuli at various loudness levels (progressing from soft to loud) and with varying degrees of warning (from full to no warning). In addition, if such attempts at facilitating adaptation to auditory startle are progressing slowly, the clinician may combine the presentation of auditory stimuli with physical restraint of the usual, rather generalized extension of the child's body parts. The goal of inhibiting infantile startle behavior is in keeping with the statement of Murphy (1964) that the "first sign of cortical function in relation to auditory stimuli is the development of selective inhibition of startle"; that is, the ability of the infant to ignore familiar sounds, while less familiar and even softer sounds may elicit startle.

FACILITATION OF AUDITORY LOCALIZING BEHAVIOR

Since localization of auditory stimuli is important to eventual auditory processing and speech perception, efforts should be made by clinicians to guide the development of this significant behavior. This may be done with the child in supine, then introducing various interesting environmental sounds on his right and left sides at adequate loudness levels in order to elicit appropriate headroll and eyeturn behavior. If the child's motor involvement does not allow for easy headroll, the clinician should utilize a partner who helps the child make appropriate movements in response to sound. With the child in a seated position, similar attempts to elicit head movements should be made with downward localization responses preceding upward, and localization toward the right preceding localization toward the left. Such activities, appropriate to the child's age, should be carried out two or three times a day by clinician or parent. A wide range of interesting environmental sounds should be used while varying direction, distance, and loudness level.

FACILITATION OF SPEECH SOUND PERCEPTION

Too often it is forgotten that speech sound perception, production, and monitoring has a prelanguage as well as a language phase and that such prelanguage speech sound functioning contributes to the later development of spoken language.

In accordance with developmental sequences, it is recommended that, as often as possible during each day of the first weeks of the child's life, an abundance of soft voice be used in conjunction with attempts to soothe or comfort the child and, of course, during feeding, bathing, and play periods. At about three months or so, the mother should vocalize a great deal and look for smile and "listening attitude" responses from her child. Then later, at six months or so, the mother and others should attempt to elicit, as often as possible, localizing responses to vocalization produced from various locations and distances from the child. At about nine months or so, daily efforts should be made at attempting to evoke some kind of response to the calling of the child's name. Also at this time, and as often as possible during each day, individuals should enter within the arms' length range of the child's communisphere and stimulate him with various speech as well as nonspeech sounds. It is hoped that such stimulation will encourage the child to imitate and engage in repetition of self-produced sounds; behavior which would indicate the capacity for speech-sound perception, production, and monitoring. Finally, at about 12 months, the child should be noted to respond quickly to his name, "give me" requests, and continue to imitate speech sounds made by others.

While attempting to elicit in the cerebral-palsied an infantile listening attitude, the recognition and localization of maternal voice, a response to name, and the imitation and repetition of self-produced speech sounds, it should be remembered that an increase in the amount and intensity of stimulation may be required and that responses may occur more slowly and at later than expected times.

Articulatory System Functioning

In the previous chapter, factors such as 1. delayed, retarded, or arrested oroneuromotor maturation—including the delay in appearance of, or the retention of infantile feeding reflexes and the lack of adequate differentiation of the articulatory system, and 2. difficulty in developing adequate intraoral breath pressure were identified as possibly contributing to speech-sound immaturity. Hence, the discussion of improving articulatory system functioning in this prophylactic section of the chapter will be confined to ways of countering such factors which may contribute to the irregular maturation of speech sounds.

FACILITATION OF ORONEUROMOTOR MATURATION

Techniques for facilitating oroneuromotor maturation were recently described by the author (Mysak, 1968a, pp. 96–97). In brief, it was pointed out that weak or absent rooting, lip, mouth opening, biting, suckling, chewing, palatal, pharyngeal, and swallowing reflexes should be stimulated by providing the appropriate stimulus and initiating and guiding the expected response. The development and strengthening of such reflexive movements is, of course, important for feeding activity, as well as for serving as precursors of the complex movements required in speech articulatory behavior.

After the feeding reflexes have served their function, and in accordance with normal developmental sequences, attempts to extinguish infantile oral activity—such as rooting, lip, mouth opening, biting, suckle-swallow and chewing reflexes—should begin. Extinction of these infantile patterns may be facilitated by providing the appropriate stimulus and be physically preventing the emergence of the expected movement. Such efforts at facilitating the extinction of such infantile oral activity should be made two or three short periods daily, and depending on the severity of the case, beginning at about a year or two of age. A further discussion of this concept may be found in the author's previously cited material.

FACILITATION OF VELOPHARYNGEAL CLOSURE

As stated in the previous chapter, Hardy (1961) believes that one indicator of an individual's physiological readiness for speech is his ability to develop sufficient intraoral breath pressure. He reported that problems in this ability may be related to palatal, respiratory, or articulatory system involvements.

At least three efforts can be made which might help the child with a malfunctioning closure mechanism buildup the intraoral breath pressure necessary for producing speech sounds. The first has been discussed by the author in connection with "voice prophylactic" techniques for the child with cleft palate (Mysak, 1966b, p. 172). As soon as it has been established that the infant's closure mechanism is functioning in a less than desirable fashion, he could be fitted, for example with an oral prosthesis, similar to that made for cleft-palate children who have experienced less than adequate surgical procedures. Such an appliance should allow for more normal suckling and swallowing, and for more normal babbling and lalling activities. Another technique involves having the parent each day gently occlude the child's nostrils during the outflow phase of activities of crying, screaming, laughing, babbling, lalling, and echolalia. Daily stimulation of palatal and pharyngeal reflexes may also be considered. It is hoped that by such techniques the establishment of an oropneumodynamic pattern for speech rather than a nasopneumodynamic pattern would be encouraged.

Phonatory System Functioning

Prophylactic considerations in voicing are necessarily linked to respiratory functioning, which has already been discussed. Possible vocal manifestations of infantile respiratory-laryngeal behavior include: interrupted, intermittent, forced, and inspiratory voicing possibly due to irregular activity of the glottic-closing reflex (i.e., involuntary, open-close or over-close activity of the glottis); delayed initiation, or short duration of voicing due to difficulty or inability to shift from vegetative to speech breathing patterns; reduced amount of voicing due to high bpm rate, and weak voicing due to shallow breathing patterns.

Effectively carrying out the techniques described in the section on respiration should make a contribution to more effective functioning of the phonatory system. It would be well, however, if specific efforts were made to stimulate the child to produce progressively longer durations of phonation, to vary pitch and loudness aspects of phonation, and to improve his ability to initiate and cease phonation with increasing rapidity.

Toward these goals, speakers in the child's environment may frequently phonate various vowels for relatively long periods and at different loudness and pitch levels, and also engage in rapid on-off vowel phonations. Spontaneous or imitative vocalization on the infant's part may be extended by gently vibrating, with an extended hand, the child's thoracico-abdominal area, or by applying slow and steady downward pressure during voicing so as to prolong the behavior. Similar techniques may be employed if the child is lying on his side or on his stomach. To facilitate louder phonation, the downward pressure in the thoracico-abdominal area may be applied more strongly and over a shorter period of time. Voicing-unvoicing activity may be stimulated by applying one hand in the thoracico-abdominal area and one over the mouth and, during the exertion of downward pressure on the thoracico-abdominal area with one hand, and while the child is phonating, covering and uncovering the mouth with the other.

It should be remembered that speech-system hygiene techniques discussed in this section are carried out by the clinician, as well as by the parents under the supervision of the clinician, and are designed primarily for the first two or three years of life. Such stimulation should be designed for the individual child and, whenever possible, should be provided for short periods of time, two or three times a day.

Research Needs

In general, there is a paucity of "controlled" studies in the area of prophylactic procedures for speech disorders. From a clinical standpoint, the speech pathologist is often concerned with possible connections between speech and language models and speech and language development in children, between parental attitudes toward developmental speech rhythm irregularities and the development of childhood stuttering, and between "misuse" and subsequent "abuse" of the voice and dysphonia. However, there is really little in the way of data of any substance on the need and value of, and what constitutes prophylactic techniques for, possible speech and language irregularities in relatively normal children, let alone for children with cerebral palsy.

Hence, a recommendation can be made to speech pathologists to show a greater interest in the study of speech hygiene in general, that is, greater interest in the study of all those factors, internal and external, which tend to promote healthy hearing, voice, speech articulation, rhythm, and language. More specifically, it is hoped that specialists would study and report on the effects of the speech prophylactic procedures, or similar ones, described here. It is the author's belief that for the child with cerebral palsy, speech prophylactic techniques are crucial, and, unfortunately, rarely if ever applied early enough and in any systematic fashion.

SPEECH ETIOLOGIC PROCEDURES

Speech etiologic procedures represent therapeutic efforts made during the speech age and aimed at those factors which appear to be directly responsible for any manifested speech symptoms. For example, the use of drugs or special surgery to counter speech symptoms falls into the category of etiologic procedures. As of this stage in our profession's history, there has been little headway made in surgical alleviation of speech disorders, except in surgery for conductive hearing loss and cleft palate. In the area of cerebral palsy speech habilitation, two interesting but preliminary reports of surgical treatment have been reported. One by Hardy et al (1961) discusses palatal surgery to increase intraoral breath pressure, and one by Myers and Smith (1958) discusses brain surgery to improve the speech of athetoid patients. Much more work will have to be done before surgical procedures of this kind become regular treatment possibilities. Also included in the etiologic category of procedures are appropriate referrals to the pediatrician, otolaryngologist, psychologist, dentist, and so on, whenever the clinician becomes aware of certain conditions in any one child which may be serving as impediments to maximum speech development.

As an example of a specific speech etiologic technique and, at the same time, as an attempt to differentiate such a technique from a speech prophylactic one, let us consider the frequently encountered problem of hypernasality in a cerebral-palsied child. If it had been determined early that deficits in velopharyngeal closure existed in any one child, speech prophylactic techniques might have included attempts to stimulate palatal and pharyngeal reflexes during approximately the first year of life in the hopes of improving their function for vegetative purposes, and indirectly for contributing to movements which are important for later speech purposes. However, if after the child learns to speak, hypernasality is detected and is traced to a still poorly functioning closure mechanism, etiologic techniques should be initiated in addition to the prophylactic techniques. Etiologic techniques may include having the child engage alternately in nasal emission vs. oral emission of the speech air stream, having the child emit the air stream nasally and quickly "shutting off" the air stream by contracting the velum, having the child voluntarily raise and lower the velum with the aid of visual clues from a mirror, and by having the child alternately produce /m-b/, /n-d/, and /n-g/ with the initial goal being good production of the nasal and non-nasal sounds (nasal pinching may be required for assistance at the beginning) and later with the goal of increasing the speed of such nasal, non-nasal sound alternations (development of velar diadochocinesis).

One obvious distinguishing feature between prophylactic and etiologic techniques is the earlier, more vegetatively oriented and involuntary nature of prophylactic tasks as compared to the later, more speech oriented and more voluntary nature of the etiologic tasks. Of course, it is hoped that when prophylactic and etiologic techniques appear successful that this would be reflected in the child's speech patterns. But as experienced speech clinicians know, this is not always the case. One reason for the disappointment is that the techniques may have been employed too late with respect to speech development, or that the effects of the techniques were slow in appearing and hence irregular speech patterns were already formed and habituated. Another reason for disappointment may be related to the fact that velopharyngeal movement patterns developed via prophylactic and etiologic techniques are not sufficient to serve speech purposes in any one child.

It is precisely because of such possibilities that speech symptomatic techniques, which are discussed in the next section of the chapter, are frequently necessary. As in the section on prophylactic procedures, this section will outline etiologic procedures as they pertain to the parents role, bipedal head-thoracic balance, and respiratory, auditory, articulatory, and phonatory functioning.

Parents' Role

The parents' role in the speech etiologic phase of habilitation is primarily an extension of their activities in the prophylactic phase.

PARENTS AS EARLY WARNING SYSTEMS

Parents continue in their role as early warning systems. However, since the etiologic phase begins when the child reaches the speech age, the time of which varies considerably with cerebral-palsied children, parents should be alerted to additional factors. For example, in the hearing area, parents should not only pay attention to their child's progress in inhibition of auditory startle and in localizing, but should begin paying an increasing amount of attention to whether the child is repeating self-produced sounds, is echoing sounds heard in the environment, and is responding to the calling of his name. Attention must be maintained for behavior which may be symptomatic of visual and emotional disturbances; continuing attention must also be paid to the development of dental occlusion and to whether infantile oral reflexes are persisting well past the first year of life.

FEEDING

In terms of oral vegetative functioning, parents should be reminded of the connections between articulatory activity for vegetative purposes and for speech purposes, and must be encouraged to provide the child with foods which require normal chewing and swallowing behavior. They should also be instructed on how to identify infantile feeding reflexes when these persist into the speech age. If such reflexes do persist, efforts must be made on the part of clinician and parents alike to suppress them. More will be said on the topic of suppressing infantile oral reflexes later on in this section of the chapter.

SOCIOEMOTIONAL DEVELOPMENT AND PERCEPTUAL ENRICHMENT

Now that the child has reached the speech age parents must also consider ways to expand and enrich the child's social and perceptual spheres. This means planned, frequent exposure to grandparents, uncles and aunts, cousins, and neighborhood friends and their children. Emphasis should be on positive encounters and on a more-frequent-than-normal basis. Individuals who respond negatively to the condition of cerebral palsy should be avoided at this early period anyway.

There must also be conscious attempts on the part of parents and friends to provide rich and varied perceptual experiences for the child. In this regard, a great deal of handling and moving about of the child is important. If the child cannot progress on his own, he should be transported daily to all rooms in the house and allowed to slowly see, hear, touch, smell and taste as much of these rooms as is possible. For example, the kitchen allows perceptual experiences with certain types of chairs, tables, cabinets, utensils, appliances, fixtures, odors, and so on. The child should be allowed the full range of "kitchen experiences." Similar perceptual exploration should be allowed in the bathroom, bedrooms, living room, and basement. Experiences should then be extended into the front or back yards (e.g., interaction with neighbors, the earth, grass, plants, insects, and animals), and then still further to various types of community shops, institutions, parks, and their personnel. Such perceptual enrichment must be planned on a daily basis, and it is important that it should be carried out by individuals other than just the parents or the immediate family.

POSITIVE SPEECH ENVIRONMENT

During the etiologic phase of treatment parents must make systematic efforts to contribute to the child's speech perceptual functioning by rewarding all of the child's attempts at speech comprehension, formulation, and expression. For example, parents should reward listening attitudes on the part of the child by responding with pleasant sights and sounds such as by singing and speaking with interesting facial expressions and body movements; and by rewarding the child with desired foods, objects, and activities if he signals appropriately. In short, parents must remember to reinforce positively all efforts by the child to produce spoken or gestured communication. In this way parents demonstrate to the child by word and deed the significant power of oral communication.

Bipedal Head and Thoracic Development

Further contributions may be made toward helping the child achieve bipedal head and thoracic balance during the speech age by having clinicians elicit reflexes and reactions that will contribute to head and thoracic balance in the standing posture. Some of these reflexes and reactions include: body righting-on-body reactions (complete rotation pattern), amphibian reaction, Landau reflex, protective-extensor-thrust of-the-arms reflex, precipitation reflex, arm walking, symmetrical chain reflex in the abdominal position, and equilibrium reactions in the kneel-standing, simian stance, and standing positions. For details on the nature of these reflexes and reactions and on the manner of eliciting them, the reader is referred to a previous work by the author (Mysak, 1968a, Ch. 2).

Respiratory-Phonatory Functioning

Since etiologic procedures are aimed at factors which appear to be directly responsible for manifested speech symptoms, respiratory and phonatory functioning will be discussed together in this section. In the previous chapter it was pointed out that the speech clinician should consider the role of respiratory dysfunctioning in voice disorders when the vocal deficits are accompanied by certain breathing anomalies. For example, when a delay in initiating phonation is associated with difficulty on the part of the child to shift from a nasal-symmetrical vegetative breathing pattern to an oral-asymmetrical speech breathing pattern; when production of only one or two syllables per expiration is associated with difficulty in modifying vegetative into speech breathing patterns; when asthenic and a reduced amount of vocalization is associated with shallow patterns and bpm's above 30; and when there is intermittent or interrupted vocalization associated with periodic, simultaneous activity of inspiratory and expiratory musculature.

Etiologic techniques for respiratory-phonatory functioning are primarily concerned with aiding the child to modify vegetative into speech breathing patterns. These techniques are differentiated from the previously described prophylactic techniques by the greater concentration on developing speech breathing patterns. Hence, the clinician concentrates on increasing the child's ability to shift from nasal to oral inspiration and to modify the regular inspiratory-expiratory phase into a quick, short oral inspiratory phase followed by a slow, extended oral expiratory phase. Such speech-breathing patterns may be facilitated by physically resisting with the hands, for a brief period, the beginning of an expiratory phase, or by following an expiratory phase and, again with the hands, applying pressure at the end of the phase so as to bring it to a deeper level. Voicing activity should, of course, be encouraged during the expiratory phase.

Auditory Functioning

Because of overlap in prophylactic and etiologic therapy categories with respect to auditory functioning, most of what could be described as etiologic considerations in auditory functioning has already been presented.

Certainly if hearing loss has gone undetected until the speech age, otologic-audiologic review must be requested as soon as possible and consideration should be given for the earliest possible use of amplification. Once amplification has been provided, the child should be stimulated as described in the prophylactic section so that he may experience the normal sequence of behaviors associated with auditory maturation.

Otologic care and speech amplification are primary etiologic considerations with respect to auditory dysfunctioning. Then efforts should be directed at facilitating the appearance in the child of body immobilization and infantile listening attitudes in response to speech signals. Recognition of the maternal voice by smile and localization behaviors, meaningful reactions to the calling of his name, and attempts by the child at reproducing speech sounds are other important behaviors to be stimulated.

Articulatory System Functioning

As mentioned in the previous chapter, adequate articulation depends on many articulators moving in appropriate directions and with appropriate range, speed, accuracy, and coordination. A program of etiologic techniques for the articulatory system can be developed for any one child once it is determined whether the phonetic lapses under consideration are due to consistent limitations in the direction and range of movements of the articulators; to inconsistency in their range and direction of movement; to problems in articulatory system coordination; to difficulty in voluntarily reproducing movements which can be effected spontaneously; to difficulty in moving separately various articulators within the system; to problems in the adequate and accurate reception of sensory feedback from the articulatory system; or to various combinations of these problems.

Of course, if the need still exists, the techniques described in the prophylactic section with respect to suppressing infantile oral reflexes and facilitating velopharyngeal closure should be continued.

LIMITATIONS IN DIRECTION AND RANGE OF ARTICULATORY MOVEMENTS

The following etiologic techniques may be utilized when certain phonemic deficits appear related to consistent limitations in the possible directions and ranges of movements of certain of the articulators.

Stimulation of speech-sound-sensorimotor patterns. In order that the child experience sensory feedbacks associated with speech-sound movements, the articulatory organs of the child should be brought through the movements and points of contact necessary for the production of the various phonemes. Bilabial movement and contact is imposed by simply bringing the lips together with the fingers, holding the lips in contact, and requesting the child to break the seal by blowing through them. Similar maneuvers can be carried out for labiodental, linguadental, lingua-alveolar, linguapalatal, and linguavelar sounds. Such activity allows the child to experience something like the actual movement and the sensory feedback associated with the various phonemes. The procedure may also stimulate the child to increase his attempts at making speech-sound movements.

Use of proprioceptive-cortical facilitation techniques. Paradoxical intention activities or resistive movement techniques should also prove useful. For example, the goal may be to help the child raise his tongue tip to the alveolar ridge. By the clinician's pressing in a downward direction (paradoxical intention aspect) and requesting the child to press upwards, suprathreshold motor units may be triggered. Then, when the clinician ceases his downward pressure the tongue may be observed to rise a little higher than previously. This technique can be used to improve mandibular flexion-extension and lip spreading-rounding movements. For a discussion on the central facilitation effects of the technique of resistance and stretch, the reader is referred to the work of Kabat (1952).

Movements in certain directions or increases in the range of certain movements may also be stimulated by utilizing the principle of resistive-movement synkinesis. Synkinesis describes the phenomena whereby unintentional movements may accompany volitional movements. In its physiologic form, it may be noted that when certain individuals are working hard at drawing, for example, various degrees of accompanying lingual protrusion and movement may be noted, or when children are asked to open their mouths wide there may be an associated extension and abduction of the fingers of the hand (mouth-and-hand synkinesia). Imitative synkinesis describes that situation whereby an involuntary movement on the healthy side may accompany an attempt at movement on the paralyzed side; whereas spasmodic synkinesis describes a movement on the paralyzed side which may accompany a voluntary movement on the healthy side. A specific example of the use of resistive-movement synkinesis in effecting certain articulatory movements follows.

In the case where tongue-tip and mandibular elevation is desired, the child's head, or head and thorax, may be ventroflexed and he may be asked to extend them. As he attempts to do so, the clinician resists the movement and by so doing hopefully triggers synkinetic flexor movements of the tongue and mandible (overflow effect). This is similar to Kabat's (1952) technique of mass movement patterns, whereby smaller movements may be facilitated through performance of larger movement patterns.

Another paradoxical-intention-movement technique could be described as the conteracting response technique. It involves the passive movement in an extreme and irregular direction of a particular articulator in the hopes that this will automatically trigger an opposite, more regular, and desired movement. To illustrate, if tongue protrusion is desired, the clinician may apply a slow and steady backward pressure on the tongue in the direction of the pharynx until the movement excites a counteracting forward movement. With respect to "still tongues," and related to the above, is the so-called "trombone" movement which is characterized by an involuntary forward and backward movement of the tongue when it is drawn out of the mouth. Similar desired counteracting responses may occur when the lips are slowly and steadily spread or when the mandible is steadily extended.

Kabat (1952) has described a procedure called "reversal of antagonists" as a facilitation technique for treatment of paralysis which could be used in treating the speech articulatory system. Kabat points out that in many activities the antagonist motion immediately precedes the main action as in the preparatory backward raising of the arm of the pitcher which precedes the forward, pitching movement, and similar preceding antagonist motions related to the golf swing or to the kicking of a football. Kabat (1952) states, "The contraction of the antagonist against resistance immediately preceding resistive exercise of the agonist is a valuable technique of facilitation . . . Reversal of antagonists is usually applied in mass movement patterns against maximal resistance . . ."

As an example of the application of the reversal of antagonists technique, let us consider the condition of "jaw droop." In the hopes of achieving more normal mandibular movements and closure, the following could be tried: 1. The mandible may be placed in a moderately extended position and the child requested to hold this position; the clinician then applies resistance alternately to mandibular flexors and extensors while the child holds. This procedure should increase the child's ability to flex the mandible. Then the child is requested to flex the mandible repeatedly against resistance. To further facilitate the movement, the clinician may have the child attempt concomitant head and/or thoracic extension from a flexed position and also against resistance. 2. The mandible is placed in a closed position and the child is requested to extend and flex it in an alternating fashion against maximal resistance. The entire range or part of the range of mandibular movement may be utilized with this technique. 3. The child is requested to extend the mandible against maximal resistance through the full range, then the mandible may be brought to a moderately open position and the child asked to hold the position against alternating resistance to flexors and extensors. 4. Finally, the child is asked to close and to hold the position of the mandible. (Kabat recommends the simultaneous use of a number of facilitation techniques, for example, a combination of resistance, mass movement patterns, and reversal of antagonist techniques.)

Use of certain reflexes as a facilitation technique. Certain oropharyngeal reflexes and desired voluntary movements can be stimulated simultaneously in the hopes that the reflex excitation will facilitate the desired voluntary movement. The author (Mysak, 1968a, pp. 96–97) has already discussed the principle of oropharyngeal reflex facilitation. For example, if hypernasality appears related to a poorly functioning velopharyngeal closure mechanism, the child may be requested to utter "ah" while the clinician simutaneously attempts to elicit palatal and pharyngeal reflexes by touch stimuli applied to the velum and/or posterior pharyngeal wall or fauces. Also, in conjunction with requests for the child to flex his mandible in the case of "jaw droop" the jaw-jerk reflex (brief reflexive elevation of jaw elicited by tapping of the mandible) may be used to facilitate mouth closure.

INCONSISTENCY IN ARTICULATORY MOVEMENTS IN SPECIFIC DIRECTIONS AND IN THEIR RANGE

When components of the articulatory system exhibit various degrees and types of involuntary and inconsistent movements, other forms of tactile-proprioceptive techniques should be applied.

Use of resistive techniques to improve balance among opposing muscle groups. For example, to help stabilize elevator-depressor movements of the tongue and to improve the range of upward movement, the child may be asked to extend the tongue and attempt to hold it while the clinician applies appropriate amounts of resistance alternately with his fingers or a tongue depressor to lingual elevators and depressors. Such activity might eventually result in improved balance between opposing muscle groups and hence to improved lingual stability. As improved stability is manifested, the emphasis of the technique may shift to the child attempting upward movements of the tongue against resistance.

"Tactile fencing" of an oscillating body part. Another technique which may prove of value when stabilization of an organ is required is tactile fencing. If, for example, the child, upon attempting voluntary movements of the lips, triggers substantial, involuntary spread-pucker activity, the clinician may bring one or two fingers of one hand in light contact with the lips during the pucker phase while he simultaneously brings one or two fingers in light contact with the rising part of the cheek during the spread phase. The child is then requested to reduce voluntarily the oscillating movement by not allowing the lips or cheek to come into contact with the clinician's fingers. As the child enjoys success, the clinician should progressively reduce the allowed range of involuntary movements. Similar maneuvers can also be carried out for the tongue. It may be found that substantial reductions in the range of oscillations of various body parts can be realized through this fencing technique.

ARTICULATORY SYSTEM DIFFERENTIATION

It may be found that certain of the child's phonemic deficits are associated with varying amounts of oroneuromotor immaturity as reflected by the persistence of infantile feeding reflexes or by incomplete differentiation of various components of the articulatory system. In the case of persisting infantile reflexes, a child when attempting to produce the /a/ in "father" may trigger the mouth-opening reflex when the mandible extends to a certain point, thus disrupting further articulation; or, in the case of differentiation deficits, attempts at raising the tongue for producing /r/ or /l/-sounds may stimulate simultaneous rounding movements of the lips and result in the often heard "bilabialized" versions of /r/ and /l/ (in younger, normal children these would be viewed as developmental sound forms). Techniques for suppressing the infantile feeding reflexes have already been discussed in the section on speech prophylactic techniques and need not be repeated here.

Toward the goal of facilitating differentiation among mandible, lips, and tongue, however, the following might be tried. The child may be asked to extend his mandible to a half-open position and then to move first his lips (spreading-rounding movements) independently of his mandible and tongue; then to extend his mandible to about a three-quarters-open position and move his tongue (protude-retrude, elevate-depress) independently of his mandible and lips; and, finally, to bring both tongue and lips to rest positions and to move the mandible (extend-flex movements) independently of his lips and tongue. If during these activities there are more than the expected amount of associated movements (i.e., more than slight movements) in the "at rest" articulators, these movements should be physically prevented by the clinician or child himself whenever possible. It is expected that with greater degrees of articulatory system differentiation will come improved speech articulation. The author discussed the concept of speech-system differentiation in a previous work (Mysak, 1968a, pp. 95–96).

ARTICULATORY SYSTEM COORDINATION

It may become apparent to the clinician that various speech symptoms such as slow and irregular rate, articulatory deterioration while using sentence and conversational patterns, difficulty with certain syllable combinations, problems in coordinating various articulatory movements with velopharyngeal closure for production of non-nasal sounds, and inconsistent articulation may be related to deficient articulatory system coordination. For such symptoms, articulatory eupraxic and diadochocinetic work is recommended.

Oroeupraxia has been defined as well-performed and coordinated movements of the articulatory system (Mysak, 1968a, p. 101). Cerebral-palsied children may engage in oroeupraxic work using one-syllable, two-syllable, three-syllable, or four-syllable combinations, depending on their capacity. For example, for the voiced-voiceless articulatory task, the child is required to produce, with assistance if necessary, /b -p/ first, and then in sequence: /və-fə/, /ðə-θə/, /də-tə/, /zə-sə/, /ʒə-ʃə/, and, finally, /gə-kə/. The aim of oroeupraxic work, irrespective of the child's present speech patterns, is accurate articulatory movements and contacts—speed of movement is not important at the beginning. Also, since the most accurate sensory feedback possible is desired, the clinician should be ready to provide articulatory movement assistance whenever needed and wherever possible. As the child progresses, the exercises proceed from the voiced-voiceless series just described to a base syllable plus a progressively receding syllable. Following is an example of the /b/ series: /bə-və/ then /bə-ðə/, /bə-də/, /bə-nə/, /bə-lə/, /bə-zə/ /bə-ʒə/, /bə-rə/, /bə-gə/. Each combination may be repeated two or three times during the work session and those which are not possible to produce even with the clinician's assistance may be temporarily avoided. Work on the two-syllable combination series should be continued until each receding syllable has served as the base syllable; for example, /və-bə/ then /və-ðə/ and so on. Three-syllable and four-syllable combination series follow next.

Following success with oroeupraxic work, the clinician may have the child return to two-syllable combinations, where he would be expected to perform the movements well but also at progressively higher speeds (addition of the diadochocinetic factor). He would then move again to all the succeeding series, but only after he reaches maximum diadochocinetic rates in each of them. Such work should be done two or three times daily, guided first by the clinician, and as soon as possible by the parent, and then by the child himself. This activity could serve as the child's daily speech-system "warm-up" or conditioning exercises.

Functioning of Speech Rhythm System

In the previous chapter, the author wrote that the discussion of cerebral palsy rhythm involvements would be confined to those associated with immaturity and pathology of the central neural mechanisms for speech rhythm control. It was pointed out that one cause of the immaturity variety could be the lack of or delay in establishing intact neuronal arrangements for percepts and their associated words, or in developing automatic and reciprocal relationships between these neuronal patterns. Another possible cause is sensorimotor integration of speech functioning at levels which do not allow for speech automaticity on phrasal and full articulatory cycle levels but rather only on phonemic or syllabic levels. On the other hand, it was indicated that disfluency symptoms related to pathology of central rhythm mechanisms included irregular rate acceleration and deceleration, inability to initiate and/or arrest speech, and out-of-phase respiratory, laryngeal, and articulatory muscle activity.

Etiologic techniques for speech rhythm regulation consist of facilitating the highest development of the central neural mechanisms of the central speech system, including the establishment of a speech-dominant hemisphere. Included in techniques which may contribute to maximum development of the central speech system are those which help to stimulate the child's overall neuromaturation. For a discussion of these techniques, the reader is referred to

Chapter Three of a previous work by the author (Mysak, 1968a).

Reducing anxiety situations such as may accompany difficulty in gaining a listener's attention, or the fear of losing his attention or interruption by a listener, or having to speak during feelings of guilt or hostility is also important. With a less stable CNS, it may be expected that such external speech stress factors may be more disruptive than usual. In this vein, it is interesting to recall the report by Dinnerstein et al. (1966) that some stuttering may be explained on the basis of an anxiety-induced delay in auditory and proprioceptive feedback.

Research Needs

As in the case of speech prophylactic procedures, there is little in the way of research data in the area of speech etiologic techniques for the cerebral-palsied. Certainly it appears logical, and it is also traditional, to consider the use of various types of exercises for the articulators when there is misarticulation and the articulators appear weak or paralyzed. However, Hixon and Hardy (1964) reported that the severity of the speech problem in cerebral-palsy is predicted better by rates of syllable repetition than by the rates of nonspeech movements; they believe, therefore, that speech development may be best promoted by eliciting actual speech movements rather than nonspeech movements in these children.

It would appear that one important factor in the effectiveness of speech etiologic techniques in modifying a child's abnormal speech patterns is the time factor. For example, attempts at improving speech-breathing patterns, stimulating speech sound sensorimotor patterns, using proprioceptive-cortical facilitation techniques to improve articulatory movements, better differentiating the components of the articulatory system, and improving articulatory system coordination, should be far more fruitful when applied during the initial stages of speech development. It might be expected that the greater the amount of speech learned with a poorly functioning speech system, and the longer these abnormal patterns have been used, the less effective will be etiologic techniques, and the greater will be the need for speech-pattern unlearning and relearning or speech symptomatic techniques.

In any case, it seems warranted and worthwhile for more specialists to consider, develop, and utilize speech etiologic techniques. It also seems warranted for them to study the effectiveness of these techniques with reference to the possible reduction of any particular speech symptom as a function of what techniques were used, and when in the child's speech history the techniques were employed.

SPEECH SYMPTOMATIC PROCEDURES

As indicated, speech prophylactic procedures are designed basically for the child's prespeech period, and the goals are to facilitate the highest possible level of speech-system maturation and to reduce to a minimum the emergence of possible secondary problems; speech etiologic procedures, on the other hand, are those used during the speech age which are designed to counter problems in the speech system which appear to be more or less directly responsible for the manifested speech symptoms. It is hoped, of course, that the more effective the speech prophylactic and etiologic procedures are, the fewer will be the manifested speech symptoms. Speech symptom techniques differ from the others since the work is concerned directly with improving the child's oral language and speech production capacities; that is, the focus is on the words and sounds themselves.

The major goal of the symptomatic phase is too ensure that the child utilizes his maximum potential with respect to speech functioning. There may be many reasons why the child may not be utilizing his maximum speech potential at any one time, for example: 1. he learned certain sounds at a time when his articulatory system was not as efficient as it may now be simply because of further growth and development; and 2. he did not automatically incorporate into his speech patterns the increased potential made possible through prophylactic and etiologic techniques.

Speech symptomatic procedures will be discussed basically as they relate to the parents' role, and to oral language functioning, phonation, and articulation during the child's speech learning period. Further, since more familiar speech symptom therapy approaches for disorders of articulation, voice, and language will be found in appropriate chapters of the Handbook, and since aspects of many of these approaches can be applied to children with cerebral palsy, these will not be repeated here. Instead, therapy will be discussed from a specific speech-system-based standpoint, that is, on the basis of developmental, speech feedforward and feedback concepts (Mysak, 1966a).

Parents' Role

In the previous sections on the parents' role, emphasis was placed on their early detection of related disorders which have a bearing on speech and hearing, on proper feeding procedures, on providing an environment conducive to socioemotional and perceptual development, and on creating a positive speech environment. The role of the parents during the speech symptom phase is related specifically to aiding the clinician in facilitating the development of particular spoken language, comprehension, formulation, and expression capacities. Of course, parents also continue efforts at providing and maintaining the most ideal environment for perceptual, socioemotional, and speech developments.

FACILITATION OF SPOKEN LANGUAGE DEVELOPMENT

In previous sections parents were asked to facilitate language development by having speakers enter the child's communisphere frequently during each day, by providing large amounts of speech stimulation during pleasant moments, and by rewarding the child's speech listening attitudes and all his efforts at gesture and spoken communication. During the symptom phase of treatment, parents may be asked to provide language stimulation in a more specific manner and to elicit more specific types of responses.

Many of the techniques that could be employed by parents and other family members have already been discussed in other places by the author (Mysak, 1966a, Chs. 3, 4; Mysak, 1968b). Examples of these techniques follow: 1. the simple procedure of labeling or naming aloud once or twice all objects within the perceptual field of the child; 2. having the child "point" with either his hand, face, or eyes to familiar persons, toys, materials, and body parts named; 3. having the parent engage in intraverbalizing behavior, that is, having her report aloud in simple phrases on her actions and what she contacts in the environment; and 4. similarly, having the parent report aloud on the child's actions and the objects in his perceptual field in the hope of triggering thereby self-talk activity in the child. 5. Individuals in the environment could also echo in a playful manner utterances made by the child in the hopes of reinforcing his attempts at oral communication. From time to time, the clinician may request the parents to emphasize certain questions in question exercises and certain sounds, words, or phrases during labeling, story-telling or self-talk activities. Emphasis of certain sounds or words, for example, may take the form of increasing their loudness, changing their pitch, repeating them, or pausing before and after they are spoken.

EXTENSION OF CLINICAL ACTIVITIES IN THE HOME

Parents should also be expected to spend some time once or twice a day reinforcing some specific goals set by the speech clinician during the formal therapy sessions. For example, reinforcing the child's ability to discriminate between standard and error forms of the /b/ phoneme as produced by someone other than the child. It is important, however, for the clinician to follow a certain procedure before actually making a specific home assignment. First, the mother should be allowed to observe the "exercise" a few times, then she should take part in the activity with the clinician and child, and finally if all goes well, she should lead the activity under the observation of the clinician. Only if this procedure has progressed satisfactorily should the therapy unit be assigned as homework.

Auditory Perception

Symptomatic techniques in the area of auditory perceptual functioning are aimed basically at developing auditory retention span, discrimination, analysis-synthesis and sequencing behavior, and preventing secondary auditory problems. As mentioned previously, for more standard approaches to hearing-aid orientation and auditory training and speech reading for those children who have hearing losses, the reader is referred to appropriate chapters in the Handbook.

SECONDARY HEARING PROBLEMS

It may be recalled that in the preceding chapter some comments were made about the concept of "auditory atrophy." Such auditory "wasting away," or "failing to grow" appears connected with lack of reward for the child for attending auditorially. Undetected or untreated acuity losses, for example, may eventually discourage the child from trying to listen to the speech around him, and hence his attempts at listening may wane. Or, if listening has little utility, that is, if it does not serve to help the child grow and adjust to his environment, there may also be a progressive lessening of the child's listening interest. Another form of secondary hearing involvement was referred to as "auditory rejection." The rejection of speech signals is usually related to the experiencing by the child of substantial amounts of noxious speech, for example, verbal punishment, anxiety-producing remarks, unhappy-appearing whisperings between parents, or between parents and physicians and parents and therapists.

The speech clinician's contribution to auditory hygiene is to counsel parents, therapists, teachers, and physicians about the concepts of auditory atrophy and rejection and to offer suggestions on how these conditions may be avoided.

AUDITORY RETENTION SPAN, DISCRIMINATION, ANALYSIS-SYNTHESIS, IMAGERY, AND SEQUENCING

As a contribution to the developments of auditory perception and speech sound and oral language, exercises for auditory span, discrimination, analysis-synthesis, imagery, and sequencing functioning are recommended.

Span may be developed by having the child, for example, point to a progressively increasing number of things named by the clinician, or by having him repeat progressively longer words, phrases, and sentences, or by having him answer questions about progressively longer and more complex questions and short stories. As the child makes progress "holding in mind" speech signals of various kinds, the clinician may introduce progressively longer lags between stimulus and response, that is, he may ask the child to withhold his response until increasing amounts of time have elapsed.

Speech discrimination activities could include having the child give yes or no responses to whether pairs of similar-sounding nonsense syllables are the same or different. Or they could include identification of the right pair of similar-sounding names of pictures or objects being uttered by the clinician.

Auditory analysis and synthesis refers to that process whereby someone analyzes words into their component syllables, or conversely, synthesizes words from hearing their component syllables. The analysis process can be extended by having the child identify the individual words that make up a certain phrase, or sentence; likewise, synthesizing can be extended by having a child put together words separated by progressively longer pauses into meaningful phrases and sentences. The synthesizing task just described also incorporates sequencing behavior which is to be discussed next.

Auditory sequencing describes that process where parts of speech signals are not only "held" but held in the proper order. For example, progressively longer series of syllables may be uttered and the child must in some way indicate that they have been heard in a certain order. Progressively longer series of objects may be named and the child must respond by pointing to them in the right order. The same kind of activity can be tried by giving the child progressively longer series of simple instructions that must be carried out in a certain sequence.

Of course, the suggestions for developing auditory perceptual functioning should be implemented with due consideration to the child's age and abilities. It may also be apparent that many of them can be carried out at home by parents.

Articulation

This section on symptomatic procedures in articulation therapy will concentrate on how to facilitate speech-sound learning in the young child. As indicated in the introduction of this section of the chapter, the ideas for this discussion are based on principles previously discussed by the author (Mysak, 1966a, Ch. 6).

SPEECH-SOUND ACQUISITION

In those instances where the child's speech-sound developmental processes are proceeding slowly or appear halted, the clinician should attempt to stimulate them directly. In this regard, attention should be given to stimulating the processes of speech-sound orienting, scanning, tracking, comparing, and approximating. As an example of such stimulation, let us suppose we have a child who consistently uses /v/ for /b/ (possibly influenced by a degree of distocclusion).

Speech-sound orienting. Orienting the child to bilabial sound production could be done in various ways. First, offering the child some simple information on how a /b/ is made and where it may appear in words, and giving demonstrations of its production could serve as introductory stimulation. Then, during conversation or oral reading by the clinician, the child is asked to signal whenever he believes a /b/-word has been uttered. The task may be made simpler by the clinician at the beginning by virtue of his repeating such words, or making them louder, or by separating them by pauses from preceding and following words. Each time a /b/-word occurs the child is required to signal its occurrence by turning toward the clinician or by signaling in whatever way he can. This type of activity should be continued until the child consistently orients toward such words.

Speech-sound scanning. Speech-sound scanning is described as exploring and selectively bringing to one's attention those features of a phoneme which distinguish it from all others.

Returning to the example, the bilabial, plosive, and voiced features of the /b/ may be simply described to the child. Next, the bilabial movement should be contrasted with the labiodental, the linguadental, the lingua-alveolar, the linguapalatal, and linguavelar movements. Voiced-voiceless sound contrasts and stop-continuant contrasts should also be made.

The child may then be asked to identify /b/-words in pairs that contrast them with words having voiceless sounds, with words having sounds made with different articulatory positions, and with words containing other than plosive sounds. In all such activities the clinician should point out those features that distinguish /b/ sounds from all speech sounds. The clinician must also gauge whether the child has come to appreciate all the distinguishing characteristics of the sound.

Speech-sound tracking. Tracking describes the child's attempts to reproduce the sound under study; tracking should be encouraged only after the child has exhibited degrees of success with speech-sound orienting and scanning. There are at least three forms of tracking: echoic, simultaneous, and imagery tracking. Echoic tracking describes the child's attempt to reproduce the sound immediately after hearing it; simultaneous tracking describes the child's attempt to produce the sound at the same time as hearing it; and imagery tracking describes the child's attempt to "hear" the sound with his mind's ear and then to reproduce it. All such efforts should be reinforced by the clinician with appropriate statements relative to the comparative accuracy of the child's attempt; that is, that's correct, or that's closer, and so on.

Speech-sound comparing. Comparing describes that process whereby the child compares the standard sound with his attempt at reproducing it, or compares his intended and actual versions of the speech sound. The child must be helped to recognize how his sound is similar in all important dimensions to the standard sound, or, if the child's version is inadequate, how it differs in the important dimensions, for example, in terms of placement of the articulators, the voiced aspect, or the plosive, fricative, and so on, aspect. The point here is that the child must become aware of all error factors present in his attempted reproduction.

Speech-sound approximating. Speech-sound approximating is that process whereby the child, once becoming aware of error factors, continues to retrack the sound hoping to reduce them.

The clinician's job is to encourage continuous orienting, scanning, tracking, comparing, and approximating until he believes that the child, within the limitations imposed by his particular speech system, is producing the best possible version of the sound. One way to keep the approximating process active is by regularly asking the child to produce all the varieties of /b/ in /b/-words that he is capable of making and reinforcing those which come closest to the standard sound. Unless the approximating process is kept active the child may cease his efforts at reducing error factors to a minimum, and hence a less-than-adequate version of the sound may be stabilized.

If an error version of the sound has been habituated, speech-sound modification procedures based on a developmental feedback approach should prove useful. The approach includes the following: 1. developing error-sound sensitivity, and measuring abilities, and thereby causing short-circuiting of error-sound production; and 2. when necessary, stimulating correct-sound seeking, approximating, and tracking processes. As already indicated, further information on this approach has been presented by the author in another place (Mysak, 1966a, pp. 76–82). Also, the reader is again reminded that discussions of articulation symptom therapy appear in other chapters of the Handbook and that many of these techniques can also be applied to the child with cerebral palsy.

SPEECH-SOUND MODIFICATION VIA SPECIAL TECHNIQUES

When increased intelligibility is desired during conversational patterns, certain individuals with neurogenic articulatory problems have made good use of speech techniques which appear to amplify sensory feedback and gear down rate. For example, asking the child to intentionally produce harder contacts during running speech, having him employ an exaggerated or an overarticulation pattern, or a slow-motion articulation pattern, or having him articulate against resistance are techniques which may prove of some value.

Spoken Language

Various techniques for facilitating the development of spoken language have already been presented in the sections on prophylactic and etiologic techniques. This portion of the chapter, therefore, will be limited to a discussion of additional ideas more specifically related to the symptomatic category of techniques. Again, the reader will find other discussions of language symptom therapy in appropriate chapters in the Handbook.

Language symptoms mentioned in the preceding chapter included delay in the appearance of first words as well as two- and three-word sentences, reduced verbal output, syllable reversals, difficulty in the use of function words, use of neologisms, irregular verbal associations, lack of meaning associated with verbalization, word-finding problems, circulocutionary verbalization, grammatical confusions, verbal perseveration, and echolalia. Suggestions for treating some of these symptoms follow.

PHYLO-ONTOGENETIC CONSIDERATIONS

The author (Mysak, 1968a, pp. 99–100) recently described how a theory of the phylogenesis of oral language in man may be applied in work with the cerebral-palsied. Four stages in the development of spoken language were presented: body-head language, hands-face language, face-hand language, and mouth language; it was also theorized that speech ontogenesis roughly reflects its phylogenesis. The clinical value of the concept of speech phylo-ontogenesis lies in utilizing it in assessing the level of communication in any one particular child, and in ensuring that each child takes full advantage of his level and makes efforts to attain the next higher level.

The earliest or body-head stage is reached by the infant in a month or two, when he communicates discomfort and hunger and is characterized by general, unorganized body and head movements plus crying and screaming (i.e., nonspecific body-head activity in association with unorganized vocalization). The second or hands-face stage is reached during the second half of the infant's first year of life, when body postures become more organized and where bilateral hand gesturing and crude facial expressions in association with more organized vocalization are manifested (e.g., in an effort to communicate he wants to be picked up, the infant may straighten and extend both arms, and may smile and lall). The third or face-hand stage is reached at about 10 months of life with the development of unilateral and bilateral hand gesturing, an increase in the range of facial expressions, plus more refined articulatory and phonatory behavior (e.g., the child in the standing position, making unilateral hand gestures, smiling and echoing heard syllable combinations). Finally, the fourth or mouth stage is reached some time during the infant's second year of life, when he uses true words in conjunction with supportive hand gesturing and facial expression.

Since even the most involved child with cerebral palsy can communicate at the lower levels described, he should be encouraged and required to do so while he works toward attaining higher levels of communication.

LANGUAGE SYMPTOM TECHNIQUES

Many of the language symptom therapy techniques to be mentioned should be familiar to experienced clinicians. However, for those who find them less familiar brief descriptions follow.

Imagery association. The clinician may present or point to an object, for example, a banana, and then have the child close his eyes and "see" it with his mind's eye. He may then utter its name and then have the child "hear" it again with his mind's ear. The clinician may then request the child to "hear" the name and to "see" the object; to "hear" the name and to "taste" the object.

It is hoped that by such techniques neuronal arrangements representing the various images and speech areas are activated and associated.

Intraverbalizing techniques. Intraverbalizing activities have already been described in this chapter. It is hoped that when the clinician describes aloud his activities he may provide meaningful, general language stimulation, as well as encourage similar activity in the child. It is often found that a reciprocal relationship exists between motor activity and words describing that activity, and that the activities may be mutually facilitatory.

Verbal exercises. There are numerous activities which the clinician could use to good advantage in trying to relieve various language symptoms. He may use sentence stubs; ask yes-no questions; request definitions or antonyms or synonyms; ask for plurals, or past or future tenses; and ask for specific or nonspecific types of verbal associations to words. Language could also be used and stimulated through the use of planned sociodramas and story continuation techniques.

Research Needs

As in the instances of speech prophylactic and speech etiologic techniques, research data on the effectiveness of various kinds of speech symptom approaches to the speech syndromes of cerebral-palsy are hard to find.

In line with the orientation of this chapter, it would be important to compare the effectiveness of a program which includes speech prophylactic, etiologic, and symptomatic techniques employed from the moment the child is identified, with various basically symptomatic approaches applied starting from the speech-age period.

SPEECH COMPENSATORY AND PALLIATIVE PROCEDURES

Concepts and use of speech compensatory and speech palliative procedures as they pertain to the child with cerebral palsy will be discussed in the last section of this chapter.

Speech Compensatory Procedures

Since the goal in speech habilitation is to ensure that each child actualizes all his potential for intra- and intercommunication, the speech clinician must be ready to assist the child in employing modified verbal and even nonverbal forms of communication in those cases where 1. there is little hope of attaining speech communication, or 2. the development of such communication is limited, or 3. the development of such communication is proceeding slowly and the child is well into the early language learning period.

Van Riper (1963, pp. 2–11) has identified at least five functions of speech: 1. as a means of formulating thought, 2. as a means of transmitting information, 3. as a means of social control, 4 as a means of emotional expression, and 5. as a means of self-identification. It is vital then that each child develop language irrespective of whether he can articulate that language. Therefore, as soon as the period of verbal expression is reached and it is believed that the child will not easily attain speech communication, plans should be made for the use of speech compensatory activities.

Some of the forms that such compensatory or "make up for" techniques may take include: 1. The use of pictures or objects which may represent important wants and needs of the child. Materials representing food, family members, pets, the various rooms of the house, and so on, should be available for the child to point to in some fashion. The child could be conditioned to come into contact with the representative materials each time he wants to express a specific need. 2. The use of some yes or no signal system (e.g., appropriate nodding of the head, or certain facial expressions or sounds) in response to expressed alternatives. 3. Spelling aloud by the child who is unable to articulate whole words adequately. 4. The use of a language or conversation board (Westlake and Rutherford, 1961; McDonald and Chance, 1964). 5. The use of morse code (Clement, 1961). 6. Finally, the use of a special typewriter. Of course, the last four suggestions can be used only after the child has developed a certain level of spoken and written language comprehension. When economically and technically feasible it would be appealing to consider the practical use of simple speech synthesizers for the severely speech-handicapped. It would be interesting to evaluate the clinical application of such a mechanism if one could be programmed to issue simple requests and social speech via some simple operation by the child.

In sum then, speech compensatory procedures should be utilized by the clinician in cases where the prognosis for speech communication is poor or where the development of speech communication is lagging. In the latter case, the clinician, of course, continues his efforts at stimulating the development of speech communication.

Speech Palliative Procedures

Palliative treatment usually refers to lessening, easing, or affording some relief from symptoms without any hope for eliminating them. In terms of speech, it is not too frequent that the clinician is involved with a case where there is little hope for any kind of progress in verbal or nonverbal communication. Such cases do exist, of course; for example, seriously retarded cerebral-palsied children, or cases of severe aphasia in geriatric patients. With respect to the adult, the clinician's job may be one of "holding the communicative line," or slowing communicative degeneration, or, when neither is possible, providing communicative support. Up to this time, clinicians have generally avoided such work or kept such work to a minimum. However, as the field grows and speech and hearing services are made available at more kinds of institutions and hospitals, such cases will appear in caseloads with increasing frequency. Almost all of the other health-related professions have been involved with such work for some time.

In the case of the child with cerebral-palsy, speech palliative techniques may include: 1. helping the parents adjust to their child's inability to use any form of verbal or compensatory communication; 2. helping the parents to comprehend any of the child's nonverbal affective communication; for example, his use of smiles, laughter, whining, crying, and nonspeech sounds; 3. helping the parents comprehend any of the child's "body language," that is, his body postures or facial expressions—of course, a careful study of the child will need to be done if the clinician is to be of any real help with the latter two suggestions; 4. finally, the parents must be counseled against behavior which may further infantilize the child or prevent him from actualizing any of his undetected potential for higher forms of communication.

Research Needs

Because of the relatively rare use of speech compensatory and speech palliative procedures in the field in general, every aspect of such procedures needs to be explored.

With respect to the child with cerebral-palsy, it would be important to gather data on the differences in perceptual, socioemotional, and language development in the child who receives speech compensatory work along with speech prophylactic, etiologic, and symptomatic activities, as compared with the child who receives work only in the three latter habilitation areas.

SUMMARY

Because of the polycausal, polymorphous, and polyphasal nature of cerebral palsy speech syndromes, wide-spectrum speech-habilitation techniques are recommended in the hopes of actualizing each child's maximum potential for speech communication. Wide-spectrum treatment means working with the total speech system, not with just the customarily recognized speech organs. It means recognizing the interrelatedness and interdependence of the child's speech development and his perceptual, motor, emotional, social, and intellectual developments. It also means beginning work with the child as soon as his cerebral-palsied condition is recognized and not waiting until the speech age. With these concepts in mind, speech habilitation is discussed in terms of speech prophylactic, speech etiologic, speech symptomatic, and speech compensatory and palliative procedures. Speech prophylactic techniques are those used basically during the prespeech stage, while etiologic and symptomatic techniques are used during the speech stage. Under these categories of procedures, the parents' role is outlined. In addition, techniques are presented aimed at stimulating bipedal head and thoracic development and at improving respiratory, auditory, articulatory, phonatory, speech rhythm, and language functioning. It was stated at the close of the preceding chapter that to become an expert speech diagnostician in the area of cerebral palsy is an accomplishment indeed. It is obvious that the statement applies to an even greater extent with respect to becoming an expert in providing speech therapy for these syndromes.

Finally, the degree of speech habilitation reached in any one case of cerebral palsy depends on the accuracy of identification of a particular speech syndrome, on the ability of the clinician to design an individualized therapy regimen, on the potential of the child's speech system, and on the ability of the clinician to motivate the child to actualize his maximum potential for speech communication.

BIBLIOGRAPHY

Berry, M., and Eisenson, J. 1956. Speech disorders. New York. Appleton-Century-Crofts.

Clement, M., Sr. 1961. Morse code method of communication for the severely handicapped cerebral palsied child. *Cerebral Palsy Rev.*, 22, 15–16.

Crickmay, M. 1966. Speech therapy and the Bobath approach to cerebral palsy. Springfield, Ill.: Thomas.

Di Carlo, L., and Amster, W. 1955. Hearing and speech behavior among children with cerebral palsy. *In* Cerebral palsy. Cruickshank, W., and Raus, G., eds. Syracuse, N.Y.: Syracuse Univ. Press, Pp. 166–255.

Dinnerstein, A., and Lowenthal, M. 1966. Anxiety, perceptual latency and behavioral disability. *J. nerv. ment. Dis.*, 142, 562–567.

Hardy, J. 1961. Intraoral breath pressure in cerebral palsy. *J. Speech Hearing Disorders*, 26, 310–319.

———, Rembolt, R., Spriesterbach, D., and Jaypathy, B. 1961. Surgical management of palatal paresis and speech problems in cerebral palsy. *J. Speech Hearing Disorders*, 26, 320-325.

Hixon, T., and Hardy, J. 1964. Restricted motility of the speech articulators in cerebral palsy. *J. Speech Hearing Disorders*, 29, 293–305.

Jones, E. 1963. Development of electrical stimulation in modifying respiratory patterns of children with cerebral palsy. *J. Speech Hearing Disorders*, 28, 230–238.

Kabat, H. 1952. Central facilitation; the basis of treatment for paralysis. *Permanente Foundation Med. Bull.*, 10, 190–204.

Lencione, R. 1966. Speech and language problems in cerebral palsy. *In* Cerebral palsy. Cruickshank, W., and Raus, G., eds. Syracuse, New York: Syracuse Univ. Press.

Mecham, M., Berko, M., and Berko, F. 1966. Communication training in childhood brain damage. Springfield, Ill.: Thomas.

Myers, R., and Smith, J. 1958. Effects of intermediate midbrain crusotomy on the speech of athetoid cerebral palsied patients. *J. Speech Hearing Disorders*, 23, 594–600.

Murphy, K. 1964. Development of articulation and hearing. *In* Learning problems of the cerebrally palsied. Loring, J., ed. London: Spastics Soc.

Mysak, E. 1966a. Speech pathology and feedback theory. Springfield, Ill.: Thomas.

———. 1966b. Phonatory and resonatory problems. *In* Speech pathology. Rieber, R., and Brubaker, R., eds. Amsterdam: North-Holland.

———. 1968a. Neuroevolutional approach to cerebral palsy and speech. New York: Columbia Univ., Teachers College Press.

———. 1968b. Disorders of oral communication. *In* Evaluation and education of children with brain damage. Bortner, M., ed. Springfield, Ill.: Thomas.

McDonald, E., and Chance, B. 1964. Cerebral palsy. Englewood Cliffs, N.J.: Prentice-Hall.

Van Riper, C. 1963. Speech correction. Englewood Cliffs, N.J.: Prentice-Hall.

Westlake, H., and Rutherford, D. 1961. Speech therapy for the cerebral palsied. Chicago: Nat. Soc. Crippled Child. and Adults.

28

Speech Defects Associated with Dental Malocclusions and Related Abnormalities

H. Harlan Bloomer

The successful diagnosis and treatment of defective speech can be achieved only by the speech pathologist who understands the relationship which exists between structure and function. It is thus that a discussion of speech abnormalities includes reference to the teeth, their development, their occlusal patterns, and the functioning orofacial complex of which they are a dynamic part. This complex of tissues determines the visual and acoustic features of all human utterance, from the most commonplace to the most profound expressions of thought or feeling.

This chapter discusses the functioning of the orofacial structures in normal and abnormal speech, the identification of certain orofacial abnormalities affecting speech (omitting cleft lip and palate), and describes the role of the speech pathologist in the examination and treatment of patients afflicted by such disorders. It provides a basis for the study of speech articulation as it is affected by the dimensions, form, and mobility of the lips, cheeks, jaws, tongue, nasal and oral pharynx, and the form and condition of the teeth, nose, and other relatively immobile tissues of the face. Reference is made to habit patterns affecting dentofacial growth and development, the effects of lingual appliances on speech, and certain aspects of the interdisciplinary relationships involving speech pathology, audiology, and the paraphoniatric disciplines of dentistry and medicine.

The relationship of anatomical structures to speech is an extraordinarily complex one in which the correspondence between structure and function is never perfect. The mobile and the supporting tissues of the face, mouth, pharynx, and nose modulate the pneumatic and acoustic events of speech to produce an almost infinite variety of qualities. The correspondence between structure and function is imperfect because some speakers are capable of compensating for seemingly insurmountable handicaps of orofacial deformity, whereas other speakers whose structures are anatomically satisfactory reveal handicapping defects of function. Other speakers possess structures which have become abnormal in form or dimensions presumably because of the distorting influence of abnormal tissue function on developing bones and cartilages. When structures are abnormal or when patterns of tissue function are distorted, they provide a dynamic milieu in which interaction of structure and function may affect not only speech, but also the physical, mental, and social health of the afflicted individual (Vocational Rehabilitation Administration 1963).

The term orofacial abnormalities includes deformities of all of the tissues of the orofacial complex—the supporting structures of cartilage and bone; the teeth; muscles and tendons; motor and sensory nerves; the glandular and relatively immobile soft tissues of the oral cavity; and the dermal coverings of the face, mouth, nose, and pharynx. It encompasses the syndromes of congenital origin, such as mandibulofacial dysostosis, first and second branchial arch syndrome, the Pierre Robin Syndrome, and several others which include distinctive clusters of abnormalities, as well as those disorders of the postnatal period created by accident, surgery, or disease. It includes *dental abnormalities* and *malocclusions*, terms which refer respectively to defects of tooth development and defects of tooth relationship. Deviations in the number, shape, texture, and position of the teeth are labeled "dental abnormalities," whereas deviations from the normal relation of the teeth to each other in the same dental arch and to the teeth of the opposing arch are referred to as "malocclusions" (Anderson, 1948, p. 18)."Orofacial abnormalities" is an inclusive term which in the context of this chapter is used in reference to those anatomical features relating primarily to speech articulation.

The emphasis on abnormalities of form in the foregoing paragraphs should not be construed to suggest that the relationship of anatomy and speech is entirely one of mechanics and acoustics in which the only determinant is the adequacy with which the structures can approximate the conditions for vowel and consonant production and the prosodic feature of speech. The effect of structure on behavior is one side only of a dynamic relationship in which speech (as a form of behavior) may in turn affect the structural environment in which it is produced. The relationship is further complicated in that a) defective speech and orofacial structures may arise from common genetic and developmental forces; b) structure and function exert mutual influences as patterns of behavior emerge and become established habits; and c) both structure and function may be changed by accident disease, or iatrogenic (medical) alteration.

As examples of these concepts, there is evidence to indicate in reference to a) that the genetic events which predispose a person to a structural deformity (e.g., a small mandible, a prognathous mandible, a macrostomia, or an incomplete temporomandibular joint) may also affect organs and functions involved in the learning of speech—vascular circulation, hearing, motor and sensory innervation of the speech organs, intelligence, and so on. As an example of b), it is postulated that muscle function (or the lack of it) influences the direction and form of bone development; and conversely, that endogenously determined patterns of bone growth may establish conditions to which the mobile tissues of the mouth and face must later adapt. With reference to c), the creation of defects of the orofacial complex by surgery, accident, or disease (e.g. glossectomy, maxillectomy) sometimes impose severely handicapping conditions to which the remaining tissues may not be able to accommodate functionally. Important as it may be for a speaker to possess resemblance to structures having normal *form*, it is of vastly greater importance to speech that the developing or modified tissues approximate the *actions* of normal structures.

THE MUSCULOSKELETAL VALVES OF NORMAL SPEECH PRODUCTION

Normal speech can be achieved only when appropriate movements of the orofacial structures occur in properly timed sequences. Abnormal orofacial structures which move maladaptively produce defective speech. It is also possible to have normal structures which move maladaptively to produce defective speech, or conversely, to have abnormal structures which function adaptively and thus produce acceptable speech. In short:

Normal structure + normal movements = normal speech.

Abnormal structures + maladaptive movements = defective speech.

Normal structures + maladaptive movements = defective speech.

Abnormal structures + adaptive movements = normal (compensated) speech.

The production of consonants and vowels requires control of a series of musculoskeletal valves which can be opened, closed, or constricted with almost kaleidoscopic variability and speed. These valves modify the channels through which the expiratory air and vocal tone must pass. They determine to a large extent the physical conditions of pressure change and air vibration which characterize the acoustic patterns which we recognize as vowels, consonants, and the prosodic features of speech.

The valves identified in the subtitle to Fig. 28-1 are designated by the following names: 1. glottal, 2. palatopharyngeal, 3. linguavelar, 4. linguapalatal, 5. lingua-alveolar, 6. linguadental, 7. labiodental, and 8. bilabial. The accessory valves are (A) plicaventricular, (B) linguapharyngeal, and (C) anterior nares.

Deviant modifications of the valves occur under conditions of malformation and maladaptive movement of the soft and mobile tissues of the mouth and pharynx in speech and in swallowing. For example, a relatively common maladaptation found especially among speakers with congenital palatal insufficiency

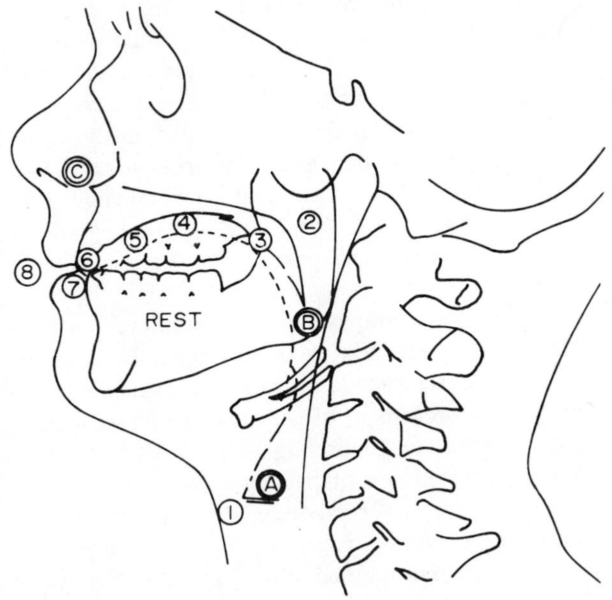

Fig. 28-1. Tracings of lateral head x-ray of normal speaker. The valves indicate respectively the following structures normally involved in phonation and articulation: (1) glottis, (2) soft palate and associated naso-pharyngeal tissues, (3) tongue and soft palate, (4) tongue and hard palate, (5) tongue and maxillary alveolar ridge, (6) tongue and anterior teeth, (7) lower lip and upper teeth, and (8) lips. The encircled letters designate respectively maladaptive valves formed by: (A) false vocal folds, (B) tongue and oropharynx, and (C) the anterior nares.

is the production of /k/, /g/, and /l/ by bringing the back of the tongue into contact or constriction with the posterior oropharyngeal wall (illustrated approximately by maladaptive valve (B). (See section on symbolization of malphones.) Another maladaptation is produced by occluding or constricting the nares at (C) to substitute for an inadequate palatopharyngeal valve. (A) represents false vocal fold constriction as in dysphonia plica ventricularis. Maladaptation of a normal valve occurs when a speaker uses the glottal valve (1) to substitute a glottal stop consonant for a plosive or other phoneme.

Although consonants are formed by a complex series of oral movements which continuously modify the sounds of speech, a critical phase of articulatory movements in consonant production can be described as an "articulatory position" and the corresponding consonants can be classified in this context according to their "place of articulation." Table 28-I presents a classification of consonant phonemes according to: 1. the presence or absence of voicing; 2. the anatomical structures by which the valve is created; 3. the degree of valve closure required to produce the phoneme; and 4. the manner of articulation. Reference to such a chart can help us understand how abnormalities of structure and maladaptive movements of the articulators may interfere with the production of satisfactory phonemes. Although this chart is relatively simple, some charts, such as the one devised by Peterson and Shoup (1966), provide elaborate and detailed information concerning the phonetic parameters of speech.

Although the form of Table 28-I suggests that the locus of the articulatory valve is the most significant factor in consonant production, the place at which the valve occurs is important only insofar as it makes possible the "manner of articulation." The manner of articulation creates the acoustic and prosodic patterns

TABLE 28-I Place and Manner of Articulatory Valving

PLACE OF ARTICULATORY VALVING	MANNER OF ARTICULATORY VALVING								
	VALVE NARROWED (GLIDES) (2) PV-c		VALVE CONSTRICTED (FRICATIVES) (2) PV-c		(Affricates)		VALVE CLOSED (STOPS) (2) PV-c		(NASALS) (2) PV-o
1. GLOTTAL			h						
2. LINGUA-VELAR							k	g	n
3. LINGUA-PALATAL	r	j	ʃ	ʒ	tʃ	dʒ			
4. LINGUA-ALVEOLAB	l		s	z			t	d	n
5. LINGUA-DENTAL			θ	ð					
6. LABIO-DENTAL			f	v					
7. BI-LABIAL	ʍ	w					p	b	m

(Note: (a) The presence of voicing is indicated by underlining.
(b) Palato-pharyngeal valve closed and open are indicated by PV-c and PV-o respectively).

which we recognize as correct for the language spoken. There are, for example, at least two acceptable ways of producing an /s/, and probably several allophonic variations of these. Reference to the palatograms and tracings of Figs. 28-2 and 28-5 indicates that the tongue is grooved in the midline, that the sides of the tongue maintain contact with the maxillary alveolar ridge laterally, and that the tongue tip contacts the palate as far forward as the alveolar-post-incisal region. In another form of /s/ the tongue tip is brought to the lingual surface of the lower incisors and the grooved blade into contact with the maxillary alveolar ridge. A study by Subtelny, Mestre, and Subtelny (1964) indicates that approximately one-third of American speakers use the latter method of articulatory placement for the /s/. An unpublished study by Bloomer based on cinematographic records of 200 school children, aged six to 10 years, indicates that approximately 75 percent use the lowered tongue-tip orientation in producing the /s/. It is possible, of course, that speakers use each method to some extent, depending on the sound which immediately precedes or follows the /s/, although Subtelny, Mestre, and Subtelny do not attach much significance to the phonetic context as a controlling factor in the choice of articulatory placement for this consonant.

Other modifications of compensatory articulatory adjustment are described in the section of this chapter dealing with orofacial abnormalities and defective speech. It is not intended to present here a complete discussion of the characteristics of the various phonemes and the requirements of their production. It is pertinent to the discussion of orofacial anomalies and defective speech, however, to present the broad outlines of the important positional relationships.

Much information can be derived from direct observation and by photography of articulatory movements. Additional information is obtainable from palatography, x-ray (still and cineradiographic), electromyography, and possibly by the use of ultrasound.

Contact palatography has been employed by phoneticians to study the areas of linguadental and linguapalatal contacts made during the articulation of discrete consonants or of consonants in combination with a vowel or diphthong (CV or VC). Shohara (1941) reported use of palatography as a means of correcting defective speech articulation. Several variant techniques of palatography have been devised, but the prototype method utilizes a thin molded palate (pseudopalate) made from a dental baseplate material (shellac, metal, acrylic, etc.) shaped to form an exact replica of the contours of the hard palate from the gingival borders of the maxillary teeth to the posterior border of the hard palate. The lingual surface is dusted with a color-contrasting powder and inserted into the mouth of the informant, who then produces the consonant to be studied. The moist surface of the tongue removes the powder from the contacted area of the pseudopalate, thereby defining the lingua-alveolar or linguapalatal pattern which is characteristic of articulation for that sound.

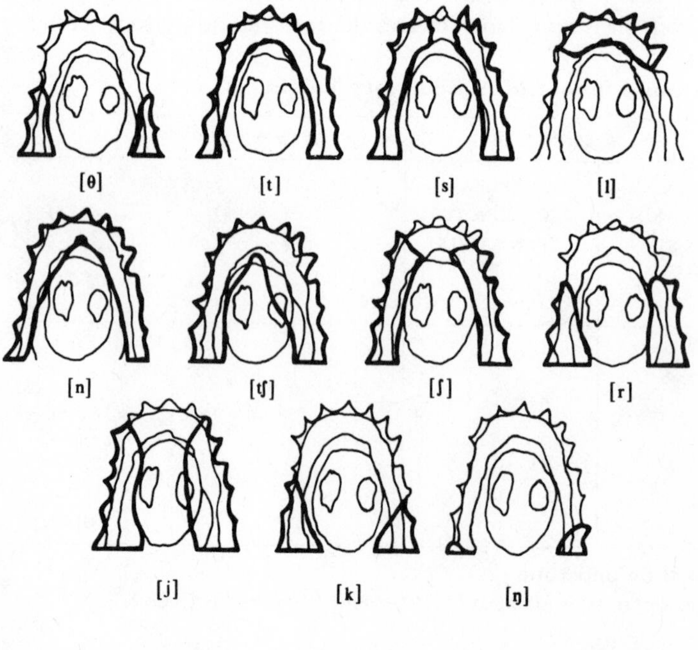

Fig. 28-2. Palatograms shown in relation to palatal contours (palatopograms). Contour lines are 5 mm apart. The areas of linguo-alveolar or linguo-palatal contact are circumscribed by the heavy lines.

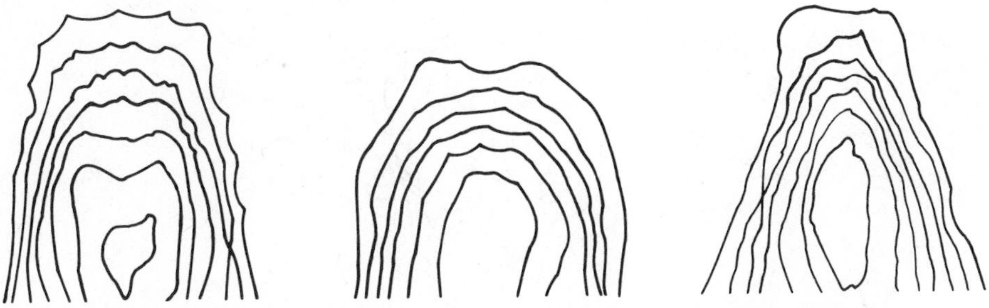

Fig. 28-3. Basic types of palatal shapes: trapezoid, ovoid, triagonal.

A direct photographic method employed by Hopkin and McEwen (1955) uses a color-contrasting dust sprayed directly on the hard palate, and a mirror placed to reflect the palatal record of lingual contacts made in normal or abnormal articulation. Kydd and Belt (1954) described an electronic display system of palatography in which the linguapalatal contact is registered as a spaced pattern of individual lights which are illuminated as the tongue contacts the correspondingly placed oral electrodes.

Palatograms ordinarily show two-dimensional patterns, thus masking the depth dimension by which steepness of alveolar slope, the height of the palatal vault, and other features of palatal configuration are defined. This limitation of palatography can be partially overcome by use of a palatopograph (Bloomer, 1943), an instrument which maps the palate contours by means of a stylus which can be set to survey the perimeters of palatal planes at selected depths. The palatograms of Fig. 28-2 present a topographical

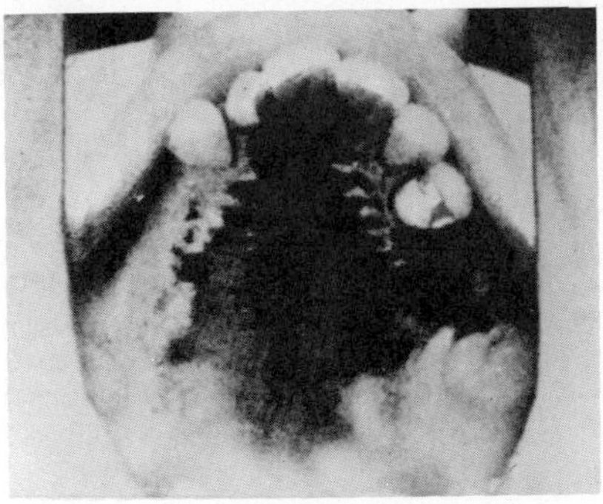

Left lateral lisp

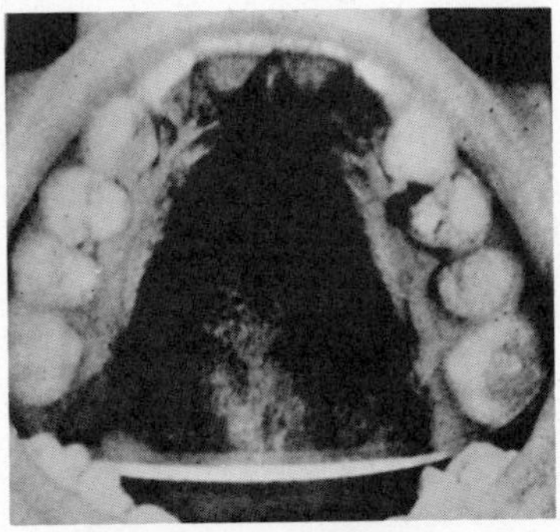

Anterior lisp in case of open-bite

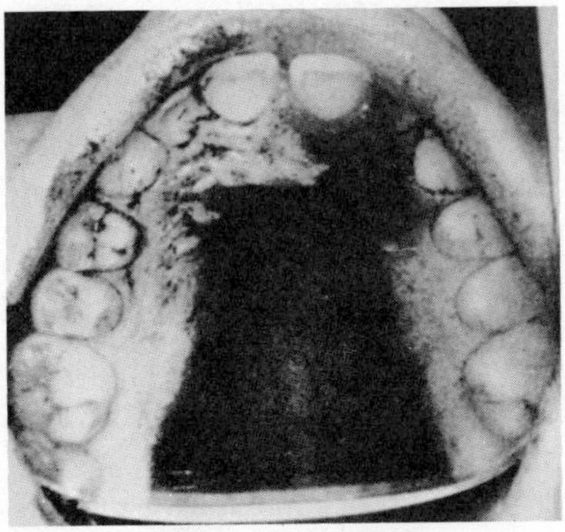

Left antero-lateral lisp
(normal occlusion)

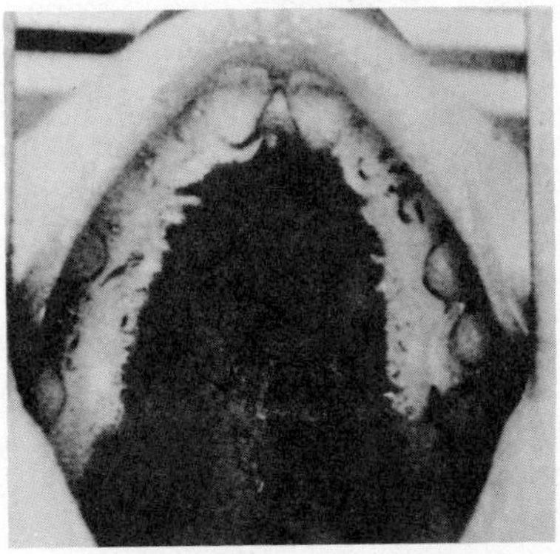

Normal /s/ in case of anterior
open-bite

Fig. 28-4. Palatograms of defective consonant articulations. *Hopkins and McEwen, 1955.*

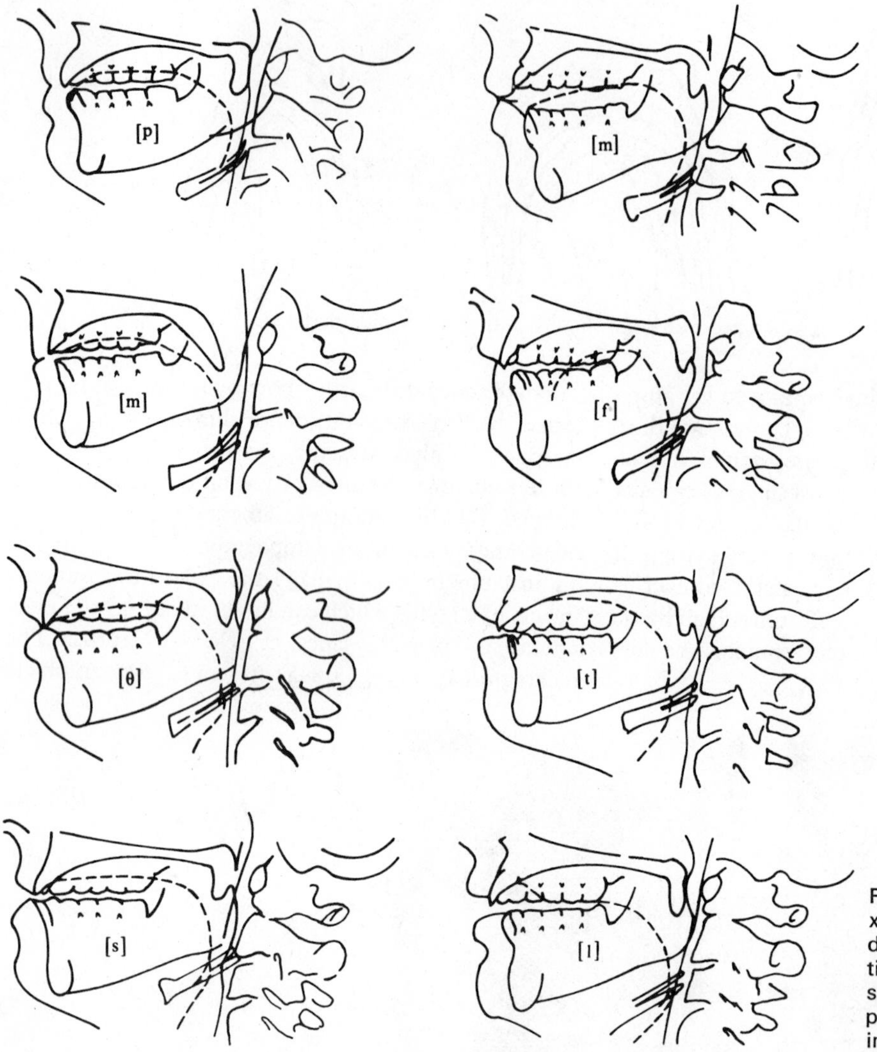

Fig. 28-5. Tracings based on x-ray films of a subject during a distinctive moment in the production of certain consonants. Exposure time .4 sec. The subject also produced the palatograms shown in Fig. 28-2.

record of the author's palate. The contours are depicted at five mm. intervals of vertical dimension. The height of the palatal vault, the angle of slope of the alveolar arches, and the area of the successively defined planes can be interpreted in much the same manner as a contour map of the earth's terrain. Starting with the gingival borders as a zero line, this palate is slightly over 15 mm. high.

Whether or not a relationship between palatal contour and lingua-alveolar contacts exists for speech has not been established. It is evident that such contacts will not depend on palatal shape and dimensions alone, but will be modulated by such factors as the mandibular-maxillary relationship and the size and general posture of the tongue in the mouth cavity. A master's degree study by Crane and Ramstrum (1943) indicates that three basic classifications of palatal shapes drawn from a population of 400 dental students can be identified according to the configuration (trapezoid, tapering, or ovoid), and the ratio of anteroposterior slope (in the midsagital plane) to the medial slope (coronal plane measured at the mesiolingual groove of the upper first permanent molar). Fig. 28-3 illustrates these basic configurations.

Photographs presented by Hopkins and McEwen (1955) do not depict all of the relevant information which is needed to study the effects of malocclusion on articulation, but they do display aberrant articulatory patterns which are of interest because of the inferences which may be drawn concerning the missing dentition and the abnormal lingual contacts (**Fig. 28-4**).

Electromyography as means of detecting the muscular contractions of the tongue, face, jaws, or palate during speech and deglutition have been reported by Moyers (1949), Pruzansky (1952), MacNeilage and

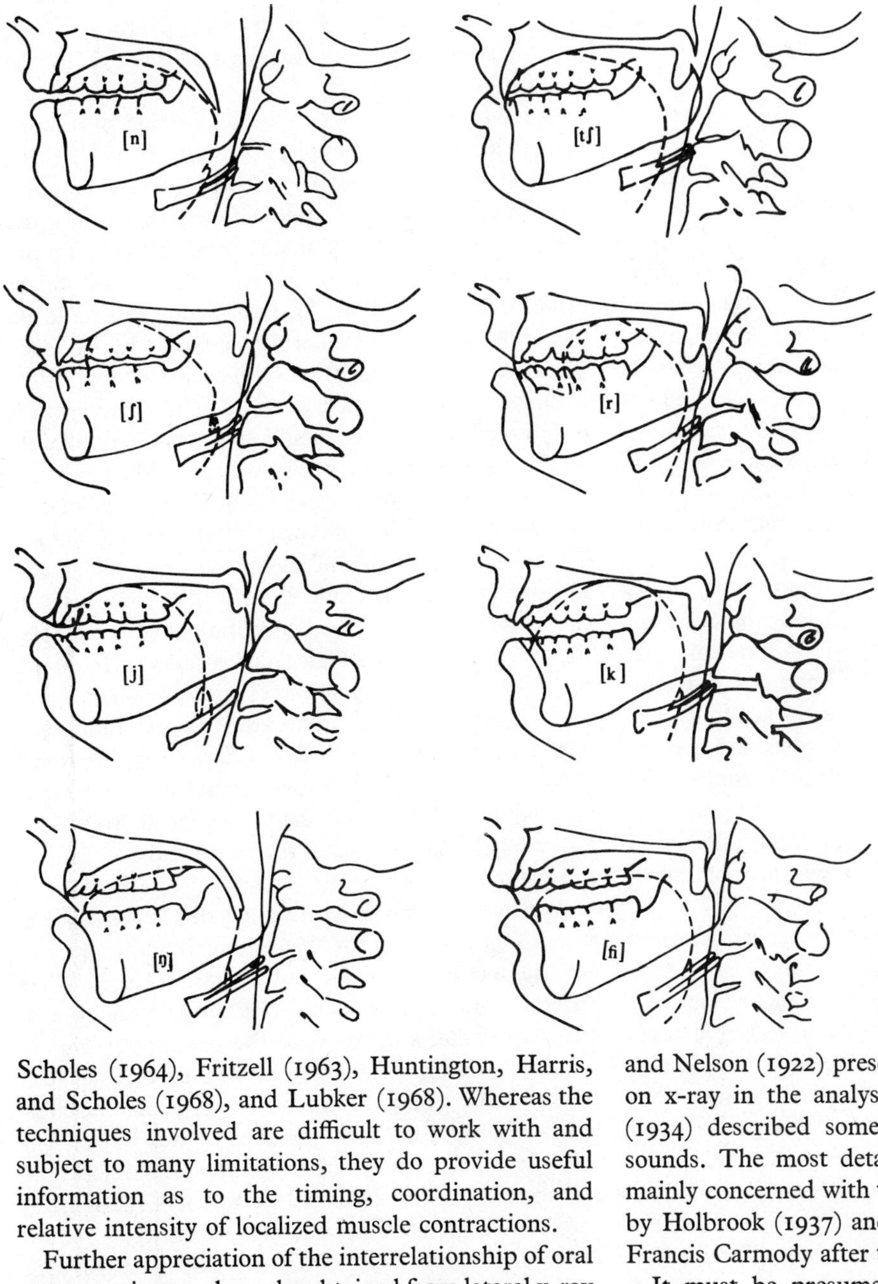

Fig. 28-6. Further tracings based on x-ray films of a subject during a distinctive moment in the production of certain consonants.

Scholes (1964), Fritzell (1963), Huntington, Harris, and Scholes (1968), and Lubker (1968). Whereas the techniques involved are difficult to work with and subject to many limitations, they do provide useful information as to the timing, coordination, and relative intensity of localized muscle contractions.

Further appreciation of the interrelationship of oral structures in speech can be obtained from lateral x-ray films of the head made during the "contact" phase of consonant articulation and from cineradiography.

Tracings outlining structures directly involved in articulation of the consonants and semivowels /p/, /ʍ/, /m/, /f/, /θ/, /t/, /s/, /l/, /n/, /tʃ/, /ʃ/, /r/, /j/, /k/, /ŋ/ and /h/ are shown in Figs. 28-4 and 28-5. The informant for the x-rays also made the palatograms shown in Fig. 28-2.

Interesting woodcuts intended to depict similar information are to be found in Kingsley (1880). Barclay and Nelson (1922) presented one of the early reports on x-ray in the analysis of speech sounds. Russell (1934) described some x-ray studies of consonant sounds. The most detailed study to date, although mainly concerned with vowel sounds, is that reported by Holbrook (1937) and assembled and arranged by Francis Carmody after the author's death.

It must be presumed that the character of the linguoalveolar and linguopalatal contacts during speech will be determined at least in part by the occlusal relationships of the maxillary and mandibular dentures and the configuration of the hard palate.

The date and study methods suggested above are adequate for the description of consonant production as it relates to average normal structures of the mouth and face. The phonetic values of an individual speaker must be studied with reference to his own peculiar physioanatomical structures. The basis for distinguishing and describing these individual characteristics of orofacial form are discussed in a section which follows.

DEVELOPMENT OF THE FACE AND MOUTH

Man's face is one of his distinguishing morphological characteristics, representing the phylogenetic end product of a long period of evolutionary development. Facial growth postnatally is sensitive to disturbances of mental and physical development. The face reflects a person's moods, his personality, his physical status. The student of human behavior learns early to search the face of his subject for the subtle nuances of expression and appearance which communicate such information.

To comprehend the relation of orofacial deformity to speech it is necessary to review briefly the composition of the orofacial complex, its framework, its musculature, innervation, the components and relationship of the dental arches, and the anatomy and physiology of the soft tissues which cover and nourish it. It is equally important to know something of the way in which the tissues of the maturing organism grow and develop. Speech is learned over a long period of time and is greatly affected by the conditions governing growth.

Whereas no attempt will be made to cover the topic of facial development completely in this chapter, it is suggested that the reader consult a standard work on human anatomy (e.g. Woodburne, 1965) or a textbook of speech science (Zemlin, 1968) for a listing of the major structures involved in speech articulation. (Also see Chapter 2 by DeuPree.) General speech anatomy, together with information concerning the development, origin of the structures will provide a useful reference for later discussion of orofacial defects related to disorders of communication. The list for study should include the major bones, cartilages, muscles, cavities and sinuses, motor and sensory nerves, glands, formina, and some of the superficial landmarks frequently identified in an orofacial examination of speech.

A majority of the occlusal abnormalities and related orofacial deformities associated with defective speech are of developmental origin; that is, they come about because of heredity or from some traumatizing condition effective during prenatal or postnatal growth of the individual. Trauma and disease also affect the mature adult, of course, as in cases of cancer of the palate, retropharyngeal tumor, and diseases of the tongue and mandible.

It is important that the speech clinician have some understanding of the etiology of certain of these abnormalities and an awareness that structural anomalies which appear to be similar may come from quite different origins—a fact which may be of great importance in the diagnosis of the speech disorder and in establishing a prognosis for treatment. He should be aware of the dynamic interplay of forces which takes place between the function of speech and the structures of the body which to some extent govern that function. The clinician should know that it is possible for the informed diagnostician to read in the teeth and their supporting structures an indelible record of certain aspects of the life history of the individual. Through a knowledge of the causes of orofacial deformity, the speech clinician may play some part in the prevention of these deformities if he recognizes the early signs of pathological development. He should realize that the etiological forces which produce structural maldevelopments may also forecast functional maldevelopments in speech. The disease or nutritional deprivation which brings about bone deformities may affect speech also through damage to the neuromuscular system, which regulates the speed and accuracy of muscle movements.

A genetic approach is much needed by specialists in our field, not only for the diagnostic and therapeutic orientation it provides, but because it can help the speech clinician understand the cooperating role of the dentist and surgeon, and the paramount importance of timing in phoniatric, dental, and surgical intervention. The brief summary of orofacial development presented herein is included by way of emphasizing a point of view, rather then to provide specific information. For an extended treatment of the subject, reference is made to such standard works as Patten (1953), or Arey (1954). An excellent summary of growth of the craniofacial complex is contained in Graber (1966), and in Hemrend and Moyers (1953).

The development of the normal structures of the face and mouth occupies a period of approximately 20 years in the life of a human being, beginning late in the first month of intrauterine life and ending sometime between the eighteenth and twenty-fifth years of adult life. By the third week in utero the fetus develops two primitive structures (the frontal process and the mandibular arch) from which the maxillary and mandibular processes grow, joining with the fronto-nasal process to become the differentiated tissues of the face and mouth.

The basic structures of the face are distinguishable by the 5th week of life, when the embryo is between five and six mm. in length. The first four of the six branchial arches are involved in facial and lingual development. Failure of this development is observed in such anomalies as the first and second branchial arch syndrome, astomia, retrognathia, and various other deformities to which reference will be made later. The branchial arches and their corresponding Cranial nerves (the trigeminal, facial, glosso-pharyngeal, vagus, spinal accessory, and hypoglossal) serve respectively the motor control of the adult muscles of mastication and the tensor tympani (V); the muscles of facial expression and the stapedius (VII); the stylopharyngeus (IX); the laryngeal and upper pharyngeal muscles involved in vocal resonation and certain aspects of swallowing (IX, X, and XI); and the tongue (XII).

The cranial skeleton develops first as a framework of connective tissue followed by the formation of cartilage, and during the second month of intrauterine life, by formation of bone. While the bony and muscular parts are developing, a concomitant development of the sense organs of the oral and nasal cavities is taking place: (Cranial nerve V to the face; general sensation through V, IX, and X to the tongue; and lingual taste through VII, IX, and X). (Woodburne, 1965, p. 250). By about the twelfth week the face assumes recognizably human features, the maxillary shelves have closed and the soft palate developed, the structures of the external and middle ear have formed, the tongue has emerged and has commenced occasional swallowing movements, the deciduous teeth have begun to calcify, the temperomandibular joints and related cartilaginous tissues are basically complete, and although the mandible is still cartilaginous (Meckel's cartilage) it has established the basic structure which will later be replaced by bone cells, commencing about the fifth month.

The genetic origins of the muscles and nerves of the orofacial region are set forth in Table 28-II.

The various parts of the head at birth are not merely small versions of parts of an adult skull but differ in proportional size and potential rates of growth. The face at birth is often less than one-eighth of the size of the cranium, whereas the adult face is one-third to one-half the size of the adult cranium. Hemrend and Moyers (1953) note that the cranium has completed 90 percent of its growth by four years of age, and maximum growth by 10 to 12 years; the nasomaxillary complex is about 90 percent complete by the age of 12 and complete by 18 years; and the mandible may continue to grow until 25 years of age. It is important to remember these facts when discussing abnormalities of facial growth and the factors which cause them, since the time at which the cause is an effective agent determines in large part the structure which is affected. Easlich and Moyers (Watson and Lowrey, 1954, pp. 254–255) note that:

> The cranial base is the most stable area of the skull during growth. Because the cranial vault and the nasomaxillary complex are attached to the cranial base, its growth is a determining or limiting factor in the growth of the rest of the skull. . . .
>
> The nasomaxillary complex at birth is farther from its adult dimensions than is the cranium. Height and length are less developed than width because they are largely dependent on alveolar growth which is yet to come. The body of the maxilla will also be increased in height and length by sutural growth. At birth the orbits have attained more of their adult size than any other portion of the face. The uppermost boundaries of the nasal cavities have also attained most of their adult size.

It is in the critical periods of fantastically rapid proliferation and differentiation of tissues of the orofacial complex that defective genes, and unfavorable gestational environment[1] or the introduction of teratogens may disturb normal growth processes and create the syndromes of orofacial deformity which subsequently may include defective speech among their functional manifestations. The varieties of orofacial deformity are thus the result not only of the tissues affected, but of the time at which they are affected. Facial growth is not achieved by uniform increase in size of its various components, but proceeds differentially in growth spurts, in which the head, then facial width, and lastly facial length and depth are completed (Graber, 1966). All parts of the orofacial complex are not equally susceptible to growth disturbance, and the various structures differ not only in the timing of critical developmental periods and maturation rates, but also in the nature of the process by which growth

[1] Lundstrom (1962) in surveying Swedish children one to three years of age, with a history of maternal rubella in the first four months of pregnancy, found that the children had 0.6 fewer teeth than those children whose mothers were afflicted at five months and thereafter.

TABLE 28-II
A General Outline of the Muscles of the Head and Neck and their Motor Nerve Supply according to their Embryonic Origin*

I. Branchiomeric Musculature. (Branchial arch musculature from mesoderm of the pharyngeal arches.)

Muscles from *First Arch* innervated by the *Trigeminal* (V) Nerve.

Muscles from *Second Arch* innervated by the *Facial* (VII) Nerve.

Muscles from *Third Arch* innervated by the *Glossopharyngeal* (IX) Nerve.

Muscles from *Fourth* and *Sixth Arches* innervated by the *Vagus* (X) and *Accessory* (XI) Nerves.

A. Muscles of the Trigeminal (V) Field. From Arch I (mandibular arch).
Innervated by fibers from the motor or third division of the V Nerve.
1. Muscles of Mastication:
   a) Temporalis
   b) Masseter
   c) Lateral pterygoid
   d) Medial pterygoid
2. Palatal Muscle:
   a) Tensor veli palatini
3. Middle Ear Muscle:
   a) Tensor tympani (attached to the malleus bone)
4. Suprahyoid Muscles: (attached to mandible)
   a) Anterior belly of digastric
   b) Mylohyoid

B. Muscles of the Facial (VII) Field. From Arch II (hyoid arch).
1. Muscles of Facial Expression:
   a) Muscles of scalp (frontalis and occipitalis)
   b) Muscles of orbit (orbicularis oculi and corrugator)
   c) Muscles of auricle (auricularis anterior, superior, and posterior)
   d) Muscles of nose
   e) Muscles of mouth (orbicularis oris, buccinator, etc.)
   f) Muscles of chin (mentalis)
   g) Muscle of neck (platysma)
2. Middle Ear Muscle:
   a) Stapedius (attached to stapes)
3. Suprahyoid Muscles: (attached to hyoid bone)
   a) Posterior belly of digastric
   b) Stylohyoid

C. Muscles of the Glossopharyngeal (IX) Field. From Arch III.
1. Pharyngeal Muscle:
   a) Stylopharyngeus

D. Muscles of the Vagal (X) Field. From Arches IV and VI (Assisted by the Accessory (XI) Nerve.) Muscles of swallowing and phonation.
1. Muscles of the Soft Palate:
   a) Palatopharyngeus
   b) Palatoglossus
   c) Musculus uvulae
   d) Levator veli palatini
2. Muscles of the Pharynx:
   a) Superior constrictor
   b) Middle constrictor
   c) Inferior constrictor
   d) Salpingopharyngeus
3. Muscles of the Larynx:
   a) Cricothyroid (innervated by external branch of superior laryngeal)
   b) Deep intrinsic laryngeal muscles:
      1) Posterior cricoarytenoid
      2) Lateral cricoarytenoid
      3) Arytenoids (transverse and oblique)
      4) Thyroarytenoid

E. Muscles of the Spinal Accessory (XI) Field. (There are differences in the literature concerning the origin and the nerve supply to the muscles listed below.)
1. Trapezius
2. Sternocleidomastoid

II. Myomeric Musculature (Somatic Musculature—from somites of the head and neck).

A. Muscles of the III, IV, and VI Fields. (From head somites)
1. Muscles of the Orbit:
   a) Levator palpebrae superioris—*oculomotor* (III) nerve.
   b) Superior rectus—*oculomotor* (III) nerve
   c) Medial rectus—*oculomotor* (III) nerve
   d) Inferior rectus—*oculomotor* (III) nerve
   e) Inferior oblique—*oculomotor* (III) nerve
   f) Superior oblique—*trochlear* (IV) nerve
   g) Lateral rectus—abducens (VI) nerve

* By permission of Alphonse R. Burdi, Ph.D., Assistant Professor of Anatomy, The University of Michigan.

TABLE 28-II (continued)

B. MUSCLES OF THE HYPOGLOSSAL FIELD (XII). (from occipital somites)

1. MUSCLES OF THE TONGUE:
   a) Genioglossus
   b) Hyoglossus
   c) Chondroglossus (sometimes described with hyoglossus)
   d) Styloglossus
   e) Intrinsic lingual musculature

C. MUSCLES OF THE CERVICAL FIELD. (from cervical somites) Innervated from cervical nerves accompanying the hypoglossal nerve.

1. SUPRAHYOID MUSCLE:
   a) Geniohyoid
2. INFRA-HYOID MUSCLES:
   a) Thyrohyoid
   b) Omohyoid
   c) Sternohyoid
   d) Sternothyroid

TABLE 28-III
Chronology of the Human Dentition

		TOOTH	HARD TISSUE FORMATION BEGINS	AMOUNT OF ENAMEL FORMED AT BIRTH	ENAMEL COMPLETED	ERUPTION	ROOT COM-PLETED
DECIDUOUS DENTITION	Maxiliary	Central incisor	4 mo. in utero	Five-sixths	1½ mo.	7½ mo.	1½ yr.
		Lateral incisor	4½ mo. in utero	Two thirds	2½ mo.	9 mo.	2 yr.
		Cuspid	5 mo. in utero	One-third	9 mo.	18 mo.	3¼ yr.
		Firs molar	5 mo. in utero	Cusps united	6 mo.	14 mo.	2½ yr.
		Second molar	6 mo. in utero	Cusp tips still isolated	11 mo.	24 mo.	3 yr.
	Mandibular	Central incisor	4½ mo. in utero	Three-fifths	2½ mo.	6 mo.	1½ yr.
		Lateral incisor	4½ mo. in utero	Three-fifths	3 mo.	7 mo.	1½ yr.
		Cuspid	5 mo. in utero	One-third	9 mo.	16 mo.	3¼ yr.
		First molar	5 mo. in utero	Cusps united	5½ mo.	12 mo.	2¼ yr.
		Second molar	6 mo. in utero	Cusp tips still isolated	10 mo.	20 mo.	3 yr.
PERMANENT DENTITION	Maxiliary	Central incisor	3–4 mo.	—	4–5 yr.	7–8 yr.	10 yr.
		Lateral incisor	10–12 mo.	—	4–5 yr.	8–9 yr.	11 yr.
		Cuspid	4–5 mo.	—	6–7 yr.	11–12 yr.	13–15 yr.
		First bicuspid	1½–1¾ yr.	—	5–6 yr.	10–11 yr.	12–13 yr.
		Second bicuspid	2–2¼ yr.	—	6–7 yr.	10–12 yr.	12–14 yr.
		First molar	At birth	Sometimes a trace	2½–3 yr.	6–7 yr.	9–10 yr.
		Second molar	2½–3 yr.	—	7–8 yr.	12–13 yr.	14–16 yr.
		Third molar	7–9 yr.	—	12–16 yr.	17–21 yr.	18–25 yr.
	Mandibular	Central incisor	3–4 mo.	—	4–5 yr.	6–7 yr.	9 yr.
		Lateral incisor	3–4 mo.	—	4–5 yr.	7–8 yr.	10 yr.
		Cuspid	4–5 mo.	—	6–7 yr.	9–10 yr.	12–14 yr.
		First bicuspid	1¾–2 yr.	—	5–6 yr.	10–12 yr.	12–13 yr.
		Second bicuspid	2¼–2½ yr.	—	6–7 yr.	11–12 yr.	13–14 yr.
		First molar	At birth	Sometimes a trace	2½–3 yr.	6–7 yr.	9–10 yr.
		Second molar	2½–3 yr.	—	7–8 yr.	11–13 yr.	14–15 yr.
		Third molar	8–10 yr.	—	12–16 yr.	17–21 yr.	18–25 yr.

SOURCE: Logan and Kronfeld (slightly modified by McCall and Schour)

occurs. Accordingly the surgeon, the orthodontist, and the speech pathologist should initiate therapeutic intervention with reference to the time-frame of the organism. For example, the growth of the mandible may be directly affected by the pressures and tensions produced by muscles, by the growth stimulus provided by the development and eruption of mandibular teeth, and by the function of the various growth areas responsible for mandibular growth (Walpole-Day, 1951). The child born with micrognathia can be permanently damaged by poorly timed and executed treatment which ultimately limits severely the extent to which the speech pathologist can later help the patient functionally (see (Fig. 28-13).

The correct identification of individual teeth, the differential recognition of deciduous and permanent teeth, and the accurate description and classification of malocclusions are areas of mystery for many students of speech pathology. Nevertheless, these features constitute such an important part of the immediate oral environment with which the speech pathologist must deal that they deserve our attention.

Formation of the teeth begins in utero and continues from the time of eruption to the ages shown for complete formation of the root (Table 28-III). The deciduous mandibular central incisors begin their formation at four and one-half months in utero, erupt about the sixth month of postnatal life, and are fully formed (root completed) at one and one-half years. The permanent lower central incisors start to form about the third or fourth month postnatally, (before the corresponding deciduous teeth erupt), erupt at six or seven years and are fully formed by the ninth year. The deciduous teeth all have their beginnings in utero. It normally takes about three years after eruption for the roots of permanent teeth to complete their formation.

TABLE 28-IV
Normal Sequences of Eruption of Permanent Teeth[2]

MANDIBLE	MAXILLA
1. First molar	2. First molar
3. Central incisor	5. Central incisor
4. Lateral incisor	6. Lateral incisor
7. Cuspid	8. First biscuspid
9. First bicuspid	10. Second bicuspid
11. Second bicuspid	12. Cuspid
13. Second molar	14. Second molar

[2] The numbers indicate the usual sequence of eruption (From Watson and Lowery, 1954, p. 260).

The chronology of tooth eruption provides an important reference from which to infer delay, acceleration, or normal growth of a child when the facts of his dental growth are compared with other facts of his physical or behavioral maturation. Reference to Table 28-III provides a basis for determining whether the teeth of a patient are on schedule.

The sequences of tooth eruption as indicated in Table 28-IV, however, are probably of greater significance for the development of normal occlusion than is the exact chronological age of eruption (Easlick and Moyers, in Watson and Lowrey, 1954). It is thought that an abnormal order in the loss or retention of deciduous teeth may result in the ectopic eruption of permanent teeth, and may thus contribute to abnormal shaping of the dental arches.

Dental Occlusion

The makeup of the deciduous and adult dental arches is illustrated in Figs. 28-7 and 28-8 respectively. There are 20 deciduous teeth, arranged in each dental arch so that the mandibular teeth normally fit within the circumference of the maxillary teeth when the jaws are closed.

There are 32 permanent teeth in the normal maxillary and mandibular dentures. Their arrangement and the standard system of numbering are indicated

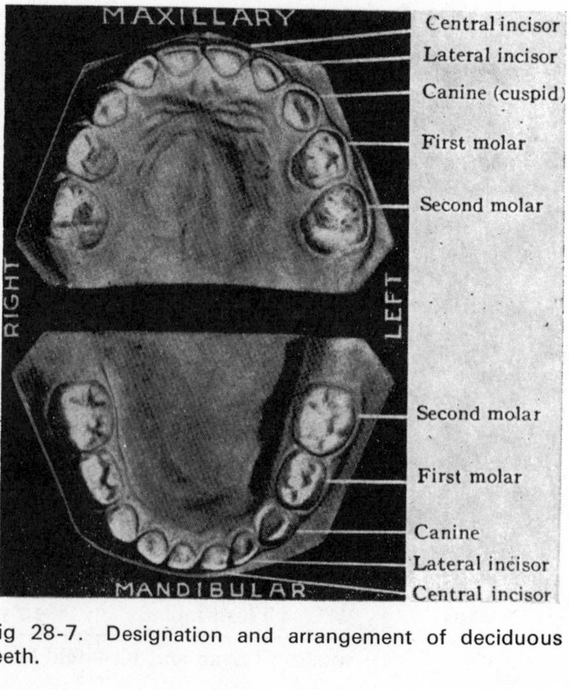

Fig 28-7. Designation and arrangement of deciduous teeth.

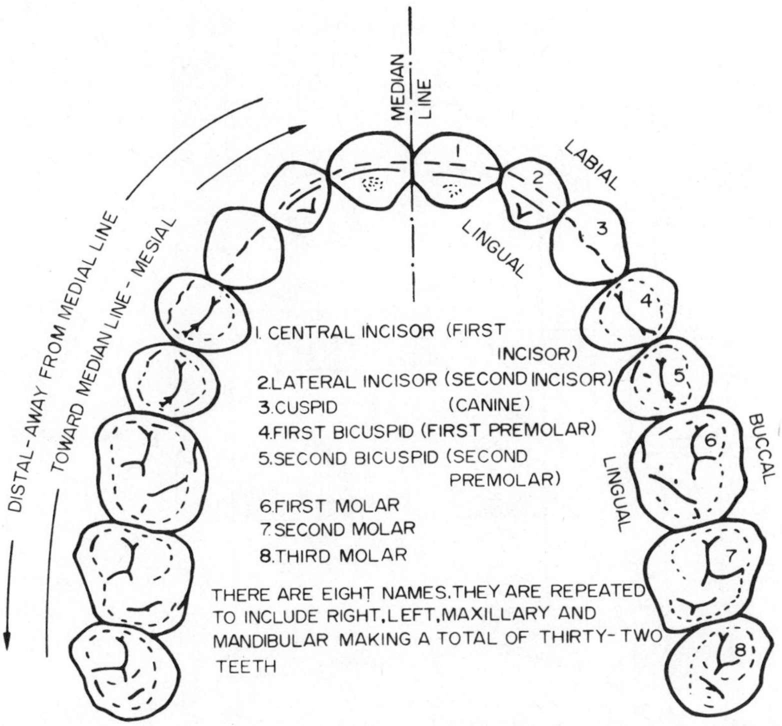

Fig. 28-8. Permanent teeth of an adult dental arch, showing arrangement and terms of orientation. *From Wheeler, 1940. TEXTBOOK OF DENTAL ANATOMY AND PHYSIOLOGY. Philadelphia: Saunders. Fig. 7, p. 7.*

in Fig. 28-8 (Wheeler, 1940, p. 7). Indicated also are the terms *distal, medial, labial, buccal,* and *lingual,* which are frequently used in describing the positional relationship of the teeth to each other and to other structures of the oral cavity.

The term *dental occlusion* has been specifically defined in many different ways. In a general sense it refers to the natural closure and fitting together of the upper and lower teeth (Wheeler, 1940). The term also implies certain concepts pertaining to 1. the alignment of the teeth in the upper and lower arches, 2. the relationship of these arches to each other, 3. the axial inclination of the individual teeth, and 4. the biting height of the teeth when the jaws are in contact relationships (Salzmann, 1950).

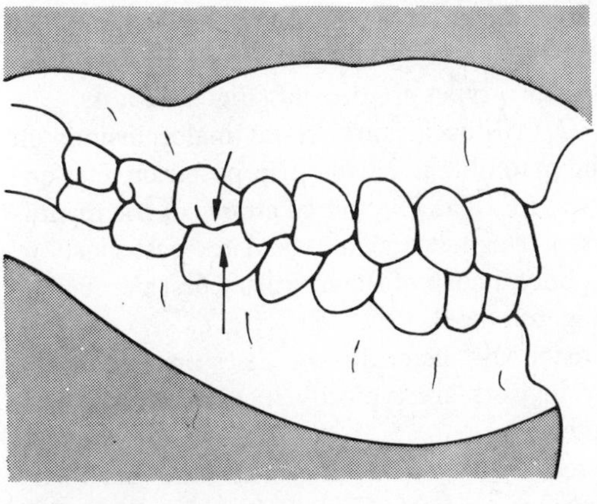

Fig. 28-9. Maxillary and mandibular teeth in normal occlusal relationship with reference to the first permanent molars.

"Normal occlusion" in the adult mouth assumes that the dental arches are arranged in concentric parabolic curves in which the outline of the maxillary arch is slightly larger than the mandibular arch (Wheeler, 1940). As a feature of this relationship between the two jaws, the mesiobuccal cusp of the maxillary permanent first molar occludes in the buccal groove of the mandibular permanent first molar (Fig 28-10). This is an important characteristic and forms the basis for various classifications of malocclusion which will be discussed later.

The teeth of the maxillary arch normally extend beyond the teeth in the mandibular arch labially and buccally—a condition described as *overjet* of the maxillary teeth when the teeth extend too far. The incisal ridges of the maxillary anterior teeth also extend below the incisal ridges of the mandibular anterior teeth when the teeth are placed in natural occlusion, a characteristic known as *overbite*. The amount of overbite is considered to be normal when the maxillary

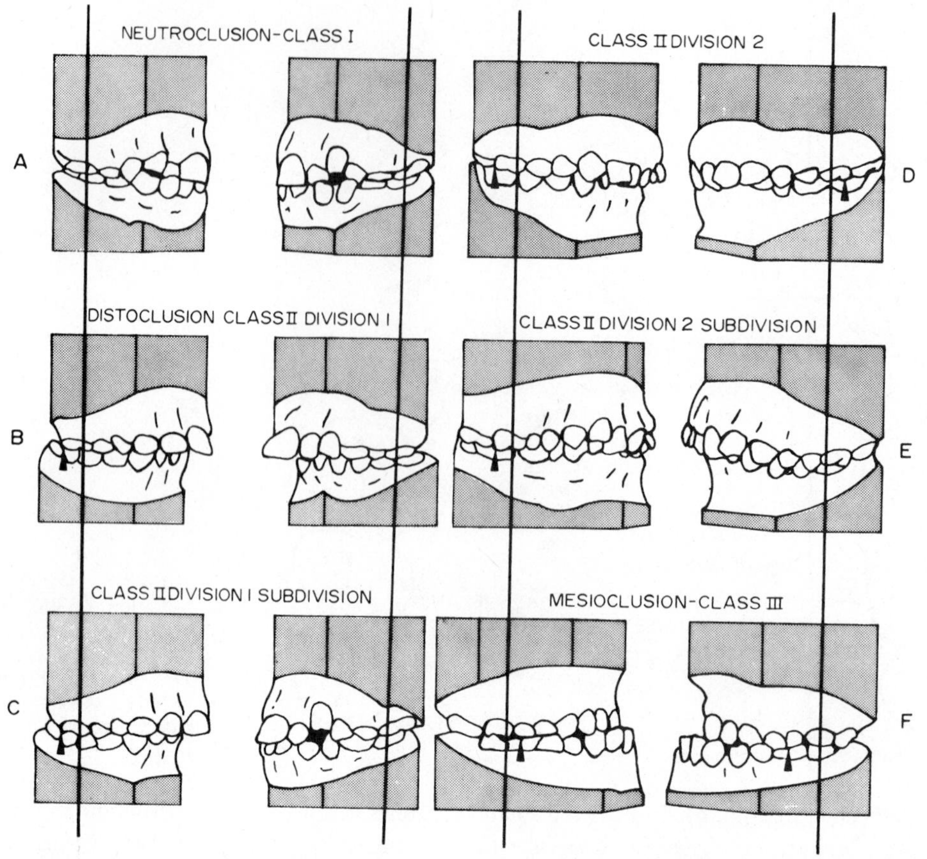

Fig. 28-10. Classification of malocclusion according to Angle. A, neutroclusion, Class 1; B, distoclusion, Class II, division 1; C, Class II division 1 subdivision; D, Class II division 2; E, Class II division 2 subdivision; F, Class III. *From Salzmann, J. A. 1950. PRINCIPLES OF ORTHODONTICS.* Philadelphia: Lippincott. p. 475.

incisors overlap the mandibular incisors one-third of the mandibular incisor crowns (Anderson, 1949). The lack of, or excess of, either overbite or overjet are considered forms of malocclusion.

Malocclusion

The classifications of malocclusion in current use are nearly all based upon a system originally worked out by Edward H. Angle (1907). In general, the system assumes a certain "normal" anteroposterior (mesiodistal) relationship of the jaws to each other. The key point of orientation is the position of the maxillary and mandibular first permanent molars, as described above. The following discussion of malocclusions is an adaptation of Moyer's (1955) restatement of Angle's original classes. The classical forms of these malocclusions are shown in Fig. 28-10.

Class I (Neutrocclusion)—those malocclusions wherein there is a normal anteroposterior relationship between the maxilla and mandible. The mesiobuccal cusp of the maxillary first permanent molar articulates in the buccal groove of the mandibular first permanent molar (Fig. 28-10). Anterior malocclusions of various types are present (Fig. 28-10, A).

Class II (Distocclusion)—those malocclusions in which the mandible is "distal" (in posterior relationship) to the maxilla. The mesial groove of the mandibular first permanent molar articulates posteriorly to the mesiobuccal cusp of the maxillary first permanent molar (Fig. 28-10, B, C, D, E).

1. Division 1—distocclusion cases in which the maxillary incisors are typically in extreme labioversion (protrusion).

2. Distocclusion cases in which the maxillary central incisors tend to be in linguoversion (retruded) while the maxillary lateral incisors are tipped labially and mesially.

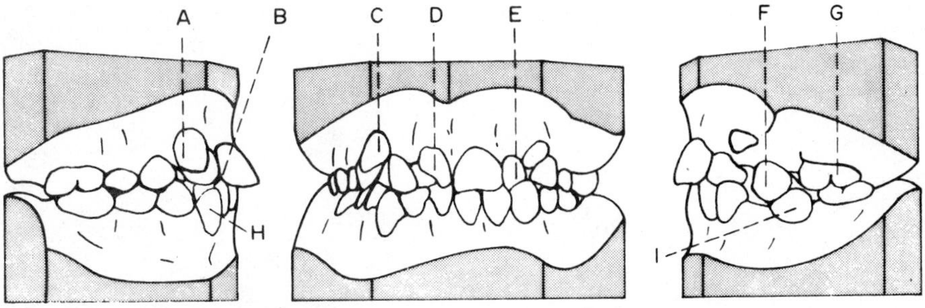

Fig. 28-11. Lischer's method of designating malposition of individual teeth. A, lateral incisor in transversion; B, central incisor in labioversion; C, canine in axiversion; D, central incisor in torsiversion; E, lateral incisor in linguoversion; F, first premolar in supraversion; G, first molar in mesioversion; H, mandibular canine in infraversion; I, first permolar in distoversion. *From Salzmann, 1950. PRINCIPLES OF ORTHODONTICS.* Philadelphia: Lippincott. p. 486.

3. Subdivisions—the distocclusion occurs on one side only of the dental arch.

Class III (Mesiocclusion)—those malocclusions in which there is "mesial" (anterior) relationship of the mandible to the maxilla. The extreme form is seen with the prognathous jaw. The mesial groove of the mandibular first permanent molar articulates anteriorly to the mesiobuccal cusp of the maxillary first permanent molar, the lower incisors protruding (Fig. 28-10, E).

In addition to the relative positions of the dental arches it is useful to the dentist and speech clinician alike to have means of indicating the positions of individual teeth in relation to each other and in relation to their position within the dental arch. Lischer (1912) has proposed the following terms (modified by Salzmann, 1950) which have won general acceptance in the field of dentistry.

a) Linguoversion—toward the tongue,

b) Labioversion (or buccoversion—toward the lip or cheek,

c) Mesioversion—mesial to the normal position,

d) Distoversion—distal to the normal position,

e) Infraversion—not reaching the line of occlusion (thus, higher in the maxilla, and lower in the mandible than the line of occlusion),

f) Supraversion—extending beyond the line of occlusion (thus, lower in the maxilla or higher in the mandible, than the line of occlusion),

g) Torsiversion—rotated on its long axis,

h) Axiversion—wrong axial inclination,

i) Transversion—wrong sequential order of position in the arch.

These malpositions of individual teeth are illustrated in Fig. 28-12.

The angle classification system tends to concentrate attention merely upon the relative position of the dental arches with respect to each other and to ignore such factors as discrepancies in the vertical or lateral planes and the general relationship of the teeth to the facial skeleton (Moyers, 1955).

The Simon system of classification takes these factors into account by utilizing cephalometric measures derived from landmarks of the cranium. This system uses three planes established with reference to cranial landmarks—the Orbital, the Midsagittal and the Frankfurt planes, from which anteroposterior, mediolateral, and vertical relationships may be ascertained and described (see Fig. 28-13 and Salzmannm 1950, p. 486, Fig. 272). A denture which is placed too far forward with respect to the orbital plane is said to be in *protraction*; a denture in abnormally posterior placement is in *retraction*. If a denture is nearer to the midline (midsagittal plane) than normal, it is said to be in *contraction*; when expanded abnormally, it is said to be in *distraction*. A denture which is abnormally high (nearer than normal to the Frankfurt plane) is said to be in *attraction*; one abnormally low with respect to that plane is in *abstraction*.

Moyers (1955) indicates that only three of these terms are in current usage—protraction, retraction, and contraction. The main advantage of the system is that it relates the dentures to the facial skeleton and thus makes possible a more accurate diagnosis of the basic dentofacial problems. From the standpoint of the speech clinician, the system's employment of anteroposterior, mediolateral, and vertical relationships is useful, especially in describing the position of the dental arches in relation to tongue positions and movements during speech.

The facial configurations depicting various mandibular malformations shown in Fig. 28-12 are also

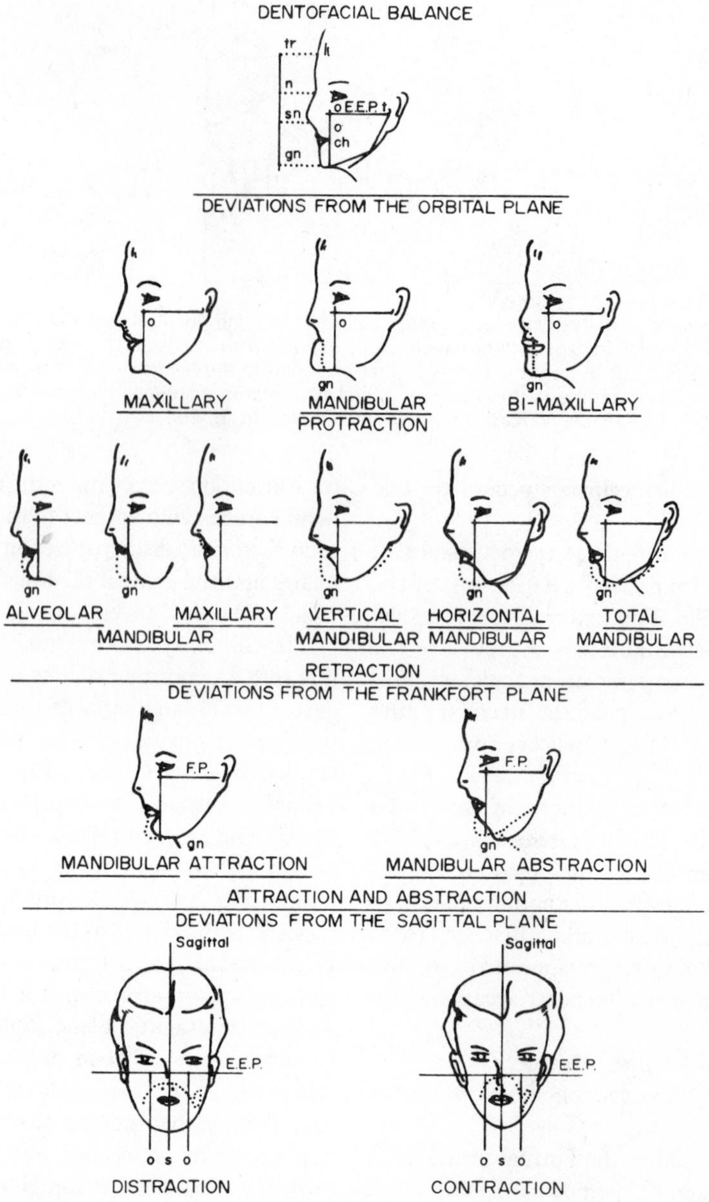

Fig. 28-12. Designations of dentofacial deviations from the three planes of space according to Simon; reading from above downward as follows:
Dentofacial balance showing the following landmarks: tr, trichion; n, nasion; sn, subnasion; gn, gnathion; ch, cheilion; op, orbital plane; o, orbitale, E.E.P., eye-ear plane; t, tragion.
Deviations from the orbital plane: protraction indicates protrusion; retraction indicates retrusion.
Deviations from the Frankfort plane: attraction indicates a shortening of the vertical dimension; abstraction indicates a lengthening of the vertical dimension from the eye-ear plane.
Deviations from the sagittal plane: distraction indicates an increase in the horizontal dimension from the sagittal plane; contraction indicates a decrease in the horizontal dimension from the sagittal plane. *From Salzmann, 1950. PRINCIPLES OF ORTHODONTICS.* Philadelphia: Lippicott. Fig. 272.

useful to the speech pathologist interested in the articulatory dynamics of patients who have these forms of jaw deformities.

The preceding sketch of orofacial growth carries the following implications for the student of speech pathology: 1. there are differential rates of growth of facial structures throughout life until about 25 years of age; 2. intervention at critical periods of growth can benefit or deter orofacial growth and subsequent orofacial function; and 3. speech diagnosis and therapy should be conceived and executed within the context of differential growth.

The face is responsive to tissue changes throughout life, whether these changes are initiated by disease, the tensions and pressures of muscle function, the effects of malnutrition, the formation, eruption, and loss of the teeth, or the response of facial tissue to the design of artificial dentures. There is nothing static about the human face, nothing stable and inalterable about the speech which it modulates, and there are no parts of the orofacial complex which exist independently of the condition of the whole.

THE TYPES AND ETIOLOGIES OF OROFACIAL ABNORMALITIES AFFECTING SPEECH

A complete list of orofacial anomalies which stand in direct or indirect relation to defects of speech would be long if all were included. Those of most immediate interest to the speech pathologist are herein limited to those demonstrably involved in speech articulation and resonation.

It would be an oversimplification and a misrepresentation of the interrelationship of defective speech and orofacial abnormalities to ascribe all manifestations of the disordered speech to anatomical causes. The ingenuity and determination of a patient and his therapist are sometimes adequate to compensate for potentially grave anatomical and functional deficits. On the other hand, surgeons and dentists who have labored carefully and skillfully to fashion or restore anatomical form are frequently disappointed to find that anatomical form is no guarantee of function. Factors of intelligence, motivation, emotional stability, auditory acuity and discrimination, and neuromotor skill are of as great importance to the final outcome as the antomical completeness of the face and mouth.

Abnormalities of orofacial tissues which affect speech may be caused by traumatic, pathological, or developmental events acting prenatally or postnatally. Moyers (1955) cites an equation attributed to Dockrell (1951) to illustrate the dynamic character of these forces of origin: Cause + Time + Tissue = Result. His further discussion of the origins of dentofacial abnormalities is reproduced in part below:

> Since investigators cannot isolate and identify all of the original causes, they may be studied best by grouping them as follows: 1. heredity, 2. developmental causes of unknown origin, 3. trauma, 4. physical agents, 5. habits, 6. diseases, and 7. malnutrition. It will be seen that there is a certain overlapping among these groups. The duration of the operation of these causes and the age at which they are seen, are both functions of time, and thus may be grouped together under this heading. The primary tissues principally involved are: 1. the bones of the facial skeleton, 2. the teeth. 3. the neuro-muscular system, and 4. the soft parts, excepting muscle. Rarely one tissue alone is involved; usually other tissues become affected, and one tissue may be termed primarily involved, and the others considered as being secondarily concerned. The result of the action of the factors is malocclusion, malfunction or osseous dysplasia; more probably a combination of all three. . . . If the primary tissues concerned involve the teeth, malocclusion is the result. If they impede the normal working of the neuro-muscular system, the result is malfunction. If they alter the growth of the bones, an osseous dysplasia is the result. Most clinical problems are a combination of these three aberrations.

In short, constitutional factors, trauma, or malnutrition may operate as causes; their relationship to time may be continuous or intermittent; the tissues affected may be dental, osseous, neuromuscular, or soft tissues; the result may be malocclusions, osseous dysplasias (abnormalities of bone development), or malfunction of muscles.

Osseous defects occur when one or more of the bones of the face develop in a perverted, delayed, advanced, or other asynchronous pattern of growth. Although each bone has a growth potential which is genetically determined, this potential may be altered by disease or by environmental forces such as mechanical interferences and habits of use, with the result that the growth of the lower jaw (mandible) or the upper jaw (maxilla and the nasomaxillary complex) may be so distorted that severe deformities of the dental arches and tooth relationships occur. Hypertrophy of the mandible due to hyperpituitarism may cause a Class III malocclusion (mandibular protraction). Underdevelopment as seen in retrognathia of the Pierre Robin syndrome may cause a Class II occlusal relationship of the jaws.

Treatment and prognosis depend upon accurate diagnosis in such cases. The alveolar bone can be shaped and altered by tooth movement or by the forces of muscular contraction; basal bone is generally unaffected by such forces. Distortions of dental-arch relationships may result from aberrent growth of either basal or alveolar bone, but only the latter can be altered effectively by orthodontic treatment or by the use of corrective muscular training.

Muscular dysfunctions which persist throughout critical periods of orofacial growth can distort the direction of facial development to cause permanent deformities of the dental arches. The musculature of the face is well defined before ossification of the face and cranium get under way (Arey, 1954). Thus the growing muscles exert a molding influence upon bone development, and in a "struggle between muscle and bone, bone yields" (Graber, 1963, p. 448). It is important to remember also that facial muscles begin to function before the muscles of mastication, that swallowing movements have been observed in the fetus and that even thumb sucking occasionally begins before birth.

Muscle groups which may affect orofacial formation include the muscles of mastication, facial expression, and the tongue. These muscles, acting in response to their motor innervators and their sensory correlates respond to innate (genetic) determiners, adapt to and modify the structures to which they are attached, and eventually develop stabilized habits of contraction, relaxation, and coordination in suckling, sucking, mastication, swallowing, and speaking. A state of physiological balance between the forces of these three muscle groups encourages normal growth and the shaping of the bones, and inclination of the teeth in the dental arches (Cooper, 1930; Winders, 1962). Distorted growth and even changes in the adult skeleton can occur if the opposing forces of the lips, cheeks, and tongue are not properly balanced (Kydd and Neff, 1964).[3]

Swinehart (1950) noted that although orthodontists agree that the tongue in habitually abnormal movement can cause a variety of malocclusions, little concerted study had been made up to that time to determine whether the tongue is an important factor in the original and subsequent forming of the dental arches. He speculated that an instance of congenital aglossia reported by Eskew and Shepard (1949) supported a contention that normal tongue function is essential to normal arch development. Since that time much work has been done to provide information on this general topic, emphasizing especially the influence of habitual patterns of sucking, swallowing, and biting.

Detrimental neuromuscular habits which are said to cause maldevelopment of orofacial structures include: abnormal patterns of mandibular closure, abnormal habits of sucking and swallowing, incompetent or abnormal lip postures, tongue- or lip-biting, the biting of hard objects (nail-biting, pencils, etc.) mouth breathing and abnormal habits of pillowing the head during sleep (Stallard, 1930).

The possible effects of thumb- and finger-sucking on occlusion have been much debated, both from the standpoint of tissue malformation and the implications which the habits and the measures employed to change them may affect personality development. There is much evidence to show that object-sucking and biting do affect occlusion, although Ruttle et al. (1953), Rakosi (1958) and de Rudder (1960), all indicate that the effect is recorded mainly on the inclination and placement of the anterior teeth. Sillman (1951), basing his conclusions on a serial study of 322 cases to 13 years of age, questions the validity of this habit as an etiologic factor except in two cases in his series. A study by Benjamin (1962) observed the consequences of digit-sucking for developing occlusion in 10 rhesus monkeys that were socially deprived and subjected to emotionally disturbing stimuli. Whereas malocclusion is not found in the dentures of wild monkeys, the deciduous malocclusions of the experimental monkeys showed a definite relationship to non-nutritive sucking habits. A less significant relationship was found between the sucking habits of these monkeys and the permanent occlusion. Although the findings on malocclusion are interesting, the development of non-nutritive sucking habits resembling those of human infants is especially striking because of the psychological implications concerning the origin of the sucking habits. Graber (Ch. 18 in Falkner, *Human Development*, 1966) concludes that finger-sucking confined to the first three years may produce damage to the occlusion in the anterior segment, but the damage is usually temporary if the child has started with a normal occlusion. Whereas Class II, Division 1 malocclusions are sometimes ascribed to the finger-sucking habit, the basic malformation is not much affected, whereas malocclusion of the anterior teeth may result. The permanence of the deformation increases if the habit persists beyond three and one-half years, and is further enhanced if perioral and lingual habits are adopted which continue to exert pressures on the teeth and dental arches. Two factors of prime importance are the frequency (constancy) of the habit, and secondly, the intensity with which it is pursued. According to this concept, if the child has sufficient feelings of security developed from early association with the mother's body and

[3] For more extensive readings on the topic of etiologies of malocclusion, the reader should consult textbooks of orthodontics such as Moyers, 1959 (Chapter 3) and Graber, 1963, 1966).

enough opportunity to satisfy his innate craving for sucking activity, there is less chance that abnormal dependency on finger sucking will develop.

Mouth breathing is also asserted to produce malocclusion. According to Moyers (1958, p. 122).

> The typical mouth-breathing syndrome is characterized by contraction of the maxillary denture, labioversion of the maxillary anterior teeth, crowding of the anterior teeth in both arches, hypertrophy and chapping of the lower lip, hypotonicity and apparent shortening of the maxillary lip and frequently marked overbite.

Salzmann (1950, p. 424) states:

> Whether or not mouth-breathing is a primary cause of malocclusion is relatively unimportant. The fact that in the mouth-breather a muscle complex is present which tends to produce narrowing, or interference with, the lateral widening of the maxillary arch. When the lower lip in the mouth-breather falls lingual to the normally erupted maxillary incisors, protrusion of the maxillary incisors and narrowing of the lateral segments of the dental arches is encouraged.

Another feature of mouth breathing of significance to both dentist and speech pathologist is lingual posture. A lowered tongue carriage not only fails to balance properly the extra oral pressures, but does not provide a posture from which accurate articulatory placement can be achieved. The tongue tends to lie between the upper and lower teeth, resting forward of the normal position. (See section on maxillary protractions for further discussion in relation to speech.)

The action of the circumoral musculature at rest and during swallowing is conditioned in part by breathing habits, and in part by the configuration of the underlying bones. One of the troublesome conditions of orthodontic treatment is the active contraction of the mentalis muscles in everting the lower lip in a Class II, Divisiion 1 malocclusion when the patient swallows. Whereas the relationship of the lower lip to the upper anterior teeth may be caused primarily by the patient's attempt to adapt to his relatively protracted maxilla, the resulting muscular pressures on the maxilla tend to exaggerate the condition and to tilt the teeth labially (Sclare, 1957; Ricketts, 1958).

In consideration of the influence of muscle action upon bone growth, it follows logically that whereas speech may be affected by the form of the face and jaws, the habits of muscular action in speech may also play a part in inflecting bone growth, an observation that has been made by Froeschels (1933), Greene (1937), Palmer (1948), and others. Henry (1937) and Jaffe (1962) suggested speech drills for the improvement of occlusion, but there is little experimental evidence to support the recommendation.

Tongue-Thrusting

The search for causes of malocclusions has led to the identification of habit patterns associated with swallowing as a possible source of maldevelopment. Straub (1960, 1961, 1962) has indicated bottle-feeding as a source of maladaptive feeding patterns of infants, and has recommended a special form of nipple as a means of avoiding the establishment of abnormal swallowing patterns. He has also described an elaborate system by which new habit patterns may be taught. Lewis and Counihan (1965), on the other hand, studied 294 newborn infants and found that 99 percent were noted to have tongue-thrust as defined by sucking or swallowing behavior in which the tongue was protruded over the lower gum pad. Ballard and Bond (1960) and a number of British orthodontists have advanced the concept that endogenous patterns of growth provide the major controlling factors, and that the modifications attributable to the influence of behavior patterns are of secondary significance. Ballard (1962) further asserts that endogenously established tongue-thrust should be distinguished from habit thrust, since the open bite associated with the former will tend to disappear at around 11 or 12 years of age, although the lingual patterns of swallowing may persist. These and many other studies have focused attention on the possible influence of muscle contraction patterns of lingual and perioral muscles on the developing structures of the mouth and face. Harvold (1968) in an ingenious experiment with adult monkeys has shown that alterations in tongue behavior induced by irritation, surgical alteration, or the use of interfering devices (for instance, a wedge wired into position in the palate to disrupt normal tongue movements in swallowing) changes the oral environment, disrupts the normal patterns of oral movement, and causes maladaptive patterns of muscle contraction which eventually lead to malformations of the jaws.

Fletcher, Casteel, and Bradley (1961) have shown that many children identified as having concurrent abnormal swallowing patterns, speech defects, and malocclusions are in a developmental stage between six and nine years of age in which the structural relationships and functional patterns will later adapt maturationally without therapeutic intervention if the child is healthy and otherwise normal. Kutt (1967) identified two types of open-bite (on the basis of vertical and anteroposterior maxillary and mandibular tooth relationships) and found that the prevalence of anterior tongue-thrust decreased significantly with age, although the prevalence of tooth-apart swallow and anterior tongue-thrust showed a less rapid decline in the children identified as having open-bite.

Bloomer (1963, 1967) has called attention to the highly complex nature of speech and swallowing, and the difficulty in defining and differentiating the significant feature of normal and abnormal swallowing. He further noted the differences in diadochokinetic performance between some speakers noted to have malocclusion, suspected abnormal swallow, and defective speech. He postulated that the observed dysdiadochokinetic patterns were due to a delay in neural maturation or possible subclinical damage to the cortico rubrocerebellar pathways or to the hemispheres of the cerebellum. The postulate of neural damage as a basis for abnormal lingual diadochokinesis has received further support from his clinical observations of patients who have demonstrable brain damage and whose swallowing and diadochokinetic patterns are altered to resemble those of children with suspected abnormal swallowing and dysdiadochokinesis.

Literature which has focused on the subject of abnormal swallowing, malocclusion, and defective speech is too vast for review and summary here. Suffice it to say that many questions are unresolved concerning the etiology of the swallowing behavior, the degree to which it conditions or is conditioned by the oral environment, the social environment, inherited mechanisms, or the effects of neural damage, or oral disease (e.g. tonsilar disease and inflammation, Moyers, 1959, p. 118). Questions concerning the diagnosis of abnormal swallowing, its significance for the developing occlusion, and the proper methods of management for persons suspected of abnormal swallowing patterns are also open to debate.

In general the viewpoints regarding tongue-thrusting cluster about two more or less opposite poles. First, muscularly induced pressures and tensions are a major cause of occlusal deformities; tongue-thrusting is a learned "habit"; and it can be eliminated by appropriate myotherapy (tongue-thrust therapy). Second, malocclusions, even in those individuals with swallowing behavior that appears to be abnormal, are due to multiple causes; dependence on a generally prescribed formula of muscle training as the principle basis of treatment is inappropriate; and treatment should be based on a program emphasizing correct diagnosis of the contributing etiological factors.

If one examines further the assumptions of those who argue for a system of tongue-thrust therapy, he will find them to run something like this:

1. There are normal and abnormal patterns of swallowing, and these can be positively identified by the use of relatively simple observational procedures (e.g., through observations of a patient's swallowing patterns in response to command while the lower lip is manually depressed by the examiner).

2. Tongue-thrusting is an abnormal feature of oral behavior which develops as a deviant response to oral stimulation, is probably learned, and will persist despite changes in the oral environment unless the behavioral pattern is corrected by training.

3. Tongue-thrust and other forms of abnormal swallowing are major causes of dental malocclusion (especially of anterior open-bite) and of defective speech (especially interdental lisping).

a) These can be demonstrated to exist concurrently and, since muscle forces are believed to affect bone growth, it can be assumed logically that lingual pressures are responsible for the special forms of malocclusion observed to exist in the individual with abnormal oral behavior patterns.

b) It is further assumed that, since the former statement is true, the malocclusions and the defective speech articulations will not be responsive to orthodontic treatment as long as the abnormal oral behavior persists.

4. Abnormal orofacial habits (especially tongue and lip habits) can be corrected by instructing the patient to swallow correctly.

a) The training will result in oral behavior which will become stabilized as a habit.

b) The retrained oral behavior will improve, or at least permit the improvement of dental occlusion and speech.

5. Speech therapists will be qualified to undertake such training of patients after the therapists have been taught (usually through a special course of relatively short duration) a prescribed method of retraining.

a) It is ethical for speech therapists to undertake this work.

b) They are justified in charging for the treatment on a "fee-for-service" basis.

c) If the abnormal oral behavior is associated with defective speech, the therapist may undertake the training without special medical or dental consultation.

The opponents of generalized, prescribed "tongue-thrust therapy" base their skepticism on the following concepts:

1. There are probably normal and abnormal patterns of swallowing, but these are often difficult to identify with certainty; their existence is not proved by one or two simple observations, and may require relatively sophisticated procedures of study such as electromyography and cineradiography.

2. Although tongue protrusion may be an abnormal feature of swallowing in the older child and the adult its origins are obscure.

a) Tongue protrusion during swallow is a "normal" behavior at some stages of human development and under certain conditions of the oral environment (e.g. during the "suckling stage" or following loss of the upper or lower central incisors).

b) Tongue-thrusting may stem from a variety of causes, including endogenously determined factors, or may be conditioned by the oral environment, and hence may not represent a learned pattern susceptible to retraining.

3. Dental malocclusions and defective speech articulation may develop from many causes (of which abnormal lingual behavior is only one), and the direct relationship between tongue-thrusting and any individual instance of dental malocclusion and defective speech must not be assumed from the observance of coexistence.

a) Coexistence of phenomena does not prove dynamic relationship.

b) The argument of "post hoc, ergo proter hoc" represents a fallacious line of reasoning.

c) Tongue-thrusting, dental malocclusions, and defective speech articulation may all represent manifestations of the same etiologic primordium.

d) The modification or elimination of "tongue-thrust swallowing" may not have a directly observable effect on occlusion or speech.

4. Tongue behavior may be changed by a variety of means, and it is difficult if not impossible to prove that tongue retraining (with or without orthodontic collaboration) is the best, or even an effective means of changing patterns of swallowing.

a) There is clinical evidence that some forms of tongue-thrust probably are not changed by exercises.

b) Some patterns change after the oral environment is changed; or other circumstances of growth and function of the orofacial complex change, or patterns change as the patient grows older.

5. Some speech therapists may become qualified to undertake the diagnosis and treatment of abnormal patterns of oral behavior.

a) The knowledge required should include much information about human growth and development in all of its complexities.

b) It is doubtful that a short course dealing primarily with a "system" for retraining lingual behavior provides adequate instruction for the would-be therapist.

c) Adequate diagnosis and treatment requires interdisciplinary professional consultation and frequently justifies medical, dental, and speech cooperation in the treatment program.

d) The ethics of undertaking treatment of a problem outside the specialized scope of the speech pathologist is questionable unless the patient understands that the treatment is experimental and that the results cannot be predicted with accuracy.

COMMUNICATION DISORDERS, MALOCCLUSIONS, AND RELATED OROFACIAL ANOMALIES

The point of view has been expressed in a variety of ways in this chapter that orofacial structures are not necessarily to be considered prime causes of defective articulation. Speakers have demonstrated that the oral mechanisms are capable of many compensatory adaptations by which intelligible speech can be produced even though the patients are deformed. The diagnostician and the therapist have responsibility for determining to what extent adaptation is not merely possible, but feasible, and to know what practicable measures can be taken to improve functional potential by seeking the assistance of the surgeon and the dentist. However, the pure mechanics of articulatory adjustment is not the only thing of importance, for the way that a patient feels about his abnormality (his acceptance of his handicap, his feeling of defensiveness and hesitancy about entering into social groups) may be of equal importance to him, and may determine to a considerable extent whether he succeeds in learning to use his speech mechanism effectively.

In the sections which follow, abnormalities which stand in potential functional relationship to the articulatory valves of speech will be described. The reader is asked to keep in mind the intricate nature of the functional interdependencies of all of the processes of speech, and to realize that there will always be exceptions to any general statement which is made.

A catalogue of the speech sounds which may be distorted by various anatomical deformities will not be very helpful to the clinician in reference to a particular patient since the variables are likely to differ for each one, defying valid generalization. A general description of the various types of speech disorder, and a consideration of the dynamics of the relationship between anatomy and speech may, however, assist the clinician in determining what to look for in his search for etiolgic factors, and in outlining his approach to treatment. It may help him decide what modifications of structure he should hope for from collaborating specialists, and in determining a prognosis for the patient's eventual development of satisfactory speech. No ethical speech pathologist would want to encourage a patient falsely, but to deny a patient realistic hope would be cruel indeed.

Defective sounds are produced if the essential valves described in Table 28-1 are not properly created because of abnormal oral structures or maladaptive patterns of articulatory movement. The nature of the articulatory defects thus caused is usually one of distortion rather than complete omission or substitution, although almost any form of defective articulation can occur. Some of the distortions are aesthetically displeasing; others will interfere seriously with intelligibility. In most instances, some improvement can be achieved.

Deformities of the Mouth Opening

ASTOMIA AND MICROSTOMIA

In rare instances children may be born without a mouth opening (astomia, or oral atresia) or with an abnormally small mouth. Since the deformity is a projection of developmental failure in the first trimester of pregnancy, it is usual for other anomalies to exist concurrently. The case reported briefly below from the records of The University of Michigan Hospital and the Speech Clinic illustrates an instance of this deformity and the nature of the speech defect associated with it.

L.W. was born with an atresia of the mouth, characterized by micrognathis, a continuous wall of mucous membrane, and congenital bilateral fusion of the mandible and maxilla and the lateral pterygoid plates. An anterior aperture was created shortly after birth by extraction of a left central incisor so that the infant could be fed. Several subsequent attempts were made surgically to give the patient a functional jaw, but after each operation heavy scarring prevented sustained mobilization of the lower jaw. Although it appears that the temperomandibular joint is potentially functional, the mandible is underdeveloped, and the range of mandibular movement at six years of age is scarcely one-fourth of an inch.

Speech evaluations on three occasions between two and six years of age showed delay in the initiation of speech and subsequent articulatory defects after functional speech developed. At six years her anterior teeth are in open-bite relationship, lingual movements are poorly controlled in both speech and deglutition, and the speech is markedly defective in articulation. She has had no speech-training and the parents have evidently made comparatively little effort to provide speech stimulation or to encourage function and growth of the oral structures.

Microstomia is often associated with micrognathia and microglossia. It has a number of manifestations, many of them of congenital origin, but some (epidermolysis bullosa, syderopenic dysphagia) appear later in life as a feature of disease (Gorlin and Pindborg, 1964). Microstomia is reported by Gorlin and Pindborg in Trisomy 21 (monogolism), Trisomy 18 (Edward's Syndrome), craniocarpotarsal dystrophy (Whistling Face Syndrome), mandibulofacial dysostosis (Treacher Collins Syndrome), micrognathia, polydactyly and genital anomalies, and oculomandibulo dyscephaly with hypotrichosis. The specific effects which these diseases have upon speech are seldom reported. In most instances of microstomia, one can assume that there are so many other maladies, including severe mental retardation, that the speech involvements directly attributable to the mouth deformity may be of minor significance in the communication disorder.

MACROSTOMIA

Macrostomia (abnormally large mouth) is usually a condition of congenital origin representing incomplete fusion of the maxillary-mandibular embrylogic processes, and is not infrequently found in association with other manifestations of oral and facial cleft. It has been mentioned as a feature of mandibulofacial dysostosis (Hunt and Smith, 1955) and of first and second branchial arch syndrome (VRA Conference on Facial Disfigurement, 1963). Speech performance will depend on the degree to which labial function is limited, and the other anomalous features present.

Case Report: A 12-year-old boy was examined with partial right facial cleft, ipsilateral mandibular micrognathia, right unilateral lingual hypoplasia and poor lingual function, microtia with associated hearing loss, and postoperative cleft palate, and malocclusion. Speech intelligibility was poor to fair, voice quality was hypernasal, and speech articulation showed distortion of consonants related to poor lingual control. The speech characteristics in general were attributable to the complex of anatomical and functional disorders rather than to specific inability to achieve satisfactory labial function.

Grabb and Smith (1968) state that the first and second branchial arch syndrome is rarely inherited but is the second commonest malformation from thalidomide ingestion during pregnancy. Included among the anomalies which characterize the syndrome are ear defects (auricular, external auditory canal, and middle ear), mandibular, maxillary, zygomatic and temporal bone underdevelopment, first branchial cleft sinus, and paralysis or hypoplasia of muscles of the face, palate, tongue, and masticatory group. The manifestations are usually unilateral, and may be associated with other skeletal anomalies and eye defects.

ANOMALIES OF LABIAL FORM AND FUNCTION

References to anomalies of the lips affecting speech and dental occlusion usually pertain to the upper lip, although both lips may be involved, and in instances of mentalis activity associated with Class II, Division 1 malocclusion, the lower lip may be at fault. Among the commonly listed lip deformities and dysfunctions (excluding cleft lip) are 1. labial underdevelopment, 2. labial deficiency from disease, trauma, or surgery, 3. restricted labial mobility from scarring or a short labial frenum, 4. immobility due to paralysis, 5. marked asymmetry of muscle contraction, 6. tumors and mucoid cysts of the lip, 7. excessive fullness (as in the Melkersson-Rosenthal Syndrome) or thickness with redundancy of lip tissues (macrocheilia) as in "double lip", protrusion and redundancy of the lower lip and median pseudocleft of the upper lip (Gorlin and Pindborg, 1964, p. 440). Even though the lips may not be deformed, they may be functionally impaired by the mechanical interference to labial closure caused by protruding anterior teeth, or because of positional malrelationship due to excessively protracted or retracted mandible or maxilla.

Quick alternate closure and release of the lips provides a pneumatic valve for the articulation of the bilabial consonants /p/, /b/ and /m/. Labial constriction has an important acoustic function in the articulation of /w/ and /ʍ/, the rounded vowels /ə/, /o/, /ʊ/, /u/, and the diphthongs /au/ and /əi/. Although these sounds can be imitated with approximate accuracy by predominantly linguadental and linguapalatal movements, the acoustic effect is qualitatively different from that which accompanies normal lip action. An effect of abnormal lip function is described by Froeschels (1940), who notes excessive tension of the lips in vocal hyperfunction Number Seven. Abnormal lip postures and malfunctions are described below in connection with the discussion on abnormal habits of swallowing. The establishment of a balance between the lips, tongue, and cheeks is especially important during the years of physical growth of the face.

In the Melkersson-Rosenthal Syndrome edematous swelling of the lips may accompany facial swelling and paralysis which is said to be clinically indistinguishable from Bell's Palsy (Gorlin and Pindborg, 1964). Plication of the tongue occurs in approximately one-third of cases, but its functional significance for speech is not mentioned in several reports describing the syndrome.

Double lip may occur alone or in combination with relaxation of the skin of the eyelid (blepharochalasis) as in Ascher's Syndrome (Gorlin and Pindborg, 1964, p. 186). The excessive tissue of the lips in macrocheilia may be evident only on smiling (Fomon et el. 1965), although a patient observed by the author showed an inner labial fold of both lips even at rest. In this patient no significant manifestations of speech disorder associated with the labial deformity were apparent.

Treatment for cosmetic reasons should be referred to a plastic surgeon for evaluation. Median pseudocleft of the upper lip is reported by Gorlin and Pindborg (1964, p. 440) to occur in orodigitofacial dysostosis. The apparent cleft is due to frenular hyperplasia, which eradicates the mucofacial fold in this area. It is not known if any speech disorder occurs.

Eversion of the lower lip is frequently associated with maxillary protraction. Whether the condition is endogenously caused or reflects persistence of a habit of early lip-sucking or biting, the patient adapts his labial postural, swallowing, and speech habits to the labially tipped maxillary anterior teeth. In such cases the lower lip pressures are thought to accentuate the already existing malocclusion. This effect of the lower lip is often further complicated by the coexistence of an incompetent or shortened upper lip so that the pressures of the tongue and lower lip on the upper dental arch are virtually unopposed by the retractive force normally provided by the upper lip. In these cases the upper lip may be congenitally short, or its structural deficiency may be exacerbated by habitual disuse. Mentalis hyperactivity and abnormal lower lip posture, together with malocclusion and a maxillo-alveolar orientation of the tongue tip may cause sibilant distortion (stridency). The distortion may be overcome by relaxation of the mentalis muscles, while simultaneously "spreading" the lips and orienting the tongue tip toward the lower incisor position for production of /s/.

Functional adaptation of the lips will probably take place if the malocclusion can be corrected. Warrer (1959) found malocclusion and mentalis hyperactivity associated in 90 percent of his subjects, whereas patients having normal occlusion showed little evidence of excessive mentalis activity. Tulley (1953, 1954, 1957, 1961, 1962) relates muscle activity primarily as an adaptation to morphology, and states that lip function will change adaptively when the occlusion becomes more nearly normal. Fortuntately for the patient and his attending speech pathologist, the resting position of the lower lip and its function in swallowing does not necessarily predict its malfunction in speech, inasmuch as the mandible can often be shifted forward during speech to bring the lower lip into satisfactory functional position with respect to the upper lip and upper anterior teeth.

An abnormally thick or short upper labial frenum can restrict movement of the upper lip. Its main consequence, however, is more likely to be seen in abnormally wide spacing (diastema) of the upper central maxillary incisor teeth. This diastema is sometimes blamed for sibilant distortion. In the author's opinion, however, this assumed cause-effect relationship is seldom a valid one, but is more likely due to deficiency of the upper lip function which in its elevated and incompetent contraction fails to cover the teeth and thus to provide a "baffle" to modulate the sibilant air stream. When the patient's lip is lowered and slightly tensed, the quality of the sibilant sound will usually improve. A similar effect of the upper lip has been observed in children who lisp after loss of the upper incisor teeth. If tongue position is essentially normal the upper lip can replace the baffle formerly provided by the teeth.

In cases of maxillary deficiency the upper lip may be so far retruded in reference to the lower lip that normal bilabial contact or labiodental contact is difficult or impossible. The major cause of the defective lip position lies in the maxillary retrusion, which fails to provide support to the lip. In such instances, if there is sufficient labial tissue and flexibility to permit, it may be possible to compensate by the use of an anterior maxillary prosthesis which will "plump" the upper lip and bring it forward. Where upper lip tissue is deficient and the lower lip is redundant, the plastic surgeon may use the Abbe flap procedure to supply extra tissue for the upper lip. Congenital shortness of the upper lip may require a lengthening procedure by surgery (Ford, 1944).

Lip function is also said to be improved by exercises. Johnson (1940) advised drills to strengthen the lips to overcome lip dysfunctions contributing the dental malocclusion and especially to eliminate hyperfunction of the mentalis muscles. Harrington and Breinholt (1963) advise counterpressure to a tongue-blade pressed against the lip. Phonetic drills involving bilabial consonants, and the practice of vigorous articulation of /oo-ee-oo-ee/ can sometimes be helpful. The author has also advised the use of a drinking straw in developing adequate lip function. Ballard (1951) warns that mere exercises will never change lip posture; the change must be achieved by reeducating the muscular system to a new pattern of behavior.

In those instances in which correction of the labial deformity is not possible, adaptations for speech can be made by substituting the upper lip for the lower, as in producing the phonemes /f/ and /v/. The lower lip may be brought into compression against the upper teeth for labial plosives. The tongue may be used to approximate the labial sound if no lip is present. A patient whose upper lip had been surgically removed (Bloomer, 1953) was able to speak with moderate intelligibility even though the upper lip, the anterior two-thirds of the maxilla, and all of the teeth were missing. Palmer (1948) describes the case of a nine-year-old boy whose face was paralyzed by bulbar polio. He was successfully trained to substitute tongue-tip for labial movements. Substitutions of this sort are basic in ventriloquism.

Dental Malocclusion, Deformities of the Maxilla and Mandible

Malocclusions and malpositioned teeth are contributory causes of articulatory defects, and are of special interest to the diagnostician of speech because of the complexity of relationship which exists between occlusal development and the motor aspects of speech and deglutition.

Anomalies of Individual Teeth and Groups of Teeth

NEUTROCCLUSION—CLASS I

The basic arch relationships as defined by Angle are normal in cases of neutrocclusion, but there may be anomalies of individual tooth position which prevent the normal valving contacts of the tongue and lips. Almost any severe interference with tongue or lip activity can cause articulatory distortions, although in actuality such distortions most frequently occur in conditions of open-bite or severe crossbite.

The condition, size, or texture of individual teeth probably has relatively little direct influence on speech. The presence or absence of teeth and the position which they occupy in the dental arches may, however, directly or indirectly affect the quality of a speaker's enunciation.

Lischer's system of designating the malpositions of individual teeth has already been described in a preceding section of this chapter (Fig. 28-11). Other useful terms, similar in function, include ectopic eruption (eruption out of normal position), supernumerary teeth, diastema (abnormal spacing of the teeth), missing teeth (whether due to extraction or failure to erupt), anodontia (congenital absence of teeth), and oligodontia (the presence of only a few teeth).

Severe labial inclination of the anterior upper incisor teeth will markedly interfere with bilabial articulation, and may cause sibilant distortion. Anterior teeth in linguoversion, especially when they distort the shape of the anterior alveolar arch of the maxilla, make it particularly difficult for the speaker to enunciate sibilant consonants with clarity.

It is doubtful that the absence of individual teeth can be considered to be a significant cause of articulatory disorder when the loss occurs in adult life. The loss of a tooth or teeth in childhood sometimes is a contributing factor in sibilant distortion, but usually is only one of two or three factors which interrelate (e.g., with maladaptive lingual grooving, abnormal labial function). As indicated above, excessive spacing of the central incisors (diastema) may affect the quality of the sibilants somewhat but should not be considered a primary cause of lisping.

Anodontia or oligodontia may be found rarely in the child with a delayed speech or a dyslalia, although it is dubious whether the absence of teeth alone can be the basic cause of the disorder. It is more likely that predisposing factors of a congenital nature are responsible for the speech pattern. Nevertheless, artificial dentures may be beneficial to speech and are esthetically important. The problem of premature loss of deciduous or permanent teeth in children should not be ignored by the speech clinician, however, since these losses may contribute to eventual malocclusion of a serious nature. The child in adapting to premature dental loss may also develop habits of lingual movement which are retained even after the second teeth have erupted. This is not so likely to be true of the child whose speech is normal before loss of the teeth, and even the loss of the central incisors often produces no noticeable effect on the child's speech (Froeschels, 1941). The significance of premature loss of teeth is related to the general health of the individual, and if the pattern of loss results in facial disfigurement, the personality of the individual may be impaired.

A completely edentulous person may have some difficulty in making fricative sounds clearly, and the /f/ and /v/ may be particularly difficult to enunciate. Properly constructed artificial dentures will usually bring a return of correct articulation if they are made with due regard to the articulatory habits of the patient and the pattern of occlusion present in his own teeth before their loss.

Maxillary Deformities

In discussing the relationship of the teeth to speech, Greene (1937) states that the ". . . existence or nonexistence of the teeth is not so important for good speech as the shape and roof of the mouth. . . . Defects in enunciation can also be caused by the condition of the arches, especially the side arches. In 92 percent of all cases of lateral lisp, the larger arch is on the lisping side." Herman (1943), in comparing the palatal configurations of lispers and normal subjects, found no significant differences between the palates of 26 lispers and 400 random selections used by Crane and Ramstrum (1943) in classifying palate shapes. Clinical observations of patients with deformities of the hard palate and alveolar arches subsequent to surgery for congenital cleft suggests, however, that there is a general tendency for the lingual groove to follow the direction of the palatal groove, and usually there is a distortion of sibilant sounds in the speech of such patients.

Luchsinger and Arnold (1965) discuss the speech symptoms of malocclusions under the term "dental dysglossia." Nine varieties of oral lisp and four varieties of nasal lisp are listed or described (p. 564 ff). Presumably most of the oral forms of lisp are subject to the influence of dental malocclusion. The authors indicate a 60–70 percent incidence of dental malocclusion among lispers, whereas normal speakers include only 25 percent with malocclusion. Their analysis of the statistical reports by several investigators leads them to the conclusion that whereas lisping is more frequent among speakers with dental malocclusion than among those with normal occlusion, the role of dentition is only a predisposing one, and other pathological conditions (e.g., hearing loss) must be considered in the diagnosis. Jaffe (1964) indicates that whereas wrong positioning of the tongue may be the primary cause of lisping, maxillary arch anomalies, especially during the period of mixed dentition, must also be included as a major cause.

Bernstein (1956) studied a group of 152 subjects of which approximately 35 percent had malocclusions. He found a realtionship between open-bite and lisping, but the severity of the lisp did not vary with the amount of open-bite nor the amount of overjet. Blythe (1959) in a study of 200 children (orthodontic patients) concluded that skeletal morphology has little if any influence on the occurrence of sigmatism because the tongue is capable of compensatory movements. He did find a close relationship between Class II, Division 1 malocclusions and interdental lisping but blamed tongue behavior rather than the incisor relationship for the speech disorder. A slight tendency for association between lateral lisp and Class II, Division 2 malocclusion was suggested. Subtelny, Mestre, and Subtelny (1964) note a tendency for the defective speakers with Class II, Division 1 malocclusion to "front" the tongue tip relative to the lower incisors, whereas the normal speakers with the same type of malocclusion adapted by retruding the tongue. Ronson (1965) identified a high incidence of "visceral swallowing" among lispers.

Maxillary Protraction (Distocclusion)

The discussion of speech defects associated with maxillary protraction includes all of those dental malocclusions in which the mandibular teeth are posterior (distal) to their normal position with respect to the maxillary teeth. This condition may be present in maxillary protraction, mandibular retraction, protrusion of the maxillary incisors, or retrusion of the mandibular incisors. Thus the anomalies affecting speech may include the various forms of Angle Class II malocclusion, those Angle Class I malocclusions in which the maxillary teeth are in marked labioversion to the mandibular anteriors, the condition of micrognathia, and certain defects of the temporomandibular joints.

The influence of maxillary protraction (or mandibular retraction) upon speech should always be considered in relation to the adequacy of tongue and lip function. A mild labioversion of the maxillary incisors may impede the correct formation of the bilabial plosive consonants if the upper lips is short of lacking in mobility, whereas a speaker with normal lip function may, under similar or even extreme conditions of labioversion of the maxillary incisors, make correct bilabial approximations for these sounds.

In general, excessive protraction tends to 1. increase the difficulty in producing normally articulated bilabial sounds (Greene, 1937), 2. make it more difficult for the speaker to form acoustically acceptable sibilants (Wolfe, 1937), and 3. modify the quality of the sibilants in characteristic ways. The acoustic effect on the sibilants has to do presumably with the difficulty which the speaker finds in directing the air current in relation to the teeth. West (1957) and others have emphasized the need to have a narrow air blade directed against the cutting edge of a tooth for the production of an /s/ sound. It can be shown, however, that the cutting edge of the teeth, although it undoubtedly contributes to sibilance, is not essential to it. It has been noted clinically that patients who have a severely protracted maxilla or who may even have lost all anterior teeth, may use the upper or lower lips to create the requisite air turbulence for satisfactory sibilant consonants (Wolfe, 1937). (See p. 738 above.)

A man whose mandibular deformity was similar to that shown in Fig. 28-13, except that the temperomandibular joint was not ankylosed, was able to produce good /s/ and /z/ consonants when the lip and tongue movements were properly coordinated during speech. When the lower lip was pulled away from the /f/ position which it characteristically assumed during the production of sibilants, the /s/ and /z/ were no longer clear.

The matter of palate height in relation to articulatory defects is sometimes mentioned as an etiological factor in dyslalia. The author recalls a case in which a dentist was so impressed by the high narrow arch of a patient that he constructed a small prosthetic palate to fill in the vault of the patient's hard palate. The prosthesis was, of course, more hinderance than help, since there is relatively little relationship between palatal height and articulation unless for some reason the range of lingual movement is abnormally small. It is usually the restriction in arch width preventing or making difficult the lingual contacts around the

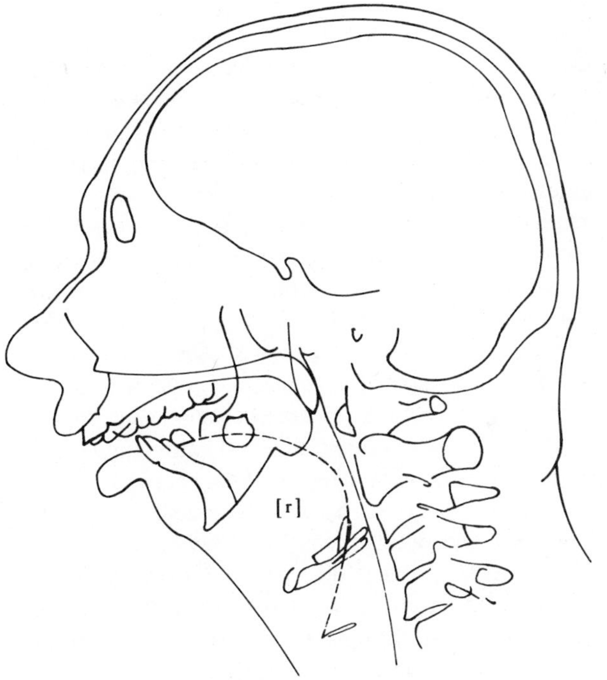

Fig. 28-13. Subject with ankylosis of the temperomandibular joints, with subsequent micrognathia and mandibular retraction.

alveolar borders of the maxillary teeth which impedes articulation. This is particularly true if the mandibular arch is of comparatively greater width, so that the tongue is able to contact only the occlusal surfaces of the maxillary teeth. If the arch is abnormally flat, the speaker can usually be taught to make the necessary lingual adaptations for clear speech.

Angle (1907, p. 413) describes a case in which ". . . the vault of the arch and bones of the nose . . . became involved until normal breathing became impossible, and as the space for the tongue was so greatly restricted, it was with much difficulty that the man could enunciate his words sufficiently to be understood." The relationship between maxillary contraction and mouth-breathing have been noted, and thus the significance of the structural defect may be useful to the speech clinician in his study of the history of his patient. As described by Massler and Schour (1946), mouth breathing leads to upper respiratory infection. The growing structures of the face are affected so that the face becomes markedly elongated and narrowed (adenoid facies), caused by dropping of the mandible into open position and by constriction of the upper arch and the palate. The nostrils are narrowed from disuse, and the facial expression becomes dull and drawn. The habit of mouth breathing and enlargement of the pharyngeal tonsils both contribute to the typical facial configuration. Correction of the deformity requires removal of the nasopharyngeal obstruction, orthodontic treatment, and muscle exercises to strengthen the lips.

The significance of mouth breathing to the speech clinician lies in the concomitant effects of the habit upon orofacial structures and their function. The lips become slack, the upper lip shortened and elevated over the maxillary incisors, the lower lip lies beneath and behind the upper incisors, and the upper teeth become spaced and protruding. There is hypertrophy of the gingival tissues. The tongue is suspended between the arches or lies on the floor of the mouth so that its molding action is lost to the upper jaw. The unopposed pressure of the check muscles gradually forces the maxillary arch to become narrowed and V-shaped, with a high palatal arch. The mandible is retruded and the mouth hangs open. The maxillary sinuses and the nasal cavity become narrowed as the upper arch is contracted. The turbinates become swollen and engorged. The nasal mucosa become atrophic from disuse and the alae nasi are red and pinched. The sense of smell is dulled, often accompanied by loss of taste sensation and decrease in appetite. Hyperplasia of the lymphoid tissues around the Eustachian tube may close it and contribute to hearing loss.

The speech of such individuals is more likely to show a composite of symptoms in which the etiology is appropriately complex. The symptoms will probably include hyponasality (Gardner 1949) or perhaps a mixed (hyper-hypo-) nasality, and articulatory distortions which result from interference with the normal mechanics of articulation and also from a loss of the normal auditory monitoring of speech.

The shaping of the alveolar arch of the maxilla can be important in the articulation of linguoalveolar sounds. The arch contours shown in Fig. 28-3 indicate clearly that there are marked differences in shape and angle of slope of the palate in adults. The speaker with a protracted maxilla or a retracted mandible (as in Fig. 28-13) will be aided in articulation of the consonants /s/ and /z/ if his maxillary alveolar arch rises gradually instead of abruptly behind the incisors.

Mandibular Deformities (Retrognathia, micrognathia, mandibular retraction)

A form of malocclusion functionally similar to that of maxillary protraction is found in the various forms of mandibular hypotrophy and retraction. The net effect for speech is much the same whether the mandible is retrognathic or the maxilla is prognathic, with the notable exception that in retrognathia (especially in micrognathia) a discrepancy in tongue size may be a complicating factor. The tongue may be too small (microglossia), in which case articulatory contacts with maxillary structures are difficult or impossible to achieve, and the mandibular arch may be abnormally narrowed due to the lack of normal pressures from the tongue to counteract those of the face. On the other hand, if the tongue is relatively too large for the small mandible (as in some early manifestations of Pierre Robin Syndrome) it will present mechanical obstruction to breathing, and perhaps to swallowing, if allowed to retract and fall back into the infant's oropharynx. Whether or not lingual size causes difficulty in articulation depends, of course, also on other factors, as indicated in the section on maxillary protraction.

Malfunction of the temporomandibular joint is often associated with micrognathia. Fixation (ankylosis) of the joint prevents normal motion, which should be a combination of hinge and gliding movement occurring at the articulation of the mandibular and temporal bones. This form of articulation permits extensive movements of the mandible for chewing and facilitates the tongue-positioning and movements required for speech. Ankylosis of the joint interferes with oral hygiene, prophylactic care and dental treatment, jaw growth, tooth alignment, and the functions of mastication and speech.

An extreme instance of fixation of the joint and distortion of micromandibular form is shown in Fig. 28-13. This patient's speech is characterized by articulatory maladaptations involving nearly all of the consonants. Vowel differentiation is impaired and the voice quality is muffled and hypernasal. Some improvement in his speech has been accomplished by careful attention to tongue and lip contacts, the use of a slower rate of speaking, and increased control of palatopharyngeal movement which is potentially adequate.

Surgical revision can lengthen the body of the mandible by sectioning it and sliding a portion of it forward. Such treatment usually requires a cooperative treatment plan from an orthodontist and other dental specialists. Although little published information has been found on the subject, verbal reports by surgeons indicate that patients are able to adjust functionally to the modified jaw and that their speech is improved.

PIERRE ROBIN SYNDROME

Congenital micrognathia is dramatically illustrated by the Pierre Robin syndrome in which the small mandible in combination with glossoptosis frequently leads to airway obstruction and feeding problems unless special care is taken to prevent this from happening. Infants with the fully developed syndrome show inspiratory distress characterized by stridor, cyanosis, and indrawing of the lower ribs and sternum (Dennison, 1965). Incomplete palatal clefts are frequently found. Smith and Stowe (1961) in a study of 39 cases note also the presence of several instances of hypotrophic tongue, enlarged tongue, short lingual frenum; ear defects including deformities and handicapping degrees of hearing loss; congenital heart defects, mental retardation; and ocular defects. Randall, Krogman, and Jahina (1965) in reviewing findings on 22 patients were able to divide them into three groups: 1. those with fairly normal mandibular growth; 2. those with persistent micrognathia with a severe Class II anterior relationship; and 3. those with persistent micrognathia who by forward positioning of the mandible and a flattening of the gonial angle were able to achieve fairly good occlusion. On the basis of these and other findings, they propose application of the term *retrognathia* rather than micrognathia in describing the Pierre Robin syndrome. Although speech information on these patients is limited, their speech has been described as hypernasal (Dennison, 1965), and articulatory defects are noted.

One patient whom the author has had an opportunity to follow over a period of several years had hypernasal speech because the palate was resected in infancy in order to provide an improved airway. Speech articulation was defective due to a moderately severe hearing loss and poor lingual coordination. Language was retarded, probably due to some degree of mental retardation and to the relatively long period of time which passed before the hearing loss was recognized and hearing amplification provided.

Another nine-year-old boy has a severe articulatory defect associated with severe hearing loss (partially compensated by bilateral bone-conduction aids). His voice is unusually high in pitch, and his stature is small. His mandible now approaches normal size.

The author has observed several patients whose tongue-tip mobility was impaired and tongue-tip consonants (especially sibilants) are affected as a result of a surgical procedure (Douglas, 1946) in which a tongue-tip adhesion is effected surgically to prevent glossoptosis and suffocation. Takagi, McCalla, and Bosma (1966) describe a procedure whereby prone feeding with the infant's neck extended, utilizing special nipples ("ducky" and "lamb" nipples fitted to a curved glass tube feeder) have permitted Pierre Robin infants to survive until sufficiently mature to feed and breathe without special assistance. Grabb (1968) states that feeding can be carried out with the child held bolt upright with the jaw held forward to avoid glossoptosis. Pruzansky and Richmond (1954) followed a series of Pierre Robin children by compiling cephalometric records of mandibular growth and concluded that where adequate nutrition for metabolic health can be provided, these children will eventually develop manidibular growth "adequate to reduce the retrognathic profile and provide an esthetically harmonious facial appearance."

The outcome of the speech of the children referred to in these reports is not known, but it must be assumed that those for whom a physiologically adaptive vegetative practice and respiratory control can be provided without surgical intervention will have a better chance of developing satisfactory articulation than those who risk the chance of lingual deformity through surgery.

TREACHER COLLINS SYNDROME

Retrognathia is also a usual feature of mandibulofacial dysostosis (Treacher Collins Syndrome). This congenital deformity affects primarily the structures derived from the first and second branchial arches, and is thought to have a strong hereditary component in etiology (Fernandez and Ronis, 1964). A unilateral form exists. In its complete from, Grabb (1968) lists antimongoloid slant of the palpebral fissures, notching of the lower eyelids, deficient or absent eyelashes of the medial two-thirds or thee-fourths of the lower lids, underdevelopment of the facial bones and of the external and middle ear, macrostomia, high palate, and malocclusion. Gorlin and Pindborg (1964) note that the mandible is almost always hypoplastic, the palate is cleft in about 40 percent of cases, and the malocclusion may be associated with open-bite. Hearing loss is found in a high percentage of cases.

Speech and language disturbances reported include delayed language development, articulatory defects (lingual and labial malarticulations), hypernasality, and central language disorder.

Two patients followed for several years at The University of Michigan, a brother and sister respectively 10 and 12 years of age when last seen, came from a mother who presented minimal characteristics of the syndrome. Both children showed most of the features described above including handicapping hearing loss. The boy had aural agenesis bilaterally with no canals. The girl had agenesis of the right canal and a small left stenotic canal and maximal conductive hearing loss. There was no cleft palate, but the girl's palate was observed to be "extremely elongated."

Description of speech: The boy's speech intelligibility is fairly good; lingual movements are somewhat slow and inaccurate; the lips function adequately; the micrognathia interferes with articulatory adaptations of the tongue; voice quality is hyponasal. Considering his multiple handicaps, he speaks surprisingly well.

The girl's speech intelligibility is fairly good; voice quality is mildly hyponasal, and there is some sibilant distortion (right lateral lisp); lip function is adequate; restricted mobility of the mandible interferes with mouth opening and hence affects voice quality and articulation to some extent, but its effects are slight.

Mandibular Protraction (Mesiocclusion)

This classification includes those cases in which the mandibular teeth are anterior (mesial) to their normal position in relationship to the maxillary teeth. It may thus include any of the Angle Class III malocclusions whether characterized by 1. macromandibular development (prognathous mandible, progenia, mandibular hypertrophy, Hapsburg jaw), 2. micromaxillary development (maxillary retraction), 3. marked labioversion of the mandibular teeth, or 4. marked linguoversion of the maxillary teeth so that they are in retroposition (distal) to the mandibular anterior teeth, 5. a pseudoprognathism caused by a patient's adaptation to insufficient vertical dimension of the maxilla, with forward thrust of the mandible as it is raised to meet the occlusal plane of the maxillary teeth, and 6. mandibular abstraction (lantern jaw) created by endogenous factors or by muscular paralysis. Most instances of prognathism are probably due to heredity, although pituitary disease is occasionally responsible. Brown and Cunningham (1961) report a Class III malocclusion in about half of a group of 80 mongoloid subjects.

Mandibular protraction may cause no difficulty in speech if the condition is relatively mild. Even a considerable deformity may cause no obvious articulatory defect if the lips and tongue can adapt to the structural handicap. Frequently, however, individuals who have this type of malocclusion have a tongue posture which is habitually low and somewhat flaccid so that a constriction of the linguoalveolar valve necessary for sibilants is not effectively produced. A further complication is often found in the relative distraction (abnormal expansion) of the mandibular arch (conversely, the relative contraction of the maxillary arch), so that the tongue is habitually brought into contact with the occusal edges of the maxillary teeth instead of being brought into proper contact with the alveolar arch and the linguodental surfaces. In such individuals the /f/ and /v/ consonants may be formed habitually by bringing the upper lip into contact with the incisal edges of the lower teeth or by approximating the two lips. The condition of mandibular protraction is oftentimes complicated by open-bite, and the speech symptoms are accentuated by missing teeth or malpositioned teeth which hamper adaptive articulatory movements.

In severe malocclusions of this general type, correction of the speech usually requires improvement or correction of the osseous or occlusal deformity. Depending on the nature and etiology of the abnormality, treatment may require osteotomy (bone surgery) such as that described by Dingman (1944), orthodontic treatment, the use of an anterior maxillary dental prosthesis, or a combination of procedures. In some cases the structurally rehabilitated patient is able to achieve clear speech without special instruction; others may require speech-training. In these instances the therapist will need to study carefully the posture of the body of the tongue, working with the patient to develop habits of mandibular position and lingua-palatal contacts which are specifically adapted to his structures.

Open-bite (infraclusion), Overbite (supraclusion), Collapsed Bite, and Cross-bite

The references to open-bite in connection with speech defects usually designate or assume an anterior open-bite relationship involving the incisors of both dental arches. There is also the possibility of a lateral open-bite which may impede linguoalveolar contact on the affected side (Greene 1937). If the anterior open-bite is extreme, it may interfere somewhat with bilabial and labiodental sounds (Gardner, 1949).

In open-bite the teeth of the upper and lower arches fail to contact. This condition can occur in a variety of ways which hold the possibility of interfering with speech articulation, especially in distortion of sibilant consonants. Some of the forms of anterior open-bite which are conducive to malarticulatory positioning of the tongue are shown in Fig. 28-14.

The most noticeable defect of speech associated with open-bite is likely to be distortion of the sibilants /s/, /z/, /ʃ/, /ʒ/, and possibly the /tʃ/ and /dʒ/. There is a tendency for the speaker to produce these consonants interdentally. Even if the tongue does not protrude interdentally, however, the sound may lack sibilance.

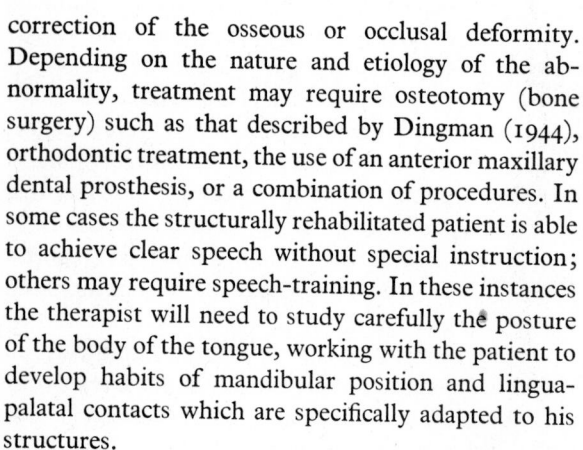

An adaptive constriction adequate to produce sibilance can be achieved, however, by placing the lower lip in relation to the air blade created by grooving of the tongue so that the requisite air turbulence is developed. Some attention may profitably be directed also to the general posture of the tongue within the mouth cavity to make sure that it occupies the best adaptive position for articulatory contact with the dental arches.

Open-bite can occur in all types of malocclusion,

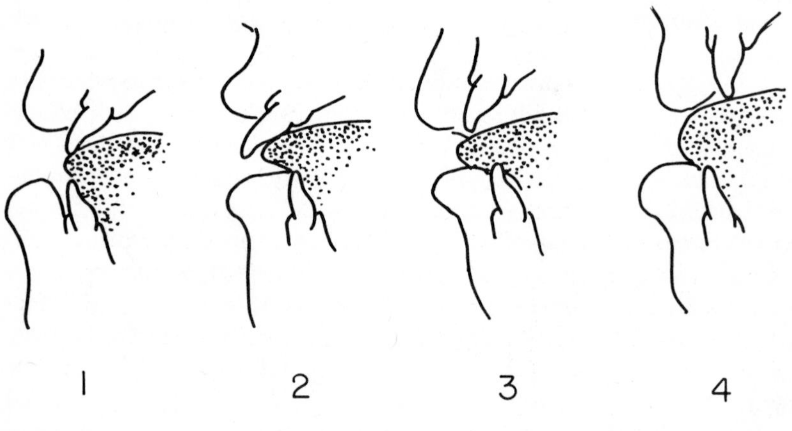

Fig. 28-14. Instances of "open bite" distorting sibilant articulation by encouraging forward positioning of lingual tip.

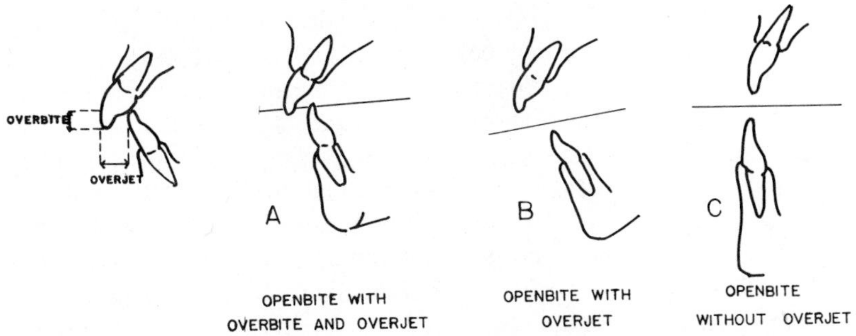

Fig. 28-15. Varieties of open bite associated with degrees of overjet.

and is often attributed to habitual interposition of the tongue, lips, fingers, thumb, or other objects between the teeth frequently enough, and with sufficient pressure, that the teeth are prevented from developing normal occlusion with the teeth of the opposing dental arch. Congenital growth factors may also be responsible. Abnormal swallowing may initiate and perpetuate the open-bite (Salzmann, 1950). Sucking habits are thought to be particularly influential in determining the forms of open-bite illustrated in (a) and (b) of Fig. 28-15.

According to Moyers (1962), however, it has not been clearly demonstrated that the magnitude and duration of tongue movements during speech are sufficient to influence the bone developments which contribute to the existence of open-bite. (Moyers, 1962, p. 72.)

Many forms of open-bite are responsive to treatment by orthodontic means, and the patient should be referred for orthodontic examination and advice as soon as the condition is recognized to exist. Inasmuch as sucking habits often are of etiological significance in such cases, proper planning in the early stages of development may prevent a disfigurement which would be difficult to treat in adult life.

There is no agreement as to a precise definition of open-bite. Two working definitions have been proposed: (A) a lack of vertical overlap of the anterior teeth; and (B) failure of the mandibular incisors to contact either the maxillary incisors or the palate when the buccal teeth are in maximum occlusion (Berger, 1961). Although not included in orthodontic definitions of open-bite, additional variations which have dynamic implications for the speech pathologist are illustrated in Fig. 28-15. In all cases, the relative positioning of the lips in reference to the teeth and the tongue are of significance in describing the articulatory patterns likely to contribute to sibilant distortion. Open-bite produces its effect on sibilant articulation not merely because of the anterior bite but because of the tendency of the tongue and lips to accommodate themselves to the relative positions of the teeth and the dental arches. That is, the acoustic distortion of sibilants /s/ and /z/ comes about because of the forward positioning of the tongue in reference to the anterior maxillary incisors.

CROSS-BITE

Extreme forms of cross-bite may interfere with lingua-alveolar contact (Palmer, 1948) and thus be a factor in the etiology of lateral and anterolateral lisp. This is particularly characteristic of cross-bite in which the entire mandible shifts so that the tongue is placed in a mechanically unfavorable position for sibilant articulation. In attempting to diagnose the basis for articulatory distortion the examiner must not overlook the possibility that other malrelationships (mild open-bite, lingualmotor problems, and malformation of the dental arches) may also be present as complicating factors.

Supraclusion (excessive overbite, or overclosure) is not generally thought to be a significant cause of defective speech, although Kessler (1953) suggests that speech may be adversely affected by inadequate lingual space in closed-bite relationship. Since the normally mobile mandible usually lowers into appropriate functional position for the tongue to make articulatory contacts, there is not much likelihood that consonants will be distorted.

The effect of "collapsed bite" in deciduous dentition is noted by Forde (1951) to prevent full eruption of the posterior permanent teeth. The collapse is said to force the tongue to a position of oral retraction, thus contributing to tonsilar and adenoidal complications.

Facial Malformations and Paralysis

Various deformities and disturbances of orofacial function accompany recognized syndromes and paralyses. Although the multiple anomalies which distinguish them may justify their inclusion under several categories of orofacial deformity, it is perhaps less confusing to present them in reference to the face itself. The categories included here are Sturge-Weber Syndrome, Turner's Syndrome, Moebius' Syndrome, progressive hemifacial atrophy, hemifacial hypertrophy, Klippel-Feil Syndrome, and Bell's Palsy. The speech symptoms which may accompany these malformations are seldom described in detail, but the nature of the deformities in their full manifestations are such that speech must certainly be affected. The deformities are included here to stimulate interest in accumulating information on the communication symptoms of the disorders.

ENCEPHALOFACIAL ANGIOMATOSIS (STURGE-WEBER SYNDROME)

The Sturge-Weber syndrome is a congenital vascular malformation affecting the brain, eyes, skin, and oral and nasal mucosa, probably originating during the sixth week of embryonic life (Peterman, 1958). It is characterized by venous angioma of the leptomeninges overlying the cerebral cotex, ipsilateral angiomatous lesions of the face (port-wine-stain facial nevi), ipsilateral calcifications of the brain, epilepsy and convulsions, mental retardation, and contralateral hemiplegia (Gorlin and Pindborg, 1964). Chao (1959) reported on seven school-age children; of these three were too retarded to speak, but those who, although mentally retarded, had speech, talked slowly, hesitantly, and speech was sluggish and incoherent. Asymmetry of the face was reported by Roizin (1959). Luc (1958) found abnormal development of the ears and a flattened nasal base in a small number of patients.

Royal (1966) and others indicate oral changes in the gingival mucosa ranging from slight vascular hyperplasia to huge masses of hypertrophied mucosa which make closure of the mouth impossible. The teeth are in ectopic eruption, and other dental anomalies are noted. Although it must be supposed that speech will be abnormal in such cases, and the size and form of the tongue may be affected, speech is not mentioned as a symptom in the references cited.

TURNER'S SYNDROME

Characteristic features of Turner's Syndrome which involve the orofacial region include small mouth with the corners drawn down by pterygium colli; high palatal vault; gingival asymmetry; asymmetry of facial bones and skull; and hypoplastic mandible. Cleft palate has also been noted (Gorlin and Pindborg, 1964).

Speech symptoms of Turner's Syndrome, when referred to, are usually described in general terms. They may be associated with hearing loss (Silver and Dodd, 1957) as well as the orofacial anomalies described above. Jackson and Sougin-Mibashan (1953) report the pitch of voice high and variable in four of six cases reported in the male version of the syndrome. The disorder is the result of a chromosomal anomaly known as the XO Syndrome, Gonadal Dysgenesis or Agenesis, Ovarian-Short Stature Syndrome or Genital Dwarfism.

MOEBIUS' SYNDROME

Known also as congenital facial diplegia, congenital nuclear agenesis, congenital oculofacial paralysis and congenital abducens-facial paralysis, between 125 and 150 cases of Moebius' syndrome have been reported in the literature (Pitner et al. 1965). Etiology of the disorder is unknown in a definitive sense, but is supposed to involve nuclear agenesis and failure of formation of facial muscles. The symptoms include a masklike face from birth, with mouth and eyes open during sleep, usually bilateral facial paralysis, unilateral or bilateral loss of abducens function, anomalies of the extremities, aplasia of brachial and thoracic muscles, and frequent involvement of other cranial nerves such as the III, V, IX, X, XI, and XII. Due to lack of lateral eye movements, the patient must turn his head to aid peripheral vision. Defective pinnae and deafness are reported, and the skin is smooth and generally shows no wrinkles. Facial movement is lacking even when crying or smiling.

The speech of affected individuals is seldom reported in detail, but is occasionally referred to as clumsy, indistinct, explosive, or difficult to understand. Sprofkin and Hillman (1956) describe the speech of two patients: a 20-year-old Negro female who could not whistle, and whose speech was indistinct, especially as to labial articulation; and a seven-year-old child whose enunciation of labial sounds was poor. Merz and Wojtowicz (1967) report a 14-year-old girl with an "ataxia of the mouth" during speech. Gordon and Brown (1933) reported monotonous voice, clumsy articulation, and lack of discriminate movement of the muscles of the lip, tongue, and throat. Fry (1920) referred to oral symptoms of lower lip eversion and short upper lip associated with otitis media in a 27-month-old female. Henderson (1939) studied a female patient from 17 months to three years, and found that she did not speak until two years, and that although vocabulary was good, enunciation was poor. He cited lingual and velar paresis and dysarthria as symptoms of the syndrome. Bonnar and Owens (1929) noted that a 15-year-old boy could be understood although labials were not pronounced, the soft palate moved sluggishly and the patient had difficulty in swallowing. Butlin in an early report (1885) noted that the tongue lies in the bottom of the mouth and may show fibrillation on attempted contraction, and that partial paralysis of the tongue may affect speech, swallowing and mastication. The sounds /s/, /sch/, /i/, /e/, /l/, /alsh/, /g/, /r/, /u/, and /w/ are described as impaired. Everbusch and Nadoleczny (1914) observed that /b/ and /p/ were replaced by labiodental and weak friction sounds, and that labial sounds were not enunciated in compound words. There was a tendency to develop vicarious articulatory movements to replace the ones rendered indistinct by the facial paralysis.

Two patients observed by the author, one a 14-year-old boy and a four-and-a-half-year-old boy, showed labial paralysis or paresis, indistinct articulation involving poor labial and bilabial consonants, and lingual maladaptations. In both instances there was a distinctive double midline grooving of the tongue on attempted protrusion. The 14-year-old could retract the angles of the mouth downward, but was unable to execute normal lip movements of elevation and eversion, and could not retract the angles of the mouth independently or for normal smiling.

It is not known just how much can be accomplished through speech therapy in these cases. Luchsinger and Arnold (1965) mention that paralytic conditions of the lips may be treated with electrotherapy, massage, and exercises of labial movements, but do not indicate specifically that these methods are useful for congenital facial diplegia. Presumably, much of what can be done for the patient may involve the development of suitable compensatory adjustments for the absence of lip, tongue, and palate movements.

HEMIFACIAL ATROPHY AND HEMIFACIAL HYPERTROPHY

Hemifacial hypertrophy is a congenital disorder which may affect the face only or may be accompanied by various hypertrophies of almost every system and organ of the body. Whereas the literature surveyed did not contain reference to speech disturbance, it must be presumed that lingual and orofacial hypertrophy will distort speech articulation.

Hemifacial atrophy may occur as a feature of a syndrome or may be present as a symptom of progressive atrophy of the facial muscles. Despite the serious disfigurement which such disease may create, speech may not be affected significantly if the wasting is confined to the lips and facial tissues. A young woman observed by the author was found to have underdevelopment of the facial and mandibular bones of the right face, without evident symptoms of speech disorder. The tongue was apparently little affected by the disease.

BELL'S PALSY

In 1829, Sir Charles Bell, a Scottish physician, gave his name to a unilateral facial paralysis that is known as Bell's Palsy. It is a relatively common neurological problem which has been noted since ancient times in the art of Mayan, Greek, and Pre-Columbian periods (Goldman et al., 1967).

The disease affects the facial nerve, paralyzing the muscles of facial expression unilaterally. The eyebrow droops; frowning and raising of the eyebrow and closing of the eye are impossible; the eyeball rolls upward and outward; and eversion of the lower eyelid hinders the management of tearing. Facial wrinkles are smoothed so that the brow and the nasolabial furrow are diminished, and the mouth is drawn to the sound side. The patient cannot retract the paralyzed angle of the mouth or purse the lips for whistling. The cheek may puff in respiration and speaking, and displacement of the mouth may create an erroneous impression of lingual paralysis as the tongue deviates toward the sound side. Loss of taste to the anterior two-thirds of the tongue, and hyperacusis from paralysis of the stapedius muscle, may also occur as a result of paralysis of the facial nerve. Often overlooked is the psychological distress which the patient experiences, sometimes under the mistaken notion that he has suffered a stroke. The cause is not known although its association with age and weather (Liebowitz, 1966), hypertension and arteriosclerosis, emotional upsets (Curran, 1965), pneumatic compression (Bennett and Liske, 1967), and inheritance (Kaker, 1966) have been noted.

The diagnosis and treatment of Bell's Palsy are medical problems which if successful will bring full return of function. Spontaneous recovery in some degree will occur in 80 percent of afflicted individuals, but in these cases Hilger (1965) pointed out that only 55 percent have satisfactory return of function, with a remainder of permanent disability varying between troublesome and tragic. A surgical procedure, involving decompression of the nerve may in some instances provide a sheath through which the regenerating nerve may grow.

In the author's personal experience, which is limited to a few cases, speech is usually not disturbed significantly but may be affected in severe cases by the immobility of the lips on the paralyzed side. According to West, Ansberry, and Carr (1957) the articulation of the bilabial and labiodental consonants may be affected, although general speech intelligibility may not be disturbed. The patient's reticence in talking may be due more to his psychological reaction to his disability than to actual physical interference with speech. West suggests that speech therapy may be needed most to assist the patient after sufficient recovery has occurred so that the effects of the palsy are apparent to him. The patient may have developed compensatory adjustments and may still feel that he does not look or sound right.

KLIPPEL-FEIL SYNDROME

This highly distinctive syndrome is difficult to forget, once seen in its full manifestations. Fusion of several or all of the cervical vertebrae causes shortness of neck, with severe limitation of head movement. It is thought to be due to "faulty segmentation of the mesodermal somities sometimes between the third and seventh week *in utero*" (Gorlin and Pindborg, 1964, p. 335). There may be facial asymmetry, the posterior hairline extends to the shoulders, and the "flaring trapezius muscles extend from the mastoid area to the shoulders, producing a pterygium-like effect." Cleft palate, a high palatal vault, cranial nerve paralysis, deafness, bimanual synkinesis, and convergent strabismus are among other anomalies listed.

A patient known to the author had speech symptoms of multiple articulatory defects, poor oral motor coordination, mandibular and maxillary asymmetry and malocclusion, limited range of ocular movement, hearing loss, and palatopharyngeal inadequacy, with hypernassal voice quality. Intelligence was normal.

There is no known treatment for the disorder, but speech may be improved by therapy.

Lingual Deformities and Malfunctions

The importance of the tongue to speech is clearly indicated in the very term language, which comes from *lingua*, the Latin word for tongue. Goldberg (1939) notes that language means tonguing, or wagging of the tongue, attributable to the observation of our remote ancestors who, by figure of speech, chose the tongue as the chief representative of all of the organs of speech. Froeschels (1933), Green (1937), and others have stated, however, that the tongue is not essential to speech, and that congenital absence or adventitious loss of the tongue need not prevent a victim of such loss from learning to talk. Despite this claim, the tongue is extremely important; and it is due to the adept action of the tongue that most of the compensatory movements of speech are achieved by those patients whose oral deformities preclude the development of normal articulatory movements. The importance of the tongue in the development of normal occlusion has already been indicated (Swinehart, 1950). The general posture and habits of lingual movement have been shown by Wright et al. (1949) to determine the stability and comfort with which artificial dentures are worn.

There are several deformities which impair movements of the tongue so that speech is distorted. There are other deformities which are of interest to the speech pathologist, not necessarily because they directly interfere with speech, but because they are of diagnostic significance as manifestations of one of the various syndromes or diseases which cause communication disorder.

Among the deformities which have been found to be directly associated with speech defects are: ankyloglossia (tongue-tie); macroglossia (large tongue); microglossia (small tongue); aglossia (absence of tongue); atrophy, or hypertrophy of all or a portion of the tongue; malignant or benign tumor (such as hemangioma); glossitis (inflammation of the tongue); ulceration, scarring, swelling, and painfulness to touch or movement; bifid, trifid, and lobulate tongue; paralysis, tremor, flaccidity, or some other form of hypo- or hypermotility caused by neural afflication; and partial or total glossectomy (extirpation of lingual tissue, through surgery, accident, or disease). Such malformations have the potential for affecting speech through prevention or impairment of articulatory movements. Indirectly they may also affect speech by distorting orofacial growth and form, and by affecting the health and psychological attitudes of the speaker.

The tongue is also an important indicator of the presence of disease in its incipient or acute phases, and as a sign of malnutrition (Spies, 1958). Some of these, such as hairy tongue (Ronchese and Kern, 1953) (reported to occur as a reaction to the oral use of certain antibiotics) and plicated or fissured tongue, may not affect speech directly but are startling to the observer when he first discovers them. Others, such as glossitis (as a manifestation of pernicious anemia) may have only temporary effect on speech, and are responsive to medical treatment. Such disorders are of little direct concern to the speech pathologist except as a basis for referral of the patient for medical consultation. Leukoplakia (smokers' tongue) may produce no direct impairment of lingual function but, since it is sometimes an early precursor of oral cancer, should be referred for medical diagnosis when its presence is suspected. Any significant alteration in the form and substance of the tongue may affect speech temporarily or permanently, but the degree of speech involvement will vary in accordance with the many other factors which are also partially determinative of the adequacy of the articulatory valves of speech.

TONGUE-TIE AND OTHER FORMS OF ANKYLOGLOSSIA

A short lingual frenum is a handicap if it restricts the range of tongue-tip mobility required for feeding or for speech, or for the maintenance of oral hygiene. Although it is frequently suspected as a cause of articulatory disorder, the indictment is seldom a valid one. Its existence can be determined by asking the patient to elevate the tongue to the alveolar ridge of the maxilla, to protrude it past the incisal edges of the anterior teeth, and to move the tip of the tongue to the right and left corners of the mouth. Indication that the frenum is abnormally restrictive is assumed if the tongue-tip is noticeably indented on protrusion; cannot contact the alveolar arch when the mandible is in normal vertical relationship to the maxilla for speech; if the tip cannot be directed to contact the angles of the mouth; or if the consonants that require linguadental and lingua-alveolar contact cannot be achieved. The fact that the frenum is prominent and clearly visible when the tip of the tongue is elevated is no indication that it should be surgically removed.

Tongue-tie is commonly diagnosed by the layman as a cause of speech disorder, and physicians sometimes resort to "clipping" the tongue as a remedy for recognized disorder of articulation. The term tongue-tie refers to abnormal shortness of the frenum of the tongue, a condition which limits the range of movement of the tongue tip. Green (1945) indicates the comparative rarity of tongue-tie as a cause of speech defects. In more than 40,000 cases examined, not more than 10 or 12 cases of real tongue-tie were recorded. McEnery and Gaines (1941) state that in observing a large number of infants and children they have never seen a tongue that had to be clipped. Inasmuch as clipping can result in infection, with subsequent ulceration and scarring, hemorrhage, or extreme mobility leading to asphyxia caused by swallowing of the tongue, they recommend that the operation, if performed, be attempted with caution. In one thousand cases of speech disorders seen in the clinic in which they worked, only four had seriously shortened frenums. In two cases of serious tongue-tie, one showed no defect of articulation and the other overcame a slight /r/ defect without surgery.

Wallace (1963) advises that no frenulum should be divided before the patient is at least four years of age, and thereafter "only if the mechanism of tongue protrusion is too feeble to stretch or rupture it." He finds persistence of tongue-tie after four years of age to be rare.

Surgery for lingual frenectomy is a moderately complicated operation involving excision of the frenum after freeing it from its muscular attachments on either side. Mere snipping of the frenum is not considered to be a useful procedure (Wallace, 1963). Cases are occasionally reported verbally by surgeons in which clipping or surgical removal of the frenum in older children or young adults is said to be followed by spontaneous correction of articulatory defects. Documented evidence of such observations is needed.

MACROGLOSSIA

Enlargement of the tongue is difficult to define since lingual size must always be viewed in reference to the size of the oral cavity and related structures. Macroglossia may be of congenital origin, existing as an isolated malformation; it may occur among a cluster of symptoms as in mongolism and cretinism; it may be acquired in connection with acromegaly or lingual hemangioma; or the tongue may seem to be enlarged only in reference to an abnormally small mandible or maxilla. Occasionally the tongue may be appropriate to the size of the mandible (as in mandibular prognathism) but entirely too large for the relative size of a retracted and constricted maxilla.

The speech distortions from macroglossia affect particularly the tongue-tip consonants. The size of the tongue renders it clumsy, so that timing and articulatory placement are impaired. The protrusive posture caused by the bulk of the tongue in comparison to the oral cavity makes it difficult to contain the tongue for normal or adaptive lingua-alveolar and linguadental contacts. Consonants /t/, /d/, and /n/ are likely to be produced with the tongue tip depressed and the blade of the tongue in contact with the upper alveolar arch, or perhaps with the tongue protruded so that the valving becomes lingua-incisal. The sibilants are characteristically distorted by interdental tongue placement.

If the lingual enlargement develops early and persists long enough, the maxillary arch will expand in response to lingual pressure, so that the teeth of the maxillary arch will be spaced widely, and normal functioning of the lips may be disturbed by the dentally interposed tongue. Treatment for the reduction of lingual size may be accomplished surgically by excision of a portion of the tongue. If the tongue is symmetrically enlarged, the central portion of the tongue may be removed as a triangular "piece of pie," and the remaining lateral segments of the tongue sutured in the midline.

Koop and Maschakis (1961) report eight cases of lingual lymphangiomas treated surgically and by electrodesiccation of hemorrhagic lymphangiectasia.

MICROGLOSSIA, AGLOSSIA, GLOSSECTOMY, AND PARTIAL GLOSSECTOMY

Microglossia and aglossia are relatively rare disorders in which the tongue may be congenitally missing, or exists in rudimentary form. Glossectomy may be employed in the surgical treatment of disease, or may occur by accident or as an effect of wasting disease.

Sulzmann and Seide (1962) ascribe microglossia to developmental failure of the anterior two-thirds of the tongue following agenesis of the mandibular process derived from the first and second branchial arches. The developmental failure occurs at the fourth week of intrauterine life when these structures normally fuse. They report the case of an eight-year-old negro girl with a narrow mandible, a Class II, Division 1 malocclusion with severe overbite and overjet, and muffled speech due to multiple articulatory distortions. The anterior two-thirds of the tongue was missing. The prescribed treatment program accomplished substantial correction of the overjet, over-bite, and a cross-bite relationship. The speech was improved by speech therapy.

The case of a 22-year-old Chinese man with congenital aglossia is described by Eskew and Shepard (1949, p. 116). The man spoke but had a definite speech impediment. "In speaking, the buccinator muscles were very noticeable in their movement, as were the muscles of the floor of the mouth. Also in speaking there was a clearly audible intake of air, and a tendency for saliva to escape from the corners of the mouth." The floor of the mouth of this patient was smooth, but could be elevated in a tonguelike structure which could contact the incisal edges of the maxillary anterior teeth. The maxillary arch was constricted and triangular in form, and in malocclusal relationship with the mandibular arch. For the /k/ sound he established contact of the buccinators and the molars; /t/ was made similarly, with some difference in breath-stream control to differentiate it from /k/. All of the vowels were made clearly except /e/ and /i/.

A 13-year-old negro girl at The University of Michigan Dental School had a small tongue which was active and functioned well in speech. The mandible was relatively prognathic and overclosed vertically, so that in occlusion the lower teeth were in labial relationship, virtually covering the upper incisors. This relationship permitted a functional vertical reduction in size of the oral cavity, and brought the tongue high enough in the mouth so that linguadental and linguapalatal contacts could be made. Speech intelligibility was adequate but there was some articulatory distortion of sibilants, and articulatory quality and vocal resonance were affected by inadequate contraction of the palatopharyngeal valve, with consequent hypernasality and slightly reduced oral air pressure.

GLOSSECTOMY AND ALTERATIONS OF LINGUAL FORM

Reference has already been made to the possibility of impairing lingual function through the deformation of the tongue tip and tongue motility which may follow use of the Douglas technique in the treatment of Pierre Robin Syndrome.

Partial excision of the tongue may be required in treatment of malignant lingual tumors. A 19-year-old female patient of The University of Michigan Hospital, Department of Oral Surgery, sustained a right hemiglossectomy, and subsequently recovered "normal" articulate speech within six months following surgery. Much of the recovery was due to the patient's own persistent efforts. She used a set of practice sentences, and followed the speech pathologist's suggestions regarding the timing and adaptive placement of the tongue. Although the patient has to speak somewhat more slowly and carefully than prior to surgery, sibilants are clearly produced and speech is fully intelligible. The tongue can be protruded and pointed approximately in the midline, can deviate to contact the left angle of her mouth, and can be moved past the midline toward the right angle of the mouth but can not contact it.

Duguay (1964) urges that patients facing a decision as to lingual surgery should be told that intelligible speech can be achieved after partial or complete glossectomy.

LINGUAL AND FACIAL PARALYSIS

Injury to the Cranial nerves V, VII, IX, X, and XII will damage lingual, facial, and palatal function, and may in time be followed by atrophy of the affected muscles as well as by impairment of mobility. Supranuclear lesions will damage muscle contraction primarily on the side opposite the lesion. Nuclear and infranuclear lesions affect the ipsilateral side. The upper face and the tongue are less subject to unilateral paralysis from cortical lesion than is the lower part of the face because of the bilateral cortical representation of the lower face. On protrusion, the tongue will deviate toward the paralyzed side, due to the relatively unopposed action of the functional portion of the genioglossus muscle. The muscles of the face will tend to sag on the paralyzed side, the wrinkles and folds will tend to be smoothed around the mouth and the eye, and it will be impossible for the patient to retract the angles of the mouth equally. Because of the differing sources of cortical innervation for voluntary and emotional smiling, the contraction of the angles of the mouth may be symmetrical for emotional smiling, but unequal for voluntary retraction of the corners of the mouth, with action diminished on the paralyzed side.

Speech symptoms of lingual paralysis frequently include lateral escape of air to the paralyzed side during speech, especially since lingual paralysis is often accompanied by facial paralysis on the same side. These anomalies of function and their attendant speech symptoms are often concurrent features of orofacial deformity. Tests of neuromuscular function should be included routinely as a part of the orofacial examination.

If paralysis occurs during the years of facial growth, the bony development of the face will be affected by unbalanced muscle contractions in unilateral facial paralysis, and in cases of bilateral paralysis (e.g., Meobius' Syndrome), the shape of the mandible and perhaps of the entire face may be altered by the unopposed weight of the attached musculature and skin, and by the pull of the inframandibular muscles. (Refer to Detection of Facial and Oral Paralysis below.)

Nasal Deformities

The shape of the nose is so important in our concept of personal beauty that any significant departure of nasal form from the accepted pattern of a race or a people provides an occasion for notice, and sometimes for consideration of plastic alteration. The size of the anterior nares, the patency of the nasal passages, and the condition of the nasal mucosa have profound influence on the quality of vocal resonance. Occasionally a child is born with choanal atresia which must be penetrated to permit nasal breathing if the child is to survive. The external shape of the nose is an important indicator of the genetic background of the individual, and various anomalies of nasal form are important diagnostic features of syndromes in which speech is likely to be affected. For instance, atresia of the nostrils may occur in oculoauriculovertebral dysplasia; saddle nose, with depression of the bridge, may occur as a feature of the Rothmund-Thompson Syndrome and Hurler's Syndrome, and as a sign of congenital syphilis; a prominent nose and small mandible are constant features of Treacher Collins Syndrome (mandibulofacial dysostosis); a thin, beaked nose found in progeria (Hutchinson-Guilford Syndrome); an enlarged nose may occur in acromegalia; and the thin nose and constricted nares of the allergic facies and the adenoid facies are often found in habitual mouth breathers. (Gorlin and Pindborg, 1964). The failure of the nostrils to flare on deep inhalation should immediately alert the orofacial examiner to the possibility that his patient is not a nasal breather. The resonance distortions of hyponasality and hyper-hyponasality are immediate signs of abnormal valve function or perhaps of some form of nasal congestion.

Although Linde-Aronson and Backstrom (1960) in a study of Swedish school children could find no direct relationship between mouth breathing and malocclusion, many observers feel that the existence of stenotic nasal passages and the patient's consequent adoption of mouth breathing contribute to the development of the collapsed, high maxillary arch so often observed in persons having a long, narrow face (Fomon et al., 1965). As described by Massler and Schour (1946), mouth breathing leads to upper respiratory infection. The growing structures of the face are affected so that the face becomes markedly elongated and narrowed, caused by dropping the mandible to an open position and by pressure of the cheeks on the sides of the upper arch. Since depression of the mandible to create an oral airway allows the tongue to drop to a lowered posture, the pressures of the cheeks are not balanced by the intraoral pressures of the tongue. The maxillary arch narrows and the high vault further encroches on nasal air space.

The nostrils become narrowed from disuse, and the facial expression become dull and drawn. The habit of mouth breathing and enlargement of the pharyngeal tonsils both contribute to the typical facial configuration of "adenoid facies."

Changes of form in the oral region may also accompany habitual mouth breathing. The lower lip may become slackened, the upper lip shortened and elevated; or if the lower lip remains active it may exert pressure on the upper teeth, forcing them labially so that they become protruding, unsightly, and malfunctional. The mandible may be retruded, and the mouth hangs open. The maxillary sinuses and the nasal cavities become further narrowed as the maxillary arch contracts, the nasal mucosa becomes atrophic from disuse and the alae nasi may be reddened and pinched. The sense of smell may be dulled, often accompanied by loss of taste sensation and decrease in appetite. Hyperplasia of lymphoid tissues around the Eustachian tubes may close them and contribute to collection of fluid in the middle ear and consequent conductive hearing loss.

The speech of such persons is more than likely to show a composite of symptoms for which the etiology is appropriately complex. The symptoms will probably include hyponasality (Gardner 1949) or perhaps a mixed (hyper-hypo-) nasality, and articulatory distortions which result from interference with the normal mechanics of articulation and from a loss of the normal auditory monitoring of speech.

The shaping of the alveolar arch of the maxilla can be important in the articulation of lingua-alveolar sounds. The arch contours shown in Fig. 28-3 indicate clearly that there are marked differences in shape and angle of slope of the palate in adults. The speaker with a protracted maxilla or a retracted mandible (as in Fig. 28-13) will be aided in articulation of the consonants /s/ and /z/ if his maxillary alverolar arch rises gradually instead of abruptly behind the incisors.

Correction of malocclusion related to mouth breathing requires removal of the causes of nasal and nasopharyngeal obstruction, orthodontic treatment to expand the maxillary arch; and perhaps training of the patient to reposture the tongue, to relearn nasal breathing, and to develop normal habits of nasal resonance and articulation. In the treatment of nasal deformities, the role of the speech pathologist should be first to identify the possible relationship between malfunction of the nose and the disturbed speech. The correction of the structural defect is, of course, the job of the surgeon and perhaps of the orthodontist, but once the structural modification has been achieved, the speech pathologist may be able to help the patient restore its function in speech. If the potential malfunction of the nose can be recognized in time to prevent adverse habits and subsequent malformations from developing, the patient may also avoid the development of related speech defects.

Diagnostic Speech Examination of Orofacial Structures

The examination of orofacial structures and functions should be conducted within the context of the total appraisal of the patient. If the examination of the orofacial complex is pursued independently and without reference to a general examination of the patient's communication abilities, the validity of the findings will be open to serious question.

As indicated in the earlier sections of this chapter, the etiologic significance of orofacial abnormality in an individual instance of defective speech must be interpreted with due regard to the total dynamics of speech and the multiple causes of speech disorders. The diagnostician must evaluate physical growth, the timing of environmental and physioatomical forces as they inflect the emerging patterns of speech, and the ways in which behavior in turn modifies the directions of physical growth. Thus he must consider not merely the effects of orofacial structure on speech, but also the possible influence of speech habits upon the formation of the dental arches and dental occlusion. He must weigh the effects of personality upon orofacial growth and speech, and the influence which the malfunctions of orofacial structures and speech have upon the personality and upon the life outlook of the individual. He should look for the clues which the physical record of dental and occlusal development can give regarding the history of the patient—as a record of his earlier nutrition, diseases, oral habits, heredity, stages of physical growth and maturation, and even as to the kind of home environment and parental concern which can be deduced from indications of oral hygiene and dental care.

The art of the diagnostician lies further in deciding how all of the multiple factors of causation interact to cause defective speech, and which factors can be modified in an appropriate sequence of interventions to improve the patient's communication. The differential diagnosis of speech disorders associated with orofacial abnormalities distinguishes: 1. those features of speech which are *directly* attributable to the deformed and consequently malfunctioning organs; 2. those that are *indirectly* affected (for example, through the traumatizing effects of a poor facial cosmesis on the social adjustment of the patient); and 3. those aspects of defective speech which are attributable mainly to other etiologic factors.

There are at least eight major categories of etiology of articulatory disorder which must be considered in the differential examination of the patient: 1. neuropathies affecting the primary motor system; 2. neuropathies affecting the sensory systems involved in communication; 3. neural pathologies affecting the cerebral integrating system; 4. myopathies affecting the muscles themselves; 5. structural defects of the face and oral cavity; 6. psychological disorders; 7. defects of environmental learning, and 8. non-specific or idiopathic maladaptations for speech. Usually more than one etiologic factor can be identified in a speaker whose speech articulation is defective.

Examination of orofacial structures in relation to speech has as a further objective the distinction between those etiologic factors which are *endogenous* (originating within the individual) and those which reflect *exogenous* (external) influences. Whereas endogenous features probably cannot be removed, if their existence is detected early and if treatment is carried out during the growth years of the individual, their harmful effects can sometimes be greatly ameliorated. Those which affect the individual from without (exogenous) can often be modified and should be identified and treated at the appropriate time.

Furthermore, the task of the examiner must include a description of the patterns of movement which produce the sounds of speech, as well as an auditory description of those sounds. Pike (1944, p. 31) calls for description based on movements of the vocal apparatus rather than mere description based on auditory acoustic judgment, "since the latter lacks sufficient points of reference which can be defined without the necessity of establishing them in relation to standards that can be duplicated only by imitation."

Description of Articulatory Disorders in Orofacial Deformities and Malocclusions

This section will not attempt a description of the complete articulatory examination, since that is adequately treated elsewhere in this book, but does introduce a system to describe *sounds* in reference to the *manner* in which malarticulations are produced by the structures which provide the articulatory environment.

In many instances, malarticulations produced in a malformed orofacial complex are distortions of the phonemes of American Speech. It is herein proposed that these distortions be labeled by the coined term "malphones" to signify that they are not allophones of a normal phoneme, nor the substitution of one phone for another accepted phone, nor misarticulations due to the omission of consonants or vowels from speech, but are abnormally articulated approximations of intended phonemes. The proposed term malphones is thus generally synonymous with "articulatory distortion" or "sound distortion."

A complete system for the description of malphonic speech has not been proposed nor adopted, although Trim (1953) has suggested a partial scheme of modifiers. I have originated and used a system proposed below as a means of describing articulatory malphones during the phonetic examination of a patient. It is based on a series of pictographic diacritics to be used as modifiers of the consonants which the speaker is evidently attempting to enunciate. Recommendation for use of the system assumes that it is not enough merely to establish that an articulatory distortion exists, but that the examiner and the therapist need to know what form of abnormal lingual valving produces the defective consonant, and how the distortion is related to the dimensions and configuration of the articulatory structures.

For example, if a patient lisps, is it a) an interdental lisp, b) addental, c) anterolateral (right or left), d) lateral (right, left, or bilateral), e) a retroflexed lisp, f) a linguapharyngeal, g) palatopharyngeal, h) linguapalatal, or i) nasal lisp? Does the patient orient his tongue tip toward the maxillary arch or toward the mandibular arch? Does the lisp seem to be related to missing teeth? Does the function of the upper lip in relation to the type of lisp, or of the lower lip, seem to provide assistance or add to the sibilant distortion? Most of the enumerated forms of lisp can be indicated by diacritical markings suggested below, to be employed at the time of the phonetic analysis of a patient's speech.

The system proposed utilizes accepted phonetic symbols of the International Phonetic Alphabet. Their use is illustrated in a table of malphones which have been frequently encountered by the author in his examination of orofacially deformed patients. The diacritics symbolize three factors which are involved in the manner of articulatory distortion:

1. Structural modifiers; 2. Airflow modifiers; 3. Resonance and phonatory modifiers. (See Table 28-V.)

In using the modifiers, the examiner should assume that the patient is in left-profile orientation, or in full-face orientation. Most of the structure and articulatory placement symbols assume the profile orientation; most of the air-flow modifiers assume the full-face orientation; the resonance features are nondirectionally oriented.

Detection of Facial and Oral Paralysis

Although paralysis of orofacial muscles may not be classed as an orofacial abnormality in the sense that we have been discussing these afflictions, it is often an accompaniment of malformation of the face and mouth. If the paralysis occurs early enough in development of the face, it may be a significant cause of orofacial deformity as well as a contributor to defective speech. It is therefore important for the examiner to be alert to common signs of facial paralysis and to compare the appearance and action of the two halves of the face during examination of a patient.

Functional indications of facial and oral paralysis include:

a) absence or diminution of wrinkles where they are ordinarily found in the adult face (about the eyes, and the nasolabial fold);
b) ptosis of one or both eyelids;
c) sagging of the skin and underlying muscles on one or both sides of the face;
d) inability to raise the eyebrows, or
e) to close the eyes tightly;
f) inability to press the lips tightly together on one or both sides;
g) inability to smile, retract, elevate, or depress the angles of the mouth;
h) drooling from one corner of the mouth;
i) inability to bare the teeth by elevating or depressing the lips;
j) inability to protrude the tongue, or to protrude it in the midline (a hemiparalyzed tongue will protrude toward the paralyzed side);
k) inability to elevate or depress the tongue tip, intra- or extraorally;
l) inability to move the tongue tip to contact the angle of the mouth on each side;
m) inability to protrude and retract the jaw in the midline;
n) inability to open, close, and bite with equal strength on each side;
o) abnormalities of lingual movement in the performance of diadochokinetic activities; (see following discussion of diadochokinetics).
p) inability to prevent air from moving through the the nasopharyngeal valve and nasal passages during blowing or speaking;
q) inability to elevate and retract the palate and associated palatopharyngeal tissues during phonation;
r) inability to maintain elevated position of the palate during sustained phonation; and
s) nasal regurgitation of liquids during swallow.

Inasmuch as the two halves of the face and mouth may not be affected equally, the examiner should commence his examination by comparing the appearance of the two sides in their structure and function. The relatively normal action of one side will serve as a basis for judging the degree of malfunction on the other side. The relative appearance, the shape, size, and degree of movement of which each side of the lips, tongue, cheeks, palate, and mandible are capable provides a basis for diagnosing the nature and etiology of the dysfunctions observed.

DIADOCHOKINETICS

Tests of oral diadochokinetics and oral stereognosis can provide important information in the evaluation of the motor and sensory systems of the mouth and face. Whereas the significance of these procedures to the speech examination has not been fully explored, enough clinical evidence concerning dysdiadochokinesis and oral astereognosis in patients with orofacial defects has accumulated to indicate their potential value as diagnostic procedures.

A number of investigators have contributed to the general information concerning rates of diadochokinetic performance for the lips and tongue in normal and abnormal speakers, according to age of subject. The information contained in Fig. 28-16 was compiled by Mr. Jack Snyder from several studies completed by students at The University of Michigan. The graph was drawn by Dr. George Herman based on the Snyder data. A slightly different curve was extrapolated for females, but the differences between diadochokinetic rates of males and females are not considered to be clinically significant.

Hawk (1967) in his unpublished doctoral dissertation at The University of Michigan, provides additional information on the developmental patterns of

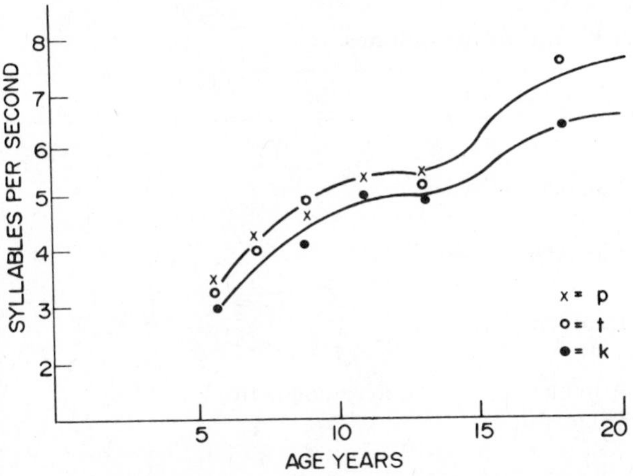

Fig. 28-16. Maximum diadochokinetic rates in males 5 to 20 years of age. *Snyder, 1955.*

lingual configuration and movement which characterize groups of children from six to 10 years of age. In general it was found that the stratified sample of normal children tested showed that alveolar lingual placements of /t/ and /l/ characterized the six and nine-year-olds, whereas linguadental contacts were more frequently encountered in the seven and eight-year-olds. Interdentalizations occurred more frequently among the few children in the samples who displayed articulatory errors. *Lingual configurations* were found to be predominantly convex in the younger age groups, with a significant increase in concavity of the tongue for the articulation of /t/ and /l/ in the older age groups. The six and nine year-olds displayed a preference for a stabilized position of the body of the tongue, with a lift of the tip to alveolar contact, whereas the seven and eight-year-olds tended toward an obtrusive movement of the tongue to the point of articulatory contact. Some associated mandibular movements are noted in all age groups, but in general the mandibular movements, when they occurred in the normal, appeared as an accompaniment of lingual movement and were not observed as a dominant behavioral feature. No subject in the sample was observed to show complete lingual dependence on mandibular movement to carry the tongue to articulatory contact, and none exhibited accompanying facial movements (grimacing, overflow, or random contraction of facial muscles).

The use of diadochokinetic tasks in the examination of speakers with orofacial defects and defective speech and patients with facial paralysis (primarily poststroke patients) indicate a number of features which differ from the patterns presumed to characterize normal speakers.

The following items of lingua-mandibulo-facial performance have been found to occur more frequently among malphonic speakers, and especially among those with some form of orofacial deformity:

1. *Predominance of lingual convexity* as the posture from which articulatory contact is made.

2. *Obtrusion to articulatory contact;* sometimes in the form of "contra-lapping" in which the tongue lifts toward alveolar contact, obtrudes and then lowers in a "counterclockwise" pattern which is a reversal of lapping movements; obtrusion with tongue-dorsum-alveolar contacts; and obtrusion to interdental lingual placement.

3. *Obvious mandibular movement* which cannot be suppressed during lingual diadochokinetic performance; mandibular movement which carries the tongue to articulatory contact.

4. *Depression of the lingual tip* during articulation of /t/, /d/, /n/.

5. *Inconsistency of movements,* displayed as imprecise lingual movements (sometimes almost "random" in appearance); tongue-tip deviations to right or left during diadochokinetics; rotational movements of tongue tip.

6. *Overflow facial movements,* lip eversions to one or both sides, grimaces, choreiform, or athetoid facial movements during diadochokinetics.

These patterns have not been encountered in persons with normal articulation, and hence are assumed to be indicative of abnormal neuromuscular behavior.

Oral Sensibility

Investigations of oral sensibility are of interest because of the assumed relationship between sensory acuity, sensory perceptions, and motor performance of articulatory movements of the lips, tongue, palate, and mandible. In addition to tactile sense which gives some awareness of position, pressures, and textural cues, proprioception guides the orofacial muscles. Even comparative temperature changes sometimes indicate the path of egress of air (as in production of sibilant sounds, or in lateral lisping) and may be used by speakers to guide the positioning of the oral structures for production of coordinated articulatory movements of speech.

Experimental disruption of sensory inputs has been shown by Ringel and Steer (1963) to interfere with accuracy of articulation. Case studies of patients who

TABLE 28-V
Diacritics for Phonetic Notation of Malphones

PHONETIC DIACRITICS		ILLUSTRATIVE MALPHONES	
STRUCTURAL MODIFIERS			
⌒ Lower lip sign	p	/p/	Labiodentalized
◡ Upper lip sign	f	/f/	Labiodental (inverted)
// Upper anterior teeth	t	/t/	Interdentalized
\\ Lower anterior teeth	d	/d/	Articulated with lowered tongue tip, lower jaw prognathic
ω Lip rounding	r	/r/	Articulated with excessive lip rounding
Unequal lip rounding	p	/p/	Articulated with unequal release, due to right facial paralysis
∘ Tongue tip sign Tongue dorsum sign	d	/d/	Articulated with depressed tongue tip, and dorsum making palatoalveolar contact
Posterior tongue sign	k	/k/	Formed by posterior tongue contacting posterior pharynx
≈ Soft palate sign	k	/k/	Formed by constriction of tongue dorsum and soft palate
(Right cheek sign	(p	/p/	With simultaneous puffing of right cheek, often seen with facial hemiparesis (prosopoplegia)
) Left cheek sign			
\ / Anterior nares sign	m	/m/	Hyponasalized due to constriction or occlusion of anterior nares
△ Maxillary dental arch	t	/t/	Formed with tongue tip deviating to patient left
▽ Mandibular dental arch	t	/t/	With tongue tip deviation to patient left, tip depressed to contact mandibular alveolar arch

TABLE 28-V *(continued)*
Diacritics for Phonetic Notation of Malphones

PHONETIC DIACRITICS	ILLUSTRATIVE MALPHONES		
AIRFLOW MODIFIERS			
/ Right anterolateral lingual grooving	/s		Right anterolateral lisp
	s		Right anterolateral lisp with tongue tip elevated
	/s or s		Right anterolateral lisp with tongue tip depressed
\ Left anterolateral lingual grooving	s\		Left anterolateral lisp with lingual protrusion
← Right lateral lingual airflow	(s		Right lateral (buccal) lisp with simultaneous puffing of right cheek
→ Left lateral lingual airflow	s		Left lateral lisp
┼ Blocked midline airflow	s┼		Addental lisp
Nasally directed airflow	s		Nasal lisp
⇓ Broad lingual groove	s⇓		Retracted lisp
	s↑		Pharyngalized lisp
	s↑		Linguapalatal lisp
+ Aspirate	+k	/k/	Aspirate
− Lacking air pressure	−p	/p/	With weak plosion
RESONANCE AND PHONATORY MODIFIERS			
∼ Hypernasality	ũ	/u/	Hypernasal
∼ Hyponasality	m̰	/m/	Hyponasal
≈ Mixed nasality	ṵ̃		Hyper-hyponasality
▽ Strident whisper	v		Strident whisper
Soft whisper	ɣ		Soft (breathy) whisper
∀ Hoarseness	−v−		Hoarse voice

manifest interrelated congenital sensorimotor dysfunctions are included in Bosma (1967) in reports prepared by Chase (Chap. 16), Rootes and MacNeilage (Chap. 17), Bosma, Grossman, and Kavanagh (Chap. 18) and Bloomer (Chap. 19). The patient described by Bloomer has subsequently developed an open-bite which is presumed to have been caused by the lack of normal orofacial muscle action in repose, deglutition, and speech.

Jerge (Bosma, 1967, Chap. 2) has postulated that disturbances in the sensory reporting systems may involve the trigeminal sensory complex and the reticular formation, as well as higher level integrating mechanisms of the cortex. Storey (Bosma, Chap. 3) discusses extratrigeminal sensory systems related to oral function, and suggests that "Proprioceptors in the trigeminal system probably alter position," (p. 95). He further postulates that in cases of "retained infantile swallow" the tongue behaves as an "intrinsic muscle" in contrast to "extrinsic muscle" behavior of the tongue in responding to the oral discomfort created by inflamed and enlarged tonsils.

Various methods of determining oral sensibility and oral perception have been proposed. Small three-dimensional geometric patterns have been constructed and presented to subjects for oral exploration in order to test "oral stereognosis" (oral recognition of shape). (McDonald and Aungst, Bosma, Chap. 11, and Shelton, Arndt, and Hetherington, Bosma, Chap. 12). Thus far, results pertinent to the clinical evaluation of patients with orofacial deformity and orofacial dysfunction are relatively meagre and inconclusive, and the investigation of disorders of sensation in persons with orofacial deformities must be considered to be in its early stages. Rutherford and McCall (Bosma, Chap. 10) report the discovery of sensory defects "with surprising frequency" in a small group of dysarthric subjects. Mason (Bosma, 1967, Chap. 15) was unable to find significant differences in the oral perceptions of cleft-palate subjects and normal subjects. Nevertheless, there are many forms of orofacial deformity in which there are manifest sensory disturbances, and in which one may logically expect to discover some relationship between oral dyscoordinations and impaired oral sensation.

Observational Outline for Orofacial Examination

An orofacial examination should be a routine part of a phoniatric appraisal of a patient. The general pattern of the orofacial examination should cover the items suggested below. The examiner must bring to the examination a knowledge of the limits of normalcy for the items which he will check.

Head: size, shape, carriage of head, hair distribution, notation of abnormal features such as frontal bossae.

Face: general appearance, skin texture, distribution and symmetry of features; indications of personality, alertness, intelligence.

Eyes: shape, spacing, indications of ocular muscle balance and eye movement; visual acuity; posture and mobility of lids, brows; presence of abnormal features (coloboma, absence of eyelashes, etc.).

Ears: shape and location of the pinnae, condition of the external canals; evidences of hearing acuity, ear pathologies, abnormalities of function.

Nose: size, shape, nostrils and nares opening, airspace in nasal passages; evidences of function (nasal breathing, resonance of voice, action of nostrils during speaking, blowing, and breathing).

Lips and cheeks: form, posture at rest, functional relationship of upper and lower lips, scarring, length, fullness; mobility in speaking, sucking, swallowing, pursing, smiling (emotional), voluntary retraction of the angles of the mouth (voluntary smiling); ability to elevate, retract, and depress angles of the mouth; control of salivation without drooling, ability to puff cheeks individually, and to inhibit puffing of cheeks during speaking and blowing; symmetry of wrinkles at eyes and mouth; presence of pits; abnormally restrictive labial frenum.

Teeth and dental arches: occlusal relationship of dental arches; spacing, presence, absence, position, and form of individual teeth; arch width, height, and configuration; hard-palate size and length; size and shape of mandibular arch in relation to maxillary; mandibular mobility in opening, closing, protrusion, and retraction in speaking and deglutition; ability to inhibit mandibular motion during diadochokinetic tests.

Tongue: size, shape, resting posture, texture of lingual surface, color; configuration in performance of specific tasks; evidences of abnormal function as shown in involuntary movement, hyper- or hypomobility at rest, or in sucking, swallowing; diadochokinetic patterning; lingual performance in speaking; inability to achieve protrusion, lateral movement to angles of mouth, or to press tongue tip hard against either cheek; ability to raise and lower tongue tip intra- and extraorally; positional relationship of tongue at rest in reference to the dental arches;

symmetry or asymmetry of the two halves of tongue, presence of abnormal grooving, texture of mucosal surface; evidences of scarring, ankylosis, abnormally restrictive lingual frenum.

Palatopharyngeal valve: shape, length, and apparent thickness of soft palate at rest, in elevation-retraction in relation to dimensions and form of nasopharynx; configuration of inferior border of palate at rest and in action; associated movements of other pharyngeal tissues during palatal action in speaking, blowing, gagging, and swallowing; shape and action of faucial arches; presence, absence, condition of tonsilar tissues related to palatopharyngeal function; ability of palate to sustain elevation and retraction during phonation; ability to control air-traffic and resonance in blowing, speaking; ability to prevent nasal regurgitation of fluids during drinking (especially when head is bent forward as in drinking from a fountain).

Effects of Malocclusion on Hearing

The claim has been made in several publications that there is a relationship between occlusion and hearing loss. Pryor (1933) in a description of the dental problems of George Washington speculates that his considerable hearing loss in his latter years may have been due to an excessive closed bite which allowed the mandibular condyles to encroach on the external auditory meatus. Costen (1936, p. 1015) describes ear symptoms which include impaired hearing, tinnitus, a stuffy sensation in the ears, pain, and nystagmous. He states:

> During the act of swallowing the tensor palatini muscle should be tensed, and effect a temporary opening of the tube. This function cannot occur during overclosure, and the result is a derangement of intro-tympanic pressure, and dizziness . . . [This] brings about a catarrhal or adhesive deafness exactly as produced by inflammation or pressure from the nasopharynx. The catarrhal deafness improves more or less after repositioning the jaw.

Ronkin (1953) notes similar symptoms but ascribes their origin to the loss of tone of the internal pterygoid muscles, which immediately cause a deviation from the norm of both the tensor palatini and the tensor tympani muscles. Treatment consists in opening the bite, thus allowing the internal pterygoid to resume its normal tone, with consequent effect on the associated muscle groups.

Harvey (1948) undertook an extensive and well-designed study of the relationship of malocclusion and ear symptoms, with particular reference to altitude changes and pain in the ears. Careful anatomical studies produced no evidence that shortening of the tensor veli palatini could have any effect on the ear, since both the tensor and levator insert into the maxilla, but not into the mandible. With respect to relaxation of the pterygoid muscles and pressure on the Eustachian tube, he found that the internal pterygoid and Eustachian tube are widely divergent in three planes, and concluded that it would be difficult to see how these structures could possibly compress the tubes. In brief, he found no support whatever for the assertions made by earlier investigators of this topic.

Artificial Dentures and Dental Appliances

Not much has been written, and apparently little study has been made, of the effect of dental appliances on speech. Van Thal (1936) states that "The wearing of an applicance appears to have little effect on speech once the wearer has got accustomed to it. Only in 13 cases (out of a total of 180 children studied) was articulation actually worse when wearing a plate or springs; and in five cases it was better . . . with the applicance than without it." Kimball and Muyskens (1937) report a case of speech improvement after prosthetic reconstruction, indicating that the placement of the bars of the supporting frame is important to the patient's speech adaptations. Palatograms illustrated how linguopalatal contacts were improved by correct denture design. Saizar (1958) cautions dentists that dental applicances do affect speech. He suggests phonetic tests which can be used to guide design of dentures and dental appliances. Bloomer (1958) has asserted the need to construct dental appliances to duplicate as nearly as is feasible the oral environment for lingual and labial movements which characterized the patient's normal production of consonants prior to dental loss. In case of asymmetry of the dental arches and open-bite, it is sometimes possible for the prosthodontist to improve the patient's chances of normal articulation by building an anterior prosthesis to produce a "normal" occlusion where none existed before and articulation was defective. Landa (1935) states categorically that the rugae should be omitted from the palatal surface except in special instances, since they add thickness to the palatal surface of the denture and thus use valuable tongue room. Pound (1951) states that the positioning of the teeth, the preservation of adequate tongue room, the correct amount of clearance between the anterior teeth, and the reconstruction of the natural plane of occlusion are all considered important. Wepman (1937) indicates that the patient should be warned ahead of time that his speech may be different with the new appliances and that the patient and dentist should discuss the possible adjustments that must be made.

In cases of inadequate palatopharyngeal function due to congenital factors, or to paralysis from bulbar polio, it is possible to restore satisfactory palatopharyngeal function by the use of a palatal lift appliance, which elevates and maintains the soft palate in a position approximating that ordinarily assumed by the palate in speaking. (Gibbons and Bloomer, 1958); Lang, 1967). Critics of this form of prosthesis have suggested that such an appliance may have an adverse effect on the supporting teeth of the maxillary arch. This author has observed, however, that a patient who wears the prototype of this lift appliance has worn it for more than 16 years at the present writing, and no adverse effects on the teeth or the soft tissues of the mouth have been found to occur. More than 50 such appliances have subsequently been constructed for other patients at The University of Michigan without deleterious effects on oral health.

Attempts have been made to use dental appliances to change the posture of the tongue and to institute a basis for new lingual habits in speech, and in the creation of an improved muscular environment for dental occlusion (Walsh, 1961). Harvold (1968) has unquestionably demonstrated that a change in lingual habits and a subsequent change in dental occlusion in adult monkeys can be achieved by the introduction of interfering dental appliances. There is some reason, however, to question the use of dental appliances in the retraining of abnormal lingual habits in humans. Children have frequently demonstrated their ability to sustain considerable discomfort and even trauma to retain old habits. Koyoumdjisky (1962) has cited a case in which "cleft palate speech" developed in a child after removal of an orthodontic appliance, and disappeared after reinstatement of the appliance. Normal speech was eventually established by speech therapy after removal of the dental appliance when treatment of the malocclusion had been effected.

There is undoubtedly much to be learned concerning denture design for speech, from the viewpoint of patient comfort, speech proficiency, and assistance of the patient in the development of satisfactory oral habits.

Dental Anomalies and Personality

One of the indirect ways in which dental and orofacial anomalies can affect speech is through their relation to personality. Personality, in turn, affects speech through the influence which anxiety, feelings of inferiority, and psychological resistance to the learning of new habits exert on the normal development and use of speech. Personality also is a factor in the development of the orofacial anomalies which affect speech.

Reference has already been made to the ways in which personal habits such as thumb-sucking, finger-sucking, nail-biting, and tongue-sucking contribute to malocclusion. Such habits are based in the personality structure and needs of the individual. Many parents and dentists feel that thumb-sucking is a habit which is to be eliminated as early as possible, without reference to its meaning to the child. This sometimes results in forcible correction of the habit or resort to methods which are more damaging to the personality of the child than the muscular habit is to the orofacial structures. Pearson (1948) reports a case of thumb-sucking in which severe restraints to thumb-sucking brought on stuttering which ceased after the father apologized to the child and permitted her to resume the thumb-sucking. Pearson states that thumb-sucking is a necessary means of gratification for young children, does not deform the mouth or face and, if stopped by punishment suddenly, affects the personality adversely. Gesell and Ilg (1943) state that its harmfulness varies greatly with the type of child and associated behavior, but doubt if it has a permanent effect upon denture and occlusion if discontinued by the age of five or six years.

The effects of sucking habits on occlusal development are well documented by Gwynne-Evans (1951) and Rix (1953). The speech clinician who is aware of the complex origins of the habit may discover as much about the etiology of the child's speech defect through an interpretation of the sucking habits in relation to personality as can be learned through a consideration of the mechanical interference which the distorted occlusion imposes upon speech.

The effect of malocclusions upon personality was noted early in the development of medical science. Walker (1941) quotes Albucasis, who lived in the years 936 to 1013 A.D. and wrote in *De Chirugia*, "When a tooth is irregularly placed or projects above the level of the others, a deformity ensues which is particularly displeasing in women." Walker is of the opinion that an inferiority complex, and attitudes of superiority, timidity, selfishness, jealousy, or over-sensitiveness all are to be found in people who have dental anomalies. Indications are strong (Glaser, 1946) that dental and surgical treatment cannot always be carried to a successful conclusion as long as the damaging forces of personality distortion persist in counteracting the beneficial effects of the surgical, prosthetic, or orthodontic treatment. Kimball and Muyskens (1937) found that the personality improved in an individual for whom speech was corrected in connection with construction of a dental prosthesis. Kempner (1943) states that carious or missing teeth, unsightly dentures, dental discoloration, malocclusions, or malpositioned teeth cause people to hide their mouths, or talk with their lips together. Gibbin (1939) reported a case of a girl, thirteen, whose morbid consciousness of a dentofacial deformity was supplanted by self-confidence, poise, and sociability after orthodontic treatment and myofunctional therapy. Speech was also greatly improved.

RESPONSIBILITIES OF THE SPEECH PATHOLOGIST IN RELATION TO DENTAL TREATMENT

The speech pathologist has a number of important functions to perform in relation to the dental specialist and to the patient. These include:

1. Speech diagnosis and professional consultation with the dental specialist.
2. Referral of speech patients suspected of having dental conditions which may currently interfere with speech, general health, or personality adjustment.
3. Speech therapy and consultation in connection with patients undergoing orthodontic treatment, the construction of artificial dentures or other dental prosthetic devices, or surgical corrections or restorations.

The average dental specialist is not a student of speech with enough detailed information about the various anomalies of speech to enable him to make an adequate diagnosis of the patient's speech problems. The speech pathologist should give a clear statement of his evaluation of the patient's speech problem, the probable etiological factors, and the importance of dental treatment in the eventual speech rehabilitation of the patient. A careful speech diagnosis can be helpful to the dentist in planning the time of corrective dental intervention and can help both the dentist and the patient to make a better prognosis of the final results of treatment.

The speech pathologist and speech therapist must be alert to the various conditions which may be present or which are incipient in the pattern of development which the individual seems to be following. Often the advice of the speech therapist will be a means of getting a child to the dentist for a preventive program which can result in the improvement of oral hygiene, the preservation of the permanent teeth, and the normal development of facial growth. The speech therapist can also be influential in letting parents know how important it is to preserve the deciduous teeth for the health and dental integrity of the growing child.

In referring the child or the adult patient to a dental or surgical specialist, it is important that the speech clinician be conservative in his estimate of the physical changes which can be accomplished. There is a tendency on the part of many individuals to "over-sell" the patient on what can be accomplished by adjunct services, with the implication that if failure in the total rehabilitation program falls short of the desired objective, it is the fault of the adjunct service rather than the referring specialist.

The patient who is a candidate for orthodontic treatment frequently will need speech-corrective work at some stage of his treatment program if he is to receive full benefit from the dental correction. A decision must often be made as to whether or not speech-correction measures should await completion of the dental treatment, should be instituted and maintained concurrently with it, or should be begun prior to dental or surgical treatment. There is merit in any of these choices for certain patients, and the determination as to which shall be chosen should be made by the speech therapist in consultation with the dentist or surgeon.

As a matter of general policy, correction of those speech defects which cannot be directly attributed to the dental or structural anomaly may be undertaken without awaiting dental treatment, but due allowance should be made for the effects which dental appliances may have upon speech. In instances in which a definite relationship between structure and speech functions can be established, it is sometimes appropriate to wait for a short time after completion of the dental work to see if the patient can successfully achieve self-correction of his speech. In some cases it may be helpful to the program of dental treatment if the speech therapist can train the patient in habits of muscle movement for speech which will accord with pressure patterns designed to promote or maintain structural changes which the dental specialist is attempting to bring about.

In the construction of complete or partial dentures the speech therapist may assist the dentist in determining the placement of crossbars and sometimes in the placement of the anterior teeth so that the /s/ sounds will not become either strident or occluded. A careful evaluation of the tongue tip movements and the labiodental contacts during speech will aid the dentist in deciding whether or not the teeth are properly positioned to enable the patients to speak properly.

BIBLIOGRAPHY

Anderson, G. 1948. Practical orthodontics (7th. ed.). St. Louis: Mosby.

Angle, E. 1907. Malocclusion of the teeth (7th. ed.). Philadelphia: S. S. White Dental Mfg. Co.

Arey, L. 1954. Developmental anatomy (6th. ed.). Philadelphia: Saunders.

Backus, O. 1940. Speech rehabilitation following excision of the tip of the tongue. *Amer. J. dis. Child.*, 60, 368–370.

Ballard, C. 1951. The facial musculature and anomalies the dentoalveolar structure, *European Orthondont. Soc.*, Report of 25th. Congress, 137–148.

———, and Bond, E. 1960. Clinical observations on the correlation between variations of jaw form and variations of orofacial behavior, including those of articulation. *Speech Pathology and Therapy*, 3, 55–65.

———. 1962. Clinical significance of innate and adaptive postures and motor behavior. *The dental Practicioner*, 12, 219–227.

Barclay, A., and Nelson, W. 1922. The x-ray analysis of sounds of speech. *J. Radiology*, 3, 277–280.

Benjamin, L. 1962. Nonnutritive suckling and dental malocclusion in the deciduous and permenent teeth of the Rhesus monkey. *Child Develop.*, 33, 29–35.

Bennett, D., and Liske, E. 1967. Transient facial paralysis during ascent to altitude. *Neurology*, 17, 194–8.

Berger, E. 1961. A cephalometric analysis of the effect of thumbsucking and associated neuromuscular habits on the craniofacial skeleton and the dentition. Ann Arbor: Univ. Mich. Press: Master's thesis. Pp. 46.

Bernstein, M. 1956. The relation of speech defects and malocclusion. *Alpha Omega*, 50, 90–97.

Bloomer, H. 1943. A palatopograph for contour mapping of the palate. *J.A.D.A.*, 30, 1053–1057.

———, 1953. Observations on palatopharyngeal movements in speech and deglutition. *J. Speech Hearing Disorders*, 18, 230–246.

———. 1958. Speech as related to dentistry. *Mich. State Dent. J.*, 40, 11.

———. 1963. Speech defects in relation to orthodontics. *Amer. J. Orthodont.*, 49, 920–929.

———. 1967. Oral manifestations of dysdiadokokinesis, with oral astereognosia. *In* Symposium on oral sensation and perception, Bosma, J., ed. Springfield, Ill.: Thomas.

Blyth, P. 1959. The relationship between speech, tongue behavior and occlusal abnormalities. *J. British soc. study Orthodont.* 11–20.

Bonnar, B., and Owens, R. 1929. Bilateral congenital facial paralysis: Review of the literature and a classification. *Amer. J. dis. Child.*, 38, 1256–1272.

Bosma, J. 1967. Symposium on oral sensation and perception. Springfield, Ill.: Thomas. P. 360.

Brown, G. 1938. The surgery of oral and facial diseases and malformations. Philadelphia. Lea & Febiger.

Brown, R., and Cunningham, M. Some dental manifestations of mongolism. *Oral Surg., oral Med. and oral Pathol.*, 14, 664–676.

Butlin, H. 1885. Diseases of the tongue. Philadelphia: Lea Brothers.

Chao, D. 1969. Congenital neurocutaneous syndromes of childhood: Sturge-Weber disease. *J. Pediatrics*, 55, 635–649.

Cheney, E. 1944. A study of embouchure adaptation as a function of the dento-facial complex. Univ. Mich.: Master's thesis.

Cooper, H. 1930. Some thoughts concerning muscle exercises. *Int. J. Orthodontia oral Surg.*, 16, 527–534.

Costen, J. 1936. Some features of the mandibular articulation as it pertains to otolaryngology. *Int. J. Orthodontia oral Surg.*, 22, 1011–1017.

Crane, E., and Ramstrum, G. 1943. A classification of palates. Univ. Mich.: Master's thesis.

Curran, T. 1965. Bell's Palsy: A modern concept of treatment. *Conn. Med. J.*, 29, 728–731.

Dennison, W. 1965. The Pierre Robin syndrome. *Pediatrics*, 36, 336–341.

Dingman, R. 1944. Osteotomy for the correction of mandibular malrelation of developmental origin. *J. oral Surg.*, 2, 239–259.

———, and Billman, H. 1947. Double lip. *J. oral Surg.*, 5, 146–148.

Dockrell, R. 1951. A classification of post-normal occlusions. London: Saward.

Douglas, B. 1946. The treatment of micrognathia associated with obstruction by a plastic procedure. *Plast. reconstr. Surg.*, 1, 300.

Duguay, M. 1964. Speech after glossectomy. *N.Y. State J. Med.*, 64, 1836–1838.

Eskew, H. and Shepard, E. 1949. Congenital aglossia. *Amer. J. Orthodont.*, 35, 116–119.

Everbusch, O., and Nadoleczny, M. 1914. Diseases of the eye and disorders of speech in childhood. London: Lippincott.

Fernandez, A., and Ronis, M. 1964. The Treacher Collins Syndrome. *Arch. Otolaryng.* 80, 505–520.

Fletcher, S., Casteel, R., and Bradley, D. 1961. Tongue-thrust swallow, speech articulation, and age. *J. Speech Hearing Disorders*, 26, 201–208.

Fomon, S., Bell, J., Lubart, J., Schattner, A., Silver, A., and Syracuse, V. 1965. *Arch. Otolaryng.*, 82, 281–286.

Ford, J. 1944. A plastic operation for lengthening the congenitally short upper lip. *J. oral Surg.*, 2, 260–265.

Forde, T. 1951. Oral dynamics. *Dent. Digest, Jan., Feb., Mar., April.*

Fritzell, B. 1963. An electromyographic study of the movements of the soft palate in speech. *Folia Phoniat.*, 15, 307–311.

———. 1969. The velopharyngeal muscles in speech (an electromyographic and cineradiographic study). *Acta Otolaryng.*, Suppl. No. 250.

Froeschels, E. 1933. Speech therapy. Boston: Expression Co.

———. 1940. Laws in the appearance and development of voice hyperfunctions. *J. Speech Disorders*, 5, 1–4.

———, and Jellinek, A. 1941. Practice of voice and speech therapy. Boston: Expression Co.

Frowine, V., and Moser, H. 1944. Relationship of dentition to speech. *J. Amer. dent. Assn.*, 31, 1081–1090.

Fry, F. 1920. Congenital facial paralysis: two additional cases. *J.A.M.A.*, 74, 1699–1700.

Fymbo, L. 1936. The relation of malocclusion of the teeth to defects of speech. *Arch. Speech*, June, 204–217.

Gardner, A. 1949. Dental oral and general causes of speech pathology. *Oral Surg., oral Med., oral Pathol.*, 2, 742–751.

Gesell, A., and Ilg, F. 1943. Infant and child in the culture of today. New York: Harper.

Gibbin, F. 1939. Macromaxillary and micromandibular development. *Amer. J. Orthodont. oral Surg.*, 25–7, 657–663.

Gibbons, P. and Bloomer, H. 1958. A supportive-type prosthetic speech aid. *J. prosthetic Dent.*, 8, 362–369.

Glaser, C. 1946. Psychotherapy in orthodontics. *Amer. J. Orthodont. oral Surg.*, 32, 341–354.

Goldberg, I. 1939. The wonder of words. New York: Appleton-Century.

Goldman, L., and Schechter, C. 1967. Art in medicine: periopheral facial palsy throughout the ages. *N.Y. State J. Med.*, 67, 1331–4.

Goldstein, M. 1940. New concepts of the functions of the tongue. *Laryngoscope*, 50, 164–188.

Gordon, R., and Brown, M. 1933. Paralysis in children. London: Oxford.

Gorlin, R., and Pindborg, J. 1964. Syndromes of the head and neck. New York: McCraw-Hill.

Grabb, W., and Smith, J. 1968. Plastic surgery. Boston: Little, Brown.

Graber, T. 1963. The "three M's": muscles, malformation and malocclusion. *Amer. J. Orthodont.*, 49, 418–450.

Graber, T. 1966. Craniofacial and dentitional development. *In* Human development. Falkner F., ed. Philadelphia: Saunders. Pp. 510–581.

———. 1966. Orthodontic principles and practice. (2nd. ed.) Philadelphia: Saunders.

Greene, J. 1937. Speech defects and related oral anomalies. *J. Amer. dent. Assn. dent. Cosmos*, 24, 1969–1974.

———. 1945. Anomalies of the speech mechanism and associated voice and speech disorders. *N.Y. State J. Med.*, 45, 605–608.

Gwynne-Evans, E. 1951. The organization of the orofacial muscles in relation to breathing and feeding. *Brit. dent. J.*, 91, 135–140.

Harrington, R., and Brienholt, V. 1963. Relation of oral-mechanism malfunction to dental and speech development. *Amer. J. Orthodont.*, 49, 84–93.

Harris, K. 1963. Behavior of the tongue in production of some alveolar consonants. *J. acoust. soc. Amer.*, Abstract, 35, 784.

Harvey, W. 1948. Investigation and survey of malocclusion and ear symptoms with particular reference to ototic barotrauma (pain in ears due to change in altitude). *Brit. dent. J.*, 85, 219–225.

Harvold, E. 1968. The role of function in the etiology and treatment of malocclusion. *Amer. J. Orthodont.*, 54, 883–899.

Hawk, A. 1967. An acoustical and physiological analysis of lingual diadochokinesis in children from five through ten years of age. Univ. Mich.: Ph.D. dissertation.

Hemrend, B., and Moyers, R. 1953. The growth of the carnio-facial skeleton. Toronto: (privately printed).

Henderson, J. 1939. The congenital facial diplegia syndrome: clinical features, pathology aetiology. *Brain*, 62, 381–403.

Henry, O. 1937. Phonetics in orthodontia. *Int. J. Orthodontia. oral Surg.*, 23, 456–461.

Herman, G. 1943. A study of palate shape and its characteristics in lispers. Univ. Mich.: Master's thesis.

Hilger, J. 1965. Bell's palsy. *Minn. Med. J.* 48, 1463–1467.

Holbrook, R. 1937. X-ray studies of speech articulations. Berkeley: Univ. Calif. Press.

Hopkins, G., and McEwen, J. 1955. Speech defects and malocclusion, Tr. Brit. Soc. for the Study of Orthodontics. 130–138.

Hunt, P., and Smith, D. 1955. Mandibulo-facial dysostosis. *Pediatrics*, 15, 195–199.

Huntington, D., Harris, K., and Sholes, G. 1968. An electromoyographic study of consonant articulation in hearing-impaired and normal speakers, *J. Speech Hearing Res.* 11, 147–158.

Jackson, W., and Sougin-Mibashan, R. 1953. Turner's syndrome in the female. *Brit. med. J.* 2, 368–371.

Jaffe, P. 1962. Speech problem and its effect on the developing dentition. *N.Y. State dent. J.*, 28, 198–200.

Jaffe, P. 1964. Lisping and malocclusion. *N.Y. State dent. J.*, 30, 279–281.

Johnson, L. 1940. Problem of the mentalis muscle in the treatment of malocclusion. *J. Amer. dent. Assn.*, 27, 1046–1054.

Juste, J. 1948. The masticatory face and the voice. *Dent. Record*, 68, 309–310.

Kaker, P., Sawhney, K., and Saharia, P. 1966, Familial Bell's palsy. *J. Laryng. Otol.*, 80, 628–630.

Kantner, C., and West, R. 1941. Phonetics. New York: Harper.

Keaster, J. 1940. Studies in the anatomy and physiology of the tongue. *Laryngoscope*, 50, 222–257.

Kempner, R., and Chock, K. 1943. Dentistry in neuropsychiatry, the significance of oral sepsis and cosmetic effects. *J. Amer. dent. Assn.*, 30, 416–420.

Kessler, H. 1953. Dentistry's part in speech production. *Oral Hyg.*, 43, 1080.

Kimball, H., and Muyskens, J. 1937. Speech reconstruction after prosthesis. *J. Amer. dent. Assn dent. Cosmos*, 24, 1158–1168.

Kingsley, N. 1880. A treatise on oral deformities. New York: Appleton.

Koop, C., and Moschakis, E. 1961. Capillary lympangiomà of the tongue complicated by glossitis. *Pediatrics*, 27, 800–810.

Koyoumdjisky, E. 1962. Speech disorder resulting from orthodontic treatment. *Dental Practicioner*, 12, 165–166.

Kremen, A. 1953. Cancer of the tongue. *Minn. Med. J.*, 36, 838–830.

Kutt, J. 1967. An epidemiologic study of open bite (with reference to aberrant swallowing and anterior tongue thrust). Univ. Mich.; Master's thesis, Orthodontics. Bloomer, H., Project director. Supported by HEW, USPH, NIDR Grant No. DE-01984.

Kydd, W., and Neff, C. 1964. Frequency of deglutition of tongue thrusters compared to a sample population of normal swallowers. *J. dent. Res.*, 43, 363–369.

———, and Belt, D. 1964. Continuous palatography. *J. Speech Hearing Disorders*, 29, 489–492.

Landa, J. 1953. The importance of phonetics in full denture prosthesis. *Dent. Digest*, 41, 154–160.

Lang, B. 1967. Modification of the palatal lift speech aid. *J. prosthetic Dent.*, 17, 620–627.

Lefkovits, A., and Kapidus, B. 1950. Hairy tongue. *JAMA*, 143, 1482.

Lewis, J., and Counihan, R. 1965. Tongue-thrust in infancy. *J. Speech Hearing Disorders*, 30, 280–282.

Liebowitz, U. 1966. Bell's palsy: two disease entities? *Neurology*, 16, 1105–1109.

Lifschiz, J. 1963. Tongue markers for cineflurographic analysis. *J. Speech Hearing Disorders*, 28, 393–396.

Linder-Aronson, S., and Backstron, A. 1960. A comparison between mouth and nose breathers with respect to occlusion and facial dimensions: a biometric study. *Odontologisk Revy*, 11.

Lischer, B. 1912. Orthodontics, principles and methods of. Philadelphia: Lea & Febiger.

Logan, W., and Kronfeld, R. 1933. Development of the human jaws and surrounding structures from birth to the age of fifteen years. *J. Amer. dent. Assn.*, 20, 379–427.

Lubker, J. 1968. An electromyographic-cinefluorographic investigation of velar function during normal speech production. *Cleft Palate J.* 5, 1–18.

Luc, J. 1958. Sturge-Weber syndrome—report of an unusual case. *Brit. J. Ophthal.*, 12, 296–305.

Luchsinger, R., and Arnold, G. 1965. Voice-speech-language. Belmont, Calif.: Wadsworth. P. 812.

Lundstrom, R., Lejsell, L., and Berghagen, N. 1962. Dental development in children following maternal rubella. *Acta. Pediat.*, 51, 155–160.

Lyonnet, R., and Morin, G. 1962. Two new cases of hydramnios co-existing with fetal malformations interfering with deglutition. *Bul. Fed. Soc. Gynec. Obstet. Franc.*, 14, 277–279.

MacNeilage, P. 1963. Motor patterns of speech production. *Acoust. soc. Amer.*, 35, 779.

———, and Scholes, G. An electromyographic study of the tongue during vowel production. *J. Speech Hearing Res.*, 7, 209–233.

McEnery, E., and Gaines, F. 1941. Tongue-tie in infants and children. *J. Pediat.*, 18, 252–255.

Massler, M., and Schour, I. 1946. Growth of the child and the calcification pattern of the teeth. *Amer. J. Orthodont. oral Surg.*, 32, 495–517.

Merz. M., and Wojtowicz, S. 1967. The Moebius' syndrome. *Amer. J. Ophthal.*, 63, 837–840.

Moses, E. 1936. Palatography, a critical study and analysis of sound-image contacts. Univ. Mich.: Ph.D. dissertation.

———. 1939. Palatography and speech improvement. *J. Speech Disorders*. 4, 103–114.

Moyers, R. 1949. Temperomandibular muscle contraction patterns in angle class II, division I malocclusions: an electromyographic analysis. *Amer. J. Orthodont.*, 35 (II), 837–857.

———. 1956. A handbook of orthodontics. Chicago: Year Book Pub.

———. 1962. The role of musculature in orthodontic diagnosis and treatment planning. *In* Vistas in Orthodontics. Kraus, B., and Reedel, R., ed. Philadelphia: Lea & Fabiger.

Muyskens, J. 1925. The smallest aggregate of speech movement, the hypha, analyzed and defined. Univ. Mich.: Ph.D. dissertation.

Noyers, F., Schour, I., and Noyes, H. 1948. Oral histology and embryology. Philadelphia: Lea & Fabiger.

Orban, B. 1944. Oral histology and embryology. St. Louis, Mo.: Mosby.

Ossi, B. 1964. Oriented cinefluorographic study of the production of certain sounds in cases of class II, division I malocclusion. *Amer. J. Orthodont.*, 50, 145.

Palmer, M. 1948. Orthodontics and the disorders of speech. *Amer. J. Orthodont.*, 34, 579–588.

Patten, B. 1953. Human embryology (2nd. ed.). New York. Blakiston.

Pearson, G. 1948. The psychology of finger-sucking, tongue-sucking, and other oral habits. *Amer. J. Orthodont.*, 34, 589–598.

Peterman, A., Hayles, A., Dockerty, M., and Love, J. 1958. Encephalotrigeminal angiomatosis (Sturge-Weber disease) clinical study of 35 cases. *JAMA*, 167, 2169–2176.

Peterson, G. and Shoup, J. 1966. A physiological theory of phonetics. *J. Speech Hearing Res.*, 9, 5–67.

Pike, K. 1943. Phonetics. Ann Arbor: Univ. of Mich. Press.

Pitner, S., Edwards, J., and McCormick, W. 1965. Observations on the pathology of the Moebius' syndrome. *J. Neurol., Neurosurgery, and Psychiat.*, 28, 362–374.

Pound, E. 1953. Esthetics dentures and their phonetic values. *Dent. J. Australia*, 25, 150–158.

———. 1951. Esthetic dentures and their phonetic values. *J. prosthetic Dent.* 1, 98–111.

Pruzansky, S. 1952. The applications of electromyography to dental research. *J. Amer. dent. Assn.*, 44, 49–68.

Pryor, W. 1933. The closed bite relation of the jaws of George Washington, with comments on his tooth troubles and general health. *J. Amer. dent. Assn.*, 20, 567–579.

Pullen, H. 1927. Abnormal habits in their relation to malocclusion and facial deformity. St. Louis, Mo.: Mosby.

Rakosi, T. 1958. Thumbsucking and malocclusion. *Bratislave. lekar. listy.*, 38: 36–40.

Randall, P., Krogman, W., and Johina, S. 1965. Pierre Robin and the syndrome that bears his name. *Cleft Palate J.*, 2, 237–246.

Ricketts, R. 1958. The functional diagnosis of malocclusion. *European orthodontic Soc.* Report of 34th Congress, 42–62.

Ringel, R., and Steer, M. 1963. Some effects of tactile and auditory alterations on speech output. *J. Speech Hearing Res.*, 6, 369–377.

Rix, R. 1953. Some observations upon the environment of the incisors. *Dent. Record*, 73, 427–441.

Roizin, L., Gold, G., Berman, H., and Bonafede, V. 1959. Congenital vascular anomalies and their histopathology in Sturge-Weber syndrome (naveus flammeus with angiomatosis and encephalosis, calcificans), *J. Neuropath. exper. Neurol.*, 18, 75–97.

Ronchese, F., and Kern, A. 1953. Hairy tongue: report of a case following use of aureomycin ointment. *A.M.A. Arch. Dermat. Syph.*, 67, 503.

Ronkin, S. 1953. Improvement of low-tone deafness and tinnitus by mandibular repositioning. *A.M.A. Arch. Otolaryng.*, 56, 669–673.

Ronson, I. 1965. Incidence of visceral swallowing among lispers. *J. Speech Hearing Disorders*, 30, 318–324.

Rousselot, L. 1910. Principles de phonetique experimental nouveau ed. Paris. Paris: Libraire universitaire.

Royle, H., Lapp, R., and Ferrard, E. 1966. Sturge-Weber drug therapy. *Oral Surg.*, 22, 490–497.

de Rudder, B. 1960. Tooth eruption and finger-sucking. *Deut. Medizinische Wochenschrift.*, 85, 1517–1520.

Russell, G. 1934. First preliminary x-ray consonant study. *J. acoust. soc. Amer.*, 5, 247–251.

Ruttle, A., Quigley, W., Crouch, J., and Ewan, G. 1953. A serial study of the effects of finger-sucking. *J. dent. Res.*, 32, 739–748.

Saizar, P. 1958. Phonétique et prosthèse, *Actualities odontostomat*, 12, 561–565 (dsh Abstracts, 1, 1960).

Salzmann, J. 1950. Principles of orthodontics. Philadelphia: Lippincott.

Schour, I., and Massler, M. 1940. Studies in tooth development; the growth pattern of human teeth (Part I). *J. Amer. dent. Assn.*, 27, 1778–1793.

Sclare, R. 1957. The trapped lower lip. *Brit. Dent. J.* 102, 398–403.

Shohara, H. 1941. Speech rehabilitation in a case of post-operated cleft palate and malocclusion. *J. Speech Disorders*, 7, 381–388.

Sillman, J. 1951. Thumb-sucking and the dentition. A serial study from birth to 13 years of age. *N.Y. dent. J.*, 17, 493–502.

Silver, H., and Dodd, S. 1957. Gonadal dysgenesis, Bonnevie-Ullrich-Turner syndrome with elevated urinary gonadotropism in the nine year old child *Amer. J. dis. Child.*, 94, 702–707.

Slaughter, M. 1945. Speech correction in full denture prosthesis. *Dent. Digest*, 51, 242–246.

Sloan, R., Ricketts, R., Brummett, S., Mulick, J., Bench, R., Ashley, R., and Hahn, E. 1963. Cephalometric-cinefluorographic diagnostic criteria utilized in cranio-facial problems. *J. S. Calif. dent. Assn.* 31, 355–362.

———, ———, Bench, R., Hahn, E., Westover, J., and Brummett, S. 1964. The application of cephalometrics to cinefluorography. *The Angle Orthodontist*, 34, 132–141.

Smith, L., and Stowe, F. 1961. The Pierre Robin syndrome; a review of 39 cases with emphasis on associated ocular lesions. *Pediatrics*, 27, 128–133.

Spannenberg, H. 1937. Effects of dental prosthetic appliances on voice quality. Chicago: Year Book Pub.

Spies, T. 1958. Some recent advances in nutrition, *JAMA*, 167, 675–690.

Sprofkin, B., and Hillman, J. 1956. Moebius' syndrome —congenital oculofacial paralysis. *Neurology*, 6, 50–54.

Stallard, H. 1930. A consideration of extraoral pressures in the etiology of malocclusions. *Int. J. Orthodontia oral Surg. Radiography.* 16, 475–526.

Straub, W. 1951. The etiology of the perverted swallowing habit. *Amer. J. Orthodont.*, 37, 603–610.

———. 1960. Malfunction of the tongue. Part I: the abnormal swallowing habit, its cause, effects and results in relation to orthodontic treatment and speech therapy. *Amer. J. Orthodont.*, 46, 404–424.

———. 1961. Malfunction of the tongue. Part II: the abnormal swallowing habit: its causes, effects and results in relation to orthodontic treatment and speech therapy. *Amer. J. Orthodont.*, 47, 596–617.

———. 1962. Malfunction of the tongue. Part III: the abnormal swallowing habit: its causes, effects and results in relation to orthodontic treatment and speech therapy. *Amer. J. Orthodont.*, 48, 486–503.

Subtelny, J., Mestre, J. and Subtelny, J. 1964. Comparative study of normal and defective articulation of /s/ as related to malocclusion and deglutition. *J. Speech Hearing Disorders*, 29, 293–306.

Sulzmann, J., and Seide, L. 1962. Malocclusion with extreme microglossia. *Amer. J. Orthodont.*, 48, 848–857.

Swinehart, D. 1950. Importance of tongue in development of normal occlusion. *Amer. J. Orthodont.*, 36, 813–830.

Takagi, Y., McCalla, J., and Bosma, J. 1966. Prone feeding of infants with the Pierre Robin syndrome. *Cleft Palate J.*, 3, 232–238.

Tarneaud, J. 1946. La voix et les affections dentaires. *Le Progres medical*, 17, 374–375.

Tench, R. 1927. The influence of speech habits on the design of full artificial dentures. *J. Amer. dent. Assn.*, 14, 644–647.

Trim, J. 1953. Some suggestions for the phonetic notation of sounds in defective speech. *Speech* (London), XVII, 21–24.

Tulley, W. 1953. Methods of recording patterns of behavior of the oro-facial muscles using the electromyograph. *Dental Record*, 43, 741–748.

———. 1954. Prognosis and treatment planning in orthodontics. *Brit. dent. J.*, 97, 135–148.

———. 1957. Muscles and the teeth. *Proceedings of the the Royal Soc. Med.*, Section of Odontology, 50, 313–30.

———. 1961. Long term studies of malocclusion. *European Orthodontic Soc.*, Report of 37th. Congress. 256–265.

———. 1962. Long-term orthodontic results, recorded by cinematography. *Dental Practicioner* and *Dental Record*, 12, 253–260.

———. 1956. Adverse muscle forces—their diagnostic significance. *Amer. J. Orthodont.*, 42, 801–814.

Van Riper, C. 1954. Speech correction, principles and methods (3rd. ed.). Englewood Cliffs, N.J.: Prentice-Hall.

Van Thal, J. 1936. The relationship between faults of dentition and defects of speech. Cambridge: Cambridge. Pp. 254–257.

Vocational Rehabilitation Administration. 1966. Facial disfigurement, a rehabilitation problem. Conference Institute Reconstructive Plastic Surg. N.Y. Univ. med. center, Mar., 1963. U.S. Government Printing Office. P. 224.

Walker, M. 1941. Psychologic effects of malocclusion of the teeth. *Amer. J. Orthodont. oral Surg.*, 27, 599–604.

Wallace, A. 1963. Tongue tie. *Lancet*, 2, 377–378.

Walpole-Day, A. 1951. The effect of the condyle on the growth of the mandible. London: Saward and Co.

Walsh, M. 1961. Breaking habits. *Dental Survey*, 456–457.

Warrer, E. 1959. Simultaneous occurrence of certain muscle habits and malocclusion. *Amer. J. Orthodont.*, 45, 365–370.

Watson, E., and Lowrey, G. 1954. Growth and development of children (2nd. ed.). Chicago: Year Book Pub.

Wepman, J. 1937. Anatomic speech defects. *J. Amer. dent. Assn. dent. Cosmos*, 24, 1799–1804.

West, R., Kennedy, L., and Carr, A. 1947. The rehabilitation of speech (rev. ed.). New York: Harper.

———, Ansberry, M., and Carr, A. 1957. The rehabilitation of speech (3rd. ed.). New York: Harper.

Wheeler, R. 1940. Textbook of dental anatomy and physiology. Philadelphia: Saunders.

Winders, R. 1962. Recent findings in myometric research. *The Angle Orthodontist*, 32, 38–43.

Wolfe, I. 1937. Relationship of malocclusion to sigmatism. *Amer. J. dis. Child.*, 54, 520–528.

Woodburne, R. 1965. Essentials of human anatomy. (3rd. ed.). New York: Oxford.

Wright, C., Strong, L., Kingery, R., Muyskens, J., Westerman, K., and Williams, S. 1949. A study of the tongue and its relation to denture stability. *J. Amer. dent. Assn.*, 39, 269–275.

Zappler, S. 1949. Dentistry and the cerebral palsied child. *J. Dent. Child.* 16, 16–18.

Zemlin, W. 1968. Speech and hearing science, anatomy and physiology. Englewood Cliffs, N.J.: Prentice-Hall.

29

Orofacial Clefts: Their Forms and Effects

Herbert Koepp-Baker

INTRODUCTION

The congenital orofacial deformity commonly identified as cleft palate, with or without cleft lip, is one of many syndromes of human developmental aberrations. Orofacial clefts may be present in the human neonate without any apparent associated anomalies. In most instances, however, other coincident disturbances of development may be clinically conspicuous, while in others they may be subtle or covert. Such attendant anomalies of development may affect one or more of the somatosystems—the skeletal, the visceral, the cardiovascular, the nervous, or the genitourinary. In these chapters, however, our discussion will be limited to the most common of congenital anomalies involving the head. We shall examine the nature of those particular deformities which are usually recognized as ceasmic interruptions, discontinuities, or impaired intactitude of critical tissues in the orofacial region; commonly identified as cleft palate and/or cleft lip. We shall also define the deleterious influences which these teratoses impose upon the processes of speech learning, speech production, and speech reception.

It is important that we assert early in this discussion that at least a modest understanding of the genetic and embryologic mechanisms which underlie both normal and abnormal development is essential to a satisfactory comprehension of the complex nature and the varied functional implications of orofacial anomalies. We are assuming here that the student already possesses or will acquire some basic biologic information and insight.

For centuries in all cultures it has been observed that these congenital dysconfigurations of orofacial anatomy operate as a severe deterrent to the acquisition of normal speech and produce one of the most profound of all speech disorders. However, circumstances dictate that contact of the speech clinician with the child with cleft palate is seldom established earlier than the age of three. Rarely, therefore, does the speech specialist have an opportunity to examine the newborn with orofacial deformity carefully, and to study him before reconstructive surgical procedures have been instituted, or oral orthopedic treatment has begun. It is for this reason that we think it imperative to first undertake a detailed description of the pathoanatomy of orofacial clefts in the neonate. Moreover, it is important to delineate the determinative influences of such congenitally deviate anatomy upon regional and total cephalic growth. It is only by a careful elucidation of the pathomorphologic features of orofacial malformations and of their peculiar effects upon growth energetics, that we are able to educe clearly the disturbing influences of these teratoses upon the physiology of speech.

THE PATHOMORPHOLOGY OF OROFACIAL CLEFTS

In a general and introductory way we may assert that a congenital cleft palate and/or cleft lip is a deformity which represents an aberrant embryologic tissue disposition, involving to some degree both the soft and dense tissues of the upper lip, mouth, pharynx, cranial base, and cervical vertebrae. Characteristically, this faulty tissue disposition takes the form of a disjunction of anatomic structures, with an associated geometric disarrangement of adjacent parts, and hyperplasia or hypoplasia. A number of systems of classification of orofacial malformations have been devised and are in present use, each having both advantages and disadvantages depending upon the particular purpose they are to serve. For our purpose we will find a scheme based upon genetic, embryologic, anatomic, and physiologic considerations as accurate and as useful as any.

Varieties of Orofacial Deformities

Based upon genetic and embryologic considerations as well as upon pathoanatomic differentials, it may be asserted that there are three general classes of congenital orofacial malformations: 1. those involving, in varying degrees, the primary palate only—the upper lip, the alveolus, and the anterior portion of the hard palate; 2. those involving in varying degrees, *both* the *primary* and the *secondary* palates—the lip, the alveolus, the anterior hard palate, the middle and posterior hard palate, and the velum palatinum; and 3. those involving the *secondary palate* only—the middle and posterior portion of the hard palate and the velum palatinum (Fig. 29-1). These three general classes, representing as they do teratotic events on genetic and embryologic levels, are displayed in a large number of individual variations, differences, and combinations in kind and in degree. It should be understood, therefore, that this broad threefold classification merely helps to bring a visualizable order to what we shall come to see is a complex and multiform clinical entity, and one reflecting great individual variability. To assume the population having orofacial malformity to be homogeneous in pathomorphologic traits is to obscure the features that need most to be understood if treatment is to be effectively specific.

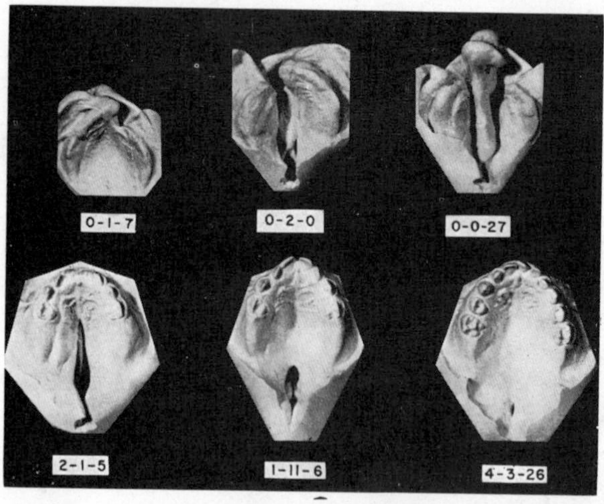

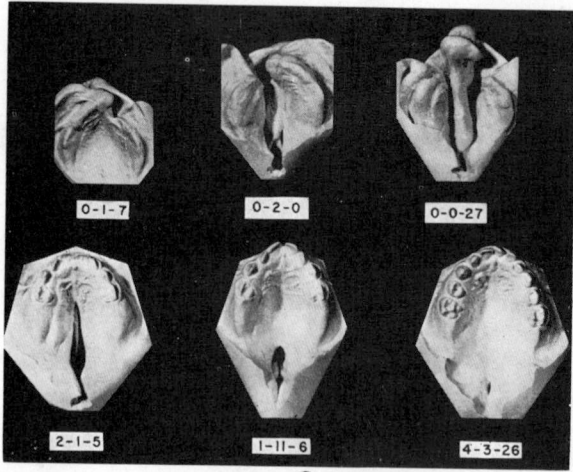

Fig. 29-1. Representative examples of common clefts of the primary and the secondary palates. The age of the patient appears beneath each figure and is stated in years, months and days. These are the photographs of casts made from impressions of the mouth before surgery or maxillary orthopedics.

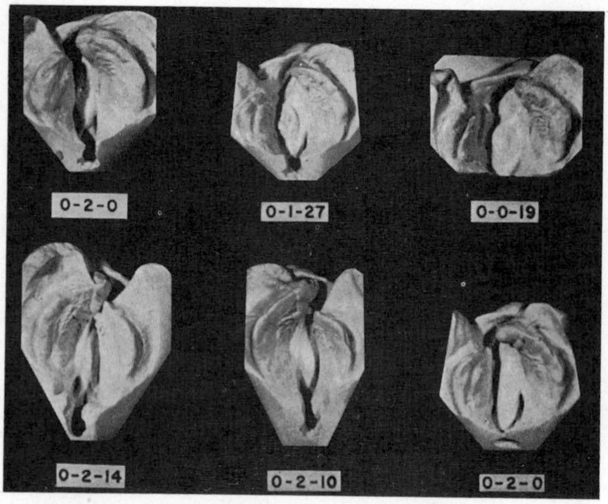

Fig. 29-2. Varieties of unilateral complete clefts of the primary and of the secondary palates. Although they are all of the one "type," they show great individual pathomorphological differences: and these differences are often more significant than is the general classification.

When the tissue disjunction is limited to one side of the midline of the lip, and/or primary and secondary palates, the clefts are designated as being *unilateral*. When some part or all of both sides of the facial complex are involved they are referred to as being *bilateral*. Another important pathomorphologic feature of clefts of the lip, hard palate, and velum palatinum, is the profound displacement of structures adjacent to the line of nonunions. This characteristic disarrangement of contiguous structures results from the absence, or from the vitiation, of the normal vectors of embryologic and neonatal growth forces which guide, stimulate, and control the architectonic organization of the facial complex (Figs. 29-2, 29-3, 29-4, and 29-5).

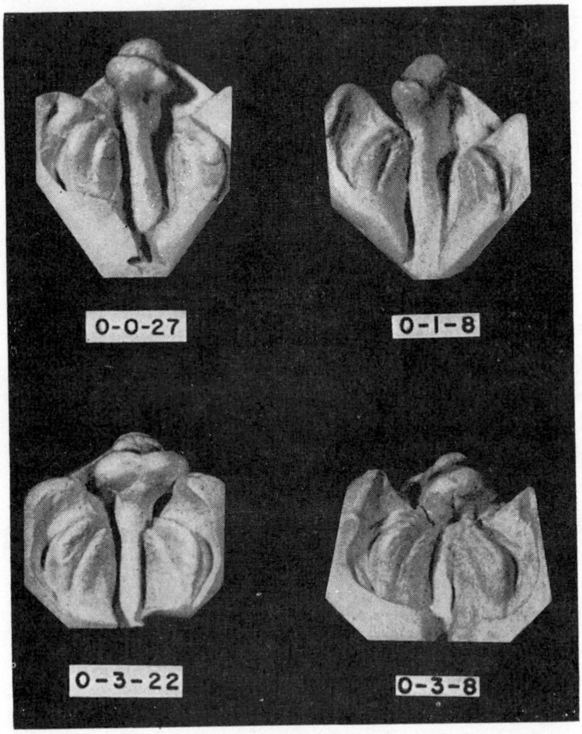

Fig. 29-3. Varieties of bilateral complete clefts of the primary and the secondary palates. The individual pathomorphologic variations are striking. The general disconfiguration of anatomic structures is characteristic.

Incidence and Teratogenesis

Orofacial malformations appear more often among children of Japanese ancestry, and less commonly in American Negroes than among Caucasians. The incidence of these teratoses also appears to vary in different parts of the world. A commonly published figure is one in 1,000 births, though some careful studies indicate that in some parts of the United States it may be as high as one in 600. About 25 percent of malformations of the primary palate are bilateral.

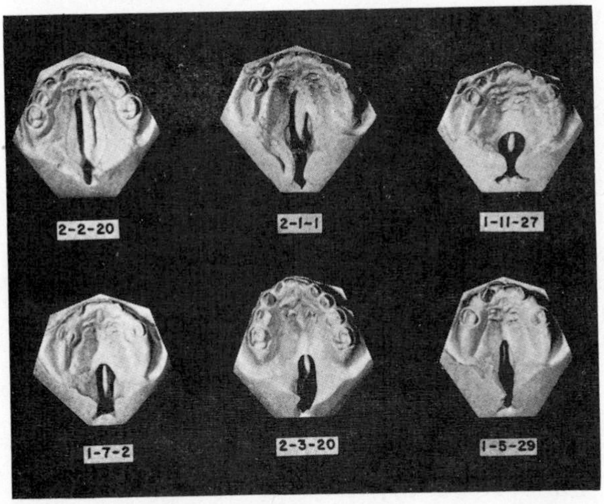

Fig. 29-4. Varieties of clefts of the secondary palate. The pathomorphological variation is noteworthy.

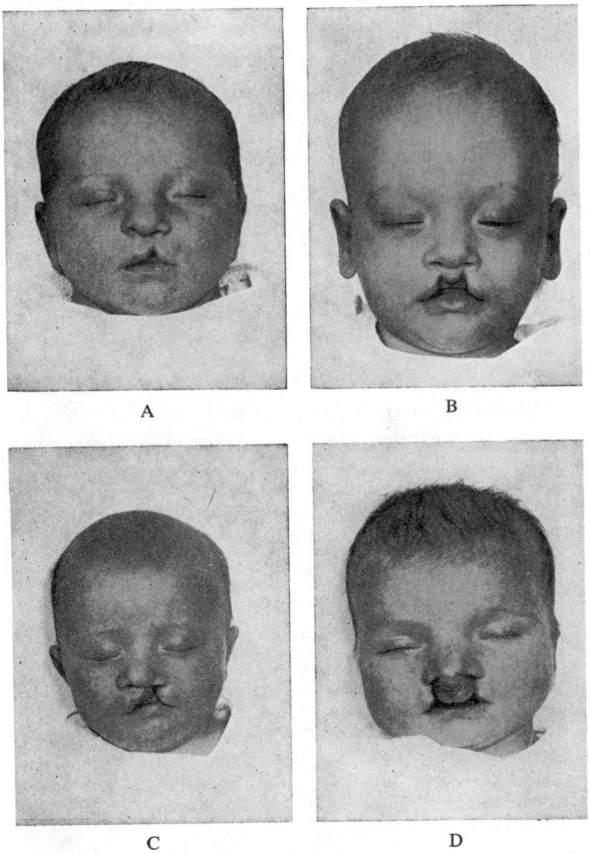

Fig. 29-5. A: unilateral incomplete cleft of the primary palate;
B: bilateral incomplete cleft of the primary palate;
C: unilateral complete cleft of the primary palate;
D: bilateral complete cleft of the primary palate.

When they are unilateral about 30 percent involve the right side, and 70 percent appear on the left. It is of special interest to note, too, that the incidence of defects of the primary palate is about twice as great in male babies as in females. It is generally asserted by clinicians that 85 percent of the bilateral clefts of the primary palate, and 70 percent of those that are unilateral, are also associated with nonunions of the secondary palates.

Teratological studies as yet provide no secure and final answer to the question: What is the cause (or causes) of orofacial deformities in man? They appear to be produced directly or indirectly by both endogenous (genetic) and exogenous (environmental) teratogenic factors. Just how these factors operate in every case is not clear, but is being illumined by studies going on in many disciplines including, more recently, molecular biology. On occasion the teratogenic factors appear to act independently and at other times interactively. It is now evident, however, that malformations of the secondary palate (often referred to as isolated clefts) are genetically at least, a quite different genetico-embryologic event from either clefts of the primary palate alone, or combined clefts of the primary *and* secondary palates. Also, they appear more frequently in females than in males (Gorlin and Pindborg, 1964).

Clefts of the Primary Palate

Tissue disunions which are limited to the upper lip, the alveolus, or the premaxillary region, may be present in varying degrees ranging from minimal defects (notches) in the vermeil portion of either or both sides of the upper lip to a complete extension into the nasal vestibule, the alveolar ridge, and the anterior nasal floor, along the premaxillary osteal sutures to the incisive foramen.

Bearing in mind that there will be great variability in individual features of any orofacial deformity, examine Fig. 29-6 as we proceed with a detailed description of a *unilateral complete* cleft of the primary palate of a newborn. Note that there is some superiolateral displacement of both divided lip segments, a lateral displacement of the nasal tip and of the columella, toward the unaffected side, a flaring and flattening of the nasal alar cartilage on the affected side, and a deflection of the cartilagenous nasal septum toward the sound side. The floor of the nose on the affected side is discontinuous, the hiatus in the body of the lip and alveolus extending posteriorward along the premaxillary-maxillary suture. The divided alveolar segments may also be asymetrically positioned.

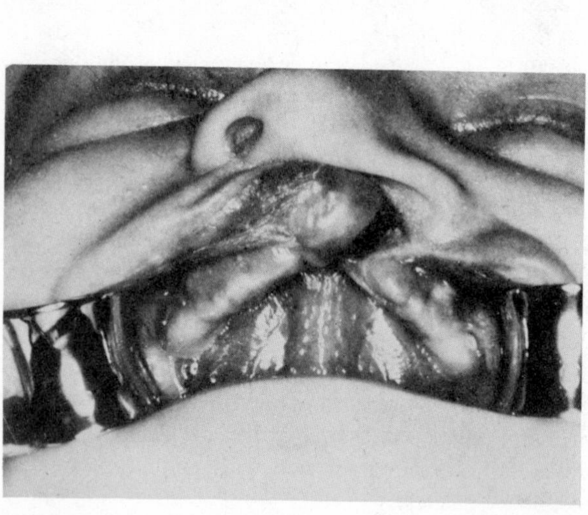

Fig. 29-6. An infant with a complete unilateral cleft of the primary palate.

The fate of the deciduous tooth buds at and adjacent to the line of nonunion is reasonably predictable. One or more may be absent, and others may be deformed. Their path of eruption may be abnormal. These may be precursors to similar conditions in the permanent dentition in that area. In a frontal view of the face the tip of the tongue may be prominent, while in profile certain areas of the middle third of the face may appear protrusive.

Examine now the salient pathoanatomic features of a *bilateral complete* cleft of the primary palate. As indicated earlier, nonunions of the primary palate may occur on *both* sides of the midline of the face. (Midline clefts of the face are very rare.) Recalling, too, that unilateral clefts may be of varying degree of completeness or differ in the extent of invasion of the orofacial tissue, so too, in bilateral clefts the disunion may be extensive or limited. Further, bilateral clefts may also be asymetrical inasmuch as the magnitude of the defect may be greater on one side than on the other (one being complete, the other incomplete).

It is an error to assume that the effect of bilaterality is merely additive—that is, that a bilateral cleft is merely the sum of two separate and individual unilateral clefts imposed upon the orofacial complex. Actually the impressive effect of bilaterality of the defect is that it produces a number of special and compounding anatomic dysconfigurations. The most significant of these is the malposition and abnormal morphology of the premaxillary bone and its soft tissue investment. Turn now to Fig. 29-7, where these features will be made clear. Note that there is a considerably greater and grosser distortion of the total orofacial anatomy than in the previous illustration of the unilateral cleft (Fig. 29-6). It will be observed that in the bilateral complete cleft of the primary palate, the integrity of *both* premaxillary-maxillary osteal sutures is violated, separating the primary palate completely from the horizontal processes of the maxillae. The continuity of the tissues of the alveolus and of the prolabium, and of the lateral labial masses, is also interrupted. The premaxillary bone with its

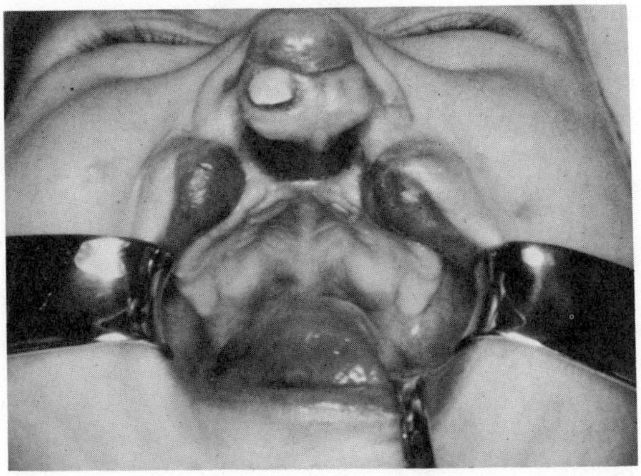

Fig. 29-7. Infant with a complete bilateral cleft of the primary palate.

overlying prolabium remains attached only to the columella, the premaxillary bony crest, and the extended vomerine stock. Upon palpation it would be noted that the whole primary palate is movable and unstable. An even more prominent feature is the elevated, severely protrusive, and rotated position of the premaxillary bone and its prolabium. The facial profile is, of course, also greatly altered. On occasion the whole premaxillary mass may be hypoplastic. Both nasal alar cartilages are flared and flattened, the tip of the nose greatly elevated, the columella shortened, and the labial philtrum obscured or absent.

Clefts of Both Primary and Secondary Palates

Pathomorphologically, this class may be conceived of as a posteriorward extension of clefts already described, throughout the full palatal axis. The disjunction involves the tissues of the secondary palate as well as those of the primary palate. This type is illustrated by Figs. 29-8 and 29-9. As in the previous class, the pattern of tissue discontinuity and structural disorder may be unilateral or it may be bilateral. That is, it may involve one or both sides of the midline of the facial complex. Fig. 29-8 shows a unilateral cleft involving both the primary and secondary palates. It will be noted that in addition to the deformities characteristic of clefts of the primary palate, this type reflects extensive deformity of the secondary palate as well. The notable features are the detachment of the horizontal process of the maxilla on the side of the cleft and the exposure of the lateral aspect of the vomer. There is, too, a superiorward displacement of the detached palatal shelf. The maxillary arch is irregular in shape with the affected portion being displaced lingually in a cross-bite position. The nonunion extends through the horizontal process of the palatal bones following the midline osteal suture. The velum palatinum is cleft throughout its length, and the two halves of that structure are reduced in size and drawn laterally. The form of the uvula is obscured. The posterior wall of the epipharynx with its lymphoid vegetation of the pharyngeal tonsil (adenoid) is exposed to view. If the tag of the velum on the affected side is elevated with a tongue blade or a dental mirror the torus tubarius and the auditory meatus may be visualized.

In the circumstance of a bilateral nonunion of both the primary and secondary palates, as shown in the photograph in Fig. 29-9, note that the horizontal processes of both the maxillary bones and of both palatal bones are detached from the vomer bone through its full length. Both nasal spaces with their turbinated walls may be seen clearly through the open mouth.

The Velum Palatinum

The classical and conventional anatomic view of the velum palatinum has been that it is an extension of the structural system forming the "roof of the mouth"; that is, that it is a part of the oral palate. Physiologically and clinically it is more enlightening to recognize that, phylogenetically and ontogenetically, the velum

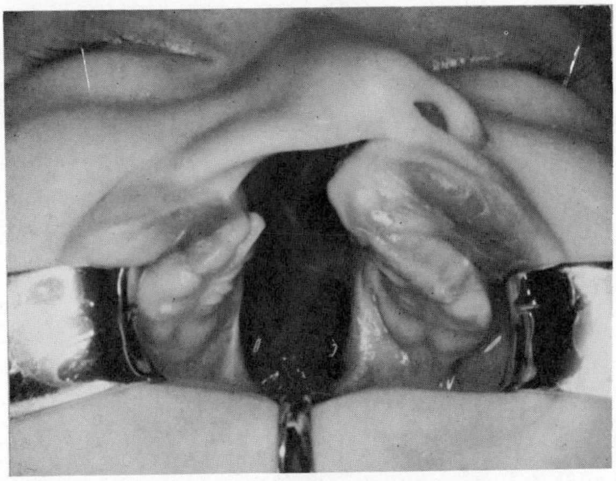

Fig. 29-8. An infant with a complete unilateral cleft of the primary and of the secondary palate.

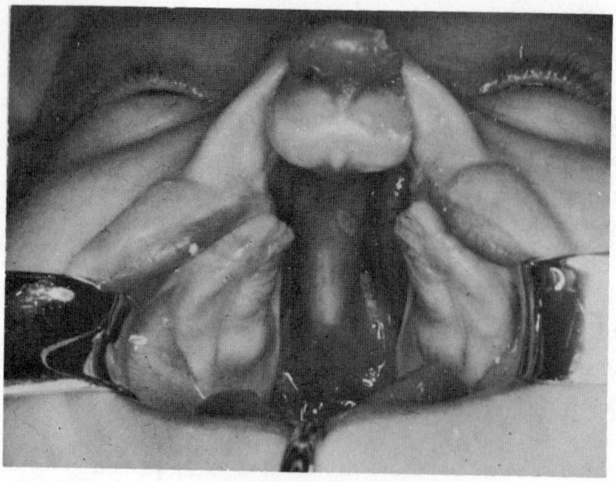

Fig. 29-9. An infant with a complete bilateral cleft of the primary and of the secondary palates.

is an intrinsic part of the pharynx and serves a pharyngeal function. Moreover, the effects of congenital discontinuity of the velum and the resulting inadequacies of that structure are more clearly discerned if it is recognized for what it is—an essential structural and functional component of the pharynx.

When the velum is congenitally divided, the complex physiomechanical system of oronasopharyngeal valving in breathing, deglutition, and speech is vitiated. Effective sphincteric action is of course, completely dependent upon the continuity and integrity of what may be conceived of as dual muscular slings—one acting superioposteriorly, the other inferioanteriorly. When the insertions of the tensor palati and the levator palati muscles in the velar aponeurosis are split, their separate contractions draw the velar remnants laterally. If the origins (or the insertions, if so viewed) of the glossopalatinus and the pharyngopalatinus are also divided in the velar aponeurosis, their contractive movements during swallowing and speech displace the divided velar segments still farther away from the midline. The existence of paired fibers of the pterygopharyngeus muscles having insertions into the velum has been questioned by some anatomists. If they are present, as they are said to be on some dissections, their defective action would be similar to other muscles of the hemisphincter (Fig. 29-10).

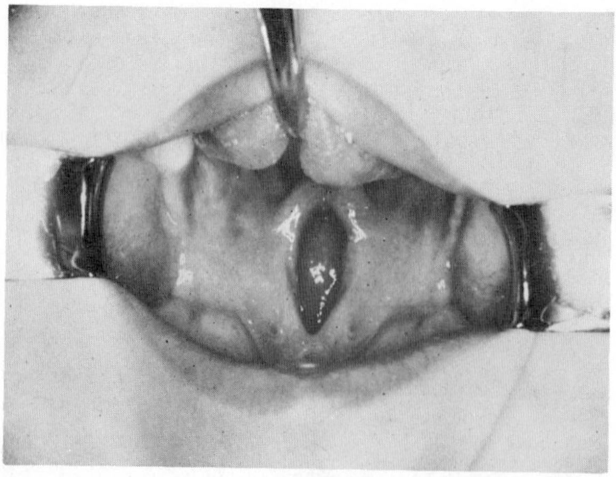

Fig. 29-10. A cleft of the velum palatinum in an adolescent. There is also some concommitant underdevelopment of the posterior borders of the palatal bones.

Individual variations in the pathomorphology of unilateral and bilateral clefts of the primary and secondary palates are almost innumerable. The following general features are of significance to the reconstructive surgeon and oral orthopedist:

1. The tissue adequacy of the divided labial parts and their positions in relation to the prolabium and premaxillary bone.

2. Asymmetry of cleft width and length—greater on one side of the midline of the palates than on the other. The lip may be divided up to or into the nasal floor. The vomer bone may be partially attached on one side and completely unattached on the other side, or unattached on either side.

3. Variant inclination of the palatal shelves. The horizontal processes of the maxillary and palatal bones may be bilaterally elevated or depressed, or one or the other may be elevated or depressed while its companion on the contralateral side may be in a reasonably normal position.

4. Adequacy of the bony palatal shelves. There may be osteal inadequacy of either or both of the horizontal plates of both the maxillary and palatal bones with a resulting increase in the lateral width of the clefts. Inadequacy may also be characteristic of their investing mucoperiosteum and mucous membrane. The total tissue inadequacy may be asymmetrical—one shelf being less developed than the other.

5. Degree of vomerine deformity. This structure may be underdeveloped or occasionally overdeveloped. The oral aspect of the vomer may be bulbous or may have a knifelike edge. It may be foreshortened or deflected from its normal position.

6. Tissue adequacy of the velum palatinum. In addition to the lateral displacement of the two split segments of the velum, one or both of its segments may be underdeveloped. There is reason to believe that

this appearance of general tissue inadequacy actually may reflect inadequacy of the muscle masses of the velum palatinum. Because the biomechanical system of the nasopharyngeal hemisphincter is violated by the embryologic midline discontinuity, it appears reasonable that the myologic components of the velum may also be growth-retarded.

We must also be aware as we study the illustrations and as we proceed with this description of the pathomorphology, that the roof of the mouth also constitutes the floor of the nose. Hence, deformity of the palatal structures, whether extensive or limited, will affect the architecture of the bounding structures of the nasal spaces. A conspicuous deformity of the inner structures of the nose is the deflected position or shape of the cartilagenous and bony septa. It may be present in either bilateral or unilateral palatal involvement. Further, intensive study of the cranio-cervico-facial structures by the refined mensurative procedures of roentgenocephalography shows that the teratogenic influences producing orofacial clefts are indeed not limited in their effects to the orofacial structures. Minimal or gross concomitant deformities are usually present in both adjacent and in remote regions of the total cephalocervical region (Subtelny, 1953; Moss, 1955; and Ricketts, 1952).

Covert Clefts of the Secondary Palate

The clefts we have so far described are clearly recognizable as tissue nonunions and disjunctions. Parts which are ordinarily united are detached from each other. There is yet another type of deformity of the secondary palate which is usually not so apparent upon peroral examination (Fig. 29-11). The mucous membrane, mucoperiosteum, and their osteal foundations of the palate appear to be intact. However, by palpation of the roof of the mouth or by transpalatal illumination, a defect in the horizontal processes of the maxillary and/or the palatal bones may be noted. The defect may range from an absence of the post-nasal spine and a slight inadequacy revealed by an atypical contour of the posterior bony palatal border, to a more extensive inadequacy which invades the palatal bones deeply along the median suture as far forward as the zenith of the palatine vault. The most noteworthy feature of these bony inadequacies, which are commonly called "submucous clefts," is the concomitant anteriorward displacement of the velar aponeurosis producing a foreshortening of the total A-P palatal axis. As in the other classes of clefts already

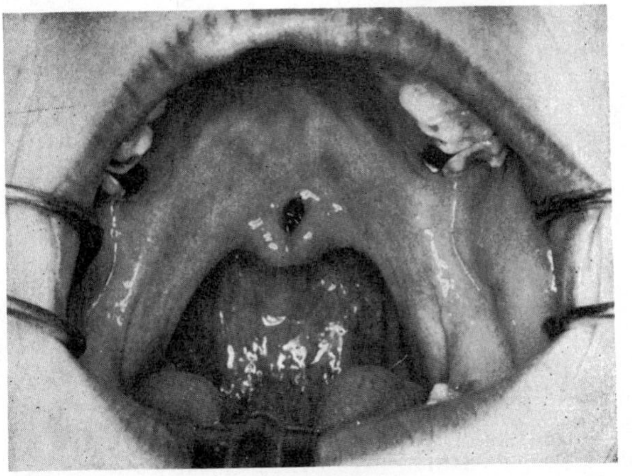

Fig. 29-11. A submucous incomplete cleft of the secondary palate. The cleft is confined to the palatal bones (covert) and the uvula. The velopharyngeal hemisphincter is incompetent.

described, the "submucosal" type presents itself in many variable forms. For example, bony inadequacies may be combined with an hypoplasia of the velum palatinum itself. The tissue of the velum, particularly in the midline, may be attenuated to a point of translucence. The levator dimples (indicating the site of insertion of the levator palati) will be located in a relatively anterior position. A deep epipharynx will complicate the situation still further. A frequent though not invariable clinical sign of submucosal cleft is a deformed or bifid uvula. This condition is also referred to (somewhat inaccurately) as "short palate."

Associated Pathomorphologies

We have observed that from a genetico-embryologic point of view it is unreasonable to assume that those teratogenic influences which produce orofacial deformities are limited in their effects to the orofacial complex, and that clefts of the primary and secondary palates are isolated defects of development. Clinically, quite the opposite is true. There are probably always at least subtle indexes of disturbed embryogenesis in adjacent or remote regions of the head. Of the many syndromes of the head and neck in which orofacial pathognomonic evidences are also present, only a few need concern us here.

One of these is mandibular hypoplasia (micrognathia), and glossoptosis, which is usually identified as the Pierre Robin Syndrome. This constellation of deformities is associated only with defects of the secondary palate. During the first few weeks of life the infant may experience respiratory embarrassment because of the retroposed tongue, but later, mandibular growth with attendant repositioning of the tongue may catch up with the growth of the rest of the head to a considerable extent (Pruzansky and Richmond, 1954).

Another syndrome which is not uncommonly associated with orofacial deformity is that of otomandibulofacial dysostosis, labeled the Treacher Collins Syndrome. Conspicuous pathoanatomic signs are antimongoloid obliquity of the eyes, microtic deformation of the auricle, atresia of the external auditory canal, malformation or absence of the ossicles, and severe dental malocclusion. Hypoplasia of the mandible and disturbances of the temporomandibular joint may also be present.

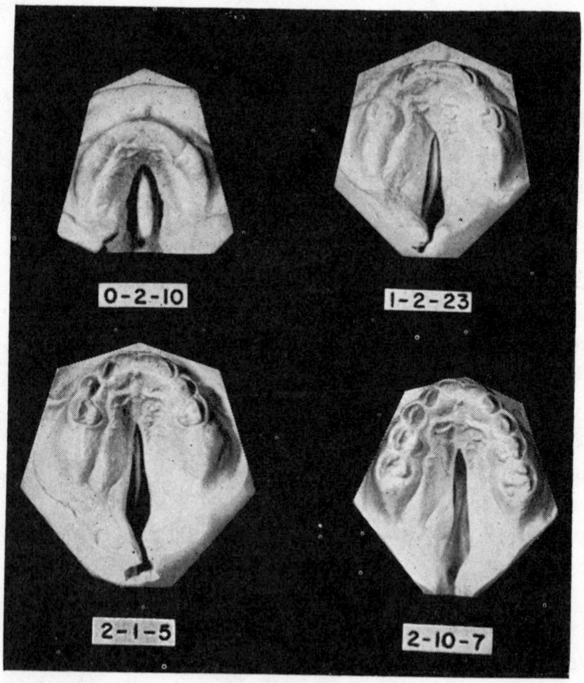

Fig. 29-12. A series of casts made from impressions of the mouth of the same child having a bilateral complete cleft of the secondary palate, beginning at the age of 2 months, 10 days, and extending to 2 years, 10 months, 7 days. Neither surgical nor maxillary orthopedic treatment intervened, nor did the child wear a temporary speech prosthesis. Note the significant decrease in the width of the cleft. Some, but not all, show such changes. Some grow wider.

The effects of Nonunions upon Orofacial Growth

In the development of the *normal* embryonic, fetal, and infant face, a number of important systems of active myologic and growth forces contribute to the ultimate alignment of the deeper structures (Fig. 29-12). The presence of an established muscular labiosphincter together with the buccal components assists in moulding and shaping the bounding structures of the oral and nasal cavities. Their external force is counterbalanced internally by the muscular pressures of the tongue. The result is the normal contouring of the maxillary and mandibular arches. The anterioinferior growth of the mandible with the coincident descent of the tongue from its intranasal position, and the earlier elevation of the palatal shelves and their union with the base of the vomer bone, confine the lingual muscular pressures within the oral cavity (Fig. 29-13).

Now let us attempt to visualize the effects of nonunions of the embryonic, fetal, and infant primary and secondary palates upon the dynamics of growth. When the mechanicophysiologic integrity of the labiosphincter is vitiated by nonunion, the divided portions of the lip will be drawn away from each other by the forces of growth and of muscular contraction. In bilateral nonunions of the primary palate, the guiding and containing influence of an intact labiosphincter being absent permits the prolabium and premaxillary structures to grow protrusively and often in superior direction and into torsive positions. In the circumstance of unilateral and/or bilateral clefts of both the primary and secondary palates, the buccal segments of the maxillary alveolar arch, being relatively unrestrained, may grow away from each other. The tongue, being unchecked because of the open palate, tends to occupy a somewhat elevated and intrusive position in the nasal space. The aberrant position of the premaxilla permits the front of the tongue to extrude from the oral cavity. The forces of muscular contraction in sucking and swallowing brought to bear upon the divided structures may encourage their further displacement.

The two parts of the divided velum palatinum are drawn laterally by the natural tonicity, the elasticity, and the contraction of the paired tensor palati, levator palati, palatopharyngeus, and palatoglossus muscles. The oral, nasal, and epipharyngeal spaces are intercommunicating. The biochemical environments of the nasal and oral cavities are intermixed. The epipharyngeal wall with its lymphoid tissue and the area of the auditory meati are exposed to the vegetative transactions in the mouth (Fig. 29-14).

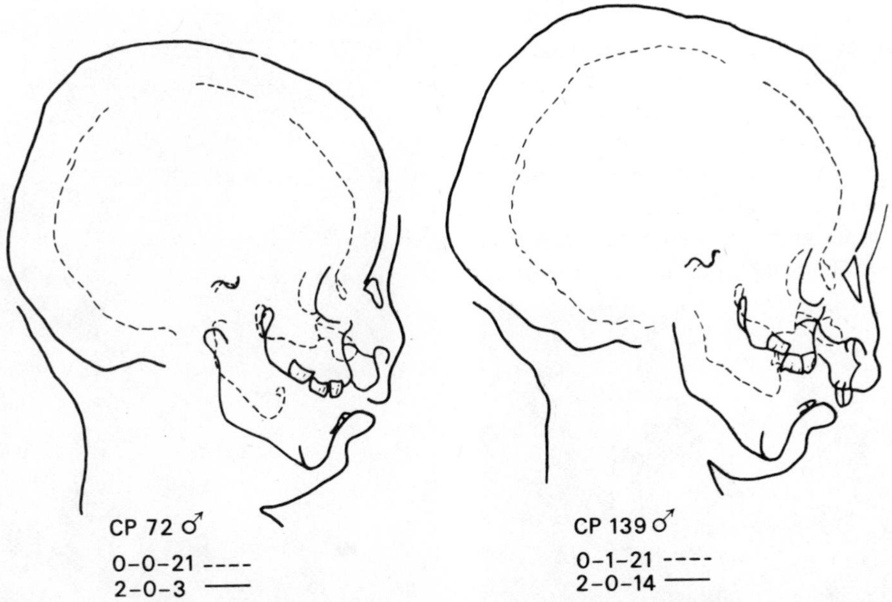

Fig. 29-13. Differences in the pattern of growth of two children with a cleft of the same "type" and each treated in a similar fashion. These are reproductions of tracings of the roentgenocephalograms made of each child at two different times, as indicated below the illustrations. The differences in growth patterns are reflected in the internal structures and in the profile.

Being again reminded that the roof of the mouth also constitutes the floor of the nasal cavities, we may expect concomitant growth deformities in the nasal structures. For example, the boundaries of one or both of the nasal choanae will be deformed or completely obliterated. The vomerine and cartilagenous septa, lacking their normally located inferior stabilizing attachments, will grow into abnormal positions. We have already seen in the pictorial displays that the external nasal configuration is profoundly altered—the change of position of the nasal tip, the flaring of one or both nasal alar cartilages—being a result of the altered dynamics of growth in the presence of bilateral or unilateral discontinuity of the primary and secondary palates.

The Effects of Surgical and Oral Orthopedic Treatments

Though we shall defer detailed discussion of surgical and orthopedic treatment, it will be useful at this point to examine the usual general effects of these treatment procedures from the standpoint of the eventual morphology of the vegetative and speech mechanisms. Examine the illustration in Fig. 29-15 as we proceed. Inasmuch as labial clefts are usually closed before the age of six months—often in the first month—we may expect to find a lip whose musculature has been restored to adequate function. There may remain perhaps, some inhibitions of lip mobility, but this does not appear to disadvantage the production of labial speech sounds. The lip will evidence some cicatricial ridges and masses, a natural and often unavoidable consequence of the plastic procedures. The degree of scarring will depend upon many factors: the type of cheilorrhaphy, the original amount and form of tissue available, the extent of undermining and transposition, the laterality of the defect, the degree of completeness of the clefts, and the eventfulness of healing. The mucodermal border may still be uneven, the cupid's bow obscured, the lip overlong or foreshortened, and the columella still binding down the inferiorly deflected nasal tip. There may be sublabial adhesions and a shallow sublabial sulcus (Fig. 29-15).

In bilateral cases the prolabium may still be protrusive until its supporting prepalate is returned to a more normal location by muscular pressure of the revised lip, or until orthopedic measures reposition the bone and the dental units it carries. Commonly either or both sides of the nose will show some residual prolapse. After the age of 12 or 14, secondary surgical revisions of both the lip and the nose may have placed the parts in proper locations and improved the cosmesis. Presurgical oral orthopedics may have realigned the clefted alveolar elements and have produced a reasonably satisfactory contouring of the anterior maxillary arch. If at the same time, or later, bone grafting of the alveolus has not been included, examination will reveal a mechanical abutment of the maxillary and premaxillary alveolar components rather than a bony union at the line of cleft. More often the segment on the affected side will still be displaced lingually to some degree. In bilateral cases having had no bone grafting, the prepalate will at times be unstable and movable on the vomerine stock.

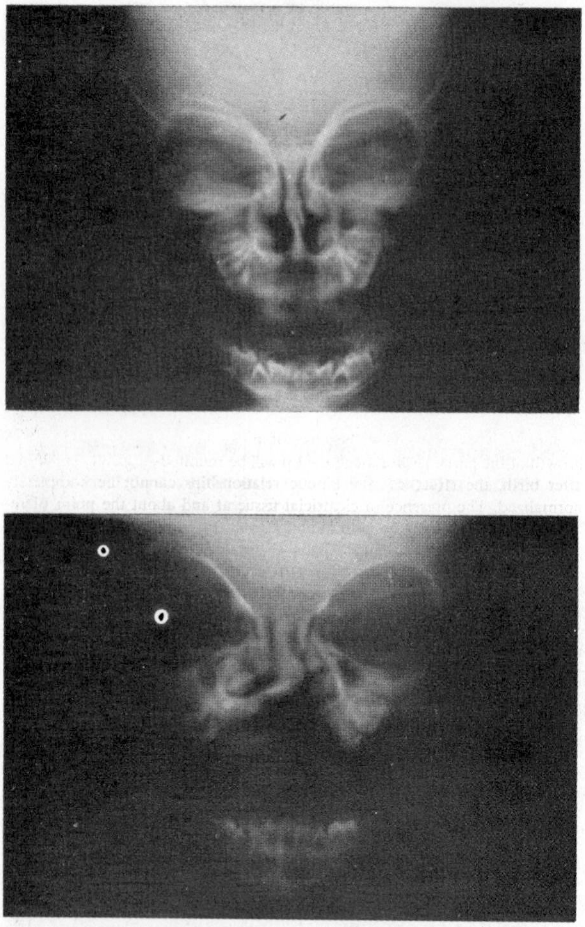

Fig. 29-14. Top, a frontal roentgenolaminagraphic projection of the deep structures of the orofacial region of a normal subject. Bottom, a similar projection of a patient with a unilateral complete cleft of the primary and secondary palates which reflects the profound alteration of these structures in many patients with congenital orofacial malformation.

Inspection of the nose in these circumstances may also reveal a remaining interruption of its floor on either side. The cartilagenous and osteal septa will still be deviate, sometimes with complete occlusion of the nasal airway on the unaffected side. Elevation of

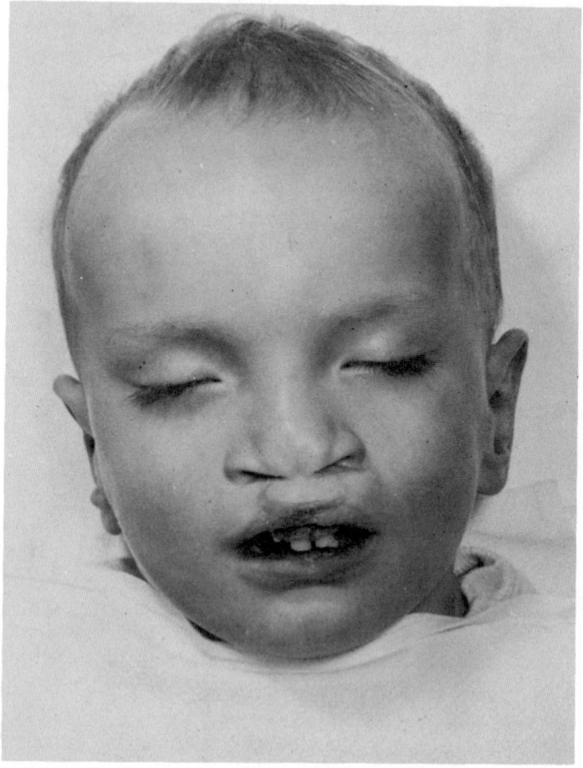

Fig. 29-15. A surgical closure of a severe bilateral complete cleft of the primary and secondary palates. Secondary surgery is required to correct the residual defects of the lip and nose. Maxillary orthopedics is employed to correct the arch form and the position of the still somewhat protrusive premaxillary bone.

the lip may show a probeable sublabial fistula into the naris. If the patient is over 12, secondary intranasal surgery may have corrected some or all of these residual intranasal defects (Fig. 29-16).

One of the more characteristic residual deformities after cheiloplastic and/or uranoplastic procedures is the evident contraction of the upper dental arch, with the teeth in bilateral or unilateral cross-bite occlusion. In bilateral clefts the prepalate and its teeth may lie in a lingual relationship to the lower anterior teeth. If the occlusion remains in this typical cross-bite relationship during the period of deciduous and permanent dentition, the mandible may also begin to show morphologic changes which contribute to the dental malocclusion (Swoiskin, 1956). Some teeth, notably the lateral incisors, may be missing or deformed, or erupting in lingual, labial, or even nasal positions.

The surface of the palatine vault will evidence the ulosis of surgical closure. Its density, amount, and location will be conditioned by the type of uranoplasty performed, eventfulness of healing, the amount of tissue available for repair in relation to the width of the cleft, and whether it was a bilateral nonunion or confined to one side.

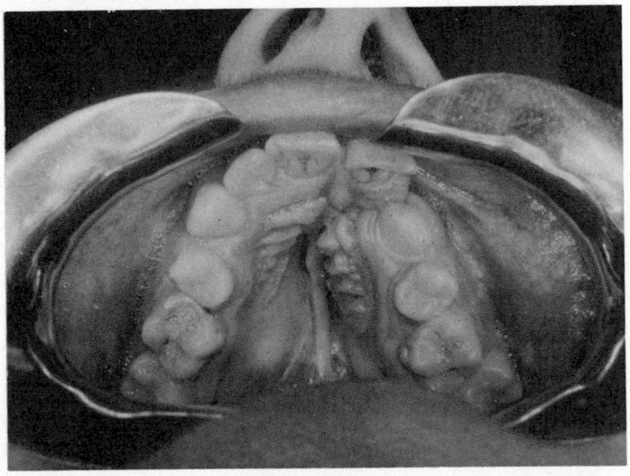

Fig. 29-16. A patient having had surgical closure of a unilateral complete cleft of the primary and secondary palates in infancy. The permanent dentition is now in place. The affected maxillary segment and its dental components are lingually disposed. The arch is contracted, and the teeth on the affected side are in crossbite occlusion.

Another usual clinical finding after surgical closure of the primary and secondary palates is the reduced palatal height and the consequently reduced vertical dimension of the oral space because of the lowered palatal vault. This further reduces lingual freeway space especially when present in association with a contracted upper arch and cross-bite.

We examine now a postsurgical morphologic condition which is one of the most vexing and in many ways one of the most difficult to revise or to correct. This is the residual structural inadequacy of the pharyngeal hemisphincter. A number of imaginative surgical techniques have been developed to reconstruct the divided palates and the velum in such a way as to restore total structural integrity of the nasopharyngeal valving mechanism. Many pathomorphologic factors militate against a universally successful achievement of this surgical goal. Many children born with orofacial malformations and who have been skillfully and conscientiously treated by surgery and oral orthopedics reach the middle and late school years with oropharyngeal structures that are still not adequate for speech production.

Upon oral examination, the anterioposterior palatal axis appears to be foreshortened. The velum palatinum may be thickened by scarring, asymetrical in form, tense, its plane of elevation improper, and the amplitude of its movement limited. Properly exposed static or cineradiographic lateral head films usually confirm the presence of these postsurgical features.

There is an unwarranted tendency on the part of the examining speech pathologist to fault the surgeon's insights and skill for the functional limits he finds after surgical procedures. If he has been made sensitive to the great individual variations, pathoanatomical differentials among types of orofacial deformities, and the varied responses of living tissues to the process of healing and to subsequent growth, he will be able to assess the postsurgical pathomorphologic features more realistically and more fairly. This is not to say that all surgery for these conditions is always done competently or with full understanding of all the implications of the surgical procedures used. But the explanation that the functional and structural limits he sees (and hears) are exclusively the result of "bad surgery" is far too simplistic. They may be, but more often they are not.

More frequently now than formerly the examiner will find that in certain patients limited or extensive modifications have been made in the anatomic organization of the velopharyngeal mechanism as a part of primary or secondary surgical procedures. The velum may show a tissue bridge (a pharyngeal flap) attaching it to the posterior pharyngeal wall. This flap may be attached low or high in the pharynx, it may be wide or narrow, located at the median line or deviate from it, and the spaces lateral to the tissue bridge may be unilaterally occluded, very small, or of moderate size. The position and form of the posterior and anterior faucial pillars may also reflect surgical manipulations. The depth of the pharynx may be great or shallow. The epipharyngeal lymphoid vegetation may be present, or the posterior wall may show the effects of its extirpation. The radiographic lateral head film will, when traced, show the contour of the wall and its spatial relationship to the posterior border of the velum in the physiologic rest position and during phonation.

The Dental State

We have already described in some detail the dental malocclusions that are commonly associated with anomalies of the orofacial structures. However, the picture would not be complete were we not to describe also the general condition of the dental tissue. Clinically one cannot but be impressed by the generalized dental breakdown of both deciduous and permanent dentition in children with cleft palate. It is to be expected that those teeth that are in, or closely adjacent to, the regions of original disunion would be atypical in position and/or in their anatomy, and hence more vulnerable to carious deterioration. But it has been demonstrated that other teeth in these mouths also show subtle and, at times, very apparent structural defects, some of which are detectable even before they erupt. Many cleft-palate patients have such serious and widespread carious lesions that many of their teeth are lost prematurely. The detrimental effects of the early loss of deciduous and permanent teeth upon the ultimate form of the dental arches, and hence upon dental occlusion, are well known to all dental specialists. In the child with orofacial anomalies these effects are especially unfortunate since they add yet another deforming condition. Often the investing tissues of the teeth will also be found to be diseased. The reluctance of these children to maintain good oral hygiene by a regular tooth-brushing regimen may be due to their sensitivity to oral manipulation, and memories of pain during recovery from oral surgery. The condition of their oral tissues, both dental and mucosal, will clearly reflect past oral hygiene practice. We shall return to this subject again when we examine the implications of diseased and absent dental tissue when oral orthopedic and prosthetic treatment is undertaken.

THE PATHOPHYSIOLOGY OF OROFACIAL CLEFTS

Our detailed examination of the pathomorphologic features of orofacial clefts has shown them to have the following general characteristics: 1. great individual variation in form and in magnitude of involvement; 2. notable potential for interference with the dynamics of growth of cephalic structures; and 3. significant potential for grave interference with motor and sensory function. It is this third characteristic which we shall now explicate.

The swallowing synergy in the normal infant has been described as "visceral" by Gwynne-Evans and differs importantly from later deglutitive behavior. It consists of strong contractions of the "buccinator mechanism" and of the obicularis oris. The tongue flattens and its anterior third is pressed strongly against the pads of the gums. The lingual action is "plunger-like," and negative intraoral air pressure is generated and maintained to draw the fluid into the mouth. The peristaltic wave begins at the lips and moves rhythmically posteriorward into the pharynx. Escape of the fluid through the nasal choanae is prevented by the action of the nasopharyngeal hemisphincter. In this synergy the velum palatinum is knuckled against the slightly bulging constrictors of the posterior wall of the pharynx while the lateral pharyngeal walls move mesially to complete the nasopharyngeal seal (Graber, 1968).

There is evidence that the primitive reflexive behaviors of sucking, swallowing, coughing, sneezing, and breathing emerge as early as the third trimester of fetal life. In the fetus and the neonate with orofacial deformities, these visceral activities must perforce be enacted with mechanisms that are not only greatly altered in form, but also in function. Their myosynergies must be expresssed through disordered architectonics.

Nursing at the breast will be nearly or completely impossible for the neonate with an extensive labial cleft. The divided lip cannot effectively embrace the natural nipple since effort to produce the necessary sphincteric contraction of the labial muscles tends only to draw the divided segments of the lip apart more widely.

When the secondary palate is also cleft, the normal linguopalatal and pharyngeal motor patterns of sucking and swallowing are even more severely disturbed. In managing the fluid flow from a modified rubber nipple, the fluid flows into the nose as the tongue propels it backward. In the semierect rather than the supine position, the infant's management of the flow is aided by gravity. Little if any negative air pressure can be generated in the mouth to draw the fluid from the bottle. The nasopharyngeal hemisphincter and tongue are unable to circumvent the flow, and it is directed into the epipharynx and nose as well as into the oropharynx. Later, when semisolid foods are swallowed, the basic motor events are little changed. However, infants with orofacial deformities may develop a variety of simple compensatory motor adjustments to accomplish sucking and deglutition with considerable success.

We have detailed the motoric events in the visceral acts of sucking and swallowing in infants with orofacial anomalies, because they clearly foreshadow the nature of the pathophysiologic conditions that will obtain in speech as well, until successful surgical reconstruction or prosthetic intervention has been provided.

The Period of Speech Learning

We may here well begin with the dictum: children with orofacial malformations are distinguished more by their differences from each other than they are by their similarities (Koepp-Baker, 1963). Each child with his subtle or obvious individual pathomorphic differences, has also been surgically treated in a different way, and has responded to that treatment in an individually characteristic way. It will not be practical to attempt a description of the children's individual functional problems. This may appear to be a contradiction of our earlier assertion that the cleft-palate and/or cleft lip population should not be regarded as a homogeneous one. For our purposes, nonetheless, it will be useful to examine as systematically as possible some of the *general* physiologic problems which may be expected in the clinical speech examination, diagnosis, and treatment of children with orofacial malformations. *Normal* children—that is to say, average children—are also similar in many respects, and different in others. Yet there are some fundamental things that we can say about normal children generally, and about the ways in which their bodies and minds work, how they respond to stimulation, which are useful in understanding them. So also some common features of children with congenital defects may have certain characteristic effects upon speech acquisition and later upon speech production. This is not to infer that their individual features are unimportant, and we shall allude to them as we proceed. There are, however, certain usual and general influences which a disturbed anatomy will have upon the behavioral responses of that anatomy. We should now be forewarned, however, that one cannot in every instance be secure in reasoning from "form to function." Yet by the recognition of certain significant details of form, certain plausible deductions regarding function may be made. Given the "same organic defect" two children may, for many reasons, *respond differently within the general limits imposed by that defect*. Let us examine these general limits.

It is time that the once-orthodox statement that "speech is an overlaid function" is put to rest. The motoric aspects of speech are in many important and even critical ways unique, specialized, and elaborated. They often bear little if any resemblance to the grosser, less specific, and slower motor behavior of the respiratory and alimentary mechanisms. On the other hand, the deterrent effects of disorder or imperfections in the structures responsible for food manipulation and ventilative management will to some extent be shared by the activities of these same organs and structures during speech. The more refined and exact motor behaviors of speech have much narrower limits of tolerance to organic disorder than do the grosser vegetative behaviors. Hence, we may expect some manifestations of the effects of organic imperfections in speech to be less evident or at least less important, in chewing, swallowing, or breathing.

The young child with congenital orofacial anomalies who is learning to talk must do so within the severe limits set by his aberrantly formed speech organs. These limits will be the product of the kind and degree of the original deformities, and of the level of adequacy which treatment has provided at a given time. It must be borne in mind that only some of these morphologic limits may be operating in a given child and that others may not. There are, however, some evident relationships between certain common features of orofacial deformations and the characteristic interferences they impose upon speech physiology.

If for some reason the surgical closure of the secondary palate has not been done, the tongue will continue to exhibit differences from normal in its rest posture, though to what extent and exactly in what way is still debated among clinicians. Cephalometrics have yielded conflicting results when tongue posture in physiologic rest has been studied. This may be due to the fact that different anatomic landmarks and their related planes have been employed. But clinical observation has long confirmed the existence of atypical myokinetic patterns of speech articulation in the presence of an hiatus in the palatal vault. The influence of early compensative visceral behavior already described is imposed upon the later learned articulatory movements and adjustments.

When surgery has closed the palates its sequelae frequently include reduced dimensions of the oral cavity because of residual arch contraction, and a lowered palatal vault. Because of this, the lingual articulatory movements in speech are likely to be reduced in amplitude, imprecise in their paths of excursion, and inaccurate in oral space-shaping. These spatial limitations may be reduced by secondary surgery or by oral orthopedic treatment. Often they will be permanent, however, and will continue to affect lingual competence adversely unless speech therapy succeeds in producing acceptable compensations within the existing organic limits—something which is often difficult to accomplish.

In untreated or unsuccessfully treated disunions of the secondary palate, the nasopharyngeal valving mechanism will be structurally inadequate and functionally incompetent. The normal dynamics of air flow and air pressure in the oropharyngeal circuit are nullified by an incompetent nasopharyngeal hemisphincter. Intraoral air pressures for speech-sound production cannot be generated levels because of the continuous oral decompression. Compensatory adjustments for inadequate intraoral air pressures and flow rates may consist of contraction of the depressor nasi muscles, increased pulmonary and tracheal pressures, and linguopalatal occluding adjustments (Fig. 29-17).

Further, the nature and degree of the deleterious influence of an open palatal vault alone, upon the balance of resonation during speech production, is difficult to assess. Careful speech testing with several different instruments may give some information. The assessment of the separate effect of an open palatal vault is difficult, and sometimes impossible, because ordinarily the nasopharyngeal valve is also incompetent. If the hiatus in the palatal vault is large it will certainly allow a large component of nasal resonance to be added to the oral resonative events. Moreover, incompetence of the hemisphincter will also result in inefficient coupling and uncoupling of the nasal and oral resonators. It is generally agreed that incompetence of the nasopharyngeal valving mechanism is the principal cause of the quality of voice which, together with malarticulation, represents "cleft-palate speech."

It has been by cineradiography that we have been able to learn much of what we know about the normal kinesiologic features of the nasopharyngeal valving function of the hemisphincter. From these observations it appears that the size of the nasopharyngeal port may vary widely and rapidly and is dependent upon physiophonetic demands of the moment of utterance. In syllabic motor sequences the normal nasopharyngeal seal is often incomplete, but research shows that a critical cross-sectional dimension of the port in a given individual cannot be exceeded without the manifestation of perceived hypernasal quality appearing in the voice. It must be made clear, however, that the speech organs represent a complete mechanicophysiologic system and that motoric events in one part of the system are interactively related to all others. The physiological nicety of temporal and spatial control, and sensitive modulation of the total system and the participation of individual motor subsystems, is impressive. It is clear, therefore, that mandibular and labial movement and position, adjustive lingual motion and posturing, will in important ways condition the motoric responses of the nasopharyngeal hemisphincter. The typical hypernasal vocal quality is, therefore, not exclusively a result of imperfect henisphincteric action, but is in reality the product of pneumatic and acoustic events in the total vocal tract.

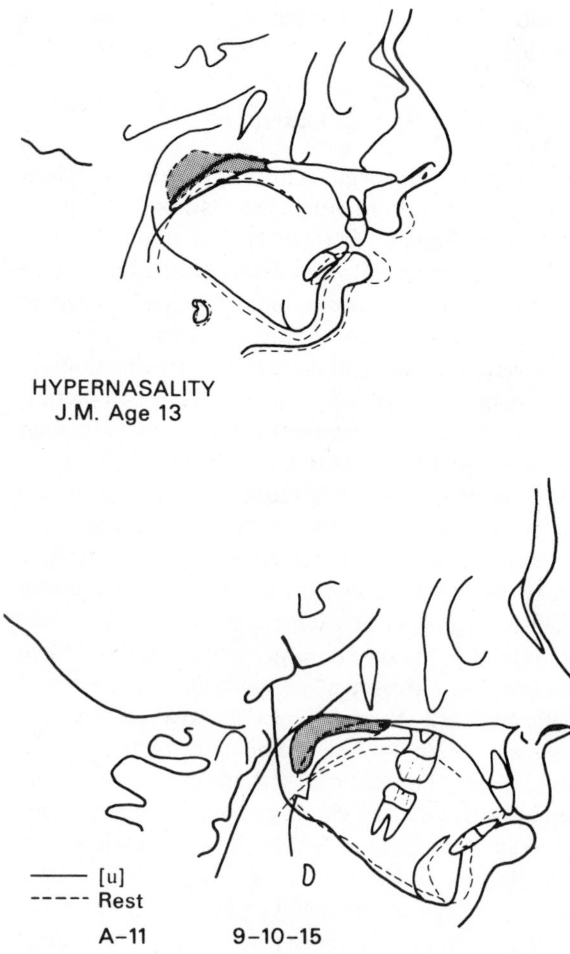

Fig. 29-17. Top, tracing of the roentgenocephalogram of a child with postsurgical palatal incompetence. The solid line indicates the structures at rest, the broken line and stippled area show the structures during phonation of a high back vowel. Bottom, a tracing of the roentgenocephalogram of a normal subject provided for comparison.

The child with congenital orofacial deformities, whether speaking with an untreated or treated speaking mechanism, will make whatever compensatory motor adjustments will help him to approximate most nearly the phonetic models around him. His success will depend upon many factors: the nature of his original deformities, the extent and effectiveness of the surgical and oral orthopedic revisions of those deformities, and his speech learning potential, facility, and aptitude. In the early and middle school years he may still be undergoing secondary surgical revisions and/or oral orthopedic treatment. The presence of orthopedic mechanical appliances will add to his speech production problems.

Otologic Concomitants

Experienced clinical observers are impressed with the high incidence of otologic disease in children with cleft palate. The details of the relationship between deformities of the secondary palate and pathology of the middle ear are not completely understood, and they are probably not as simple as first assumed. Presence of fluid behind the tympanic membrane of newborns with clefts of the secondary palate is a very common finding. Pediatric otologists and surgeons suspect that this may be due to a congenital interference with the ventilative function of the salpingopharyngeal system. A relatively shorter Eustachian tube lying in a more horizontal position, and with a larger orifice located in a somewhat lower position in the rhinopharynx, is anatomically *normal* in the infant. We may reasonably assume that in the infant and young child whose secondary palates are open, or in whom the surgical or prosthetic treatment has not importantly improved the competence of the nasopharyngeal valving mechanism, the epipharynx is subject to considerable abuse because of the presence of fluid or solid foods during eating. Certainly food and the usual secretions of the oral cavity are alien to this sensitive region and to the Eustachian tubes opening into it. The health of the otoventilative system is probably threatened by these unnatural conditions.

Surgical closure of the secondary palate (especially the velum palatinum) ordinarily involves a manipulation and repositioning of the divided muscular elements of the pharynx. Interference with, or at least modification of, the usual position and action of the tensor palati in pharyngoplastic procedures has also been indicated as the cause of Eustachian dysfunction in children with cleft palate.

(For bibliographic references *see* Bibliography at end of Chapter 30.)

The illustrations appearing in this chapter have been provided by the Cleft Palate Clinic of the Colleges of Medicine and Dentistry of the University of Illinois, Chicago, Illinois.

30

The Treatment of Orofacial Clefts: Surgical, Orthopedic, and Prosthetic

Herbert Koepp-Baker

There are a number of valid reasons why the speech pathologist should possess a good understanding of the *principles* of surgical, orthopedic, and prosthetic treatment procedures that are currently employed in the treatment of children and adults with orofacial malformations. This is not to imply that *all the technical details* of these procedures require elucidation for the speech pathologist, though there is no reason at all why he couldn't comprehend them, should this on occasion be necessary. The purpose of the discussion which follows in this section is not to make "half-baked, pseudo-physicians-and-dentists" out of earnest speech pathologists, but rather to encourage the development of speech specialists who can communicate comfortably and effectively with other specialists with whom they work or associate. Regrettably there has been, for many speech pathologists and clinicians, a kind of mystic, unapproachable quality about the medical specialties of pediatrics, surgery, and dentistry which causes them to relate to the specialists of these branches with awe and consequent tentativeness. Speech pathologists are often unaware that medical and dental specialists may also be made uneasy when the speech specialist discusses problems with his characteristic phonetic, linguistic, and psychosocial jargon. But, by their increasingly frequent association with biologically oriented speech pathologists, more and more medical and dental specialists are overcoming the suspicion that concepts in speech and the procedures used in its treatment are superficial or overelaborated. No one is served by such misinterpretation, least of all the patient.

It might be contended that being informed about medical and dental matters "doesn't really make any difference" in the practice of clinical speech. Actually it may make a great deal of difference. The processes and procedures of the speech clinician involve modification of speech behavior through learning. The child with orofacial deformity acquires his speech with a mechanism that is abnormal in varying degrees. He must depend upon that abnormal speech machine for his principal communication throughout childhood and perhaps even into adolescence. Though surgery and dentistry may indeed provide a much-improved speech mechanism, it is rarely ever made wholly normal. These residual organic interferents may be minimal, but they will be present nonetheless. Often they operate as severe deterrents to the acquisition and development of acceptable speech. Therefore, in our judgment it is highly important that the speech pathologist understand clearly and appreciate fully what has been done to the speech mechanism in the processes of surgical and dental revision and reconstruction, for it is with that mechanism that the child must talk—he has no other.

Treatment is an interdisciplinary process. It is now universally recognized that the habilitation of the child with congenital orofacial anomalies requires the insights, skills, and experience of a number of different specialists. The treatment is often a long-term process, extending into late childhood and adolescence. The precise way in which the skills of the several specialists are integrated and coordinated is determined by factors in the local situation. Whether it is accomplished by a formal and fully organized scientific-clinical "team" which functions as a panel of experts for examination, study, treatment, and follow-up; or whether some other device for the facilitation of interdisciplinary consultation is employed, the need for interspecialistic communication is clear.

The role of the speech pathologist in the interdisciplinary clinical setting has become an important one. The demands it makes are different from those of the past. Not only must the speech pathologist know in a general way what his colleagues are talking about, but he must have sufficient specific information and insight in fields other than his own to share responsibly in clinical decisions. This makes demands upon him which transcend his own narrow, specialistic concerns.

PLASTIC AND RECONSTRUCTIVE SURGERY FOR OROFACIAL DEFORMITIES

The plastic surgeon has usually first trained as a physician, then often as a general surgeon (or in another specialty), and finally has specialized in what is commonly called plastic and reconstructive surgery. In a few places in the United States and in some other countries, specialists whose basic training is dentistry may have specialized in stomotologic surgery, and on occasion perform reconstructive procedures on a child whose deformities are limited to the oral cavity.

Plastic surgery has been described as an art as well as a science. Primarily its aim is the restoration of function and appearance of patients afflicted with congenital anomalies or defects resulting from accidental or man-made trauma, or physical imperfections (Stark, 1962).

Let us at this point examine in a broad way the nature of the task which the surgeon sets for himself in his treatment of the patient born with an orofacial malformation, and the biologic limits within which he must perform that task. As we have learned in the preceding chapter, he is confronted with an infant or young child whose orofacial structures are abnormal in configuration, and disordered in functional relationships. To bring the parts into shape and alignment in such a way as to assure that they will look well and function properly, involves surgical procedures which are as delicate as they are formidable. Moreover, the living material which he manipulates, reforms, and reorganizes is not static. The child's face and mouth will grow, and the surgeon's technical maneuvers must not in themselves, or in their results, interfere with growth of individual structures or of the systems of structures. Though recognizing that any surgical procedure is in a sense "controlled injury" to tissue, he must nonetheless keep such injury within the narrowest of limits to assure that there will not be necrosis and loss of tissue, or unusual amounts of cicatrization. He cannot interfere seriously with tissue respiration, or nutrition, if he expects healing to proceed uneventfully. Further, his patient is not a diminutive adult. Infants and young children respond to anesthesia and surgical procedures differently from adults. His little patient may have other anomalies which operate as stringent limitors to what may be done, how much may be done, when it may be done, and expectations of success. His preoperative and postoperative care also poses special problems and, finally, the parents expect the child to look well and to talk well. The possibility of achieving these goals depends, of course, upon a variety of factors, some of which are far more amenable to control than are others. Since clefts and their associated deformation of structure are not traumatic avulsions or accidental mutilation but are embryologic in origin, the plastic and reconstructive problems are in many ways unique in surgery.

Our earlier discussion tried to make it apparent that no two orofacial deformities are alike, that there are many different "kinds" or types, and that even within these classes there are great individual differences. This wide spectrum of pathomorphic features requires that to a considerable extent each surgical and orthopedic treatment must be individualized. Important determinative individual differences will be reflected in, 1. the extent of hypoplasia of the parts (sometimes hyperplasia), 2. the pattern and degree of geometric and topologic disorganization of the affected parts, 3. idiosyncratic healing, 4. the basic recoverable functional potential of the revised structures, and 5. the kind and degree of concomitant defects.

The actual techniques employed in surgical reconstruction of orofacial anomalies are numerous. From time to time some are more popular than others. It is now generally agreed, however, that the *primary* purpose and goal of any surgical and orthopedic procedure for cleft palate is the improvement of speech. The individual surgeon's view of these matters and the techniques he employs are greatly affected by the mentors he has had and the experience he has had with various approaches. It is acknowledged that the same technique may yield two quite different results in the hands of two different plastic surgeons. All "classic" operations tend to be modified in some small or large respect by each individual surgeon. It is probable that no other branch of surgery has had a more impressive history of resourcefulness, ingenuity, inventiveness, experimentation, and responsible search for supporting genetic and embryologic facts than has surgery for orofacial anomalies. It has also had more than its share of failures and of brilliant successes. This history is long and complex and cannot be reviewed here, but the student who would understand and appreciate modern plastic surgery for congenital orofacial deformities will profit greatly from an acquaintance with it.

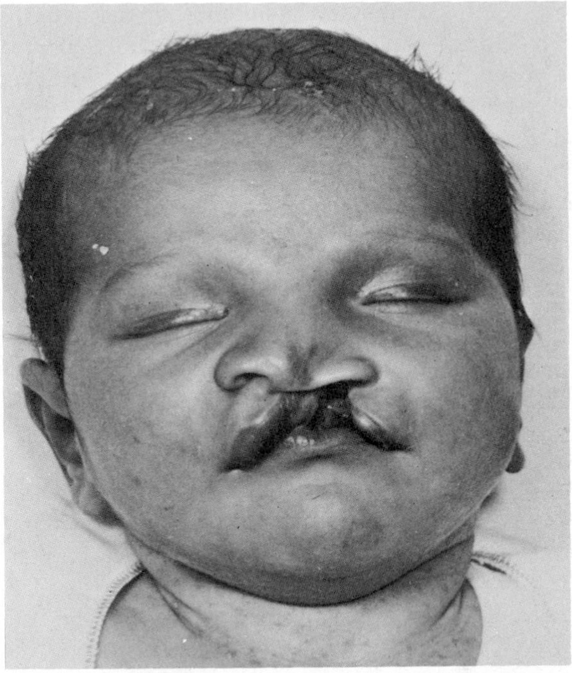

Fig. 30-1. This infant face shows the tissue disarrangement and discontinuity often present in orofacial deformity.

Some Basic Principles Involved in Plastic Surgery

At this point let us turn our attention to the baby in Fig. 30-1. It is clear that if this baby's face is to be made to *look* normal, 1. certain parts of the face which are now in improper locations in relation to the face in general and to other parts in particular must somehow be brought into more normal anatomic locations, 2. parts which would ordinarily be united are separated and must be brought into contact and united, and 3. parts of the face which, though located in relatively normal locations with respect to other parts, are as individual structures twisted, bent, stretched, contracted, flattened, or otherwise misshapen, must somehow be made to conform more closely to normal shape and form.

How can and how will these things be accomplished? When they are accomplished, will the parts function within reasonably normal limits? Will the pattern and rate of growth of the parts of the whole face be affected as the child's face (and body) matures? There is a tendency for the nonmedical specialist to describe and to evaluate surgical procedures almost exclusively from the standpoint of those events occurring in the surgical suite. He is not unlike the layman whose pride in "his operation" and in its results is directly proportionate to "how long he was on the table." What is done and what goes on in the surgical suite are indeed critical and determinative. From the standpoint of the surgeon and his associates, however, these minutes or hours in the operating room and the manipulative procedures and maneuvers, are only *a part* of the total surgical event. Outcomes of the surgery may only in a limited way be determined in the operating room, no matter how intelligent, sensitive, and dextrous the surgeon is. The operation viewed in its fullest perspective begins hours and often days before the patient's transfer to the operating area. It may end days, weeks, or months afterward.

One of the impressive evidences of the advancement of surgery for congenital defects has been the notable reduction in mortality, and in the once common complications that followed surgical procedures. Many things have contributed to these improved conditions. Important among them are more careful preoperative preparation of the patient, early recognition of subtle associated anomalies of the visceral, skeletomuscular, cardiovascular, and nervous systems, improved anesthesiologic equipment and control, continuous monitoring of the patient's physiologic state during the operation, and improved aftercare. Better understanding of the histochemistry of wound healing and recognition of the limits of antibiotic therapy as well as its advantages, have reduced breakdown of reconstructed tissues and assured better functional and cosmetic results. Very important, too, is the deepened insight of the surgeon into the genetic and embryologic bases of the structures he revises.

Turning now to the actual surgical manipulation of the tissues of the face and mouth, it is necessary for us to set forth and elaborate upon several important facts and principles which are basically biological. The living body is not merely an assembly of anatomic structures. The parts (tissues and organs) are organized into structural and functional systems. Parts are not only physically attached to each other, they are also systemically interdependent. Hence to manipulate one part is often to affect adjacent and even remote parts in significant ways. Since the surgeon cannot in the usual sense "make" new tissue, he must use, re-form, or transpose what is available to him. This may be much or little, and it is a characteristic of deformities that the tissue which would be useful is often located in less than advantageous positions.

Let us first examine those general principles that are involved in plastic repair and revision, and then provide details of their application in the repair of clefts of the primary and secondary palates. For the most part, plastic surgery involves the transposition of soft tissues—skin, subcutaneous tissue, mucous membrane, facia, and sometimes muscle, cartilage, and bone. This is accomplished mainly by the preparation and manipulation of pedicled flaps of tissue. The flap is given form by an initial semicircumferential incision of a selected adjacent area. Its important feature is the reserved and undisturbed connection of the flap with its original site through a bridge of tissue. This tissue bridge (pedicle) provides vascular service to the flap so that its vitality can be maintained until it heals in its new location. Such pedicled flaps, undermined and freed from their supporting substructures, may then be advanced or rotated to cover an adjacent lesion or area of embryonic defect.

Let us turn now to the application of pedicle flaps to the repair of the unilateral or bilateral clefts of the primary palate (lip and premaxilla). The preparation of such flaps in the repair of the lip requires that careful nasal and labial measurements be made using the anatomic landmarks as points and lines of reference. Guided by these precise measurements the lines of incision are marked upon the surface of the lip segments, so that triangular or quadrilateral flaps will result. The advancing margins of the flap are usually cut in a Z-form, and two opposing flaps may be incised, elevated, and advanced toward each other with interdigitation of the flap margins. The advantage of this pattern of flap construction is that the undesirable contractive effects of straight-line healing are obviated or greatly reduced. Adjustments are also made at that time in the floor of the nose and the sill of the nasal vestibule and the alar cartilages (Fig. 30-2).

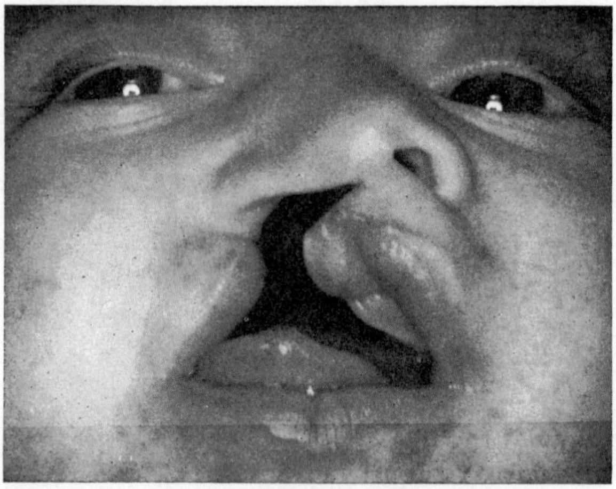

Fig. 30-2. In the surgical closure of the lip in this infant, triangular flaps on both sides were first measured, marked on the skin, incised, freed, and interdigitated. The closed lip brought the divided alveolus into good position. There was no presurgical maxillary orthopedics. The floor of the nose was repaired, and the nasal alar cartilage was revised during the second operation for the closure of the secondary palate. Secondary revision on the lip and nose was done at age 15.

A completely satisfactory surgical solution of the problem of the unilateral or bilateral nonunion of the alveolus is yet to be found. It is compounded in difficulty by the malposition of the premaxillary bone in bilateral deformities. The conventional surgical view is that the reunited lip will bring the divided alveolar segments into a relatively normal position by its physiologic pressures and the molding action of its muscles, and thus restore adequate arch form. However, the instability of the affected maxillary bone often permits an overcorrection or mesial collapse of the segments, and the arch ends up in a cross-bite relationship. Some surgeons bring the divided alveolar segments into apposition by manual force, closing the lip over the digitally remolded alveolar arch. In some surgical hands a flap is lifted from the anterior vomerine area, advanced, rotated, and used to close the remaining hiatus or point of abutment. Since postsurgical sublabial fistulae at the point of alveolar interruption are relatively common, these are usually closed by an everted gingival or sublabial flap in the secondary surgical procedures.

In recent years considerable attention has been directed to the use of bone grafts in the correction of alveolar nonunions. During the lip closure, a bone graft from the rib, iliac crest, or tibia is applied to the prepared site of the divided alveolus and covered with a flap of adjacent soft tissue. The histologic fate of these bone grafts is not yet clear. Some believe that the graft serves as a matrix for stimulation and support of osteoblastic activity. It has been reported that teeth have erupted in the graft site. Under this surgical scheme the usual practice in bilateral clefts is to close one side at a time after the premaxillary segment has first been brought into its proper position by means of an orthopedic appliance. There has been only limited acceptance of presurgical orthopedic treatment followed by bone grafting and surgery, and these procedures have raised highly controversial questions. Many surgeons feel that the additional surgical trauma to which the infant is exposed, as well as other considerations, outweigh the value of these procedures. If they are more carefully documented by future longitudinal growth studies we shall be better able to evaluate the results in adolescence and adulthood.

Closure of the Secondary Palate

The basic principle of pedicled flap manipulation is also applied in the repair of clefts of the secondary palate. Though the exact procedure of flap measurement, outlining, elevation, and transposition may be modified in different surgical hands, the present practice is to create flaps from the mucous membrane and its attaching mucoperiosteum of the palatal shelves, which are then mobilized and reflected from the osteal substratum, advanced, rotated, or retroposed and interdigitated, to cover the fissure in the palatal vault and close the velum palatinum. Another common procedure is to create flaps from the tissue covering the vomer bone and articulate them with flaps from the opposing palatal surfaces. However, even the most atraumatic manipulation of the tissue flaps in closing the palatal hiatus may be attended by some foreshortening of the anterioposterior palatal axis (Fig. 30-3).

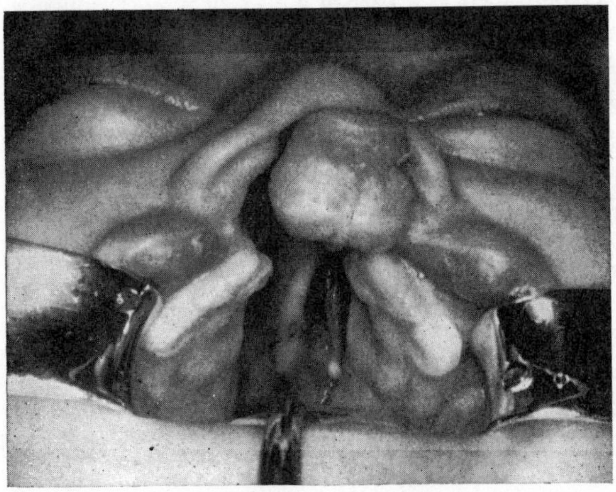

Fig. 30-3. This photograph of an infant reflects the formidable and delicate task assumed by the plastic surgeon and the maxillary orthopedist in treating infants and children with orofacial deformities.

The goals of all conventional surgical procedures for the closure of clefts of the secondary palate may be summarized as follows: 1. to achieve a closure of the fissure in the palatal vault and velum without wound disruption, 2. to obtain closure with minimal ulosis and freedom from tensions in both the palatal vault and in the anterior portion of the velum palatinum, and 3. to place the velum in the most advantageous position for its effective participation in velopharyngeal closure in speech. Some modification of the Dieffenbach-Warren-von Langenbeck procedure, when done expertly, accomplishes these goals, with the notable exception of the last—the effective functional reestablishment of the velum in the complex velopharyngeal hemisphincter. The common velopharyngeal incompetence that exists after the classic operations for closure of the secondary palate is the bane of speech pathologists and plastic surgeons alike.

A variety of pharyngoplastic and modified palatoplastic procedures have been devised to resolve the problem commonly called "short palate." It cannot be overemphasized that the final *location* of the velum is not the *only feature* of velopharyngeal incompetence which requires consideration from the speech standpoint. The total muscular arrangement within the velopharyngeal complex must always receive sensitive attention. Many modern operators combine the classic initial closure with one or more of the following palatovelar and velopharyngeal procedures: 1. retropositioning of the palate. This is usually accomplished as a part of a V-Y or a W-Y advancement of dual palatal flaps with protective attention to their denuded nasal surface, fracture of the pterygoid hamuli, or section of the tensor tendon; 2. the repositioning of the pharyngeal walls. This may consist of narrowing the oro-nasopharyngeal isthmus by tissue reorganization or the use of implants. These procedures are yet to be fully evaluated; and 3. tethering the posterior pharyngeal wall to the velum, commonly referred to as a "pharyngeal flap." This involves the elevation of a flap of mucous membrane, underlying muscle and facia from the midline of the posterior pharyngeal wall. The pedicle is hinged either in the nasopharynx or in the oropharynx, and the freed flap is then attached to the nasal surface of the foreshortened velum, inserted between divided layers of the velum, or attached to its oral surface (Fig. 30-4).

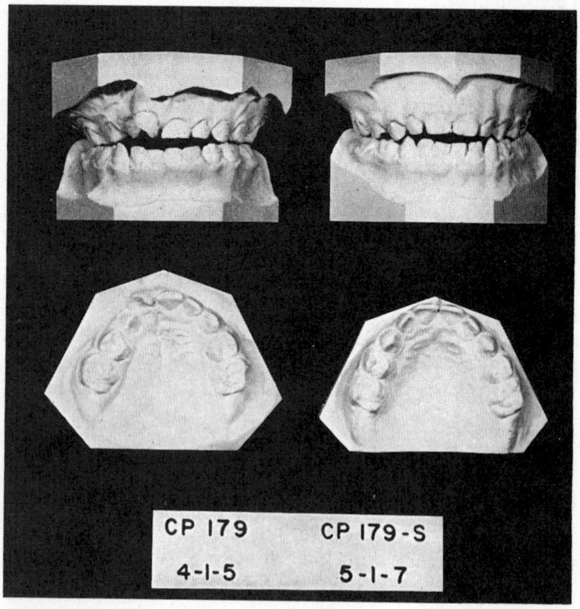

Fig. 30-4. Results of oral orthopedic treatment of a child in deciduous dentition and with a surgically corrected moderately severe unilateral cleft of the primary and secondary palates. The dental occlusion before and after orthopedic treatment is shown in the pictures at the top. A palatal view of the maxillary dental arch is depicted below. The typical crossbite has been corrected.

MAXILLARY ORTHOPEDICS

Biomechanical treatment occupies an important place in habilitation of patients with orofacial deformities. Its goals and procedures fall into the province of the oral or maxillofacial orthopedist. He is a specialist who is trained as a dentist and then usually as an orthodontist or pedodontist. The treatment of orofacial deformities, however, goes beyond the correction of purely dental irregularities. Special training and experience in this field are imperative. In addition to the regularization of individual teeth and improvement of the occlusive relationship of the dental arches, this treatment modality involves the correction of abnormal configurations of the premaxilla, and the alveolar and palatal segments of the maxillae.

These ends are accomplished through the use of individually designed mechanical appliances which apply controlled mechanical forces on individual teeth, groups of teeth, or upon segments of bone and their investing mucous membrane and mucoperiosteum.

At this point the speech pathologist may be inquiring as to why, after the various surgical procedures have been done, it is necessary for still other treatment processes and procedures to be employed. The facts are that regardless of how skillful and successful the surgery, how excellent the recovery, and how little the interference with growth, slight or serious residual deformities remain in a large number of children. Some of these residual defects may actually be the unavoidable result of the surgery itself. After primary surgery has been completed there may yet remain 1. defects of the lip, 2. defects of the nose, 3. defects of the alveolar arch, 4. defects of the palatal vault, and 5. defects of the nasopharyngeal hemisphincter. The residual defects of the lip, nose, and velum are usually greatly improved by secondary surgical procedures at the age of 12 to 16 years.

However, the common postsurgical malposition of the premaxillary bone in bilateral clefts and the lateral alveolar segments in both bilateral and unilateral defects are generally not amenable to surgical correction. The use of mechanical measures antecedent to closure of the lip for the management of the cleft alveolus is a comparatively new development. Such presurgical procedure has earnest and zealous advocates and equally earnest opponents. We shall describe it here because it is being employed in some centers in the United States and is popular in Europe.

Presurgical Maxillary Orthopedics

In recent times the problem of the alveolar defect in bilateral and unilateral nonunions has been attacked in a somewhat different manner. Before the lip is closed, an impression of the infant's mouth is made, usually under the controlled conditions of the hospital operating room and with an endotracheal tube in place. A working model of dental plaster and/or stone is poured and trimmed. On this model a small plastic appliance is designed to cover the divided alveolus.

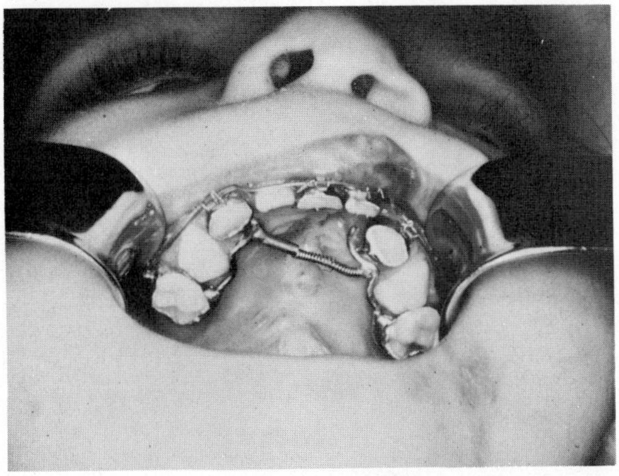

Fig. 30-5. Illustrating one of a number of techniques and devices used in maxillary orthopedics. The lingually disposed affected maxillary segment and its teeth are being moved into proper position by bio-mechanical force applied in a predetermined direction and rate. The anterior teeth of the unaffected segments are being moved to correct positions by orthodontic procedures.

If it is a bilateral involvement, the appliance is designed to receive the free premaxillary segment as well. It is placed in the infant's mouth and retained by a cloth band attached to a cloth cap or similar arrangement (Fig. 30-5). Since the appliance covers the palatal vault as well, the child finds sucking on a nipple much easier. Infants appear to make a rapid adjustment to the appliance and frequently do not wish to be without it. It may help to contain the tongue at rest and during eating, controlling the tendency for it to extrude through the alveolar fissure and widen it. The function of the appliance is to guide the separated parts to more normal positions. By certain adjustments in the appliance from time to time the widely divided parts may be brought more closely together; or, if the alveopalatal segments are lingually disposed, it may expand the arch. These orthopedic steps are designed to facilitate the surgical closure of the lip with less tension and better form. It is assumed that it makes later postsurgical maxillary orthopedic, and orthodontic treatment less difficult, more effective, or perhaps even unnecessary. It is a usual practice of those surgeons preferring such presurgical orthopedic treatment, to prepare, place, and cover a bone graft in the alveolar gap before closing the lip.

Postsurgical Maxillary Orthopedics

The contracted upper dental arch is so common a residual deformity after surgical closure of the primary and secondary palates that further mechanico-orthopedic measures for its correction are usually required. These procedures are included as a part of the orthodontic or pedodontic care provided for most children with congenital clefts. The speech pathologist will discover that, just as in plastic surgery, a variety of philosophies and techniques prevail. Just as we have described surgery as "controlled injury," so oral orthopedics has been described as "a pathologic process from which the tissue recovers." The basic principles governing all oral orthopedic treatment are reviewed here.

It has long been known that a mechanical force continuously and lightly applied to a tooth will cause it to move through its bony support in the alveolus in the direction of the vector of force. This force is usually applied through metal bands embracing the crown of the tooth. To these bands, wires, ligatures, elastics, etc., are attached and so arranged as to provide controlled forces in specific directions and at predetermined rates. The molar and premolar teeth are frequently used as the fixed structures for providing reciprocal force and anchorage. Individual teeth or groups of teeth may be moved in a straight line, tipped on their vertical axes, or rotated.

In patients having clefts of the primary and secondary palates, the maxillary arches are less stable because of the absence of a strong union at the midline osteal suture. Therefore it is possible for the type of controlled mechanical pressure generally used in orthodontics, to move not only the teeth, but the entire horizontal processes of the maxillary bones in which they are imbedded. Hence the palatal shelves and their alveolae may be rotated buccally and retained in these new and correct positions with special retention appliances. Because of the irregularity of individual teeth or groups of teeth in these cases it is often impossible to achieve the usual satisfactory self-retaining occlusive relationship between the upper and lower dental arches. Therefore there is a tendency for the active forces of the buccal and labial musculature to return the structures to their earlier improper positions. Extensive cicatrization of the palatal vault following surgical closure of the secondary palate may, through its very powerful contractive influence, make such arch expansion difficult. If no retaining appliance is used, the segments of the arch may again drift or collapse. A number of biomechanical schemes are employed to open up contracted dental arches and to move their bony maxillary supports. These consist essentially of the application of tissue-moving forces in lateral directions by adaptation of the labial or palatal arch-wire or by a turnscrew which can be gradually adjusted by the parent or the child himself. While the maxillary segments are thus rotated and moved buccally, there may be some concern that such total movement of the alveolar bone and palatal shelves may cause the healed suture line to reopen. If, however, the repositioning of the parts is done gradually, the ulotic area on the palate will stretch and readjust. If a palatal fistula does appear it is closed surgically.

The general dental needs of the child with congenital cleft lip and/or palate have already been referred to in our earlier discussion. It must be made clear, however, that before orthodontic or maxillary orthopedics are initiated, the carious teeth must be restored and strict oral hygiene measures instituted. Conventional orthodontic procedures for the straightening of individual teeth and generally improving dental arch form and occlusion are usually necessary. The orthodontic and maxillary orthopedic treatment of these children presents special problems. Being deeply concerned with the child's speech improvement, the dental specialist is eager to provide adequate lingual freeway space by dental arch expansion, and by the correction of dental irregularities and malocclusions as early as possible. We have already noted that presurgical maxillary orthopedics is carried out in the edentate infant mouth. Conversely, postsurgical orthopedic procedures are done in early and middle years of childhood after some useful deciduous teeth have erupted, during the stage of mixed dentition, or when most permanent teeth are in place. This means that the corrective appliances must be modified as deciduous teeth are shed, or treatment temporarily discontinued until permanent dental units have erupted sufficiently to be clasped or banded. This tends to interrupt and to prolong orthodontic or maxillary orthopedic treatment and to delay the time when the child's mouth is significantly improved for speech (Fig. 30-6). Nature being what it is, however, it is the best he can do, and he must bow to its dictates. The pedodontist is accustomed to providing preventive and interceptive orthodontics during the stage of deciduous or mixed dentition. Generally orthodontists also include these preventive and interceptive steps in their total program of dental care for the child with congenital orofacial malformations.

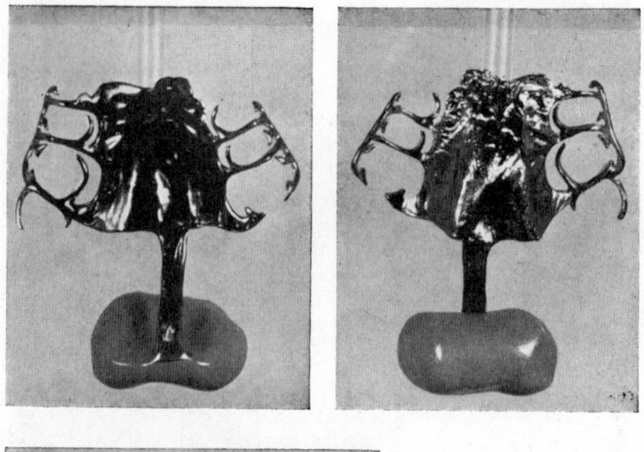

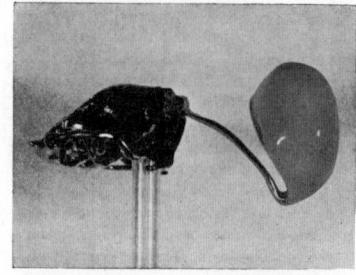

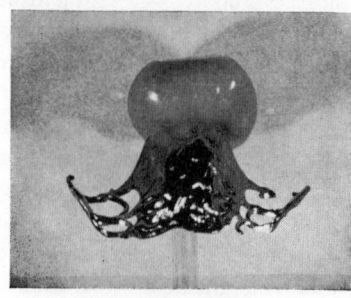

Fig. 30-6. Prosthetic speech aid for an adolescent. Top left, the lingual aspect; top right, the nasal aspect; middle left, the lateral aspect; bottom left, the labial aspect. The component parts are clear: the cast-metal dental clasping system, the palatal portion, the pharyngeal section and its carrier.

PROSTHETIC TREATMENT

There are patients whose oral deformity is so extensive that surgical closure of the cleft in the secondary palate is not recommended because of the likelihood of a resulting velopharyngeal hemisphincter inadequacy and incompetence. There are, too, patients whose surgery has ended in failure both cosmetically and in the ability to produce sufficiently intelligible speech. For such patients the use of prosthetic devices has long been recommended. Despite the improved techniques of modern cleft-palate surgery and its better speech and cosmetic results, there is still a sizable group of patients for whom cosmetic and speech improvement is available only through prosthetic treatment (Fig. 30-7).

orofacial malformation is determined by the nature and extent of the residual deformities for which it must compensate. Harkins (1960) has described a prosthesis for the person born with cleft palate as "a device whose principal purpose is the separation of the oral and oropharyngeal spaces from the nasal and nasopharyngeal spaces" and, it may be added, to provide artificial teeth, and a lip plumping section where it is required.

The production of a prosthesis is a highly technical and exact procedure requiring a good understanding of pathomorphology and pathophysiology of orofacial malformations. Here we shall deal only with the underlying principles rather than with all of the technologic details (Fig. 30-8).

An oral impression of the maxillary (and sometimes the mandibular) region is taken and study models are made. Such models reproduce the anatomic details of

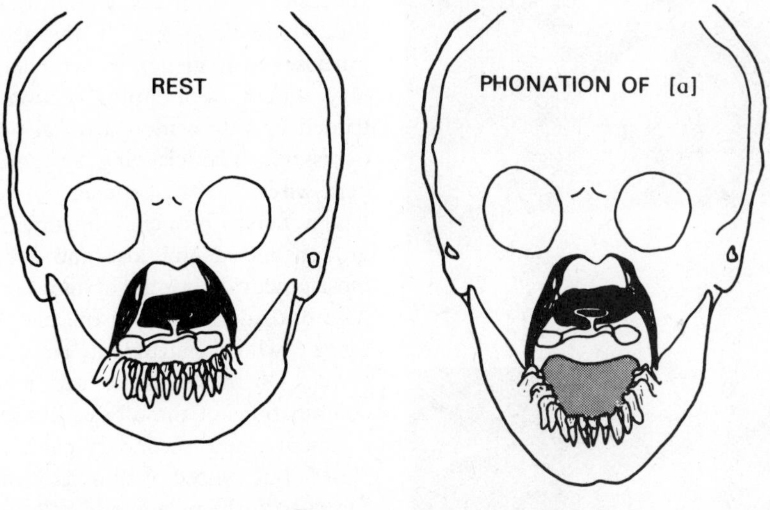

Fig. 30-7. Reproduction of a tracing of a frontal roentgenolaminagraphic projection of a patient wearing a prosthetic speech aid, showing the role of the lateral pharyngeal walls in phonation of a vowel.

A prosthetic device may serve to improve a number of conditions: 1. the disturbed facial profile, 2. absent teeth in the anterior dental arch, 3. severe hypernasality of voice, and 4. severe air loss through the nose. Still another important application of a prosthesis is in those circumstances in which surgery of the secondary palate must, for one reason or another, be postponed. The use of a prosthesis makes it possible to help a child to improve his speech meanwhile, and until surgical intervention is appropriate.

The actual form of a prosthesis for patients with

the normal and defective areas of the hard palate and the dental arches exactly. Since the velum palatinum is mainly muscle and not supported by bone, the task of obtaining good registration of its structural details is more difficult. It is upon the study models and perhaps a later master model that the complete design of the instrument is completed (Fig. 30-9).

The instrument may be fabricated of metal (gold or steel alloy), or from metal and plastics (e.g., acrylic resins) combined (Fig. 30-4). The typical instrument consists of the following parts or sections: 1. a palatal section which covers the vault of the hard palate

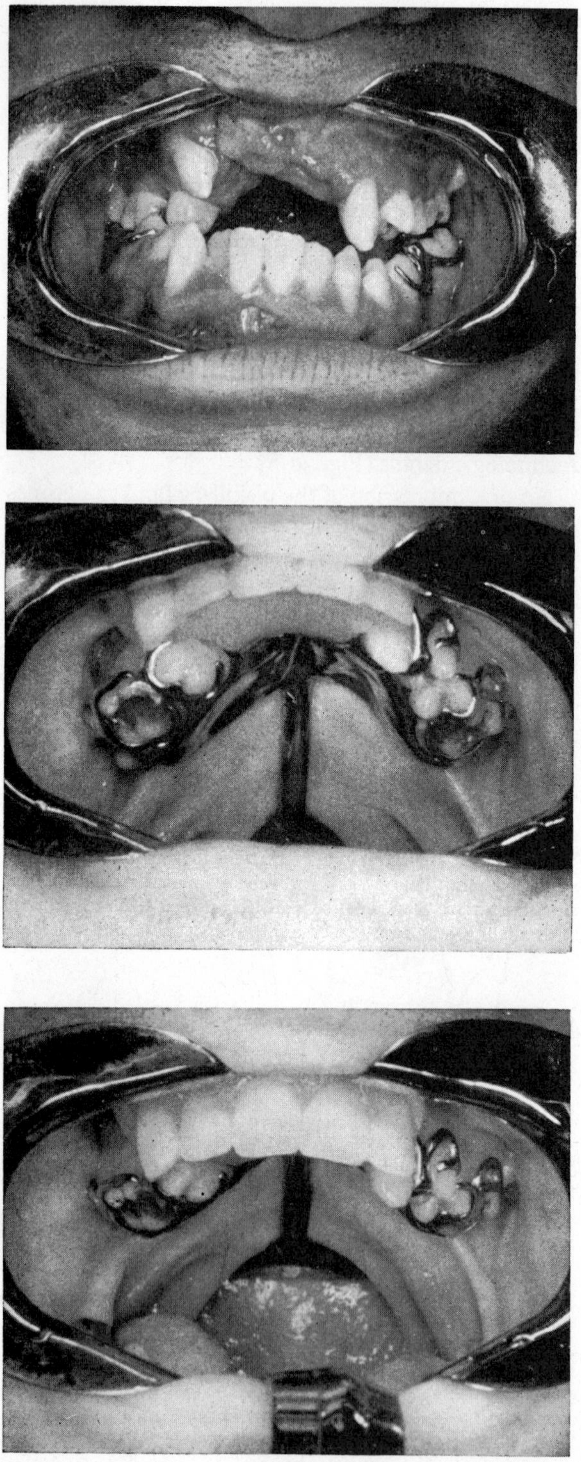

Fig. 30-8. Prosthetic treatment of a patient with a previously surgically treated unilateral complete cleft of the primary and secondary palates, and in whom poor speech persisted because of an inadequate and incompetent nasopharyngeal hemisphincter, contracted mandibular arch, and absent anterior teeth. A, the patient without the prosthesis; B shows the cast metal clasping system embracing the supporting teeth, the palatal section which also carries anterior teeth and plumps the lip, and the carrier bar supporting the pharyngeal section is shown in position in C.

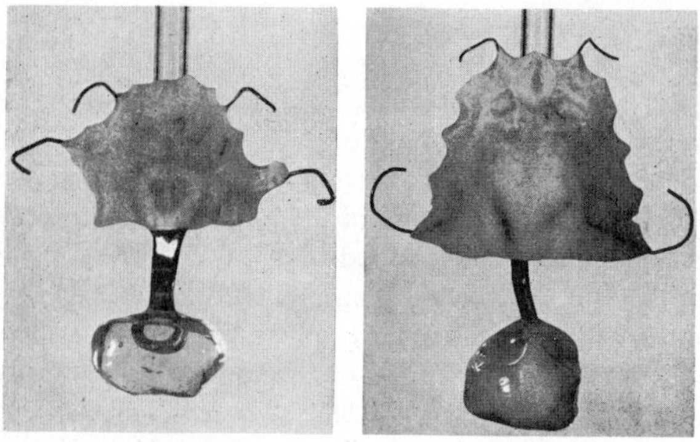

Fig. 30-9. Two children's ad interim speech aids. These have bent-wire clasps that are retained by lugs soldered on orthodontic bands which have been fitted and cemented to the deciduous teeth.

partly or completely, 2. a velar section which either covers the velum or passes between its still-divided segments, 3. a pharyngeal section in the shape of a spheroid bulb, 4. a clasping system which anchors the whole appliance to the teeth (removable for purposes of hygiene), 5. artificial teeth when necessary, and 6. a plumping section for bringing a retruded lip into a more natural position when this is necessary. The clasping system may be either of bent wires or of cast metals. In younger children for whom fairly frequent adjustments are required as growth and dental loss and eruption proceed, the most practical clasping system is usually of the bent-wire design. Later both the clasps, and the skeleton for the whole instrument, are usually made of cast metal. Obviously there are many variations and combinations of these basic designs. For example, in a patient whose secondary palate has been surgically closed but whose velum is foreshortened and incompetent, the palatal and velar sections may consist only of a metal skeleton to which the plastic pharyngeal section is attached. To make provision for the continuing growth of the orofacial complex in children the prosthetic speech aid must occasionally be modified or adjusted. Such adjustments may involve the redesign of the clasping system when critical deciduous teeth are lost and the required permanent teeth are not yet sufficiently erupted.

Speech aids may be designed, made, and fitted by prosthodontists, pedodontists, and by orthodontists, depending upon the pattern of specialistic association in a given treatment center. There are occasional treatment programs for a child in which the diastema in the hard palate is closed by surgical procedures, but the velum remains undisturbed. A prosthetic aid is then fitted for permanent use. Some oral orthopedists elect to combine certain of their stages of correction within the design of the prosthesis.

The rationale for the function of a prosthetic device as a speech aid is based upon the principle of making the compensatory movements of the pharynx available and effective for the regulation of pneumatic and acoustic traffic during speech. It may also replace teeth and improve the appearance of the lip. A speech aid is most successful in those patients in whom the lateral pharyngeal walls are active or whose pharyngeal myokinetics can be developed by speech therapy.

SPEECH CONSIDERATIONS IN THE TREATMENT OF OROFACIAL MALFORMATIONS

It would be a serious error to assume that there is, or always must be, a direct relationship between each feature of defective speech in the child born with orofacial malformation and each of his structural anomalies. One of the notable features common to both functional and organic speech disorders is inconsistency and variability (Winitz, 1969). No two children having what appear to be the same organic defect, will exhibit the same degree or form of speech disorder. Intelligence, speech learning aptitude, social and language experience, and emotional development and status are also important determinators of the kind and severity of speech defects which result from morphologic disorder. Yet the general deleterious influence of defective speech organs on speech learning is universally acknowledged. The organically based interference may be displayed in speech in different ways, at different times, in the same child and in different children. Nor can it be disputed that children born with orofacial disorders have some common features of speech production and that their characteristic speech behavior may, in a general way at least, be related to the nature of their structural defects. We shall here describe the varied influence of orofacial deformity on speech behavior.

For convenience of the present discussion, the important characteristic features of the uncorrected speech of the person with orofacial deformities will be described as disturbances of articulation and of voice quality. Such a division of the speech syndrome labeled "cleft-palate speech" is, of course, in some ways artificial, since the speech act cannot be fractioned. The processes of phonation, resonation, and articulation are so intimately interrelated that a disturbance in one is reflected to some degree in the others. The close physiologic unity of these speech processes is made apparent by this speech disorder.

The Articulatory Disturbances

Practically all of the articulatory movements in these speakers are subject to defect to a greater or lesser degree. With the exception of the nasal sounds, a large number of consonantal release-and-arrest movements of syllables are modified by the congenital organic deformity. The plosive sounds are commonly absent, weak, or distorted. If the palate is open or the velopharyngeal hemisphincter is incompetent, and no obturation by a speech aid is present, it is impossible to impound the required air pressure within the oral cavity for the implosive phase of consonant production. Even if intactness of the palatal vault has been produced by surgical repair, but the velopharyngeal hemisphincter remains inadequate and incompetent, it will still be impossible to produce sufficient air pressure within the mouth. The usual substitution for plosive sounds is a nonphonetic laryngeal or pharyngeal stop. The relative ease of producing an occlusion at a lower level in the airway and at a point ahead of the usual and normal point of articulatory contact for the plosive encourages this type of substitution. Because of differences in presurgical and postsurgical pathology there is considerable variation from speaker to speaker in omission or substitution in plosive production. The resulting speech lacks the sharp definition characteristic of normal syllable boundaries. In some speakers, sufficient reduction of the nasopharyngeal port can, in deliberate and careful speech, be achieved by compensatory pharyngeal movement so that weak or transient oral occlusives can be produced. In syllable production at normal or more rapid rates, however, the plosives drop out or glottal or pharyngeal stops are substituted.

When the consonant movement does occur in the mouth rather than lower in the airway, phonokinesiographic and palatographic records of the speaker show extensive variation as to the loci of oral occlusive contacts and of the temporal features of organ movement. The total consonant coordination appears to be modified. There is also some modification of voicing and unvoicing of consonants with a tendency toward partial voicing.

The fricatives, in cleft-palate speech, are either absent or suffer distortion because of the substitution of characteristic pharyngeal fricatives or the improper posture and movement sequences. The loss of air pressure by leakage into the nasopharynx and nose during the production of fricatives is very apparent in this speech at normal and rapid rates. In some speakers, the compensatory pharyngeal and posterior lingual adjustments reduce air leakage sufficiently so that weak fricatives are heard in some articulations. However, their acoustic qualities are usually changed. The voiceless fricatives may become voiced under effort of production or stress.

Many clinical observers feel that the lingual synergies for both plosives and fricatives reflect characteristic malhabits. These have been described as 1. a reduced activity of the anterior tongue and tongue tip and 2. atypical postures and movements of the dorsum of the tongue. Some studies suggest that the tongue is habitually retroposed and lowered. Subtelny and Subtelny (1962) have produced evidence that a dependable skeletal frame of reference is important in making accurate measures and judgments of tongue positions in these speakers. There is little doubt, however, that the mode or manner of tongue behavior is basically variant and affects practically all articulations to some degree. This generalized lingual disturbance also affects the articulation of vowels, and the vowel-to-consonant and consonant-to-vowel transitions.

Nor should the effects of mandibular adjustments in consonant production be neglected. Clinically, the reduced vertical and horizontal intraoral space and the concomitant reduction and interference with lingual movement appear to be related. In chronic cleft-palate speech, the degree of mandibular depression during consonant production is also often reduced. Whether this mandibular depression is due to a continuing compensatory malposition of the tongue which restricts the mandibular movement is not known. There are good phonetic reasons why this relationship may exist. There are, however, other organic factors which may also affect mandibular habits. As has been pointed out earlier, the cleft-palate speaker frequently has gross alterations of upper dental arch form, dental occlusion, and form and height of palatal vault. These variations in the areas of occlusive contact available to the tongue, particularly anteriorly, impose limitations upon tongue movement. Wide individual differences make generalizations of the effect of these maxillary factors difficult or impossible. Size of tongue and individual characteristics of lingual dynamics also play a role in determining how, in a given speaker, the maxillary deformities will affect the range and character of tongue movement and posture.

In the early years of the life of many cleft-palate speakers, after surgery and before maxillary orthopedic correction, it is not unusual for the mandibular dental arch to lie outside the maxillary arch. This may operate to modify the characteristic lingual and mandibular rest position as well, and hence affect the position from which lingual movement sequences start and to which they return. That this may encourage lower or more retroposed tongue positions has been suggested by some speech clinicians.

The function of repaired lips is probably not wholly normal. The degree of disturbance is determined by the extent of the original labial deformity, the inadequacy or superfluity of muscle tissue, and the final results of surgical reconstruction. The repaired lip is often less flexible, and its range of movement reduced. Since lip movement in the articulation of bilabial and labiodental sounds is, in the normal person, relatively gross, the effect of lip deformity is probably less critical than is often assumed. However, dental irregularity in the anterior region of the upper dental arch, common to cleft-palate persons, may be a disturbing factor in articulation of the labiodental as well as the linguadental sounds.

Because of the generalized malarticulation of both plosives and fricatives, it is to be expected that affricate production is also modified. If the implosive movement of the affricate is omitted, the entire affricate will be omitted or executed with an extensive acoustic change. The semivowel and glide articulations are thought to show less phonetic change in cleft-palate speakers than those of the fricative and plosive groups. A more detailed and useful discussion of the dynamics of speech production in the speaker with orofacial deformities is provided by Brackett in Chapter 17.

The principal handicap to an understanding of the variations of consonant production in cleft-palate speakers is the difficulty of obtaining adequate *dynamic* records of these movements in the release and arrest of the breath pulse. The full implication of disturbance of movement cannot be seen on conventional palatograms or on static radiographs which record only a moment in time in the occlusive-contact phase of consonant production. Cinefluoroscopic records are of some help, but reliable measurement techniques are not yet refined enough for highly exact description. This technique, and especially that of sagittal x-ray have, however, added considerably to our understanding of vowel articulation in these speakers.

Disturbances of Vowel and Consonant Resonation

The disturbance of vowel quality in these speakers is one of the most conspicuous features. The quality is usually described as "hypernasal." The phenomenon of nasality in speech is a highly complex acoustic matter. Our understanding of the relationship between organ position, physiologic function, and the acoustic pattern of vowels is by no means clear. It appears tenable that basic physiologic mechanisms are important determinants of vowel quality. In recent years much attention has been directed to the nasopharyngeal valve and its role in normal speech production. There is some evidence through radiography and air-flow-and-pressure registration that for the production of consonants requiring steep intraoral pressure gradients, the valve must be closed or nearly closed. The degree of occlusion of the nasopharyngeal airway appears to be dependent upon the kind of consonant, the function of the consonant, its phonetic environment, the rate of speech, and the syllabic stress.

In the *normal* production of vowels or vowellike sounds, the patency of the nasopharyngeal airway also appears to be variable. The degree of closure for a sound of any class is related to the total synergic adjustments of the palatopharyngeal and palatoglossal systems, the muscles of the superior constrictor, and the lingual and mandibular adjustments. It is generally assumed that the normal vowel quality is the product of the combined effects of the pharyngeal, oral, and nasal resonators upon the laryngeal tone. In the presence of complete or partial stenosis of the nasal airways, the vowel quality may become "hyponasal."

From clinical observation and experimental studies it has been inferred that, in the normal speaker, the epipharynx and nasal cavities contribute characteristic components to the acoustic spectrum of the normal vowel. The adjustment of the velopharyngeal valve that is necessary for the proper oronasal acoustic balance is one of great physiological nicety. It must provide appropriate regulation of pneumatic traffic and, at the same time, be sensitively responsive to the phonetic and phonatory needs through rapid coupling and uncoupling of the oral and nasal resonators. In cleft-palate speakers the extent and character of the original oral and pharyngeal deformity must be taken into full account, if the disturbance of resonation is to be understood. The character and the effects of reconstructive surgery or of prosthetic intervention are also significant conditioners of the kind of resonator relationships that will be available to the speaker during the period of speech learning.

Three types of postsurgical conditions of the secondary palate are usual. The first is a closed hard palate and closed velum palatinum in which the disturbance of the architecture of the palatal vault and arch form is slight, the vault being of normal or near-normal height; and the velum united, of adequate length, and of satisfactory mobility. In these patients the internal nasal anatomy is also usually relatively normal. The faucial pillars are in normal position and their mobility is unaltered.

The second type is that in which extensive changes in the arch form and palatal vault dimensions are present. These also present a partially closed or closed velum, but the tissue in the velar region is under tension, attenuated, and the velum inadequate in length. The pillars may also be in an abnormal position and changed in form. The nasal septa are often deflected and the columellae shortened.

The third class of postsurgical states is that in which the lip and alveolar process have been closed, with much or little residual deformity in the dental arch, but the palatal vault and the velum palatinum are still cleft. It is obvious that each of these classes produces different effects upon the mechanism of resonation. It is of interest to note, however, that in the first class described the voice may still be strongly hypernasal even though all the structures of the mouth and pharynx appear to be relatively normal.

We have asserted earlier that though a variety of secondary surgical procedures have been devised and advocated for providing more mobile and adequate vela for improved velopharyngeal function, their speech value may sometimes be questioned. Their sequelae of extensive cicatrization sometimes actually produces velar shortening, immobility, and other inhibitions to hemisphincteric function. Merely lengthening or retroposing the velum frequently appears to leave unaffected the residual inadequacies in the total musculature of the *pharynx*. Further, the malarticulations have often been so thoroughly habituated that little change in the hypernasality of the patient can be detected following this type of surgery. In some cases, attempts are made to ameliorate the hypernasality and air emission by pharyngoplasty or by the introduction of a prosthetic speech aid. Other conditions assuring optimum success of a prosthesis in this type of patient are not always present. In recent years, oral prosthetists have devised a variety of aids to assist these speakers in controlling hypernasality and air loss, but the margin of success is less than ideal.

From the standpoint of speech improvement, one of the most promising surgical procedures in selected cases is palatopharyngoplasty of the "pharyngeal flap" type. Though different surgeons may vary the technical details, all have as their intent the improvement of the function of the velopharyngeal hemisphincter for acoustic and pneumatic control during speech. Since this procedure is sometimes included in initial closure of the secondary palate and combined with adequate retropositioning of the palate, it may provide the patient with an early functioning nasopharyngeal closure mechanism. When successful it obviates the need for a prosthetic speech aid. Its use is strongly advocated by some surgeons because it is a relatively simple procedure, and can be done as a primary procedure or as a part of secondary surgical revisions of the secondary palate. Its proponents advocate this palatopharyngoplastic procedure for the following reasons: 1. the child need not be exposed to the troubling experiences in the dental chair of impression taking and multiple fittings of a prosthetic aid, 2. there is no need to revise a prosthesis as growth proceeds, 3. it is more hygienic than having to wear an alien apparatus in the mouth, and 4. it produces better speech. Nonetheless, there are cogent reasons why this surgical procedure cannot be viewed as a panacea. The speech effect of the pharyngeal flap is not always significant. There are occasional difficulties produced by the reduction of the lateral ventilative space at the sides of the flap. If the procedure is not done carefully, or anatomic conditions are unfavorable, there may be interferences with Eustachian function. The production of an effective tether to the velum is sometimes made difficult because the flap may be based in the densely lymphoid area of the epipharynx. The flap does not always heal in a predictable way and its ultimate form may not provide the presumed advantages for improvement of velopharyngeal hemisphincteric action. There are occasions in which a pharyngeal flap actually appears to interfere with acoustic and pneumatic control. Some patients find that they cannot breathe comfortably through their nose. In children who have frequent upper respiratory infections this condition may assume distressingly acute proportions. Good residual mesial movement of the lateral pharyngeal walls is requisite for speech improvement.

The second class (that in which the serious alterations of arch form, dental occlusion, and vault dimension together with a partially closed or closed velum exist) may be more amenable to pharyngoplastic or prosthetic treatment for control of hypernasality. In cases of this class speech improvement may be achieved by surgically retroposing and relaxing the entire palate and proceeding with some type of pharyngoplastic procedure which will establish the functional integrity of the velopharyngeal valve. The pharyngeal flap may be the procedure of choice in this situation. If the prosthetic route is elected, the design of the speech aid must take into account the fact that the velar section of the prosthesis will have to be so placed as not to interfere with the downward movement of the velum in deglutition. Otherwise this velar movement in swallowing will dislodge the clasping system or place unusual strain on the anchoring teeth. If the circumstance of a partially divided velum exists, the velar section may carry the pharyngeal bulb directly to that plane in the epipharynx where it will be most effective in controlling air and sound. The speech aid may include additional features for the improvement of dental occlusion, better maxillomandibular and lip relationships, and facial contour. These help to improve speech in specific ways.

When, as in the third postsurgical class, the secondary palate is open and clinical judgment dictates no further surgical intervention of any kind, a prosthetic speech aid is the only means by which the patient may be prepared for effective speech reeducation. In this instance the prosthetic speech aid can be so designed as to provide satisfactory obturation of the cleft of the hard palate, as well as providing prosthetic assistance for oronasopharyngeal valving. Some speech clinicians and speech-oriented surgeons feel that in many cleft-palate children, surgery of the secondary palate should be delayed beyond the time of closing the lip and restoring continuity of the alveolar arch. This, then, should be followed by prosthetic treatment. Speech improvement, by these combined limited surgical and prosthetic procedures, is sometimes obtained more quickly and effectively. It is essential to point out that prosthetic assistance, if it is to be used at any stage, should not be unduly delayed. (Satisfactory speech aids can be designed for, and worn comfortably and usefully by young children who are in the stage of deciduous or mixed dentition.) It is also often practical to use a speech aid as an *ad interim* assistance in patients for whom further palatal surgery is projected but, for good reasons, is postponed. There is at present no complete agreement among maxillofacial surgeons as to how much surgery should be performed on patients with clefts of the secondary palate, nor at what age it should be done. Therefore, there are perhaps good clinical speech reasons for occasionally employing prostheses in young children. This makes it possible to intervene early with speech training and decelerate or prevent the establishment of the profound speech malhabits which attend cleft palate.

Longitudinal radiologic cephalometry provides an excellent basis for more secure diagnosis and encourages a more specific and adaptive surgical and/or prosthetic treatment. Moreover, it increases greatly the accuracy of prediction of the outcome of a selected treatment. It underscores the clinical significance of individual anatomic differences and reveals how unsafe any casual and routine surgical solution may be. Cephalometric growth-and-development research provides abundant evidence that children with orofacial deformity are more often distinguished by their anatomic and physiologic differences from each other than by their similarities. It is these individual variations of skeletal and soft tissue growth which are clinically more significant than the general fact that they have been "born with cleft palate and/or cleft lip."

The Physical Examination

The clinical examination made by the speech pathologist includes a systematic study of the patient's speech organs at rest and, insofar as possible, in use; and making a careful record of these observations.

The mouth and its contiguous facial structures are, for the cleft-palate child, often highly charged with fear, anxiety, and embarrassment. Previous medical, surgical, and dental treatments of these regions have often been painful and emotionally upsetting. Hence, examination of his speech structures requires adequate and sensitive preparation. Sudden or rough manipulation of his mouth will be threatening and will defeat the purposes of a satisfactory physical examination. Preparatory contact with young children with congenital orofacial defects through friendly, indirect play situations will build up the young patient's confidence. The structures of the facial mask may, in a young child, be examined without in any way making physical contact with him. The shape and contour of the external nasal structures will be apparent and should be recorded. The extent and character of tissue displacement should be noted. The external disfiguration will, in many patients, be related intimately to internal nasal deformity. When the light is adequate and when the head of the patient is slightly tilted backward, the nasal vestibules may be inspected. The speech clinician may not be experienced in the use of a nasal dilator or speculum, but this is not necessary. Any marked stenosis caused by displaced or deformed alae, columella, cartilagenous septum, or the anterior nasal floor will be manifest without dilation of the nasal vestibule.

In recording the observations, the correct and specific anatomic designation should be used. If the observations can be even grossly quantified it will be useful. The amount of cicatricial tissue present in the lip, its location and its distribution, should be described. The general mobility and length of the upper lip should be assessed. The nose and lip must be studied from both cosmetic and functional standpoints. The labial rima and the mucodermal border will provide the most important observational landmarks. When the child has sufficient confidence in the examiner, the dental structures and the interior of the oral cavity may be examined. One of the most important observations is that of dental occlusion. The child should assume a natural bite relationship for this inspection. It is usual for a child to protrude his lower jaw when asked to "bite his teeth together." Sometimes the mandible may be gently guided in its upward path to proper position. If the child is asked to place the tip of his tongue as far back on his palate as possible and to press it firmly while he moves his jaw into a bite position, his habitual maxillomandibular relationship is more likely to be produced. A wooden tongue depressor will be useful in retracting the buccal surfaces for examining the relationship of the teeth in the molar and premolar areas.

The speech clinician is not expected to make as experienced and detailed examination of the jaw and dental relationship as would the dentist, but he certainly should be sufficiently acquainted with normal external tooth anatomy, and interdental and jaw relationships to make reasonable judgments of irregularity. The most obvious deviations will be on the side of the line of cleft in unilateral cases, and on both sides in bilateral. Cross-bite occlusion on either or both sides is not uncommon. In addition, in bilateral deformities the premaxillary segment which carries the two central incisors may show marked deviation of position and shape. Presence of an alveolar disunity and its size should be noted as well as the character of the tissue at its closure. Individual teeth at the line of cleft and on the cleft side should be included in the general inspection. General health of the teeth and their investing tissue should be noted, even though carious areas on the teeth need not be counted or detailed, since this is done expertly by a dentist when he examines the mouth, explores the teeth, takes intraoral x-rays, and charts the carious regions. It is, however, highly important that the speech clinician determine the general extent of dental disease, for the health of the teeth and the need for restorative and peridontal treatment is a critical determinant in a child's speech recovery, especially if he is to receive orthodontic and maxillary orthopedic care, or be fitted with a temporary speech aid.

A simple way to make a preliminary inspection of a child's palate is to ask him to look up at a point on the ceiling and to open his mouth as he does so. The child's mouth will not need to be touched at this stage. This head posture places the palate in direct view. A flashlight is a convenient source of light. An orderly sequence for examining the palate is to observe first the general upper dental arch form as a palatal boundary. Degrees of arch contraction and any asymmetricality should be estimated. The height and shape of the palatal vault should be studied next. The amount and distribution of cicatricial tissue and the degree of depression of the zenith of the palatal vault are important points for observation. As inspection proceeds posteriorward, the location of the point of muscular flexion and of the levator dimples will suggest how far forward the anterior border of the velum is placed. Extensive scarring in this region may obscure this point. Asking the patient to phonate the vowel /α/ or /a/ while the tongue is lightly depressed will usually cause sufficient elevation of the velum for this observation. Care should be exercised with regard to the degree of depression of the mandible and of the tongue with the tongue depressor. The movements of the velum in surgically operated cleft-palate children are often apt to be limited at best. If the mouth is forced open too widely and the tongue depressed too much or too forcibly, it will produce marked tension in the faucial pillars and restrict the upward and backward movement of the velum. Minimal movement of the velum may thus be obscured and the degree of its mobility misjudged. Placing the patient in front of you with his head resting on your body and with the *washed* middle finger, the posterior border of the palatal bones may be palpated and its outline and contour determined. The presence of defects of the uvula should not be missed. Frequently a bifid uvula may be unmasked by placing a dry wooden tongue depressor under the structure and drawing it forward. A fissure will be displayed if one is present.

The oropharyngeal region can be examined best if the patient is placed high enough so one obtains a fairly direct line of vision into his posterior oral cavity. If he is not so seated and is asked to tip his head back to "improve" the view, his cervical structures are retroflexed and serious inhibition or distortion of the pharyngeal movements is produced. He should be seated with head erect. The muscles of the tongue, of the velum, of the lateral walls of the oropharynx, and the posterior pharyngeal wall are so intimately related mechanically that any marked displacement of one changes the postures and range of movement of the others. Peroral inspection of the form and functions of the velopharyngeal hemisphincter is limited to its oral aspect, and information provided by this view is limited. Hence, it is important that the cervical supports and the cranial base be so positioned as to cause the least possible distortion of the pharyngeal tube and its contiguous structures. If necessary, stimulation of the dorsum of the tongue to elicit the gagging reflex will also elicit maximal elevation of the velum. It is difficult to see this fleeting movement unless the patient's head is stabilized with one hand and the tongue depressor firmly held. The examination of the posterior of the oral cavity should be extended to include the position, form, and movement of the palatoglossus and palatopharyngeus muscles. In certain surgical procedures the anterior faucial pillars are united with each other superiorly or with the free posterior borders of the velum, in order to reduce the lateral dimensions of the oropharyngeal or nasopharyngeal isthmus. Of particular interest is the amplitude of mesial movement of the anterior and posterior pillars and lateral pharyngeal walls.

The estimation of the extent and character of occlusive movement of the total nasopharyngeal valve is a difficult one to make by peroral inspection. Static or dynamic radiography may be usefully employed. Especially difficult is any objective estimate of the completeness of closure during continuous speech. About all that can be accomplished in this direction, without cineradiography or a static x-ray projection, is to examine the valve by reflected light during phonation of a low mid or back vowel. The best instrument for such visualization is a nasopharyngeal mirror of generous diameter. The tongue is controlled but not depressed with a metal tongue depressor, and the mouth only slightly more open than it is in the rest position. The illumination must be directed upon the mirror's face. If the examiner is skilled in the use of the head mirror it is even better. The nasopharyngeal port can be viewed if the mirror is held at the appropriate angle. Care must be taken to reduce the possibility of the patient's gagging. Even under the best conditions with the most skillful instrumental manipulation and posture and cooperation of the patient, the view obtained is not always adequate or meaningful. If the nasopharyngeal port is wide during phonation of a low vowel, the vowels /i/ or /u/ should be tried. The elevation of the front of the tongue must be controlled, however. X-ray projections of velopharyngeal closure of normal subjects suggests that the maximum closure on the vowel series is for /i/ and /u/. It is then, with experience, possible to educe in a general way the extent of velopharyngeal closure from direct observation of the velum, pillars, and posterior and lateral pharyngeal walls during deglutition (with the tongue controlled) and during phonation. In many ways, the most significant picture is that of the general lateral dimensions of the oropharyngeal isthmus and the distance between the posterior margin of the velum and the posterior pharyngeal wall in rest. The description of examinative procedure so far has been limited to the patients with clefts of the secondary palate that have been closed by surgery.

When the hard palate and velum are open, a direct view into the inferior regions of the nasal spaces and the epipharynx is available. This examination should include an estimate of cleft length, width, and shape, as well as a description of the inferior turbinates, and should reflect an impression of the location, shape, and size of the vomer bone. In these cases also, careful study of the extent and path of movement of the divided velar remnants is necessary. The adjustment of these velar tags, together with that of the palatoglossus and palatopharyngeus and the posterior pharyngeal wall are important in visualizing their adaptation to a pharyngeal flap or the bulb of a speech aid. This judgment will also be useful in predicting the length of the palatal axis and ultimate velar size and shape following classical surgical closure.

A thorough physical examination of the patient by the speech pathologist should include an observation and report of any associated structural anomalies of the head. The general shape and size of the auricles, deformities of the tragi and helices or the lobes, and asymmetry in the location of the ears on the head are features of embryologic and clinical significance. The presence of atresia of the external auditory canals will be missed if the external auditory meatuses are not examined. An atypical path of excursion of the mental point of the mandible upon opening the mouth widely may suggest a disordered temporomandibular joint or inequality of length of the corpora of the mandible, or variation in the angulation and form of the rami. The position of the whole head on the neck and shoulders should be noted. Evidences of a foreshortened neck with limited movement on flexion and extension, or restricted rotation of the head may signal the presence of associated deformities of the cervical bones. The implication of such osteal defects of the cervical vertebrae in the shape and adjustments of the pharyngeal tube are of clinical importance to the speech pathologist. They are, too, evidences of the close teratologic relationship between many subtle and overt anomalies involving the whole cephalocervical complex. It does no harm but may improve an understanding of congenital anomalies to also examine the hands, fingers, and feet of the patient. These structures may also show morphologic differentials which, when recorded, provide a better picture of the whole problem of habilitation, of which the correction of orofacial deformity is only a part.

BIBLIOGRAPHY (*Chapters 29 and 30*)

Brackett, J. Chap. 17, this vol.

Dorrance, G. 1933. The operative story of cleft palate. Philadelphia: Saunders.

Fogh-Anderson, P. 1942. Inheritance of harelip and cleft palate. Copenhagen: Nyt Nordisk Forlag—Arnold Busck.

Gorlin, R., and Pindborg, J. 1964. Syndromes of the head and neck. New York: McGraw-Hill.

Graber, T. 1968. Orthodontics, principles and practice. Philadelphia: Saunders.

Harkins, C. 1960. Principles of cleft palate prosthesis. New York: Columbia.

Kirkham, H. 1931. *Quoted* by Peyton, W. The dimensions and growth of the palate in the normal infant and in the infant with gross maldevelopment of the upper lip and palate. *Arch. Surg.*, 22, 704–737.

Koepp-Baker, H. 1963. Cleft palate: multidisciplinary management. Univ. Iowa: *Conference Report*, 21–29.

McCarthy, M. 1925. Preliminary report of studies on the nasopharynx. *Ann. Otol., Rhinol., Laryng.*, 34, 801–813.

Moss, L. 1955. Postnatal growth of the human skull base. *Angle Orthodontist*, 1, 25(2), 155–162.

Pruzansky, S. 1953. Description, classification, and analysis of unoperated clefts of the lip and palate. *Amer. J. Orthodont.*, 39, 8, 590–611.

———, and Richmond, J. 1954. Growth of the mandible in infants with micrognathia. *Amer. J. dis. Child.*, 38, 29–42.

Psaume, J. 1950. Contribution a l'étude du squelette du Bec de lièvre et de la division palatine non-opérés. Thése Doctorat en Médecine. Paris.

Ricketts, R. 1952. The significance of variation in the cranial base and soft structures. Amer. Assn. Cleft Palate Rehabilitation: newsletter, 3, 5–6.

Schüller, A. 1929. X-ray examination of deformities of the nasopharynx. *Ann. Otol., Rhinol., Laryng.*, 38, 108–129.

Sicher, H. 1949. The development of the face and oral cavity. *In* Orban, B., Oral histology and embryology (2nd. ed.). St. Louis: Mosby.

Stark, R. 1962. Plastic surgery. New York: Hoeber.

Subtelny, Joanne, and Subtelny, J. 1962. Roentgenographic techniques and phonetic research. *Proceedings of the Fourth International Congress of Phonetic Sciences*. The Hague: Mouton.

Subtelny, J. 1953. Width of the nasopharynx and related anatomical structures in normal and unoperated cleft palate children. Univ. Ill.: Master's thesis.

Wardill, W. 1928. Cleft palate. *Brit. J. Surg.*, 16, 127–148.

Winitz, H. 1969. Articulatory acquisition and behavior. New York: Appleton-Century-Crofts.

31

Communication Disorders in the Mentally Retarded

Jack Matthews

INTRODUCTION

Terminology

In citing studies from the field of mental retardation, we do not find a consistent terminology employed. The same term may be used by two different investigators to describe two different degrees of mental retardation. Even the same degree of retardation may be designated by different writers in different terms. Wallin (1949) has suggested terminology that is widely but by no means uniformly employed. He lists the following terms to represent the range from high degree of retardation to average or normal intelligence: idiot, imbecile, moron, borderline, backward or dull, retarded, and average.

Among many workers in the field of mental retardation, the term *idiot* became widely accepted to designate individuals whose retardation, as measured on intelligence tests, placed them in the I.Q. range below 25. Individuals in the I.Q. range of roughly 25–50 were frequently referred to as imbeciles. The term *moron* was often applied to the I.Q. range of approximately 50–70.

In May of 1960 the American Association on Mental Deficiency approved an official manual on terminology and classification in mental retardation. This official manual was published as a monograph supplement to the *American Journal of Mental Deficiency* (Heber, 1961).

> Mental retardation refers to subaverage general intellectual functioning which originates during the developmental period and is associated with impairment in adaptive behavior.

This 1961 definition is consistent with the usage suggested by the Nomenclature Committee of the American Association on Mental Deficiency (Sloan, 1954).

While the latter conditions (defects in the psychological and sociological spheres) are recognized as causative mechanisms in their own right, they may also, and frequently do, play significant roles in influencing the degree and nature of the mental retardation resulting from cerebral defects. The implication of this premise also involves the conception of mental retardation as a dynamic rather than static condition, amenable in many cases to treatment through therapeutic procedures even though the basic cerebral defect is irreversible.

The terms *speech therapist*, *speech clinician*, *speech correctionist*, and *speech pathologist* are used interchangeably. The term *communicologist* is used to designate clinicians dealing with communication disorders of language, speech, or hearing. *Communicology* is employed as a general term to include areas commonly designated as *audiology*, *speech pathology*, and *language pathology*.

The Role of the Speech Pathologist

Lillywhite and Bradley (1969) suggest "the necessity for the communication specialists to be able to function as members of multidiscipline diagnostic and management terms." This suggestion is in keeping with recommendations made by the Presidents' Panel on Mental Retardation (1962). Such recommendations would make the diagnosis and interpretation of mental retardation to parents the responsibility of community-centered clinics. In such a center the communicologist would be a member of a diagnostic, interpretation, and research team composed of specialists from the fields of medicine, psychology, social work, and education, as well as communicative disorders.

In many communities such clinics are not available and the communicologist is often one of the first professional persons to evaluate the mentally retarded child.

Frequently a child may first be recognized as mentally retarded when his inability to express himself becomes obvious. The speech pathologist may not treat the speech problem per se but may initiate the series of referrals to physician, psychologist, social worker, educator, and so on, which results in parents coming to understand that they have a mentally retarded child. Often the chief contribution of the speech pathologist is an intelligent sympathetic interpretation of the diagnosis of mental retardation. Such an interpretation may help parents to take their focus off the communication problem and to place it on other problems which must be recognized and dealt with in mental retardation. Some of these other problems often need attention before consideration can or should be given to the communication problem.

The role of the speech pathologist in the area of mental retardation is certainly not limited to that of diagnostician, interpreter, and referring agent. We feel there is also an important role for language and speech therapy in the field of mental retardation. The decision as to whether or not a given speech pathologist wishes to work in the field of mental retardation will of course have to be made by him.

The first edition of this chapter (Matthews, 1957) suggested that although communicology as a profession may not have actively discouraged speech therapy for the mentally retarded, there had been little encouragement given by the profession to devote attention to communication disorders associated with mental retardation. One of the most significant developments we can report in this 1971 revision is the great increase in the interest of communicologists in the field of mental retardation.

As long as communicologists deal with problems of language and speech retardation, they will almost of necessity be confronted with problems of mental retardation. In our own clinical experience, mental retardation has been one of the most frequently encountered factors associated with language and speech retardation. With the increased attention currently being given to mental retardation will come more and more pressures on communicologists to devote greater attention to communication problems associated with mental retardation. This will require that communicologists increase their knowledge not only of communication disorders of the mentally retarded, but of the broader field of mental retardation itself.

LANGUAGE AND SPEECH RETARDATION

The dependence of language on intelligence can be illustrated by observing the frequent absence of language and speech in the severely mentally retarded. Absence of these functions has actually been employed as a basis of classification of the mentally retarded. Binet and Simon (1914) employed this principle in defining the idiot.

> An idiot is any child who never learns to communicate with his kind by speech—that is to say, one who can neither express his thought verbally nor understand the verbally expressed thought of others, this inability being due solely to defective intelligence, and not to any disturbance of hearing, not to any affection of the organs of phonation.

Tredgold (1947) has observed that in idiocy "Speech is usually absent, although a few do learn to articulate such simple monosyllables as man, cat, eat, etc., but none of them can form sentences."

Few statistical studies have been made to determine the relationship between intelligence and speech retardation. We have little accurate information concerning the average age at which individuals with varying degrees of mental retardation begin to babble, use words meaningfully, combine words into phrases and sentences, and so forth.

In her examination of the speech status of 32 idiots (I.Q.'s below 20 and chronological ages from seven years nine months to 38 years), Kennedy (1930) found 22 were altogether mute, nine could produce only jabbering, and only one produced recognizable words. In this one instance, however, the words were used in nonmeaningful and irrelevant contexts. Kennedy reported that some idiots gave evidence of understanding simple commands.

TABLE 31-I
Language Development of Idiots (Town)

LANGUAGE CHARACTERISTICS OF IDIOTS	% PRESENT IN 17 LOW-GRADE IDIOTS	% PRESENT IN 8 MIDDLE-GRADE IDIOTS	% PRESENT IN 25 HIGH-GRADE IDIOTS
Understand gestures	2	2	23
Imitate gestures	0	1	20
Make voluntary gestures	4	2	22
Understand a few words	1	3	14
Speak a word or two	0	1	10

Town (1913), studying 50 idiots, divided his sample into low-, high-, and middle-grade intelligence levels. His data (Table 31-I) suggest that among idiots, the degree to which language develops is directly dependent on intelligence. At all levels, more children used voluntary gestures than imitated them. Town observed that where voluntary gestures develop before ability to imitate gestures develops, the voluntary gestures seem to be limited to prehension or a direct need for expression of repulsion. Many of the high-grade idiots who could say nothing except perhaps "mama," "yes," and "no," understood the names of many familiar objects.

Lapage (1911) noted that high-grade defectives acquired speech at 20 months compared with 41 months for low-grade defectives. In this study neither "high-grade" nor "low-grade" defectives is defined.

In an investigation of 1,000 boys and girls whose I.Q.'s ranged from 10 to 159, Abt, Adler, and Bartelme (1929) correlated age of speech onset (time child first associated a word with an object) with intelligence (Stanford-Binet). The correlation between age of speech onset and intelligence was —.41 for boys and —.39 for girls.

Mead (1913) studied 92 feeble-minded children (not defined in terms of I.Q.) and reported that the "typical" feeble-minded child uses a word meaningfully at 34.44 months and that this behavior may have its onset at 12 months or up to 156 months.

Karlin and Strazzulla (1952) investigated age of babbling, word use, and sentence use in three groups of mentally retarded. Their data are summarized in Table 31-II. Karlin and Strazzulla's data on the use of the first word by children in the I.Q. range of 51–70 are in substantial agreement with the earlier work of Mead (1913).

TABLE 31-II
Age of Speech Acquisition
(Karlin and Strazzulla)

ACTIVITY	I.Q. 15–20	I.Q. 26–30	I.Q. 51–70
Babbling	25 mths	20.4 mths	20.8 mths
Word use	54.3 mths	43.2 mths	34.5 mths
Sentence use	153 mths	93 mths	89.4 mths

Meader (1940) compared the age of speech onset of a mentally retarded group with the group of gifted children studied by Terman (1925). In Terman's genius group the incidence of delayed speech was one percent. In Meader's group with I.Q.'s of less than 66, the incidence of delayed speech was 44 percent. In the group with I.Q.'s of 67 and higher the incidence was 25 percent.

Wallin (1949) examined 272 "subnormal" children and found that this group used single words at an average age of one year and eight months. Sentences were used at two years six months. "Mentally defective" children (164 in number) used single words at two years and sentences at three. Morons used words at 1.6 years and sentences at two years and three months. Imbeciles used single words at two years and three months and sentences at three years and seven months.

Ingram (1935) and Gesell and Amatruda (1937) present some general tables outlining the progress that a mentally retarded child can be expected to make. Although these tables contain items concerned with the onset of speech, no information is given about the sample from which these norms were derived.

Table 31-III summarizes the findings of studies of the time of use of the first word in groups of mentally retarded.

During the past decade there has been a greater interest in the language aspects of retardation than in any similar time span. For a sampling of this recent literature the reader is directed to presentations found in Spradlin (1963), Spreen (1965a, 1965b), and Jordan (1966). In December 1963 a conference on language and mental retardation was held at Lawrence Kansas. The papers of this conference formed the basis of "the first book to explore the importance of language in both research and clinical work with the mentally retarded" (Schiefelbusch, Copeland, and Smith, 1967).

TABLE 3-III
Summary of Studies on Use of First Word by Mentally Retarded

INVESTIGATOR	TYPE POPULATION	TIME OF USE OF FIRST WORD
Karlin & Strazzulla (1952)	I.Q.'s from 15–20	54 mths
Karlin & Strazzulla (1952)	I.Q.'s from 26–30	43.2 mths
Lapage (1911)	Low-grade defectives	41 mths
Karlin & Strazzulla	I.Q.'s from 51–70	34.5 mths
Mead (1913)	Nondefined retarded population	34.44 mths
Wallin (1949)	Morons	18 mths

The studies concerned with time of speech and language acquisition in mentally retarded children do not provide us with normative data we can accept with confidence. Various indices of speech and language acquisition have been employed by different investigators. Definitions of intellectual levels of subjects are not always presented, nor are they comparable from study to study. The sampling procedures and statistical treatment are subject to question. In spite of these limitations, the studies do point out clearly that on the average the mentally retarded child acquires language and speech considerably later than the child of normal intelligence.

INCIDENCE OF SPEECH PROBLEMS

Not only is speech frequently delayed in the mentally retarded, but when it does emerge it is often defective. The incidence of speech problems among the mentally retarded has been reported in a number of studies, and the incidence figures vary widely. Variations in the incidence figures are probably due to differences in criteria of what constitutes a speech defect and to differences in the composition of the mentally retarded groups studied.

Sir Cyril Burt (1937) studied the speech of children in typical schools in London and Birmingham. In the group with I.Q.'s 70–85, he found nine percent of the children with mild speech defects and five percent with severe speech defects. In the group with I.Q.'s 50–70 there were 13 percent with mild speech defects and 11 percent with severe defects. Burt estimated that at least 25 percent of retarded children are speech defectives.

American incidence statistics are considerably higher than those of Burt. However, most of the American studies have been carried out in institutionalized populations and have included the speech of children too retarded to have ever entered regular schools. Such a population would never have been part of that on which Burt's figures are based.

Lewald (1932) investigated 533 patients in an institution and found that 56 percent of all the patients had speech defects. Sirkin and Lyons (1941) examined 2,522 institutionalized mentally retarded. They reported that 50 percent had speech defects and 17 percent had no speech at all. Schlanger (1953c) found that 68 percent of 74 children in a private school for retarded children had speech defects. Kennedy (1930) studied speech defects in an institution population and found that 71.87 percent of 27 imbeciles had dyslalic speech. Of 249 morons 42.57 percent had speech disorders ranging from slight to severe in nature. All of 32 idiots studied lacked language beyond jabbering, crying, and utterance of isolated words.

Sachs (1951) examined 210 morons and imbeciles who were inmates at the Lynchburg State Colony in Virginia and found that 57 percent had speech defects. Eighteen percent of the borderline group were defective in speech, whereas 44 percent of the moron group and 79 percent of the imbecile group had defective speech. Sirkin and Lyons (1941) found 31 percent of the institutionalized mentally retarded with I.Q.'s over 69 had speech defects. In the moron group 47 percent had speech defects and in the imbecile group 74 percent had speech defects.

In the present decade Tarjan (1961) reported the incidence of communication disorder as 94 percent among the first admissions of the mentally retarded in a state hospital. Steinman (1963) estimated an incidence of 57 percent articulation errors in a population of 1,000 educable retarded children. Wilson (1966) found 53 percent of a group of educable mentally retarded had articulation errors. Sheehan et al. (1968) reported that more than 50 percent of the patients in five wards at Porterville State Hospital had no speech or severely delayed speech.

An examination of Table 31-IV indicates that incidence figures vary from five percent to 94 percent. Such variations are attributable in part to differences among investigators' definitions of speech defects and to differences in the various populations studied. Although the incidence figures reported in Table 31-IV vary greatly, the data permit us to conclude

TABLE 31-IV
Summary of Studies on Incidence of Speech Defects Among Mentally Retarded

INVESTIGATOR	TYPE POPULATION	INCIDENCE OF SPEECH DEFECTS (%)
Kennedy (1930)	Institutionalized imbeciles	71.87
Kennedy (1930)	Institutionalized morons	42.57
Lewald (1932)	500 institutionalized defectives	56
Burt (1937)	Mentally backward school children (I.Q.'s 70–85)	9 mild 5 severe
Burt (1937)	Severely retarded school children (I.Q.'s 50–70)	13 mild 11 severe
Sirkin and Lyons (1941)	2,522 institutionalized defectives	67
Sirkin and Lyons (1941)	Institutionalized defectives (I.Q.'s over 69)	31
Sirkin and Lyons (1941)	Institutionalized imbeciles	74
Sirkin and Lyons (1941)	Institutionalized morons	47
Sachs (1951)	210 institutionalized imbeciles, morons, border liners	57
Sachs (1951)	Institutionalized borderliners	18
Sachs (1951)	Institutionalized imbeciles	79
Sachs (1951)	Institutionalized morons	44
Schlanger (1953)	74 private school retardates	57
Tarjan (1961)	First admissions in state hospital	94
Steinman (1963)	1,000 educable retarded children	57
Wilson (1966)	777 educable (I.Q. 48–78)	53
Sheehan, Martyn, and Kilburn (1968)	5 wards of Porterville State Hospital	50

that the incidence of speech defects in populations of mentally retarded is high—considerably higher than in the general population.

TYPES OF SPEECH PROBLEMS

We have established that the mentally retarded are slower than the normal in acquiring speech and language. We have also shown that when speech is acquired, it is likely to be defective in the mentally retarded. We can now ask if the speech defects found among the mentally retarded are essentially different in kind from those found in nonretarded populations. Irwin (1942) is one of the few investigators who feel that the mentally retarded child is not only delayed and defective in speech but that his entire course of development of sounds is different from that exhibited by normal children. Irwin studied 10 children having I.Q.'s (as measured by the Kuhlman and the Binet) ranging from seven to 48. He made transcriptions of their speech sounds twice with an interval of a year between times of testing. He found these children used back vowels more infrequently than front vowels. In this respect their speech resembled that of infants more than that of adults. Since the chronological ages of the children ranged from two to five years, one would expect to find back vowels in greater use. The retarded children showed concentration in the labial, postdental, and glottal sounds; whereas infants show the greatest piling up among the glottals and adults among the postdental sounds. The ratio of vowels to consonants in the speech sounds of this retarded group was 1:1; whereas the adult ratio is 1:2. The ratio for newborns is 3:2. Irwin's study of infants is the only one of its kind and suggests that in the mentally retarded the course of development of sounds is different from that found in normal children. However, most investigators of the speech of older mentally retarded children find that speech defects in the mentally retarded are similar in kind to those found in a nonmentally retarded population of speech defectives.

Karlin and Strazzulla (1952) listed consonant defects in order of occurrence in a population of retarded. The most frequently occurring defective consonant was /s/ followed by /z/, /l/, /r/, /tʃ/, /dʒ/, /ð/, /ʃ/, and /θ/. This is similar to the order of occurrence of articulation errors that would be found in a nonretarded population. Karlin and Strazzulla's findings are similar to those reported by Kennedy (1930), Lapage (1911), Lewald (1932), and Sachs (1951).

The most systematic study of the kinds of substitutions, omissions, and additions in the speech of mentally retarded was made by Bangs (1942). He selected a homogeneous group of primary aments from an institution and gave them articulation tests by using 65 picture cards as stimuli. Bangs's data in general indicate that the speech of primary aments tends to correspond closely to that of normal children insofar as sounds avoided and sounds most frequently substituted are concerned. Bangs concluded that the speech of the primary ament shows the same retardation as all of his other functions. Bangs noted that the aments differed from normal children in the great number of omissions made in the final position. Normal children generally do not leave off their final consonants as frequently as the aments do. Bangs suggested that the omissions may be due to the inability of the ament to concentrate on one act until full completion. He further noted that although in general there were no significant differences between the sort of errors made by normal and ament children, sometimes the retarded children made minor substitutions which were bizarre and not of the sort ever found among normal children.

Using phonellegraphic techniques Neelley, Edison, and Carlile (1968) compared the fundamental frequencies of 14 retarded adults ages 17 years, six months to 18 years, two months with 14 normal adults ages 18 years, one month to 19 years, five months. They found a statistically significant difference between the means and medians of the two groups in their fundamental frequencies. The difference was 1.35 tones higher for the retarded group, but it is questionable if any perceptual differences could be detected.

In special syndromes of mental retardation such as mongolism, cretinism, or microcephaly no special speech pattern or particular type of speech has been reported in any systematic investigation. There is, however, a certain amount of opinion expressed in the literature concerning speech problems "typical" of certain syndromes. West, Kennedy, and Carr (1946) note that mongols have very hoarse voices and that they are frequently afflicted with nerve deafness. Their voices are supposed to be loud and inflectionless. Mongols are supposed to have difficulty in the articulation of /k/, /g/, /ij/, and the back vowels. No data are presented to support any of these contentions. Benda (1949) states that mongoloid children often have deep voices and that these are so typical of the syndrome that often a diagnosis of mongolism can be made on the basis of hearing the child speak. The voice is raucous, low in pitch, and sounds masculine and mature. Again no data are presented to support these conclusions.

In one of the few objective studies of the speech of mongoloids, Gottsleben (1955) reported the incidence of stuttering in a group of 36 mongoloids to be 33 percent. In a control group of nonmongoloid mentally retarded the incidence of stuttering was only 14 percent. The high incidence of stuttering in mongolism found by Gottsleben is consistent with observations made by Travis (1931), Gens (1951c), Schlanger (1953), Schlanger and Gottsleben (1957), and Schaeffer and Shearer (1968).

Hollien and Copeland (1965) found that the fundamental frequency of a group of nine female mongoloids did not differ significantly from that of a normal group. They concluded, "Their apparent voice abnormalities must be explained by other relationships." Michel and Carney (1964) found no differences in speaking pitch and mean pitch levels between a group of eight to 11-year-old mongoloid and normal boys.

Zisk and Bialer (1967) reviewed recent literature dealing with speech problems of mongoloids. Nothing reported in the Zisk and Bialer (1967) review changes our earlier conclusion (Matthews, 1957).

Although there is some evidence to suggest that the incidence of stuttering in mongoloids is higher than that in the nonmongoloid mentally retarded population, there is no evidence to suggest that mongolism could be recognized on the basis of the speech symptoms alone.

Gens (1950) studied the speech of a group of 1,252 epileptics. He found that 73.6 percent had defective speech. He did not find any typical epileptic pattern of speech, but instead found the same disorders that are found in a nonepileptic population.

Although one may find in the literature references which attempt to describe the "typical" speech of certain syndromes in mental retardation, there are no systematic studies to bear out such a contention. There is clear-cut evidence to indicate that the incidence of speech disorders among the mentally retarded is considerably higher than in a nonretarded population. There is, however, no evidence to suggest that the speech defects of the mentally retarded differ in kind from those of a nonretarded speech-defective population.

RELATIONSHIP TO OTHER FACTORS

Intelligence

In studies which have related I.Q. and onset of speech, or I.Q. and speech proficiency, low correlations have been reported. Abt, Adler, and Bartelme (1929) studied 1,000 children excluding those with I.Q.'s below 70 and those who did not begin to talk until after five years. The correlation between age of onset of speech and Binet I.Q. was —.41, indicating that the earlier the onset of speech is, the more intelligent is the child. Bangs (1942) found that when chronological age was held constant there was a correlation of .39 between speech proficiency and mental age. In a study of 12 birth-injured children with defective speech, Doll (1932) reported a correlation of .02 between I.Q. and severity of the speech defect. Schlanger (1953c) found a correlation of .37 between mental age and articulation proficiency. Although all of the correlations just cited are low, they do point to a relationship between intelligence and degree of speech involvement.

Since the original edition of this chapter was written (Matthews, 1957) little has been reported on the relationship between intelligence and degree of speech or language deficit. This stems in part from the more recent concept of mental retardation as a multiple handicap in which an intelligence quotient is only one of a number of factors entering into the diagnosis and treatment of mental retardation.

Handedness

Karlin and Strazzulla (1952) reported 16 percent of the mentally retarded children they studied were left-handed as compared to three percent in a normal population. The percentage of established handedness increased with I.Q. level. Lewald (1932) found approximately 20 percent of 466 mentally retarded either left-handed or without hand dominance. Hawk (1950) in a study of 53 cases of dull normal children found that next to the speech handicap the most frequently occurring difficulty was with establishing handedness and poor use of the right hand. Burt (1937) reported that 7.4 percent of the mentally deficient children in Birmingham and 12.3 percent of those in London were left-handed. Left-handedness and lack of hand dominance is reported more frequently in populations of mental defectives than in the normal population.

Hearing Loss

Kodman (1958), Moss, Moss, and Tizard (1961), Lloyd and Frisina (1965), Watkins, Stewart, and Ryan (1966), Reneau and Mast (1968), Lamb and Graham (1968), and Lloyd, Spradlin, and Reid (1968) have described techniques for audiometric testing of the mentally retarded. These techniques include the GSR and the EEG as well as operant procedures and more conventional audiometry.

Reports of Birch and Matthews (1951), Kopatic (1963), Lloyd and Melrose (1966), Fulton (1967), and Lloyd, Reid, and McManis (1968) support the contention that it is possible to secure reliable audiometric thresholds from mentally retarded subjects.

A high incidence of hearing loss is found in populations of mentally retarded. Tredgold (1947) has stated:

> Defects of hearing are fairly common in the aments and include complete deafness, tonal deafness, and word deafness. Some of these conditions may be due to developmental anomalies or disease of the peripheral organ, but others are of central origin. Even where no actual deafness is present the acuity and range of auditory perception are usually below normal.

Burt (1937) reported that slight hearing defects were present in four percent of the normal school children in London. In backward children, hearing defects were present in six percent and these defects were severe in nature. Twelve percent of the backward children had slight hearing defects. Burt also records the fact that boys who are backward seemed to have more hearing defects than girls who are in a similar I.Q. group.

Abernathy (1938) administered pure-tone audiometer tests to children with I.Q.'s ranging from 20 to 69 and with chronological ages ranging from seven to 20. Children with ear pathologies or who were deaf or extremely hard-of-hearing were excluded from the study. He computed the median thresholds (in sensation units) for 373 subjects for eight frequencies. His results are summarized below.

Frequency	64	128	256	512	1024	2048	4096	8192
Sensation Unit Loss	10	15	15	20	10	10	15	10

Birch and Matthews (1951) found that over half of a mentally defective population of 247 persons from

10 to 39 years of age had hearing losses. Of this group with hearing losses, 32.7 percent had severe enough losses to be handicapped in some activity. Depending upon which frequency was being used for comparison, the incidence of hearing loss was two and one-half to 18 times greater than that found in a normal population. Schlanger (1953c) in a study of 70 mentally retarded children reported data on hearing loss in substantial agreement with Birch and Matthews.

MacPherson (1952) sent questionnaires to various institutions for the mentally retarded and inquired about the status of deaf patients committed for mental retardation. He found that 22 schools considered 50 percent of their patients to be either deaf or very hard-of-hearing. Fourteen schools estimated that about 50 percent of their patients had at least moderate hearing losses.

Johnston and Farrell (1954) studied 270 mentally retarded with mental ages from prekindergarten to fifth-grade levels of functioning. The mean chronological age of his population was 12 years nine months. He found that 24 percent of the children had hearing losses greater than 20 dB. This percentage, according to the author, is five times the percentage of hearing loss found in an audiometer survey made in the public schools in Massachusetts.

Foale and Paterson (1954) measured the hearing loss of 100 juvenile patients at Lennox Castle Institution for Mental Defectives in Scotland. The mean I.Q. of the patients was 66. Of the boys tested 67 percent had good hearing in both ears and approximately 13 percent were handicapped by their hearing impairment. Although the incidence of hearing impairment at Lennox Castle was lower than that reported by Birch and Matthews (1951) at Polk, the incidence of hearing loss in the retarded children at Lennox Castle is considerably higher than that found in normal populations surveyed in Scotland.

Rittmanic (1959) reported that 40 percent of a population of institutionalized mentally retarded patients had hearing losses which were considered a significant number in need of medical or other types of assistance.

Rigrodsky, Prunty, and Glovsky (1961) found that approximately 25 percent of the residents of Vineland Training School had a hearing loss. Twice as many males as females had impaired hearing. About half the hearing-loss population was in the age group of 11 to 30 years.

Dansinger and Madow (1966) found that approximately 13 percent of 967 testable retarded children and adults had sufficient hearing impairment to interfere with communication. They reported the relative frequency of hearing loss among retarded children to be two to six times greater than among normal children.

Lloyd and Reid (1967) obtained complete pure-tone audiograms on 482 children (ranging in age from six to 22 years old) at Parsons State Hospital and Training Center. Approximately 29 percent were reported as having some hearing loss with the more severely retarded having more hearing impairments.

Fulton and Lloyd (1968) reported an incidence of hearing loss of approximately 42 percent in a group of 79 children and young adults classified as having Down's Syndrome and residing at Parsons State Hospital and Training Center.

Table 31-V summerizes studies of hearing loss in mentally retarded children.

TABLE 31-V
Summary of Studies of Hearing Loss in Mentally Retarded Populations

INVESTIGATOR	HEARING LOSS
Burt (1937	6 percent severe, 12 percent slight
Abernathy (1938)	Median thresholds 10–20 sensation units below normal
Birth and Matthews (1951)	50 percent some loss, 32 percent severe loss
Macpherson (1952)	50 percent severe loss
Schlanger (1953c)	30 percent
Foale and Paterson (1954)	33 percent some loss, 13 percent severe loss
Johnston and Farrell (1954)	24 percent loss greater than 20 db
Rittmanic (1959)	40 percent
Rigrodsky, Prunty and Glovsky (1961)	25 percent
Dansinger and Madow (1967)	2 to 6 times greater than in normals
Lloyd and Reid (1967)	29 percent
Fulton and Lloyd (1968)	42 percent

Although there is not complete agreement among all the investigators as to the incidence of hearing loss in mentally retarded cases, there is a clear-cut indication that the incidence of hearing loss among the mentally retarded is considerably greater than that in a nonretarded population.

Differential Diagnosis

During the past decade several batteries of tests have been developed for the evaluation of language. The Parsons Language Sample (PLS) (Spradlin, 1963) contains six subtests which depend heavily on Skinnerian concepts (Skinner, 1957). The Illinois Test of Psycholinguistic Abilities (ITPA) (McCarthy and Kirk, 1963) is made up of nine subtests, all of which can be administered to a subject who gives only single-word responses. These instruments make a distinction between the expressive and the receptive aspects of language. In spite of the limitations of each of these test batteries they show promise of contributing significantly to the diagnostic task of the communicologist on the mental retardation team.

In view of the high incidence of speech and hearing problems among mentally retarded children, it is not surprising that communication disorders are often thought to result from mental deficiency. The well-trained clinician should recognize that there may be many explanations of delayed or defective speech which have no relation to intellectual retardation. Brain injury, glandular dysfunction, emotional disturbances, hearing loss, and lack of stimulation all may cause retardation in the development of language or result in poor articulation. Becky's (1942) study of 50 children with delayed speech revealed a number of constitutional, environmental, and psychological factors other than mental retardation.

The lack of understanding or the rejection of ghetto language and speech on the part of white middle class teachers and clinicians may be an inhibiting factor in the development of communication skills in the child who is culturally different.

Kanner (1948) believes there are groups of individuals who may be called "pseudo-feeble-minded," since their overall abilities may not be retarded. He includes in this group individuals with delayed speech but well-developed nonverbal abilities. Matthews and Birch (1949) have pointed out some of the problems encountered in evaluating the intelligence of speech- and hearing-handicapped.

The responses required in many tests are verbal. Children with speech defects often are very self-conscious about speaking. They will sometimes feign ignorance rather than make a speech attempt that will lead to their embarrassment. Often the responses of a child with defective speech cannot be understood by the examiner. This difficulty is especially noticeable in testing individuals with severe articulatory problems or with delayed speech; both conditions often found in severely involved cerebral palsy cases.

These problems can be overcome in part by making use of tests requiring nonverbal performance. Many such tests, however, depend almost exclusively on verbal directions for administration. For the child with a hearing loss such directions have an obvious weakness. In certain cases, e.g., in delayed speech, speech may be a relatively unimportant entity. A child may be habitually inattentive to the speech of others. In certain instances there may actually be a negative reaction to speech. Under any of these circumstances the use of verbal instructions may place the speech and hearing clinic case at a disadvantage; he may not get from the directions of the test an adequate knowledge of what is expected of him.

In administering intelligence tests to the hearing-handicapped, psychologists have attempted to replace verbal instructions with pantomime. When the tester is able to use pantomime freely—and many psychologists find it hard to do so—it is difficult to standardize. Matthews and Birth (1949) suggested some of the requirements of an adequate intelligence test for use with individuals with speech and hearing problems.

Such a tool while meeting the usual requirements of objectivity, reliability, and validity should also conform to additional specifications. It should not require verbal responses. The instructions should not involve speech or complicated pantomime on the part of the test administrator. The test should be relatively free from time limits and scoring based on speed. The test should impose as little penalty as possible on the handicapped child when he lacks experiences which are commonplace to normal youngsters.

Hardy (1948) feels that the child with hearing loss in certain frequencies who presents a picture of inconsistent responses to speech along with delayed speech or defective articulation may be superficially diagnosed as feebleminded. Jellinek (1941) has described phenomena resembling aphasia, agnosia, and apraxia in mentally retarded children and adults. Myklebust (1954) describes a number of clinical-observational techniques which may be employed in the differential diagnosis of hearing loss, aphasia, mental retardation, and emotional disturbance. Nance (1946) devised a scale in which an attempt is made to differentiate aphasia and mental retardation. The directions are given in pantomime and the scale includes items from well-known standardized intelligence tests. Strauss and Lehtinen (1947) have developed tests which attempt to differentiate brain damage from mental deficiency.

Morrow (1959) suggests that mentally retarded children can be differentiated from psychotic children on the basis of 1. signs of retardation such as late walking and sitting; 2. physical stigmata of retardation; and 3. presumptive evidence of additional congenital deformities. The retarded child compared to the psychotic child relates more quickly and usually warmly. Even if he is hostile, this is considered by Morrow as a manner of relating different from that of the psychotic child.

Most of the differential diagnosis techniques referred to are based on rich clinical experience. There is little validation information about any of the procedures. The speech pathologist should remember that in mental retardation we are dealing with a symptom complex which may result not only from defects of the central nervous system, but from defects "in the psychological and social spheres" (Sloan, 1954). Defects "in the psychological and social spheres" can themselves be causative mechanisms and can also influence the nature and degree of mental retardation caused by cerebral defects. This implies that mental retardation is "amenable in many cases to treatment through therapeutic procedures even though the basic cerebral defect is irreversible" (Sloan, 1954). The communicologist must be alert to the roles of aphasia, hearing loss, and emotional disturbance in influencing both the nature and degree of mental retardation. Mental retardation is no vaccination against emotional maladjustment, brain damage, or hearing loss. The speech pathologist must be equally careful that the role of mental retardation as an etiological factor be considered in all cases of language and speech retardation even though the primary problem may appear to be aphasia, hearing loss, or emotional disturbance. It is all too easy to forget that the child we have labeled psychotic or aphasic may also be mentally retarded. In the realm of mental retardation it is extremely important for the speech pathologist to recognize the role of the pediatrician, audiologist, psychologist, neurologist, psychiatrist, and other specialists in making a differential diagnosis.

THERAPY

Prevailing Attitudes

For some years good educational practice has called for the exclusion of the mentally retarded children from the regular classroom. This has not meant total exclusion from formal education. Instead special classes have been established for the mentally retarded. These classes have been set up to meet their special needs. Techniques have been developed for teaching the mentally retarded. Today we no longer ask, "Is it possible to educate and to rehabilitate the retarded child?" Instead our questions are concerned with developing the most effective techniques of education, training, and rehabilitation.

In the original edition of this chapter (Matthews, 1957) we reported that in many speech clinics, little provision was made for the mentally retarded child with a speech problem. In many clinics, no cases with an I.Q. of less than 70 were admitted. West, Kennedy, and Carr (1946) state that "the true mongol is particularly unresponsive of speech rehabilitation and it is practically useless to attempt such training." In the introduction to Stinchfield and Young (1938), Immel gives a similar opinion: "Mental subnormality is still a fact and when a child fails to learn to talk because of real mental deficiency hope is still an illusion and must remain so under the limitations of our present knowledge." Backus (1943) has pointed out that a low I.Q. is not necessarily a "death warrant" for a child and that the child's handicap may be lessened by improving his articulation. At the same time, she implies that working with a severely retarded child who has an I.Q. below 70 is likely to be a waste of time. In the last 10 years this attitude has undergone considerable modification. There has been an increase in the number of published articles which describe or evaluate attempts to initiate language and speech programs for the retarded. The annual conventions of the American Speech and Hearing Association reflect an increasing interest in the field of mental retardation. The American Association on Mental Deficiency has organized an interest group in the area of speech pathology and audiology parallel to interest groups in administration, psychology, medicine, etc. An increasing number of communicologists are devoting a large portion of their professional time to communication problems of the mentally retarded.

Evaluation of Therapy

One of the earliest attempts to evaluate speech therapy with mentally retarded children was that of Sirkin and Lyons (1941). They selected 169 institutionalized patients for a three-and-one-half-year therapy program. The mean length of treatment was five months with two or three sessions weekly. Patients were selected on the basis of intelligence, cooperation, and likelihood of receiving parole. Nineteen borderline, 104 moron, and 4 imbecile patients were in the therapy group. Seventy patients achieved satisfactory speech levels and 17 cases were still under treatment and progressing well at the time of the writing. These 87 cases comprised 52 percent of the therapy group. Seventy-three cases, or 48 percent of the group, had to be dropped from the program because they had insufficient intelligence or were too uncooperative to make any progress. At the end of three and one-half years, 44 of the cases had retained the improvement. Thirty out of the 44 cases had retained this improvement from one to three years or more. Ten of the cases had retrogressed, and 14 cases could not be contacted by the authors. Two cases had died. The I.Q.'s of those who had retained the correction ranged from 43 upward, but only eight of this group had I.Q.'s below 50. In those who had retrogressed, I.Q.'s ranged from 48 to 67, but only five had I.Q.'s above 53. In percentage terms, 52 percent of the total group benefited from the therapy; 79 percent of the borderline group, 59 percent of the moron group, and 26 percent of the imbecile group had profited by their experience. Because no control group was used, it is difficult to determine how much of the improvement may have been due to factors other than speech therapy.

Schlanger (1953b) carried out speech therapy with 62 mentally retarded children in special classes in Madison, Wisconsin. The mean chronological age of the group was 11 years 11 months, and the mean mental age was seven years and two months. The I.Q. range extended from 39 to 77. Significant improvement was noted in articulation, mean sentence length, and percentage of complete sentences used. No significant improvement was noted in number of words spoken per minute or in sound discrimination. The speech therapy program included many activities structured to encourage spontaneous conversation and listening. Schlanger felt that desirable changes in attitude, responsiveness, self-confidence, and so on, were brought about not entirely because of speech therapy but also as a result of establishment of group unity and the influence of the therapist. Because Schlanger employed no control group, it is difficult to separate the improvement which came as a result of Schlanger's program from the improvement which may have come from maturation or other factors in the total school program.

Schneider and Vallon (1955), at the end of one year of a speech therapy program carried out at the Westchester School for Retarded Children, concluded: "On the basis of our experiences, there is definitely a place for speech therapy in the educational or training programs for the moderately and the severely retarded child." The Schneider and Vallon (1955) program involved a small number of cases and did not utilize a control group.

Arnold (1955) reported a public school speech program for the mentally retarded which extended over a period of two and one-half years. Children improved in articulatory skills, rhythm of speech, and language growth. No control group was reported. Lubbman (1955) described a nine-month speech program for 93 children in the I.Q. range 19–50 and concluded that 62 children had improved their articulation. No control group was employed. Mecham (1955) reported that after eight weeks of speech therapy his experimental group of 21 children improved over his control group in articulation, auditory discrimination, auditory memory span, and average sentence length.

Donovan (1957), Rittmanic (1958), Kolstoe (1958), Schlanger (1959), Lassers and Low (1960), Rigrodsky and Steer (1961), Spragge (1962), and Peins (1967) describe programs and studies in which mentally retarded children benefited from speech and language therapy.

Shubert, Heuval, and Fulton (1966, 1967) reported two studies in which a traditional public school speech therapy program was applied to treatment groups at Fort Wayne State Hospital and Training Center. Results indicated that articulatory skills did not improve as a result of treatment. The authors reported, "The subjects seemed to be more aware of individual speech sounds and displayed a modified attitude toward communication in general."

Wilson (1966) studied educable mentally retarded children drawn from special education classes within the Special District of St. Louis County. The experimental group received phoneme-oriented articulation therapy for two half-hour periods per week. A placebo group received general communication therapy but not articulation therapy. A control group received no speech therapy but was tested for articulation errors at the same times as the other groups. The reduction in articulation errors for the respective groups was 5.9, 4.6, and 4.3. None of the differences was statistically significant.

Although these studies do not rest on as firm an

experimental and statistical basis as one might desire, they do not differ significantly in this respect from studies evaluating therapy with nonretarded populations. Available research data suggest that speech therapy with the mentally retarded can produce beneficial results. The author's clinical experiences suggest that language therapy is of greater benefit than articulation therapy, in particular with younger retarded children.

Approaches to Therapy

The communicologist must learn to accept and to strive for language and speech appropriate to mental age rather than chronological age. Prognosis for the severely retarded is not favorable. We can turn to no studies which have compared the effectiveness of various types of speech therapy in working with the mentally retarded. Our therapy guides for the present come largely from the techniques employed by teachers of the mentally retarded. To these techniques might well be added the speech improvement procedures which speech correction has developed for use in kindergarten and elementary grades. We have developed a set of materials which we have been able to turn over to teachers, teachers' aides, and parents for use in stimulating language and speech (Birch, Burgi, and Matthews, 1966). Our early work with programmed instruction (Holland and Matthews, 1963) and other aspects of operant conditioning (Spradlin, 1963) show promise for work with the retarded. Clinicians will have to plan activities suited to the mental age of the child and which will be appropriate to his short attention span. Rote memory drills will probably have little value. Group activities can no doubt be profitably employed. Principles of mental hygiene will be applicable. Language and speech simulation and correction programs integrated with the entire educational and training program of the retarded child will probably be more successful than programs lacking such integration. These suggestions represent the author's clinical judgments. A sampling of other judgments, some of which are based on research findings, may be suggestive of additional procedures.

Wallin (1924) has stressed the importance of developing a speech therapy program in which the mentally retarded child is accepted with all his limitations for what he is. His personal problems and needs must be attended to instead of routinely giving him practice in speech improvement.

As early as 1932 Twitmyer and Nathanson stressed the importance of integrating speech training with other aspects of training for the mentally retarded.

> The employment of technical speech training alone yields scanty results. On the other hand in those cases of amentia where the general condition improves through education, environmental control, and the like, the employment of specific speech training incidental to the general training is indicated and is usually followed by improvement in speech and increased ability to enjoy communication with fellow human beings.

West, Kennedy, and Carr (1946) stress the importance of simplifying directions for the mentally retarded child. They feel that motivation and praise of the child may be factors determining the success or failure of the program. The therapist is warned that improvement if it comes at all will come slowly.

Kirk and Johnson (1951) try to improve the child's language facility by discussion of situations within the child's range of experience. The weather, the home, and personal activities including walks the child has taken, the pictures he has seen, and the stories he has heard are all topics of discussion and part of a program of increasing vocabulary and concepts.

Schlanger (1958) believes that since the goals of speech therapy may be limited, therapy should concentrate on the reduction of negative interpersonal interaction and attempt to make communication rewarding.

Plotkin (1959) advocates a speech program for the trainable cerebral-palsied child based on recreational therapy, physical therapy, and arts and crafts or occupational therapy. The speech therapist is a part of the overall daily training program, the goal of which is to initiate enough speech or language to aid in developing useful communication. Speech correction is only a subordinate goal. All members of the staff must aid in the speech and communication activities. The program begins with informal comments such as "good morning," and "how are you?" which set the tone for the day and establish a routine. Subsequent speech activities might center around toileting, which could help speechless children develop regular toilet habits. Children should be encouraged to respond during roll call and saluting the flag even if only by an unintelligible grunt. Playtime and lunchtime provide opportunities for speech and language development. During song- and story-time the therapist has an opportunity to do some individual work.

Harrison (1959) describes a program in which developmental language activities are integrated with an education program for the mentally retarded children. Curricular experiences are utilized as motivation for communicative behavior through both separate and combined efforts of teachers and the language developmentalist. Teachers, parents, and language specialists must take into consideration the child's readiness, and stress relationships and relaxation. The same problem should be restated in a variety of forms and experiences should be rotated. Activities for language development are derived from interests of the children as reflected in free play activities—block building, bicycle riding, removing or putting on clothing, etc.

Renfrew (1959) reports an experiment in which nine children (aged six to nine, I.Q. 45 to 64) with markedly poor speech were taken in groups of three with their teacher and speech therapist working together thirty minutes once a week. Study of tape recordings of these sessions revealed that both teacher and therapist talked too much and impatiently supplied the missing word so that the child barely had a chance to think of it. The tempo of the sessions had to be reduced in order for the children to set the pace.

Mecham and Jex (1962) feel that motivation and communication interaction in structure life situations between children in a group are of primary importance in oral communication training. Segmented practice drills should be avoided. There should be repeated opportunity to engage in whole speech responses such as words and phrases with a good model always present.

Friedlander presents a rationale for speech and language development which may account for the high incidence of communicative disorders of the mentally retarded (1962).

> When the mentally retarded child is born, the stigmata of his 'difference' are sometimes evident at birth or shortly thereafter. As the child presents his 'differences' to his environment, a growing concern and anxiety develop in the parents. We have found that as the retarded child's lack of awareness and responsiveness to the parent's daily attempts to establish contact become increasingly evident, changes in the relationship occur which are emotionally unwholesome and contribute to attitudes and practices which in turn further impede the development and growth of language and communication. Some parents withdraw from further involvement with the child except to minister to his physical needs. There is no longer the warmth which forms the foundations of interpersonal reactions and communication for the child. Consequently the mentally retarded child is deprived of the normal sustenance for further growth without which even the intellectually unimpaired child will suffer delay and impairment of growth. On the other hand parents may bombard the child in frenzied anxiety to elicit speech and language far beyond his capabilities. This, too, results in failure. The parent-child relationship in these examples must be altered.

The Parsons Project (Schiefelbusch, 1963) has focused its attention on the interpersonal variables of the environmental setting, assuming that mentally retarded children may be subjected to interpersonal processes which tend to perpetuate a low level of behavioral functioning, particularly verbal behavior. The speech and language assessment is described as follows:

> The system for analyzing language behavior in developing the Parsons Language Sample was the Skinnerian model. A classification was made according to whether language is vocal or non-vocal, and according to the situations which control the occurrence of the language. Seven subtests were developed out of the Skinnerian rationale. These tests include tact, mand, echoic, intraverbal, comprehension, echoic gesture, and intraverbal gesture. One hundred twenty three test items are used. The studies relate to three broad areas of ongoing language research. These areas are concerned with language measurement of mental defectives; dyadic and small group studies where language output was investigated as a function of group composition; and the relationship of reinforcing variables to language performance and learning. (Spradlin, 1963.)

A study by Horowitz (1963) was designated to investigate types of reinforcing stimuli that were most effective in increasing the frequency of a correct vocal response among retarded subjects, the nature of the effectiveness of vocal and nonvocal components of social reinforcement, and the demonstrability of the partial reinforcement effect with retarded subjects. The main conclusion of this study was that a partial reinforcement effect was not significantly operative. Though partial reinforcement has been found to be effective in other situations, the learning of a complex vocal task for mental retardates may require longer periods of continuous reinforcement before switching to partial reinforcement or higher percentages of partial reinforcement.

Richardson (1967) has described a series of techniques for teaching language development to retarded children. The procedures employ early sensorimotor training and draw heavily from the Montessori system (Montessori, 1912).

Carrier (1967) has indicated that as educable retardates were reinforced for using successively higher numbers of words in describing pictures, the nature of their language, in terms of parts of speech, grammatical complexity, and types of errors, changed to more closely approximate that of nonretarded children of the same chronological age.

An examination of the various suggestions for speech therapy for the mentally retarded indicates that many of the recommended procedures might be difficult to carry out in the traditional one-or-two-sessions-per-week kind of individual therapy offered in many speech clinics. Much of the suggested speech correction program may not be carried out by the speech therapist but by parents, teachers, and others who spend considerable time with the retarded child (Birch, Burgi, and Matthews, 1966). Perhaps the pessimism about the success of speech and language therapy with the mentally retarded is based to a large extent on the failure to apply to the retarded therapy procedures suited to their needs and capacities.

Justification of Therapy

If we grant that speech and language procedures can be successful with the mentally retarded, we still must make a value judgment as to the value of such activities. There is now, and will continue to be, a shortage of communicologists to work with children with normal intelligence. Should we add to the shortage by diverting speech pathologists to work with the mentally retarded? In making a decision it would be well to remember that in high-grade defectives adequate communication may make a difference between self-sufficiency and dependence—between a lifetime in an institution at taxpayers' expense and vocational adjustment in society. Blanton and Blanton (1924) raised the question as to the amount of time the speech teacher is justified in spending on the mentally retarded. Their answer, given almost half a century ago, seems to this writer equally valid today.

> This (the amount of time the speech teacher is justified in devoting to the mentally retarded) must be decided on the merits of each individual case and of the learning ability and temperament of the child. While with the present scarcity of trained teachers in the speech field it would hardly be wise that the abnormal should be cared for and the normal child not; still, the speech defect may be the one added handicap that makes of the high-grade deficient a pauper or a criminal.

To the research-oriented communicologist the field of mental retardation offers an excellent laboratory. The institutional setting in which many retarded children grow up provides unusual opportunities for experimentally manipulating environmental factors. In classrooms for the retarded child there is freedom from pressure to "stick to the curriculum." Such freedom makes possibles types of experimentation which might be considered too disruptive of established routine in the normal class.

We have learned that the normal child can benefit from many of the techniques which were originally developed many years ago for teaching the exceptional child. It is equally possible that research in the area of language development in the mentally retarded will make valuable contributions to our knowledge of normal language development and to the field of communicology in general.

SUMMARY

Our survey of current research and clinical judgments has shown that in the population of mentally retarded there is a high incidence of communication disorders. Even though the communicologist might wish to avoid contact with the field of mental retardation, it is unlikely he will be able to do so. The speech pathologist often performs the first evaluation which leads parents to recognize that what appears to be a communication problem is actually a more basic problem of mental retardation. Many communicologists provide no time for the retarded child. Such an exclusion of the retarded child grows out of pessimism concerning the feasibility of therapy for the mentally retarded. There is no research evidence to show the inability of the mentally retarded to profit from language and speech therapy. The literature does contain studies showing the effectiveness of speech and language therapy with the mentally retarded and a number of suggestions for modifying traditional speech therapy techniques to meet the needs of the mentally retarded. For the communicologist who is careful in diagnosis, adapts techniques to the capacity of cases, and sets realistic goals, there can be challenges and successes in working with the mentally retarded. For the profession of speech pathology and audiology we feel an obligation to explore further the field of communication disorders in the mentally retarded.

BIBLIOGRAPHY

Abel, T., and Kinder, E. 1942. The subnormal adolescent girl. New York: Columbia.

Abernathy, E. 1938. The auditory acuity of feebleminded children. Ohio State Univ.: Ph.D. dissertation.

Abt, I., Adler, H., and Bartelme, P. 1929. The relationship between the onset of speech and intelligence. *JAMA*, 93, 1351–1355.

Anderson, V. 1953. Improving the child's speech. New York: Oxford.

Arnold, R. 1955. Speech rehabilitation for the mentally handicapped. *J. except. Child.*, 22, 50–52.

Backus, O. 1943. Speech in education. New York: Longmans.

Baker, H. 1945. Introduction to exceptional children. New York: Macmillan.

Bangs, J. 1942. A clinical analysis of the articulatory defects of the feeble-minded. *J. Speech Disorders*, 7, 343–356.

Barr, M. 1904. Mental defectives. Philadelphia: Blakiston.

Becky, R. 1942. A study of certain factors related to retardation of speech. *J. Speech Disorders*, 7, 223–249.

Benda, C. 1949. Mongolism and cretinism. New York: Grune & Stratton.

———. 1952. Developmental disorders of mentation and cerebral palsies. New York: Grune & Stratton.

Bennett, A. 1932. A comparative study of subnormal children in the elementary school grades. *Teach. Coll. Contr. Educ.*, No. 510, New York: Teachers College, Columbia Univ.

Berry, M., and Eisenson, J. 1942. The defective in speech. New York: Appleton-Century-Crofts.

———. 1956. Speech disorders. New York: Appleton-Century-Crofts.

Berry, R., and Gordon, R. 1931. The mental defective. New York: McGraw-Hill.

Best, H. 1943. Deafness and the deaf in the United States. New York: Macmillan.

Bibey, M. 1951. A rationale of speech therapy for mentally deficient children. *Train. Sch. Bull.*, 48, 236–39.

Bijou, S., and Werner, H. 1945. Language analysis in brain injured and non-brain injured mentally deficient children. *J. genet. Psych.*, 66, 239–254.

Binet, A., and Simon, T. 1914. Mentally defective children. London: E. Arnold.

Birch, J., and Matthews, J. 1951. The hearing of mental defectives: its measurement and characteristics. *Amer. J. ment. Defic.*, 55, 384–393.

Birch, J., Burgi, E., and Matthews, J. 1966. Manual for effective use of the best speech series with special pupils. Pittsburgh: Stanwix House.

Blanton, M., and Blanton, S. 1924. Speech training for children. New York: Century.

Brodbeck, M. 1941. Remedial speech in a special school curriculum. *Amer. J. ment. Defic.*, 45, 598–601.

Buck, P. 1950. The child who never grew. New York: John Day.

Burt, C. 1937. The backward child. New York: Appleton-Century.

Cabanas, R. 1954. Some findings in speech and voice therapy among mentally deficient children. *Folia Phoniat.*, 6, 34–37.

Carrell, J., and Bangs, J. 1951. Disorders of speech comprehension associated with idiopathic language retardation. *Nerv. Child*, 9, 64–76.

Carrier, J., Jr. 1967. Changes in language of mentally retarded children as a function of increased length of verbal response. Univ. Pittsburgh: Master's thesis.

Dansinger, S., and Madow, A. 1966. Verbal auditory screening with the mentally retarded. *Amer. J. ment. Defic.*, 71, 387–392.

Descoeudres, A. 1928. The education of mentally defective children. Chicago: Heath.

Doll, E. 1940. The nature of mental deficiency. *Psychol. Rev.*, 47, 730–780.

———. 1941. The essential of an inclusive concept of mental deficiency. *Amer. J. ment. Defic.*, 46, 215–217.

———, Phelps, W., and Melcher, R. 1932. Mental deficiencies due to birth injuries. New York: Macmillan.

Donovan, H. 1957. Organization and development of a speech program for the mentally retarded children in New York City public schools. *Amer. J. ment. Defic.*, 62, 455–459.

Dorcus, R., and Shaffer, G. 1945. Textbook of abnormal psychology. Baltimore: Williams & Wilkins.

Eisenson, J. 1940. The psychology of speech. New York: Crofts.

Foale, M., and Paterson, J. 1954. The hearing of mental defectives. *Amer. J. ment. Defic.*, 59, 254–258.

Friedlander, G. 1962. A rationale for speech and language development for the young retarded children. *The Training School Bull.*, 59, No. 1, 9–14.

Fulton, R. 1967. Standard puretone and Békésy audiometric measures with the mentally retarded. *Amer. J. ment. Defic.*, 72, 60–73.

Fulton, R., and Lloyd, L. 1968. Hearing impairment in a population of children with Down's syndrome. *Amer. J. ment. Defic.*, 73, 298–302.

Garrison, K. 1950. The psychology of exceptional children. New York: Ronald.

Gens, G. 1949. Let's be realistic about aphasics. *Train. Sch. Bull.*, 46, 49–57.

———. 1950. Correlation of neurological findings, psychological analyses, and speech disorders among institutionalized epileptics. *Train. Sch. Bul,.*, 47, 3–18.

———. 1951. The speech pathologist looks at the mentally deficient child. *Train. Sch. Bull.*, 48, 19–20.

———. 1952. Congenital aphasia: a case report. *J. Speech Hearing Disorders*, 17, 32–38.

Gesell, A. 1926. The mental growth of the preschool child. New York: Macmillan.

———, and Amatruda, C. 1937. Developmental diagnosis and supervision. *In* Practice of pediatrics. Brennemann, J. ed. Hagerstown, Md.: W. F. Prior.

Giannini, M., Snyder, E., Smith, H., and Slobody, L. 1954. Home training program for retarded children. *Pediatrics*, 13, 278–282.

Goddard, H. 1914. Feeblemindedness: its causes and consequences. New York: Macmillan.

Goldenberg, S. 1950. An exploratory study of some aspects of idiopathic language retardation. *J. Speech Hearing Disorders*, 15, 221–233.

Goldstein, M. 1939. The acoustic method for the training of the deaf and hard of hearing child. St. Louis: Laryngoscope Press.

Gottsleben, R. 1955. The incidence of stuttering in a group of mongoloids. *Train. Sch. Bull.*, 62, 209–217.

Hardy, W. 1948. The relations between impaired hearing and pseudo-feeblemindedness. *Nerv. Child*, 7, 432–445.

Harrison, S. 1959. Integration of developmental language activities with an education program for mentally retarded children. *Amer. J. ment. Defic.*, 63, 967–970.

Hawk, S. 1950. Speech therapy for the physically handicapped. Palo Alto: Stanford.

Heber, R. 1961. A manual on terminology and classification in mental retardation. *Monogr.* Suppl. *Amer. J. ment. Defic.* (2nd. ed.).

Holland, A., and Matthews, J. 1963. Application of teaching machine concepts to speech pathology and audiology. *Asha*, 5, 474–482.

Hollien, H., and Copeland, R. 1965. Speaking fundamental frequency (SFF) characteristics of mongoloid girls. *J. Speech Hearing Disorders*, 39, 344–349.

Hollingworth, L. 1921. The psychology of subnormal children. New York: Macmillan.

Horowitz, F. 1963. Partial and continuous reinforcement of vocal responses using candy, vocal, and smiling reinforcers among retardates. *J. Speech Hearing Disorders*, Monogr. Suppl. No. 10, 55–69.

Ingram, C. 1935. Education of the slow learning child. New York: Ronald.

Irwin, O. 1942. The developmental status of speech sounds of ten feebleminded children. *Child Developm.*, 13, 29–39.

———, and Spiker, C. 1949. The relationship between the IQ and indices of infant speech sound development. *J. Speech Hearing Disorders*, 14, 335–43.

Jellinek, A. 1941. Phenomena resembling aphasia, agnosia, and apraxia in mentally defective children and adults. *J. Speech Disorders*, 6, 51–62.

Johnson, W., Brown, S., Curtis, J., Edney, C., and Keaster, J. 1948. Speech handicapped school children. New York: Harper.

Johnston, P., and Farrell, M. 1954. Auditory impairments among resident school children at the Walter E. Fernald State School. *Amer. J. ment. Defic.*, 58, 640–643.

Jordan, T. 1966. The mentally retarded (2nd. ed.). Columbus, Ohio: Merrill.

Kanner, L. 1948. A miniature textbook of feeblemindedness. New York: Child Care Pub.

Karlin, I., and Strazzulla, M. 1952. Speech and language problems of mentally deficient children. *J. Speech Hearing Disorders*, 17, 286–294.

Kastein, S. 1951. The different groups of disturbances of understanding language in children. *Nerv. Child.*, 9, 31–42.

Kennedy, L. 1930. Studies in the speech of the feebleminded. Univ. Wis.: Ph.D. dissertation.

Kirk, S., and Johnson, G. 1951. Educating the retarded child. Boston: Houghton Mifflin.

Kolstoe, O. 1958. Language training of low grade mongoloid children. *Amer. J. ment. Defic.*, 63, 17–30.

Kopatic, N. 1963. The reliability of pure tone audiometry with the mentally retarded: some practical and theoretical considerations. *Train. Sch. Bull.*, 60, 130–137.

Lamb, N., and Graham, J. 1968. GSR audiometry with mentally retarded adult males. *Amer. J. ment. Defic.*, 1968, 721–727.

Lapage, C. 1911. Feeblemindedness in children of school age. Manchester: Univ. Press.

Lassers, L., and Low, G. 1960. Symposium on assessing and developing communicative effectiveness in mentally retarded children. *Asha*, 2, 377.

Leherfeld, D., and Nertz, N. 1955. A home training program in language and speech for mentally retarded children. *Amer. J. ment. Defic.*, 49, 413–416.

Lewald, J. 1932. Speech defects as found in a group of five hundred mental defectives. *Proc. Amer. Assn. Study Feeblemindedness*, 37, 291–301.

Lillywhite, H., and Bradley, D. 1969. Communication problems in mental retardation: diagnosis and management. New York: Harper & Row.

Lloyd, L., and Frisina, R. 1965. The audiologic assessment of the mentally retarded, proceedings of a national conference. Parsons, Kan.: Parsons State Hospital and Training Center.

———, and Melrose, J. 1966. Reliability of selected auditory responses of normal hearing mentally retarded children. *Amer. J. ment. Defic.*, 71, 133–143.

Lloyd L., and Reid, M. 1967. The incidence of hearing impairment in an institutionalized mentally retarded population. *Amer. J. ment. Defic.*, 71, 746–762.

———, ———, and McManis, D. 1968. Pure tone reliability of a clinical sample of institutionalized mr children. *Amer. J. ment. Defic.*, 73, 279–282.

———, Spradlin, J., and Reid, M. 1968. An operant audiometric procedure for difficult-to-test patients. *J. Speech Hearing Disorders*, 33, 236–245.

Lubman, C. 1955. Speech program for severely retarded children. *Amer. J. ment. Defic.*, 60, 297–300.

McCarthy, D. 1954. Language development in children. *In* Manual of child psychology. Carmichael, L., ed. New York: Wiley. Pp. 492–631.

McCarthy, J., and Kirk, S. 1963. The construction, standardization and statistical characteristics of the Illinois test of psycholinguistic abilities. Madison, Wis.: Photo Press.

MacPherson, J. 1952. The status of the deaf and/or hard of hearing mentally deficient in the United States. *Amer. Ann. Deaf*, 97, 375–386.

Maknen, G. 1898. Training of speech as a factor in mental development. *Bull. Amer. Acad. Med.*, 3, 501–505.

Martinson, B., and Strauss, K. 1940. Education and treatment of an imbecile boy of the exogenous type. *Amer. J. ment. Defic.*, 45, 274–280.

Matthews, J. 1957. Speech problems of the mentally retarded. *In* Handbook of speech pathology, Travis, L., ed. New York: Appleton-Century-Crofts. Pp. 531–551.

———, and Birth, J. 1949. The Leiter international performance scale—a suggested instrument for psychological testing of speech and hearing clinic cases. *J. Speech Hearing Disorders*, 14, 318–321.

Mead, C. 1913. The age of walking and talking in relation to general intelligence. *Pedagogical Seminary*, 20, 461–484.

Meader, M. 1940. The effect of disturbances in the developmental processes upon emergent specificity of function. *J. Speech Disorders*, 5, 211–220.

Mecham, M. 1955. The development and application of procedures for measuring speech improvement in mentally defective children. *Amer. J. ment. Defic.*, 60, 301–306.

Mecham, M., and Jex, J. 1962. Training mentally retarded children in oral communication. *Asha*, 4, 441–442.

Michel, J., and Carney, R. 1964. Pitch characteristics of mongoloid boys. *J. Speech Hearing Disorders*, 29, 121–125.

Montessori, M. 1912. The Montessori method. *Trans. by* George, A. New York: Stokes.

Morrow, J. 1951. A psychiatrist looks at the nonverbal child. *J. except. Child.*, 25, 348–349.

Moss, J., Moss, M., and Tizard, J. 1961. Electrodermal response with mentally defective children. *J. Speech Hearing Disorders*, 4, 41–47.

Myklebust, H. 1954. Auditory disorders in children. New York: Grune & Stratton.

Nance, L. 1946. Differential diagnosis of aphasia in children. *J. Speech Disorders*, 11, 219–223.

Neelley, J., Edison, S., and Carlile, L. 1968. Speaking voice fundamental frequency of mentally retarded adults and normal adults. *Amer. J. ment. Defic.*, 72, 944–947.

Nehem, S. 1951. Psychotherapy in relation to mental deficiency. *Amer. J. ment. Defic.*, 55, 557–572.

Peins, M. 1967. Client-centered communication therapy for mentally retarded delinquents. *J. Speech Hearing Disorders*, 32, 154–161.

Plotkin, W. 1959. Situational speech therapy for retarded cerebral palsied children. *J. Speech Hearing Disorders*, 24, 16–20.

Presidents' Panel on Mental Retardation. 1962. A proposed program for national action to combat mental retardation. Washington: U.S. Government Printing Office.

Reneau, J., and Mast, R. 1968. Telemetric EEG audiometry instrumentation for use with the profoundly retarded. *Amer. J. ment. Defic.*, 72, 506–511.

Renfrew, C. 1959. Speech problems of backward children. *Speech Pathology and Therapy*, 2, 34–38.

Richardson, S. 1967. Language training for mentally retarded children. *In* Language and mental retardation. Schiefelbusch, R., and Copeland, R., eds. New York: Holt, Rinehart and Winston.

Ridenour, N. 1943. Mentally retarded preschool children: suggestions to doctors and nurses in well-child clinics. *Amer. J. ment. Defic.*, 48, 72–78.

Rigrodsky, S., Prunty, F., and Glovsky, L. 1961. A study of the incidence, types and associated etiologies of hearing loss in an institutionalized mentally retarded population. *Train. Sch. Bull.*, 58, 30–44.

Rigrodsky, S., and Steer, M. 1961. Mower's theory applied to speech habilitation of the mentally retarded. *J. Speech Hearing Disorders*, 26, 237–243.

Rittmanic, P. 1958. An oral language program for institutionalized educable mentally retarded children. *Amer. J. ment. Defic.*, 63, 403–407.

———. 1959. Hearing rehabilitation for the institutionalized mentally retarded. *Amer. J. ment. Defic.*, 63, 403–407.

Saiijenga, H. 1954. Do's and dont's for speech correctionist. *J. except. Child.*, 20, 322–324.

Sachs, M. 1951. A survey and evaluation of the existing interrelationships between speech and mental deficiency. Univ. Va.: Master's thesis.

Sarason, S. 1953. Psychological problems in mental deficiency (2nd. ed.). New York: Harper.

Schaeffer, M., and Shearer, W. 1968. A survey of mentally retarded stutterers. *J. Speech Hearing Disorders*, Monogr. Suppl. No. 10.

Schiefelbusch, R. 1963, ed. Language studies of mentally retarded children. *J. Speech Hearing Disorders*, Monogr. Suppl. No. 10.

———, Copeland, R., and Smith, J. 1967. Language and mental retardation. New York: Holt, Rinehart and Winston.

Schlanger, B. 1953a. Speech measurements of institutionalized mentally handicapped children. *Amer. J. ment. Defic.*, 58, 114–122.

Schlanger, B. 1953b. Speech therapy with mentally retarded children in special classes. *Train. Sch. Bull.*, 50, 179–186.

———. 1953c. Speech examination of a group of institutionalized mentally handicapped children. *J. Speech Hearing Disorders*, 18, 339–350.

———. 1953d. Suggested practices for developing speech in speech handicapped children in institutions. (Unpublished manuscript.)

———. 1958. Speech therapy with mentally retarded children. *J. Speech Hearing Disorders*, 23, 298–301.

———. 1959. A longitudinal study of speech and language development of brain damaged retarded children. *J. Speech Hearing Disorders*, 24, 354–360.

———, and Gottsleben, R. 1957. Analysis of speech defects among the institutionalized mentally retarded. *J. Speech Hearing Disorders*, 22, 98–103.

Schneider, B., and Vallon, J. 1955. The results of a speech therapy program for mentally retarded children. *Amer. J. ment. Defic.*, 49, 416–424.

Sheehan, J., Martyn, M., and Kilburn, K. 1968. Speech disorders in retardation. *Amer. J. ment. Defic.*, 73, 251–256.

Shubert, O., Heuvel, C., and Fulton, R. 1966. Effects of speech improvement on articulatory skills in institutionalized retardates. *Amer. J. ment. Defic.*, 71, 274–278.

———, Jansen, B., and ———. 1967. Effects of speech improvement on articulatory skills in institutionalized retardates: II. *Amer. J. ment. Defic.*, 72, 212–214.

Shuttleworth, G. 1900. Mentally deficient children. London: H.K. Lewis.

Sirkin, J., and Lyons, W. 1941. A study of speech defects in mental deficiency. *Amer. J. ment. Defic.*, 46, 74–80.

Skinner, B. 1947. Verbal behavior. New York: Appleton-Century-Crofts.

Sloan, W. 1954. Progress report on special committee on nomenclature of the *Amer. Assn. ment. Defic.*, 59, 345–351.

Smith, M. 1935. A study of some factors influencing the development of the setence in the preschool child. *J. genet. Psychol.*, 46, 182–212.

Spradlin, J. 1963. Assessment of speech and language of retarded children: the Parsons language sample, *J. Speech Hearing Disorders*, Monogr. Suppl. No. 10, 8–31.

Spradlin, J. 1963. Language and communication of mental defectives. *In* Handbook of mental deficiency. Ellis, N. ed., New York: McGraw-Hill. Pp. 512–55.

Spragge, C. 1962. Speech therapy for the mentally handicapped child. *Speech Pathology and Therapy*, 5, 79–87.

Spreen, O. 1965a. Language functions in mental retardation: a review I: language development, types of retardation and intelligence level. *Amer. J. ment. Defic.*, 69, 482–94.

———. 1965b. Language functions in mental retardation: a review II. language in higher level performance. *Amer. J. ment. Defic.* 70, 351–62.

Steinman, J., Grossman, C., and Reece, R. 1963. An analysis of the articulation of the educable mentally retarded child. *Asha*, 5, 791.

Stinchfield, S., and Young, E. 1938. Children with delayed or defective speech. Palo Alto: Stanford.

Strauss, A., and Lehtinen, L. 1947. Psychopathology and education of the brain injured child. New York: Grune & Stratton.

Tarjan, G., Wright, S., Dingman, H., and Eyman, R. 1961. Natural history of mental deficiency in a state hospital: III. selected characteristics of first admissions and their environments. *Amer. J. dis. Child.*, 101, 195–205.

Terman, L. 1925. Mental and physical traits of a thousand gifted children. Genetic studies of genius, I. Palo Alto: Stanford.

Town, C. 1913. Language development in 285 idiots and imbeciles. *Psychol. Clinic*, 6, 229–235.

Travis, L. 1931. Speech pathology. New York: Appleton.

Tredgold, A. 1947. A textbook of mental deficiency. Baltimore: Williams & Wilkins.

Twitmyer, E., and Nathanson, S. 1932. Correction of defective speech. Philadephia: Blakiston.

Van Riper, C. 1947. Speech correction principles and methods. Englewood Cliffs, N.J.: Prentice-Hall.

Wallin, J. 1916. A census of speech defectives among 89,157 public school pupils—a preliminary report. *Sch. and Soc.*, 3, 213–216.

———. 1921. Problems of subnormality. New York: World.

———. 1924. The education of handicapped children. Boston: Houghton Mifflin.

———. 1949. Children with mental and physical handicaps. Englewood Cliffs, N.J.: Prentice-Hall.

Watkins, E., Stewart, J., and Ryan, M. 1966. A novel hearing test for retardates with mental ages below four years. *Amer. J. ment. Defic.*, 71, 396–400.

Weiss, D. 1951. Speech in retarded children. *Nerv. Child.*, 9, 21–30.

West, R., Kennedy, L., and Carr, A. 1947. The rehabilitation of speech (rev. ed.). New York: Harper.

Wilson, F. 1966. Efficacy of speech therapy with educable mentally retarded children. *J. Speech Hearing Research*, 9, 423–433.

Zisk, P., and Bialer, I. 1967. Speech and language problems in mongolism: a review of the literature. *J. Speech Hearing Disorders*, 32, 228–241.

32

The Psychopathology of Articulation and Voice Deviations

Clyde L. Rousey

Most current textbooks in speech pathology pay some attention to the fact that there may be emotional disturbance in some individuals sustaining articulation and voice disorders (cf. Van Riper, 1963, Van Riper and Irwin, 1958, Berry and Eisenson, 1956, Brain, 1965, and Travis, 1957). The primary thesis in most of these references is that individuals may sustain a psychological disturbance as a secondary result of a communication disorder. The thesis that the voice and articulation disorder may itself be symptomatic of a primary psychological disturbance is usually not proposed.

It is the purpose of this chapter to present assumptions and hypotheses which advocate that, with the exception of blatant organically caused voice and articulation disturbances,[1] the speech behavior itself is symptomatic of a primary psychological disturbance and should be so treated. An earlier presentation of this notion was published by Rousey and Moriarty (1965). Before presenting these hypotheses, and some applications of their usefulness in clinical practice, we should first clarify some of the terminology as well as outline the data used in the present formulation. In so doing, we shall examine critically aspects of looking at nonorganic voice and articulation difficulties primarily as disturbances in learning.

Of initial importance is the clarification of the terms *speech* and *language*. These terms, in the context of this chapter, will be used as defined by Rousey and Toussieng (1964).

> Speech is meant to refer to the sounds . . . which when used together in certain accepted ways then produce verbal language. *Verbal language* refers to the symbolic meanings attached to these sound groupings.

In the present chapter we shall confine our attention to speech as it has been defined[2] and not talk about language per se. That the distinction we are advocating is not universally held can be seen by surveying the literature of various psychological writers. For example Mowrer (1950), in his classic paper on the "Psychology of Talking Birds" which proposes an autistic theory of language development, freely interchanges the words "speech" and "language" throughout his theory. Precisely because Mowrer does interchange the terminology freely and

[1] By this the author refers to speech disorders secondary to such conditions as cerebral palsy, cleft palate, paralyzed cords, parkinsonism, etc. The majority of articulation and voice problems occur in individuals not sustaining such obvious organic disorders.

[2] In the current chapter the author contends that even sounds made by animals or sounds uttered reflexively by humans who for example would be stung by a bee are within the realm of what is defined as speech. This is so because acoustically they can be described as vowels. The reason they are not customarily so defined is that they are considered from the viewpoint of whether or not they are language. And, of course, they are not.

because of the dynamics which he postulates as necessary for evoking speech in his parakeets, it is possible that in effect he may have produced speech as we have defined it rather than language. This tendency to use speech interchangeably with the concept of verbal language also occurs in more recent American literature. For example, McNeill (1966) is obviously talking about verbal language as it has been defined, but uses the term "speech" instead. That this terminology problem is not specific to American authors is evident from examination of such widely diversified writers as Luria and Yudovich (1966), Luria (1961), Anna Freud (1965), and Brain (1965). These writers interchangeably use the terms "speech" and "language."

The next important term to define is *symptom.* Disorders of speech and voice without organic causation are understood as symptoms in the current chapter. A symptom is presumed to have dynamic, adaptive, economic, and social meanings. Thus a symptom 1. contains elements centering around hidden libidinal needs, 2. serves as an aggressive discharge in an external sense, 3. also has elements of self-directed aggression, 4. is a compromise between the aforementioned items and reality, 5. serves as a salvaging device to maintain one's equilibrium, and 6. is a distress signal to individuals in the environment.[3] All of these elements are thus to be found in a nonorganically caused voice and articulation disorder. This definition is preferred over the term "symptom" being defined as merely indicating the presence of a pathological condition (English, H. and English, A., 1957), or the differentiation made by Jackson (1884) of the positive and negative sides of a symptom (cf. the discussion of symptom as provided by Menninger et al., 1963, and Freud, 1959).

CRITICAL FACTORS REGARDING SPEECH DEVELOPMENT WHICH ARE RELEVANT TO THE CURRENT THESIS

Initially, one should be aware of the early and monumental studies of Irwin (1947, 1948) and his associates regarding the speech utterances of youngsters from infancy to two and one-half years of age. These provide some extremely important data for the proposal contained in this chapter. The outstanding finding reported by this investigator and his associates was that there was a clear preponderance of vowel sounds uttered during the first part of the first year of a child's life which gradually changed so that by the end of the first year all of the consonant sounds had been uttered which would be later used in the child's verbal language. This finding is significant irrespective of the fact that Irwin's transcription probably dealt more with allophones than with the specific phonemes which he lists.

Secondly, recent data casts doubt on the historically treasured idea that speech development proceeds through a specific maturation sequence. For example, Hall (1962) and Healey (1963) point out that there is simply no apparent standard pattern for sound acquisition in children. That is, many children never have sound substitutions in their articulation patterns, whereas some have sound substitutions which persist long after the age of seven or eight when, historically, speech development is supposedly completed. Templin's data (1957) allude to this possibility by the fact that her norms are presented in terms of 75 and 90 percent cutoff levels for correct articulation in the groups she studied. A later paper by Templin (1966) reports that although she had originally anticipated terminating her study of the development of articulation of children by the time they had reached the second grade, unfortunately, a fairly large-sized group of the children of her original study still had inadequate articulation scores (i.e., errors) in the second grade. Templin also reports that there is no consistency in terms of the type of misarticulation among children seen by public school speech pathologists. Finally, the data presented by Rousey and Toussieng (1964), Cozad and Rousey (1966), Rousey and Averill (1963), Green (1962), Grimes (1962), Shervanian (1959), Weber (1964), and Walle and Morris (1967) point to the fact that in psychiatric patients above the chronological age, where the so-called developmental process should have been finished, there exists a significant and unusually high incidence (up to 60–80 percent) of voice and articulation problems. All of these findings lend credence to the possibility that the developmental hypothesis accounting for articulation problems in the first seven to eight years is insufficient. An alternative hypothesis would be that errors in articulation of consonants reflect developmental failures in personality rather than reflecting stops or arrests in the normal maturation process of speech articulation.

This hypothesis would, of course, run counter to

[3] The author is indebted to Dr. Paul Pruyser for his clarifying discussion of the various aspects of meaning a symptom may have.

the views of many individuals who contend that articulation is a learned skill and should be so treated. A sophisticated statement regarding the "learning" of speech has been provided by Winitz (1966). He proposed two stages in the development of infant vocalizations prior to the acquisition of language: "1. fractional anticipatory goal response (from birth until about three months)" and "2. secondary reinforcement (three months to about twelve months)." The key assumption in the first period is that vocalizations associated with the activity of feeding are conditioned to the sequence of events occurring around the feeding situation. In his second period, which he calls the period of secondary reinforcement, there occurs the so-called babbling period wherein the infant engages in repetitive verbal behavior. This repetitive verbal behavior is explained as persisting because it serves as "secondary reinforcers for the motor responses necessary for the production of vocal sound or babbling." One of the difficulties with this theory is the immensely complicated task of specifying the parameters that are involved in any given situation which are sufficient to explain both the later normal or later abnormal articulation patterns. For example, Butt (1965) suggests that even in a controlled laboratory setting preliminary training in auditory discrimination interferes with the acquisition of a new (unfamiliar) sound.

Perhaps even more significant in terms of questioning the assumptions used by Winitz are studies reported by Lenneberg, Rabelsky, and Nichols (1965) and Lenneberg (1967). These authors report studies concerning the emergence of vocalization during the first three months of life in children with congenitally deaf parents. If Winitz's assumptions are correct, especially relating to the period he labels as fractional anticipatory goal responses, one would expect to see a significant difference in vocalizations of children born to congenitally deaf parents as compared to children born to hearing parents. The findings of the aforementioned studies were that the children born of deaf parents went through the same sequence of vocalizations as did the control group where the parents had normal auditory sensitivity for speech sounds. Of signal importance is the finding reported by these authors that the deaf mothers even had trouble telling from the child's facial expression and gestures whether there was accompanying silence or noise.

Diedrich's (1966) unpublished paper provides a straightforward presentation with reference to treatment. His approach assumes the error is perpetuated because of faulty learning or that the individual is still maintaining a bad habit long after it has met any psychological need. Thus, most articulation and voice problems are conceived of as persisting because of mislearning. No room is provided in the theories suggested by Diedrich and Winitz for dynamic moti-vational hypotheses. It is the author's contention that, far from being a circumscribed acquired function, speech production reflects basic personality issues which are common to all children and which are relatively independent of later verbal language patterns.

DATA REGARDING THE PSYCHOLOGICAL ASPECTS OF SPEECH

To appreciate the possibility that articulation and voice disorders may by symptomatic of nonlinguistic dimensions of personality, one needs to recall that, as early as 1925, Sapir (1926) suggested that sounds might be related to psychological factors. For example, he wrote:

> One of the most interesting unwritten chapters in linguistic behavior is the expressively symbolic character of sounds, quite aside from what the words in which they occur mean in a referential sense. On the properly linguistic plane sounds have no meaning, yet if we are to interpret them psychologically we would find that there is a subtle, though fleeting, relation between the "real" value of words and the unconscious symbolic value of sounds as actually produced by individuals.

Since 1925 other authors have produced experimental evidence which has been published in psychological journals relating the production of sound to psychological factors (cf. Sapir, 1929, Jakobson, 1960, Miron, 1961, Alpert, Kutzberg, and Friedhoff, 1963, Ostwald, 1961, Heinstein, 1963, and, most recently, Paves, 1965). These authors, utilizing either experimental or descriptive research studies, have contended that there may be some psychological meanings inherent in sounds. One needs to look at the psychoanalytic literature for helping in assessing this possibility. Perhaps the clearest remarks have been made by Greenson (1954 and 1961), who proposed that sound serves a discharge function for both pleasure and pain and both accompanies instinctual activities and is an indicator of affects. He postulates that sounds have both erotic and aggressive components and that the use of sounds serves a tension discharge function. Of special interest, in view of our differentiation between the concepts of speech and language, is Greenson's notion that "great emotions are wordless but not soundless." He seems to state in a succinct manner that language is not necessary for the transmission of affect, but rather that affect can be and usually is transmitted through sound.

As further support for our thesis that sounds have primarily affective rather than cognitive meaning, we refer to Freud's (1901) discussion of slips of the tongue. In his *Psychopathology of Everyday Life*, he wrote:

> Among the slips of tongue that I have collected myself I can find hardly one in which I should be obliged to trace the disturbance of speech simply and solely to what Wundt (1900) calls the "contact effect of sounds." I almost invariably discover a disturbing influence in addition which comes from something outside the intended utterance; and the disturbing element is either a single thought that has remained unconscious, which manifests itself in the slip of the tongue and which can often be brought to consciousness only by means of searching analysis, or it is a more general psychical motive force which is directed against the entire utterance.

In general, psychological writers have held the notion that speech is a primary reflector of cognitive development rather than affective development. This in part has been caused by the lack of a distinction being made between speech and language. Thus, psychoanalytic writers such as Hartmann (1951) customarily consider language or, as it is sometimes called, speech, as an autonomous ego function which is only secondarily related to conflictual material. For example, he writes:

> I am certainly not implying that these [he refers among other things to speech and language] and other pertinent childhood activities remain untouched by psychic conflicts nor do I imply that disturbances in their development do not give rise to conflicts, or are not woven into other conflicts. On the contrary, I want to emphasize that their vicissitudes play a great role in the well-known typical and individual instinctual developments and conflicts in that they may facilitate or inhibit the individual's ability to master such conflicts.

Anna Freud (1965) implies much the same in her discussion of the relationship between sensation and perception and language:

> Speech and with it the introduction of *reason* and *logic* into the thought processes mean in themselves an enormous advance in socialization. They imply the understanding of *cause* and *effect*, which has been missing before and without which environmental rules were merely confusing to the child, as extraneous influences enforcing mechanical submission. They also introduced trial action in thought, i.e., make it possible for the child to insert reasoning between the arising of an instinctual wish and the behavior aimed at its fulfillment.

If the terms speech and language are differentiated as previously defined, and speech is assumed to reflect affects whereas verbal language reflects primarily cognitive and only secondarily conflictual material, it is possible to make assumptions regarding speech which heretofore have been impossible to make. Speech behavior then becomes theoretically an indicator of one's emotional life rather than of one's cognitive life alone. Used in this fashion it may be understood as a symptom and be understood from the earlier mentioned aspects of a symptom. Use of speech behavior in this way is not at odds with the conviction of either Hartmann (1964) or Anna Freud (1965 and 1966). For example, Hartmann (1964, p. 102) states:

> Such studies will of necessity lead to a growing awareness of the sign—or signal—function which behavior details may have for the observer, that is, to a better and more systematic understanding of how data of direct observation can be used as indicators of structurally central and partly unconscious developments—in a sense that by far transcends the possibilities of sign interpretation accessible to the various methods of testing.

Also, Anna Freud (1966) states:

> Personally I can see no difficulty in extending this conviction of certain fixed relationships existing between surface appearance and id content from the mental phenomena named above to particular items of behavior, especially, of children, as they can be observed in the areas of play; in hobbies; in the attitude of illness, food, clothing, etc. I believe what deters the majority of analysts from accepting this suggestion is not so much a disbelief in the validity of the material, but a reminder of certain phases in the history of psychoanalysis when such items were used profusely and disadvantageously for the purpose of symbolic interpretation within analysis, which is a technical mistake, of course.

This same view is expanded in another of Miss Freud's separate publications (1965).

CLINICAL RESEARCH RELATING VOICE AND ARTICULATION PROBLEMS TO PERSONALITY DEVIATIONS

Unfortunately there is little specific clinical research relating voice and articulation problems to personality deviations. McWilliams (1960) reported on the process of speech therapy with a six-year-old boy hospitalized because of frequent psychosomatic illnesses. His articulation pattern was characterized by the omission of /s/ and /h/ sounds. After a session wherein a connection between the sounds and an external third stimulus was discovered, McWilliams reported that the therapy seemed to progress more adequately. She suggested:

> It becomes increasingly apparent that certain children may have psychologically determined speech symptoms and that these may well be the children who, after years of speech therapy, retain their symptoms in unaltered form.

Solomon (1961), in writing of personality and behavior patterns in children with functional defects of articulation, said:

> Speech problems of this type, apparently are not isolated phenomena but part of a total adjustive pattern. It is suggested that an underlying stress may be common to the diverse symptomatology here presented and that the infantile and nonassertive behavior could very well serve as anxiety-reducing devices to meet environmental pressure.

A study by Ostwald and Skolnikoff (1966) of an adolescent schizophrenic patient indicated that along with other disturbances in his communication some of his vowel and consonant sounds were disturbed. By using spectrograms they provided a visual indication of the disturbance. Weiss (1964) has also referred to this possibility in an account of his work in a mental hospital. Moses (1954) has offered some hypotheses regarding persistent speech problems which, while not tied specifically to a theory, nevertheless point out in a clinical style some of the psychological meanings which may become attached to sounds. For example, he writes with regard to lisping:

> Lisping at this age [he probably refers to early childhood, although he gives no specific ages] is a simple continuation of infantile oral gratification. Playing with saliva, touching mucus membranes with the tongue are among the earliest sources of pleasure. Children like to lisp because it involves a similar kind of enjoyment.

Other clinical research relating use of speech to feelings has been reported by Freud and Burlingham (1944), Spitz (1957), Rheingold (1956), and Provence and Lipton (1962). These authors emphasize the fact that the speech of institutionalized children is more unintelligible than speech of noninstitutionalized children. If one assumes that the affective life of institutional children described by these authors was different and not as adequate as of those living at home, one would have every reason to infer that this disturbance in articulation patterns reflects primarily a disturbance in the children's emotional conditions.

A PROPOSAL RELATING ARTICULATION AND VOICE PROBLEMS TO PSYCHOPATHOLOGY

Certain assumptions must be made to interpret the psychological meanings which articulation and voice problems may have. It will be recalled that *sounds* are assumed primarily to reflect feelings and only secondarily to reflect cognitive content. This is in contrast to *verbal language*, which reflects cognition first and transmits feelings only secondarily and in cognitive form. Some of the hypotheses of psychoanalytic theory provide the basis for spelling out the implications of these assumptions. Of special help are the hypotheses relating to the dual instincts and psychosexual development. In regard to the so-called "dual-instinct theory," Freud (1920) proposed that there are two psychological drives which influence affective relationships between individuals: the sexual and the aggressive drives (cf. Brenner, C., 1955). Theoretically these drives are supposed to be present from birth but undifferentiated as to object during the early part of life. They become modified by their own momentum and with the emergence of the functions ascribed to the ego.

It is interesting that the predominant sounds which occur in the child's first few months of life are vowels. Since vowels as opposed to consonants require only minimal amounts of contact between the speech articulators, one might make the assumption that the production of vowels is similar to the early expression of these drives, i.e., there is a relatively uncontrolled discharge of sounds. The well-known clinical fact to most speech pathologists that vowels are rarely distorted in later life would be understood as further evidence of their basic nature from a personality sense. The fact that Shervanian (1959) reports that vowels are distorted in the speech of the so-called autistic (psychotic) child would seem to support the possibility that they are related to the early stages of libidinal and aggressive drive organization. To sum up, then, vowels have psychological significance in the sense of their being a means of the earliest vocal expression of libidinal and aggressive drives.

The next assumption to be made is that the emergence of the consonant sounds reflects the onset or controls over these drives. It is of no small matter that the major use of consonants in an infant's life begins in the latter half of the infant's first year. At the same time such functions of the ego as language, increasing motility, and the development of memory as evidenced by the so-called eighth-month anxiety (cf. Spitz, 1965) begin to be important. It is also of significance that there is a parallel in the emergence of speech viewed from the maturational hypothesis and the classical pattern of psychosexual development proposed up to the latency period. Thus, the developmental notion regarding the emergence of normal articulatory patterns holds that all consonantal sounds are mastered by all children by around seven to eight years of age.

From the standpoint of psychosexual development, it is usually held that early relationship difficulties are experienced, worked through, and resolved by approximately age seven or eight. If this correlation between speech development and psychosexual development is not accidental but meaningful, it might be interpreted as signaling a parallel sequence. Thus, the struggle with the conflicts and difficulties appropriate to the various psychosexual stages may be reflected through the struggle with the mastery of the various consonantal sounds at the various age levels.

A consistent sound substitution is understandable as a fixation to an earlier level of psychosexual development, whereas an inconsistent sound substitution occurring in periods of stress would be understood as a regression. For example, in a person who substitutes /f/ for the voiceless /th/ sound, the /f/ sound is understood as a dynamic residual from an earlier level of psychic development. Because consonants are either voiced or voiceless, even further distinctions can be made. Voiced consonants are thought to reflect more active ego control whereas voiceless consonants reflect more passive ego control. This position is taken on the basis that, if voicing of voiced consonants is vowel like, then voiced consonants represent the most complete amalgamation of the psychological functions that are postulated for both vowels and consonants. Since by definition voiceless consonants are not endowed with voice, they would have none of the psychological derivatives ascribed to voiced consonants and would be more passive. Sound substitutions then become symptomatic of difficulties the child is sustaining in his psychosexual development rather than solely in auditory discrimination or in learning. Such an assumption allows the inference that a child who is progressing without undue stress in his psychosexual development would never manifest sound substitutions.

The aforementioned assumptions provide the basis for making further speculations as to the level of psychosexual development to which a sound belongs. If the assumption is correct that there should be no difficulty with the articulation of sound in speech development, then the customary age level of mastery of sound (Templin, 1957) may provide us with an index of delayed mastery in psychological development as it is reflected through speech. Precisely because it would be a lag in development rather than a normal sequence, if speech development turns out to occur in groups of sounds, we may have reason to suspect it to be related to the stages of psychosexual development.

We have already seen that the traditional developmental viewpoint of speech contends that the process of speech development is completed by approximately age seven. It is also known that this corresponds roughly to the onset of latency in the psychoanalytic theory dealing with psychosexual development. Now, there are essentially three large groupings of times when sounds are mastered which precede this time (Templin, 1957). In the present paper we make the assumption that this grouping is not accidental and that it will be useful to designate these chronological groupings as being related to three broad areas of psychosexual development which precede the latency period.

Knowledge of physiological activities which might be related to specific sounds is of further help in the categorization of sounds. Thus, because the /m/ sound is made with the lips closed together and since the closing of the lips around the nipple is obviously an accompaniment of the physiological act of nursing, one would expect to see this sound fall with the earliest grouping of sounds which are mastered. This is in fact the case (note below). Similarly, if one views a thrusting motion of the tongue as being in some way related to activity of the phallus, and if, as is the case, the /th/ sound is made in such a manner, then according to the foregoing theory it should be in the last grouping of sounds which are mastered. This again is the case.

Now, keeping in mind the useful discussion of infantile sexuality by Erikson (1950), and the foregoing discussion, the sounds /m/, /p/, /w/, /h/, /y/ as in *y*ellow, /l/, /n/, and /t/ seem to belong in the oral respiratory-sensory stage, while /b/, /f/, /k/, /g/, and /d/ seem to belong in what Erikson calls the oral-biting stage. Similarly, it is hypothesized that /s/, /r/, /sh/, and the /z/ as in azure may be placed in the anal-retentive stage, and /ch/ and /j/ as in judge are most closely related to the anal-expulsive stage. Finally, it is proposed that the voiceless /th/, /v/, the voiced /th/, and /z/ are sounds most likely to be associated with the phallic period. Thus, utilizing the aforementioned assumptions, certain working hypotheses can be made regarding the clinical meaning of misarticulations of these sounds.

WORKING HYPOTHESES RELATED TO CONSONANTS

The Substitution of the /f/ for the Voiceless /th/ Sound is Related to a Disturbance in Early and Significant Relationships with the Child's Father

If the assumption that the voiceless /th/ sound is related to the phallic stage of psychosexual development is correct and if one assumes the phallic stage of psychosexual development is related to one's feelings about masculinity and inferentially one's father, then the inability of a child to produce the voiceless /th/ sound becomes obviously related to the feeling about the father and masculinity in general. Further, the substitution of the sound of /f/ in this case for the voiceless /th/ sound would then represent the use of an earlier sound assumed to be characteristic of the oral-biting period. If this in fact does represent difficulty in an adequate relationship with one's father, and if working through this relationship is important in a sense of attaining a satisfactory identity, then it is also appropriate to infer that individuals (male or female) who sustain this substitution might be expected to persist in some confusion over their sexual identity. Indirect evidence for this hypothesis may be gathered both in clinical experience and from such an apparent divergent source as the comic strip.

The character of Mammy Yokum in the Li'l Abner comic strip is well known. Her questionable feminine appearance and actions are also well known. If one assumes that part of a comic strip's continued appeal is based on the adequate and correct portrayal of the character, and that the foregoing hypothesis is correct, then it is not surprising that she routinely substitutes /f/ for the voiceless /th/ sound.

Deprivation Disturbances in Mother-Child Relationships are Reflected Through Difficulties with the /l/ Phoneme

Since the /l/ phoneme has been placed in the oral respiratory-sensory stage, and since physiologically it is a sound which may be heard as one swallows, the assumption here is that a distortion in this sound would reflect some disturbance in terms of the nurturance and giving to a child which is customarily provided by the mother. There are numerous variations in the /l/ phoneme which may occur in pathological speech deviations. It is also important to note that the /l/ phoneme is sometimes labeled as a semivowel and/or as a consonant. It represents, thus, a transitional stage between the expression of both libidinal and aggressive drives through vowels and the ego controls as expressed indirectly by consonants. The speculation is offered that the so-called "dark l" ("backthroated l") occurs primarily in individuals where there has been some gross disturbance in early psychological nurturance from their mother. If this is so, then one should expect to find a preponderance of this difficulty occurring in individuals who from a clinical viewpoint manifest certain so-called predominantly oral needs. These might include, for example, individuals where alcoholism occurs primarily as a manifestation of a fixation at an oral stage.

Another variation in difficulty with the /l/ phoneme is the substitution of /w/ for /l/. Inasmuch as both the /w/ and the /l/ are sounds which have earlier been speculated as belonging to the oral respiratory-sensory period, it would be hypothesized that the persistence of this difficulty represents a kind of accentuated statement of the deprivation which occurred in that individual's psychic life. The strong statement of this deprivation by these individuals via speech thus would lead one to infer that they would be demanding in their attempts to satisfy their earlier lack of nurturance.

The Substitution of the /d/ for the Voiced /th/ Sound is Related to an Oral Expression of Aggression

In looking at the earlier suggested placement of the consonant sounds at various psychosexual levels, the voiced /th/ sound was believed to emerge at a time sequence related to the phallic stage, whereas the /d/ phoneme was designated as appearing in the oral-aggressive stage. If this is the case, then the substitution of the /d/ for voiced /th/ sound would be symptomatic of an oral expression of aggression toward a masculine figure. Stereotypically, this substitution is associated with the verbal expression of aggression typical of the speech and verbal language patterns utilized by "tough guys." The speculation would be that the aggression would be more verbal than any specific acting out.

Persistence of the Frontal Lisp Occurs in Individuals who Prefer to Maintain Earlier and More Infantile Levels of Development While at the same time giving Passive Indications of more Maturity

If one assumes the voiceless /th/ sound is typical of the so-called phallic period of psychosexual development, and if the /s/ phoneme is associated with the anal period of psychosexual development, the substitution of the voiceless /th/ for the /s/ sound is then indicative not only of failure to pass totally through the anal stage but also an attempt to passively assert oneself. In other words, there is an attempt to be assertive in a manner less than appropriate. The inference would be made that individuals with this particular substitution would be infantile and unwilling to engage in more mature interaction with others. Such an interpretation is not inconsistent with the clinical behavior seen in individuals manifesting a frontal lisp.

The Occurrence of the Lateral Lisp is a Manifestation of Difficulty in Psychosexual Development Occurring Earlier During the Anal Period than is the case with the Front Lisp

The lateral lisp is not one of the usual phonemes which is typically described in the development process. It is often referred to as a sound distortion. It comes close to the /sh/ sound which, if we refer to the speculations regarding the meaning of consonants, occurs in the anal period. Since this is a sound which is not a substitution of one usual phoneme for another, it is thought in a sense to be a more unusual and more primitive substitution. If this is so, the speculation is offered that it falls at the beginning of the anal period and would be manifested through such behavior as messiness in general physical appearance and behavior, and in having a good deal of difficulty in surrendering any of oneself to others.

A Whistle which Accompanies the Articulation of the /s/ Phoneme is Felt to Reflect Anxiety

Since, by definition, the /s/ sound is felt to be related to the anal period, the specific anxiety the individual experiences is felt to center on the shame and doubt he experiences in resolving his conflicts over retaining and expelling his feces. Clinical observation of individuals who are anxious, either on a clinical or situational basis, demonstrates that there is often a marked whistle which occurs on sibilant sounds. This phenomenon was initially noted by the present author during routine screening of students with speech disorders in a college population. The complaint for which they were sent to the speech clinic was the manifestation of a sharp whistle while articulating the /s/ phoneme. It soon became obvious that these referrals involved mostly students new to college life, or students having some difficulties in their college experience. It also became apparent that as the new students became accustomed to college life, and inasmuch as these other students resolved their school and/or personal difficulties, the whistles accompanying the production of the /s/ phoneme diminished markedly.

Bradford and Rousey (1961) demonstrated that the amount of whistling accompanying the articulation of the /s/ phoneme could be increased by creating the stress of failure and inferentially anxiety. This phenomenon is also frequently noticed in individuals giving reports or speeches in strange environments. The individuals who manifest a persistent whistle on their /s/ phonemes, as opposed to individuals whose whistle accompanying sibilant sounds is only transitory, obviously make up two groups. On the basis of the theory presented to date, one would assume that a chronic whistle accompanying the sibilant sounds represents a persistent anxiety over the issues of giving of himself and entering into interaction with others in his environment. The transitory whistle is a signal of the momentary revival of the shame and doubt that was struggled with long ago.

The Articulation of the Consonantal /r/ and Vowel /r/ Reflect Both Early Lack of Impulse Control and Inappropriate Discharge of Aggression

Since the vowel /r/ and the consonantal /r/ are closely related in phonetic sense, it is hypothesized that they may also be related in a psychological sense. To begin with, if one assumes that the consonantal /r/ occurs primarily in Erikson's anal-retentive period, then one would hypothesize that it has to do principally with deciding whether or not the waste should be shared. The substitution of /w/ for /r/, such that the word "rabbit" becomes "wabbit," would represent the interaction of the /w/ sound with the /r/ sound. Inasmuch as the /w/ sound is a sound characteristic of the earlier oral-incorporative stage, one would speculate that the conflict that is expressed through the /w/ for /r/ substitution is one centering around both taking in in an oral sense, and retaining in an anal sense. Clinically such a symptom suggests that individuals manifesting this difficulty would have difficulty with letting go of acquired information, while at the same time taking in all the new information that they can. Thus one might expect to see this symptom occurring in the bright person who nevertheless has difficulty sharing the knowledge that he has. Behaviorally, this could take the shape of an underachieving person or a person who, because of this particular constellation, is irritating to individuals in his environment. That is, he would always be taking from them without ever giving anything in return. This would represent a rather subtle discharge of aggression which, while not always perceived by individuals as aggressive, is nevertheless irritating to them.

The distortion of the vowel /r/, according to the earlier assumptions relating to vowels, would place the person back at the earliest stages of his development where the instincts of aggression and sexuality are predominant. Since this vowel /r/ is in the same family as a consonantal /r/, and since the consonantal /r/ has to do, from a theoretical viewpoint, with the anal period, it would therefore be hypothesized that it has to do with aggression rather than sexuality. Clinically, one would expect individuals sustaining difficulty with the vowel /r/ to have major difficulties in the control of their aggression, and to impulsively and unexpectedly discharge this energy. Thus, individuals whose hyperactivity is a result not of cerebral dysfunction but of increased energy as the result of unexpressed aggression, may be expected to manifest this difficulty. Further, patients who are given to episodic dyscontrol would also be expected to manifest this difficulty. Individuals with a distortion of the vowel /r/ and the substitution of /w/ for /r/ would be expected to manifest the characteristics hypothesized for both substitutions. If the pressure to give of oneself were sufficiently great the individual might impulsively discharge his aggression toward himself or others. If this is so, this combination of substitutions should occur with the greatest frequency in persons who are high homicidal or suicidal risks.

Interchange of Sounds Believed Characteristic of the Oral Period Indicates an Early Fixation in Psychosexual Development

It is probably no accident that the child who says *titty* insteady of kitty is popularly characterized as using baby talk. In line with the assumption made as to the psychosexual level of the sounds involved in this substitution, one would be constrained to speculate that a person manifesting such substitutions would indeed be infantile. Experimental evidence for the meaning that seems to be tied up in such substitutions can also be obtained from the speech patterns of adults who are trying to talk "baby-talk." In other words, the sounds which would be substituted would be sounds of the oral-respiratory-sensory stage for sounds of the oral-biting stage. The fact that these substitutions usually do not persist once the child is in school is undoubtedly a function of the tremendous individual push toward maturation.

WORKING HYPOTHESES RELATED TO VOWELS

Persistent Hoarseness in the Absence of Significant Laryngeal Pathology Occurs in Individuals who Attempt to Manifest Both Sexual and/or Chronologically Inappropriate Striving

Since hoarseness can be simulated by lowering one's pitch, and since the lowering of one's pitch is closer to a masculine than to a feminine voice, one would hypothesize that the occurrence of a hoarse voice occurs primarily because of an attempt to be masculine. Thus, hoarseness in a girl would represent an attempt to be more masculine and identify herself more with the father than with the mother, whereas hoarseness in a boy would represent a premature attempt to be as masculine as the father. Transitory hoarseness might then be expected during the height of the normal oedipal struggle.

Deviation from Culturally Accepted Pitch Levels is Related to Distortions in Sexual Identity

Culturally, women are expected to have higher pitched voices than males even though there are variations in the pitch level that individuals may use. Since vowel sounds may be identified in the pitch of one's voice and since vowels are assumed to express sexuality, it is hypothesized that the pitch a person uses reflects his sexual identification. The well-known illustration of the football player with the high feminine voice or the woman with a low masculine voice are common examples of the general belief that such individuals are psychologically different from other members of their sex. What can be said of the woman who voluntarily states that a low-pitched voice is adopted because it sounds "sexy"? One could speculate that the woman who openly admits adopting a low voice in order to sound sexy has a stronger drive toward overt as opposed to latent homosexuality. In other words, she is attempting to be sexy not primarily for the purpose of attracting a male but to be sexy by adopting a male-sounding voice to seduce other women.

Finally, in this discussion some mention should be made of the psychological meanings which this theory would ascribe to the pubertal change of voice. While in the popular conception this event is supposedly a dramatic episode accompanied by creaking and groaning, in practice this notion probably is more romantic than real. Weiss (1950) lends support to this statement when he writes: "Most frequently the normal mutational change in the voice proceeds gradually. . . ." While the usual reason offered for a child's sudden loss of control in his voice is that there is a physiological growth spurt which temporarily makes him physiologically unable to control the functioning of his cords, to the present writer's knowledge there has been no substantiation of this belief. The hypothesis offered on the basis of the speculations advanced in this chapter is that the loss of control of pitch represents difficulty in controlling the emergence of the sexual drive with the onset of puberty.

In Cases of Breathiness, Dysphonia, or Aphonia the Primary Meaning of the Symptom is the Individual's Attempt to Deny or Repress Sexuality

In a breathy voice, it is hypothesized that the mechanism of denial is operative; while, in the case of dysphonia or aphonia, the main defense mechanism employed is repression. Breathiness as a social phenomenon is not unusual and is often seen in teenage girls identifying themselves with popular singers of one sort or another. Its popularity among teenage girls then is understood as their attempt to deal with the normal emergence of sexual wishes which at that age cannot be gratified.

The Vocal Quality of Harshness, Whininess, and Nasality is a Manifestation of Aggression

It has been demonstrated repeatedly that consistent identification of the phenomenon of nasality even by trained listeners is difficult (cf. Bradford, Brooks, and Shelton, 1964). This also speaks to the fact that the inconsistency of labeling someone's voice as being nasal and/or harsh is probably a function not only of the vagueness of the concept but also of the wide tolerance for what is nasal or what is harsh. Why should this be so?

Barring the presence of organic deviations causing nasality, the notion is advanced that the sounds of harshness, nasality, and whininess are all aspects of aggression which is portrayed through an individual's voice. This hypothesis thus offers new light in understanding why it is so difficult for trained listeners to identify vocal quality such as nasality. That is, their inconsistency in judgments is not necessarily because the concept itself is vague, but more because their individual tolerance for what is an acceptable discharge of aggression varies substantially. The continuum along which these three aspects of vocal behavior are viewed is as follows. The whininess in a person's voice is believed to go along with the more immature, demanding, and childish aspects of the person, whereas nasality is a more characterological manner of discharging agression.

Harshness is conceived as being an open display of aggression and would presumably occur primarily in individuals manifesting overt cruelty.

The Spread in the Individual's Pitch Range is Related to the Available Variations in his Affective Life

Psychiatric personnel are prone to insist that an individual with little affect has a dull, monotonous voice. If there is little pitch range available then one could understand the reason for the monotony and also follow the hypothesis which has been made. In a sense one may look at the ability to make variations in pitch as ability to delineate variations in feelings.

Tongue-thrusting Occurs where there is an Excessive need to Compete in an Aggressive Sense

The phenomenon of tongue-thrusting is speech behavior about which speculation is also possible. In recent years it has received much attention by both speech pathologists and orthodontists. A number of alternative theories have been offered as to its etiology, ranging from purely neurological and/or physiological to strictly psychological cases (cf. Palmer, 1962). The most sophisticated dental description of the problem of tongue-thrusting has been presented by Moyers (1962). He felt that there could be a tongue-thrust as a result of abnormal posture of the tongue or what he calls a simple tongue-thrust, a complex tongue-thrust or, finally, a retained infantile swallow. The resulting malocclusion usually ascribed to the tongue-thrust may be, in his opinion, a function of the other musculature surrounding the teeth and lips. He does emphasize in his discussion of the retained infantile swallow the psychological aspects of the person as causative agents.

In this chapter the position is taken that tongue-thrusting may be viewed primarily as evidence of inappropriate attempts to compete and to discharge aggression. Thus among individuals manifesting a tongue-thrust, whether men or women, one should expect to find a good deal more competition and striving than in individuals who do not manifest a tongue-thrust. Taking the data presented by Fletcher, Casteel, and Bradley (1961), wherein the authors note a high incidence early in life of tongue-thrusting with a rapid decline as a child grows older, it would be contended that the reason for this early and high incidence of tongue-thrusting is precisely that the individual concerned has not sublimated his aggressive and competitive urges in a satisfactory manner. The fact that the incidence drops dramatically at around age five is of interest inasmuch as by around this age the child should have passed through and achieved some degree of resolution of his oedipal conflicts and inferentially channeled his competitiveness and striving into more appropriate areas.

COMMENTS REGARDING RECEPTION OF SOUND

Finally, it should be noted that nothing has been said in the current chapter regarding the receptive aspect of sound. While the expressive aspect has been emphasized, it would stand to reason that there might be an equally important element in the psychological meanings of sounds as experienced by the listener. This possibility might explain some of the misperceptions which occur on such auditory discrimination tests as the Harvard Lists of Phonetically Balanced Words, etc. Errors on such tests are explained by utilizing the construct of auditory discrimination. Generally some organic factor is assumed to be the causative agent for the discrimination difficulty. Klein and Schlesinger (1949) suggest the importance of psychological factors:

> In the careful research on seeing, hearing, feeling, the see-er, the hearer, the feeler are somehow obscured or lost. The person himself, the pivot of all these sensations, the source and root of motives whose influences are sought, is ignored as a determinant of his own perceptual behavior.

Further, it could be speculated that psychological meanings might be attached to sounds which are heard early in life. The capacity for sensitivity to sound by infants has most recently been demonstrated by Spiegler and Ourth (1967). It is also known that there are receptive disturbances for sound among psychiatric patients. Recent articles by Baker (1964), Billingberg and Jonsson (1965), and Briskey, Jansen, and Merklen (1966) all comment on the problem. As yet no studies utilizing the hypothesis presented in this chapter have been presented. In the spirit of the hypotheses proposed in this chapter one would consider that the relationship between auditory discrimination and articulation problems which is periodically demonstrated (e.g., Sherman and Geith, 1967, Luterman, 1960, and Kronwall, 1959) may in reality be the effect on discrimination of the psychological meanings of sounds. If this is so, then the receptive aspect (auditory discrimination) becomes a counterpart of the expressive aspect (voice and articulation problems).

CLINICAL APPLICATIONS OF THE THEORY

In the following section two cases will be presented to illustrate how data obtained in the speech examination allow for complementary inferences to what is reported in the case history and the examinations of the psychiatrist and psychologist.

CASE NUMBER 1

Historically, this child's past psychological difficulties included such things as hyperactivity from infancy on, aggressive behavior at home and at school, including biting, scratching and kicking doors, picking his nose and eating the contents, persistent enuresis, nightmares, using foul language, and lifting up the dresses of little girls. The history of the mother's pregnancy with this child was normal until about the seventh month of gestation, when there was a mild leaking of amniotic fluid which lasted two days with no apparent complications. The patient was born full-term, with an essentially normal birth weight and duration of labor. The patient was bottle-fed, and in addition there was full-time help with housekeeping. Sometime during the first five months of the patient's life the mother had a miscarriage, became depressed, and required some hospitalization. Speech development was always considered slow, and the patient did not use sentences until the age of three. Between six months and one and one-half years, the patient was quite often left alone with a baby-sitter and reportedly always created a fuss. Enuresis persists at nighttime at the present time. At age one and one-half years the patient began to get into everything, in a destructive, uncontrolled way. This behavior supposedly persists to the present time. The child was seen prior to the current examination by a neurologist and the findings, including the electroencephalogram, were reported as normal. He had been in speech therapy for approximately two and one-half years with little or no improvement.

At the time of the present examination the following sound substitutions were noted: /f/ for the voiceless /th/, /w/ for /l/, and /d/ for the voiced /th/. In addition there was also the presence of a lateral lisp, occurrence of the "dark l" and distortion of the vowel /r/ as in bi*r*d. In addition there were numerous sound omissions in his articulatory pattern. The pitch range to his voice was only one-half of one octave in spread. There was a tongue thrust in the swallowing pattern and a mild lateral open bite. The examination of the peripheral speech mechanism was negative with the aforementioned exceptions. Although his voice quality at times was nasal, palatal movement and length were adequate and there were no signs of any submucosal cleft. Tests of his auditory sensitivity for pure tone stimuli were within normal limits.

Solely on the basis of the speech data taken in the context of the aforementioned theory, one would infer that this is a child who manifests significant emotional difficulties. This statement is made inasmuch as there is a major cluster of what has been speculated as being pathognomonic difficulties with speech. To begin with, the occurrence of the so-called "dark l" and /w/ for /l/ in the child's speech patterns would suggest that there was significant early disturbance in the normal nurturing relationship with his mother from which this child is attempting to obtain some restitution. This inference is based on the assumption that the "dark l" sound when it occurs has reference to a disturbance in the early nurturing relationship between mother and child. If one remembers that the /l/ phoneme is also a semivowel, one could date the psychological difficulty back to a period somewhere in the first half of the child's first year of life, at a normal period for nursing and/or close nurturing by the mother. One would expect to find in the clinical history of this patient evidence of interpersonal disturbance between mother and child during the first year of his life. The presence also of the /w/ for /l/ substitution suggests that this child is attempting himself to obtain from this environment some of this early nurturance which he missed. This is based on the assumption that the /w/ sound is a sound associated with the child's early attempts at incorporating this nurturing. If the child is attempting to do this at his current chronological age, one expects to find that individuals in his environment may feel that they are being devoured by his omnipresent needs and wants.

In addition to the primary disturbance with the mother, there is datum in the speech examination to indicate a similar early disturbance with the father. This inference is based on the substitution of the /f/

for the voiceless /th/ sound. It will be recalled that we have assumed the voiceless /th/ sound is associated with the phallic period of psychosexual development and the /f/ phoneme is associated with the discharge of early oral aggression. The persistence of this substitution pattern suggests that, instead of coming to grips with the realistic concept of the father, the child maintains instead an early orally aggressive type of relationship with him. Since effective interaction with both parents is necessary for forming an adequate self-concept, one would expect that this boy had never made any firm masculine identification.

Another indication from the speech data that the psychological disturbance dates back to the child's early life is a persistence of the distortion of the vowel /r/ as in the word "bird." This distortion, it will be recalled, occurs on a vowel which is hypothetically believed to be related primarily to the early undifferentiated discharge of sexual and aggressive instincts. Specifically, the discharge of the vowel /r/ has been hypothesized as related primarily to the aggressive instinct and only secondarily to the sexual instinct. Thus, in addition, one infers that there is the likelihood of impulsive, misdirected, and unexpected discharges of aggression. In view of the fact that it has been inferred on the basis of the speech data that significant interaction traumas have been sustained with both his mother and father, one would expect a relatively undifferentiated discharge of aggression against both masculine and feminine figures in his environment.

In addition to these speech difficulties, the patient sustained a tongue-thrust in his swallowing pattern. It will be recalled that our hypothesis related this to an excessive need to compete and achieve at a level which is beyond both this individual's chronological and sexually appropriate age level. This inference necessitates the assumption that a tongue-thrust represents phallic strivings on the part of the person who manifests it and that in its normal occurrence does not persist after the resolution of the oedipal conflict. Since this child is nine years of age and still persists in this difficulty, one would be able to hypothesize that psychosexual development has never progressed through the oedipal stage. This reasoning is not inconsistent at this point in terms of the aforementioned inferences, for we have already speculated that early and significant conflicts occurred at or below the level of one year of age.

The persistence of a lateral lisp in this patient is the basis for speculating that some significant disturbances occurred in the anal period of psychosexual development. Utilizing Erikson's constructs about this period, it would be inferred that the struggle was around the development of a sense of autonomy and was never completed. Further, one would expect that in much of his behavior there would be evidence of his messiness and reluctance to enter into any but a most superficial relationship with a person.

How might this child attempt to organize some level of equilibrium out of the chaos that is inferred in his life? Once again the speech data allow us to arrive at some idea of one of his maneuvers. The marked constriction in the pitch range of his voice is approximately one-half of what, in our experience, is a normal pitch range for a child of this age. If, as we have already mentioned, the amount of spread in pitch range is related to the amount of affect that a person allows himself to experience, one would be able to say that this child is very constricted in his affective life. In someone at least theoretically so tormented by his impulsive life and early traumas, one way to keep some semblance of control would be to narrow his affective life, thus allowing little or no feelings to impinge on him or become important to him.

The composite picture drawn from the current speech examination, utilizing the theory presented in this chapter, is that the child is unsure of his own sexual identity, has sustained early and significant psychological traumas from both his mother and father, is subject to sudden and unrestrained discharge of impulses, has an inability to trust anyone other than himself, and is probably a child whose thought processes would be grossly disturbed. Finally, if the speech is really symptomatic of all of the features which have been discussed, one could see why conventional speech therapy procedures focusing on auditory discrimination drills would be unlikely to effect any significant shift in the speech disturbance.

During the current psychiatric examination the child was again seen by a neurologist with the impression that there were some minimal nonrelated neurological findings such as inability to close one eye alone, mixed dominance, and some mild asymmetry in the placement of the ears. The electroencephalogram was still normal. The usual laboratory examinations were noncontributory. The results of the examination by the psychiatrist and psychologist revealed that the patient's thought processes were disorganized, characterized principally by concreteness and rapid shifts between opposite, extreme ideas. His emotions were considered as primitive and not well modulated. Anger was expressed in banging, kicking, breaking, angry words, swearing, and pronoucements of hatred and desires to hurt or kill. His affect was blunted and inappropriate and the child was restless, hyperkinetic, and expansive. His concept of his body and of himself was unclear and unsteady. Sexual identity was confused and he was uncertain of his age and size. His general level of common sense and reality contact was poor. On formal psychological tests it became abundantly clear that he was flooded with primitive impulse pressures and representations which repeatedly disrupted and dominated his thinking and threatened to gain access to motor expression. Outstanding in his productions was intrusion of material dealing with anger and destruction, together with the lack of constancy, stability, and predictability. The father was most often pictured by the boy as a frightening, powerful, and destructive figure who is at times an all-devouring creature. The mother was pictured by the social worker as confused in her own mind about her desire for him to have been a girl, as well as feelings about coping with pregnancies and resulting miscarriages during his first year of life. The final psychiatric diagnosis of this child was that he manifested a syndrome best labeled as schizophrenic reaction, childhood type.

This patient is of more than passing interest in that he manifests a speech disturbance obviously felt within the realm of treatability by speech therapy, which was tried without success for approximately two years. While most speech pathologists would characterize this child's articulation difficulties as severe, most would have been unlikely on the basis of his articulation problem to have viewed this child as being this seriously emotionally disturbed. Certainly, the conventional hypotheses regarding the etiology of articulation problems would not lead to this conclusion.

CASE NUMBER 2

The child was a 15-year-old boy who came for a psychiatric examination because his grades in school were becoming increasingly poor. He was becoming irresponsible and frequently lied, was enuretic, and his dress and personal habits seemingly had deteriorated. This child was one of four children. The oldest sibling received brief psychiatric treatment. A younger sister had not had any apparent difficulties, but a younger brother had undergone ten operations for a cleft palate and for a hearing loss.

Both the pregnancy and birth of this child were normal. Bowel training was completed by 36 months with occasional soiling persisting until the age of 10. Enuresis still occurs. The frenulum was clipped when he was two and one-half years of age. The mother believed that she was close to the patient for the first several years, while the father openly remarked that it was not until he was four years old "that he became my son." Approximately from the age of four through seven, the mother spent a good deal of time attending to the youngest boy, who sustained a cleft palate. School all along has been a situation where the patient continued to learn in spite of poor attention and increasing disruptive behavior in school. In school he complained of school sickness, headache, and stomachaches. The patient told one psychiatrist that he had been constantly fighting his parents without letting them know how much he had been hurt by them in the hopes that he would win and be left alone by them. As he became older, around age 13, his behavior became more self-defeating as he failed in activities in which he wanted to do well. Also at age 13, it was recommended that his parents supervise him so closely that in effect he would be "put in jail." It was at this time that he committed a delinquent act involving shooting out the lights on a Little League baseball field.

The speech evaluation noted the presence of a lateral lisp, a frontal lisp, substitution of /f/ for the voiceless /th/, substitution of /w/ for /r/, substitution of /d/ for the voiced /th/, a nasal voice, a hoarse voice, and a whistle accompanying articulation of sibilant sounds. The spread in pitch range of his voice was approximately age adequate. A tongue-thrust existed in his swallowing pattern. Audiometric testing indicated a bilateral apparent sensorineural loss at 4,000 and 8,000 Hz. The other frequencies were within normal limits.

There are some significant articulation problems which interact to give us an entirely different clinical picture from the previous case. If one starts with the substitution of /f/ for the voiceless /th/ sound, one would infer that the primary disturbance in this child's life has been a totally unsatisfactory relationship with the father. It will be recalled that this inference is based on the assumption that the voiceless /th/ sound is a sound which is related to the phallic period of psychosexual development while the /f/ sound is believed related to the oral-biting stage. Thus it is hypothesized that this child's primary way of relating to masculine figures is by oral aggressive means. Further it would be expected that since this conflict with his father was never resolved, there would be some confusion in the patient's sexual identity.

In addition to the failure to successfully resolve the psychosexual conflicts of the phallic stage, one would also have to infer that the child's problems date back at least to the anal period in view of the persisting substitution of /w/ for /r/. It will be recalled that the /w/ is a sound hypothesized to be associated with the oral incorporative period, whereas the /r/ sound was believed to be related primarily to the anal retentive stage of psychosexual development. Thus, the child would be pictured as someone demanding in the sense of taking from others, but reticent in giving back of himself. In a behavioral sense in a child of this chronological age, one might expect him to be in major difficulties in terms of his school achievement and performance. The hypothesis might also be offered that since there is the capacity to take in and to retain this child is probably not a retarded child, but instead bright and an underachieving child.

The child additionally presented the sound difficulties of a frontal and lateral lisp. It will be recalled that the lateral lisp was specified as occurring at the anal stage and suggested a failure to develop a sense of autonomy. The persistence of a frontal lisp in addition would suggest that there is some tendency to push on in his psychosexual development while at the same time hanging onto more infantile traits. This may be viewed as a positive indication for growth mixed in as it is with all of the earlier negative indications.

Another positive sign in the speech behavior is the presence of a whistle accompanying the articulation of some of the sibilant sounds. In this case it appears that this child is capable of experiencing shame and doubt and, inferentially, the hope would be that the child would be motivated to change. Finally, another indication of the child's desire to move onward in his psychosexual maturation is the presence of the hoarse voice. This is believed to indicate an attempt to be and act more masculine than the child is realistically able to manage. Nevertheless, the persistence of the hoarse voice in this case may be a harbinger of the child's desire to move beyond his hypothesized current low level of psychosexual immaturity. Also the persistence of the tongue-thrust is interpreted as but another indication of the child's wish to compete and strive and again may be viewed in this context as indicating some potential for growth on the part of the child. However, the nasal voice in the absence of organic pathology suggests the possibility of a somewhat characterological manner of handling aggression. Because of the child's chronological age one would be hesitant to say how much of the misdirected aggression could be rechanneled as a result of any therapeutic intervention. The approximately age-adequate spread of the pitch range of the voice suggests that most of the affect which should be available to the child is there and that his psychological disturbance has not taken too great a toll in this respect. The apparent bilateral sensori-neural loss for sensitivity for pure tones was considered noncontributory at the time inasmuch as the audiometric study failed to suggest any major loss for speech reception or speech discrimination ability. In view of the child's chronological age, the possibility of there being a more or less characterological way of handling anger and the hypothesized problems in psychosexual development relating to the anal stage, one would hope that the other balancing signs in the speech examination (i.e., the hoarse voice, tongue-thrust, and whistle accompanying the sibilant sounds) will be sufficient basis for expecting some psychological change to occur during the process of treatment.

This child had two speech examinations, the first of which has been reported in detail and on which one can make both some diagnostic and prognostic remarks. Before checking the results of the second speech examination, let us review the impressions of the examining psychiatrist and psychologist.

The current physical and neurological examination was within normal limits. In the psychiatric and psychological examination he demonstrated essentially appropriate affective range and manifested no evidence of any disordered thinking. He showed no anxiety or guilt about lying and expressed the belief that he is fated to die in an automobile accident or in combat before he is 50. He gives the picture of a person who can control himself when he wants. He manifests ability to avoid environmental demands comfortably without apparent guilt. His general appearance was dirty and disheveled. His intellectual ability as measured on the Wechsler-Bellevue Test of Intelligence was in the bright-normal range. The examining psychologist felt that this estimate was an underestimate of his actual potential. During the course of the evaluation he became increasingly aware how much he was revealing personal aspects of himself. He gave the impression to the examiners that he was painfully aware of his vulnerability and his needs and was considered a good candidate for treatment.

The diagnosis was made of the patient sustaining an adjustment reaction of adolescence.

Approximately one year after the first examination, this child's speech was reevaluated. There had been no intervening speech therapy procedures. The substitution of /s/ for the voiceless /th/ sound and an occasional omission of /s/ and /w/ on triple consonant combinations remained. Whereas in the previous examination there was a nasality and hoarseness in the voice, these did not occur in the present examination. The pitch range of the patient's voice remained at the same spread as at the time of the prior examination. The tongue-thrust was still present in the swallowing pattern. There was also no significant findings in terms of functioning of the peripheral speech mechanism. The auditory sensitivity at 4,000 and 8,000 Hz was now some 20 to 30 dB better than at the time of the first examination.

The significant change in the voice and articulation pattern and somewhat curious gain in sensitivity for pure-tone stimuli at 4,000 and 8,000 Hz would speak in a general way to the fact that this patient probably has made significant gains as a result of his psychiatric treatment. The remaining consistent substitution of /s/ for voiceless /th/ sound as in the word "bathtub" is a reversal of the usual pattern of a frontal lisp. Since the patient still maintains a tongue-thrust in his swallowing pattern, one might expect that this is still clearly an indication of his excessive need to compete and achieve. If one assumes that the /s/ sound is associated with the anal period and the voiceless/ th/ sound with the phallic period, then one would be able to say that the substitution of /s/ for the voiceless /th/ sound is a continuation of the anal level of psychosexual development into the phallic stage. The fact that some of the substitutions characteristic of earlier psychosexual developmental stages have dropped out, e.g., the /w/ for /r/ substitution, speaks to the fact that many of the earlier conflictual levels have been resolved sufficiently to allow substantial psychological growth to occur. Further confirming data would be the disappearance of the hoarseness in the patient's voice even though there is still a persisting tongue-thrust. Thus, one would say that although there is still competitiveness which is inappropriate in both an age- and role-level sense, there has been growth toward a more appropriate degree of competitiveness. Further, one would suggest also that this patient has developed a better self-concept on the basis of the disappearance of the /f/ for the voiceless /th/ substitution and has learned how to channel his open expressions of aggression in a more suitable fashion. While one would not infer that all of the patient's emotional difficulties have been solved, one would expect the final summary of his psychological status should reflect considerable change.

At the time of the discharge, the patient was in a public school on a full-time basis and was seen by everyone associated with him as quiet and functioning in a socially accepted manner. His grades, however, had still not risen to the level that he theoretically should have been capable of attaining. Even though he had regard for certain strong masculine figures involved in his treatment process, he nevertheless had few close friends, appearing to his peers as superficial and distant though outwardly pleasant. His character structure was considered only moderately changed, although his social adjustment was such that he no longer was involved in grossly disturbing antisocial behavior.

The partial improvement in this child's speech disturbance parallels in similar ways his partial though not complete improvement in his psychological adjustment. The persistence of some speech disturbances is in good agreement with the fact that his psychiatric treatment was never completed in its total sense. This is not only an example of how the speech disturbance in the beginning was symptomatic of the psychiatric disturbance, but also how its remission paralleled closely the remission of the psychiatric problem.

SUMMARY

This chapter has focused on presenting theoretical constructs for the psychopathological meaning of speech disturbances with specific reference to articulation and voice defects. A theoretical framework is proposed wherein these defects are conceived as manifestations of the psychological drives of aggression and sexuality, and of the developmental issues arising in the course of psychosexual development. A sharp distinction is made between the terms "speech" and "language," emphasizing that speech reflects emotions whereas verbal language expresses primarily cognition and only secondarily feeling.

To illustrate the usefulness of this theory in clinical practice two examples were presented. Each child sustained speech disturbances concomitantly with their psychiatric disturbance. One child was evaluated at both the beginning and end of his psychiatric treatment, and one child was discussed only in terms of the initial evaluation. Like all theories, one would expect that certain hypotheses which have been offered will need revision and further clarification, but they offer nevertheless a reasonable place to begin to look at voice and articulation problems as symptoms of significant psychological disturbance. This theory also makes it possible for speech pathologists to contribute to the work of psychiatrists and psychologists with the emotionally disturbed individual. If the theory is valid, it obviously has broader implications in terms of diagnosis, treatment, and assessment of change in treatment for the emotionally disturbed person. Perhaps it is even more significant to the field of speech pathology in general since it would necessitate a critical reassessment of our current academic and clinical training programs.

BIBLIOGRAPHY

Alpert, M., Kutzberg, R., and Friedhoff, A. 1963. Transient voice changes associated with emotional stimuli. *Arch. gen. Psychiat.*, 8, 362–365.

Barker, F. 1964. Impaired hearing in psychotic patients. *Mental Hospitals*, 434–438.

Berry, M., and Eisenson, J. 1956. Speech disorders. New York: Appleton-Century-Crofts.

Billingberg, O., and Jonsson, C. 1965. The ability of schizophrenic patients to interpret intonation. *Acta Psychiat. Scandinavica*, 41, 218–226.

Bradford, L., Brooks, A., and Shelton, R. 1964. Clinical judgment of hypernasality in cleft palate children. *Cleft Palate J.*, 1, 329–335.

———, and Rousey, C. 1961. Psychological implications of the whistling /s/. (Unpublished manuscript.)

Brain, Lord. 1965. Speech disorders: aphasia, apraxia and agnosia (2nd. ed.). Washington: Butterworth.

Brenner, C. 1955. An elementary textbook of psychoanalysis. Garden City, N.Y.: Doubleday. Pp. 16–32.

Briskey, R., Jansen, R., and Merklein, R. 1966. Listening problems of the mentally disturbed. *J. auditory Res.*, 6, 379–383.

Butt, D. 1965. The effect of preliminary training in phoneme discrimination on the articulation of an unfamiliar sound. Univ. N. Mex.: Ph.D. dissertation.

Cozad, R., and Rousey, C. 1966. Hearing and speech disorders among delinquent children. *Corrective Psychiat. J. Soc. Therapy*, 12, 250–257.

Diedrich, W. 1966. Assessment of the treatment process. Unpublished paper presented at Rehabilitation Workshop. Parsons, Kan.: Parsons State Hosp. and Training Center.

English, H., and English, A. 1957. A comprehensive dictionary of psychological and psychoanalytical terms. New York: Longmans. P. 540.

Erickson, E. 1950. Childhood and Society. New York: Norton. Pp. 44–92.

Fletcher, S., Casteel, R., and Bradley, D. 1961. Tongue-thrust swallow, speech articulation and age. *J. Speech Hearing Disorders*, 26, 201–208.

Freud, A. 1966. Links between Hartmann's ego-psychology and the child analyst's thinking. *In* Psychoanalysis—a general psychology. Loewenstein, R., Newman, L., Schur, M., and Solnit, A., eds. New York: Int. Univ. Press. Pp. 16–27.

———. 1965. Normality and pathology in childhood. New York: Int. Univ. Press.

———, and Burlingham, D. 1944. Infants without families. New York: Int. Univ. Press.

Freud, S. 1955. Beyond the pleasure principle. *In* Standard edition. Strachey, J., ed. London: Hogarth. Pp. 3–64.

———. 1959. Inhibitions, symptoms and anxiety. *In* Standard edition. Strachey, J., ed. London: Hogarth. Pp. 87–91.

Green, A. 1962. Speech of psychiatric patients: A hospital survey. Purdue Univ.: Master's thesis.

Greenson, R. 1954. About the sound "MM." *PSA. Quart.*, 23, 234–239.

———. 1961. On the silence and sounds of the analytic hour. *J. Amer. psychoanalytic Assn.*, 9, 79–84.

Grimes, J. 1962. The status of speech and language of emotionally disturbed children. Kansas Univ.: Master's thesis.

Hall, W. 1962. A study of the articulatory skills of children from three to six years of age. Univ. Mo.: Ph.D. dissertation.

Hartmann, H. 1951. Ego psychology and the problem of adaptation. *In* Organization and pathology of thought. *Trans. by* Rapaport, D. New York: Columbia. Pp. 362–396.

———. 1964. Psychoanalysis and developmental psychology. *In* Essays on ego psychology. New York: Int. Univ. Press. Pp. 99–112.

Healey, W. 1963. A study of the articulatory skills of children from six to nine years of age. Univ. Mo.: Ph.D. dissertation.

Heinstein, M. 1963. Behavioral correlates of breast-bottle regimes under varying parent-infant relationships. *Monogr., Soc. Res. Child Developm.*, 28, 4.

Irwin, O. 1947. Infant speech: consonantal sounds according to manner of articulation. *J. Speech Disorders*, 12, 402–404.

———. 1947. Infant speech: consonantal sounds according to place of articulation. *J. Speech Disorders*, 12, 397–401.

———. 1948. Infant speech: development of vowel sounds. *J. Speech Hearing Disorders*, 13, 31–34.

Jackson, H. 1965. On dissolution of the nervous system. *In* Source book in the history of psychology. Herrnstein, R., and Boring, E., eds. Cambridge: Harvard.

Jakobson, R. 1960. Why mama and papa. *In* Perspective in psychological theory. Kaplan, B., and Wagner, S., eds. New York: Int. Univ. Press. Pp. 124–134.

Klein, G., and Schlesinger, H. 1949. Where is the perceiver in perceptual theory? *J. Personality*, 13, 32–47.

Kronwall, E. 1959. An investigation of some of the factors frequently suggested as causes of articulation disorders. Univ. Ky.: Ph.D. dissertation.

Lenneberg, E. 1967. Biological foundations of language. New York: Wiley.

———, Rabelsky, F., and Nichols, I. 1965. The vocalizations of infants born to deaf and to hearing parents. *Vita Humana* (Human Development), 8, 23–37.

Luria, A. 1961. The role of speech in the regulation of normal and abnormal behavior. Elmsford, N.Y.: Pergamon Livwright.

———, and Yudovich, F. 1966. Speech and the development of mental processes in the child. London: Staples.

Luterman, D. 1960. The relationship between speech-sound discrimination ability and articulation of the /s/ phoneme. Penn. State Univ., Ph.D. dissertation.

McNeill, D. 1966. Development psycholinguistics. *In* Genesis of language, Smith, F., and Miller, G., eds. Cambridge: M.I.T.

McWilliams, B. 1960. Psychological implications of consonant sounds. *J. Speech Hearing Disorders*, 25, 89–91.

Menninger, K., with Mayman, M., and Pruyser, P. 1963. The vital balance. New York: Viking.

Miron, M. 1961. A cross-linguistic investigation of phonetic symbolism. *J. abnorm. soc. Psychol.*, 62, 623–630.

Moses, P. 1954. The voice of neurosis. New York: Grune & Stratton.

Mowrer, O. 1950. Learning theory and personality dynamics. New York: Ronald. Pp. 688–726.

Moyers, R. 1962. The role of musculature in orthodontic diagnosis treatment planning. *In* Vistas in orthodontics. Kraus, B., and Riedel, R., eds. Philadelphia: Lea & Febiger. Pp. 309–328.

Ostwald, P. 1961. Humming, sound and symbol. *J. aud. Res.*, 3, 224–232.

———, and Skolnikoff, A. 1966. Speech disturbances in a schizophrenic adolescent. *Postgraduate Medicine*, 1, 40–49.

Palmer, J. 1962. Tongue thrusting: A clinical hypothesis. *J. Speech Hearing Disorders*, 27, 323–333.

Paves, L. 1965. A study to determine relationship between voice qualities and attributed states of personality. N.Y.U.: Ph.D. dissertation.

Provence, S., and Lipton, R. 1962. Infants in institutions. New York: Int. Univ. Press.

Rheingold, H. 1956. Modification of social responsiveness in institutional babies. *Monogr., Soc. Res. Child Developm.*, 21, No. 2, 2:2.

Rousey, C., and Averill, S. 1963. Speech disorders among delinquent boys. *Bull. Menninger Clinic*, 27, 177–184.

———, and Moriarty, A. 1965. Diagnostic implications of speech sounds. Springfield, Ill.: Thomas.

———, and Toussieng, P. 1964. Contributions of a speech pathologist to the psychiatric examination of children. *Mental Hygiene*, 48, 566–575.

Sapir, E. 1929. A study in phonetic symbolism. *J. exper. Psychol.*, 12, 225–239.

———. 1926. Speech as a personality trait. *Mental Health Bull.*, 5, 1–7.

Sherman, D., and Geith, A. 1967. Speech sound discrimination and articulation skill. *J. Speech Hearing Res.*, 10, 277–280.

Shervanian, C. 1959. The speech development level of precommunicative psychotic children. Univ. Pittsburgh: Ph.D. dissertation.

Solomon, A. 1961. Personality and behavior patterns of children with functional defects of articulation. *Child Developm.*, 32, 731–738.

Spiegler, D., and Ourth, L. 1967. Factors involved in the development of prenatal rhythmic sensitivity. Paper presented at the Soc. Res. Child Developm. meeting.

Spitz, R. 1945. Hospitalism: An inquiry into the genesis of psychiatric conditions in early childhood. *Psychoanalytic Study of the Child*, 1, 53–74.

———. 1965. The first year of life. New York: Int. Univ. Press.

Templin, M. 1957. Certain language skills in children. Institute of Child Welfare, Monogr. Series No. 26.

———. 1966. The study of articulation and language development during the early school years. *In* Genesis of language. Smith, F., and Miller, G., eds. Cambridge, Mass.: M.I.T. Pp. 173–180.

Travis, L., ed. 1957. Handbook of speech pathology. New York: Appleton-Century-Crofts.

Van Riper, C. 1963. Speech correction (4th. ed.). Englewood Cliffs, N.J.: Prentice-Hall.

———, and Irwin, J. 1958. Voice and articulation. Englewood Cliffs, N.J.: Prentice-Hall.

Walle, E., and Morris, P. 1967. Hearing and speech research and therapy with sociopathic criminals. *Hearing Speech News*, 2, 8–12.

Weber, J. 1964. Speech therapy with emotionally disturbed children. *Canada's mental Health*, 6, 16–19.

Weiss, D. 1964. Logopedic observations in a mental hospital. *Folia Phoniat.*, 16, 130–138.

———. 1950. Pubertal change of the human voice. *Folia Phoniat., Separatum*, 2, 126–159.

Winitz, H. 1966. The development of speech and language in the normal child. *In* Speech pathology. Riever, R., and Brubaker, R., eds. Amsterdam: North-Holland Pub. Pp. 42–76.

Wundt, G. 1900. Vokerpsychologie, 1, Part 1, Leipzig: W. Engelmann (Pp. 60–61, 81, 131–132) as cited in Freud, Sigmund (1901): The Psychopathology of Everyday Life. (Standard Edition Vol. VI), London: Hogarth Press, 1960, 53–105.

33

Functional Disorders of Articulation—Symptomatology and Etiology

Margaret Hall Powers

GENERAL CONSIDERATIONS

Articulation problems have long been recognized as the most prevalent of all the disorders of speech. Because this is true and since only a small fraction of articulation cases are organically based, functional articulation problems constitute a highly significant group of disorders in the total field of speech pathology. They merit serious study and much greater scientific investigation than they have yet received, not only because they are so common but also because they are by no means so simply explained and treated as many people have assumed.

How can *functional articulation disorders* be defined? Let us examine the words of the term separately. *Articulation* can be defined as the production of speech sounds by the stopping or constricting of the vocalized or nonvocalized breath stream by movements of the lips, tongue, velum, or pharynx. *Disorders* of articulation are faulty placement, timing, direction, pressure, speed, or integration of these movements, resulting in absent or incorrect speech sounds. *Functional* is more difficult to define. The term originated in the field of medicine but has been widely adopted in speech pathology, where it has come to have a meaning practically synonymous with *nonorganic*. Some speech pathologists use it in such a way as to suggest the even narrower meaning of *nonstructural*, though most prefer to think of it as having physiological and neurological connotations as well as anatomical significance.

A functional articulation disorder can be defined as an inability to produce correctly all of the standard speech sounds of the language, an inability for which there is no appreciable structural, physiological, or neurological basis in the speech mechanism or its supporting structures, but which can be accounted for by normal variations in the organism or by environmental or psychological factors. In reality there can be no strict separation between *organic* and *functional*. There are probably few, if any, cases which are purely organic or purely functional.

Many of the so-called *functional* cases have subtle organic factors in their pattern of etiology, particularly when the past history of the case is considered. For example, a child may have developed a lisp because of irregular dentition which has been corrected before we see him. The lisp continues and should be diagnosed as *functional*, although it might originally have been diagnosed as *organic*.

It has become customary to diagnose a case on the basis of the etiological factors operating at the time the diagnosis is made. Any sensible clinician will naturally give consideration also to factors which have been operative in the past in order to understand the problem as thoroughly as possible. However, it is the causal pattern operating at the time the case presents itself for study which will largely determine the diagnosis and the program of therapy.

It should also be emphasized that *functional* is an etiological, not a symptomatological term. It is frequently seen that the same acoustic effect may be produced by either an organic or a functional cause. Two cases with lisps, for example, may sound almost identical but may have very different causes.

Still another issue arises in the *organic* versus *functional* dilemma. Many *functional articulation* cases are so labeled unjustifiably through what this writer calls "diagnosis by default," meaning that an assumption is made that a speech defect must be functional if no obvious organic deviations are found to account for it. The term *functional* is used as a catchall for speech problems which cannot be explained in other terms. This is not a legitimate procedure. It is necessary for the speech diagnostician to demonstrate positive evidences of functional etiology as well as to eliminate negative ones.

The term *functional* does not exclude the normal variation within the population of almost all physical and psychological traits. Indeed, the greater part of the research which has been done on functional disorders of articulation has been devoted to investigating the presence or absence of systematic differences between functional articulation cases and normal speakers in a series of traits, ranging from structural differences of the speech mechanism to motor dexterity, auditory memory span, sound discrimination, and others. Such differences when found have not often been of the order of pathological variations but merely of normal variations. It is important to distinguish between *pathological variations* and the *normal variations* which are to be expected of most human physical and psychological traits. The former, if present in an articulatory case and causally related

TABLE 33-I

Incidence of Functional Articulatory Defectives as Reported in Various Studies*

STUDY	POPULATION STUDIED	TOTAL NO. OF SPEECH DEFECTIVES	AUTHOR'S DIAGNOSTIC CLASSIFICATIONS	NO. OF CASES	% OF TOTAL CASES	PROBABLY CLASSIFIABLE AS "FUNCTIONAL ARTICULATORY" NUMBER	%
White House Conference (1931)*	Ages 5–18 in 48 U.S. cities over 10,000	Reduced to basis of 10,000 cases	Sound substitutions	4,623.80	46.2	5,770.24*	57.7
			Oral inactivity	1,146.44	11.5		
ASHA Comm. report of	Ages 5–21	2,000,000 (assumed)	Functional articulatory	1,200,000	60.0	Same	60.0
White House Conference (1951)	All ages	7,500,000 (assumed)	Functional articulatory	4,500,000	60.0	Same	60.0
Louttit and Halls (1936)	Grades 1–12 County schools	3,049	Articulatory	2,434	80.0	Same	80.0
	City schools	4,258	Articulatory	3,354	79.0	Same	79.0
Burdin, L.G. (1940)*	Grades 1–4	106	Indistinctness	—	42.45		67.9
			Baby talk	—	14.15		
			Lispers	—	11.32		
Mills and Streit (1942)	Elementary children	473	Dyslalia	326	69.0	Same	69.0
Powers, M.H. (1951) Chicago Public Schools	Elementary and high school	8,391	Functional articulation disorders	6,713	80.0	Same	80.0
Black, M.E. (1950–51) Illinois State Program	Elementary and high school	26,416	Articulatory	20,800	78.7	Same	78.7
MacLearie, E.C. (1953) Ohio State Program	Elementary and high school	12,323	Articulatory	10,028	81.3	Same	81.3

* In starred entries the published data have been rearranged or combined by this writer. For original references, see bibliography at end of Chapter 34.

to the speech deviation, would lead to a diagnosis of *organic*. The latter, being normal, would be encompassed within the diagnosis of *functional*. Variations of physical, sensory, and other factors *within the normal range* are expected in functional articulation cases as in other types of cases and in normal speakers as well.

Probably more than any other type of speech disorder, with the possible exception of those often classified as *delayed speech*, functional articulation cases are intimately associated with all dimensions of the individual's growth. They are to be understood only in terms of the dynamics of physical, intellectual, emotional, and social growth patterns, the relationships among these patterns within the individual, and the the modifications produced in them by the environment.

Functional articulation disorders can, therefore, be complex as well as simple. There may be many etiological factors involved or only one or two. The complexity of etiology is not always related, either, to the extent of speech involvement. A relatively limited speech symptom such as a lateral lisp may be difficult to explain. Every experienced clinician knows that there are some articulation cases which seem to defy explanation.

It is perhaps helpful to consider that causal factors may be of three types: predisposing, precipitating, and perpetuating. All may be involved. Although, as stated earlier, only presently-operating factors determine a diagnosis of *organic* or *functional*, factors in all of the above categories should be investigated. It is more important to understand than to label.

It is sound clinically to assume multiple causation of functional articulation cases—indeed, of all cases—so that we will force ourselves to examine all possibilities. Fewer mistakes or oversights will be made than if we start out with the easy assumption that an obvious causal factor is all-effective in a given case and are thus led into overlooking contributing factors. It is good clinical wisdom to operate with the concept of *causal pattern* rather than *cause*.

Incidence

Functional articulation disorders are the most numerous of all speech disorders. Their importance as a therapeutic problem is suggested by Table 33-I, which presents a summary of the incidence of these disorders taken from some of the major survey reports published. Examination of this table shows clearly the high incidence of this type of disorder among speech problems in general. The final three entries are of particular significance because of the large numbers of cases involved and because the figures given are based not upon estimates or questionnaires, but upon diagnoses by trained speech-correction teachers in public school programs, using fairly uniform criteria. It is also significant that there is remarkably close agreement in the percentages reported in the three studies. Upon the basis of these results, it is safe to say that functional articulation defectives represent between 75 and 80 percent of all speech defectives in the school population.

SYMPTOMATOLOGY AND CLASSIFICATION

General Description

The term *functional articulation disorders* encompasses a wide variety of deviate speech patterns. These can all be described in terms of four possible types of acoustic deviation in the individual speech sounds; omissions, substitutions, distortions, and additions. An individual may show one or any combination of these deviations.

Functional articulation disorders may range in severity from mild misarticulation which is hardly noticeable except to the trained ear, through various degrees of severity to complete unintelligibility at the other extreme. Articulation disorders may involve only one or two sounds, they may involve certain groups of sounds, or they may involve all or nearly all the speech sounds of the language. Errors on one or two sounds, while often conspicuous and unattractive, do not usually affect seriously the intelligibility of the individual's speech. Intelligibility is related to the number of different sounds misarticulated. The particular sounds which are defective will also determine to some extent the obviousness of the disorder and the degree to which it interferes with communication. Some consonants are more critical for intelligibility than others.

Another factor determining the conspicuousness of the defect is the frequency with which the individual's defective sounds occur in speech. Travis (1931, p. 223) found consonant sounds occurring in the following rank order of frequency in the conversational speech of children: /t/, /n/, /r/, /s/, /l/, /d/, /m/, /k/, /z/, /w/, /ð/, /h/, /b/, /p/, /g/, /f/, /v/, /ŋ/, /j/, /ʃ/, /θ/, /tʃ/, /dʒ/, /ʌ/, /ʒ/. Henrikson's study (1948) showed approximately the same order of frequency. From this ranking it can be seen, for example, that a defective /ʒ/ is relatively unimportant, a defective /s/ conspicuous because of its frequent occurrence.

Articulation disorders also vary in the degree of consistency of the misarticulations. Some individuals make the same acoustic errors consistently regardless of the word or the position of the sound within the word. Others vary greatly, using the sound correctly in some words, omitting it in others, and using substitutions for it in others. It is not uncommon for a sound which occurs twice within one word to be given differently in the two positions.

The degree of articulatory defect, therefore, has to be evaluated in terms of the degree of misarticulation, the consistency of misarticulation, the importance for intelligibility of the specific sounds involved, and the number of different sounds involved.

Classification

Functional articulatory disorders share in the general confusion which has existed and still exists in speech pathology in regard to what labels to attach to various speech symptoms. Some authors have tried to classify and name speech disorders on the basis of etiology, some of the basis of symptomatology. Most of the commonly used terminology has a foot in each camp. This is the case with the disorders under discussion here—*functional articulatory*, in which *functional* is an etiological term and *articulatory*, a symptomatological term.

Some writers (Ainsworth, 1948); Johnson et al., 1948; and others) describe functional articulation problems quite simply in terms of the four basic types of misarticulation mentioned earlier: omissions, substitutions, distortions, and additions. Others have ranged from elaborate subclassifications (Seth and Guthrie, 1935, who list *dyslalia*, *logorrhea*, *idioglossia*, *audimutitas*, and *rhinolalia* as varieties of articulation disorder) to general categories of a descriptive type such as Van Riper's (1963) *infantile perseveration*, *lalling*, *lisping*, *delayed speech*, and *oral inaccuracy*.

Prins (1962a) has made an impressive attempt to classify functional articulation defects into subgroups by means of a detailed analysis of errors and an intercorrelation study of 30 factors. Children of three to six years of age were given an original picture articulation test. Four subgroups were found: I, variables correlated with interdental lisping; II, variables correlated with the omission error score; III, variables correlated with phonemic sound substitutions in which one articulation feature—place, manner, or voicing—is altered; and IV, variables correlated with nonphonemic distortions in which all articulation features are changed.

The classification preferred by this writer is based on speech symptomatology and makes no assumptions concerning etiology except the obvious one that all disorders encompassed within the term are primarily *functional*. It has the merit of simplicity and does not overreach our present stage of knowledge. Future research may help us to refine this classification considerably.

Functional disorders of articulation can be divided into two general categories and the first of these into several clinical types. The classification given below is followed by a description and discussion of each type:

1. **Misarticulation of specific speech sounds or groups of sounds (sound omissions, substitutions, distortions, additions).**
   Infantile perseveration (baby talk, infantile speech).
   Lisping (misarticulation of one or more of the sibilant consonants: /s/, /z/, /ʃ/, /ʒ/, /tʃ/, /dʒ/.
   Lalling (distortion of /r/ or /l/.
   Misarticulation of other miscellaneous sounds.
2. **General oral inaccuracy.**

1. Misarticulation of Specific Sounds or Groups of Sounds

Defective articulation can be analyzed in terms of one or more of the four types of deviation listed above: omissions, substitutions, distortions and additions. In *omissions* the individual leaves out a phoneme at a place where it should occur. It is not replaced by any other sound. Examples of this are found constantly in the speech of young children, as *tep* for *step*, *pay* for *play*, *daw* for *dog*. Omissions are particularly likely to occur in consonant blends, as in the first two examples above.

In *substitutions* the individual substitutes one standard speech sound for another or may substitute consistently a nonstandard speech sound, such as a glottal stop, for a standard speech sound. Usually, though not always, the substituted sound is one of the sounds earliest acquired in the normal sequence of speech development. A /w/ is often substituted for /r/ or for /l/ as in *w*an for *r*an, a*w*ound for a*r*ound, *w*ady for *l*ady. In mu*vv*er for mo*th*er /v/ is substituted for /ð/; in *t*itty for *k*itty /t/ for /k/; in bu*t* for bu*s* /t/ for /s/.

In *distortions* the production of the speech sound

is modified in some way so that the acoustic result only approximates the standard sound and is not accurate. The individual might be said to aim at the sound and miss it. Distortions vary in degree, some being extreme mutilations, others varying only slightly from the standard sound. Distortions are likely to be fairly regular and consistent while substitutions and omissions are often highly inconsistent. Distortions cannot be described easily in writing because they are often sounds for which we have no printed symbol even in the phonetic alphabet.

Additions are a less frequent form of misarticulation than the others. Sounds which are not part of the words are interpolated or added, as in wa*r*sh for wash, p*uh*lease for please, and p*uh*retty for pretty. In the last two examples a vowel is interpolated between the two consonants of a blend.

All misarticulations can be described in terms of the four error types just discussed. However, there are *patterns* of misarticulation which we recognize as clinical types. They are seen so frequently, and the cases within one type are so similar, that it is important to identify and describe them. The types to be described are by no means mutually exclusive; in fact, they are often overlapping. Specific cases may show characteristics of more than one type. Yet there is a clinical reality to these types which warrants discussion.

Infantile Perseveration (*Baby Talk, Infantile Speech, Pedolalia*). The terms *baby talk* or *infantile speech* do not refer to the type of speech heard in very young children during the early stages of normal speech development, but rather to the persistence of some of these early characteristics beyond the age at which correct speech sounds should have been acquired. Infantile perseveration is characterized mainly by the omission and substitution of sounds and is frequently but not always associated with immaturity in language development. The child who says, "Me do in tah" (Me go in car), is using immature grammatical forms (*me* for *I* and omission of *the*) as well as sound substitutions, /d/ for /g/ and /t/ for /k/, and omissions (/r/ in c*ar*). Another characteristic of infantile perseveration is the marked inconsistency with which sound omissions and substitutions are often made. A child may substitute /f/ for /θ/ in one word, /t/ or /s/ for /θ/ in another word, or a sound may be substituted for a second sound and that one in turn substituted for still a third. Sound omissions may be similarly inconsistent, with the same child giving a sound correctly in some words and omitting it in others.

Normal developmental order of sounds. In order to judge whether a child's misarticulations are normal for his age or are perseverations of speech characteristic of an earlier age level, we must be aware of the developmental order of sounds and the ages at which the various speech sounds normally appear. Table 33-II summarizes some of the principal investigations on genetic development of the voluntary use of English consonant sounds. Careful study of this table will show that there is considerable agreement among the studies in regard to the developmental *order* of the different sounds. There is less agreement on the age levels at which the different sounds appear. The Wellman, Case, Mengert, and Bradbury study (1931) shows a considerably earlier appearance of sounds than do the other studies, but these results are doubtless influenced by the evident fact that the children in this study were a superior group (average I.Q.—115.9).

Bricker (1967), studying articulation of young children from 3.0 to 5.9 years of age, found that "the errors made were inversely related to the frequency of the sounds in the repertoires of infants, and to the frequency of the sounds in the English language." Pendergast et al. (1966) studied the articulation of 15,000 unselected first-grade children and found that slightly more than one-fourth of them misarticulated one or more sounds.

It is interesting to compare the common misarticulations found in cases of infantile perseveration with the developmental pattern as shown in Table 33-II. Van Riper (1938) studied 60 cases of baby talk, ages eight to 29, and found that 68 percent of the errors were on blends, such as /str/, /thr/, and involved, particularly, blends with /r/, /s/, /l/, and /th/. The nine most frequently missed single consonants were, in this order, /s/, /r/, /l/, /ch/, /th/, /k/, /g/, /f/, and /v/. Berry and Eisenson (1942, pp. 89–90) list the sound substitutions which, in their experience, are most frequently made in *baby talk:*

[w]	for	[l]	[f]	for	[s]
[j]	for	[l]	[θ]	for	[s]
[p]	for	[f]	[t]	for	[k]
[ʔ] (glottal stop)	for	[l]	[d]	for	[g]
[ʔ] (glottal stop)	for	[t]	[t]	for	[tʃ]
[f]	for	[θ]	[d]	for	[dʒ]
			[s]	for	[ʃ]

TABLE 33-II
Development of the Purposive Use of Consonant Sounds*

INVESTIGATOR	AGE IN YEARS 2	2½	3	3½	4	4½	5	5½	6	6½	7	7½	8
Wellman, Case, Mengert, and Bradbury (1931, pp. 50–52) Given correctly by 75% or more of the children.	p– –p– b– –b– t– d– m– –m– n– –n– w– –w– h		–b f– –t –f– –d– –f k– –z– –k– –z g– –g– –m –n –ŋ–		–p l– –d –l– –k –l –g –r– –v –ɹ –tʃ j– dʒ– –j– –dʒ–		–t– v– –v– θ– ð– –ð– s– –s– –s z– ʃ– –ʃ– –ʃ ʒ	tʃ– –tʃ– r–	–dʒ	(The authors do not list the following by 6:) –ŋ ʍ– –ʍ– –θ –θ– –ð			
Poole (1934)				p b m w h		t j d n ŋ k g		f		v ð ʃ ʒ l		s θ z ʍ r tʃ dʒ	
Roe (in Johnson, Editor, 1950)			p b m		t k d g n ŋ		f v		l r ʒ dʒ tʃ		s z ʃ sl pl st		
Templin (1952) Percentage of correct utterance.			90% (vowels and diphthongs) 2/3 (consonants) ½ (2-cons. blends) 1/3 (3-cons. blends)		80% (cons.) 70% (2-cons.) 60% (3-cons.)				90% 80% 70%		90% 90% 90%	Not uttered correctly by 90%: Initial ʍ, sl Medial: ʍ, ʒ Final: ʒ, z, r, θ, nt, kt, skr, str, dʒ, tl, tr	
Templin (1957)** Earliest age at which 75% of children gave correctly. (Only single consonants included—initial, medial and final positions)			I: m, n, p, t, k, b, d, g, f, h, w M: m, n, ng, p, k, b, d, g, f, h, w F: m, n, ng, p, t, f	I: y M: s, z, y F: r	I: s, sh, j, r, l M: v, r, l F: k, b, d, g, sh	I: ch M: sh, ch F: s, ch	I: — M: j F: —		I: th, v, th M: t, th F: th, v, l		I: z M: th, zh F: th, z, zh, j	Not produced by 75% of subjects: hw– –hw–	

* Some of these data have been rearranged by the present writer. For the original data, see the references listed in the bibliography.

** For detailed results, see Templin, 1957, p. 51. Standard letters, not phonetic symbols, are used.

Sex differences should also be considered in evaluating infantile perseverations of young children. As the result of a thorough investigation of speech-sound acquisition, Templin (1952, p. 284) reported: "The girls reach about 95 percent correct articulation, probably practically adult articulation, at about seven years while boys take another year in which to reach the same degree of perfection."

Consonant sounds are most likely to be omitted when they occur in final or medial positions in words or initially as a member of a consonant blend. This position differential is also true of normal speech development. Irwin (1951), in a prolonged and intensive investigation of normal infant speech-sound development, found that the development of initial consonants is linear during infancy, of medial consonants decelerating, and of final consonants accelerating. He found that the occurrence of initial consonants is greater than medials and medials greater than finals in infant vocalization. Final consonants are infrequent during the first half-year of life. Thus, the inferiority of medial and final consonants as compared with initial is seen to be as true of normal speech development as it is of consonant production in infantile perseveration.

In extreme cases of infantile perseveration, nearly all consonants are omitted and the resulting speech is a series of vowel sounds, sometimes interspersed with glottal stops. In other cases several of the early consonants are made to substitute for all the others. The preponderance of vowels in these extreme cases again shows the perseveration of sound patterns which are typical of early stages of speech development. Chen and Irwin (1946) found that at two and a half the infant possesses practically all the vowel types used in adult speech and about two-thirds of the consonant types. Metraux (1950) confirms this with her finding that vowel production in the child's speech is more than 90 percent correct by 30 months, but that consonant production does not reach 90 percent correctness until 54 months.

Lundeen (1950) has shown that the diadochokinetic rate of the different speech sounds tends to follow the developmental order. He found that the diadochokinetic rate for /t/, /d/, /p/, and /b/ is faster than that for /s/, /z/, /k/, and /g/, with /f/ and /v/ occupying an intermediate position. The diadochokinetic rank order of sounds corresponded closely with the developmental order reported by Poole (1934) and shown in Table 33-II.

To summarize the misarticulations characteristic of infantile perseveration, we can say that children tend to substitute more visible for less visible sounds, sounds acquired early in normal speech development for those acquired later (see Table 33-II), diadochokinetically faster sounds for slower, and phonetically easier, less precise sounds for phonetically harder sounds requiring more precise coordination and timing. In short, the pattern of speech-sound production which research has shown to be typical of normal speech development in the first several years of life is reflected at later age levels in cases of infantile perseveration.

There are two general types of disorder which both fall within the broad category of speech immaturity. These are *delayed speech*, which is a more complex and profound disorder, and *infantile perseveration*. Delayed speech is the more inclusive of the two. Indeed, infantile perseveration can be thought of as the articulatory aspect of delayed speech, but there is no sharp distinction between the two. If a child's speech immaturity is confined largely to sound omissions and substitutions, if he has learned to rely mainly on speech as his means of communication, if there is considerable output of speech, if the onset of speech has been fairly typical, if he attempts sentences as well as words and phrases, his speech deviation can best be referred to *as infantile perseveration*.

If, however, there has been little or no attempt at speech until past two years of age, if gestures and nonspeech vocalizations are used extensively, if speech is limited mainly to nouns, with little use of qualifying, connective, or auxiliary words, if vocabulary is meager, if single words are used for sentences or phrases, most speech clinicians would tend to call the disorder *delayed speech*. The distinction between *infantile perseveration* and *delayed speech* is thus both qualitative and quantitative, but there is considerable overlap between them in symptomatology. Of the two, *delayed speech* is usually the more serious and complex. It is a language as well as a speech disorder and is usually more difficult to diagnose and to treat.

Lisping (*Sigmastism*). Lisping can be defined as misarticulation of one or more of the six sibilant consonants, /s/, /z/, /ʃ/, /ʒ/, /tʃ/, /dʒ/. Some individuals have difficulty with all six, but many misarticulate only /s/ and /z/. Occasionally a person has difficulty with only /ʃ/ and /ʒ/ or with /tʃ/ and /dʒ/. The /s/ and /z/ sounds are among the most frequently misarticulated of all the speech sounds, probably because the requirements for their production in terms of muscular adjustments are so exacting that minor variations can easily occur. Minor distortions are also more easily heard in these sounds than in most others.

Most writers in speech pathology agree in defining *lisping* essentially as it is defined here, though there is considerable variation in their manner of classifying and describing various types of lisping. Three types of defective sibilant articulation are described, however, by nearly everyone: *lateral*, *lingual protrusion* (also called *interdental*, *frontal*, or *central* by some authorities), and *nasal* (called *recessive* by Berry and Eisenson, 1942).

Because of the tongue's unique capacity for assuming an almost endless variety of positions and shapes, sibilant distortion can be equally varied. However, it seems meaningful and useful to identify only three principal types of lisping, based upon the direction of breath emission, and one subclassification within the first of these. These three types are: *central* (with *interdental* or *tongue protrusion* as a subtype), *lateral*, and *nasal*.

In a *central lisp* the tongue functions in the midline as it should and breath is emitted centrally through a groove, but the tongue position is faulty in either the vertical or the anterior-posterior plane or in both. The tongue may be carried too high so that the air stream is partly or entirely occluded against the upper incisors, alveolar ridge, or hard palate, producing a sound resembling /t/ or /d/ or a dull, weak, distorted sibilant. If the tongue-tip is too high and also retracted, a whistling, overly sharp /s/ is produced. The position of the tongue may be too low, flat, or relaxed in the mouth so that the sound produced lacks sibilance and sounds dull or "mushy." In the anteroposterior plane the tongue may be too retracted so that the /s/ sound is more like /ʃ/, or it may be placed too far forward so that it touches the upper incisors or protrudes between the upper and lower incisors.

This latter *tongue protrusion or interdental* distortion is so common that it merits special designation as a subtype of the *central lisp*. It is frequently heard as one characteristic of infantile perseveration cases, often as a residual lingual habit formed when the upper deciduous incisors are lost and a space is left temporarily before the permanent incisors erupt. In this type of lisp, /s/ approximates /θ/ and /z/ approximates /ð/. All of the varieties of distortion just described as coming under the *central lisp* category have in common a faulty midline tongue position. Although the tongue is usually bilaterally symmetrical and emission of air centralized, the tongue is incorrectly positioned vertically, anteroposteriorly, or some combination of both.

In a *lateral lisp* the tongue-tip is pressed against the upper central incisors or alveolar ridge much as it is for the /l/ sound. The air stream cannot be emitted through a central groove but is divided and escapes at the sides of the mouth. In other cases the tongue moves to one side or the other of the midline and lifts or twists to touch the lateral teeth, forcing the air out over the opposite side of the tongue. The *lateral lisp* is so named because of this essential characteristic of unilateral or bilateral rather than central emission of breath. The acoustic result is conspicuous and highly unpleasant. It has a "slushy" sound as though an excess of saliva were present. This type of lisp is persistent and usually one of the most resistant to corrective training of the functional articulatory problems. Lateral lisps often have their origin in early irregularities or lateral spaces in the upper dental arch. Incorrect lingual habits are formed and often persist after the dental problem has been corrected. Most cases of lateral lisp have to be classified, therefore, as functional.

The third type of lisp, the *nasal lisp*, is relatively rare compared with the others. It is produced by a relaxed soft palate and retracted tongue which fail to effect a nasopharyngeal closure and allow air to escape through the nose. The result in some cases is a voiceless nasal fricative for /s/ and in others a more conspicuous and unpleasant snort.

Sibilant distortion can be produced by, or accompanied by atypical lip movements. Since good sibilant articulation depends upon the air shaft's passing between the incisal edges of the teeth, any approximation of the lips to the teeth constitutes an obstruction to the free passage of this air shaft. The lower lip may touch the upper teeth in a manner similar to the production of the /f/ sound and do this either symmetrically or to one side. Less often the upper lip is involved. These labial habits are unattractive visually as well as acoustically.

Lalling (*Distortion of /r/ or /l/*). *Lalling* is less well defined than *lisping* and yet represents a type of case encountered quite often clinically. The sounds affected are usually /r/ or /l/ or both, but other consonants for whose production the tongue-tip is important, such as /t/ or /d/, may also be involved. No clear-cut substitutions are made for these sounds. Rather there is a distortion of them in which the tongue is mainly at fault. The tongue-tip instead of being raised to the alveolar ridge for /l/ or approximating the alveolar ridge for /r/, is kept low in the mouth, the tongue is flat and lax, tongue movements are weak and sluggish, and the back of the tongue may be retracted and humped. Articulatory movements occur farther back in the mouth than normally. A sound resembling /w/ but without lip action may replace /r/ and /l/ or the result may more resemble a /j/ or the vowels /ə/ or /ɔ/.

Lalling resembles *general oral inaccuracy*, to be described later, in that tongue movements are sluggish and insufficiently energized. *Lalling* refers, however, to the distortion of this limited group of sounds whereas *general oral inaccuracy* involves most or all of the speech sounds.

Lalling, though usually functional, may also have an organic basis, past or present. Like the lateral lisp, it may have had its origin in an organic deviation which may or may not be present when the case comes to our attention. In cases where the lingual frenum has been tight, raising the tip of the tongue has been prevented. Even with surgical correction, if there is no subsequent speech training, the tongue may fail to develop the activity of which it is now capable and lalling speech continues on a functional basis. Damage to the nervous innervation of tongue muscles may also produce lalling. Cases of cerebral palsy with mild speech involvement often show this characteristic. In cases of lalling, therefore, both functional and organic possibilities must be explored.

Misarticulation of Other Miscellaneous Sounds. Most of the functional articulation cases will fall into the three groups just discussed or the one to follow. There are occasional cases which have difficulty with other sounds. A description of the possible forms of misarticulation of all the sounds will not be attempted here, but a few of the more common are: the labiodental fricatives /f/ and /v/, the linguadentals /θ/ and /ð/, the velar plosives /k/ and /g/, and the nasal /ŋ/.

For a detailed description of types of misarticulation of these and other speech sounds the reader is referred to Nemoy and Davis (1937), Koepp-Baker (1936), and Gray and Wise (1946). Perhaps the most detailed and clinically useful description in the literature on types of articulatory errors is given by Van Riper and Irwin (1958, Chapter 4).

2. General Oral Inaccuracy

In the types of articulatory disorder we have been discussing, the case can be expected to have difficulty with certain sounds or groups of sounds while his other sounds will be produced with relative accuracy. There are certain cases, however, in whom distortion and other forms of misarticulation seem general rather than specific. All or nearly all sounds are affected. The degree of severity of *general oral inaccuracy* can vary over a wide range. There are individuals whose articulation, though generally inaccurate, is only mildly so. Though their speech is unattractive it is perfectly understandable and no important communication handicap exists. At the other extreme are some of the most severely handicapped individuals to be seen in clinical practice, those whose speech, though possibly adequate enough in output or fluency, is nearly or completely unintelligible. In many cases of *general oral inaccuracy* there are obvious organic factors responsible. There are also, however, many cases where even the most careful study fails to reveal organic factors and which appear to be entirely functional in etiology.

To understand general oral inaccuracy it might be helpful to consider briefly what the motor requirements are for accurate articulation. First there must be *precision* of movement. Contacts or approximations of parts of the speech mechanism must be made at the right *place*, in the right *direction*, must involve the right *amount of contact surface*, and the right *shape*. Second, articulatory movements must be made at the right *speed*. Third, they must be made with sufficient *energy* or *pressure*. Finally, there must be *synergy* of the sequential movements of speech, an optimum temporal-spatial integration of movements.

In cases of general oral inaccuracy any or all of these aspects of articulation may be inadequate. Movements are approximate rather than precise, broad rather than small surfaces are sometimes contacted, and contacts are made at the wrong place. In some cases movements are fairly accurate but are slow, weak, or underenergized, so that, though contacts are made, they are not tight or firm. The speech is spoken of as "careless," "lazy," "sluggish," in its milder forms; "indistinct," "confused," "mutilated," "distorted," "unintelligible," in its more severe forms.

Writers in speech pathology have described certain of the characteristics of *general oral inaccuracy* in other terms. Van Riper (1963), the 1931 White House Conference report, Anderson (1953), and others speak of *oral inactivity* as one type of articulation problem. Another term used by several writers, *cluttering*, might well be classified here, too. *Cluttering*, as used by most, implies a rate and rhythm aspect as well as an articulation aspect to the deviate speech pattern.

Anderson (1953, p. 44), describing *oral inactivity*, says:

> In general, the speech of individuals exhibiting oral inactivity is either of the slow, sluggish type, or it is characterized by a rapid, slurring, often irregular, tempo sometimes described as "hitting the high spots." In both types many speech sounds are either omitted or are imperfectly formed, speech becomes unclear and distorted, and intelligibility is reduced.

Anderson is describing here as a form of *oral inactivity* what some have called *cluttering*.

In Prins' study (1962a), cited earlier, his Group IV was characterized by correlation of the variables studied with *nonphonemic distortions* in which *all articulatory features*—place, manner, voicing—were changed, either individually or in combination. This experimentally identified group appears similar to those cases the present writer describes as *general oral inaccuracy*. Basically, though varying in degree and kind, the defective speech patterns have an all-pervasive deficiency rather than one which is limited or specific. It seems appropriate, therefore, to group them together under the designation *general oral inaccuracy*.

Analysis of Misarticulation

Scientific analyses of misarticulation, whether made in connection with genetic studies of normal speech development or in connection with studies of deviate speech, are remarkably consistent in their findings. Some of the principal facts and conclusions are summarized briefly below.

SPECIFIC SPEECH SOUNDS MOST OFTEN DEFECTIVE

Comprehensive studies of defective articulation were made by Roe and Milisen (1942) and by Sayler (1949) working under Milisen's direction. In both studies large, unselected school populations were tested for articulation. Roe and Milisen studied the first six grades; Sayler, grades seven through twelve. Roe and Milisen (1942, p. 43) rank single consonants in the following order according to frequency of error (after eliminating minor voicing errors): /θ/, /s/, /t/, /ð/, /z/, /dʒ/, /tʃ/, /r/, /v/, /k/, /d/, /ʃ/, /g/, /f/, /p/, /l/, /b/, /ŋ/, /ʍ/, /w/. Of the ten most frequent in this list, six (/θ/, /s/, /ð/, /z/, /tʃ/, /v/) are also found among Sayler's 10 most frequent errors. In both studies two *s*-bends, /st/ and /sk/, ranked high among the single consonants in frequency of error, Roe and Milisen also ranking /str/ high. It is interesting that /r/, /l/, and /ʃ/, which most writers list as frequently defective, do not appear prominently in either of these lists. Van Riper's observations (1947, p. 152) that the most frequently mispronounced sounds are: /s/, /z/, /θ/, /ð/, /r/, /ʒ/, /l/, /tʃ/, /dʒ/, /ʃ/, /f/, /v/, with substitutions of /t/ for /k/ and /d/ for /g/ in young children, are typical of those of most authorities in speech pathology.

Hall (1938) found the most frequent errors among school children to be in rank order these nine: /s/, /z/, /ʃ/, /tʃ/, /dʒ/, /ʒ/, /ʍ/, /θ/, /r/; among college freshmen these seven: /s/, /z/, /dʒ/, /ʃ/, /tʃ/, /ʍ/, /ʒ/. Fairbanks and Spriestersbach (1950) found the same seven sounds heading the list for the college students in their study, though in slightly different rank order.

Pendergast and her associates (1966) gave an articulation screening test to 15,255 first-grade children, followed by a phonetic inventory for all children who had any errors on the screening test. The order of misarticulation of specific sounds and the percent of the total group who misarticulated each sound were as follows:

[s]	15.8	[l]	5.8
[θ]	14.4	[tʃ]	5.5
[z]	12.8	[dʒ]	3.5
[ð]	9.2	[f]	1.4
[r]	8.4	[k]	1.1
[v]	6.7	[g]	.8
[ʃ]	6.0		

Among the 10 most frequent errors in each of the five studies of school-age children cited above all five listed: /s/, /z/, /θ/, /tʃ/; four of the five listed: /ð/, /r/, /dʒ/; three of the five listed: /v/, /ʃ/; and two of the five listed: /l/, /ʒ/, /ʍ/.

TYPE OF SOUND MISARTICULATED

Genetic studies show that at any given age level among young children vowels are most correctly articulated, consonants next, and consonant blends least. Analysis of errors in articulation cases shows essentially the same result. Templin (1957, on the basis of an extensive study of articulation and other language skills in young children, states (p. 58), "In the early years, diphthongs, vowels, consonant elements, double-consonant blends, and triple-consonant blends are produced in that order from most to least accurate. This holds for both sexes and socioeconomic status groups, and other studies are in substantial agreement."

Although the progression from vowels and diphthongs to consonants and then to consonant blends is found both in the genetic development of articulation and in the errors characteristic of articulation cases at various ages, these stages are overlapping and increasing attention is being given to the exceptions to this rule. For example, Spriestersbach and Curtis (1951), reporting detailed studies of /s/ and /r/ articulation, show that these sounds are sometimes produced better in certain consonant blends than when preceded and followed by vowels.

MISARTICULATIONS IN RELATION TO MANNER, PLACE, AND VOICING

Numerous analyses have been made of the type of consonant most likely to be defective, from the standpoint of both *manner* of articulation and *place* of articulation. A finding of the Wellman et al. study (1931) was that in young children nasal consonants are easier than plosives (stops) and plosives easier than fricatives. No differences were found between voiced and voiceless consonants. Templin and Steer (1939), studying preschool children, also found nasals most correct, then plosives, semivowels, and fricatives in decreasing order, with consonant blends most defective. Backus (1943) observed that nasals are rarely defective; some glides, /w/ and /j/, rarely; others, /r/, often; that the most common plosive errors are /t/ for /k/ and /d/ for /g/; and that fricatives are the most frequently defective of the speech sounds. It can be said, therefore, that there is close agreement among the various writers that fricatives account for the great majority of articulation errors.

Pendergast et al. (1966) found that, contrary to some previous studies, voiceless sounds were defective more frequently than voiced sounds. Bricker (1967, p. 67) concluded from an analysis of specific articulation errors of young children "that more errors were associated with the place of articulation than with either the manner of articulation or the voiced-voiceless dimension."

TYPE OF MISARTICULATION

Sound substitutions and omissions are common in preschool and primary children and grow less frequent with increase in age. Sound distortions are relatively less frequent at these early age levels but tend to be the predominant type of misarticulation with increase in age. Wellman et al. (1931), reporting on consonant blends in children from two through six, found that substitutions and omissions decreased with age while approximations (distortions) and inconsistencies increased with age. Substitutions were more frequent in consonant blends than in single consonants, but omissions and inconsistencies less frequent.

Repeated testings of children as in the Roe and Milisen study (1942) have shown that sounds omitted or substituted for in the first test often show up as distortions in later tests, if still defective at all.

These results were substantiated by Wilson's (1966) study of the articulatory abilities of mentally retarded children, in which omission and substitution errors tended to decrease and distortion errors to increase with increasing mental age.

There is general agreement in these studies that omission errors are common at the early age levels and diminish with increasing age, that substitutions are also common early and diminish with age, and that distortions become the predominating error type with increasing age. This suggests that distortions are a transitional phase of articulation learning. It further suggests that for many children the learning of a consonant sound may progress through a sequence from omission to substitution to distortion, with the *degree* of distortion becoming less and less until the sound is mastered. McDonald (1964, pp. 97–99) has diagrammed this progression and described it in detail.

ERRORS IN RELATION TO POSITION IN WORD

Again there is a parallel between genetic development of speech and errors made by articulatory defectives. As cited above in connection with infantile perseveration, initial consonants tend to develop first, medials next, and finals last. Templin and Steer (1939), in their study of preschool children, found speech sounds most often correct in the initial position, next in the medial, and least in the final. Considering substitution errors alone, fewest were made in the initial position, with about equal numbers for medial and final positions. Omissions were less frequent than substitutions, and they occurred most often in the final position, next in the medial, and least in the initial position.

Templin (1943) in a later study of sound discrimination in elementary school children found more *discrimination errors* when a consonant or combination was in a medial or final position than when it was in an initial position. This suggests that the greater difficulty in discriminating medial and final sounds may account for the greater difficulty of articulating sounds in these positions.

INCONSISTENCY IN MISARTICULATION

Infantile perseveration cases are notoriously inconsistent in their misarticulations. A young child often omits a sound in some words, uses it correctly in others, and uses one or more substitutions for it in other words. Wellman et al. (1931) found that within the age range they studied, two through six, inconsistencies tended to increase with age.

Spriestersbach and Curtis (1951) cite several studies of misarticulation done under their direction at the State University of Iowa. A study by Amidon (1951) of 100 first-grade children found that on the average only 36.5 percent of the articulation errors observed in the responses of a given child occurred in all three positions in the words tested. Nelson (1945), Hale (1948), and Buck (1948) each tested a specific sound intensively in functional articulation cases; Nelson tested /s/ in children in the first six grades; Hale tested /s/ in children from kindergarten through third grade; and Buck tested /r/ in the same age range. From the data reported by Spriestersbach and Curtis (p. 484) the following summary can be made:

	PERCENTAGE OF SUBJECTS		
	NELSON [s]	HALE [s]	BUCK [R]
Consistent (sound normal in neither blends nor singles)	46.6	26.7	5.5
Inconsistent (sound normal in some phonetic contexts, misarticulated in others)	53.4	73.3	94.5

From these results, inconsistency appears to be typical rather than unusual or exceptional. Spriestersbach and Curtis concluded that inconsistencies in speech-sound production cannot be attributed to chance but are governed by variables which operate in a systematic, lawful fashion.

Perkins (1952), in a study of /s/ and /z/ articulation, also reached the conclusion that sound combinations are more influential than the position of the sound on the type and frequency of errors on /s/. For /z/, position had more importance. Nelson found less inconsistency of misarticulation in his older age group than in his younger, from which Spriestersbach and Curtis concluded that older children have become so strongly conditioned to the faulty sound production that maturation processes are no longer effective in producing improvement, the transitional state is past, and misarticulations are, therefore, more consistent.

The dependency on phonetic context demonstrated in these studies accounts to some extent for the inconsistencies which we observe in misarticulations. These research results also point up the importance of making a thorough evaluation in every case of functional articulation disorder, not only of the specific sounds misarticulated but also of the *specific phonetic contexts* in which misarticulations occur and in which the sounds are produced correctly.

Templin and Darley (1960) in their tests of articulation make provision for detailed analysis of misarticulation inconsistency. McDonald (1964) in his discussion of articulation problems bases his diagnostic and therapeutic approach largely on the facts of articulatory inconsistency and dependence upon phonetic context.

Factors Related to Misarticulation

MISARTICULATION IN RELATION TO AGE OR MATURATION

The relationship of age to growth in articulation at the lower age levels has already been discussed in connection with infantile perseveration. Results of studies on early speech-sound acquisition were summarized in Table 33-II. A number of investigators have also reported on misarticulations at the elementary and secondary school levels, in relation to age.

One of the earliest studies relating articulation difficulty to age was made by Root (1925). Data on the incidence of various disorders were secured by questionnaires. He found 2.6 percent of the total school enrollment to have problems of lisping and lalling, and these problems accounted for 41.2 percent of all speech defects found. Root did not give separate percentages for those labeled "indistinct speech" or "thick speech" but, if included, these would have increased the percentage of children who might be classified as *functional articulatory* cases. The incidence by grade of *lispers* and *lallers* is shown in Table 33-III. The decrease is rapid from grade to grade at first, then more gradual. There is an 82 percent decrease between grades I and IV.

Dawson (1929) investigated the development of *rate* of articulation with a series of six tests, such as repetition of numbers, of the alphabet, and so on. He found that children have not mastered all the articulation skills when they enter school; that there is a rapid increase of rate during the first three grades and then a more gradual increase above that level.

Francis (1930) surveyed school children for speech defects and found that functional articulatory defects amounted to 51.8 percent of all speech defects.

TABLE 33-III
Investigations on Misarticulation in Relation to Age*

GRADE	ROOT (1925) % OF SCHOOL POPULATION WITH LISPING OR LALLING	FRANCIS (1930) % OF SCHOOL POPULATION WITH ORAL INACCURACY	ROE AND MILISEN (1942) (GRADES I THROUGH VI) SAYLER (1949) (GRADES VII THROUGH XII)			WHITE HOUSE CONFERENCE REPORT (1931) NO. OF SOUND SUBSTITUTION CASES	
			ARTICULATION ERRORS				
			MEAN NO.	DIFFERENCE	CRITICAL RATIO	BOYS	GIRLS
Kindergarten		27.8					
I	5.70	19.3	13.30			3,854	2,533
II	3.60	11.5	9.99	3.31	6.89	2,684	1,725
III	2.50	9.9	8.85	1.14	2.71	1,916	1,042
IV	1.04	3.1	7.62	1.23	2.91	1,223	738
V	2.70	3.6	7.61	.01	.02	848	538
VI	1.01	2.1	8.01	−.40	−1.21	657	402
VII	0.60	2.6	3.92			277	175
VIII	1.00	4.7	4.31	.39	.72	190	108
IX		2.6	4.54	.23	.77	} 82	71
X		6.7	4.39	.15	.54	}	
XI		2.1	3.34	1.05	3.75	} 28	25
XII		4.7	3.25	.09	.32	}	
Number of cases		191	Grades I–VI, 1,989 Grades VII–XII, 1,998				

* Some modifications have been made here in the form of presentation of the data from the presentation in the original publications. In each case the author's own diagnostic terms are given in the table. The data presented in Table 33-III, all show misarticulations in relation to grade level though all are not comparable as to the measure used. Root and Francis report percentage of defectives in the school population, Roe and Milisen, and Sayler report mean number of errors made by unselected children and the White House data give numbers of speech defectives.

Percentages for the different grades are given in Table 33-III. Mills and Streit (1942) made a survey of speech defects in a school population and reported *dyslalia* as having the following percentages of incidence: grade one, 28.9; grade two, 22.2; grade three, 22.1; and grades above three, 0.9—a marked falling-off from the first to the upper grades. The White House Conference report of 1931 also gave incidences by grade and sex of "sound substitution" cases. These data are given in Table 33-III.

Notable among the studies of articulation defects in relation to age are the two investigations carried out at Indiana University under Milisen's direction—Roe and Milisen (1942) and an extension of this study by Sayler (1949). Unselected school populations were tested for articulation by trained speech therapists. The statistical results by grade for both studies are given in Table 33-III. Roe and Milisen found that a decreasing number of children make articulatory errors in each successive grade and that those who do make errors make fewer.

Morley (1952) has reported the results of speech tests given to incoming and transfer students at the University of Michigan over a 10-year period. There are minor fluctuations of incidence from year to year, but the incidence for the whole period is 3.85 percent classified as "clinical cases" out of the 33,339 tested. Articulation defects account for 50.7 percent of the "clinical cases," an incidence of 1.9 percent of the university enrollment tested.

Study of Table 33-III shows that in all sets of data included there is a decrease in misarticulation with increase in grade level up through at least grade four. With the exception of the White House data, the studies show only small decreases or no decreases at successive levels above grade four and up through grade 12. Misarticulation decreases rapidly from grade to grade from kindergarten up through grade four.

At that point it levels off and there is little further decrease due to maturation alone. The White House Survey report, based upon very large numbers, is less subject to chance errors of sampling. It shows an abrupt, then a more gradual but still continuous, decrease in numbers of articulation defects for all grades up through 12.

We can conclude that maturation and the speech stimulation provided by the school are effective for most children in producing rapid improvement in articulation during the early grade levels, that they are of only mild effectiveness from grades four through six, and above that level cease to be noticeably effective in improving articulation.

MISARTICULATION IN RELATION TO SEX

According to clinical experience and the findings of most investigations, the same preponderance of boys over girls holds true for functional articulation problems as for speech defects in general. In studies of early genetic development of articulation, sex differences have been found rather consistently. Wellman et al. (1931) found girls superior to boys on consonant elements, though sex differences on vowels were inconclusive. Poole (1934), Irwin (1952), and Templin (1952) all report sex differences in favor of girls in the development of articulatory skill.

Templin (1957) found that by eight years of age children reached essential maturity in articulation but that boys take about one year longer than girls to reach this level. Winitz and Lawrence (1961) found kindergarten girls superior to boys of the same age in learning unfamiliar, non-English speech sounds.

For school-age children, few satisfactory sex comparisons are available. Although numerous investigations report on sex differences for speech defects in general, few report on sex differences for functional articulation defects separately.

Root (1925, p. 537) reported sex ratios separately for each type of speech defect found. For the types which might be considered as coming within the general category of *functional articulatory* the ratio of boys to girls was as follows: *indistinct speech*, 2.5 to 1.0; *thick speech*, 1.4 to 1.0; *lisping* and *lalling*, 1.1 to 1.0. The sex ratio for all defects was 1.5 to 1.0.

Dawson (1929) found that girls articulated at a more rapid rate than boys and developed more rapidly in articulation up to 12 or 13 years of age. Then boys articulated more rapidly, reaching a higher level than girls in grade 12.

From the data reported by Mills and Streit (1942) it can be calculated that among *dyslalia* cases in the first three grades, 62 percent were boys and 38 percent girls. Above third grade the percentages were 70 and 30 respectively. School enrollment of boys and girls is not given, however, and these percentages would be of significance only if the enrollments of the two sexes were approximately equal. The authors concluded that boys exceed girls in all categories of articulatory defect, but that there is least difference in *sigmatism*.

Roe and Milisen (1942) found no significant difference between the mean number of articulation errors for boys and for girls in their tests of unselected children in grades one through six. Their study differs from most in that they report on *unselected* children, while most investigations are on children identified as speech defectives. Sayler (1949) in a continuation of this study into grades seven through 12, found no differences in the mean number of errors made by boys and girls but found, however, that slightly more boys than girls made errors in all grades but 12.

The present writer (Hall, 1938) found that among the grade two through six population used for her study, 8.4 percent of the boys and 3.3 percent of the girls had functional articulatory defects; and that at the college freshmen level 8.8 percent of the men students and 6.3 percent of the women had low ratings on articulation. Current data from the speech correction program in the Chicago Public Schools, under the writer's direction, show that, of the 132,211 boys in schools receiving speech correction service, 5.8 percent have been identified by the school speech therapists as having functional articulation disorders. Of the 129,136 girls, 3.5 percent have been so identified. This is a highly significant contrast, based as it is upon numbers of such size. Combining both sexes, the incidence of functional articulation disorders is 4.7 percent of the school population.

Morley's study of college students (1952) reports that, of the articulation cases found, 61.4 percent were males, 38.6 percent females, a ratio of 1.5 to 1.0. The number of men students tested, however, was considerably in excess of the number of women. Additional calculations on Morley's data by this writer show that the percentage of articulation defects among all men tested (19,730) was 1.95 percent and among all women tested (13,609) 1.78 percent. There is thus a slightly higher percentage of articulation cases among these men college students than among women. The difference, though small, may be significant in view of the very large number of cases involved.

Although there is some inconsistency in the conclusions reached in these studies, the weight of evidence supports a sex difference in favor of girls, both in the normal development of articulatory skill during the early years and in the smaller percentage of functional articulatory defects among girls throughout the entire educational range from preschool through college.

ETIOLOGY OF FUNCTIONAL ARTICULATION DISORDERS

Functional articulation disorders until recent years received little attention from research workers as compared with other disorders of speech. Lately there has been a mounting number of research studies, most of them—like most of the earlier ones—directed mainly toward the investigation of etiology. Although many good studies are now available to the student of speech pathology, their results are still inconclusive and often mutually contradictory.

Research has succeeded mainly so far in eliminating certain factors from consideration as causally related to articulatory defects rather than in showing what factors do have a causal relationship. In short, our research results to date are of more value for their negative than for their positive significance.

Textbooks in speech pathology are liberal in advancing many and diverse physical, mental, environmental, and emotional variables as underlying causal factors in these disorders. The factors suggested range from simple physical variables such as tongue size, lip mobility, *diadochokinesis* of the jaw, on through more complex variables such as auditory perceptual variations, to complex emotional problems reflecting child or parental maladjustment, at the other extreme.

The writer will review systematically the principal studies supporting or refuting the many etiological possibilities and will then attempt to integrate and evaluate them and to draw what conclusions are possible as to our understanding of functional articulation disorders at the present time.

The studies reported in the literature are, of course, of varying merit. Some have been done with little attention to sound research method and are little better than casual observation liberally salted with opinion. Others have been done with careful experimental design and results are presented in precise statistical form with proper attention to measures of reliability and significance of results. Some writers, in presenting their results, confuse *concomitant* factors with *causal* factors. The reader should keep this difference in mind so that unwarranted conclusions will not be drawn as to relationships between articulation problems and some of the variables studied.

Physical and Psychophysical Variables

The reader must bear in mind that, since we are considering *functional* articulation problems in this chapter, most of the physical variables discussed are to be thought of as in the order of *normal variations*, not *pathological variations*. If pathological variations are present and related causally to the speech deviation, the disorder would be *organic* rather than *functional* and would not come under discussion here.

ANATOMICAL FACTORS

Various writers have suggested the possibility of systematic differences between functional articulation cases and normal speakers in such anatomical variables as size and shape of the oral cavity, size and shape of the tongue, length of the lingual frenum, dental structure, relationship of upper and lower jaws, size of lips, and other more obscure variables. Actual research on anatomical variables has been meager.

Dental structure and palatal dimensions have been mentioned frequently in connection with articulation problems, but research results are inconclusive. Carrell (1936) studied the population of a children's institution and found no differences between a speech defective and a normal speech group in palatal malformations, dental abnormalities, or status of dental health.

Fymbo (1936) studied the relationship of malocclusion of the teeth to defective speech and found the severity of the speech defect varied directly with the severity of the dental anomaly. The following dental factors were found to be significantly related to defective speech: abnormal vertical relations of the jaws, edentulous spaces, especially those occurring among the eight anterior teeth, spacing of the teeth, and unusually high or low palate. Fymbo's speech-defective group, of course, was not limited to "functional" cases.

It is of equal significance, too, that Fymbo found that malocclusion of the teeth existed in 35 percent of his superior speech cases and 62 percent of his average speech cases as well as in 87 percent of his defective speech cases. Poor articulation is not a necessary consequence of all malocclusion, nor is it to be assumed that malocclusion is present in all articulation disorders.

A carefully designed study by Fairbanks and Lintner (1951) compared two groups of college students, one with superior consonant articulation and one with inferior consonant articulation, on four anatomical measures: cuspid width, molar width, palatal height, and maximum mouth opening. Their results support Fymbo in finding that marked dental deviations were significantly more numerous among the inferior speakers. Open-bite and close-bite were more numerous in the inferior group, open-bite being the greater factor in the difference. However, their results do not support Fymbo in other respects. Their superior and inferior ability groups did not differ significantly in the number of atypical anteroposterior relationships (overjet or undershot conditions) or in molar occlusion, anterior occlusion, anterior alignment, or anterior spaces. Neither were significant differences found in dimensions of the dental arch and hard palate (width and height).

Dental anomalies have been mentioned particularly in relation to lisping. Fymbo found the sibilant sounds /s/, /z/, /ʃ/, /ʒ/, /tʃ/, /dʒ/, and /θ/ and /ð/ most difficult for malocclusion cases. Froeschels and Jellinek (1941) found, however, that even in cases of interdental lisping with open-bite, the dental anomaly did not usually cause the lisping. In 800 such cases only three protruded the tongue through the opening formed by the abnormal teeth, all others lowering the jaw to make room. The authors suggest that the interdentality in speech produces the dental anomaly rather than the reverse.

Snow (1961), studying the articulation of /f/, /v/, /s/, /z/, /θ/, and /ð/ in children six to eight years of age, found that a significantly larger proportion of children with missing or abnormal upper central incisors misarticulated these sounds than children with normal teeth, although there were many exceptions. Bankson and Byrne (1962) studied articulation in relation to missing teeth in young children. Children who had produced sounds correctly on a pretest, on retest after a four-month period were more affected by loss of teeth during that period than were children who had produced sounds incorrectly on the pretest. More children changed from correct to incorrect initial and final /s/ following the loss of two or more teeth than did not change.

Tongue size and shape are other factors which have often been suggested as related to adequacy of articulation, particularly as the tongue relates to the size of the dental arches and the oval cavity as a whole.

Fairbanks and Bebout (1950) estimated size and shape of the tongue in the superior and inferior groups of college speakers referred to in the preceding section. Size was classified as small, average, or large, and shape as flat or bulged. The tongue tip (distance forward from the anterior margin of the frenulum) was also measured. They found no statistically significant difference in length of tongue-tip between their superior and inferior groups, and comparisons of tongue size and shape were inconclusive though primarily negative.

The size of the mouth opening and *thickness and shape of the lips* have also been mentioned as possibly related to articulatory efficiency. Again Fairbanks has included precise measurements of these factors as part of the study already mentioned in which speakers with superior and inferior articulation were compared. Fairbanks and Green (1950) measured the following: thickness of upper lip, thickness of lower lip, horizontal spread from corner to corner, and vertical length of upper lip in the midline. Although expected sex differences were found, no statistically significant differences were found between ability groups. The conclusion is drawn that lip dimensions are unrelated to articulatory ability. Estimates were also made of the anteroposterior and inferosuperior relations of the lips. Instances of protrusion of both lips and incomplete inferosuperior contact between the lips were more frequent among the inferior group, but this result was considered only tentative because of the small number of cases involved.

General anatomical comparisons, not limited to the speech mechanism, have also been made. Carrell's study (1936) referred to above, on comparison between defective and normal speech groups in a children's institution, included these anthropometric measurements: standing height, sitting height, weight, right and left grip, and vital capacity. The slightly speech-defective group did not differ significantly from the control group in any of these measures, but the severely speech-defective group was significantly inferior to the control group in all but standing height. The greatest difference occurred in vital capacity, a speech-related measure. The author concluded that the speech-defective children tended to be physically "weak" and deficient in their ability to make use of their physical possibilities.

SUMMARY OF ANATOMICAL FACTORS

The results of the studies cited on anatomical factors as related to articulation do not encourage us to feel that there is any systematic relationship. While all studies are fairly consistent in finding more anomalous jaw, dental, and tongue conditions among defective than among average speakers (and these would be considered organic, not functional cases), they are also remarkably consistent in finding no differences of significance in normal variations of any part of the speech mechanism. Functional articulation cases do not differ systematically from normal speakers in tongue size or shape, length or height of palate, or size of lips.

Then too, the human speech mechanism has remarkable compensatory capacities. Many individuals make adaptations, even without special training, to anomalies of the speech mechanism. If an individual can produce a speech sound correctly in any context at all, it is probably safe to assume that his misarticulations of the sound are not due primarily to an anatomical deviation he may possess. We should be cautious in assuming that when anomalies are present and articulation is defective, the speech is necessarily a result of the observed anomaly. It is always wise to evaluate other causal possibilities as well.

MOTOR COORDINATION

Another area in which the explanation of functional articulatory problems has been pursued even more vigorously is that of motor coordination, both of the body as a whole and within the speech mechanism specifically. Since speech is admittedly a complex process of delicate muscular adjustments, it has been natural to suppose that cases in which articulation was defective might have less than average precision, speed, strength, or control of movement. A substantial number of investigations has attempted to throw light on this problem.

General bodily coordination and control have been investigated as possibly related to articulatory defectiveness. Wellman et al (1931) found in children two to six years of age a correlation between number of sounds correctly articulated and performance on a tracing path and a perforation test. With age held constant, however, this might not have been found since both abilities are highly correlated with age.

Carrell (1937) compared a speech-defective with a control group on a number of tests, including a tapping, a tracing, and a "tensiometer" test. The latter tested "kinesthetic imagery" and involved the arms. For all tests the control group was superior to the speech defectives (sound-substitution cases), but the differences had low statistical reliabilities. Differences were greatest between the controls and the most defective subgroup of the speech-defective group.

Major (1940) found that speech defectives (all types mixed) tended to be inferior to normals on thirteen tests, including simple and multiple choice, reaction time, rhythm, speed of tapping, and eye-hand coordination. The results, however, were recognized as not applying to speech defectives as a whole because of the large number of stutterers included. They were inconclusive so far as articulation cases are concerned.

Bilto (1941) tested 34 stutterers and 56 articulation cases (organic problems excluded) between nine and 18 years of age and children without speech defects, on three tests: the Brace Motor Ability test battery, the Nielsen and Cozens' Jump and Reach test (which measures ability to develop power), and his own eye-hand coordination test. Both the stuttering group and the articulation group were inferior to the normal speech group on all three of the tests.

Mase (1946) investigated six factors commonly cited as causes of articulatory defects. One of them was coordination of gross muscles, which was tested by means of a rail-walking test. Boys in grades five and six with articulatory problems were carefully matched with normal speakers for age, I.Q., and socioeconomic status. He found no reliable difference between the groups in general muscular coordination as tested by the rail-walking test.

Albright (1948) and Maxwell (1953) made a particularly detailed and careful investigation of the relation between articulation ability and motor coordination and control, both in the gross, skeletal musculature and in the speech mechanism itself, the latter during both speech and nonspeech activities. Albright found significant differences between good and poor college speakers on three of the tests of motor skill (synchronometer, Miles speed rotor, and speech-rate test) and on three of the four tests of articulatory skills (/lɑ/, /tʌkə/, and /mu/, but not the teeth-click). The greatest difference was found on the synchronometer, and Albright accounts for this by pointing out that this test involved a factor of auditory-motor coordination in addition to the rhythm factor found in other tests. Positive but low intertest correlations were found, indicating that the skills measured were relatively independent.

Maxwell (1953) also studied the relationship between both general and specific motor skills and articulation. He used 13 boys with defective articulation at each of three age levels, seven, eight, and nine years, and an equal number of control boys at these levels, with good speech. His battery included tests to measure the following: 1. speed of diadochokinetic movements of tongue, lips, and jaws, using the number of repetitions in two seconds of /pɑ/, /tɑ/, /kɑ/, /lɑ/, and the combination /pɑtɑ kɑ/; 2. speed of diadochokinetic movements of the hand, measured by tapping, and a ball-bounce test; 3. accuracy of eye-hand coordination, measured by dotting, tracing, putting pellets in a bottle, and a form board; 4. hand steadiness, measured by a cube-stacking test; 5. station, as measured by eight tests from Variable One of the Oseretsky scale; and 6. gait, as measured by four walking tests.

Maxwell found reliable differences between his good and poor articulation cases on only the following: repetition of /pɑtɑkɑ/; of /lɑ/ (at eight- and nine-year levels only); speed and accuracy of movement required to perform the tracing and the pellet and bottle tests with the nonpreferred hand; tapping and bouncing tests (seven-year level only), and steadiness, as measured by the cube-stacking test. He concluded (p. 50), "There was no difference between the children with normal speech and children with articulatory speech defects in their ability to repeat /tɑ/, to dot rapidly, to perform the pellet and bottle test with the preferred hand, to perform the Seguin Form Board test, and in their ability to control the coordination required to perform tests of station and gait."

Dickson (1962) compared 30 children in grades one through three who had spontaneously outgrown functional articulation errors with a similar group who had retained their errors. On the Oseretsky Tests of Motor Proficiency the children who retained errors were inferior in gross motor tasks to those who outgrew them.

Laterality was studied in relation to articulation by Johnson and House (1937), who compared articulatory defective children with normal speakers on tests of ocular and hand dominance. Their conclusion was that handedness, as measured, tends to be related to severe functional articulatory defects, but that the findings with regard to eyedness were not significant. In opposition to these results, Everhart (1953) found no significant relationship between articulatory defectiveness and handedness in children in grades one through six.

Motor coordination and control within the speech mechanism have been approached specifically in a number of studies, as well as included as part of some of the studies cited above.

Karlin, Youtz, and Kennedy (1940) concluded from a small study comparing speech-defective with normal-speaking children that motor speed, among other factors, may operate to produce dyslalia. Mase (1946), in a well-controlled study of boys in grades five and six, compared articulatory defectives and normal speakers on a number of tests of various functions. Included were five tests for speed of various actions of the speech mechanism: moving tongue from corner to corner of mouth, opening mouth and closing lips alternately, touching a tongue depressor with the tongue-tip, stretching and rounding the lips alternately, and repeating "daddy" rapidly. He found no significant differences on any of these tests between his defective and his control groups. Lip mobility was the only test in which a significant difference was approached.

Fairbanks and Spriestersbach (1950), in part of a larger study under Fairbanks' direction, cited earlier, compared college students with superior and with inferior articulatory ability on the rate at which they could perform the following repetitive movements: approximation of upper and lower lips, vertical movement of the mandible, tongue to alveolar ridge, and tongue protrusion. Only small differences were found between ability groups. A significant difference was found only for lip movement and only for the male. These results agree almost perfectly with those of Mase, reported above. In speed of movement the speech structures ranked as follows in descending order: lips, mandible, tongue-alveolar, tongue protrusion.

In another part of the same study Fairbanks and Bebout (1950) measured maximum length of tongue protrusion, tongue force, and percentage of error in duplicating a tongue position. Again no differences between ability groups, sex constant, were significant. A significant sex difference in favor of males was found only for tongue force.

Palmer and Osborn (1940) in an earlier study found results contradictory to those of Fairbanks and Bebout. Within a larger group of individuals used for their experiment was a group of 44 articulatory cases, ages six to 36, from which cases with known organic defects were excluded. They were matched for age and sex with normal speakers and both groups tested for tongue pressure. A significant difference was found in favor of the control group. No significant sex differences were found in either group. A factor which may partially account for the difference in results from those of Fairbanks and Bebout is the greater frequency of malnutrition, febrile and wasting diseases which Palmer and Osborn report among their articulatory cases, as compared with their controls. As the authors themselves indicate, it is known that in all lowered physiological conditions there is diminished tongue strength.

SUMMARY OF MOTOR COORDINATION AND CONTROL FACTORS

The results of these studies on motor coordination, viewed as a whole, are discouragingly contradictory and inconclusive. For nearly every type of motor skill investigated, some studies have found differences between good and poor articulation groups, some have been inconclusive, and others have found no differences.

For motor abilities not involving the speech mechanism, fewest differences seem to have been found in general bodily control, strength, and speed (Mase and Albright rail-walking and Maxwell's tests of station and gait), though Bilto's results contradict this (Brace Motor Ability tests and the jump and reach test). Tests of hand speed and reaction time have been inconclusive or negative in regard to differences for the most part (Major, reaction time; Major, Albright, and Maxwell, tapping; Albright, writing rate, hand steadiness).

The tests which have seemed to show most difference are those involving eye-hand or auditory-hand coordination, rather than simple speed, strength, or steadiness (Albright's synchronometer and speed rotor; Bilto's eye-hand coordination test; the tracing tests used by Wellman et al., Carrell, and Maxwell; and Maxwell's cube-stacking test). The inconsistency of even these results is exemplified, however, by Maxwell's finding of a difference between ability groups for the pellet-and-bottle test when the non-preferred hand was used but no difference when the preferred hand was used.

One would perhaps expect logically that if any differences in motor coordination were present in relation to articulatory skill, these differences would show up most in the motor skills involving the speech mechanism itself. Here again we find highly contradictory and inconclusive results. Let us first mention a few points of consistency. Neither Fairbanks and Spriestersbach nor Albright (teeth-click test) found a difference between ability groups in vertical movements of the mandible. Mase and Fairbanks and Spriestersbach found no difference for any type of nonspeech tongue movement (speed or extent). Apparently no investigator has so far been able to demonstrate significant differences in tongue movements in articulatory defectives apart from speech. Both Mase and Fairbanks and Spriestersbach found slight differences between ability groups in lip movements only.

Results have been more likely to show differences when actual speech movements have been tested. Both Albright and Maxwell found significant differences between articulatory defectives and normal speakers for rapid repetition of syllables such as /lɑ/, but particularly for more complex patterns, /pɑtɑkɑ/ or /tʌkə/. Even here differences were not striking and there was much overlapping of ability groups.

In regard to tongue pressure or force, the results of Palmer and Osborn and of Fairbanks and Bebout are contradictory. The former found a significant difference, the latter did not.

The many discrepancies in the studies reviewed can be accounted for in part by differences in methods, in the tests used, in the way cases were selected for comparison, in the success with which other variables than the one being measured were eliminated, and by the rigor with which statistical tests of significance were applied. All of these explanations together, however, do not account for the lack of a more unified picture emerging from such an impressive mass of scientific research. A more probable explanation is that there are actually not any great and consistent motor differences between individuals with superior and with inferior articulation skill. When we are dealing with small differences anyway, then differences in research methodology, which in this field lacks the precision of the physical sciences, can be expected to yield inconsistent results. Even in those studies which found significant differences between ability groups, the differences were neither large nor consistent. Within the functional articulatory groups there were always some cases whose performance was average or superior. There is not even one motor variable which is reported by all investigators as showing a consistently negative deviation for all articulatory cases. When the means for groups barely reach significance criteria the test in question has little predictive value. Obviously the clinician cannot assume negative deviation in any motor skill for a given case but must study each case independently.

It is possible that certain types of functional articulation defectives, if separated out, might show more marked differences in motor skill than have been shown for the group as a whole. Most investigators have realized that it is unprofitable to lump together all types of speech defectives in making comparisons with normal speakers. It is probably also unwise to lump together all types of functional articulation cases in making such comparisons. There would seem to be a strong possibility, for example, that the type of case designated earlier in this chapter as *general oral inaccuracy* might show more marked and consistent negative deviations in motor skill than cases of lisping or infantile perseveration. The possibility seems well worth investigating.

Many speech pathologists have postulated a weakness of the intrinsic muscles of the tongue, particularly the longitudinal muscles, as responsible for various forms of misarticulation. Inability to groove the tongue by raising its edges has been advanced as a reason for lateral and interdental lisping by Froeschels (1933). This motor skill has apparently been neglected in exact, scientific investigation in spite of its frequent mention in clinical observations. It was not tested in any of the research studies reviewed above but may be another possibility worth investigation.

TONGUE-THRUST OR VISCERAL SWALLOWING

In recent years many clinicians have shown interest in the possible relationship between a visceral or tongue-thrust pattern of swallowing and failure to develop correct articulation. Both etiological and practical therapeutic aspects of this issue have been widely discussed. A few research studies throw some light on the subject.

Fletcher et al. (1961) studied swallowing patterns and sibilant articulation in 1,182 children in grades one through four, and 433 in upper grades and high school. The subjects with tongue-thrust swallowing were found more likely to have sibilant distortion than those without such a swallowing pattern. It is of interest that tongue-thrust swallowing was still found in 21 percent of 18-year-olds.

However, most of the studies show less, if any, relationship between swallowing patterns and articulation. Ward et al. (1961) studied 358 children in grades one through three. Visceral swallowing was found in 75 percent of the group, dental malocclusion in 47 percent, and articulation variations in 64 percent. They concluded that visceral swallowing is typical of children at these age levels. They identified a syndrome of forward placement of the tongue-tip sounds, tongue-thrusting in swallowing, and incipient malocclusion, a syndrome which may be significant in persistence of articulation variations and in determining the optimum age for speech correction.

Bell and Hale (1963) in evaluating 353 five- and six-year-old children, found 82 percent tongue-thrust swallowers, and concluded that this is the normal pattern. Of the tongue-thrusters 89 percent, and of the nontongue-thrusters 92 percent, articulated the test sounds in a dental or interdental position.

Jann et al. (1964) studied 281 unselected children in grades one to three over a two-year period. The tongue-thrust syndrome was found in the majority of the group; and, maturation alone did not appear to reduce this incidence appreciably over the two-year period of the study. Lewis and Counihan (1965) observed 294 newborn infants, finding 286 (97 percent) to have tongue-thrust. Eight infants without tongue-thrust were considered to have feeding problems. They raised the question as to what causes the abnormal *persistence* of tongue-thrust which, they conclude, is a normal condition in infants.

Subtelny et al. (1964) did an elaborate radiographic study of subjects with normal occlusion and normal speech, with malocclusion and normal speech, and with malocclusion and defective speech. Their study resulted in many interesting findings, one of which is pertinent here. Tongue-thrust and malocclusion were found to coexist with both normal speech and defective speech.

Hoffman and Hoffman (1965), in their comprehensive review of tongue-thrust and deglutition, stated (p. 117): "Tongue-thrusting is a speech problem: 1. if it interferes with or prevents the proper production of speech sounds when the child is able to make the necessary tongue movements and placements to improve or correct these sounds; 2. when tongue-thrusting persists after space is available in the oral cavity for the tongue; or 3. when tongue-thrust is observed as a concomitant of a condition which ordinarily responds to speech therapy." One of their conclusions was that tongue-thrusting may be a speech or an orthodontic problem or both or neither. They advise the speech pathologist to decide on the merits of each case whether or not training in compensatory tongue movements and placements is possible or advisable.

SENSORY FACTORS: AUDITORY

Because of the known closeness of relationship between speech and hearing, most writers in speech pathology have regarded auditory processes as the most promising direction in which to search for factors which might explain functional articulatory disorders. Every aspect of audition—basic acuity for pure tones, acuity for the higher frequencies, pitch discrimination, speech-sound discrimination, auditory memory span, perception for complex auditory patterns—has received attention. There is hardly an aspect of auditory behavior which has not been investigated in at least several research studies. Audition has been the most thoroughly explored of all the causal possibilities advanced to account for functional articulation disorders. Despite this, our information about the relationship of hearing processes to articulation remains equivocal. However, the past 10 years have produced some new approaches to the study of auditory factors which seem fruitful.

Auditory Acuity. Since serious hearing loss is known to affect the development and maintenance of good articulation, many speech pathologists have thought it possible that functional articulatory cases might have slight degrees of hearing loss, not observable behaviorally. Hearing loss, perhaps, at certain frequencies only, particularly high frequencies, has been considered also as a possible factor in these cases. These hypotheses have been subjected to several experimental tests.

Barnes (1932) tested university freshmen on the Western Electric 4-A Audiometer and on an articulation test. He found no relation between their articulation ratings and their hearing test results. Carrell (1936) compared sound substitution cases with normal speakers on the 4-A Audiometer and found the sound substitution group inferior. He stated, however, that though suggestive, it could not be concluded from these results that hearing defects have etiological significance in the consideration of speech disorders.

Hall (1938) administered individual threshold tests on the Western Electric 2-A Audiometer to articulatory defectives and their matched normal-speaking controls at two age levels, university freshmen and elementary-school children in grades two through six. At both age levels studied there were slight differences between speech-defective and normal speakers at every frequency, but the differences were not statistically significant. All composite auditory measures—average of middle frequencies, average of lower four, average of upper four, and average of all eight—also showed differences in favor of the control groups, but none of statistical significance.

Karlin, Youtz, and Kennedy (1940) found hearing loss, especially at higher frequencies, in a group of six articulatory defectives, as compared with matched controls, but their cases are too few to give their results significance.

Sullivan (1944, p. 128) reported results of Maico D6 pure-tone audiometer tests of 25,708 Minneapolis school children. "A hearing loss was defined as a diminution of ten decibels from the normal sensitivity in either ear." Percentages of children with hearing loss were as follows: without speech defects, 18.8; all speech-defectives, 22.2; functional articulatory cases alone, 20.3. Measures of significance are not given, but from the above results it is obvious that the slight difference between normal speakers and functional articulatory defectives is probably without significance. It is interesting and may be significant that the small group of 56 "oral inactivity" cases had a higher percentage, 25.0, of hearing loss.

Mase (1946) compared boys with functional articulation disorders and their matched controls on the Maico D5 Audiometer. Differences between the two groups did not reach the critical one-percent level of significance, though four measurements were within the questionable one- to five-percent level. Differences were more pronounced when the upper three frequencies were analyzed. His results, therefore, are inconclusive in regard to auditory acuity.

Rossignol (1948) investigated the relationships among hearing acuity, speech production, and reading performance of unselected children in grades 1A, 1B, and 2A. She found a zero correlation between articulation of speech sounds in familiar words and hearing acuity. She found, however, a low but statistically significant correlation between hearing acuity and ability to repeat nonsense syllables, which tested ability to produce new sound combinations. She also found low but significant correlations between hearing acuity and reading and between reading and articulation. Rossignol says (p. 30), "It is possible to infer from these data that hearing acuity is more important when the child is learning to say a new word than when he is articulating a word that is familiar to him. It is also possible that hearing acuity is more important in the earlier stages of acquiring speech than in the stage investigated in the present study."

To summarize, the results of the studies cited are inconclusive as to the relation between auditory acuity and functional articulation problems. Karlin, Youtz, and Kennedy, who studied very few cases, and Carrell found differences in auditory acuity in favor of normal speakers. Barnes, Hall, Mase, Sullivan, and Rossignol did not find significant differences, though

Mase's results suggest the possibility of more incidence of high-frequency loss among functional articulatory defectives. Sullivan's results raise the possibility, furthermore, that "oral inactivity" cases may possibly be an exception.

The weight of evidence, therefore, is against there being a significant deficiency in auditory acuity in functional articulatory cases. At least we can conclude with confidence that there is no general tendency for these cases to show hearing loss and, therefore, that this appears not to be a major etiological factor. This does not eliminate the ever-present possibility of hearing loss in individual cases, however, and it remains our obligation to exclude this possibility in the examination of every functional articulation case for whom therapy is undertaken.

In an attempt to probe still further into the auditory processes as they relate to speech, several investigators have compared normal and defective speakers on the Seashore Measures of Musical Talent. Travis and Davis (1927) administered three of these measures, pitch, intensity, and tonal memory, to college freshmen in inferior, standard, and superior speech groups. The inferior group included various types of speech defectives. They concluded that certain types of speech-defective cases as a group have lower scores than normal speakers and greater variability. All groups overlapped, however, and had a similar range of distribution.

Stinchfield (1927) and Gilkinson (1943), also using Seashore tests, found little difference between good and poor speakers. Mase (1946), using the rhythm and tonal memory tests, also found no reliable difference between boys with good and with poor articulation. A more recent study (Mange, 1960) used three of the Seashore tests (pitch, loudness, and timbre), a test of auditory flutter fusion rate, and a test of word synthesis with matched groups of children with functional misarticulation of /r/, and with normal speakers. He found a low but significant partial correlation between phonetic word synthesis ability and number of articulation errors but no significant relationship between the other auditory abilities tested and number of errors. The control group was significantly higher than the experimental group on pitch discrimination.

Sommers et al. (1961) gave the pitch subtest of the Tilson-Gretsch Music Test to matched groups of children with /r/ or /s/ errors and normal speakers and found the defective speech group inferior in mean pitch discrimination.

The above studies which have explored discrete auditory discrimination skills have shown little or no difference between groups with good articulation and groups with poor articulation. The one exception is pitch discrimination, which several of the studies found inferior in the misarticulation group.

SPEECH-SOUND DISCRIMINATION

Of all auditory factors suggested as having a possible causal relationship to functional articulation defects, the most generally advanced is a specific deficiency in speech-sound discrimination. Most writers have considered this factor to have at least some importance both in the development of articulation defects and in the retraining program for individuals with functional articulation problems. Speech-sound discrimination has been investigated as a *normal* developmental skill and as a factor which may be deficient in certain children.

Templin's classic study (1957) established beyond doubt that improvement in speech-sound discrimination ability is a function of chronological age. She found a fairly consistent increase in this ability up through eight years of age, the highest age studied. She found a tendency for girls to exceed boys and children of upper socioeconomic groups to exceed children from lower groups in this ability. Numerous other writers have supported Templin's finding of increased ability with age, notably Wepman (1960) and Weiner (1967). Both of them consider slowness in developing speech-sound discrimination a factor in articulation defects.

Lupella (1967) found in children ages three through seven that analysis and synthesis of speech sounds improved with chronological age. However, overlapping of age groups indicated that performance was not primarily a function of chronological age as such but of the relative maturity of the perceptual functions involved.

Schlanger and Galanowsky (1966) related increase in discrimination ability to mental as well as chronological age, finding intellectually normal children, though several years younger chronologically, superior to mentally retarded children of the same mental ages.

The relationship of speech-sound discrimination ability to functional defects of articulation has been extensively investigated experimentally over the years. Until recent years most of the studies involved a comparison of matched groups of functional articulation defectives with normal speakers. Various age levels have been studied and a variety of techniques used.

Travis and Rasmus (1931) developed an original test of speech-sound discrimination and compared normal and defective speakers at the elementary school level and at university freshman level. At every age level their articulation cases made significantly more errors than the normal speakers. Carrell (1937), using a modification of the Travis-Rasmus test, found defective speakers somewhat inferior to normals, but the two groups were not so clearly differentiated as in the Travis-Rasmus study. Barnes (1932) used the same test but found no relation between speech-sound discrimination and articulation in university freshmen.

The present writer (Hall, 1938), also using the Travis-Rasmus test, compared functional articulatory cases with carefully matched good speakers at two age levels, university freshmen and elementary school children. At neither level was a significant difference found. The two groups were also compared on an original test requiring sound discrimination in more complex auditory patterns. Again no differences were found between good and defective speakers.

Several other careful studies have failed to find differences between functional articulation cases and normal speakers. Mase (1946) compared boys in grades five and six with articulation defects with matched normal speakers on original tests of discrimination. There was no significant difference between groups although both groups showed great variation in skill. Hansen (1944) applied a vowel-discrimination test, the Seashore test of timbre, and a short form of the Travis-Rasmus test to three groups of college students: untrained functional articulatory defectives, functional articulatory defectives who had received speech therapy, and normal speakers. He found no differences between any of these groups for any of the three measures used. Dickson (1962) found that the Templin Short test of Sound Discrimination did not differentiate between children in primary grades who had outgrown functional articulation errors spontaneously and children who had retained their errors.

On the other side of the ledger there have been a number of studies, similar in method and subjects, in which differences *have* been found between functional articulatory defectives and normal speakers. Donewald (1950) compared functional articulatory defectives with normal speakers in first and second grade on a test consisting of 100 paired sounds. A significant difference was found between groups. Kronvall and Diehl (1954) compared 30 children with functional articulatory defects and matched controls on the Templin Speech Sound Discrimination Test. The controls made significantly fewer errors than the articulation cases. This result was supported in a later study involving one of these authors (Cohen and Diehl, 1963), again using the Templin test. A group of 30 children in grades one through three with severe functional articulatory defects were compared with 30 normal controls. Speech-sound discrimination ability tended to improve with grade level, but at all levels the controls were superior to the defective articulation group.

Farquhar (1961) found in a study of kindergarten children that auditory discrimination tests did not have much prognostic significance. However, children with mild articulatory defects were more proficient in discriminating and imitating the correct form of a misarticulated sound than the children with severe articulatory defects.

Schiefelbusch and Lindsay (1958) studied speech-sound discrimination in a new and interesting way, using three methods of presentation of pictures: naming of pictures by the tester, naming aloud by the child, and silent identification by the child. Two groups of first- and second-grade children were compared, one a group of articulatory defectives, the other normal speaking controls. Tests involved three types of discrimination: rhyming, initial sounds, and final sounds. Articulation cases were inferior to their controls in the discrimination test as a whole and in each of the three types of discrimination. The comparison of the various methods of presentation produced inconclusive results but no evidence that speech-defective children have greater difficulty than normal speakers in discerning self-monitored sound patterns.

Haller (1967) compared first- and second-grade functional articulatory defectives with matched normal speakers on nonsense syllable and word discrimination tests presented in a quiet environment and under three levels of background speech. Background speech affected both groups adversely, but the defective speakers showed a greater decrement under the most unfavorable condition of background speech.

Sherman and Geith (1967) approached the study of speech-sound discrimination in relation to articulation from the opposite direction. They began by testing speech-sound discrimination in 529 kindergarten children, then selected the 18 with the highest and the 18 with the lowest discrimination scores. These two discrete groups were then compared on the Templin-Darley Picture Articulation Test with the conclusion that low speech-sound discrimination ability is in general causally related to poor articulation.

The results of the numerous studies reviewed are conflicting and inconclusive though the weight of evidence may be somewhat on the side of an inferiority in speech-sound discrimination in functional articulation defectives as compared with normal speakers. It still appears doubtful to this writer that a *systematic, generalized* inferiority exists in *all* or most articulation cases. More probable is the concept of speech-sound discrimination inferiority in severe cases.

Even more probable is the concept, increasingly stressed in recent years by speech pathologists, that functional articulation cases may have speech-sound discrimination problems with *specific sounds* or *sound groups* even though not with all. It has been repeatedly emphasized in both theoretical discussions and some research studies that inferiority in speech-sound discrimination may be specific for the sounds an individual misarticulates himself. In other words, he may misarticulate certain speech sounds because he does not discriminate them.

This concept is not inconsistent with a conclusion that a *group* of functional articulation cases may not differ significantly from a *group* of normal speakers over the whole gamut of speech sounds. Group results may have masked a relationship in individual cases between discrimination errors and articulation errors.

Templin (1943) investigated the relation between discrimination errors and the position of the discriminative element in syllables. She found that children in all grades made more errors when the element to be discriminated was in the medial and final position. As reported earlier, articulation errors are also more frequent in those positions.

Spriestersbach and Curtis (1951, p. 486), recognizing that individuals with defective articulation have no generalized inability to discriminate speech sounds, go on to say, ". . . the assumption is nevertheless logical that certain individuals who misarticulate a given sound may not have developed fully effective awareness of that particular phonetic entity." They report a study by Anderson (1949) done under their direction in which children, kindergarten through fourth grade, judged to have defective /s/ articulation were given an articulation test involving /s/ in different word positions and phonetic combinations, and a speech-sound discrimination test using the same words. She found a difference between the percentage of /s/ discrimination errors in contexts in which the subjects misarticulated /s/ and the percentage in contexts in which they had no articulation difficulty, more errors being made in the former. Sound-omission errors tended to be more related to discrimination than sound-substitution errors.

Summers (1953) investigated the relationship between the ability to perceive the different speech sounds and to analyze and produce these sounds, using normal speakers as subjects. He found that sounds are perceived most accurately in the initial position but are analyzed and produced most accurately in the final position. Those sounds perceived most accurately were also most accurately analyzed and produced. Speech-sound discrimination was correlated with speech-sound perception but not with speech-sound analysis-production.

Winitz and Lawrence (1961) found that kindergarten children with good and with poor articulation were equally facile in learning new, non-English sounds. This finding, they felt, contraindicated the presence of any factor, physical or psychological, which would inhibit learning of sounds. Organic factors could have been operative but were clearly no longer operative. When learning conditions were made similar, differences between children with good and poor articulation were not apparent in rate or level of sound learning.

Prins (1963) analyzed articulation errors and speech-sound discrimination errors of six-year-old children with functional articulation defects and normal speaking controls. He found a significant correlation between the sound discrimination test score and articulation errors in which only one feature of the intended phoneme was altered and in which the place of articulation was altered one degree. Children who tended to confuse place of articulation (bilabial, linguadental, etc.) during production also had difficulty in discriminating minimal word pairs in which place of production was altered in a single phoneme. Prins concluded that poor speech-sound discrimination could be regarded as an effect of disturbance in the total language learning process rather than as a primary limitation of etiological significance in defective articulation.

Aungst and Frick (1964) studied children with misarticulation of /r/ alone, applying four discrimination tests. They found that ability on the Templin Test of Auditory Discrimination was unrelated to ability to judge the correctness of their own speech production; that ability as measured on traditional sound-discrimination tests was unrelated to consistency of articulation; and that ability to judge their own production *was* significantly related to consistency of articulation.

To summarize, although there is considerable doubt as to the existence of generalized inferiority in speech-sound discrimination in functional articulation defectives, the studies just reviewed demonstrate clearly that functional articulation defectives probably have at least limited and selective difficulties in sound discrimination, particularly in relation to the speech sounds they themselves misarticulate. On the other hand, some writers have reversed the causal sequence and have suggested that poor discrimination of specific sounds may be the result, not the cause, of misarticulations of these sounds.

Auditory Memory Span. Over a long period of years the texts in speech pathology have stressed the hypothesis that functional articulatory defects may be determined in part by deficiencies in auditory memory. Most authors suggest specific tests for measuring this ability and some give suggestions for retraining which take this factor into account.

Robbins and Robbins (1937) suggest methods for improving poor auditory memory span, which they consider an important cause of articulation defects. Backus (1943, p. 133), speaking of short auditory memory span as a cause of articulatory defects, says: "This condition does not predicate poor hearing in the usual sense of that term. It means that the child's range of memory for the time order of sounds has not developed normally for his age." West, Kennedy, and Carr (1947) mention short auditory memory span as a possible factor in dyslalia and suggest remedial measures. Van Riper (1963) suggests several tests for auditory memory span and several remedial procedures, indicating that some individuals, though not most, have difficulty in this area. Anderson (1953) stresses the importance of auditory memory span in speech development and points out that memory span is a product of maturation, and that in some children it develops more slowly than in others. He feels that where memory span is delayed in maturing, speech development is also likely to be retarded.

A number of experimental investigations have also been made of auditory memory span in functional articulation cases. Anderson (1938) developed two tests to measure auditory memory, one composed of vowels, one of consonants, and established norms for college students. He found that memory span for speech sounds, especially vowels, seemed independent of phonetic training. He found no relationship between auditory memory span and either pitch discrimination or auditory acuity but found a relationship with ability in learning a foreign language. He considered the vowel test particularly satisfactory for measuring auditory memory span. In 1939 Anderson reported that the memory span for speech sounds is lower than accepted norms for digits.

Metraux (1942 and 1944) used an adaptation of Anderson's tests and developed age norms. She found an increase with age in auditory memory span for both consonants and vowels, found no difference between boys and girls in auditory memory span, and found no significant correlation between mental age and auditory memory span.

Robbins (1942) published results of a study of auditory memory span for digits, phonemes, and syllables, comparing cases of sound substitution, of sound omission, and of delayed speech. He found a consistent increase with age in memory span for phonemes and syllables and found the span for syllables highest, phonemes next, and digits shortest. Short auditory memory spans were found in 13 percent of sound-substitution cases, 33 percent of sound-omission cases, and 45 percent of the delayed-speech cases. The factor of intelligence is not controlled in this study and comparative results for normal speakers are not given.

Beebe (1944) summarized the age norms for auditory memory span published by other authors and added her own. She concluded that auditory memory span for meaningless syllables increases with age, but differences between age groups are small. Like Metraux, she found no sex differences.

Hall (1938) found no difference in auditory memory for speech sounds between groups of functional articulatory cases at a university and at an elementary school level and carefully matched groups with good speech. Mase (1946) also found no differences in auditory memory span between normal-speaking and functional articulatory defective boys in grades five and six.

Irwin et al. (1966) found auditory memory span for vowels one of the factors predictive of speech improvement in second-grade children over a seven-month period. Locke (1969) found children with high scores on auditory memory better than children with low scores on auditory memory in imitating non-English speech sounds.

These studies of auditory memory span are inconsistent but, in general, the more carefully controlled ones in which functional articulatory defectives and good speakers were matched for age and intelligence show no differences in auditory memory span between speech ability groups. Auditory memory span, however, may have predictive value for speech improvement.

Few studies have made much attempt to *interrelate* various auditory factors. Most have studied these factors one at a time. Stitt and Huntington (1969) used correlational techniques to investigate relationships among articulation and other variables, including a variety of auditory abilities and memory. A wide range battery of tests was applied to college students. The investigators found articulation significantly related to auditory abilities, memory, college aptitude, and language abilities. Auditory abilities and memory accounted for 61 percent of the variance in articulation.

SENSORY FACTORS: TACTILE AND KINESTHETIC

Another of the hypotheses concerning the causation of functional articulatory defects has been that individuals with these defects have less than average sensitivity to position, movement, and degrees of muscular tension within the speech mechanism. Muscle movements in the articulators are hypothesized to be inaccurate because of inadequate feedback from the oral surfaces and the muscles involved in articulation. Lack of kinesthetic sensitivity in the tongue has been considered especially important. The possible relation of deficient tactile or kinesthetic sensitivity to articulation, however, has been studied little experimentally.

Patton (1942) tested 214 elementary school children with functional articulatory defects and an equal number of normal-speaking children on seven tests of kinesthesia, none of which involved the speech mechanism but rather the gross skeletal muscles. A statistically significant difference was found in favor of the control group, and the author concluded that the speech cases have less kinesthetic sensibility than the controls.

Fairbanks and Bebout (1950) measured percentage of error in duplicating a tongue position, a skill which depends primarily upon kinesthetic sensitivity. Comparisons between college students with inferior and superior articulation yielded no statistically significant difference. These two studies found conflicting results but used very different types of tests and involved quite different parts of the body. The question of whether deficient tactile or kinesthetic sensitivity is a causal factor in functional articulatory defects remains open and requires study.

In recent years a different aspect of intraoral sensitivity—oral stereognosis—has been advanced by various speech pathologists as a basic requirement for articulation development. As yet, however, little research on this has been done. Locke (1969) found that children with high scores on oral stereognosis were better than children with low scores in imitating non-English sound presented to them. Ringel et al (1970) studied intraoral sensitivity in relation to articulation, testing children on the ability to distinguish objects of different shapes placed within the mouth. Sixty children with so-called functional disorders of articulation, in grades one through five, were compared with normal-speaking controls on discrimination of 65 pairs of three-dimensional stimuli. The speech-defective group made more errors than the controls and there was also a tendency for errors to increase with increase in the severity of the articulation problem. Two groups of adults were also compared with similar results except that both adult groups made fewer errors than the groups of children. The authors raise the interesting question of whether sensory discrimination abilities and speech development exist in a cause-effect relationship or whether both are related to more general factors of neurological and/or perceptual skill development.

SENSORY FACTORS: VISUAL

Visual skills are not usually thought of as having much relationship to speech, but several authors have mentioned speech defects in children with visual deficiencies. The relationship merits some consideration. Eisenson (1938) mentions that articulatory defects are frequent among even the mature blind. He accounts for it by their lack of visual cues and by the disinclination others show to correct their speech.

Rossignol (1948), in studying relationships among hearing acuity, speech production, and reading performance in primary children, found higher scores on a sound-repetition test when the children were able to look at the tester while listening as compared with listening alone. She also found that the examiners were more consistent in their phonetic ratings when watching the children as against listening to their recorded speech. The author infers that it is important for children to look at the speaker when learning to produce consonants in new words and even earlier when learning to form the consonant sounds.

Brieland (1950), in a comparison of the speech of blind and sighted children, reported one incidental finding, a difference in favor of the sighted group in degree of lip movement. It may be that visual factors should receive more attention than they have heretofore.

OTHER PHYSICAL VARIABLES

Writers in speech pathology have mentioned a variety of additional physical factors which may have etiological importance in functional articulatory disorders. Such factors as general physical debility and poor health, a history of frequent illnesses, especially during the speech-learning years, developmental slowness, glandular deficiencies, "heredity" or "biological inferiority," and others.

Some writers appear to regard such factors as having a direct physical relationship to speech in that they produce a weak and inefficient speech mechanism. Others discuss these factors as having a more indirect relationship. Physical disability restricts a child's activities and experiences and thus deprives him to some extent of both speech stimulation and of motivation for producing speech himself. More subtle factors may also enter the picture, such as the greater emotionality and overprotectiveness which is frequently engendered in parents by an ill child, or a failure on their part to exact normal communicative effort from the child.

Although much discussed, such physical factors have been little studied for functional articulatory defects specifically. Carrell (1936) reported the results of medical examinations and medical histories of 61 sound-substitution cases and normal speakers to show no statistically significant differences between the groups in either health history or medical examination items. Karlin, Youtz, and Kennedy (1940) found more endocrine dysfunction in six articulatory cases as compared with six normal speakers, but this result is no more than suggestive because of the small number involved.

Beckey (1942) made a thorough investigation of possible factors differentiating retarded speech cases from normal speakers. Although she studied retarded speech cases, not functional articulatory cases, the results may have some significance for the latter. Detailed histories were taken and a battery of tests applied to 50 young children with retarded speech and 50 with normal speech. Of the many items investigated, Beckey found statistically significant differences to the disadvantage of the speech-defective group for only the following: mothers who had had abnormal pregnancies and birth complications, children who had had asphyxia at birth, poor motor control, two or more infectious diseases, measles, slow physical growth, diseased or removed tonsils, and presence of adenoids. Although these factors would be expected logically to have more relation to retarded speech than to functional articulatory defects, they may be of interest as possible causal or concomitant factors in functional articulatory defects as well.

Everhart (1953) compared 110 children with articulatory defects in grades one through six with 110 normal-speaking controls on a battery of tests and developmental data secured from a questionnaire filled in by parents. No significant relationship was found between articulatory defectives and the following: Onset of holding head up, of sitting alone, of crawling, of walking, of talking, of voluntary bladder control, and eruption of first tooth. Differences, but of low significance, were found for onset of sitting alone and of holding head up. He also found no significant relationship between articulatory defectiveness and grip, height, weight, or handedness.

De Hirsch et al. (1964) compared 51 premature with 55 full-term children matched for I.Q., race, sex, education of parents, both groups having a mean age of 5.8 years. Tests of 15 oral language skills were given. No differences were found on eight tests, including consonant articulation, auditory discrimination, and auditory memory span. The premature group was inferior to the maturely born group on seven tests: tapped patterns, language comprehension, word finding, number of words used, mean of the five longest sentences, sentence elaboration, and definitions.

Too little research has as yet been done on growth and health factors in relation to articulation skills to enable us to reach definite conclusions. It seems clear that large and generalized differences will not be found. At the same time it would seem profitable to investigate these factors further and especially—as with auditory factors—to investigate the interrelationship or *patterning* of growth and health factors as they may relate to the development of articulation.

Intellectual Variables

The solution to functional articulatory disorders has been sought by many speech pathologists in differences in general intellectual endowment or in the present of certain special mental abilities or specific disabilities. Thus a great deal of attention has been given to studying the general intelligence of speech defectives and of evaluating their possible deficiency in "verbal intelligence" as against "nonverbal intelligence." Texts in speech pathology all stress the importance of evaluating the intelligence of a case as part of the basic diagnostic examination, both as an aid to diagnosis and as a significant factor in planning therapy.

The relationship between speech and other language functions—vocabulary, reading achievement, spelling achievement—has also received considerable attention. It has been suggested by many that certain types of abilities tend to vary together, so that, for example, individuals deficient in speech would tend to be deficient in reading skill and that other individuals would tend to be superior in these supposedly related abilities. This is a tantalizing subject for thought and for research. Here it can occupy us only to the extent of discussing the possible relation these variables may have to functional articulatory defects.

INTELLIGENCE

The relationship of intelligence to articulation development and to defects of articulation has long intrigued the interest of speech pathologists. Intelligence has been felt to have such a basic influence on speech that investigators have considered it an important factor to control in studying other variables. Thus, in the many studies in which matched groups of articulatory defectives and normal speakers have been compared for possible differences, intelligence has usually been one of the bases on which the matching was done.

The relationship of intelligence to articulation skill has been approached in three principal ways. Some investigators have studied articulation growth in relation to intelligence in normal, unselected children. Others have compared intelligence of articulatory defectives with that of normal speakers. Still other investigators have started with intelligence as the independent variable and have compared the speech of mentally deficient with mentally normal individuals.

One of the first studies to relate articulation development to intelligence was that of Wellman, Case, Mengert, and Bradbury (1931), who studied children from two to six years of age. They found a correlation of .80 between articulation skill and chronological age, and of .71 between articulation skill and mental age on the Stanford-Binet; but with chronological age held constant, little relationship was found between articulation and mental age. In other words, articulation development had a closer relationship to chronological than to mental age.

Irwin (1952), reporting on studies of speech development in infants up to 30 months of age, concluded that the relationship between speech-sound development and intelligence is not very dependable at 18 months, but that from the twentieth to thirtieth month there are reliable correlations between various indices of speech-sound development and both the Kuhlmann and Cattell intelligence tests. Dawson (1929), studying rate of articulation, found a tendency toward more rapid articulation in pupils with high I.Q.'s than in those with low I.Q.'s.

Several studies have compared intelligence ratings of functional articulatory defectives and normal speakers. Carrell (1936) reported that speech defectives as a group had a lower intelligence level than normal speakers and that articulatory cases (oral inaccuracy) had the greatest deficiency in intelligence. Speech defectives were also below normal speakers in school achievement, the oral inaccuracy group again showing the most retardation.

Beckey (1942) found that retarded speech cases usually made inferior ratings on intelligence tests as compared with children who had normal speech. Hall (1938) found a zero correlation between articulation ratings of college students and their composite percentile rank on the Iowa Qualifying Examination. Everhart (1953) found that a real difference in intelligence exists in favor of children with normal articulation as compared with children with defective articulation in grades one through six. Sperling (1948) compared children with functional articulatory defects on verbal and nonverbal intelligence tests and found that they had significantly higher performance scores than verbal scores. She concluded that more than one intelligence test should be used in making a prognosis for speech training with articulatory cases.

The third approach concerns itself with the speech proficiency of children with known mental retardation. Ingram (1935) found speech defects in about 12 percent of mentally retarded children as compared with two or three percent of children in regular grades and found that speech defects also tend to persist longer in retarded children in spite of remedial instruction. Sirkin and Lyons (1941) found that only a third of institutionalized mental defectives speak normally and that the lower the intelligence rating the lower the incidence of normal speech.

Bangs (1942) made a careful study of the speech deficiencies of mentally defective children and concluded that mental age has much greater predictive value for speech than does chronological age. He found that, except for more frequent omission of final sounds, the speech of these children does not differ very much *qualitatively* from that of children with normal intelligence. Misarticulations followed essentially the same pattern as they do in functional articulation cases of the same mental age but of normal intelligence.

Karlin and Strazzulla (1952) concluded after studying 50 children with I.Q.'s below 70 that language defects are even more striking than speech defects and in some cases resemble aphasia. Irwin (1952) tested children with I.Q.'s from seven to 48 at age three years and again at four. He found almost complete identity of vowel and consonant curves for the two tests, showing little growth. Vowel profiles were comparable to those of normal one-year-old infants.

Schlanger (1953) studied 74 mentally handicapped children between the ages of eight and 16 years and found 56.7 percent of them to have articulatory problems. The children were found to have a marked deficiency in auditory memory span for vowels and in sound discrimination. Higher correlations were obtained between mental age and articulatory proficiency than between chronological age and speech proficiency.

Wilson (1966) studied the articulatory abilities of 777 educable mentally retarded children six to 16 years of age. In those with speech deviations (53.4 percent), substitution and omission errors tended to decrease with increasing mental age, but distortion errors increased. The speech-deviant group was divided into three subgroups and followed over a three-year period: one group received direct speech therapy, one group nonphoneme-oriented speech and language therapy, and one group no therapy, only testing. Development of consonant sounds extended well beyond the seven and a half to eight-year level commonly accepted for normal children. Group differences, though not statistically significant, tended to show more decrease in speech errors for the direct therapy group, less for the indirect therapy group, compared with the no-therapy group.

What can we conclude about the relationship of intelligence to articulatory deficiences? The relationship has certainly not been shown to be so close that it has much predictive value except within broad limits. At the same time results of research are consistent in showing a gross relationship, particularly for the low end of the intelligence range. Except for the greater incidence of articulatory deficiency among mentally retarded individuals, intelligence appears to be relatively unimportant as a determining factor in articulatory disorders, at least above the age range during which most speech learning takes place. In short, during infancy and the preschool years intelligence appears to be an important factor in articulation growth. Above that level intelligence bears only a general relationship to articulatory proficiency except when intelligence is below normal limits, when it unquestionably affects speech adequacy.

It is interesting again, as with other etiological factors previously discussed, to consider the possibly greater relationship of intelligence to certain types of functional articulatory defects, notably general oral inaccuracy, than to others.

READING AND OTHER LANGUAGE SKILLS

Articulation problems have been mentioned frequently as a cause of reading disability. It has been assumed by many that reading and articulation, both being language-related functions, are interdependent and that a deficiency in one tends to be associated with a deficiency in the other. Other writers have stressed not a direct causal relationship between speech and reading deficiency but rather the possibility that other more basic skills, such as auditory acuity, auditory memory span, and sound discrimination, are fundamental in both reading and speech, and, if deficient, retard both. If this were true, speech and reading disabilities could be said to have a concomitant rather than a causal relationship. The possibility of a relationship between reading and articulation has interested both educators and speech pathologists and has been approached experimentally from both aspects.

Monroe (1932) was one of the first to discuss defective speech as a causal factor in reading disability or, at least, as a factor associated with reading disability. She found that among her reading defect cases there were many more speech defects than among her controls. She considered inaccurate articulation particularly effective as a factor in retarding reading. Since then Moss (1938), Bennett (1938), Witty and Kopel (1939), Hildreth (1946), Betts (1946), and Eames (1950), to mention but a few, have written more or less in support of this view or have presented data which support it. Jones (1951) found experimentally that speech training accelerated the reading achievement of one group of children as against their matched controls who received no speech training.

Bond (1935) studied speech characteristics of good and poor readers and found no difference between them in incidence of speech defects. However, when skill in oral and in silent reading were considered separately, he found that 35 percent of children retarded in oral reading but good in silent reading had speech defects. The children who were retarded in silent reading but not in oral reading showed no speech defects. Everhart (1953) found some tendency for boys with normal articulation to have higher reading achievement than boys with functional articulatory difficulties. Hall (1938) and Moore (1947) both found articulatory cases equal to normal speakers in silent reading achievement.

Robinson (1946) made a particularly searching investigation of possible causes of reading disability, including speech defects, and a careful analysis of previous investigations. Previous studies led her to conclude (p. 99): "On the basis of the evidence available, articulatory defects may be conceded to be important in oral reading but of little significance in silent reading." She found dyslalia in 20 percent of her 30 reading disability cases but stated that its effect as a cause of reading failure could not be determined in many of the cases and that in others no direct relationship could be either established or denied. Her conclusion is that speech difficulties may be causal factors in reading difficulties but that the mere presence of a speech defect does not necessarily mean that it is causally related to the reading difficulty.

Artley (1948) reached much the same conclusions in reviewing the literature on some of the factors presumed to be associated with reading and speech difficulties. He concluded that speech defects may be the cause of reading defects, the result of reading defects, or that both defects may result from some common factor. He also concluded that such factors as reduced auditory acuity, auditory discrimination, and auditory memory span, may be related significantly to reading retardation, but that they do not appear to be significantly related to speech defects.

A few later studies have continued to explore a possible relation between reading and articulation. Weaver et al. (1960a and 1960b) found a significant relationship between articulatory skill and reading readiness. Sommers et al. (1961) found that reading comprehension was not significantly better for first-grade children with misarticulations than for children with normal articulation after a period of speech-correction measures. An exception was a group of children with severe articulation problems. Irwin (1963) in a wide-range study of linguistic skills, reached essentially the same conclusions.

Many studies have investigated the development of vocabulary, sentence use, length of sentence, and other language skills as a function of age, but few have related these skills to articulation. Templin's basic study (1957) established age norms for each language skill separately. She found a (p. 140) "substantial interrelationship among the language skills measured, but the magnitude of the relationship varies with the skill measured." The intercorrelations she found among the verbalization measures and articulation were not high and tended to decrease with age.

Darley and Winitz (1961), in a review of research on the age of the first word, stated among other conclusions that there is no evidence to indicate that age of the first word has any utility for predicting severity of articulatory defectiveness at some later date.

Carrell and Pendergast (1954) investigated another language function—spelling—in relation to articula-defects in children. A comparison of functional articulation cases with matched controls showed no significant difference between the groups either in spelling ability or in the types of spelling errors which occurred. They concluded that there is no underlying phonetic disability.

Vandemark and Bann (1965) compared a group of 50 children with defective articulation in grades three through six with a matched group of 50 normal speakers. Language samples of the 100 children were analyzed for mean length of response, structural complexity, and several other skills. The only significant difference between the groups was on structural complexity, in which the normal speakers were superior. They conclude (p. 412): "It appears that children with defective articulation are not inhibited in terms of the amount of verbal output, but they do perform less well in the areas of grammatical completeness and complexity of responses."

Shriner, Holloway, and Daniloff (1969) compared 30 children, grades one through three, with severe articulatory problems with 30 normal-speaking controls on development of syntax, as shown in storytelling. The children with articulation problems were significantly inferior in grammatical usage and they used shorter sentences.

The nature and degree of interrelationship between articulation and other language-related functions is still little understood. Results of past studies are inconclusive and often contradictory. This area offers challenging problems for future investigation.

Environmental Variables

Much attention has been given by speech pathologists to factors which do not lie within the individual himself but which, though external to him, influence his development and his learning of speech. A child's speech adequacy is conditioned by the speech patterns surrounding him. These patterns in turn are thought to be conditioned by other factors such as the educational and cultural level of the parents, urban versus rural living, and foreign language background or bilingualism. Other factors in the speech environment alleged to be influential are the number of siblings and their ages relative to the child under consideration, speech defects in members of the family, and, to a lesser degree, speech defects in playmates and teachers. Blanton (1936), for example, stressed the "bad habit" origin of speech defects and attributed over 50 percent of lisping in children with a normal speech mechanism to mothers who lisp.

The methods of child training used by parents, particularly their methods of speech training, parental attitudes toward speech, the degree and kind of attention given the child's speech, are all mentioned frequently as being of great influence in determining the various aspects of his speech and language development. At one extreme we find parents who are indifferent and neglectful of the child's speech. They spend little time reading to the child, telling him stories, or just talking with him. They fail to expect speech of the child, to train him in good speech habits, or to correct his errors, either because of indifference or through a belief that errors will be outgrown. At the other extreme are the parents who overcorrect the child's speech so that he becomes discouraged, self-conscious, or negativistic about his own speech attempts.

Other parents offer poor speech patterns either consciously through the use of "baby talk" or mimicry of the child's own immature expressions and errors, or inadvertently because of foreign or native dialects or actual speech defects. Parents sometimes encourage the prolongation of infantile speech habits by rewarding them with attention and admiration. The child whose infantile speech wins him the delighted approval of an admiring family circle is ill-motivated to develop mature speech.

Speech develops in response to a need to communicate and the pleasure experienced in communicating. Some children seldom feel a need to talk. Their communicative urges are anticipated or they succeed at a simple communicative level, such as gesture or pantomime. Other children have ever-willing brothers, sisters, or parents ready to interpret for them when their immature speech is not readily understood. They are deprived of the need to improve their intelligibility.

A few children experience more serious deprivation of speech stimulation. Children who are left alone much of the time because parents are working or otherwise preoccupied, children who have little contact with other children or with adults, who hear little speech, who have no one to talk to or little urge to talk because of a dearth of experiences may be critically handicapped in speech development. The handicap is probably greatest if the deprivation comes during the speech-learning years. It has been observed, for example, that children brought up in institutions during their early years are often slow in speech development. They hear relatively little adult speech. They lack individual parental attention to speech and the constant speech interaction provided by the typical parent-child relationship.

Many possible factors which violate good speech-learning conditions have been mentioned above. They represent the pooled clinical experience of speech pathologists. Some of them have the support of research findings as well; others remain still unverified.

EDUCATION AND CULTURAL STATUS OF PARENTS

A number of studies have compared the speech development or incidence of speech defects among children of different socioeconomic groups. Occupational status of parents has been used as an index of parental education and culture. Davis (1937) found a considerably higher percentage of children with good articulation among upper occupational groups than among lower. Beckey (1942) also found that significantly more children with retarded speech belonged to lower socioeconomic groups. Parents of children with normal speech represented most frequently the professional and managerial occupations. Parents of children with delayed speech also had an inferior educational background as compared with parents of children with normal speech.

Irwin (1948, 1952), studying infants up to 30 months of age, found a marked difference between infants reared in homes of professional and business parents and infants reared in homes of laboring parents. Differences in both frequency and type of speech sounds were negligible for the first year and a half, after that were in favor of the former. Irwin concluded that the factor of parental stimulation is an important variable in speech development. McClure (1952) found that "factory working parents" was one of the items in common for children with articulatory and reading defects.

Templin (1953) found a significant difference between children of upper and lower socioeconomic groups (according to the Minnesota Scale of Occupations) on both screening and diagnostic tests of articulation, the difference being in favor of the upper group. She stated that children of the lower socioeconomic group take about a year longer to reach essentially mature articulation than those of the upper group. In her later and more comprehensive study (1957) Templin found children of upper socioeconomic status parents superior to children of lower socioeconomic status parents in all of the language skills she studied. A difference, though, in intellectual ability between the two groups may also have had some influence. The greatest superiority of the upper socioeconomic group was (p. 148) ". . . concentrated in articulation of vowels, medial and final consonants, in the grammatical complexity of the verbalizations, and in the vocabulary of recognition at the older ages."

These findings are further verified by Weaver et al. (1960b), who found paternal occupation significantly related to early speech maturation. Among their cases a greater proportion of children without dyslalia fell at the upper end of the occupational scale and with dyslalia at the lower end. Andersland (1961) found that children in lower socioeconomic groups who participated in kindergarten speech improvement achieved articulation success approximating that of upper class groups.

These and other studies are consistent in finding that upper socioeconomic status homes tend to provide a more favorable linguistic environment for the child, particularly during his speech-learning years, than homes of lower socioeconomic status. This is reflected in the smaller incidence of children with defective articulation from upper level homes and the superior rate of their speech and language development. Upper group parents, in general, present better speech patterns to their children. They create a more stimulating speech environment and for the most part do more and better articulatory training of their children.

RURAL VERSUS URBAN ENVIRONMENT

Rural as compared with urban living has been considered by some to be related to articulatory development, presumably because of differences in the quantity and quality of speech stimulation provided in these two environments. Louttit and Halls (1936) found a greater incidence of speech defects in county school systems than in city school systems. Articulatory defects specifically had a slightly higher ratio than other speech defects among rural children. Wilson (1952) on the contrary found a slightly higher incidence of articulatory defects among urban children than among rural children. In neither study was the difference very large, so that the relative effects of urban and rural environments on articulation are still in doubt. It seems unlikely that the urban or rural variable in itself would be a factor but rather the educational-cultural level of parents regardless of location.

EFFECT OF SIBLINGS, TWINS, BIRTH ORDER

Wellman et al. (1931) found no relationship in children two to six years of age between articulation skill and number of older children in the family. Davis (1937) found twins considerably inferior to singletons and to only children in articulation skill. This supports the common clinical observation that twins tend to be deficient in articulation and to show highly similar patterns of misarticulation. Beckey (1942) found no significance in birth *order* as related to delayed speech but found that the child with speech retardation tended to be the youngest child. Irwin (1952) reported practically no differences in speech-sound development for infants with older siblings and infants without siblings. However, his studies included only infants under 30 months of age when the influence of other children could perhaps be expected logically to be less effective one way or another than above that age.

Conflicting notions have been proposed regarding the influence of siblings on a child's articulatory development. One opinion is that siblings tend to stimulate speech. Another and opposing view is that siblings tend to provide less perfect articulation patterns to a child than do adults. An only child or oldest child (while he remains the only child) receives nearly 100 percent of his speech stimulation from adults, his parents. The child with siblings receives a considerable proportion of his total speech stimulation from them, whose speech is likely to be less mature than that of adults. The extreme example of this is the case of twins, who hear much of their speech from each other. The emotional ties of twins, too, are likely to be closer than those of single siblings, which further augments their interdependence in speech.

POOR SPEECH PATTERNS

Bilingualism has often been said to retard speech development, but both McCarthy (1930) and Beckey (1942) failed to find such a relationship in the children they studied. Similarly, speech defects in parents and older siblings are often mentioned as an influential factor and most clinicians would agree on the basis of their experience. There is little exact statistical evidence, however, to either support or refute this relationship. It is probable that a child's speech patterns are adversely affected by an articulatory defect in a parent or in an older sibling. It is further probable that his specific misarticulations will resemble those of the defective speaker. It is also probable that the degree of influence of the defective speaker upon the child will depend upon the emotional relationship existing between them. If the child strongly identifies emotionally with, for example, an older brother who has a speech defect, the chances are probably greater that his own speech will be adversely affected than if he does not have this positive identification. There is strong motivation, though often at an unconscious level, to become like those we admire.

LACK OF SPEECH STIMULATION OR TRAINING

Beckey (1942) found a significantly greater number of children among her retarded than among her normal speech group whose wants had been anticipated by parents without speech or from whom gestures had been accepted and speech not required, factors considered to handicap speech development. She also found that children of her delayed speech group had too much isolation for the encouragement of speech. Carrell (1936) who made a study of speech in an institution for dependent children, considered the incidences of speech defects found at various age levels relatively high. He accounted for this by the fact that the children lived in groups, which made their contacts with adults more limited than is the case in a family of normal size. Irwin (1952) reported speech-sound development for orphanage babies below that for home babies. The present writer, during her experience as a psychologist in a children's institution, made the same observation. Preschool and kindergarten children, particularly, were markedly deficient in speech output, vocabulary, and articulation as compared with noninstitutional children. They did poorly, for example, on vocabulary items of the Stanford Binet scale.

Mason (1942) cites an extreme example of a child who did not learn to talk until she was six and a half years of age because she had been living alone until that age with a mute and uneducated mother.

Irwin (1960) compared the speech-sound development of 24 infants whose mothers were instructed to read to them daily with a similar group whose mothers were not so instructed. There was little difference between the groups of infants until the seventeenth month of age. After that the infants who were read to had consistently higher phoneme frequency scores than the infants not read to.

Andersland (1961), cited above, found that low socioeconomic level children gained in articulation with a kindergarten speech-improvement program. Pendergast et al. (1966) carried out a study which is of special interest because of the vast numbers involved. Articulation tests were given to 15,255 entering first-grade children. Those who had attended kindergarten did not appear to have fewer articulation errors than those who had not attended kindergarten. The rank order of defective sounds for the two groups was almost identical.

From the point of view of both research and clinical experience it is obvious that the amount and kind of speech stimulation in the home is a powerful determinant of the child's articulation and language development. Certain environmental conditions and certain types of interaction between the child and his environment are necessary for the development of mature speech. To develop normal patterns of speech a child must hear normal patterns of speech, must have a need and desire to talk, must experience pleasure in hearing speech and in responding with speech, must have sufficient variety in his day-by-day experience to stimulate a communicative urge and to provide communicative content, and his speech must be reacted to constructively by others. The influence of such out-of-home experiences as kindergarten attendance are less certain but are clearly less crucial.

Emotional and Personality Variables

Speech pathology has shown increasing interest during the past two decades in personality characteristics and the emotional and social adjustment of individuals as effective determinants of their speech patterns. The emotional and interpersonal life of the young child as it relates to his developing speech and language concerns not only the speech pathologist, but also the child psychologist, psychiatrist, and educator. The variables of personality and emotional adjustment have received growing emphasis, both as possible etiological factors and as factors of significance for the success of speech therapy and for determining the types of speech therapy to be employed in each specific case. In relation to stuttering, the importance of emotional factors has long been recognized by even the most somatically minded. Functional articulatory disorders, too, are belatedly receiving more attention as possibly symptomatic of personality structure and emotional adjustment. The interpersonal and self-expressive nature of speech makes it a vulnerable point for difficulty or breakdown in the developing behavioral complex of the child.

In the field of emotional and personality growth and adjustment, cause-and-effect relationships are perhaps more difficult to determine than in other aspects of growth. Even if we could, for example, demonstrate that functional articulation cases are significantly less well adjusted emotionally than normal speakers, we would still be left with the chicken-and-egg dilemma. Has the emotional maladjustment "caused" the articulatory problem, has the articulatory problem "caused" the emotional maladjustment, or is there a more complex reciprocal relationship between them? We are in no position at the present time to give a satisfactory answer to such a question. Both theoretical and clinical discussions in the writings of speech pathology are replete with confident statements about the paramount importance of emotional and personality factors in the etiology and treatment of speech disorders, including functional articulatory disorders. Research, however, has barely nibbled around the edges of this intriguing area. There is little to show of an objective nature, and that little is inconclusive.

PERSONALITY TRAITS AND ADJUSTMENT OF THE CHILD

Some writers have raised the question as to whether functional articulatory disorders tend to develop more in individuals with certain normal personality traits than in individuals with other normal personality traits. Anderson (1953) even related specific traits to specific speech characteristics. For example, he stated that the slow-moving, sluggish, phlegmatic individual is likely to speak with a slow tempo, with poorly formed sounds and words; the nervous, high-strung, hyperactive person is likely to talk fast and thus omit or distort sounds, and display irregular rhythm, etc. Other writers, too, have assigned specific speech deficiencies to specific personality traits. These relationships remain unverified and little has been done to investigate them experimentally.

Wellman et al. (1931) found no relationship between speech-sound development in young children, two to six years old, and introversion-extroversion ratings. Davis (1937) found that normal-speaking children tended to rate higher on "talkativeness" and "spontaneity" than children with defective articulation. The latter were more shy and negativistic than good speakers.

Templin (1938) tested college speech-defective and normal-speaking groups on the Moore-Gilliland Test for Aggressiveness and found the speech-defective group significantly less aggressive than the normal-speaking group. Of the speech defectives, the articulatory group were the lowest in aggressiveness. Articulatory cases tended to be more aggressive as their defects were more severe. The results of the Davis and Templin studies are fairly consistent, though done on widely separated age groups.

Beckey (1942) found that children with retarded speech tended to play alone, to cry easily, and to be less demanding of attention than children with normal speech. She found no difference between the groups in incidence of temper tantrums, thumb-sucking, or enuresis. The retarded-speech group had more instances in its histories of severe fright.

Anders (1945) found children of six to 12 years with functional articulatory defects to be above average in adjustment as measured by the California Test of Personality. McAllister (1948), using the same test, found no difference in adjustment between children in grades one through eight, with articulatory defects and matched children with normal speech. She also found no significant differences between the two groups on her speech-attitude scale, though there was a tendency for the speech-defective children in the upper grades to compare less favorably with their controls on reactions to speech than speech defectives in the lower grades. The author concludes that emotional instability is not substantiated as a causal factor in articulatory defects and that speech defects do not cause emotional instability or malattitudes toward speech.

A significant study on this problem was done by Wood (1946), who studied the emotional adjustment of both children and their parents. He gave the California Test of Personality and the Aspects of Personality Test to 50 elementary school children with functional defects of articulation, with some also receiving the Murray Thematic Apperception Test.

The 50 pairs of parents were given the Bernreuter Personality Inventory and the California Test of Personality. He found that the speech-defective children did not fall below test norms in personality adjustment. The Thematic Apperception Test results, however, suggested a sense of frustration in 66 percent of the children, withdrawing tendencies in 65 percent, and lack of affection in 30 percent. Other elements suggested by the results were anxiety-insecurity, lack of belongingness, lack of achievement, aggressiveness, hostility, and escape. The results on the parents are reported below in the next section.

Perrin (1954) made sociometric ratings of 37 children. Nine percent of them were receiving speech therapy, most of them being functional articulatory cases. More of the isolates came from the speech-defective group, no leaders were selected from that group, and the speech-defective children were found to be not readily accepted into the classroom group.

Spriestersbach (1956) reviewed all the studies up to that time—nine—relating articulation disorders and personality. Some studies dealt with articulation disorders as a *cause* of maladjustment and tended to show articulation defectives as less aggressive and less accepted. Other studies, dealing with articulation disorders as a *result* of maladjustment, were about evenly balanced between positive and negative evidence of such a relationship. Spriestersbach points out that many of the articulation cases were mild so that a lack of maladjustment was not surprising.

Goodstein (1958a) reviewed 12 studies of the relationship of functional articulation disorders to the personality and adjustment of children with these disorders. Five of the studies reported a positive relationship, four reported no relationship, and three reported results which were internally contradictory. Goodstein's review reached essentially the same conclusions as the earlier one by Spriestersbach just cited.

PARENTAL ADJUSTMENT AND ATTITUDES

What about the effect of *parental* adjustment, attitudes, and personality on the development of articulation in children? Most speech pathologists have considered these factors vitally important both in the etiology of functional articulation problems and in their remedial management. Research on these relationships is still meager.

In Wood's study (1946) referred to above more significant differences in adjustment were found for parents of articulation cases than for the children themselves. Maternal Bernreuter scores differed significantly from test norms, showing that the mothers as a group were more neurotic in tendency, more submissive, and more self-conscious. Fathers as a group did not differ significantly from test norms. No correlation was found between personality test scores of children and their parents. Seventy-two percent of the 50 speech-defective children had at least one parent above the 60th percentile in neurotic tendency.

On the California Test of Personality maternal scores again differed significantly from test norms, indicating that mothers were lower in self-adjustment, social adjustment, and total adjustment. Fathers rated significantly lower in self-adjustment. Social standards of mothers were very high in comparison with other adjustment scores and Wood concluded that the speech-defective children had imposed upon them a set of very high standards in an atmosphere of habitual emotional outbursts from the parents.

Case history data revealed 13 home environment factors which would militate against a satisfactory emotional life for the child, or would predispose the parent to neglect and mishandle the child (p. 272). "The most frequent factors were lack of recreational outlet for the parents, ignorance of child behavior problems, overly severe child discipline methods, and defective home membership."

The children whose mothers were clinically treated improved in speech more rapidly with speech correction than did the children whose mothers were not so-treated. Wood's conclusion was that (p. 272): ". . . functional articulatory defects of children are definitely and significantly associated with maladjustment and undesirable traits on the part of the parents, and that such factors are usually maternally centered."

Egbert (1955) held clinical interviews with mothers of two matched groups of articulation cases, one group which had made superior progress with speech therapy and the other which had made below-average progress. Mothers of the successful cases had more information about speech therapy and were more active as auxiliary therapists. Mothers of the low group used more frequent and injudicious punishment and methods of training.

Swenson (1956) administered a parental attitude scale to parents of functional articulation cases and parents of normal speakers. Parents of the articulation cases had significantly less favorable attitudes towards certain aspects of children's behavior than the control parents.

Moll and Darley (1960) compared mothers of functional articulation cases, delayed speech cases, and normal speakers on two parental attitude scales. On the Wiley "Attitude Toward the Behavior of Children" scale there were no group differences. On the Schaeffer and Bell "Parental Attitude Research Instrument" there were differences on three of the scales. It was found that mothers of speech-retarded children offer their children less encouragement to talk and that mothers of articulatory impaired children have higher standards and are more critical of their children's functioning than are mothers of non-speech-impaired children.

In a study by Marge (1965) 140 preadolescent children were evaluated on 40 speech and language measures. Their parents were also evaluated. He found that children of permissive mothers achieved higher scores on language maturity and that parental demands and greater use of techniques of speech training in the home related to general speaking ability as assessed by teachers.

The few studies reviewed, while differing in the degree of relationship found between parental—especially maternal—attitudes and adjustment and children's articulation, are reasonably consistent in showing such a relationship. Few speech clinicians on the basis of their experience would fail to attach great importance to parental attitudes and emotional adjustment as factors in the failure of their children to develop good articulation. Even fewer would fail to deal with parental attitudes and adjustment in speech therapy.

Mowrer (1952) has given a good account of the specific learning mechanisms by which the emotional atmosphere surrounding a child becomes effective in influencing his speech development. When the mother is a love object for the infant, a source of gratification and pleasure, the sounds made by her, including speech sounds, become pleasurable stimuli. The sounds are associated with basic satisfactions and thus become positively conditioned, they become *good sounds*. The human infant, being vocally versatile, in the course of random vocalizations will make sounds similar to those of the mother. Since these sounds have already acquired pleasant connotations for him, he will try to repeat and refine them (p. 265). "Soon, however, the infant discovers that the making of these sounds can be used not only to comfort, reassure, and satisfy himself directly but also to interest, satisfy, and control mother, father, and others." He then begins to speak purposively. It is thus that speech development is motivated by a favorable emotional environment.

The implication of this analysis is that when the mother is not a source of pleasure and gratification to the child the sounds associated with her become negatively conditioned and the child tends to reject and withdraw from them. He is not motivated, as in the first instance, to produce sounds himself and is thus delayed and handicapped to various degrees in his own speech development.

SUMMARY

In the developing field of speech pathology many factors have been considered as having a possible effect on the development of articulation and on the failure of some children to develop good articulation at a reasonable age. An extensive review has been presented of these factors, categorized arbitrarily as physical, sensory, intellectual, environmental, and personality and emotional adjustment variables. The research results which tend to support or refute these factors have been evaluated and an attempt made to draw meaningful conclusions from them.

The review of studies on anatomical variables concluded that there is no systematic relationship between functional articulatory disorders and the dimensions or shape of any part of the speech mechanism. The studies on motor coordination for the body as a whole and within the speech mechanism specifically are less conclusive and leave open the possibility that future research may establish differences. It seems unlikely, however, that large and systematic differences will be found between functional articulatory cases and normal speakers for any motor function. Similarly, it appears unlikely that there are consistent, significant differences between the two groups in various growth and physical health factors.

A form of intraoral sensitivity—oral stereognosis—has received some attention in recent years. It offers an interesting possibility for continuing investigation, both as a skill possibly basic for normal articulation growth and as a possible factor in defective articulation.

The largest amount of research effort has been directed toward the study of various *auditory* factors. Because it is well established that hearing loss has adverse effects on articulation, it has been an appealing thought that this sequence could be reversed and that articulation defectives could be assumed to be deficient in various auditory processes or skills. With several probable exceptions, this has not proved to be the case.

For each of the auditory skills reviewed, there is some evidence both for and against a systematic difference between normal speakers and functional articulatory defectives. For each auditory factor, however, with the possible exception of speech-sound discrimination, the weight of evidence is against a significant, generalized difference. The weight of evidence is even stronger if we consider only those studies which have been carefully designed, where the factors of age and intelligence have been controlled, where defective and normal speakers have been carefully matched, and where tests of statistical significance have been applied.

Articulation cases appear to have about the same range and distribution of auditory abilities as normal speakers, group for group. This means that we cannot predict a probable degree of inferiority in any of the auditory factors for a specific functional articulatory case. It also follows that we cannot theoretically rule out a possible inferiority in any auditory factor for this specific case without examination. It remains possible for any functional articulatory case to have a deficiency in any one or combination of the various auditory factors discussed.

Though single, simple auditory factors do not seem to distinguish functional articulatory defectives from normal speakers, a possible etiological factor in the auditory area which has yet to be investigated experimentally is that of the *patterning* of auditory factors. It is quite possible that different *patterns* of auditory ability may be found in articulatory cases than in individuals with good articulation. There is need particularly for investigation of how various aspects of the auditory process develop *genetically* and whether the developmental patterns are different in those children who later develop good articulation from those who do not. The investigations up to now have dealt largely with the elementary school age and older. Is it not possible that some children are slow to develop skill in speech-sound discrimination, auditory memory, high-frequency acuity, or other skills, and that they are, therefore, deficient in these skills at the age range most crucial for speech development? Even slight deficiencies may make a difference during the speech-learning period. To hypothesize further, such children may eventually reach average or superior skill in these factors so that the earlier and temporally critical deficiency is masked and does not show up in comparative studies at older age levels.

A further essential concept in evaluating the role of auditory factors is that of *utilization* of a skill as contrasted with possession of the skill. It has long been this writer's clinical observation that many functional articulatory cases are *inattentive* to sound differences. If pushed, they can usually discriminate as well as normal speakers, as shown in the many comparative studies done, but they do not *habitually* do so. We, therefore, have to evaluate not only auditory capacities but also auditory habits or—more accurately—*attentional habits* as related to sound.

Another promising emphasis resulting from recent research is the pinpointing of *auto*-discrimination deficiency in functional articulatory cases. Even though interpersonal speech-sound discrimination is not in general inferior, many studies have found a deficiency in discrimination of self-produced sounds or intrapersonal discrimination. There seems to be general agreement among speech pathologists that this is an important area for diagnostic evaluation and for remedial training.

Still another area of needed investigation is the possible relation of auditory abilities to specific types of functional articulatory defects. It is possible that real etiological differences may exist in some types, such as general oral inaccuracy, but be masked by the absence of differences in the much larger group of functional articulatory defectives as a whole.

In summary, the evidence of the accumulated research on auditory factors in relation to functional articulatory disorders calls for a much more sophisticated approach to the role of audition in all of its ramifications. Certainly the simple deficiency in any single auditory skill is largely ruled out. The comparison of group with group, usually at age levels where speech is already established, has perhaps masked the interrelationships and patternings which take place within the single individual as his speech-hearing-language system develops. Comprehensive, longitudinal studies of young children will be needed if we are to understand the role of auditory factors in the failure of some individuals to develop good articulation.

Intelligence has been shown to have only a gross relationship to articulation and is not a helpful index, except at low I.Q. levels, for the prediction of probable articulatory skill.

The relationship between articulation and other language-related functions, such as reading, spelling, vocabulary, sentence structure, and others, is still in doubt. Although research results are mutually contradictory, there is again in this area little evidence of large, consistent differences between functional articulatory defectives and normal speakers. There is need for more comprehensive, longitudinal approaches to the problem of interrelationships among linguistic skills if they are to be better understood.

Environmental factors show more evidence of a positive relationship with articulation. The socio-economic, educational, and cultural level of parents, the amount and kind of speech stimulation provided in the child's home environment, and the general management of the child's speech learning all seem to be causally related to defects of articulation. There is both research and clinical verification of such relationships.

The area of personality traits and emotional adjustment of the child as related to inadequate articulation has been explored only meagerly by research, and with inconclusive results. There is some evidence that children with functional articulation problems are more shy, submissive, anxious, insecure, and withdrawn than children with normal articulation. It has not been established, however, whether these traits are contributory to or result from articulation problems, or whether there is a circular or reciprocal relationship.

Parental attitudes and adjustment appear, from both research and clinical experience, to be more clearly related to the child's articulatory development and adequacy than his own personality and adjustment. Or, perhaps it would be more accurate to say that parental attitudes and adjustment are primary factors in the child's articulatory development, with the child's own adjustment a secondary outcome. Parents, especially mothers, of functional articulatory defectives appear to have more neurotic traits than the norm, tend to be demanding and critical, to have excessively high standards, and to show poor attitudes toward the child's speech. It seems probable that in a rejecting, overcritical, punitive, or emotionally disturbed atmosphere a child may develop a *protective inattention* to the speech surrounding him and be handicapped in developing speech himself.

What general conclusions can we reach then about the etiology of functional disorders of articulation? It would be reassuring if we could say that even one factor has been demonstrated to be associated always —or even nearly always—with these disorders. This is not the case, however. These cases have no general, systematic deficiency in any factor which is of sufficient size to have predictive value. Similarly, there is no factor which is consistently absent in all functional articulatory cases. All are found in some cases; all are absent in some cases.

The speech-hearing-language system is the most complex function which the human being develops. It is subject to a wide range of hazards and disruptive possibilities which may be physical, environmental, or emotional. Any disruptive factor will probably have, not a discrete effect on a limited aspect of the developing system, but an effect upon the total system to some degree. It seems reasonable to assume that a child's developing speech-hearing-language system is more vulnerable to disruption during the first few years of life when it is developing rapidly, and relatively less vulnerable after the fifth or sixth year of age. This may be the reason for the negative or, at best, inconclusive results of research in this field, most of which has been done on school-age children.

Another reason for our lack of success in identifying causal factors stems from our oversimplied approach to the investigation of what is an enormously complex system. Cross-sectional studies of single, specific factors or certain categories of factors have been disappointing.

It seems to this writer more productive to think of functional disorders of articulation as determined by a *causal pattern*, a combination of causal factors, and by the *temporal relationship* of the various aspects of the causal pattern to the developing speech-hearing-language system of the child. The causal pattern may occasionally be simple, uncomplicated, obvious, and may consist of only one or two of the many factors mentioned. Far more frequently, however, we are likely to find a causal pattern of greater complexity, with several factors operating successively or simultaneously. Thus the causal pattern for a single case may involve predisposing, precipitating, and perpetuating factors and these factors may lie in any or all of the areas mentioned—physical, sensory, intellectual, environmental, and emotional.

Let us cite several hypothetical cases in which various factors might combine to produce a functional articulatory disorder, although any one of them alone would not be sufficient. For example, a child might have intelligence in the 70 to 85 I.Q. range. This deficiency in itself would not produce an articulatory problem, but it might act as a predisposing factor which, in combination with such precipitating factors as marked lack of speech stimulation and a feeling of inadequacy and insecurity, would retard his articulatory development. A brighter child might override the environmental and emotional factors to develop good speech. Low intelligence then would act as a predisposing or augmenting factor which would require the presence of other factors to be effective.

Another child might be clumsy in his movements and have less than average skill in tongue coordinations. This minor deficiency would act as a predisposing factor. If this child is subjected to a bilingual home environment or to a severe articulation disorder in a parent, he will in all probability have trouble in mastering articulation skills. If, in addition, the child is shy and withdrawn, his difficulty will be still further increased. A child with normal motor dexterity in the same environment might succeed in developing good articulation in spite of poor parental speech, through the incidental stimulation received from playmates and others outside the home.

Still another child might have a slight hearing loss or an unusually short auditory memory span. This would be a predisposing tendency, but the extent to which it would handicap him, if at all, would depend upon the further factors with which it might combine. If the parents were emotionally disturbed, rejecting, or indifferent, so that he developed serious insecurity in the parental relationship, then his slight auditory handicap might make the crucial difference which would produce an articulatory disorder. With calm, approving, encouraging parents, it would probably have little effect.

Each factor present, though noneffective alone, increases the probability that any other factor or factors, also noneffective alone, will in combination produce a functional articulatory problem, particularly if they occur during the crucial speech-learning years. Anatomical, motor, sensory, and intellectual variables probably operate most frequently as predisposing factors. Environmental, learning, personality, and emotional variables probably act as precipitating and perpetuating factors which are superimposed on the predisposing factors. The more predisposing factors there are present and the more severe any such factor is, the more chance there will be for any one environmental or emotional factor to become effective.

There is a great challenge to be seen in a different type of research approach to functional articulatory disorders. Most studies have approached the problem piecemeal. They have not been sufficiently comprehensive to permit a study of the *patterning* of factors. There is need for extended, longitudinal programs of research to study large numbers of children from infancy over extended periods of time to speech maturity, measuring a wide variety of factors and studying many kinds of interrelationships. Only then will the reasons become clear for the failure of some children to develop mature articulation.

In the meantime, before we have this understanding, the careful speech clinician will be obligated to make a thorough evaluation of most of the possible etiological factors discussed if he is to evolve the causal pattern for each case he studies. It seems likely, too, that there will always be an occasional case which will defy us, the case for which even the most experienced and thorough clinician will find no satisfactory explanation. Such a case serves a useful purpose in its own way as a deterrent to complacency.

(For bibliographical references, see end of Chapter 34.)

34

Clinical and Educational Procedures in Functional Disorders of Articulation

Margaret Hall Powers

In the preceding chapter we were concerned with the more theoretical aspects of functional articulation disorders—their symptomatology, nature, and causation. In this chapter we will be concerned with aspects of more immediate clinical importance—the evaluation and diagnosis of these disorders and the planning and management of speech therapy. Throughout the previous chapter it was emphasized that much of what we think we "know" about the etiology of functional articulation problems lacks a secure research foundation. When we come to the consideration of the relevance or reliability of current diagnostic procedures or of the efficacy of commonly used therapeutic procedures, research has even less to offer. The inherent difficulty of planning controlled studies of the dynamic and complex therapeutic process has been a deterrent. Recently more investigators have been challenged by this area, and research studies are appearing with increasing momentum.

In the meantime speech clinicians are still operating more out of experience and judgment than out of scientific security. The experience and judgment of well-trained, thoughtful speech pathologists have great value but they must be verified, corrected, and refined by objective, scientific study if the profession of speech pathology is to advance.

It is too early even yet in the development of speech pathology to be wholly supportive of any one point of view to the exclusion of others, whether we are considering the etiology of articulation disorders, their diagnosis, or the therapy approaches which give most promise of success. This chapter, therefore, will attempt to bring together the research and clinical contributions of speech pathologists in the field to both the task of evaluation and diagnosis and the even more difficult task of planning and managing speech therapy. It is hoped that this chapter will present an eclectic viewpoint.

EXAMINATION AND DIAGNOSIS

The examination and diagnosis of any speech case are designed to answer essentially three questions: What kind of person has the speech disorder? What kind of speech disorder does he have? Why does he have it? These questions must be answered to the best of the clinician's ability as a basis for finally developing therapy objectives and a plan for reaching them. The purpose of the diagnostic operation is clearly not for mere categorization but, rather, for understanding so that rehabilitative efforts will be appropriate and successful.

The examination of functional articulation cases follows the general outline of clinical examination procedures which would be followed for any case. In fact, a case would be diagnosed as having a "functional articulation" disorder only following the completion of such an examination program (see Chapters 24 and 25 for details of examination procedures). Here a suggested general examination program will be given merely in outline form, and only those aspects of it which pertain to functional articulation disorders particularly will be amplified. The following outline organizes the examination procedure around the three questions given above.

In a large speech clinic, various individuals may be involved in the study of the case, each assuming responsibility for specific parts of the examination. In some clinics, for example, a social worker is available for case history taking, a physician to secure the medical history and give the physical examination, and a clinical psychologist to administer psychological tests and to make the evaluation of personality and adjustment. More commonly the speech pathologist works alone and merely utilizes reports sent him by other specialists who are not actually part of the clinic organization. The necessity for seeking the collaboration of other professional persons in obtaining the general picture of the case will be determined by the training of the clinician making the examination. The ethical speech pathologist will not attempt to perform the parts of the examination which must be done by a physician or a clinical psychologist unless he has had these additional types of training.

WHAT KIND OF PERSON HAS THE SPEECH DISORDER?

The purpose of this part of the examination is the understanding of the child or adult with whom we are dealing, as an individual, different from all other individuals. Too often only lip service has been paid to the accepted doctrine of "understanding the whole child." Information from various sources and of various kinds must be integrated into a meaningful picture of the person. We need such a picture of the dynamics of the individual before we can construct a sound and appropriate therapeutic program. We need to see him clearly as a unique person, which means that we must understand his history, the environmental setting in which he lives, his physical, mental, social, emotional, and communication characteristics, his aspirations, anxieties, motivations, strengths, weaknesses, areas of insecurity, and areas of confidence.

Getting a general picture of the person—as a background for the study of his disordered speech—involves the following major types of investigation and examination.

The Case History

A carefully taken case history can contribute significantly to the total study of a case; a perfunctorily taken one may be a waste of time. An account of the individual's past development and present status should be obtained from the person or persons best able to give the information, usually the parents in the case of a child, or the person himself, in the case of an adult. Information from several sources is often valuable by adding detail and by revealing discrepancies at times which may be significant. The case history should include the following principal areas:

- Family history and present status.
- Birth and developmental history.
- Health history and present status.
- Educational (and occupational) history, present status, and plans.
- Personality, emotional, and social development and present status.
- Adjustment problems, especially in relation to members of the family or peers.
- Interests and recreational activities.
- History of speech and language development.
- History and present status of the individual's specific speech problem.

Evaluation of Physical Health and Developmental Status

As distinguished from the health information secured in the case history, this part of the study involves a physical examination by a physician, preferably one who works on a continuing basis with the speech pathologist and who has developed special interest and competence in evaluating cases of speech disorder. The physician will also contribute birth and developmental data.

A dental examination is also useful to supplement the speech clinician's own evaluation of the speech structures and their functioning. This is particularly true when anomalous conditions exist which may have a bearing on the articulation disorder.

Further and more specialized evaluations, such as neurological or otological, should be sought when appropriate. With the increasing proportion of multiple-handicapped children who are appearing in our clinics and schools, the question of subtle neurological deficits is becoming of more concern.

Evaluation of Intellectual Capacity and Academic Achievement

The speech clinician should have available the results of standardized intelligence tests or should be able to refer cases to a qualified clinical psychologist for this type of study. With children handicapped in speech it is necessary to be cautious in interpreting intelligence test results. Even when an articulation problem is not severe enough to interfere with intelligibility, it may still inhibit the child sufficiently so that he fails to make a maximum effort in giving test responses. The intelligence of speech-handicapped children is frequently underestimated on standardized tests. On the other hand, it cannot be assumed that, merely because he has a speech problem, his intelligence is higher than the obtained result.

It is always advisable to check the results of a "verbal" type of test, such as the Stanford-Binet, with a "nonverbal" or "performance" test. A test such as the Wechsler Intelligence Scale for Children (Wechsler, 1949) has the advantage of including both a verbal and a performance scale, each yielding an independent rating. This test can be applied to children from five years of age through adolescence. The newer scale, Wechsler Preschool and Primary Scale of Intelligence (Wechsler, 1963), extends the scale downward to ages four through six and a half, and also yields a verbal, a performance, and a full-scale I.Q.

Many clinicians find the Illinois Test of Psycholinguistic Abilities of great value in analyzing strengths and weaknesses in various language processes. This test series, developed at the Institute for Research on Exceptional Children of the University of Illinois, (McCarthy and Kirk, 1961), is based upon a comprehensive theory and model of language acquisition and use. It includes nine tests—six at a "Representational level (Auditory decoding, Visual decoding, Auditory-vocal association, Visual-motor association, Vocal encoding, and Motor encoding)," and three tests at an "Automatic-sequential level (Auditory-vocal-automatic, Auditory-vocal-sequencing, and Visual-motor-sequencing.)" Age norms from two to nine years are provided for each of the separate tests. The Peabody Picture Vocabulary Test (Dunn, L. M., 1959, 1965) is also a useful instrument to supplement other tests in clinical appraisal.

With children or adolescents it is advisable also to have available the results of standardized achievement tests in the principal school subjects. These test results are helpful in gaining insight into the nature of the speech problem and its possible relationship to other language functions. From an even more practical standpoint, this appraisal of academic strengths and weaknesses is helpful in planning therapy.

Evaluation of Personality and Emotional Adjustment

This is one of the most essential parts of the clinical study of a case. The person's emotional characteristics and modes of adjustment may have a causal relationship to his speech problem and, in any case, are important to the therapeutic management of the problem.

Personality and adjustment can be studied in a variety of ways. The personal interview with the case reveals much information to the observant and psychologically trained clinician. Young children should be observed in a free-play situation, particularly one involving other children. The interaction between the child and his parents as observed in the clinic is of considerable clinical interest. Observation of the child in his schoolroom often yields valuable insights. The case should be observed in as wide a variety of situations and with as many different people as is feasible.

There are also various more formal ways of evaluating personal characteristics—the standardized personality schedule, such as the Bernreuter Personality Inventory, and the various projective techniques such as the Rorschach or the Murray Thematic Apperception Test. Symond's Picture-Story Test (1948) is a projective test of a thematic apperception type similar to Murray's but for adolescents. Bellack and Bellack (1961) in their Children's Apperception Test (CAT) have extended the projective type of test to a still younger age range than even the Symonds test for use with adolescents. These tests require special training to administer and interpret and under no circumstances should be used without such training. For children the Vineland Social Maturity Scale developed by Doll (1947) gives valuable insight into personal and social adjustment.

When adjustment problems of any seriousness are uncovered, the assistance of a clinical psychologist or a psychiatrist should be sought.

Evaluation of Communicative Behavior as a Whole

Since the speech clinician is interested in understanding the whole person with whom he is dealing, it follows that he must study what is such an important part of the person's total behavior and adjustment, his mode of communicating with the world around him. An articulation disorder cannot be seen in realistic perspective or in its full context without evaluation of all facets of the person's patterns of communication. An articulation problem may or may not be associated with other deficits in communication. Therefore, all aspects of speech should be appraised systematically, preferably under conditions where the individual is conversing naturally and is unaware of being evaluated. Observations can be made with the greatest objectivity and accuracy if the clinician considers only one aspect of speech at a time and each aspect independently of the others. These aspects can be analyzed as follows:

Motivation for interacting with persons in his environment—degree of communicative urge.

Fluency of self-expression in speech; output or flow of speech; ease in formulating and expressing ideas.

Intelligibility—degree to which the speech can be understood.

Vocabulary—level and extent in relation to age.

Level of language organization in relation to age; use of single words; phrases, sentences; length of sentences; complexity of sentences; use of various parts of speech, of various tenses.

Grammar and pronunciation.

Foreign or regional dialect.

Articulation (See below for detailed examination procedures).

Voice—pitch, loudness, or quality deviations; inflectional patterns.

Rate—habitual use of too slow or too rapid speech.

Rhythm—hesitancy; stuttering; irregular or staccato rhythm.

Visible accompaniments of speech—facial expression and gestural patterns; bodily tension or relaxation; posture.

Emotional reactions accompanying speech.

Person's evaluative reactions to speaking and listening.

WHAT KIND OF SPEECH DISORDER DOES THE PERSON HAVE?

From a study of the child or adult as a total personality we now need to narrow our focus of attention to a study of the dimensions and characteristics of his specific disorder of speech. Since this chapter deals with functional articulation disorders, we are concerned here with techniques for studying only this type of problem.

A convenient scheme for describing and analyzing articulation is the following: 1. degree and consistency of the communication handicap; 2. a systematic phonetic inventory; and 3. an analysis of misarticulation.

Degree and Consistency of the Communication Handicap

The clinician needs to listen to the person's articulation in the context of his communicative behavior as a whole. Does his intelligibility vary with the speaking situation, or with the person to whom he is talking, or with the type of speech task engaged in? Careful observation of variations in articulation contributes to an understanding of the problem and to an estimate of probable response to therapy. Observe his articulation in the following contexts:

OFF-GUARD, CONVERSATIONAL SPEECH

Listen to the child or adult when he is talking freely, unaware that his speech is under observation. This can be done best at the beginning of the diagnostic examination before the more formal tests have made him conscious of his speech. Engage the adult, adolescent, or older child in friendly conversation about topics which interest him. Enter into a play situation with the younger child or, better still, observe him at play with others. Notice his speech as he talks with his parents or siblings. Observe each case also, if possible, in a stress situation, as well as in a pleasant, relaxed situation.

The objective in this observation is to get the "feel" of the problem, to evaluate the person's intelligibility under normal speaking conditions, to evaluate the conspicuousness of the defect, and the degree to which it is a communication handicap. A distinction must be made between *intelligibility* and *conspicuousness* of defect. Unintelligible speech will always be conspicuous but the converse may not be true. For example, a lateral lisp is usually very conspicuous but seldom interferes with intelligibility.

Intelligibility can be roughly graded from one extreme to the other as follows: speech easily and completely understood, speech understandable except for some words, speech understandable only when the topic is known to the listener, speech unintelligible even to members of the family. If the person is not understood by his listener and is asked to repeat, can he improve his intelligibility?

ORAL READING

Have the person read continuous material which is well within his reading level and offers no problem in word recognition. Does the response to visual symbols and the higher level of awareness produce any improvement in articulation over the conversational speech situation?

REPETITION OF LEARNED SERIES

Have the person count, name the days of the week, the months of the year, or recite a well-known nursery rhyme or poem. Is articulation the same or better than in the preceding situation? Have the person try the above series again with a deliberate attempt this time to speak as carefully as possible. Is there any improvement?

When the person is able to control his articulation to some extent, it indicates often that he is in a transitional phase in learning the sound, either through maturation or through training, and that the outlook is good for eventual habituation of the correct pattern.

EVALUATION OF ARTICULATION CONSISTENCY

The systematic phonetic inventory will be described in the next section. However, the word-by-word response given on a test of articulation may vary considerably from articulation in connected, conversational speech. Differences should be identified and evaluated.

Some individuals will show the same articulatory errors in all situations—from the most off-guard to those in which they are trying to articulate carefully—and will show them with all the people to whom they speak and in all phonetic contexts. Other cases will show some variation; others much variation. Variations in misarticulation in relation to the person to whom the case is speaking may be important. Some children speak better or less well to their parents than to others; some speak better to one parent than to the other. Twins or siblings close together in age, in speaking to each other often use speech which is more or less unintelligible to others, but in speaking to adults use a considerably better level of articulation. Articulation cases also commonly vary considerably in articulatory adequacy in relation to their emotional state.

The Phonetic Inventory—A Systematic Analysis of Articulation Proficiency

METHODS OF TESTING ARTICULATION

A number of investigations have been concerned with identifying the most useful types of materials for articulation testing and the most effective methods of presentation. All clinicians would agree that test materials must be of interest to the subject and within his vocabulary range, and must lend themselves to objective evaluation and recording. However, there are differing findings and opinions as to which test materials and methods do in fact provide the truest picture of a subject's articulation. Such issues as spontaneous versus imitative responses, single-word versus connected-speech testing, and others have been studied, but with equivocal results.

Templin (1947a) found that in articulation testing of young children similar results are obtained when pictures are named spontaneously as when their names are repeated after the examiner. Snow and Milisen (1954a), however, found that children in both the primary and upper grades gave better responses to oral tests than to picture or reading tests. They concluded, therefore, that in articulation testing a picture test is preferable in order to avoid influencing the child's response. Snow and Milisen further reported (1954b) that the difference in a child's response to a picture as compared with an oral test may be a valuable prognostic clue. In their study the sounds made better in response to the oral than to the picture test showed most spontaneous improvement over a six-month period.

Siegel et al. (1963), using 50 unselected kindergarten children, compared imitative and spontaneous methods of response to pictures and found significant differences in favor of the imitative method for only eight of the 40 sounds tested. They concluded that the method does alter significantly the articulation responses of normal children but that the effect is small in magnitude.

The probable conclusion to be drawn from these studies is that the spontaneous method gives the most typical picture of the subject's articulation at the time tested, but that oral prompting by the examiner on pictures or printed words not recognized quickly will not greatly affect the results and will save time in a practical testing situation. More will be said about this issue later in discussing stimulability testing.

MATERIALS FOR USE IN A PHONETIC INVENTORY

Picture or object tests should be used with children who have not yet learned to read, who read little, or who have difficulty with reading for any reason. It is articulation, not reading, which is being tested, so care should be taken not to introduce artificial barriers to natural speech responses. In most such tests pictures are printed or mounted on cards and the cards assembled in packs or in a ring booklet. Pictured objects should be familiar, realistic, interesting, clearly depicted, and designed to produce the desired word or phrase. Any clinician can make up his own set, keeping these criteria in mind.

The clinician can develop a picture or reading test which calls for a single-word response or can arrange such tests so that a phrase or longer unit of speech is produced. Picture tests are usually of the single word type, reading tests of the phrase or sentence type. For use with individuals well able to read the clinician can construct or find in the literature series of words, phrases, or sentences, often at several levels of difficulty. It is useful to have available reading tests at at least two levels so that the test used will be appropriate to the vocabulary, reading, and interest level of cases ranging from the middle school grades to adults. Tongue twisters should be avoided and sentences kept short and constructed so that test words will be heard easily by the examiner.

Diagnostic tests of articulation should include items to test all of the vowels, diphthongs, consonants, and some at least of the consonant blends, as listed below. The list of consonant blends given here includes only those which occur most frequently in speech or which are most likely to be defective. A key word is given for each sound. The consonants should be tested in initial, medial, and final positions in words when they occur in all of these positions.

Vowels

[i]	(feet)	[ɚ]	(car)	[ɑ]	(father)
[ɪ]	(fish)	[ɝ]	(bird)	[ɔ]	(ball)
[ɛ]	(bed)	[ʌ]	(cup)	[ʊ]	(book)
[æ]	(hat)	[ə]	(above)	[u]	(school)

Diphthongs

[eɪ]	(play)	(ɑʊ]	(cow)	[ɔɪ]	(boy)
[ɑɪ]	(pie)	[oʊ]	(snow)	[ju]	(use)

Consonants

[p]	(pencil)	[ð]	(mother)	[tʃ]	(chair)
[b]	(baby)	[t]	(table)	[dʒ]	(jump)
[m]	(man)	[d]	(dog)	[r]	(rabbit)
[w]	(window)	[n]	(nest)	[l]	(leaf)
[ʍ]	(wheel)	[s]	(soap)	[j]	(yellow)
[f]	(fork)	[z]	(zipper)	[k]	(cat)
[v]	(vegetables)	[ʃ]	(shoe)	[g]	(gun)
[θ]	(thumb)	[ʒ]	(television)	[ŋ]	(ring)
				[h]	(house)

Partial List of Common Consonant Blends

With [s]:		With [r]:		With [l]:	
[sk–]	(skate)	[pr–]	(pray)	[pl–]	(play)
[skr–]	(scratch)	[br–]	(bread)	[bl–]	(blue)
[skw–]	(squirrel)	[dr–]	(dress)	[fl–]	(fly)
[sl–]	(sled)	[fr–]	(frog)	[kl–]	(clock)
[sm–]	(smoke)	(gr–]	(green)	[gl–]	(glove)
[sn–]	(snake)	[kr–]	(cry)	[–ld]	(cold)
[sp–]	(spoon)	[ʃr–]	(shrub)	[–lk]	(milk)
[spl–]	(splash)	[tr–]	(tree)	[–lt]	(salt)
[spr–]	(spring)	[θr–]	(three)	[–lz]	(dolls)
[str–]	(street)	[–ɚd]	(hard)		
[st–]	(stove)	[–ɚk]	(fork)	With [w]:	
[sw–]	(swing)	[–ɚn]	(corn)	[dw–]	(dwarf)
[–ks]	(box)	[–ɚt]	(heart)	[kw–]	(queen)
[–ns]	(fence)	[–mɚ]	(hammer)	[tw–]	(twins)
[–ps]	(cups)	[–tɚ]	(butter)		
[–ts]	(hats)	[–ðɚ]	(mother)		

METHODS OF RECORDING RESPONSES

Record forms are usually published with commercial tests of articulation. Each clinician can also develop an original record form for his own clinic or school program. For ease in recording it is important that speech sounds on the record form be arranged in the order in which test items will be presented. The most convenient arrangement provides for a list of sounds in a column down the left side of the blank, with three lines to the right of each sound to record responses on initial, medial, and final consonants, on vowels, on diphthongs, and on at least the most important consonant blends. The examiner will achieve the most accurate record if he listens for only one sound at a time, temporarily disregarding others.

It is further recommended that an extra space or spaces be provided at the right of each item so that the examiner, after completing the inventory, can go back over it and record the subject's response to stimulation on the sounds he had misarticulated.

Clinicians vary in the system used for recording misarticulations on the record form. However, in the interests of bringing about a desirable degree of standardization in the professional field, it is strongly recommended that all clinicians use the system described by Johnson, Darley, and Spriestersbach (1963, p. 90.) It is as follows: For a correctly articulated sound record a check (√), for a substitution of one sound for another record the phonetic symbol of the sound substituted, for a sound omission record a dash (—), and for a sound distortion record X. This type of precise recording of misarticulations provides a basis for analysis of the articulation problem and a permanent record for comparison with later results after therapy.

Upon initial examination of a case it is desirable to make a tape recording of the individual's speech, sampling both conversational speech and the responses to an articulation inventory. Periodic recordings provide a more objective and accurate record than even the best written record and can be evaluated by other clinicians. They are a check on examiner reliability and are useful clinically in evaluating progress with therapy objectively. For the case himself they are useful for motivation and self-appraisal.

SPECIFIC TESTS OF ARTICULATION

The selection of an articulation test will depend upon the purpose to be served and the age and reading ability of the subject. If only a rough estimate of articulation is desired, as in a screening survey of school-age or adult populations, or in the articulation evaluation of cases referred for other types of speech disorders, only the speech sounds more frequently defective need be tested. These are: /s/, /z/, /ʃ/, /ʒ/, /tʃ/, /dʒ/, /ʍ/, /θ/, /ð/, /r/, /l/. For young children /f/, /v/, /k/, and /g/ should also be included.

The most commonly used and commercially available screening tests are the *Templin-Darley Tests of Articulation* (Templin and Darley, 1960) in which 50 of the 176-item diagnostic test items are used for screening purposes. The series includes both picture and sentence tests. Van Riper and Erickson (1969) developed a predictive screening test of articulation which can aid the school speech clinician in identifying those first grade children who are likely to require professional help if they are to develop mature articulation.

For purposes of diagnostic examination of cases of articulation disorder a much more systematic and thorough examination of articulation is called for than can be provided by a brief screening test. Such a diagnostic test should include all the speech sounds listed earlier. The thorough articulation inventory serves the dual purpose of furthering understanding of the nature and possible cause of the disorder and of establishing a basis for planning an effective sequence of therapeutic steps.

The most widely used, commercially available diagnostic tests of articulation to appear in recent years are those of Templin and Darley (1960), referred to earlier, and McDonald's *Deep Test of Articulation* (1964). Both of these series have great merit although they differ considerably in form and in the theoretical bases on which they were developed. Both series include picture tests for younger children and sentence tests for those who can read easily. McDonald emphasizes the overlapping, ballistic nature of speech movements and rejects what he regards as the fallacy of analyzing articulation of single sounds or of testing consonant sounds in initial, medial, and final positions in words. His tests, therefore, attempt to identify the specific phonetic contexts in which misarticulations occur, as well as the specific phonetic contexts in which sounds are correctly produced. The tests of Templin and Darley and of McDonald are in extensive current use for both research and clinical purposes.

Other speech pathologists have developed articulation tests which are less well known than the above but which are of utility for certain purposes. These tend to be shorter than the Templin-Darley or McDonald tests. A brief but clear picture test for initial consonants, as well as reading tests of articulation at two difficulty levels, are given in Anderson (1953, pp. 51–61).

The Buck and Perritt Test (Carter and Buck, 1958) contains subtests for spontaneous and imitative responses to pictures, and for imitative responses to nonsense syllables.

Hejna's *Developmental Articulation Test* (Hejna, 1955) tests consonants in all positions and some blends and is arranged by developmental level. Goldman and Fristoe (1967) developed a filmstrip articulation test which they consider better than Hejna's because it can be given in less time, elicits more sounds, and produces fewer ambiguous responses.

In the *Arizona Articulation Proficiency Score* (Barker and England, 1962) sounds are arranged and tested in developmental order, and a numerical score and an "articulation age" are obtained.

Irwin and Musselman (1962) developed the *Compact Picture Articulation Test* which attempts to shorten the required time for application by testing more than one sound per word. The test uses 27 words (pictures) and tests 61 phonetic elements. No consonant blends are included. The authors compared their own test with other articulation tests and found a high correlation with even the longer articulation tests.

Unusually well-prepared test sentences in large type for the primary reader are given in Schoolfield (1951, pp. 2–5). For adult readers excellent test sentences for vowels, diphthongs, and single consonants will be found in Fairbanks (1940, pp. xii-xv).

STIMULABILITY TESTING

As a basis for planning therapy no procedure can be more useful than testing the subject's ability to respond to oral stimulation from the examiner by improving his articulation of the sounds he misarticulated on the articulation test. His response to stimulation also adds to an understanding of the nature of his articulation problem and its probable etiology. Milisen (1954) was one of the first to stress the importance of this type of evaluation, but most writers in the field are now in thorough agreement as to its importance. Degree of stimulability has been shown to be closely related to later articulation development without therapy and also to response to speech therapy. This has been demonstrated in numerous studies such as those of Irwin et al. (1966), Kisatsky (1967), and Sommers et al. (1967).

When the clinician has completed the articulation testing of an individual he should go back over the defective sounds to determine the subject's ability to produce the sounds correctly by imitation of the examiner. The stimulability of a sound should be tested by presenting the isolated sound, then the sound in initial, medial, and final positions in nonsense syllables and in words. The sound should be presented in words where it occurs singly and then in various blends. The subject should be able to both see and hear the examiner easily when the stimulability test is given. The clinician should record responses to stimulation as precisely as he records responses on the articulation test. The record form for an articulation test should provide spaces after each sound to make convenient the later recording of responses to stimulation.

When the individual can correct his misarticulations fairly readily in response to stimulation from the examiner, it suggests, for one thing, that organic factors—structural, motor, or sensory—are probably not contributing importantly to the problem. Diagnostic light is shed on the articulation problem and a prognosis as to the probable response to speech therapy is aided.

The relative ease with which the case can produce his various defective sounds by imitation will also be indicative of a good place at which to begin articulatory training. Other factors being equal, it is profitable to begin training with the sounds which the individual can correct most easily. A trial of the person's response to retraining, therefore, is well worth making from a diagnostic, a prognostic, and a therapeutic point of view.

Analysis of Articulation Test Results

The administration of an articulation inventory and stimulability test is only a first step in analyzing the individual's articulation proficiency. From the test responses it is important for the clinician to go further and to make both a quantitative and a qualitative analysis.

QUANTITATIVE ANALYSIS

Over the years many investigators have attempted to quantify articulation, to measure it by precise degrees, even to come up with a single score or index which would indicate degree of communication handicap. Some of the investigations have been directed toward developing articulation scales by precise psychological scaling methods, mainly for research rather than clinical purposes. Notable among these are the numerous studies carried out by Sherman and her associates at the State University of Iowa, such as Morrison (1955), Sherman and Morrison (1955), Prather (1960), and Sherman and Cullinan (1960).

More clinically oriented attempts have been made to quantify articulation. Some, such as Templin and Darley (1960), Barker and England (1962), and others, have done this through constructing articulation tests which yield a quantitative measure of articulation proficiency in terms of number of correct responses. Others have utilized a scoring system which assigns different weights to the various types of errors. A study of this type is that of Snow and Milisen (1954b), who derived an articulation score based upon assigning a value of 1.0 to 5.0 to each speech sound in each position. A value of 1.0 indicates correct articulation, 2.0 a mildly distorted sound, 3.0 a severely distorted sound, 4.0 a substitution, and 5.0 an omission. The articulation score is the mean of these rank order values for all sounds in all positions.

Wood (1946 and 1949) described an *articulation index* which takes into consideration the relative frequency with which the different speech sounds occur in speech and the different positions in which they occur in words. He developed an inventory of 70 consonant sounds, counting each of the positions of the 25 consonants (phonetic alphabet) as a separate sound. Five of the consonants occur in only two positions; the remainder occur in three positions. Each consonant was given a weighting, in relation to its frequency of occurrence as established by Travis (1931, p. 223). The weighting for each consonant was prorated among the three (or two) positions in which it occurs. The total of all weightings is 100. The *articulation index* is obtained by subtracting from 100 the weight of each sound misarticulated. The index takes into consideration the obvious fact that all sounds do not have equal value but that misarticulation of frequently occurring sounds is more of a handicap than misarticulation of sounds which occur but rarely.

Henrikson (1948) has objected to Wood's prorating of each consonant's weight equally among the positions, on the ground that sounds do not occur with equal positional frequency. Wood, however, has defended this technique as the only one feasible and has pointed out that position in words is relatively meaningless anyway in connected speech. Pettit (1952) evolved an extension of Wood's technique, securing an articulation index at each of five levels of articulatory difficulty, yielding a maximum score for perfect articulation of 504.15 and permitting articulatory differences to be more finely differentiated.

Each clinician should derive a quantitative score from whatever articulation test he uses. The commercial tests yield such a score. For a self-constructed test a simple score of number right out of a standard total number of stimuli presented will at least permit comparison between cases and comparison of the same case at different testings.

It is to be hoped that efforts toward precise measurement of articulation proficiency will continue. It is clear that a valid, reliable, and quantitative index of articulation would have wide application to both research and clinical problems through facilitating the statistical handling of articulation data.

QUALITATIVE ANALYSIS

It is not sufficient for clinical purposes to find out the number of speech sounds misarticulated. The clinician must go further and analyze the *types* of misarticulations made and the *phonetic contexts* in which they occur, as well as the phonetic contexts in which the same sounds may be articulated correctly. In the preceding chapter research bearing on misarticulation types was cited. From both research and clinical experience it appears that misarticulation types follow a rough hierarchy, with omissions the most extreme form of misarticulation, substitutions next, and distortions the closest to correct articulation. The learning of a speech sound often seems to pass through stages of approximation to the attempted sound, with distortions indicative of an about-to-emerge sound or transitional phase of the sound. Snow and Milisen (1954b) based a quantitative articulation score on this misarticulation heirarchy.

In analyzing the articulation test results on a specific case, therefore, the clinician must identify the *types* and *phonetic consistency* of misarticulations and the specific phonetic character of the misarticulations. What sounds are used to substitute for the desired sound? If distortions are produced, what is the exact manner of producing the distortion? In what positions in words, in what phonetic contexts, and in what motor and auditory sequences do errors occur? As Van Riper and Irwin (1958), Curtis and Hardy (1959), and many others have stressed, a thorough phonetic analysis of misarticulations is valuable to an understanding of the problem and to planning a remedial program.

McDonald (1959, 1964) has particularly stressed the need to analyze sensorimotor *patterns* in misarticulation and in his test provides for the testing of each sound in approximately 50 phonetic contexts.

The results of stimulability testing, together with the analysis of misarticulations recommended above, will provide the clinician with valuable diagnostic information and will assist him in planning the entire therapeutic program as well as in deciding where to "take hold" of the problem first.

The reader is referred to Van Riper (1963), Van Riper and Irwin (1958), McDonald (1959, 1964), and Johnson, Darley, and Spriestersbach (1963) for particularly thorough and helpful discussions of both principles and techniques for diagnostic testing and analysis of articulation cases.

WHY DOES THE PERSON HAVE THE ARTICULATION DISORDER?

All of the examination procedures already described contribute to the eventual attempt to explain the "why" of the specific problem under consideration. The study of the various facets of the individual's personality and the detailed examination of his speech, as described in the preceding sections, will have led the clinician to tentative conclusions as to the factors which have produced the articulation disorder. Certain specific etiological possibilities will have to be investigated further, however, always with the double purpose of explaining the problem and of getting clues as to how it can best be approached remedially.

In the preceding chapter the various etiological possibilities were reviewed and the conclusion was reached that there is no factor which is always associated with functional articulation problems. However, until future research conclusively rules out some of these factors, it is expedient to explore them. Any one or combination of them *may* be present in a case we are examining.

Examination procedures are for the most part common to the diagnostic study of all types of speech disorders. (These are described adequately in Chapters 24 and 25. The reader is also referred to the diagnostic manual by Johnson, Darley, and Spriestersbach (1958) for examination techniques and record forms.) Only a few supplementary techniques which are of special significance for functional articulation cases will be described more fully here.

Speech-Sound Discrimination

Although the research reviewed in the preceding chapter on speech-sound discrimination led to the conclusion that it is doubtful that a generalized deficiency in speech-sound discrimination exists in functional articulation cases, it also seemed clear that these cases probably have—or many of them have—at least selective difficulties in sound discrimination, particularly on the specific sounds they themselves misarticulate. Moreover, it seems probable that many functional articulation defectives have more difficulty with intrapersonal than with interpersonal discrimination. In other words, even with little or no difficulty in discriminating speech sounds produced by others, they may have difficulty discriminating sounds in their own speech. Therefore it is important that speech-sound discrimination be thoroughly tested as part of the complete diagnostic evaluation of functional articulation cases.

SPECIFIC TESTS OF SPEECH-SOUND DISCRIMINATION

Pronovost and Dumbleton (1953) published a report of a picture test of speech-sound discrimination suitable for young children. For each test item, the child is confronted with three pairs of pictures involving only two different words, a "like" pair for one word, a "like" pair for the other word, and an "unlike" pair depicting both words. The child points to the pair of pictures which he thinks the examiner has named. Test data were gathered on first-grade children. The authors consider the test a useful diagnostic instrument.

Templin (1957) developed what are the most widely used tests of speech-sound discrimination, based upon her earlier studies (1943). Out of 200 stimulus items consisting of same or different pairs of nonsense syllables she selected the 50 most discriminating pairs and developed norms for children six to eight years of age. She also developed a paired-picture test of 59 items and norms for testing speech-sound discrimination in children three to five years of age. Templin's tests have had wide application for both research and clinical purposes.

Wepman's *Auditory Discrimination Test* (1958) has also been used extensively. It contains two parallel forms, each consisting of 40 same or different pairs of words. The words in the "different" pairs vary by only one phoneme and within the same phoneme category. Norms are given for ages five through eight.

Some of the techniques to be described later for training in auditory discrimination can be used on a trial basis in the diagnostic examination to permit still further observations of the individual's present level of skill and his capacity for developing skill.

Following the application of one of these standardized tests of speech-sound discrimination, all of which are based upon interpersonal discrimination of speech sounds in general, explore informally the subject's discrimination for those sounds which he himself misarticulates.

For example, have the person turn his back or close his eyes. Present him with two, three, or four (depending on age) repetitions of the same word. Make an error in one of them and have him identify the order in which the incorrect word occurred. Present a series of words in this manner, the position of the incorrect stimulus being varied at random. The error made by the clinician should simulate the person's own error on that sound. If the case has difficulty, for example, with /s/, present a series of *s*-words, the sound occurring in various positions in the different words. If several sounds are defective, more extensive testing of this sort will be necessary. Does the subject have more difficulty discriminating in the examiner's speech those sounds he misarticulates himself? As Spriestersbach and Curtis (1951) have reported, there tends to be a relationship between a person's discrimination errors and his articulation errors.

Since discrimination of speech sounds as produced by another person (interpersonal discrimination) may be discrepant with the person's discrimination of his own speech sounds (intrapersonal discrimination), it is important to carry the testing one step further. Various simple techniques can be used. For example, have the subject read a word or name a picture. Immediately after, say the same word to him twice, once correctly and once with an imitation of his error. Ask him which of your repetitions was like his. Try this with a number of words containing his defective sounds. Training in autodiscrimination is a thread which runs through all articulation therapy, particularly when the diagnostic evaluation of the case shows this to be a problem.

Auditory synthesis or the ability to identify a word from hearing its component phonemes is another aspect of discrimination which the clinician may want to explore. Van Riper (1954, pp. 195–196) describes and gives rough norms for a simple test of this skill. He refers to it again in his later revision (1963, p. 480) He has found that individuals who have difficulty in thus synthesizing sounds tend to have difficulty also in analyzing words into their component sounds.

Auditory Memory Span

Auditory memory span also fails to show a consistent relationship to functional articulation disorders but may be a factor in a few cases. There are standardized memory-span tests available using digits, nonsense syllables, vowel sounds, consonant sounds, or nonsense words. Anderson (1939) experimented with digits, vowels, and consonants but found vowel sounds to be the most suitable material for testing auditory memory span. His vowel test is reproduced also in Berry and Eisenson (1942, p. 411).

Metraux (1944) used adaptions of Anderson's tests and published norms for vowel and for consonant tests. Van Riper (1963, p. 477) gathers together the norms given by various authors, including Metraux.

Since Irwin et al. (1966) found initial scores on auditory memory span for vowels predictive of improvement in intelligibility of connected speech, emphasis is given to the usefulness of testing this skill in a diagnostic examination.

Diadochokinetic Rate

As indicated in the preceding chapter, tests of motor speed and dexterity have shown no consistent relationship to functional articulation disorders. Individual cases, however, may have a deficiency in motor coordination, so it is important to rule in or rule out this factor in making a diagnostic examination. As concluded in the last chapter, the tests which have seemed most promising, among the many tried, are those in which movements of the speech mechanism itself, during a speech act, have been utilized.

Irwin and Becklund (1953, pp. 156–157) give tentative age norms, for ages six through 15 years, and for boys and girls separately, on the number of repetitions per second of /pə/, /tə/, and /kə/, as well as for hand-tapping.

TABLE 34-I
Irwin and Becklund's Data on Number of Repetitions in One Second*

	[pə]		[tə]		[kə]	
AGE	GIRLS	BOYS	GIRLS	BOYS	GIRLS	BOYS
6	3.67	3.49	3.51	3.33	3.28	3.18
7	4.38	4.34	4.33	4.14	3.88	4.02
9	4.40	4.56	4.32	4.49	3.94	4.19
11	4.88	4.80	4.84	4.75	4.46	4.52
13	5.44	5.17	5.22	5.09	4.76	4.84
15	5.44	5.86	5.38	5.77	5.00	5.27

* These figures are the mean number of repetitions of the syllable in one second. Their table also gives the standard deviation of each mean.

Maxwell (1953) found that, of a number of motor tests used to compare articulatory-defective and normal-speaking boys, repetition of /lɑ/ and of /pɑtɑkɑ/, of the tests involving the speech mechanism, distinguished best between the two groups. These two tests also showed the most consistent increase with age for the control group.

TABLE 34-II
Maxwell's Data on Number of Repetitions in Two Seconds

AGE	[lɑ]	[pɑtɑkɑ]
7	11.77	9.23
8	13.08	9.69
9	13.54	10.62

In evaluating the subject's patterns of coordination within the speech mechanism the clinician may want to note the presence or absence of a tongue-thrust or visceral pattern of swallowing, even though the relationship of this to articulation is uncertain. As in the preceding chapter the reader is again referred to Hoffman and Hoffman (1965) as the most authoritative reference on this topic.

DIAGNOSTIC AND PROGNOSTIC EVALUATION

The Diagnostic Summary

The entire diagnostic operation should be therapy-oriented. Throughout the various evaluative procedures he uses the clinician must be constantly asking himself what the implications are for the selection and sequencing of therapeutic techniques. He tries to come to a diagnostic conclusion about his case, but a final conclusion about the nature and cause of the speech disorder is not always possible at the time of the diagnostic examination. Sometimes only trial speech therapy reveals the true extent of the problem and the factors which have been responsible for it. In fact, many clinicians consider what can be called "diagnostic therapy" an integral part of the total diagnostic process.

However, the sooner a reliable diagnosis can be reached the less will time be wasted in inappropriate procedures and the more quickly and dependably can a constructive therapeutic program be initiated. The desirability of an early diagnostic conclusion about a case, however, should never preclude the modification of this conclusion by new insights gained through therapy.

To reiterate a statement made in the preceding chapter, a diagnosis of "functional" should be made on the basis of the factors operating at the time of the examination. However, a genuine understanding of the problem will be reached only by careful study of factors—organic or functional—operative in the past as well as in the present. It is easy to be misled by the presence of a major organic factor—such, for example, as a cleft palate—into assuming that the speech characteristics noted are due to that factor. They may or may not be, or they may be only in part. The mere presence of a factor does not mean that it necessarily has a causal relationship to the speech disorder. This needs to be evaluated carefully in each case.

We cannot stress too much the desirability of thinking in terms of a *causal pattern* rather than a *cause*. Seldom is etiology single and simple in a function so complex as speech. The careful clinician evaluates systematically the factors in all of the possible etiological areas—structural, motor, sensory, developmental, health, intellectual, learning, environmental, emotional—before trying to identify the particular ones which, in combination, have produced the problem as it is now seen. The diagnostic pieces should be integrated into a meaningful whole. The outcome of the diagnostic procedures should be a unified picture of the person and his speech problem and at least a tentative answer to the question of whether and how it can be treated.

DEGREE OF COMMUNICATION HANDICAP

As part of the diagnostic summarization of a case the clinician should evaluate the degree of communication handicap experienced by the person. The extent to which the individual's functional articulation disorder constitutes a handicap for *him* specifically will be related to:

His degree of intelligibility.
The number of different sounds defective in his speech.
The specific sounds which are defective—frequency of their occurrence in speech.
The consistency with which these misarticulations occur.
The age of the individual.
The general speech standards prevailing in the individual's environment.
The importance of good speech for the individual's personal career or social needs.
The attitudes of family and friends, the significance they attach to his speech disorder, and
The individual's self-attitudes, and, specifically, his attitudes about his own speech.

Prognosis—Predicting the Response to Speech Therapy

It is clinically useful to attempt to make a prognosis for each case examined, an estimate of probable outcome, both without therapy and with therapy. We should evaluate the extent to which the speech disorder can probably be remedied and the future conditions which will have a bearing on its correction. We should also attempt a conservative estimate as to the amount of time which the treatment of the problem will require.

The speech clinician should be extremely cautious in discussing the outcome of the therapy with the case himself or with his parents. The relative crudeness of even present-day diagnostic and therapy techniques and the many variables which enter into a successful therapeutic outcome preclude the placing of a definite time limit on speech therapy. At the same time, the person who is entering upon speech therapy wants and should have some idea of how long it will probably take—a month, a year, five years. The clinician should be prepared to discuss in at least general terms the speech outcome to be expected and indicate at the same time the factors which will tend to hasten or retard speech improvement.

For his own private benefit the speech clinician can afford to be less cautious. Excellent professional discipline and important clinical learning are gained by writing down for oneself or one's colleagues only a careful estimate of the final speech outcome and an estimate of the amount of therapy which will be required to reach that outcome. Later comparison of the actual and the prognosticated progress adds to and refines clinical judgment.

RESEARCH CONTRIBUTIONS TO PREDICTION

A number of investigators have contributed to our knowledge of at least some of the factors which contribute to the prediction of speech therapy outcome.

The severity of the disorder, in terms of number of sounds misarticulated, was found to have predictive value by Pettit (1952), Steer and Drexler (1960), Sommers et al. (1961), Sommers et al. (1967), and Irwin et al. (1966). Steer and Drexler also found the type of error to have some predictive value, especially errors in the final position, and most of all omissions in the final position. Various writers have reported that distortion errors are most responsive to therapy, substitutions next, and omissions least.

Results are conflicting regarding the predictive value of mental age or intelligence. Steer and Drexler (1960) found the intelligence of kindergarten children unrelated to articulation status five years later, but speech improvement was given the experimental group for only 12 weeks and no therapy thereafter to either group. This finding does not negate a possible relation of intelligence to the outcome of therapy. Irwin et al. (1966) did find that improvement in articulation of second-grade children could be predicted from mental age.

Auditory skills have been explored as predictive factors. Farquhar (1961) compared kindergarten children with mild and severe articulation problems on tests of auditory discrimination and on stimulability. The auditory discrimination tests had no prognostic significance for status of spontaneous speech seven months later, but the imitative ability or stimulability did have. Irwin et al. (1966) tested second-grade children with articulation disorders and normal controls on a wide battery of tests. They found Wepman's Auditory Discrimination Test, auditory memory span for vowels, and a stimulability test for consonants in nonsense syllables all predictive of proficiency or improvement in speech for children with articulation problems.

Other investigators also are virtually unanimous in finding stimulability a highly predictive factor. In agreement with the above studies are Carter and Buck (1958) and Kisatsky (1967). In the latter study a "high stimulability" group of kindergarten children corrected 59 percent of its original articulation errors in six months, as compared with 10 percent for a "low stimulability" group; neither group had speech therapy. Sommers et al. (1967) point out that subjects with low stimulability scores benefit more from therapy than those with good stimulability scores. Presumably the good stimulability group improve without therapy because of their sensitivity to environmental speech stimulation, but also presumably they would respond rapidly to therapy if it were offered.

Van Riper and Irwin (1958, pp. 66–67) offer a useful set of workable criteria for determining when a child will achieve good articulation.

GUIDELINES FOR PREDICTING THE OUTCOME OF SPEECH THERAPY

The clinician will have to weigh a number of factors in estimating the success which articulation therapy can be expected to have and the probable length of time it will have to continue. These factors are closely related to some of the factors which determine the present degree of communication handicap. The following are the most important to consider in functional articulation cases:

> Severity of the speech disorder, number of sounds defective, and the nature of the misarticulations. In general, the greater the number of defective sounds the greater the evidence of improvement per unit of therapeutic time, but the longer the total amount of therapy required. Types of misarticulations, their phonemic similarity to the correct sounds, and their consistency in connected speech.

Stimulability—the degree to which misarticulated sounds can be produced correctly by imitation.

Intelligence of the individual.

Age of the individual. Other factors being equal, the younger the person, the more easily can his misarticulation be corrected.

Frequency with which therapy sessions can be given.

Impeding physical factors such as poor health or low vitality.

Impeding personality or emotional characteristics.

Degree and quality of cooperation to be expected from family, teachers, and associates.

The individual's own motivation for speech improvement.

SPEECH THERAPY FOR FUNCTIONAL ARTICULATION DISORDERS

Therapy has even less research evidence to support it than have other aspects of speech pathology. It is still largely a product of clinical experience. Speech pathologists have only in recent years begun to develop their own rationale and methodology for articulation therapy, to add to or modify the earlier synsthesis of techniques taken over from the speech arts, education, and psychotherapy. Articulation therapy still reflects—and possibly always will—each clinician's personal background and bias, even though he builds upon the accumulated experience of his colleagues. There are encouraging signs that more attempts are being made to subject approaches and techniques for therapy to scientific scrutiny.

In the pages which follow an attempt has been made to bring together the points of view and the practices concerning articulation therapy which have common acceptance. Notable divergences in viewpoint are indicated in some cases. It is urged that the statements made in the remainder of this chapter be thought of as tentative formulations awaiting experimental verification and modification. Nearly every principle of articulation therapy discussed—from the mechanical aspects of therapy structuring to the selection of therapeutic method—should make a profitable subject for future research investigation.

Planning Speech Therapy for the Functional Articulation Case

The organization of the therapeutic program for a case follows logically from the diagnostic evaluation. Within the causal pattern which has been identified, the clinician will want first to distinguish between those causal factors which he can hope to affect or eliminate and those which he cannot. He will have to minimize or compensate for the latter or at worst accept them and work around them. The therapeutic program should be concerned mainly with the causal factors which *can* be eliminated or modified. For example, if low physical vitality is contributing to a child's articulatory retardation, obviously efforts should be made at the outset to reduce this factor by advising medical care. If parental attitudes are contributing to the problem—as is so often the case—immediate measures should be instituted in the direction of parental guidance or, if necessary and possible, psychotherapy. A first step, then, in therapy is the evaluation and management of the various factors thought to be contributing to the speech problem.

THE THERAPY PLAN FOR EACH INDIVIDUAL

A clinical plan should be developed for each case. This plan should encompass, first, a statement of long-term objectives; second, a general outline of the clinical procedure to be followed; and, third, a listing of the immediate steps to be taken. It is worthwhile to state final objectives explicitly because they are the goals at which therapy will be directed. They should include the specific speech objectives to be reached and objectives in areas other than speech, such as personal adjustment, improved health, or improved academic progress. The final objectives represent the balanced, multisided approach to therapy which is necessary for a successful outcome.

The outline of clinical procedure will indicate the kind of approach to be followed with the case, the sequence of therapeutic stages to be presented, what problems or aspects of the problem will be worked on first, next, last. Part of this procedural plan with an articulation case would be a decision as to which of his defective sounds should be corrected first and which should be deferred until later. In this ordering of sounds the clinician should take into consideration the possibility of further modification of some of them by maturation and environmental stimulation alone.

If only one sound is defective there is no problem of selection. If a number of sounds are defective, it is usually advisable to work with only one at a time. The following considerations should determine the best sound with which to begin: 1. the most defective or conspicuously handicapping sound, 2. the one which occurs most frequently in speech, 3. the one in which the misarticulation is in the form of a distortion, rather than a substitution or omission, and 4. the one which the individual produces most readily with stimulation. The greatest observable difference in the subject's speech will take place most quickly if these criteria are followed. With younger children the developmental order of sounds should also be considered. Other things being equal, a sound of less rather than greater phonetic complexity should be selected first. For example, most clinicians would not begin with the /r/ unless it was the only sound defective. When working with groups of cases, as in public school programs, practical considerations of grouping may also have to enter into the selection of the sound to be corrected. Informal exploration by the clinician with his case will also yield useful clues as to an effective point of attack. A sound correctly produced in one phonetic context may serve as a bridge to its production in other phonetic contexts.

When the first sound has been brought to the point of voluntary mastery and partial carry-over into conversational speech, work with a second sound can be started. The same criteria apply to the selection of a second sound as to the selection of the first.

The procedural plan should include the general methodology to be followed, the consideration of group or individual therapy or a combination of both, the frequency of therapeutic sessions, and the types of therapeutic activity which will be used.

The third aspect of therapeutic planning is the decision as to where to begin and how to begin—the planning of the first therapy sessions. Detailed planning cannot be done far ahead because of the need for flexibility and constant modification of methods in relation to the individual's response and his progress in speech. Therapeutic sessions should, though, be planned in advance and not left to the ingenuity of the moment. One of the therapist's first decisions will concern the possibility of plunging directly into speech work or the desirability of using a more indirect, unobtrusive approach. With shy, withdrawn children a period of play-therapy activity may be necessary before the child achieves sufficient confidence and responsiveness to profit by direct speech training. In all cases, however responsive, some attention needs to be given initially to establishing rapport and securing the child's understanding of and motivation for the speech training which is being undertaken.

The Structuring of Articulatory Training

Such considerations as frequency, length, and spacing of therapeutic sessions, the use of group therapy, individual therapy, or a combination of both, and the size and composition of therapy groups are determined to a considerable extent by circumstances. Clinical judgment, unfortunately, cannot dictate the structuring of therapy as much as would be desirable. Structuring is likely to be determined by the type of organizational setting—public school, clinic, private practice—within which the therapy is carried out, and by time, space, and staff limitations. To the greatest extent possible, however, certain principles should guide the structuring of therapy. Experimental research so far as had little to contribute to these. They are, rather, the result of the accumulated clinical experience of many therapists.

ARRANGEMENT OF THERAPY SESSIONS

For children below the age of eight, therapy sessions should probably not exceed half an hour. Longer sessions are effective only if the type of activity is varied considerably after the first half hour. Older children can usually work effectively at one type of task for 40 minutes or more. Even adults should probably not be expected to give close attention or sustained effort for longer than an hour at a time.

There is some experimental evidence to add to clinical experience that the more frequent therapy sessions are the more effective they will be. Sommers et al (1970) compared the relative effectiveness of group articulation therapy four times a week, group therapy once a week, and a control group who received no speech therapy at all, using mentally retarded children with misarticulations. Those who received group articulation therapy four times a week improved their articulation significantly compared with the control group. The group who received once-a-week therapy did not improve significantly compared with the control group. Much good work has been done by skillful therapists, however, on a once-a-week basis.

GROUP AND INDIVIDUAL SESSIONS

Increasingly with experience most clinicians would consider group therapy the method of choice for articulation cases rather than a necessity. It is timesaving for the clinician, for most cases it does not sacrifice any advantages, and it has its own overwhelming advantages. Sommers et al. (1966) compared the relative effectiveness of individual and group therapy with 240 children with articulation problems over a treatment period of eight and a half months and concluded (p. 219), "Group therapy was found to be as effective as individual therapy, regardless of the severity of speech defectiveness or grade levels of the children."

The alleged advantages of individual therapy may result from the sterile way in which group therapy has too often been handled. The clinician who stimulates a dynamic interaction among the children in a group and who sees that all children are constantly involved, rather than passively awaiting a turn, can find a powerful clinical tool in the group structure.

The optimum program for most articulation cases below the adult level would provide for a combination of group and individual procedures. Groups should probably not exceed six children and are preferable with only three or four. For effective group interaction the age range within one group should not usually exceed three years, though comparable intellectual and social maturity are more significant than chronological age. In group work the desire of children to communicate through speech, the amount and variety of material they have to communicate, and their motivation to improve in speech are all more easily secured than in working with one child alone. Children stimulate each other, so that even a therapist of modest ability has little difficulty in developing keen interest in speech activities. Group therapy provides a natural situation for speech practice and carry-over of newly learned speech habits.

On the other hand, individual sessions with the therapist are preferable for some cases when their speech problems are so unique that they would profit little from the type of training provided for other children. For example, many speech therapists find that cases with lateral lisps, unless they can be grouped with other lateral lispers, can be handled best alone, rather than with lispers of other types. Even with children who are being handled effectively in a group, there should be some opportunity for occasional individual sessions. Children learn at different rates and the child who makes conspicuously slower progress than other members of the group should have additional help by himself. The therapist's schedule should be flexible enough to permit this individual supplementation of group work.

COMPOSITION OF THERAPY GROUPS

An issue to be considered in organizing groups for articulation therapy is the relative desirability of homogeneous or heterogeneous grouping of cases. A few speech therapists, notably Backus and Beasley (1951, p. 43), advocate the inclusion of cases of various types within one group, even cases as different as articulation, cleft palate, and stuttering. In expressing this view they explicitly reject what they regard as the older practice of grouping cases by type of disorder on the assumption "there there is a different type of therapy for each type of disorder." They protest against what they evidently regard as the general assumption of workers in speech therapy that all cases with one type of disorder are exactly alike and have identical needs. They attack also what they consider a common practice, drilling on specific speech habits out of the context of actual communicative needs and an ignoring of interpersonal relations as related to speech behavior.

Most clinicians, however, seem to feel that therapy methods can be more appropriate and specific to needs if cases are grouped homogeneously. Most clinicians have apparently experienced no difficulty in utilizing interpersonal relations and children's communicative needs and drives and are still working with homogenous rather than heterogeneous groups. Most clinicians, too, while recognizing the many overlapping needs of speech cases of all types, also recognize the necessity for a considerable degree of differentiation of therapy depending upon the type of disorder involved. Because of this need for differentiation, it is usually found most effective to group individuals for therapy according to the specifics of their speech problems. The emotional and interpersonal aspects of the therapy program can be furthered fully as well by grouping several lispers together, or several stutterers, or several cleft-palate cases, as by mixing these types of cases in a single group. At the same time, the highly differentiated aspects of therapy for these different cases will not be sacrificed.

Major Approaches to Articulation Therapy

Speech pathologists who have written on functional articulation disorders or who work clinically with these cases tend to rely primarily on one or another basic concept of therapy. However, their differing viewpoints as to the most productive approaches to therapy are often more apparent than real. Apparent differences may be more a question of differing *emphasis* than of fundamental disagreement. As one peruses the modern literature in speech pathology he can hardly escape the conclusion that a growing eclecticism and communality of viewpoint is developing. Most clinicians seem to do most of the same things in articulation therapy regardless of their expressed theoretical viewpoints. They vary chiefly in the importance they place on certain aspects of a common program of therapy or on certain techniques in the armamentarium common to most clinicians They differ most when they talk or write about their practices, least when they sit down with a treatment case.

In the early days of speech pathology great emphasis was given to the phonetic-placement method (Scripture, 1923; Cotrel and Halsted, 1936; Mulgrave, 1939, Raubicheck, Davis, and Carll, 1932; and Raubicheck, 1952). In this approach, the individual is given training in the specific placement of the articulators for the production of each sound. He is shown where the position of his tongue, or other parts of his speech mechanism, is faulty and what changes in positioning are required to produce the sound correctly. Speech training is based upon a knowledge of phonetics. The phonetic-placement approach is based upon the assumption that there is a standard way to produce each sound. Doubt has been thrown upon this, however, by modern phonetic research, which has tended to show that a given acoustic result can be achieved by a considerable variety of positionings in different individuals. What may be an optimum placement for one may not achieve a satisfactory result for another. The production of speech sounds is a dynamic and highly individual process. Overawareness of the mechanics of sound production, moreover, is apt to create an artificial, unnatural attitude about speech and have an inhibiting effect. The most serious objection, however, to relying heavily upon the method of phonetic placement is that it gives the individual little help in judging his own speech. It is a technique which has limited usefulness in carry-over. Incidental use should be made of phonetic methods, of course. With older children and adults particularly, incidental description of the production of the sound in question helps to shorten the training process.

A motor-kinesthetic method was described by Stinchfield-Hawk and Young (Stinchfield and Young, 1938; Hawk, 1942; Young and Hawk, 1955), though this method was never widely used. In the motor-kinesthetic method the therapist manipulates the articulators of the case, so that—passively—he produces the correct sound. The individual thus is presumed to receive the correct kinesthetic pattern for each sound and is enabled eventually to reproduce it himself. The therapist accompanies his manipulation with auditory stimulation. Some observers of this method have felt that it was the auditory stimulation, rather than the kinesthetic, which was the effective element in the therapy. Few therapists have been willing to rely primarily upon the motor-kinesthetic method, though nearly all make incidental use of kinesthetic cues. In teaching the less visible sounds, the individual can be helped to develop the "feel" of the correct positioning. Kinesthesis, however, is a relatively crude and undifferentiated sense and cannot assist much in fine discrimination.

An auditory training approach, the so-called "stimulus method," was developed over 30 years ago, particularly at the State University of Iowa (Travis, 1931). This approach over the intervening years has gained increasingly wide acceptance in the profession as the most effective basic method for working with functional articulation cases. Today most clinicians use auditory stimulus methods as the core of their therapy with these cases, though recognizing the incidental utility of the phonetic placement and kinesthetic approaches and also of visual aids in the learning of new sounds.

Hearing is the primary sensory basis for the natural acquisition of speech in early childhood. Hearing is an infinitely more complex and highly differentiated sense than the tactile or kinesthetic and, therefore, permits of finer discriminations. There is a rich source of possible training techniques and materials utilizing audition, whereas touch and kinesthesis are very limited. Visual techniques are useful mainly for the more visible sounds.

Most important of all, audition provides the person with a permanent monitoring system for his own speech. If he develops reliable auditory discrimination, especially self-discrimination, through training, it carries over to all situations—away from the speech therapy session as well as in it—and permits auto-evaluation of speech-sound production. Auditory training becomes, therefore, a powerful technique for habituating the correct production of speech sounds.

AN ECLECTIC, MULTISENSORY APPROACH TO ARTICULATION THERAPY

In recent years speech pathologists seem less and less inclined to limit themselves to any single approach to therapy. Although strong auditory stimulation is still the core of a therapeutic program for most clinicians, because of the obvious advantages described above, they make use of other sensory channels as well. The subject is given visual cues to the correct production of a sound, particularly when the sound has highly visible characteristics. He is also helped to identify kinesthetic cues and uses these both for discovering the way to produce a sound and for monitoring later productions of the sound. Such writers as Milisen (1954), Van Riper (1963), McDonald (1964), and many others, though differing in their individual emphases, have given support to an eclecticism of viewpoint which did not exist earlier.

Clinicians are almost unanimous in stressing primarily auditory methods, but these methods have been greatly modified and amplified. There is less emphasis than formerly on developing auditory discrimination for speech sounds as a generalized skill, though the present writer still considers this a valuable activity as part of a total articulation therapy program. There is increasing emphasis on training for discrimination of the sounds misarticulated, both when these sounds are produced by the therapist and when they are produced by the subject himself. In short, the emphasis has shifted from training in interpersonal to training in intrapersonal discrimination.

Throughout therapy the objective is first to help the subject identify his defective sound by hearing it, seeing it if possible, and feeling it, and then to produce the sound correctly as a result. The second objective is to so train him in self-monitoring skill that he will be able to proceed from few or no correct productions of the sound to ever larger percentages of correct productions, and finally to mastery of the sound in all phonetic contexts and in all types of speech activity.

Another issue which has to be faced in an eclectic approach to articulation therapy is that of reconciling the divergent viewpoints on what constitutes useful and appropriate speech tasks to be used as therapy material. Though all clinicians would surely agree that speech tasks in therapy must be meaningful to the child, they vary in defining what is meaningful. Such writers as Hahn (1960, 1961), Backus and Beasley (1951), and Low et al. (1959) feel that all therapy must be communication-centered, that it must be real communication, not artificially abstracted samples of speech for drill. Some feel that drills are meaningless and valueless because speech is not motivated and corrections do not carry over. Others feel that real communicative situations must be developed first, that units of speech can then be abstracted from these situations for practice, but that these units must then be brought back into the original communicative context.

However, most clinicians seem to feel themselves able to achieve a reasonable compromise between the use of natural, nonspecific speech activities, which are time-consuming, and specific even though artificial drill-type activities. The issue seems to hinge on the ability of the individual clinician to keep interest and motivation at a high level but, at the same time, to proceed as quickly to the point as possible. Well-motivated drills, with the child participating in the selection of topics and words for practice and thoroughly informed and accepting of the purpose of the activity, is a useful and efficient means of achieving clinical ends.

Perhaps most of all the eclectic approach stresses the need to plan therapy which is unique for each case and is based upon a thorough, painstaking analysis of the individual's difficulties, needs, and patterns of articulation and misarticulation. The specific procedures and speech tasks to be used in therapy will then emerge logically from this analysis. Therapy must begin where the individual is now and carry him forward from there. No approach, however eclectic, will suit all cases equally well. No technique can be evaluated in isolation but only in terms of its appropriateness for the specific individual at a specific point in time. The wise clinician will experiment constantly with his case and use what works.

A Program for Articulation Therapy

The process of correcting a misarticulated speech sound can be said to have three phases though these phases are not end-to-end but, rather, are overlapping or even concurrent. These phases are: learning to identify and discriminate the sound (auditorially, visually, kinesthetically, and tactilely), learning to produce the sound at will in a variety of phonetic contexts, and learning to use the sound more and more widely until it is established in connected speech under all conditions. More briefly, these phases can be designated as 1. identification and discrimination, 2. production, and 3. carry-over or habituation.

Discrimination training should play a relatively large part in initial stages of therapy, less as the sound production phase is undertaken, except for continuing emphasis on *auto*discrimination. Activities designed to secure carry-over to habitual speech should begin as soon as the individual has attained some degree of voluntary mastery of the sound in even a few words. The emphasis on auditory training is in no way inconsistent with the absence of clear-cut evidence that a relationship exists between auditory deficiencies and functional articulation problems, since the purpose of giving auditory training is to develop a *positive skill*, an *awareness* of speech sounds, rather than to overcome a deficiency.

The detailed objectives and a few typical activities for each phase of training are described below. In both auditory discrimination and articulatory production the progression in therapy is from the simple, specific, easily identified, highly conscious, and easily controlled toward the more complex, less specific, less easily isolated or identified, less conscious, and less easily controlled listening or speaking behavior. Throughout the following discussion, the sound /s/ is used for illustration. Similar procedures would be used with other sounds.

For purposes of convenience in the pages which follow each phase is discussed separately. However, it is again emphasized that an arbitrary separation of phases is not intended. They will overlap and intermingle differently for each case.

AUDITORY DISCRIMINATION TRAINING

1. Identifying and naming the sound. The therapist should introduce the new sound, particularly for young children, in some interesting and dramatic manner, such as telling a story in which the sound is featured. The sound should be given a "name" to establish its identity clearly for the child, such as for /s/ the "snake sound" or the "steam sound," whatever is appropriate for the stories or pictures used. The child should be stimulated abundantly with the sound, the therapist naming pictures or objects in which the sound appears in the initial position.

2. Learning to discriminate the stimulus sound from other speech sounds. The therapist can then present to the child a series of consonant sounds in random order, such as: /s/, /t/, /k/, /b/, /s/, /m/, /k/, /s/, /g/, /l/, /s/, /s/, /r/, /t/, etc. Have the child tap the table or clap or make some other agreed-upon response every time he hears *his* sound. At first avoid consonants easily confused with /s/, but as the child gains skill in discriminating these should be included, too, as a further refinement of his discrimination.

Very young children may need some preliminary training to establish the concept of listening and discriminating by starting with nonspeech sounds such as noise-making toys. For each auditory activity, first let the child watch you so that he will be aided by visual cues. Later arrange the presentation so that the discrimination will be entirely auditory.

3. Discriminating the sound in more complex contexts. Train the child to discriminate the sound in single words, later in longer speech units such as phrases and sentences read by the therapist. Begin with discrimination between words which start with his sound and words which start with other sounds. Research has shown that discrimination of initial sounds is more accurate than of medial or final sounds (Templin, 1943).

Prepare a supply of cards with pictures mounted or drawn on them. Mix those whose names begin with /s/ with some whose names begin with some easily distinguished sound, such as /l/ or /g/. Leave out one key picture for each sound, such as *soap* for /s/ and *ladder* for /l/. As the therapist names each picture the child decides whether it should be placed under *soap* or under *ladder*. When the child can perform this discrimination reliably, introduce one or two more sounds so that he has three or four choices to make for each word given.

This type of activity provides an excellent opportunity to train the child in a specific discrimination between the sound he is misarticulating and the substitution he is using. For example, children who substitute /w/ for /r/ should be given practice in sorting pictures beginning with these two sounds; similarly for a /θ/ substitution for /s/.

When discrimination of initial sounds is developed, a logical next step is learning to identify the sound when it occurs in *any* position in words. Pictures can be named or words read by the therapist, the child deciding whether each word does or does not contain the /s/ sound. The therapist can motivate such activities by varying the response asked of the child from one session to another. The child can move a marker along a "track" or up a "ladder," place a chip on various pictures, "break a balloon" by covering a series of pictured balloons, or respond in one of the many other possible ways.

Discriminations should be easy in early stages but should increase in difficulty so that the child can finally identify reliably words which contain /s/ in such series as: buzz, bus, zoo, shoe, sew, show, sip, chip, ship, mouth, mouse, etc.

Another activity useful in developing discrimination is the presentation by the therapist of pairs of words or nonsense syllables, in some of the pairs giving the same word or syllable twice, in some giving two different words or syllables. The child is asked to indicate after each pair whether the two words (or syllables) were alike or different. Again, discriminations should be relatively gross at first but become more subtle and demanding as skill is developed.

4. Identifying the position of the sound in words. This skill needs to be developed as a preliminary to enabling the child later to produce the sound correctly himself in all positions. As the therapist names pictures or reads words from a list (all of which contain /s/), the child indicates whether /s/ comes at the beginning, in the middle, or at the end of the word. He can place a mark in one of three appropriately labeled columns on paper or on the blackboard, can put a chip under the "engine," "car," or "caboose" of a pictured train or into a real toy train, or can use any one of many possible response methods. For older children, a simple verbal response is probably most efficient.

5. Discriminating the correct from the incorrect production. If the earlier stages of auditory training have been well done, it will be relatively simple for the child to learn to discriminate between correct production of *his* sound by the therapist and varieties of misarticulation of the sound. It is useful for the therapist to attempt to reproduce accurately the individual's own form of misarticulation and then help him to discriminate reliably between this and the correct sound. The therapist can, for example, read a list of /s/ words or name pictures, giving some correctly at random and in the others using the child's error-type. The child indicates in some manner when he hears an error or checks errors on a numbered list.

A variation of these activities was described earlier in the section on diagnostic techniques. The therapist repeats a word three or four times, the child then indicating which, if any, contained errors. Present a series of words in this manner.

6. Evaluating his own speech. It is of fundamental importance to train the child to apply the auditory discrimination skill he has developed to the monitoring of *his own speech*. One might say that this is the ultimate purpose of auditory training, yet it is an aspect of therapy which is often omitted or inadequately stressed. Too often the therapist continues to do the evaluating for the case, who remains passive and accepts the therapist's verdict as to whether the speech response he has just given was satisfactory or not. It is probably safe to say that habituation of new speech habits, assuming good motivation, will proceed rapidly or not in relation to the individual's self-monitoring skill. It is not safe to assume that skill in identifying errors in the therapist's speech will be applied by the case to his own speech. It is probable that this specific self-application of auditory discrimination skill needs to be given special attention—at least in all but the most alert and highly motivated individuals. How can this be done?

After some articulatory production training has been given and the person has gained a fair degree of voluntary mastery of his new sound, techniques such as the following can be used. These are but several of numerous possibilities:

Have the child name a series of /s/ picture cards, placing each one after he names it in a "good" or a "poor" pile, depending upon his own judgment of his articulation of /s/. When the series is finished discrepancies between the case's judgment and the therapist's may be discussed and some words repeated, if necessary. The same practice can be given through having the child read a list of /s/ words, placing a chip in a "good" or "poor" box or below a smiling or a frowning clown face, or by tallying his judgments on paper or on the blackboard. For older children it may be preferable to have three-degree rather than two-degree evaluation, such as "good," "fair," "poor."

Another and more demanding activity is making up a sentence about each picture or word, the case after each one identifying any errors he has made. In a group situation a high degree of motivation can be secured by having one child at a time read or talk and the others keep a record of his errors. Any errors he notes and corrects spontaneously are not counted. A premium is put on autoevaluation, because the child with the fewest unnoted errors "wins."

TRAINING IN ARTICULATORY PRODUCTION OF A NEW SOUND

Research on the production aspects of articulation training is meager, but a few studies provide some hints as to the most effective ways to proceed. It is probably the most common and accepted practice in articulation therapy to begin training in production with the sound in isolation. On logical grounds it seems probable that an individual can most easily learn to produce that which is highly identifiable and specific and which least involves already established habits. The coordinations involved in producing a single sound, though complex, are less so than those involved in producing a whole word in the context of a sentence.

Research by Scott and Milisen (1954a and b) supports this. In studying 64 elementary school children with functional articulation problems, they found that consonant sounds were produced more often correctly in isolation than in any position in nonsense syllables or words. Furthermore, sounds were made more often correctly in nonsense syllables (any position) than in the corresponding position in words. In nonsense syllables and words, sounds were produced most correctly in the initial position, next most correctly in the medial, and least in the final position, with a few minor exceptions. These results lend strong support to the general clinical practice of beginning with the isolated sound and proceeding to nonsense syllables, then to words, and finally to more complex speech contexts. The individual learning a new sound is thus led by easy stages through an increasingly complex heirarchy of speech configurations. However, most clinicians would agree that, when the subject can produce a correct sound in some contexts, practice on the isolated sound is usually unnecessary.

Milisen's findings also support the common clinical experience that results are best—when the syllable and word stages are reached—if practice is given first with the initial position of the sound, later with medial and final positions.

A few investigators have studied the effectiveness of various methods of stimulus presentation. The findings of Milisen and his associates again give support to the general practice of utilizing the therapist's own speech as his principal clinical tool. The individual learning a sound listens to and watches the therapist saying the sound and then tries to reproduce it. Scott and Milisen (1954a and b) and Humphrey and Milisen (1954) found that combined auditory and visual stimulation was more effective in producing correct responses than either auditory or visual stimulation alone. These results are supported by Huffman and McReynolds (1968).

Webb and Siegenthaler (1957) compared six auditory training methods and found the most effective to be auditory stimulation followed by evaluation of the child's response, including verbal instruction on how to make the sound.

OUTLINE OF THE ARTICULATORY PRODUCTION SEQUENCE

The following outline of procedural stages in articulatory production training summarizes and extends what has already been said. The steps indicated are suggestive only. No outline can be followed rigidly and inflexibly but must be adapted to the needs and responses of the individual case. It is assumed that several sessions on auditory discrimination training will have preceded the sequence here presented and that such training will continue to form part of therapy sessions.

Assuming that the clinician has carried out a careful analysis of the case's articulation, has decided upon the speech sound with which to begin remedial training, and has given the case discrimination training on the sound, what techniques can he use to get correct production of the sound? If the subject is able to produce the sound correctly in any context, this context should be used as a starting point to secure production in other contexts. The subject should be helped to hear, see, and feel how the sound is produced, the clinician also calling his attention to aspects of phonetic placement which will help him identify the specific set of movements involved. The auditory-kinesthetic-tactile feedback from a correct production will be the basis for his duplicating the same set of movements again.

1. **Sound in isolation.** The therapist gives several productions of the sound, asking the child to listen and watch carefully. The child then gives the sound once and his production is evaluated by the therapist. This process is repeated a number of times, if necessary adding descriptive clues as to placement. When the sound is a visible one the child will often be helped, too, by the use of a mirror. This practice should be carried beyond one or two correct responses, so that the child will become secure in just how the sound is produced. For young children interest can be held easily by allowing the child to "climb a ladder" or go "around a track" or simply receive a chip or other token for each correct response he gives.

2. **Sound in nonsense syllables.** The therapist continues with the multiple auditory-visual stimulation and single-response technique but presents the sound followed by a vowel, as /sɑ/, giving practice with the sound preceding the other principal vowels or diphthongs, /sɑ/, /so/, /si/, /sɑɪ/, /su/, etc.

Stimulation practice should next be given with the medial position of the sound, as in /ɑsɑ/, /osɑ/, etc., and then with the final position as in /ɑs/, /is/, /os/, etc. Extended training at the nonsense-syllable stage is seldom necessary, but it is usually a helpful intermediary between the learning of the sound alone and the use of it in the complex context of a whole word. Motivational devices can easily be developed to interest and challenge even young children.

3. **Sound in short, simple words.** It is usually best to begin again with the initial position and to avoid consonant blends. Words such as sun, soap, sit, soup, sing should be used. With some individuals—and with occasional sounds—production is more easily controlled with the sound in the final or medial position. Occasionally, too, blends are more easily handled than the single consonant. Good clinical observation and flexibility in procedure are essential.

Some cases are highly inconsistent in their misarticulations and will need practice only on those words in which the sound occurs in the phonetic contexts which are difficult for them. These contexts will have been identified in the diagnostic examination.

Practice in using the sound in words can be given through such activities as naming pictures or words after the therapist, climbing word ladders, competing with others in the group to be first around a race track made up of words, hanging word *ornaments* on a Christmas tree, putting word *eggs* in a basket, pulling word *petals* from a flower, and innumerable other variations. Many suggestions for speech games and activities at this and other levels of training will be found in "Speech Correction Techniques and Materials," prepared by speech therapists in the Chicago Public Schools, under the writer's direction.

The writer has coined the term *core vocabularies* to designate the concept of selecting for practice words which are meaningfully related to each other. Clinical experience—if not yet research—indicates that more rapid learning of a sound takes place through the mutual reinforcement of words which have been learned in relation to a "core" topic or experience, as compared with practice situations in which the words employed are selected at random and are unrelated. Thus practice will probably be most effective if the vocabulary involved centers around a "core" or theme familiar to the child. To illustrate, core vocabularies for /s/ can be developed around: 1. things in the home (house, stove, sink, bookcase, sofa, fireplace, toaster, etc.); 2. things to wear (sweater, skirt, blouse, slip, socks, dress, pants, scarf, etc.); 3. things at school (school, principal's office, desk, books, pencils, erasers, waste basket, etc.); 4. things children do for fun (skating, swimming, sliding, skipping, singing, baseball, tennis, etc.); 5. things at the grocery store (store, grocer, spinach, celery, lettuce, salt, spaghetti, soup, cereal, rice, etc.), and many other topics. A core vocabulary developed at the single-word level can and should be utilized repeatedly in the more advanced stages of training indicated below.

4. **Phrases and sentences.** The child is given practice in using his sound in larger speech units than words. For example, instead of naming pictures or reading single words, he can make up a sentence for each one. The same "games" used at the word level, such as ladders, race tracks, object or picture-placing, can be used equally well at the phrase or sentence level. Activities utilizing "carrier phrases" featuring /s/ can be employed. A perennial favorite of speech therapists and one which never loses its fascination for children is the guessing game in any of its many variations. For example, ten or twelve core vocabulary pictures can be laid out and each child asked to guess which one the therapist is thinking of. The phrase can be, "I guess it is the—(guessing one of the pictures)." The therapist replies, "No, it isn't the—" or "Yes, it is the—." Guessing continues until the right one is found. Children take turns in thinking of a picture for the others to guess. Throughout the activity only correctly produced /s/ words are counted. Another carrier phrase could be, "Please pass the—" in imaginary dinner table situations, with pictured foods and objects.

Question and answer activities, quiz games, adaptations of the game of "Authors," using animal, flower, food, clothing, and other categories, the game "Taking a Trip" in which the child says "I went to St. Louis and in my suitcase I took a—," naming an /s/ word, and each child, in turn, repeating what has gone before and adding his own /s/ word—are but a few of the many activities which utilize the sentence level.

5. **Controlled conversation.** This is a step further in the direction of the less specific, less conscious, less identifiable, and less easily controlled speech toward which we aim in articulation therapy. Situations should be created in which the child, though constantly encouraged to use his sound correctly, is able to give only marginal attention to articulation and must give more attention to content and action.

Among typical activities at this stage are the following: a) interviewing each other about hobbies, about sports, about future plans, etc.; b) simple dramatizations such as the role of a shopper and a clerk in a grocery store, a clothing store a sporting goods store, a post office, or a travel agency; c) a person seeking information at an employment office; d) a policeman and a traffic violator; e) a door-to-door salesman and a housewife, to mention but a few. Situations and roles can be adjusted to the age and specific interests of the cases involved.

Oral reading should not be overlooked as a means for securing excellent articulation practice. It can be adapted to all the levels of training, from single words to continuous text. It can be made more or less easy for the case to control his articulation by premarking of the sound being practised or by spontaneous reading of new material. The visual cue provided by the printed letter is a needed temporary aid in many cases.

6. **Free, off-guard speech.** There is no sharp distinction between this and the preceding stage. The therapist will need to move constantly—as the individual gains reliability in the use of his sound—toward creating situations which approximate as closely as possible nontherapeutic, real-life situations, maintaining at the same time the individual's awareness of good articulation and his effort to control his sound. To this end activities should involve more continuous and rapid speech and more distraction resulting from emotionally toned content or keen competition. Utilize such activities as impromptu speeches, telling of experiences or stories, telling jokes, discussions between members of the group, preferably on topics which will generate strong feeling. For example, when there are both girls and boys in the therapy group, such emotionally charged discussion topics as "Are girls brighter than boys?" "Should boys have more freedom than

girls?" will put newly acquired articulation habits to a severe test. Many additional suggestions for group speech activity are given in the Chicago pamphlet mentioned above.

CARRY-OVER TRAINING

The term *carry-over* is used by most therapists to refer to the habitual use of the new sound in real-life speech situations, outside of the speech therapy sessions. All of the auditory discrimination and articulatory production training which has just been described is actually part of the carry-over training, in that the correct sound is gradually becoming habituated and is making its appearance in non-therapy situations. However, it seems necessary in most cases to give specific and serious attention to promoting this carry-over in order to insure that it will take place. Many a speech therapist who has been pleased at a child's consistent and accurate use of his new sound in the therapy session has been disillusioned and discouraged a few moments later to overhear him on the playground using his old substitution or distortion, apparently untouched by the speech therapy he has undergone. Carry-over might be said, therefore, to be the "eating" which is proof of the therapeutic "pudding."

The rapidity, thoroughness, and permanence of carry-over are largely a function of motivation. Other factors being equal, the child or adult who has a strong personal desire to improve in speech will profit more readily from speech therapy than the individual who is passive or complacent about his own speech, however cooperative with the therapist he may appear to be superficially. The problem of motivation is fundamental, therefore, to successful articulation therapy, particularly at the level of carry-over.

The effectiveness of carry-over is also a function of the soundness and thoroughness of the training given at the earlier stages of therapy. Particularly crucial is the degree to which self-monitoring of speech has been stressed and has become habitual. The most highly motivated person conceivable will hardly learn to articulate accurately if he is unable to identify his own errors, either because of poor sound discrimination or because of inattention to his own speech. This is the basic rationale for stressing training in auditory discrimination.

When should emphasis on carry-over begin? Should the therapist await near-perfect reliability of the child's sound in the therapy sessions themselves before beginning to concern himself with his use of the sound in other situations? Most therapists would answer an emphatic "No!" Carry-over can begin as soon as the child has gained voluntary control of his sound and is able to produce it correctly at will. Before a child *can* produce a correct /s/ it is manifestly useless to expect him to use it in words. As soon as he *can* produce it, carry-over efforts can and should begin. They should be a part of every therapy session, since it is urgent to assist the child to communicate better as soon as possible.

Techniques for Securing Carry-over. At each lesson some time should be devoted to helping the child to produce his sound correctly in one or two words and expressions he has to use frequently, such as: his name, address, telephone number, names of brothers, sisters, parents, his birthday, age, name of his school his grade, his teacher's name. Early attention should be given to common utilitarian and social courtesy words and expressions such as *yes, no, please, thank you, May I please—?, Will you please . . .?*, the numbers, at least up to 10, the days of the week, the months of the year, and others which are pertinent to the particular case. These words and expressions are so frequently used that they are likely to have become sore points because of teasing or parental criticism. Their mastery is, therefore, correspondingly gratifying to the child and his parents.

Words for practice should be selected in part from the subject matter currently being taught in the child's classroom. Carry-over will be aided by the opportunity thus afforded to practice words newly learned in speech therapy, particularly if the classroom teacher is alerted to the need for reinforcing the child's new and uncertain learning with a word of praise for the word correctly said. Vocabularies surrounding holidays and special events are good practice material. The use of core vocabularies, discussed earlier, will also tend to accelerate carry-over.

Since awareness of speech and motivation for better speech are large factors in carry-over, the following techniques are suggested to assist in motivating and increasing speech awareness:

1. Give the individual a clear understanding of his problem at the beginning of therapy. He should know which of his sounds are defective, the nature of his errors, and the stages which are involved in the correction of each sound. A clear knowledge of the problem tends to challenge and motivate.

2. Objectify the individual's progress. Be sure he understands how far he has come and what his next task will be. His progress may be evident to you as therapist but may not be evident to him and, therefore, not effective in motivating him. At all ages the use of

periodic recordings of the person's speech help him to trace his progress.

With children, graphs and charts are often helpful. Colored stars for speech work well done are displayed proudly by children and stimulate them to further efforts.

3. Speech workbooks are a highly effective device to enhance motivation. At each lesson new words or pictures can be added for home practice and serve later as evidence of words already mastered. Children should be encouraged to find pictures containing their sound. These should be used in therapy and then pasted into the workbook. The child who is on the lookout for /s/ pictures in the magazines around home is thinking about his /s/ sound and apt to begin using it at least part of the time. Children can also be encouraged to write sentences or stories which feature the sound they are learning and to be ready to read them with good sounds at the next session.

Workbooks help to make the child conscious of his speech task between lessons and to increase his awareness of *his* sound in the speech he hears around him. He can be asked to collect in his speech-book the words containing his sound which he has heard other people say. Attentiveness to speech is thus spread over the interval between therapy sessions. Speech workbooks interest not only the child himself but also his teacher and his parents. They are often stimulated to do a considerable amount of incidental encouragement of correct articulation and calling of attention to lapses.

4. When voluntary mastery of a sound has been achieved it is helpful to establish a weekly quota of words to be "remembered" and uttered correctly whenever they occur in the intervals between lessons. Each week's quota is added to the speech workbook. Two or three words are usually sufficient for primary age children, five to ten for older children. Core vocabularies are useful as a source for the word quotas.

Parents and classroom teachers, sometimes older brothers and sisters, can be helpful by having a copy of the child's quota for that week and assisting him, in a friendly spirit, to use these words consistently. They can even ask questions or create situations in which the quota words will have to be used.

One therapist on the writer's staff invented the highly stimulating device of calling each therapy group a "speech club," with "passwords" or "secret sentences" which had to be articulated correctly in order to gain admission to the next "meeting of the club." The club "members" took delight in asking each other for the passwords between therapy sessions. Ingenuity can harness powerful motivational forces to speech carry-over.

5. Participation by children themselves in the selection or invention of speech techniques, in the selection of the words for the next week's quota, and in the finding of pictures and reading material, is a strongly motivating factor. Interim assignments will be carried out with more interest and reliability if children—or adults, for that matter—have helped to set up their own goals and to find or devise their own practice material.

6. Propaganda for good speech will be an aid to motivation and carry-over. The speech therapy room should suggest "speech" from the moment the individual enters it. "Good Speech" posters may be made by children and hung up in the room. A pinup board can be used to display magazine or newspaper articles on speech, items about people who have outstandingly good speech or who have overcome speech problems, or speech materials prepared by children. These all help to interest and challenge the individual who is working on his own speech problem or the parent who comes in for a conference with the speech therapist.

The speech therapist will need to verify the reliability of the individual's carry-over of the corrected sound by checking with teachers and members of the family and, if possible, by himself listening to his case in an off-guard speaking situation when the individual is unaware of his presence. The final test of the clinical result is consistent, accurate use of the new sound in rapid speech under somewhat emotional or stress conditions.

Further suggestions for articulation-training techniques and activities will be found in the Chicago pamphlet, *Speech Correction Techniques and Materials* (Revised 1968), in Ainsworth (1948), Anderson (1953), Berry and Eisenson (1942), Koepp-Baker (1936), Van Riper (1963), Van Riper and Irwin (1958), and in some of the other texts listed in the bibliography. Excellent practice material for children in the form of word lists, sentences, or stories, will be found in Ainsworth (1946), McCullough (1940), Nemoy (1954, Nemoy and Davis (1937), Schoolfield (1951), and Zedler (1955). For adolescents and adults practice material will be found in Fairbanks (1940) and Fisher (1966). Engel et al. (1966) discuss motivation for carry-over and suggest useful techniques.

Principles of Good Articulation Therapy

The formulation which follows restates and emphasizes some of the points implied in the foregoing outline of articulation therapy:

1. Articulation therapy should be carefully planned but should also be flexible so that it can adapt itself to the individual's needs and responses as these manifest themselves during the course of therapy.

2. Articulation therapy cannot be standardized for all cases. It is not rigid, routinized, or stereotyped, but is adapted to the individualized needs and deficiencies of each case.

3. Articulation therapy in its various phases—auditory discrimination, articulatory production, and carry-over—proceeds from the simple, the highly specific, the conscious, the easily identified, the easily controlled toward the more complex, less specific, less conscious, less easily identified and less easily controlled.

4. Articulation therapy utilizes all appropriate sensory avenues and intellectual aids to understanding, but is probably most effective when it places major emphasis on auditory training, as the process most basic to speech learning.

5. Articulation therapy must begin with the individual *where he is*—at the point where the normal process of speech acquisition was stopped or disrupted. This means that new habits must be learned to replace incorrect ones. This in turn usually involves a considerable amount of drill or repetitive practice. Drill is a sound psychological concept when it also implies *motivation* and *purposefulness*.

6. Even from the initial stages, where drill is used to develop mastery, articulation therapy is probably most effective when it utilizes practice materials which have interest and meaning to the individual and when it relates and integrates practice with real-life speaking situations.

7. A technique or activity for auditory discrimination, articulatory production, or carry-over should be selected with certain criteria in mind:

It should be of interest and meaning to the case with which it is to be used, and appropriate for his maturity level.

It should be appropriate to his intelligence, experience, and reading level.

It should be appropriate to the *stage* of therapy which has been reached.

It should be simple to explain and to understand so that therapeutic time is not wasted in mere preparation for practice.

It should provide a maximum opportunity for speech practice, which is the fundamental purpose of the therapy session. Motivational aspects of the situation, such as "winning the game," should not obscure the more basic objective of using good articulation. Motivation should be harnessed to good speech, not irrelevant to it.

8. At all stages, articulation therapy must be oriented psychotherapeutically. Attention must be given, not only to the development of accurate articulation but also to the individual's security and pleasure in speaking, to improvement of his communicative attitudes and habits, and to his motivation for personal speech improvement.

9. Articulation therapy is not a simple, didactic relationship between the therapist and his case. It is a cooperative enterprise in which the case is an active, informed participant, aware of his problem, of the stages involved in speech learning, and of the progress being made. Articulatory improvement should be a conscious, self-selected goal, and a process to which the case contributes ideas, materials, and evaluations, as well as deliberate effort.

10. The cooperative nature of articulation therapy implies not only the participation of the case but also of his family, teachers, and even associates. When an appropriate point in therapy has been reached, their active assistance—guided by the therapist—will to a considerable degree determine the rapidity and effectiveness of carry-over.

The Role of Parents in Articulation Therapy

Most speech clinicians today try to involve parents as much as possible in the program of articulation therapy for children. A few research investigations of parental attitudes and involvement in speech therapy lend support to this practice. Swenson (1956) compared the attitudes of parents of functional articulation cases and normal controls on a parental attitude scale. He found the parents of functional articulation cases to have less favorable attitudes than control parents toward certain aspects of children's behavior, and that mothers' attitudes were more favorable than fathers' attitudes. The implication was that parental reeducation was called for, especially for fathers.

Egbert (1955) found that mothers of functional articulation cases who made good progress with therapy were better informed about speech therapy and were more active as auxiliary therapists than were the mothers of matched cases who made poor progress.

Shea (1957), on the other hand, had somewhat less favorable results. Parents of experimental group children were asked to assist with homework on speech at the carry-over stage; children in the control group had only speech therapy at school. Only about half of the parents were willing to commit themselves to working with their children and these parents tended to be above average in intelligence. Shea concluded that we cannot assume parental willingness to help. Even the most motivated parents gradually decreased the amount of time per day for this activity during the experimental period. The conclusion was that public school speech therapists cannot rely heavily on regular, systematic supplemental teaching by parents.

Tufts and Holliday (1959) studied three matched groups of moderate functional articulation cases from four to six years of age. Group A received no training of any kind, Group B received speech therapy twice a week, and Group C received no therapy from a speech therapist but their mothers were trained one hour weekly for seven months. Groups B and C gained significantly in speech compared with Group A, but no difference was found between Groups B and C. They concluded that trained mothers are effective in improving moderate articulation cases.

Several studies of maternal attitudes and training as related to articulation disorders have been done by Sommers and his associates (Sommers et al., 1959, 1962, 1964). Good and poor maternal attitude groups were compared, and groups of mothers who were given training in working with their children's speech compared with groups who were not. It was found that both maternal attitudes and maternal training are important. Children of mothers with "healthy" attitudes improved more than children of mothers with "unhealthy" attitudes. Children of trained mothers improved more than children of untrained mothers. The main conclusion seems to be that the most improvement in articulation takes place when both conditions, "healthy" attitudes, and training of mothers, are present and that time spent in training mothers is clinically valuable.

HOW SHOULD PARENTS BE INVOLVED?

Two quite different issues are constantly confused in discussions of the pros and cons of involving parents in articulation therapy. One issue concerns the effectiveness of parental guidance and education as related to the child's speech. The other issue involves the degree to which a parent should be asked to carry out direct, specific, supplemental speech training of his child.

On the first issue there can be little difference of opinion. Since parents are involved with their children anyway, whether we like it or not, we should make every effort to channel their interest and activity along constructive lines, to inform them about the child's speech problem, to improve their attitudes about it, to solicit their active support and encouragement of the child's efforts to improve his speech—including his between-session assignments at home, and to show a positive and supportive rather than critical attitude toward the child's speech. Techniques for carrying out such work with parents range from occasional individual conferences with the speech clinician to intensive, systematic series of group conferences.

The issue of direct involvement of the parent as an auxiliary speech therapist is much more complex and controversial. Here the clinician must be more selective. To ask a critical, tense, rejecting parent to carry out speech work with his child is to invite disaster. The child can only suffer. However, if the parent-child relationship is warm, friendly, and mutually trustful, and if the parent is intelligent enough and motivated enough to learn good techniques and carry them out with reasonable regularity, the child will progress in speech far beyond what he would do with only therapy from the clinician. The clinician must evaluate each case—both child and parent—carefully. All parents should receive guidance and information. More intensive involvement of the parent should depend upon the complexity of the child's problem, the stage of therapy which has been reached, the quality of the parent-child relationship, and the intelligence and motivation of the parent.

Termination of Articulation Therapy

An important question in clinical treatment of functional articulation disorders is that of how long to go on with therapy in each individual case. Should an individual remain under treatment until his every speech sound is produced correctly at all times, even under stress? This goal may be ideal but is seldom practical. In public school programs in particular the pressure of numbers of cases waiting for therapy leads the speech clinician to dismiss children before this ideal objective is reached in many cases. The cost of clinical or private fees may also lead to termination before complete correction is attained. On the other hand, dismissal too early may mean regression and a loss of what has already been accomplished.

There is obviously no convenient rule for determining the point at which therapy should be terminated. The motivation and standards of the case will enter into the decision, as well as the clinician's prognosis as to how much more improvement is likely to take place.

Termination of therapy seems logical when most of the individual's misarticulations have been corrected and correct production of sounds is carrying over to habitual speech under most conditions. Aside from this general rule of thumb, the clinician will have to be guided by specific issues in each case.

The Results of Articulation Therapy

Little information is available in the professional literature concerning the effectiveness of articulation therapy. Precise evaluation of articulation changes resulting from therapy is dependent upon application of exact measurement criteria before therapy begins and after various durations of therapy. Seldom has this been done. Elbert and Shelton (1967) administered a 60-item sound-production task to their subjects before therapy began and after every second therapy session. They concluded (p. 288) ". . . the technique of frequent task administration holds promise of measuring articulation change in such a way that the learner can be used as his own control." In most clinical situations, however, less precise evaluation takes place.

For purposes of practical program evaluation the writer annually collected data on dismissal of cases as "corrected" in the large program of speech correction in the Chicago Public Schools. These data, shown in Table 34-III are of interest because they represent a large number of cases, even though criteria are subjective and variable from one staff member to another. In the table the term "corrected" means the clinician's judgement that the child had reached a level of reasonable speech adequacy and no longer needed speech therapy.

TABLE 34-III
The Effectiveness of Speech Therapy
The Division of Speech Correction
Chicago Board of Education

TYPE OF CASE	NO. ENROLLED FOR SPEECH THERAPY YEAR 1966–1967	NO. DISMISSED AS "CORRECTED" DURING THE YEAR	% OF CORRECTION FOR EACH TYPE
Stuttering	2,073	346	16.7
Functional articulation	14,038	3,868	27.6
Cleft palate	183	23	12.6
Neurological	275	10	3.6
Hearing loss*	364	34	9.3
Voice disorders	321	75	23.4
Miscellaneous	353	32	9.1
Total	17,607	4,388	24.9

* Not including children in special classes for deaf or hard-of-hearing.

It is clear from the table—and not surprising—that a higher percentage of functional articulation cases is corrected and dismissed from speech therapy than of any other type of case. For all types of cases together the dismissal rate is 24.9 percent, and functional articulation cases exceed this with 27.6 percent. This does not tell us what the ultimate percentage of correction might be since these data refer only to one school year. The ultimate percentage of functional articulation cases corrected, however, would undoubtedly be much higher.

BIBLIOGRAPHY (*Chapters 33 and 34*)

Ainsworth, S. 1948. Speech correction methods. Englewood Cliffs, N.J.: Prentice-Hall.

Albright, R. 1948. The motor abilities of speakers with good and poor articulation. *Speech Monogr.*, 15, 164–172.

Amidon, H. 1951. A statistical study of relationships among articulation errors made by one hundred first grade children. Univ. Iowa: Master's thesis.

Anders, Q. 1945. A study of the personal and social adjustment of children with functional articulatory defects. Univ. Wis.: Master's thesis.

Andersland, P. 1961. Maternal and environmental factors related to success in speech improvement training. *J. Speech Hearing Res.*, 4, 79–90.

Anderson, P. 1949. The relationship of normal and defective articulation of the consonant (s) in various phonetic contexts to auditory discrimination between normal and defective (s) production among children from kindergarten through fourth grade. Univ. Iowa: Master's thesis.

Anderson, V. 1938. The auditory memory span for speech sounds. *Speech Monogr.*, 5, 115–129.

———. 1939. Auditory memory span as tested by speech sounds. *Amer. J. Psychol.*, 52, 95–99.

Anderson, V. 1953. Improving the child's speech. New York: Oxford.

Artley, A. 1948. A study of certain factors presumed to be associated with reading and speech difficulties. *J. Speech Hearing Disorders*, 13, 351–360.

ASHA Committee on the Midcentury White House Conference. 1952. Speech disorders and speech correction. *J. Speech Hearing Disorders*, 17, 129–137.

Aungst, L., and Frick, J. 1964. Auditory discrimination ability and consistency of articulation of (r). *J. Speech Hearing Disorders*, 29, 76–85.

Backus, O. 1943. Speech in education. New York: Longmans.

———, and Beasley, J. 1951. Speech therapy with children. Boston: Houghton Mifflin.

Bangs, J. 1942. A clinical analysis of the articulatory defects of the feebleminded. *J. Speech Disorders*, 7, 343–356.

Bankson, N., and Byrne, M. 1962. The relationship between missing teeth and selected consonant sounds. *J. Speech Hearing Disorders*, 27, 341–348.

Barker, J., and England, G. 1962. A numerical measure of articulation: further developments. *J. Speech Hearing Disorders*, 27, 23–27.

Barnes, H. 1932. Diagnosis of speech needs and abilities of students in a required course in speech training at the State University of Iowa. Univ. Iowa: Ph.D. dissertation.

Beckey, R. 1942. A study of certain factors related to retardation of speech. *J. Speech Disorders*, 7, 223–249.

Beebe, H. 1944. Auditory memory span for meaningless syllables. *J. Speech Disorders*, 9, 273–276.

Bell, D., and Hale, A. 1963. Observations of tongue-thrust swallow in preschool children. *J. Speech Hearing Disorders*, 28, 195–197.

Bellak, L., and Bellak, S. 1961. Children's apperception test (C.A.T.) (4th. ed.). Larchmont, New York: CPS Co., Box 83.

Bennett, C. 1938. An inquiry into the genesis of poor reading. *Teach. Coll. Contr. Educ.*, No. 755. New York: Teachers College, Columbia Univ.

Berry, M., and Eisenson, J. 1942. The defective in speech. New York: Appleton-Century-Crofts.

Betts, E. 1946. Foundations of reading instruction. New York: American Book.

Bilto, E. 1941. A comparative study of certain physical abilities of children with speech defects and children with normal speech. *J. Speech Disorders*, 6, 187–203.

Black, M., compiler. 1952. The Illinois plan for special education of exceptional children. The speech defective. Circular Series "E" No. 12, Revised. Springfield, Ill. Issued by Superintendent of Public Instruction.

———, and Ludwig, R. 1956. Analysis of the games technic. *J. Speech Hearing Disorders*, 21, 183–187.

Blanton, S. 1936. Helping the speech handicapped school student. *J. Speech Disorders*, 1, 97–100.

Bond, G. 1935. The auditory and speech characteristics of poor readers. *Teach. Coll. Contr. Educ.*: No. 657. New York: Teachers College, Columbia Univ.

Bricker, W. 1967. Errors in the echoic behavior of preschool children. *J. Speech Hearing Res.*, 10, 67–76.

Brieland, D. 1950. A comparative study of the speech of blind and sighted children. *Speech Monogr.*, No. 17, 99–103.

Buck, M. 1948. A study of the misarticulation of (r) in children from kindergarten through third grade. Univ. Iowa: Master's thesis.

Burdin, L. 1940. A survey of speech defectives in the Indianapolis primary grades. *J. Speech Disorders*, 5, 247–258.

Carrell, J. 1936. A comparative study of speech defective children. *Arch. Speech*, 1, 179–203.

———. 1937. The etiology of sound substitution defects. *Speech Monogr.*, No. 4, 17–37.

———, and Pendergast, K. 1954. An experimental study of the possible relation between errors of speech and spelling. *J. Speech Hearing Disorders*, 19, 327–334.

Carter, E., and Buck, M. 1958. Prognostic testing for functional articulation disorders among children in the first grade. *J. Speech Hearing Disorders*, 23, 124–133.

Chen, H., and Irwin, O. 1946. Infant speech vowel and consonant types. *J. Speech Disorders*, 11, 27–29.

Cohen, J., and Diehl, C. 1963. Relation of speech-sound discrimination ability to articulation type speech defects. *J. Speech Hearing Disorders*, 28, 187–190.

Cotrel, E., and Halsted, E. 1936. Class lessons for improving speech. Boston: Expression Co.

Curtis, J., and Hardy, J. 1959. A phonetic study of misarticulation of (r). *J. Speech Hearing Res.*, 2, 244–257.

Darley, F., and Winitz, H. 1961. Age of first word: review of research. *J. Speech Hearing Disorders*, 26, 272–290.

Davis, E. 1937. The development of linguistic skill in twins, singletons with siblings, and only children from age five to ten years. Minneapolis: Univ. Minn. Press.

Dawson, L. 1929. A study of the development of the rate of articulation. *Elem. Sch. J.*, 29, 610–615.

DeHirsch, K., Jansky, J., and Langford, W. 1964. The oral language performance of premature children and controls. *J. Speech Hearing Disorders*, 29, 60–69.

Dickson, S. 1962. Differences between children who spontaneously outgrow and children who retain functional articulation errors. *J. Speech Hearing Res.*, 5, 263–271.

Doll, E. 1947. Vineland social maturity scale, manual of directions. Minneapolis: Educational Test Bur.

Donewald, M. 1950. The relation of speech sound discrimination to functional articulatory defects in children. Purdue Univ.: Master's thesis.

Dunn, L. 1959. Peabody picture vocabulary test. Minneapolis: American Guidance Service.

———. 1965. Expanded manual, Peabody picture vocabulary test. Minneapolis: American Guidance Service.

Eames, T. 1950. The relationship of reading and speech difficulties. *J. educ. Psychol.*, 41, 51–55.

Egbert, J. 1955. The effect of certain home influences on the progress of children in a speech therapy program. Stanford Univ.: Ph.D. dissertation.

Eisenson, J. 1938. The psychology of speech. New York: Appleton-Century-Crofts.

Elbert, M., and Shelton, R., Jr. 1967. A task for evaluation of articulation change: 1. development of methodology. *J. Speech Hearing Res.*, 10, 281–288.

Engel, D., Brandriet, S., Erickson, K. Gronhovd, K., and Gunderson, G. 1966. Carryover. *J. Speech Hearing Disorders*, 31, 227–233.

Everhart, R. 1953. The relationship between articulation and other developmental factors in children. *J. Speech Hearing Disorders*, 18, 332–338.

Fairbanks, G. 1940. Voice and articulation drillbook. New York: Harper.

———, and Bebout, B. 1950. A study of minor organic deviations in "functional" disorders of articulation: 3. the tongue. *J. Speech Hearing Disorders*, 15, 348–352.

———, and Green, E. 1950. A study of minor organic deviations in "functional" disorders of articulation: 2. dimensions and relationships of the lips. *J. Speech Hearing Disorders*, 15, 165–168.

———, and Lintner, M. 1951. A study of minor organic deviations in "functional" disorders of articulation: 4. the teeth and hard palate. *J. Speech Hearing Disorders*, 16, 273–279.

———, and Spriestersbach, D. 1950. A study of minor organic deviations in "functional" disorders of articulation: 1. rate of movement of oral structures. *J. Speech Hearing Disorders*, 15, 60–69.

Farquhar, M. 1961. Prognostic value of imitative and auditory discrimination tests. *J. Speech Hearing Disorders*, 26, 342–347.

Fisher, H. 1966. Improving voice and articulation. Boston: Houghton Mifflin.

Fletcher, S., Casteel, R., and Bradley, D. 1961. Tongue-thrust swallow, speech articulation, and age. *J. Speech Hearing Disorders*, 26, 201–208.

Francis, J. 1930. A survey of speech defectives of Iowa City, Iowa. Univ. Iowa: Master's thesis.

Froeschels, E. 1933. Speech therapy. Boston: Expression Co.

———, and Jellinek, A. 1941. Practice of voice and speech therapy. Boston: Expression Co.

Fymbo, L. 1936. The relation of malocclusion of the teeth to defects of speech. *Arch. Speech*, 1, 204–216.

Gilkinson, H. 1943. The Seashore measures of musical talent and speech skill. *J. applied Psychol.*, 27, 443–447.

Goldman, R., and Fristoe, M. 1967. The development of the filmstrip articulation test. *J. Speech Hearing Disorders*, 32, 256–262.

Goodstein, L. 1958a. Functional speech disorders and personality: A survey of the research. *J. Speech Hearing Research*, 1, 359–376.

———. 1958b. Functional speech disorders and personality: methodological and theoretical considerations. *J. Speech Hearing Res.*, 1, 377–382.

Gray, G., and Wise, C. 1946. The bases of speech (rev. ed.). New York: Harper.

Hahn, E. 1960. Communication in the therapy session: a point of view. *J. Speech Hearing Disorders*, 25, 18–23.

———. 1961. Indications for direct, nondirect, and indirect methods in speech correction. *J. Speech Hearing Disorders*, 26, 230–236.

Hale, A. 1948. A study of the misarticulation of (s) in children from kindergarten through third grade. Univ. Iowa: Master's thesis.

Hall, M. 1938. Auditory factors in functional articulatory speech defects. *J. exper. Educ.*, 7, 110–132.

Haller, R. 1967. Effect of background speech on phoneme discrimination abilities of children with normal and defective articulation. *J. auditory Res.*, 7, 77–84.

Hansen, B. 1944. The application of sound discrimination tests to functional articulatory defectives with normal hearing. *J. Speech Disorders*, 9, 347–355.

Hawk, S. 1942. Moto-kinaesthetic training for children with speech handicaps. *J. Speech Disorders*, 7, 357–360.

Hejna, R. 1955. Developmental articulation test. Madison, Wis.: College Printing and Typing.

Henrikson, E. 1948. An analysis of Wood's articulation index. *J. Speech Hearing Disorders*, 13, 233–235.

Hildreth, G. 1946. Speech defects and reading disability. *Elem. Sch. J.*, 46, 326–332.

Hoffman, J., and Hoffman, R. 1965. Tongue-thrust and deglutition: some anatomical, physiological, and neurological considerations. *J. Speech Hearing Disorders*, 30, 105–120.

Huffman, L., and McReynolds, L. 1968. Auditory sequence learning in children. *J. Speech Hearing Res.*, 11, 179–188.

Humphrey, W., and Milisen, R. 1954. A study of the ability to reproduce unfamiliar sounds which have been presented orally. *J. Speech Hearing Disorders, Monogr. suppl.* No. 4, 58–69.

Ingram, C. 1935. Education of the slow-learning child. Yonkers-on-Hudson: World Book.

Irwin, J., and Becklund, O. 1953. Norms for maximum repetitive rates for certain sounds established with the sylrater. *J. Speech Hearing Disorders*, 18, 149–160.

———, and Duffy, J. 1951. Speech and hearing hurdles. Columbus, Ohio: School and College Service.

Irwin, O. 1947a. Infant speech: consonantal sounds according to place of articulation. *J. Speech Disorders*, 12, 397–401.

———. 1947b. Infant speech: consonant sounds according to manner of articulation. *J. Speech Disorders*, 12, 402–404.

———. 1948a. Infant speech: development of vowel sounds. *J. Speech Hearing Disorders*, 13, 31–34.

Irwin, O. 1948b. Infant speech: the effect of family occupational status and of age on use of sound types. *J. Speech Hearing Disorders*, 13, 224–226.

———. 1948c. Infant speech: the effect of family occupational status and of age on sound frequency. *J. Speech Hearing Disorders*, 13, 320–323.

———. 1951. Infant speech: consonantal position. *J. Speech Hearing Disorders*, 16, 159–161.

———. 1952. Speech development in the young child: 2. some factors related to the speech development of the infant and young child. *J. Speech Hearing Disorders*, 17, 269–279.

———. 1960. Infant speech. effect of systematic reading of stories. *J. Speech Hearing Res.*, 3, 187–190.

———, and Chen, H. 1943. Speech sound elements during the first year of life: a review of the literature. *J. Speech Disorders*, 8, 109–121.

———, and ———. 1945. Infant speech sounds and intelligence. *J. Speech Disorders*, 10, 293–296.

———, and ———. 1946. Infant speech: vowel and consonant frequency. *J. Speech Disorders*, 11, 123–125.

Irwin, R. 1949. Speech and hearing therapy in the public schools of Ohio. *J. Speech Hearing Disorders*, 14, 63–68.

———. 1953. Speech and hearing therapy. Englewood Cliffs, N.J.: Prentice-Hall.

———. 1963. The effects of speech therapy upon certain linguistic skills of first-grade children. *J. Speech Hearing Disorders*, 28, 375–381.

———, and Musselman, B. 1962. A compact picture articulation test. *J. Speech Hearing Disorders*, 27, 36–39.

———, West, J., and Trombetta, M. 1966. Effectiveness of speech therapy for second grade children with misarticulations—predictive factors. *J. except. Child.*, 32, 471–479.

Jann, G., Ward, M., and Jann, H. 1964. A longitudinal study of articulation, deglutition, and malocclusion. *J. Speech Hearing Disorders*, 29, 424–435.

Johnson, W. 1950, ed. Speech problems of children. New York: Grune & Stratton.

———, Brown, S., Curtis, J., Edney, C., and Keaster, J. 1956. Speech handicapped school children (rev. ed.). New York: Harper.

———, Darley, F., and Spriestersbach, D. 1963. Diagnostic methods in speech pathology. New York and Evanston: Harper and Row.

———, and House, E. 1937. Certain laterality characteristics of children with articulatory disorders. *Elem. Sch. J.*, 38, 52–58.

Jones, M. 1951. The effect of speech training on silent reading achievement. *J. Speech Hearing Disorders*, 16, 258–263.

Jordan, E. 1960. Articulation test measures and listener ratings of articulation defectiveness. *J. Speech Hearing Res.*, 3, 303–319.

Karlin, I., and Strazzulla, M. 1952. Speech and language problems of mentally deficient children. *J. Speech Hearing Disorders*, 17, 286–294.

———, Youtz, A., and Kennedy, L. 1940. Distorted speech in young children. *Amer. J. dis. Child.*, 59, 1203–1218.

Kisatsky, T. 1967. The prognostic value of the Carter-Buck tests in measuring articulation skills of selected kindergarten children. *J. except Child.*, 34, 81–85.

Koepp-Baker, H. 1936. A handbook of clinical speech. (Vol. 2.) Ann Arbor: Edwards Brothers.

Kronvall, E., and Diehl, C. 1954. The relationship of auditory discrimination to articulatory defects of children with no known organic impairment. *J. Speech Hearing Disorders*, 19, 335–338.

Lewis, J., and Counihan, R. 1965. Tongue-thrust in infancy. *J. Speech Hearing Disorders*, 30, 280–282.

Locke, J. 1969. Short-term auditory memory, oral perception, and experimental sound learning. *J. Speech Hearing Res.*, 12, 185–192.

Louttit, C., and Halls, E. 1936. Survey of speech defects among public school children of Indiana. *J. Speech Disorders*, 1, 73–80.

Low, G., Crerar, M., and Lassers, L. 1959. Communication centered speech therapy. *J. Speech Hearing Disorders*, 24, 361–368.

Lundeen, D. 1950. The relationship of diadochokinesis to various speech sounds. *J. Speech Hearing Disorders*, 15, 54–59.

Lupella, R. 1967. Maturational patterns of certain auditory skills. Ill. Speech and Hearing Assn. Newsletter, 7, 5–11.

MacLearie, E. 1953. The Ohio plan for children with speech and hearing problems. Columbus: Ohio Depart. Pub. Instr.

Mader, J. 1954. The relative frequency of occurrence of English consonant sounds in words in the speech of children in grades one, two, and three. *Speech Monogr.*, No. 21, 294–300.

Major, C. 1940. A comparison of the performance of speech defectives and normal speakers on certain motor tests. Purdue Univ.: Master's thesis.

Mange, C. 1960. Relationships between selected auditory perceptual factors and articulation ability. *J. Speech Hearing Res.*, 3, 67–74.

Marge, M. 1965. The influence of selected home background variables on the development of oral communication skills in children. *J. Speech Hearing Res.*, 8, 291–309.

Mase, D. 1946. Etiology of articulatory speech defects. *Teach. Coll. contr. Educ.*, No. 921. New York: Teachers College, Columbia Univ.

Mason, M. 1942. Learning to speak after six and one-half years of silence. *J. Speech Disorders*, 7, 295–304.

Maxwell, K. L. 1953. A comparison of certain motor performances of normal and speech defective children, ages seven, eight, and nine years. Univ. Mich.: Ph.D. dissertation.

McAllister, M. 1948. A study of the relationship between defects of articulation in speech and emotional instability in elementary school children. Univ. Wash.: Master's thesis.

McCarthy, D. 1930. The language development of the preschool child. Minneapolis: Univ. Minn. Press.

McCarthy, J., and Kirk, S. 1961. Illinois test of

psycholinguistic abilities (examiner's manual, test materials, and record forms.) Urbana, Ill.: Institute Res. Except. Child., Univ. Ill.

McClure, H. 1952. A study of the existing relationship between articulatory speech defects and related disabilities including reading. Ball State Teacher's College: Master's thesis.

McCullough, G. 1940. Speech improvement work and practice book. Boston: Expression Co.

McDonald, E. 1959. Rationale for a "deep test" of articulation. *Asha*, 1, 103.

———. 1964. Articulation testing and treatment: a sensory-motor approach. Pittsburgh: Stanwix House.

Metraux, R. 1942. Auditory memory span for speech sounds of speech defective children compared with normal children. *J. Speech Disorders*, 7, 33–36.

———. 1944. Auditory memory span for speech sounds: norms for children. *J. Speech Disorders*, 9, 31–38.

———. 1950. Speech profiles of the pre-school child 18 to 54 months. *J. Speech Hearing Disorders*, 15, 37–53.

Milisen, R. 1945. Principles and methods of articulation testing. *Speech and Hearing Therapist*, Bloomington: Ind. Univ. Speech Hearing Clinic, Feb., 6–10.

———. 1954. A rationale for articulation disorders. *J. Speech Hearing Disorders*, *Monogr.supple* No. 4, 6–17.

Mills, A., and Streit, H. 1942. Report of a speech survey, Holyoke, Mass. *J. Speech Disorders*, 7, 161–167.

Moll, K., and Darley, F. 1960. Attitudes of mothers of articulatory-impaired and speech-retarded children. *J. Speech Hearing Disorders*, 25, 377–384.

Monroe, M. 1932. Children who cannot read. Chicago: Univ. Chicago Press.

Moore, C. 1947. Reading and arithmetic abilities associated with speech defects. *J. Speech Disorders*, 12, 85–86.

Morley, D. 1952. A ten-year survey of speech disorders among university students. *J. Speech Hearing Disorders*, 17, 25–31.

Morrison, S. 1955. Measuring the severity of articulation defectiveness. *J. Speech Hearing Disorders*, 20, 347–351.

Moss, M. 1938. The effect of speech defects on second-grade reading achievement. *Quart. J. Speech*, 24, 642–654.

Mowrer, O. 1952. Speech development in the young child: 1. the autism theory of speech development and some clinical applications. *J. Speech Hearing Disorders*, 17, 263–268.

Mulgrave, D. 1939. Speech for the classroom teacher. Englewood Cliffs, N.J.: Prentice-Hall.

Nelson, J. 1945. A study of misarticulation of (s) in combination with selected vowels and consonants. Univ. Iowa: Master's thesis.

Nemoy, E. 1954. Speech correction through story-telling units. Boston: Expression Co.

———, and Davis, S. 1937. The correction of defective consonant sounds. Boston: Expression Co.

Ness, A. 1932. A comparison of the response and stimulation methods in the re-education of speech defectives. Univ. Iowa: Master's thesis.

Palmer, M., and Osborn, C. 1940. A study of tongue pressures of speech-defective and normal-speaking individuals. *J. Speech Disorders*, 5, 133–139.

Patton, F. 1942. A comparison of the kinaesthetic sensibility of speech-defective and normal-speaking children. *J. Speech Disorders*, 7, 305–310.

Pendergast, K., Soder, A., Barker, J., Dickey, S., Gow, J., and Selmar, J. 1966. An articulation study of 15,255 Seattle first grade children with and without kindergarten. *Except. Child.*, 32, 541–547.

Perkins, W. 1952. Methods and materials for testing articulation of (s) and (z). *Quart. J. Speech*, 38, 57–62.

Perrin, E. 1954. The social position of the speech defective child. *J. Speech Hearing Disorders*, 19, 250–252.

Pettit, C. 1939. Diadochokinesis of the musculature of the jaw during puberty and adolescence. Univ. Wis.: Master's thesis.

———. 1952. The predictive efficiency of a battery of speech diagnostic tests for the articulatory development of a group of five-year-old children. Univ. Wis.: Ph.D. dissertation.

Poole, I. 1934. Genetic development in articulation of consonant sounds in speech. *Elem. Eng.*, 11, 159–161.

Powers, M. 1953. Speech correction in the Chicago public schools. *In* Special education in the Chicago public schools (rev. ed.). Chi. Bd. Educ.

Prather, E. 1960. Scaling defectiveness of articulation by direct magnitude-estimation. *J. Speech Hearing Res.*, 3, 380–392.

Prins, T. 1962a. Analysis of correlations among various articulatory deviations. *J Speech Hearing Res.*, 5, 152–160.

———. 1962b. Motor and auditory abilities in different groups of children with articulatory deviations. *J. Speech Hearing Res.*, 5, 161–168.

———. 1963. Relations among specific articulatory deviations and responses to a clinical measure of sound discrimination ability. *J. Speech Hearing Disorders*, 28, 382–388.

Pronovost, W. and Dumbleton, C. 1953. A picture-type speech sound discrimination test. *J. Speech Hearing Disorders*, 18, 258–266.

Raubicheck, L. 1952. Speech improvement. Englewood Cliffs, N.J.: Prentice-Hall.

———, Davis, E., and Carll, L. 1932. Voice and speech problems. Englewood Cliffs, N.J.: Prentice-Hall.

Reid, G. 1947a. The etiology and nature of functional articulatory defects in elementary school children. *J. Speech Disorders*, 12, 143–150.

———. 1947b. The efficacy of speech re-education of functional articulatory defectives in the elementary school. *J. Speech Disorders*, 12, 301–313.

Ringel, R., House, A., Burk, K., Dolinsky, J., and Scott,

C. 1970. Some relations between orosensory discrimination and articulatory aspects of speech production. *J. Speech Hearing Disorders*, 35, 3–11.

Robbins, S. 1942. Importance of sensory training in speech therapy. *J. Speech Disorders*, 7, 183–188.

———, and Robbins, R. 1937. Correction of speech defects of early childhood. Boston: Expression Co.

Robinson, H. 1946. Why pupils fail in reading. Chicago: Univ. Chi. Press.

Roe, V. 1948. Follow-up in the correction of functional articulatory disorders. *J. Speech Hearing Disorders*, 13, 332–336.

———, and Milisen, R. 1942. The effect of maturation upon defective articulation in elementary grades. *J. Speech Disorders*, 7, 37–50.

Root, A. 1925. A survey of speech defectives in the public elementary schools of South Dakota. *Elem. Sch. J.*, 26, 531–541.

Rossignol, L. 1948. The relationships among hearing acuity, speech production, and reading performance in grades 1a, 1b, 2a. *Teach. Coll. Contra. Educ.*, No. 936. New York: Teachers College, Columbia Univ.

Sayler, H. 1949. The effect of maturation upon defective articulation in grades seven through twelve. *J. Speech Hearing Disorders*, 14, 202–207.

Schiefelbusch, R., and Lindsey, M. 1958. A new test of sound discrimination. *J. Speech Hearing Disorders*, 23, 153–159.

Schlanger, B. 1953. Speech examination of a group of institutionalized mentally handicapped children. *J. Speech Hearing Disorders*, 18, 339–349.

———, and Galanowsky, G. 1966. Auditory discrimination tasks performed by mentally retarded and normal children. *J. Speech Hearing Res.*, 9, 434–440.

Schoolfield, L. 1951. Better speech and better reading. Boston: Expression Co.

Scott, D., and Milisen, R. 1954a. The effect of visual, auditory, and combined visual-auditory stimulation upon the speech responses of defective speaking children. *J. Speech Hearing Disorders*, *Monogr. suppl.* No. 4, 38–43.

———, and ———. 1954b. The effectiveness of combined visual-auditory stimulation in improving articulation. *J. Speech Hearing Disorders*, *Monogr. suppl.* No. 4, 52–56.

Scripture, E. 1923. Stuttering, lisping and correction of the speech of the deaf. New York: Macmillan.

Seth, G., and Guthrie, D. 1935. Speech in childhood. Oxford Univ. Press. London: Humphrey Milford.

Shames, G. 1957. Use of the nonsense-syllable in articulation therapy. *J. Speech Hearing Disorders*, 22, 261–263.

Shea, W. 1957. The effect of supplementary parental corrective procedures on public school functional articulatory cases. Univ. Fla.: Ph.D. dissertation.

Sherman, D. and Cullinan, W. 1960. Several procedures for scaling articulation. *J. Speech Hearing Res.*, 3, 191–198.

———, and Geith, A. 1967. Speech sound discrimination and articulation skill. *J. Speech Hearing Res.*, 10, 277–280.

———, and Morrison, S. 1955. Reliability of individual ratings of severity of defective articulation. *J. Speech Hearing Disorders*, 20, 352–358.

Shriner, T., Holloway, M., and Daniloff, R. 1969. The relationship between articulatory deficits and syntax in speech defective children. *J. Speech Hearing Res.*, 12, 319–325.

Siegel, G., Winitz, H., and Conkey, H. 1963. The influence of testing instrument on articulatory responses of children. *J. Speech Hearing Disorders*, 28, 67–76.

Sirkin, J., and Lyons, W. 1941. A study of speech defects in mental deficiency. *Amer. J. ment. Defic.*, 46, 74–80.

Snow, K. 1961. Articulation proficiency in relation to certain dental abnormalities. *J. Speech Hearing Disorders*, 26, 209–212.

———, and Milisen, R. 1954a. The influence of oral versus pictorial presentation upon articulation testing results. *J. Speech Hearing Disorders*, *Monogr. suppl.* No. 4, 30–36.

———, and ———. 1954b. Spontaneous improvement in articulation as related to differential responses to oral and picture articulation tests. *J. Speech Hearing Disorders*, *Monogr. suppl.* No. 4, 46–49.

Sommers, R. 1962. Factors in the effectiveness of mothers trained to aid in speech correction. *J. Speech Hearing Disorders*, 27, 178–186.

———, Cockerill, C., Bowser, D., Fichter, G., Fenton, A., and Copetas, F. 1961. Effects of speech therapy and speech improvement upon articulation and reading. *J. Speech Hearing Disorders*, 26, 27–38.

———, Copetas, F., Bowser, D., Fichter, G., Furlong, A., Rhodes, F., and Saunders, Z. 1962. Effects of various durations of speech improvement upon articulation and reading. *J. Speech Hearing Disorders*, 27, 54–61.

———, Furlong, A., Rhodes, F., Fichter, G., Bowser, D., Copetas, F., and Saunders, Z. 1964. Effects of maternal attitudes upon improvement in articulation when mothers are trained to assist in speech correction. *J. Speech Hearing Disorders*, 29, 126–132.

———, Leiss, R., Delp, M., Gerber, A., Fundrella, D., Smith, II, R., Revucky, M., Ellis, D., and Haley, V. 1967. Factors related to the effectiveness of articulation therapy for kindergarten, first, and second grade children. *J. Speech Hearing Res.*, 10, 428–437.

———, ———, Fundrella, D., Manning, W., Johnson, R., Oerther, P., Sholly, R., and Siegel, M. 1970. Factors in the effectiveness of articulation therapy with educable retarded children. *J. Speech Hearing Res.*, 13, 304–316.

———, Meyer, W., and Fenton, A. 1961. Pitch discrimination and articulation. *J. Speech Hearing Res.*, 4, 56–60.

———, Schaeffer, M., Leiss, R., Gerber, A., Bray, M., Fundrella, D., Olson, J., and Tomkins, E. 1966.

The effectiveness of group and individual therapy. *J. Speech Hearing Res.*, 9, 219–225.
———, Shilling, S., Paul, C., Copetas, F., Bowser, D., and McClintock, C. 1959. Training parents of children with functional misarticulation. *J. Speech Hearing Res.*, 2, 258–265.
Speech correction techniques and materials. 1968. (revised). Chi. Bd. Educ.: Div. Speech Correct., Margaret Hall Powers, Director.
Sperling, S. 1948. A comparison between verbal and non-verbal test results of children with articulatory speech defects. Univ. Mich.: Master's thesis.
Spriestersbach, D. 1956. Research in articulation disorders and personality. *J. Speech Hearing Disorders*, 21, 329–335.
———, and Curtis, J. 1951. Misarticulation and discrimination of speech sounds. *Quart. J. Speech*, 37, 483–491.
Steer, M., and Drexler, H. 1960. Predicting later articulation ability from kindergarten tests. *J. Speech Hearing Disorders*, 25, 391–397.
Stinchfield, S. 1927. Some relationships between speech defects, musical ability, scholastic attainment, and maladjustment. *Quart. J. Speech Education*, 13, 268–275.
———, and Young, E. 1938. Children with delayed or defective speech. Palo Alto: Stanford.
Stitt, C., and Huntington, D. 1969. Some relationships among articulation, auditory abilities, and certain other variables. *J. Speech Hearing Res.*, 12, 576–593.
Subtelny, J., Mestre, J., and Subtelny, J. 1964. Comparative study of normal and defective articulation of (s) as related to malocclusion and deglutition. *J. Speech Hearing Disorders*, 29, 269–285.
Sullivan, E. 1944. Auditory acuity and its relation to defective speech. *J. Speech Disorders*, 9, 127–130.
Summers, R. 1953. Perceptive vs. productive skills in analyzing speech sounds from words. *J. Speech Hearing Disorders*, 18, 140–148.
Swenson, G. 1956. An experimental study of the relationship of parental attitudes to functional disorders of articulation in children in two different cultural environments. Univ. So. Calif.: Ph.D. dissertation.
Symonds, P. 1948. Symond's picture-story test. New York: Teachers College, Columbia Univ.
Templin, M. 1938. A study of aggressiveness in normal and defective speaking college students. *J. Speech Disorders*, 3, 43–49.
———, 1943. A study of sound discrimination ability of elementary school pupils. *J. Speech Disorders*, 8, 127–132.
———. 1947a. Spontaneous versus imitated verbalization in testing articulation in preschool children. *J. Speech Disorders*, 12, 293–300.
———. 1947b. A non-diagnostic articulation test. *J. Speech Disorders*, 12, 392–396.
———. 1952. Speech development in the young child: 3. the development of certain language skills in children. *J. Speech Hearing Disorders*, 17, 280–285.
———. 1953. Norms on a screening test of articulation for ages three through eight. *J. Speech Hearing Disorders*, 18, 323–331.
———. 1957. Certain language skills in children. Minneapolis: Univ. Minn. Press.
———, and Darley, F. 1960. The Templin-Darley tests of articulation. Iowa City: Bur. Educ. Res. and Services, Ext. div., Univ. Iowa.
———, and Steer, M. 1939. Studies of growth of speech of pre-school children. *J. Speech Disorders*, 4, 71–77.
Travis, L. 1931. Speech pathology. New York: Appleton.
———, and Davis, M. 1927. The relation between faulty speech and the lack of certain musical talents. *Psychol. Monogr.* 36, 71–81.
———, and Rasmus, B. 1931. The speech sound discrimination ability of cases with functional disorders of articulation. *Quart. J. Speech Educ.*, 17, 217–226.
Tufts, L., and Holliday, A. 1959. Effectiveness of trained parents as speech therapists. *J. Speech Hearing Disorders*, 24, 395–401.
Vandemark, A., and Bann, M. 1965. Oral language skills of children with defective articulation. *J. Speech Hearing Res.*, 6, 409-414.
Van Riper, C. 1938. Persistence of baby talk among children and adults. *Elem. Sch. J.*, 38, 672–675.
———. 1947. Speech correction principles and methods (2nd. ed.). Englewood Cliffs, N.J.: Prentice-Hall.
———. 1963. Speech correction principles and methods (4th. ed.). Englewood Cliffs, N.J.: Prentice-Hall.
———, and Irwin, J. 1958. Voice and articulation. Englewood Cliffs, N.J.: Prentice-Hall.
———, and Erickson, R. 1969. A predictive screening test of articulation. *J. Speech Hearing Disorders*, 34, 214–219.
Ward, M., Malone, Sister H., Jann, G., and Jann, H. 1961. Articulation variations associated with visceral swallowing and malocclusion. *J. Speech Hearing Disorders*, 26, 334–341.
Weaver, C., Furbee, C., and Everhart, R. 1960a. Articulatory competency and reading readiness. *J. Speech Hearing Res.*, 3, 174–180.
———, ———, and ———. 1960b. Paternal occupation class and articulatory defects in children. *J. Speech Hearing Disorders*, 25, 171–175.
Webb, C., and Siegenthaler, B. 1957. Comparison of aural stimulation methods for teaching speech sounds. *J. Speech Hearing Disorders*, 22, 264–270.
Wechsler, D. 1949. Wechsler intelligence scale for children. New York: Psychological Corp.
———. 1963. Wechsler preschool and primary scale of intelligence. New York: Psychological Corp.
Weiner, P. 1967. Auditory discrimination and articulation. *J. Speech Hearing Disorders*, 32, 19–28.
Wellman, B., Case, I., Mengert, I., and Bradbury, D. 1931. Speech sounds of young children. Univ. Iowa Studies in Child Welfare, 5, No. 2.

Wepman, J. 1958. Auditory discrimination test. Chicago: Language Res. Associates.

———. 1960. Auditory discrimination, speech, and reading. *Elem. Sch. J.*, 60, 325–333.

West, R., Kennedy, L., and Carr, A. 1947. The rehabilitation of speech (rev. ed.). New York: Harper.

White House Conference on Child Health and Protection. 1931. Section III: education and training. Report of the committee on special classes. The defective in speech. 349–381. New York: Century.

Wilson, F. 1966. Efficacy of speech therapy with educable mentally retarded children. *J. Speech Hearing Res.*, 9, 423–433.

Wilson, M. 1952. A comparative study of the defective speech of children found in the rural area of Van Buren County and the urban area of the city of Muskegon. Mich. State College: Master's thesis.

Winitz, H., and Lawrence, M. 1961. Children's articulation and sound learning ability. *J. Speech Hearing Res.*, 4, 259–268.

Witty, P., and Kopel, D. 1939. Reading and the educative process. Boston: Ginn.

Wood, K. 1946. Parental maladjustment and functional articulatory defects in children. *J. Speech Disorders*, 11, 255–275.

———. 1949. Measurement of progress in the correction of articulatory speech defects. *J. Speech Hearing Disorders*, 14, 171–174.

Young, E., and Hawk, S. 1955. Moto-kinesthetic speech training. Palo Alto: Stanford.

Zedler, E. 1955. Listening for speech sounds. Garden City, N.Y.: Doubleday.

35

Psychotherapy in Public School Speech Correction

Lee Edward Travis and LaVerne Deel Sutherland

The great majority of speech-defective children in the public schools of America are not suffering from any determinable form or degree of organicity. They present no known organic impairment of either the sensory or the motor structures used in the acquisition and the maintenance of speech. In the absence of any structural deficiency of a clinical nature, these children are diagnosed as functional cases and commonly classified as articulatory, stuttering, and delayed-speech defectives. With articulatory and delayed-speech cases the common approaches in speech therapy are the phonetic-placement, the motokinesthetic, and auditory training. These methods assume that speech therapy involves the teaching of correct or normal speech habits to replace the defective or abnormal ones. Could we not make a further valid assumption that these methods would be more effective if they were practised in conjunction with psychotherapy which would deal with emotional problems either underlying the speech symptoms or aggravating them? Our current stance is that for stuttering, psychotherapy of the type described in this chapter is the best approach to the problem.

THE THERAPY SESSION

The Therapist as a New Parent

Some speech symptoms may be considered as the advertising camouflage of the speaker's inadmissibility of certain of his thoughts and feelings. This denial is a learned response from his early years when his "old parent" was his only source of recognition, warmth, love, and physical sustenance. The condemnation of some of the acts of the child by the parent was interpreted by the child to include the condemnation of himself as a person. What were those basic acts? They were acts of love, hostility, sensuality, orality, messing, aggression, dependency, sibling rivalry, and child-parent rivalry. These acts and their associated feelings become the troublesome ones which need now to be "unlearned."

The child soon knows that he can count on coming regularly to the therapy room which becomes and is labeled a "special time" and a "special place." He is repeatedly encouraged by the therapist, a "special person," to express himself freely verbally while engaging in potentially anxiety-provoking acts such as finger-paint messing, clay smashing, sucking and blowing on a modified spirometer, picture drawing, storytelling, and dramatizations. While he is doing these things he may be using puppets, plastic figures, and Travis Story Pictures. These clinical techniques are being used in speech therapy in the public schools quite successfully by setting limits on acting out, but none on verbalizations. They provide safe disguises under which the child may more honestly express his disabling fears, hostilities, and loves in the "unlearning" process.

The primary process that results in behavior change is communication, free and open, between the child and the therapist. The purpose of therapy is to improve the communication of the child with himself and with others, to improve him intrapsychically and interpersonally. He must admit his feelings to himself and accept them and then dare share them in the safe and sheltered relationship of the therapy situation.

In the periodic company of his insightful new parent, the child models his behavior, including speech, after that of the therapist, and largely "grows up again" to feel good and talk well. Coming to therapy originally he talked as he felt—not good, not sure, not clear, not self respectful, not free. Through the hours, generally not really enough, of sharing the presence of an authentic person who loves him and literally lives his life with him, the child of poor speech talks better, and finally, maybe, perfectly.

Introducing the Child to Therapy

At the outset the therapy session is given definition. "This is your special time, special place, and I'm a special person with whom you may say anything you feel like saying, in any way you feel like saying it, and everything is all right. We may not do anything we feel like, but we may talk about it. Everything we say here, and do here, or make here, stays here." Here then is the beginning of a new experience for each child, an opportunity to learn to talk about himself freely, to explain himself to his welcoming therapist, to his group therapy associates, and to himself.

As the therapy progresses in the months to follow, the therapist occasionally reinforces the simple standards and limits regarding the fact that the productions of the therapy sessions are "strictly saved for this place." "When you are away from here and have upset feelings save your acting them out until you are here with me, and we'll talk about your feelings and learn safe ways to get rid of them without hurting you or anybody else."

At the end of each session, before the children leave the therapy room, the therapist is responsible for bringing them back to the reality of the school world outside which they will reenter through the door into the hall. She does this essentially by reminding them again that this is a "special place." "We haven't many rules, but we respect those few we do have. You get to do special things that you may not do outside, but here they're all right. I love you and accept your angry, upset feelings whenever you have them. But everyone else can't understand and accept them. Remember?" Or the therapist may say, "Do we live alone? No, we live with many other people every day. We may not hurt another or destroy another's property. I love you too much to let others hurt you. I love you too much to let you hurt yourself by making trouble."

Eliciting the Child's Verbalizations

As a "special person" the therapist is different from any authority figure the child has ever known. She is a mature, well-adjusted person who speaks little, but who speaks simply and intelligently; who listens attentively and with an open mind; who is warm, acceptant, patient, supportive; who is respectful of the child's status and self-regard; who is not disturbed by the child's expressions of raw emotions; who is trustworthy of rare confidences; who is consistent with regard to set limits; and who is able to identify with the child by having great self-knowledge. The therapist must impress the child with her own authenticity, her strength for emphatic responses, and her unconditional love for him.

The child finds in the therapist the most effective listener he has ever known. She listens with calm attention. The more dramatic or rare the child's verbalizations, the more quietly serious is the therapist's interest. The shock value of a story is wasted on this "special person" in this "special place." The child learns that he must admit his feelings to himself aloud and thus share them with this keen but kindly listener in the safe and sheltered relationship of the therapy session. A slight nod from the therapist, a thoughtful or puzzled look, lifting the head, cupping the chin and other minimal gestures serve to reassure the child in his struggling efforts to be open with himself, with her and with others.

The therapist is an expert in the ways of eliciting verbal responses. She conveys genuine interest rather than prying curiosity. To stimulate a child who is faltering in his attempts to create a story, the therapist allows a reasonable time at each searching pause (which is not a stuttering block), then softly and slowly speaks with a gently questioning tone of rising inflection, "and then . . . ?" thus indicating an invitation to continue his unfinished remark. Perhaps she repeats his last phrase: "so the little boy . . . ?", or she guides him on with his verbalization: "When he ran away he felt . . . ?" or, "he ran away because . . . ?" The threateningly bold questions: "What did he do?" "Why did he do it?" "How did he feel?" so defensively answered with the finality of "I don't know," are avoided whenever possible in the initial, vulnerable stage of therapy. Some of the children's projections which follow later in the chapter will include additional examples of the therapist's verbalizations.

When tape recording is introduced, a child might test the therapist with some silly behavior. To the child's surprise, the therapist reacts as if the child were in earnest. The therapist's responses are made with consistent and increasing courtesy, seriousness, and interest in what the child is saying or doing. At a later time the child might be helped to recall his behavior for discussion in regard to the feelings which prompted it.

This new relationship is not an attitude to be assumed. The therapist is a healthy person who has become an enlightened communicator with children, a relationship requiring both science and art. The children quickly discover any falseness in "performance" as compared to the integrity of an honest interpersonal relationship. To lessen the schoolroom atmosphere, the therapist uses a table only when furniture is required for an activity. It is preferable to sit in fairly close proximity to the children so that the therapist may reach the child comfortably with voice, vision, and perhaps, a gentle touch.

TALKING ABOUT SELF

The Family

To set the children upon a course of talking about themselves, it is wise to lead them out of their familiar and possibly restrictive home setting into creative and spontaneous self-disclosures. A few pages from the illustrated book, *A Book About Me* (Jay, 1952) are useful for initiating verbal responses from children. "Here are some mothers. This mother is washing dishes. Here's a mother cooking. See this mother is . . . etc." "Now Johnny, tell us about your mother. What does your mother do?" As Johnny, perhaps hesitatingly, begins, the therapist is obviously relaxed but interested, assuming that Johnny has something to say. The therapist's comments are brief, spoken in a pleasant voice, and often ending with a rising inflection, indicating an invitation to continue.

The picture pages "My Daddy" and "My Family" follow "My Mother" for setting the pattern of respectful listening and speaking.

The next session affords the children opportunities to work on a deeper level with "When I sleep, eat, and play"; "Things I do at home . . . or don't do"; "Things I can do all by myself . . . or can't do", and "People I see, know, like . . . or don't like." At this point it is enough that they can admit there are some hush-hush areas and dislikes without delving into the "why" before the children feel real security in the environment.

Feelings

When enough security has been established, discussion about the page "Real Animals I have Seen" is a good introduction to "Things I am afraid of." The therapist sits close to the children, showing the pictures, and speaking in calm, matter-of-fact tones. "We are all afraid at times. We are all afraid of different things." Now showing pictures the therapist continues. "Some of us are afraid of fire, some of us are scared of spankings. Mary, you're afraid of . . . (rising inflection) . . . ?" When it is his turn, perhaps Bill will claim, "I'm not afraid of nuthin'." The therapist, in quiet surprise says, "You're not afraid of anything? Most everyone has some fear, perhaps a little one? No? Then you will tell us about the fears you used to have." With the reassurance that it is all right for a boy to have had fear, he usually admits to some current fears as well.

Over the years it has been interesting to note that this session on "Things I'm afraid of" marks a turning point in the therapy. Through gentle guidance and consistent fairness the therapist earns the children's trust and they are ready to talk about their fears. The group responds with a good sense of unity.

Reinforcement of gains may be assured at the next session. "Last week we talked about things we're afraid of. We found that all of us have been afraid. What is fear? How do you feel when you are afraid? I'll be your secretary and we'll see how many ways we can tell about fear. Marshall, sometimes when you're afraid it feels like . . . ?"

The following are examples of the children's descriptions of fear: "shaky," "scary," "hot," "cold," "nervous," "real weak," "can't move," "real pale," "my tonsils break all to pieces," "heart pumps, pounding very fast, then slows down, slower and slower so it would stop," "hands kind of puffed up bigger, bigger, bigger," "no power in your hands," "weakened," "breath is much more harder," "lost my legs, paralyzed or shaky and after it's over they're ticklish."

Toby[1] (stutterer, seven years): "You want to fight back and if you can't they have you there. You think you're going to die . . . or live? You do some things while you're afraid and don't realize it until later."

Harry (stutterer, eight years): "I feel I'd like to be locked up in a room. I would be safer from harm. My family makes me feel safer. If they are not there I'd still feel safer because it would be home."

Lanny (stutterer, 11 years): "I'm nervous . . . stumble . . . drop everything . . . shaky . . . I can't even talk . . . 'cause I'm thinking 'is he goin' to spank, yell, or what?' . . . Dad is mad and sometimes he hits me . . . I cry so hard . . . I feel like I can't hardly breathe . . . like . . . (gasping) . . . uh . . . uh . . . He gives me a spanking and a lecture . . . and then a day later he gives me a dollar . . . if he keeps feeling bad then I feel worse."

In talking about the feeling of anger, Saul, an eight-year-old stutterer, explained:

"Its kinda like you're not going to let the 'scare' get you . . . 'cause you're gonna do somethin' about it (clenching fists in lap) . . . and that's 'angry' and that's 'mad' . . . you're not gonna let the 'scare' get inside you and make you run away . . . 'cause that's when the fear shows inside you."

A bright 10-year-old youngster, Esther, who was no longer stuttering much, observed:

"We get very mad at our father and mother, maybe they're the first people we ever get mad at because they were the first people we ever knew . . . it's kinda hard to explain . . . well it's easier to get mad at your brother and sister, because, well, anyway, they got mad at us . . . We live with them all the time and they get over it, and don't take it like other kids might take it . . . They get over it easier . . . You get mad at them easier and get over it easier."

Children of all ages respond to the therapist's invitation to talk about themselves through definitions. She may say, "Remember one time we talked about fear and another day we talked about what anger is. Today we'll talk about many other feelings. Like what "happy" means. Linda, to you happy means . . . ?"

Children have given some of the following definitions of feelings:

Happy: "Jumpy," "Bumpy," "Feel good."
Mixed-up: "You want to but you don't want to, all mixed-up together 'till you're all upset."
Calm: "Empty of upset."

[1]It must be realized that some children did not stutter with the therapist.

Nervous: "Shaky inside." "Full of upset."
Love: "Warm," "Close," "Somebody wants you," "Holds you soft," "Tucks you in," "Likes you anyhow."
Lonesome: "Want someone to want you."
Excitement: "Whee!" "Wow!" "You have to zoom!"
Sad: "So bad there's inside tears."
Strong: "Can do anything you want to, like Superman."
Weak: "Like a baby." "Like need help."
Beauty: "Pretty, a happy-pretty, like a smile."
Ugly: "Real, real bad. All bad, upset."
Laughing: "Feel good sounds." "Bubbly, feel good."
Selfish: "You don't want nobody to have it but you."
Jealous: (after much thought) "A kind of 'selfish'."

Experiences

The therapy situation often lends a new dimension to the child's concept of self in his recall of trying experiences. Ten-year-old Nikolo's memories incorporated several of the problems which children recall of that first day in school. While the therapist was familiar with his multiple problems of noncommunication, stuttering, articulation, and harsh voice quality, she had not witnessed his chronic vomiting which was suspected of being psychosomatic.

Therapist: "Tell us about your first day in school Nikolo. You felt . . ."
Nikolo: (tentatively) ". . . shy, nervous . . . (voice trembling). My mom taked me to the office and I didn't know what was it . . . I thought it was a place you eat . . . then I went in . . . then I saw Mrs. Marton . . . an' I didn't know what to say . . ."
Therapist: "She's the lady in the office . . . Then you went to the kindergarten room . . . did you talk there?"
Nikolo: ". . . a little . . ."
Therapist: "You felt . . ."
Nikolo: ". . . Nervous . . . I played sick."
Therapist: "You played sick . . . You mean sick throw up, sick tummy ache?"
Nikolo: "Stomach ache."
Therapist: "When you were with the youngsters and the teacher you felt . . ."
Nikolo: ". . . shy . . ."
Therapist: "By shy, you mean . . . afraid to talk?"
Nikolo: "Yeah."
Therapist: "Afraid to talk because you felt if you did . . ."
Nikolo: "She'll clobber me."
Therapist: "You mean the teacher or the children or . . . ?"

Nikolo: "The children and the teacher."

Therapist: "What do you suppose parents or teachers could do to help children feel better about going to school?"

Nikolo: "Going home."

Therapis: "Who should go home?"

Nikolo: "Me."

Therapist: "Then the next morning?"

Nikolo: "I wouldn't want to go."

Therapist: "And when you didn't want to go . . ."

Nikolo: "I got sick again."

Therapist: "Is it their feelings that make children sick, or is it somebody else who thinks they're sick, or is it their stomachs that are sick?"

Nikolo: "Their feelings."

Therapist: "Are you saying that if your feelings are sick, then your body would start to act sick? In what way?"

Nikolo: "All of it . . . could throw up."

Therapist: "Could throw up. I'm sure that's happened to people. Has it happened to you?"

Nikolo: "Yeah."

Therapist: "Does it happen anymore?"

Nikolo: "No."

Therapist: "Some of the feelings that would make you feel sick are . . . ?"

Nikolo: "Names."

Therapist: "Somebody calling you names?"

Nikolo: (nodding).

Therapist: "Like . . . ?"

Nikolo: "He's a bad drawer."

Therapist: "Oh, someone . . ."

Nikolo: "I was in kindergarten."

It is interesting to note that with the advent of therapy Nikolo's chronic vomiting had lessened and from the day he haltingly told of his misery there has been no recurrence at school (two years) and he has made marked improvement in his speech.

Carlton (stutterer, eight years): "I was crying my head off. I didn't want to go to kindergarten. I wanted to stay home 'till I was more grown up, about eight years old. I didn't know the teachers. I thought they'd hit me if I talked. She'd ask a question and I'd know the right answer, but I'd think I was wrong. So I was too scared to talk. Afraid I'd be wrong. Boy was I scared of the teacher and all the things I didn't know . . . because I was too little and I didn't know yet that it was all right and she was nice and friendly."

Taking tests, receiving grades and report cards are usually dreaded.

Rebecca (stutterer, 10 years): "I'm sure glad we don't have to take tests in speech class. My mother doesn't care what grades I make and neither does my father, but it's scary because everybody else is scared. It's catching and when you don't know something you 'uh, oh, what's going to happen now?' I don't really expect to do well. In fact I'm surprised when I get good grades. I know I put pressure on myself. Lately I haven't been trying half so hard and I've been making better grades, because before I'd get so scared I wouldn't know which way was up. When I'm at home I can do anything. But when I'm at school I can't do it so good. So I think I'm just awfully tight about it."

Admission of Speech Problems

In speech therapy, the therapist waits for the children to approach the subject of their stuttering. She avoids giving direct answers to the children's questions. The questions are about themselves, and so are the answers. Both the questions and the answers should be worked through by the child in interaction with the therapist.

A child responded:

"When you're talking it's kinda like a (hands circle throat) hurt inside. When you cry you feel better and then you kinda forget. You get all the stuff in your system out. Other people probably feel the same bothered way I do about the way I talk. It sounds stupid, the way I talk. It worries me. When I hear myself talking I feel horrible and embarrassed . . . the way I'm saying it. I'd like to talk different so I didn't stutter. The 'stutter' is like an interruption. There are not too many kids who have the problem. When they make fun of you you feel real bad. It's no fun to be criticized about it all the time.It's different in speech class. I speak better because I don't worry about being criticized. When you try so hard to keep from stuttering the trying hard makes you talk worse sometimes. The harder you try the worse you do. I don't stutter nearly so bad as I did. When I have to say something in front of the class I get upset and I don't say it out good . . . I can't. No one tells us what to say here. You learn how to talk better and you don't get cri-cri-criticized in here because everybody has the same problem. People really listen to you here. No kids will make fun of you here. Well, when you're upset you can come here to speech class and talk here and get rid of your upset feelings and you won't be so scared when you go to the room."

IMAGINARY CREATIONS

Imagery is the primary mental process used in working with these young children. In expressing their troubled feelings through lively and rich imagination in a therapeutic climate, unlearning and relearning are allowed to take place. The therapist introduces pictures to trigger the process of imagination and to furnish the child with purpose. Rehearsing his problem through shared imagination with his insightful therapist leaves him with better potential for growing, sharing himself with people, and talking better.

A projective picture provides the child with a stimulus situation that may give him an opportunity to impose verbally upon it his consciously guarded secret needs. It may be used to elict interpersonal relationships of both overt and hidden forms. The use of this procedure in speech correction is not so much for diagnosis as for therapy. By involuntarily revealing feelings and thoughts that are below the surface and otherwise incapable of exposure by questions and suggestions, the child may come to recognize, express, and more wholesomely manage them. The speech therapist can develop her own projection test or she can use those already developed. The Travis Story Pictures were found to be good for speech therapy, since the pictures were drawn to portray adults and children in situations and relationships centering in the important and potentially troublesome areas in the socialization of the child. The areas pictured are sibling rivalry, child-parent rivalry, discipline, eating, sleeping, toilet training, cleanliness, and sexual development.

The great majority of the children will respond well verbally to the pictures. Occasionally a child will refuse to respond to a given picture. One nine-year-old boy showed great anxiety in saying, "I'm not going to tell a story." Later he wanted to talk, started a story five different times, finally stopped and could not go on. The child is told simply to tell a story about the picture. The therapist can make the situation a group or an individual one as time and circumstances warrant. The speech therapist can use one picture only, or a choice of two representing different areas of development, or she can present a picture while the child is doing something else, such as working with clay, playing with puppets, or playing a role in sociodrama.

Travis Story Pictures[2]

In response to the picture in Fig. 35-1, Clifford (stutterer, seven years) said:

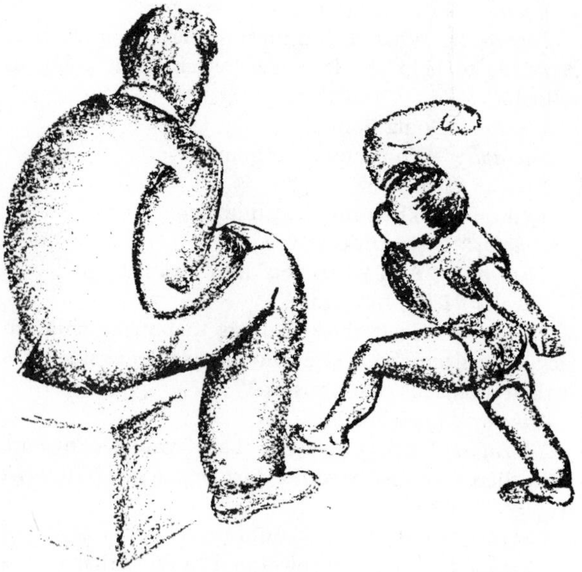

Fig. 35-1. Picture 23 of the Travis Story Pictures.

"His dad is teaching him how to fight and he's not putting his head up . . his hand up . . . and he . . . and he's gonna . . . he's gonna fall . . . and he wants his dad to pick him up and show him once more . . . and he . . . he . . . he (clears throat) said he didn't want to and he went in his room and played with his toys and he wants to play with his toy rifle . . . then his daddy came and called him for dessert. That's all."

Therapist: "Clifford, when the little boy fell down and wanted his dad to help him try again to learn how to fight properly, who was it who didn't want to try again?"

Clifford: "It was the boy."

Therapist: "The boy doesn't want to try again . . . the father wanted him to try again?"

Clifford: "Yes."

Therapist: "How does the boy feel about learning to fight?"

Clifford: "He . . . he . . . he . . . feels good about it but . . . but . . . but after he got . . . got. . . fell . . . fell he don't feel . . . feel good about it."

Therapist: "Does he want to learn to fight because his father wants him to learn, or because he wants to learn?"

Clifford: "He wants to fight because he wants . . . his dad wants him to fight."

Therapist: "His dad wants him to fight so that's the reason he wants to learn . . . but when he tried, and he didn't do it the right way, then he felt . . ."

Clifford: "He . . . he felt . . . uh . . . sad."

Therapist: "um hmm . . . and then his dad wanted him to try again?"

[2] The set of 29 pictures may be obtained from Dr. Lee Edward Travis, 3412 Red Rose Drive, Encino, California, 91316.

Clifford: (nods)

Therapist: ". . . yes? . . . but the boy didn't want to try again because . . ."

Clifford: "Because he . . . he . . . he . . . fell and he didn't fee . . . feel good after that because he banged his head."

Therapist: "How was it that he banged his head, Clifford?"

Clifford: "His father hit and then he fell and banged his head and he was bleeding . . . and he got a cloth over his head upstairs . . . and . . . and then he came down with a big bump. He had to eat dinner with a big bump on his head . . . and . . . and his de . . . dessert was ice cream and cake . . . and he . . . he went back upstairs to play with his game . . . and he . . . started blooding again . . . and . . . he got blood all over his carpet . . . and then he got another towel . . ."

Therapist: ". . . Another towel . . . ? Uh hmm . . . so he felt . . ."

Clifford: "He felt sad about that . . . that he went went back downstairs. That's all."

Therapist: "When he went downstairs did he see someone there?"

Clifford: "Mmmm . . . yes . . . he saw his grandma."

Therapist: "And his grandmother felt . . ."

Clifford: "His grandma and mother didn't feel very good when she saw that big bump on his head with blood all over it."

Therapist: "And father felt . . ."

Clifford: "And father felt sad about his grandma not feeling good."

Therapist: "Then it was grandma that daddy was worried about not feeling good?"

Clifford: (nodding hopelessly).

It is interesting to note that Clifford's paternal grandmother did live with the family. His stepfather was very much older than his mother. Both Clifford and his mother had strong feelings that the grandmother received primary attention in the home, ahead of the mother and the children. In his story he had the grandmother's worry of greater concern to the father than the child's injury.

Barney (articulation, voice, nonfluency, nine years) lived with his father and brother. His mother had deserted the family when Barney was an infant. His hostility is expressed with similar stories to two different pictures (Figs. 35-1 and 35-2). To the first picture he said:

"The boy learns judo . . . lives alone with his father . . . he wraps father around his finger . . . throws him to Hong Kong . . . the boy sprouts wings on his bicycle . . . flies to Hong Kong . . . throws father again and again through the air . . . the father hits a bird . . . falls and is drowned . . . the boy is eaten by a shark . . . the boy had no mother because he ate his mother up . . . because he got hungry . . . because mother would not feed him . . . after eating his mother he lost his appetite."

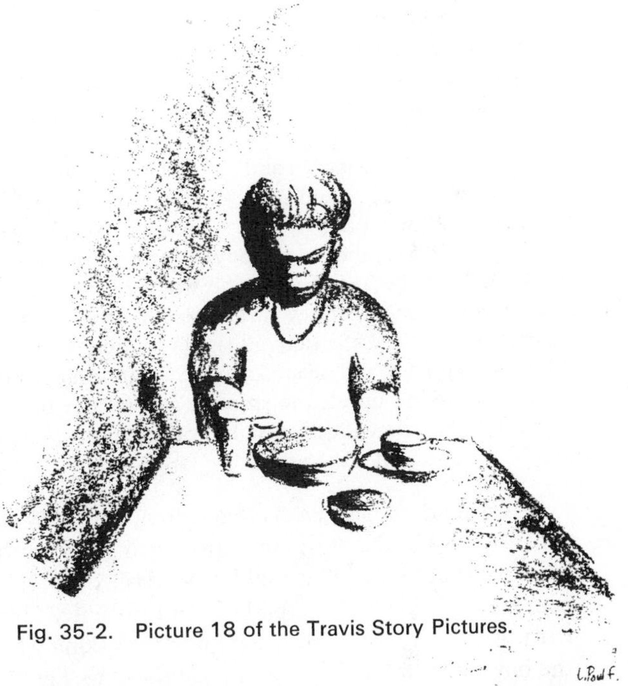

Fig. 35-2. Picture 18 of the Travis Story Pictures.

To the second picture he said:

"The boy's mother gave the boy bad food . . . worms were too good for him . . . he should have the garbage . . . mother ate regular, good food . . . the boy got used to bad food."

A year later Barney was considered to have normal speech. He was making a successful interpersonal relationship and had initiated some interest in his academic work.

Pablo (stutterer, seven years), in responding to the picture in Fig. 35-2, provides an example of reality combined with fantasy, and also of delayed language. English is Pablo's second language marked by grammatical errors.

"a boy . . . and . . . and . . . he didn't want to eat . . . and . . . and . . . and . . . he was . . . he looked like a monster every time he didn't want to eat and his mother punish him . . . when he went to bed wi . . . th no eating . . . and . . . and then . . . and then . . . and then the boy and he jumped out in the window . . . and he runned away to his friend's house . . . and the mother said 'you can't go' and . . . and . . . and then he turned out of a . . . a . . . a . . . a . . . a bird and . . . he flied up in the sky . . . and . . . and . . . and . . . and then . . . and he bought something with his money . . . and . . ."

Therapist: "It was a . . ."

Pablo: ". . . a . . . hat . . . and . . . and he bought some clothes too . . . so . . . and so . . . and he bought a jacket because he didn't bring none . . . (cough-cough) and then . . . (sniff) . . . the . . . the boy . . . and he wanted to go back home because he . . . he was hungry and he didn't have no more money . . . and said 'mother, I want to eat now' . . . and she said 'all right' . . . and she gave him some spinach and he ated it up . . . and he ate some more and he ate up all the spinach and all the bread and all . . . all the coffee 'cause he was hungry . . . and that's . . . and that's the end."

When children have been offered an opportunity to use imagery, the therapist must enter their world with sensitivity and care. She could have dashed Pablo's courage, quenched his sparkle, and forfeited his trust by overtly correcting his grammar or asking why the boy could not fly home as he had flown to Texas; or why he bought a hat since he had become a bird. Pablo returned his boy to reality when he finished his flight into fantasy and was ready to return.

Pablo responds to another picture (Fig. 35-3):

"A mother was socking the little boy in . . . in the pants because he . . . he . . . he make pee in bed and . . . and he said him to . . . to . . . make in the night time you gotta wake up and go in the bafroom and then . . . and then . . . he said and when I'm asleep I can't wake up . . . w . . . wake up and then she said . . . but anyway . . . but wake up or I'm gonna hit you and . . . and the little boy . . . and him went to bed and then the mother came and gave the boy . . . gave him a little bit of food . . . because he wanted him to eat and then the father came . . . and . . . and . . . he brought some ice cream for him and . . . and . . . he ate some . . . and then he ate some tea . . . and because nobody want to . . . and then last night he didn't make pee in his bed and he didn't get a whipping and he gets to play outside and . . . and . . . he . . . and . . . and . . . he's . . . and he's a little boy . . . and he makes pee in his pants."

Therapist: "Do you remember when you were little, when you wet the bed? Did you ever get punished for it?"

Pablo: (shaking his head)

Therapist: "You don't remember this?"

Pablo: "I don't make *tea* in bed."

Therapist: "Not anymore?"

Pablo: "That's the end."

Therapist: "Yes, Frank?"

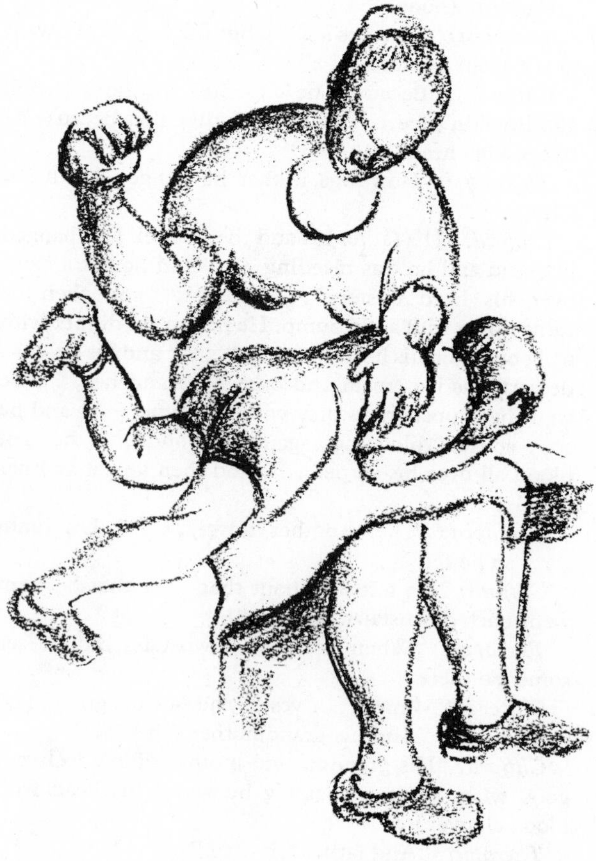

Fig. 35-3. Picture 25 of the Travis Story Pictures.

Frank, as a member of the group, had indicated his desire to interrupt. He was a seven-year-old stutterer.

Frank: "I . . . I . . . I . . . sometimes uh . . . when I was a baby . . . then uh . . . uh . . . I make pee in the bed . . . and my . . . m-m-m . . . mom doesn't do nothin' . . . she just clean up m-m-my bed . . . and my mom already has a baby."

Therapist: "Your mother already had another baby . . ."

Frank: "Uh . . . hmm . . ."

Therapist: "Do you remember being punished for it?"

Frank: "Huh . . . uh . . . I never . . . I was a baby. If my mother gave me a good . . . a good . . . spanking . . . I'd die."

Therapist: "If your mother gave you a good spanking?"

Frank: "A hard one . . ."

Pablo: "Can I hear my story?" (it was being recorded).

Therapist: "A hard one? You think you'd die?"

Pablo: "Yeah and you're a little baby you will."

Frank: "M hum . . . not . . . not . . . now."

Therapist: "But then you think you would because . . . You think it would hurt too much?"

Frank: "To me it would, if I be a baby."

Therapist: "mum . . . hum . . ."

Frank: "I'd cry . . . I . . . I . . . I . . . I . . . I will . . . yell or something."

In this example of collaboration by two children Frank became involved in Pablo's production and a mutually supportive interaction followed.

Timmy was an eight-year-old boy whose father also stuttered. He was his father's favorite of three children and also the oldest. He was admittedly rejected by his mother, and the father had repeatedly deserted the family from the time Timmy was a few months old. When he looked at the picture (Fig. 35-4) he said:

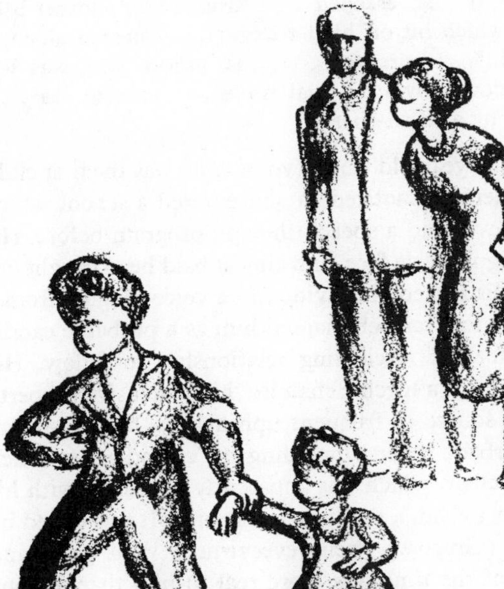

Fig. 35-4. Picture 1 of the Travis Story Pictures.

"F-f-f-father and m-m-m-mother tried to plan how to get money for a h-h-h-h-h-ome. F-f-f-f-ather worked and saved and bought a h-h-h-h-ouse. M-m-mother worked and bought clothes. B-b-brother sold newspapers and bought furniture to put clothes in. The h-h-h-ouse had no roof. S-s-sister worked and bought a r-r-roof for the h-h-h-h-ouse. B-b-brother and s-s-s-sister went to the store to get milk and cookies which they all ate. They went to b-b-bed (pause). The h-h-h-h-ouse disappeared (pause). The furniture disappeared (pause), and the r-r-r-roof. S-s-so they . . . they had nothing (pause). Then they . . . they wakened (pause). It was a dream."

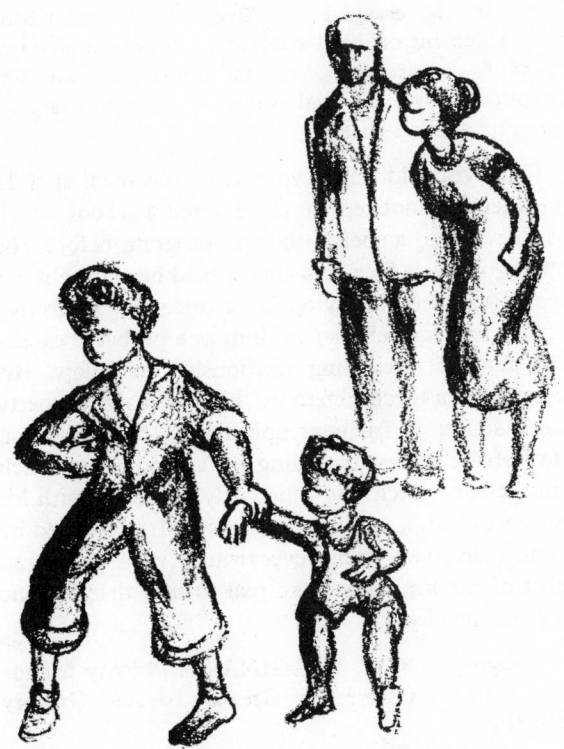

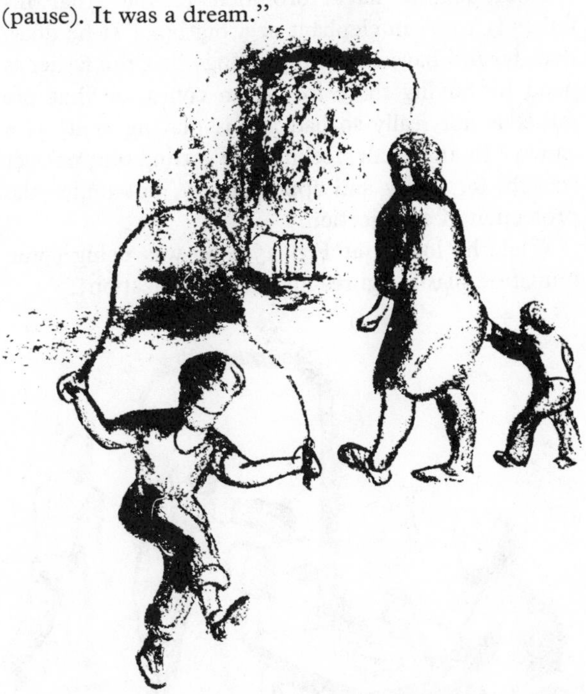

Fig. 35-5. Picture 2 of the Travis Story Pictures.

It seems clear that Timmy was projecting his own feelings into the picture. His troubling insecurities caused him great difficulty in acquiring and keeping a roof. Even his fantasy was frightening, so fearsome in fact that he had to call it a dream. Really, he had to give a dream within a fantasy to tolerate his feelings.

When the picture (Fig. 35-5) was presented to him, he said:

"B-b-big b-b-brother went to the a-a-attic to see the rats. The f-f-f-ather was there (pause) but no one knew it. B-b-b-brother was q-q-q-quiet so as not to s-s-s-scare the rats. H-h-he came back down and said a b-b-big huge rat was in the a-a-a-attic. M-m-m-mother went up and came back and said an e-e-e-elephant with a s-s-small nose was up there. L-l-little b-b-brother went up and came back and said a b-b-big b-b-box shaped like a m-m-man was up there. They decided to cut the r-r-roof off and find out. They started s-s-s-sawing around the r-r-r-roof. F-f-f-ather heard it and thought the rats were beginning to ch-ch-chew the r-r-r-roof off. While the f-f-f-family was inside, the f-f-f-ather s-s-s-s-sneaked downstairs and out the garage. H-h-h-h-e bought three ice cream cones and put a b-b-box in the a-a-a-ttic shaped like a m-m-m-man, a r-r-rat and an e-e-elephant (pause). They brought it downstairs (pause) and out jumped a funny clown."

Does Timmy have forbidden feelings that his father is a rat, an elephant or a big box? If he does, does he also have offsetting feelings that the father is good by buying three ice cream cones, or that the father is not really so bad but is playing at it, as a clown? In any event, feelings are getting out, not yet straight forwardly and appropriately, but under the protection of a projection.

While he looked at Fig. 35-6 he was using some miniature plastic figures for his dramatization:

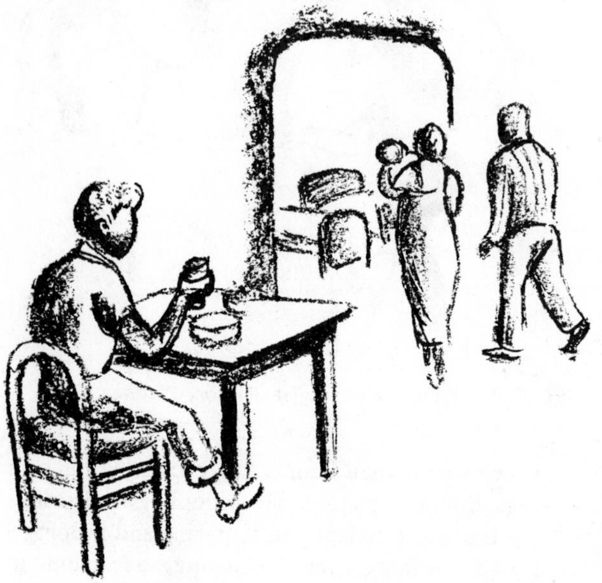

Fig. 35-6. Picture 17 of the Travis Story Pictures.

"The title of this story is 'A-a-a-anyone can be a S-S-S-Spirit' (holding doll figure of father in hand). Barry and Timothy's f-f-f-f-ather had h-h-heart trouble and he f-f-f-fell over on the ground (dropping father figure). (Holding two boy figures in one hand while flying the father through the air to the boys.) H-h-h-h-e appeared to the boys and s-s-s-said 'anyone can be a Spirit' (pause), and killed the boys (gently hit boys and they fell down). (Picking up all three figures in one hand and soaring through the air upwards.) They all went *up* (pause) and lived happily through their death."

Timmy felt that his only permanency was death. Happily he believed there was hope after death. The most certain way he knew that he could be assured of his father's companionship was through companionate death. He was even willing to share this beautiful spiritual relationship with his younger brother. He even used their actual names. His actions with the figures were gentle; the killing scene tenderly enacted. It is interesting to note that he chose to make the father bring death to the children. Timmy's vivid and stimulating experiences of a religious nature were evidenced in many of his productions.

Rennick (10 years) had problems of harsh voice quality, articulation, and stuttering. He was resentful of the divorce of his attractive and dynamic parents. His story of Fig. 35-5 was one of great courage, disaster, and futility.

"A child hit his m-m-mother with a j-j-jump rope and didn't have a chance to explain the accident . . . he was sent to b-b-bed . . . He ran away . . . became l-l-lost in a forest . . . attacked b-b-by a b-b-bear . . . escaped . . . attacked by another b-b-bear which bit off his f-f-finger . . . beated alone to Hawaii . . . wrecked . . . cast ashore . . . was s-s-swept away by a t-t-tidal wave . . . out to sea . . . eaten by a sh-sh-shark."

Eight-year-old Colin (voice case) was the first child the therapist noticed as she entered a school which had never had a speech therapy program before. His frail figure, pale face, and almost bald head caught her eye. His frenetic behavior and a voice ranging from a squeak to a screech marked him as a probable candidate for the fascinating relationship to follow. His selection of a specific chair as "his" exclusive property was a source of frequent upheaval in his classroom. He forbade others, including the custodian, to touch "his" chair, which was apparently identified with his fantasy friend, a prehistoric monster. It was called by name (Gregory), went everywhere with him, and most of the time was more real to him than anyone or anything else.

"Gregory is NOT IMAGINARY! ! ! ! My friends have even been scared by Gregory because Gregory yelled! !"

All of Colin's early verbalizations were about Gregory and Stormy, his real cat.

"He's a cat that talks. He can say all the words that I can say."

As therapy progressed he was gradually less threatened by reality. His voice, though sometimes strident when excited, developed a more mature quality and he made more friends. His former wispy tufts of hair were now lost in the crop covering his head, which made fair growth considering the years he had torturously pulled and twisted it from his scalp. The last recording made of him was an individual session in which he referred only to people. The one exception was in answer to a question about Gregory. His simple explanation was that he "didn't need that child stuff anymore."

In answer to a request for his age he chuckled and dramatically changed voices for each character in his story using Fig. 35-7.

"I'm thirteen. No, I'm twenty-five or I wish I were. I'm one. Now add a zero and that's my age, ten . . . well, he's just playing in a little dirt pile."

He then continued an elaborate story of a child whose mother shamed him about wearing shorts when his younger brother didn't. The next day he continued:

"Hey, I like these long pants and I hate those shorts and that's the end of the story. He liked the shorts because he felt so childish. He got into trouble at school . . . he has little boy feelings. His last birthday he left only four candles on his cake. He took seven off! . . . He's just the opposite of me. I don't like to be called a CHILD . . . ugh!! Last week on my spelling test after the word 'child' I wrote BAH! . . . He made F's in arithmetic and I make A's . . . Mother is shamed of the way he acts. She says 'listen here, you're a big boy and not a little imp!' . . . He thinks his mother expects too much of him because he thought he was only four . . . He wore the long pants at home, but he was bound and determined to wear shorts at school. He was twenty-five when he got out of grammar school and fifteen years of high school. He never did really grow up. His body grew up but his feelings didn't."

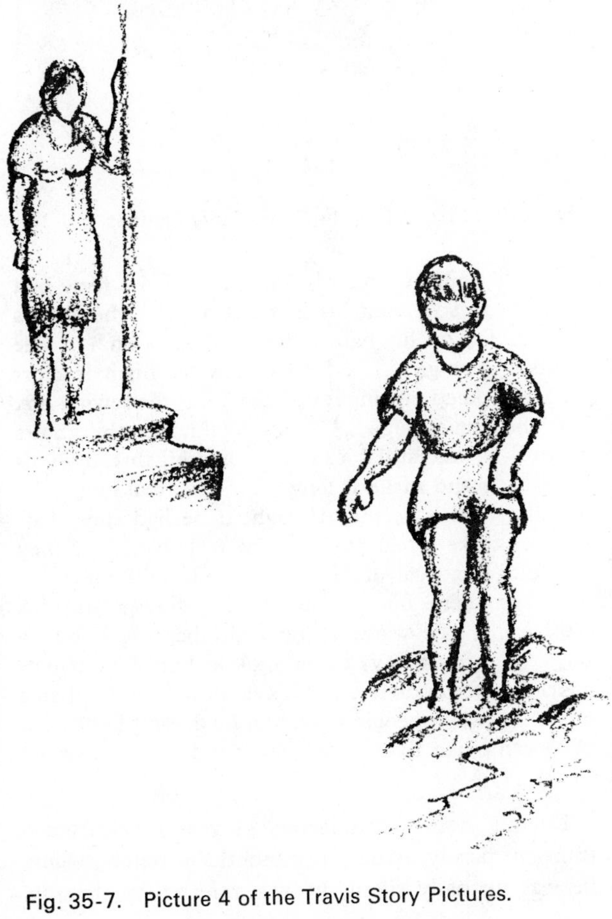

Fig. 35-7. Picture 4 of the Travis Story Pictures.

Colin's ambivalence about growing up was depicted in his story. But he is struggling to grow up, although he may think that his little-boy feelings will always be a part of him.

Manuel and Rudolfo were 10-year-old stutterers. Both were members of ever-increasing but fatherless families on welfare. With Fig. 35-6 they reacted as follows:

Manuel: "A m-m-m-mother went to the hospital and while she was u-u-u-unconscious gave b-b-b-birth to lots and lots of children. While she was st-st-still unconscious they t-t-t-took her home and put her in a chair. She 'came to' and saw a ch-ch-ch-child, then another . . . and many . . . until she saw h-h-h-hundreds and th-th-th-thousands. She didn't have a house and b-b-b-beds big enough . . . so she d-d-d-dug a h-h-h-hole in the ground for them. Then she used a derrick for f-f-f-feeding milk, putting p-p-p-pipes from it to the ground where the children were. On each p-p-p-pipe was a (pause) you know 'n-nipple.' When the b-b-b-babies were thirsty, they just went to the n-n-n-nipple and drank their milk without b-b-b-bothering their m-m-m-mother. Finally she ran out of milk, so she bought a farm. When the cows died she t-t-t-took the children to an orphanage (pause). When she got home, the b-b-b-b-babies were b-b-b-back in the h-h-h-hole in the ground."

Rudolfo: "Mmmmay I go on with your story?"

Manuel: "Sure."

Rudolfo: "The mooooother got a big house for them (pause), biiiiig enough for them."

Manuel: "The ch-ch-ch-children got too b-b-big for the house and then the m-m-m-mother took them to Alcatraz, but they couldn't take care of them there (pause), so they d-d-d-dumped them in the ocean. They made so m-m-m-many children in the ocean that the steam ships could not move through the waves (pause), so she p-p-pushed them all d-d-d-down to the b-b-bottom of the ocean where they p-p-p-poured cement on them to make them s-s-s-stay down."

Rudolfo: "Buuuuut the cement didn't cover all the sides and the chiiiiildren got out that way and got back to land safely."

Once again Rudolfo kept softening Manuel's expressions.

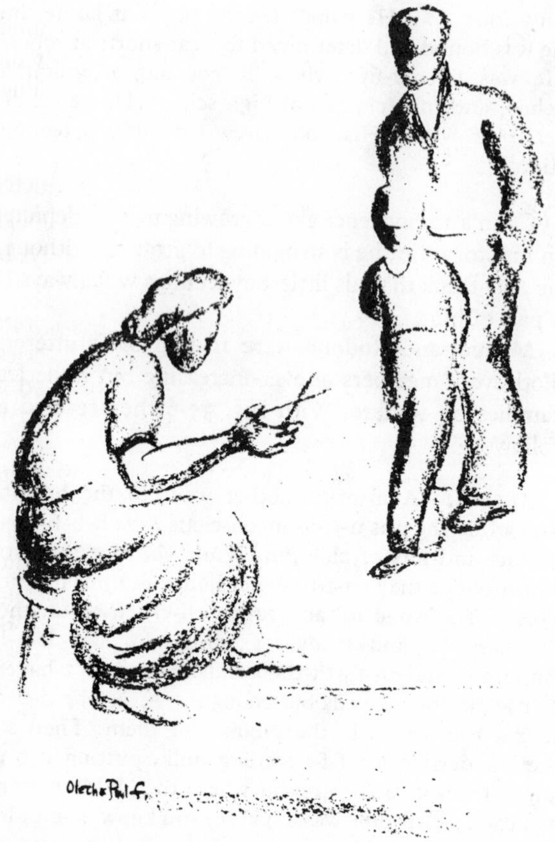

Fig. 35-8. Picture 27 of the Travis Story Pictures.

What is reported here may occur in a group. One child can speak more honestly or tolerate more anxiety than another child, so that the second child will have to "doctor" the story. Manuel's tale was too raw for Rudolfo. It produced too much anxiety in him. He handled his fears by softening the relationships between the people of the picture. One might speculate that Manuel was further along in his therapy than Rudolfo, or that he had more severe problems.

Kenton (noncommunicator, five years) was an emotional little boy who refused to talk at school. After a semester of therapy he asked to use two pictures, Figs. 35-8 and 35-9, to tell his story.

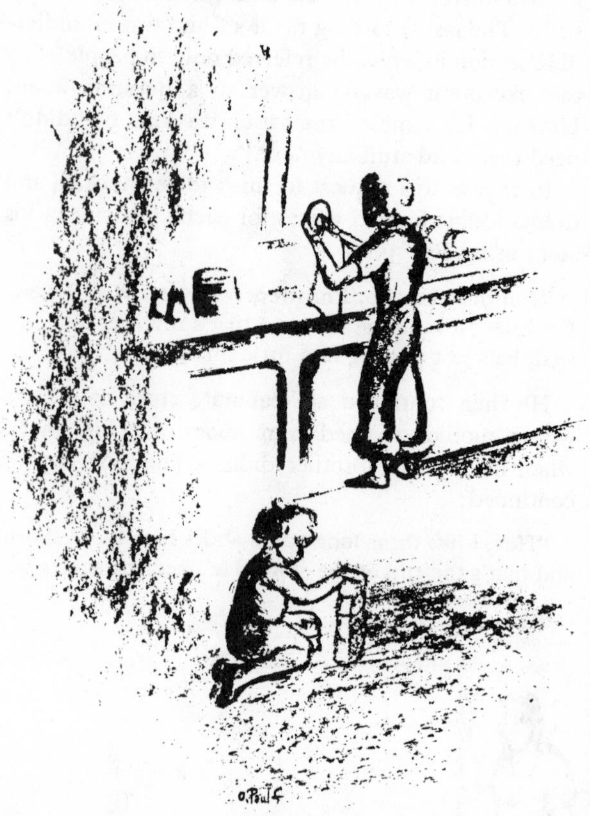

Fig. 35-9. Picture 5 of the Travis Story Pictures.

"She's going to cut his hair off . . . he feels bad . . . he doesn't want his hair cut off . . . he always sews thread on his hair and puts dresses on . . . he wants to be a girl . . . his father wants his hair short . . . they keep putting it up high . . . the sewing box and the chairs high . . . but he knocks the chairs down . . . and still does it . . . and his thread on his head . . . and make it long . . . real, real long . . . and they cut . . . they thought if he had short hair he'd look like a real boy . . . he feels bad . . . they won't let him wear dresses . . . but he still does . . . he takes them out of his sister's drawer and his mother . . . he wants to be a girl because if he's a boy . . . girls always throw junk at him . . . if he's a girl they won't do it . . . it's easier to be a girl than a boy . . . when people tease him he doesn't fight . . . he doesn't like to . . . he never did try . . . afraid to . . ."

Roland (noncommunicator, 11 years) was from a transient family. After a few months at school, where he was virtually silent, he was referred to therapy.

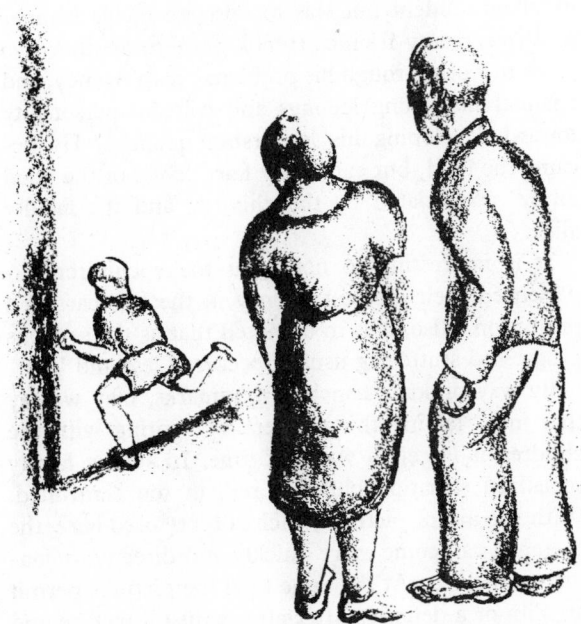

Fig. 35-10. Picture 10 of the Travis Story Pictures.

Several months later he responded to Fig. 35-10 in the following way:

"They want him to go and he doesn't want to go to the store . . . He spent some of the money on something he wanted . . . he doesn't think he has a fair allowance . . . He had slammed the door in place of something else I wanted to do. . . . Slamming helps get the angry out of you. . . . I wish I could go back in and argue with them some more. . . . Slamming the door let them know how mad they made you. . . . I'd like to have another chance to win. . . . I've felt the same way playing with another boy, a younger boy at his house . . . he accused me of cheating . . . when I left I wanted to go back and have another chance to win the argument . . . (sighing deeply) *Sometimes it's not so easy to be a child.*"

Roland's statement was made with insight rather than complaint. His rarely-used voice became more intelligible as he continued to share his history of feeling inadequate and ineffectual. In reaction to the picture in Fig. 35-11 he said:

"He sneaked out of apartment . . . Mother dragged him back. . . . He doesn't like to sleep as late as mother . . . feels embarrassed lots of times . . . I've felt embarrassed lots of times . . . like going to a new school . . . I changed pretty often . . . I'll feel bad I guess when I go to junior high in a few months . . . I like first grade . . . that was hard . . . I walked out and was going home when the principal came after me . . . I didn't even go into the room . . . just stood there . . . can't remember if I ever went to kindergarten. . . . Father had taken me to school . . . we shared the playground with sixth graders . . . felt I couldn't get out of their way . . . they bossed little kids . . ."

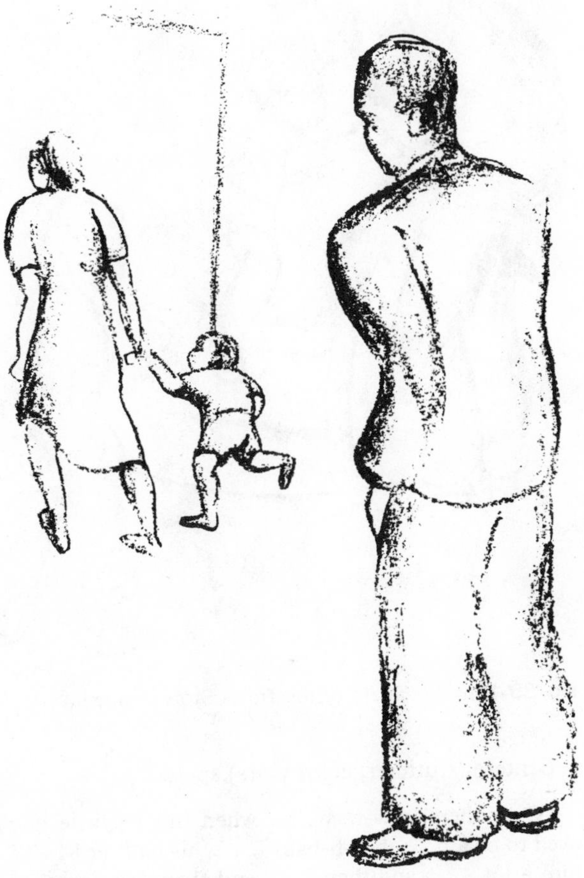

Fig. 35-11. Picture 7 of the Travis Story Pictures.

Two boys, Stanley and Santero, gave their stories to a picture depicting sibling rivalry (Fig. 35-12). Stanley expressed jealousy while Santero pictured rejection, hostility, aggression, antisocial behavior, and punishment to the boys and vengeance on their parents.

Stanley (stutterer, nine years) said:

"This little brother was a baby . . . f-f-feels comfortable. The bigger br-br-brother feels he was kin . . . kinda jealous because she gave all the l-l-loving to the little b-b-b-baby . . . soooo . . . he's jealous (much clearing of throat) . . . the m-m-m-mother gives the baby m-m-m-more attention . . . and if they h-h-h-have another baby and if . . . and if they don't give *him* the attention that's wh-wh-what jealousy is . . . he wishes m-m-mother would give him the attention *and* the ba-ba-baby . . . *both*."

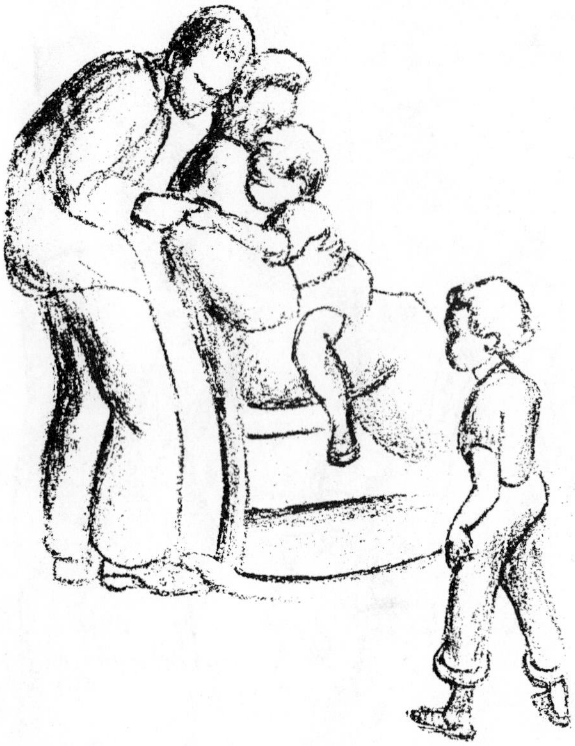

Fig. 35-12. Picture 11 of the Travis Story Pictures.

Santero (stutterer, eight years) spoke up:

"Over there w-w-was . . . when this l-l-little boy used to be a . . . b-b-b-baby . . . his mother l-l-like him a lot . . . and then . . . and then . . . another b-b-baby came into the world . . . and then the mother didn' like her big boy any more . . . baby grew up . . . and he . . . and he was s-s-six and the b-b-boy who wasn' liked by mother ran away . . . then he joined this p-p-place . . .a . . . a . . . club . . . then he grew up. He was fourteen . . . he was a-a-a-gangster . . . he . . . he . . . he didn't do a rob right . . . and when he . . . when he didn't do it right . . . they tied him to the railroad tracks . . . the club members . . . and the train came and-and-and ran right over him . . . and . . . and flattened him . . . and the mother and father came to his funeral . . . and that's all . . ."

Stanley's speech was soon fluent and he became an excellent student but was too precise in his manner to attract many friends. It took Santero another two years to work through his problems, gain fluency, and channel his strong feelings and colorful personality toward developing his leadership qualities. He became the loud, but extremely fair, "chief of the good guys," appreciated by the children and the faculty alike.

It is interesting to note that many children experienced their greatest fluency in the last part of a projection. Also, it is to be noted that as the sessions progressed stuttering usually occurred less and less.

By way of some concluding remarks, may we say that just "talking things over" or visiting with the children is largely a waste of time. In such a highly socialized situation children remain too controlled. With the aid of pictures, such as those used here, the therapist can come more quickly and directly to conflictual feelings. At the same time the pictures permit an alibi or a defense. After all it is just a picture and just a story.

Through and around the defense, however, true feelings and thoughts get out and are recognized and generally accepted and managed.

Possibly the therapist could use just one picture per session. She can assure the children that each one will have a chance to tell his story or to add to another's story. Children may benefit not only from their own stories but from listening to the stories of others as well. The therapist should be alert and sensitive to the expressions of feared and antisocial feelings and attitudes in order that she may encourage their revelation. She must take care not to react to the child's fear and anxiety by expressing criticism or condemnation. Such expression has been the response the child both feared and expected. It has no place in the therapy situation, a new growing-up relationship.

Purposeful Fantasy

To speak fantasies aloud in group therapy may be achieved by asking the children to play an imaginary or make-believe game. The therapist may cue the children: "If I were someone else, I'd be . . .," or "if I could not be I, but were an animal, I'd be . . .," or "when I grow up, I'd like to . . ." Or she may have them dictate a dream that they have actually had. As children tell their fantasies or their dreams they sometimes decode their symbolic messages into terms of present reality.

George (articulation, eight years), said:

"I'd choose to be a lion. I wish I had my home back . . . my dog back . . . my brother's broken arm to get well."

Betsy (noncommunication and articulation, nine years) said:

"I'd choose to be a bird. I wish a genie was my mother . . . that I had my own pet, and I had no sisters."

Her divorced mother was quite ineffectual. Her maternal grandmother, with whom the family lived, was extremely aggressive. Betsy did not wish her mother to become a genie, but rather that a genie should be her mother. She resented having no privacy. She anticipated success in relating to a pet while shrinking from her formidable sisters and grandmother. She frequently identified with a pet from the time the therapist brought her own to the therapy session.

Therapist: "At times we have talked about when you were little. About experiences you have had. About your feelings and how they sometimes change. You are all growing taller, larger, and having birthdays. So we know you are growing up and up and that someday you will be a Grown Up. I want you to think about it and then tell us what you would like to be when you grow up. Winona, when you grow up . . . ?"

Winona (stutterer, 11 years) ". . . when I grow up I-I-I-want to b-b-be a stewardess on a . . . on a . . . plane. I heard when a p-p-p-plane crashes and you're on it, they give you a nice funeral. The f-f-funeral lasts a long time before it ends (slapping her legs repeatedly). The r-r-reason I want to be a s-s-stewardess on a plane . . . I never been on a plane before . . . I th-th-think it's going to be lots of fun."

Toby (delayed speech, stuttering, mental retardation, eight years): "Not . . . me . . . I not . . . grow up. My dad . . . won't let . . . me. Me-not-be-man. Me be . . . b-b-boy. My dad won't let me . . . be . . . m-m-man. My dad s-s-say I be . . . fireman . . . play like fireman . . . n-n-not real fireman . . . my d-d-dad don't let me . . . my dad give me . . . money . . . I not get m-m-married . . . stay home . . . I w-w-want . . . some children . . . one boy . . . one girl."

Pietro and Gordon wanted to be world-renowned scientists. Both were normally intelligent but educationally retarded. Each was receiving speech therapy and remedial reading help for the first time. It is interesting to note how each incorporated his learning problem, and even its removal, into his projections. Pietro was eight years old when he first came to therapy with unintelligible speech. One year later he said:

"I want to be a scientist . . . find out what happens . . . discover the world . . . I would tell everybody . . . and they would like to know about everything . . . and I'd tell them . . . then they would . . . everybody . . . come to me when they want to be a scientist . . . so they would have a head-start . . . I wouldn't let them just sit there. If some of them . . . are poor at learning . . . I would help them . . . help them catch up with the rest . . . then they would like to come where I was . . . everybody who wanted to be a scientist . . ."

Gordon (stutterer, 10 years) named 24 different professions that he wanted to pursue when he grew up. They included numerous scientific fields and the writing and publishing of scientific books and "books for children, easy enough for them to understand." He also wanted to be a "rocket explorer about this galaxy, and the other planets."

"I'd put the new planet animals in a zoo . . . and people . . . if they'd come . . . and they'd be treated careful . . . and nice . . . the surface samples I'd put in a big building and give them and the new planets names . . . and I . . . I wouldn't have time to get m-m-married . . . I have a br-br-brother . . . he can have sons . . . and . . . and pass on the f-f-family name . . . on from one . . . generation to another generation . . . I'd have a special f-f-fuel so my rocket ship would never . . . would never go out of fuel . . . it would go in water . . . in land . . in space . . . I'd make f-f-friends of all p-p-people on all the . . . all the planets. I'd be famous from generation to generation . . . and I'd never die . . . I'd take food and b-b-books to other p-p-planets . . . pub-pub-published in their language. I'd never die . . . I'd never die . . I'd never die!!" (gesturing expansively).

Marna (stutterer, 10 years): "I w-w-want to be a . . . get married . . . but I don't want any children . . . not unless I adopt ten. No! Not have them myself! (holding stomach) . . . I want to . . . to . . . to be a pastor's wife . . . and be a Sunday School teacher . . . on Sunday. . . . On weekdays . . . I'd . . . I'd . . . like to be an artist . . . with my own room with supplies . . . or maybe a h-h-half time nurse at a c-c-convalescent home . . . I want to h-h-have beautiful paintings . . . I'd need to-to-to work some, because p-p-pastors don't make that much . . . and I'd have ten children to-to-to support."

Betsy (noncommunication, nine years): "I'm going to be a speech teacher . . . get a tape recorder . . . get a pet . . . take the pet to the Speech room . . . so the children can see it . . . buy a car . . . get married . . . and have happy children . . . a boy and two girls."

One child, Kitti (stuttering, delayed speech, five years) was troubled by her father's aggression and her parents' divorce. She responded to a dream.

"O . . . nce dere be a little g . . . host and h . . . im turn my light off and him . . . him . . . him . . . h . . . im put me in bed and den a b . . . ig black g . . . host . . . . him . . . him . . . h . . . im took me and t . . . ook me way from my mom . . . mom . . . mom . . . mommie . . . h . . . im took mom . . . mom . . . mommmmmie too . . . h . . . im b . . . roke my window and h . . . im to-to-to-toook my toys away . . . D . . . en de g . . . host get me in h . . . im house and p . . . put me in bed. . . . Me . . . e got up and called mom-mom-mommie a . . . nd d . . . addy and say. . . . 'A g . . . host open my window and turn off my light.' . . . My mom-mom-mommie and d . . . addy be in de g . . . host house too. . . . Me saw a m . . . onster and me say 'Take dat cover off your face, Mommy! . . . de g . . . host be re . . . really my mom-mom-mommie and de m . . . onster be really my d . . . addy. . . . No! D . . . addy be de g . . . host and mom-mom-mommie be de m . . . monster . . . when de g . . . host break my window and jump in . . . me call 'Mommie, Mommie, Mommie, Daddy, Daddy help me, help me, help me.' When me saw mommie in de castle . . . me say 'Mommie . . . Mommie me glad to see you home!'"

An abnormally small boy, Winston (six years), who felt crippled by his stuttering blocks, harsh voice quality, and general unintelligibility, reported the following dream:

"I don' 'member all the . . . dream . . . but it wath true too . . . an happen juth lath Thurthday. We dot two baby ratth . . . one ob dem . . . bit de oder oneth . . . tail . . . I took one ob dem out to play wif an-an- he tried to . . . bite my . . . noth . . . dat all I 'member of it . . . I dreamed de dream 'fore we dot d . . . reth . . . but I had theen dem at my friend houth an' I . . . want thome . . . but my . . . dad firth had to make a cadth . . . I wathn't for thure I'd . . . det dem . . . .Dey thure had loth of . . . babieth. . . . Thomething woth wrong wif one ob dem. . . . It had two feet in de back and . . . only . . . one in de front. . . . I di not wanth . . . dat one. It woth white, ith tail pink and ith eyeth de darketh wed. . . . In my dream, it woth . . . one ob de . . . two rath I had . . . It woth de one . . . dat tried to . . . bite my noth . . . It ith the one . . . dat bit de odder rat'th tail . . . in my dream . . . an' lef' only . . . de bone an' loth an' loth of blood."

Sherry (noncommunication, five years) said: "I' wa' a dood d'eam. Mommie work. Me p'ay. Te 'top wok a' p'ay wi' me. Te p'ay howth. Te wa' Mommy . . . a' me wa' debi' ti-ah. Te di wha I wan' te do. Te p'ay a' wuv me, bof("

George (articulation, eight years) spoke as follows: "One time I was in the back yard in my dream and I looked up up in the sky and I saw a man on a bike and he was flying in the air. What made the bike fly in the air was soft dirt and a formula. I said to him that if you will give me some of the formula for my bike . . . and then he told me where he lived. He lived in the clouds and I flew up there on my bike. Then I heard that he died and there was not any formula left. In the bike there was no way to get down and his wife told me where I could get some of the formula. It was across to the next cloud, and I had only a little fuel left so I said that I will try to reach the other cloud. I just barely made it and I got home safe and the next day I told everyone in school about it and I tried to make them believe me but they did not believe me so I put some in each room (formula) and I said the magic words and the school flew in the air and the school crashed and that was the end. They all died and I did too."

This dream occurred after George had moved from his former home due to the divorce of his parents. He had suffered greatly from this separation from his father, home, pets, and friends. He often complained of the little yard he had now compared to the great yard and fields surrounding his former home. He also could have no pets in the apartment.

Fumi (noncommunication, 11 years) revealed her Japanese heritage in her dream as follows:

"I had a dream and it was a beautiful, also strange garden. There were lots of beautiful trees and flowers growing. I enjoyed it very much. I found a cherry tree (pause) and I was just about to eat them (pause) that it looked so good (pause) and I saw a big shadow. I was too afraid to look who it was, but I looked and it was a witch (pause) and I was very scared (pause) and I tried to run (pause) but I couldn't (pause) and that witch caught me (pause) and took me to a small cabin (pause) and I woke up. I felt very safe in my bed. The end."

Rick (stutterer, 10 years) whose speech was hardly audible when he entered therapy, dreamed that:

"O-o-o-one time I dreamed there was a b-b-b-big beautiful cake and j-j-j-just as I was about to t-t-t-take a b-b-b-bite I woke up. I always dream things like that (disappointed tone). I also always dream that I'm t-t-talking real l-l-l-loud and making l-l-l-lots of n-n-n-noise and my d-d-d-dad is always y-y-y-yelling at me to be q . . ." (he wanted to say quiet).

Dramatization

STAGE AND PUPPETS

A small portable puppet stage is available to the speech therapist (Figs. 35-13 and 35-14.) With it come scenery and miniature puppets which are extremely simple to manipulate because they require no strings. Each puppet is mounted on a spring-covered spindle. The floor of the stage has horizontal and vertical slots through which the tiny spindle slides as it is moved by a hand under the stage floor. As many as four puppets may be handled simultaneously when the spindles are held between the fingers of one hand.

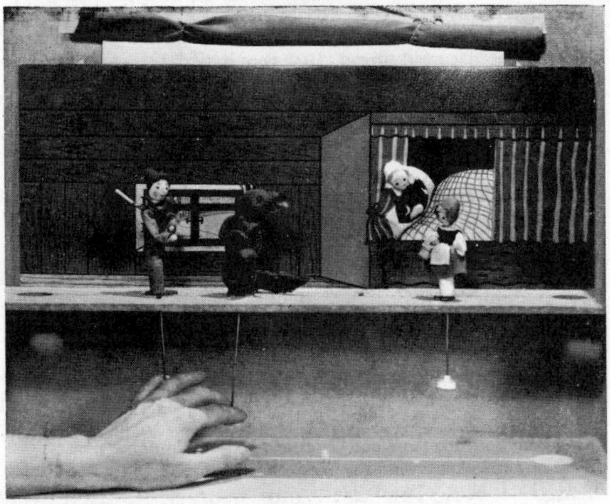

Fig. 35-13. A small, portable puppet stage with scenery and miniature puppets showing how the puppets may be manipulated by the spindles extending through the stage floor. *"Baps" die neuen Nürnberger Puppenspiele, Nürenberg, Germany.*

In this fashion the puppets are moved about on the stage, jiggled up and down when talking, and turned this way and that. Simplicity of maneuverability is important in puppetry, so that interest and activity may be focused in the expression of feelings through characterization. To that end the therapist may have a larger stage constructed of lightweight plywood in which the slots are arranged to provide triple the amount of puppet-slide space. While it has no curtain or superstructure, it affords ample opportunity for two children to work in a joint dramatization. This stage has a metal ring attached to each slide on which a sturdy strap hooks, converting the stage into a carryall for the therapist's supplies. Less elaborate but effective puppets may be fashioned by attaching metal washer weights on the end of a metal spindle stuck into each of an assortment of small plastic (toy) figures.

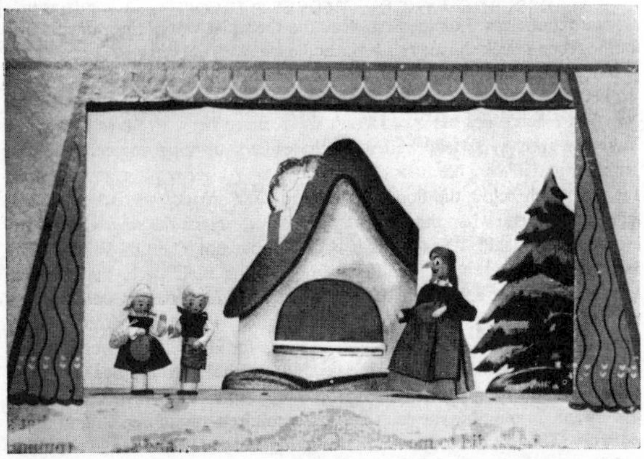

Fig. 35-14. Characters and scenery for "Hansel and Gretel."

The puppets may be introduced to the group as a "show." The therapist works the puppets while the children verbalize the activity. The children's interest is immediate and strong. "How does it work?" "Bet we could do it," and so on. After some experimenting on their parts, the children are promised the return of the stage and characters for the next session. The second session begins immediately with the children choosing parts. Often a child will take several parts. Rarely does a boy reject a girl's role when there are no girls in the group. Later it may prove more satisfactory for one child to take one scene or act, and play all the parts. This plan not only eliminates confusion in back of the stage, but it leaves someone besides the therapist in the audience. Then too, children are better able to express more feeling in their characterizations.

Three sets of storybook puppets have been found useful. In the "Three Little Kittens Who Lost Their Mittens," the "naughty" kittens progressively lost, found, soiled, and then washed their mittens. The role-reversal technique is particularly effective in this medium. The favorite character with the children is the vacillating Mother Cat who alternately scolds, rewards, chastises, and kisses the kittens.

In producing "Little Red Riding Hood" the children vie for the parts of the Big Bad Wolf and the Wood Chopper who slew him. Thus they express feelings of aggression toward the Wolf and the love of Little Red Riding Hood toward her father, the Wood Chopper.

"Hansel and Gretel" proves a favorite. The horrible Old Witch of the Gingerbread House is used so vigorously that it is necessary for her crooked nose to be replaced frequently. The stage and one set of puppets may provide two successive weeks of activity in order to give the children ample time to express themselves.

The first time the puppets are introduced to the children the therapist demonstrates them, setting the limits on their use and on time. "Anything you want your puppets to say or do is all right as long as you keep them on or inside the stage and handle them by their sticks. I'll give you a signal one minute before your time is used up." When the puppets are then provided only a brief reinforcement of the standards is needed. Very soon the children move away from a formal folk story to pure, spontaneous creativity. Indeed the activity is now introduced on this basis alone. From a changing variety of about 10 puppets each child selects four or five to use when it is his turn. If two children work together each is limited to three and he plays all those parts.

Mary (noncommunicator, six years), who had finally been able to speak of her mistreatment by her mother, was made extremely anxious by the appearance of the Witch puppet.

"Oh I don't like her . . . I don't want to see her . . . Take her away . . . she's mean . . ."

She was screaming, squirming uncomfortably in her chair and holding her hands in front of her eyes. At her request the therapist put the Witch below the floor of the stage. Her anxiety was accepted. When the promise was made to return the stage the following week she said, "yes . . . bring it back . . . but not the Old Witch."

The following week when the children were dividing their parts by complete acts, Mary lost her reluctance to see the Witch. In fact, she insisted on playing the final act where the Witch tries to bake Hansel and Gretel. She worked the puppets enthusiastically and spoke for both Hansel and Gretel.

"Push . . . and push . . . and push . . . the mean Old Witch into the oven . . . and bake her into a gingerbread cookie. So there! And I'm glad . . . cause she was mean . . . and now she can't hurt little children anymore . . . and that's what my mommie did to me . . . and she burned me . . . and see . . . (pulling her socks down to show her scarred feet) . . . that's what she did . . . and it hurt . . . and hurt . . . bad . . . and I cried . . . and cried . . . and then the hospital . . . and now she can't hurt me any more and . . . (sigh) . . ."

DOLLS, FURNITURE, AND MINIATURE ANIMALS

Family relationships in the dining room (eating problems), in the nursery (problem of the new baby), in the bedroom (sleeping and dressing problems), in the bathroom (cleanliness and toilet training problems), and in the living room (parent-child and sibling rivalry) can be dramatized with these objects. A child may live through or live out or even correct his perception of members of his family and their interrelationships, and his role in the family grouping. Dinner time, bath time, nighttime, weekends, can all be portrayed and acted out, frequently with the discovery, acceptance, and channeling of troublesome and handicapping feelings. Some children may find it easier to begin with the animals. It is usually more acceptable to give an animal animalistic feelings than it is to give a human being, even an inanimate representation of him, such feelings. Later a child may be able to be more honest and use the dolls. Through a representation of himself (doll or animal) the child may be able to reevaluate and reintegrate his cathartic preoccupations.

Judy (stutterer, six years), choosing the little calf and moving it about, said:

"The li-li-little calf wa-wa-wa-was hungry for h-h-her dinner and sh-sh-sh-she went to the Muh-Muh-Muh-Mo . . . ther Horse. 'Wi-wi-wi-wiiiill you give m-m-m-m-me m-m-m-my dinner'? 'I'm not your Mmmmmmother!' (indignantly). Then sh-sh-sh-sh-she went to the Muh-muh-muh-mother sheep. 'Wi-wi-wi-wiiill you please give m-m-m-m-me m-m-m-my dinner?' 'No, I'm not your m-m-m-mother. Why don't you go where you belong? I'm not your m-m-m-mother. Why doesn't your own m-m-m-mother take care of her child?' Then the calf went to the Muh-muh-muh-mo . . . ther Hen. 'Wi-wi-wi-wiiill you give m-m-m-m-me m-m-m-my dinner please? I-I-I-I'm hungry and n-n-n-no one will help m-m-m-me.' No, I'm not your m-m-mother. I have many baby chicks to care for as you can see. What kind of a m-m-m-mother do you have anyhow, to let her ba-ba-baby go hungry? I take care of my ba-ba-ba-babies as I should. Besides yo-yo-yo-you couldn't eat the food I scratched up for my ba-ba-babies. You should find your m-m-mother soon.' (Judy went to the Mother Cat, Dog, etc.) Then the Li-Li-Li-Little Calf went to the Muh-Muh-Muh-Mother Cow (which had a conspicuously full udder and distended teats). 'Wi-wi-wi-will you give m-m-me m-m-m-my dinner?' 'Yes mmy Bbbbaby, I will give you your dinner. I have lots of warm milk for yyou. Come close to Mmmmother and drink all you wwwant because it's all for you!' And the little calf drank. When sh-sh-she was full she lay down right next to her Mmother. I've got to lay the Mmmother down too. So they can be close together . . . and went to sleep."

The other children of the group who had listened and looked attentively during Judy's performance sat back in their chairs and sighed deeply at the ending. Some held their stomachs contentedly. The action, the story, the choice of central character, all reveal the child's problems and the attempted management of them. It has been noted, for example, that an obese child will usually place a pig in the leading role. Might it not be equally revealing if a child chose a horse, or dog, or cat, or hen or rooster? Does this central figure then want love and warmth, or food and succor, or status and power, or death and destruction? Everything the child says and does in these little lands of make believe is useful to him and his insightful helper.

Is is not significant that Judy's repetitions and prolongations of sounds occurred in words referring to herself and her mother as well as when making a polite request for fulfillment of basic need? Also, as Judy's story progressed her stuttering became less pronounced. This is a feature frequently noted in children's projections.

Spontaneous Word Games

RHYTHMICAL HAND CLAPPING

The children, including the therapist, sit in a circle. A four beat rhythm is established, using open hands. For each of the first three beats, everyone pats his hands on his knees. On the fourth beat he brings his hands together in a soft clap:

1	2	3	4
knees	knees	knees	clap together

The children soon learn that the activity is a quiet one so that the verbalizations may be heard. The therapist begins a four-word sentence with the rhythm. As each child has his turn he supplies the fourth word, preferably one not previously used. This game goes somewhat rapidly when the beat is kept constant. Hence, the word supplied by the child is fairly spontaneous. Of course a child will sometimes "block" or "draw a blank," When this occurs, the rhythm is continued until the child can supply the last word. Reinforcement is supplied by the group repeating immediately in unison the statement completed by each child. The statement, "The body can ———," holds great opportunity for the exploration and expression of the child's feelings. The whole group (led by the therapist) begins the hand-clapping rhythm in silence. The word "body" having two syllables, is allowed two beats, thereby producing a five-beat rhythm in this instance.

knees	knees	knees	knees	clap

When the rhythm is well established, the therapist says, "The body can see," speaking the words in time with the five beats of the clapping:

Group:	knees	knees	knees	knees	clap
Therapist: (clapping)	The	bo	dy	can	see
Group: (clapping)	The	bo	dy	can	see
John: (clapping with group)	The	bo	dy	can	walk
Group: (clapping)	The	bo	dy	can	walk
Jane: (clapping with group)	The	bo	dy	can	eat
Group: (clapping)	The	bo	dy	can	eat

And so on around the group.

The game may begin with such seemingly disarming last words as *look, run, drink,* and so on. However, by the therapist's adventuring forth in taking her turn as a member of the group, the children are encouraged to advance to more threatening words: The body can feel, hear, smell, speak, hurt, ache, cry, fear, laugh, touch, love, hate, fall, squeeze, sleep, bite, kick, hit, dream, taste, chew, swallow, fight, live, hope.

BALL-TOSS AND WORD-TOSS

With the children seated in a semicircle and the therapist in front, she "tosses a word" with the toss of a ball. The child immediately tosses the ball back to her, simultaneously saying the first word that comes to his mind. Any word is acceptable to the therapist, thereby encouraging its acceptance by the speaker and the group. The therapist chooses words with an ever-increasing threat in meaning: *house, drink, sit, eat, spank, gun, kill.* She can select a string of words that explore one area at a time (sibling rivalry, hostility, messing, sex, and so forth) or she can use words that cover all areas in one setting. Group members should sit fairly close together and be instructed to toss with an underhanded motion to the lap. A soft, sponge-rubber ball is preferable to an inflated or hard ball, since it has little bounce and roll should it be missed by one of the group. Skill in catching or throwing is not the issue. The activity serves merely as an adjunct to free expression. It is best to advance around the group at the start. When the children become more accustomed to the mechanics and the spirit of the sessions, the therapist can toss the ball to the children at random.

One round of word-and-ball tossing went as follows:

Therapist:	House	*Therapist:*	Eat
Tom:	Live	*Mary:*	Don't
Therapist	Drink	*Therapist:*	Run
Sue:	Milk	*John:*	Away
Therapist:	Sit		
Joe:	Still		

In one session the therapist noted that Gloria, an eight-year-old girl, was muttering words to herself when it was the therapist's turn to supply the word. Taking her cue, the therapist asked the child if she would like to "start it." With eager acceptance she told the therapist: "Now you say what I say." She was asking for reinforcement and approval by requesting repetition of the words she would choose. Gloria kept a fast pace of simultaneous ball-and-word tossing while the therapist echoed the word as she returned the toss. Here is the parade of Gloria's words which may be telling a significant story: "Little . . . Sister Mean . . . Big . . . Sister . . . Hit . . . Mother . . . Mad . . . Daddy . . . Whip . . . Bed . . . Cry . . . Crib . . . Hate . . . Glad . . . Hit . . . Mad . . . Sad . . . Glad Mad . . . Sad . . . Glad . . . Mad . . . Sad . . ."

Variations in the word-ball-tossing sessions may be introduced. One is to toss the ball and a word to the first child. The child is instructed to toss the ball and the same word back. To the same child the therapist will then toss the ball and the first word's opposite, and the child will toss them back. A different word and its opposite are tossed to the second child and so on. After a bit of this play the children usually want to do their own choosing of words and their opposites. Such freedom and courage are heartily supported. The therapist can again progress to more vulnerable areas by her choice of words. Our progression may be: eat-drink; big-little; happy-sad; glad-mad; love-hate; save-kill. Another one could be: smooth-rough; soft-hard; warm-cold; pretty-ugly; dry-wet; clean-messy.

ORIGINAL DRAWINGS

Family

Early in the school year when the children are being initiated into learning to talk about themselves they talk about people, those that they know best—their families. Then very soon their therapist provides each child with a sheet of plain paper and a box of primary size crayons. "Draw your family—all of your family." As they proceed the therapist will frequently speak with each child about the people he is drawing, marking each with a number to indicate the order in which they were drawn. An initial system may also be used to identify each figure (F.—father, Y.B.—young brother, etc.) and any comments are noted. The drawings are significant in relation to size, placement, posture, and color of figures. The verbalization which takes place is as revealing as the illustrations. *The children literally "talk their way" through their drawings.* This procedure tends to get the children involved in communicating about their relationship with this basic unit of people with whom they must strive daily to develop their selfhood.

Trent (stutterer, five years) drew a complex figure of a house with a lone figure standing inside.

"I-I-I-don't want to m-m-make any more of m-m-my family. M-m-my br-br-brother is real b-b-big. M-m-my sister is b-b-big and m-m-m-mother. They're all b-b-big and I-I-I don't w-w-want to m-m-ake them. It's raining. The rain is c-c-coming through a h-h-hole in the h-h-house. It goes up a p-p-pipe and c-c-omes out in the h-h-house. Comes out on the f-f-father . . . and h-h-he gets c-c-cold."

Martha (stutterer, 10 years) first drew her house, then a yard with flowers, and then her father and mother.

"D-d-do I h-h-have to make the r-r-rest?"
Therapist: "There are others in your family and now you wonder if you have to make them?"

Martha sat thoughtfully for a while and then reluctantly finished.

Therapist: "Is this your whole family?"
Martha: "Yes . . . all b-b-but m-m-me . . . I don't w-w-want to m-m-make m-m-me . . . Well, I'll m-m-make m-m-me . . . but w-w-way . . . away here. (turning to the therapist with her drawing) I-I-I-put s-s-some grass under m-m-me so I won't f-f-fall."

Martha's feelings of estrangement, difference, and rejection, and of a responsibility over being the eldest child to three younger brothers were depicted in her drawing of the family. A new and confused pride in early pubic development also appeared in the drawing. She pictured herself, in profile, alone, apart, and walking away from the house and its members. Yet at the same time she gave herself the security of a family foundation in her separateness. In such manner she risked a daring ambivalence to find herself.

Bright, eight-year-old Hun Fook had never vocalized a sound at school. His father reported that he rarely spoke at home. On those occasions he made minimal use of Chinese and English and stuttered severely. He was the eldest child and his parents practised the old-world tradition of his acceptance of heavy familial responsibilities. In the course of four months he persistently maintained his silence in spite of all efforts of the therapist and his peers. This attitude even persisted when the children used the tape recorder. When the children left Hun Fook alone with his therapist he finally made his first sound, a minute whistle. After this experience he would giggle a great deal or whistle softly while drawing, modeling, or carrying on other activities. This was all preceded by a rituallike behavior of repeatedly blowing on his hands with pursed lips, and then rubbing them together, grinning widely, and feigning a look of devilish mystery.

In February he drew a family picture. He made the house and the outdoor buildings and plantings first. Then he drew two younger brothers outside together. Next he put himself inside with his mother, who was across the room holding the baby brother with prominent arms. Last, and with some reluctance, he placed his father looking out a big window. In March he repeated the same picture when messing with finger paints, and again in April with clay. The classroom teacher and the school psychologist reported that he produced identical pictures for them.

When the therapist saw him for the last time in June, the children were given a choice of several activities. Hun Fook selected paper and crayons. He began to whistle as he drew his father as a strong figure in the center of the page. Lower on the page he put his fat baby brother with his big arms out, one toward trembling Hun Fook, the other toward the young brother, who was also trembling while urinating and defecating. At last he drew Mother next to Father. Then he wrote the names for each member of the family except for Mother. The shaky lines used to indicate Hun Fook and his brother showed that they were afraid . . . afraid the baby would hit them.

His mother spoke no English and was too embarassed to come to school. His father spoke only minimal English but closed his little business to meet the therapist's request for a conference before his "Number One Son" was enrolled. He came again five months later after Hun Fook's last session. He was extremely concerned as he listened to the vain attempts of the therapist who was trying to tell him that it had been impossible to elicit any verbalization from Hun Fook even though he seemed ready to talk. He then disclosed that he had been looking forward to this encounter because of the remarkable change in his son. Hun Fook was happier, had developed better relationships with members of the family, was accepting responsibility with more courage, and was, above all, talking fluently. He was interpreting conversations between his mother who spoke only Chinese, and her neighbour, who had recently arrived from Mexico and knew little English. The prime disclosure made by the father was that his son was no longer stuttering in any language! Follow-up within the next school year revealed that Hun Fook was considered to have gained fluent speech.

Self-Image

In "telling himself" to his therapist, the child, as well as the therapist, is gaining insight into his self-image.

Therapist (Handing out material which the children take and proceed to use, talking all the time):

"Here is one paper for each of you and a pencil. There are no erasers because you are going to draw yourself. Just yourself. And any way you draw yourself is all right. So we won't need any erasers."

Despite their youth and inexperience they drew pictures that showed remarkable likeness to their own personal characteristics. Frequently seen were straight and tight or sad and tense lips and self-conscious smiles. Noted also were worried, frowning, or puzzled eyes, and a weary and downcast posture. Often a figure of meager size appeared on the large sheet.

Marna (stutterer, noncommunicator, 10 years) (Fig. 35-15) pictured herself stiffly. She put a mark on each side of her lips and "sewed" them tightly together. Then she drew deep, dark circles weighting her eyes. It was an excellent self-portrait.

Todd (stutterer, seven years) (Fig. 35-16) drew himself without arms or feet. There was a prominent

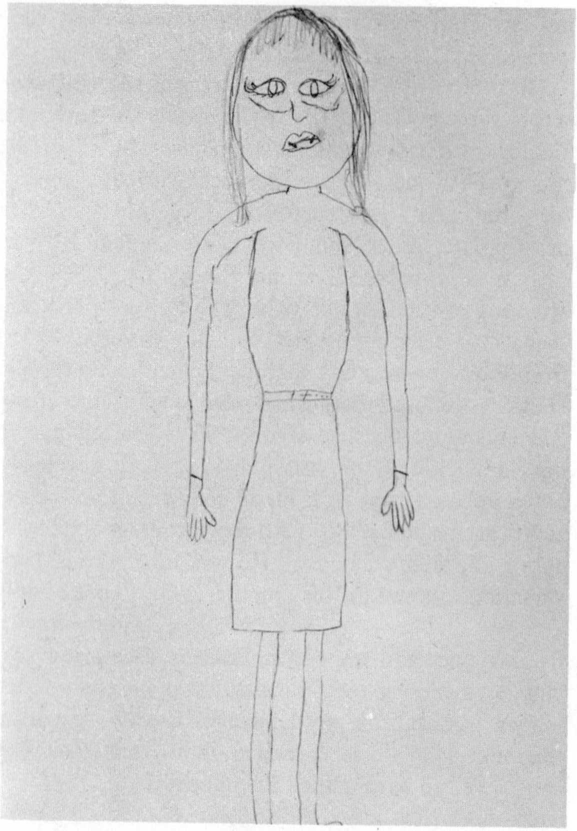

Fig. 35-15. Marna's self-portrait.

viscera. He was wearing a crushed hat, a twisted smile, and one of his eyes peeked out from beneath a black patch. Pale, frail, and inffectual, he actually had one eye patched from corrective surgery. His stuttering and his high-pitched, squeaky voice came from his mouth which always had a crooked, embarrassed smile.

Later, as some of the children finished, all were given a second sheet of paper.

Therapist: "When you're finished use this second paper to draw how you feel when you are talking. Then I'll write on the back anything you want to say about it."

Chang (stutterer, noncommunicator, 10 years) drew an attractive self-portrait. He worked as an artist might, taking care to develop proper proportions in his sketch and using two thirds of the paper, seven and one half inches. When depicting his speaking, however, his small stick figures measured one quarter inch and the ball was almost as large.

Chang: "I-I-I-broke the w-w-window. My m-m-mother was t-t-talking to me. Sh-sh-she asked me 'w-w-why?' I-I-I-told her b-b-ut had t-t-trouble t-t-telling her. I-I-I-felt l-l-like everyone w-w-was against me. I-I-I-felt v-v-very l-l-little."

Todd (Fig. 35-17) drew a circle. In the center of it he placed a heart, a darkly submerging part of it. The upper half of the circle was heavily marked with scratches.

"This is m-m-my f-f-food. This is m-m-my heart and up h-h-here this is all m-m-my stutter, stutter, stutter." (His drawing of the upper portion was accompanied by his repeating "stutter, stutter, stutter.")

Marna (Fig. 35-18) created a grotesque female figure in great detail.

"Well . . . w-w-when I'm talking . . . especially in f-f-front of t-t-the class . . . m-m-my eyes f-f-feel popping. M-m-my head f-f-feels flat . . . l-l-like I didn't even have a t-t-top of m-m-my head. M-m-my heart f-f-feels like it k-k-keeps jumping out . . . I-I-I- have to c-c-catch it. It h-h-has the measles . . . spots on . . . on . . . it . . . l-l-like my l-l-legs have w-w-warts all over. That s-s-spider is crawling up m-m-me . . . I-I-I- keep l-l-looking d-d-own . . . I-I-I- shake and shiver

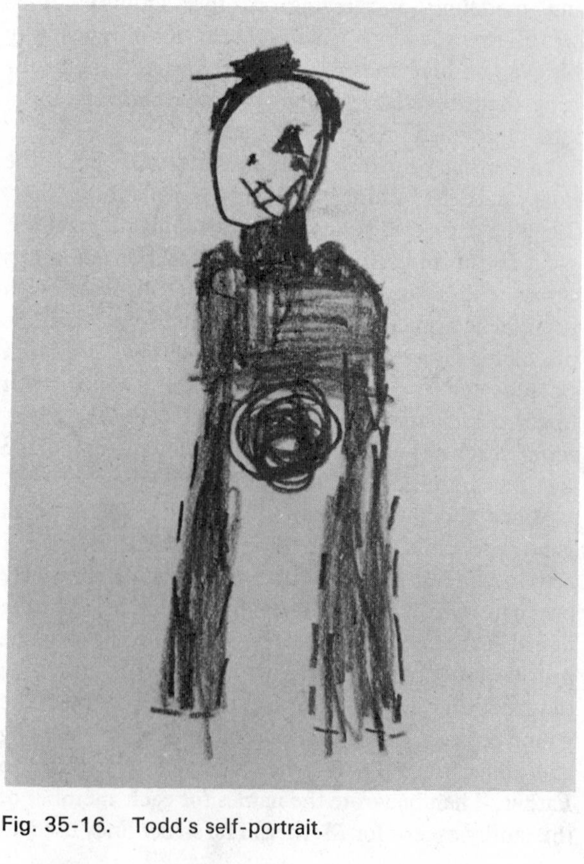

Fig. 35-16. Todd's self-portrait.

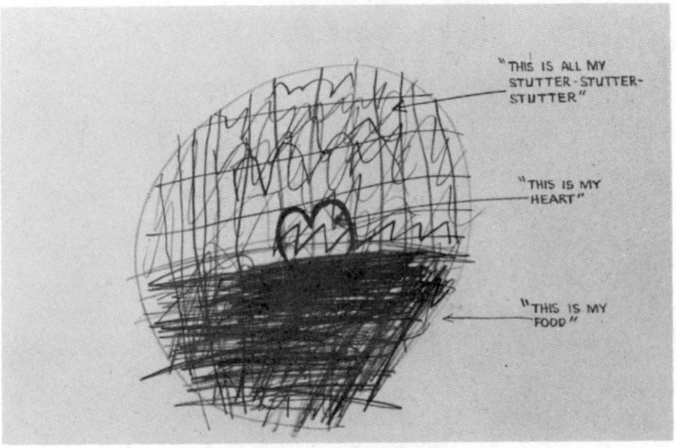

Fig. 35-17. Todd's drawing of his stuttering.

inside . . . I-I-I-I keep s-s-stumbling on m-m-my words . . . Oh yes . . . m-m-my toes keep on f-f-feeling big."

Sean (secondary stuttering, six years) (Fig. 35-19) said:

"When I s-s-stutter . . . the f-f-feelings are in my h-h-head . . . that's w-w-where the s-s-stutter is . . . one p-p-picture is the h-h-happy me . . . the other is the s-s-sad me. It's s-s-sad because of . . . because of . . . you know . . . the s-s-stutter . . ." (He gestured to his head at this point).

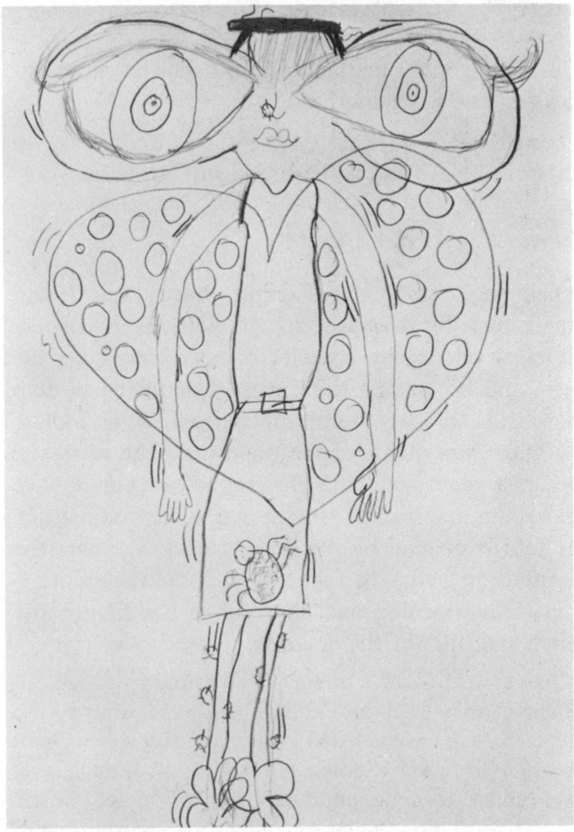

Fig. 35-18. Another self-portrait by Marna.

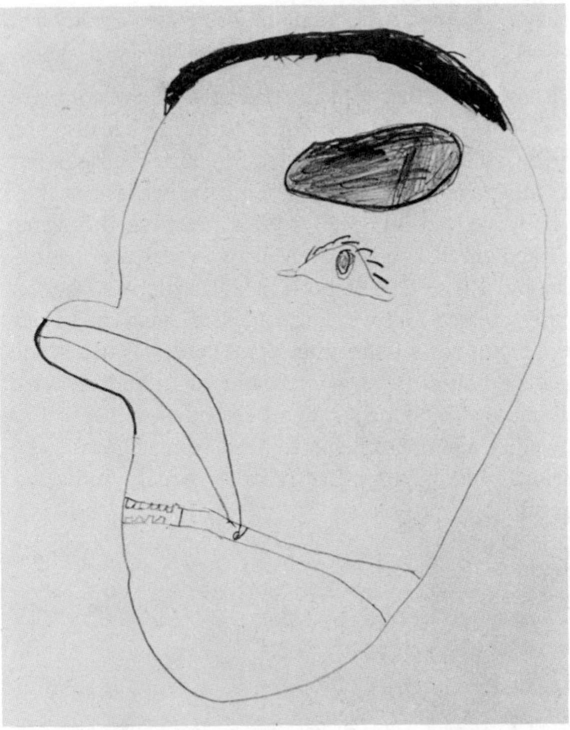

Fig. 35-19. Sean's self-portrait during stuttering.

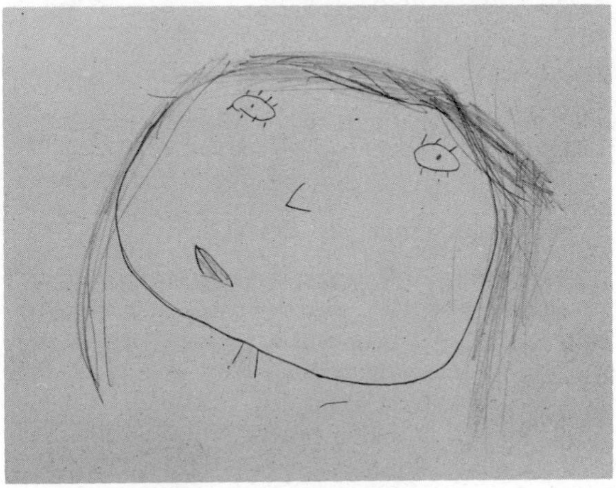

Fig. 35-20. Sangel's self-portrait.

Sangel (noncommunication, nine years) (Fig. 35-20) said:

"I want to talk . . . but I don't want to talk."

Enrico (noncommunication, nine years), while drawing just his head in profile, put a dark cloud above the eye, the nasal and oral cavities, the uvula and the teeth and said:

"It bothers me up here in the head. It feels afraid . . . buzzy . . . heavy. After I talk it goes away. Then I feel better."

Russett's mother told the therapist that she understood how her child felt when stuttering because she herself still stuttered at times. She also realized that she must make a change and not have her sister act as a baby-sitter while she worked because the sister "picked on" Russett. However, two years later, eight-year-old Russett's self portrait aptly depicted her as neatly dressed and wearing a look of concern. In her next picture of talking (Fig. 35-21) she was in a scene inside a house. Two women and two children were talking to a small forlorn figure seated on a chair, head bowed. Coming from the four standing figures were various hieroglyphic-like marks which indicated speech.

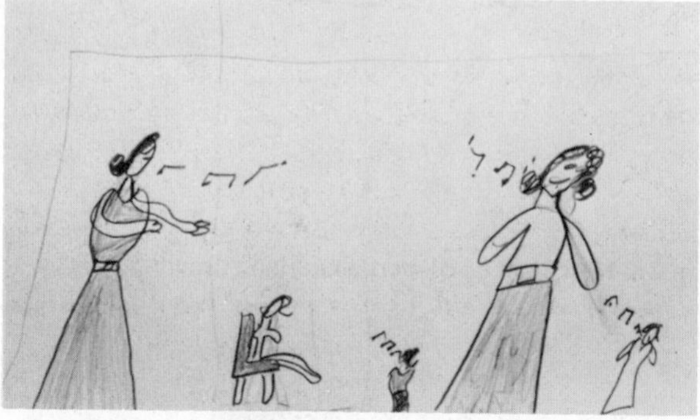

Fig. 35-21. Russett's drawing of talking with her mother, her aunt (the baby sitter) and her cousins.

Russett (in describing her drawing) said:

"This is m-m-my mother and m-m-my aunt . . . she's m-m-my bb . . . baby sitter . . . and m-m-my cousins . . . They are t-t-talking to m-m-me . . . and making m-m-me say things I-I-I- can't s-s-say . . . and they are l-l-laughing at m-m-me. . . . Sounds c-c-come out . . . but I-I-I- couldn't say it right . . . and they were l-l-laughing at me . . . I-I-I- felt real b-b-bad. . . . May I-I-I-have another p-piece of paper ?" (Her voice was very sad.)

Her last picture (Fig. 35-22) shows a heart-shaped chest and a prominent heart (broken), and hieroglyphics different from those of her mother and aunt. Her characters are repetitive in form but increase in size,

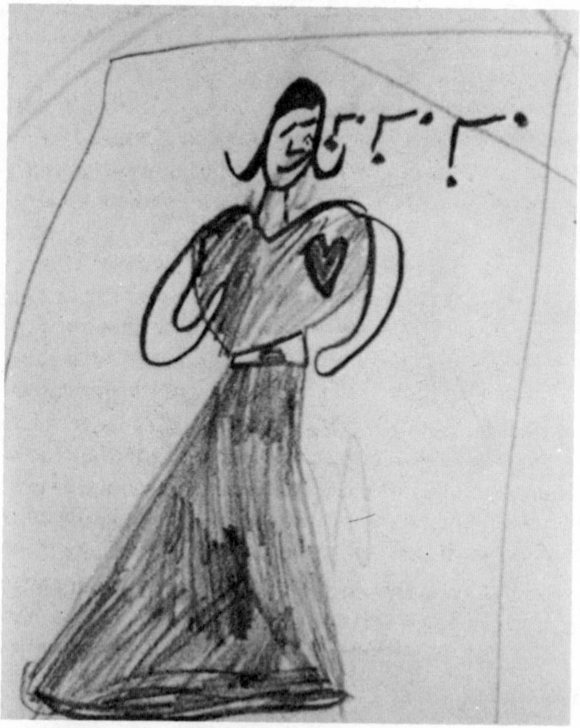

Fig. 35-22. Russett's second self-portrait while talking.

while those of her mother and aunt showed variations in form, one from another.

"Inside me. I-I-I-feel real b-b-bad and . . . real embarrassed . . . and it b-b-breaks my h-h-heart."

Paper-Bag Hand Puppets

Paper bags, sizes six or eight, have been found satisfactory for use as puppets. Various characters (in black and white or color) can be drawn on the bags, and by curling the fingers around the bottom fold inside the bag, mouth movements can be indicated with movements of the fingers. At the start, the therapist may show the children. She should have drawn the mouth only so that it is at the fold. When the fold is opened by the fingers inside the bag, the mouth is opened, when the fold is closed the mouth is shut. This opening and shutting of the mouth becomes realistic for the children.

Therapist: "Make a puppet of anything you wish . . . a person, an animal, or a 'thing.' It is to be yours to use in speech class only. I will keep it for you and we will use them at times when we tell stories or act our plays. You can see that the mouth must be on the fold of the bag if it is to move when you open and close your hand. Put your name and age on the back of the bag."

Many of these puppets reveal clearly the child's troubled feelings and focal anxieties.

Gene (stutterer, eight years) gasped when he finished a full-length two-gun cowboy and turned the bag over to write his name.

"Oh! I-I-I-must c-c-cover me up in b-b-back . . . someone will s-s-see me without my c-c-clothes on my . . . (pause) Oh! W-w-what if a g-g-girl . . . (pause)."

There was "Mr. Two Face," a cramped, double-faced puppet made by a very disturbed boy of twelve who later freely expressed his quandary over his identity. In his case the puppet definitely afforded the way for the discovery and better management of his basic problem.

When the activity has gotten underway the therapist may write on the back of the puppet the remarks of each child in answer to her question, "Tell us your puppet's name and what it's like."

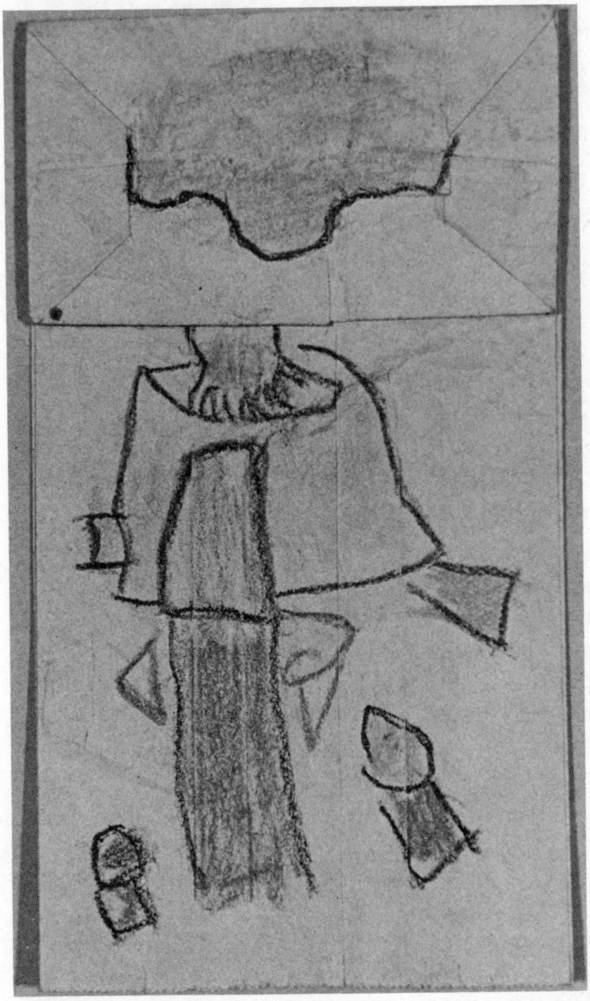

Fig. 35-23. Burt's paper-bag hand puppet.

Through the drawing and the subsequent characterization of his puppet in acts and speech the child works out, in his new family (therapist and children), his disturbing feelings and thoughts.

Burt was a stutterer having articulation problems. At five years of age he drew his puppet and also a little figure on each side below the puppet's knee level (Fig. 35-23).

"That n-n-naughty . . . n-n-naughty . . . n-n-naughty bank robber . . . and the two g-g-goodies who will b-b-bite his head off . . . and his arms off and h-h-him legs (touching buttocks) . . . and b-b-bite his-t-tummy off . . . and bite him g-g-gooey off (indicating buttocks) so n-n-no potty can come out of h-h-him . . . and s-s-stink come out of his g-gooey . . . b-b-bite him legs off . . . and down h-h-here . . . (gesturing across pelvic area) and c-c-cut him's tongue off . . . and h-h-him can't ever t-t-talk." (He scissored his fingers on his lips and pointed two fingers at his larynx.)

Page (stutterer, eight years) drew a picture of his hurts (Fig. 35-24). During the three years he was in therapy there was rarely a time when his family was free from serious illness.

"This is the d-d-devil . . . with a b-b-big hurt on him and lots of h-h-hurts . . . he gave himself the h-h-hurts . . . l-l-like this." (He stood up and hit the puppets on the wall.)

Hun Fook (stutterer, noncommunicator, eight years) (Fig. 35-25) drew his paper-bag puppet simply, bearing little resemblance to himself. When asked its name he pointed nevertheless to himself. He took delight, along with the other children, in working its mouth open and shut. They urged him to speak when working with his puppet. He left the group quickly and used the crayons to add an arm with one finger touching the tongue. He returned to the group and added red flame to the finger point. He often used pantomime to insure the group's understanding.

Jose (stutterer, nine years) was feeling much better about himself. This was shown in his improved fluency and in his puppet (Fig. 35-26). It bore large smiling lips and was surrounded by a blue sky.

"It's n-n-name is 'A Flower' . . . it's h-h-happy because it thought that it wouldn't g-g-grow. But n-n-ow it is outside . . . it c-c-can get sunshine and water and g-g-grow . . . others were in h-h-his way . . . always . . . always in h-h-h-his way . . . and so he c-c-could not see v-v-very good . . . but now h-h-he can . . . because the others are g-g-gone . . . people pulled t-t-them out. . . . Now he c-c-can live and be h-h-happy."

The stutterers used strong colors in making their puppets, indicative possibly of their own strong feelings.

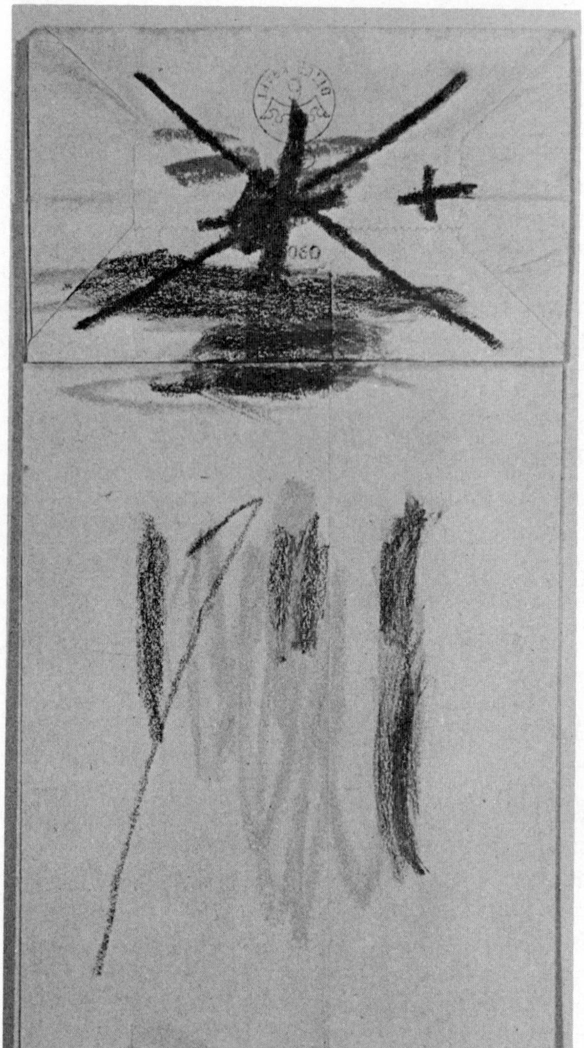

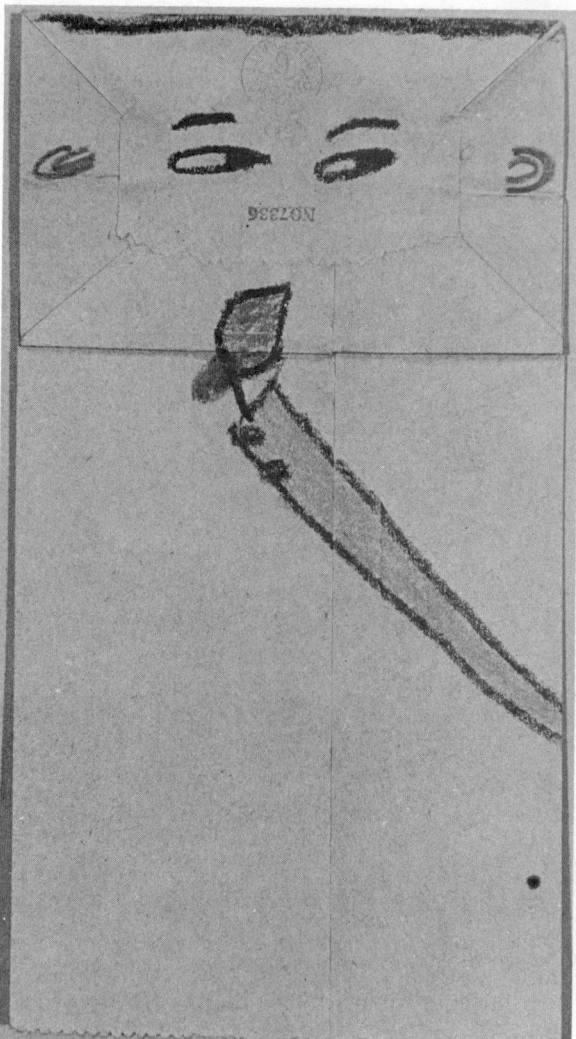

Fig. 35-24. Page's drawing of his hurts on his paper-bag puppet.

Albert (nine years), who was exceedingly anxious, depicited a sad-mouthed worry-lined boy (Fig. 35-27). Chet (six years) drew a lady with a large round mouth (Fig. 35-28). "Th-th-this is the most b-b-best puppet I can make . . . 'cause it is you" (indicating speech therapist).

The definition and the airing of his view of him-

Fig. 35-25. Hun Fook's drawing on his paper-bag puppet.

self, when given in this "special" atmosphere, offers the opportunity to the child for acceptance of feelings and the modification of them. He learns that he can feel miserable about and with himself and that he is not too "different" in suffering from his feelings of inadequacy. Finally, he may find self-value in the opinion of the therapist and his peers.

INFANTILE ORAL ACTIVITY

Spirometer

There is reason to assume that children with functional speech troubles (stuttering, delayed speech, faulty articulation) could profit from the recapture and the channeling of their disavowed infantile oral activities such as blowing, sucking, tongue-lolling, babbling, licking, biting, and chewing. In honor of this assumption an effort was made to adapt some conventional means already recognized in speech correction to elicit some possible shameful feelings about the mouth and its functions. The spirometer was chosen as affording a possible approach to the problem

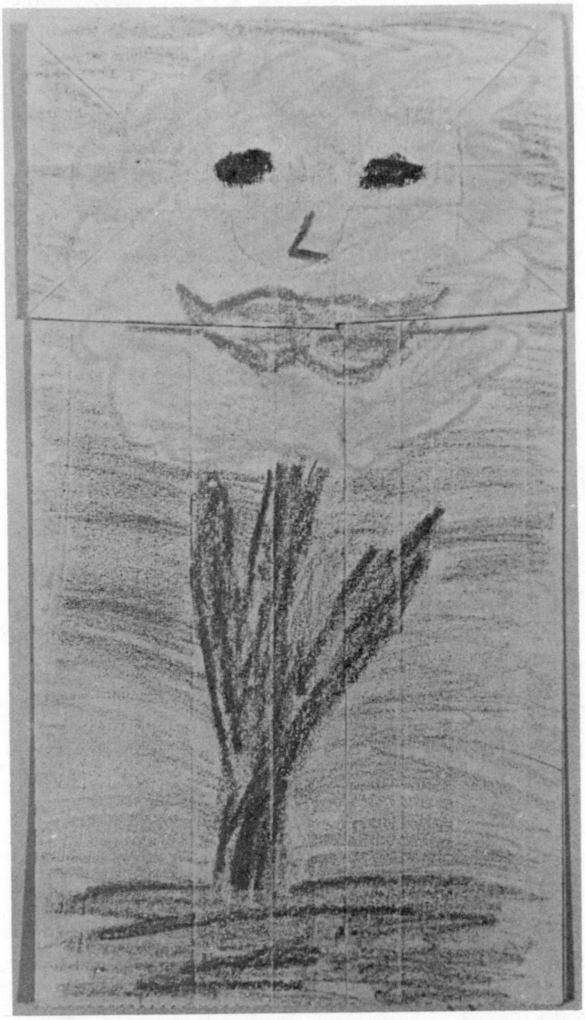

Fig. 35-26. Jose's drawing on his paper-bag puppet.

(Fig. 35-29). Essentially, it is a small and portable pressure device consisting of two bottles joined by a hollow glass bridge. From each bottle there extends a length of small plastic tubing with a removable mouthpiece. To eliminate the annoyance of sterilization, a mouthpiece can be a short length of 3/16-inch fountain straw given to each child for his own indi-

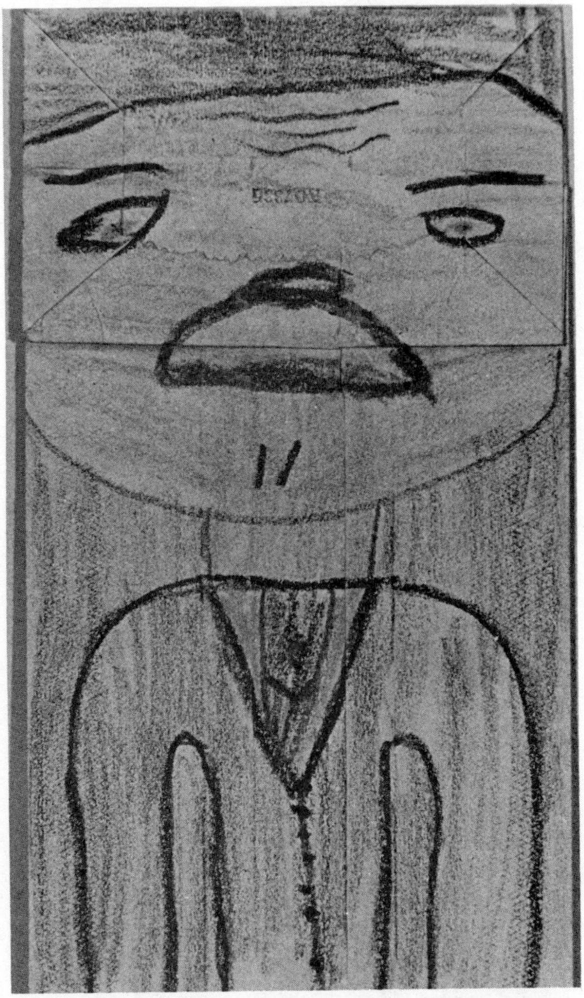

Fig. 35-27. Albert's drawing on his paper-bag puppet.

vidual use. One bottle is filled three-fourths full with colored water. A tiny pellet or two of commercial water purifier may be dropped in the water periodically. This could require the occasional addition of a drop of vegetable color.

By the application of air pressure (blowing or sucking) through the straws and tubing, the water is transposed from one bottle to the other through the interconnecting bridge of tubing. The base of the box is a separate piece of wood having three grooved circles for securely holding upright the two bottles and the bottle for straws. The rest of the box is in one piece which fits over the base just described. A handle on the top and hooks on the sides hold the two pieces together securely for easy transportation.

Two children use the spirometer at a time. The other children are grouped next to them at the table.

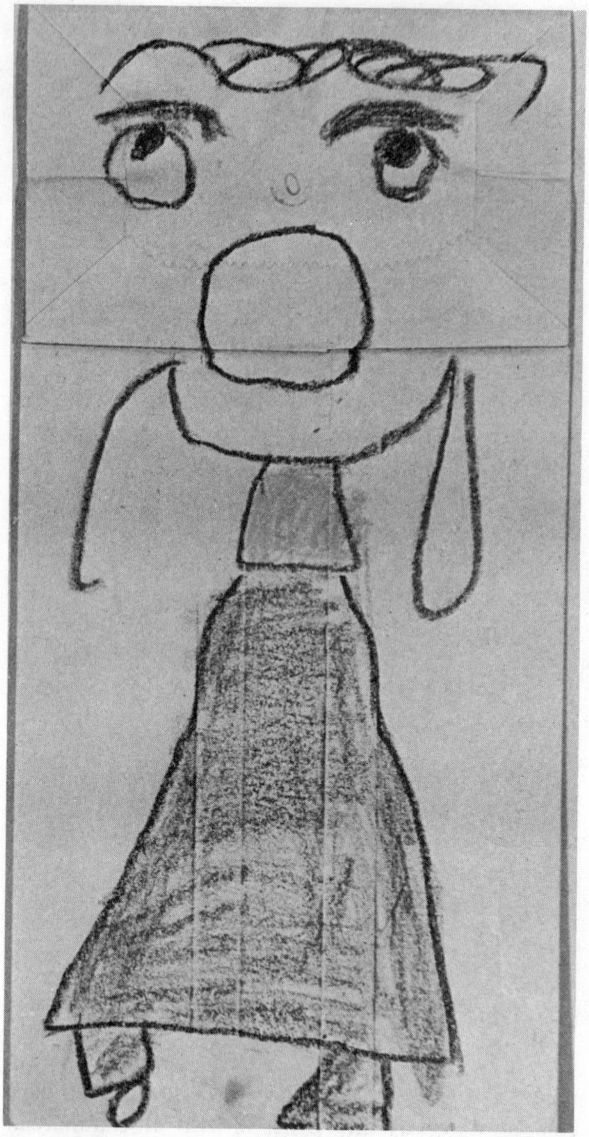

Fig. 35-28. Chet's drawing on his paper-bag puppet.

Each of the two selects a straw and inserts it in the end of a tube. The remaining children join in the verbal-echo part of the game speaking in unison while the two children at the spirometer take turns in performing the activity:

Group: "Blow . . . Rest . . . Blow . . . Rest . . . Blow Rest," etc.

Child: Blows . . . breathes . . . blows . . . breathes, in rhythm to the verbalization of the group, displacing one-half of the water in his bottle.

The second child then blows while the first joins the group in speaking. They take turns again while the directions and activity are changed to: "Suck . . . Rest . . . Suck . . . Rest," etc. As the bottle nears emptiness, they use pressure gently so as to capture bubbles in the glass bridge. The "nursing" movement may be well insured by the variation of the blowing and sucking activities: "Blow, blow, blow, rest; Blow, blow, blow, rest," etc.; and "Suck, suck, suck, rest; Suck, suck, suck, rest," etc.

Therapist: "Now see if you can keep these bubbles in the tube and jiggle them by your *speaking* gently on the straw while it is in your mouth. Take turns saying what I say: (one phrase at a time)

Therapist:	"Bah—Bah—Bah"
First Child and Group	"Bah—Bah—Bah" (Bubbles jiggle in tube)
Second Child and Group:	"Bah—Bah—Bah"
Therapist:	"Bay—Bay—Bay"
First Child and Group:	"Bay—Bay—Bay"
Second Child and Group:	"Bay—Bay—Bay"

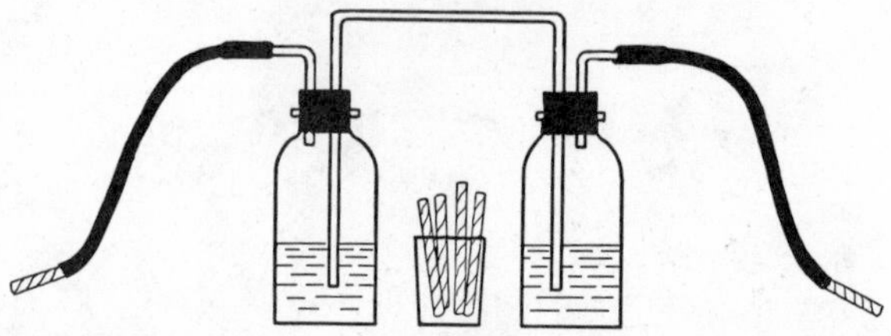

Fig. 35-29. Modified spirometer.

Then may follow the *b* and *p* sequences in full:

Bah—Bah—Bah	Pah—Pah—Pah
Bay—Bay—Bay	Pay—Pay—Pay
Bee—Bee—Bee	Pee—Pee—Pee
Bie—Bie—Bie	Pie—Pie—Pie
Boh—Boh—Boh	Poh—Poh—Poh
Boo—Boo—Boo	Poo—Poo—Poo

These in turn may be followed with brief phrases suggestive of infantile expression and "loaded" with *b* and *p*. Because these particular sounds jiggle the bubbles, the potential emotional content of the phrases is softened somewhat:

Bye-bye Baby	Baby plays pat-a-cake
Baby Bobby's bottle	Baby blows bubbles
Baby Bobby's buggy	Baby plays peek-a-boo

The older children accept the use of this "baby-talk" and jabberwocky when they are prepared for it by the explanation that only *b* and *p* sounds will jiggle the bubbles and yet not lose them down the tube. Even sixth-grade boys show great enthusiasm over this oral play. Indeed, some of the phrases given above are the suggestions of older boys. At first there were a few snickers and occasional sidelong glances when "Pee—Pee—Pee" or "Poo—Poo—Poo" was verbalized. When the therapist showed no negative response to the term or to their reactions, some shrugged their shoulders and accepted it.

Upon occasion, when it seemed relevant and timely, the therapist used this opportunity to ask the children to analyze their spontaneous reactions. This discussion led to interesting realizations, such as "Yeah, I laugh when I really don't mean funny- ha-ha." "Sure, I sorta laugh too, but I really mean I'm embarrassed. Why? Because we said . . . you know . . . that word." In subsequent use of this activity, the few children having the initial reaction of embarrassment regarding the term have come to use it noncommittally.

MESSING ACTIVITIES

Purpose

The child seeks to protect himself against the frustration of his primitive impulses. He is resentful of restraint and because of his immaturity is given readily to outbursts of rage and anger when he is inhibited. Often these reactions of frustration get him into still deeper water, since they are as antisocial as his primitive feelings and drives, so that they in turn have to be restrained. The restrictions and inhibitions of the culture that do not follow the orderly development of the total child produce tensions, repressions, fear, and guilt in him. As a consequence he may feel rejected, unworthy, and incompetent, or develop overcompensatory and symptomatic behavior. One area of the child's development, fraught with much danger to future well-being, is that of toilet and cleanliness training.

The purpose of having groups of children with functional speech disorders work with paints and clay is to give substitute satisfactions through the free acting out of messing impulses, opportunity for sublimative activity (painting pictures and making clay models), gratifying experiences, group status, recognition of achievement, and unconditional love and acceptance from an adult (speech therapist). With these beneficial results as a foundation, speech training may proceed with sureness and speed.

Organization and Limitations of Group Activity

The general, prevailing atmosphere is permissiveness. This spirit is stated and exuded by the therapist *especially* in relation to the children's verbalizations. Limitations, control, and denial will arise as members infringe upon the rights and convenience of others, and upon the integrity of school property.

The speech therapist may say: "We are using paints today just for the fun of messing in them. These papers are staying with me, but smear them to suit yourself. You may mess your hands all the way up to your wrists (demonstrating). Of course it would be fun to cover more of ourselves, but though we can't do that we can talk about it."

This statement may receive a wholehearted response from some children. Others may reveal a great deal of anxiety which they usually verbalize freely. Starting with one finger of one hand, while holding the other hand behind his back, a child may gingerly stir the paint and starch. Usually, before the period is ended, he will have both hands actively working in the paints up to his wrists while he verbalizes what he might *like* to do. At first, the therapist should emphasize the "messing in paints" for the fun of it. When the frightenening, messing impulses have been worked through, the child may go on to the sublimation or channeling of them in making a picture.

When the children walk into the room, they find a large piece of wrapping paper on the floor. On it is a smaller piece of paper for each child and one for the therapist. She is sitting on the floor holding a bottle of liquid starch in one hand and calsomine in the other. The children immediately take their places and await the blob of starch. A bit of calsomine paint is added which the children mix with the starch. It has been found that this method is more satisfactory and quicker than mixing the paints ahead of time. Any smear of paint on the floor is ignored; a smear on their clothing is dismissed with "It will wash out." When the children indicate a need for more starch, they hold cupped hands to receive it, commenting on the good "squooshy' feeling. They then cover their hands completely with the starch before using it on the paper. Some children work so vigorously that they actually wear through the tough paper. It is important that the therapist anticipate and plan avoidance of anything which might bring negative reaction or penalty to a child because of his activity in the speech class. The acceptance and release he has experienced in the therapy session must be protected. To spare the child the puzzlement and possibly even the criticism of parents if he should take his messy paper home with no picture on it, the therapist expresses her pleasure of his product and reminds him gently "remember that everything we do here and make here stays with me."

Another procedure has been developed and found to have some merit. The therapist uses a pencil, chalk, or eyebrow pencil to draw a rectangular space directly on the table or the chairs so that a "no-man's-land" surrounds all four sides of each space. The children stand beside the table or kneel beside a chair on which his limits are drawn. "We will each use our space for messing the starch while staying inside our squares. We have limit lines, because that is the way life is. We have limits at school and at home, and we have limits here. Having so few limits here makes it easy to remember them." The therapist indicates the limits by drawing her finger well within the limit-lines of the squares. The pleasant, calm, sincere voice of the therapist sets the tone for the acceptance of freedom within fair limits.

The matter of the child's spattered clothes may be a matter of concern to the parents or other teachers who in turn might react unfavorably upon his therapy. If there are no washing facilities at hand the children are sent to the lavatory in staggered rotation in order that they do not react to their free activity by "whooping down the hall," thus incurring the possible censure of other authorities in the school. The therapist may instruct, "Jimmy, here's a paper towel to dry as much paint as possible from your hands. Now I'll open the door for you so you can walk down the hall and then back yourself through the lavatory door. You will find that the paint cleans off better if you use just water before you use soap. I'll see you next week. Goodbye. Now George, here's your towel. When you're ready I'll open the door for you."

Any offer on the part of a child to help clean up the paints is appreciatively declined. The large paper for floor protection may be folded, rolled, and carried, or stored for repeated use. Many papers for individual use may be cut at one time. If table tops or chair seats have been used instead of paper it is best to wipe them off quickly with dry paper towels and finally a damp sponge.

All of the materials for messing (paper, starch, calsomine, clay) are usually available at each school for the asking. While it may be a good therapeutical technique to give the children a choice of colors in the paints, this could prove impractical because of cost or the problem of packing and handling. If only one color can be used, terra-cotta is recommended because of its close resemblance to mud and soil.

The practical factor of the therapist's clothing has importance, too. If she is to enter into the activity of the children and yet quickly move on to another group or school appearing well groomed, she must provide for a quick change. A full belted and printed nylon coat dress is found to be suitable as it can be slipped on and off easily over her street clothes. If it becomes spotted by paint, it can be quickly spot-washed and dried between sessions with groups of children in the same school. Or it can be rolled up and stuffed into a bag with the other speech materials and carried to another school. Apparently the children do not suspect that this coat-dress is not the therapist's regular garment for the day. Some therapists no longer find such preparations are necessary. On days when they will be using messing techniques they plan to wear clothing of printed fabric, avoiding long sleeves and, in the event they might be seated on the floor, straight skirts. If the therapist is a man it is suggested that he wear a cobbler's apron, sport shirt, or some such masculine attire.

With clay, the general plan is the same as that for the use of paints. For each child and the therapist there is a blob of wet modeling clay on the individual sheets (they are of plastic this time), or directly on the table or chairs within a marked rectangle. Both the clay and the sheets can be used many times. The plastic is light and easily washed. The table may be quickly cleaned with a sponge and paper towels.

Reactions to Finger Painting and Clay

Children identified their finger paintings as "A Tornado," "A Cyclone," "The Sea," "A Rope," "A Worm," "Roads," "The Freeway," "A Dirt Cave-In," "Lightning," "Water Waves," "Bones," "A Jail," "A Junk of Strings," "Hair," "Mud," "Quicksand," "My Old Man is Sinking in Quicksand," "My Design of Finger Nails," "Witch," "Making a Cake," "Washing my Hands with Messy Mud," "Magic . . . making Something Disappear," "Slopping," "Oooey-goooey-skwooshy Mud," 'Gishy-Gooey," "Cool," "Cold." Their activities were sometimes accompanied by reversion to infantile speech or humming such tunes as "Row, Row, Row, Your Boat," "Swanee River," and "Skater's Waltz."

Sally (stutterer, eight years): "I'll m-m-make my brother and t-t-then smear him away b-b-because h-h-he's a tease."

Cecil (noncommunication, 10 years, whose father had deserted the family): "I'm making a giant spider web . . . with a man caught in it . . . he got eaten up by the giant spider . . . It was a *she* spider."

He softened the man's face as he made the next picture.

"This is a rough river . . . with a trout in it. . . . The man doesn't know there's a giant waterfall . . . ten feet ahead. . . . A giant log stopped him."

At the end of the school year a group of six-year-old stutterers were recalling their experiences in their speech class.

Bart: ". . . and we got all g-g-gooey with starch."

Therapist: "Jamie was just using his fingers and saying some words. What is it Jamie?"

Jamie: "Squash . . . Squash . . . You know . . . when I say that w-w-word . . . I think I'm squoooooooo."

Therapist: "Your eyes are all squinchy, and your face is all squinchy. Your hands are gripping. . . . You mean that this bothers you?"

Jamie: . . . "Yeah . . . "

Bart: "It b-b-bothers me! I f-f-feel like I'm st . . . uck!" (He was squirming his buttocks on his seat.)

Therapist: ". . . You feel as though you're stuck . . ."

Bart: "Yeah . . . And I can't moooove."

Therapist: ". . . . like you can't move. . . . Is this a sort of frightening feeling? . . . How do you feel about it, Page?"

Page: "Ju . . . Ju . . . just . . . just fine. 'Course . . . just fine . . . like a normal boy."

Therapist: "You like to mess in paints and get good and gooshy. You like having a special place where it's all right to get messy and feel good about it?"

Suzie was a ward of the court. She has been hospitalized for months following cruel mistreatment by her mother. She has been able to verbalize her fears only to the extent of saying: "I have two mommies. I did have a bad mommie but now I have a good mommie."

At the seventh session she participated in the use of finger paints and clay for the first time. The use of these materials triggered her anxiety regarding the final traumatic experience, being placed in a tub of scalding water. She told of this experience and for the first time her speech, which had been severely infantile, was clearly intelligible. She started her story by saying: "I'm not afraid of the tub . . . not anymore . . . " She ended on a happy note, telling of what she was doing and her happiness in her new home.

AGGRESSION ACTIVITIES

Games

A game that may be entitled "You're Gone" is designed to offer the children an opportunity to express hostility and aggression without destruction of school property and without disturbing the peace of the school. The materials used consist of:

1. A plastic toy of the weapon type. A small, inflated baseball bat and a Davy Crockett, soft-headed, plastic axe. Any similar toy which is unbreakable and noiseless when used will do.

2. A small pillow or preferably a piece of sponge rubber to place on the chair to muffle any sound.

3. A set of cards made up of pictures from magazines, each mounted on durable tag board paper and especially selected to illustrate and symbolize people, objects and relationships such as the following:

Man or a fierce animal (preferably of the ape family)
Woman (attractive), or an article of intimate feminine attire
Male child
Female child
Woman holding an infant
Bed
Child and bottle
Animal nursing its young
Soap
Bathroom including the toilet
A mother bathing an older child (both sexes)
Dirty-faced and dirty-handed child
Knife, scissors, firecracker
Fire and flames.

The idea is to acquire pictures that portray the more common socializing areas in family living. Pictures may be chosen on the basis of both realism (mother nursing baby) and symbolism (scissors or knife for hostile cutting). The pictures may be presented with no story at all but with the purpose candidly stated.

"We have talked about the ways in which we can get rid of our upset feelings safely. Now I've brought something for you to use and find out one way to make it work. Will you come close to the table and study the pictures so that you may know them quite well." (Allow time for them to become familiar with the pictures and to then return to their seats). "You will take turns choosing any card you wish. Put it on the chair." (A small chair is placed beside the table.) "Use the plastic bat or axe on it and say whatever you need to say. Here are two sponge cushions on the chair. Choose the picture you want and then place it between the two cushions and hit or pound it with your fists."

After one turn around the circle with each child hitting one card, he may take another turn, with each one now choosing two cards to hit. The third time around each child may choose three cards. It is interesting to note the high percentage of repetition of cards from a particular area that will be chosen consistently by a child. Many children choose only cards bearing symbolic illustrations at the beginning of the game. As the game progresses they grow less defensive and gradually dare to choose "reality" pictures.

Agression with Clay and Pictures

Instead of prepared pictures of such objects as axe and bat, resistant butcher paper or plastiline clay and the child's own bare hands may serve well in playing out aggressive feelings.

"Here are some balls of clay (or paper and crayons) for each of you. You may make anything or anybody you like who makes you angry, or frightened, or upset, and we'll talk while we work."

The therapist places a small ball of clay in front of each child and encourages him in his crude modeling of something which he hates or fears. Then demonstrating with her own model she says:

"You may place on the table the thing which you have made. Now say anything you feel like saying and *smash* it!

Freddie: "You mean it? We can SMASH it?"

Jerry: "Of course, you dope. Didn't you just hear her SAY so?"

Freddie: ". . . Well . . . (He vigorously did).

If the children drew pictures the therapist says:

"Now that you've finished follow me over here. (She moves to the wastebasket.) You may hit the picture, smash it, or tear it into bits." Usually each child smashes and tears his clay model or picture with a growing vengeance.

The children were discussing these activities when Phyllis (eight years) said:

"You get out your tensions and nerves . . . the nervous in your mind . . . and get your mad out."

Scott (six years): "Like if you have a brother and he did something to hurt you and you want to smash him in the face . . . you just get a big glob of clay . . . and make a face . . . and smash that instead. You don't have to smash him . . . and get into trouble . . . but you sure can *tell* him how you feel!"

Page (six years): "Tear . . . tear . . . tear . . . tear it up. The reason why is . . . *much more safer* . . . MUCH! MUCH!

Therapist: "What can you do at home if you don't have clay to use like we have here."

Page: "Uh . . . uuhm . . . uh . . . um . . . uh . . . Cardboard box . . . and . . . and . . . and . . . and . . .m . . . n . . . n . . . and . . . and . . . and draw . . . draw on the outside and the . . . and the . . . (blocking) . . . and the inside . . . (blocking)."

Therapist: "Then you could . . . "

Page: "I'd un . . . (blocking)."

Therapist: "You just used your fist in showing me."

Scott: "I would jump on it!"

Phyllis: "Smash it down!"

Burt: "I'd just jump on it and just . . . whom! . . . 'til it breaks!"

Therapist: "Usually you have a paper you could hit. What else could you use at home that's soft that you could hit?"

Scott: "A pillow!"

So the children learn to handle their feelings safely when they are not with the therapist.

Gordon (stutterer, 10 years), in reacting to his clay figure (Fig. 35-30), said:

"When m-m-my mother grabs m-m-me and punishes m-m-me in front of l-l-l-lots of people . . . l-l-like in a s-s-store. . . . Oh man! . . . She seems l-l-like a giiant size with h-h-horn ears and I-I-I-feel like when . . . when I-I-I-was a little bitty baby . . . only it's w-w-worse . . . even n-n-now . . . Oh man! It's awful!"

Scott (noncommunication, 11 years) had begun to express himself as he looked at his clay model (Fig. 35-31):

"My big brother is a snake in the grass . . . a rattle snake . . . always lies . . . and gets me into trouble . . . It's no use saying I didn't do it!"

The foregoing children reacted to overt aggression, Gordon to physical and Scott to verbal.

Kiti (secondary stuttering, five years) interpreted apparent passivity as active, hostile rejection (Fig. 35-23.).

"D . . . is here be Mom . . . Mom . . . Mommie. D . . . is be me. Mom . . . Mom . . . mommie . . . h . . . er say . . . 'Not talk' . . . Me say . . . 'Mom . . . Mom . . . mommie . . . please talk me.' . . . H . . . er say . . . 'Not talk!' . . . A . . . ll time. . . . 'Not talk' . . . Her

. . . her . . . her . . . her watch TB all . . . all . . . all time. H . . . er not talk. . . . H . . . er say 'Not talk . . . me want Mom . . . mom . . . mommie talk. . . . Me want talk my Mom . . . mom . . . mommie TB a . . . ll time. . . . Me want Mommie like m!"

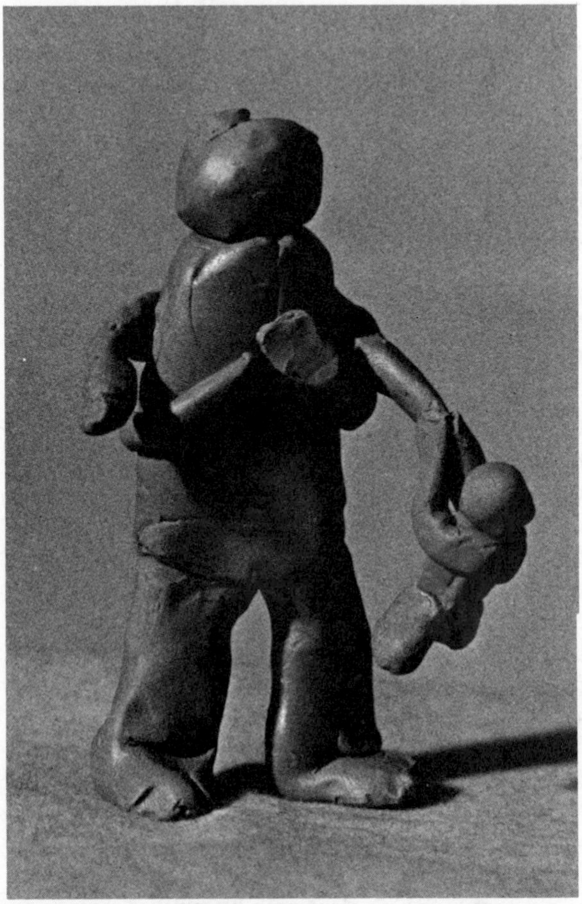

Fig. 35-30. Gordon's Clay Figure.

Gina (stutterer, 11 years) effectively avoided talking. She was obese, the only girl in the group, and was extrenely shy about hitting the resistant paper. At this point Carlos said:

"Here let me help you. I'll hold the paper on both sides and you give it a hard karate chop in the center. . . . That's a good start. . . . Now . . . chop again . . . again . . . again. Bet you didn' know you were so good!"

Gina responded tentatively, then with a surprising show of strength demolished the paper, growling all the time.

"Chop . . . chop . . . chop . . . CHOP!"

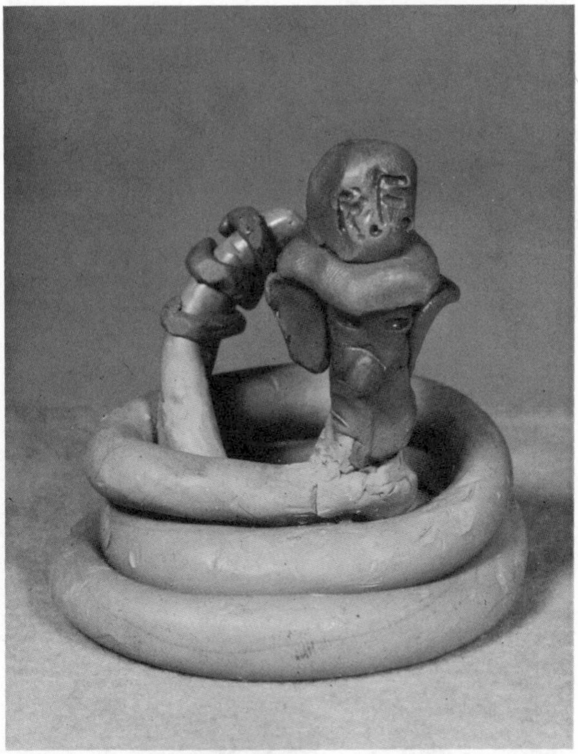

Fig. 35-31. Scott's Clay Figure.

Her face was flushed from her unusual physical and emotional behavior and she simply beamed with her surprising success. She left the session talking quietly with her new friends.

Donald (stutterer, 10 years), as he was drawing a picture depicting an experience he had had of fear, said to the therapist:

"I w-w-want you to w-w-write my story too. I w-w-w-was about one or two years old w-w-when my

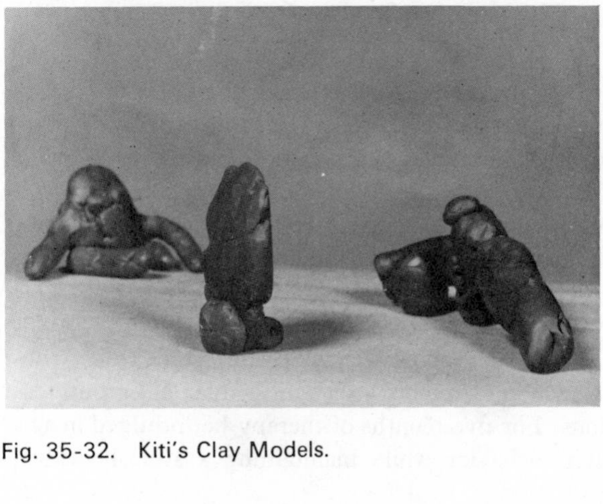

Fig. 35-32. Kiti's Clay Models.

m-m-mother had a f-f-fight and I was in the c-c-crib . . . I remember w-w-when someone . . . I d-d-don't know who it was . . . threw a c-c-catsup . . . a b-b-bottle of catsup . . . and m-m-my Uncle Bobby told me 'Don't cry' because I saw m-m-my mother f-f-fighting with my f-father. My m-m-mother had a pan in her h-h-hand and almost . . . almost h-h-hit my father . . . and j-j-just in time m-m-my Uncle Bobby stopped her . . . I saw . . . I saw . . . I saw some other p-p-people fighting . . . but I . . . I don't remember w-w-who they were."

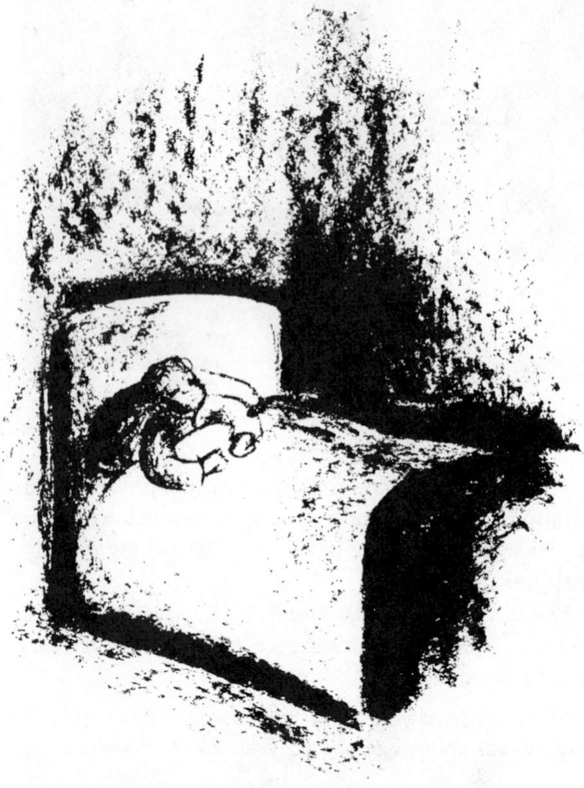

Fig. 35-33. Picture 21 of the Travis Story Pictures.

It is not too important when the child is relating such a memory to discover the validity of every statement. He is recalling his fears felt at the time of the experience and his childhood interpretation of them. Acceptance of his current feelings about them is important if he is to lower the degree of fear and put the ordeal in its proper place in his new-found value system.

Hun Fook (noncommunication, eight years) developed keen interest in his individual and group sessions. For five months of therapy he indulged in agitated behavior while maintaining a stoical silence.

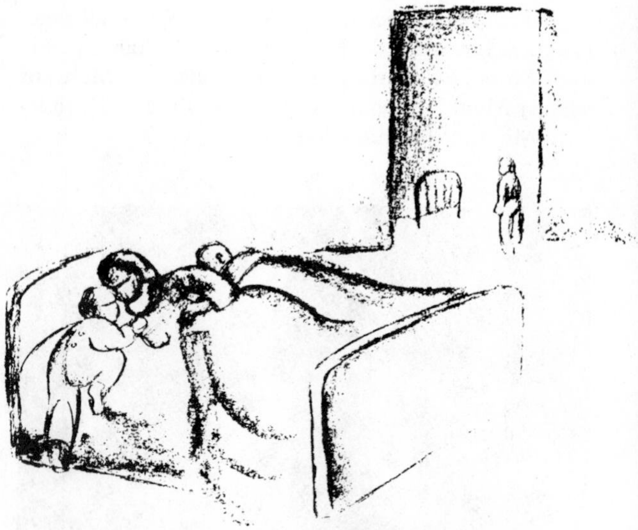

Fig. 35-34. Picture 20 of the Travis Story Pictures.

Using clay he made a dinosaur devouring a boy. Next he made a tiger leaving a dead boy. He then erected a war scene with a fort containing machine guns, three enemies, and numerous bullets. His final model was of two fathers throwing a boy to a snake. Upon finishing each of the four scenes made with clay he removed the boy figure safely before smashing the rest. A week later he combined the use of plastiline clay, pliable family figures, and two story pictures (Figs. 35-33 and 35-34). The therapist started the story by saying: "The child had a dream. He told his mother and father that . . ." Hun Fook enthusiastically grabbed the clay and rapidly made a snake. He then had the snake bite the boy on the arm. Then the boy slept with the father. The next dream that he enacted was of a dinosaur, which slept with his mother, breathing fire. His last dream was of a tiger which bit a boy. The father kicked, slapped, and spanked the boy, finally kicking him out of the house. The boy returned and kicked the father out. The father, then the boy, alternated in kicking one another out. Finally the boy slept with the father and the girl with the mother. Then babies arrived and the family was all together.

Another group of children was modeling and smashing the clay figures when the new boy in the group suddenly asked:

Jim: (stutterer, nine years) "Why are w-w-we doing this?"

The therapist thought about his question and then referred it to the group.

"Why are we smashing clay figures?"

Ruth (stutterer, 12 years): "We're getting r-r-rid of some of our *big feelings*!"

Jim: "Why?" (Smashing his clay vigorously.)

Ruth: "So those f-f-feelings won't *bother* us so much!

Jim: "How d-d-does smashing clay th-th-things do that?"

Ruth: "Well . . . you see . . . I-I-I-'ve been making and sm-sm-smashing Mary . . . because she m-m-makes me *so mad* . . . I'd like to just s-s-s-smash her . . . but I-I-I- know I can't. Now . . . in th-th-this room . . . it's d-d-different. . . . The clay isn't really h-h-her . . . but I c-c-can *feel* like it is . . . and do to it . . . and . . . say to it the things and do to it the th-th-things I really want to d-d-do . . . I don't know what h-h-happens to my *mad* at h-h-her . . . I guess I just use it up. . . . When w-w-we leave here . . . I'll see her and and I c-c-can be nice to her . . . I'm n-n-not saying I'll *love* h-h-her . . . but I can b-b-be *nice to her without being mad at myself*!"

Jaime (stutterer, 12 years) "Wouldn't t-t-that be funny . . . if you 'c-c-came here' until you *d-d-did love her*?"

Ruth (laughing softly) "Wouldn't t-t-that be something? . . . Well . . . could be . . . maybe!"

When Ruth said, "I can be nice to her without being mad at myself," is she also saying, "I do not feel so guilty about disliking Mary. I like myself more?" In becoming more communicative with herself and with others, her severe stuttering showed great improvement.

THE ROLE OF SPEECH THERAPY

Milisen and Johnson (1936), Bryngelson (1938, 1943), and Glasner and Rosenthal (1957) agree in reporting that either remission or improvement occurred in about one half of stutterers, both children and adults, without benefit of public school speech therapy. Glasner and Rosenthal (1957) state that 54 percent of 153 stuttering children were reported by their parents to have stopped stuttering sometime before they were seven years old. From their data one may assume that the majority of their children overcame stuttering before five, since their sample at the time of interview was at least five but not yet seven years old. Further, one may assume that 46 percent of the stuttering children still stuttered, at least to some degree.

To compare the results of what we may call "home treatment" of stuttering as indicated in the studies just cited with the results of public school therapy with stutterers, we devised the following questionnaire for the classroom teacher. This instrument was used for six consecutive years to obtain a fair degree of sophisticated judgment, that of the child's teachers, of the effectiveness of therapy for stuttering. Data were collected on 235 children, 154 stutterers, and 81 noncommunicators, from many ethnic backgrounds, attending eight elementary schools in a large metropolitan area. Six of the schools were located in definitely lower socioeconomic neighborhoods (179 children), while two schools were in mixed middle to lower class areas (56 children). These children were originally identified and referred to the speech therapist by classroom teachers, parents, and various other school personnel. The stutterers were diagnosed on the basis of blocks and repetitions, and the noncommunicators on the basis of verbal unresponsiveness. The noncommunicators were without determinable organic etiology.

There was no purposeful selection of cases except that each one had to have at least a total of eight therapy sessions. At the end of every semester the questionnaire was sent for all children diagnosed as stutterers and noncommunicators who had been in therapy with Mrs. Sutherland. The data presented here were compiled from the most recently completed reports on the children (one per child). In those children with dual problems, each child was counted only once, either as a stutterer or as a noncommunicator, depending on which type of speech trouble was the more severe.

A child was considered to have achieved normal speech when no trouble occurred over a minimum time of one year which usually included a semester of reinforcement therapy. Each child's progress was evaluated periodically by Mrs. Sutherland and by his teachers during his entire enrollment in the school, up to six years. If he were transferred to another school, information on his speech condition was obtained from the speech therapist in the new school. The results of the study of effectiveness of speech therapy (group therapy) in a large metropolitan area are presented in Tables 35-I, 35-II and 35-III.

Table 35-I reports the results of research efforts involving six years, eight schools, 97 teachers, and 154 stutterers. Sixty-six percent of these stuttering children gained normal speech from an average of 32 therapy sessions; 32 percent experienced significant improvement from an average of 36 sessions; and two percent made little consistent improvement from an average of 41 sessions. Of the latter three children, one was severely mentally retarded from brain injury, while the other two were victims of deplorably bad home situations.

QUESTIONNAIRE FOR CLASSROOM TEACHERS IN EVALUATING CHILD'S SPEECH

Date...

This is a confidential report for my own personal guidance only; it is **not** for the cumulative file.

As part of my longitudinal evaluation of the children with whom I work in speech therapy I greatly need your specific opinions on several items. Since you see this child under a variety of conditions will you please use a checkmark on the following scales to show your estimate of the change in the child's communication abilities this past year. Please return in the manila envelope to my box before...

Thank you.

La Verne Sutherland, speech therapist.

SCHOOL ROOM GRADE CHILD

1. Do you notice the problem of (The child's speech problem)

   Always ....|....................|....................|....................Never

2. How would you score the child's (Speech problem)

   No improvement....................|....................|....................|....................Great improvement

3. How would you score child's communication of a formal nature—when called upon in class for a specific answer, for example?

   No improvement....................|....................|....................|....................Great improvement

4. How would you score child's communication of a spontaneous, voluntary nature?

   No improvement....................|....................|....................|....................Great improvement

5. How would you score child's communication in playground situations?

   No improvement....................|....................|....................|....................Great improvement

6. How would you score child's general social adjustment—making friends, growth in sharing self with others, etc.?

   No improvement....................|....................|....................|....................Great improvement

7. How would you score child's opinion of himself?

   No improvement....................|....................|....................|....................Great improvement

   Is there a personal comment you would like to offer?

   Would you like to arrange a personal conference regarding this child?

....

Teacher's name

Table 35-II reports the results of research efforts involving six years, eight schools, 55 teachers, and 81 noncommunicators. Sixty-one percent of these children achieved normal speech from an average of 21 sessions; 36 percent made improvement from an average of 21 sessions; and three percent made no consistent improvement from an average of 16 sessions.

Table 35-III presents data on the improvement of the stutterers and the noncommunicators in several communication situations, in social adjustments, and in self-esteem. The number of children enjoying some degree of improvement in relating to others through speech and in self-esteem is great, and this improvement is probably related to their improvement in speech itself.

If we compare the results of what we may designate as "home treatment" for stutterers as reported by Glasner and Rosenthal (1957) with our results with stutterers (Table 35-I), we will be concerned with 54 percent of 153 children reported by their parents to have stopped stuttering and 66 percent of 154 children reported by their teachers to have stopped stuttering.

TABLE 35-I
Results of Speech Therapy in Public Schools for 154 Stutterers

	% OF CHILDREN GAINING NORMALCY				% OF CHILDREN IMPROVING FLUENCY				% OF CHILDREN WITH NO CONSISTENT IMPROVEMENT			
GRADE	M	F	TOTAL	NO. OF SESSIONS	M	F	TOTAL	NO. OF SESSIONS	M	F	TOTAL	NO. OF SESSIONS
Kdg. M=11 F=6	36	83	53	18	64	17	47	22	0	0	0	0
I M=19 F=10	63	90	73	27	32	10	24	28	5	0	3	15
II M=23 F=4	65	75	67	33	35	25	33	38	0	0	0	0
III M=23 F=6	48	66	52	28	52	17	45	47	0	17	3	89
IV M=21 F=3	81	67	80	29	19	33	20	32	0	0	0	0
V M=8 F=5	63	80	70	43	37	0	23	41	0	20	7	19
VI M=14 F=1	71	0	67	47	29	100	33	44	0	0	0	0
Total 154 M=119 F=35	61*	66	66	32	38	29	32	36	1	5	2	41

Number of Elementary Teachers Reporting = 97
Number of Schools in Study = 8
Number of Years of Reporting = 6
*Average

The difference between these two values, 66 percent and 54 percent, is significant at the .05 level of confidence. But the public school speech therapy is probably much better compared to home treatment than these figures would indicate. We must assume that the samples of stutterers compared are different in several ways. The home treatment sample is younger, and presumably in a more flexible period of speech maturation. Related to this thought is the statement by Glasner and Rosenthal that of the 996 children in their sample, 15.4 percent or 153 stuttered. According to Johnson (1955, p. 351) of 22,976 school children in grades one to 12 inclusive, only 0.55 percent stuttered. Does this obviously great reduction in the incidence of stuttering from the preschool to the school years indicate that the schools get the failures of the home program? Do they get the "hardened" cases, the recalcitrant ones, the ones who have been impervious to change under home rule? Yet in spite of the possibly more difficult cases the speech therapist does better than the parents. Could we guess that should the speech therapist apply her skills in the home before the children ever go to school there would be no need for her to ply her trade in the schoolroom. Might the thinking of Shames, Egolf, and Rhodes (1969) be expanded to include experimental programs in stuttering therapy in both the home and the school.

CONCLUDING THOUGHTS

We have not intended to present a complete exposition of the modifications and adaptations of the psychotherapeutical process for use in public school speech correction. Rather, we have wanted to indicate procedures that might prove provocative of further exploration and testing. The order of procedures, the length of a single session, the number of sessions for each procedure, the number of children in a group, the types of speech cases used, and the training of the speech therapist are points to be settled by further study. Our strong clinical impression is that those

TABLE 35-II
Results of Speech Therapy in Public Schools for 81 Noncommunicators

	% OF CHILDREN GAINING NORMALCY				% OF CHILDREN IMPROVING COMMUNICATION				% OF CHILDREN WITH NO CONSISTENT IMPROVEMENT			
GRADE	M	F	TOTAL	NO. OF SESSIONS	M	F	TOTAL	NO. OF SESSIONS	M	F	TOTAL	NO. OF SESSIONS
Kdg. M=4 F=4	75	50	63	16	25	50	37	15	0	0	0	0
I M=13 F=8	85	75	81	22	15	25	19	16	0	0	0	0
II M=8 F=5	38	100	61	28	50	0	31	26	12	0	8	17
III M=12 F=4	50	75	56	28	42	25	38	19	8	0	6	15
IV M=4 F=4	50	100	75	23	50	0	25	32	0	0	0	0
V M=4 F=7	75	29	45	13	25	71	55	23	0	0	0	0
VI M=3 F=1	33	100	50	15	67	0	50	16	0	0	0	0
Total 81 M=48 F=33	58*	75	61	21	39	24	36	21	3	0	2	16

Number of Elementary Teachers Reporting = 55
Number of Schools in Study = 8
Number of Years of Reporting = 6
*Average

TABLE 35-III
Results of Speech Therapy in Public Schools in Reference to Specific Communication and Interpersonal Situations

	STUTTERERS (154)			NONCOMMUNICATORS (81)		
	GREAT IMPROVEMENT	AVERAGE IMPROVEMENT	NO CONSISTENT IMPROVEMENT	GREAT IMPROVEMENT	AVERAGE IMPROVEMENT	NO CONSISTENT IMPROVEMENT
Formal Communication	69%	25%	6%	68%	28%	4%
Voluntary Communication	70%	24%	6%	67%	28%	5%
Communication on Playground	73%	23%	4%	76%	23%	1%
General Social Adjustment	71%	21%	8%	73%	26%	1%
Self-Opinion	77%	18%	5%	68%	30%	2%

Stutterers:
Number of Elementary Teachers Reporting = 97
Number of Schools in Study = 8
Number of Years of Reporting = 6

Noncommunicators:
Number of Elementary Teachers Reporting = 55
Number of Schools in Study = 8
Number of Years of Reporting = 6

procedures discussed here have been sufficiently helpful to deserve further consideration. In using only these suggestions, some children (both functional articulatory and stuttering cases) overcame their speech troubles entirely. Other children improved markedly. Our current feeling is that some form of psychotherapy is the only approach, even in the public schools, to the problem of stuttering, and an important supplementary tool with functional articulatory disorders. We know that some people may want to quibble over psycotherapy. What is it? Is not any good interpersonal relationship a psychotherapeutical one? Are not ear-training and speech exercises really psychotherapeutical? These are hard questions to answer definitively. As we see it, the core of psychotherapy is the resubmission of feared and anxiety-producing feelings and thoughts to the integrating forces (ego) of the person in the presence of a new parent (therapist) who rewards the discovery, acceptance, and channeling of these dreaded feelings and thoughts and does not reward the fear of them. This is not the place to argue the dynamics of the functional speech and voice disorders. It may be enough to state that clinical evidence is piling high to support the worth of psychotherapy as a method of choice with these cases.

BIBLIOGRAPHY

Bryngelson, B. 1938. Prognosis of stuttering. *J. Speech Disorders*, 3, 121–123.

———. 1943. Stuttering and personality development. *Nerv. Child*, 2, 162–166.

Glasner, P., and Rosenthal, D. 1957. Parental diagnosis of stuttering in young children. *J. Speech Hearing Disorders*, 22, 288–295.

Jay, E. 1952. A book about me. Chicago: Science Res. Associates.

Johnson, W. 1955. Stuttering in children and adults. Minneapolis: Univ. Minn. Press.

Milisen, R., and Johnson, W. 1936. A comparative study of stutterers, former stutterers and normal speakers whose handedness has been changed. *Arch. Speech*, 1, 61–86.

Shames, G., Egolf, D., and Rhodes, R. 1969. Experimental programs in stuttering therapy. *J. Speech Hearing Disorders*, 34, 30–47.

36

Preparation in Speech Pathology: Matter and Matrix

Robert Gillen

Here in this room we meet and face each other for the first time. I am the speech pathologist and he is my patient. He is a child or a teenager or an adult. He came voluntarily or he was brought or he was sent for. We regard each other. I have had training and he looks to me for help in the matters I have been trained in. I am confident, yet somewhere between my navel and the base of my trachea I may feel uneasy. Perhaps we chat. I perform appropriate diagnostic tests and I observe him with studied casualness. I know that he is monitoring me, and from our respective ignorance of each other as individuals old primitive cautions may be felt through the mesh of civilized convention. What does he see when he looks at me? A doctor, a healer, a mystic? Will he test me, will he want to outwit me? What is there about me to give him confidence in me, that I am one who can help him? I have my degrees and my certificates. Do I have, should I have, something more than learned theories and practised methods? I have those qualities, just what are they? Would he recognize them, need them, want them? If they exist, might they somehow enhance the therapeutic relationship?

I look past his features, through his skull, at the pink-gray brain beneath, pulsing with sensations and images, cased in quiet darkness, marvelously aware of the sounds, colors and dimensions of the world it will never know directly. Might the basic trouble lie somewhere there in the Gordian circuitry of his brain?

Yesterday in town I passed a shoeshine stand and the man looked at my shoes.

I have studied the tongue and its jumping muscles . . .

My father was a roofer. On Sundays we'd go for a ride. All he seemed to look at were rooftops.

My patient is an association of operants, one or more of them out of joint . . .

A barber looks at me and sees the cut of my hair.
A tailor looks at me and sees the cut of my jacket.
But another person looks, then knocks at his bosom and asks his own heart what *it* knows of me.

INTRODUCTION

The proper study of Man is perhaps not man himself but his words, how he fashions them to explain himself, to deceive himself, to inform others, to amuse them, woo them, shock them, manipulate them, and to fool them. Gaps between generations, between people or within an individual, have to do with words and their meanings, those ones we choose, the ways we inflect them, dole them out cautiously, spend them lavishly or withold them, and the ways we listen to and interpret them. Leaving out organic pathology, most of man's disorders come from the clumsy use of his greatest gift, symbols which he devised and employs so imperfectly. He is hoist by his own ingenious petard. Symbols physical, arithmetic, chemical, semantic, nuclear, and in the computer are no longer tools, they are his partners and, if he is lazy, one day may become his master.

Speech is language written on a breath. Enough time to be born in, to die in, to love, to utter a phrase that shakes the world. Yet this fleeting span of time and all the physical and linguistic processes which occupy it is what holds the interest of the speech pathologist. He examines and practises the ineffable business of man's principal difference from all other animals. His epitome would fill more pages than there are in this book for he is a man for all moods, ages, and circumstances. He is one who impossibly strives to be man's most perfect clinician.

To give line, form, and hue to this person, to see him in all his many planes, is to sum up the measure of everyone in the table of contents and to plot that aggregate three-dimensionally. In this chapter I will only suggest some guidelines for those interested in entering the field, for those who engage in the training of these earnest, ambitious people, and for those who are curious as to how one prepares for so protean a profession.

THE NEED FOR PERSONNEL

To learn the value of a service or a product go to the marketplace. Buyers of speech and hearing services must exist to stimulate training institutions to initiate programs, to support them, and continually to review and revise them in the light of changing times. Are there buyers? Just what is the state of that old law of supply and demand?

In 1965 the population of the United States was 194,583,000, in 1970 it was 207,127,000, in 1975 it will be 222,952,000 (Census Bureau, 1966). In those 10 years the nation's net gain of births over deaths will be more than 28,000,000 persons.

According to a conservative estimate published by the Office of Vocational Rehabilitation in 1960, approximately 20,000 speech and hearing personnel would be needed by 1970, and to attain that goal at least 1,500 clinicians would have to be trained in each of those ten years. By 1965 the estimated number ot needed speech pathologists and audiologists had risen to 40,194. For 1975 it will be 44,000 (Castle, 1967b). These figures may be modest. Trends in government support of public medicine seem to point to everincreasing services for the aged and for preschool children, as well as for school-age children. Those are the needs, as nearly as they can be projected.

How many personnel are being trained? In 1960 about 400 trained speech and hearing people were graduated from all qualified training institutions in the United States. In the academic year 1967–68, about 1,500 students with master's degrees and about 150 doctorates were produced (Lawrence, 1969).

Not only are trained personnel in short supply, but a swelling population moves the required number ever higher. There are more than 9,000,000 Americans in need of speech and hearing services as this is written. Where will the healers come from? Recruitment efforts certainly have paid well since June of 1948 when only 22 persons came into the field with the academic requirements for professional membership in the American Speech and Hearing Association (Palmer, 1948). Recruitment however remains one of the front-ranking problems facing the profession, a profession too few even know exists.

Clearly the jobs are there waiting to be filled by competent people. Crucial as the need for clinicians is, however, inextricably tied to the matter is the quality of their training. It is impossible at present to develop the quantity of clinicians needed and yet hold to high standards of training. Faced with that, the American Speech and Hearing Association and all leading training institutions have elected to maintain uniformly high training standards.

ACADEMIC PREPARATION

Minimally, the speech pathologist-audiologist is trained in basic sciences and humanities relating to speech, language, and hearing; he is familiar with the nature and causes of speech, language, and hearing disorders; he has mastered the clinical procedures appropriate to these disorders; he sees communication problems as central to the radii of dentistry, education, medicine, psychology, and social work, as well as his own discipline; and finally, with all of this, he must be willing and prepared on occasion to work as a member of an interdiscipline team in diagnosing and treating those persons impaired in the ways of his special interest and preparation.

On January 30, 1971 the American Speech and Hearing Association had 13,659 members. Forty-eight hundred were employed in elementary and secondary schools, including schools and classes for the deaf; 2,500 were employed in colleges or universities. The remainder were employed by community rehabilitation centers, clinics and hospitals, in private practice, or were unemployed (Logan, 1971).

Regardless of his ultimate work setting, however, with respect to his training the speech pathologist-audiologist follows the medical model; on the undergraduate level at a given training institution all students take nearly the same program. Just as the medical student obtains a general preparation and then studies for his specialty board, the speech and hearing student may go on to the master's or doctorate degrees, specializing in subject matter which interests him and which will be appropriate to his later employment.

Though course titles differ from school to school, the undergraduate will receive upper division training in such as the following:

SCIENCES
Human Development
Genetics
Biology
Speech and Hearing Science

SPEECH
Introduction to Speech Disorders
Advanced Speech Disorders: Organic
Advanced Speech Disorders: Nonorganic
Phonetics
Language Development
Group Techniques in Speech and Hearing
Diagnostic Methods: Speech Disorders

HEARING
Psychoacoustics
Principles of Audiology
Speechreading
Hearing and its Measurement
Diagnostic Methods: Hearing Disorders

PSYCHOLOGY
Psychology of Speech
Abnormal Psychology
Psychology of Personality
Educational Psychology
Child Psychology
Mental Hygiene

OTHER
Linguistics
Semantics
Tests and Measurements
Speech and Hearing Services in the Schools

Graduate work may include electives, seminars, and courses in:

Psycholinguistics
Voice and Articulation Disorders
Stuttering
Neurological Disorders of Speech
Dysphasia and Symbolic Disorders
Instrumentation
Cleft Palate

Practicum

Clinical training in speech, language, and hearing disorders is usually offered at on-campus facilities in both the undergraduate and the graduate programs. The American Speech and Hearing Association's Certificate of Clinical Competence (the CCC) requires a minimum of 275 clock-hours of experience among three age groups: preschool children, school-age children, and adults. By January of 1971 ASHA had issued the CCC in speech pathology to 8,528 members and in audiology to 1,703 members. Exposure to disorder types is as broad as is feasible and will include techniques appropriate to individual and group therapy. Other practicums, however, are carried out at rehabilitation centers, community service centers, and clinics. Fieldwork may take the form of internships in hospitals and other medical facilities. At the more advanced levels internships, under supervision, may carry stipends.

Post-doctoral programs in special studies are offered from time to time by leading institutions.

DISSOCIATION AND OVERLAP

With each passing year the list of required subjects grows longer, the number of required units increases, and course titles reveal a large and growing disparity between speech pathology as a healing art and speech pathology as the study of other peoples' disciplines. Has this not grown from our frustrated need to prove our value as respected members of the *scientific* hierarchy? Are we perhaps a bit embarrassed by the Joseph's coat nature of our professional training and by the general absence of "hardware" in our practice? Would we be more comfortable in scientific company if all speech and language were reducible to numbers or, better yet, to a simple binary radix, either "on" or "off"?

Training institutions erect academic towers. Like all towers they are meant to be seen from afar. They are advertisements to attract trainees, to be noticed by the competition and hopefully admired.

Students attending accredited training institutions are now well prepared academically. On the other hand they need, more than ever in an increasingly technical world, training in how to be a human being. Perhaps we are easily seduced by our own fawning admiration of other sciences but we should never lose sight of our real purpose: that the real essence of our profession is working with *people* who neither know nor care about muscles or nerves but who have adaptability for change regardless of structures or environments, past or present. For a student to learn all that he is now required to learn in the advanced arts and sciences of this profession is, for him and for us, to receive less and less return for the time and energy spent.

The basic structure of the American high school and college was formed over 100 years ago. It was called liberal arts because it was designed to educate a small number of children of the elite. These young people would be called on to supervise family fortunes and business interests, to travel, and to be at ease among the *cognoscenti* of the day. The curriculae laid down then, and the philosophies behind them, linger on in our schools today despite the absence of Greek and Latin and the emphasis on adjustment to others.

In this chapter I am most concerned, not with general curriculae, but with preparation in the highly complicated field of human communication and its disorders. I ask, then, if from time to time we should not call into question all of our curriculae in speech pathology. Periodically should we not seriously question our educational *purposes*, our origins, the routes we take, our implementations, and even our vocabularies?

Might our purposes be better served via an imaginatively different route? As it is, students must study in lockstep, for a prescribed number of years, a prescribed curriculum designed around a prescribed concept of what speech disorders are, what causes them, how to treat them. They must do this largely when they are young, since most of them go on into the public schools and traditionally the new teacher is a young person.

Is this wise in the long run? The student who comes along, drifting, looking for an identity, a way to be helpful, and still make a living, is caught up on the endless belt and processed; required to take, and learn something from, a certain curriculum whether he or she is ready for the course content or not.

Suppose the credential or the diploma were eliminated as a necessary prerequisite to employment? Suppose, instead, a student were entitled to gainful employment as an apprentice or as an intern after 16 semester units of preprofessional training beyond the general education requirements and given several more years in which to complete another 16 semester units. Certification would be required for permanent positions, but in the meantime the student will have supervised practicum mixed with formal training and will have measured both of these against his own continuing maturity.

Evidence shows that true learning occurs best when spaced out over some years and that mature students profit much more from their education when permitted to season at their own rate. A good example of this was the influx of veterans who flooded the campuses after World War II under the GI Bill. Educators everywhere pronounced that these savages would adulterate academic standards. Instead, the savages turned out to be superior students; they asked questions their professors could not answer and made the dean's list more often than their younger contemporaries. Drucker (1969) points out that in management, in law, in medicine, in engineering, in education, in architecture, in many other fields, there are areas of study that the inexperienced youngster can hardly learn and the beginner rarely needs.

In terminology are we not imperfectly married in common law to the term Pathologist? If we understand this term in its accepted meanings then we are, at best, laboratory oriented and only advisory to those who actually work with speech disorders in people. Of course, in another sense of the word Pathology we are specialists in the speech of dead people. Nomenclature remains a problem for us.

The lion's share of academic preparation is research oriented, and if carried along to a logical conclusion with more course work in statistics and experimental design would deposit the speech pathologist in the laboratory; he would indeed then be a pathologist in an advisory capacity. Is that what we want? Is this a big part, a small part, or any part of what we want? Do we even want the right things? Are we still in touch with language as it is used? Is word-language communication necessarily our only or primary concern as speech pathologists? What of the other communicative avenues that speak to our hearts and minds in our culture—architecture, dance, art, dress—all of them influenced by, and influencing this society we live in of which word-language is only one part?

Should there be two general approaches to training for the profession? One curriculum for the person preparing to be truly a speech pathologist, and another curriculum for those whose motives for entering the field originate in a simple, uncomplicated, generous wish to help others? There would be commonality between the two groups, and overlap, but emphasis in the second group would be on linguistics, child development, language development, perception, the problems of language deprivation in cultural pockets of our society where a child has an ice cream bar for breakfast on the way to school and who does not know what a knife and fork are because they are not used in the home. This group would enter practicum early so as to begin developing their clinical 'feel.'

Black and Brown Language were until recently almost unknown in current training programs, as were other ethnic language studies. The black man uses the white man's language as a starting point and goes on to fashion an incredibly creative, emotive, and gut language of his own. It is a whole communication system apart, two-level, slangy, full of action, terribly direct and honest. It has been going on under our noses all these years, yet many training programs have yet to notice it. The black speech clinician, working with black speech problems, can "say it Black." Shouldn't the white clinician?

At this writing Body Language is a fashionable topic, with premises and assumptions perhaps better explained in orthopedic terms than those advanced. Many of the blacks in our country, on the other hand, have incredibly expressive ways of moving. May I describe it as danceform, a true body language. How many other ethnic groups have such a somalinguistic language?

If our professional concern is with all forms of communication should we be involved in this form of 'talk' too?

FROM THE LABORATORY

Only three things excite a student professionally: discovering himself, discovering someone else, and discovering the future. Rehearsal of dead issues and long-known facts is necessary as academic study, but only as a background against which to measure and relate the now to the yet to come. One of Man's more persistent mistakes seems to be his secure belief that the future will be like the present, only more so. Military leaders are perhaps best examples of this. The fool sees the future as an extension of the past and the present; the wise person knows that the future is largely unknowable, particularly in the humanities. In the technical sciences, however, a bit of the near future is constantly being revealed to us. In this area speech pathologists need to be iconoclasts, to think bigger and more imaginatively. Is it laughable to wonder if the synthesis and physiology of synaptic chemistry, microminiaturization, and advances in techniques to block the body's rejection of foreign matter may yet come together to permit attachment of an exquisitely tiny electronic grid directly to the proximal surface of a sectioned optic nerve, permitting persons with certain kinds of blindness to "see" by means of small video cameras mounted in the eye sockets? If all things are possible, then that is possible. And, if that example has little to do with speech pathology, might something similar be done for the deaf person who has an intact auditory nerve and cortex? Is it quixotic to ask why cryosurgery should not do for the cerebral palsied what it has done for Parkinsonism?

The two-point threshold for touch is very fine in the oral areas, the lips, nose, and chin, both internally and externally. With specific training a man wearing an intraoral or extraoral electronic mask over these facial parts could be directed by a distant observer by means of a small transmitter-receiver. Tiny electric stimulations, singly and in combinations, in varying strengths, would inform the wearer what manual task to do next. Such a noncoded, nonlinguistic communication might be useful to the military under certain circumstances. Industry might find such a method useful in high-noise situations. And what possibilities might such an arrangement yield in research studies in stuttering?

In a few years color neutrography will show us far more about velopharyngeal competence than X-ray or cinefluoroscopy show us now.

Man has been fairly described as a machine whose parts, though made of different materials, do the same sorts of things that metallic and plastic machine parts do. They process, transduce, use fuel, give off wastes, and yield some product or service. Logically, analogies are made between man and the computer designed in his image with man coming out second best. And yet the information explosion which will transform all our lives within the next ten years will not be dependent on the computer-man but rather on neighborhood, or even household, programming inputs which will feed into and get from *regional* time-shared master computers, in a few seconds, information which will make our lives many times more simple from a data-handling standpoint than our lives are today. In this way man the communicator will control, not compete. The most trivial, the most inaccessible bit of information stored deep in the farthest library will be available to any beginning graduate student at any time of day or night. There will be no months or years of waiting to verify findings. The creative student will know nearly in an instant if he is on the right track and, if he isn't, how to control and direct his inquiry. As Drucker says, the computers exist now in large numbers; all that is lacking is the equivalent of Edison's lightbulb. Computers are the local and regional power plants; all each of us needs is a small, easy-to-operate, analog or digital feeder-printer to make use of that central information bank.

Everything in the above paragraph has to do with speech pathology. The Machine, science-fiction bugaboo and subject of countless dire predictions by sociologists, feared by workingmen afraid for their jobs, suspected by the educator afraid for *his* job, is with us, upon us, among us, and ahead of us. But, the machine works only with what it is given; it receives information from a human source (or his surrogate), processes these data, and then either stores it or transmits it to another human (or his surrogate) for useful translation or application.

It is all speech pathology, if speech pathology means concern with data—gathering, processing, transmitting, and use. The analogy with man the listener, thinker, speaker, and acter, is attractive. There is no reason—none—why the speech pathologist should not be concerned in these matters. Communication is the affair of the speech pathologist and these affairs are the future of communications. Sophisticated hardware means nothing without language, and a speaker and an understander of that language: coded, electronic, verbal, analog, binary, or waveform.

And then, further ahead, if man is to hold onto his soul he must come to grips with the machine as at least a partner in the intimacy of living. Even now machine talks to machine. Machines also talk to man, now limitedly. Before long machines will be talking to man in his many aspects much more than the individual man now talks to machine. Here, then, is a philosophical, even a theological, concern of the speech pathologist. Might a machine eventually have feelings? And if so, may there be feelings without a soul? Might a conglomerate of levers, cams and memory drums eventually possess the one thing that all men have thought confidently was uniquely human, a soul beyond consciousness?

Fritz Zwicky of the California Institute of Technology describes invention as "morphological thought." If one were to set out to invent a new kind of telescope, he says, one would lay out on a long table every known part of every known telescope. Then, alert to any fresh implication, one would methodically fit parts together which had not gone together before, being constantly receptive to any new application of the already known. This is what the speech pathologist and clinician can do and should do, whether he works in a school or a laboratory.

The dancer is thought to be mad by those who can't hear the music. The broadly trained speech specialist is an educated humanist with a child's uncomplicated vision, who sees and may even foresee the possibilities of his profession in all of its relationships to the arts and the sciences. As John Muir said, "When we try to pick out anything by itself, we find it hitched to everything else in the universe."

DIRECTED TEACHING

It may be appropriate here to emphasize gender. In January 1971 the American Speech and Hearing Association reported 13,659 members, of whom 10,239 were women, presumably mostly in the schools. When one adds to that figure the unknown but probably large number of people (estimated 9,000) not affiliated with ASHA and who are employed in the public schools, the typical person under discussion in this section is decidedly female.

In addition to the academic requirements, the clinician who intends to practise in the public schools will do approximately 150 clock-hours of student teaching in the public schools, working directly with children. Directed Teaching in speech disorders is a weaning period serving to link academics with the realities of public school employment; it is the climax of the preservice phase of teacher preparation. Often the student leaves Academe with a high muzzle velocity, brimming with enthusiasm, ready to go to work, and is shocked and bewildered by what is, for him, an entirely different way of doing things. Here for the first time he confronts PTA meetings, scheduling problems, in-service training, bells, sometimes poor physical facilities, interruptions of all kinds, and the dawning realization that public school is hard work. She learns something of what professionalism means, the responsibilities of being a teacher in the schools. To what degree, for example, does she involve herself in the home life of a child? Should she join a union? What are the ethics of trade unionism? Should she strike? Cross a picket line? Should she take part in political activities and, if so, to what degree? As Purpel says (1967), "Where does dedication leave off and exploitation begin?"

Only in directed teaching does the student learn how important public relations are to her program, how important it is to educate teachers, administrators, and parents in what she is doing and what she is trying to do. Only in directed teaching does she see, as Garbee (1967) points out, how speech and hearing therapeutic techniques must take second place to the child's total language communication and perceptual development.

There is little or no preprofessional training in these matters; as mentioned, college programs are based on the hospital model and the special needs, demands, and opportunities, and rewards of career work in the schools tend to be slighted. This may be only a venial sin; the feeling is general at the college level that for a student to become a professional he must know all about theory. And theory is where the professor shines.

A review of the prior art in directed teaching reveals a rich lode of references concerned with the public school classroom. There are few, however, which deal specifically with directed teaching in speech pathology in the schools. Andrews (1964b) says:

> Nowhere are the vast extremes between excellence and inadequacy in student teaching more striking and more shocking than in the dimension of quality. Some student teachers have a skillfully guided growth experience which leads them to an artistic and professionally effective performance in directed learning, while others have a continuously frustrating, emotionally disturbing experience during which they receive little positive direction or assistance, and may in fact learn unwise and professionally unsound procedures . . .
>
> Unless all signs fail, the fears of many directors and coordinators seem well founded—that the quality of student teaching will not improve generally, actually will decline in various places, unless and until the profession as a whole recognizes the dimensions of the problem and takes effective action.

Although in 1964 Andrews is lamenting the problems of elementary and secondary classroom directed teaching, Mac Learie anticipated Andrew's plea for quality in directed teaching 16 years before. As long ago as 1948 Ohio required 200 hours of clinical training for state certification in speech and hearing therapy, at least 100 clock hours of which were done in practice teaching.

> In such (training) clinics, for the most part, children are handled individually. In the schools, opportunity is given to acquire skill in handling a group. Practice teaching in speech differs from practice-teaching in any regular school subject in respect to the average size of the group, which is usually rather small, averaging five to eight pupils . . . (MacLearie, 1947).

Powers (1956) sees additional problems:

> . . . Educational administrators, under whose jurisdiction the school speech therapist works, tend to underestimate the highly technical and specialized nature of the work and the preparation needed for it. They tend to see it as essentially the same in preparation and function as classroom teaching, with a little extra specialization in and responsibility for the area of speech. On the other hand, college professors who train young people for public school speech correction too often lack direct experience in this work themselves. They tend to see the school speech therapist's work as being essentially the same as any other clinical speech therapy, except that it happens to go on within the organizational framework of a school, a difference which actually makes a very large difference.

There is no doubt that one of the major problems is the shortage of qualified public school supervisors —master teachers, critic teachers. (As an aside, each of these two terms appears to me to be either supercilious or presumptuous. I recommend Training Teacher as a suitable substitute; she is in fact a qualified therapist-teacher, with experience in the field, who is helping to train another on-coming teacher.) Purpel and others feel that much of the aggravation of this shortage is due to the failure of the teacher-training institutions to provide the necessary resources for the desired improvement.

> Typically, the situation for local school supervisors is . . . ludicrous. These teachers [it must be remembered that Purpel speaks for the classroom], usually already overwhelmed with a teaching load, are often given the

de facto responsibility for supervision. Teacher-training institutions are in this case taking the cost of supervision out of the hides of teachers since there is little, if any, compensation for their supervisory duties. When there is, it is usually in the form of a free course, a gift, or a nominal sum of \$100.00 or \$200.00. In these cases, although the acceptance of the principle of compensation is to be applauded, the actual value to the teacher approaches an insult. Hollow indeed is the noble cry that teacher training is part of a teacher's professional responsibility and merits no extra compensation. (Purpel, 1967.)

If there is to be monetary compensation at all, certainly it should be substantial enough to be given, and received, without approaching insult. Since 1951 the State of California for example has paid each school district five dollars per semester hour. This is passed on to the training teacher and nets her, after taxes, a few cents under \$20.00 (Andrews, 1964a), thereby achieving insult.

Training teachers and supervisory personnel I talk with believe that it is part of a teacher's professional responsibility to bring on the next generation. In 15 years of professional acquaintance with training public school speech and hearing personnel I have found no training teacher who took her responsibility for the money it paid. I have found instead a general eagerness among these dedicated people to take on fledglings, to get them started, to pass on the essence of accrued experience. On the other hand it hardly needs to be pointed out that federal and state aid to education has increased markedly since 1951.

The issue then is one of principle: if we reject the principle of compensation for Training Teachers who supervise beginning speech specialists, that is one thing. Most, I suspect, would say that they do not need or want the money. But if we accept that principle of payment, then that payment should be worthy of those whose worthiness we exalt by selecting them for their superior service.

How easy it is to beat a tired horse with a new stick. If it needs servicing, what are some ways in which directed teaching in speech and hearing might be improved? Here are some suggestions:

1. Directed teaching should begin in the fall of the year. In many school districts this is the only time in the school year when certain procedures are carried out: screening, case selection, grouping, and scheduling. It is also the best time to get acquainted with other staff members.

2. College course work specifically related to speech and hearing services in the public schools is suggested. This may be required of the student at any time approaching directed teaching. Preferably this course would be taught by a public school person with a valid state public school credential to do a speech clinician's work in the public schools, the ASHA Certificate of Clinical Competence (CCC), and at least three years' experience in the public schools.

3. Training institutions might close the gap further with workshops on campus to include training teachers and prospective practice teachers, offered prior to directed teaching.

4. More observation in the schools as corollary to course work.

5. Work to change state codes so that qualified training teachers are fairly compensated for their work. This could take the form of money, release time, or a combination of the two.

For the majority of persons employed in speech and hearing services, directed teaching is the bridge from clinic to classroom. In this burst of exposure to the communication problems of many children, the clinician is introduced to the exhilaration, dilemmas, and all the rewards of the career she has chosen. It is here too that she sees how important to her work are such human qualities as warmth, empathy, enthusiasm, and potential for growth.

It is time too precious and fleeting to be squandered.

THE UNMEASURABLE PREPARATION

Having pledged ourselves and prepared academically and clinically to be communicators, it is of course imperative that we be able to do personally what our degrees and credentials say that we do. Especially is this true for those who work directly with individuals with speech and communication problems.

The experienced clinician knows that with a certain type of case, with a certain individual, at some certain time, a forward step was taken almost despite the techniques or instrumentation which were used. It may have come as a surprise to both the clinician and to the patient, but it was immensely satisfying. It was as if some X factor were operating, some unseen member of the therapeutic team, working along with the flesh and blood participants for the common good. This subtle *something* often seems to be related to the clinician's personality, his ethos, the kind of total person he is. Imparted is a quality of secondary communication beyond the known channels. This reinforcement is very likely the plus factor of the inspired and inspiring clinician who, using ordinary tools and methods, succeeds where another does not. It seems especially operative in nonorganic disorders such as articulation, stuttering, nonverbal children, infantile speech, and those with psychological overlays on organic disorders. Because articulation disorders make up some 81 percent of the public school speech clinician's caseload, those of us engaged in training would do well to consider these parameters not taught in the usual academics.

The clinician-in-training is taught to look at the "whole child." Should we, reciprocally, look at the *clinician* as a whole: *his* personal, physical, intellectual, social, and cultural inventory, and acknowledge that perhaps these matters add fully as much to a clinician's qualifications and effectiveness as the subjects he has studied?

The inward view

The clinician's honest relationship with his patient is equaled only by the demand that he be honest with himself.

It is worth noting that at professional conferences, in learned treatises and texts dealing with stuttering, for instance—everyone in the patient's environment who has a "role" to play is discussed thoroughly. If the patient is an adult his parents may be discussed. His wife counseled. The patient himself is discussed, tests and diagnoses are discussed in detail. If the patient is a child his teachers, school nurse, his peers, his siblings, his parents, all are discussed. The child himself is probed tirelessly. Often he is talked about as if he were an instrument panel which will give the right answers if only the right combination of dials and switches can be found. A short list of typical questions asked *about the child* by clinicians would include:

How does he perceive himself?
How does he express himself?
Can he express his feelings?
Can he reveal himself to others? Can he share with others?
Can he come close to another person? Can he reach out, touch, be touched?
Is he spontaneous?
What motivates him?
Does he like being yelled at?
How does he respond to praise?
He is asked to answer the question: What kind of person am I?

The one person we omit, the one whose assignment is to palliate the problem at hand, *is the clinician himself*. It is assumed that his academic and clinical training plus his experience and maturity are sufficient to the task. That may be a shaky assumption, however. It may be that he is not equal to the job and no one knows it, not even he himself.

Should the clinician ask the above questions not only of the child, but also of *himself*? Might he ask question number one: How do I perceive *myself*? Question 2: How do I express myself? Questions 3, 4, and 5: Can I? Question 6: Am I? And what motivates me? How do I respond to praise, or to being yelled at? What kind of person am I?

The answers are important on both sides. Someone (the clinician) must observe the child, consult his own feelings and reactions, then reach some kind of decision about how that child must feel in a given set of circumstances. The clinician's internal state of affairs then becomes most important if he is successfully to set up a feeling loop between himself and his patient. Of course there should be as little static, as little interference as possible, as the child's feelings are processed through the examiner's feelings.

We all know from our studies in physics that a conducting medium imparts distortion to the energy moving through it, a distortion determined by the medium's mass, density, molecular structure, temperature, and so on. The speech clinician looking at his patient is seeing a complex of conducting media, the sensory avenues of sight, hearing, touch, taste, smell, heat, cold, plus all of the learned associative responses to those stimuli, plus their qualitative and esthetic correlates: one person hates the sound of a clarinet, for another the feel of silk on the skin raises goosebumps. The sound of fingernails scratched on a blackboard sends wild shivers through one person while another person seemingly is unaffected. Beyond the physical and chemical rationales, each maturing individual is an accreting interweave of experiences colored by the distortions of his equipment, and the influences of his own idiosyncrasies and those of the culture he inhabits. Pure oriental music does not speak to the occidental ear because the western ear is tuned to the octave, the fifth, the major third. To the western ear, aperiodic sounds are noise.

But again, here we are, the two of us, in this first of perhaps many meetings. I look at this troubled person and I ask myself: In his time what significant things have his senses told his mind which my senses might echo? What is treasured in his feelings? What caskets are buried in that reliquary? What fuschia pleasures has he known? What sweet winds of special insight have blown among the stored, aging cheeses bequeathed to him by his parents and teachers? In what important ways have his senses, his intellect, and his feelings used him or failed him here or there so that he has seen himself and learned about himself in special ways?

As he speaks to me I listen to myself listening to him. Always there is the Me Between, mediating, filtering, choosing from what he says and making it agree in some Procrustean way with what I already understand. For his message to arrive on the inside of me at a moment when I am ready to be altered by it is to describe insight, that temporal flash in which a trenchant perception occurs.

And so I view his *reports* of his own perceptions through the distortions of my own perceptions, trained as these are to be objective. All diagnosis and treatment becomes, then, to one degree or another a collaborative effort between therapist and patient in which a workable goal is worked toward, with allowances and corrections being made for the distortions as they are mutually recognized.

Every practising speech clinician should have a personal analysis. It is the necessary corollary to all his other preparation. It opens the doors to which academic preparations have no keys. It is a singular, extra step he takes, beyond the legal and ethical requirements of his calling. In this most personal experience the clinician learns of himself, and through himself he learns of others. Making this special demand of himself the speech clinician becomes a special person. He is one who has explored the far limits of the self, discovered and brought back insights, someone who knows far better than before what it is to be human. He becomes an interesting person because he is interested in the world and more aware of it. With blind Homer he can study his thumb and see new marvels in it from moment to moment. This person knows his own feelings, knows the language of his own abdomen, and has learned to use these feelings and to understand them in others.

Most of us are governed at least as much by our feelings as by our intellects. Often something will please us or shock us without our knowing why, and the "reasons" for our reaction come to us only later. Reason acts slowly. As Pascal says, reason is constantly falling asleep or going astray for want of having all its principles present. Feeling, on the other hand, acts right now. This immediacy, though it has its flaws, can tell us quickly and honestly the state of our true beliefs, before rationalizations and defenses arrive to cloud matters. None of this is taught in the classroom or the clinic, nor can it be taught there; it can only be discussed. Autorevelation can come only through individual initiative accompanied by another person, or others who are the therapists, and in whose reflecting presence the individual sees himself unfold as he more truly is. As a rule we are more firmly convinced by reasons which we discover for ourselves than by those which occur to others. It is all very well to memorize science's proven verities in the curriculum, but someone else made those discoveries and wrote them down for us to study. Optimally, no one can know me better than I, and these discoveries—so personal, so unique—will be written in my brain, not in a book. They will then write themselves on the phrases I speak and the ways I speak them. I will recognize their universality in the speech of others because I discovered them in the laboratory of myself.

Custom tends to convince us better than scientific proofs. Custom and habit are for us easily the strongest and most readily accepted proofs in our dealings with ourselves and with others. Here is a dollar bill. Every one knows what it is: it is a symbol, a stand-in, redeemable in goods or services. But is that all? If I can look at it freshly, as if I hadn't seen one before and habit hadn't made my perception of it stale, I see other possibilities. It might make a good coaster for a wet drink. Or fold it in half and it will make a fine shoehorn.

Shoehorns and coasters may not seem at first to have much to do with speech pathology, but the speech clinician who is both scientist and humanist, and who can see himself and his patient and the world they occupy together illuminated more clearly, will be less likely to generalize, to stereotype. He will be more likely to see his patient freshly, inventively, more likely to "find the parts that seem to want to go together" and in ways not yet revealed to the patient himself.

A hearing aid worn in a certain way, for a certain purpose, by someone who doesn't hear well, is how we all think first of a hearing aid. It helps someone to hear. The creative speech clinician looks at a hearing aid and sees something else: a marvelous opportunity in his work with a normally hearing child who has a speech defect. In his blindness would

Homer have enjoyed listening to ants and beetles at work under the garden leaves with an electronic hearing aid?

This special person is a listener, a noticer, someone who sees that the lanes up a mountain road are darker than the ones down and who *wonders*, someone who is transcendentally tuned to nature and all its wonderful contents, able to look at a field and see that there is also in that field a town, and in that town houses, and in the houses people and pets, and in the walls of the houses ants and other creeping creatures, and in the people veins and arteries and pulsing needs. He is able to look at a patient and see beyond the diagnostics and test results. He looks, knocks at his own bosom, and asks his own heart what it knows of that person. The speech clinician who has taken this extra step, who in psychotherapy has looked into himself and weighed his own humanity, knows that reasons and reasoning amount to little more than giving way to feelings.

Fundamentally the speech pathologist knows clearly that he is dealing with language. He is wise enough to know that language is plural; that Man explains himself and shows himself to others in many media. Nations have no territorial claims on the verities of the scientific communities. Spain does not control physical laws and license them out to others; there are no Norwegian laws of chemistry. But there is a Spanish tongue, there are Norwegian dances, there is a black African art, a Mexican culture. The truly prepared and seasoned speech pathologist is acquainted with all of the ways men speak to each other; he is most truly an acculturated, compassionate person.

As Nuttall points out (1968), the speech pathologist sees himself and his work in the broadest perspective of mankind and nature. Where the psychologist studies speech as behavior, and the neurologist sees it as a potassium-sodium reaction to stimuli, and the radiologist sees it as a shadowplay, the speech pathologist studies speech as a unified field. This is what we are, this is our exceptional contribution.

The qualifications for the ideal speech and hearing pathologist are higher by far than for any other discipline. In a large part this is because our profession is frustratingly amorphous, indescribable, bold and unsure, mercurial, narrow and obtuse, eager but diffident, both old and young. But then this is Man, and so, in short, preparation for the practice of speech pathology is the study and treatment of Man as his language expresses his condition. To prepare as fully as possible for that heroic task should give every undergraduate some pause.

BIBLIOGRAPHY

Andrews, L. 1964a. State and federal aid for student teaching—now? *J. Teacher Educ.*, 15, 165.

———. 1964b. Student teaching. New York: Center for Applied Res. Educ.

Baisinger, W. 1968. Preprofessional education in speech pathology and audiology. *Asha*, 10, Sept., 375.

Bloomer, H. 1968. Preprofessional education in speech pathology and audiology. *Asha*, 10, June, 255.

Castle, W. 1967a. The 1966 membership of ASHA. *Asha*, 9, June, 219.

———. 1967b. Employment opportunities in speech pathology and audiology: fact and prophesy. *Central States Speech J.*, Feb. 27–31.

Census Bureau. 1966. Revised projections of the population of the United States by age and sex to 1985. United States Publishing House, Mar. 48.

The clinician. 1961. *J. of Speech and Hearing Disorders: Mongr.* Supplement No. 8, Part II.

Conant, J. 1963. Education of American teachers. New York: McGraw-Hill.

Darland, D. 1967. Needed: new models for learning. *J. Teacher Educ.*, 18, 4.

Drucker, P. 1969. The age of discontinuity. New York: Harper & Row.

Fleming, J. 1953. Role of supervision in psychiatric training. *Bull. Menninger Clinic*, 17, 157–168.

Garbee, F. 1967. New directions in planning for the provision of services for children with communication disorders. *The Voice*, 16, Nov., 91–98.

Gayles, A. 1968. The director of student teaching. *Improving Col. Univ. Teaching*, Spring, 144–147.

Halfond, M. 1964. Clinician supervision—stepchild in training. *Asha*, 6, Nov., 441.

Improving supervision of clinical practicum: a symposium. 1967. *Asha*, 9, Dec.

Johnson, K., and Newman, P. 1961. Trends in the profession. *Asha*, 3, April, 109–114.

Logan, E. 1971. Amer. Speech Hearing Assn. Personal correspondence.

MacLearie, E. 1947. Suggestions for supervised teaching in speech correction. *J. Speech Disorders*, 12, 369–372.

Norton, M. 1968. Preprofessional education in speech pathology and audiology. *Asha*, 10, Nov., 473.

Nuttall, E. 1968. Preprofessional education in speech pathology and audiology. *Asha*, 10, Oct., 442.

Palmer, M. 1948. Students and graduates in speech correction in the United States. *J. Speech Hearing Disorders*, 13, 267.

Powers, M. 1956. What makes an effective public school speech therapist? *J. Speech Hearing Disorders*, 21, 461–467.

Professional standards of training. 1961. *J. Speech Hearing Disorders*, supplement No. 8, part 8.

Purpel, D. 1967. Student teaching. *J. Teacher Educ.*, 18, 20.

Rees, M., and Smith, G. 1967. Supervised school experience for student clinicians. *Asha*, 9, July, 251–256.

Sezak, W. 1968. Student teaching: the shakedown cruise. *Leadership*, 25, April, 646.

Van Riper, C. 1965. Supervision of clinical practice. *Asha*, 7. Mar., 75.

Winitz, H. 1968. Preprofessional education in speech pathology and audiology. *Asha*, 10, July, 294.

37

Communications Disorders in the Public Schools

Clayton L. Bennett

INTRODUCTION

It is acknowledged that the disciplines of speech pathology and audiology are of relatively recent origin. As young professionals the practitioners are as yet much concerned with identity, terminology, and other concerns of an emerging profession (Perkins, 1962; Peterson and Fairbanks, 1963; Spriestersbach, 1965; Doerfler, 1968; Moeller, 1968). The reach for maturity is expressed in frequent articles and extended discussion of these topics at professional meetings. The training programs of our universities strain to accommodate the increasing demands made upon them for relevant curricula in these communications disciplines.

A large and growing segment of these professions is engaged in serving the communication-handicapped in the public schools. In 1956, 32.5 percent of the membership of the American Speech and Hearing Association was made up of public school clinicians.[1] The proportion of all clinicians in the public school setting who are members of the American Speech and Hearing Association is unknown, although Summers (1959) reported that two-thirds of his population were not ASHA members. In the analysis of the 1966 membership of ASHA according to "environment," 44 percent were reported in elementary and secondary schools, including schools or classes for the deaf. The role of the public school speech and hearing clinician as an application of the disciplines of speech pathology and audiology also has been subject to considerable discussion and some debate. Two statements on this topic have been released by the American Speech and Hearing Association: "Services and Functions of Speech and Hearing Specialists in Public Schools" (1962) and "The Speech Clinician's Role in the Public School" (1964). Ainsworth (1965) has also considered this issue. Attitudes of clinicians in the public schools have been reported by Weaver (1968). Further changes are reported by O'toole (1969).

It is this public school environment and the range of services rendered to the communication-handicapped within it that constitutes the focus of this chapter (Monog. Suppl., No. 8, 1961).

PATTERNS OF SERVICES

Large City School Systems

Services to the communication-handicapped in the public schools emerged early in this century, appearing first in large cities where a substantial population and broader base of financial support rendered such services feasible. To determine configurations of services currently rendered and to infer directions, it would appear logical to examine program descriptions derived from such settings. Ten large city school systems representing various geographical areas of the United States were solicited for program descriptions.[2] Responses were received from all 10

[1] Report of the Convention, *Journal of Speech and Hearing Disorders*, Volume 22, 1957.

[2] Atlanta, Boston, Chicago, Detroit, Los Angeles, New Orleans, New York, Philadelphia, San Francisco, Seattle.

cities. The pattern of having itinerant speech and hearing specialists serve several schools appears well established. Optimally, three or four buildings are served, but service to as many as six buildings is occasionally noted. Case finding is typically done by surveying at one or more grade levels, usually in the primary school. Procedures for referral by the teachers and other staff are designed to reach cases at levels not routinely screened.

Some communication disorders found are so severe that the traditional once or twice a week therapy sessions offer limited prognosis for recovery or amelioration. Referral to outside agencies except for supportive care is not usually regarded as the most fruitful way to dispose of such cases. In order to provide the frequent intensive treatment these children require, Chicago has developed a center school concept. Children who have particularly severe speech, voice, or language disorders are transferred from adjacent areas to one of the two center schools. A full-time speech clinician is assigned to each center providing daily therapy to fifteen such cases. The children are enrolled in the grade to which they belong. More detailed consideration of this concept is given in this book by Powers. Other school systems undoubtedly will consider this type of service, but it would appear that a school population of about thirty thousand would be necessary to justify one center school. Transportation could present considerable difficulty.

In some large school systems, children may be referred to a district-operated speech and hearing clinic. Detroit Public Schools have for a number of years provided diagnostic and consulting services in this manner in facilities at Wayne State University. The clinic is open daily during the school year for pupils from preschool to high school. Although located in the same building, the hearing and the speech clinics function as distinct units. Otological examinations are available to a limited number of children by a physician from the Department of Health.

Since many serious speech and hearing impairments can be identified and treated before children enter school, larger school systems have begun to offer preschool speech and hearing programs. Detroit Public Schools have three such programs. One speech and hearing clinic operates as a part of the Department of Speech Correction and Hearing Conservation of the Detroit schools. This unit includes, in addition to a therapy room with one-way mirrors, a sound suite for clinical audiometry. Referrals of preschool children with speech, language, or hearing problems are received from physicians, pediatricians, otologists, otolaryngologists, agencies, nursery schools, psychologists, and others. These children are seen diagnostically and most are worked with along with their parents on a monthly basis. Selected cases in each of the three categories are given intensive therapy in two or three 45-minute appointments per week as time permits. Some deaf and hard-of-hearing babies ranging in age from 13 months to three years are also scheduled three days a week with a clinician. Detroit also has a federally funded preschool intensive language therapy experimental program. In addition there is a preschool education program primarily for disadvantaged children for whom a language development emphasis is fundamental.

Case finding in the hearing conservation program may be done through Department of Health technicians, freeing the certificated hearing specialists to do the intensive follow-up indicated. In some areas the schools are cooperating with nearby training facilities to provide supervision for student speech and hearing clinicians, but furnishing increased guidance to classroom teachers for work in speech improvement is much more common.

School administration also looks increasingly to the speech and hearing specialist for consultation and direction in language development programs. In Detroit, speech and hearing staff are being assigned to Manpower Retraining Projects since speech handicaps are often a significant factor in securing employment. Under state law these staff members are also supplying proportionately equal correction services to nonpublic schools.

Larger systems with well-developed special education programs serve communication-handicapped individuals who are enrolled in special schools and classes. Thus, children having a major educational problem requiring special consideration may receive, in addition to these services, the help of speech and hearing specialists. Categorical programs for the educable mentally retarded, the trainable mentally retarded, the emotionally disturbed, the neurologically handicapped, the visually handicapped, the orthopedically handicapped, and the cerebral-palsied are most common. These classes are in addition to programs, long a part of public education, for deaf and hard-of-hearing children, who present communication disorder as a primary component. More recently, programs for "childhood aphasia" have begun to appear.

Although public schools are not often a research agency, the population served does provide an ideal setting for certain kinds of investigations. The staff of the Seattle public schools has made an important contribution to program research. This system has pursued a research study on the articulation of 15,255 first-grade children concerned with the effects of kindergarten experience on speech development (Pendergast, 1966). Recently the United States Office of Education has funded a five-year study of children with protrusional lisps which may provide a means of differentiating those children who will require speech therapy from those who will not.

It is generally acknowledged that the Horace Mann School for the Deaf, founded in 1869 in Boston, was the first public day school of its kind in the United States. The oral method of communication is used so that children are enabled to follow the Boston course of study as soon as possible. The goal of high school attendance with their hearing peers is uppermost in this program. Graduate students from the Boston University School of Education spend a day a week at the school. Boston's classes for the correction of defective speech were named "speech improvement classes" as a less stigmatizing title, the year following establishment of the program. A speech improvement program for grade one classrooms was introduced in 1957. This program provides a 20-minute lesson once a week and is credited with the correction of many slight defects. Speech correction is available at all levels but not in all schools in Boston, so car tickets are provided for necessary student travel. The cerebral palsy class at Patrick O'Hearn School is assigned a full-time speech teacher. Itinerant lip-reading teachers serve those hard-of-hearing children for whom this service is recommended in any part of the city. Tutorial instruction in the development of language concepts is projected for the near future.

The Atlanta public school system has a significant population of underprivileged children. Recognizing the enormous task faced by classroom teachers in providing adequate communication skills to these children, the administration involves speech and hearing specialists in various ways. In Atlanta's Headstart programs, the specialists created six units of instructional media for teachers to use in promoting language and speech development. Another group compiled a list of books and materials for the school libraries to make available to classroom teachers. In-service instruction was provided these teachers in using the materials. A television program—"Speech Improvement for Kindergarten and First Grade Classrooms"—was produced by a staff of five speech therapists under the direction of the staff of the school system's Educational Broadcasting Facility. Speech and hearing services are being extended in Atlanta public schools to provide for children enrolled in classes for the mentally retarded and in the local Child Treatment Center (Juvenile Detention). The involvement of speech therapists in the Learning Problems Center is also anticipated. Communication Skills Laboratories, a program supported through federal funds, provides remedial services at the eighth-grade level, the beginning year in Atlanta's high schools. The program provided approximately 50 percent coverage during the 1966–67 school year.

In New Orleans public schools, communications disorders are handled through the Corrective Speech and Hearing Section. All elementary schools are served, and pupils are scheduled for two periods of instruction per week. Children enrolled in classes for the crippled receive speech therapy, but the service is not offered in the classes for the mentally retarded. However, one specialist has been assigned to assist teachers in these classes to evaluate their pupils' needs and to set up a program of speech improvement. In 1966–67, speech correction was offered at the junior high school level during afterschool hours in those junior high schools serving underprivileged areas.

In the San Francisco Unified School District, children from regular classes in kindergarten through grade 12 are served by rotating teachers of speech correction and teachers of lipreading. In addition there are "Contact Classes" for the severely hard-of-hearing, the deaf, the partially seeing, the blind, the orthopedically handicapped and cerebral-palsied, a day school for the deaf, and health classes. There are also teachers of home-bound and hospitalized children. The Langley-Porter Neuro-psychiatric Clinic is also served by the public school speech and hearing program, whose supervisor is considered to be in an advantageous position to coordinate many nonschool agency services to school-age children.

Speech and hearing services in the San Francisco Unified School District were augmented in February 1966, when a Speech Development and Correction Program was established as part of a Compensatory Education Plan funded under Title I of the Elementary and Secondary Education Act. As modified in May of that year, four speech and hearing specialists were assigned full-time in each of four schools to provide "saturation" services. A fifth specialist was assigned to coordinate the services as they relate to all of the compensatory schools in the district. This concentration of services made many additional program modifications possible, such as earlier identification of prekindergarten children with severe communications disorders, intensified parent conferencing, more effective coordination with classroom work, more flexibility in the scheduling, and more opportunity for therapy innovations. Speech and hearing specialists also have provided significant support in the referral and differential study of candidates for the Educationally Handicapped Minors program.

The regular district case-finding program in San Francisco consists of screening all first-grade children and receiving referrals from classroom teachers, nurses, administrators, parents, and doctors. In addition, the four target school specialists screened each child. Case finding in the secondary schools is by referral only. Many children with communication handicaps undoubtedly escape detection and service due to the limited time the specialist has available. When the ESEA program and Sunshine School, which have full-time specialists, are deleted from the computation, San Francisco has a ratio of one specialist to about 3,000 pupils. From nine to 11 percent of elementary pupils have usually been identified as communicatively handicapped. Under the more intensive services in San Francisco's four target schools, approximately 12 percent have been so identified. Another disproportionate statistic which is a common finding in public school speech and hearing programs is San Francisco's ratio of 15 percent of specialist time assigned to junior and senior high schools, the enrollments of which represent about 45 percent of total district attendance. To estimate the adequacy of coverage in the speech and hearing program, it should be noted that the mean number of pupils served by each specialist is approximately 120. Of the total number of pupils presently identified as having communication impairment, only 64 percent are being served. As one criterion of program effectiveness, it may be pointed out that the Speech Development and Correction Program in San Francisco is increasingly perceived as an essential part of the basic school program rather than as an ancillary service.

Patterns of speech and hearing services in the large urban community are well illustrated by examples from the School District of Philadelphia. This is one of the older continuous operations, and functions along the principles outlined in the text by Black (1964) and by Powers (1956). Itinerant speech therapists provide service to children with speech and language problems in the regular school setting. A speech-correction program handbook has been developed which sets forth basic procedures, gives some specific instructions, and contains enriching materials. A guide is under consideration which will direct therapists to the most adequate commercial materials and materials prepared by other school systems. Several series of programmed therapy procedures are also contemplated for the guide.

Children are served in various special settings, including the Martin Day School for the Deaf and Hard of Hearing and the Widener Memorial School for Crippled Children. Exceptional teamwork among staff members, including those specializing in speech, occupational therapy, physical therapy, and other areas has been applied to the needs of those with multiple handicaps. Children who are blind and visually handicapped are served in the Logan Day School and in 36 classes for the emotionally disturbed, whose incidence of speech and language problems has been found to be no greater than in a normal school population. In Philadelphia, with its extensive medical care facilities, autistic and schizophrenic children are considered to be better treated in hospital clinics than in school-operated facilities. The itinerant speech therapy service is doubled in schools where the educable mentally retarded are housed. For the trainable mentally retarded, however, the classroom teacher works under the direction of a speech therapist and develops daily training procedures. The highly developed music therapy program is also considered a valuable adjunct to the daily training.

One group of "aphasic" children (who also have hearing loss) is treated by modified Association Method techniques in the school for the deaf. More recently formed are classes for children with learning disability. The speech and language needs of these pupils will be assessed specifically. Philadelphia also has a substantial cultural deprivation problem and seeks to serve the communication needs of this group with federal funding assistance through incorporation of special programs into the language arts curriculum.

The Board of Education of the City of New York serves the communication-handicapped under a Bureau of Speech Improvement and refers to its specialists as Teachers of Speech Improvement. A detailed handbook has been prepared to guide new Teachers of Speech Improvement. The handbook includes master plans for dealing with lingual protrusion, lisping, lalling, lateral emission, and other handicaps. Steps for organizing a program in schools previously served as well as for schools not previously served are laid out in detail. Simple screening procedures are suggested primarily to locate serious disorders. Individual diagnostic testing follows. Speech improvement teachers arrange with the principal to test children who will enter second grade in the fall, during late May or early June of the school year. They confer with teachers of kindergarten classes for referrals. Case selection hierarchies suggest the highest priority be given all stutterers regardless of grade and including kindergarten. Cleft palate, hearing loss, spastic, or other severe cases are next, with the lowest priority given "baby talk" and other sound substitutions found in children above the second grade.

Group speech therapy is considered a necessity in New York City schools. Basic principles for conducting group therapy are set forth; group size recommended is from 10 to 15 pupils. In several school districts there are speech centers for intensive therapy. The purpose of such centers is to provide training for the severely handicapped pupils who have been unable to progress satisfactorily in a weekly clinic program and to provide a setting for experimental study of therapy for severe speech handicaps. Units for complete therapy of pupils severely handicapped by cerebral palsy are maintained in several school districts. A Teacher of Speech Improvement is an integral part of the therapy team in each unit.

A special program for speech development is conducted in most schools for Children of Retarded Mental Development (CRMD). Teachers of Speech Improvement are requested to accept for clinical help only pupils referred to them by the special speech teacher assigned to the CRMD Speech Program in their schools.

Whenever feasible, pupils in classes for the physically handicapped who are in need of speech help are scheduled for speech classes. In some schools a speech development program for physically handicapped pupils is being carried out by a specially assigned Teacher of Speech Improvement. Referrals are made to outside agencies through the principal's office, but if a child attends a speech clinic outside of the school, he may not attend the speech class in his school.

Intermediate Units

Many children attend school in relatively small, geographically dispersed schools or school districts. Educational services to these schools are frequently the responsibility of a county or intermediate unit (Isenberg, 1964; Bennett, 1965). Not all county systems are highly organized and well staffed; there are some, however, which have become well known for their elaborate programs. Services to handicapped children in particular would often be nonexistent in smaller school systems were it not for a well-developed intermediate service unit. To examine program characteristics in this setting, a number of well-known county school organizations were asked to supply descriptive materials. Again, different areas of the United States were interrogated.[3] It should be noted that some of these are actually operating school systems whereas others are more properly designated as service units.

In Montgomery County (Maryland) Public Schools, itinerant speech and hearing therapists serve each public school in the county on a weekly schedule. Children in special as well as in regular classes are served. Caseloads range from 80 to 100 students weekly, seen individually or in small groups for periods of about 30 minutes. Children are found through both routine screening and referral. Although the number of schools assigned to one itinerant speech and hearing specialist depends upon school location, projected caseload, and specific competencies of the therapist, no therapist serves more than five schools. During the fiscal year 1966 the grade level distribution of cases averaged about 14 percent per grade in kindergarten through grade three, about seven percent in grades four through six, and about two percent in grades seven through 12. Special classes accounted for 6.5 percent of caseloads. Kindergarten Roundups are scheduled for the purpose of identifying and making referrals of severe problems. Diagnostic evaluation and summer therapy often follow as a result of this early identification program.

In the Montgomery County program, children with hearing impairment are sought through audiometric testing of pupils referred for speech and hearing therapy, as are all pupils enrolled in special education programs excepting those in the severe auditory program, the crippled and chronic health

[3] Erie County (New York), Montgomery County (Maryland), Polk County (Iowa).

program, those with known moderate auditory handicap, and those previously tested in the annual Health Department hearing screening program. Children failing established criteria are referred to the Montgomery County Health Department for further evaluation.

In the fiscal year 1965, third-grade screening became a part of the regular duties of the speech and hearing staff. Over 11 percent were found in need of therapy. The following year 8.7 percent were designated in need of therapy. Whether or not it constitutes a trend, it may be noted that over a three-year period the proportion of total caseloads coming from kindergarten and first and second grades dropped, probably due to the change in screening pattern. The percentage of third-graders increased. Speech therapy enrollments from the fourth through twelfth grades remained essentially unchanged over the same period. In terms of the number of pupils served above grade four, the reduction in the proportion of the caseload contributed by grade is essentially linear, falling to just over one percent in senior high school. The caseload distribution according to category approximates 75 percent with functional articulation problems, 12 percent with delayed language, four percent with hearing loss, five percent with stuttering, two percent with voice disorders, and two percent classified as organic.

For pupils with special disabilities, school-based therapists provide daily speech and hearing therapy to children with moderate to severe hearing losses, to pupils with orthopedic or chronic health conditions, and to pupils with severe auditory handicaps. Itinerant hearing specialists provide speech and hearing therapy and academic support for pupils with moderate hearing losses who are enrolled in their home schools.

The program for pupils with severe auditory handicaps in Montgomery County Public Schools is described briefly. In the introductory phase the emphasis is on auditory training, listening skills, and patterns of responses to language. As these skills develop, pupils are introduced to curricular activities appropriate to their academic communicative and/or developmental level of achievement. When feasible, students are assigned for a part of the day to regular classes to participate with their normally hearing peers in a particular activity such as art or science. This program also utilizes the services of the Captioned Films for the Deaf Program.

Student therapists from George Washington University and the University of Maryland have been assigned for 10 weeks of field experience in the public school setting since January 1965. Support for this program comes from the Training Grants Program of the United States Office of Education. Under Title I of the Elementary and Secondary Education Act, speech and hearing therapists have been employed to serve in the public and parochial schools assigned that assistance. A special summer program for students with severe auditory impairment was also funded under this Title. A Title III research project has also been concerned with speech and hearing services. As noted in other settings, speech and hearing therapists have been active also in Project Headstart.

In connection with the Montgomery County Health Department, diagnostic services have been provided, and in addition to grade level screening, follow-up service in the ear clinic. Recently, a jointly prepared medical referral letter has facilitated work with voice problems. School medical advisors of the Health Department are readily available for assistance with diagnosis and referral. In addition, these advisors frequently request therapist opinion on speech, hearing, and language problems under study.

Therapy schedules will be increased in Montgomery County to twice-weekly sessions when staff permits. In April 1967 a pilot program was offered in one high school, offering speech and hearing therapy from four until six p.m. two evenings a week. This program served children who were not served during the regular day or whose schools were not served or who needed other kinds of assistance. It appears to be a program filling an otherwise unmet need.

Freeman (1969) describes the Oakland Schools Plan, a speech and hearing clinic developed in the special education department of an intermediate unit.

The Polk County, Iowa, Board of Education serves an area with a school enrollment of about 65,000. Staffing to serve the communicatively handicapped in this county poses some real difficulties. During 1966–67 there were only five speech clinicians to serve 18,000 pupils. Each clinician carried a caseload of 50 to 56 pupils per week in six to 12 centers. Most pupils were seen individually on a twice-a-week basis. Other children were seen in groups, most usually of two, for a single half-hour session per week. Incidence was listed as from 3.4 percent to 7.2 percent. From 3 to 10 percent of pupils with identified speech problems were referred to other specialists.

In the effort to reach larger numbers of children and effect their speech and language development, a television series, "Speech Time," has been programmed for kindergarten and grade one. This is a 15-minute language development series broadcast morning and afternoon on Tuesdays, and afternoon on Tuesdays and Fridays each semester.

It was estimated that the hearing conservation program of Polk County was reaching only about one-third of the student population. During 1966–67, one hearing clinician supervised parents and nurses in the screening of 6,021 pupils from first, third, sixth, and ninth grades. Threshold audiometry was administered to 736 pupils in the follow-up testing. As a result, 111 children or about 1.7 percent were found in need of further study. The need for services thus demonstrated stimulated the submission of a two-year pilot project to study and implement the hearing conservation program for Polk County.

In New York State the Supervisory District is an interdistrict organization composed of one or more towns, which may be in different counties. Although it is now possible to include cities with 125,000 pupils as components, the usual population range is from about 2,000 to 65,000 pupils. Boards of Cooperative Educational Services were legislated in 1948, thus providing a new source of support from the state for shared programs. This arrangement permits more effective programs for children with special needs even though they may reside in small communities. The Board of Cooperative Educational Services in the First Supervisory District, Erie County, New York, may be cited. The Board has moved recently to the concept of a "language consultant" whose functions are conceived as broader than the correction of defective speech. (That language functions are becoming increasingly the concern of speech and hearing personnel in the schools cannot be questioned. Even the American Board of Examiners in Speech Pathology and Audiology (ABESPA) of the American Speech and Hearing Association has considered the possibility of needing to add the *L* for language in that program.)

The Board of Cooperative Educational Services has also employed speech correctionists to work with 45 classes of retarded youngsters. This reflects the trend in services to children with other handicaps previously often unserved by a speech and hearing clinician. In this program, the Board's Director of Special Educational Services plans to change gradually the designation of specialists from "speech-specialists" to "language-specialists" and eventually to "communication-specialists."

INFLUENCES IN PROGRAM DEVELOPMENT

The patterns of services to the communication-handicapped in the schools are subject to other influences. Those which affect the school setting change the working relationships within it. For example, major effects may be traced to federal influences.

Directions in which services to the speech and hearing handicapped are moving have been suggested by Haines (1965), who received replies to a questionnaire directed to all 50 State Departments of Education, the District of Columbia, and Puerto Rico. By 1963, four of five states which had certification under study previously, had now adopted certification standards. By mid-1963, 45 states required the public school clinician to hold a bachelor's degree or its equivalent. Only four reported that they required some work beyond the baccalaureate level. In 31 of the 45 states, the clinician is required to qualify for a regular teaching credential, on either the elementary or secondary level. In addition to his specialized preparation in 13 of the 45 states certifying speech clinicians, the requirements are judged to be equivalent to the 1964 ASHA standards for Basic Clinical Certification. The number of states using clinicians in their public schools has risen from 38 percent in 1953 to 86 percent in 1963. The requirement that a speech clinician also qualify for a teaching credential remained essentially constant—about 70 percent during the same period. The most significant trend reported by Haines was in the direction of qualitative improvement. All states using clinicians in their public schools now require the possession of a bachelor's degree or its equivalent, while two-thirds have requirements equalling ASHA standards for Basic Clinical Certification. There were, however, neglected areas in preparation for the management of voice disorders, organic disorders, and stuttering. Of 168 training institutions surveyed, 24 percent did not offer work in voice disorders, 15 percent offered none in organic disorders, and 18 percent offered none in stuttering. A more recent survey shows that the upgrading trend has continued (Causey, et al. 1971).

Black (1966) has noted that a large majority of

school children are not yet served. Since the greatest number of clients are to be found in the schools, she views the school clinician as a perennial pioneer. In tracing the origins and history of the profession, she also observed the growing awareness that speech programs for children must become preventive as well as rehabilitative. In a comment on the effectiveness of speech therapy, Black points out that in school populations where clinicians have worked ten or more years there is a reduction in the proportion of speech problems. Most of the caseload is below the fourth grade. The type of defects now reported also reflects a change. In Illinois the 1953 percentage for stutterers served was 7.4; 12 years later it was only three percent. Another change which underscores a vitally needed training objective is the increasing proportion of caseloads contributed by children with retarded language development. This shift undoubtedly reflects the move on the part of the schools to enroll more mentally retarded children and to begin substantial programs for the culturally disadvantaged. Black's discussion of the programs abroad provides some interesting contrasts as well as food for thought.

The Federal Government

Of the major influences upon education which have made their mark upon speech and hearing programs in the last decade, certainly actions of the Congress, must be given particular notice. Federal government influence has been felt directly as well as indirectly. During a national convention of the American Speech and Hearing Association, Spriestersbach spoke of "ASHA and Federal Programs: A Review of a Marriage" (1965). He commented, particularly, on federal programs designed to improve communication skills of culturally deprived children and asked whether the profession was doing all that it could and should do in the language area.

Since 1963 regional research centers have been conducting research into ways of achieving more effective pupil personnel services in the schools. These projects, under the Interprofessional Research Commission on Pupil Personnel Services (IRCOPPS) (1966), are located at several university sites in the United States. The Central Office collected information from more than 600 elementary and secondary schools to gain information about current practices in the use of various types of workers including speech and hearing personnel. In the center at the University of Maryland they have been concerned specifically with determining the kinds of problems, including speech, hearing, and language, with which teachers need help, and the types of help they desire. A major effort has been made to measure the effectiveness of the different types of pupil personnel members at the elementary school level.

When the National Association of Pupil Personnel Administrators was formed, speech and hearing services were included as one of the six services covered along with guidance, health, psychology, and social work. During 1964–65, the staff of IRC on PPS conducted a nationwide survey of role perceptions including those of speech and hearing specialists (*Asha*, 1967). Of 303 elementary principals participating, 77 percent said that they had speech and/or hearing specialists (only nurses were more often present). Of 289 secondary principals, 58 percent reported speech and hearing personnel. Nurses, counselors, and attendance personnel were more common. Of 248 speech and hearing specialists participating, 41 percent served elementary schools exclusively, 14 percent served secondary schools, and 45 percent served both levels. Twenty-eight of the respondents were male, almost one-half had master's degrees, and only one-third reported less than 10 hours of graduate work. It is an interesting professional note that speech and hearing personnel were more often affiliates of a national professional organization than were other pupil personnel workers. In terms of accessibility, 78 percent of speech and hearing specialists saw themselves as readily available to children and teachers needing their assistance. A like proportion of directors of pupil personnel services surveyed foresaw an expansion in the number of speech and hearing specialists. The directors also rated these services more highly than any other of the pupil personnel services.

With respect to the desirability of teaching experience, elementary principals gave it high value for all pupil personnel services, but of the teachers queried, only one-third felt teaching experience was mandatory for speech and hearing specialists, one-half thought it was desirable, but 18 percent thought it was not of great importance.

Speech and hearing personnel apparently meet with others for case conferences less often than the other pupil personnel workers responding. As compared with counselors, social workers, and psychologists, speech and hearing personnel more often see themselves as persons with a specific helping function which they usually carry out without need for a major amount of interprofessional communication.

They also receive direct referrals from teachers more frequently than do psychologists and social workers.

Public Law 89–10 may prove to be the most significant congressional act of the decade in its influence on the schools of the United States. The various titles of this legislation have been considered in professional journals (*Asha*, 1966). Project Headstart in particular motivated ASHA's executive secretary to issue a statement to stimulate speech and hearing personnel and ASHA established an *Ad Hoc* Committee on Guidelines for Speech and Hearing Services in Project Headstart (*Asha*, 1966). Since the Office of Economic Opportunity publications are not specific regarding the activities of speech and hearing personnel in Project Headstart, the ASHA *Ad Hoc* Committee has prepared a booklet, *Guidelines*, for use as an elaboration of existing OEO guides. Mackie (1966) has also outlined opportunities available for the handicapped under Title I of PL89–10.

It would not be feasible to relate specific accomplishments under Project Headstart directly bearing on the speech- and hearing-handicapped. The impact of this program beginning in the summer of 1965 in 2,398 communities and affecting more than one-half million children remains to be seen. After three years, some two and one-half million children, and about 800 million dollars, however, enough research data are available to accomplish evaluation. We do know that Headstart children gained significantly on such measures as the Peabody Picture Vocabulary Test and the Columbia Mental Maturity Scale, as well as on several tests of intellectual ability. There are, however, questions about the durability of such gains. Some evidence suggests that Headstart children entering middle class schools continue to show improvement while those entering ghetto schools seem to level off.

Two other titles of PL89–10 which have considerable potential for affecting the speech- and hearing-handicapped in the schools are Titles III-A and VI. Fifteen percent of the allocation to Title III is earmarked for projects concerned with the handicapped, and all of Title VI is so allocated.

Research efforts and services to the handicapped were assured more substantial support with the creation of the Bureau of Education for the Handicapped in the United States Office of Education. Current bureau programs support training for speech pathologists, audiologists, teachers, and other professional personnel. Grants for research in this field are provided as well as immediate services, including the Captioned Films for the Deaf Program. Marge (1968) considers the impact of five years of effort on the part of the Research and Demonstration Program.[4] Thirty-one projects funded to over three million dollars have been initiated in the area of speech and hearing. The Research and Development Grant awards in speech and hearing reflect clearly the stable growth in research in this area.

The types of research and development projects supported are discussed under four broad classifications:

1. Screening and longitudinal studies
2. Evaluations—tests and measurements
3. Automated and programmed instruction
4. Instructional media and prototype programs

Brief reference may be made to some representative projects which illustrate research and development efforts pertinent to these concerns.

Representative of projects under the first classification is the four-year National Prevalence Survey of Speech and Hearing Disorders in School Children being conducted by the Colorado State University. Illustrative of a project in the second category is the recently completed four-year project to develop a Predictive Screening Test for Children with Articulatory Speech Defects, under the direction of Van Riper. The development of a computer-assisted instruction terminal input for use in the training of audiologists will have as an additional end product a set of programmed materials suitable for computer storage.

"Training Speech Sound Discrimination in Children Who Misarticulate" is a three-year study to demonstrate the use of teaching machine techniques in speech correction. One of the five objectives of the study is an evaluation of the practical aspects of such a program for use in a clinic or a public school. Another project will develop, apply, and evaluate an automated speech-correction program designed to correct functional defects of articulation in elementary school children. Habilitation of the cleft-palate child is the objective of another demonstration project considering the feasibility of initiating remedial speech training as early as 18 months of age. At the State University of Iowa, a two-year study has attempted to develop a model speech program for children who stutter. A part of this project involves working with public school clinicians in defining problems of and developing procedures for an effective therapy program in the schools.

Federal support contributing to the ultimate benefit of the communicatively handicapped has

[4] Michael Marge, Research and Demonstration Projects in the Area of Speech and Hearing Supported through the United States Office of Education. Draft of paper for the 1968 convention of ASHA.

been reviewed by the late Congressman John E. Fogarty (Rhode Island) (1967). Fogarty describes the way federal programs are developed and briefly notes support under the National Institutes of Health, Vocational Rehabilitation Administration, the Children's Bureau, and the Neurological and Sensory Disease Service. Specifically relevant are the Model Secondary School for the Deaf at Gallaudet College, the National Institutes of Health Program in Human Communication, and the extramural, intramural, and cooperative, and field research, under the aegis of the National Institute for Neurological Disease and Blindness.

The Vocational Rehabilitation Administration Amendments of 1967 are of particular interest to the profession of speech pathology and audiology. Notably, a plan calls for the establishment of a National Center for Deaf-Blind Youth and Adults. This handicapped group will be provided with an intensive program of specialized services to prepare them for adult responsibilities and pleasures, and employment whenever possible. The Center will also conduct extensive programs of research, professional training, family orientation, and education, and will also provide an information service (*Asha*, 1968).

The Social Security Amendments of 1967 which became effective in January 1968 will also influence the schools' programs for handicapped children. The amendments consolidate the Maternal and Child Health Program and Crippled Children's Services into one program. The changes related to health manpower which extend the services of obstetric and pediatric medical personnel with various levels ot training presage new working relationships for speech and hearing specialists. Every state is now required to make services, including case finding, diagnoses, medical care, and hospitalization available to children in all areas of the state by 1975. The Child Health Act of 1967 consolidates existing authorizations and allocates one-half of the total for formula grants, 40 percent for project grants, and 10 percent for research and training. The 250,000 dollars apportioned for 1969 increases to 450,000 dollars in 1973 and thereafter.

Professional Associations

There is good reason to believe that public school clinicians will become increasingly involved in and contribute more effectively to research in their field. Anticipating this, and to build increased confidence and understanding in the design of research, a conference was held in New Orleans in January 1966 (*Asha*, 1966). In cooperation with ASHA, six lectures were presented to a subcommittee of ASHA and 40 speech pathologists and audiologists from the public school setting. Discussion groups explored a wide range of topics appropriate for research in public schools and considered problems involved in writing proposals and implementing research projects.

A Joint Committee on Audiology and Education of the Deaf held a series of regional meetings to strengthen the relationships between audiologists and educators of the deaf, encourage enlargement and improvement of audiological services to the deaf, and develop recommendations for improved services to a full range of hearing-handicapped persons. The Office of Education approved a 59,200-dollar grant for a study of current practices in the education of hard-of-hearing children. ASHA's continuing concern with professional development was reflected in the sponsorship of five regional workshops with special emphasis on school programs, early in 1971.

Tangible support for a continuing problem—appropriate accommodation of the speech and hearing program in the schools—was indicated in ASHA's Executive Council report (*Asha*, 1968). The Council recommended publication of the report "Recommendations for Speech Facilities in the Schools" and approved open meetings to explore in depth those problems related to speech and hearing services in the schools. School systems were also urged to eliminate minimum caseload standards and to set maximum caseload standards.

An influence of increasing significance to school programs for the speech- and hearing-handicapped are the state Speech and Hearing Associations. Marge (1967) has described some of their characteristics and notes their potential as both a professional and political force. Some examples of state Speech and Hearing Association actions illustrate the range of their influence. In California the cooperation of the California Speech and Hearing Association and the State Department of Education resulted in a new credential eliminating the previous requirement that personnel be trained both as classroom teachers and as speech and hearing clinicians. In Alabama members actively recruit promising professional workers as well as promising students for the profession. The Nebraska Association has established a library service for its members. Georgia members have taken an active interest in state and federal legislation. In Ohio members are encouraged to do more writing for state and national professional journals. Oregon's Association succeeded in obtaining the backing of the

Oregon Association of School Administrators and School Boards for the designation of a statewide day for professional meetings. In Vermont, the Association presented a caseload recommendation that includes consideration of the severity of speech problems making up a caseload rather than simply a specific number of cases.

State Departments of Education

In each of the states, departments of public instruction have been created and have developed to various degrees of elaboration. Within these departments are bureaus or divisions having responsibility for speech and hearing services which consult with county and local units of education. One of the roles of the state department of public instruction is that of assuring that local programs meet prescribed standards.

An examination of trends in state planning for children with communicative disorders was the subject of a conference sponsored by the United States Office of Education (Marge, 1966). Two elements of the conference relevant to this chapter are: 1) manpower needs of speech and hearing programs in the schools and 2) new directions in state planning for the provision of services for children with communication disorders. The conference addressed itself primarily to the traditional role of the speech and hearing clinician. Public school speech and hearing programs were perceived as being most effective when integrally related to the total educational program. Recognizing that the status of the speech and hearing programs is in transition from new and increasing demands with proportionately fewer personnel, the report sets forth guidelines for growth. The use of state consultants in the continuing professional development of local speech and hearing personnel is also considered.

The broadened scope of the school speech and hearing program is exemplified in this statement from the Commissioner of Education, Commonwealth of Pennsylvania:

> Programs directed toward speech and language development, improvement, and correction must be carried on as basic educational activities. Responsibilities for communication work with children who have delayed speech, retarded vocabulary development, and problems noted by the terms dyslexia, aphasia, brain damage, and minimal cerebral dysfunction, must be undertaken by the knowledgeable educator . . . We feel that the therapist serving a school performs his complete role only when he participates as a member of the educational staff.

In this same report, Garbee suggests that the profession will build new directions in state planning based on successes. Enumerating the successes, he notes first that speech and hearing services are now an integral part of the public school system. Commenting on the positive and unique characteristics of the schools as a setting for these services, he cites successes in particular with certain communication disorders, such as articulation problems and as members of cleft-palate teams. Gains in credentialing requirements are another favorable development at the state level. Some success is also reported in reducing caseloads. We appear to be more aware of the need for a thorough assessment and appraisal of children. As a basis for providing new directions, Garbee also mentions several of our failures. The major thesis of this paper is that planning for new services must be based on genuine respect, understanding, support, and complementation of the total educational program for the individual child without dissipation or sacrifice of the specialized services of the speech and hearing program. Especially noted are the needs for interprofessional rapport and for interpretation to administrators of the speech and hearing program contribution to the education of children.

If clinicians are unprepared for their roles in the schools, appropriate in-service should be provided and meaningful preservice training initiated. Garbee would also encourage college personnel to apply for federal funding for special study institutes and training grants. Research activity among public schools is considered not just a help but a "must" in determining adequate services for children. Adequate supervision must be provided for local programs. School clinicians must keep informed about various channels of support. The development of complementary diagnostic centers will be efficacious in some regions. Future directions may also include the services of speech and language development specialists. Very important to the full development of speech and hearing services in the schools is the achievement of coordination of all pupil services.

Ohio's program for hearing-handicapped children is described by Hartwig and Jones (1966). School districts in Ohio are permitted under statutory provisions to provide for the education of hearing-impaired children. Those which can provide and maintain adequate programs are encouraged to do so. The day school programs for the deaf consequently become "centered," usually in the larger metropolitan areas. If a local school district cannot provide the special education services, placement may be requested in another school district.

Children with hearing impairment which may necessitate special education may be identified in the hearing screening program of the local school or through clinics conducted by a Health Department, privately financed speech and hearing centers and clinics, speech and hearing centers in colleges and universities, social welfare agencies, outpatient clinics of hospitals, or through programs of the Society for Crippled Children.

Appropriate placement for eligible children may be found in programs of the local school system, or in some instances, in the Ohio School for the Deaf. A child with normal hearing may be appointed to assist a hearing-impaired child in classroom participation, in locating correct pages, in writing assignments, and in checking his understanding of oral directions. It is considered desirable that one system of teaching speech, language, lipreading, auditory training, and all regular subject matter be adopted. Children with mild hearing impairment, not eligible for special class placement, are enrolled in regular classrooms. The speech therapist often includes these children in her caseload and consults with the classroom teacher. Supportive services usually emphasize lipreading, drill, and practice, auditory training, and language improvement.

The Ohio plan for children with speech and hearing problems is described by MacLearie (1964). The legal basis for the establishment of speech and hearing therapy programs is found in the Ohio Revised Code. For financial support the state provides that special education units for speech and hearing therapy are additional units above the number of teaching units to which a district may be entitled under the foundation program. Minimum standards have been adopted by the State Board of Education. Administrators are encouraged to set goals for their programs beyond these minimums. MacLearie also discusses the evaluation of professional growth and teaching effectiveness of the speech and hearing therapists and their qualifications.

CONTRIBUTIONS OF RESEARCH

Case Selection

The determination by the speech clinician of those children who will be enrolled in a therapy program remains one of the most important and demanding tasks. The efficacy of various procedures has been extensively considered. The literature contains references to professional opinion and some research for use as guidelines. Considered a controversial issue, the problem of case selection in the public schools was deliberated by seven established clinicians (Allen et al., 1966). They were asked: "What guidelines do you use in determining which children should be enrolled in a clinical speech program?" and "What tests of articulation have you found to be appropriate and predictive for children in the primary grades?" Briefly summarized, it may be reported that in general, single-element testing, such as testing the ability of a child to produce a sound in isolation, was not regarded as an adequate diagnosis of need.

It was apparent however, that clinicians had favorite instruments which were used in combination with some other information. One respondent found the Carter-Buck Nonsense Syllable Test reliable for prognosis. Although most standard articulation tests were regarded as weak predictors of speech growth, the McDonald Deep Test was thought to approach the ideal. The clinicians also felt it necessary to consider the type of program available for the child when considering case selection.

The problems involved in case selection and differences in procedures followed by clinicians in the schools are described by Webster and others (1966). The wide range of criteria employed is clearly shown and the cruciality of case selection in the public schools is underscored. The prognostic value of the Carter-Buck test in selecting kindergarten children is considered by Kisatsky (1967). Requiring the .01 level for rejection of the null hypothesis he found over a six-month period without speech therapy that the high stimulation group made a significant improvement in articulation skills. This group had corrected 59 percent of their original errors.

In the continuing search for timesaving devices in case selection, Fristoe and Goldman (1968) compared traditional articulation tests with a condensed version, examining the same number of sounds. Recorded speech samples were presented to judges under two listening conditions: listening for only one sound per sample word compared to listening to one, two, or three sounds. It was concluded that speech clinicians can listen effectively for more than one sound per word. Thus a condensed test of articulation is a useful addition to existing speech evaluation materials. Goldman and Fristoe (1966, 1967) have given additional consideration to this problem.

Henrikson (1968) suggests another criterion for case selection, that of "learning by the clinician," and evaluates a rationale for considering such a criterion. He observes that the school clinician functions in patterns and operates under time pressures which are different from those prevailing in colleges and universities. He argues that continuing growth as a clinician is a valid criterion for such a suggestion. In this provocative proposal, self-learning becomes consciously a primary goal at times, and the clinician systematically conducts a series of experiments.

In a further effort at reducing time spent in articulation testing without sacrificing reliability, Irwin and Musselman (1962) devised a picture articulation test to check more than one sound per word. The test of 27 words includes all of the consonants in the initial and final positions, all of the vowels, and all of the diphthongs. The study procedure provided for applications by experienced as well as inexperienced examiners. It was concluded that the tests devised for the study may be used to evaluate more than one error in a word with reliability by both experienced and inexperienced judges. Moreover, the test required only one-half as much time to administer as the equivalent items from a conventional test.

Although the typical caseload of the public school clinician contains a large proportion of children from the primary grades, there remains the need to screen carefully in the upper elementary grades. Avant and Hutton (1962) constructed a passage which could be read with ease by most fourth-graders. Vocabulary for the passage was drawn from the Row-Peterson basic primer and first- and second-grade readers, and from the first 1,000 words of the Rinsland list (1945). Consideration was given to frequency of occurrence and frequency of error of speech sounds. The 123-word passage was read quickly and without difficulty by the fourth-grade subjects in the study. The mean reading time was one minute, 14 seconds. Six scoring procedures were evaluated.

Public school clinicians frequently depend upon the classroom teacher's opinion for referral and as a criterion for gauging improvement in articulation. Differences between articulation test measures and other listeners' ratings of speech are often noted. Jordan (1960) attempted to evaluate relationships between measures of defectiveness of articulation obtained from articulation test responses and those obtained from listener ratings of short samples of connected speech in a multiple regression analysis. The dependent variable was the scaled severity of articulation defectiveness while the independent variables were 22 measures obtained from articulation test responses and the age of each subject. The conclusions merit the attention of the school clinician: 1) articulation test responses under the conditions of the experiment provide valid information on articulatory behavior in connected speech; 2) reactions of listeners to articulation effectiveness are primarily dependent on two factors—frequency with which articulatory deviations occur and degree of articulatory deviations; 3) to the listener, omissions are more deviant than substitutions and substitutions more deviant than distortions; and 4) articulation test measures of number of defective items and number of defective single sounds are both highly related to measures of defectiveness of articulation derived from listener responses to connected speech.

The selection of children whose articulation competence indicates a need for therapy and for determining some priority for assignment requires the clinician to render a judgment on the basis of a limited amount of information. Typically, some form of articulation test—either one of those commercially produced or a homemade version—constitute a primary instrument. It has been observed that these tests differ in the choice and order of sounds tested as well as in the stimulus that is used and method of stimulus presentation. Siegel and others (1963) investigated the influence of the test instrument used on the responses of the children. Forty test sounds, each tested in two words, were selected as the test items. The sounds selected were those frequently misarticulated according to Templin (1947) and Roe and Milisen (1942). Sounds were included only if they could be presented in pictures that would be familiar to kindergarten children. The subjects were 50 children drawn randomly from a population about to enter two kindergarten classes, who were free from gross physical abnormality, and who came from monolingual homes. Of the 40 chi-square values, only three (final /l/, initial /sw/, and initial /θ/) were significant, that is, these words cannot be considered equal in difficulty. All phi-coefficients were significantly greater than zero except those for medial /dʒ/ and /l/. In a second experiment with 100 kindergarten children, imitative and spontaneous methods of word presentation were compared during articulation testing. The method of stimulus presentation was related to accuracy of production in eight of the 40 sounds tested.

It would seem obvious that there are differences between children who outgrow their misarticulation spontaneously and those who do not do so. Differentiating between these populations is a demand made routinely upon the public school clinician. Dickson (1962) examined for differences in first-, second-, and third-grade children who the year before, as kindergarten, first- and second-grade pupils, had been judged to have functional articulation defects. He studied differences in the performance of 30 children who outgrew spontaneously their functional articulation errors and 30 children who had retained some of the errors. Measures were obtained from the Oseretsky Tests of Motor Proficiency and the Templin Short Test of Sound Discrimination. The Minnesota Multiphasic Inventory was administered to the parents of the children. The results indicate that children who retain speech errors are inferior in gross motor tasks to those who outgrow errors. Speech-sound discrimination ability did not differentiate between the two groups. There are some indications that mothers of children who retain errors tend toward "emotional immaturity and instability" more than do the mothers of children who outgrow their speech errors.

Articulation-Discrimination

Equivocal findings are not uncommon in research relating to poor auditory discrimination and functional articulation disorder. Bearing in mind certain criticisms of previous research, Aungst and Frick (1964) designed a study to investigate the hypothesis that for children eight years of age or older and who misarticulate the /r/ sound only, consistency of articulation is more directly related to the ability to judge one's own speech productions as correct or incorrect than the ability to discriminate between paired auditory stimuli presented by another speaker. Subjects who met the experimental criteria were obtained from caseloads of public school clinicians. A 50-item "deep test" of articulation for /r/ was used for subject selection. Four different tests of auditory discrimination constructed for this study were administered to each subject. It was concluded that for subjects who meet the criteria used that: 1. the ability to discriminate between paired auditory stimuli presented by another speaker is unrelated to the ability to judge one's own speech productions as correct or incorrect; 2. the ability measured by the traditional tests of speech sound discrimination is not related to consistency of articulation; and 3. the ability to judge one's own speech productions is significantly related to the consistency of articulation. Tests of the ability to judge one's own speech production should therefore prove valuable in diagnosis, therapy, and research.

Using a control group design and children from grades one, two, and three having severe functional articulation problems, Cohen and Diehl (1963) attempted to replicate a previous study which had shown a reliable relationship between auditory discrimination and articulation. In general, the results were confirmatory. As a group, first-, second-, and third-grade children with severe functional articulation type defects show significantly more errors in speech-sound discrimination than a matched group of children with normal articulation. Speech-sound discrimination ability tends to improve with grade level; however, a speech-defective group at equivalent grade levels continues to perform inferiorly to a group of normally speaking children. Sherman and Geith (1967) studied this relationship with a kindergarten population. The experimental subjects were selected on the basis of high or low scores on the 50-item speech-sound discrimination test of Templin. The 18 high scorers selected and the 18 low scorers were given the Templin-Darley 176-item Picture Articulation Test. The children with high speech-sound discrimination scores were significantly (.001 level) superior to the low group in articulation skill. The authors conclude that it is a reasonable assumption that low speech-sound discrimination ability is an etiological factor in articulation disorder and therefore valuable information in the diagnostic process. They do not feel that the significant difference between the two groups on the Peabody Picture Vocabulary Test scores is necessarily indicative of a meaningful relationship between articulation and intelligence. Two explanations are offered: 1. taking only the very top discriminators from a large group is a highly selective device, and 2. poor speech-sound discrimination may result in perceptual confusion of some dictated words which lend themselves to such confusion.

Pitch discrimination also may contribute to articulation proficiency. Sommers and others (1961) investigated pitch discrimination in school children with functional articulation errors in grades three through 12. Subjects having articulation errors on either /r/ or /s/ were matched to a group of normally speaking subjects on the basis of I.Q., sex, and grade.

The pitch subtest of the Tilson-Gretsch Music Test was administered to each subject following standard procedures. Children with functional misarticulations were found to be poorer in mean pitch discrimination than normal subjects. No evidence was found of a difference between the group misarticulating /r/ and the group misarticulating /s/ on mean pitch discrimination scores. Matching variables were found to be ineffective in increasing the precision of the experimental design.

The relationship between articulation and speech-sound discrimination was studied within a learning framework by Winitz and Bellerose (1962). The subjects were 72 fourth-grade public school children. The English sound /sh/ and the non-English sound /ç/ were selected as test stimuli. Discrimination learning was studied as a function of three pretraining conditions: 1. correct reinforcement, 2. incorrect reinforcement, and 3. no reinforcement of a speech sound (control group). Discrimination learning involved a two-bar successive discrimination of the /sh/ and the /ç/ sounds. No evidence was obtained to support the hypothesis that discrimination was reduced following incorrect reinforcement. It was noted, however, that subjects assigned to the pretraining condition of incorrect reinforcement continued to utter the incorrect response when it was reinforced. This finding suggests that the study of articulation behavior from a learning model might have implications for both the teaching and understanding of articulation modification. In a subsequent study (1963) using 200 first- and second-grade children, the pretraining conditions were so constructed as to permit the correct and incorrect learning of the syllable /vrou/, that is /vrou/ for /vrou/ and /brou/ for /vrou/. Findings indicate that discrimination learning was significantly impaired following incorrect learning of the chosen syllable. A significant difference favoring the second grade was obtained when pretraining groups were combined. Sex differences for grades and for groups were not significant. From the evidence it appears that tests of speech-sound discrimination may measure in addition to developmental skills the learned equivalents and distinctiveness of speech sounds.

In an article bearing on this issue, Locke (1968) developed a paradigm of defective sound learning and its subsequent correction, which can be entered at several points for study. Fundamental to this position is his statement that "From an acoustic point of view, disordered articulation is best considered in terms of ease of articulation." This is to say that defective articulation may be a problem of production rather than perception. The theories of acquired equivalence and acquired distinctiveness of cues are presented as particularly effectual models in terms of their capacity to explain certain normal and deviant articulation learning. Articulation therapy is considered then as an application of the acquired distinctiveness model. The effect of distinctive feature pretraining in phoneme discrimination learning was studied by Winitz and Preisler (1967). Procedures that might prove to be effective in teaching difficult sound discriminations were considered in two separate experiments; primary emphasis was placed upon distinctive stimuli pretraining. In addition, the effect of verbal unit and the effect of distinctive stimuli order was studied. Subjects in Experiment I were first- and second-grade children who would be classified as coming from families of "middle" socioeconomic status. Subjects in Experiment II were second-grade children coming from families of "lower-lower" socioeconomic status. In Experiment I, groups were pretrained on sounds that differed markedly in phonetic features but which did not provide a graded sequence of progressively smaller phonetic differences. In Experiment II the effectiveness of distinctive stimuli pretraining was replicated with different sounds and with a different set of children. In the second experiment, the subjects pretrained on markedly different sounds significantly outperformed a group not so trained. All tasks were administered by automatic programming devices. Findings indicate that pretraining procedures can be used to increase effectively the learning of difficult discriminations.

THE EVOLVING ROLE OF THE SCHOOL CLINICIAN

The role of the public school clinician is clearly one that is undergoing progressive modification. One of the most pervasive influences is the rapidity with which special programs have been developed in the last twenty years. The statement drafted by the 1963 Committee on Speech and Hearing Services in the Schools and approved by the Executive Council of ASHA clarifies this role (*Asha*, 1964). The needs of children with inadequately developed speech and language skills are differentiated from those with speech-handicapping disorders. Clinical speech services are viewed apart from speech improvement. The functions of the speech clinician in special services are:

> To identify the children who require special services; provide these services through identification and selection of children for therapy and a clinical program of diagnosis, direct and indirect remedial methods, and consultative services . . . In addition the speech clinician may have some responsibilities for the development and conduct of research and for assistance in the training of other personnel for the field. (p. 190.)

Although he will serve as a consultant to the speech improvement program, the primary responsibility is in clinical speech services. The statement is extended to include the importance of collaboration with other disciplines.

> In providing for these needs, the professional knowledge and skills of several disciplines are used. The effectiveness with which the needs of children are met depends to a large degree on how advantageously the special skills of the various groups of professional workers are used . . . The basic responsibilities of the speech clinician do not differ whether these are discharged in a hospital, a community clinic, a rehabilitation unit or a public school. (p. 191.)

Even though there are more speech specialists in the public schools than in other work environments, there are as yet serious disagreements concerning the appropriate responsibilities of these specialists. Ainsworth (1965), using two previous articles as a point of departure, outlines two points of view—the clinician as a "separatist" and the clinician as a "participant." He notes that the former view has logical appeal when we look at the way other professionals see us. Some fear that the "participant" view may lead to further identification as a kind of "teacher." He suggests that the "separatist" point of view appears essentially negative and restrictive while the "participant" model provides constructive possibilities for leadership. He draws some implications for training, offers content and experiences for work in the schools, points out evidences of need, and makes suggestions for ways to include training for clinical speech in schools.

Van Hattum (1966) has proposed that the effectiveness of the school programs for communication handicaps may be influenced by the self-concepts held by the clinicians. Five issues are examined which he considers the concern of the clinician working in the public elementary and secondary schools. In brief, these issues are that his training is not appropriate for the tasks confronting him, some of the training is inadequate, he does not get research help or practical advice, he feels that the association he supports does not meet his needs, and he feels that his professional colleagues do not respect him. Several courses of action are offered for consideration.

The attitudes of speech clinicians in the public schools were investigated by Weaver (1968), who mailed questionnaires to various school districts in a dozen states. A 62 percent return was achieved. In ranking positions according to their importance, 89 percent ranked the classroom teacher first, the public school clinician second, the college instructor third, "other" speech clinicians fourth, and special education teachers fifth. However, in selecting "level of importance" on a five-point scale, 41 percent reported feeling that public school speech therapy was of the "highest importance"; 52 percent reported a feeling of "significant importance." Sixty-nine percent believed themselves capable of working with language disorders. Eighty-six percent reported that the public school clinician was capable of doing research and 89 percent felt that he should do so. Caseload requirements were the most consistently suggested problem, but the need for adequate facilities and the shortage of required personnel were also noted.

The Clinician's Training

Training programs must of course be modified continuously if they are to prepare persons properly for the role of the public school clinician. The status of education and training programs in speech pathology and audiology was reported by Castle, Johnson, and Neuman (1966). When the 1966 survey information is compared to earlier data, increases in both number and size of programs is noted. There has been expansion in graduate level training—40 percent of earned degrees in speech pathology and audiology were at the graduate level compared to 24 percent in 1960. Most existing programs felt an immediate need for further growth. Federal legislation has contributed to the growth and is expected to alleviate some current drawbacks. Oyer and Davis (1967) conducted a dialogue on education and service needs in the profession. Both general and specific needs were dealt with. The recent series of Special Reports (*Asha*, 1968) on preprofessional education in speech pathology and audiology serve as an excellent roundup of existing training efforts at that level.

The Effectiveness of the Clinician

The effects of speech therapy on school children have been studied from different points of view and with mixed results. Irwin (1962) was specifically interested in the effects of speech therapy for second-grade children with functional misarticulations upon 1. articulatory adequacy, 2. reading readiness, 3. word recognition, and 4. word meaning. Criteria were differences between pretest and posttest scores over an experimental period of seven months. She found no evidence from which to draw definite conclusions. In a subsequent study of the effectiveness of speech therapy on linguistic skills of first-grade children (1963), Irwin's findings were in agreement with the previous investigation. Although trends favored the children receiving therapy, the measured effects of a twice-a-week program administered over a seven-month period were not statistically significant, that is, the linguistic skills considered were not significantly affected.

Since every clinician must at some time make a judgment to continue or dismiss from therapy each client served, these criteria become an important program attribute. The time at which dismissal is considered may not always be the point at which completely normal speech patterns have been acquired. Although the clients involved are adults, a study by Siegenthaler and others (1962) has relevance for the work of the public school clinician. In this investigation of the relationships obtaining between the speech status of patients and the recommendations made by clinicians regarding dismissal, it was found that factors other than speech status contribute to the decision to terminate therapy.

Sommers and others (1966) were interested in the effectiveness of group and individual therapy for articulation disorder with two factors involved: 1. the degree of speech defect—total number of misarticulated phonetic contexts using McDonald's Deep Test (1959) and 2. the grade level of the subjects. It was also postulated that subjects enrolled in the second grade would profit equally from group or individual therapy. There were 12 experimental groups. Group articulation therapy consisted of one session of 45 minutes weekly, and individual articulation therapy was provided once weekly for a 30-minute period. It was concluded that individual and group therapy were equally effective, independent of either the grade level or the degree of articulatory defect. Generally, children with "moderate" speech problems were found to improve more than those having "mild" problems.

Sommers and others (1967) also studied factors related to the effectiveness of articulation therapy for kindergarten and first- and second-grade children. Subjects were selected for inclusion in the study by 20 speech clinicians. Children selected were those who had prognostic scores of 25 percent or less (modified Carter-Buck), 60 percent or better, half with "mild" defectiveness, and half with "moderate" defectiveness. Classes in the study received one 45-minute session of group articulation therapy weekly during the eight and one-half months of the study. Groups ranged in size from three to five. On an average, children received 29 speech therapy lessons during the period and clinicians served 12 subjects. Although the variables of grade level and severity of defectiveness did not interact to influence the effectiveness of therapy, the significant interaction of Therapy by Stimulability proved to be in the hypothesized direction, that is, subjects with poor stimulability scores improved significantly as a result of speech correction compared with subjects having good stimulability scores. It is also apparent that regardless of stimulability scores, subjects who received speech therapy improved significantly compared with those who did not. It appears that the effectiveness of correction was dependent neither upon the grade level of the subjects nor the severity of their speech problems. Stimulability was found to be a significant factor in articulation improvement for all second-grade subjects and one group of first-grade subjects.

The articulation program, which typically constitutes the greatest time commitment in the school's speech therapy program, has been under scrutiny frequently to justify its emphasis as well as to develop its effectiveness. Nichols (1964) has examined the time allocation in the articulation program. He reviewed research showing the effects on children's articulation from the use of "supplementary" clinicians such as classroom teachers and parents. He also noted that prognostic testing shows promise of allowing the clinician to concentrate on those children most in need of therapy. He observes that children have been shown to improve their articulation without therapy and cites the predictive validity of the Steer and Drexler approach. In relation to Carter-Buck testing, he points out the considerable amount of time required for administration and that even in the first grade the group that was not stimulable did not respond to speech therapy. He concludes that: 1. participation of teachers in the articulation therapy program via speech improvement routines may contribute to the effectiveness of therapy and shorten the time needed for correction of faulty articulation; 2. parents may be effective as supplementary clinicians (although further research is indicated here); and 3. prognostic testing offers the opportunity to accept for therapy children who would probably not improve without help.

Pronovost (1966), concerned with case selection in the articulation program, suggests an inconsistency when clinicians screen to detect misarticulations which teachers would miss but who then settle for helping most stutterers to live with their stuttering. He proposes that we differentiate between "impairment" and "handicap" and shows preference for definitions found in the Rehabilitation Codes. He infers that therapists may have lost their perspective on what constitutes a "speech problem." He recommends a test battery for those primary-grade children with low articulatory proficiency scores, that is, with three or more misarticulated sounds.

PROGRAM EVALUATION

The considerable investment in professional effort and financial support for speech and hearing programs requires that their effectiveness be subjected to study. As a professional organization most concerned, the American Speech and Hearing Association, through its Research Committee, applied to the United States Office of Education for grant support to conduct an appropriate study. The product of the subsequent research effort is reported in the document "An Evaluation of Speech and Hearing Programs in the Schools" (Rees, 1967). The long-range objective of the study was to conduct an intensive longitudinal evaluation of selected speech and hearing programs located in a variety of cultural settings throughout the United States. Acknowledged as one of the unresolved issues in school therapy programs is the age or grade level at which a child should receive assistance. This issue is pertinent primarily to children with functional articulation deviation in the primary grades. It is significant in relation to the efficiency and effectiveness of school programs in which average caseloads are comprised of 81 percent articulation problems and in view of the fact that about three-fourths of school clinicians work mainly with children in kindergarten and first and second grades.

The literature review contained in the report reveals that developmental norms leave much to be desired. Most are based on chronological age and do not account adequately for other variables affecting learning. Also, failure to identify subgroups within the broad category of articulation deviations may introduce conflicting data about relations between speech and other language disabilities. Objective data about the effects of therapy on articulatory skills are not extensive enough to furnish guidelines for results that might be expected in school speech and hearing programs.

Among the conclusions drawn from the exploration of this problem were: 1. a tremendous body of information must be developed before school speech and hearing programs can be evaluated with respect to standards for efficient and effective practices; 2. surveys are not suitable for deriving this information; 3. standard research procedures are difficult to implement in schools; and 4. new ways of meeting a problem of this magnitude need to be explored.

Section II of the report considers an alternate procedure for resolving some of the issues. A research center designed specifically to encourage and assist school clinicians to engage in research appears to be potentially a partial solution to these problems. The second phase of this project is devoted to a process of evolving and testing a model for such a center. Two kinds of results are reported. One set pertains directly to the model itself; the second set consists of the research projects completed or the plans and procedures developed for research still in progress. The projects illustrate that a research center for school clinicians is a feasible approach to research related to school speech and hearing problems. Such a center has the potential for developing a unified and coordinated approach to resolving many of the issues pertaining to these programs. It is a practical and workable concept.

THE USE OF NONPROFESSIONALS

The limited supply of professional speech and hearing personnel, a condition which is likely to persist, requires that other means of program extension be explored. The use of mothers trained as aides offers some promise as a therapy adjunct. Sommers

(1962) describes the effects obtained from training mothers of children with functional misarticulations. Support was found for the observation that the trained mothers can be effective adjuncts in the therapy process. The data do support the contention that training mothers may be a more valuable clinical procedure than attempting to arrange articulation therapy for each child on an individual basis. Evidence was also found to support the efficacy of training mothers of slow-learning children.

Following suggestions by other investigators that attitudes toward childrearing practices tend to be less favorable in parents of children with functional misarticulations, Sommers and others (1964) studied a population of 80 children and 80 mothers. Time spent training mothers to assist in the correction of articulatory error was found to be clinically valuable in the correction of such problems. It was also concluded in part, that:

training was as effective for mothers with "unhealthy" attitudes as it was for mothers with "healthy" attitudes. Children of mothers with "healthy" attitudes improved significantly compared with children of mothers with "unhealthy" attitudes. Children of mothers trained by a speech clinician to assist in speech correction improved significantly compared with children of mothers not trained.

In view of a limited amount of time the speech and hearing specialist has for direct work with children, the utility of using inexperienced examiners in the program needs consideration. Siegel (1962) reports an investigation in which he found it not only expedient but practical to train inexperienced examiners to a satisfactory level of proficiency. He found that the inexperienced examiners not only agreed with themselves but correlated well with more experienced and trained examiners. The Templin-Darley screening articulation test was used. The subjects used were institutionalized mentally retarded children. It was noted, however, that reliability did not necessarily guarantee examiner equivalence since examiners did tend to differ significantly in absolute scores assigned to the children. Student therapy "teams" may offer some relief for service problems common in rural situations (Wingo, 1970).

In an excellent discussion of the parameters of the issue of supportive personnel in speech pathology and audiology, Irwin (1967) cites the report of the 1959 ASHA Committee on Legislation. Even using Linder's conservative estimate (three percent), the need for the 1970 projected population of 217,127,000 would be 27,500 specialists. He concludes that "the real supply has not met the real demand and cannot meet the potential demand." Education and training facilities cannot meet the need. Among the more promising alternative solutions for alleviation is the use of supportive personnel. Irwin considers some of the problems to be faced and notes the urgent need to study the problem and to come up with appropriate decisions. He urges that tentative standards be set quickly but proposes study and discussion as immediate goals, rather than setting of rigid standards.

Ptacek (1967) discusses supportive personnel as an extension of the professional worker's nervous system. He notes certain advantages over machines as well as some distinct disadvantages. A primary advantage is that through proper selection and training they can extend the "systems" in ways not possible for machines to duplicate. As warm, responsive, compassionate human beings they can provide the professional worker with a crucial extension by the establishment and maintenance of a relationship with a person in need. Ptacek also observes that the federal government is committed to the concept of supportive personnel. A pilot project on the use of supportive personnel in speech correction was undertaken in Colorado during 1967–68 and reported by Alpiner (1970).

In September 1967 the American Speech and Hearing Association, in cooperation with the University of Maryland, sponsored, with support from the United States Office of Education, an Institute on Utilization of Supportive Personnel in School Speech and Hearing Programs. Comprehensive work sessions centered around actual and potential roles, including problems in defining the role or designing job descriptions for such personnel, relationships between supportive personnel and the professionals, and qualifications needed in supervisors.

Another extensive treatment of this topic appears in a Special Report (*Asha*, 1967) which contains condensations of speeches presented at the Conference on the Use of Non-professionals in Mental Health Work, Washington D.C., May 3–5, 1967. In the overview it is noted that in spring 1967 there were 75,000 new nonprofessionals. The Scheuer-Nelson Sub-Professional Career Act appropriates 70 million dollars to hire and train more unemployed persons in public service. Some of the issues needing study are outlined by Goldberg (Information Retrieval Center on the Disadvantaged). Bertrand Beck, Executive Director, Mobilization for Youth Incorporated, talks about a professional approach, noting that no consensus has been reached on the role of the social welfare worker without full formal education. Robert Reiff (Albert Einstein College of Medicine) considers the social consequences of professionalism and nonprofessionalism. He warns that if the professions resist these developments, the new careers movement is in danger of being aborted.

INCREASING RESPONSIBILITIES FOR SCHOOL SPEECH AND HEARING PERSONNEL

The influx of more severely disabled groups in the schools will increase the need for more concentrated therapy programs. Clinicians will undoubtedly need more opportunity for refresher courses and will probably be more often involved in experimental studies. Jerger and Speaks (1967), in a review of research, report a trend toward increased participation and an apparent willingness on the part of researchers to tackle some of the problems speech clinicians face daily in the public schools.

Serving the Mentally Retarded

The number of mentally retarded individuals attending public schools will continue to increase. Probably all except the ultimate fraction of "custodial" types will spend some portion of their first 21 years in a special education school setting. The extent of communication disability among the mentally retarded has been adequately documented in the reviews by Matthews (1957) and Spradlin (1963).

Even though the evidence suggests a significantly greater incidence of speech defects among institutionalized mentally defective children than among those enrolled in the public schools, these pupils will provide substantial caseloads. The research reported in Monograph Supplement No. 10 (1963) provides useful information. The section prepared by Spradlin (pp. 8–31), on the assessment of speech and language including the Parsons Language Sample (PLS), is especially pertinent to public school personnel. The PLS is described as an objective instrument that does not require an examiner with extensive training or background for its administration. It gives evidence of being a reliable instrument with validity for predicting nontest language behavior in retarded children.

Much direct help as well as supportive aid will be rendered to the mentally retarded pupil by his teachers. Freeman and Lukens (1962) describe a speech and language program for educable mentally handicapped children. A coordinated interdisciplinary offering has been developed for the schools. Essentially it provides for the individual diagnosis of speech problems by the speech specialist and the formulation and direction of a plan for improving communication skills. Speech and language are taught as a part of the regular classroom curriculum. It is a responsibility of classroom teachers to cooperate in the formulation and execution of a curriculum for oral communication. A salient feature of the curriculum provided is that it must provide many "opportunities for extremely frequent repetition of meaningful communication experiences."

Speech through color as an aid in speech improvement for the mentally retarded has been proposed by Wood (1965). Since no more knowledge of speech than the classification of consonants as breath, voiced, and nasal is needed, the special class teacher should be able to apply this procedure.

One part of a two-phase study of articulation among educable mentally retarded children in a public school setting serves to emphasize the lack of a simple relationship between articulatory ability and mental age. Wilson (1966) found that substitution and omission errors tended to decrease with increasing mental age, but distortion errors increased in phase two of the study. The effects of articulation therapy on sound-error production over a three-year period proved nondifferentiating for experimental, placebo, and control groups.

The growth of programs for trainable mentally retarded children has resulted in new demands for speech therapy requiring consideration in the school speech and hearing program. Clinicians would do well to note the literature review prepared by Zisk and Bialer (1967). The research and theory on speech problems of mongoloid retardates are considered under four major headings: symbolization, articulation, rhythm, and phonation. An attempt is made to link possible predisposing mongoloid stigmata with specific deviations. In a study of auditory discrimination, Schlanger and Galanowsky (1966) found that institutionalized mentally retarded children performed significantly more poorly than normals matched for mental age on all tests given both as a total group and in mental age groups.

A speech and hearing program conducted under a state agency jurisdiction is described by Rittmanic (1966). Surveys were conducted in representative

State Schools and Hospitals in Illinois to determine the need for and feasibility of providing comprehensive speech and hearing services for the institutionalized mentally ill and mentally retarded. Results of the speech examination in the state schools for the mentally retarded and brain injured revealed that 90 percent of the 4,437 patients tested at Dixon and Lincoln State Schools had speech and/or language disorders ranging from mild articulation defects to severe problems of delayed language and mutism. Fifty-one percent of the 3,700 testable patients had hearing losses which were medically significant ranging from borderline to profound deafness. Twenty percent of the hearing-impaired subjects did require a program of speech, language, and/or hearing therapy. In the various mental hospitals, 31 percent had speech and language disorders ranging from mild to severe. The incidence of auditory impairment was approximately 12 percent.

At Dixon State School the clinical program includes speech examinations, audiological evaluations, speech and hearing therapy, and speech improvement and language development activities conducted within both academic school setting and in certain rehabilitation wards, nurseries, and halfway houses. At the Charles Read Zone Center, the first of eight planned, the speech and hearing program is an important part of the overall comprehensive multidisciplinary program which minimizes rigid distinctions among the various specialities.

Serving the Emotionally Disturbed

As more seriously deviant children become more frequently enrolled in the public schools, the need for increased awareness and sensitivity on the part of the school staff becomes critical. Communication problems are frequent concomitants in disturbed youngsters, and speech and hearing personnel offer an important resource. Schulz (1965) provides some suggested responsibilities in relation to the autistic child in the school. She notes that speech development may be late, of nonsense pattern, and meaningless. Echolalia or parroting is common. Extremely literal use of concepts or terms is found. These children are often thought to have a hearing loss, and mental retardation is often suspected. Where there is no retardation, the child may compensate readily. Stamp (1966) lists nine behavior characteristics usually observed in autistic children and suggests ways a teacher may begin communication with the child on a nonverbal basis. She states that an autistic child should be in a group only as long as the teacher can watch for opportunities for contact. Ignoring the child may only increase his tendency toward isolation.

The incidence of emotional handicap in schools is not known with any real precision. Children are identified as such, however, in various ways, and the public has determined that special education programs will be created. These may be justified on various grounds; for example, academic retardation, severe behavioral problems, or as devices to exclude the disturbing influence from a regular classroom. In a series of brief screening studies aimed at determining the extent of emotional handicaps in school children, Stennett (1966) states that "about five to ten percent of the children enrolled in elementary schools can be identified as having adjustive difficulties of sufficient severity to warrant professional attention." School clinicians who have been alerted to certain verbal cues may also be in a position to suggest intervention procedures for anxious children. Barnard and others (1961) report that the verbal behavior of anxious children can be differentiated on several dimensions from that of nonanxious children. When Zimbardo and others (1963) subjected the data on 40 third-grade boys to more thorough analysis, further support was found for Mahl's measure of speech disturbance as a sensitive indicator of anxiety. It appears that "high anxious" children are more disturbed under evaluative than permissive conditions while the opposite is true for "low anxious" children. While emotionally disturbed children are frequently hospitalized at some time in the course of their illness, many writers suggest that there are substantial benefits to be derived from placement approximating a "normal" environment. Reinhold and Farragher (1967) describe specialized services designed to maintain severely disturbed children in public schools within the community. Raab (1967) has made suggestions for developing appropriate classroom behaviors in a severely disturbed group of kindergarten-primary children utilizing a behavior modification model. Gold (1967) discusses the use of a clinic's psychoeducational facility for new programming in the public schools.

Serving the Hearing-Impaired

CASE FINDING

Case finding in the hearing conservation program may be the responsibility of health personnel or an integral part of the school's speech and hearing program under the direction of a speech and hearing specialist. Although conditions for audiometry are seldom ideal in the school environment, it is here that case finding may be most crucial. In a study related to this problem, Eagles and Doerfler (1961) evaluated acoustic environment control and audiometer modification and performance. They concluded that "rigid criteria for control of acoustic environment can be met in the field and that audiometers can be modified to test accurately levels well below the American Standard audiometric zero." They also state that audiometric testing alone cannot identify physical abnormalities of the ear which may have predictive value.

With the decline in the use of group audiometry for case finding in schools, time demands for individual pure-tone audiometry brought about consideration of limited-frequency screening. Ventry and Newby (1959) investigated the validity of the one-frequency screening principle for public school children. Pure-tone air-conduction threshold tests were conducted on every fourth subject failing a standardized five-frequency sweep test. The results of the threshold analysis indicated that there were significant differences between the mean threshold losses from 500 through 8,000 cps. Further statistical analysis provided evidence that the mean threshold loss at 4,000 cps was greater than the mean threshold loss at any of the other four frequencies tested. It would appear that the validity of a single-frequency principle, at least under the conditions of this study, was established. The authors indicate, however, that one-frequency screening needs further evaluation to determine the efficiency of this approach in detecting medically significant hearing loss in children.

Glorig and House (1957) have previously reported that single-frequency screening is 99.5 percent as effective as the customary "sweep" check method. Furthermore, since the school audiometric environment is often unfavorable for the use of pure tones at 500 and 1,000 cps, it would seem that 4,000 cps provides some hedge against false positive referrals. Hanley and Gaddie (1962) studied the single-frequency procedure with inexpensive equipment in a regular public school setting. The subjects were second- and fourth-grade children screened at 15 dB. Validating threshold tests were conducted for each child on the same day. The authors conclude that a single-frequency screening test using a 4,000 cps pure tone may be used adequately to predict with a high degree of accuracy the subsequent audiometric measures obtained on second- and fourth-grade children. A high level of interest was obtained and the time required for this procedure averaged less than 30 seconds per pupil. A comparison of the pass-fail scores indicates that the single frequency test correctly classified 90 percent of the hard-of-hearing ears and overselected 2.8 percent of the normal ears.

Downs, Doster, and Weaver (1965) consider the identification audiometry dilemma. Procedures, standards, frequency of screening, and grades to be screened are discussed. The following recommendations are offered: 1. the presently recommended screening level of 10 dB adequately fulfills the goals and responsibilities of educational programs at the present time; 2. the medical aspects of the hearing problems of school children should be attacked vigorously with special emphasis on obtaining an examination by an otolaryngologist of every child found to have a hearing problem; and 3. more intensive search should be concentrated on the lower grades. Lloyd (1966) also comments on this dilemma and, based upon his critical review of recent literature, rejects the use of limited frequency audiometric screening for school identification programs except as a last resort. For primarily service programs, he would employ either four- or five-frequency screening depending on the screening environment. He also suggests that conversion of screening level based on the 1951 American Standards Association standard to one based on the International Standards Organization 1964 standard should not be lightly passed off with the suggestion of adding a consistent amount to each frequency.

One of the outcomes of the National Conference on Identification Audiometry (1960) was a proposal of basic procedures for a program for school-age children. Melnick, Eagles, and Levine (1964) conducted an investigation to evaluate some of those recommended procedures. Children from kindergarten through the eighth grade participated. The results of the study show that the recommended screening program was successful in characterizing the hearing sensitivity of the participating children. Ninety-six percent were correctly identified as having either normal or decreased hearing sensitivity when a threshold test was used for validation. The screening test incorrectly indicated normal hearing sensitivity in 2.5 percent of the children subsequently shown to have some hearing loss by threshold measures. The remaining 1.5 percent were falsely identified as having decreased hearing sensitivity. The screening program was made more effective by using failure on two sweep checks as an indication for more thorough threshold testing. The frequency most often failed by the children was 6,000 cps. The use of audiometric test results to identify those children with otologic problems was not adequate.

Another approach to school audiometry which has been considered is Békésy audiometry. Price and Falck (1963) used as subjects public school children who ranged in age from six through 11 years and whose hearing levels were 10 dB or better at octave intervals from 125 through 8,000 cps. The criterion used to select subjects was chronological age (C.A.). Classroom teachers were asked to refer normal children within the appropriate age limits. All children tested who had a minimum C.A. of seven years produced clinically useful results using the Békésy audiometer. The nonuseful clincal results were all within the six-year C.A. group. However, five of the nine children in the six-year C.A. group produced clinically useful results. Thus, clinically useful information was obtained from 50 subjects, and from all subjects whose C.A. was at least seven years, from all children whose M.A. was at least seven years, and from all children but one whose I.Q. was at least 100.

For very young children, screening with verbal stimuli may be preferred. Mencher and McCulloch (1970) describe the use of Verbal Auditory Screening for Children (VASC).

CLASSES FOR THE HARD-OF-HEARING

Children who are found to have significant hearing impairment in the schools' case-finding programs may, after suitable follow-up, prove to be candidates for speechreading services, special education for the hard-of-hearing or consideration for enrollment in special classes for the severely hard-of-hearing or deaf.

Building toward optimum relations with normal-hearing peers, public school classes for the hard-of-hearing usually attempt some integration into the regular program as soon as possible, and for the length of time deemed feasible. Determining readiness for limited participation in regular classes, however, is not always a simple matter. Usually integration will be gradual, following intensive training, will be cautiously entered into, and will provide opportunity for frequent evaluation. Kowalsky (1962) reports on the findings of a study in the integration of a severely hard-of-hearing six-year-old in the first grade of a public school. The account covers a successful integration for one child and suggestions are offered for subsequent study. The author feels that a fully developed facility for speech and lip reading is not always a prerequisite for success in regular school. Caution is advised by Van Wyk (1960), who recommends no integration until speech and language skills are well established. He believes that the candidates should be carefully screened prior to admittance into an integrated program.

Early identification of children with hearing impairment is universally approved. Approaches to habilitation for the young deaf or hard-of-hearing child, however, reflect no such unanimity of opinion. Some would place hearing aids on children in infancy if hearing loss is detected (Griffiths, 1966). The more conservative school of thought is represented in the philosophy of the preschool training program at Albany Hospital (Landoli, Winkler, and Barton, 1960). It is believed there that individual aids should not be worn until a child is able to recognize amplified sounds and begins to produce sounds. The parent program is considered an integral part of the preschool setting. Stewart, Pillack, and Downs (1964) aver that the auditory sense is the most suitable perceptual modality by which a child learns speech and language. They describe the theoretical basis for a clinical program for acoustically handicapped children, utilizing a unisensory approach. The assumptions underlying the program are: 1. the auditory residual in most limited-hearing children merits the use of early amplification and unisensory training; 2. the traditional emphasis on lipreading may tend to limit the usefulness and effectiveness of auditory training; 3. the development in infants of awareness of sounds, voice, and speech is best conducted in the home under the supervision of the hearing center; and 4. effective preschool education can be structured as for the totally hearing child, rather than for the "exceptional" child.

CLASSES FOR THE DEAF

Special classes for the deaf in the public schools are now commonly found in systems where the population within the area to be served is large enough to provide an adequate number of pupils, regardless of the number of school districts involved. In the preschool and early school years, speech and language problems are the essential focus of the educational effort. Deaf children of all ages whose residence is in rural or sparsely populated areas may need to attend a residential school. Deaf students of secondary school age are more frequently enrolled in state residential schools due to their greater dependence on manual communication (not commonly used in public day schools) and their need for the well-developed vocational training programs.

In "Education of the Deaf in the United States," a report to the Secretary of Health, Education and Welfare, an 11-member committee reported dissatisfaction with educational provisions for deaf students (*Volta Review*, 1965). The inadequacy was attributed in part to "failure in attacking language problems agressively" and in part to inadequate programs for educating the deaf at all levels. This concern about language instruction is reflected in the emphasis of several periodical publications (Jordan, 1964; Quigley, 1966) in which whole issues are devoted to the topic.

Morkovin (1968) reviews research in the Soviet Union on language of the preschool deaf child. Experiments at the Moscow Institute of Defectology comparing oral versus finger-spelling approaches are described. Also considered are the systems of rearing (Vospitanie) and teaching (Obuchenie) found in the highly enriched residential environment. Work at the level of the first signal system and the second signal system (Vygotsky), the creative power of language, and language as an instrument of personality development are discussed.

An historical overview of language instruction for the deaf in Europe and the United States is offered by Schmitt (1966). He notes particularly in the United States the contributions to language instruction made by the Fitzgerald "Key," Buell's Outline of Language for Deaf Children, and Vinson's "Logical System of Language Teaching and an Analysis of the English Language, with a Course of Study in Language: A Manual for Teachers." The Deaf Language Outline at Central Institute for the Deaf and the appearance of Groht's "Natural Language for Deaf Children" are noted. Promising advances are seen in programmed language instruction, Project LIFE sponsored by the United States Office of Education, and Language Development in the Home (Lowell). Schmitt believes that the future holds promise in applications of linguistics and learning theory in addition to programmed instruction.

Olson (1967) studied the relation between speed of visual perception and language abilities in deaf adolescents. The correlation coefficients and the 10 factors extracted from the matrix show the measures of visual perception and the language tasks used in the investigation to be positively related.

Odom, Blanton, and Nunnally (1967) applied "Cloze Technique" to comparative studies of language capability in deaf and hearing subjects. Their results indicated that the two deaf groups performed similarly but much lower than either of the hearing groups. There was no general effect of span between deleted words; only the deaf increased in ability to predict the correct form class of function words with increasing span between deleted words. It was suggested that the deaf use different types of rules in constructing a sentence than do hearing subjects, particularly with regard to function words. When 40 deaf adolescents were compared with 40 sixth-grade hearing students on a multiple-choice sentence-completion test, the deaf subjects' scores were significantly lower than the hearing subjects' scores, particularly for adjectives, prepositions, and conjunctions.

The report of the Advisory Committee to Health, Education and Welfare, summarized by Morton (1965), outlines an "adequate system for the education of the deaf." The Committee stated its belief that the states and their political subdivisions should, wherever feasible, be the basic unit of education of the deaf. The Committee recommended that Congress authorize funds for assisting and encouraging the states to develop their individual programs and that the United States Commissioner of Education hold a national conference of federal, state, and local governmental and professional leadership to find ways of encouraging the development of state plans. In 1966 the California State Department of Education initiated the development of a plan for the improvement of the education of the deaf in that state. Hayes and Griffing (1967) describe the present status of public school education of the deaf in California.

In the continuing oralism versus manualism controversy, Cornett (1965) suggests that "cued" speech may be the answer. He explains the method as a compromise that permits early acquisition of language and early communication between parents and child. The method is said to be learned quite readily by both hearing and deaf persons. It has been used successfully at Gallaudet College and is being used experimentally by the New York School for the Deaf at White Plains in the first large-scale employment of the method with deaf children. Cornett believes that if a child's earliest communication is in the visual equivalent of spoken English, it will do much to help him develop to the fullest his capabilities in speech, speechreading, and language.

In a study of categorization behavior and achievement, Silverman (1967) used the Triple Mode Test based on the work of Vygotsky. She concluded that deficiencies in categorization behavior may contribute to deficient language performance in the deaf child. The developmental guidelines hold up well in the analysis of both deaf and hearing children's categorization responses. The use of an achievement instrument standardized on hearing children, however, is said to have little validity in measuring achievement in deaf children.

Any system which may contribute to speech development in deaf children warrants consideration. Speech through color is a system developed in an experimental program at the Lexington School for the Deaf (Wood, 1965). It is now quite widely used and has been adapted for use in speech improvement for the mentally retarded. Color-form attitudes of deaf children were investigated by Doehring (1960). School-age deaf children and nursery school hearing children and hearing adults were studied. Results indicate that "deaf children as compared with their hearing peers showed a greater tendency to differentiate visual stimuli on the basis of differences in color. There was no change in the distribution of color-form attitudes between the nursery-school group and the adult group."

More extensive use of programmed instruction in the teaching of deaf seems certain. Different skills lend themselves to this approach. The development of skill in written language continues to be a matter of concern for teachers of the deaf. Rush (1966) considers a programmed application with a group of deaf students in the intermediate grades. It appears that training in short-term memory for small units of meaningful language visually presented assists the deaf child in "establishing memory traces" for language patterns. The orderly progression of programmed instruction is one medium through which the kind and frequency of meaningful units can be visually presented, controlled, and extended. Through reinforcement of correct responses, the learner can be trained to recall longer and longer units of sentence patterns. Other language-handicapped people may also benefit from the application of these programmed techniques.

Programmed instruction in picture-sound association with deaf children was studied by Doehring (1968). The learning task involved tape-recorded presentations of a meaningful nonverbal sound in conjunction with three pictures projected on the response windows of a viewing-response device. The subjects ranged in age from four to 10 years. The results indicate that even profoundly deaf children may benefit from such auditory nonverbal perceptual training.

Serving the Multiple-Handicapped

Although deafness undoubtedly presents one of the most serious challenges to educators and to speech and hearing specialists, the existence and possible increased incidence of children with associated handicaps poses even more difficult management problems. The recent outbreak of maternal rubella has already thrust a new population of multiple-handicapped children upon the nation's schools. Education along strict categorical lines seems unlikely to be a productive approach. Multidisciplinary consideration is clearly necessary.

Rh-factor origins constitute another source of multi-involved children. This complication represents a leading perinatal cause of deafness, accounting for about 3.1 percent of all profound hearing loss among school-age deaf children. Vernon (1967) states that there is strong evidence of a high prevalence of brain damage among Rh deaf children. In his *in situ* research he attempts to establish the behavioral correlates of such neurological damage. Of direct significance for special education and psychology is the fact that profound hearing loss is only one manifestation of the extensive central nervous system damage resulting from Rh factor complications. In 71 percent of the cases studied, deafness is one of two or more disabilities.

In addition to the language and communication problems of deafness, there is a high percentage of aphasia in Rh-involved children. Thus, education is presented with the task of developing techniques which overcome two major factors contributing to language pathology—deafness and aphasia. Cerebral palsy, which is present in over half of Rh children and in even a higher proportion of those with aphasia, poses still other management problems. Vernon asks whether it is realistic to expect understandable speech from a child with these combined handicaps. The functional value of the hearing which pure-tone audiometry reveals to be present in Rh cases must be questioned since those children who had the most hearing of any of the groups tested did not reflect this in their written language, speech, and speechreading. There appears to be pathology of auditory perception or integration and symbolization to sound that reduces the effectiveness of the ability to respond to auditory input. It is proposed that Cloze Procedure be used with Rh-deafened children to determine their language problems.

In an extensive discussion of language acquisition, Withrow (1966) considers deaf children having other disabilities. He describes methodology applicable to young aphasic children, the cerebral-palsied deaf, the emotionally disturbed deaf, the mentally retarded deaf, and the deaf-blind. He notes that the literature on multiple-handicapped deaf is characterized by a lack of specific research or educational programs. There is apparently little insight into the real needs of the mutliple-handicapped deaf.

As a demonstration of what may be attempted in the way of service to multihandicapped and culturally deprived children, the pilot speech and language program at Hunter College may be cited. Doob (1967) describes this program, which was established in 1966, and serves children with multiple handicaps for six weeks during the summer session. This laboratory school, supervised by the Hunter College Department of Education, functions as an advanced training center for speech and hearing clinicians. The school includes classes for aphasic, deaf and hard-of-hearing, partially blind, trainable and educable mentally retarded, cerebral-palsied, and culturally deprived children, as well as a class for the gifted. Three one-hour demonstrations of speech and language therapy given during the six-week session are planned to give graduate students, interns, and teachers of special education opportunities to observe.

Serving the Aphasic Child

Only relatively recently have children whose communication problem was diagnosed as aphasia been accepted in special education classes in the public schools. The transition is due, at least in part, to a broadening of traditional definitions of the problem and recognition of the beneficial effects to be derived from a stable, dependable learning environment. Not to be minimized is the effect on these children's behavior of a "normal" learning situation. Some programs which enroll aphasic children operate under the rubric of "severe language disability."

In California, programs for dysphasic children are authorized in the California Education Code and governed by regulations contained in the California Administrative Code, Title 5, "Education." Problems of identification are acknowledged and an accurate diagnosis is stressed. A plan which allows for selective and objective placement as well as separation from the special program is recommended. Enrollment limits are specified: eight pupils, or six when the age range is greater than four years. School personnel are expected to develop a sound system of guidance and instruction. What the child is taught and how he is taught constitute the essential ingredients of this objective. Although there are no California public school credentialing regulations that apply specifically to teachers in this program, all teachers of such children are expected to hold a valid credential in the specialized area of speech and hearing. A valid standard teaching credential is also required. The applicable definitions appear in the California Administrative Code (Title 5, Article 7 of sub-chapter 5.5, Section 1320(c)):

> An aphasic pupil for the purpose of this article is a pupil with respect to whom all of the following are true: 1. The child has severe speech (oral language) disabilities (other than those speech disabilities associated with deafness, mental retardation, or autism) of an expressive receptive and/or integrative character stemming from central nervous dysfunction or central nervous impairment or both. 2. The dysfunction or impairment is diagnosed by each of the following persons as aphasia or probable aphasia: a physician who has training and experience working with children who have neurological defects; a certified psychologist; a person who holds a credential authorizing the teaching of exceptional children in the area of speech and hearing handicapped or speech correction and lip reading in remedial classes. Each diagnosis shall be evidenced by a written statement subscribed by the persons making the diagnosis. 3. The disabilities require enrollment in a special day class and transportation to a special day class.

Classes for aphasic children must accommodate, in addition to the traditional learning needs, the range of communication problems usually presented. These dimensions are considered in the Proceedings of the Institute on Childhood Aphasia (1962). These serve to identify crucial elements in the school program. Auditory discrimination learning, for example, represents one such feature. Wilson, Doehring, and Hirsch (1960) have compared aphasic and nonaphasic children on their ability to discriminate among four sounds differing in two acoustic dimensions. The subjects were primarily sensory-aphasic children. More than half of the aphasic children learned the task in about the same number of trials as did the nonaphasic children. The difference in learning ability within the aphasic group was unrelated to age, I.Q., or amount of hearing loss.

Doehring also examined visual spatial memory in aphasic children and found that the aphasic group was significantly less accurate than both the deaf and the normal groups in terms of total amount of error, which suggests that aphasic children are retarded in some, but not all, aspects of visual perceptual ability. Operant conditioning was employed for investigating speech-sound discrimination in aphasic children (McReynolds, 1966). Subjects were children between the ages of four and eight. The results suggest that applying unqualified and generalized phrases such as "poor auditory discrimination" to aphasic children is unwarranted. The study results support the third hypothesized cause of auditory perceptual disorders —poor reinforcement contingencies. Alternative explanations may account for differences found for sounds-in-context tasks. This may be related more to an inability to retain and sequence the sounds of language or the inability of the aphasic child to use one perceptual skill efficiently when it is necessary to use two or more skills in combination, as in this case —discrimination, retention, and sequencing.

Lowe and Campbell (1965), in a study of temporal discrimination, found significant differences between aphasoid and normal children on their "order" task. They suggest that temporal ordering malfunction of the aphasoid child may be a major factor contributing to his communication problem. Alterations of prosodic features seem to affect the sequencing performance of aphasic children. Five out of eight subjects studied by Stark, Poppen, and May (1967) had difficulty with sequences of three. It appears that their sequencing difficulty is due largely to forgetting the first item in the sequence. When the initial item was stressed, recall of the entire sequence was enhanced. When other features of the sequence were altered, recall was disrupted. These effects were not observed in the normal group.

McWilliams (1965) discusses the language-handicapped child as he actually exists and is viewed by clinicians. She notes the difficult task of translating clinical observations in terms understandable to the teachers who will meet the language-handicapped child in the classroom. She argues for descriptive approaches as opposed to specific diagnostic labels. The classroom teacher is viewed as an individual competent to devise teaching methods applicable to the peculiar requirements of widely differing children.

The teaching of aphasic children is considered by McGinnis, Kleffner, and Goldstein (1956). Following a discussion of characteristics, the authors describe the speech and language training regimen at Central Institute for the Deaf.

Serving the Brain-Damaged

When a diagnosis of aphasia is not sustained or when a categorical program for "brain-damaged" children is not available, children presenting behaviors usually ascribed to brain injury appear in different special education classes as well as in regular classrooms. The communication disorders associated with neurological impairment have been an accepted responsibility in classes for the cerebral-palsied for many years. In this setting, the "ideal" approach has frequently been considered the team approach. The unique contributions of occupational therapy, physical therapy, and speech therapy are conjoined with those of the teacher in a coordinated attack on the child's communication and learning problems. Although children usually are seen for individual remedial assistance as well, the team approach calls for close planning and frequent case conferences to assure truly collaborative efforts.

The lack of general agreement on what constitutes a "brain-damaged" child has created a potpourri of terminology. Some authors conclude that the term "brain damage" simply cannot be used as a unitary construct. Following a three-year study, Schulman, Kastar, and Thorne (1965) reported that the only behavioral variable which even approached unequivocal support as a correlate of brain damage, regardless of extent or location of damage, was distractability. No evidence was accumulated to support the hypothesis that hyperactivity is a correlate of brain damage. In a comparison of visual and auditory perceptual functions, however, Deutsch (1966) found that the brain-injured group which she studied demonstrated less differentiated functioning in the auditory modality than did her intact comparison group. She also discussed the susceptibility of auditory functioning to attentional disorders.

Since learning problems often exist in the apparent absence of an organic substrate, considerable effort has been directed to develop tests which could expose reliably any tissue pathology. Gross neurological study in the fashion designed for use with injured adults is generally unproductive. In recent years the emergence of pediatric neurology as a medical speciality has brought some competence in the interpretation of so-called "soft" signs. Proponents of psychometric evaluation suggest that psychological tools may in the long run prove more sensitive and more practicable in the screening of school populations.

An extensive treatment of this topic is inappropriate here, but a few exploratory references seem indicated. The "hyperactive child syndrome" is the focus of a report by Stewart and others (1966). Greenburg (1967) has also considered the development of assessment techniques for brain damage. Early "minimal brain damage" is discussed by Pollack (1967). Consensually validated behavioral correlates in the hyperkinetic child have been examined by Schrager and others (1966). The use of the well-known Purdue Pegboard as a screening test for brain damage is evaluated by Rapin, Tourk, and Costa (1966). The test appears insensitive to the presence of chronic convulsive disorders unassociated with mental retardation or other evidence of brain damage. It does indicate lateralized damage and is sensitive to the syndrome of clumsiness, hyperactivity, and visual motor dysfunction. However, the test does not discriminate between brain damage, mental retardation, psychosis, and severe emotional disturbance.

While it is obvious that we have become more aware of the existence of children who may be called "brain-injured" or something else, their efficient identification and appropriate educational management is only now emerging. Since language, and in particular language deficits, are important clues to the identity of "brain-damaged" children, the role of the speech therapist must be considered important. The subsequent reeducation and training will constitute another task for the communications specialist in the schools.

GENERALIZATIONS

Among the more obvious trends observed is the growth of public school programs for more seriously involved children having speech and language disorders. The consistently increasing range of recognized communication disorders implies the need for broader knowledge on the part of the public school speech and hearing clinician. As this need for a greater range of competence increases, more specialization seems inevitable. The "general practitioner" may be found only in rural areas.

More specific responsibilities in relation to language disability and language development programs are already being demanded. Since the demand will undoubtedly continue to exceed the supply of specially trained clinicians, the use of nonprofessionals working under the direction of the specialist will surely emerge rapidly. More clinical "centers" will be established to serve the most seriously involved. For the primary school, richer communication environments are in order. The communications specialist is destined to be in the education mainstream of the public school.

BIBLIOGRAPHY

Ad hoc committee on guidelines for speech and hearing services in project headstart. 1966. *Asha*, 463–464.

Ainsworth, S. 1965. The speech clinician in the public schools: "participant" or "separatist"? *Asha*, 7, 495–503.

Allen, E., Black, M., Burkland, M., Byrne, M., Farquhar, M., Herbert, E., and Robertson, M. 1966. Case selection in the public schools. *J. Speech Hearing Disorders*, 31, 157–161.

Alpiner, J., Ogden, J., Wiggins, J. 1970. The utilization of supportive personnel in speech correction in the public schools: A pilot project. *Asha* 12, 599–604.

The American boards of examiners in speech pathology and audiology. 1966. *Asha*, 8, 109–113.

Andersland, P. 1961. Maternal and environmental factors related to success in speech improvement training. *J. Speech Hearing Res.*, 4, 79–90.

ASHA executive secretary's statement to stimulate speech and hearing personnel. 1965. *Asha*, 7, 162–163.

Aungst, L., and Frick, J. 1964. Auditory discrimination ability and consistency of articulation of /r/. *J. Speech Hearing Disorders*, 29, 76–85.

Avant, V., and Hutton, C. 1962. Passage for speech screening in upper elementary grades. *J. Speech Hearing Disorders*, 27, 40–46.

Bankson, N. 1968. Special reports: report on state certification requirements in speech and hearing. *Asha*, 10, 291–293.

Bennett, C. 1965. Educating children with learning differences. Dept. Rural Educ. Co. and Intermediate Unit Superintendents. Gen'l. Session Address. San Diego.

Berlin, C., and Dill, A. 1967. The effects of feedback and positive reinforcement on the Wepman auditory discrimination test scores of lower-class negro and white children. *J. Speech Hearing Res.*, 10, 384–389.

Black, M. 1964. Speech correction in the schools. Englewood Cliffs, N.J.: Prentice-Hall.

———. 1966. The origins and status of speech therapy in the schools. *Asha*, 8, 419–425.

Bloomer, H. 1968. Special reports: preprofessional education in speech pathology and audiology. *Asha*, 10, 255–256.

Bradley, B., Maurer, R., and Hundziak, M. 1966. A study of the effectiveness of milieu therapy and language training for the mentally retarded. *Except. Child.*, 33, 143.

Calvert, D., Redell, R., Donaldson, R., and Pew, L. 1965. A comparison of auditory amplifiers for the deaf. *Except. Child.*, 32, 247–252.

Castle, W., Johnson, K., and Newman, P. 1966. The status of education and training programs for speech pathology and audiology—1966. *Asha*, 8, 447–456.

Causey, L., Johnson, K., and Healey, W. 1971. A survey of state certification requirements for public school speech clinicians. *Asha*, 13, 123–129.

Cohen, J., and Diehl, C. 1963. Relation of speech-sound discrimination ability to articulation-type speech defects. *J. Speech Hearing Disorders*, 28, 187–190.

Comments on education of the deaf in the U.S. by a Finnish visitor. 1965. *Asha*, 7, 193–196.

Committee on language development and disorders. 1967. *Asha*, 9, 273–274.

Committee on speech and hearing services in schools. 1965. *Asha*, 7, 477–478.

Conference on research for public school speech and hearing personnel. 1966. *Asha*, 8, 242–243.

Cornett, R. 1967. Oralism versus manualism—cued speech may be the answer (and) The method explained. *Hearing Speech News*, 35:5, 6–9.

Deutsch, C. 1966. Comparison of visual and auditory perceptual functions of brain-injured and normal children. *Perceptual and motor Skills*, 22, 303–309.

Dickson, S. 1962. Differences between children who spontaneously outgrow and children who retain functional articulation errors. *J. Speech Hearing Res.*, 5, 263–271.

Doehring, D. 1960. Color-form attitudes of deaf children. *J. Speech Hearing Res.*, 3, 242–248.

———. 1960. Visual spatial memory in aphasic children. *J. Speech Hearing Res.*, 3, 130–137.

———. 1968. Picture-sound association in deaf children. *J. Speech Hearing Res.*, 11, 49–62.

Doob, D. 1967. A pilot speech and language program in the vacation demonstration school at Hunter College. *Asha*, 9, 304–306.

Downs, M., Doster, M., and Weaver, M. 1965. Dilemmas in identification audiometry. *J. Speech Hearing Disorders*, 30, 360–364.

Eagles, E., and Doerfler, L. 1961. Hearing in children: acoustic environment and audiometer performance. *J. Speech Hearing Res.*, 4, 149–163.

Education of the deaf in the United States. 1965. *Volta Rev.*, 67, 345–351.

Elliott, L. 1967. Descriptive analysis of audiometric and psychometric scores of students at a school for the deaf. *J. Speech Hearing Res.*, 10, 21–40.

An evaluation of speech and hearing programs in the schools. 1967. *Asha*, Final report, proposal number R-054. Grant number 32-18-0000-1026.

Executive council report. 1968. *Asha*, 10, 158–159.

Ferrier, E. 1966. An investigation of the ITPA performance of children with functional defects of articulation. *Except. Child.*, 32, 625.

Freeman, G., and Lukens, J. 1962. A speech and language program for educable mentally handicapped children. *J. Speech Hearing Disorders*, 27, 285–286.

———, 1969. Innovative school programs; the Oakland Schools plan. *J. Speech Hearing Disorders*, 34, 220–225.

Fristoe, M., and Goldman, R. 1968. Comparison of traditional and condensed articulation tests examining the same number of sounds. *J. Speech Hearing Res.*, 11, 583–589.

Furth, H. 1961. Visual paired-associates task with deaf and hearing children. *J. Speech Hearing Res.*, 4, 172–177.

Glorig, A., and House, H. 1957. A new concept in auditory screening. *A.M.A. Arch. Otolaryng.*, 66, 228–232.

Gold, J. 1967. Child guidance day treatment and the school: a clinic's use of its psychoeducational facility for new programming in the public schools. Digest issue. *Amer. J. Orthopsychiat.*, XXXVII, 276–277.

Goldman, R., and Fristoe, M. 1966. Film strip articulation test. *Except. Child.*, 33, 42–43.

———. 1967. The development of the filmstrip articulation test. *J. Speech Hearing Disorders*, 32, 256–262.

Greenberg, E. 1967. The development of assessment techniques for the brain damaged adolescent. Digest issue. *Amer. J. Orthopsychiat.*, XXXVII, 213–214.

Griffiths, C. 1966. Once children hear. *Hearing Speech News*, 34, 8–10.

Haines, H. 1965. Trends in public school speech therapy. *Asha*, 7, 187–190.

Hanley, C., and Gaddie, B. 1962. The use of single frequency audiometry in the screening of school children. *J. Speech Hearing Disorders*, 27, 258–264.

Hartwig, J., and Jones, C. 1966. Ohio's program for hearing handicapped children. Ohio State Dept. Educ., Columbus.

Henriksen, E. 1968. Case selection in the schools—an addendum. *J. Speech Hearing Disorders*, 33, 232–235.

Hull, F., and Timmons, R. 1966. A national speech and hearing survey. *J. Speech Hearing Disorders*, 31, 359–361.

Irwin, J. 1967. Supportive personnel in speech pathology and audiology. *Hearing Speech News*, 35, 32–40.

Irwin, R. 1962. Speech therapy and children's linguistic skills. *J. Speech Hearing Res.*, 5, 377–381.

———. 1963. The effects of speech therapy upon certain linguistic skills of first-grade children. *J. Speech Hearing Disorders*, 28, 375–381.

———, and Musselman, B. 1962. A compact picture articulation test. *J. Speech Hearing Disorders*, 27, 36–39.

Isenberg, R. 1964. Various approaches to developing area programs. *Cooperative programs in special education*. Lord, F. and Isenberg, R., eds. Joint Publication, Council for Exceptional Children and Department of Rural Education, National Education Association.

Jenkins, E., and Lohr, F. 1964. Severe articulation disorders and motor ability. *J. Speech Hearing Disorders*, 29, 286–292.

Jerger, J., and Speaks, C. 1967. Annual review of JSHR research, 1966. *J. Speech Hearing Disorders*, 32, 107–111.

Joint committee on audiology and education of the deaf. 1966. *Asha*, 8, 243.

Jordan, E. 1960. Articulation test measures and listener ratings of articulation defectiveness. *J. Speech Hearing Res.*, 3, 303–319.

Jordan, J. ed. 1964. Whole issue devoted to teaching language to the deaf. *Except. Child.*, 30, 333–371.

Kisatsky, T. 1967. The prognostic value of Carter-Buck tests in measuring articulation skills of selected kindergarten children. *Except. Child.*, 34, 81–85.

Koplin, J., Odom, P., Blanton, R., and Nunnally, J. 1967. Word association performance of deaf subjects. *J. Speech Hearing Res.*, 10, 126–132.

Kowalsky, M. 1962. Integration of a severely hard of hearing child in a normal first-grade program: a case study. *J. Speech Hearing Disorders*, 27, 349–358.

Landoli, E., Winkler, P., and Barton, L. 1960. Preschool training program. *Volta Rev.*, 62, 63–65.

Language studies of mentally retarded children. 1963. Monograph supplement No. 10. *J. Speech Hearing Disorders*.

Lloyd, L. 1965. Use of the slide show audiometric technique with mentally retarded children. *Except. Child.*, 32, 93.

———. 1966. Comments on "dilemmas in identification audiometry." *J. Speech Hearing Disorders*, 31, 161–165.

Locke, J. 1968. Discriminative learning in children's acquisition of phonology. *J. Speech Hearing Res.*, 11, 428–434.

Lowe, A., and Campbell, R. 1965. Temporal discrimination in aphasoid and normal children. *J. Speech Hearing Res.*, 8, 313–314.

Mackie, R. 1966. Opportunities for education of handicapped under title I, PL 89-10. *Except. Child.*, 32, 593.

MacLearie, E. 1964. The Ohio plan for children with speech and hearing problems. Ohio State Dept. Educ., Columbus.

Mandell, T. 1967. Public schools and the community hearing and speech agency. *Hearing Speech News*, 35, 30–32.

Marge, M. 1966. New directions in state planning for school children with communicative disorders. Office of Education (DHEW), Washington, D.C.

———. 1967. The emergence of state speech and hearing associations. *Asha*, 9, 343–347.

Matthews, J. 1957. Speech problems of the mentally retarded. *In* Handbook of speech pathology. Travis, L., ed. New York: Appleton-Century-Crofts. Pp. 531–551.

McGinnis, M., Kleffner, F., and Goldstein, R. 1956. Teaching aphasic children. *Volta Rev.*, 58, 239–244.

McReynolds, L. 1966. Operant conditioning for investigating speech sound discrimination in aphasic children. *J. Speech Hearing Res.*, 9, 519–528.

McWilliams, B. 1965. The language handicapped child and education. *Except. Child.*, 32, 221–228.

Melnick, W., Eagles, E., and Levine, H. 1964. Evaluation of a recommended program of identification audiometry with school-age children. *J. Speech Hearing Disorders*, 29, 3–13.

Mencher, G., and McCulloch, B. 1970. Auditory screening of kindergarten children using the VASC. *J. Speech Hearing Disorders*, 35, 241–247.

Menyuk, P. 1964. Comparison of grammar of children with functionally deviant and normal speech. *J. Speech Hearing Res.*, 7, 109–121.

Merow, E. 1965. Speech and the "below 50's." *The Instructor*, XXIV: 8, 46.

Monog. Suppl., No. 8, 1961. *J. Speech Hearing Disorders*, July.

Monsees, E., and Berman, C. 1968. Speech and language screening in a summer headstart program. *J. Speech Hearing Disorders*, 33, 121–126.

Morkovin, B. 1968. Language in the general development of the preschool deaf child: a review of research in the Soviet Union. *Asha*, 10, 195–199.

Morton, D. 1965. Education of the deaf. *Asha*, 7, 108–111.

Moser, H. 1961. Distance and fingerspelling. *J. Speech Hearing Res.*, 4, 61–71.

Moss, J., Moss, M., and Tizard, J. 1961. Electrodermal response audiometry with mentally defective children. *J. Speech Hearing Res.*, 4, 41–47.

Nichols, A. 1964. Allocation of time in the articulation program: applications of research. *Asha*, 6, 8–12.

Odom, P., Blanton, R., and Nunnally, J. 1967. Some "cloze" technique studies of language capability on the deaf. *J. Speech Hearing Res.*, 10, 816–827.

Olson, J. 1967. A factor analytic study of the relation between the speed of visual perception and the language abilities of deaf adolescents. *J. Speech Hearing Res.*, 10, 354–360.

O'toole, T., and Gaslow, E. 1969. Public school speech and hearing programs: things are changing. *Asha*, 11, 499–501.

Oyer, H., and Davis, G. 1967. Educating hearing and speech personnel. *Hearing Speech News*, 35, 18–26.

Pendergast, K., Soder, A., Barker, J., Duckey, S., Gow, J., and Selmar, J. 1966. An articulation study of 15,255 Seattle first grade children with and without kindergarten. *Except. Child.*, 32, 541.

Pollack, C., and Sher, N. 1967. Extending clinic resources: a remedial therapy program in a school Digest issue. *Amer. J. Orthopsychiat.*, XXXVII, 277–278.

Pollack, M. 1967. Early "minimal brain damage" and the development of severe psychopathology in adolescence. Digest issue. *Amer. J. Orthopsychiat.*, XXXVII, 213–214.

Prehm, H. 1966. Concept learning in culturally disadvantaged children as a function of verbal pretraining. *Except. Child.*, 32, 599.

Price, L., and Falck, V. 1963. Békésy audiometry with children. *J. Speech Hearing Res.*, 6, 129–133.

Prins, T. 1962. Motor and auditory abilities in different groups of children with articulatory deviations. *J. Speech Hearing Res.*, 5, 161–168.

Pronovost, W. 1966. Case selection in the schools: articulatory disorders. *Asha*, 8, 179–181.

Ptacek, P. 1967. Supportive personnel as an extension of the professional worker's nervous system. *Asha*, 9, 403–405.

Pupil personnel services as seen by the speech specialist. 1967. *Asha*, 9, 43–44.

Quigley, S. ed. 1966. Language acquisition. *Volta Rev.*, reprint number 852.

Raab, E. 1967. Developing appropriate classroom behaviors in a severely disturbed group of institutionalized kindergarten-primary children utilizing a behavior modification model. Digest issue. *Amer. J. Orthopsychiat.*, XXXVII, 313–314.

Raph, J. 1967. Language and speech deficits in culturally disadvantaged children: implications for the speech clinician. *J. Speech Hearing Disorders*, 32, 203–214.

Rapin, I., Tourk, L., and Costa. 1966. Evaluation of the Purdue-Pegboard as a screening test for brain damage. *Developm. Med. Child Neurol.*, 8, 45–54.

Reinhold, P., and Farragher, M. 1967. Specialized services for maintaining severely disturbed children in public schools within the community. Digest issue. *Amer. J. Orthopsychiat.*, XXXVII, 314.

Resolution presented to the executive council by the committee on speech and hearing services in the schools. 1967. *Asha*, 9, 88.

Rinsland, H. 1945. A basic vocabulary of elementary school children. New York: Macmillan.

Rittmanic, P. 1966. Special report. *Asha*, 8, 182–187.

Roe, V., and Milisen, R. 1942. The effect of maturation upon defective articulation in elementary grades. *J. Speech Disorders*, 7, 37–45.

Rush, M. 1966. Use of visual memory in teaching written language skills to deaf children. *J. Speech Hearing Disorders*, 31, 219–226.

Sayre, M. 1966. Report on educators' conference. *Asha*, 8, 67–69.

Schiefelbusch, R. 1963. Language studies of mentally retarded children: a report of the Parsons project in language and communication of mentally retarded children. *Monogr. suppl.* No. 10. *J. Speech Hearing Disorders.*

Schlanger, B., and Galanowsky, G. 1966. Auditory discrimination tasks performed by mentally retarded and normal children. *J. Speech Hearing Res.*, 9, 434–440.

Schmitt, P. 1966. Language instruction for the deaf. *Volta Rev.*, 68, 85–105+.

Schrager, J., Lindy, J., Harrison, S., McDermott, J., and Killins, E. 1966. The hyperkinetic child: some consensually validated behavioral correlates. *Except. Child.*, 32, 635–637.

Schulman, J., Kaspar, J., and Throne, F. 1965. Brain damage and behavior. Springfield, Ill.: Thomas.

Schulz, E. 1965. The autistic child in the school and the school-nurse teacher responsibility. *J. Sch. Health*, XXXV, 396–398.

Sherman, D., and Geith, A. 1967. Speech sound discrimination and articulation skill. *J. Speech Hearing Res.*, 10, 277–280.

Siegel, G. 1962. Experienced and inexperienced articulation examiners. *J. Speech Hearing Disorders*, 27, 28–35.

———, Winitz, H., and Conkey, H. 1963. The influence of testing instrument on articulatory responses of children. *J. Speech Hearing Disorders*, 28, 67–76.

Siegenthaler, B., Davis, A., and Christensen, N. 1962. Speech ratings and dismissal from therapy. *J. Speech Hearing Disorders*, 27, 47–53.

Silverman, R. 1967. Categorization behavior and achievement in deaf and hearing children. *Except. Child.*, 34, 241–250.

Sommers, R. 1962. Factors in the effectiveness of mothers trained to aid in speech correction. *J. Speech Hearing Disorders*, 27, 178–186.

———, Leiss, R., Delp, M., Gerber, A., Fundrella, D., Smith, R. II, Revucky, M., Ellis, D., and Haley, V. 1967. Factors related to the effectiveness of articulation therapy for kindergarten, first, and second grade children. *J. Speech Hearing Res.*, 10, 428–437.

———, Meyer, W., and Fenton, A. 1961. Pitch discrimination and articulation. *J. Speech Hearing Res.*, 4, 55–60.

———, Schaeffer, M., Leiss, R., Gerber, A., Bray, M., Fundrella, D., Olson, J., and Tomkins, E. 1966. The effectiveness of group and individual therapy. *J. Speech Hearing Res.*, 9, 219–225.

———, Shilling, S., Paul, C., Copetas, F., Bowser, D., and McClintock, C. 1959. Training parents of children with functional misarticulation. *J. Speech Hearing Res.*, 2, 258–265.

Special Report. 1966. *Asha*, 8, 182–187.

Special report: use of nonprofessionals widely discussed. 1967. *Asha*, 9, 442–445.

Speech and hearing programs, organizational and administrative manual. 1966. Montgomery Co. Public Schools: Rockville, Md.

The speech clinician's role in the public school. 1964. *Asha*, 6, 189–191.

Spradlin, J. 1963. Language and communication of mental defectives. *Handbook of mental deficiency.* Ellis, N., ed. New York: McGraw-Hill.

Spriestersbach, D. 1965. ASHA and federal programs: a review of a marriage. Presidential address—1965 national convention.

Stamp, I. 1966. Teachers look at autism. *Australian Pre-School Quart.*, 7, 12–14.

Stark, J. 1966. Performance of aphasic children on the ITPA. *Except. Child.*, 33, 153.

Stark, J., Poppen, R., and May, M. 1967. Effects of alterations of prosodic features on the sequencing performance of aphasic children. *J. Speech Hearing Res.*, 10, 849–855.

State associations. 1966. *Asha*, 8, 337–340.

———. 1967. *Asha*, 9, 143.

Stennet, R. 1966. Emotional handicap in the elementary years: phase or disease. *Amer. J. Orthopsychiat.*, XXXVI, 444–449.

Stewart, J., Pillack, D., and Downs, M. 1964. A unisensory program for the limited-hearing child. *Asha*, 6, 151–154.

Stewart, M., Pitts, F. Jr., Craig, A., and Dieruf, W. 1966. The hyperactive child syndrome. *Amer. J. Orthopsychiat.*, XXXVI, 861–867.

Summary and recommendations of the advisory committee's report to secretary, HEW. 1965. *Volta Rev.*, 67, 345–351.

Summers, R. 1959. Private practice of public school therapists in Indiana. *J. Speech Hearing Disorders*, 24, 51–54.

A symposium: improving supervision of clinical practicum. 1967. *Asha*, 9, 471–481.

Templin, M. 1947. Spontaneous versus imitated verbalization in testing articulation in preschool children. *J. Speech Disorders*, 12, 293–300.

Vandemark, A., and Mann, M. 1965. Oral language skills of children with defective articulation. *J. Speech Hearing Res.*, 8, 409–414.

Van Hattum, R. 1966. The defensive speech clinicians in the schools. *J. Speech Hearing Disorders*, 31, 234–240.

Van Wyk, M. 1960. Integration—a look at the total picture. *Volta Rev.*, 62, 69–70, 82.

Ventry, I., and Newby, H. 1959. Validity of the one-frequency screening principle for public school children. *J. Speech Hearing Res.*, 2, 147–151.

Vernon, M. 1967. Rh factor and deafness: the problem, its psychological, physical, and educational manifestations. *Except. Child.*, 34, 5–12.

Weaver, J. 1968. An investigation of attitudes of speech clinicians in the public schools. *Asha*, 10, 319–322.

Webster, E., Perkins, W., Bloomers, H. and Pronovost, W. 1966. Case selection in the schools. *J. Speech Hearing Disorders*, 31, 352–358.

Weinberg, B. 1968. A cephalometric study of normal and defective /s/ articulation and variations in incisor dentition. *J. Speech Hearing Res.*, 11, 288–300.

West, R. ed. 1962. Childhood aphasia: proceedings of the institutes on childhood aphasia. San Francisco: Calif. Soc. Crippled Children and Adults.

Wilson, F. 1966. Efficacy of speech therapy with educable mentally retarded children. *J. Speech Hearing Res.*, 9, 423–433.

Wilson, L., Doehring, D., and Hirsch, I. 1960. Auditory discrimination learning by aphasic and nonaphasic children. *J. Speech Hearing Res.*, 3, 130–137.

Wingo, J. 1970. Student speech and hearing "terms" in the public schools. *Asha* 12, 605–606.

Winitz, H. 1963. Effects of pretraining on sound discrimination learning. *J. Speech Hearing Res.*, 6, 171–180.

———. 1963. Temporal reliability in articulation testing. *J. Speech Hearing Disorders*, 28, 247–251.

———. 1968. Harris Winitz on preprofessional education in speech pathology and audiology at the University of Missouri—Kansas City. *Asha*, 10, 294–295.

———, and Bellerose, B. 1962. Sound discrimination as a function of pretraining conditions. *J. Speech Hearing Res.*, 5, 340–348.

———, and Lawrence, M. 1961. Children's articulation and sound learning ability. *J. Speech Hearing Res.*, 4, 259–268.

———, and Preisler, L. 1967. Effect of distinctive feature pretraining in phoneme discrimination learning. *J. Speech Hearing Res.*, 10, 515–530.

Withrow, F. 1966. Acquisition of language by deaf children with other disabilities. *Volta Rev.*, 68, 106–115.

Wood, D. 1965. Speech through color as an aid in speech improvement for the mentally retarded. *Except. Child.*, 31, 492–494.

Zandoli, G., Winkler, D., and Borton, L. 1960. Preschool training program. *Volta Rev.*, 62, 63–65.

Zimbardo, P. 1963. The measurement of speech disturbance and anxious children. *J. Speech Hearing Disorders*, 28, 362–370.

Zisk, P., and Bialer, I. 1967. Speech and language problems in mongolism: a review of the literature. *J. Speech Hearing Disorders*, 32, 228–241.

38

Symptomatic Therapy for Stuttering

C. Van Riper

In the decade that has passed since the first edition of this Handbook was published, a basic change seems to have occurred in the acceptance of symptomatic therapy not only for stutterers but for many other ills that afflict the human race. At the time that this chapter was first written, any therapy which dealt directly with maladjustive behaviors was immediately suspect and it was necessary to defend it strongly. Both the stutterers and their therapists tended to feel that any treatment which did not base itself upon removing the essential and original causes of the disorder should be treated with skepticism. The influence of Freud, who equated symptom formation with the need to protect oneself against the pain of anxiety, had pervaded all forms of psychotherapy. Freud (1920) wrote that there was a "very important connection between anxiety development and symptom formation. It was that the two are interchangeable." Since the anxiety was considered to be a response to deep-seated emotional conflicts of long standing, psychoanalysis insisted that these conflicts must be attacked rather than the symptoms. As a result, symptomatic therapy has been not only de-emphasized but viewed with more scorn than it deserves. If current medical practice may be used as a criterion, symptomatic therapy has certain virtues of its own. Of all the thousands of drugs being used by physicians at the present time, only a very few are *specifics* (Thorne, 1950). Most of them merely attack the symptoms and reduce their distress, thereby providing *time* for the homeostatic or recuperative powers of the organism to take care of the real causes of the illness. Other procedures, such as bedrest, reassurance, and specified routines of diet merely help the individual by creating favorable conditions for such recuperation. Digitalis never cured a cardiac case, but it often helps to tide the person over a crisis which might otherwise result in death. Symptomatic therapy then can be *time-gaining* and *palliating* (distress reducing). In this sense at least it can assist all other forms of therapy. In treating the stutterer who comes to us greatly troubled by his inability to communicate, who must meet one verbal crisis after another, all full of penalty, threat, and trauma; in order to gain time enough to teach him to control not only his stuttering but himself, symptomatic therapy is vital. Whatever their etiological beliefs or therapeutics may be, few speech therapists fail to use it.

At the present time, due largely to the behavioral theorists (Skinner, 1963), the therapists (Wolpe, 1958; Eysenck, 1960), and the experimenters (Goldiamond, 1965), symptomatic therapy is no longer in such ill repute. We have come to see that verbal behaviors can be maintained, that they can be shaped, and that they even can be extinguished by differential reinforcement. Those who have treated stuttering have always known this. The view is not new; it has merely begun to become respectable.

Perhaps a brief historical review of the sorts of procedures used in treating stuttering symptomatically would be useful here. In recounting them, it may be tempting to assume that because they were used so long ago or far away they were completely ineffective, but anyone who has investigated either the literature or the testimony of self-recovered stutterers cannot be so certain. We find it hard to escape the conclusion that some stutterers have become freed from their stuttering behaviors (which is all that we mean by symptoms) by undergoing an almost incredible variety of treatments, self-imposed or administered to them by others.

If we examine some of these older treatments for stuttering we note that some of them probably owed their efficacy to the way in which the stuttering behaviors were punished. For example, in the 1800's much surgery was performed on the tongues of stutterers. These were cut horizontally and vertically, and wedges removed from them (Burdin, 1940). Although such procedures soon were discarded, those of us who have read the original reports recognize that some stutterers were temporarily benefited and a few were evidently cured thereby. Why? Apart from the reassurance effect which decreases anxiety when such drastic treatment is carried out, or the absolution of presumed guilt acquired by paying such a penance, or the powerful suggestion that doubtless accompanied such surgery, it is also possible that many stutterers, especially during the period of ther convalescence, would find that strong contacts and pressures with the tongue would be most painful. After such surgery hypertensed postures with the tongue could not be maintained without contingent hurt. Sudden movements, hard contacts, and tremors would make a sore tongue shriek with immediate discomfort. In such a situation some modification of the usual struggling stuttering behavior would certainly occur, and that modification would probably be in the direction of decreasing severity. When the consequences of a bit of abnormal behavior are immediately punishing, that behavior is attentuated. In ancient times, stutterers have had their tongues burned with hot irons, painted with caustics, and scarified by strong spices, probably because each of these produced some of the same decrease in stuttering for the same reasons. We are also reminded of the British physician who prescribed croton oil, a profound cathartic. Stutterers who took their croton oil did not dare to struggle when they talked lest they fill their robes. If they stuttered, they would have to stutter easily and without pressing.

As a disorder, stuttering has always been subject to social penalties, but these penalties are seldom response-contingent in any systematic way. They are not applied immediately or consistently, or according to the sort of scheduling which might be used in a psychological laboratory. Often, indeed, the stutterer finds a bit of stuttering behavior more rewarding than painful, since his spasmodic struggle ends his communicative gap and also results in the furtherance of communication. It enables him to continue. Many a sudden jaw jerk or other contortion has been habituated by negative reinforcement. The noxious stimulus of a frustrating repetition or prolongation is terminated by that jaw jerk. Since these instrumental responses often make up the bulk of the stutterer's abnormality, we should not scoff too much at the possibility that some stutterers got some relief by undergoing such procedures. Indeed the present scheduling of electric shock or the application of delayed auditory feedback or loud masking noises by such operant investigators as Goldiamond (1965) demonstrates that a reduction in frequency and severity of stuttering can be procured, at least in the laboratory, by pairing these aversive stimuli with stuttering responses.

Another group of techniques used frequently in the past (and which still find some usage today) had their focus in attempting to alter, weaken, or remove the stimuli to which stuttering behavior was presumably the learned response. There are many such stimuli in the confirmed stutterer. Some are phonemic or morphemic, the stutterer fearing certain sounds and words. These stimuli have visual, auditory, and postural features. In addition to these, the position of the sound in the word, or the word in the sentence, the load of propositionality or meaningfulness, borne by that word or its history of past stuttering unpleasantness, all of these features and many more may be scanned by the stutterer for signals of approaching unpleasantness. When these stimuli are discriminated as indicating a high probability of stuttering the stutterer often then resorts either to avoidance or to covert or overt rehearsal behaviors preparatory to speech attempt. When this occurs, these rehearsals themselves can then become cues which increase the certainty. The stutterer cocks his mouth for stuttering. He assumes articulatory and phonatory postures and increases in the tension of these musculatures which almost guarantee trouble.

Many of the older methods used in treating stutterers probably found their utility by preventing the stutterer from scanning his speech for such stimuli or by preventing the preparatory rehearsal behavior. The stutterer who resorted to Demosthenes' pebbles or Madame Leigh's pad of cotton (Klingbeil, 1939) or used the Stammercheck wires (patented as recently as 1957) found it much more difficult to scan for stuttering in the same fashion that he did before. They interfere with his stereotyped preparatory sets to stutter in his old way. If you have a mouthful of pebbles you tend to concentrate more on keeping from swallowing them than on getting set to stutter. They alter the whole complicated stimulus configuration and tend to mask out the subtle stimuli to which stuttering or the expectation thereof has been conditioned.

Another set of techniques used by some therapists of the past (and present!) seeks to accomplish the same end by training the stutterer to speak in a monopitch, or regular rhythm often aided by finger pinching, arm swinging, or electric metronomes which tick their regularity into his ears. Simultaneous talking and writing, syllable tapping, and speaking in unison have a similar rationale. Why do these methods reduce stuttering? It is certain that they do, though the relief is usually temporary. Our explanation is that by altering the prosodic features of utterance so drastically and artificially, and by making all words or syllables motorically alike in their timing, these procedures reduce the stimulus value of the cues to which the expectation of stuttering has been conditioned. No sound, no syllable, no word can stick its head up long enough or far enough to be feared when such procedures are used. When stimuli are reduced in their visibility or potency, they become weakened or masked, and then the responses to which they have been conditioned will tend to occur less frequently. In learned behavior, the strength of the stimulus is as important as the strength of the response. For a thousand years distractions of a hundred kinds have been deliberately used by stutterers and their therapists to reduce the probability of stuttering by masking the verbal stimuli that lead to stuttering. Unfortunately, most of these distractions give small permanent relief because once their novelty is lost their interference with the stuttering stimuli becomes less effective. Indeed, through the reinforcement they achieve, distracting motor rituals can become incorporated into the abnormality.

Another group of techniques long used for treating stuttering owes its effectiveness to desensitization, not so much to the verbal stimuli we have last described, but to the interpersonal and communicative conditions which generate stuttering fears. There are situational fears as well as word or phonemic fears. Sheehan has described some of them in his six levels of approach-avoidance conflict (1957). Stuttering is not simply a disorder of speech; it is a disorder of communication, and the latter implies that the relationships between speaker and listener (as well as the conditions of communication) are the source of stimuli to which the stuttering behavior can become conditioned. Stutterers scan much more than the linguistic features of their forthcoming utterance; they also program into their internal computers a host of bits of information regarding the communicative situation as a whole before assessing the probabilities that they will stutter or not, or stutter mildly or severely. Such stutterers survey the approaching communicative situation with all their antennae quivering, searching for stimuli that might indicate trouble.

Many workers in the field of stuttering have devised methods which seek to weaken the potency of such situational stimuli. Suggestion in all of its forms, including hypnosis, has been used repeatedly to assure the patient that he could speak without stuttering. Prayer, exhortation, incantation, breath-chewing, rituals of many kinds, the two-room technique, and perhaps all therapeutic regimes have been employed to the same end. We are certain that some suggestible stutterers have been thereby reassured enough or convinced enough to enable them to stop attending to the situational stimuli connected with the stuttering response. When they are so reassured, their stuttering will markedly decrease or, temporarily at least, disappear. Self-recovered stutterers often tell us only that somehow they gained confidence and stopped fearing that they might stutter.

Another common set of therapeutic procedures devised to accomplish this same goal of minimizing or weakening the strength of situational stimuli are those in which the stutterer is gradually led from safe speaking situations, devoid of threatening stimuli, by a progression of steps into those which formerly were full of such threat. Stutterers have begun with pantomime, progressed through whispering into phonated speech, first when reading aloud to themselves, then when speaking to themselves, then in unison with the permissive therapist, then alone with him, then with other listeners gradually introduced into the speaking milieu, then to the telephone, and finally into the outside world. They have also been trained to progress from grunts, to vowels, to syllables, to words, to rhymes, to memorized sentences, to propositional speech. The old commercial schools for stutterers and summer camps, yes, and many a speech clinic, exploited this process of desensitization to situational stimuli, often with excellent though again temporary results. Some behavioral therapists have similarly used desensitization programs, as witness Meyer (1963), who shows how the dreaded telephone can lose its power to evoke stuttering by having the stutterer go through a series of programmed approximations while remaining completely relaxed, beginning by silently looking at a picture of a telephone and ending with the actual performance of phoning, and not moving on to the next step until each one has been scanned without tension or anxiety.

We find the same therapy now being advocated by Brutten and Shoemaker (1967). It is indisputable that such desensitization procedures are effective. The trouble with them is that the constellations of situation stimuli are so complex and extensive in the life of the usual confirmed stutterer that one would need a lifetime of therapy to scotch all the stimuli which might set off stuttering again. And, it is sad but true that stimulus generalization, so far as the dread of speaking situations is concerned, can proceed almost as rapidly as cancer. Many a stutterer has been led carefully up the desensitization ladder of increasing communicative stress only to fail to make the top rung and then to fall hard to the bottom. Once this happens it is difficult to get him to start climbing again.

Still another symptomatic approach to stuttering therapy which has been employed for many years is relaxation. Whether induced by hypnosis, strong suggestion, training in the methods pioneered by Jacobson, or as a by-product of psychotherapy the result, at least in the therapy room, is an immediate decrease in stuttering frequency and severity. In essence, relaxation is incompatible not only with tremors but also with fear, since the latter always generates tension. If, through systematic counter-conditioning, the situational and verbal cues can be programmed to evoke states of relaxation rather than tension, we have here a technique of real promise. But the *if* is a big IF. As Martin Palmer once remarked, it is hard to be a rag doll in a steel world. Moreover, the stimuli to which stuttering fears have been glued for so many years are many and various. They have their roots in the past history, in the self-concept, in the language, and in interpersonal relationships. They have been strongly and intermittently reinforced. Avoidance responses are notoriously hard to extinguish even in the laboratory where conditions can be rigorously controlled. In the real communicative life of a confirmed stutterer such controls are lacking. One would be hard-pressed to remain calm and relaxed in such a world as ours even if one did not stutter. Nevertheless we are sure that some individuals have found relief by reducing their states of hypertension. We are not impressed, however, with the results of relaxation training as the core of stuttering therapy. It has failed too often with too many stutterers.

In all of the foregoing techniques, the emphasis is upon *not stuttering*. To the extent that they reduce the frequency of the symptoms they serve as palliatives. Even though these methods may afford only temporary relief, as is usually the case, they may be thought to gain time enough for psychotherapy, for easing environmental changes, or for homeostasis to occur. Some therapists use repressive symptomatic therapy of the kinds mentioned for this very purpose, and with full knowledge that all that is gained is time. Unfortunately, most of those who use the distraction, suggestion, speech-alteration, or postural-set manipulations are less sophisticated. Often no therapy other than these palliative devices is given, and when relapse comes the therapists either go around the same old clinical bush another time or discharge the patient with the accusation that he has failed to follow instructions in some way. The resulting feelings of guilt, frustration, and inadequate helplessness render the case even more resistant to future therapy.

Now let us examine a typical example of repressive symptomatic therapy, first in terms of its ability to facilitate psychotherapy, and secondly in terms of learning theory. Froeschels (1950) describes the technique somewhat as follows: First the patient is instructed impressively concerning the importance of articulatory movements as modifiers of phonation. During this instruction, the therapist manipulates the stutterer's lips to produce different vowels. The case is then "told that voice and sighing are essentially the same function" and, if phonation seems blocked, to sigh. The stutterer is then required to read aloud "with opened mouth, but to move neither the lips or tongue." Then he is asked to make minimal movements of those structures as does the ventriloquist in utterance. No complete closures are permitted. Both therapist and patient then practice ventriloquizing. To quote specifically (p. 337):

> The stutterer is then told to use this method whenever possible, but certainly always at home. The parents, brothers and sisters should be trained in

ventriloquism in order to remind him how to speak. For some days he is required to read several times a day alternating "singing the speech melody" with ventriloquizing. After that time he is permitted to move lips and tongue a little more extensively, yet avoiding every closure and every narrow passage (fricatives). Still he should go back from time to time to ventriloquism and even to the pure speech melody.

Normal articulation is reached step by step, slowly or rapidly, according to the clinical picture. The patient is taught by steps which are only slightly different from the preceding one, i.e., progressing from pure speech melody to ventriloquism or from just avoiding every closure to normal articulation. Therefore, difficulties are avoided.

Since Froeschels in the same article refers to stuttering as a severe neurosis, let us examine this form of treatment to see how it agrees with the general principles of psychotherapy. Kanner (1942) says, "Any remedial program will depend on the knowledge of that which is to be relieved, namely, the *patient* rather than a detached organ or habit." Dollard and Miller (1950, p. 231) describe the therapeutic process as follows:

In addition to permissiveness, to skill in decoding conflict, and to the ability to aid the patient to label and discriminate, the therapist has skill in "dosing" anxiety. Others have tried to punish the symptoms or force the patient to perform the inhibited act. Both of these methods tend to increase the fear and the conflict. The therapist concentrates on reducing the fears and other drives motivating repression and inhibition, or in other words on analyzing "resistance." He tries to present the patient with a graded series of learning situations. He realizes that the patient must set his own pace and learn for himself; that it is the patient not the therapist who must achieve insight. He does not try to force the patient into any preconceived mold but helps him to develop his own potentialities in his own way within the limits imposed by our culture.

Freud says, "When we undertake to cure a patient of his symptoms he opposes against us a vigorous and tenacious resistance throughout the entire course of therapy" (1920, p. 253). Mowrer states (1950, p. 567):

One of Freud's earliest and most revolutionary contentions was that symptom therapy is futile. He believed that neurotic symptoms are essentially habits which the disturbed individual acquires as a means of reducing or avoiding anxiety. Thus by means of suggestions, authoritarian command, or other procedures, it may be possible to make a compulsive handwasher or an agoraphobiac give up his particular eccentricity, but the underlying problems remain and substitute symptom formation is very likely to occur.

According to Brown (1940, p. 76), "A symptomatic cure is concerned with removal of the symptom itself and is at best a temporary procedure. A dynamic or causal cure attempts to remove the basis of underlying maladjustment so that the symptoms disappear automatically." He goes on to say, "If there is one basic rule which may be laid down for all psychotherapy, it is the rule that symptoms are always helped by being admitted and faced."

The basic principle of psychotherapy, according to Alexander (1946) is "to re-expose the patient, under more favorable circumstances, to emotional situations which he could not handle in the past." That this reexposure is deep rather than superficial is indicated by Maslow and Mittelmann (1951, p. 248):

The special therapeutic aim is extremely thoroughgoing recasting of those reaction patterns which are responsible for the patient's difficulties. Not only are the symptoms relieved, but there are also changes in some aspects of his relationship with others, his evaluation of himself and others, his goals and the way in which he seeks to attain them.

For those who feel that the treatment of choice is nondirective counseling, Rogers (1942, p. 929) has these things to say:

Therapy is not a matter of doing something to the individual or of inducing him to do something about himself. It is instead a matter of freeing him for normal growth and development, of removing obstacles so that he can again move forward. . . .

Pennington and Berg (1947, p. 445) summarize these points of view as follows:

Most would agree, however, that the byproducts of the therapeutic process should incorporate for the client a long-range understanding of himself, the development of more satisfactory modes of adjustment, the objective acceptance of his thoughts, feelings and impulses.

The question before us is this: Will the ventriloquism techniques as a form of symptomatic therapy tend to aid or interfere with accompanying or subsequent psychotherapy? The answer seems to us to be definitely unfavorable for the following reasons: 1. If ventriloquism is successful, it immediately reduces motivation for any other therapy; if unsuccessful, it casts strong doubts on the therapist's ability. 2. By its tricklike simplicity, it tends to minimize the patient's true feelings concerning the seriousness of the disorder. 3. By its immediate effect, it tends to give the patient the feeling that basic therapy should also be of brief duration. 4. The technique itself may become a substitute symptom incorporated into the stuttering abnormality. 5. Because of the strong factor of suggestion implicit in the technique, it would tend to create attitudes of overdependency rather than self-sufficiency. 6. It places too great an immediate burden of responsibility upon the case for monitoring his speech in the presence of situation and word cues which must still be as potent as ever so far as fear and anxiety are concerned. 7. Finally, it is technique-centered rather than client-centered with all the disadvantages to psychotherapy which such an attitude would produce. All of these observations lead us to the inescapable conclusion that this form of repressive symptomatic therapy is unwise, even when attendant psychotherapy is being provided. When employed as the sole form of therapy, and nothing in Froeschel's article leads us to feel that this is not the case, the technique would seem to be even more contraindicated. It should be stated immediately that the same criticisms and objections hold for all of the other forms of repressive symptomatic therapy, of which ventriloquism is but a chance example.

Happily, in recent years speech therapists have begun to use a different type of symptomatic therapy, that which we have earlier labeled as expressive or dynamic. It probably had its origin in Freud's early interest in getting the patient to express rather than to inhibit his symptoms and in using the symptoms as barometers of the basic conflict. Symptoms became useful in therapy, and although symptom analysis and interpretation did not lead to complete solution of the patient's emotional problems, psychoanalysis stressed expression of symptoms rather than inhibition and repression. The fundamental permissiveness of the psychotherapist also led to a changed attitude toward the behavioral peculiarities of the case. It became apparent that before the devils could be cast out of the swine, they must be observed and worked with.

Dunlap's *beta hypothesis* (1932) also contributed to the development of the dynamic type of symptomatic therapy. Instead of using various ways of getting the stutterer to speak without stuttering, the case was required to practice duplicating his own symptoms, a process which the author termed *negative practice* (Dunlap, 1944). Although Dunlap conceived the stuttering symptoms to be merely habits which, when the stutterer became highly aware of them, could be brought under voluntary control and discarded, a good amount of psychotherapy was inherent in the process.

With Bryngelson's development of the therapeutic concept of "voluntary stuttering" (1935), symptomatic therapy, and psychotherapy became combined. Historically, he combined the beliefs of Travis (1931) —that the higher cortical (voluntary) centers can dominate the lower ones responsible for emotional behavior—with the mental hygiene point of view of Blanton (1936). In his therapeutic regime, Bryngelson (1943) stressed both the objective and subjective confrontation of self. The moments of stuttering were seen as the battleground in the struggle for control. The case was required to demonstrate in social situations his acceptance of self as revealed through stuttering. A repetitive symptom pattern was taught as the vehicle for these psychotherapeutic interactions. Group therapy was stressed. The stutterer was trained to stutter voluntarily, using the repetitive pattern whenever he felt under threat. If "voluntary stuttering" proved too difficult under these conditions, the case was taught to let the symptoms appear openly without attempts to avoid or inhibit them. Willingness to stutter openly became a goal of therapy. The contrast between this and the repressive form of symptomatic therapy is obvious.

Johnson, in several publications (1944, 1948), has presented another variety of expressive symptomatic therapy having many similarities to "voluntary stuttering" but also some important differences. In accord with his diagnosgenic or semantic theory of stuttering, he stresses the importance of nonfluency as an essential characteristic of stuttering and normal speech alike. The stutterer, through parental anxieties and semantic misinterpretations, has learned to react to these moments of nonfluency or the threat thereof by avoidance. He "hesitates to hesitate." The stuttering symptoms are merely the overt sign of a semantically fixed, approach-avoidance conflict. The basic psychotherapy is nondirective counseling at first, then training in semantics. But it is the accompanying symptomatic therapy with which we are here concerned.

As in the preceding treatment, the stutterer is urged to express and exhibit his stuttering under all kinds of communicative conditions and in all situations. The stutterer must not avoid or inhibit his symptoms but must use them for semantic analysis.

Since, according to Johnson, the stutterer's troubles stem from his attempt to avoid nonfluency, he should be willing to stutter openly, realizing at the same time what he is doing and why he is doing it. Observing that the normal speaker's nonfluency is characterized by effortless repetition, he sets up a similar pattern called "the bounce," which the stutterer should attempt to use instead of his avoidance reactions, contortions, hesitations, and other vocal abnormalities. In using the bounce, the stutterer responds to the feared stimulus by simply repeating the first syllable or sound of the word he is trying to say. This repetition is done fairly swiftly, effortlessly, and almost automatically. There is no struggle to make each repetition a highly voluntary act as is done in Bryngelson's "voluntary stuttering." There is no battle for control; the stutterer merely lets the repetitions bounce along until the word comes out. Other forms of "easy stuttering," such as the effortless prolongation of a sound or posture, are also acceptable. It is apparent that such a symptomatic therapy harmonizes much better with semantic psychotherapy than would any of the types of repressive symptomatic therapy described earlier.

Another type of symptomatic treatment has been evolved by the author through his continuing experimenting with therapy for adult stutterers. Since, in this chapter, he has been highly critical of other symptomatic therapies, he submits his own to the same objective inspection.

Briefly, the theoretical foundation for this therapy is based upon two assumptions: First, that most of the abnormality of the stutterer consists of a) avoidance responses to various phonetic, situational, and semantic cues; and b) habitual escape and struggle responses to self-initiated *tremors* in the structures dealing with articulation, phonation, or respiration. Second, he assumes that most, if not all, secondary stutterers present the picture of neurosis. The author feels that this neurosis is *occasionally* primary, the symptoms being pregenital conversion reactions with both anal and oral components, but much more often it is *secondary*, that is, the neurotic behavior originates as a defensive reaction to the penalties which our highly verbal culture imposes upon those individuals whose nonfluency is excessive. In either event, some form of psychotherapy seems absolutely necessary.

But what kind? The author has referred his cases to psychiatrists and psychoanalysts. He has employed nondirective counseling, vocational rehabilitation, socialization, psychodrama, and other types of psychotherapy extant. He has used these alone without any symptomatic therapy; he has employed them concurrently with or prior to speech therapy, and also as terminal therapy. The results were generally unsatisfactory. Some stutterers improved in their basic personal adjustment and personality but very few in speech. When psychotherapy was used concurrently with speech therapy, the best results were obtained, although each was affected by the other in both positive and negative ways.

Following up this empirical lead, we tried to develop a therapy which, while masquerading as symptomatic therapy, would actually be a psychotherapy. It was felt that the laws of learning and unlearning apply to neurotic behavior in general much in the same fasion as they do to a habitual lip protrusion conditioned to the perception of an approaching labial sound in particular. If this is true, then a combination symptomatic psychotherapy might possibly be evolved, not by repressing the symptoms but by manipulating them in the interests of the healing process. If the self could be equated with the stuttering, then by working with the stuttering we might be able to alter the self. The fact that the case accepts the self-concept and label of "stutterer," and conceives of himself as playing that dominant role, tends to render such a hypothesis tenable at least. Moreover, each moment of stuttering can be envisaged as a miniature neurosis in itself, with a surrender of responsibility, compulsive behavior, and anxiety reduction as important features. The symbolic nature of many symptoms is quite apparent. Symbolically, stutterers soil, whimper, bite, gag, and recoil from themselves and their listeners as they stutter. The choice of symptoms in a disorder whose symptomatology varies so widely as it does in stuttering is probably due to both availability and need (Rotter, 1942). If the basic response to cultural penalty or frustration is aggression, the symptoms are explosive in nature. As one of many possible illustrations, one of our cases spat upon his listener in the throes of his verbal struggle. The internalized symptoms described by Douglass and Quarrington (1952) may be viewed as inwardly turned aggression. Whatever the symptoms may be, they can become highly revealing to the case and therapist alike.

But even more revealing than the presenting symptoms is the general behavior of the stutterer when, in the course of speech therapy, he begins to display and to manipulate and modify his stuttering reactions. As in psychoanalysis, where there occurs strong initial resistance to the method of free association as demanded by the analyst, so too there is usually found a similar resistance to free uninhibited stuttering as demanded by the speech therapist. As the case finds his stuttering offerings accepted permissively by the therapist without penalty but with interest, a transference relationship comes into being as it does in analysis. With this supportive relationship existing and in part due to the presence of similar reinforcement from the other members of the group receiving therapy, the stutterer begins to get interested in his stuttering as revelatory of self. He begins to assign himself large cathartic doses of real and pseudo-stuttering. As his tolerance of himself as a stutterer increases, he begins to use the therapist and other members of the group as parental or sibling figures, and a process very similar to abreaction takes place. At this stage the stuttering becomes much more frequent and severe. Much emotional heat is generated and discharged upon the therapist, the other stutterers receiving group therapy, and upon certain innocent auditors in the world outside the speech clinic. A good amount of reality-testing takes place. Since the basis of the therapeutic method is the collection by the stutterer of a certain quota of stuttering in self-chosen speaking situations each day as a vehicle for the exploration, understanding, and control of the self, the choice of auditors becomes of great significance. Instead of conjuring up a father image verbally on the psychiatrist's couch, the case finds a flesh-and-blood yet symbolic one in the traffic policeman on the corner. With him he can interact. He can confront his anxieties, his compulsions, and defenses in his moment of stuttering and recount these to the therapist in his report, or the therapist can be with him at the time to observe, protect, and occasionally to interpret. If he finds the situation too threatening, he has the perfect right to retreat, providing he attempts to understand why he must do so. Even as the analyst and later the case learn much from trains of thought which become blocked, refused, or diverted into safer channels, so the therapist and stutterer achieve much insight from these experiences. Active analysis, such as that described by Herzberg (1945) in which graded tasks performed by the patient during treatment contribute much to insight, gives us some precedent for using this type of symptomatic therapy in the interests of self-understanding.

In any psychotherapy, there is a need not only to understand one's impulses toward socially reprehensible behavior, but an equally important need to assess the self-punitive aspects of our beings. How stutterers feel about their moments of stuttering can reveal much about how they feel about themselves. At any rate, a marked change in attitude occurs during the early stages of therapy toward both self and stuttering. Most cases magnify and exaggerate the penalties they have received and those they expect to receive. As they try to achieve the goal of stuttering openly and freely they tend to whittle their blown-up superegos down to size. They find that the less they punish themselves, the less punishment they receive from others. The permissiveness of the therapist transfers to permissiveness in the case and this attitude in turn transfers to many of his auditors. By actively displaying their free stuttering in communicative situations, much reality-testing is accomplished in this area as well.

It is no easy task to confront oneself; and when the stutterer tries to stutter willingly without avoidance or recoil, that is what he is attempting to do. The rejecting ghosts of his parents and associates find reincarnation in every present listener. Fortunately, in the therapist and in his fellow stutterers he finds enough acceptance and reward to permit him to make the tentative attempts necessary to progress in solving the approach-avoidance and avoidance-avoidance conflicts (Mowrer, 1950) that comprise his neurosis and beget his symptoms.

In order to stutter freely, the case must surrender many of the defense and disguise reactions which themselves are part of the symptomatology. He can do this only insofar as he finds acceptance and reward on the part of the therapist and others. By rewarding the approach tendency and failing to reward the avoidance, the therapist helps the case get out of the oscillating or fixating behavior so characteristic of his abnormality. As the stutterer finds that his anxiety is not followed by punishment, it tends to decrease. This is especially true when the anxiety reduction is the result not of avoidance but of adaptation training or of testing the formerly noxious stimulus. All psychotherapy, including this, can be formulated in these terms (Dollard and Miller, 1950).

In the daily collection of a quota of attempts to stutter freely, the therapist and case not only become aware of the emotional states involved; they also come to a better understanding of the case's ability to formulate and carry out and evaluate an unpleasant task. Not only his performances but also his aspiration levels are scrutinized. Through the discussion of both, the case comes to a more realistic concept of self. Clarification of the essential attitudes toward oneself comes swiftly when the case is actively attempting to modify his behavior, but only if he is protected and supported by the therapist or the group at the same time. Our experience with purely passive and verbal forms of psychotherapy, as we have said before, is that they often help the case with his other problems but leave the stuttering problem intact. The reason for this, we believe, is that the stutterer so closely identifies his *self* with his stuttering. Psychiatrists have considered stuttering to be a very difficult disorder to treat if not to understand. Were they to use free stuttering in the same revealing way that they do free verbalization, they would lessen their difficulties.

As time goes on, the stutterer finds it increasingly possible to stutter uninhibitedly and openly in situations which formerly were filled with great anxiety. He also finds that, uncomplicated by struggle and avoidance, the severity of his stuttering is lessening. He can stutter with more muscular as well as mental ease. He becomes interested in and curious about both his fluency and nonfluency. He has regained contact with his listener and himself. His insight has grown in every sphere. He has increased his frustration tolerance. He has behind him a good backlog of partial successes in self-acceptance and control. His feelings make sense. He does not seem to need the therapist's or the group's support as much as he did formerly. He has begun to experiment a little with his interpersonal relationships and with his stuttering.

When this point is reached in therapy, the case is given a new tool of adjustment, a technique called *cancellation*. This consists of coming to a complete halt after the stuttered word has been finally uttered, pausing a moment and then attempting to say the word again with even less struggle and avoidance. The case is not to try to say the word without stuttering. Even when the fear and threat is gone and he knows he can say it without having any symptoms, he deliberately does some pseudostuttering on the cancellation. This pseudostuttering should not be a facsimile of the original symptoms, but represent a modification of them in the direction of normal nonfluency.

The pause in cancellation is used for scrutinizing the symptoms and feelings existing during the preceding blocking in the light of his newly-found insight into self. In the pause the case also evaluates his preceding behavior in terms of its adjustive pertinence to efficient communication. For example, he may say to himself, "That was a silly reaction, trying to utter the word 'business' with my mouth wide open. Can't be done. Why did I just give up?" During the interim between the original stuttering and the new cancelling attempt, the stutterer finds himself altering his sets and making plans for the subsequent modification of symptoms.

From the point of view of psychotherapy, what have we in this cancelling technique? First of all we have provided an opportunity for self-confrontation and evaluation. We have also prevented the repression that usually takes place immediately after a moment of stuttering. Most stutterers verbally flee the site of the crime. They distract themselves. They try to avoid contemplating their fiascos. Much of the self-reinforcing value in stuttering is due to this immediate repression of auditor hostility or self-revulsion. The pause and new attempt are valuable in yet another way; by deliberately interrupting the communicative process they allow the stutterer to test his independence of auditor penalty and his own strength. In effect, he says to the world, "Behold! I stutter, but I am working with it, trying to conquer it. If this bothers you, I'm sorry, but I've a job to do." It also gives the stutterer an opportunity for discovering his new potentialities for controlling his emotions and behavior. It enables him to test the reality of his evaluations.

From the point of view of learning theory, cancellation has these advantages. It takes advantage of the moment of reaction inhibition, the point in time at which the old stuttering response is weakest. It interferes with the self-reinforcing tendency of stuttering symptoms to terminate the fear. It increases the strength of the approach factor in the approach-avoidance conflict. It facilitates discrimination of the phonetic and other cues. It provides a substitute response which society in general rewards. (People generally approve of an individual who shows evidence of wrestling with his problem.) Finally, it provides a symbolic goal. The stutterer realizes that a form of stuttering similar to that which is demonstrated in the cancellation would be tolerable to both himself and other people. It demonstrates to the stutterer that it might be possible to stutter in another way, that he might be able to stutter and still communicate, that stuttering need not be catastrophic. When such reassurance comes from one's own behavior rather than from the verbalizations of the therapist, it is an extremely potent force in psychotherapy.

Let us point out again the parallel between this

"symptomatic technique" and what happens in psychoanalysis. In the latter, as a result of the intensive exploration of self, there comes a stage in which the victim of a compulsion, such as the urge to scrub the hands fiercely, has gained considerable insight into the origins and dynamics of this behavior, yet finds himself still doing it as soon as certain cues appear. In any specific instance, however, it is only after handwashing has taken place that he can analyze and understand why he did what he did, and what else he might have done under the same circumstances. In a very real sense he is doing the same thing our cases are doing when they cancel.

Later on, the insight and understanding move forward in time and take place *during* the compulsive handwashing which is interrupted at that point and replaced by behavior which is more adaptive. Similarly, in our symptomatic therapy, once cancellation has become a fairly common practice on the part of the stutterer, we provide another technique called "*pull-out*." In pulling out of blocks, the stutterer does not let the original blocking run its course as he does in cancellation. Instead, he makes a deliberate attempt to modify it before the release occurs and before the word is spoken. The same analysis and insight which in cancellation took place *subsequent* to the stuttering now takes place *during* it. Again, he tries to modify the symptoms in the direction of normal nonfluency. Again, we find a real battle against his neurotic tendencies. Gradually the insight comes to dominate the resistance, and a further resolution of the conflict occurs. The struggle for control of conflicting impulses is the heart of all psychotherapeutic healing. We have it here.

At this point let us describe something of the mechanics of the pull-out process. Many workers in the field of stuttering (Johnson and Knott, 1936; Wischner, 1950; Sheehan, 1953) see only one side of the stuttering problem, viewing it as a clear example of the approach-avoidance conflict. With them, we agree wholeheartedly so far as this describes symptoms of avoidance, postponement, and disguise which precede the actual speech attempt. But we feel there is something else equally as important. In most but not all moments of stuttering we find a *tremor* to which the stutterer reacts maladaptively and with feelings of helplessness and inability. This tremor is similar to *intentional tremor* in many ways, though we do not consider the stuttering tremor to be organically caused.

In order to occur, this tremor requires a sudden surge of localized tension in a certain area of the speech musculatures and is triggered by a posture or contact differing from those used in normal speech. The assumption of these trigger postures can be envisaged as being conditioned to certain phonetic cues, for example, the perception of the *b* in the word *busy* as threatening stuttering. The old terms *clonus* and *tonus*, formerly used to classify stuttering symptoms, were probably due to recognition by early observers of these tremor and trigger-posture states.

Once in stuttering tremor, the case is caught in a physiological trap. He may stop it at will (Van Riper, 1938), but only by giving up his intention to utter the word. If he attempts the word again, the same trigger posture may be assumed and a new tremor started. When this fails to solve the problem, his response to the renewed tremor is a natural one. He starts struggling, thereby increasing the tension. This unfortunately merely increases the tremor amplitude and/or frequency and renders release more difficult. The same mechanism can be seen in athetosis and other tremors. With enough effort, the tremor speeds up until it creates the tonic state of contraction so familiar in severe stuttering.

The picture of oscillation and postural fixation as a result of the organism being confronted by two equally punishing alternatives is well known. Avoidance-avoidance conflicts produce them routinely. A long gap of silence in the midst of important communication can be extremely punishing. When speaking and nonspeaking are both punishing, tremor and tonic fixation tend to appear.

How then, does the stutterer ever get out of the trap? The author (1939), using a pneumatic recording device, examined jaw tremors of nine stutterers in an effort to determine what happened at the moment of release from block. All stutterers showed three basic patterns: the tremors decreased in amplitude or they decreased in frequency or a large sudden movement of the jaw out of phase with the tremor occurred. When the large movement was in phase, no release took place. We would explain these tentative findings as follows: in approaching a feared word, the stutterer expects *a certain amount* of unpleasantness. The more the fear, the greater is the unpleasantness expected. Milisen and Van Riper (1934) showed that stutterers could predict the duration of their stuttering with a fair amount of accuracy. The point we wish to make here is that once the amount of expected abnormality has taken place, the fear is satisfied and tension reduction takes place. This in turn causes a decrease in the amplitude and frequency of the tremor and the alteration of the trigger posture, and release results. This occurs in some of the blockings. In other blockings, random struggle and repeated attempts to jerk out of the tremor may shift the focus of tension, alter the trigger posture, or break the oscillation by an out-of-phase movement of the tremored structure. But, at best, this is relatively the poorest of the three ways of releasing oneself from tremor. Not only does the effort to jerk out of the tremor result in bizarre symptoms which the subsequent release rewards and fixates, but in many cases (if in phase) it merely bounces the stutterer back into his tremor. Trying to pull out of a tremor by any out-of-phase movement calls for precise timing and a good deal of luck. Observation of any severe stutterer will yield many instances in which syllables and whole words are actually uttered during the throes of his struggle only to have the stutterer continue stuttering.

When the stutterer, during the course of his symptomatic therapy, begins to pull out of his blocks, he learns to discard this third way and instead he spends his efforts trying to smooth out the tremor and slow it down. By this time, the moment of stuttering no longer is the shaking experience it was formerly. He can experiment with it, varying the tension, altering the trigger contacts and postures. At this point the therapist suggests the possibility of learning how he can deliberately throw himself into tremors. Again resistance is found and overcome and out of the experience comes a marked gain in his feeling of control and self-responsibility. No longer does the symptom control the stutter; instead he is the master.

In terms of learning theory, the pull-out technique has effectiveness because the release (the utterance) rewards not the uncontrolled abnormality which formerly preceded it but the voluntary smoothing out and slowing down of the tremor. The anxiety reduction has its greatest potency at this moment. Guthrie (1935) and others have shown that the behavior immediately preceding release from punishment gets the strongest reinforcement. The gradient of reinforcement is steepest at this point. At any rate, in therapy it is interesting to observe how swiftly the stutterer gains an ability to take charge of his tremors and to effect a controlled release. Even more interesting is the change in the approach-avoidance features of the conflict. The awareness of approaching stuttering no longer repels. Instead, it signifies an opportunity for winning a new battle. The cases go out to look for trouble. They hunt for feared words and situations. It is axiomatic, of course, that this desired result is the consequence of a long learning process with many unsuccessful trials along the way. Even if the case fails in his attempt to pull out of a block, however, he can still cancel; and in any event he learns a good deal about himself. All therapy is structured in terms of the question: what did you discover about yourself when you stuttered? The therapist is always interested and permissive and he is supportive to the degree required by the case. Often he is able to clarify an experience, to interpret a bit of behavior on the part of either the stutterer or his listener. He is always far more the psychotherapist than the dog-trainer.

To describe the dynamics of the terminal stages of therapy is always difficult. The case has less need for the therapist; he "feels like a different person"; he loses interest in his symptoms; his emotions are less intense; he becomes involved in new fields of endeavor; he begins to accept responsibility for his own failures and difficulties; he learns to monitor his behavior in terms of the realities that exist; he can both venture and control. Viewed from the vantage point of learning theory, new competitive responses have become conditioned to the stimuli which formerly set off the whole stuttering volley of behavioral and emotional reactions. These have moved forward in time so that they now exist as *preparatory sets*. With enough experience in pulling out of tremors of fairly long duration, the stutterer finds himself able to get this control sooner. The tremors get shorter. The case can take charge earlier. He soon finds himself preparing in advance to smooth out and slow down his tremors and when this happens preparatory sets are being used.

At this point the stutterer becomes able to control the duration of his abnormality, to stutter so briefly that his listener will not react to it with penalty. The symptoms become tolerable. Indeed, they become normal non-fluency. What happens is that the stutterer learns to stutter fluently. This can be a pleasant experience. The approach-avoidance and the avoidance-avoidance conflicts have turned into an approach-approach situation. The vicious circle is broken. No longer does the tension subside only when struggle results in verbal utterance. No longer does anxiety reduction reinforce the unpleasant symptoms. Stuttering has lost its threat and its usefulness.

The author is highly aware of the fact that much of

the foregoing presentation is based upon assumptions urgently in need of experimental verification. They have been derived primarily from experimental therapy and clinical observation. If they can do no more than to jar stuttering research out of its present sterile doldrums, they will have served a vital purpose. But the basic concept, that some type of "symptomatic" therapy can also be viewed as a form of effective psychotherapy, we feel, has been demonstrated. Our cases do not only find an amelioration in their symptoms; they change as persons. Moreover, we do not feel that such symptomatic therapy is at all incompatible with other forms of psychotherapy. Used concomitantly, subsequently, or prior to the traditional forms of psychotherapy, it has proved extremely facilitating. In many cases, especially with those whose neurosis seems to have arisen as a result of audience penalty or verbal frustration, it can be used alone.

SUMMARY

In this chapter we have described two types of symptomatic therapy for stutterers, that which attempts to inhibit the symptom and that which exploits the symptom as a vehicle of psychotherapy. Examples of each are examined in terms of their congruence with basic psychotherapy and in terms of learning theory. It is concluded that symptomatic therapy of the latter type can facilitate psychotherapy or serve as a vehicle of psychotherapy.

BIBLIOGRAPHY

Ainsworth, S. 1945. Integrating theories of stuttering. *J. Speech Hearing Disorders*, 10, 205–210.

———. 1949. Present trends in the treatment of stuttering. *J. except. Child.*, 16, 41–43.

Alexander, F., and French, T. 1946. Psychoanalytic therapy, principles and application. New York: Ronald.

Appelt, A. 1929. Stammering and its permanent cure. London: Methuen.

Blanton, S. 1931. Stuttering. *Ment. Hyg.*, 15, 271–282.

———, and Blanton, M. 1936. For stutterers. New York: Appleton-Century.

Bloodstein, O. 1949. Conditions under which stuttering is reduced or absent; a review of the literature. *J. Speech Hearing Disorders*, 14, 295–302.

Bluemel, C. 1935. Stammering and allied disorders. New York: Macmillan.

Boome, E., and Richardson, M. 1932. The nature and treatment of stuttering. New York: Dutton.

Brown, J. 1940. The psychodynamics of abnormal behavior. New York: McGraw-Hill.

Brutten, E., and Shoemaker, D. 1967. The modification of stuttering. Englewood Cliffs, N.J.: Prentice-Hall.

Bryngelson, B. 1935. Voluntary stuttering. *Proc. Amer. Speech Correction Assn.*, 5, 35–38.

———. 1943. Stuttering and personality development. *Nerv. Child.*, 2, 219–223.

Clark, R. 1948. Supplementary techniques to use with secondary stutterers. *J. Speech Hearing Disorders*, 13, 131–134.

Cypreasen, L. 1948. Group therapy for adult stutterers. *J. Speech Hearing Disorders*, 313–319.

Dollard, J., and Miller, N. 1950. Personality and psychotherapy. New York: McGraw-Hill.

Douglass, E., and Quarrington, B. 1952. The differentiation of interiorized and exteriorized secondary stuttering. *J. Speech Hearing Disorders*, 17, 377–385.

Dunlap, K. 1932. The technique of negative practice. *Amer. J. Psychol.*, 55, 270–273.

———. 1944. Stammering: its nature, etiology and therapy. *J. comp. Psychol.*, 37, 187–202.

Eysench, H. ed. 1960. Behavior therapy and the neuroses. New York: Pergamon.

Fenichel, O. 1945. The psychoanalytic theory of neuroses. New York: Norton.

Fletcher, J. 1928. The problem of stuttering: a diagnosis and a plan of treatment. New York: Longmans.

Freud, S. 1920. A general introduction to psychoanalysis. New York: Liveright.

Froeschels, E. 1950. A technique for stutterers—ventriloquism. *J. Speech Hearing Disorders*, 15, 336–337.

Gifford, M. 1940. How to overcome stammering. Englewood Cliffs, N.J.: Prentice-Hall.

Goldiamond, I. 1965. *In* Research in behavior modification. Krasner, L., and Ullmann, L., eds. New York: Holt, Rinehart and Winston.

Greene, J. 1931. Stuttering: what about it? *Proc. Amer. Speech Correction Assn.*, 1, 165–175.

Gustavson, C. 1944. A talisman and a convalescence. *Quart. J. Speech*, 30, 465–571.

Guthrie, E. R. 1935. The psychology of learning. New York: Harper.

Hahn, E. Stuttering: 1943. Significant theories and therapies. Palo Alto: Stanford.

Herzberg, A. 1945. Active psychotherapy. New York: Grune & Stratton.

Jackson, B. 1950. An on the spot survey of stuttering therapies. Univ. Denver, Master's thesis.

Johnson, W. 1944. The Indians have no word for it. *Quart. J. Speech*, 30, 456–465.

———. 1946. People in quandaries. New York: Harper.

———, Brown, S., Curtis, J., Edney, C., and Keaster, J. 1948. Speech handicapped school children. New York: Harper.

Johnson, W., and Knott, J. 1936. The moment of stuttering. *J. genet. Psychol.*, 48, 475–479.

Kanner, L. 1953. Child psychiatry. Springfield, Ill.: Charles C Thomas.

Klingbeil, G. 1939. The historical background of the modern speech clinic. *J. Speech Disorders*, 4, 115–132.

Lemert, E., and Van Riper, C. 1944. The use of psychodrama in the treatment of speech defects. *Sociometry*, 7, 190–195.

Maslow, A., and Mittelmann, B. 1951. Principles of abnormal psychology (rev. ed.). New York: Harper.

Meyer, J. 1963. A new technique to control stammering: a preliminary report. *Behavior Res. Therapy*, 1, 251–254.

Milisen, R., and Van Riper, C. 1934. A study of the predicted duration of the stutterer's blocks as related to their actual duration. *J. Speech Disorders*, 4, 339–345.

Moore, W. 1946. Hypnosis in a system of therapy for stutterers. *J. Speech Disorders*, 11, 117–122.

Mowrer, O. 1950. Learning theory and personality dynamics. New York: Ronald.

Pennington, L., and Berg, I. 1947. An introduction to clinical psychology. New York: Ronald.

Rogers, C. 1942. Counseling and psychotherapy. Boston: Houghton Mifflin.

Rotter, J. 1942. A working hypothesis as to the nature and treatment of stuttering. *J. Speech Disorders*, 7, 263–288.

Schultz, D. 1947. A study of non-directive counseling as applied to adult stutterers. *Speech Monogr.*, 14, 206–207.

Sheehan, J. 1953. Theory and treatment of stuttering as an approach-avoidance conflict. *Amer. J. Psychol.*, 35, 24–49.

———. 1957. *In* Stuttering, a symposium. Eisenson, J. ed. New York: Harper.

Skinner, B. 1963. Operant behavior. *Amer. Psychol.*, 18, 503–515.

Steer, M., and Johnson, W. 1936. An objective study of the relationship between psychological factors and the severity of stuttering. *J. abnorm. soc. Psychol.*, 31, 36–46.

Thorne, F. 1950. Principles of personality counseling. *J. clin. Psychol.*

Travis, L. 1931. Speech pathology. New York: Appleton-Century.

———. 1940. The need for stuttering. *J. Speech Disorders*, 5, 193–202.

Van Riper, C. 1938. A study of the stutterer's ability to interrupt stuttering spasms. *J. Speech Disorders*, 3, 117–119.

———. 1939. An investigation of stuttering tremors. Unpublished paper read at the national convention American Speech Correction Association.

Wilton, G. 1950. How to overcome stuttering. New York: Harper.

Wischner, G. 1950. Stuttering behavior and learning: a preliminary theoretical investigation. *J. Speech Hearing Disorders*, 15, 324–355.

Wolpe, J. 1958. Psychotherapy by reciprocal inhibition. Stanford: Stanford.

39

The Unspeakable Feelings of People with Special Reference to Stuttering

Lee Edward Travis

Stuttering is the consequence of the young child speaking with his mother and father. In his words he sought their appraisal of him. In his utterances he asked to be known and to be understood. In their reply they told of his unacceptability in his current verbalized form. He would need to change, either in his deep parts or in the verbal expression of them. As he continued to talk, not knowing quite what to do about himself, he began to hesitate and to stumble a little and to repeat. Now his mother and father were no longer so critical and rejecting of him and his telling, but were actually supportively concerned. He must need their love and they would give it to him. He must need their attention and they would give that also. He did need these things, their love and their attention, but not for the reason his parents gave them, not because he stuttered.

GENERAL STATEMENTS

May I propose that stuttering is based upon an interchange between the speaker and the listener, an interaction between what is in the speaker's mouth to say and what is in his listener's ear to hear. The main troubles of the stutterer are derived from the complimentarity and mutual exclusiveness of orders of opposite sign given simultaneously by an authority. By every seemingly normal and natural appearance the parents want their child to talk early and to talk well. It may be really that they are too ambitious for him in these areas. Yet by a frown and a glance and even by a verbal message he is asked if not ordered not to talk now, or that way, or about that subject matter. As the parents and the child define a relationship between them they work out together what type of communicative behavior is to take place in the relationship.

In the beginning of speech in the child, was not speech meant to be pure impulse perfect in every motion like the walk of the cat? The child did not know that he talked, let alone how he talked. One day his mother called his attention to his speech, however, and he knew for the first time that he talked, and never again would he not know that he knew. From then on he was responsible, and possibly terribly responsible, too responsible for his speech revelations. He was initiated young into the monitored ways of life and his confidence and simplicity were checked. Something had gone wrong, something possibly undefined, but something in some way was his fault; he had done it. He was to blame. He was responsible. From now on he must make speech happen. No longer or ever again will it just happen of itself. He must through pain of thinking and choice decide the course of his declarations. Always now he will move with some anxiety, because he can never know what is right and when something will go deeply and strangely wrong.

Stuttering may be considered as an advertisement of some form and degree of placing the speaker under taboo (Frank, 1961). In stuttering, the speaker is experiencing an interdiction laid upon his performance in saying words to another. In his speech blocks he is signaling his ostracism imposed upon him by his company of listeners. Stuttering is a special case of the universal conflict between closeness and distance, involvement and autonomy, intimacy and autism. His experiments in closeness have been too painful to stand and he has suffered a reaction of self-banishment. He has settled for a minimum relatedness which does not include free talking about his thoughts and feelings. Rightly or wrongly he has interpreted the responses of another as adversive.

In a significant way parents place the child in a paradoxical position in teaching him to talk. Conflicting levels of message occur when the verbal statements of parents qualify their tone of voice, body movement, or contextual situation incongruently (Haley, 1963). Stuttering is the reciprocal to the parents' verbal requests. They ask the verbal symptom of their child, thereby participating in its appearance and its maintenance. Their verbal demands contain qualifications of themselves. Saying this another way, the parents teach the child how (by his stuttering) to circumscribe their management of his behavior, particularly of his verbal behavior. Stuttering is thus responsive behavior occurring in an interpersonal context. It will not stop on command because it is a style of maneuvering other people, although the results may be stressful to everybody.

Like all other developmental deviations, stuttering tends to be self-perpetuating. The interpersonal pattern between child and parent that flowered the stuttering originally trained the stutterer to prefer his stuttering relationship with other people as well. His experiences with all people continually confirm his stuttering reactions to them, for his stuttering is not dependent only upon an intrapsychic deviation, but also upon current interpersonal experience. Between people who speak and those who listen, stuttering tells of excuses and explanations in the preservation of the speaker's self-esteem. The symptom is the advantage enjoyed by the stutterer in gaining control of what is to happen in a relationship with someone else. The obvious trouble in speaking may represent considerable distress to the stutterer subjectively, but much distress is preferred to living in an unpredictable world of social relationships over which he may otherwise have little or no control.

In the control of a relationship stuttering is symptomatic because neither the stutterer nor the listener necessarily senses this to be true. On the contrary, the stutterer circumscribes the behavior of the listener while denying that he is doing so. The stutterer denies responsibility in the control of the listener, but nonetheless controls him, blaming his control on something else, the stuttering, over which he insists he has no control. Stuttering is assured since parents and others, including speech therapists, dance to the stutterer's tune of stuttering and thereby perpetuate his stuttering behavior. What works now started the stuttering in the first place. The start was when the child speaker was told either implicitly or explicitly by his parents to try to say something that he had been told not to say. And he would never be quite clear what it was that received such paradoxical treatment. What exactly was it that he should and should not say? His guilt was all the more disquieting since the nature of his crime was usually unstated. "You know what I mean," "you know very well what you have done," "you know why I punish you," "we both know your problem," are all common statements to the child facing reprimand. He has an obscure and gnawing sense of being profoundly in the wrong, though for no discernible reason. May he avoid if possible the feeling that his very existence is an effrontery to his parents and even to others. Finally, may he avoid the feeling that just to be alive is both a fault and his own fault.

THE CORE PHENOMENON OF STUTTERING[1]

Neurophysiologically, speech is a modification of expiration. In the organism at rest, normal breathing movements consist of an active inspiration followed by a passive expiration. It is evident, however, that with speech, an inspiration which is always active is followed also by an *active* expiration. The speaker regulates the rate and amount of expiration and properly modifies it to form sounds and sound combinations to suit best the purposes of his speaking. In modifying the outgoing breath stream for goals of vocalization and articulation, the speaker does one essential thing—for varying periods of time he partially or completely obstructs this breath stream by the partial or complete approximation of juxtaposed structures in the pathway of the outgoing air column. The primary structures used in this process of modification are the vocal cords, tongue, velum,

[1] This section, The Core Phenomenon of Stuttering, and the next section, Stuttering as Learned Behavior, are based upon the author's article, A Theoretical Formulation of Stuttering, which appeared in *Western Speech*, 23, Summer, 1959.

hard palate, alveolar ridge, teeth, and lips. In one sense, these structures used in relationship to each other present a series of air valves which may completely or partially block the passage of air. The movements of these and other structures in proper temporal and spatial relationship to each other constitute the so-called speech movements—the movements necessary for the production of speech sounds. When the speaker is performing normally, the alteration and control of the outgoing breath stream are appropriate to the intention of communication.

As we have noted, the speaker is constantly blocking the outgoing breath stream in various degrees and for varying lengths of time. The length and completeness of the blocks determine, partially at least, the rate and rhythm of speech. If juxtaposed structures, such as the vocal cords, back of the tongue and velum, middle of the tongue and hard palate, tongue tip and upper front teeth, upper front teeth and lower lip, or the two lips were to continue the approximation beyond certain time limits, speech would be altered in rate and rhythm. Some sounds would be prolonged if the approximation of juxtaposed structures were of the improper length for the production of that sound, and other sounds would be completely absent if the approximation of the juxtaposed structures involved was complete. For example, if a speaker continued the correct approximation of the structures involved in the formation of (s) beyond the desired or standard time limit, a continuous hissing sound would be produced. If, on the other hand, he carried the approximation of these same structures too far, made a complete block and held it, then no sound at all would be forthcoming.

These examples pertain to the prolongation or the complete blocking of a single sound. The repetition of a sound, a syllable, a word, or even of a phrase may occur as an expression of the same fundamental overmodifying process. May it be concluded, then, that the core of the phenomenon known as stuttering may be conceived neurophysiologically as an overmodification of the outgoing breath stream by a series of air valves? This overmodification is, essentially, a prolongation of the proper degree of approximation of juxtaposed structures or a prolongation of the complete approximation of these structures, resulting in varying degrees and kinds of blocking of the forward flow of speech. The stutterer experiences a perseveration or an exaggeration, or both, of the functioning of the speech valves. It is as though he were unable to manage the air stream by means of these valves; they close too tightly, or too long, or repetitively in violation of his purposes. Crudely, the defect may be described as "sticky valves." To the discomforture of the stutterer the valves stick. This is unintentional or involuntary, and it interferes with and interrupts the stutterer's management of the valves. When it is occurring, the stutterer may struggle with it and manifest the well-known secondary symptoms. After this uncontrollable sticking has occurred sufficiently often in interpersonal relationships, the stutterer establishes anticipatory reactions to possible future occurrences. As a consequence of the anticipatory, current, and consequent reactions, a whole constellation of thoughts, feelings, and acts are built around the core phenomenon of "sticky valves." Thoughts of suicide, feelings of inadequacy, and acts of grimacing are family members of this constellation.

The word "stuttering" then can be used to denote the overmodification of the outgoing breath stream by a series of air valves. It would seem that explanations of anticipatory, current, and consequent reactions to the nuclear phenomenon are not too difficult. Although the core phenomenon itself is difficult to explain etiologically, we shall concentrate our main efforts to do just that.

STUTTERING AS LEARNED BEHAVIOR

The basic assumption is made that stuttering is established and maintained by learning. According to current learning theory as I am able to understand it (Hilgard and Bower, 1966), this assumption appears to be logically tenable. Too, in paying deference to learning as a psychoneurological process, one is paying deference to psychology, and to glands, nerves, and muscles; in short, to psychophysical issues. In the simplest possible statement, some cue or set of cues is bound with stuttering in such a way that the appearance of the cue evokes the stuttering. The process binding the cue and the stuttering response is gearlike. The following formula should clarify this:

(1) Cue (listener, real or imaginary)———→Activation of unadmitted feelings and thoughts———→Fear of the revelation of these inadmissibles———→Defense against revelation of these inadmissibles (stuttering)———→Reactions to stuttering (secondary stuttering).

On occasion, possibly on many occasions, the stutterer will want to talk, to say or reveal some thoughts or feelings to another person. He will want to tell his mother something, something of his observations or feelings; and in these instances the communication process originates from within; the process has an intrapsychic origin. On other occasions the sight, sound, or presence of his mother or her verbal relationships with him will stimulate him to talk to her. The communication process now has an interpsychic origin. In the first example, the drive or need or anxiousness to speak may arouse the unadmitted feelings and ideas which, in turn, would arouse the fear of them, the fear of their revelation, and the child will honor the fear and defend against the threat of telling by saying nothing. This idea may be expressed in the following formula:

(2) Need or desire to communicate——→Activation of unadmitted thoughts and feelings——→Fear of revelation of these inadmissibles——→Defense against the revelation of these inadmissibles (silence)——→Shyness, delayed speech, unsociability (secondary symptoms).

Although clinically we consider this second child to be a delayed-speech case, in a sense he is a stutterer. Under pressure to talk, from both within and without, his symptom may change, superficially, from speechlessness or delayed or unintelligible speech to stuttering as a defense. Whether the first factor in formulae (1) and (2) is intrapsychic or interpsychic, the defense is the same: a defense, silence or stuttering, against the revelation of feared thoughts and feelings.

Although the stimulus to speak may be an inner desire (intrapsychic), it may lead to the cue (another person) that in turn starts the chain reaction leading to stuttering. This idea may be formulated as follows:

(3) Need or desire to communicate——→Cue-producing response (noting another person)——→Activation of unadmitted thoughts and feelings——→ Fear of revelation of these inadmissibles——→Defense against revelation of these inadmissibles (stuttering).

The real significance of the cue (parent, sibling, friend, teacher, lover, anybody, or any number of people) is its vigilance. It must first of all be alive (stutterers have little, if any, trouble addressing inanimate objects); in addition it needs to be human (stutterers have little or no trouble addressing animals); and finally, and above all, it needs to listen. The listener is the trigger for most stuttering. Possibly the deeper meaning of listening is that it implies understanding, discovery, and detection on the part of the listener of that which may lead to punishment and condemnation of what was understood about the speaker. Notoriously, the stutterer is relatively untroubled when speaking in unison with others where everyone is talking and no one is listening. Conversely he is troubled, relatively very much, before an audience where everybody listens and only he speaks. The audience multiplies the danger that the speaker will be found out. The stutterer may have trouble even when speaking alone, for he is speaking to an imaginary listener, or listeners, or to himself. We must realize that a speaker is also his own listener and at times his most vigilant one, affording an evaluation often more severely critical than that afforded by others. So regardless of whether the vigilance is from within or from without, we hold it to be the provocation of stuttering.

Too, we believe that stuttering itself—the overmodification of the outgoing breath stream—is not, in the ordinary sense, learned by the child or taught by the parents. The stutterer does not "imitate" the stuttering of others. He never hears it, or hears it so infrequently in relation to relatively fluent speech, that to assign any importance to the idea that stuttering is learned by empathizing with other stutterers is absurd. Equally absurd is the thought that parents or siblings give the young speech-learner examples of stuttering to imitate. Even those few stuttering parents whom we know have little or no difficulty in communicating verbally with their children. Stated more technically in terms of learning theory, parents do not make stuttering speech as such worthwhile. It is not rewarded and hence learned in this simple fashion. Instead parents actually punish stuttering; or more accurately, they punish the child for stuttering almost as though it were a naughty act. Yet stuttering occurs in the first place without example, and more puzzling still keeps on occurring, even increasing in frequency and severity without example and without obvious reinforcement. The answer to this enigma is to be found in the stand that stuttering is not an excitatory or release response, but an inhibitory one, and that the punishment it incurs is less than the punishment the inhibited response would have received had it not been inhibited. In this sense stuttering is rewarded, relatively, as being the lesser of two pains. The stutterer accepts the punishment for his stuttering in order that he will not receive a greater punishment for speaking the truth. Punishment of stuttering is a reward for not revealing the guilty secrets which one has judged to be dangerously threatening. Punishment of stuttering may make the stuttering worse as a symptom to the listener but really better to the speaker in the sense of developing it as a defense. This is to say that stuttering when punished is a success (reward) in that it keeps the punitive agents off the track of the really dreaded feelings and thoughts seeking expression through speech. The more severe and the more obvious this camouflage (stuttering) becomes, even by being attacked and condemned, the more effective it will be in reducing the fear and anxiety cued by the arousal of the real culprits—hate, lust, exhibitionism, voyeurism, etc. Punishment and even certain kinds of would-be therapy may increase the tendency for the punished act (stuttering) to occur, since in a real sense stuttering is being rewarded thereby, in shifting the vigilance of the listener (self or another) away from the detection of the really dreaded feelings and thoughts of the speaker.

Current theory presumes that drives, feelings, and thoughts seek release through responses. When these responses, including speech, are punished, fear will be learned and will act consequently to motivate its own responses to keep these punished acts from occurring. Now the person has two opposing sets of drive-response dynamics. One set is composed of a wish, a feeling, or a thought and an appropriate response for the realization of the wish, feeling, or thought. The other set is composed of the fear of the appropriate response and some response for the realization of the fear. More concretely, the child has a wish, feeling, or thought to express verbally. He speaks his mind and is punished for doing so. The pain scares him, scares him for speaking simply and plainly what he felt and thought. He is now trapped. He is caught in a dilemma. If he wants to say something and cannot for fear of being punished, what is he to do when both the need to speak and the fear of speaking either persist throughout the day or are being activated constantly by his surroundings? If he speaks he is punished and frightened. If he does not speak he is frustrated. Either condition is, relatively speaking, untenable. There is, however, a way out: a compromise between speaking the truth and keeping silent. He can guard, monitor, and screen carefully his verbal output, to honor somewhat both the need to speak his mind and the fear of speaking it.

The responses motivated by fear have a central core of flight. To reduce the fear which produces an unpleasant tension one seeks to separate himself from the fear-producing stimulus. The separation need not always mean fleeing literally from something. At important times it may mean the inhibition of acts, including thoughts and feelings, that may lead to something. One need not always retire from a frightful situation; one may simply inhibit the thoughts and feelings about it and remain there physically. In a manner of speaking the thoughts and feelings flew away, were chased away, or possibly more revealing still, one flew away from them. Of the many ways to think about the significance of stuttering, in a real sense it is a partial success at telling the truth and simultaneously a partial success at silence. Tragically, in the end one learns to fear his own wants, feelings, and thoughts, and he acts to flee from them or to destroy their expression by various means, including stuttering. The conflictual relationship between responses motivated by such drives as aggression, sex, and messing, and those motivated by fear intensifies the struggle of all drives for expression and leaves the host in possession of soil fertile for the fostering of symptomatic behavior.

Possibly too obviously we have not come to grips with today's most perplexing question about stuttering—its selection by the child as his choice of symptom. Why exactly does anybody, the child in his early days and the adult in his more mature ways, tell everyone of his troubled soul by settling for such a personally and socially handicapping means as stuttering? Why does not this child, along with all children, reveal his misgivings about himself in some other language—in enuresis, asthma, lying, or stealing. He could wet in the dark, wheeze behind a cold, or lie or steal in relative inconspicuousness. But he must always stutter in public, in plain sight and sound of a vigilant listener. In some way and by somebody who mattered dearly he must have been convinced that the cost of stuttering was relatively reasonable. Some extremely significant person told him so clearly by word, by inflection and quality of voice, by lifting an eyebrow, by a pained expression, by seeking a speech teacher, or by some other unmistakable sign that what now was perceived only as nonfluency, but what later would come to be known as stuttering, had a peculiarly misleading value. Three absolutely necessary ingredients had to be present simultaneously to form stuttering: fearfully disavowed thoughts and feelings, nonfluency, and a diagnostician. The expanded concept may be expressed in the following formula:

(4) Need to speak (internally or externally aroused) ——→Activation of disavowed feelings and

thoughts———→Fear of these feelings and thoughts ———→Non-fluency———→Internalization of diagnosis of stuttering———→Stuttering.

When a child is convinced that his parents are convinced that he is just stuttering, then a certain relief follows in the stuttering. The stuttering is misleading the diagnostician and successfully serving the purpose of obscuring, if not entirely covering, the really dreaded preoccupations with speaking the truth. Really stuttering is a manifestation of a fear to speak the truth to oneself or about oneself to another. It occurs most frequently in those families that place a high premium upon the truth and then punish its verbalization. To the extent that a child can be self-conscious comfortably, he will not stutter.

THE PEOPLE OF THIS STUDY

This chapter reports a picture of some people obtained from the psychotherapeutic situation. The therapist is given a unique opportunity to view and to experience the mental life of another person who is in the throes of a struggle to solve vital intrapsychic and interpersonal problems. The psychotherapeutic relationship affords a naturalistic approach to an increased understanding of the magnificent mental processes of man. Before some of the manifestations of these processes, the therapist stands in awe and in humility. Before others he stands in sheer ignorance. Even at a time when there are those who feel that little is left to learn in therapy, the present writer believes that only an humble beginning to an immensely significant approach to humanity's problems has been made. It seems true that some main highways have been cut through the forest, but it seems equally true that untold riches remain as mysterious as ever away and beyond the beaten paths.

Some people have enough misery to drive them to enter into therapeutic negotiations. In their misery they have sufficiently high motivation to get them to talk long enough and honestly enough to explore the wonderfully intricate details of themselves in relatedness. Imagine the average person who is indistinguishable from the mine-run of people spending three or four hours a week for two to three years talking freely and almost interminably about himself. He just would not do it because he has no need or motivation to do it. Mainly, he is not miserable enough. Then, too, there will have to be someone who has the motivation and the patience to listen for all of these hours and months and years, one who has the training and experience to understand and accept what he hears.

In most instances where human behavior is studied, in the laboratory, at the party, in the parlor, motives are slight and the situation is trivial. In psychotherapy just the opposite is true. Not only are motives strong, but the situation is crucial. For the patient it is either a continued life of sickening anxiety and misery or a new life of peace and happiness. Such urgency brings every resource of the patient and therapist into play in the interpersonal relationship of therapy where the patient will reveal and sense himself more completely than he ever has in the past and more than he ever will again in the presence of another. The patient must tell all and the therapist must cope with the most vexing and vital issues of interpersonal relationships.

The label of "patient" misleads many people. For the purpose of this chapter, the patient is one who is so anxious and miserable that he seeks help. According to other criteria, he may not be as maladjusted as others who do not go into therapy, but the way *he* sees and feels himself makes him a patient. Our patients should not be considered basically different from other people. Rather, they are a group of people who differ from other people in the degree of motivation for psychotherapy.

The clearest common feature of the people we studied was misery. In a way and to a degree they were all miserable. Their misery was enough to drive them to seek help. They expressed their misery in the various complaints of irrational fears and anxieties, stage fright, distaste for life, homosexuality, sexual frigidity, alcoholism, primary hypertension, asthma, ulcer, and stuttering. Some had more of one complaint than another, but all were miserable. In a word, their lives did not agree with them. Psychological burps and belches threatened to expose their emotional indigestion.

Actually 65 people were studied, and their productions and reactions form the basis for the materials of this chapter. These people were observed in the psychotherapeutic situation for a total of approximately 13,000 hours. Some were seen for as little as 10 hours and some for as much as 400 hours. The average number of hours was about 200. Thirty of these people complained mainly of stuttering. Thirty-five complained of the other conditions listed above. Further breakdown of these people seems unnecessary for the main theme of this chapter. All of these people were adults ranging in age from 16 to 50 years. There were 27 females and 38 males.

Our special respect will be paid to those 30 individuals who complained of stuttering. Most of them felt severely handicapped in speech, and not only undertook therapy but persisted in the therapeutic relationship up to 400 hours for some individual cases. Some stutterers for one reason or another, including insufficient motivation, discontinued therapy early. No statistical comparisons will be made between those who came for stuttering and those who came for some other reason, such as homosexuality or sexual frigidity. Some broad comparisons will be noted and evaluated, mainly to stimulate further study rather than to draw any final conclusions.

We are impressed with the obvious: that stutterers are human beings and that as such they have a great deal in common with other people, even in the manner of speaking. Both introspective and objective observations convince us that most people stutter. Only a few people are sufficiently miserable over their speaking relationships, however, that they bring their problem to therapy under the label of stuttering.

THE OLD CONDITIONS OF LEARNING

A symptom is a remark about the culture in which that symptom developed. It is a reflection upon the nurturing influences of the home and community in which the person was reared. According to his lights, the patient was right in adopting a response or a set of responses known as a symptom. He found along the way that to react symptomatically reduced drives and tensions. His symptom was thus rewarded or reinforced, and in this sense learned (Dollard and Miller, 1950, p. 15).

Our people came to us because of what happened to their basic needs and drives as they grew from birth. Originally, *in utero*, their environment was relatively perfectly comfortable and complete. It met relatively perfectly and completely their growing demands. There were no discomforts, deficiencies, or frustrations. And then they were born: physically, mentally, and emotionally helpless. They were extremely weak in every way but one, the need to live. Their desire to eat, to eliminate, to breathe, and to be comfortable was great. Their means of satisfying these living needs were utterly dependent upon those who cared for them. Their very existence was entirely at the mercy of their elders, at the mercy of the physical, emotional, intellectual, economic, and social conditions of the adult giants around them. Only in infancy and childhood were our people's own capacities to control their lives so meager, ineffectual, and pitiful.

It ought not to be surprising, then, that acute emotional conflicts occurred in the earliest days of our people. These people, as children, had no tolerance for delay of the satisfaction of their needs. They could not yet learn to wait, to reason, to hope, to plan. Rather, they were compelled by all-consuming drives, tensions, and discomforts to action—crying, twisting, flaying. They could not think, talk, or reason, or control either themselves or their environment. Between them and their adult teachers was a tremendous gap. They had to be fed, picked up, hauled around, cleaned, and protected. And how were these things done? Here was the critical issue. At this time what may be done for good or for bad may never be undone. What was lacking may never be made up. What pain was given may never again be taken completely away. These possibly tumultuous interpersonal relationships furnished the soil for unverbalized and hence unconscious emotional conflicts. Only when these people learned to talk and to think could the impact of these circumstances be reduced.

Had our people, as helpless children, been handled with the greatest indulgence, they would not have served as subjects of this chapter. Could they have had the greatest support from parents during the earliest weeks, months, and years of their lives, they would not have stuttered. Their savage drives should have been kept at the lowest possible level by the attentiveness of their parents. Every supportively encouraging effort should have been made by the parents to teach the child to talk and to think in order that he might in turn learn to wait, hope, reason, and plan.

But the parents of our people did not keep the strongest drives of their children at a low level of urgency and they did not know how or they did not resolve to impose the burdens of a civilized life in a tolerable and reasonable way. Instead our people, as children, were treated as emotional and intellectual little adults. Adult powers to control their drives and feelings were assumed. Incompatible demands were made and utterly impossible checks and tasks were set. Unlearned and at times unlearnable discriminations were expected. Heavy sanctions were applied for mistakes and failures.

The conditions of the stutterer's early life created his stuttering. They proved hostile and painful to the expression, verbal and otherwise, of his drives, and he feared rejection and punishment if he tried honestly to express himself. He feared criticism of his true thoughts and words. He felt that others expected him to be unbearably good in thought and in word. Too, through his failure to be received for what he was, he had suffered wounds to his self-esteem. He had generalized from specific, unacceptable thoughts and words to the unacceptability of himself as a whole. Not only were his expressions unworthy, but he himself was unworthy as well. His old repressions were continually reinforced by the current contempt of others. No one understood him and he was not capable of understanding himself. In listening to their stuttering child, parents might have felt deservedly miserable in realizing that they were listening to themselves.

Stuttering may be defined as an advertisement of strong, dimly admitted motives of which the stutterer is deeply ashamed. Repression falls on the verbal expression of these motives and may fall on all words and sentences lest they might lead to these motives. When any person stutters, he is blocking something else besides what you and he might think he is trying to say; something else that is pressing for verbal expression but which will be intolerable to you and to him alike should it be uttered.

A SKETCH OF SOME OLDER TRAINING SITUATIONS

With our stutterers, the culture took a position on their various infant and child needs. It took the position, a traditional one, that their drives should be tamed relatively early and firmly. This was accomplished mainly by setting up in the child, fear, shame, and guilt in opposition to drives, urges, and wants. This opposition of forces, such as fear against drive, resulted in dilemmas which produced acute emotional conflicts. Then our people as children inhibited many cue-producing responses which would have mediated thinking, feeling, and talking. In short, they repressed the conflicts. Unfortunately, this learned management of conflicts (repression) did not solve the dilemmas permanently. The emotional paralysis of repression had to be continually maintained in the face of environmental factors which kept threatening to reactivate the conflicts. As these situational stimuli pecked away at these children, rewarding drive one time and fear another, the children were constantly taxed to keep the painful and anxiety-producing conflicts low. One manifestation or advertisement of this taxing effort was stuttering. Before the eyes and ears of their parents, our people showed in stuttering speech the operation of opposing feelings: sexual curiosity and the shame of it, hostility and the fear of it, and desire to mess and the embarrassment over it.

Possibly there are innumerable ways and combinations of ways by which society imposes its will through the acts of the parents. Yet it seems clear that we can group these ways into a certain limited number of clusters. We may be accused of overemphasizing these relatively few situations. Our excuse for seeming to do so is that the situations listed are clinically and experimentally documented (Travis and Baruch, 1941, Ch. 7; Dollard and Miller, 1950, Ch. 10). Certainly our general thesis will not be altered by substituting or adding other situations.

Crying

Crying is the child's first powerful response. It is assumed to be a response to some need or discomfort. The baby's or child's cry is also a powerful stimulus to its elders, producing empathically anxiety in the mothering ones (Sullivan, 1953, Ch. 3). It amounts to a demand or command upon those who are in a position of responsibility to the child. The culture takes the position that a child should not cry, at least not much. The members of the culture vary in their ways of meeting this position, and the way it is met determines important habits and traits in the child.

Crying may be thought of as the first cue-producing response. Its purpose is to attract stimuli that will relieve tension. In general, it should be honored as the one simple thing the child can do to get results and as the first small unit in the child's control of the world. Not to reward or reinforce crying is to teach the child that there is nothing it can do to relieve tensions, discomforts, and pain of the moment. Such training may lay the foundation for apathy and not trying something else, such as speech, when in need or in trouble. Too frequently a child is recognized only when its cry is violent. It may learn from this to respond all out of proportion to its needs and to become excessively demanding. It will fail to learn such discriminations as small needs are met by smaller demands. Possibly most important of all, when a child is left to "cry itself out" or is slapped for crying, it may learn too well that it is unloved and unwanted and that its world, the parents or family, is hostile and spiteful. Further, the fear, anxiety, and hostility existing with the futile crying will become associated with the original need for crying; to the darkness, the isolation of the nursery, the absence of parental stimuli, and other current things, acts, and relationships. So the child may become anxious when hungry (the original drive for crying), afraid of the dark or of quietness, nervous or angry when left alone, and so on. And as it grows, the parents may complain of a shy, or apathetic, or excessively demanding, or retarded and inhibited child, and later on of a socially handicapped adolescent and adult. To cry when in need, when hurt, lonely and devastated, and to fail to get available help will leave long and lasting adverse effects.

Feeding

Hunger is probably the strongest living need. Everything else depends upon the satisfaction of the hunger drive, which is an urgent, incessant, all-consuming, and timeless force producing intense activation. In the early years of life, the hunger drive and the strong responses it excites are completely incompatible with the child's ability to cope with them. He is utterly dependent upon somebody else for the management of his problem. He cannot wait, or talk to himself, or hope, or plan. He can only cry, now.

The culture takes a stand here, too. Mainly it is that the child shall be fed, but fed predetermined amounts of food, on schedule. In addition, the child shall be fed, but only under certain conditions (i.e., being alone, or after being good, or only if he will eat quickly and neatly). For rigid cultural standards governing the satisfaction of the hunger drive, the child has little or no tolerance. He cannot tell time. He cannot distract himself with feelings and thoughts and words about the future. He cannot understand the meaning of delay, or the limited amount of milk, or the conditions of its forthcoming. But he is acquiring much important learning. He may be learning that effort, particularly vocal effort, does not pay. He may learn that he is not wanted or loved. He may learn to fear the dark or being alone. He may learn to "overreact" because he is fed only after his most violent responses. On the other hand, the feeding experience can be the occasion for the child to learn to like others and to be with them; to learn that he is desirable and wanted; to learn that his needs are appreciated; and to learn that his reactions, particularly his vocal ones, are helpful. The seemingly "natural" and innocuous feeding situation is fraught with important and emotional consequences. Too many people, including parents, do not see this. They see little if anything at all to worry them. Yet observant students may see the child becoming apathetic, apprehensive, and shy, and failing to develop appropriate verbal skills. The tragedy is that much of this learning is secret. The child cannot label the experiences which it is having at this time. It cannot talk about them or talk them out. It portrays them in ways that we label as apathy, or speechlessness, or fearfulness, or sociability, or confidence. What was not labeled and not verbalized at these early times cannot well be reported later. In therapy only shadows and echoes of these early and deep feelings appear. Patient and therapist glimpse only their contrails. They emerge mutely interwoven into the fabric of conscious expression.

Toilet and Cleanliness Training

Although possibly not as strong as the hunger drive, the drive to eliminate is nevertheless persistent and commanding and at times takes precedence over every other need. Bowel and bladder tensions may exert a priority right upon the interests and efforts of the organism.

The child begins with an innocent interest in his feces and urine. He may handle and play with fecal material. There is no evidence of an innate revulsion toward the acts or the products of elimination. Quickly, in some instances during the first few months of life, his natural and naive eliminative behavior runs into the cultural patterns lying in wait. These patterns will demand that he deposit his excretory materials only in a prescribed and secret place and that he keep his body clean in doing so. These patterns will demand, too, that he limit to the bare essentials any verbal reference to these issues so that this subject matter is closed out and excluded from social reference for life.

More often than not, instead of the child being led gently and supportively by example into meeting the cultural goals of elimination and cleanliness, it is doused with hostile, punitive, and loathing parental attitudes when it displays its naiveté or fails to honor cultural demands. The culture sets its task as the building within the personality of the child barriers of loathing and disgust for urine and feces. To construct these inward barriers, the child must put himself in a conflict situation. He must pit one set of feelings against another set. He must desire and loathe the same thing at the same time. A swelling bladder or bowel produces a strong drive that the child wishes to honor. The pain of losing the parents' love and of their punishment if he does honor this drive naturally places the child in a state of great anxiety. To salvage something from this dilemma, the child has to turn on the drive or on the parents or both. This management of a conflict situation is loaded with possible future emotional sickishness. If he turns on the drive with fear, loathing, and disgust, he will repress it in certain ways and to certain degrees. In the future he may become constipated, he may cry when eliminative demands call him, or he may become afraid of the toilet itself. If he turns on the parents, he may become defiant and stubborn, or furtive and sneaking, or attempt struggling with them, or possibly resort to biting and slapping them.

Whatever course or combination of courses the child may select to follow in the face of harsh and hasty toilet and cleanliness training, he will be the loser. On the basis of a pursuing, all-seeing, punishing parent, the child may be making as few responses as possible, certainly not adventuring forth. Being unable to discriminate between parental loathing for his penis and anus and their excreta, and loathing for himself, he adopts feelings of unworthiness, insignificance, and hopeless sinfulness. These feelings and reactions are of particular interest to the speech pathologist. Any child laden with guilt, fear of its guardian, loathing for its excretory organs and their functions, and feelings of wretched awfulness cannot be expected to acquire and risk verbal, adventuresome communication. It has too much that it must not talk about. It will learn to speak less well or not at all because it does not remain close and warm and free in a give-and-take relationship to those very people who could teach it to talk well.

Sex training

Sex is an ever-recurring conflict element. Hourly feelings, reactions, and words confirm this statement. This is not so because sex is the strongest drive. Certainly under specific circumstances, pain, fear, and hunger outrank it. Even some secondary drives such as ambition and pride can be stronger than sex. It appears that sex is so universally implicated because it is so universally attacked and inhibited. In no other instance is an individual asked to block completely the expression of such a strong drive for such a long period of time; the culture demands for all practical purposes a completely sexless child.

Conscience and custom weigh most heavily upon sex. Too many people do not guess that children have a sex life and that guilt and shame are a crushing burden to lay on a child's mind. But the guilt will not always crush or hold. Although there are taboos which dare not be broken, children and adults learn interesting ways to break them. They lie or cheat; become impotent or inverted; develop anesthesia or paralysis; and speak not at all or block in their attempts at verbal utterance. It is around sex that the culture builds its biggest moral junk pile. Sex, or rather its place, has been cast in the leading role in interpersonal relationships. Society is split into boy and girl, man and woman, male and female, masculinity and femininity. Sex typing becomes inextricably involved with sex rejection and sex acceptance. Is the baby a boy or a girl; is the child a sissy or a tomboy; is the adult a homosexual or a Lesbian? That there is such wondering is telltale.

Cultural management of sex often ends in the greatest misgivings that the individual can have in regard to himself and others. His sexual feelings can come to evoke intense anxiety. They can come to arouse loathing and nausea for his sexual anatomy and physiology. They can lead him into feared relationships with others where defensively he may close up and escape. The individual can come to despise and reject parts of himself and to generalize from the parts to the whole.

The extensions of his feelings may become puzzling if not amazing. Because of masturbation taboos he may dread to be alone. Because of homosexual taboos he may be afraid of men. Because of incest taboos he may be fearful of women. These fears may lead him to be afraid to be. And even if he should try, he will have trouble in talking his way out. His teachers have been niggardly about giving him names for sexual organs, sexual feelings, and sexual acts. What names they may have given him were powerfully emotionally loaded. But, anyway, he was harshly intimidated relative to talking or feeling or thinking about sex at all. It became remote, inscrutable, and maleficent. Some way or other, though, he did learn something. He did acquire some words and thoughts. When they occurred to him, however, especially when the possibility of doing anything about them occurred to him, his conflict was keener both by arousing drives and by cueing off the anxiety attached to them. He was pained when he thought about sexual matters and relieved when he stopped. The result was repression. This was just not good management. The person was victimized. He lost, possibly forever, the opportunity to use higher mental activities in solving conflicts involving sex and authority. In the future he could see the unreasonableness of his sexual inadequacies and his crippled interpersonal relationships based upon those ineptnesses, but he could not do anything about them. No amount of reasoning, or logic, or pleading helped. Some people find that help through the renaming and reestablishment and re-evaluation of these bygone feelings and events can come only by succeeding in the weary work of psychotherapy. Some people find in therapy that sex conflicts lurk behind the all-too-innocent appearing speech block. They may also find it possible to accept cheerfully and amiably a degree of authority and threat without the defensive measure of stuttering.

Anger-Fear Situations

We may assume that anger responses are produced by the innumerable and unavoidable frustration situations of child life (Dollard, Doob, Miller, and Sears, 1939). We could certainly recommend a regimen of child care to minimize frustration situations, but our big quarrel here is with the management of anger responses when they do occur. Society takes a firm and consistent stand toward the responses of anger in inhibiting them by fear and pain and allowing them reign only in a few circumstances of play and self-defense. Parents resent and fear the anger and rage of a child; and the culture, since it is dominated by parents, accepts and even rewards the virtuous chastisement of the rebellious youngster. Possibly it would not be so harmful if anger and anger alone could be inhibited or extinguished by fear and pain. But universally anger is associated with toilet and cleanliness training, eating, sleeping, sex, and all the other learning situations in the home. So we come to have such combinations as anal and oral sadism, and sexualized aggression. The fear and pain that was meant for the anger and its responses became attached to all feelings, drives, thoughts, and words that were in the child's consciousness at the time. Too, those people and things and relationships that were present became connected to the fear and anxiety responses of the child. Thus fear and anxiety became attached not only to anger, but to all the other emotional responses which the child might have been making at the time, and to all the cues of the situation in which the responses were occurring. After this learning has occurred, the cues produced by any emotion of anger may set off anxiety responses which will outstrip not only the emotional responses of anger themselves but all the associated feelings and emotions. This produces conflict, and repression results to relieve the situation. When anger with its partners in pluralistic marriage is repressed, it is constantly exposed to reactivation, and as it stirs to subject the person to pain and humiliation, the counterforces of fear and guilt arise to hold it down. Among other evidences of this fear is stuttering, the inhibition of speaking for fear of revealing anger and its several associates.

Summary of Some Older Training Situations

We have sketched some training situations where conflicts abound in our culture. In these situations particularly, the child's drives meet frustration, condemnation, and derogation. At first, the conflicts are between the wanting child and society, especially his parents. The conflict is quickly internalized, however; it is between two of the child's incompatible drives or between the two contradictory sets of responses to these drives. Parents and the culture instill fear, anxiety, shame, and the need to please in the child to block his sex, anger, and messing responses. Thus their child comes to own pairs of conflicting motives, drives, and responses. He will have such pairs as sex-anxiety, anger-fear, and messing-shame. Society is on the side of the second member of each pair. It not only induces anxiety, fear, and shame; it acts to perpetuate them. These feelings are not pleasant to the child. They are unpleasant. They are to be avoided. But how? It appears that the child need make only one response to relieve or reduce his fear and anxiety: *stop thinking* (Dollard and Miller, 1950, p. 203). He stops thinking about anger, or sex, or messing. He is aided in this response by the fear and anxiety which seem to have an innate tendency to stop thinking and speaking. With awareness of sex or anger or messing gone, unpleasant fear is likewise gone, and the child is learning or has learned to forget or to repress. His stopping thinking or his forgetting or repressing has been rewarded by the removal of an unpleasant feeling and the installation of a feeling of well-being once again. Repression is really not "good" learning, however. It is a deficit development. Stopping thinking and feeling are costly. Repression leaves gaps, holes, and deficiencies in the personality structure; importantly in social relationships. As stimuli, especially social ones, arouse feared and

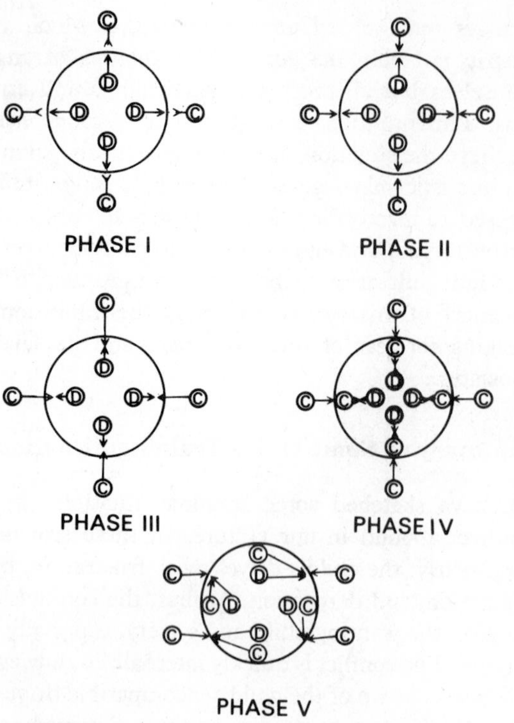

D – Drives, feelings, even thoughts of child
C – Cultural forces of fear, pain, condemnation
C – Cultural acceptance of infant's wants

Fig. 39-1. Crude schematic representation of the internalization (introjection) of the cultural forces of fear and condemnation and their inhibition (repression) of the drives, feelings, and thoughts of the child. The compromise expressions of these opposing systems may result in symptoms including stuttering. Phase I—The needs of the very young infant gain satisfaction from the culture. The very young baby's wants are generally met. Phase II—The beginning of the taming or domestication of the older infant's biological drives, generally by fear and pain. The conflict is between the baby and his environment, between the inside and the outside. Phase III—To cope better with the internal-external conflicts of Phase II, the child (one to three years of age) begins to adopt the negative attitudes and values (internalize, introject) which the culture has expressed relative to his wants and feelings. The conflict is beginning to be internalized, to be between action systems within the child. He is beginning to be split. Phase IV—By three, the child has made the inhibitory forces of fear and condemnation which originally belonged to the culture more completely his own to oppose his drive and feeling system. He is now more split, having parts of himself disavowed by other parts. External cultural inhibitions still help his internal inhibitory forces to control his now repressed wants and feelings and thoughts. Phase V—Through the ever-waxing and waning of both sets of the internal oppositional forces in their relation to environmental factors, compromise or symptomatic expression may occur (including stuttering).

dreaded responses, the repressed person exhibits hesitancies, blocks, and awkwardness. The range and richness of his responses will be lessened. Rigid, repetitious, and tried-and-true responses will predominate his repertoire. Repression falls alike on all responses, including speech, that may arouse fear and anxiety. When it is impossible to avoid speaking, consistently for some people, and at times for all people, stuttering blocks will be necessary lest the sentences lead to strong motives of which the speaker is deeply ashamed or terribly frightened. (Reference to Fig. 39-1 may help clarify these concepts.)

NEW CONDITIONS OF INTERPERSONAL RELATIONSHIPS

As we have seen, there is the strongest likelihood that the conditions of the stutterer's early life created his speaking difficulties. The main conditions were the methods of his parents in transmitting the spirit of the culture to him. The parents not only induced in the child the drives of fear, guilt, and shame as checks on the child's primary drives, but they and their helpers in society perpetuated these checks. The parents and society aligned themselves behind not only the establishment of fear and its derivatives but the continuation of these inhibiting and anxiety-producing forces. So the patient not only had effective help in acquiring or learning conflicts and repression within himself but strong support in maintaining them. Under these conditions his stuttering, the manifestation of his conflicts, was likewise fostered. In his search for help with his speech, the necessary conditions of unlearning and new learning were usually not found and he continued in his stuttering ways. On the basis of principles and practices borrowed from psychoanalysis and learning theory, our stutterers were subjected to conditions which reversed essentially the old conditions of their rearing. We offered the stuttering individuals conditions which in certain crucial respects were in striking contrast with those of their previous life.

The New Parent

The patient entered into interpersonal relationships with a person of prestige who paid strict, favorable, and sympathetic attention and who held out strong hope of help. This person felt and showed exceptional permissiveness, no condemnation, total tolerance, and complete composure. He made one important demand: the patient must do his best to say everything that came to his mind, to strive for complete self-revelation. For failing to do this at times the patient was not condemned but constantly encouraged to be under high obligation to succeed. This person, the therapist, was a new experience for the patient. He loomed large in contrast with the patient's parents, teachers, relatives, bosses, and other fellow members of society. He never became frightened or punitive or ashamed of anything that the patient said. He never gossiped, or became impatient. He set his patient free from the restraint of logic, and cross-examination; and when the occasion demanded, he fearlessly stepped in and said things which the patient could not say for himself (see Chapter 9 for a more complete exposition of these points).

The Extinction of Repressing Forces

The patient talked about frightening topics. He talked about shameful and embarrassing feelings and experiences. He expressed anxiety. For these revelations he was not punished. The feared and shameful motives and feelings were completely accepted. The fear, shame, and guilt were not rewarded by words or expressions from the therapist of condemnation or nonacceptance. Therefore they were extinguished. The extinction generalized to weaken the motivation to repress other related topics that were too frightening and shameful to discuss or even contemplate before. On the other hand, sexual, angry, and messing feelings were rewarded. They came back and out easier and easier to be channeled for future usefulness. The patient was helped to place these helpless past conditions of childhood and contrast them with his present interpersonal relationships. As fears were reduced by reassurance and extinction (unrewarded), at first the most lightly repressed thoughts and feelings began to appear. In generalizing, the patient adventured further to risk greater fears, and since they too went unreinforced, more strongly repressed and inhibited responses occurred.

The Reward of Discovery and Admission

Simultaneously with the unrewarding of fear and consequently its extinction, there is the reinforcement of the discovery and admission of repressed thoughts and feelings. The patient is accepted, even praised, for his painful and anxiety-producing revelations. Whereas before he has received severe disapproval (reward of fear and consequent further repression of primary drives), he now receives calm approval. The rewarding of his repressed materials and the unrewarding of his repressing forces bring him great relief and the feeling of a striking intervention in his life of conflict and anxiety.

Concluding Thought

Under these conditions, admittedly sketchily and schematically presented, the unspeakable feelings of the stutterer were discovered. It is hard, if not impossible, to be fair to the great richness, wide variety, beautiful intricacy, and strict lawfulness of the phenomena to be reported. In the author's attempts to present these matters to students and colleagues, he has met with awe, doubt, and even hostility on the part of his listeners. Two colleagues doubted that human beings could possess, let alone express, such thoughts and feelings. Our reaction was that we had not in any way given the materials to the patients; that the productions were their very own. Of course our reaction could have been that even had we suggested the unbelievable thoughts and feelings, they still would have had to come from a human being. Our purpose in reporting findings obtained under the conditions of certain new interpersonal relationships is to spur thought and research in the area of impaired communication between people.

THE UNSPEAKABLE FEELINGS

Through the processes we have delineated, the child comes to a day when he has strong and important feelings that are conflicting and ambivalent. In a general way, these feelings may be grouped into two opposing camps; the primary drives and their derivatives in one camp, and fear and its derivatives in the other. Assigning to fear both an inherent and an acquired function of inhibition of thought, feeling, and action, it is the basic repressing force. Its victims are primary drives of eating, elimination, sex-curiosity, and anger, and their elaborations. Large constellations of behavior become built up around these opposing camps. The child becomes to a degree split. He is racked with wanting and fearing the same thing. Into interpersonal relationships he carries his civil warfare. First one and then the other of his opposing feelings are tugged and pulled. If inhibited wanting is enticed out of hiding, fear and anxiety arise to hold it down. If fear is enhanced, the child becomes all the more paralyzed in thought, feeling, and action. In either instance, fear is the predominately felt drive and all responses, particularly thinking and speaking, are thwarted. Out of this soil stuttering flowers. Thoughts must not be thought; feelings must not be felt; and words must not be spoken.

In what form and complexity do the uncommunicable thoughts and feelings reside within the person? Are they familiar to our senses and understanding? Do they conform to logic and to space and time-binding? Some of the answers to these questions will appear in the materials that follow. More important than the answers may be the puzzles that emerge. Could we hope that to be puzzled might lead not necessarily to the right answers but to the right questions?

In discovering and expressing unspeakable feelings and thoughts, the patient approaches his task gingerly. Anxiety and fear make it impossible for him, even with the therapist's heartiest support, to realize easily and quickly the existence and operation of his most important feared and condemned forces. He has suffered greatly in putting away naughty, childish behavior and he is not about to release it. He has paid dearly for what self-esteen he now possesses, and it will take great patience and effort on the part of both him and his therapist to get him to risk his present painfully gained position. But bit by bit, advancing a little and slipping a little, risking and testing, he learns more and more who he is, what he really wants, and how to discriminate, label, and channel.

The patient's first successes are in sharing conscious misgivings. He is guilty over his socially disrespectful thoughts. He is ashamed of some of his anger and sex feelings. Fear plagues him. These he tells, and they are accepted. He, too, is accepted. He risks more of his known frailties, meannesses, and littlenesses. Over and over these are accepted and he is honored for his honesty of expression. As fear is unrewarded and consequently reduced relative to these more lightly inhibited feelings, more heavily repressed feelings share in the fear reduction and commence to stir. They stir and rise up into the dim light of recognition. It is not enough that they move in the shadows. They carry protective armor against even the recognition that might occur in the dusk. To continue the simile, as fear is reduced, the light of recognition increases and the opaqueness of the armor decreases. The result is a clearer understanding of what the patient really is saying. An example may help to clarify this. Relatively early in therapy an adult male stutterer spoke slowly and painfully as follows.[2]

Now I'm in my old room at home and some long object is here. Over at the opposite wall is a large hump. It is a large woman's body lying there. It has no head, but arms and legs. An extraordinary thing is, it has large breasts. I have an idea it ought to have a head but I won't let that head be there. Now head comes and it has long black hair hanging down and it is my mother. I remember away back in the old days that my mother had this long black hair, three feet long. Everything now looks very far off. Huge objects all around, but very far off. I feel small and one object moves in close. I'm afraid it is going to crush my legs. I didn't have time to mention that when I saw my mother lying there naked I felt guilty and uneasy. That huge object over there I'm afraid is going to crush my legs. What am I afraid of? That huge object? I'm lying there so small. Hands are here somewhere. I feel terribly empty and hungry.

From this production, neither he nor his therapist knew what the long object was. Both of them came to know what it was, however, that began as the large hump. Against the inhibitory forces of the patient it could appear first only as an indistinguished hump. In this form, not too much anxiety was raised over it and consequently the force of the repressed thoughts and feelings pushed further to reveal a woman. For the moment, who she was, was too much. The patient's anxiety could tolerate her nudity and her

[2] The author is sensitive to the likelihood of the reader's resistance and reactions of anxiety and even disgust to some of the recorded utterances of stutterers in therapy. Could it not be that both the author's sensitivity and the reader's disturbance focus the significance of unspeakable thoughts and feelings in the etiology of stuttering? Might there not be a positive relationship between the unreadability and the unspeakability of certain materials? If the reader has trouble in reading another's words, how much more trouble must the speaker have had in speaking them. It is to be hoped that we, the author in presenting and the reader in accepting communications from areas in interpersonal relationships, will share a deeper understanding of the stutterer's problem.

Then, too, the author has purposely adopted an objective and scientific attitude in reporting accurately samples of the raw data from which his implications and conclusions were drawn. If he makes an inference that people may stutter as a defense against the possibility of saying certain customarily unspeakable things, it becomes important to know what these things are. He could have reported simply that the stutterer has thoughts and feelings of which he is deeply ashamed and the possibility of their verbalization causes him to stutter. Is it not more honest that the author report what he found under certain conditions (therapy) and let the reader have the opportunity to draw his own conclusions?

breasts but not her identity. So she was headless. The struggle between the opposing camps of feelings continued with the repressed thoughts and feelings getting the better of the repressing forces of anxiety. And then the head with its long black hair hanging down appeared. With this much out, the identity of the woman who formerly was headless and originally appeared as just a hump became clear. She was his mother. For the discovery of this fact, he paid a price. Threats assailed him. He became small and afraid, empty and hungry. His inhibiting fears were not wont to resign without a struggle and they left him with a knowledge all right, but a guilty knowledge. He knew something now that he should not have known. He knew that once consciously and more recently unconsciously he had desired his mother in a socially unacceptable and dreaded manner. With the therapist's support and his own good discriminating powers, however, he held his knowledge to use in the future to gain more understanding still.

Repressed feelings rarely emerge singly. They generally come in two's and three's. Sexual and messing preoccupations may appear together, or one or both may accompany anger. And essentially always fear and anxiety are present. Later in his therapy, the same stutterer whose production was used above said:

There is a place here with a lot of gravel. Water running through a river bed. A man comes walking along through this water which comes from a cave. It runs in between two ridges of ground. These two ridges turn into two legs. The rest of the body that was lying there now sits up. Now it stands up and leaves a little pile of feces on the ground. Then a hand throws a basket of feces over the head of this person. I grab his hands and pull on his arms and try to throw him over. We wrestle and I throw him over into this water. He gets up all covered with light and dark spots. I grab his head and throw him in again. He comes out all black this time with a long, black, catlike tail. I throw him in again and he comes out a bear. I rush out and he tries to bite me. But I throw him in again. This time it's very thick mud and he has a hard time climbing out. I note that his legs have become very slender and pretty and I pull him out and he becomes a woman. She also has a long, thin tail like a cat. I try to clean the mud off her and hold her close to me and stick my penis into her. She shrivels up and disappears. Then I look up and there's a house looking like army barracks. She's in the doorway of this house and she has a long tail, long ears, and web feet with hair all over her. She turns into an ugly animal. Queer thing—there's a tree here and a large window and other things, but always in front of me is this ugly animal. Everywhere I look, she's there. I look down at my legs and they have turned into the hind legs of a horse. I have long ears like a horse. Dog here too like a French poodle, long, thin, and queer. I grab the dog by the throat and shake him and throw him down on the ground. He turns into my brother.

Hostile feelings arose against the man (father?), the woman (mother?), and the dog (which turned into his brother). Actually, he did have a younger brother. Messing and sexual feelings emerged. Fear and anxiety existed throughout this production. To help make the repressed hostile, sexual, and messing feelings palatable, the father and mother were not clearly recognizable. Further, they and his brother were given animal characteristics, because bestial feelings deserve only bestial objects. Even he had to become animallike, with the legs and ears of a horse, in order to tolerate or excuse his primitive feelings.

The young man whose productions we have been citing was the older of two boys. He was two years old when his brother was born and was held out of school until his brother was old enough to enter with him. On the patient's part, the rivalry between the two brothers was keen. We never saw the younger brother. The parents, especially the mother, were strong, exacting, and highly monitoring. Their attitudes toward the sex, eating, and toilet training of their boys were strict and inflexible. Their social goals were high and no effort was spared to attain them. The patient began to stutter early, about a year after the birth of his brother, and developed a very severe stuttering. He was practically speechless when he came to us, being able to produce around 50 words an hour during continual efforts to speak in his early hours of therapy. His primitive feelings were strongly repressed and fixated at an early developmental level. They remained infantile and childish because of being repressed so early and harshly, and they could not be modified and channeled by the subsequent experiences of later childhood and early adulthood. Upon coming to us at 25, he was generally constipated, picky in his eating habits, and had never had a date.

This short historical background has been given in order that we might better appreciate the following productions. They were his total verbal output for fifty minutes of continuous effort to speak. The bulk of the time was occupied in stuttering blocks which were characterized by an extremely tight pursing of the lips. The therapist could write down easily every word the patient said.

Large object, man's legs. He has loose pair of pants on. I reach up under his pants and grab his penis. It is large and soft. I pull on it and pull it off. This man stands up and reaches out as though asking for his penis back. I don't want to let him have it. He reaches out and tries to grab it. I put my hand on his face and push him away. He opens his mouth and cries. All this happens on the lawn of our old home. Across the field mother comes running. She is real large, larger than the house. This man is my brother. She comes over and I hold out my hand with the penis in it to show her what I had. He's over there hollering and waving his arms. Suddenly I squat down and take a crap and feces come out in a long ribbon—like toothpaste being squeezed out of a tube. I look up and overhead is a long, thin lamp post. It walks in and out among tangled ribbons of feces. It almost trips. It does trip and falls over with a crash. I leap on it. This ribbon of feces still hangs out of my anus. The lamp post has arms and I hold them. It also has a penis and I kick that and break it off. It also has hair and I reach up and grab a handful and pull it off. A hat comes off with the hair. On the upper end of the post are eye glasses like father's. I hit it in the head that is made of glass. The whole front of the head is broken in. I run my hands over the lamp post looking for other protuberances that I can break off. I roll it over and it has a pair of buttocks and between them an anus. I run my hand and arm up the anus and spread my fingers out inside and grab intestines and tear them out through the anus. I shake my fist in front of father's face and cram fistfuls of intestines into his face and say "how do you like that?" I grab him by the throat and order him to stand there. He tries to fall over but I hit him so hard that the lamp post is bent. He stands up there bent over. His head is low enough that I hit him in the head if he does anything wrong. He cries and wipes intestines out of his eyes. All over the place are trees standing around with their hands on their hips with the attitude that I should be ashamed of myself. A head floats in the air. I grab for it. It has long black hair that I hold in my arms. It's only a head. I stick my penis into the neck. The lips on the head kiss me. Liquid runs out between the lips and all over my front. I put my thumbs into the eyes and pull out the eyeballs and play with them in my hands. But they are hooked onto the head with two long white cords. The head isn't angry at me for playing with the eyes. I replace one eye and try to pull the other one off completely by breaking the cord. The head opens its mouth and shows lots of teeth. It tries to bite my penis off but I believe it can't. As I look at the head it becomes very ugly. A hole is through its lower jaw so that by looking into the mouth I can see out the bottom. I grab the ears and throw the head to the ground and stamp on it. It rolls around on the ground, all covered with blood and dirt. I try to clean if off but it's hard to do since the dirt is in the eyes, hair, and mouth. I want to wash it off but there is no water. So I urinate on it but this doesn't clean it very well. Besides, it turns yellow. I look up and there is father, very large and heavy and angry. He has a club. I look closely at the club and it is my brother. Father brandishes my brother like a club and I feel he is trying to hit me. I try to strike my father but he holds my brother out real close to me so that I can't get at my father. I reach out and pull out two large handfuls of hair from my brother's head. The places where I pulled the hair out are bleeding. I try to replace the hair but I get it on crooked and it grows like that and my brother has these two uneven places on his head pointing up like horns. His ears are pointed and his nose is long and he's like an elf that I thought of as a kid. He has wings. All this time father has been holding my brother out at me. Father has a long pencil between his fingers. I grab it and stab him through the penis and push the pencil on all the way through until it comes out the other end. His legs shrivel up and turn into a horse's legs. He turns into a horse hooked onto a wagon with its wheels all broken. The horse looks queer too, as though made out of a fluid, and he's not firm. He keeps changing his shape.

At first blush, the feelings and acts revealed in such products are unacceptably raw to our conscious selves. And this is exactly the point. Many people, including stutterers, are numbly and dumbly involved in such culturally unbearable mental materials that are repressed and, therefore, consciously undetectable. Nevertheless, their presence is felt in a gnawing anxiety that has its peak moments handled by some symptom, including stuttering. Before therapy our stutterer did not know that he wanted to bite off his brother's penis and show it to their mother as if to say, "Look what I have done. Now you have only one whole son. Brother is weak and impotent, I am strong and potent. Only I can deserve your complete respect." Before therapy he did not know that he had equally strong if not stronger feelings of aggression and destruction against his father. He wanted to destroy him in a most thorough and brutal manner. And as it was with his brother, his father too would snivel and beg for mercy in the face of our stutterer's pent-up rage. After each savage but successful attack upon his competitors, brother and father, his mother would appear. Is it not true that she is the real issue? With the brother she appeared clearly as the mother. Her only distortion was her enormous size, "larger than the house." Her role here was not too important, mainly to see what he had done. With the father, she appeared only as a head floating in the air. Here her role was extremely important. She was made to receive his primitive, sexualized aggression. In proportion to the importance and unacceptability of his casting of his mother, she was distorted, finally ending as an ugly, yellow, dirty head.

Finally, to justify the venting of his spleen in one fell swoop, our patient has the father threaten him with a club that is the brother. Our patient's wrathful retaliation is so right now since both of his competitors are a menace to him. He can justifiably save his life and strikes out to do so. To get at the father he must destroy his weapon, the brother. The outcome is humiliating to his antagonists. The brother becomes an elf with horns, pointed ears, and a long nose; and the father, a formless, spineless horse hooked to a broken-down wagon.

It is our contention that these strong anal and sexual aggressions of antisocial quality grew out of the important training situations of infancy and early childhood. Because of the pain and anxiety meted out by the parents in temporal and spatial relation to the patient's expression of early instinctual drives, he repressed (drive reduction by stopping thinking and feeling) these drives and the interpersonal relationships connected with them and henceforth carried them as unconscious, motivating forces. When these forces taxed the patient's repressing or inhibiting forces (fear and anxiety) to the limit, other defenses were called into action. When these defenses in turn could not hold, a final stand was made through stuttering. Stuttering may be conceptualized then as a final defense or block against the threatening revelation through spoken words of unspeakable thoughts and feelings. It may be visualized as a sieve through which some materials and force can pass, emerging in reduced amount and altered form. Both the repressed feelings and the restraining force (sieve or stuttering) derive some satisfaction. The former does get out, albeit in reduced amount and altered form, and the latter does hold even if it has to give a little. Certainly it held to the extent that few, if any of the listeners really knew what the stutterer said when he stuttered. If the unspeakable thoughts and feelings of the stutterer are strong and plentiful, his stuttering will be severe, because as a defense it must be equal to or better than the forces defended against.

According to clinical observation stutterers, both children and adults, are well-spoken. That is, they speak words that are highly socially proper and acceptable. As a group they do not speak "mean" thoughts and feelings to others or about others. They are polite and respectful. They are "good" people. What they say in the interpersonal relationships of everyday life is in sharp contrast with what they say in the interpersonal relationships of therapy. This great incompatibility of conscious and unconscious mental content may be a factor in the stutterer's problem.

Mr. Brown, 45, was a brilliant businessman with legal training and experience. To others his stuttering appeared inconsequential. To him it was catastrophic. His professional life was being ruined by his unbearable anxiety in verbal communication which was an absolute essential in his business. All his life he has had an ineluctable need to please and be loved and respected and he has succeeded, at least as far as others are concerned, in realizing this need. Indeed, by all others he is a most admired and respected man. In therapy, impressing upon him the attitude that nothing is to be feared or hated but only understood, he communicated many times the following content and feeling:

> I'm chopping wood with an axe. I shudder. Splinters hit me in the eyes and that gave me a shudder. Two of us chop off our toes and this makes me shudder. We look alike and act in unison. We dig a V-shaped ditch and plant radishes and they grow up very rapidly. We have to plant them very quickly and get away because they grow so fast. I kick this other guy in the rear and this gives me a shudder. I want to split him in half and this gives me a shudder. I do it and each half turns into a whole person. Branches grow out of the ears and I cut them off and I shudder. I see a penis and it is sliced lengthwise. Cut-off, smaller penises are marching towards me and I fight back at them with a stick or sword but they get bigger and bigger, too big to subdue. Some of them urinate like a shower and I run away but a big man catches me and brings me back and I have to sit there. Finally, penises all lie down and I can get up and walk over them. Big man doesn't care, but I mustn't get too far out of his sight. If I go too far a big penis rises up in front of me. He puts a big penis to watch over me. I shudder. I feel hemmed in. I walk away and come to that V-shaped ditch and a person is lying in it. I cross over and climb stairs and big man sees me. I'm still within his reach. I'm washed off and someone urinates on me. All this makes me wince. I hide inside the branches of a tree. I get out and penises are all around me like a fence and I shudder. They start spraying. I can't get away. I slide down into a river and wash off and feel safer. I swim under logs like penises lying on water. I go into a cave and a nude woman is there, and I feel secluded

and safe. Animals are roving outside but I feel safe. They look in but it's dark and they can't see me. I have to defecate and I do it right there. This makes me shudder. A messy deal. Snakes come out of rock. I feel antagonistic.

I'm in a train, and instead of going into a tunnel, it goes into a large reptile's mouth. We back up and try again and go into another reptile's mouth. I'm surrounded by reptiles wagging their tails. They get closer and closer and I go up a tree, safe for awhile but someone chops the tree down. I'm still safe like in a womb. Wish I could get away, out into the sun. I'm getting awfully tired. Another reptile is after me. I'm getting worn out. This is awfully hard. That's the way it used to be. I shouldn't feel that way now. Snake comes up and I'm too tired. It grabs my hand. I run up a tree but that's a snake too (breathing hard). I want to give up but I can't. Remember running home from school when I had defecated in my pants. Remember a man who approached me with his penis out. Don't remember what we did. Other boys there. Maybe we touched his penis. Maybe with our mouths. Don't remember. See a vision of this. I'm so tired. This is so hard (breathing heavily). One big penis I'm particularly afraid of. Wish I could sleep. I try not to see it. I just wish it would let me alone.

There is a treasure-trove of exquisite design in this production. We should be remindful that it, as well as every other similarly obtained projection, is not a production of intellection. Mr. Brown did not consciously construct this adventure. He did not know what he would say during the therapeutic hour. He had no plans for the hour, other than to be there. Under the obligation to speak absolutely freely, the feelings, ideas, and words given above came to him. They came at about the rate of slow conversational speech. He did not look ahead, or plan ahead, or structure what came. Rather, he simply reported what came into consciousness as it came. His attention was focused upon his stream of consciousness, which seemed to flow involuntarily. Some anxiety existed throughout. Anxiety peaks occurred at those times when he would say, "this gives me a shudder," or "this makes me wince."

This stutterer adds exemplification of the almost monotonous regularity of the existence, in these people, of raw and culturally disowned feelings and ideas in the areas of sex, elimination, and hostility. The presence and influence of these unconscious preoccupations were afflictive and uninviting in interpersonal relationships, particularly in communication. In stirring from their servile state, to which they never willingly submitted, they gum the gears of verabl output. Too full of such terrorizing longings, it is no wonder that Mr. Brown dared not speak fluently. His fear and anxiety were not over the possibility of stuttering speech. They were over the threat of the telling in talking, of giving himself away in his words. He was never afraid of his stuttering per se. Really, he was afraid that his stuttering, as a defense, would not hold. He was afraid of possible loopholes in his stuttering and the consequent probability that his blocking utterances were not capable of fulfilling their purposes of defending against words conveying unspeakable feelings and thoughts.

Conflicts and defenses incident to the attempted achievement of sex-typing were seen frequently in the productions of Faith, a relatively severe stutterer of 20. She reported:

I see a man walking toward me with a child under each arm—a boy and a girl. I call to him and he drops the children and I see he has a very large sexual apparatus in his pants which frightens me and which he is going to use against me as a weapon. The children are for a "come-on." I use pubic hair as a weapon of defense against him but it is futile. So I cut half my hair off my head to make me have half of a man's haircut and I put hair on my chest and it grows so that I'm part man to defend myself. Then I become half male and half female, with half a penis and half a vagina and these halves make love to each other. The right half of me is man and the left half of me is woman. The man-half bends over onto the woman-half which doesn't do anything, just remains passive. The right hand which is the man's hand starts tickling the sole of the left or woman's foot, and goes on up over the leg, mostly over the back of the legs and on up over buttocks, especially around the anus and then continues the tickling all over the woman-half.

Somewhat later in therapy she found herself swimming into shore with a strong, overhand crawl stroke executed by her long, strong arms (in reality she is small and does not swim). Waves beat against her but she got into shore strong and fresh and with a penis. Her breasts were exposed like a man's chest. As she stood there she lost the penis and a brassiere covered her breasts. But as she continued to stand there on the shore she became more and more interested in the girls and developed a penis again. She went into the toilet and her penis melted away and she sat down and urinated like a woman. These reversals in sex-typing kept occurring: a penis would appear and then disappear; hair on her breasts would come and go; a butch hair-cut and long hair would alternate. She would be first a woman, then a man; or half female and half male. Sometimes her sex role, whether male or female, was in relation to others; while at other times she was complete within herself, her male half relating to her female half. A third variation was for her to have complete male and complete female sexual organs at the same time and to relate to a similar person, each person behaving at the same time both as a male and as a female.

Actually, this girl's father was not a strong masculine figure. But from an early day the mother had instilled within her daughter the feeling that for a woman sex was cruel and painful and that man was a bestial creature preying upon women for his own selfish satisfactions. The patient has had three husbands and has never experienced orgasm. Her latest husband often calls her his little man.

Brimful of ambivalence in a most important interpersonal relationship with both men and women, it may be surprising that her only apparent trouble was stuttering. To have the larger force of her unacceptable preoccupations funnel through oral communication, rather than through some other expressive avenue, might account for the original severity of her stuttering. As her anxiety was reduced as she discovered, accepted, and realigned these conflictual feelings, her speech became remarkably improved and her role as a woman more firmly established.

Repeatedly, our stutterers engaged in anthropomorphism. Time and again they would ascribe human characteristics to things not human. They would express feelings, words, thoughts, and acts of a conflict in the form of objects and object relationships. Unacceptable feelings and desires would be concentrated in objects, their location, and their movement. This process may be clearer if we give some examples.

Glass tube filled with tiny microbes lowered into my throat. A swab saturated with argyrol is inserted down my throat. Steady flow of talk keeps flowing from me like accumulation of junk. A mass of gold trinkets is in my mouth, back of my lower teeth. I am a storage house, a vault. I expectorate a ball-like object that remains rolling in my throat. A dentist's mirror probes my teeth and enters my throat. I'm crying and between sobs, toffee-like substance moves back and forth in my mouth. Orifices and tubes and the words vital and potent. Now I'm pushing something up in my throat, using both hands. It's a window and I can't, it's too heavy. Hot stove pipe and a big boat in my throat. Honeycomb in my throat. Cells of the honeycomb are really breathing cells. A broom sweeps my throat. Spitting out and vomiting coins, muddy water and junk such as nuts and bolts. I want to explode all the antiquated things—junk, old coins, chewing gum, a lump of coal, horseshoe. It was necessary to stifle everything and choke to death all my life. I've been afraid of expelling anything, as though I took a deep breath and held it all my life. I've inhaled, but I've never exhaled. I've sucked in all my desires and cravings. I'm a volcano erupting and pitching all the junk out.

Many hours later, the patient whose examples we have been citing did not need to use so much anthropopathy as a defense against the realization and expression of her feelings. She could speak more directly as follows:

I'm raring to go places emotionally. I'm not scared like I used to be. You kissed me and put your tongue into my mouth and I had an orgasm. It felt just like a stuttering spasm except the fullness and constriction was in the vagina instead of in my throat. I feel that in order for me to speak I must take my panties off and keep my vagina uncovered. It's crazy to hesitate to say anything now. My breasts have grown up. They're full and I'm happy. They're not flabby like they used to be. Hair around my vagina is no longer unclean. It is sweet and wanted. I have no need for stuttering anymore. I'm grown up. My breasts and vagina feel so good. Once when we started I made a vow I'd never discuss sex or religion with you. I exhale through the vagina pure, clean air. I cough up not coins which are obsolete but circles—little emotional feelings and sexual cravings. They come up from my vagina and out through my mouth. I open up the orifices and tubes of my body and feelings, desires and cravings come out. I'm burning up, I'm on fire, I'm alive. I don't have to stutter anymore. Damn it, I can talk as well as you. All my life I thought my body was well but my speech organs were sick. Now the most normal part is the speech part.

This person, in her early forties, came into therapy with a very severe stutter. She was an uneducated, restricted, and economically and socially limited virgin. As she dwelt in the protective shadow of her aging mother, life was passing her by. A combination of external circumstances, including the death of her mother and the remarriage of her father, and internal forces, drove her to seek help, first in a speech clinic and finally in individual therapy. Considering many factors, her age, the severity and duration of her stuttering, her highly restricted upbringing, her limited physical and educational capabilities, her success in therapy was phenomenal. From a halting beginning she progressed to a fluent conclusion. For example, toward the end she said:

Suddenly I see my father and I hate him. He is responsible for me having no husband, no home, and no children. Now I see my hairline structure [pubic hair] and it doesn't disgust me anymore. I'm riding nude on a bare-back horse and the horse becomes my father and I hate him and I hate you too, terribly, sitting there coldly trying to figure me out in a professional way. I lie here on the defensive. I've been belching him up for years, my hate for him. I don't need to stutter him up anymore. Through lip service I was supposed to love him but I didn't, I was lying. It was sinful to hate your father. It was a commandment to love thy father and thy mother. This lie I stuttered.

Still closer to the end she proclaimed:

I can go up to a prominent person and talk without any feeling of ill-at-ease. I just don't care. He and I are just two human beings. Used to have an internal fight, now it's an external fight. I'm ready to go and no home and no education hit me. Formerly when I had a speech spasm or any other trouble I ran home. Now I don't want to hide, I want to come out, to expand, to make my debut. A debut among people. But certain people push me back and I find no refuge in the corner anymore. If my father should die tomorrow I'd cry for the father I used to know or the father he might have been. I feel that Sally is my little sister instead of me being really her little sister. She's away back down the road, so simple and prejudiced. I approach you, I can walk with you.

And at the end:

All the junk and surplus and debris have left me. I'm free and pure. I think of grit and a mouthful of dung and I'll spit it out, defecate through my mouth. I've been defecating and urinating all the years of my life out through my mouth. I was saying all the nasty things through stuttering. I was saying my father was a son-of-a-bitch and my mother was a deluded fool. You held my hand and taught me to talk and I never knew just when you let go and I talked alone.

Eight years have passed since these last words were spoken. During those years her job, which she has handled very successfully, has demanded the meeting of the public at a teller's window and over the phone. Not once, she reports, has she stuttered. Would it be presumptuous to think of her as a "cured" stutterer?

From unexpected people, the expression and communication of the interaction of opposing feelings (want and fear) frequently reveal the magnificence of the mental processes of man. The feelings themselves may be simple, simple want and simple fear of wanting; but the revelation of the conflict is often strangely penetrating and thought-provoking. Our surprising source of the production to follow was a 17-year-old lad who had stuttered severely since early childhood. In literature, psychology, philosophy, and the social sciences he was extremely naive. His entire life had been spent in activity to satisfy his interest in hunting, ranching, and livestock. He read practically not at all, worked and played mainly alone, and was unsocial, if not antisocial. He knew nothing of such concepts as symbolism, the unconscious, repression, and the like. Theories, principles, and practices of psychotherapy were foreign to him. He did know, of course, what was expected of him; an absolutely free and complete verbalization of his thoughts and feelings. One hour, after he had learned relatively well how to relate in therapy, he spoke as follows:

I see a large body of water. The surface is calm and very smooth, and green and very clear. Then as I see deeper it gets very dark. There seems to be no bottom to it. It gets blacker and blacker the deeper you go. Something is in there like a huge snake. He is very long and winds around and swims along. There are things like weeds, very dense, but no bottom. This eel, or snake, or whatever it is, is the key to something, the guard to a whole new land. The snake goes through an opening that leads to something like a tunnel, and disappears. As I look on the other side, the tunnel comes out into an uncivilized place, with huge reptiles and prehistoric monsters of all sorts in a tangled and dark forest. There is no sky. There is ground with very dark ponds around. All these creatures seemed worried about something. There have been men here before who tried to conquer the animals, to build up civilization but they have all been destroyed. One man is here now. He wears hunting clothes like we have today. He has a rifle but he is just walking along among the animals which are of tremendous height and size, as big as our buildings. The animals are all respectful because the man thinks he is the master of them; and the animals have the same feeling, not because he is cruel but because he has broken them. Something in the animals wants to fight back, but something else in them is like horses that have been ridden and broken and know there is no sense in resisting. That's the way this whole setup seems to be. The animals seem to have a feeling of respect but if the man were ever to weaken, or to show by some means that he was not the master of the situation, they would destroy him immediately. This man seems to feel that he wants something harder to break, something that will offer resistance but will be useful after it is broken. But also, he has the feeling that he is afraid to tackle this other situation until he has acquired more confidence by proving that he is master of things that can fight back and have sense, not human sense, but animal sense. He knows that these things can hurt him physically but can never command him. In these animals once they are broken, as it is with all animals, there is that loyalty of feeling that their master can do no wrong to them. There is a big problem appearing on the scene. It is the girl he wants. He knows that she can never be completely broken because he is afraid of trying to conquer her like he has conquered the animals. There is always the possibility that he might lose control of the situation, and then he would have somebody who would tell HIM what to do. In other words he is afraid that he will not receive from her the same faith in himself that he received from the animals. The question seems to be does he want this human companionship enough to give up his freedom and the respect of the animals?

With our present understanding of the human mind, we would be presumptuous to attempt a full explanation of this communication. Possibly we will be rash to pretend any comprehension of this young man's meaning here, but with the encouragement from the findings of other workers and from this patient's own clearer subsequent communications, we are encouraged to venture some translations of his language into forms more familiar to our current understanding. May we speak for him then as follows?

On the surface I am very calm and unruffled and easily understood. I am quiet and my wants are simple—to be left alone, not to be bothered, to come and go as I please, no fuss, no trouble, no demands upon me. But really, down deeper, I am not so simple and clear to myself or to others. Feelings stir, rebellious feelings, male feelings, conquering feelings. They are powerful and hard to hold in check and ever pressing for expression. I have to be always on the alert to contain them. They are not very smart as human beings go, but they have animal wisdom and demand my constant vigilance to manage their sexual hunger. Only my superior intelligence gives me an advantage. Were it not for this leverage their size and strength would overpower me. I cannot risk any diminution of my already slight superiority. I cannot tackle any other job. I must keep all my energies mobilized to manage my raw, animal-like, male feelings; my maturing feelings of maleness, of being a man. If I gave in to these feelings they would weaken me, even destroy me. Yet I do want to grow more. I want to reach out with my maleness. I want to test my powers. But as I think this way I become frightened. My feelings go a little too fast. They want to conquer a girl now. This is something different. With great effort I can manage my own sexual feelings. I can control them as long as they are all mine, just mine. But if I let them flow out to another, to a female, can I rule them in relation to her? Can I hold in check both her and me? What will she do to me? I'm fearful that she, being human, will not submit to my will. She may not be mine, all mine. I can keep my feelings all mine. Had I better live alone with them or risk trying to live with her too? I don't know now.

In exploring his big new land of big feelings, he knew that other men had been there before and that they had failed in their conquests. Were not these men the men of his family, or rather his own feelings of the men of his family? He felt that they had failed to crush his feelings, even had been destroyed themselves. (Actually his father was dead.) One man, himself, remained alive. And with great exertion he was not only living but reigning over his feelings. But when his feelings expanded to include women, fear assailed him. Had he not met with trouble, even failure, in controlling his mother, or his feelings about her? Was this trouble or failure to be repeated? So our patient spoke in a strange tongue about his great perplexities; and as he spoke more often, he spoke more plainly until even he understood his speech and his speech troubles.

Before he came into therapy, Allen, a severe stutterer of 16, had the following recurrent dream:

I feel as though I have awakened suddenly. When I look up a huge gorilla is standing over me and reaching out toward me. Then I get out of bed and start running around the room with it chasing me. Although it gets me pretty well cornered, it never quite gets hold of me. I try to go over to my desk to get a knife to kill the gorilla, but it always blocks me. After it chases me awhile I run out into the hall. Although there are people downstairs I am afraid to call them. I fear they will be very angry with me. But downstairs they hear me running around so they come up. As they come up I go into my room to hide from them.

This dream of nightmarish proportions reveals the dreamer's bare management of some of his powerful and dreaded feelings. During the day, conscious control conceals their being; but at night during sleep, with a weakening of his inhibitory forces, they are able to attain an outlet in disguised form. The gorilla is his fearful evaluation of warm, affectional feeling toward his father. When these feelings strive for expression, his fearful learned appraisal of them casts them in monstrous form, and even affords him strength to make an ineffectual attempt to fight. In simplest language, he wants the warmest, most affectional responses from his father. But these wants, he has learned well, are dreadful and when they gain the relative force in sleep to advertise themselves, they are permitted recognition only in caricatural outline. It is informative that in the dream he feared the people (parents) downstairs more than he did the gorilla in his room. He knew in a subtle, subliminal way what the gorilla was; that it was his own wants which had to be concealed from others at all costs. The others were the punitive mentors of his past who had instilled and maintained his fear and dread of his wanting the sexual love of his father.

During the hours of therapy Allen would have thoughts and feelings similar to those expressed in the dream. For example:

> Now I'm thinking of a huge octopus. It's in a glass cage. It's an awful looking thing. I wouldn't want to be in there with it, although I might as well be. Why do I think of this? It just popped into my head. That is, I might as well be in there with him. Let me think. There is a resemblance between it and my father. The long arms of parents and the long arms of the octopus.

Allen was a brilliant lad whose stuttering was so severe that he was practically speechless. He sucked his thumb and pulled his hair out when he first entered therapy. His parents were exceptionally fine, able, and strong people who enjoyed upper class socioeconomic status. Allen was in continual and futile conflict with them, his school, and constituted law and authority. These conflictual issues came up time and again in his spontaneous and unminded verbalizations.

> A bee is on a streetlight. He's flying all around it trying to get in. He finally finds a hole in it and gets in and sits on the light and it burns him. He gets mad and stings it only it burns his stinger off and that scares him. He tries to get out only he can't find that hole so he dies in there. There's this man and he wants to join the underground in France. He doesn't know how to get into it but finally finds out where they meet and goes there. They grab him and torture him to find out if he's German. He convinces them he isn't so they let him join. He's supposed to blow a bridge with dynamite. He lights it wrong and it blows up too fast and kills him. There's this elephant and he wishes that he were smaller. I don't know why but he does. Finally, somehow he gets to be a tiny elephant. Only then all the big ones kick him around and he wants to be big again, only he can't. There's this flower and it wants to be wheat. It's changed into wheat and is very happy until a horse comes along and eats it. There's a man and he liked to go into the freezing compartment in a store. The store owner finally lets this man go in and look around. When he goes in he closes the door behind himself and it locks automatically and he freezes in there. When they find him, he's frozen so they cut him up and sell him as steak. The person who eats him dies from some poison that was in him. There's a dog and he wishes he were a man, so he's turned into a man. On the first day he's drafted into the army and killed in training. Now there's this person who has his hand caught in a washing machine, in those rollers. He tries to get it out but can't and figures it will be easier if he pushes his arm through. He starts to push but finds his arm is attached to his body and he will have to push his body through. He does this and all gets through but his head which he can't get through. He's stuck there. Now there's a person who's a terrific wire walker. He always wears shoes when he is doing this. The manager tells him not to wear shoes this time because people think he has something on his shoes that holds him on the wire. He starts out without shoes and the wire tickles his feet and he falls. There's this man and he swings a sledgehammer around and around, faster and faster. The hammer is tied to his hands and as he swings it too fast he is pulled off his feet into a swamp where there are crocodiles which kill him.

With a plant, an animal, or a man, it is always the same. They want to do something else or be something else and regularly disaster befalls them in the attainment of their wants. In his family of high standards, so very much of his wanting had been blocked with disapproval, fear, and pain. Now at 16 he carries uneasily the repressed conflict of urges and their omnipresent and obdurate counterfeelings of fear and guilt. In the acceptant atmosphere of therapy, his repressed urges and wants were beckoned into being. It appears that they were essentially explorations into new and forbidden roles and relationships and as they enjoyed even disguised realization, their associated, oppositional feelings appeared also. And in every instance the latter won. But this outcome will not always be so. The now maligned feelings will get stronger under the new conditions of learning and simultaneously the restraining and punitive feelings of shame, fear, and guilt will get weaker. His ambivalence of roles, to be this or to be that, is further unmasked in the next day's productions.

> There are two people on horses and they have a rope tied around their necks connecting themselves. They want to go in different directions and kick their horses. The two people look exactly alike. They kick their horses and are pulled off and they try to run in opposite directions, only they can't get apart and can't agree on where to go. I think one is trying to go toward a swamp

where there are all kinds of birds, crocodiles, and stuff. The one that doesn't want to go to the swamp has a black mask over his face. But he still looks exactly like the other one. These Siamese twins here. One wants to bathe and the other hates to bathe. He won't let the other one take a bath. There is a book and one of the pages wishes it were a different page. If it were a different page it would mix up the book, but still it wants to be a different page. There's this colt that was just born. Its belly button is still attached to its mother and he wants it separated, but mother doesn't because she wants her colt around her. There are two people and they are handcuffed together and they hate each other. They kill each other because they can't get away from each other. There's this spring and it's being kept together, only it wants to get open and can't. Now there's a person driving a black Ford up in the mountains where there are curves. He didn't like to go around the turns so he goes straight over the mountains and smashes into a tree. He had been in prison before and had promised to go straight. He went straight—that's how he interpreted it. There are two people standing on a fence, and each wants the other one to get off but neither will, so one starts shaking the real thin fence and then the other one starts to shake the fence and they both fall off. There's a person with three arms and he didn't like one of them, so he puts it into a vise and squeezes it thinking it will fall off this way. He succeeds only in crushing the bone. There's a person riding a bicycle and the front wheel wants to go backwards but can't. When he's in the middle of the road, the front wheel comes off and the bike falls and a truck comes along and runs over the man. There's a person in an airplane and he takes off all right, but once he's up the propellers start going in the wrong direction and he flies backwards. He can't see where he's going so crashes into the Empire State Building. He bails out, but his chute catches on a flagpole and his chute is torn. He's held up there. The trouble is, though, that the ropes were tangled around his own neck and he was strangled by his own weight. There are two people with their belts tied together and they hate each other and start hitting each other and both get bloody noses. They are in the ocean and the sharks smell the blood and come and kill both of them.

Toward the end of therapy when her stuttering had become of no consequence, a young woman who had stuttered so severely, spoke as follows:

A geyser is blowing up in the air. A volcano is erupting molten stuff and it's dangerous. People better watch out. Out comes lava, lavatories, bowls and, toilets. Volcano is like an anus sticking up in the air and out shoots all this stuff. Feces, all the insides, like this is anger. All the insides shoot out, tremble all over. All of one gets mad, not just a part. Volcano keeps shooting and spitting up, and feces roll down the side and bury all the houses. I'll go over and tell my mother that I don't need to stutter any more because I know all those words that I saw written on the sidewalks when I was little and wanted to ask her, but was afraid, afraid to know, afraid I was bad, afraid I was naughty. I felt an urge this afternoon to go over and tell her all that has happened. How stuttering is gone and why it's gone.

Throughout therapy, a chief area of concern for her had been elimination. Like any other child, she must have begun the same naive interest in her feces and urine that she had in other parts and products of her body. Undoubtedly she handled and played with fecal material. Without a shadow of a doubt in her case, the day arrived when her mother found her innocent child smearing feces over her own little sweet body, into her beautiful curls and on her clean crib, with vocal abandon. Sharp, punishing, and fear-producing management followed. The baby experienced strong anxiety in relation to her feces and her interest in them. On pain of losing the mother's love and on the further pain of punishment, this baby girl repressed her messing interests and activities. She also learned to repress verbal reference to these matters, except for slanting and oblique allusions, with the consequence that what began innocently and openly ended up closed out and excluded from the interpersonal relationships of the future. Although repressed, these interests did not die. Their life was partly saved by the eternal cues of swelling bladder and bowel, odors, noises, and sights. But words must not be spoken. Naughty words, dirty words they became, and they must not be uttered. These words married other words which in turn became contaminated by connubial connection and they too could not be said. Well, where do we end? It is reasonable to assume that in her case we ended with stuttering.

CONCLUDING THOUGHTS

We have used 16 productions of our 30 stutterers. These few were chosen as typical from literally thousands of originations. Every one of our stutterers used the larger share of his therapy in expressing his conflictual feelings through these forms. We have not yet attempted to compare our 30 stutterers with our other group of 35 patients in regard to these productions. We cannot state now that our stutterers gave more, or longer, or more complete, or more diversified originations than did our other group of people. It is our strong clinical feeling, amounting almost to a certainty, that the type of materials we have been presenting is practically exclusively paradigmatic of our stuttering group. The largest proportion of our other patients did not give any such materials. A few gave scattered projections. Those who gave the most did not approximate those stutterers who gave the least. If our feelings stand the test of further study, we may have here an important differentiating factor. It would appear that until such a difference might be established, we should refrain from any consideration of its possible significance.

With almost monotonous repetition our stutterers advertised their unconscious preoccupation with the salvaging of some remnants of their early physical enjoyment. They revealed endlessly a nostalgia for their culturally disavowed, biologically rooted pleasures of sucking, eating, evacuating, and exploring. So frequently their revelations told of their lonely longing for the most primitive, raw, and earthy sensory and motor enjoyments and delights. When early training began its attack upon these pleasures of the flesh, our stutterers must have had three purportful reactions: anger, which met with triumphant counter-anger and which ended in being repressed by fear; a loss of oneness with themselves; and finally, a crippling of interpersonal relationships, significantly with the parents. Their productions portrayed these early reactions. They, the stutterers, did release in therapy hostility; they showed disabling vacillation about themselves, and they manifested fears about others. We were not there to see for ourselves when the parents made their attacks and the stutterers made their reactions, but under the conditions of therapy, the stutterers provided proof that the attacks and the reactions had occurred.

As seen through the feelings and thoughts of our stutterers, the parents, particularly the mothers, were highly monitoring of their children's behavior. In the stutterers' productions or originations, and in their conscious and recovered memories, the mothers were felt as harsh disciplinarians who held their offspring to excessively high standards of conduct and who used shaming and anxiety-dousing tactics in the socializing of their children. The accuracy of our stutterers' feelings are borne out by the studies of Moncur (1951, 1952) who found that the mothers of stutterers were more dominant than the mothers of nonstutterers. In the therapeutical process with our stutterers there emerged clearly, possibly a still more significant implication. It was that the father was relatively weak and passive. We may express this feeling more poetically and say that the stutterer's mother sang an operatic aria while his father hummed a lullaby. It is possible that this relatively greater strength of the mother operated adversely in the sex-typing of the child. An ambivalence of the sexual role was a constant worry at the unconscious levels of our stutterers.

Note may be made of the clinical outcome of psychotherapy with our stutterers. It must remain at this writing, however, as only a note. Our study can hardly be considered as proving anything—most of all, favorable clinical results. We may say though that those stutterers who recovered and expressed what we have termed unspeakable feelings and thoughts did enjoy increased speech fluency and less anxiety over speech blocks. Eleven adult stutterers (seven men and four women) had at least 150 hours each of psychotherapy with us. Of these, five (four men and one woman) were helped greatly; and six (three men and three women) were "cured." We may put psychotherapy in the worst possible light by stating that just as good results might be forthcoming if a stutterer talked to anybody about anything for at least 150 hours. We do not feel that it deserves this harsh dismissal. From the day-to-day, anxiety-producing recoveries and expressions and the consequent reductions in anxiety and speech blocks, we feel on the contrary that therapy was a dynamic, curative process for those stutterers who had the motivation and courage to drive them on.

BIBLIOGRAPHY

Dollard, J., Doob, L., Miller, N., and Sears, R. 1939. Frustration and aggression. New Haven: Yale.

———, and Miller, N. 1950. Personality and psychotherapy. New York: McGraw-Hill.

Frank, J. 1961. Persuasion and healing, Baltimore: Johns Hopkins.

Haley, J. 1963. Strategies of psychotherapy. New York: Grune & Stratton.

Hilgard, E., and Bower, G. 1966. Theories of learning. New York: Appleton-Century-Crofts.

Moncur, J. 1951. Environmental factors differentiating stuttering children from non-stuttering children. *Speech Monogr.*, 18, 312–325.

———. 1952. Parental domination in stuttering. *J. Speech Hearing Disorders*, 17, 155–165.

Sullivan, H. 1953. The interpersonal theory of psychiatry. New York: Norton.

Travis, L., and Baruch, D. 1941. Personal problems of everyday life. New York: Appleton-Century-Crofts.

40

A Two-Factor Learning Theory of Stuttering

Gene J. Brutten, and Donald J. Shoemaker

Learning theoreists concern themselves with the conditions under which organisms learn and unlearn stimulus-response relationships. They are interested, therefore, in examining the environmental phenomena that affect learning and unlearning and in developing effective procedures for changing behavior. Some learning theorists are also interested in the organismic processes that affect learning. Such an interest has led them to the study of individual differences among members of a species or to the study of differences among the organisms of different species. It is appropriate, therefore, to say that learning theorists are concerned with both environmental events and internal processes that influence the acquisition and extinction of stimulus-response relationships.

As a result of their investigations, learning theorists generally agree that the acquisition, maintenance, and modification of stimulus-response relationships depend on the contingent stimulation[1] the organism receives from its environment. Classical or Pavlovian conditioning is a training procedure that involves the contingent relationship between conditioned and unconditioned stimuli. Instrumental or Thorndikian conditioning is a training procedure that involves the contingent relationship between responses and subsequent stimuli. Classically conditioned learning can be modified or retrained by the repeated presentation of the conditioned stimulus in the absence of the unconditioned stimulus (deconditioning) or by the repeated presentation of the conditioned stimulus in the presence of an unconditioned stimulus that leads to a competing response (counterconditioning). Instrumental learning can be modified or retrained by the repeated evocation of the response in the absence of response-contingent stimulation (nonreinforcement), by the contingent presentation of aversive stimulation (punishment), or by the learning of a competing response through reinforcement.

Theorists who see stuttering within a learning theory framework consider it either a learned response or the result of learned behavior. Stuttering occurs and is maintained, from their view, as a result of the stimulus conditions that precede and follow its occurrence. Theorists influenced more by the Pavlovian approach to learning consider stuttering a disorganization of normal speech that occurs as a part of the organism's total reaction to stress-producing conditions. From this point of view stuttering is maintained when noxious events in the environment act as unconditioned stimuli that reinforce an existing relationship between conditioned and unconditioned stimuli. On the other hand, theorists influenced more strongly by the Thorndikian approach to learning consider stuttering a response that is a maladaptive attempt to avoid the aversive reactions of the environment to stuttering. Stuttering is maintained, according to these theorists, because it is followed immediately by some reinforcing stimulus.

[1] Contingent stimulation, as used here, means the delivery of a stimulus as a consequence of either a stimulus or a response.

Approaches to stuttering that can be strictly described as learning theory positions should be distinguished from approaches that include among their assumptions the idea that stuttering represents a change in speech behavior resulting from experience, and is thus learned, but which do not use the basic concepts and assumptions found in learning theories. Although Johnson (1967), for example, suggested that stuttering is learned, and although fundamental aspects of Johnson's positions have been translated into learning theory terms, his basic framework was semantic. Johnson was concerned with the relationship between stuttering and certain linguistic or verbal events, namely, the mislabeling of "normal disfluency" as stuttering. He hypothesized, of course, that if disfluency is consistently followed by the use of a term such as "stuttering" and the implications of unacceptability that such a term conveys, the individual will attempt to avoid disfluency. Although this set of events has been reconstrued in learning theory terms, Johnson did not do so and never appeared to consider his position as anything other than a semantic theory. In general, Johnson focused on the idea that mislabeling or misdiagnosis is the source of punishing circumstances that eventually lead to stuttering. Although he pointed out that individuals learn to stutter as a result of the anxiety engendered by punitive reactions to disfluency, he did not specify the type or types of learning (classical or instrumental) involved in establishing the relationship between social rejection of speech and stuttering. He did not, furthermore, specify in learning theory terms how a child learns to respond with anxiety when listeners correct or criticize his speech, how the child learns to produce the specific speech phenomena known as stuttering when he experiences anxiety, or how the learned relationship between the stimuli of speech situations and the response of stuttering is reinforced in a way that would account for the maintenance of stuttering. Johnson's diagnosogenic theory thus utilized the idea of learning in a general sense, but it was not specific enough in saying how the learning takes place to be thought of as a learning theory approach to stuttering.

Psychodynamic approaches also imply that learning is involved in the development of stuttering, but they, too, do not specify either the conditions that determine whether learning will take place or the parameters of acquisition. Most psychodynamic theorists have been strongly influenced by the psychoanalytic position and have taken the approach that behavior patterns, including speech, result from personality development and functioning. From this point of view, it is the stutterer rather than the behavior of stuttering that is of critical importance. Stated differently, these theorists take the position that the stutterer, as a result of his unique life experiences, has developed an inadequate personality in which conflict or weakness interferes with the normal act of speaking. Fenichel (1945), for example, considers stuttering a symptom of an anal sadistic personality. Stuttering is the result of the conflict between the unconscious wish to speak in an anally obscene and aggressive manner and the necessity for suppressing this behavior. Fenichel (1945, p. 312) further points out that:

> The anal-erotic nature of speech is seen best when, in analysis, a specific situation, which either provokes or accentuates stuttering, proves to be an anal temptation. Unconsciously, speech in general or in certain situations is thought of as a sexualized defecation. The same motives which in childhood were directed against pleasurable playing with feces make their appearance again in the form of inhibitions or prohibitions of the pleasure of playing with words. The expulsion and retention of words means the expulsion and retention of feces, and actually the retention of words, just as previously the retention of feces, may be either a reassurance against possible loss or pleasurable autoerotic activity. One may speak, in stuttering, of a displacement upward of the functions of the anal sphincters.

Though this explanation of stuttering is uniquely Fenichel's, other dynamically oriented theorists have suggested that stuttering is symptomatic of a conflicted personality. Travis (1957), for instance, hypothesized that the early environment of stutterers punishes the expression of various powerful drives. The conflicting impulses of expression and inhibition create a deficient personality structure in which stuttered speech represents but one aspect of repressed thought, feeling, and action. It is obvious that not all psychodynamic theorists agree with Fenichel's or Travis' conception of stuttering as symptomatic of the repression of unspeakable impulses, but they do tend to agree that personality deficiencies lead to stuttering because there is a conflicting demand both for speech and for the protection that is inherent in not speaking. Nearly all of these theorists, in addition, assume that personality develops in the way it does as a result of experience and is thus a result of learning. *What* is learned, however, is a personality configuration, not a behavior such as stuttering. Thus, the concept of learning in such theories is used in a vague and abstract manner that is unlike the use found in contemporary learning theory.

Many theorists who have developed a physiogenic explanation of stuttering have also, surprisingly, incorporated the concept of learning into their approach at some level. West (1958), for example, has considered the primary antecedent of stuttering to be epileptiform seizures that produce involuntary interruptions of the automatic control of speech. He has also suggested that when speech is impeded by the loss of automatic control, the stutterer

> . . . tries consciously to establish the continuity of his speech. He is caught in a conflict between voluntary control of individual movements of speech on the one hand, and voluntary initiation of automatic serial responses, on the other. At such times, he repeats phrases, words, syllables, or individual sounds; or he prolongs vowels or other continuants; or he lengthens abnormally the "hold" of the implosion of plosive sounds (West, 1957, p. 255).

Thus, according to West, the individual who experiences stuttering as a result of such seizures often develops additional symptomatic behaviors in an attempt to produce fluent speech. Although these secondary behavior patterns are initially voluntary and purposive, they may become a stereotyped or involuntary part of the stutterer's behavior if they serve to facilitate his speech.

West distinguished, therefore, between primary or basic stuttering, whose antecedent is an organic (unlearned) condition, and secondary stuttering, which involves learned, overlayed attempts on the part of the stutterer to speak more adequately. Most physiogenically oriented theorists make this distinction. They may differ as to the hypotheses they make concerning the organic conditions that create stuttering, but they generally assume that the stutterer develops secondary symptoms or adjustments that become a fundamental part of the stuttering constellation. Karlin (1959), for example, attributed the repetition and prolongation of sounds and syllables in stuttering to delayed myelinization of the cortical association areas that are involved in the production of speech. Karlin, however, like many other physiogenic theorists, suggested that the stutterer does not begin to employ behaviors for escaping and avoiding the circumstances associated with stuttering until he becomes aware of and anxious about his speech difficulties. Karlin further acknowledged the importance of learning when he indicated that stutterers develop, as they mature, both a pattern of speech that produces a minimal amount of stuttering and an attitude that permits them to live more easily with their speech difficulty. Finally, Karlin emphasized the role of learning in stuttering when he suggested that if stuttering does result solely from delayed myelinization, it should stop altogether when the individual achieves maturity. The fact that this does not generally occur suggested to Karlin that stuttering depends ultimately on learned as well as organic antecedents.

This brief overview of representative psychogenic and physiogenic theories makes it evident that many theorists think that learning plays a meaningful role in the occurrence of stuttering. Learning is common to each of these theories, although theorists vary in the emphasis that is placed upon it. They have, however, consistently used learning in a broad and unspecified manner. No specific or definitive statements have been made by any of these theorists about the type or types of learning that are involved in stuttering or how this learning is like the learning of responses generally. The role of learning has been acknowledged in a general sense, but the theories have not been elaborated in a way that permits ready and direct use of the present information on conditioning procedures and learning processes.

Learning theory approaches to the development of stuttering, on the other hand, have usually been explicit about *what* is learned in stuttering and about *how* the learning takes place. Wischner (1950), Sheehan (1958), Shames and Sherrick (1963), and Brutten and Shoemaker (1967), for example, have all dealt directly and at length with the issue of whether or not stuttering can be construed meaningfully as a response and with the types of relationships that exist between stuttering and stimulus circumstances. These approaches, in other words, have placed major emphasis on examining whether or not predictable relationships develop between stuttering and measurable stimulus conditions and on experimentation to determine the specific nature of these relationships. Furthermore, since experimental psychologists have long dealt with similar issues, those using learning theory approaches to stuttering have been able to borrow heavily from a well-established bank of relevant experimental data. Perhaps most importantly, many of the theorists who have examined the data on both learned behavior and stuttering have agreed that the relationships between many aspects of stuttering and stimulus contingencies are similar to the stimulus-response relationships acquired through classical and instrumental training procedures. They have, therefore, concluded not only that learning is somehow involved in stuttering, but also that this learning is not significantly different from that involved in the acquisition of other responses.

LEARNING THEORY APPROACHES TO STUTTERING

The notion that learning is involved in a general way in the development of stuttering has, as we have seen, occupied a place in both early and contemporary theories of stuttering. Relatively few theorists, however, have tried to place this learning within the framework of formally stated psychological learning theories. Historically, learning theory approaches to stuttering have been developed as a result of 1. the failure of physiogenic theorists to demonstrate an undeniable link between constitutional factors and stuttering, 2. the sharply increased interest in learning theory that occurred when it appeared that this approach permitted psychologists to explain existing data and predict the direction of new data parsimoniously, and 3. the striking resemblance of the data from experiments on stuttering to data from experiments on learning. There was thus good reason to explore the possibility that learning, as defined by learning theorists, was involved in the development of stuttering. This idea was especially provocative in light of the information concerning behavior that had already been gathered by experimental psychologists. If, indeed, a reexamination of stuttering justified its conceptualization in learning theory terms, a gigantic forward step would be taken. The results of many years of labor by experimental psychologists would become relevant to stuttering, a direction for future research would be clearly illuminated, and there would be a marked increase in the understanding and control of this behavior. It is not surprising, therefore, that there followed an upsurge in research that was designed to determine if stuttering was similar to other learned behaviors. The results of this research often gave the experimenter reason to conclude that stuttering could be considered a form of learned behavior (Flanagan, Goldiamond, and Azrin, 1958; Jones, 1950; Shulman, 1944).

As more and more experimental data came in supporting the contention that learning plays a role in the development of stuttering, it became inevitable that efforts would be made to bring the data together within the framework of one or more of the then current learning theories. The first approach to such a systematic integration of the data on stuttering was made by Wischner (1947). Wischner used the Hullian (1943) mathematico-deductive system that had shown itself to be a meaningful and generally encompassing approach to the understanding of learned behavior. For Hull, an organism's response potential is primarily a function of the multiplicative interaction between drive stimulation and habit. Drives result from an organism's needs, and responses that reduce these drives are habituated. On the basis of this framework, Wischner hypothesized that stuttering is a learned instrumental response that is typically, though not necessarily, motivated by the learned drive of anxiety about the normal disfluencies of speech. He thought stuttering was learned because it was, at least temporarily, instrumental in avoiding the punishment originally associated with normal disfluency. The avoidance of anticipated, though not necessarily existent, punishing circumstances resulted in drive reduction that reinforced the instrumental responses of stuttering.

Wischner apparently chose the Hullian learning theory as a model because much of the data concerning stuttering were consistent with Hull's approach and because this approach had already been shown to be generally productive. The utility of Hull's system also influenced some psychologists to reinterpret the clinically based statements of Freud and his followers in the more stringent language of learning theory. Dollard and Miller (1950), for example, maintained the dynamic concepts of analytic theory in their approach to personality, but they restated them in the language of Hull's reinforcement theory of learning. Such amalgamations of dynamic and behavioristic concepts were attractive to many psychologists. On the one hand, the so-called mechanistic attitude of behavioristic theory derived in the laboratory was tempered by an approach that had its origin in the clinical setting. On the other hand, the vague and highly abstract concepts of analytic theory were now defined in ways that permitted controlled exploration of theoretical predictions. Sheehan (1958), for example, recognized the apparent experimental and clinical advantages of such a *rapprochement* between dynamic and behavioristic approaches to the understanding of stuttering. He used the Miller and Dollard postulations concerning conflict as his explanatory model. Sheehan maintains, in his approach, that the repetitions and prolongations of stuttering are the symptomatic expression of an approach-avoidance conflict whose most likely source is guilt. The inner turmoil of opposing impulses produces oscillations and fixations that are displayed in disrupted speech. The conflict is heightened by the shame, frustration, and secondary guilt that are the consequences of stuttering. While, according to Sheehan, the oscillations and fixations that result from conflict are directly predictable from Dollard and Miller's conflict theory, the "secondary" symptoms that tend to develop as the result of increased emotion require dynamic explanation. These secondary symptoms reflect the individual stutterer's personality and the dynamics of his unique manner of defending himself during the stress of conflict. They are not, thus, simply responses that are learned because they have, by chance, been instrumental in avoiding punishment.

Both Wischner's and Sheehan's approaches to stuttering were dependent, at least in part, upon Hullian learning theory. The other learning theories that were in vogue during the 1940's, such as those of Guthrie (1935) and Tolman (1932), were not employed by speech pathologists as a means of integrating the data on stuttering. As a matter of fact, no other learning theory approach to stuttering was formally proposed until Shames and Sherrick (1963) used the Skinnerian (1938) system to describe the circumstances under which stuttering occurs. Skinner was a contemporary of Hull, but unlike the major theorists of that era he came to the conclusion that it was premature, unnecessary, and unwise to make assumptions about how unobserved events, such as drives, that may occur within the organism help determine the course of behavior. Skinner proposed that such hypothetical constructs be dropped in favor of a more rigorous and thorough examination of dependent and independent variables. Specifically, Skinner suggested that it would be better at this time to direct attention to measured responses, stimuli, and their relationships rather than to use hypothetical constructs to explain why organisms behave the way they do.

Shames and Sherrick have suggested that the disfluencies emitted by children are not typically followed by differential responses from listeners in the environment. When no differential stimulation is made contingent upon the presence or absence of disfluent responses, there are no changes in their base rate or form. When disfluencies are contingently punished by listeners, however, the child modifies his typical speech behavior in order to avoid continued aversive stimulation from the listener. The changed or degenerate form of speech is stuttering, according to Shames and Sherrick, and this manner of responding increases in frequency because the termination and avoidance of aversive stimulation is negatively reinforcing. The pattern of stuttering displayed by an individual speaker is momentarily stabilized when positive reinforcement for these responses is more potent than aversive stimulation for further behavior change.

While there are basic differences in the theories of Wischner, Sheehan, and Shames and Sherrick, there are also noteworthy similarities that should be highlighted. For example, both Wischner and Shames and Sherrick have stated that stutterings are learned avoidance responses to the punishing or aversive stimulation that is the listener's contingent reaction to disfluency. Sheehan, too, stresses the importance of the relationship between avoidance responses and stuttering. Moreover, Sheehan (1958), like Wischner (1952b), has suggested that the responses of stuttering are typically learned as a result of the reinforcement of drive reduction. Shames and Sherrick are also reinforcement theorists, although they do not suggest that the occurrence of a response depends on drive reduction, personality dynamics or other intervening variables. Finally, each of these theorists would contend that the fundamental laws that underlie the acquisition, maintenance, or modification of one particular response would hold for all responses. They would state, in other words, that stuttering is a response that holds in common with all responses the fact that its occurrence and course are determined by the principles of learning.

THE EFFECTS OF RESPONSE-CONTINGENT STIMULATION[2] ON MOMENTS OF STUTTERING

The results of experiments constantly affect the understanding of learning. The principles or laws of

[2] Response-contingent stimulation refers to the procedures used in the acquisition and modification of instrumentally conditioned responses. Instrumental conditioning depends on some scheduled relationship between a response and consequent stimulation.

learning are not static; they are affected by current data. This is true even for those lawful relationships that, with some modification, have seemingly withstood the test of time. The law of effect, for example, which was first enunciated clearly by Thorndike (1911), remains a basic tenet of learning even though research has pointed up certain predictive difficulties that have limited its usefulness and have led to its recasting. This law served as a fundamental principle in the learning theories of Hull, Miller and Dollard, and Skinner, and these theories, in turn, provided the frameworks for the learning theory approaches to stuttering of Wischner, Sheehan, and Shames and Sherrick, respectively.

The law of effect is essentially a statement of the relationship between responses and their consequences: the probability of occurrence of responses is increased or decreased as a function of their consequences. Thorndike went on to point out that satisfying consequences strengthen stimulus-response bonds while annoying consequences decrease the strength of connective bonds. A more current statement of this relationship posits that when a response made to a stimulus is followed by reward, the tendency to produce the response to that stimulus in the future is increased and when a response made to a stimulus is punished, the tendency to produce the response to that stimulus in the future is diminished.

Learning theory approaches to stuttering, as we have seen, are in agreement that stuttering depends, at least in part, on learning. Because of this, it was anticipated that positive or negative contingent stimulation of stuttering would result in changes predictable by the law of effect and that these modifications would serve as partial validation of the assumption that stuttering is a learned response. It was anticipated, in other words, that rewarding stuttering would result in an increased occurrence of this behavior and punishing it would result in its decrease. Unfortunately, these predictions have not been explored fully even though they are vital to an evaluation of stuttering as a learned response. There do not appear to be any published studies in which positive reinforcement was made contingent upon stuttering in order to determine if the occurrence of rewarding stimuli would lead to an increase in this behavior. In addition, there have been only a few studies reported that investigate the effect of negative reinforcement (offset of an aversive stimulus) on stuttering (Felty, 1959; Flanagan, Goldiamond, and Azrin, 1958; Frederick, 1955; Goldiamond, 1965).[3] In contrast to this paucity of research on the positive or negative reinforcement of stuttering, there has been a substantial number of clinical reports and experiments investigating the effect of the onset of contingent negative stimulation (punishment) on stuttering. The results of these observations and studies, however, do not provide consistent and unequivocal support for the assumption that stuttering is a learned response. Neither clinical experience nor experimental data, in other words, provide clear support for the presence of the predicted lawful relationship between stuttering and punishment; the punishment of stuttering has not invariably led to its decrease. As a matter of fact, a majority of the published reports of speech therapists indicate that the punishment of stuttering leads to an increase rather than to the decrease that would occur if it acted in accordance with the law of effect (Bloodstein, 1958; Johnson, 1956; Sheehan, 1958).[4]

As research has progressed, it has become more evident that punishment of stuttering produces inconsistent effects. Some of the experiments done since Van Riper (1937) first attacked the problem have indicated that punishment can lead to an increase in stuttering instead of a decrease. Other investigators have observed that punishment has no apparent effect on the frequency of stuttering. Still others have found that punishment can result in at least a temporary decrease in the frequency of stuttering. This diversity of findings overtaxes all present explanatory systems, but, regardless of the explanation offered, the data do not permit the secure assumption that stuttering is a response invariably reduced by punishment. Furthermore, this assumption was placed in jeopardy by the data from the very first experiment on the effect of threatened punishment on stuttering. In this study, Van Riper (1937) fastened electrodes on his subjects' necks and had them read the same passage aloud three consecutive times. The subjects were then given a sample electric shock and informed that they would be given one shock at the conclusion of the next reading of the passage for each stuttering spasm that occurred during that reading. Shock was not actually delivered following this reading. As far as the subjects

[3] In these investigations "stuttering" tended to increase when the subjects could temporarily terminate or escape a continuous aversive stimulus by producing dysfluencies.

[4] Speech therapists have generally contended that stuttering increases when punished because the punishment increases negative emotion (fear, anxiety, tension, stress).

knew, however, the threatened punishment, although deferred, was to be contingent on each moment of stuttering.[5] The results of this study indicated that stuttering increased under this condition in all but one of the 16 subjects. The subjects displayed an average increase of 5.2 stutterings over the frequency observed during the preceding reading when shock had not been threatened as a contingency for each spasm.

It is possible, of course, that the increase in stuttering obtained in this study resulted from the general fear of shock rather than from the threatened contingent relationship between stuttering and shock. Van Riper introduced two additional consecutive readings of the same material in an attempt to control for this possibility. The fifth reading of the passage was like the first three oral readings in that no shock was threatened. In the sixth reading the subjects were informed that although they had not been shocked before, this time they *would* be shocked once at the conclusion of the next passage for each spasm that had occurred during their *first* reading of the passage. The negligible average increase of 1.5 stutterings that occurred in this final reading, when noncontingent negative stimulation was threatened, was significantly less than the increase of 5.2 stutterings that occurred during the fourth reading, when the threatened punishment was contingent upon stuttering.

The results of the Van Riper experiment represented a major contribution to the investigation of the relationship between punishment and the frequency of stuttering. The implications of this research are clouded, however, by the fact that the punishment was not actually delivered following the occurrence of the behavior, even though it had been threatened as a contingency. It is possible, on the one hand, that the instructions and the demonstration shock heightened the negative effect of the stuttering itself so that its occurrence became more punishing. Seen in this way, the results would describe the effects of punishment on stuttering. It is also possible, however, to consider this experiment in terms of a classical conditioning or stimulus-contingent procedure, and we shall discuss it again when we deal with the effects of preresponse stimulus conditions on stuttering.

Frick (1951) attacked the problem created by Van Riper's experimental strategy by designing a study in which the frequency of stuttering displayed during control readings of a passage was compared to the frequency displayed when 1. shock was delivered immediately following each stuttered word, 2. the shock was delivered at the completion of the reading, with the number of shocks being dependent upon the number of stutterings that occurred during the reading, and 3. shock was delivered immediately following each word spoken regardless of whether it was spoken fluently or dysfluently. Punishment was thus a factor in each of these experimental conditions. However, the behavior punished and the delay of punishment were varied. In any event, these experimental conditions did not produce significant differences in the frequency of stuttering. Stuttering was not decreased significantly more when negative stimulation was both contingent and contiguous than when it was either contingent but delayed or immediately contingent on all spoken words. Moreover, punishment immediately following each stuttered word not only failed to bring about less stuttering than the other punishment conditions, it also failed to produce less stuttering than the nonpunishment, control condition. Indeed, the frequency of stuttering in this condition ". . . was greater on every reading than in the control condition . . ." (Frick, 1951, p. 74). Once more, therefore, the data ran against the prediction that is consistent with that aspect of the law of effect concerning the punishment of responses; stuttering was neither reduced nor extinguished by punishment.

As a part of a more ambitious study of positive and negative contingencies, Frederick (1955) compared the mean number of stutterings in punishment and control conditions. In the control condition the subjects read a word list orally while they received a steady electric current of twice the individual threshold. In the punishment condition each subject's shock

[5] Some say that the threatened negative stimulation in Van Riper's experiment was not response-contingent because the stimulus did not immediately follow each stuttering moment. This is a rather limited definition of contingency even if, contrary to current data (Webster, 1968a), it were possible to deliver punishment consistently prior to the production of the next word. Stimulation is contingent upon a response if it is consistently delivered as a consequence of that response. A delay in the delivery of the punishment may reduce its effectiveness (Kamin, 1959; Warden and Dymond, 1931) but it would not eliminate its contingent relationship to the response. Moreover, a number of recent investigations indicate that a limited delay in the presentation of punishment has no significant effect on the course of behavior in experiments with lower animals (Azrin, 1956; Estes, 1944; Hunt and Brady, 1955). A limited delay in the anticipated delivery of contingent stimulation apparently has even less of an effect with mature, human subjects. In the Van Riper experiment, for example, the subjects were told that the shock would be delivered after a short delay. The fact that there was a significant increase in stuttering suggests that this anticipated delay was bridged by the subjects.

level was increased by one-third when he stuttered. The increase was maintained until each fluency failure was terminated. Stuttering was significantly more frequent in the punishment condition than in the control condition ($p = .001$). A further analysis of this difference indicated that the higher frequency of stuttering in the punishment condition was related to the preexperimental anxiety level of the subjects as measured by questionnaires; the medium- and high-anxiety subgroups showed a greater increase ($p = .001$) than the low-anxiety subgroup ($p = .003$). In any event, stuttering increased in the presence of punishment.

Hansen (1955) also studied the effect of rewarding and punishing contingencies on the frequency of stuttering. Instead of shock, however, he used the presumed reaction of an audience as the negative consequence. Each subject read two different passages orally and described two different photographs to an audience. Lights and numerical indicators were used to communicate supposed audience reaction to the speaker. The audience reaction to periods of stuttering and fluency were rigged by the experimenter without the knowledge of either the speaker or the listeners. Stutterings were followed by "unfavorable" audience indicators and fluency by "neutral" indicators in one of the conditions of the study. Fluent speech was followed by "favorable" indicators and stuttering by "neutral" indicators in a second condition. No "favorable" audience reactions were presented to the speakers in the first of these two conditions and no "unfavorable" reactions were presented in the second. Speech during these two experimental conditions was compared to that during a control condition in which the speakers were given no evidence of the audience's reaction. Although Hansen did not submit his results to significance tests, the data indicate slight increases in observed stuttering when it was punished. Thus, the contingency of "unfavorable" reaction to stuttering did not result in the decrease that the law of effect would predict.

Daly (1964) also investigated the effect of punishment on stuttering. Daly, like Frick, varied the delivery of response-contingent electric shock. In the Daly study, however, the shock was reportedly delivered immediately *after* each moment of stuttering in one condition and *during* each moment of stuttering in the other. The mean percentages of stuttering during the oral readings under the experimental conditions were compared with the mean percentage of stuttering during a control condition in which the subjects were wired for shock but none was administered. An analysis of the frequency of stuttering under these conditions indicated that they were not significantly different. This study, therefore, indicated that response-contingent electric shock had no significant effect on the frequency of stuttering.

Cady and Robbins (1968) investigated the effect of verbally delivered punishment (the word "wrong") on the fluency failures of stutterers and nonstutterers. The negative stimulus was contingently delivered in the second of three seven-minute oral reading segments. This stimulus was not delivered during the first (base rate) or third (extinction) segments. These controls were supplemented by separate conditions in which the subjects' fluency failures were contingently followed by the stimulus "right" or "tree." The data of this study revealed that in each of these three conditions the contingent use of verbal stimulation resulted in a significant reduction of the frequency of fluency failures. It is noteworthy, however, that the extent of this reduction was not significantly different for the conditions involving verbal stimuli considered to be "negative," "positive," and "neutral." Because of the similar effect produced by these different contingent stimuli the experimenters concluded that ". . . there might be a situational factor involved in the presentation of the stimuli and that any stimulus presented would obtain the same results. It does not appear that the affective content of the word presented is the critical factor." (p. 2).

Timmons (1966) also found that punishment did not produce a significant reduction in the frequency of stuttering. In this study the spoken word "wrong" was made contingent upon stuttering. This stimulus was delivered contingently to an experimental group of stutterers during the middle five of 15 oral readings of the same passage. A control group of stutterers received no contingent stimulation during readings of the same passage. The experimenter concluded that further study of verbally delivered punishment appeared warranted even though its effect was not statistically significant in this study.

Hegde (1970) was concerned because the data from studies like those we have been discussing conflicted with evidence that stuttering is suppressed by contingent negative stimulation. He compared the effect on stuttering of conditions in which his subjects merely read orally with those in which they were contingently shocked. In the shock condition, this negative stimulus was made contingent upon hesitations, repetitions, and prolongations whether or not they were accompanied by "secondary" behaviors. For each subject, the no-shock and shock conditions were counterbalanced during the four experimental sessions that were held on two consecutive days. Then the number of words stuttered in the two shock conditions were averaged and compared with the frequency displayed during the no-shock conditions. For each of the subjects more stuttering was evidenced during shock than during its absence. In the averaged shock conditions, 1,992 words were stuttered while in the no-shock conditions, 1,532 words were spoken dysfluently. This significant difference occurred even though the subjects were reportedly aware of the presence or absence of the contingency. Moreover, the subjects reported that the contingent shock provoked anxiety. As a result, Hegde stated that stuttering might best be seen ". . . within the context of traumatic emotional conditioning and learning. Stuttering does not seem to behave like an operant response under punishment, particularly when shock isused as a stimulus" (p. 4).

The contention that investigating the effects of contingent stimulation is worthwhile and should be continued has come from a number of sources. Such a position results in part from the fact that the issue to be resolved—whether or not stuttering is a learned response—bears importantly on our understanding and control of it. The studies to which we have just referred do not lend support to the contention that stuttering behaves in a manner that is consistent with the basic predictions of the law of effect. On the contrary, in almost all of these studies, stuttering either increased or did not significantly decrease when it was followed by a punishing consequence. In the rest, the decrease in stuttering could not be attributed to punishing stimulation. We have already stated, however, that experiments on the punishment of stuttering have been noted for the inconsistency of their findings. The call for further research has been made by a number of people, such as Timmons (1966) and Hegde (1970), because the results of some studies have supported the contention that stuttering *does* diminish as a function of punishment. Martin and Siegel (1966a), for example, studied the effect of punishment on various verbal and nonverbal behaviors of three stutterers. They contingently shocked nose-wrinkling and vocalized "uh-uh-uh" in one subject, tongue protrusion and /s/ prolongations in a second subject, and "moments of stuttering" in a third subject. These moments, which occurred an average of five or six times per two-minute period, were characterized by word repetitions and by ". . . a short, jerky, holding and releasing of the breath" (p. 348). Martin and Siegel reported a marked decrease in all of these behaviors when they were contingently followed by electric shock. The relationship between the contingent stimulus and the decrease in these behaviors was demonstrated by the fact that their frequency returned to base-rate level when the contingent stimulus was removed. Here, then, is a study in which the results clearly imply that certain behaviors which are among those traditionally labeled as stuttering were temporarily reduced by punishment in at least three subjects.

As early as 1959, Wingate expressed concern with what he felt was the unsupported assumption that listener disapproval (punishment) of stuttering would lead to an increased disruption of speech. His investigation of this theoretical contention involved a trial-by-trial count of stuttering during eight massed oral readings. The reading materials were instructions as to how a listener should complete simple tasks. No contingency was provided in the control condition for the act of speaking or the speech product. In one of the experimental conditions, however, the speaker's voice contact was cut off as a consequence of the *beginning* of each stuttering moment. Each time this occurred, the speaker was signaled that voice contact was disrupted. He had previously been instructed that contact would not be reinstituted until the word was spoken fluently. In a second experimental condition each speaker was instructed, prior to speaking, that he should be as fluent as possible and was signaled, without further consequences, each time he stuttered. The mean frequency of stuttering on each of the eight oral reading trials in both of the experimental conditions was significantly less than that displayed in the control condition.

Wingate's finding that stuttering decreased when the speaker had to achieve fluent production before communication would be continued is consistent with data previously reported by Sheehan (1951).[6] The

[6] In both Sheehan's and Wingate's studies the subjects repeated the stuttered word as often as they had to in order to be fluent. As a result, the stuttered words were produced more times than the same words in the control readings. In effect, then, there were more oral readings in the experimental conditions than in the control conditions. Since the number of stutterings during repeated readings of the same material is known to be a dependent function of the number of times the words are spoken (Golub, 1951; Yensen, 1947) and the extent to which the word repetition is massed (Dancer, 1966; Shulman, 1944), the significant differences found may be accounted for by the inequality inherent in the experimental design.

results of these two studies were consonant even though the interruption of the forward flow of speech occurred at the *beginning* of a stuttering moment in Wingate's study and at the *completion* of the stuttered word in the Sheehan study.[7] Wingate, however, also found a comparable decrease in stuttering when the subjects were instructed, prior to the speech attempt, to speak fluently and were signaled, without further consequences, when they did stutter.

More recently, Goldiamond (1965) has reported a series of studies in which he investigated the effects of response-contingent stimulation on stuttering. Although the procedures varied from subject to subject, Goldiamond most consistently used a short period of delayed auditory feedback as a contingent stimulus. The four stutterers described were subjected to the response-contingent delayed feedback and control conditions five days a week, 90 minutes per day, over a period of up to nine months. All of the subjects showed a reduction in stuttering under the response-contingent condition. The specific effects of the contingent stimulations were indicated by the fact that the rate of stuttering typically returned to approximately the base-line level upon removal of the contingency.

Goldiamond also found, however, that stuttering was not consistently increased in a predictable way when the removal of delayed auditory feedback was used as negative reinforcement. The removal of the aversive stimulus at first produced an increase in stuttering, as would be predicted. That is, when DAF was left on, except for .10 of a second immediately after each stuttering, the stuttering increased. However, the continued use of DAF in a negative reinforcement procedure produced marked verbal prolongations, a reduction in oral reading rate, and a striking reduction in "stuttering." The continued use of DAF, in other words, appeared to play a more important role as a disrupter of the stutterer's typical speech pattern than as a reinforcer for stuttering. In this sense, an *alteration* in speech behavior was produced by Goldiamond's use of DAF as it was by Sheehan's (1951) and Wingate's (1959) use of forced repetition of a stuttered word until fluency is achieved. It is of interest in this regard that Goldiamond, himself, raised the question of whether straightforward instructions to a stutterer to alter his speech pattern by prolonging words might not be as effective in establishing this new speech pattern as was the use of DAF.

Quist and Martin (1967) have reported a recent experiment in which the word "wrong" was used as a response-contingent stimulus with three stutterers. The target behavior in the first stutterer was any repetition or prolongation. An interjected "Uh" and an interjected, prolonged "n-n-n" sound were the contingently stimulated behaviors of the second and third subjects, respectively. The subjects were run for 50-minute periods in a laboratory situation. In each session, base rates for these behaviors were established, and the response-contingent condition followed immediately. Quist and Martin reported that, in general, there was a 30 to 40 percent reduction in the frequency of the target behavior in the first and third subjects and a reduction to near zero for the second subject. The target behaviors returned to base-rate for all subjects when the response-contingent stimulus was removed from the situation.

This group of studies clearly implies, then, that certain aspects of stuttering behave in accordance with the predictions of the law of effect under some experimental conditions. Significant reductions of stuttering have been reported when it was immediately followed by stimulus conditions such as electric shock, forced repetition until fluency was achieved, delayed auditory feedback, and the spoken word "wrong." At first glance, the data collected by Sheehan (1951), Wingate (1959), Martin and Siegel (1966b), Goldiamond (1965), and Quist and Martin (1967) appear to be diametrically opposed to those of Van Riper (1937), Frick (1951), Frederick (1955), and Hegde (1970), and unsupported by the data of Daly (1964), Hansen (1955), Cady and Robbins (1968), and Timmons (1966). Behavior traditionally labeled as stuttering decreased when followed by punishment in one group of studies, increased in another group of studies, and remained unchanged in a third. Obviously, the issue of whether stuttering should be considered a learned response has not yet been resolved and demands further, more careful experimentation.

Such differences among the results of experiments examining the same issue are by no means restricted to research on stuttering. The history of the physical and behavioral sciences is full of similar concern and dispute over apparently conflicting research results. Typically, such disputes have led either to changes

[7] Wingate (1959, p. 328) ". . . required that the subject's communications be interrupted whenever he began to stutter . . .," and Sheehan (1951, p. 56) gave his readers the instructions: ". . . do not interrupt yourself in the middle of a block. That is, be sure to finish the word first before repeating it, and be sure to repeat it until you can say it without stuttering before going on to the next word."

in theoretical structure, refinement of experimental procedures, or both. Clearly, adequate research on the question of whether or not stuttering is controlled by environmental consequences requires that the experimental operations be consistent among the studies compared. Variations in research results suggest either that the experimenters are using different measurement procedures or that they are actually measuring different phenomena even though they are using the same label. In such a situation, therefore, it becomes crucial that the experimenters specify and describe the measurement procedures clearly enough to allow exact replication. This level of sophistication has not been reached in the research on stuttering as often as desirable. Webster's (1968a) data, for example, indicate that it is extremely difficult to be accurate and consistent in presenting contingent stimulation immediately after fluency failure. Quite often, in other words, the stimulus that is a consequence of a specific stuttering moment is more contiguous to fluent speech than it is to fluency failure. Experimenters should specify, therefore, not only the accuracy with which the contingent stimulus is applied, but also the degree to which it is contiguous with the critical behavior.

An even more fundamental issue in experiments on stuttering, however, involves the definition of the events that are to be followed by contingent stimulation. Usually, the experimenter must determine whether or not the subject has stuttered in order to deliver a contingent stimulus. This apparently simple task requires that the experimenter be able to define stuttering in observable or measurable terms. Theorists and experimenters have not always agreed, however, on what behaviors they will call stuttering. Some, like Johnson and his students (Bloodstein, 1958; Johnson, 1967; Wischner, 1950), have contended that stuttering is an avoidance reaction motivated by environmental rejection of "normal disfluency." Stuttering, then, is what the speaker does so as not to be disfluent. Using this definition, the experimenter would have to stimulate contingently the adjustive reactions that the speaker has made to avoid "disfluency." It would not necessarily lead him to stimulate disturbances in the speech signal. Williams (1962), for example, electrically shocked prespeech adjustments such as tensing of the mandibular muscles, breath-holding, and rate changes. He did not contingently stimulate the speakers for their fluency failures. This distinction between avoidance reactions and fluency failure has not usually been so finely drawn, however. Johnson's contention that stuttering is what the speaker does to avoid disfluency has led many experimenters to apply contingent stimulation to 1. speech disruptions, such as repetitions and prolongations, and 2. nonspeech behaviors, such as eyeblinks, arm movements, nose wrinkling and foot tapping. This heterogeneous approach to the definition of stuttering appears to have been used, for example, in the Frick (1951) experiment, which we have already discussed. Specifically, in the response-contingent condition, Frick's subjects were stimulated with electric shock for stuttering moments that consisted of many different speech and nonspeech behaviors.

A similarly molar definition of stuttering has been used by most of the operantly oriented experimenters concerned with stuttering. Martin and Siegel, in their studies, have contingently stimulated both speech and nonspeech behaviors and have called both types stuttering. This is consistent with the operant viewpoint expressed by Shames and Sherrick (1963), who have pointed out the similarity between Johnson's view of stuttering as a listener-created avoidance reaction and the operant view of stuttering as a response whose form is determined by the environment's punishment of "normal disfluency."

Van Riper (1963) and his students, at least at the theoretical level, have maintained that a distinction should be made between primary and secondary aspects of stuttering. For them, the primary "symptoms" of stuttering are the repetitions and prolongations of sounds and syllables. This abnormal interference in the forward flow of speech is viewed as not necessarily dependent on the environment's rejection of "normal disfluency" and is not necessarily, therefore, either an anxiety-motivated avoidance reaction or an operant response to aversive stimulation. On the other hand, Van Riper considers the secondary symptoms to be the struggle reactions that develop as the speaker becomes aware and concerned about his disordered speech and as he attempts to improve it. Despite this theoretically relevant distinction, however, both primary and secondary symptoms are thought to be indicative of stuttering, and no attempt was made to differentiate between them in Van Riper's study of threatened punishment. As a result, in this investigation and in most of those that followed, the stuttering measured was an inseparable compound of primary and secondary behaviors. There is similar confounding in the punishment experiments conducted by Sheehan (1951) and his student

Frederick (1955). On a theoretical level Sheehan, like Van Riper, seems to suggest that a significant difference exists between primary and secondary reactions. The primary reactions of oscillation (repetition) and fixation (prolongation) stem from the basic conflict. These reactions, however, do not generally comprise the main body of what the listener receives. Sheehan contends that the secondary symptoms predominate and are *defensive* reactions to the moments of conflict. In his experiments on stuttering, however, he recorded a moment of stuttering whenever a primary symptom, a secondary symptom, or a combination of the two, was observed.

Wingate (1964) recognized that the diverse definitions of stuttering have hampered the theoretical integration of the accumulated research findings. He consequently proposed that we acknowledge our ignorance about the etiology of stuttering and limit its definition to observable events, at least for the present. For Wingate, stuttering is fundamentally characterized by unitary repetitions and prolongations that are either audible or silent. He considers these speech disruptions to be the cardinal characteristics of stuttering because one or both of these features is found among all stutterers. He also points out, however, that these disruptions, whose immediate source is some speech-expressed incoordination, are often accompanied by 1. accessory features that appear to be struggle activities and which some theorists have called secondary symptoms and 2. the associated features of arousal that range from general tension to specific negative emotional states. This definition is thus similar to those of Van Riper and Sheehan, at least to the extent that it relates to the measurement of stutterings. There are, of course, nuances in this definition that might well cause Wingate to count stutterings differently than other experimenters. Wingate, however, despite his emphasis on particular types of repetitions and prolongations as the necessary "kernel" that distinguishes stuttering from normal dysfluency, counted the accessory features or "secondary symptoms" as stutterings in his experiments. In other words, integral speech characteristics and accessory features, or some combination of the two, were all reported as moments of stuttering. Clearly, then, Wingate's experimental operations have implied a definition that is molar in nature.

We have seen that although there have been noteworthy differences in theoretical emphasis, a molar operational definition of stuttering has been used in almost all of the experiments of response-contingent stimulation. As a result, the experimenters have counted as stutterings a considerable mixture of various speech disruptions and so-called accessory or secondary mannerisms. In this circumstance, it is not surprising that the data are diametrically opposed and inconclusive about the effect of punishment on stuttering. Even when the data have indicated that response-contingent stimulation reduced the frequency of these complex moments of stuttering, it has not been possible to tell whether the speech disruptions and the accessory mannerisms of the molar movement have been equally affected. It is possible, as we have contended repeatedly, that a molar definition of stuttering masks inherent differences in these classes of behavior and that failure to recognize this is one significant reason for the confusion that we have been discussing (Bloodstein and Brutten, 1966; Brutten and Shoemaker, 1964, 1967). This contention gained initial support from those experiments in which punishment of molar moments of stuttering did not completely suppress the measured behaviors. The contention was further supported by certain results from a study by Martin, Brookshire, and Siegel that we have discussed in another context (Brutten and Shoemaker, 1967). In this study the experimenters directed their attention to the effect of punishment on specific molecular aspects of stuttering rather than on the more complex molar moments. They designed their study to determine, in part, if specific molecular aspects of the stuttering moment could be suppressed by shock and, if so, whether or not this decrease was associated with side effects on other aspects of the moment. More specifically, they contingently shocked their subject for, first, his nose-wrinkling responses, and then, after this behavior had been markedly reduced, they successfully suppressed the frequency with which the interjection "ah-ah-ah" was produced. The occurrence of these responses approached zero without any immediate evidence that the behavioral modification was accompanied by a decrease in the subject's verbal output. But, the continued use of punishment ultimately depressed the rate of verbal output. There was also a dramatic change in one of the nonexperimental aspects of the molar moments of stuttering: the number of prolongations of initial sounds increased in the ninth session to more than eight times what it had been in the first session. This increase in prolongations persisted until the final nonshock (extinction) period of the eleventh session.

Webster (1968b) directly tested Brutten and

Shoemaker's (1967) hypothesis that molar moments of stuttering are composed of at least two different classes of behavior. Webster used two adult stutterers as subjects. These subjects defined the behaviors they exhibited during stuttering moments as either voluntary or involuntary. Behaviors chosen for study were those that occurred frequently and that could be filmed. For subject A, the behaviors chosen were: involuntary part-word repetitions and voluntary complete headturns, partial headturns, interjections, and word manipulations. For subject B they were involuntary part-word repetitions and voluntary head-jaw movements.

The punishment of involuntary part-word repetitions for subject A resulted in increases in this behavior in three out of the four contingency segments. The first two of these increases were statistically significant (see Fig. 40-2). There was, moreover, no significant decrease in part-word repetitions during the contingency period. In addition, the voluntary behaviors showed fundamentally no change as the part-word repetitions significantly increased.

Subject B's voluntary head-jaw movements reduced significantly to zero *before* the contingent stimulation was introduced and remained essentially at that level throughout the entire contingency period. There was,

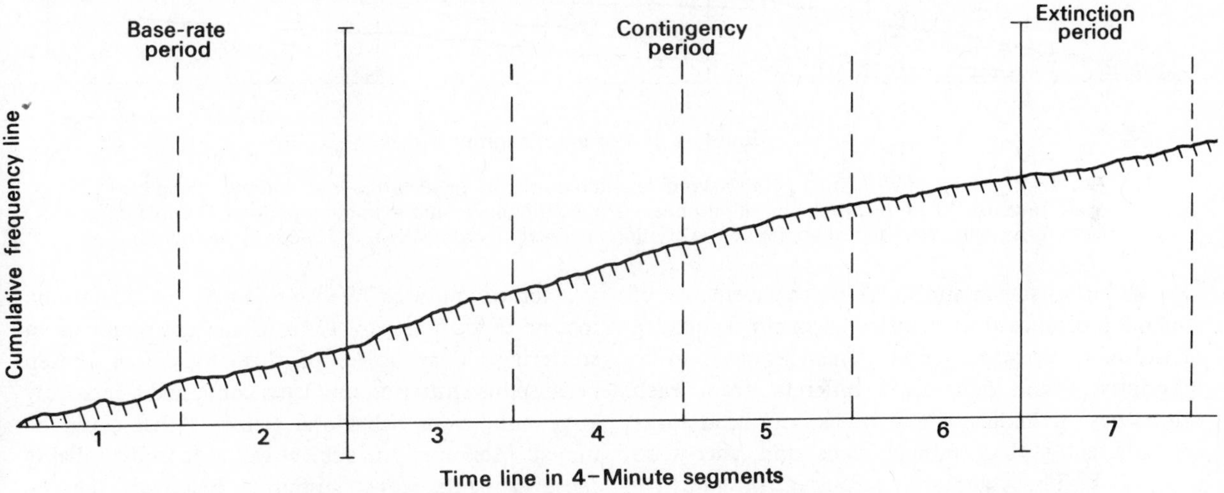

Fig. 40-1. Cumulative graph of part-word repetitions during base-rate, contingency, and extinction periods. *From Webster, 1968b, by permission.*

Sound motion pictures were taken of these two subjects during a base-rate session and two counterbalanced experimental sessions. During one experimental session, a voluntary behavior was punished with the verbal stimulus "wrong." During the other, an involuntary behavior was punished with the same stimulus. Each experimental session was followed by an extinction period. The base-rate, contingency, and extinction periods were divided into four-minute segments. The voluntary complete headturn of subject A was chosen for response-contingent stimulation. Punishing this response produced a statistically significant decrease and its frequency approximated zero during the entire contingency period. As can be seen in Fig. 40–1, however, the other voluntary responses and the involuntary behavior measured increased significantly during the same contingency period.

therefore, little opportunity for this subject to experience punishment and no way to determine the effect of punishment on this response. Involuntary part-word repetitions increased nonsignificantly in two of the four contingency segments and did not decrease significantly in either of the two remaining segments.

Considering the data from both subjects, the distinctive difference between the effect of response-contingent stimulation on voluntary and involuntary responses led Webster to conclude that there is strong support for the ". . . contention that two different classes of behaviors are embodied in what has traditionally been called stuttering." (p. 96).

The data from these experiments bear importantly on a number of issues with which we have been concerned. It is evident now that the molar moment of stuttering is not unitary. Neither is it a compound

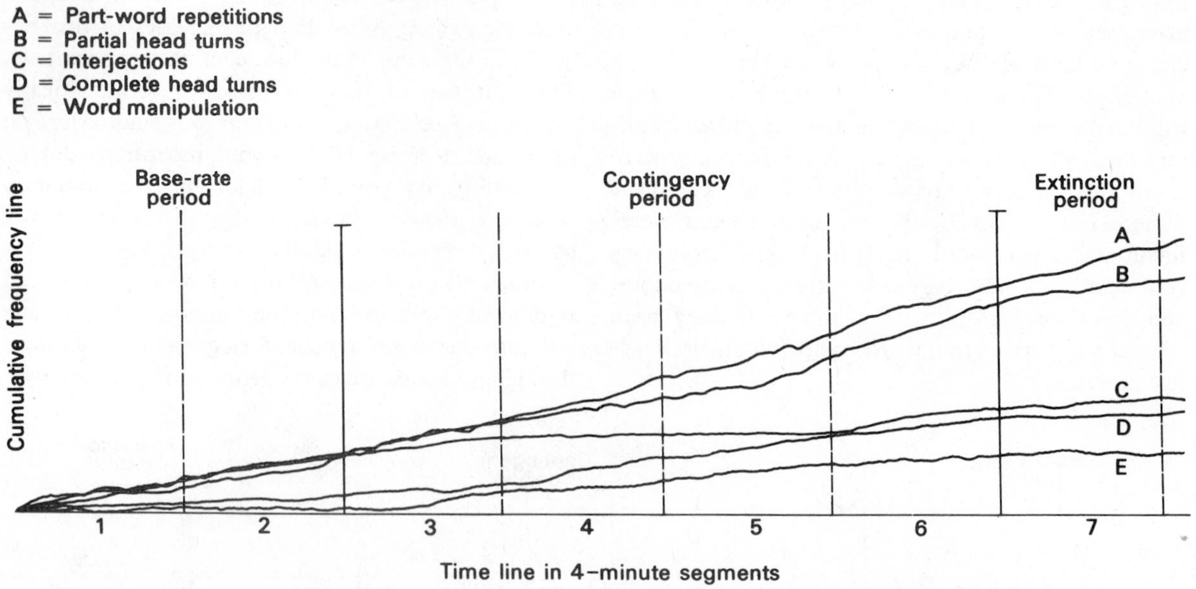

Fig. 40-2. Cumulative graphs of part-word repetitions, partial head turns, interjections, complete head turns, and word manipulation during base-rate, contingency, and extinction periods. Complete head turns, only, were punished during the contingency period. *From Webster, 1968b, by permission.*

that differs characteristically from the elements of which it is composed. It is, instead, a complex mixture of isolatable elements. These elements appear to be descriptively and generically different from each other; nose wrinkling, interjections, and head turns act differently than prolongations and part-word repetitions. The voluntary, purposive, or adjustive nature of responses such as nose-wrinkling, interjections, and head-turns has been repeatedly noted by speech pathologists. Part-word repetitions and prolongations have often been considered as both different from the obviously voluntary responses and more definitive of stuttering (Sheehan, 1946; Van Riper, 1963; Wingate, 1964). Moreover, nose-wrinkling and interjections seem to belong to a class of behavior that is decreased by punishment. Involuntary repetitions and prolongations, on the other hand, belong to a class that is increased by such stimulation. Therefore, if the moment of stuttering is made up largely of "primary," "universal," "kernel," or involuntary elements, its frequency as a whole will be increased by punishment. If the so-called secondary, accessory, or voluntary responses predominate, however, there will be a decrease in measured stuttering. If these two classes of behavior are in equal mixture, there will be no significant change in frequency.

The distinction between the two classes of behavior that make up a stuttering moment can be seen clearly in another study by Webster (1966). In this study, too, he used motion pictures to analyze moments of stuttering. The subject of this study was chosen because his stuttering moments contained a relatively large number of behavioral elements that could be filmed. Moreover, the subject was able to list reliably those elements of his stuttering behaviors that he thought were involuntary and those that he thought were voluntary. The experimenter selected part-word repetitions as the behavior for analysis from the list of involuntary elements and eyeblinks as the behavior from the list of voluntary responses. He also selected two other behaviors that were not reported by the subject but were observed to occur during his moments of stuttering. These two unreported behaviors were repetitions of whole words (predominantly single-syllable words) and interjections. Counts of these four behaviors during six oral readings of the same material revealed that there was no significant correlation between the reportedly involuntary part-word repetitions and voluntary eyeblinks (−.20). Neither was there a significant correlation between the "kernel" repetitions of whole words and the "secondary" or "accessory" interjections (+.22). In contrast, part-word repetitions and repetitions of whole words that were predominantly of one syllable correlated significantly (+.80), as did eyeblinks and interjections (+.84). These data suggest again that for this subject the so-called kernel elements of stuttering moments (repetitions of a sound, syllable, or one-syllable word) and the secondary or accessory elements represent different classes of behavior. Moreover, these data are consonant with the results of Martin, Brookshire, and Siegel (1964) and the Webster (1968b) data already referred to. In these studies, negative stimulation had differential effects on voluntary and involuntary behaviors.

The study by Quist and Martin (1967), which we have already discussed, also bears meaningfully on the distinction we are making. In this study the stimulus "wrong" was made contingent upon specific aspects of stuttering moments that were displayed by three different subjects. Quist and Martin's subject B reportedly interjected a strained and somewhat prolonged "uh" sound prior to certain speech attempts. In the first session the average number of these interjections was reduced as a result of contingent negative stimulation from a base-rate of 18 to a rate of 11 for each two-minute segment. By the end of four sessions, the base-rate average was 14.8, and interjections were decreased to 2.4 as a result of the contingent stimulation. This decrease occurred even though the number of words spoken was reported not to vary systematically as a function of the contingent stimulation. This dramatic decrease of more than 85 percent was not matched by a similar reduction in stuttering behaviors for their subject A. For this subject, stuttering was defined as any repetition or prolongation. The mean base-rate of these combined behaviors was 11 for each two-minute period in the first session. These behaviors were not contingently stimulated during the first session. The mean base-rate of measured stuttering increased to 12.8 in the second session. In the contingency period of the second session, the average of 11.9 stutterings was greater than that displayed in the base-rate period of the first session and only .9 stutterings less than that displayed in the base-rate period of the second session. It is apparent from these data that the contingent stimulation had little or no effect on the rate of stuttering during these two sessions. Moreover, in the seven sessions that followed the decrease in measured stuttering averaged only about 30 to 40 percent. Response-contingent "wrong," in other words, apparently produced no meaningful behavior change in the first punishment session, and only a limited amount of change in subsequent sessions (three to four stutterings per unit). Furthermore, some of the few repetitions and prolongations that did decrease may have been voluntary responses, since some speakers use certain kinds of repetitions and prolongations as avoidance responses.

Subject C of this experiment interjected a prolonged nasal sound ("n-n-n") before many different words. Prolongations of this type have typically been viewed as purposive, "secondary" mannerisms unless they are limited to words that begin with this sound. The base-rate of this response in the first session was 26 for each two-minute period, and the initial use of the contingent stimulus "wrong" reduced this average frequency to about 16. Subject C's decrease of about 40 percent in the first session contrasts sharply with subject A's decrease of only nine percent in the first session for which data were reported. Perhaps it was this lack of initial change, as much as the limited absolute change in all of the sessions involving subject A's repetitions and prolongations, that led Martin and Siegel (1966b) to point out that ". . . for two of three subjects used in the experiment, the presentation of 'wrong' resulted in a reduction of stuttering frequency." (p. 467). In any event, these data are consistent with the findings of the other studies that we have reviewed.

Starkweather (1970) recently completed a study in which he specifically limited his measures to involuntary repetitions because of their apparent difference from the voluntary responses often associated with the speech of stutterers. He used a factorial design to investigate the simple, main, and interactive effects of contingent and noncontingent stimulation of high and low intensity on the frequency of involuntary repetitions. The four conditions that resulted from these factors were counterbalanced among the four subjects of this experiment. For the first time in an experiment of this kind, awareness and the number of punishing stimuli presented were held constant. Awareness was controlled by presegment instructions which indicated the possible events that might follow. The total numbers of shocks delivered to the subjects as a group during the contingency and noncontingency conditions were exactly the same.

An analysis of the simple effects involved a comparison between the no-stimulation (base-rate and extinction) and the experimental periods. This represented a punishment study when either the low- or high-intensity shock was made contingent upon repetition. Starkweather reportedly anticipated that the effect of these punishment conditions would be suppressive. He found, instead, that as a group his subjects did not significantly reduce the frequency of repetitions as a result of the contingent delivery of the negative stimuli, whether of high or low intensity. Moreover, he found that withdrawal of either stimulus during the extinction period produced a significant *decrease* in the repetitions displayed by the group. Some essentially similar results were obtained when the main effects were analyzed. These results concerned the effect of introducing and withdrawing a punishing stimulus regardless of its intensity. When the high- and low-intensity conditions were combined, it became apparent that these stimuli had no significant group effect; repetitions were not decreased. Unlike the analysis of the simple effects, however, the withdrawal of the combined high- and low-intensity shock stimuli did not bring about a significant decline in the frequency of repetitions displayed during the extinction period.

Since there is no nonparametric statistic for assessing the significance of an interaction effect, Starkweather was unable to determine if the interaction between the high/low intensity variable and the contingent/noncontingent variable was a meaningful or chance occurrence. He did approximate this test, however, by comparing each of the simple and main effects. These evaluations led him to point out cautiously that, contrary to what one would expect if the involuntary repetitions were instrumentally (operantly) conditioned responses, high-intensity contingent shock was less likely to reduce these behaviors than was low-intensity punishment.

In summary, Starkweather contends that the most likely explanation for the discrepancy between the simple and main effects of his study and the results of past studies which have indicated that stuttering is suppressed by punishment ". . . is that in the experiments done previously, no attempt was made to distinguish between voluntary and involuntary behaviors. This suggests the possibility that when 'stuttering behaviors' have been found to decrease under contingent negative stimulation, they have consisted wholly or partially of voluntary behaviors." (p.390). On the basis of the interactive data he was led to conclude that these ". . . involuntary repetitions did not respond to different punishment intensities in a way that would have been predicted for behavior that had been learned by instrumental conditioning." (p. 401).

Taken as a whole, these investigations indicate that the use of a molar approach to the measurement of stuttering moments leads to ambiguity and confusion in interpreting research results. What has been traditionally defined as stuttering usually includes a complex of involuntary and voluntary behaviors. The involuntary behaviors, as we have seen, have been generally described as the "primary" or "kernel" elements of stuttering that affect fluency directly. The voluntary behaviors have been generally described as "secondary" or "accessory" characteristics, which often have no direct effect on the fluency of the speech signal. Moreover, these two classes of behavior have been observed to act in distinctly different ways when followed by punishing stimuli: the involuntary behaviors tend to increase, and the voluntary behaviors tend to decrease. This interpretation of the data also implies that these two behavior classes are not the result of the same conditioning procedures and that they need not follow the same laws of learning.

THE EFFECTS OF STIMULUS-CONTINGENT STIMULATION[8] ON MOMENTS OF STUTTERING

Up to this point, we have discussed only those experiments that have dealt with the effects of response-contingent stimulation on measures of stuttering behavior. These investigations, though of great import, represent a relatively small number of the experiments that have been done on stuttering. Much of the research on stuttering has emphasized the stimulus conditions that set the occasion for stuttering (Berwick, 1939; Dixon, 1947; Shulman, 1944; Van Riper and Hull, 1955; Wischner, 1952a). This research has made it clear that stuttering does not occur randomly; stuttering is cued off by stimulus circumstances that have been associated with noxious stimulation in the past. Fluency, on the other hand, seems to occur in stimulus circumstances that have a history of positive rather than noxious stimulus associations. Stated differently, the tendency for stuttering or fluency to occur in a particular stimulus situation depends on whether the situation has a history of contingent negative or positive stimulation. Among nonstutterers, also, the stimulus occasions for

[8] Stimulus-contingent stimulation refers to the procedures used in the acquisition and modification of classically conditioned responses. As the data of Rescorla (1967) indicate, classical conditioning depends on some scheduled relationship between the conditioned and unconditioned stimuli rather than on their random association.

fluency or fluency failure are determined strongly by the stimuli that make up the speech situation; in other words, by stimulus properties that are contingent upon the speech situation (Hill, 1954; Savoye, 1959; Stassi, 1961). We have contended, on the basis of such observations, as have Bluemel (1932) and Wischner (1947), that classical conditioning plays a vital role in the onset, development, and maintenance of stuttering. Our contention was also stated in the evaluative review by Bloodstein and Brutten (1966), in which a call was made for ". . . research that is concerned with the modification of stuttering through stimulus manipulation, change, or desensitization." (p. 395). It needs to be reemphasized here because the data suggest that changes in stuttering and associated behaviors result both from alterations in stimuli that are contingent upon the speech situation and from alterations in stimuli that are contingent on responses. These data have led us 1. to attend to *both* the classical and instrumental conditioning that seem to be involved in what has been traditionally defined as stuttering, 2. to be aware that different aspects of stuttering moments can be modified by the extinction of the classically conditioned and the instrumentally conditioned components, and 3. to realize, more fully than before, that the acquisition and extinction of the classical and instrumental responses of stutterers are often interdependent and interactive.

The reduction of stuttering moments through the counterconditioning of word stimuli has been investigated by Brutten and Gray (1961) and by Adams and Brutten (1968). In the first of these studies the subjects, who were stutterers, read aloud two different lists of words that had been printed on white cards and placed on a display board. In the control condition, words that had been stuttered during each of the five oral readings were eliminated at the end of each trial by turning the word card to its blank yellow side. In the experimental condition, previously stuttered words were completely removed from the display board after each trial, and the remaining word cards were spatially rearranged to minimize the topographical effect of removing cards from the board. Significantly less stuttering, that is, greater fluency, was found in the experimental condition than in all but the first oral trial of the control condition.

The procedure in this experiment was considered to be an analogue of Johnson and Millsapps' (1937) blacking-out method that produced a significantly greater reduction in stuttering than was found in the traditional adaptation sequence. In the Johnson and Millsapps study, however, words adjacent to the blacked-out words showed a distinct tendency to be stuttered, and this indicated that the blackouts themselves interfered with adaptation. It would seem, then, that the adjacency between the previously nonstuttered words (conditioned stimuli) and the noxious environmental signs that stuttering had occurred before at the point of the blackouts (higher-order unconditioned negative stimuli) led to classical conditioning that set the occasion for new stuttering. This difficulty was obviated in the Brutten and Gray study since, in the experimental condition, all of the words stuttered were completely removed from the display board at the completion of each oral reading. As a result of this procedure the remaining word stimuli were placed in a contingent and contiguous relationship with environmental stimuli indicative of previous fluency (higher order positive unconditioned stimuli). Moreover, this contingent relationship between stimulus events set the occasion for significantly greater fluency than that found in the control condition where cues of the previous stuttering were present. In other words, in this situation the proportion of positive stimuli, words that had previously been spoken fluently, was increased by removing word stimuli that were associated with previous fluency failure. In addition, clinical exploration with this procedure indicated that previously stuttered words would soon be spoken fluently if they were selectively reintroduced one by one into a list of fluent words. The order of reentry was an inverse function of the trial on which the word was stuttered: words stuttered on the first oral reading trial were the last to be introduced into the fluent word list while those stuttered on the last oral reading trial were the first to be reentered and contingently stimulated by word stimuli indicative of fluency. Brutten and Gray have suggested that the counterconditioning that occurs may be seen in terms of "positive adjacency."

One of the control conditions of the Adams and Brutten (1968) study also reflects upon what Brutten and Gray called positive adjacency. In this investigation, printed word cards were used to construct three decks that contained the same common nouns. Though the same 75 nouns appeared in each of these three decks, their specific order was randomized. The subjects orally read each deck once, so that each noun was read three times. The experimenters then removed from each deck those words that had been stuttered two or more times during the three oral readings. The remaining words were those that had been spoken fluently at least two times during the three oral readings. As a matter of fact, almost all of the remaining words had been spoken fluently on each of the three oral readings. Half of the stuttered words that had been removed were reinserted into each of the three decks. In the silent control condition, these consistently stuttered words were inserted into the predominantly fluent decks after the subjects had rested for about 30 minutes. In the desensitization condition, an equal number of words, matched for consistency of stuttering, was presented auditorily to the subjects 30 times in quick succession. Following each of these conditions the three decks were orally read again. The frequency of stuttering on the reinserted words reduced significantly in both the silent control and the desenitization conditions. The decrease in the silent control condition could not be attributed either to an experimental variable or to adaptation, since, in this condition, no experimental manipulation was introduced. Furthermore, adaptation studies have indicated that a 30-minute rest period leads to a marked spontaneous recovery in stuttering (Gray and Brutten, 1965; Maxwell, 1965; Shulman, 1944). It was assumed, therefore, that the significant decrease resulted from inserting a small number of stuttered words (negative conditioned stimuli) into a larger context of words that had a recent history of relative fluency (higher order positive unconditioned stimuli). In other words, it was theorized that the negative valences of the conditioned stimuli were modified because of their contingent relationship with a preponderant number of positively valenced stimuli. The counterconditioning that resulted from positive adjacency was demonstrated by a significant reduction in stuttering when, after the silent period, the previously stuttered words were read three more times.

In both the Brutten and Gray study and the Adams and Brutten study, then, a reduction in stuttering occurred when the proportion of stimuli associated with fluency was increased relative to stimuli associated with fluency failure. In each of these studies, stuttering decreased significantly when words previously stuttered were presented in the stimulus context of an increased proportion of word spoken fluently. In conditioning terms, the stimulus situation was changed by a reduction in the stimuli that evoked negative emotional reactions and a relative increase in the stimuli that evoked positive emotional reactions. This particular alteration of the stimulus contingencies apparently led to counterconditioning of the negative emotional reactions previously evoked by the situation.

The valence of stimuli that set the occasion for stuttering has been modified in a number of studies by a variety of counterconditioning procedures. The studies that we have just been discussing, and some others that we will consider, were designed to investigate the effect of stimulus-contingent stimulation on stuttering. Others, like Van Riper's (1937) study of the effect of threatened punishment on the frequency of stuttering, were apparently designed to investigate the effects of response-contingent stimulation. Even Van Riper's study, however, involved methodological manipulations that, in part, served to alter the stimulus value of the situation in which speech took place. Remember that the subjects of this study first read a passage three times. Then, *before* the next oral reading of the same passage, they were shocked and told that they would receive a similar shock for each moment of stuttering in the trial that followed. Since this oral reading had not yet occurred, it is apparent that the shock and the instructions were contingent upon the speech situation and not upon words already stuttered. It is of more than passing interest, therefore, that the average frequency of stuttering increased significantly in this stimulus circumstance. It is not possible to determine what part, if any, of this increase in stuttering is attributable to stimulus-contingent stimulation, however, since each time the subjects stuttered, they must have realized that the punishment count had increased. In other words, the expected negative stimulation was also contingent upon each moment of stuttering. This confounded experimental procedure makes it impossible to comment upon the effect on stuttering of either stimulus- or response-contingent stimulation alone.[9]

[9] The stimulus valence of the speech situation may well have been altered even if 1. the subjects of this experiment had not been given instructions about a threatened and demonstrated penalty prior to responding and 2. the negative stimulus had been immediately delivered as a contingency of stuttering. Response-contingent stimulation is necessarily also contingent upon the stimulus situation. Learning theorists have repeatedly pointed out that it is not logically possible ". . . to perform an instrumental conditioning experiment without also arranging the conditions for a classical conditioning one. To obtain instrumental conditioning it is essential to reinforce a subject for performing some act. Obviously this reinforcement must occur in some situation. Thus the situational cues are conditioned stimuli regularly associated with reinforcement, after the manner of classical conditioning" (Kimble, 1961, p. 78). It is noteworthy, in contrast, that the unconditioned stimuli of classical conditioning need not serve as contingent consequences of instrumental responding.

The same confounding between stimulus- and response-contingent stimulation exists in the third condition of Frick's (1951) experiment. As in Van Riper's experiment, the subjects were told that they would receive an electric shock for each word stuttered during a forthcoming oral reading. This experimental condition produced considerably more stuttering than the nonshock, control condition. On the last conditioning trial, for example, the group that anticipated delayed response-contingent shock displayed a mean of 9.00 stutterings, and the control group showed a mean of .25 stutterings.[10]

One condition of Wingate's (1959) experiment also involved the use of both stimulus-contingent instructions that negatively conditioned the stimulus circumstances and response-contingent consequences that appear to be aversive. Remember that the subjects in this experiment were required to communicate task instructions to an assistant who would carry them out. They were advised, however, that the microphone connection would be interrupted each time they stuttered and that they could not continue with their communication until they said the stuttered word fluently. The combination of these instructions and the actual interruption of communication as a contingency of stuttering was associated with a significant reduction in the frequency of this behavior. Fortunately, one condition of this experiment involved stimulus-contingent stimulation without response-contingent consequences that would generally be regarded as aversive. In this condition, the stutterers were told to speak as fluently as possible. They were also told that each instance of stuttering would be recorded on an electrical counter placed before them. This condition resulted in less stuttering than was found in an unstimulated control group. Moreover, the combination of instructions and cumulative count of stutterings produced as great a decrease in the mean number of words stuttered as did the response-contingent consequence of interrupting communication until the stuttered words were spoken fluently. This similarity may, of course, have resulted because stimulation was contingent upon stuttering in both conditions: in the one, speech was interrupted, and, in the other, the counter advanced. It is possible, of course, that the contingent stimulation from the counter was aversive for the subjects since they had been instructed to speak as fluently as possible and they failed to carry out the instructions when they stuttered. It seemed to Wingate, however, that the counter simply reminded the subject of the instructions. Moreover, the "reminder" may have served as additional instructions about those behaviors that needed to be changed to achieve the requested fluency. He proposed that the improvement in fluency may well have come about because the instructions developed a set to speak fluently. Sheehan (1951) raised a similar hypothesis while discussing another study. He suggested that some children continue to stutter because they do not follow parental instructions to repeat stuttered words until they are spoken fluently. Sheehan felt that such children simply experience the instructions as a penalty. It is not unlikely, in other words, that Wingate's subjects who were simply instructed to speak fluently decreased their stuttering as a result of stimulus-contingent stimuli that were presented before responding. To repeat, the changes on the counter, from this point of view, would remind the subjects of the original instructions and help define for the subjects which specific behaviors the experimenter wanted modified. A similar interpretation could be made for Wingate's subjects who read task directions to an assistant and were instructed that the communication would be interrupted for each stuttering and would not be continued until the stuttered word was spoken fluently. The interruption could be considered as a reminder that the ultimate requirement was to speak fluently and as a way of clarifying which behaviors the experimenter defined as fluency failure. The primary effect of the response-contingent stimuli, from this point of view, would be to give the subjects information about the nature of the stimulus situation instead of suppressing the behavior as a direct effect of punishment.

Certainly, it is often difficult to separate clearly the effects of stimulus- and response-contingent stimulation. Most frequently, the stimulation is contingently associated with both aspects of stimulus-response chains. However, there are experiments in which the only observable stimulus manipulated is contingent

[10] Frick analyzed the differences between the group anticipating response-contingent shock, the control group, and two other shock groups on the tenth trial by means of a simple analysis of variance. The assumptions of this parametric test were not met, however, because the distribution of stuttering moments is markedly skewed to the right (Soderberg, 1956) and is noncontinuous (Lindquist, 1962) and not representative, then, of an interval scale (Siegel, 1956). Consequently, we analyzed the data of the tenth trial with the Wilcoxon Signed-Ranks Test, a nonparametric statistic. This two-tailed analysis revealed that the difference between the group that anticipated the punishment of shock and the control group was significant ($p = .05$).

upon the stimulus circumstance. Perhaps, the clearest example of such pure stimulus-contingent stimulation is found in one aspect of a study by Siegel and Martin (1966). This investigation was designed primarily to study the effect of three response-contingent auditory stimuli on the fluency failures of nonstutterers. Siegel and Martin found that the word "right" had no effect but that fluency failures[11] were reduced during oral reading by the contingent use of the verbal reprimand "wrong." They also discovered, however, that a presumably neutral buzzer produced a significant decrease in fluency failures, although they had no reason to assume that the buzzer was negative and would be punishing. It was not painful, nor did it have a history of indicating disapproval. To explain these results, Siegel and Martin hypothesized that fluency failures may be punishing to the normal speaker because of their frequent association with "tension" and "uncertainty" and thus *any* ". . . events that call the speaker's attention to his disfluencies might serve to decrease their occurrence" (Siegel and Martin, 1966, p. 215). They went on to suggest that if, in fact, the buzzer was not a punishing stimulus,[12] the reduction in fluency failures occurred because the buzzer "alerted" the speaker to his mistakes. If this were the case, of course, it should also be possible to alert the speaker *before speaking* with stimulus-contingent instructions about his speech. This is exactly what Siegel and Martin found in a final experimental condition of the same study. In this condition, they told 10 nonstutterers that they had displayed a number of fluency failures in the initial oral reading segment, and they instructed them, before the next segment, to ". . . try not to repeat or interject words, that is, try not to make mistakes (Siegel and Martin, 1966, p. 216)." The result was a significant decrease in fluency failures. In fact, the average decrease after instructions to avoid mistakes was considerably greater than the decrease for the subjects who received the verbal reprimand "wrong" and for the subjects who were contingently stimulated by the buzzer. Furthermore, the decrease following the instructions was maintained even though they were never repeated and no response-contingent stimulus was used to "remind" the speakers of the "mistake" they had just made. We can thus say with some certainty that this reduction in fluency failures cannot be attributed to any observable response-contingent stimulus. Indeed, the only independent variable was the stimulus-contingent instruction to avoid repetitions and interjections, and this stimulus was delivered only before the subjects began to read.

The instruction not to stutter need not be given verbally. If a nylon band or a blue light (Martin and Siegel, 1966a) is consistently present in a stimulus situation in which the speaker is selectively punished (electric shock) for stuttering and not punished for fluency, it can become a classically conditioned stimulus that signifies the valence of certain modes of behaving. It is not surprising, then, that these conditioned stimuli decreased the frequency of at least certain instrumental aspects of measured stuttering. It is not unexpected, either, that these conditioned stimuli failed to remain effective suppressors when the unconditioned stimulus of electric shock was no longer contingently paired with them.

Brookshire (1967) has used various forms of stimulus-contingent stimulation in his clinical work with stutterers. He thought it inadvisable to use response-contingent negative stimulation with one of his patients who had been diagnosed as a paranoid schizophrenic. Instead, he trained the subject to identify and describe the rapid repetition of an initial sound and the occasional repetition of an interjected vowel. He then instructed the patient to move from the repeated initial sound to the following sound of those words on which stuttering occurred. This new manner of behaving was verbally reinforced by the clinician, and fluency was attained in seven sessions. The patient was then discharged from speech therapy, and informal checks of his speech on the ward indicated that the behavior change was maintained. Brookshire also used stimulus-contingent stimulation

[11] In this experiment Siegel and Martin (1966, p. 210) defined fluency failure broadly ". . . as an interjection or repetition of a sound, syllable, word, phrase, etc." They did not report any attempt to distinguish these forms of fluency failure from each other or to analyze the effectiveness of the contingent stimuli in modifying these separate behaviors.

[12] Siegel and Martin have in the past contended, as operantly oriented researchers do, that a punishing stimulus is defined, post hoc, by the response reduction that follows its contingent presentation and by the increase in rate that occurs when it is removed. But Dulany (1961, p. 251) has pointed out in his review of studies on verbal operant conditioning that various kinds of stimuli have produced significant effects and that although "mm-hmm" under several circumstances could be a pleasant thing to hear, ". . . it is unclear how a buzzer or a flash of a 75 watt bulb would activate any of the processes variously assumed to be the basis for a law of effect that is more than empirical." He went on to suggest that response-contingent consequences do not automatically determine learning. He contended, instead, that the relationship between a response class and certain consequences lead the individual to form behavioral hypotheses and that the resulting self-instruction sets determine the response selection.

with another stutterer whose fluency failures were reduced but not eliminated by response-contingent noise. Much of the remaining fluency failures were eliminated by having him read in time to the clicks of a metronome. This improvement was maintained outside the clinic where the stutterer used a transistorized pocket metronome. Apparently as a result of the fluency experienced in various speech situations, the stutterer reported that he became less and less dependent on the metronome.

The behavior change brought about in these two stutterers was apparently dramatic and relatively stable. In one case the increased fluency occurred with no previous attempt to use punishment and in the other when response-contingent stimulation failed to produce complete fluency. It was undoubtedly these clinical experiences, among others, that led Brookshire (1967) to point out that ". . . the major tasks in the treatment of stuttering are first, to find or create a situation in which the client is fluent, and second, to manipulate stimuli so that this fluency may generalize. Punishment of stuttering or reinforcement of fluency may be only incidental to these concerns." (pp. 6–7). In other words, the valence of the stimulus circumstance in which speech takes place is a vital conditioner of fluency or fluency failure. The stimulus-contingent events are probably at least as vital, if not more so, as the response-contingent stimulation. In any event, the data at hand suggest that at least certain aspects of stuttering or fluency failure have been modified by stimuli that precede the speech attempt as well as by stimuli that are a consequence of disrupted speech. This, of course, vitiates the contention that stuttering and fluency failure are exclusively instrumental responses that are shaped *only* by their consequences. Their would appear, instead, to be at least two types of training procedures or learning conditions involved in the development of what has been traditionally labeled as stuttering—classical conditioning (stimulus-contingent stimulation) and instrumental conditioning (response-contingent stimulation). Although theorists have distinguished, in the past, between the primary and secondary behaviors of stuttering, they have not, unfortunately, distinguished between the learning conditions that produce these two types of behavior. The result, as we have seen, has been conceptual and methodological confusion. The hypothesis that at least two types of learning are involved in molar stuttering holds considerable promise for reducing this confusion by allowing theorists, experimenters, and therapists to deal differentially with behaviors acquired under different learning conditions.

A TWO-FACTOR THEORY OF STUTTERING AND ASSOCIATED BEHAVIORS

Two-factor theories of learning have existed in the psychological literature for more than 50 years (Mowrer, 1947; Rescorla and Solomon, 1967; Skinner, 1937; Thorndike, 1911). These theories typically differentiate classical conditioning or stimulus-contingent learning from instrumental conditioning or response-contingent learning. Although theoretical variations exist, classical conditioning is generally thought to describe conditions under which the organism learns to be motivationally or emotionally stimulated by previously neutral stimuli. Classical conditioning, in other words, increases the number of stimuli that can motivate, arouse, or drive the organism. In contrast, instrumental conditioning is generally thought to describe conditions under which the organism learns coping responses as a means of modifying the learned or unlearned drive states that are associated with particular stimulus circumstances. Thus, for most two-factor theorists, classical conditioning leads to the development of relationships between stimuli and motivational states or emotional responses, and instrumental conditioning leads to the development of relationships between stimuli and relatively specific, goal-oriented behaviors.

Two-factor theorists typically postulate that there is a difference in the training procedures and in the response systems of classical and instrumental conditioning. With regard to the training procedures, classical conditioning occurs when a conditioned stimulus is contingently followed by unconditioned stimuli regardless of the organism's behavior. Instrumental conditioning occurs when a response is contingently followed by a stimulus that either reduces a negative drive state or increases a positive one. With regard to the response system, classical conditioning is often thought to involve the autonomic nervous system that innervates primarily involuntary, smooth muscle activity. Instrumental conditioning, on the other hand, is thought to involve divisions of the central nervous system that mediate voluntary, striate muscle activity. Although these distinctions are usually made with the awarenesss that the response systems, and possibly even the training procedures that effect them, are not mutually exclusive, the general position of two-factor theorists is that classical conditioning involves responses that are more reflexive and less voluntary, and instrumental conditioning involves responses that are more adaptive and less involuntary (Mowrer, 1950; Rescorla and Solomon, 1967).

Furthermore, most two-factor theorists have developed specific hypotheses about the functional relationships between classical and instrumental responses. It is generally accepted, for example, that conditioned emotional responses can serve as learned drive states that motivate instrumental responding. In this way, classically conditioned emotional responses are thought to function as secondary or learned drives that affect the activity level of the organism. Most two-factor theorists maintain, in addition, that the learning of instrumental responses is determined by changes in classically conditioned drive stimuli. More specifically, it is assumed that the learning of specific approach and avoidance responses to given stimulus conditions is reinforced if the behaviors are contingently followed by an appropriate increase or decreased in positive or negative conditioned emotion. In other words, emotional conditioning is thought to serve as both an instigator of instrumental responding and as a potential source of positive or negative reinforcement for instrumental responses.

The relationship between conditioned negative emotion and instrumental behavior seems to serve a useful survival function for the organism. Unconditioned stimuli, such as strong electric shock, that produce negative emotional conditioning are noxious to the organism and represent threats to survival. Instrumental behaviors that lead to successful escape from or avoidance of such unconditioned stimuli can thus be considered adaptive or consistent with the continued survival of the organism. Learning to respond to a conditioned stimulus in such a way that interaction with the unconditioned stimulus is reduced or avoided is similarly adaptive. Such learning, however, can become useless or self-destructive under certain circumstances. This can be exemplified in the classical shuttle-box experiment with animals (Solomon, Kamin, and Wynne, 1953). In this type of experiment, animals are shocked in one side of a divided box immediately following presentation of a conditioned stimulus. They can escape the shock by engaging in some instrumental activity such as jumping across a barrier into the other side of the box where there is no shock. After a number of contingent presentations of the conditioned stimulus and the shock, many animals jump to the nonshock side of the box when the conditioned stimulus is presented and thus avoid the shock altogether. This instrumental responding is adaptive so long as the shock does, in fact, follow the conditioned stimulus. Once established, however, the avoidance behavior may become maladaptive. Such responses, for example, often persist long after the experimenter has disconnected the shock (Solomon, Kamin, and Wynne, 1953), and in some experiments avoidance behaviors have even driven animals away from a highly desirable goal object such as food (Massermen, 1943; Wolpe, 1958). Thus, instrumental behaviors that were formerly adaptive may become maladaptive because they lead the organism to expend energy wastefully or because they block the organism's movement toward reinforcements that are available in the situation. Usually it is hypothesized that the reinforcement for the maintenance of such maladaptive responding is the contingent reduction of the drive stimulus of fear. It has also been hypothesized that, all things being equal, escape or avoidance responses will be maintained even if they are punished, as long as the reinforcement of fear reduction is in closer temporal proximity to the instrumental response than the punishment is (Mowrer and Ullman, 1945). Thus, the alcoholic continues to drink in spite of the physical and social punishment that comes the morning after, and the stutterer continues to jerk his head to one side in spite of the rejecting glances of his audience.

Another functional relationship hypothesized by some two-factor theorists is that instrumental responding affects the course of emotional conditioning. This interaction occurs when an instrumental response evokes positive or negative reactions from the environment. These reactions may produce or strengthen emotional conditioning by serving as unconditioned stimuli in relation to the stimulus conditions that evoked the instrumental behavior. Under at least one set of circumstances, such interaction between instrumental and classical responding can produce maladaptive behavior. Some instrumental behaviors, for example, that are initially effective in reducing a negative drive state come to be punished by the environment. Thus, although the punishment may lead to modifications in the instrumental behaving, it can also function to strengthen the emotional conditioning that originally motivated instrumental responding. As a result, although punishment may lead to the modification of a specific instrumental behavior, it may also increase the frequency and strength of instrumental behaving. This seemingly paradoxical effect of punishment on instrumental responses that are motivated by negative emotional conditioning can be seen in the difficulty that Solomon, Kamin, and Wynne (1953) had in extinguishing avoidance responses through punishment. It can also be seen in the development of "side effects" during the punishment of instrumental aspects of stuttering moments by Martin, Brookshire, and Siegel (1964) and by Webster (1968b). The effect of response-contingent punishment on both the instrumental and classical aspects of stimulus-response chains has been discussed at length by Mowrer (1960).

In general, postulating a two-way interaction between classically and instrumentally conditioned behaviors helps in dealing with complex behavioral phenomena because, as in the case of response-contingent punishment, it makes both the experimentalist and therapist sensitive to the possibility that a stimulus in a given situation may cause a modification of *both* the classically and instrumentally conditioned responses of the organism. While the two-factor approach is thus not as parsimonious as a monistic reinforcement theory and presents more difficult measurement problems, it does seem to be more comprehensive and to avoid, at least potentially, the confusion created by an oversimplified attack on complex events. Moreover, the data on classical and instrumental conditioning have generally supported two-factor theory rather than a monistic approach to learning. As Kimble (1961) has pointed out, ". . . the bulk of the evidence suggests that classical and instrumental conditioning *are* different forms of learning . . ." (p. 98). Of course, there is not complete agreement among behavior theorists that there are two types of learning. As Kimble has noted, it ". . . is more than barely possible" for the processes underlying classical and instrumental conditioning to be basically the same. Miller (1969) is one of those who would take this stand. He contends that classical and instrumental conditioning are two procedures for activating a single learning process. He believes that this position is supported by recent data from his laboratory which indicate that autonomically mediated responses can be modified by instrumental procedures. Since there are many experimenters on each side of this issue, it appears that concern about one-process versus two-process learning approaches will stimulate considerable research in the next few years. Hopefully, this research will help to clarify the nature of learning.

Turning now from a general discussion of two-factor theory to a consideration of stuttering, the role played by classical conditioning in the development and maintenance of this disorder seems to depend primarily on the effects that conditioned negative emotional responses have on speech. Both naturalistic observation and experimental data indicate that an organism's behavior during a negative emotional state is similar to its behavior during a pain state. Under conditions of either pain or negative emotion, organisms exhibit a heightened degree of sympathetic autonomic activity and vigorous escape behaviors, both of which tend to disrupt ongoing behavior patterns. The emotional reaction is defined by a large number of physiological changes that result in the activation of effector organs that may be smooth or striate. Typically, the coordination or integration of muscular activity is less effective under heightened emotional states. If the escape behaviors are successful, the organism usually returns to a coordinated behavior pattern. If the escape behaviors are not successful, however, the disruption or disorganization continues and the organism's behavior may become more severely uncoordinated or even totally disintegrated. Such disintegration can be seen clearly in animals or humans subjected to an intensely painful or fear-provoking situation (Dollard and Miller, 1950; Wolpe, 1958). The disintegration of instrumental behaviors, including speech, under such conditions is hardly surprising. Even under less intense noxious stimulation, however, certain activities, such as speech, may become disrupted even though gross motor behavior remains relatively coordinated. This is not really surprising if we consider the high level of cognitive and motor coordination required for the production of fluent speech. Behaviors requiring high levels of coordination are usually disrupted to a measurable degree by stimulus conditions that represent a threat to the organism. It should be no great cause for wonder, then, that speech pathologists have consistently postulated a relationship between negative emotion (fear, anxiety, stress, etc.) and certain forms of fluency failure.

The disorganizing effect of a conditioned noxious stimulus on the speech of adult nonstutterers was clearly delineated in an experiment by Hill (1954). He repeatedly presented an originally neutral stimulus (red light) with a noxious unconditioned stimulus (electric shock) to his subjects. Following this stimulus-contingent stimulation, the subjects described TAT cards for brief periods while the red light was on. The subjects were also asked to perform complex manual activities at the same time they were speaking. The manual activities were constant in all phases of the experiment. A qualitative comparison of the speech was made between the trials that occurred after and those that occurred before the classical conditioning. Hill rated severity of speech "disorganization" in the pre- and post-conditioning trials and reported a statistically significant increase in disorganization after conditioning. Moreover, he described the resulting speech disorganization of clonic vocal reactions and prolonged vocalizations as often indistinguishable from stuttering.

Two other experiments, by Savoye (1959) and Stassi (1961), also demonstrate the disruptive effects of conditioned noxious stimuli on speech. Savoye studied the effect of a classically conditioned stimulus on the speech of nonstutterers. While her subjects were reading aloud, she presented 30 trials of a 10-second, 500-Hz tone, whose termination was followed immediately by an electric shock. Fluency failure was measured during the 10-second period midway between the electric shocks, during the 10 seconds immediately preceding the tone onset, during the 10-second tone presentation, and during the 10 seconds immediately following the shock. The results indicated that, as predicted, the experimental subjects had more fluency failures than the controls in all of the intervals measured except the one midway between the electric shocks. The experimental subjects also had more fluency failures in the intervals preceding and during the tone than in the interval midway between the shocks.

Stassi studied the effect of prescheduled stimulus-contingent stimulation on the speech of nonstutterers as they repeatedly spoke a set of eight nonsense words. He used the words "right" and "wrong" as stimuli which were delivered in four schedules of reinforcement: 1. 100 percent reward, 0 percent punishment; 2. 66 percent reward, 33 percent punishment; 3. 66 percent punishment, 33 percent reward; 4. 100 percent punishment, 0 percent reward. The judges' rating of fluency failure indicated that schedule four produced significantly higher fluency failure scores than any of the other schedules and that schedule three produced higher scores than schedule one. In other words, the consistent or predominant use of negative stimulation produced significantly higher fluency failure scores than the consistent use of positive stimulation. Stassi also found that males received significantly higher fluency failure scores than females under condition 4), the condition in which they were negatively stimulated 100 percent of the time.

On the basis of data from studies such as these we have hypothesized that negative emotional responses tend to disorganize or disrupt the cognitive and motor processes that mediate speech behavior. The observable effects of these disruptions are typically in the form of involuntary phonemic repetitions and prolongations which have been described by most speech pathologists as the primary elements of stuttering. The pattern of disorganization, at both the neurological and motor levels, is largely unlearned and strongly affected by constitutional factors that produce individual differences in the observed behaviors. Similarly, constitutional factors are probably important in determining whether or not given stimulus conditions will produce enough disorganization to lead to observable failure in fluent speech. However, the relationship between the eliciting stimuli and the emotional responding that produces disrupted speech is learned through classical conditioning. In other words, it is emotional conditioning that is learned, not the specific pattern of disorganization; the stutterer learns *when* to respond with disruptive emotion, not *how* to stutter. Through stimulus-contingent stimulation, conditioned stimuli become capable of evoking negative emotional responses with predictable regularity, and the related fluency failures attain the consistency and dependence on learned stimulus-response relationships that differentiate stuttering from fluency failures that occur on an unlearned basis. In essence, then, it is hypothesized that when an individual exhibits what has been called "primary" stuttering, he is experiencing learned negative emotion and that this emotion disrupts his normally fluent speech. This hypothesis is supported by the research on non-stutterers, indicating that noxious stimulus-contingent stimuli tend to disrupt speech in a way that has been considered indistinguishable from stuttering (Hill, 1954).

We have already pointed out, however, that *both* emotional conditioning and instrumental conditioning are involved in the development of a complex of behaviors such as that found in stuttering moments. It has been clear to most speech pathologists that stutterers usually develop a number of verbal and nonverbal responses that are associated with, but basically different from, the involuntary repetitions and prolongations of stuttering. Voluntary responses such as word changing, facial grimacing, head tilting, eye closing, finger snapping, intensity or pitch shifts, and even gross avoidance of speech situations are examples of these behaviors. These responses are best construed as instrumental attempts on the stutterer's part to escape or avoid the noxious quality of the eliciting stimulus situation or the punishing consequences of stuttering. Thus, the stutterer develops a changing, usually complicated, pattern of behavior in an attempt to escape from or avoid the noxious stimuli that elicit disruptive negative emotional reactions, the punishing reactions of the environment, and, later, the stuttering itself. Stuttering itself can become a noxious stimulus for the stutterer after it consistently produces negative reactions from the external listening environment.

Instrumental escape and avoidance responses become a part of the individual's behavioral repertoire when they are associated with a reduction in negative emotion. In the case of gross avoidance of a feared speech situation, of course, the reinforcement obtained by reducing negative emotion is obvious. It is also easy to see the reinforcement obtained by backing away from a speech situation when an approach to that situation in the past has produced a marked increase in emotional tension. It is often difficult, however, to see how the more molecular responses, such as voluntary eyeblinks, facial grimacing, or tongue protrusions are reinforced. Most of the stutterers with whom we have worked reported that behaviors of this type were initiated "by accident" or upon advice and were originally maintained voluntarily because they seemed to help reduce stuttering. It is likely that the original success of these behaviors in reducing negative emotion and stuttering is often related to the "distraction effect" reported frequently by stutterers and demonstrated by several experiments in which new stimuli are introduced (Barber, 1939; Johnson and Rosen, 1937; Maraist and Hutton, 1957; Sternberg, 1947). Similarly, almost any new response the stutterer voluntarily inserts into his repertoire may temporarily reduce his stuttering. It would appear that the reduction in stuttering in these circumstances occurs because the stimulus field is changed by the introduction of a set of instructions to produce the response or by the new response itself and because the emotional impact of the field is reduced in the process. Wischner (1947) has already pointed out that this reduction in stuttering can be considered as resulting from what Pavlov called *external inhibition*. Pavlov (1927) demonstrated that a new stimulus brought into a training situation would reduce the strength of the conditioned response. It is interesting to note in this regard that both Evans (1925) and Winnick and Hunt (1951) found that the effectiveness of an external inhibiter was reduced with its repeated presentation. A similar reduction in effectiveness appears to occur when stutterers persist in using behaviors that at first produced a noticeable reduction in stuttering. Stutterers often report, however, that many of these responses become "automatic" and are maintained even though they no longer appear to have a beneficial effect. It is likely, in this regard, that since the responses tend to develop in sequences or chains, reinforcement of the last, or most recent, segment of the chain influences the response units found earlier in the chain. As a result, responses that no longer produce successful escape or avoidance can be maintained for considerable periods.

There has been much discussion among theorists and therapists about whether instrumental responses are or are not stuttering. Johnson (1967) and his students (Bloodstein, 1958; Wischner, 1950) have defined stuttering as an avoidance or struggle response. Bluemel (1932), Sheehan (1958), Van Riper (1963), and Wingate (1964), on the other hand, have differentiated behaviors that they consider definitive or basic to stuttering from those that they consider to be secondary behaviors of stuttering. We have hypothesized, in contrast, that there are *not* two types of stuttering; that stuttering is limited to those fluency failures that result from conditioned negative emotion. We have thus taken the position that the instrumental escape and avoidance responses are *not* denotative of stuttering. For us, then, stuttering and associated instrumental behaviors are based on different conditioning procedures and response systems. We have taken this position because we believe that stuttering is most adequately seen as the result of involuntary and reflexive responses that are not affected by the manipulation of response-contingent punishment in the same way that instrumental responses are. We consider stuttering to be the reflexive disorganization of ongoing speech that is precipitated by conditioned negative emotional reactions, and we consider instrumental escape and avoidance responses to be what the stutterer *does* in order to cope with this disorganization, the punishing reactions to this disorganization, and the noxious speech situation. Considerable data suggest that these two classes of behavior are differentially responsive to stimulus-contingent and response-contingent stimuli, and a comprehensive approach to stuttering requires consideration of both classes of events. It is our contention that this discrimination holds considerable promise for resolving much of the confusion that is found in the interpretation of experimental results and that it will provide a basis for a more adequate design of diagnostic and therapeutic strategies.

FLUENCY AND FLUENCY FAILURE

For many years most speech pathologists have viewed the speech of non-stutterers as "normally disfluent." Evidence for this position came from experiments indicating that the speech of normal children and adults shows various forms and amounts of fluency failure (Branscom et al., 1955; Davis, 1939; Hughes, 1943; Johnson, 1956). Saying that normal speakers have fluency failures, however, is different from saying that they are "normally disfluent." Furthermore, it is grossly inaccurate to state that the speech of nonstutterers is characteristically, typically, or "normally" disfluent. Although these experiments show that normal speakers *may* exhibit fluency failures, they also make it abundantly clear that fluency failures are not characteristic of normal speakers' speech. In nonstuttering children, for example, the data show that repetitions occur on less than five percent of the words spoken and that fluency failure, of any kind, is far less common than fluency (Davis, 1939; 1940a; 1940b). Thus, fluency rather than fluency failure abounds in children. But, fluency is not characteristic of just children. It is also characteristic of adults. It is even, as Johnson (1961) pointed out, characteristic of the average stutterer. It should be evident, therefore, that the speech of both nonstutterers and most stutterers is best seen as normally fluent rather than "normally disfluent."

The acceptance of the position that speakers are "normally disfluent," even in the light of contrary evidence, may not have been a mere oversight. It served a purpose; it permitted speech pathologists to consider the repetitions, prolongations, and hesitations of speech as merely benign or nonsignificant events. The alternative, that the speech of nonstutterers is normally fluent, places greater demands on the speech pathologist. It requires that he recast his view of speech *dys*fluencies.[13] If dysfluency is a failure of a normally fluent state, it becomes the speech pathologist's responsibility to determine the conditions under which fluency fails to occur and the relationship between these conditions and fluency failure. In other words, if fluency is normal, the disruption of fluency is a significant rather than a benign event. This position, although it is a different and more demanding framework, is also a more fruitful one. We are suggesting, therefore, that the occurrence of fluency failure should not be defined away or made meaningless by the use of a term such as "normal disfluency." As a result, we have chosen to emphasize the importance of the disorganization or disruption of normal fluency by referring to involuntary repetitions and prolongations as fluency failures or dysfluencies rather than as disfluencies.

FLUENCY FAILURE AND STUTTERING

The normal fluency of most children is evident whether the words used are of a repetitive nature, like ma-ma- and da-da-, or not. The repetition in the cry of infants or the occurrence in language of words whose structure is repetitive is not adequate evidence that the absence of fluency is normal (Chen, 1946; Winitz, 1961). All words, whether inherently repetitive or not, are spoken fluently as long as the organism's functioning is not disorganized by internal or external stimulus events. Fluency, then, depends on the relatively normal operation of the organism's physiological and psychological processes. Using a psychological variable as an example, speech is fluent when the stimulus situation in which it occurs elicits an emotional response that is either positive or relatively neutral. In other words, if the physiological and psychological functioning of the organism is adequate, a relatively pleasant or benign emotional climate will facilitate fluency. This momentarily facilitating emotional climate is the net result of both the past conditioning in this and similar situations and the present contingent environmental stimulation of the stimulus situation.

The emotional climate is not always positive, however, and, as a result, the organism's behavior is not

[13] It is to be noted that *dys*fluency (fluency failure) rather than *dis*fluency is employed to denote the failure of normal fluency. The prefix *dys-* appropriately reflects the tone that we wish to set; when placed before the word fluency it indicates *ab*normality. Though this prefix *dys-* shares some meanings with *dis-*, because they both indicate the absence of, opposite, or reverse—in this case of fluency—the former prefix is preferred because it emphasizes our contention that fluency is the normal state of affairs and that dysfluency is the faulty one.

always facilitated. Fluency failure tends to occur, for example, in speech that is elicited in a noxious or overstimulating environment. This effect has been reported both experimentally and clinically. We have already discussed the experiments of Hill (1954), Savoye (1959), and Stassi (1961) that support this hypothesis, and these are only some of the experiments demonstrating that fluent speech is disrupted by noxious stimulation such as electric shock. Indeed, we have referred throughout our discussion to the experimental evidence that electric shock is a stimulus that, under certain circumstances, has been associated with the fluency failures of both stutterers and nonstutterers. Electric shock, however, is only one stimulus that disrupts normal fluency, and an experimental laboratory is only one situation in which fluency failure has been produced. Johnson (1967) pointed out, on the basis of his clinical interviews, that stimuli other than primary pain-inducing ones will lead to fluency failure. One of his major contributions is the proposal that verbal stimulation and secondary punitive reactions of the environment can affect the normal speaker emotionally and ". . . inhibit and disrupt his speech reactions in various forms and to varying degrees . . ." (p. 239). This proposal has been supported by many clinical observers (Bloodstein, 1960b; Van Riper, 1963; Wischner, 1947). Moreover, these and other observers have pointedly stated that not just the verbal stimulus "stuttering," but many noxious or overintensive stimuli will disrupt fluency. In other words, there are undoubtedly many stimuli and possibly even several classes of stimuli that can, in one way or another, disrupt a speaker's normal fluency. Thus, as we have already implied, fluency failure is not limited to those stimulus situations in which fear, anxiety, or stress is reported. Fluency may also be disrupted, at any particular moment, if the organism is overstimulated. Whether overstimulation evokes negative emotion or whether noxious stimulation is a form of overstimulation may be an issue, but it is apparent, in either case, that an organism's normal speech can be disrupted by stimulus circumstances that are observably noxious or overstimulating.

A fundamental question of long standing in speech pathology is whether or not there is a difference, quantitative or qualitative, between the fluency failures of nonstutterers and those of stutterers. If there is such a difference, it could be used as the basis for differential diagnosis. Johnson (1967) held that there were no meaningful differences between the "disfluencies" of nonstutterers and at least those of stutterers who have recently been labeled as such. Moreover, Johnson indicated that frequency distributions of disfluencies displayed by nonstutterers and stutterers overlap to some extent. He pointed out also that both nonstutterers and stutterers show the same types, if not the same frequencies, of disfluency. His position that the disfluencies of stutterers and nonstutterers are similar is supported by the experimental finding that speech pathologists were unable to distinguish between the tape-recorded speech of relatively fluent stutterers and relatively disfluent normals (Johnson, 1961). Similarly, Hill (1954) has reported that he could not distinguish the fluency failures elicited from nonstutterers by the use of noxious stimulus-contingent stimulation from the fluency failures of stutterers.

Van Riper (1963) has disagreed consistently with Johnson's position and has suggested that the apparent similarity between the fluency failures of these two groups was caused by grossly lumping together all types of disfluency. Van Riper pointed out that the predominance of specific kinds of fluency failures, such as part-word repetitions and prolongations, differentiates the nonstutterer from the stutterer. Van Riper has acknowledged, of course, that even nonstutterers occasionally show the sound and syllable repetitions and prolongations that he considers to be a fundamental sign of stuttering. From his point of view, however, stutterers show an excessive number of these specific types of fluency failure. To distinguish, then, between stutterers and nonstutterers it would be necessary to determine that specific forms of fluency failure are "excessive." The problem of determining what constitutes "excessive," however, makes such a criterion extremely difficult to apply.

It is not entirely clear at this time whether or not there are any readily observable differences between the fluency failures of nonstutterers and those of stutterers. Whether or not fluency failures may be differentially identified, however, the *primary* difference is the absence or presence of conditioned negative emotional responding. The primary distinction between nonstuttering and stuttering, then, is that the fluency failures of stuttering are tied to conditioned stimuli through emotional learning. In other words, the fluency failures of nonstuttering are a function of *unconditioned* responding or physiological malfunction, while the fluency failures of stuttering are a dependent function of *conditioned* emotional responding. When classical conditioning has taken place fluency failure occurs consistently in the presence of stimuli that were previously "neutral" and did not evoke a disruptive negative emotional response. That is, stuttering is the consistent speech disruption that results from stimulus-contingent emotional conditioning. Such conditioning leads, of course, to an increase in the number of stimulus situations that evoke negative emotional responses and probably, therefore, to an increase in the frequency of fluency failures.

The distinction between fluency failure based on unconditioned responding and fluency failure based on conditioned emotion is one that has not been made clearly before. From this point of view, the fluency failures that result from unconditioned stimulation are not stutterings. Unconditioned stimulation tends to occur infrequently and inconsistently in the environment and the fluency failures that result from it are consequently also infrequent and inconsistent. In short, the fluency failures that result from unconditioned stimulation tend not to be consistently associated with specific speech situations, words, individual listeners, or audiences, to name a few of the stimulus circumstances to which emotional conditioning may develop. If a nonstutterer occasionally displays fluency failures in the presence of stimuli such as these, he is being affected either by unconditioned stimuli that happen also to be present in the total stimulus situation or by biologic or physiologic factors that limit his functioning. In these circumstances, moreover, there is no evidence of emotional conditioning. Emotional conditioning does not occur until and unless a stimulus-contingent relationship develops between the conditioned and unconditioned stimuli. Once such conditioning has occurred, and the fluency failures become consistent because they depend on the learned stimulus-response relationship, we would call the fluency failures stuttering. Therefore, the primary distinction is not that the fluency failures of nonstutterers are *necessarily* different from those of stutterers. It is, instead, that the fluency failures of nonstutterers are correlates of stimulus-response relationships that are unlearned rather than learned. We do not mean to imply by this emphasis on conditioning that unconditioned stimuli are unimportant in stuttering. *Any* environmental stimulus that interrupts normal fluency can set the stage for emotional conditioning and the consequent disorganization that is stuttering. In other words, primary or higher order unconditioned stimuli are a necessary element of the stimulus-contingent stimulation that creates emotional conditioning. The fluency failures caused by unlearned constitutional factors can also be important to the development of stuttering. These fluency failures are an ultimate consequence of a biological condition or of physiological malfunctioning and are not related directly to conditioned stimulation. Indeed, they may well be independent of any environmental stimulation. It should be noted, however, that the environment may react contingently to these constitutionally based fluency failures in a way that leads to emotional conditioning and the disorganization of speech.

It should also be pointed out that the probability of an individual displaying a fluency failure in a given stimulus situation is undoubtedly affected by genetic and nongenetic constitutional factors. Although we have stressed the relationship between stimuli, negative emotion, and fluency failures, it should be obvious that individual differences among speakers determine, in part, whether a stimulus of a given nature and intensity will lead to a fluency failure.[14] Individual differences in autonomic reactivity, conditionability, and coordination, among others, could be expected to contribute to the variance in fluency failures even if stimulus characteristics were held constant. It is also important to keep in mind that although some of these constitutional factors are constant and thus affect speech consistently over time and across situations, others are variable and affect speech inconsistently. Thus an individual might respond differently to the same or similar stimulus circumstances on two different occasions because of temporary changes in his neurological or physiological functioning. Variability in the production of fluency failures, therefore, depends on both stimulus characteristics and individual differences.

To repeat, the fluency failures of stuttering, at least at onset, do not appear to be observably different from those caused by unconditioned stimulation. We must, however, distinguish between the chronic nature of stuttering and the generally sporadic nature of fluency failure that results from unconditioned stimulation. Stuttering is tied to specific stimuli as a result of emotional conditioning. It thus occurs rather consistently with respect to these conditioned stimuli. Without emotional conditioning, fluency

[14] Brutten and Shoemaker (1967) have reviewed elsewhere the data concerning the relationship between constitutional factors and fluency failure.

failures will occur only when unconditioned stimulation is present. Since unconditioned stimulation occurs inconsistently in most situations fluency failures dependent on unconditioned stimulation will occur inconsistently. The critical distinction, then, between the fluency failures of stuttering and those that depend on momentary unconditioned stimulation does not rest primarily on the number of speech disruptions, although they tend to increase with emotional conditioning, or on the form of fluency failure, although they usually change slowly as a result of emotional conditioning. The primary distinction is between the generally inconsistent occurrence of fluency failures that depend on organismic responses to unconditioned stimuli and the generally consistent occurrence of fluency failures that depend on emotional responses to specific conditioned stimuli.

The critical difference, then, between stuttering and other forms of fluency failure is that stuttering depends on emotional conditioning. Because of this conditioning, situational and word stimuli consistently evoke the emotional responses that are disruptive of normal fluency. From this it should be seen that it is the disorganizing emotional response that is the learned result of stimulus-contingent stimulation, not the stuttering. Stuttering is the disorganization of normally fluent speech that is a consequence of conditioned emotion. Thus, the consistency of stuttering reflects the strength of emotional conditioning rather than the extent to which stuttering has become instrumentally habituated. The consistency of stuttering does not indicate that it is an instrumental response any more than the consistency of pupillary dilation or eyeblinking would indicate that these behaviors were acquired through instrumental rather than classical training procedures (Kimble, 1961). Stuttering is not a response; it is the fluency failure that results when conditioned stimuli evoke a disruptive emotional response.

This disorganizing conditioned emotional response results from the contingent relationship between originally "neutral" stimuli[15] and negative unconditioned stimuli that are present in the same stimulus situation. This response is generally considered to be an emotional reaction that is the conditionable part or a fractional component of the unlearned response to unconditioned stimulation. Thus, as a result of classical conditioning, the organism responds consistently with negative emotion to a stimulus event even when negative unconditioned stimulation is no longer present.

A negative conditioned emotional response can disrupt the normal manner in which an organism responds. It can effect an organism's behavior in various ways. The effect of negative emotion on the functioning of the organism is not limited to the disorganization of normal fluency. Indeed, many aspects of the conditioned emotional response have no direct bearing on fluency. In other words, through classical conditioning, the speaker may learn to respond emotionally to situations in ways that do or do not directly interfere with fluency. Breathing disturbances, extraneous vocalization, and muscular rigidity in the muscles of articulation are examples of emotionally based responses that *do* interfere with fluency. Pupillary dilation, nasal dilation, and eyeblinks are a few of the emotionally based responses that *do not* interfere with fluency. These responses are involuntary and must be distinguished from those grossly similar voluntary reactions that the speaker may ultimately make as instrumental adjustive responses to noxious stimulus situations or punishing environmental reactions. In other words, we consider it vital that a clear distinction be made between these emotionally based responses and instrumentally conditioned "avoidance responses," "struggle reactions," or "secondary symptoms" that may be displayed by stutterers. An eyeblink, for example, is not necessarily an instrumental response. It may be the result of either classical or instrumental conditioning. Classical and instrumental conditioning are defined by their training procedures and by differences in response characteristics. An eyeblink is defined as a classical (involuntary) rather than an instrumental (voluntary) response if its acquisition is based on stimulus-contingent stimulation, rather than on response-contingent stimulation. This determination may also be made on the basis of response characteristics such as latency and form (King and Landis, 1943; Marquis and Porter, 1939; Spence and Ross, 1959).

The kinds and number of stimuli that are capable of evoking a conditioned emotional response change with experience. An increase tends to occur when negative emotional learning is enhanced through

[15] These stimuli are considered neutral because there is no evidence, prior to conditioning, that they elicit a conditioned emotional response that disorganizes fluent speech. Through classical conditioning the neutral stimuli in a situation take on the valence of the contingent unconditioned stimuli and become capable of evoking a response that is similar to the unconditioned response.

higher order conditioning and stimulus generalization. The stimulus circumstances in which stuttering occurs and the frequency of stuttering tend to be progressive rather than static because stimuli that have become capable of eliciting conditioned emotion can then serve as higher order unconditioned stimuli. In other words, once conditioning has taken place, the conditioned stimulus can be used to modify the valence of neutral stimuli in the same way that an unconditioned stimulus can. Moreover, because of stimulus generalization, conditioning is not limited to just those stimuli that were present during the original emotional conditioning. Stimuli that are conditioned through a contingent relationship to unconditioned stimuli are similar to other stimuli along a generalization gradient. This similarity is based on components shared by the conditioned and the generalized stimuli. The more components they share the greater will be their similarity and the more likely it will be that the generalized stimuli, like the conditioned stimuli, will be able to elicit a conditioned emotional response. What we are saying, then, is that the conditioning of specific stimuli indirectly affects the valence and the emotion-evoking potential of a wide range of stimuli.

Higher order classical conditioning and stimulus generalization are not limited only to the negative emotion that disorganizes fluency (Adams, 1966; Brutten and Gray, 1961). Classical conditioning and generalization also occur for the positive emotion that facilitates normal speech fluency. Indeed, positive emotional conditioning seems to predominate since the speech of the average stutterer contains more fluency than fluency failure. The unconditioned stimuli in positive emotional conditioning evoke an unconditioned response that is pleasurable rather than painful. Positive emotional conditioning results from the contingent relationship between these positive unconditioned stimuli and previously neutral conditioned stimuli. The valence of the conditioned stimuli is changed to positive because of this contingent relationship, and they evoke a conditioned emotional response that is the conditionable part of the unlearned positive reaction. Moreover, these positive conditioned stimuli, like their negative counterparts, can serve as higher order, unconditioned stimuli. The number of positively valenced stimuli is further increased by the generalization of the conditioning to those stimuli that share common components. Through stimulus generalization, then, the positive emotional conditioning in one stimulus situation can have an effect on several relatively similar situations. Of course, the generalized conditioning weakens along a gradient as the similarity between the conditioned stimuli and the generalized stimuli decreases. Nevertheless, through higher order conditioning and stimulus generalization the speaker experiences an increasing number of stimulus situations and stimulus words on which he tends to be fluent.

Individuals learn to react with negative or positive emotion to various stimulus circumstances as a result of emotional conditioning. The nonstutterer's emotional conditioning to speech is generally positive, so the few fluency failures that do occur are the result of unlearned factors. The stutterer, on the other hand, is conditioned to react negatively to specific speech-associated stimulus events. This differential conditioning of negative and positive emotion increases with experience. In an absolute sense, then, both fluency and fluency failure increase with conditioning. In a relative sense, however, the stutterer may become neither more fluent nor more dysfluent. The ratio of positive and negative conditioning can remain relatively constant even though the absolute quantities of fluency and fluency failure increase. As a result, the stutterer tends to remain more fluent than dysfluent in stimulus situations in which speech occurs. Johnson's (1967) summary of the Iowa studies on fluency supports our contention that the ratio relationship between fluency and fluency failure tends to remain relatively constant. In these studies, the percentages of fluency failures displayed by young stutterers and by adult stutterers during extemporaneous speech are similar. The children, who ranged in age from approximately two to eight, showed an average of 16.1 fluency failures for every 100 words spoken in conversation with the experimenter or in describing pictures. The adult stutterers showed a median of 17.5 fluency failures for each 100 words they used to discuss a job they had or hoped to have. Stated positively, the measures indicated that both young stutterers and adult stutterers were fluent approximately 83 percent of the time.

Obviously, there are stutterers for whom the ratio relationship between positive and negative conditioning is not constant. The environment of a particular speaker, for example, may be more likely to react negatively to the absolute increase in stuttering than positively to the absolute increase in fluency. Changes take place in the ratio relationship between positive and negative conditioning as a result of this differential reaction. A marked increase in fluency failure, relative to fluency, then develops. Occasionally, this change in the ratio relationship between fluency and fluency failure is the result of an unusually low tolerance to even minimally punishing stimuli and not the result of a particularly pernicious environment. In any event, more and more stimulus circumstances elicit negative emotion and fewer and fewer are associated with positive emotional reactions, so that stuttering increases relative to fluency.

Stutterers' experiences with fluency and fluency failure are reflected in their positive and negative anticipations about speaking situations and words. Experimental investigations of these anticipations have shown that stutterers are relatively accurate in predicting the degree of fluency or fluency failure that will occur in various speech situations (Berwick, 1939; Dixon, 1947). Stutterers have also shown a notable accuracy in predicting the specific words on which they will stutter (Knott, Johnson, and Webster, 1937; Milisen, 1938; Van Riper, 1936). This accuracy is not greatly diminished when up to a week separates the prediction and the oral reading (Johnson and Solomon, 1937). Not only are stutterers relatively accurate in predicting fluency or fluency failure, but they are also successful in predicting the duration of their stuttering (Van Riper and Milisen, 1939). In addition, removing the words on which stuttering is anticipated or has previously occurred results in a marked increase in fluency relative to fluency failure (Brutten and Gray, 1961; Johnson and Millsapps, 1937; Johnson and Sinn, 1937). Stated differently, stutterers tend to be fluent on words that have previously been spoken fluently or on which they do not anticipate stuttering. The anticipations of fluency or fluency failure have been shown to be consistent even when their reliability is assessed as much as a week later (Johnson and Ainsworth, 1938).

The emotional conditioning of stutterers is not limited to whole words or situations. The stutterer can also learn to respond emotionally to parts of the words he uses and the situations he meets. He may react positively or negatively to the element sounds and the articulatory movements required to speak words or to the specific stimulus elements of complex situations he meets. Many stutterers, as a result, are able to discriminate between the molar and molecular aspects of words and situations that elicit positive or negative emotion. It is these differential emotional reactions to words or situations that allow stutterers to predict the stimulus conditions under which they are likely to speak fluently and those under which they are likely to stutter (Bloodstein, 1949). This emotional polarization is a continuing function of the stutterer's experiences with situational and word-associated fluency and fluency failure. In other words, the classical conditioning that results from the stutterer's experiences heightens the emotional dichotomy and determines the probability that the speaker will exhibit normal fluency or *ab*normal dysfluency.

The words that a speaker uses and the situations that he meets are not a random sample of all possible stimulus events. Stimulus words and situations do not have an equal probability of occurrence. Some words, for example, occur more frequently as a function of the language structure. These stimulus words are more likely, therefore, to be contingently stimulated and emotionally conditioned than are those that occur less frequently. In other words, the probability of stuttering on a given word is partly determined by the frequency with which it occurs in language. Thus, as Bloodstein and Gantwerk (1967) found in their study of young stutterers, ". . . the amount of stuttering associated with a given part of speech appears to be determined by little more than how often it is represented in the individual's speech" (p. 789). Wischner (1956) has shown that this same relationship between frequency of usage and frequency of stuttering exists for adults. A similar correlation may well exist between stuttering and the frequency with which the speaker meets different situations. If the findings for words may be applied to situations, it would appear that the probabilities with which stuttering occurs in given speech situations depends on the frequency with which those situations are met by the stutterer. Therefore, stuttering is partly a dependent function of the conditioning that results from situational experiences; the more frequently a noxious situation is met the greater is the probability that it will be associated with stuttering.

STUTTERING AND THE CONCEPT OF DEVELOPMENT

There are a number of ways of looking at the development of stuttering. Johnson (1967), for example, distinguished between nonstutterers and stutterers but did not propose developmental stages of stuttering. Van Riper (1963) and Bloodstein (1960a, 1960b,

1961), in contrast, have taken the position that stuttering should be viewed in developmental terms. Van Riper has indicated that the form of stuttering changes as it develops, and Bloodstein (1960a) has suggested that changes ". . . take place in stuttering as it grows from a phenomenon of early childhood into a disorder of adolescence and adulthood" (p. 219). Both of these theoreticians have suggested, furthermore, that different developmental stages require different treatment procedures. Indeed, Van Riper has suggested that stuttering might be exacerbated by attempts to modify it with methods that are inappropriate to the developmental stage. Luper and Mulder (1964) considered this point of view in designing a therapeutic program for children that is based on Bloodstein's developmental phases.

A somewhat different concept of the development of stuttering is derived from the medical point of view concerning the course of pathological disorders. Medically, stuttering, like pneumonia or cancer, would be assumed to follow a course that is regular and predictable from stutterer to stutterer. This view of stuttering as a progressive pathology differs from the maturational approach to development because it involves the assumption that the course of the disorder is roughly the same regardless of the individual's age. Both of these approaches imply, however, that stuttering increases with time and that it changes in all stutterers in essentially the same general pattern.

The idea that stuttering is a developmental disorder is inherently attractive. Stuttering typically changes over time, and an approach that would allow speech pathologists to predict these changes accurately could be helpful in planning therapeutic strategies. Such prediction would be possible because, according to either a maturational or pathology approach to development, the changes which take place in stuttering are dependent upon some factor that is common to all stutterers and are thus consistent from stutterer to stutterer. Given such consistency, it would be possible to measure the developmental pattern in a sample of stutterers and to use this pattern to predict the course of stuttering in other stutterers. In other words, if stuttering develops in an orderly manner and if the stages of development could be delineated, the future course of a given individual's stuttering could be predicted simply by determining the stage represented by the present behavior. A speech pathologist would thus know what to expect and how to alter the future course of the disorder. The fact that certain aspects of stuttering tend to change, however, is not sufficient evidence that it follows either a maturational or pathological course of development. Stuttering is not static. It tends to change in individuals over time. But, even those speech pathologists who have been most concerned with uncovering regularities and order in these changes have been dissatisfied with their descriptive systems. Typically, they have been forced to recognize that the stages or phases of development that they have proposed are only generalized statements of trends and have not generated valid predictions about the course of stuttering in individual cases. These difficulties became evident through the criticisms (Bloodstein, 1961; Glasner and Vermilyea, 1953; Johnson, 1956) of the early two-stage system of "primary" and "secondary" stuttering. Partly as a result of such criticism, Van Riper (1954, 1963) proposed a three- and then a four-stage description of its course. Even these adjustments did not halt the criticism, however, because the distinctions between stages are less than definitive and the varied behavior patterns of individual stutterers do not consistently fit predictions based on them. Van Riper himself has pointed out that "The beginning and terminal stages of the disorder differ greatly in terms of both the overt and covert symptoms. The stages in between are less clearly definitive and all stutterers do not seem to follow the same pathway." (p. 327). Bloodstein's (1960a, 1960b) schema also involves a four-phase description of the course of stuttering. He has made it clear, however, that the developmental phases of stuttering can be only roughly delineated. He observed that the age ranges of various behaviors are relatively large and that even the most advanced "symptoms" of stuttering may be found in young stutterers. In a similar vein, Brutten and Shoemaker (1967) have pointed out that developmental stages should ". . . be seen as representative of a tendency rather than inviolable occurrences." (p. 32). In short, attempts to conceptualize behavior changes in stuttering, in terms of either developmental stages or a universal course, have been unsuccessful. Stuttering is not separable into *discrete* stages, and many individual stutterers do not follow the predicted course.

Support for the developmental position rests heavily on data obtained through cross-sectional observation of stutterers of different ages and through interviews with stutterers and their parents. Van Riper (1963), however, has pointed up the limitations of a cross-sectional approach, and Johnson (1967) has demonstrated the questionable reliability of data about stuttering that are obtained through interview rather than through direct observation. It may be that these procedural difficulties account for some of the differences in the developmental systems that have been proposed by speech pathologists. From our point of view, however, it is more likely that the primary difficulty with the developmental approach to stuttering is the concept that stuttering follows a consistent course among individual stutterers that is independent of their specific and differing experiences. The conditioning that is fundamental to the occurrence of stuttering and to the acquisition of instrumental adjustive responses does not occur in a longitudinal pattern that is more than roughly consistent among individual stutterers. Because of this, statements about the development of stuttering have always required the disclaimer that individual stutterers do not necessarily follow the proposed developmental sequence. The necessity of such disclaimers and the high probability that any given stutterer may display behaviors representative of several stages at the same time damages severely the assumed utility of developmental approaches. Further damage has been done by the inference that developmental stages and severity are equated. In other words, it has been suggested that the severity of stuttering increases as the stutterer moves through the developmental stages. Clearly, however, there are a number of individuals who may be descriptively classified as stage-one or stage-two stutterers even though they show a high probability of stuttering in a profusion of stimulus situations. Conversely, there are those individuals who have been classified as stage-three or stage-four stutterers even though their fluency failures occur infrequently and in a limited number of situations. There is no *necessary* relationship, therefore, between the stages and the frequency of stuttering. In a developmental sense, severity depends more on the behaviors displayed than on the frequency of stuttering. Indeed, the presence of instrumental adjustive responses rather than the frequency of stuttering has been used to define the third and fourth developmental stages. And yet, as we have already seen, these instrumental responses are neither the *sine qua non* of stuttering behavior, nor are they exclusively limited to only certain specific developmental stages or phases.

From our point of view, stuttering is not a developmentally based disorder. The developmental concept is demonstrably brittle because there are no recognizable stages of phases through which stutterers may be said to pass in a predetermined sequence. The involuntary repetitions and prolongations of stuttering are a dependent function of emotional conditioning. At any given time a stutterer may display more or less fluency failure, varying levels of intensity, and differing degrees of consistency as a result of many different kinds of conditioned stimuli. There is no type of fluency failure, intensity level, or source of stimulation that is exclusively characteristic of one period in the life of a stutterer. In other words, one cannot determine, with any accuracy, how long an individual has stuttered or in what ways he will stutter in the future simply by classifying his present stuttering. Stuttering, even if broadly defined, does not develop horizontally. That is, stutterers do not develop all possible "stage-one" behaviors before those of subsequent stages. Instead, like other behaviors based on learning, stuttering develops vertically; that is, in terms of specific stimulus-response relationships. It is for this reason that it is common to find stutterers of any age exhibiting behaviors that are considered characteristic of all the stages of development. In evaluating the responses of stutterers, the vertical approach is more fruitful than the horizontal approach. In the vertical approach one determines such factors as the frequency and intensity of specific classically and instrumentally conditioned responses to particular stimuli, while in the horizontal approach one tries to place the stutterer in an appropriate developmental stage. If these responses are based on learning, as most of the data we have reviewed seem to indicate, they should change in ways that learned responses change rather than in the way which either maturationally based behaviors or pathological conditions develop. Stated differently, if the changes in a stutterer's emotional and adjustive behaviors are the result of learning they should be fundamentally dependent on specific stimulus-response experiences rather than on developmental age or pathological process. The experiences of stutterers differ and lead to conditioning that produces an individualistic pattern of responding rather than one that is representative of stutterers generally. It is much more useful, therefore, to observe and chart an individual stutterer's classical and instrumental response patterns than to attempt to force his behavior into a predetermined set of developmental stages. It is the examination of these classical and instrumental responses and their interactive relationships that leads to an understanding of a stutterer's behavior.

Both types of responses are dependent functions of contingent stimulation and are not direct products of maturational growth or pathological development. The behavior of stutterers is best dealt with, then, by charting the acquisition and modification of classical and instrumental responses rather than by classifying the behaviors in terms of developmental stages.

From a behavioral point of view, then, the course of emotional and adjustive behaviors in any given stutterer is determined by changes that occur in learned stimulus-response relationships. These changes occur as a result of experience and involve the development of new stimulus-response relationships and the modification of established relationships. The changes take place in both conditioned emotional responding and instrumental learning. In other words, in the face of changing experience the stutterer responds emotionally to a shifting array of stimuli and exhibits a changing pattern of adjustive responses. His individual experiences, then, determine the specific stimuli to which he learns to respond emotionally and the particular instrumental escape and avoidance responses that he will develop and use in any given stimulus circumstance. The pattern that a stutterer's behavior follows over time is thus a result of learning experiences and not the result of an unfolding of an internally predetermined sequence of events. Furthermore, any similarity of patterns among stutterers is much more likely to result from common experience than from an equivalent sequence of maturational or pathological development.

SUMMARY

Learning theorists describe stuttering in terms of the acquisition and modification of relationships between stimuli and responses. Learning theorists differ among themselves, however, as to the nature of the learning involved in stuttering. Some emphasize classical conditioning (stimulus-contingent stimulation), others emphasize instrumental or operant conditioning (response-contingent stimulation), and still others the interaction between these two types of conditioning. Those theories in which it is assumed that classical and instrumental conditioning represent two different, though interactive, types of learning are known as two-factor theories.

In two-factor theory, the complex of behaviors that has traditionally been called stuttering, is considered to involve the classical conditioning of negative emotional responses *and* the instrumental conditioning of adjustive responses. Negative emotional conditioning disrupts or disorganizes normally fluent speech and creates the involuntary fluency failures that define stuttering. The escape and avoidance responses frequently associated with the stuttering are acquired through instrumental conditioning. In other words, stutterings are the involuntary disruptions of speech that result from negative emotional responding that is classically conditioned. Escape and avoidance are the instrumentally conditioned responses of stutterers to noxious and punishing stimulation. Individual differences in emotional responsivity and in the tendency for speech to become disrupted contribute to the determination of the specific individuals who will develop constant and lasting stuttering.

A two-factor approach to conditioning allows a number of important issues in the field of stuttering to be clarified. First, many of the contradictory findings among studies on the punishment of stuttering can be explained as resulting from the failure of the experimenters to discriminate between responses that have been classically conditioned and those that have been instrumentally conditioned. Learning theorists have typically assumed that stuttering is an instrumental (operant) response. If stuttering is an instrumental response it should obey the law of effect, a major principle of such learning. Specifically, rewarding or punishing stuttering should increase or decrease its frequency, respectively. Although little work has been done on the effect of reward on stuttering, much has been done on the effect of punishment. The results of the punishment studies, however, have been inconsistent—some indicating that stuttering increases when punished, some that it decreases, and some that it is not affected. A careful analysis of these studies indicates that the inconsistencies result primarily from definitions of stuttering and experimental procedures that are too molar and fail to discriminate between classically and instrumentally conditioned responses. In other words, a discrimination has not been made between the involuntary repetitions and prolongations that are a consequence of classically conditioned negative emotion and the voluntary escape and avoidance responses that are instrumentally conditioned. Only the latter responses appear to behave in a way that is consistent with the law of effect.

A two-factor theory also throws light on the relationship between fluency, fluency failure, and stuttering. Although fluency failures are found in nonstutterers, normal speech is characterized by fluency, not by fluency failure. Even the average stutterer is fluent most of the time. Fluency is normal and the failure of fluency is *ab*normal. Fluency failure will occur if physiological functioning is inadequate, if unconditioned responses disorganize motor functioning, or if conditioned negative emotion disrupts fluency. Only the last of these, however, is stuttering.

Finally, two-factor theory suggests the need to reevaluate the developmental concept in stuttering. From the point of view of two-factor theory, behavior changes in stutterers are seen in terms of classical and instrumental conditioning and are a function of individual experiences. It is not considered meaningful to suggest that stutterers go through a fixed sequence of developmental stages, each of which precedes the next. Behavior change is primarily a function of stimulus- and response-contingent stimulation rather than a function of either maturational development or progressive pathology. Behaviors are best classified and dealt with, therefore, in terms of the classical or instrumental conditioning through which they were acquired rather than in terms of a series of developmental stages.

BIBLIOGRAPHY

Adams, M. 1966. An exploratory investigation of the effect of an auditory extinction procedure on the consistency of stuttering. Unpublished doctoral dissertation, Southern Illinois University.

———, and Brutten, G. 1970. Auditory extinction and reinforcement procedures for modifying stuttering and instating fluency. *J. Communication Disorders*, 3, 123-132.

Azrin, N. 1956. Effects of two intermittent schedules of immediate and nonimmediate punishment. *J. Psychol.*, 42, 3–21.

Barber, V. 1939. Studies in the psychology of stuttering: XV. chorus reading as a distraction in stuttering. *J. Speech Disorders*, 4, 371–383.

Berwick, N. 1939. Stuttering in response to photographs of listeners. Unpublished master's thesis, University of Iowa.

Bloodstein, O. 1949. Conditions under which stuttering is reduced or absent: a review of the literature. *J. Speech Hearing Disorders*, 14, 295–302.

———. Stuttering as an anticipatory struggle reaction. *In* J. Eisenson (ed.). 1958. Stuttering: a symposium. New York: Harper. Pp. 1–69.

———. 1960a. The development of stuttering: I. changes in nine basic features. *J. Speech Hearing Disorders*, 25, 219–237.

———. 1960b. The development of stuttering: II. developmental phases. *J. Speech Hearing Disorders*, 25, 366–376.

———. 1961. The development of stuttering: III. theoretical and clinical implications. *J. Speech Hearing Disorders*, 26, 67–80.

———, and Brutten, E. Stuttering problems. *In* R.W. Reiber, and R. S. Brubaker (eds.). 1966. Speech pathology. Amsterdam: North-Holland. Pp. 354–402.

———, and Gantwerk, B. 1967. Grammatical function in relation to stuttering in young children. *J. Speech Hearing Res.* 10, 786–789.

Bluemel, C. 1932. Primary and secondary stammering. *Quart. J. Speech*, 18, 187–200.

Branscom, M., Hughes, J., and Oxtoby, E. Studies of non-fluency in the speech of preschool children. *In* W. Johnson (ed.). 1955. Stuttering in children and adults. Minneapolis: Univ. of Minnesota Press. Pp. 157–180.

Brookshire, R. Behavior modification in treatment of stuttering. Paper presented at the 43rd. Annual Convention of the American Speech and Hearing Association, Chicago, November 1967.

Brutten, E., and Gray, B. 1961. Effect of word cue removal on adaptation and adjacency: a clinical paradigm. *J. Speech Hearing Disorders*, 26, 385–389.

———, and Shoemaker, D. 1964. Stuttering: conditioned disintegration of speech behavior. Unpublished manuscript, Southern Illinois University.

———, and Shoemaker, D. 1967. The modification of stuttering. Englewood Cliffs, N.J.: Prentice-Hall.

Cady, B., and Robbins, C. 1968. The effect of the verbally presented words, "wrong," "right," and "tree" on the disfluency rates of stutterers and nonstutterers. Unpublished manuscript, University of Alabama.

Chen, H. 1946. Speech sound development during the first year of life, a quantitative study. Unpublished doctoral dissertation, University of Iowa.

Daly, D. 1964. Rate of stuttering adaptation under two different electro-shock conditions. Unpublished master's thesis, Ohio University.

Dancer, J. 1966. Stuttering adaptation under conditions of massed and distributed practice. Unpublished master's thesis, Southern Illinois University.

Davis, D. 1939. The relation of repetitions in the speech of young children to certain measures of language maturity and situational factors: Part I. *J. Speech Disorders*, 4, 303–318.

Davis, D. 1940a. The relation of repetitions in the speech of young children to certain measures of language maturity and situational factors: Part II. *J. Speech Disorders*, 5, 235–241.

———. 1940b. The relation of repetitions in the speech of young children to certain measures of language maturity and situational factors: Part III. *J. Speech Disorders*, 5, 242–246.

Dixon, C. 1947. The amount and rate of adaptation of stuttering in different oral reading situations. Unpublished master's thesis, State University of Iowa.

Dollard, J., and Miller, N. 1950. Personality and psychotherapy. New York: McGraw-Hill.

Dulany, D. 1961. Hypotheses and habits in verbal "operant conditioning." *J. abnorm. soc. Psychol.*, 63, 251–263.

Estes, W. 1944. An experimental study of punishment. *Psychol. Monog*, 47, whole No. 263. Pp. 1–40.

Evans, C. Recent advances in physiology. 1925. London: Churchill.

Felty, J. 1959. The operant nature of stuttering behavior of adolescent boys. Unpublished master's thesis, University of Washington.

Fenichel, O. 1945. The psychoanalytic theory of neurosis. New York: Norton.

Flanagan, B., Goldiamond, I., and Azrin, N. 1958. Operant stuttering: the control of stuttering behavior through response contingent consequences. *J. Exper. Anal. Behav.*, 1, 173–177.

Frederick, C., III. 1955. An investigation of learning theory and reinforcement as related to stuttering behavior. Unpublished doctoral dissertation, University of California at Los Angeles.

Frick, J. 1951. An exploratory study of the effect of punishment (electric shock) upon stuttering behavior. Unpublished doctoral dissertation, State University of Iowa.

Glasner, P., and Vermilyea, F. 1953. An investigation of the definition and use of the diagnosis, "primary stuttering." *J. Speech Hearing Disorders*, 18, 161–167.

Goldiamond, I. Stuttering and fluency as manipulatable operant response classes. *In* L. Krasner, and L. P. Ullmann (eds.). 1965. Research in behavior modification. New York: Holt. Pp. 106–156.

Golub, A. 1951. The influence of constant and varying word stimuli on stuttering adaptation. Unpublished master's thesis, University of Iowa.

Gray, B., and Brutten, E. 1964. The relationship between anxiety, fatigue, and spontaneous recovery in stuttering. *Behav. Res. Ther.*, 2, 251–259.

Guthrie, E. 1935. The psychology of learning. New York: Harper.

Hansen, H. 1955. The effect of measured audience reaction of stuttering behavior patterns. Unpublished doctoral dissertation, University of Wisconsin.

Hegde, M. 1954. The effect of shock on stuttering. Unpublished Manuscript, 1970.

Hill, H. An experimental study of disorganization of speech and manual responses in normal subjects. *J. Speech Hearing Disorders*, 19, 295–305.

Hughes, J. 1943. A quantitative study of repetitions in the speech of two-year-olds and four-year-olds. Unpublished master's thesis, State University of Iowa.

Hull, C. 1943. Principles of behavior. New York: Appleton.

Hunt, H., and Brady, J. 1965. Some effects of punishment and intercurrent anxiety on a simple operant. *J. comp. and physiolog. Psychol.*, 48, 305–310.

Johnson, W. 1961. Measurements of oral reading and speaking rate and disfluency of adult male and female stutterers and non-stutterers. *In* Studies of speech disfluency and rate of stutterers and non-stutterers. *J. Speech Hearing Disorders, Monograph* 7, Pp. 1–20.

———, et al. 1956. Speech handicapped school children (2nd. ed.). New York: Harper.

———, et al. 1967. Speech handicapped school children (3rd. ed.). New York: Harper.

———, and Ainsworth, S. 1938. Studies in the psychology of stuttering: X. constancy of loci of expectancy of stuttering. *J. Speech Disorders*, 3, 101–104.

———, and Millsapps, L. 1937. Studies in the psychology of stuttering: VI. the role of cues representative of past stuttering in the distribution of stuttering moments during oral reading. *J. Speech Disorders*, 2, 101–104.

———, and Rosen, L. 1937. Studies in the psychology of stuttering: VII. effect of certain changes in speech pattern upon frequency of stuttering. *J. Speech Disorders*, 2, 105–109.

———, and Sinn, A. 1937. Studies in the psychology of stuttering: V. frequency of stuttering with expectation of stuttering controlled. *J. Speech Disorders*, 2, 98–100.

———, and Solomon, A. 1937. Studies in the psychology of stuttering: IV. a quantitative study of expectation of stuttering as a process involving a low degree of consciousness. *J. Speech Disorders*, 2, 95–97.

Jones, E. 1950. An investigation of stuttering viewed as learned behavior with special reference to experimental extinction and spontaneous recovery. Unpublished doctoral dissertation, University of Iowa.

Kamin, L. 1959. The delay of punishment gradient. *J. comp. and physiolog. Psychol.*, 1959, 52, 434–437.

Karlin, I. 1959. Stuttering: basically an organic disorder. *Logos*, 2, 61–63.

Kimble, G. 1961. Conditioning and learning (2nd. ed.). New York: Appleton.

King, H., and Landis, C. 1943. A comparison of eyelid responses conditioned with reflex and voluntary reinforcement in normal individuals and psychiatric patients. *J. exper. Psychol.*, 33, 210–220.

Knott, J., Johnson, W., and Webster, M. 1937. Studies in the psychology of stuttering: II. a quantitative evaluation of expectation of stuttering in relation to occurrence of stuttering. *J. Speech Disorders*, 2, 20–22.

Lindquist, E. 1956. Design and analysis of experiments in psychology and education. Boston: Houghton Mifflin.

Luper, H., and Mulder, R. 1964. Stuttering: therapy for children. Englewood Cliffs, N.J.: Prentice-Hall.

Maraist, J., and Hutton, C. 1957. Effects of auditory masking upon the speech of stutterers. *J. Speech Hearing Disorders*, 22, 385–389.

Marquis, D., and Porter, J., Jr. 1939. Differential characteristics of conditioned eyelid responses established by reflex and voluntary reinforcement. *J. exper. Psychol.*, 24, 347–365.

Martin, R., Brookshire, R., and Siegel, G. 1964. The effects of response contingent punishment on various behaviors emitted during a "moment of stuttering." Unpublished manuscript, University of Minnesota.

———, and Siegel, G. 1966a. The effects of simultaneously punishing stuttering and rewarding fluency. *J. Speech Hearing Res.*, 9, 466–475.

———, and ———. 1966b. The effects of response contingent shock on stuttering. *J. Speech Hearing Res.*, 9, 340–352.

Masserman, J. 1943. Behavior and neurosis. Chicago: University of Chicago Press.

Maxwell, D. 1965. A palmar sweat investigation of stuttering adaption and spontaneous recovery under two conditions of audience complexity. Unpublished master's thesis, Southern Illinois University.

Milisen, R. 1938. Frequency of stuttering with anticipation of stuttering controlled. *J. Speech Disorders*, 2, 207–214.

Miller, N. 1969. Learning of visceral and glandular responses. *Science*, 163, 434–445.

Mowrer, O. 1947. On the dual nature of learning—a re-interpretation of "conditioning" and "problem-solving." *Harvard educ. Revue*, 17, 102–148.

———. 1950. Learning theory and personality dynamics. New York: Ronald.

———. 1960. Learning theory and behavior. New York: Wiley.

———, and Ullman, A. 1945. Time as a determinent in integrative learning. *Psychol. Rev.*, 52, 61–90.

Pavlov, I. 1927. Conditioned reflexes. Oxford: Clarendon Press.

Quist, R., and Martin, R. 1967. The effect of response contingent verbal punishment on stuttering. *J. Speech Hearing Res.* 10, 795–800.

Rescorla, R. 1967. Pavlovian conditioning and its proper control procedures. *Psychol. Rev.*, 74, 71–80.

———, and Solomon, R. 1967. Two-process learning theory: relationships between Pavlovian conditioning and instrumental learning. *Psychol. Rev.*, 74, 151–182.

Savoye, A. 1959. The effect of the Skinner-Estes operant conditioning punishment paradigm upon the production of non-fluencies in normal speakers. Unpublished master's thesis, University of Pittsburg.

Shames, G., and Sherrick, C., Jr. 1963. A discussion of non-fluency and stuttering as operant behavior. *J. Speech Hearing Disorders*, 28, 3–18.

Sheehan, J. 1946. A study of the phenomena of stuttering. Unpublished master's thesis, University of Michigan.

———. 1951. The modification of stuttering through non-reinforcement. *J. of abnor. and soc. Psychol.*, 46, 51–63.

———. Conflict theory of stuttering. *In* J. Eisenson (ed.). 1958. Stuttering: a symposium. New York: Harper. Pp. 123–166.

Shulman, E. 1944. A study of certain factors influencing the variability of stuttering. Unpublished doctoral dissertation, University of Iowa.

Siegel, G., and Martin, R. 1966. Punishment of disfluencies in normal speakers. *J. Speech Hearing Res.*, 9, 208–218.

Siegel, S. 1956. Nonparametric statistics. New York: McGraw-Hill.

Skinner, B. 1937. Two types of conditioned reflex: a reply to Konorski and Miller. *J. of gen. Psychol.*, 16, 272–279.

———. 1938. The behavior of organisms: an experimental analysis. New York: Appleton.

Soderberg, G. 1962. What is average stuttering? *J. Speech Hearing Disorders*, 27, 85–86.

Solomon, R., Kamin, L., and Wynne, L. 1953. Traumatic avoidance learning: the outcomes of several extinction procedures with dogs. *J. of abnor. and social Psychol.*, 48, 291–302.

Spence, K., and Ross, L. 1959. A methodological study of the form and latency of eyelid responses in conditioning. *J. of exper. Psychol.*, 58, 376–385.

Starkweather, C. 1970. The simple, main, and interactive effects of contingent and noncontingent shock of high and low intensities on stuttering repetitions. Unpublished doctoral dissertation, Southern Illinois University.

Stassi, E. 1961. Disfluency of normal speakers and reinforcement. *J. Speech Hearing Res.*, 4, 358–361.

Sternberg, M. 1946. Auditory factors in stuttering. Unpublished master's thesis, University of Iowa.

Thorndike, E. 1911. Animal intelligence. New York: Macmillan.

Timmons, R. 1966. A study of adaptation and consistency in a response-contingent punishment situation. Unpublished doctoral dissertation, University of Kansas.

Tolman, E. 1932. Purposive behavior in animals and men. New York: Appleton.

Travis, L. 1957. Handbook of speech pathology. New York: Appleton.

Van Riper, C. 1936. Study of the thoracic breathing of stutterers during expectancy and occurrence of stuttering spasm. *J. Speech Disorders*, 1, 61–72.

———. 1937. The effect of penalty upon the frequency of stuttering spasms. *J. of gen. Psychol.*, 50, 193–195.

———, and Hull, C. The quantitative measurement of the effect of certain situations on stuttering. *In* W. Johnson (ed.). 1955. Stuttering in children and adults. Minneapolis: University of Minnesota Press. Pp. 199–217.

Van Riper, C. 1954. Speech correction: principles and practice (3rd. ed.). Englewood Cliffs, N.J.: Prentice-Hall.

———. 1963. Speech correction: principles and practice (4th. ed.). Englewood Cliffs, N.J.: Prentice-Hall.

———, and Milisen, R. 1939. A study of the predicted duration of the stutterer's blocks as related to their actual duration. *J. Speech Disorders*, 4, 339–346.

Warden, C., and Dymond, S. 1931. A preliminary study of the effect of delayed punishment on learning in the white rat. *J. gen. Psychol.*, 39, 455–461.

Webster, L. 1966. An audio-visual exploration of the stuttering moment. Unpublished master's thesis, Southern Illinois University.

———. 1968a. Response-contingent stimulation: a methodological note. Unpublished study, Southern Illinois University.

———. 1968b. A cinematic analysis of the effects of contingent stimulation on stuttering and associated behaviors. Unpublished doctoral dissertation, Southern Illinois University.

West, R. An agnostic's speculations about stuttering. *In* J. Eisenson (ed.). 1958. Stuttering: a symposium. New York: Harper. Pp. 169–222.

———, Ansberry, M., and Carr, A. 1957. The rehabilitation of speech (3rd. ed.). New York: Harper.

Williams, D. 1962. Modification of stuttering behavior by the use of shock. Abstract, *Asha*, 4, 408–409.

Wingate, M. 1959. Calling attention to stuttering. *J. Speech Hearing Res.*, 2, 326–335.

———. 1964. A standard definition of stuttering. *J. Speech Hearing Disorders*, 29, 484–489.

Winitz, H. 1961. Repetitions in the vocalizations and speech of children in the first two years of life. *J. Speech Hearing Disorders, Monograph Supplement*, 7, 55–62.

Winnick, W., and Hunt, J. 1951. The effect of an extra stimulus upon strength of response during acquisition and extinction. *J. exper. Psychol.*, 41, 205–215.

Wischner, G. 1947. Stuttering behavior and learning: a program of research. Unpublished doctoral dissertation, University of Iowa.

———. 1950. Stuttering behavior and learning: a preliminary theoretical formulation. *J. Speech Hearing Disorders*, 15, 324–335.

———. 1952a. An experimental approach to expectancy and anxiety in stuttering behavior. *J. Speech Hearing Disorders*, 17, 139–154.

———. 1952b. Anxiety-reduction as reinforcement in maladaptive behavior: evidence in stutterers' representations of the moment of difficulty. *J. of abnor. and soc. Psychol.*, 47, 566–571.

———. 1956. An experimental study of some verbal cues as instigators to stuttering behavior. Unpublished manuscript, University of Pittsburg.

Wolpe, J. 1958. Psychotherapy by reciprocal inhibition. Stanford, Calif.: Stanford.

Yensen, E. 1947. Stuttering adaptation and the role of cues. Unpublished master's thesis, University of Iowa.

41

Stuttering Therapy for Children

Dean E. Williams

INTRODUCTION

The problems of elementary-school-age children who stutter have received relatively little attention in the literature compared to those of adults and of preschool children. The explanation appears to lie, at least in part, in the fact that adults more often than children seek help for extended periods of time at a university clinic. They are therefore more accessible for observation and for use as subjects in studies by the persons in our profession most concerned with research and theoretical formulations concerning the onset and the development of the stuttering problem. A few investigators have turned their attention to the child from three to six years of age, but, because the questions asked by these investigators mostly have concerned factors related to the onset of stuttering, the investigators usually have observed parents rather than children. Consequently, clinical attention for the most part has been directed toward developing 1. effective therapy procedures for the adult and 2. preventative measures for the youngster of three to six years of age.

Little systematic attention has been directed toward the principles and procedures of therapy for the child of approximately seven to 12 years of age. Because the problem is not thought to be serious enough to require removing these children from their schools and school clinicians often are available in their home locale, the most common source for help is their local school speech clinician. Sometimes "summer clinics" are available at a university or community center for this age child, but these ordinarily are of such short duration that concentrated therapy is necessary and systematic observations over an extended period of time are not possible. Data are not available, but it is probably safe to guess that approximately 75 percent to 85 percent of all the elementary-school-age children in the country who receive help with stuttering receive that help from the school clinician. Yet these clinicians are trained through university programs in speech pathology and audiology where their clinical practicum experience concerning stuttering is mainly with stuttering adults and with counseling parents about prevention of the problem. According to an unpublished study (Williams, Melrose, Silverman, and Cox, 1968), of 89 Iowa school clinicians trained at 33 different institutions, 72 percent had less than 10 hours of supervised experience with elementary-age stutterers. In certain instances, the "supervised experience" consisted solely of observing another clinician work with a child of this age. The extent to which these data are applicable to other states has not been ascertained. It is assumed, however, that comparable data would be obtained in many states throughout the country. Thus, in many instances the school clinician is asked to work with a stuttering child of an age with which the clinician has had little experience, and concerning whose stuttering problems and therapy procedures little has been written.[1]

There is seldom a question with a child from seven to 12 years of age as to whether his disfluencies are "normal" or whether he is "really stuttering." He is usually tensing and struggling to a certain degree as he talks and he will tell the clinician that he "stutters." Hence, preventive measures such as the parent-counseling procedures suggested by Johnson (1961) are no longer applicable as a sole means of therapy. In most instances, direct therapy with the child is indicated. Too often, however, the clinician approaches a child in therapy by superimposing on him the therapy procedures developed mainly by working with adults. Such an approach toward therapy can create confusion and feelings of inadequacy for the clinician—as well as for the child—because the child usually does not react as an adult would or evaluate his problems in the ways a clinician has learned to expect from the adult stutterer.

The fears, embarrassments, shame, avoidance reactions, etc., with which one is concerned in adult stuttering therapy are developed by the so-called "stutterer" during the process of growing up. These reactions should not be thought to "exist" within a child the moment that people tend to agree that he is "stuttering." Stuttering is not a problem that has fully developed the moment people agree that he is "stuttering"; it is a problem that is *always* in the process of developing. If, through the years of growing, a person filters his experiences through faulty beliefs and erroneous information, he is continually developing a more complex problem. To assume that the complex problem of an adult exists in the child can lead to obvious difficulties in therapy. This point will be illustrated by the use of several examples.

In adult therapy, a clinician often examines the ways a person feels about his problem, the situations in which he has most difficulty talking, and the ways other people react to him. In a therapy session with an adult, a topic for conversation is seldom a problem because the adult is willing to discuss these topics at great length. The clinician is somewhat taken aback, then, when he asks a child how he feels about stuttering and the child shrugs his shoulders and says, "I don't know." He asks the child whom he is scared to talk to and the child replies, "I don't know." The clinician fails to realize that the child, knowing little about his problem, has little to talk about if the focus of conversation is on "his stuttering." "Stuttering" is a word that other people use in referring to the ways he talks, and he knows little about the ways he talks. An adult stutterer, on the other hand, will talk about his experiences and his feelings during the many years he has been talking the ways he talks because, to him, these experiences and feelings are, in large part, his problem.

An approach that another clinician might take is to ask the child what sounds or words he is more likely to have difficulty with. The young child will reply that he doesn't know. However, if the clinician wishes, he will be glad to watch and see what words or sounds give him trouble. Undoubtedly, after a few days' watching, he will find some that do. At this point the clinician "knows" how to begin therapy. He discusses with the child the fact that no sound is any more difficult than any other and that he should practise using the sounds and words with which he has "more" difficulty. If the clinician is particularly skilled, he will help the child get back to the point where he was when the clinician brought up the point about "hard sounds" and "hard words."

A common observation made with adult stutterers is that they do not talk much. Therefore, it is not uncommon for a clinician to suggest to the adult that he do more talking in more situations than he has in the past. At times the same suggestion is made to a child without checking the extent to which he already is talking. This can create difficulty for teachers or parents of a child who is talking "too much" already. Such are the problems that one can get into by dealing with a child in ways that one is accustomed to use with an adult in therapy.

From seven to 12 years of age, children vary markedly in the ways they react toward stuttering. One child may profess little concern about the ways he talks. He may become momentarily concerned because he "stuttered," but then he becomes so interested in other activities that it is difficult even to discuss with him the ways he talks. He is outgoing and mixes easily with other children and with adults. He speaks, for the most part, spontaneously. He may talk so frequently at home or at school—even though he "stutters" considerably—that parents and teachers are baffled as to how to handle him. Generally, he does not act in a way that stutterers are "supposed" to act. The next child may represent the opposite end

[1] A few of the more recent discussions of therapy for the elementary school-age stutterer include: Luper and Mulder, 1964; Emerick, 1965; Chapman, 1959; Fraser, 1964; Williams and Roe, 1960.

of the reaction continuum. He is considerably embarrassed by the ways he talks. He is afraid to play with other children for fear they will tease him about the ways he talks and he grasps every opportunity to be excused from reciting in class.

Most children of this age group, however, fall between these two extremes and, more importantly from the standpoint of therapy, they oscillate between the two extremes. They are at a stage of development in which their speaking behavior, their reactions to others, and the reactions of others to them are changing rapidly, and in a ragged, zigzag manner. The clinician is often unprepared for such changes. For example, the child may show considerable bodily tensing and struggle behavior one day and demonstrate almost none the next. Moreover, he may demonstrate the bodily tension and struggle behavior in only one situation during the day. Or, he may recite freely in class one day and be reluctant to do so the next. Or, he may be reluctant to perform during "show and tell time" but be willing to read aloud in class. Talking privately with the clinician the child may do an adequate job of talking, yet it is reported that at other times he is relatively disfluent.

The clinician must do a careful analysis involving the people with whom the child talks to discover when and where he is talking satisfactorily and when and where he is struggling in varying degrees. Before the clinician begins therapy with the child, he not only should evaluate carefully the nature of the child's interpersonal relationships, but he also should realize that one of his major responsibilities is to be alert to the changing aspects of these relationships from day to day and from week to week.

The clinician must be aware that the child is struggling to cope with the ways he talks, with the increasingly disturbing effect he has on his listeners and with the decreasingly positive concept he has of himself as a speaker and as a person. The child is becoming confused about the ways he talks and is increasingly developing a feeling of "copelessness."

The emphasis in therapy cannot be the same for a child within this age range as it is for an adult. Ordinarily, major attention in adult therapy is directed toward 1. reducing, modifying, and in a sense breaking down the person's embarrassments and fear reactions toward speaking and 2. reshaping the distorted interpersonal relationships that developed during his years of growing up. In the child, however, these faulty beliefs and related reaction patterns are just beginning to develop. One of the major purposes of therapy, therefore, is to *prevent* them from spiraling in intensity and complexity until they reach a level at which a child feels he can no longer cope with them. This, then, is one of the problems that faces the clinician.

In this chapter the writer will describe a stuttering retraining program for children approximately seven to 12 years of age. The program was designed in accordance with the theory that stuttering is a learned reaction pattern involving speaker and listener. No lengthy theoretical discussion will be presented but, in the main, the program will be permitted to explicate the theory.

The therapy program was developed over a period of approximately 10 years. Its development was speeded up considerably, however, in 1965 when the writer received a research grant from the U.S. Office of education which permitted implementation of the program in selected public school systems of Iowa and which enabled the clinical staff to keep systematic records of the summer residential stuttering therapy program at the University of Iowa.[2]

The viewpoint about the nature of the stuttering problem assumed by the writer and hence the one upon which the therapy program is based, is expressed essentially by Johnson (1961). The assumption is made that stuttering is a problem that is learned. In most cases, it is learned when the child is quite young. Specific in this learning is the disruption in interaction between the child and his listening environment. This interaction hypothesis assumes that the child, at approximately three or four years of age, is repeating or prolonging sounds to a degree that bothers the important listeners in his environment. They react adversely to him as a speaker and he in turn reacts to their reactions. This promotes a feeling and belief on his part that the ways he talks—and even possibly he as a person—are not acceptable to them. As a result, he begins to develop a cautious, hesitant way of talking that is highlighted by increased tensing behavior with undue efforts to "talk right." "Talking right" is often construed to mean "not talking wrong." It is the wrongness that receives attention. The child begins to do things behaviorally to "not talk wrong." He begins to develop beliefs about the reasons that he talks the way he

[2] The writer is particularly indebted to Philip R. Cox, formerly a research associate, who participated in this aspect of the research program for three years and to William Yovetich and Margaret Evans Joyce who participated in the experimental therapy program for two years.

does—and begins to act accordingly to do something about them in the only way he knows how—by trying harder not to do things wrong! As this way of talking continues, he begins to associate his internal feelings with the occurrence of "talking wrong." Therefore, with increasing frequency, when he is called upon to talk he attends to his internal feelings for "cues" as to whether he can or cannot say acceptably what he wants to say, and then acts accordingly. These ways of attempting to talk are reinforced in inappropriate ways by the important listeners in the environment because of their own beliefs about the nature of the problem. These beliefs vary from person to person but essentially contain several assumptions. One of them is that he "has trouble getting certain words out," and the other one is that he needs to do something special to help himself (by this it is meant things that other people do not have to do) "get the words out." The more he tenses, struggles, and does "special things to help him talk" the more that people—and, *he*—evaluate this as "talking wrong," and therefore seemingly the only thing left to do is to "try harder." This process can be illustrated by examples from interviews with a number of second-grade boys who were referred to the writer because they "stuttered." They related that they "used to stutter" but that they didn't any more. They went on to point out that when they were in first grade they used to stutter a great deal but had gotten over it. When the writer inquired as to what they did in first grade that they called "stuttering," they reported that they repeated a great deal. During the discussion it was noted that they tensed and struggled slightly as they talked. When they were asked what they had done to get over the stuttering, they said if they were careful, talked slower, and tried harder they could say the words. Furthermore, they related that if there were any times when they thought they would "stutter" (repeat) they simply would not talk. Now, they were somewhat confused because they had been referred for "stuttering." According to their own belief, they were no longer stuttering (as they understood the meaning of the word) and the tensing behavior was their successful manner of coping with the stuttering. Now, people were calling the tensing "stuttering." It was confusing to them.

On the assumption that the child is attempting to solve the problem in what to him is a logical manner and, too, that he is increasingly developing a self-concept of a person with "something wrong with him" we designed a therapy program which seeks to help the child learn about the normalcy of his speech mechanism and of his feelings and to help him learn *how* to learn to talk the way he wants to. We find that it is important for a child to learn how to learn. In his school work he is traditionally learning "new" things, things that he did not know before. This learning experience is ordinarily positive. The other way of learning is to unlearn, relearn, or whatever one wants to call it, some behavior that he has already learned—but has learned in an inappropriate way. Our society, in the main, approaches this kind of learning with negative instructions, such as "don't do that" or "stop that," with the hope that if the child avoids the inappropriate behavior, the correct behavior will appear. It is assumed too often that correct behavior will emerge by itself—that it is there all the time but is being blocked by incorrect behavior. So with the adults in the child's environment, who too often use a "don't do that" approach apparently on the assumption that if the "stuttering" can be reduced, "normal speech" is there inside the child and will emerge by itself.

The therapy program which is to be described emphasized a positive approach to learning: 1. by examining the child's basic assumptions about stuttering and what, as he thinks, causes it, 2. by providing considerable information about talking (not only about stuttering—but primarily about the total process of talking), 3. by helping him understand and accept his feelings, 4. by helping him become more aware of the purpose of talking, that is, of verbal communication, 5. by helping him to experiment with and to explore the versatility of his behavior that we call talking, and 6. by demonstrating and then reinforcing the things he can do to talk easily and spontaneously in any situation where he is called upon to speak. By these means we provide a framework within which the child can meet new experiences tomorrow, next week, or next year in ways that will allow him to view them, evaluate them, and behave in them more informatively and realistically. The emphasis is broadly on talking and communicating, not narrowly on controlling his "stuttering."

Two variations on the therapy program will be described, one developed during six-week summer clinics at the University of Iowa and the other developed in the public schools of Cedar Rapids and Iowa City, Iowa. The basic concepts of the therapy were the same in both settings, but methods of implementation differed. The concepts covered in therapy, with examples of techniques used to develop them, will be described in the section entitled "Therapy in a Residential Clinic Setting." How these concepts were adapted to the public schools will be described under the heading, "Therapy in the Elementary Schools."

THERAPY IN A RESIDENTIAL CLINIC SETTING

Organization of the residential clinic program and the number of children participating varied from year to year. The least number of children attending at any one time was four and the most was 12. Some years the children were scheduled for three one-hour group sessions a day, five days a week. These included: Session I, Learning About Talking; Session II, Talking in an Informal Situation; and Session III, Talking in a Formal Situation. Most of the basic information was given in Session I. The other two sessions were designed to provide control situations in which the children applied the concepts learned and experimented with behavioral changes made in Session I.

Other years we used two one-hour group sessions and one half-hour individual therapy session a day, five days a week. Session A was similar to Session I mentioned above, and Session B combined the activities of Sessions II and III. The individual sessions provided an opportunity for a clinician to work with the child on whatever had not become clear during group discussions or on aspects of behavioral change which required additional demonstration. In this chapter the use of three one-hour group sessions a day will be discussed. The reader will easily see how the program can be adapted to fit other types of scheduling that may seem desirable.

Session I. Learning About Talking

The concepts presented in Session I were basic to the entire therapy program. They included: what we mean by stuttering, how we learn to say words, how we talk words into sentences, how we use words to carry meaning, how we observe what we do, how we learn new ways to do things, how feelings of being afraid or embarrassed can interfere with doing the things we want to do, how we change the way we do things, how we change the way we talk, and how we use talking to help us get to know people.

It was necessary to present certain information by explanation and by the use of examples; however, as much as possible, concepts were built by guiding discussions, by asking questions, by reformulating questions asked by the children, by developing ideas which resulted from discussions, and by suggesting alternatives to problem solutions presented by the children. Every attempt was made to help the child learn by experiencing things for himself. In practice, the information presented was never as neatly divided, unit by unit, as might be suggested by the listing here. To relate the concepts and behavioral changes discussed and demonstrated at one time with those discussed and demonstrated at another time, it was often necessary to repeat, to return to a point already discussed, to discuss other points related to the chief topic of the moment. The process of therapy, therefore, involved not only the planned content of three sessions, but also considerable repetition and amplification and experimentation as these were needed.

A. WHAT DO WE MEAN BY STUTTERING

Early discussions were concerned with what the children thought was meant by "stuttering" and what they considered to be involved in "being a stutterer." They were encouraged to talk about their feelings and reactions during times when they stuttered. One of our procedures was to ask a child to stop talking immediately after *he* considered that he stuttered and tell the group how he felt at that time. Inasmuch as the child knew that he was attending the group because he stuttered, it was considered advantageous to begin immediately by discussing, looking at, and reacting to the behavior that he called his stuttering. The clinician, assuming a relatively passive role, obtained during these discussions an evaluation of each child's emotional reactions toward his stuttering behavior, the variability of the behavior, and of the degree to which the child was willing or able to express his feelings. The clinician also had an opportunity to begin establishing an atmosphere in which the child was more willing than usual to express his feelings, reactions, and opinions.

One of the most interesting things we found about children of this age group is that few people have ever talked to them about *talking*. About what to do to "not stutter," *yes*—about talking, *no!* The child is left to speculate about what is wrong with him, some mysterious thing that he should try not to do. He receives such instructions as, "Words are getting stuck, aren't they?" and "If you relax they will come out." Or, "They won't come out because you're nervous." Or, "You're having trouble because you are talking too fast." We believe it is particularly important to ask the child what *he* thinks is wrong. The clinician raised questions about certain statements the children made, such as "the words won't come out," "I can't talk right," or "the words get stuck and I go l-l-l-l-like that." At times the child "parrots" statements he has heard—"I am nervous," "I talk too fast," etc., but at other times the explanation the child offers derives from his observation of his own behavior. One child said that he knew that he could not talk because his throat "gets dry." His talking behavior consisted of swallowing and wetting his lips and trying to get saliva in his mouth before he started a word. This was the behavior classified by an observer as his "stuttering." He merely was trying to do what he thought would be helpful in relation to what he thought was wrong. Another child said that his trouble was that he could not say words—"particularly those that have consonants or vowels in them." One is fairly safe to predict that he soon will have a great many "hard sounds" and "hard words" because he is placing the trouble "in" the words. Another child said that he could not talk right because two little men were fighting in his throat and wouldn't let the word come out. While speaking, he tensed and struggled in the chest and throat area to try, as he said, "to force the word out past them." The child was acting as he believed he had to act in relation to the explanation of his problem he had given to himself.

From discussions of what different children thought caused their stuttering, it was relatively easy to make the point that their opinions differed and generally no one in the group knew much about it. This provided a foundation from which the clinician could discuss and demonstrate that a person can more readily understand what he is doing wrong and what he can do about it if he first understands much more about how a person learns to talk and what we do when we talk. By providing information about the behavior involved in talking, we equip the child with a reference point against which he can check what he is doing to see what is wrong and what he can do that is right.

B. HOW WE LEARN TO SAY WORDS

(The following two paragraphs contain the essence of the information presented and also the kind of language used in explaining it to the children.)

We must *learn* to talk. Talking is not something we have completely learned by the time we are three years of age. We go on learning to talk better and better about more and more things, using more words and longer sentences, perhaps throughout our whole lifetime. As a part of learning to talk better, we make mistakes—that is, we bobble, we repeat some, we get tangled up. We do a great many things that interfere with talking smoothly. Yet, this is normal talking. Learning to talk, like learning to do anything else, involves making mistakes. By learning from the mistakes we make, we can improve the ways we do things. This point can be made clear by comparing the way we learn to talk with the way we learn to do other things.

We learn to read, to play ball, to swim, to ride a horse. As part of learning to do these things, we make mistakes. We mispronounce a word, we drop the ball, yet we expect to do this, to a degree, because we realize it is part of learning. On the other hand, as we talk and make the normal mistakes—bobbling or repeating sounds—some of us may regard these mistakes as something "wrong" rather than just as a normal part of learning. So, we feel ashamed and we tense our muscles in an effort to fight against our mistakes. We fight in order to keep the bobbles from happening because we believe that when they do happen something is wrong with us. The fighting and the struggling we do in order to keep from making mistakes is a part of what we call "stuttering." Learning to speak is not too different from, for example, learning to catch a baseball. If we worry about what someone might say or how he might look at us, or that he might think that it is somehow wrong if we drop the ball, we are likely to tense and fight hard not to drop it. In all probability, then, we will drop it more often than we would if we just thought, "Here comes the ball. I had better catch it."

To demonstrate the process of learning to say words, new and somewhat difficult words such as "aluminum" and "statistics" were introduced. The children took turns learning how to pronounce them. Ordinarily a child made various attempts on the word, some of them incorrect, others more nearly correct. It was pointed out that by *attempting* the pronunciation and by learning from the mistakes he made, he eventually learned how to pronounce the word and, further, that fighting a mispronunciation by stopping as soon as it was spoken did not help at all. We acted out this point. Several children were instructed to tense their jaw muscles and "fight" as soon as they became aware that they were mispronouncing the word. When they did this, it became obvious to everyone that this procedure interfered not only with pronouncing the word, but also with their ability to talk at all. This demonstration was followed by one in which the child, as he began mispronouncing a word, was instructed to accept calmly the mispronunciation, to learn from it, and to try to come closer to the correct pronunciation on the next trial by changing—rather than by *struggling to stop*—what he was doing. It was pointed out that this is the basic procedure followed in learning to talk under any circumstances. These demonstrations led naturally into a discussion of how we learn to produce what we call "sounds" and "words," how, ordinarily, a person listens to and watches the speaker and then tries to imitate with his voice, tongue, lips, jaw, the sound or sequence of sounds. The clinician illustrated by producing many different sounds, then asking the children to try to imitate them. Certain sounds were grouped together in ways that were recognized as a "word." Other sounds were grouped together in ways that resulted in nonsensical jargon. Thus we demonstrated that what we call "words" are created by the movements we make with our tongue, lips, and jaw muscles. One cannot expect to open his mouth and wait for the "word" to come out, nor can he "push it out of" his mouth.

The procedures described above help the child understand that the "words" do not come from a person's throat or stomach. He is armed against beliefs so common among adults who stutter—and, as has been discussed, among some children,—that "the word gets stuck in one's throat" or "the word won't come out." Such beliefs on the part of an adult distract his attention from his speaking behavior and center it on techniques to "get the words out without having trouble on them." A person, with this faulty orientation, easily assumes that when a "stutter" occurs as he is trying to say a "word," it is the *word* that is at fault. That is, the difficulty's assumed to be somehow *in* the word. Out of this faulty assumption develops the belief that there are "hard sounds" or "hard words." One comes to view the word as an enemy that somehow "possesses" the "trouble"—that *causes* one to stutter. This animistic thinking creates considerable difficulty for a person who stutters. Instead of being able to use words to assist him in communication, he finds that the words themselves with ever-increasing frequency determine what he does or does not say.

C. HOW WE TALK WORDS INTO SENTENCES

The discussion about talking moved from the production of sounds and words to the complexity of the total process of talking. We demonstrated the continuous movements, the amount of tension necessary, the use of breath involved in talking normally. Emphasized here was the "ongoingness" of the talking process.

Talking does not ordinarily mean saying one word and then the next word and then the next. Rather, words spill and tumble in such a way that they have no clear beginnings or endings. They blend into a continuous process of making sounds and of making movements. More importantly, we do not *talk* words; we talk ideas, observations, needs, and feelings. In learning this kind of talking, we again are bound to make mistakes, just as we do in learning sounds and words. We repeat sounds, words, phrases. We hesitate because we are not sure of what we want to say or what word to use to say what we mean. We start one sentence, stop, and start another one, and generally get tangled up.

This learning process was compared to learning other activities which require rapid and continuous performance. Examples from the children's own experiences such as typing, playing the piano, and hitting a baseball were used. The following paragraph represents the information presented and the language used.

When we get tangled up while typing, we accept our blunders as part of learning how to type. We do this for talking, too. We are likely to think that we are supposed to know how to talk "right" and so we feel ashamed of our talking mistakes and try to hide them. Making mistakes is a perfectly normal part of learning and so we can use our mistakes to learn in talking as well as in typing or batting a ball or whatever.

At this point considerable time was devoted to a discussion of the children's attitudes and feelings about making mistakes while reciting in class or while learning a new game where people were watching. It was pointed out that there is a difference between "learning how" and "knowing how." We cannot expect to know how to perform a certain task until we spend time learning how. The more we practice learning how, the fewer mistakes we make, and hence, the closer we approach "knowing how." Even when we think we know how to do something well, we must realize that we will make mistakes from time to time. This is an important part of learning—and learning is normal.

Many children in these groups appear to function with the belief that they should *know how* to accomplish a task; they appear not to realize that they first must learn how. Making a mistake embarrasses and shames them. Obviously, this attitude results not so much in *striving* for perfection as in the need to be perfect the first time one attempts a task. This felt need to be right the first time extended to many activities other than speaking, for example craft work in Session II, described later. This belief, of course, is not unusual in our society, but it becomes a problem that must be resolved, at least partially, when a person is faced by the need to change a well-learned behavior pattern.

The children discussed the feelings they had when they made mistakes while speaking and while performing nonspeech tasks. They discussed what they thought were the reactions of people present when they made mistakes and compared these supposed reactions to their own reactions to mistakes of others. This comparison was deemed important for two reasons: through it the children could become aware of the many and varied mistakes other people make and begin to understand that their own mistakes do not always seem so bad to others.

Throughout the discussion, the point was made that if a person fights making mistakes *because* he feels that to make them is wrong, he is reluctant to try new games or tasks. When he becomes afraid to try, it is difficult for him to learn. Again, examples were used. For instance, a child who is afraid to try to ride a bicycle will have difficulty learning to ride it. It may be said that such a child has no self-confidence. Yet, self-confidence is not a feeling inside the child that will enable him to know how to ride a bicycle perfectly the first time he tries. Self-confidence is not a state in which a person is always sure of success. It is one of being willing to try, of being willing to make mistakes, and even to fail, and of being willing to learn by trying again.

The children discussed their experiences in learning new tasks at home and at school. They talked about the times when they were most afraid to make mistakes and the times when they were least afraid, the times when they did not try because of fear of criticism if they failed, the times when they tried even though they were afraid. From these discussions the children then could go on to observe and evaluate more meaningfully the imperfections in their speaking behavior and their feelings, fears, and confusions about speaking. Using as a foundation the material on what a person does to talk, and within the context that mistakes are normal, the clinician led the discussion to what the children were doing at times to interfere with talking.

The discussion was supplemented by observation and demonstrations of what any person can do to help talking and what he can do to interfere with it. These activities were turned into verbal games. One child tried to talk while holding his tongue to the roof of his mouth. Another tried to talk while holding his breath. A third tried to talk while tensing his jaw muscles as much as possible. Each child tried to originate new ways to interfere with talking. As one child talked, the others observed and then tried to describe what he was doing. These activities were not only entertaining but also beneficial in helping the children become aware of and describe talking behavior. The "games" provided an excellent setting, it was felt, in which the child could learn what he is doing to interfere with the talking that he calls his "stuttering." Not uncommonly a child observed another one tensing his jaw muscles and said, "That's what you do when you stutter, too."

In conjunction with these activities, the clinician introduced what was called "belief in magic." This referred to the relatively common belief that some "special" behavior will help a person say certain words. For example, a child may hesitate before a feared word, blink or shut his eyes, or swing an arm or foot, because he believes that this will "help" him say the word. The clinician demonstrated that a person may or may not do these things while he talks. They do not interfere with *or* facilitate talking. To think they "help" is to believe in magic.

D. HOW WE USE WORDS TO CARRY MEANING

Many words used in the discussion were defined. It was necessary, for example, to explain the meaning of such words as "process" and "behavior." Not only did the clinician explain what he meant by certain words, but he also encouraged each child to inquire about the meaning of the words he heard used in these sessions that he did not understand. Through these discussions about the meaning of words the child was helped to become aware that a speaker tries to convey meaning by the words he uses but that the meaning is not *in* the word.

Here is an example of the discussions held about the meaning of words:

"Cod-liver-oil" tells us nothing about the smell or taste or color or feel or use of the liquid inside the bottle to which the label is attached. There are other words like that—"label" words which tell the listener very little. To say that we "stuttered" does not tell us much of what we did. Certainly such words as "stuck," "block," "force out," do not help us understand what we do that interferes with or facilitates talking. But, to say we repeated words or stopped when we felt we were about to make a mistake, or tensed our lips, or held our breath, helps us understand what we did that interfered with our talking.

Words were discussed in terms of their usefulness and their meaning. The children were encouraged to ask what words meant whenever they were in doubt. Every effort was made to use words which were descriptive and specific and within the child's own active vocabulary.

E. HOW WE OBSERVE WHAT WE DO

There are reasons to use descriptive words other than those discussed in the previous section. If the word "stuttering" is used and the child is trained to "work on his stuttering," he learns to observe and attend to his speaking behavior only at those times when "stuttering" is thought to occur. A "stutter" is all he is watching for. It is difficult then, if not impossible, for him to view the total process of talking behavior if the instructions we as clinicians give him focus his attention on only certain minor aspects of this total process. Of equal, if not more, importance is to help the child observe, get the feel of, play with, and have fun with the talking he does that is not regarded as "stuttering."

To help the children become more aware of the process of talking, the concept of time-space was introduced. Each child took turns describing a sequence of behavior. One performed a series of acts, both verbal and nonverbal, and another then described the acts in the sequence in which they were done. The children enjoyed these activities and became proficient at describing sequences of behavior. This kind of introduction prepared the children for the next step—discussions and demonstrations of talking behavior as a continuous process. The point about continuity was made so the child could see the talking he is doing *as* certain behavior that interferes with and certain behavior that facilitates the kind of talking he wants to do. This orientation helps to short-circuit the development of the erroneous belief common to most adults who stutter—that a person stops talking when he begins "to stutter," and hence, he must stop "stuttering" before he can begin talking again.

F. HOW WE LEARN NEW WAYS TO DO THINGS

As the child began to understand how to describe sequences of behavior, he began to develop a sense of the forward motion in these sequences. Next, he could go logically to a consideration of how changes in specifics of such a sequence could be made without interruption of sequential continuity. With this foundation, he comes to understand that, if he makes a mistake during sequencing of behavior, he should *change* what he is doing but continue with the sequence instead of stopping the sequence by tensing.

Many examples were used to help the child understand the idea of "change." Illustrations were selected to coincide with the child's interests: a batting stance, a particular swimming stroke, or a dance step. If, for example, one wants to learn a batting stance that is different from the one he has been using, he must first study what he is doing and then experiment with what he can do to change certain aspects of it. He must become acquainted with the similarities and the differences between what he "had been doing" and what he "wants to begin doing." Again, however, the clinician emphasized that one does not learn to change the way he is doing things by "fighting to stop" or by "struggling to keep from doing" the old behavior. Specifically, if a child has learned to swim by using the "dog paddle" but now desires to learn the crawl, he will not master the new stroke by jumping into the water and trying as hard as he can *not* to dog-paddle. If he did, he would tense his entire body in his effort *not* to dog-paddle and as a result would sink. He would have stopped doing what it is necessary to do to stay afloat, let alone to do the crawl.

By comparison, if one desires to learn a more forward-moving, easy way of talking he will not learn by trying as hard as he can "not to repeat sounds," or "not to stutter," or "not to have trouble." If he proceeds in this way, he probably will tense the oral muscles, perhaps even his entire body, and stop doing the things he must do in order to talk. In short, he will stop talking. Often it is found that a child—or an adult, for that matter—believes or acts as though he believes, that "his talking will go on all by itself" if he uses his muscles to "keep the trouble from happening." This is similar to a situation in which a person assumes that the crawl "will continue by itself" if he tenses his muscles hard enough "to keep the dog paddle out." These kinds of illustrations were acted out by children in the group. The children were then encouraged to *do* things to *talk* instead of to "not stutter." If, as a child was talking, he did certain things that began to interfere with talking, he was to *change* them *as* he continued talking. Swimming again serves to clarify the point. If, as a person is first learning the crawl, he becomes frightened by a mouthful of water and reverts to his best-learned response, which is dog paddling, his task is not fighting "to stop" the dog paddle; it is *changing* what he is doing *as* he is swimming so he again will be swimming the crawl. A child can be helped to understand that changing what he does while he is speaking is like that.

G. HOW FEELINGS OF BEING SCARED OR EMBARRASSED CAN INTERFERE WITH DOING THE THINGS WE WANT TO DO

Throughout the entire therapy program an attempt was made to help the children come to an understanding of feelings such as fear, guilt, and embarrassment.

Although it is necessary to help the children of this age group learn to accept, i.e., not to feel guilt about, various feelings, it was considered particularly important to assess and to understand feelings of fear. Fear and the inability to deal with it become so entwined with speaking behavior that the result is one indivisible thing called "stuttering." Then, fear and its dreaded consequence, disrupted speech, generate feelings of "copelessness."

In our society, fear is considered generally to be "bad" because it is a sign of weakness or of inadequacy. Our cultural mores particularly condemn fear in boys. As a result, it is not unusual for a child to believe that one should not have such feelings, and most certainly if he does have them, he should make every effort to "hide them" so people cannot "see them." The child becomes afraid of being afraid, which results in becoming more afraid. He believes that any time he begins to experience fear, he must take corrective action to prevent it, and if he cannot prevent it, he must hide it, and if he cannot hide it, he must "get over it" quickly. These reactions to fear make it difficult for the child to react constructively to the people or to the events of his situation. He is too busy fighting his own feelings.

The results of these reactions are obvious in working with the adult who stutters. During the years of growing up with the stuttering problem, he has observed that when he is "by himself" or when he is "relaxed"—generally he means when no "feelings of fear" are present—he stutters much less or is even fluent. Therefore, he believes that the solution to his problem lies in getting rid of these "feelings of stuttering." In fact, he ties these "feelings" so closely to the occurrence of stuttering that any time he is called upon to speak, his first task is to evaluate the way he "feels." If he feels a little afraid, it never occurs to him to try to do things to talk. From experience he is convinced he cannot. Therefore, *once again* he does not try; instead, he gets set by tensing his muscles, and by hesitating to talk in order to avoid, to control, or if need be, to fight the "stutter" that he is convinced will follow. The child should learn, therefore, not only to understand these feelings but also to cope with them in a realistic way. Instead of trying to convince the child that he should *not* be scared or that he should "get over" being scared when he talks, he was encouraged to feel that it was all right to be scared. This point of view was discussed and illustrated in relation to many nonspeech experiences as well as those involving speech. The discussion with the children on this point was put in the following context:

> Fear is not only a very normal feeling, but also an extremely healthy one. It is a feeling that we all experience, and furthermore, we are better off because we do. Fear of a hot stove can keep us from burning our fingers. Fear before a football game or a dance recital can help us to be more alert and to do a better job. Feelings of fear before an examination can help us study harder and get a better grade. Fear can be a very useful thing. In growing up, our job is to learn to use it instead of to be afraid of it. We should not be afraid of becoming afraid. When this happens it gets in our way. We begin to stop doing some of the things we want to do for no other reason than because we are becoming afraid. We come to believe that the way to stop the fear is to stop doing the kinds of things that make us afraid. Before long, we are convinced that when we begin to feel fear, we cannot continue doing what we are doing. Instead, we must stop it. When we feel very sure of ourselves we don't stop what we are doing or become embarrassed. It is just as normal to be afraid or to feel unsure at times as it is to feel sure and to be filled with courage. In either event it is possible for us to continue doing the kinds of things we want to do regardless of how we feel.
>
> Just as we usually consider fear as bad, so we also consider it as unpleasant. There are circumstances in which the feeling of fear is not at all unpleasant; in fact, it is very enjoyable. When we see a football or basketball game in which the score is close and we are afraid our team will lose, we consider it an exciting game. We go to a so-called horror movie and we do not feel that the show is very good unless we have been scared.

The purpose of this discussion was to prepare the child to *experience* fear willingly and to evaluate it calmly. The children described and discussed how they felt when they were afraid, the kinds of situations in which they were likely to be fearful, the ways they act in these situations, and how they think other people react to them at these times.

These discussions were augmented by assignments in which each child was to perform some nonspeech act that he was afraid to do. His task was to plan his actions carefully and then to perform them as calmly as possible even though he was afraid. These procedures invariably led into discussion of fear in speaking situations such as talking to a group or to an adult or to a stranger.

To emphasize the fact that to feel fear at times while speaking was a normal reaction experienced by everyone and not unique to "stutterers," normal-speaking children and adults were invited to the group to discuss and to evaluate their own speaking fears. The children discovered that normal speakers experience fear in many of the same situations as do the children who stutter; they simply evaluate it and react to it differently. It was then possible to point out that our goal in therapy is not to eliminate speaking fears. It is to calmly change the ways we talk when necessary even though we are afraid.

H. HOW WE CHANGE THE WAYS WE DO THINGS

Because the children had been introduced to the idea of behavior changes in the preceding sessions, it was now productive to direct their attention to behavior change as a process and to talk with them about the problems of changing any kind of behavior that has been well learned.

They discussed and then practised changing certain instances of nonspeech behavior and of speaking behavior other than that associated with "stuttering." They participated in deciding what behavior each was to change. Some were to sit straight instead of slouching in a chair, some were to stand tall instead of stooping as they walked; others were to say "yes" instead of "yeah," or "pardon?" instead of "huh?"; others were to look at people when they talked with them instead of looking at the floor. Generally, an attempt was made to select behavior that would improve their appearance or that would bring about a more favorable reaction from other people during communication. It was not long before they began complaining that their old way of behaving was so natural that they used it without even thinking, and that the new behavior seemed strange and made them feel or sound funny.

The clinician explained that when a person first tries to change his behavior, he feels strange about it and uncomfortable; moreover, it is difficult to remember to act in the new way. Sometimes one hesitates to try a new way of acting because he thinks that people are noticing his efforts to do something different. If he continues to practise, however, his new behavior soon feels natural. It was suggested that the children schedule daily periods during which they were to experiment with the changes they were learning to make.

The schedule served not only as a reminder but also as encouragement because, in effect, it broke up the learning task into small pieces, and in this form the total task appeared manageable. A person is ordinarily more willing to attend closely to a new task and to experiment with the new feelings and related reactions for a short time than to go at the job full-time at once. Besides, without a schedule he is likely first to forget and then to proceed in a haphazard way, remembering his new behavior only *as* or *after* he performs the old. If this pattern is followed very long, he not only becomes discouraged, but he is also increasingly convinced that he cannot change the way he acts; he reinforces an erroneous belief that he just has to act the way he always has acted—that he is just the way he is, and nothing can be done about it.

Considerable time was devoted to helping each child learn *how* to change the ways he acts; in brief, to learn how to learn to change behavior. This experience served a) to introduce procedures for changing aspects of general behavior and b) to provide a framework for introducing the child to the idea that since talking is behavior, these procedures apply equally to changes in talking.

I. HOW WE CHANGE THE WAY WE TALK

For a child to begin making positive changes in his speaking behavior, he had to observe what he did to interfere with and what he did to facilitate the ways of talking that were normal. A child observed his total talking behavior and not just certain small instances of "stuttering" within the total talking behavior. During the time a child did specific things to interfere with talking, he was generally "holding back" in his overall talking behavior. Often he began to "hold back" even before he began to talk. On the other hand, when the child was doing things to help himself talk, his total talking behavior was forward-moving. The differences between "holding-back" behavior and "moving-forward" behavior were demonstrated and imitated until the children began to get the feeling of the difference between the two. Each child worked to get the feeling on a motoric, muscle-tensing level, of holding back as he talked, and to observe how different degrees of holding back interfere in differing degrees with talking. For example, he was asked to begin to talk and then increasingly to tense his jaw muscles and his abdominal muscles as he continued talking. He soon observed that after he had tensed them to a certain degree, he stopped talking entirely. Or, he might tense them, holding back to a lesser degree, and manage to keep a certain part of the talking process operating. Finally, it was demonstrated that the child can hold back a little as he talks and continue talking in a way that most listeners would agree was fluent speaking, even though it was not normal, forward-moving talking. For example, he might hold back by tensing his abdominal or jaw muscles slightly or by slowing down or speeding up his speaking rate even though there was no obvious interruption in speech fluency. Ordinarily, the child believes that he is not "stuttering" at these times. As a consequence it is easy for him to believe that he did not "stutter" because he held back to a certain degree. Through this belief, he reinforces belief in the holding-back behavior.

Next, the child observed the things he did, and could do, to move forward easily and effortlessly as he talked. As each child worked to get the feeling of moving forward the clinician repeatedly pointed out the continuous lip and jaw movement and the degree of tensing necessary. The clinician emphasized that, as one moves forward in his talking, he may repeat or interject certain sounds or make mistakes in other ways; however, he should accept these mistakes calmly and continue moving forward easily. This represents the way that most "normal speakers" talk.

Each child practised and compared the two ways of talking, i.e., holding back and moving forward, until he became so familiar with the differences between them that he could institute each upon command in the clinical situation. To reinforce in every way possible, by as many cues as possible, the difference between these two ways of talking, we asked the children to talk in front of a mirror and watch themselves, talk into a tape recorder and hear themselves, and to talk to each other. Then, to make clearer our conversations about the things the child was doing as he talked, we labeled one way of talking as "talking hard" and the other way of talking as "talking easy." These labels enable the clinician to give instructions such as, "When you begin to talk, begin to talk easily and then continue talking easily. If you bobble or get tangled up as you are talking, bobble or get tangled up easily as you go on talking." This language, it was felt, enabled the clinician to give positive suggestions about what the child could *do* as he began to talk and to reinforce a child's behavior both positively and negatively. As each child began to carry over the easy talking into situations outside the clinical room, the clinician could remind him before he started to "talk easily as you begin to talk and then continue to talk easily." After the child performed the task, the clinician could say, "Fine. You did a good easy job of talking." Or, he could say, "You began talking easily but then you began to do things to make talking hard for yourself." Another advantage of our dichotomy was that it helped the child cope with his feelings while he talked. The clinician could bring the child to see that, even though he had feelings of fear—or as the child might say, he "felt funny in his stomach"—he could still talk easily.

In summary, a person learns to improve the ways he talks by learning 1. what is involved in talking and how to perform the necessary acts easily, 2. that as he makes mistakes while talking, he can do them "easily," 3. that if he gets feelings of fear, he can continue talking easily in spite of the feelings, and 4. that he will learn to talk easily to different people in different situations by practising at scheduled times.

J. HOW WE USE TALKING TO HELP US GET TO KNOW PEOPLE

One of the most important concepts interwoven through the entire therapy by discussion and illustration was the *reasons* that we talk. At times there is so much emphasis in speech therapy on attempting to help the child speak efficiently that we fail to help him learn, to any measurable degree, to talk effectively. The child who is likely to become increasingly concerned with the *ways* he talks needs to learn that the major purpose of talking is to communicate with people—to get to know them and to help them get to know him.

The clinician led discussions in which the children were to think of all of the reasons that a person might want to talk: to let people know the way you feel, to let people know what you want, to help people by giving them information, to help people by warning them if something is about to happen to them, to ask questions so that one can learn more, etc., etc.

Verbal communication involves both talking and listening. The children practised listening. They were assigned to engage in conversations with other children who lived in the dormitory. In these conversations, they were to practise being a good listener. They were to observe that when they listened attentively and when they reacted to what the other person was saying, it encouraged the person to say more and more. They learned that by asking questions about what the other child talked about, they got to know the child well. They found that in certain respects he had the same kinds of interests that they had. Also, they found that when they inquired about and were interested in what another child did and the ways he felt, they came to like the child and, what is more important, the other child came to like them.

After the organized discussions of this topic, the reasons why we talk were pointed out throughout therapy when situations arose that would illustrate the point. Several such situations arose in Sessions II and III.

Session II. Talking In An Informal Situation

Session II was structured as an informal group situation to provide an opportunity for the child to discuss his talking behavior, his reactions to attempted behavioral changes, and his feelings about talking to people. The emphasis was on activities other than speech—soap carving, developing exhibits, making nonobjective sculptures, finger painting, creative painting, and drawing—but discussion was organized as a natural part of the activity.

As points were discussed in Session I, they were carried over and applied to the nonspeaking behavior in Session II. For example, at the time the child was learning to describe his speaking behavior in Session I, he was learning also to describe the project on which he was working in Session II. Similarly, when the children discussed in Session I the mistakes they made while speaking, they discussed in Session II the mistakes they made on their projects and the feelings they experienced while making them. The children were encouraged to undertake activities that they were interested in but that they had had little experience in doing. Thus they had an opportunity to begin to learn how to do things that they did not know how to do. After they had selected their projects, we proceeded as follows:

The children discussed among themselves ways to undertake each project. Children in the group who had experience with a particular activity were asked to help the child who had chosen that activity. If none of the children had had any appropriate experience, each child was instructed to ask the clinicians supervising in Session II whether they could provide help. If none of the clinicians had had relevant experience, a person from outside the clinic was brought in to help. First, the child was asked to find out through discussion as much as he could about ways to do the job. Next, he was to begin on the project while his "teacher" observed and discussed with him ways to proceed. Then the child practised the skills that he needed to make an adequate job of his project. As he made mistakes he was counseled not to get upset and not to quit because he made mistakes. Instead, with the help of the person teaching him, he was to learn from his mistakes until he improved his skill. Finally, he was to continue to practise until he achieved mastery. This procedure was discussed as a "problem-solving" approach. Willingness to "try" in face of the possibility that mistakes would be made was emphasized; the children were told that if they made mistakes they were to learn from them. The "problem-solving" attitude was related to working on his speech.

As the child worked on a project, the concepts dealt with in Session I in relation to learning to talk more easily were emphasized. The project situation provided a setting in which communication was meaningful and a child could see that a problem-solving attitude is important in attempting to learn anything new. Later on in therapy, new projects were undertaken. The same procedures were followed except that the child was asked to demonstrate increased independence in finding out how to help himself learn. This requirement parallels, of course, the expectation later on in therapy that the child accept the responsibility to do more and more things to help himself talk. Visitors were encouraged to come to this group session and to ask the children to describe what they were doing and the steps they had followed in doing it. The children were encouraged to tell the visitors about the mistakes they had made in learning, how they felt about the mistakes, and what they did about them.

During the entire six-week therapy period, the children were encouraged to talk with each other as they worked. In this way, they found an opportunity to make the changes in their speaking behavior that they had learned and had been practising in Session I.

Session III. Talking In A Formal Situation

This session was to help the child to continue learning about talking and to carry over into a more formal speaking situation what he had learned in Session I and Session II. It is particularly important for a child of this age to learn to express himself verbally in the variety of situations our society presents. The normal-speaking child of this age customarily receives considerable instruction about "speech manners." On the other hand, it is not uncommon for the child who stutters to receive little or no instruction in the procedures of making introductions, of talking on the telephone, or organizing and delivering speeches in front of a group—or for that matter, even how to behave nonverbally in front of a group. Too often, he has been excused from these activities because he "stutters." This omission places a tremendous burden on the child as he becomes older. Generally, these more formal speaking situations are the more difficult ones for normal speakers. They also in later life typically become the more difficult situations for the person who stutters.

In Session III, therefore, the child learned to present a speech in front of a group. He was helped to organize his speech and he was instructed in proper methods of delivery. He practised looking at his audience, maintaining good posture, and using appropriate gestures. He was taught to look at his audience, not because "one is to maintain good eye contact when he stutters," but because this is good speaking procedure for anyone. He learned to organize and to give different kinds of speeches: descriptive, argumentative, humorous, etc. He learned that the important thing in making speeches is to provide information and to communicate ideas. Most certainly the purpose is not "seeing how many words one can say fluently."

The children learned proper procedures for making introductions. They took turns introducing one person to the next. They received instruction about telephone manners and practised making telephone calls. They were told how to conduct group discussions. They were given topics to discuss as a group. A discussion leader named for the day was coached in leading the discussion and in encouraging other people to talk. It was easy to point out that most people are reluctant to talk in a group. Therefore, a group member has a responsibility to help others feel comfortable and willing to express their ideas, and one of the best ways is to listen attentively, showing interest in what the person has to say.

Toward the end of the six-week summer session, visitors were encouraged to attend the formal speaking situations to serve as an audience for the children. The visitors discussed with the children their own speaking fears. The children learned that most people experience speaking fears in front of a group and have to make themselves go ahead and talk even though they are somewhat scared. Children in the nine-to-12-year age group are becoming increasingly aware of themselves as individuals, and more concerned with what other people think about them than they ever were before. It is easy for a "stutterer" of this age to assume that his increased fear in speaking situations is a consequence of "stuttering" and not a normal reaction for anyone at those ages. This type of session provided an opportunity to reassure the child about the normalcy of his feelings and stress that he could talk easily and conduct himself in an appropriate manner *even though* he was experiencing feelings of fear or embarrassment.

Discussion and Evaluation of the Therapy Program

At the end of the therapy period, a two-day conference was held with the parents of the children. The purpose was to help the parents become familiar with the activities in which the child had been engaged and the kinds of things that the parents could do to be helpful after the child's return home. The parents' child was present at these conferences, an active partner in the discussions. He demonstrated to his parents what he had done to learn to talk easily. A detailed letter was sent home after the conference in which the therapy program was outlined, the child's progress was described, and ways that the parents could help ensure continued progress were set forth.

There are two considerations in evaluating the success of such a therapy program: how the children are talking at the end of the therapy, and the degree to which they maintain the progress they made or improve on it after they return home. In developing the retraining program it was decided to take one criterion at a time. The initial concern of the clinical research staff was to evaluate changes that had been made in speaking behavior by the end of the therapy. As the therapy program was developed and refined each succeeding summer session, more children who attended during any one summer either were greatly improved or were talking normally within the environment of the dormitory, the clinic, and the city. By the end of the therapy period in 1965, most of the children who attended that summer would have been rated either one or two on a seven-point scale where one represented no stuttering and seven represented most severe stuttering. There were always a few each summer who improved some but had brought with them to the summer clinic problems so complex that, although their behavior may have improved in many ways, six weeks was not long enough to make possible all the desired changes in their speech.

Up to 1966, personnel, time, and financial support were not sufficient to permit us to follow up the children systematically to determine the extent to which progress maintained after they returned home. Among those who were followed we found generally encouraging, although mixed, results. Some of the children continued to talk normally, according to the reports of their parents. Others regressed somewhat but not back to the severe disfluency of their speech before therapy began. Others regressed considerably upon returning home and then after a time began to improve again without any concomitant speech therapy in the interim. Still others were referred to school clinicians in their home communities for more help and, therefore, assessment of the effect of the summer clinic was difficult. Up to this point, we had not been discouraged by the nature of the speaking behavior after they returned home. We operated on the assumption that if a program could be established which sent the child home talking in the ways that he wanted to at any time under any conditions, the next step would be to develop follow-up procedures to insure the continuation of this kind of speaking behavior.

In the fall of 1965, the writer received a research grant from the U.S. Office of Education to continue development of the therapy program, to develop follow-up procedures, and to begin development of an experimental therapy program in the public schools. The public school program and the rationale for it will be described in the next section of this chapter.

Beginning in the fall of 1967 we obtained information at regular intervals concerning the children seen in the summer clinic of 1967. A clinical research associate visited the home community of each child twice, in the fall of 1967 and in the spring of 1968. The child, the parents, and the teachers of the child were interviewed.

We are still assessing the best kinds of information to obtain, the most efficient ways to obtain it, and the most effective ways to deal with problems in the home community. The findings to date indicate that soon after the termination of the summer clinic, the parents tend to forget or become confused about what they can do to be helpful. The teachers have little or no idea of what we have done or what they can do to be helpful. As a result, it is not uncommon for the child to lose his perspective toward what he can do to help himself talk easily.

In the fall of 1968 we adopted a procedure somewhat different from that followed in the previous year. In the early fall, as soon as possible after school began, a visit was made to the home community. During this visit a conference was held with the child's classroom teacher about what the child had done in therapy, the progress he had made, and what the teacher could do to help. At a conference with the parents the concepts of therapy and the helpful procedures they can use were reviewed. The clinical research associate met the child and, if necessary, worked with him for an hour or two, reviewing the therapy process and giving him practice at talking easily. This visit was intended to assist the child to carry over into the school environment the progress he had made and to refresh the parents and the child about what to do to talk easily.

After the visit to the home community, phone calls at regular intervals were made to parents to discuss the progress their child had made and to answer any questions they might have about how they react to the child. A visit was made again to the home community during the early spring of 1971.

The new procedures followed in 1968 arose from a change in philosophy concerning just what one should do in a follow-up. We now view the visit to the home as one of "continuing therapy" instead of "follow-up" to a therapy program that has been "completed." We observed that in previous years children who maintained normal speech or who continued to improve after they went home were those whose parents were clear in what they could do to help and continued to maintain that relationship with the child. These parents had talked to the classroom teachers and explained to them what the child was doing and what the teacher could do to help. The therapy program had, in effect, been continued by the important people in the child's environment.

STUTTERING THERAPY IN THE ELEMENTARY SCHOOLS

Operating with the assumption that stuttering is a problem of disturbed interaction between the child and the important persons in his environment, the school has advantages over the clinic as a locale in which the child learns to improve the ways he talks. In school, the clinician can be much more aware of the child's normal daily environment and his interactions with other children, his teachers, and his parents, than he can when the child is in a clinic removed from contact with these important persons. The clinician can observe the child interacting with these persons and they with him. As such, he can be alert to the reactions of others to changes the child begins to make in the ways he interacts and the changes he makes in the ways he talks. The clinician then has the opportunity to reinforce appropriately desirable changes and to restructure or redirect behavior that brings about inappropriate responses. The child is able to make further changes which are subsequently reinforced according to their consequences. Through close contact with the important persons in the child's environment, the clinician is in a position to promote and to develop an environment in which the child can afford to—can feel free to—change constructively the ways he acts. The concepts and the procedures used to help the child learn to change the ways he talks gain considerable meaning for him when they are illustrated by and related to the many facets of the learning that takes place daily in school. Yet, school clinicians often report considerable difficulty in adapting the principles and procedures of stuttering therapy they have learned in a clinic environment to fit the school environment.

As a part of the experimental stuttering therapy program mentioned previously, two one-day conferences were held with groups of Iowa public school clinicians and one one-half day conference was held with principals and classroom teachers in Cedar Rapids, Iowa. The major purpose of these conferences was to determine what, according to the clinicians, constituted the major problems in conducting the stuttering therapy program within the school environment and possible ways to resolve them. Problems appeared to center around five points.

1. *Lack of Understanding by the School Personnel About the Stuttering Problem.* Elementary school personnel naturally have considerably less understanding of the stuttering problem than persons who work in a speech clinic. In fact, school personnel often appear to be uneasy, or puzzled, at times even frightened, about stuttering problems and in many instances not even aware that they can do anything to be helpful. Instead, their attitude is one of "taking it easy" on the child so his stuttering will not become worse than it is. On the other hand, most people within the clinic possess a general knowledge of the nature of the problem and what they can do to help the child as he learns to change the ways he talks. Many school clinicians reported a feeling of being "overwhelmed" by the dual problem of a stuttering child and an environment where few persons, if any, are aware of what they can do to help the child improve the ways he talks. There is a helpless feeling of not knowing where to begin. Too often the clinician resolves this problem by working with the child alone in a therapy room and then by hit-and-miss methods attempting to "educate" the school personnel generally about the problem of stuttering. Therapy can, and must, be offered on a broader, more systematic basis than this. For important persons in the child's environment to learn how to be helpful and to reinforce appropriately the child's efforts is one of the most effective ways to bring about stable changes in the child's speaking behavior. Rather than constituting a limitation to an effective therapy program, it is one of the strengths of a therapy program within the elementary schools.

2. *Lack of Flexibility in the Daily School Schedule.* Inasmuch as there are a great many children in the typical elementary school and a great many activities to include in any given day, school administrators must enforce strict scheduling. This situation, of necessity, prevents the clinician from carrying on a program of therapy for a given child independent of school activities. The lack of flexibility in the school schedule is reported by the clinicians to induce a feeling of lack of freedom to carry out clinical procedures. For example, they report that often there are "school rules" which prohibit a child from walking in the halls between classes, or going on the playground during class, or entering the gym during an unscheduled period, or a ban on visits by parents to school during class except at specified times of the year.

The principals and the teachers at the conference reported, however, that even though there must be a routine schedule for each day, modifications can be made in this schedule if the administrators see the reasons for doing it. Too often the clinicians do not communicate effectively with school administrators. They do not have a positive program planned for a child and therefore find it difficult to explain to a principal just what the "special" needs will be. Under these circumstances, it is difficult for the school administrators to work out with the clinician the special allowances, whatever they might be in a specific school, that need to be made. Exceptions to these rules usually can be made when the persons involved understand the necessity of permitting a child and his clinician, for example, to walk down the hall to talk to a janitor or a secretary in order to reach some goal in therapy. School personnel are interested in helping children. However, when a particular activity is going to inconvenience them or disrupt in some way the operation of the school, they desire to know in what ways the activity will be helpful. This is only reasonable.

3. *The "Transient Status" of Most School Clinicians Within a Particular Elementary School.* Most school clinicians provide therapy in more than one school during a given week, and they report difficulty in becoming a part of any school environment. Many problems may arise from this situation, but reportedly one fairly common result is that their schedules and their clinical rooms are likely to be changed upon short notice. Adaptability then becomes a requisite for the school clinician: he must have a basic understanding of the goals of therapy so that he can adapt on short notice the things he does in therapy to meet the goals on a particular day for a stuttering child. If the clinician knows the goals he wants to reach, he will realize that there are various ways to reach them.

4. *The Role of the Clinician in Parent Counseling.* A common complaint was that the school clinician is at a disadvantage in counseling parents because he has to *go to* the parents rather than the parents coming to the clinician, as in a clinic. It is held that the matter of where the initiative lies markedly affects the parents' attitude. A common complaint of school clinicians is that the parents "will not cooperate." Through careful discussions with approximately 85 Iowa school clinicians and through observations in working in a variety of schools, we came to believe that this problem may have been overemphasized. Most parents want their child to do the best he can in every way possible. They may fail to understand that they as parents need to be involved in any way in helping the child to talk better. They assume that is the "job" for the clinician. When they understand what they can do to help and when a positive program is explained to them they are ordinarily more than willing to do everything they can. There are always a certain number of parents who either cannot understand what they can do or, because of their own needs, cannot bring themselves to do what they should do. However, the same situation exists in the clinic.

5. *Lack of Time to Conduct a Meaningful Stuttering Therapy Program in the Schools.* The biggest problem reported by school clinicians was lack of time. In certain states, the law requires that a clinician work with such a large caseload that little time is available to give a child individual attention. This situation is unfortunate. When there is insufficient time for adequate individual attention, a clinician's expectations of the progress a child with any speech problem can make are restricted. In the case of a stuttering child, the clinician must evaluate what progress can be expected within the time available to work with a child and then decide whether it is advisable to include the child in his therapy schedule.

In the state of Iowa, there is no minimum caseload required of the clinician. They still reported that "lack of time" was a major problem. One of the main reasons for this was that they viewed the structure of the therapy program in the same way as they had observed it in the clinic. In this environment the child often has four or five clinical sessions a week and these are supplemented by lengthy and often frequent conferences with his parents. It must be remembered, however, that considerable time is spent in the clinic structuring situations in which the child can practise changing his speaking behavior. In the school situation, these situations are available during his daily routine activities. Furthermore, lengthy conferences are necessary in the clinic environment in order to ascertain, as best one can, the problems the child encounters in interacting with persons in his environment. In the school situation, it is possible to observe his interacting behavior and to supplement these observations by holding short conferences with important persons in his environment.

During our three-year experimental therapy program, we scheduled the child for two half-hour therapy periods a week. Before we began seeing the child regularly, we spent approximately one-half to three-quarters of an hour talking with each of the following: 1. the child's teacher, 2. at least one of the child's parents, 3. the principal—if the principal knew the child well enough, and 4. the child. After the first interviews with the important people in the child's environment many of our conversations with them could be held by phone or in the hall between classes. If there was a need to see the mother longer, she came in the child's place on a particular day. If there was a need to observe the child in the classroom, this was done during his regularly scheduled therapy period. The amount of "time" outlined above does not seem unreasonable in most school situations.

Implementation of the Stuttering Therapy Program in the Schools

The stuttering therapy program for a child begins by defining and describing the scope of the problem, by determining the important people involved in the problem and its consequences to them. We operate on the principle that one of the most effective ways to change the manner in which one interacts with another person is to determine what the person likes, what he dislikes, and what he would like to change about the other person. Much of what bothers Person A about Person B is a difference between the way Person B is acting and the ways that Person A would like to see him act. Therefore, the important persons in the child's environment, usually the teachers, the parents, sometimes the principal, and the child are interviewed. We establish a "problem profile" for each person in relation to the child, and for the child in relation to himself. Our goal is to define the problem as it is *perceived* by the teacher, parents, etc., so that as a part of therapy the clinician can work to bring about changes in the child's talking and interacting behavior that will be viewed as "improvement." For example, if the child's teacher reports that she becomes particularly uncomfortable during his stuttering behavior when he holds his breath, this is one of the first behaviors that receives attention in therapy. We consider it important for the teacher to learn that the child can change his talking behavior in ways she will view as "improvement." Similarly, if the teacher reports that the child frequently creates disturbances in the classroom by tripping other children and she *perceives* this behavior as being related to his stuttering problem, we consider it important to work with the child on this aspect of his behavior. As the frequency of this behavior is reduced, the teacher will view this as improvement and is likely to begin interacting with the child in a more positive way than she had in the past. Therefore, the following information is obtained from each person:

1. *Description of the speaking behavior of the child.* First, we determine insofar as possible what the person believes to be "wrong" with the child, that is, what he believes about the cause of stuttering. As one works with the child to help him learn to change his talking behavior, the important persons must be shown that there is a problem here that involves *learning*. If the person continues to believe that something is basically "wrong" with the child, he either will think there is not much that one can do or that there is something the clinician has to "take out of" the child. Hence, he will find it hard to see that he has a role in helping the child learn to talk better.

Next, the person is asked to describe what the child does when talking that bothers him as a listener. A statement such as, "he just stutters," or "he has trouble" is not generally accepted. The person is encouraged to be more descriptive and to mention such things as feelings of discomfort when "he tenses so much," or when "he holds his breath," or when "he squirms and blushes." Behavior like this can be changed and its disappearance readily noted. The person is asked to describe the ways in which, in that person's opinion, the child would have to change his talking behavior to improve. This statement becomes a reference point for later discussions with the person of the degree to which and the ways in which he observes the child improving.

2. *Description of the ways the child interacts with his environment.* We ask each person to discuss and to describe the way the child interacts with other children in the classroom, on the playground, in the home, etc. Then, we ask them to tell how they would like to see the child change in these respects. This information is obtained for two reasons. First, the clinician can determine the ways in which these persons relate the child's nonspeech behavior to the "stuttering problem," and secondly, the ways the child is behaving that promote a negative reaction by the person toward the child. Then, either by counseling to change the person's attitude toward the behavior, or by working with the child to change his behavior, or both, the clinician works to develop a positive interaction between the child and the important persons in his environment. Also, as with the information obtained about the child's speaking behavior, the statements made about his interacting

behavior serve as a reference point for later discussions with the person of the ways the child has improved.

The Therapy Program

After the interviews described, direct therapy is begun with the child, employing concepts and procedures similar to those used in the clinic situation and outlined earlier in this chapter. As one discusses learning to talk, learning to make mistakes, learning new nonspeech behavior, and learning to accept one's feelings, these concepts are related to and implemented through his daily experiences and activities in the classroom, in the halls, on the playground, and in the home.

Nonspeech behavior often is used to help parents or the teachers learn how to help the child learn new behavior. For example, if the mother is concerned that the child will "never clean up his room," and "always leaves it in a mess," we suggest things she can do to help him learn to pick up his room instead of "just expecting him to do it." We advise her to explain to him what she *expects* him to do; if necessary, show him how to do it, then to compliment him as he does a little more each day. We point out to the mother that what we are doing in therapy to help him learn to talk "easier" is much like that.

A similar kind of parallel can be used with the teacher. The teacher might report that he is "a very messy and careless writer." The clinician can help the child learn to improve his writing skills, relating his problems in doing this to the problems involved in learning to talk more easily. Assignments can be made for execution in the classroom, where, at a particular time, he will work at doing a better job of writing than he had done in the past. The teacher is told of the penmanship practice so she can take note and compliment him for this. These kinds of activities provide an environment in which the child comes to feel free to change the ways he does things. Moreover, when he does change them, he observes that the important persons in his environment notice and are pleased by his new ways.

As the child learns to do things to talk easily in the therapy situation, we use considerable role-playing in which the clinician takes the role of his mother, the teacher, etc., and role-plays a variety of speaking situations while the child practises talking easily. A conference is then held with the teacher and the child during which the clinician has the child demonstrate for the teacher what he can do to talk easily. In this way the teacher comes to learn what to expect from him, and the child knows what the teacher will expect. After this, when the child is assigned to talk easily at some specific time in class, and the teacher is forewarned, she can by a smile, a wink, or words (whichever the child prefers) reinforce him immediately for the easy talking he did. This same procedure is followed with the parents.

In addition to the mother and teacher, the clinician may enlist in the therapy the janitor, the school secretary, or several of the child's playmates. The main objective is to get as many people as possible involved in reinforcing positively the easy talking he does.

The language used in talking about the child's speech behavior within the school environment is in terms of "talking easy" and "talking hard." The persons reinforcing the ways the child is talking are not required to react to either "fluency" or "disfluency," but instead to observe the behavior of talking easy regardless of whether there is fluency or minor disfluency. Talking easily is readily discernible by untrained persons and therefore lends itself to consistent reinforcement. The emphasis of the therapy program described above is on helping the child do positive things to "talk easy." As these attempts meet with increased acceptance by the people in his environment it results in a spiraling circle of positive interaction. This promotes increased spontaneity in speaking behavior as well as in social interaction and this, in turn, increases the ways of talking we call "normal speech."

Discussion

The function of an experimental therapy program is to revise, expand, and delete certain aspects of the therapy program as one assesses the results and as one evaluates research information as it becomes available. This we are doing.

During the 1966–67 school year we provided therapy for five children in the public schools of Cedar Rapids, Iowa (Cox and Williams, 1968). In the fall of 1967, we felt that four of the five children had improved sufficiently to warrant discontinuing a systematic therapy program. The evaluation of "satisfactory speech" was arrived at in the following ways: 1. we obtained speech samples which were compared to the pretherapy and post-therapy speech samples for each child; 2. we interviewed the child and persons in his environment, such as parents and teachers, and compared these interviews to the pretherapy interviews.

Analysis of the speech samples obtained from the children showed an increase in acceptable speaking behavior and a decrease in unacceptable speaking behavior. For example, the stuttering pattern of one child, a fifth-grade boy, before therapy was characterized by tense prolongations and broken words while reading, and whole-word repetitions, tense prolongations, and broken words while conversing. The speaking behavior at the time of the post-therapy evaluation consisted mostly of easy, part-word repetitions of one or two syllable duration when conversing and zero stutterings while reading. His parents and his teacher considered that he had improved sufficiently that he had little or no problem of "stuttering." They reported that they now "were treating him just like anyone else."

Another example concerns a third-grade girl. Before therapy, the child's stuttering pattern was characterized by tense prolongations and broken words while reading and conversing and specific sound, word, and situation fears. After therapy, her speech showed a decrease in prolongations and broken words while reading and conversing and a decrease in sound, word, and situation fears. During the school year of 1967–68, the clinician met with the child approximately once a month in order to discuss the kinds of progress she was making and to evaluate any problems that arose. She continued to improve and, more importantly, she felt confident about her ability to say *what she wanted to say*, but still on occasion she felt she made talking difficult for herself. However, this did not seem to bother her particularly; consequently, we were interested in why these occasional interruptions in speech did not apparently seem to merit much concern on her part. We concluded from talking to the child and persons in her environment that she was basically *optimistic* concerning her speech, and her ability to speak, and this optimism was characterized by the following: 1. she knew what she could do to change her speaking behavior; 2. she felt confident in her ability to make these changes; and 3. there was no doubt in her mind that if she continued to make the appropriate changes, *she would improve*. Hence, even though there were some reminiscences of the original overt "stuttering behavior," she felt that she could *cope* with it. She was not reluctant to talk in any situation. Furthermore, her parents and her teachers were pleased with the ways she talked.

The other two children for whom therapy had been discontinued were judged to be "talking satisfactorily." The other of the five children continued in therapy during the next academic year. He had improved to a certain degree but not sufficiently to warrant discontinuing therapy.

Measurement of "improvement" for these children was a difficult task. Instead of relying solely on counting the number of disfluencies still existent in the child's speech, it seemed to us that it was more important to determine the attitudes and evaluations of the child and the important persons in his environment toward the ways he talked. We considered that a child was "talking satisfactorily" when he reported that he was satisfied with his speech in different environments; he felt self-confident in his ability to say what he wanted to say when he wanted to say it; he was unafraid to talk to different people; he was willing to take part in class discussions and group activities; and he felt proud of the changes he had made in his speech, interaction, and self-concept behavior. This seems to be a meaningful operational definition of "improvement." The child is fulfilling his responsibility as a verbal communicator.

By describing in this chapter a stuttering therapy program in a residential clinical setting and in a public school environment, the intent was not to provide "the answer." Rather, the purpose was to describe the development of a therapy program based on certain assumptions about the nature of the problem. Every attempt was made to develop therapy concepts that were consistent with the hypothesis that stuttering develops as a result of disturbed interaction between speaker and listener. Hopefully, it will stimulate others to develop therapy programs specifically related to their hypotheses about the nature of stuttering. Also, it is hoped that it will encourage others to raise researchable questions about the nature of the problem, or about the children of this age group who present the problem. At least, as of 1969, it was a start.

BIBLIOGRAPHY

Bloodstein, O. 1960. The development of stuttering: I. changes in nine basic features. *J. Speech Hearing Disorders*, 25, 219–237.

———. 1960. The development of stuttering: II. development phases. *J. Speech Hearing Disorders*, 25, 366–376.

———. 1961. The development of stuttering: III. theoretical and clinical implications. *J. Speech Hearing Disorders*, 26, 67–82.

Bradford, D. 1964. A survey of contemporary American literature in stuttering speech rehabilitation. *Asha*, 6, 13–16.

Chapman, M. 1959. Self-inventory: group therapy for those who stutter. Minneapolis: Burgess.

Cooper, E. 1965. Structuring therapy for therapist and stuttering child. *J. Speech Hearing Disorders*, 30, 75–78.

Cox, P., and Williams, D. 1968. Follow-up procedures for use in the public school setting for the child who stutters. Paper presented at the Nat. Conv. Amer. Speech Hearing Assn., Denver, Colo.

Emerick, L. 1965. Therapy for young stutterers. *Except. Child.*, 31, 389–448.

Fraser, M. 1964, pub. Treatment of the young stutterer in the school. Memphis, Tenn.: Speech Foundation of Amer.

Johnson, W. 1961. Stuttering and what you can do about it. Minneapolis: Univ. Minn. Press.

Luper, H., and Mulder, R. 1964. Stuttering therapy for children. Englewood Cliffs, N.J.: Prentice-Hall.

Murphy, A., and Fitzsimons, R. 1960. Stuttering and personality dynamics: play therapy, projective therapy and counseling. New York: Ronald.

Williams, D. 1957. A point of view about "stuttering." *J. Speech Hearing Disorders*, 22, 390–397.

———, Melrose, B., and Cox, P. 1968. Problems of stuttering therapy in the schools as viewed by school clinicians (unpublished manuscript).

———, and Roe, A. 1960. Teachers, parents, and "stutterers." *Education*, 80, 471–475.

Wyatt, G., and Herzan, H. 1962. Therapy with stuttering children and their mothers. *Amer. J. Orthopsychiat.*, 32, 645–659.

42

Methods for Integrating Theories of Stuttering

Stanley Ainsworth

The process of attempting to provide a way of integrating the multiplicity of ideas and facts concerning the nature and sources of stuttering continues to be frustrating and fragmentary. The student is faced with an array of divergent concepts, many of which appear to be mutually exclusive. Sometimes one wonders if two "authorities" are discussing the same problem. At the same time, there is a virtual necessity to arrive at some manageable framework upon which to structure a basic rationale for therapy and further study. Ideally, an integration should pull things together in such a fashion that a fundamental unity and relative completeness is recognizable in the midst of complexity. The knowledge of stuttering has not yet progressed to this level, but periodic evaluations can be made of contributions of various theories to improved understanding and their specific points of divergence. Only in this way can we proceed systematically toward more effective therapy based on a sound rationale. In the meantime, each professional must find a way to arrive at his own integration.

This chapter is an attempt to provide a framework for continuing analysis and synthesis of theoretical constructs of stuttering. No attempt will be made to review all the theories or to summarize the state of the knowledge in the field. The types of approaches to integration and the problems encountered will be discussed. Examples of various aspects of theories will be presented to illustrate elements within the suggested integrative organization. In this way attention can be focused on the process for analyzing and evaluating any specific theory with the expectation that the reader can apply the method more broadly.

APPROACHES AND PROBLEMS IN INTEGRATION

Every author who attempts to present a comprehensive discussion of stuttering has found it necessary to devise a way of talking about a mass of divergent ideas and overlapping theories in the literature. In response to this need, a variety of ways have evolved, each with some element of integration or classification that was presumed to be helpful. A brief review of some representative approaches should provide some clues as to the problems of any framework for integration.

Review of Approaches to Integration

One of the ways to classify the theories is to group them by "types." Travis (1933) provided the headings of educational, psychological, neurological, neurotic, imagery, and inhibitory theories. Van Riper (1939 and 1947) used these same groupings but also presented more extensive discussion under another system in his second edition. In 1954, Van Riper discussed the following as possible sources of stuttering: emotional conflict, low frustration tolerance, speech environment filled with fluency disruptors, poorly timed dysphemia, parental labeling of normal nonfluencies as abnormal, and stress from being driven to master too quickly the art of talking. Berry and Eisenson (1942) grouped etiologies under the headings of biochemical, neurological, psychological, and genetic. In their 1956 edition the headings used were heredity, neurology, psychosomatic factors, perseveration, and learning. Robinson (1964) used the following topics: cerebral dominance and dysphemia, servo theory, conflict theory, stuttering as a neurosis, the self-process theory, and evaluational theory. These, and other similar classifications, provided a way to organize the many points of view for discussion, understanding, and comparison. This approach has tended to leave the student aware of the divergence of, and differences among, theories rather than provide a basis for any personal integration of concepts—except for the obvious approach of "multiple causation" which will be discussed below since it creates problems of its own.

A step toward integration is represented by a different method of classifying theories. This approach involves determining what seem to be basic, underlying concepts which cut across several theories or groups of theories. Ainsworth (1945) presented three fundamental differences in theories of stuttering: those which see stuttering as due to severe emotional conflict (neurosis); those which denote a constitutional or organic basis (dysphemia); and those which assume a physically and psychologically normal child who develops stuttering in responses to environmental pressures and circumstances (developmental). Variations of these three basic differences appear in many discussions of stuttering. Van Riper (1947 and 1963) used three major groups: *learning* theories, *neurotic* theories, and theories of *constitutional difference*. Brutten and Shoemaker (1967) described the traditional theories of stuttering as falling into three classes based on physical or neurological concepts, psychological concepts, and interaction of physiogenic and psychogenic factors. They proposed that these theories have one underlying point of view—that stuttering is a disorder of the processes that integrate the activities of the speech mechanism. These traditional theories were then used as a basis for discussing the authors' behavioristic approach which does not imply a *type of person*. In *Stuttering: Training the Therapist* (Van Riper, 1966), a syllabus or course of study, theories were classified for study under organic, neurosis, learned behavior, and multiple origins.

A somewhat different statement of underlying concepts was suggested by Bloodstein (1958). There are three major explanations of what stuttering "is." The first is a "repressed need" hypothesis (a temporary failure in the complex sequence of neuromuscular activity needed for fluent speech). The second is a "breakdown" hypothesis (a temporary failure in the complex sequence of neuromuscular activity needed for fluent speech). The third is the "anticipatory struggle" hypothesis (the stutterer exerts himself in various ways on the assumption that he must do so in order to speak). In the introduction to *Stuttering: A Symposium*, Johnson (1958) further reduces the basic considerations to two. The first (the "speech" theory) takes two forms—the speaker is characterized by either a physical or a psychical flaw. The second (the "interaction" theory) functions on a continuum on the preceptual and evaluational reactions of the listeners, which may include the speaker himself.

Another step toward integration was presented by Hill (1945), who brought together a number of studies within a particular framework (Kantor's interbehavioral system). This represents a true integration limited to one point of view. Brutten and Shoemaker (1967, and Chapter 41) also developed an approach which considers many elements of traditional theories of stuttering. They recognize the role of possible organic factors in creating fluency failure (as different from stuttering) and interpret the psychological elements in stuttering within a learning theory framework (as opposed to the concept of personality structure and dynamics). This represents another approach to integration rather than classification.

Discussion of Integration Approaches

It sometimes seems that attempts at integration of theories create more problems than they solve. Each of the three approaches to integration has limitations and, in most cases, does not actually "integrate." The approaches tend to encourage the student of stuttering to make choices as to which theory or classification is "right" or "most important." This choice does not improve his understanding—it is similar to his position before learning of the classifications—but he now has a grouping of theories. As an additional source of inaccuracy, this approach tends to create the idea that theories in the same category are essentially the same. Any thoughtful study of the different theories will demonstrate that this assumption is erroneous. For instance, a comparison of the ideas of Johnson (1958), Johnson, Brown, Curtis,

Edney, and Keaster (1967), and Brutten and Shoemaker (1967) reveals profound differences, and yet they would be placed in the "learning" category.

Proponents of a "constitutional" basis provide an even wider range of variation. Some have been content with general statements about the nervous system, such as increased irritability and diminished capacity (Greene and Wells, 1927) or supersensitivity. There are frequent references in the literature to constitutional predisposition, biochemical or neurological factors, or motor inadequacies as causes for stuttering. An early Travis theory (1931) attempted to pinpoint the cause as a lack of cerebral dominance. (See Travis, 1940 and 1946, and Chapter 40 for more recent formulations by him.) A contribution by Karlin (1947) proposed that the basic physiological cause is a delay in the myelinization of cortical areas concerned with speech. West (1958) stressed pyknolespy as a possible primary source of stuttering, while Eisenson (1958) proposed that more than half of the stutterers have trouble because they are constitutionally inclined to perseverate. Mysak (1960) presented a servo theory discussion of stuttering as a disorder of verbalizing automaticity; while Stromsta (1959) found evidence that phonation blockage may be directly related to distortions in the auditory feedback mechanism.

In theories which support a neurosis as the basis for stuttering, there is a similar range of diversity. It is possible to consider stuttering as a symptom of: a negative compulsion (Krausz, 1940); a neurotic anxiety (Cobb, 1943) or an anxiety which is not sufficient to be labeled as neurotic (Murphy and FitzSimons, 1960); or a compulsive, narcissistic neurosis (Coriat, 1931 and 1943). Stuttering may be described as a "nervousness," as a problem of "emotional maladjustment," or, in contrast, as a problem involving fundamental and deep-seated inadequacies in personality organization. The psychoanalytic concepts go the farthest of this group of theories in presenting explanatory elements of causation (Travis, 1940; Chapter 40; and Glauber, 1958). Barbara (1954) offered a different description and explanation of the neurotic character of stuttering based on Horney's theory of neurosis. Van Riper (1954, 1963, and Chapter 39) proposed that in some cases a neurosis may be causative, but that in most stutterers the neurotic aspects develop after the onset of stuttering and as a result of it. Stuttering as an approach-avoidance conflict (Sheehan, 1953) contains some psychoanalytic concepts, but this theory includes learning theory concepts and is often identified in that grouping.

The wide range of possible sources of stuttering, even within the same general conceptual area, raises a further question. Is it possible that "stuttering" does not represent a unitary entity? If "stuttering" is used to represent several disorders that may have some similar symptoms but which, on the other hand, involve fundamentally different causes that produce a group of disorders which have significant differences, then any unitary integration of present theories may not be appropriate. The possibility of this is suggested by several writers who present summary discussions of stuttering. Van Riper (1954), for instance, proposed several "possible sources of stuttering." Adler (1966) adapted material from Robinson regarding five possible causes of nonfluencies. Eisenson (1958) definitely divided stutterers into two groups: "organic" and "non-organic" stutterers. Johnson et al. (1967) have approached this problem of the multiple nature of "stuttering" by limiting the term and differentiating the disorder from other speech problems which might be mistaken for it. These problems include mechanical repetition related to certain kinds of brain injuries, "neurotic stuttering," and "cluttering." (It should be observed that the first and third types fall into, but are not inclusive of, the "constitutional" theories; the second would be identified with the various theories that regard stuttering as a neurosis.) Brutten and Shoemaker (1967) approached this problem with some similarities to and some differences from other writers. They proposed that fluency failure may result from various forms of organismic stress, and that stuttering is but one class of fluency disruption due to learned emotional and instrumental responses through the operation of several causative factors. Clearly, the present theoretical formulations do not provide a clear answer to the question of the unitary nature of "stuttering."

Another problem revolves around the frequently invoked concept of "multiple causation" in reference to stuttering or to predisposing factors. (Van Riper, 1954 and 1963; Robinson, 1964; Adler, 1966; Brutten and Shoemaker, 1967, are examples.) The paragraph above suggests one dilemma presented by this concept—it seems to thrust us into a choice between accepting many types of stutterers or one type with all others classified as something other than stuttering. As the term is used by many individuals, particularly in lectures and casual conversation, there is also some confusion as to their meaning(s) of "multiple causation." This term can have at least five different interpretations. First, it can mean that for different stutterers, each may be stuttering for a different reason. Or it can mean that several causes may be simultaneously or sequentially operative within the same individual. This syndrome also might be patterned differently for different stutterers. Fourth, there may be different predisposing, precipitating, and maintaining causes. Finally, all blockages would not need to be the result of the same immediate cause or causes. That is to say, in one sentence various blocks may be caused by basic fluency failures (each deriving from varied sources), by specific word fears, or by generalized anxiety—or by a combination of these. Thus immediate causes of blocks may be multiple and also different from the original or initiating causes. The most eclectic workers will probably hold that all meanings are probable—but this creates a complexity that needs some systematizing process if we are ever to become definitive about stuttering and its causes. It is reasonable to assume that there are at least five types of causal factors—predisposing, precipitating, maintaining, intensifying, and complicating. The conditions, situations, events, and interactions contributing to stuttering might well subsume all of the possible categories of causes however they may be organized; but the struggle to encompass them meaningfully, to identify pertinent elements, to understand the interactions and exceptions, and to evolve an approach which will lead directly and reliably to alleviation of the problems due to stuttering apparently cannot be accomplished satisfactorily by a glib reference to "multiple causation."

INTEGRATION BY CONTRIBUTIONS TO BASIC QUESTIONS

It would appear that the pathways offered for integrating theories of stuttering, instead of illuminating and clarifying, lead to problems, limitations, and frustration. Until our knowledge is much more nearly complete, we need a framework *within* which divergent elements of theories may be discussed in relation to each other and to the basic understandings necessary for the solution of the problems of stuttering.

The earlier edition of this chapter (Ainsworth, 1957) proposed a way of doing this by determining the way in which a theory answers three basic questions.

1. What are the contributions to the *description* and *definition* of the physiological, behavioral, social, and psychological concomitants of stuttering? (This question is a rewording of the original question for use in the present revision, but its intent remains the same.)
2. What are the contributions to understanding the *process* of *development* of stuttering?
3. What contributions toward *explaining* these phenomena are offered?

The present revision proposes to further develop this framework in order to allow for more complex concepts and interactions as reflected in our developing knowledge and more sophisticated procedures for research. The framework suggested by the three questions needs two major additional features to enhance its usefulness. The first is the addition of a "depth" dimension to each question. The second involves further elaboration of the question on contributions to the development of the problem.

The three questions, as originally proposed, essentially provided a one-dimensional framework, and some basic differences among theories had no way of being expressed. An examination of theories reveals that they tend to order themselves along a continuum which can be identified as differences in the degree to which they focus on factors relatively near the surface of consciousness or on underlying mechanisms (either psychological or physiological). We can, then, "place" them along a "depth" dimension. This dimension can be conveniently divided into four levels or categories and ordered so that "deeper" segments undergird the more superficial levels. On this basis, the continuum would be divided as follows:

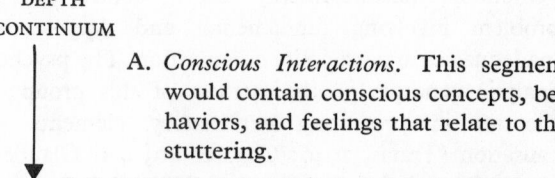

DEPTH CONTINUUM

A. *Conscious Interactions.* This segment would contain conscious concepts, behaviors, and feelings that relate to the stuttering.

B. *Unconscious Interactions.* This area would range considerably from assumptions, attitudes, and feelings that are relatively "close" to the conscious level (and can be fairly easily elicited) to deeper anxieties, conflicts, guilt feelings, and conditioned processes.

DEPTH
CONTINUUM

C. *Personality Structure.* Personality theory includes concepts of a structuring in some form or another which is, in turn, created by constitutional characteristics and the experiences of the organism.

D. *Organic (Constitutional) Structure.* This involves the biochemical, neurophysiological basis for existence and function.

The levels presented are not mutually exclusive and do not represent rigid categories. The lines between levels are dotted to indicate that they are stages along a continuum. Many theorists will agree on the existence of factors within all levels of depth for behavior as complex as stuttering, but feel that only one level may be of *critical* importance for the understanding and treatment of the problems. (It will be noted, however, that some theories shift levels as they move from causes to therapy.) The illustrations to be discussed below will demonstrate the use of this continuum for differentiating important components of various theories.

The second feature (on contributions to the development of stuttering) may involve a sequence of events over a period of years in the life of a stutterer. Therefore, some method for denoting different stages in this sequence is needed. It is proposed that contributions to the development of stuttering may be studied and described under the following divisions of a hypothetical time sequence for each stutterer.

1. *Before Stuttering Appears.* This is concerned with such concepts as constitutional "subsoil," personality characteristics of the "incipient" stutterer, environmental syndromes conducive to the initiation of stuttering, and interactions of the speaker with his environment.

2. *The Onset of Stuttering.* This stage involves immediately precipitating factors, descriptions of the process of transition from "normal" to a "disorder" behavior or condition, and the nature of the "primary" symptoms or characteristics of stuttering.

3. *Development After the Onset.* Here are the maintaining factors, the development of secondary activities and interactions, and changes in personality related to this problem.

4. *The Therapeutic Period.* Obviously not all stutterers go through a formal therapy period, and "treatment" may take place before or during any of the stages listed above. However, the study of any theory must include analysis of recommended therapeutic procedures to determine how they relate to and what they reveal about theory of causation.

5. *The Post-therapeutic Period.* Here again, this is hypothetical for many stutterers, but the nature of assumptions about, and the attention to, this stage must be the concern of anyone who is searching for a way to integrate theories. This period may involve the nature of speech behavior changes, social and personal changes, and personality alterations.

The total framework for the analysis and synthesis of theories of stuttering is summarized in Table 42-I. The remainder of this chapter will provide some illustrations of ways that theories may be placed within it and discuss some additional factors which relate to it.

The following discussion of the basic questions will make no effort to fill in all possible segments of the framework or to provide a complete picture of what is available in the literature. Selected examples will be used to illustrate ideas under the three questions and the subdivisions of development at various "depth" levels. The reader should then be able to study these and other theories in detail in a similar manner.

I. What Are the Contributions to Description and Definition of Stuttering?

It would seem difficult to develop any respectable theory of causation without some concepts or assumptions regarding *what* is caused. Therefore, it is not surprising that we can find a wealth of material providing contributions toward describing stuttering more definitively. The literature is full of clinical observations of stuttering behavior, most of which we recognize easily in the cases that come to our attention. It is when the descriptions become interspersed with assumptions about the stutterer that we begin to take exception. The first sentence of a lecture on Elocution delivered by Andrew Comstock in 1837 was not far from a present-day description. "Stammering or stuttering is a hesitation or interruption of speech, and is usually attended with more or less distortion of feature." He goes on to talk about two types, recognizable as clonic and tonic blocking. (Incidentally, he offers three levels of causes—predisposing,

TABLE 42-I
Summary of Framework for Analysis of Theories of Stuttering

DEPTH CONTINUUM	I. DESCRIPTION AND DEFINITION	II. DEVELOPMENT OF STUTTERING					III. EXPLANATION
		1. Before Stuttering	2. Onset of Stuttering	3. After Onset of Stuttering	4. Therapeutic Period	5. Post-Therapy	
A Conscious Level							
B Unconscious Level							
C. Personality Structure Level							
D. Organic (Constitutional Level							

exciting, and proximate—this last being "a spasmodic action of the muscles of speech.") The research of the last 30 or 40 years has added many more subtle details and refinements to the symptoms than could be obtained by the observant therapist in his swivel chair. We not only know that the breathing is often disturbed, but the fantastic disorganization of the whole mechanism has been explored in detail. (See Travis, 1931, 1933, and 1936 for reports of some of the earlier studies.) The locations and degrees of muscular tensions have been similarly studied. Steer (1937) reported on symptomatologies of young stutterers.

Not satisfied with purely physiological characteristics, workers have made numerous studies of psychological factors. One series, "Studies in the Psychology of Stuttering," by Wendell Johnson and his students, is particularly noteworthy for providing a detailed and accurate picture of the phenomena. Several of these researches have been published in the *Journal of Speech Disorders* and the *Journal of Speech and Hearing Disorders*. Further descriptive studies are found in volumes edited by Johnson (1955 and 1959). Recent summaries of many of these studies are available in Robinson (1964), Adler (1966), and Johnson et al. (1967). Stuttering has been found to be not only a wide variety of postures, tensions, and vocal patterns which accompany an interruption in speech, but it also is a pattern of behavior which varies in frequency and severity under particular circumstances (Bloodstein, 1949 and 1950) and is usually accompanied by a fairly representative group of attitudes about speech and stuttering by the person who stutters. Another approach to description plus an understanding of the relationships of factors in stuttering has been made by Hill (1945). He presents an "avenue of systemizing" many aspects in an interbehavioral framework.

Many of the studies are concerned with elements which may be placed in the conscious and unconscious levels of the depth continuum. The various behavioral signs of stuttering with their irregularities in occurrence and severity, the variation in degrees of awareness of them by the stutterer, the situations which relate to these variations, the feelings and self-concepts of the older stutterer are elements which have general acceptance, even though there are disagreements as to their meaning and importance.

As the studies progress further into the nature of the stutterer, toward the personality structure level, there is disagreement as to the nature or actual existence of identifiable personality characteristics. The most noticeable departure from the importance of these descriptive findings arises in the theories that identify stuttering as having origins in a neurosis. (Glauber, 1958, is an example.) If stuttering behavior in all its complexities is a reflection of a disordered personality structure, the important elements lie within the person, and elaborate study of the behavior itself is irrelevant.

Some of the elements in the nature of stuttering still have not been resolved. The "something" that is "wrong" seems to be a different entity in the varied theories. Some of the disagreements concerning stuttering as a disruption of fluency illustrate this difference. Disfluencies are part of the speech of all of us. Young children usually produce them more often than older children or adults. Johnson (1957) and Johnson et al. (1967) looked upon repetitions and hesitations of young children as "normal" and believed that stuttering is a behavior that develops in response to unfavorable reactions to these normal disfluencies. Brutten and Shoemaker (1967) took direct issue with the "normalcy" concept. They advocated that fluency failure is evidence of disturbance of functioning in the organism, and that stuttering is but one class of fluency disruption. Van Riper (1963) and Wingate (1962) supported the idea that stoppages on a sound and repetitions of syllables and sound represent different kinds of hesitancies than those occurring in normal speech. Glauber (1958) believed that repetitions of the first syllable are normal at first, but that in the second year they begin to reflect anxiety, thus giving a different psychological significance to disfluencies. West (1958) stated that in response to interruptions that are the result of an organic condition, repetitions may be attempts to retain fluency rather than a break in fluency. Thus we have theories representing various levels on the depth continuum and some within the same levels with divergent ideas concerning the nature and role of disfluency in stuttering.

An important development which concerns the nature of stuttering involves two different points of view. Older theories have stressed what stuttering "is"—some kind of entity which is characteristic of the individual apart from behavior—something which *causes* the behaviors (blocking, hesitations, etc.) that indicate its existence. Williams (1957), on the other hand, proposed that stuttering should be understood as something that the stutterer "does"—a focus on the behavior rather than something which is "part of him" and thus implies a certain kind of person who stutters. This behavioral point of view, in one form or another, has been utilized by others and is most recently illustrated in the writings of Brutten and Shoemaker (1967).

Description leads inevitably to definition, in fact or by implication. *Stuttering Words* (Fraser, 1963) provided several from which to choose. These range from several descriptive, behaviorally oriented definitions, to expression of anxiety, to identification with the whole person, to emphasis on the involuntary nature of the act. Wingate (1964) supplied what he considered to be a three-part "standard" definition which includes a number of descriptive statements. All who write at length about stuttering present a personal or quoted statement. With the possible exception of some theorists who look on stuttering as a neurosis, the definitions reflect the complexity of stuttering by outlining more than one basic component.

II. What are the Contributions to Understanding the Process of Development?

An understanding of the process of development of stuttering is important for formulating any theory as to its source. It is difficult to conceive of such a complex entity as springing "full-blown" into being, and throughout the years it exists, significant additions and alterations occur which need some explanation. That stuttering usually begins in early childhood after speech begins, but that it also can appear in later years (according to some definitions of stuttering), are facts which emphasize the developmental character of the disorder. In general, this concept has been recognized, as witnessed by "primary" and "secondary" stuttering and the "stages" or "phases" of stuttering. Perhaps the most critical judgments of the value and acceptability of a theory can be made from a study of how it treats this entire question of development. Some examples of discussions of development are presented below under the five divisions of the time sequence and with reference to different levels on the "depth" continuum.

BEFORE STUTTERING

Many theories give attention to the reasonable assumption that, since stuttering usually begins at some point in time after the beginnings of speech, "something" must precede and lead up to the event. This attention may focus on several aspects of the environment, on the child himself, or on the elements of interaction. It is possible to identify most of the ideas with a particular level on the depth continuum.

Factors identifiable at the conscious or marginally conscious levels involve high standards of fluency, intolerance of nonfluencies (Bloodstein, 1958), and listening erratically to imperfections in speech. Overprotective and perfectionistic behavior on the part of the parents may be important bases of stuttering (Barbara, 1954). At the unconscious level, there may be parents whose anxiety and conflict from a variety of sources (Glauber, 1958) may create conditions conducive to stuttering. Sheehan (1958) referred to primary guilt in the stutterer as a constellation of feelings behind the original appearance of stuttering. Murphy and FitzSimons (1960) felt that stuttering developed from anxiety arising from a variety of sources such as threats to self-autonomy, inconsistency, and belittling by adults. From another point of view, the work by Schuell (1946 and 1947) suggested possible culture influences which create additional pressures in males, with resulting anxiety and insecurity.

It should be recognized that the division of concepts into "unconscious" and "personality structure" categories may sometimes be an artificial dichotomy that does an injustice to the writers. However, a careful review of theories seems to indicate that they are talking about different levels. The important and difficult task is to determine what the writer identifies as the *critical* factors in stuttering. Does he focus on the *behaviors* of parents or others, or on the unconscious but readily available *feelings*, or on the underlying *personality structure*, or on some *combination* as being the important elements for attention in precipitating stuttering?

At the personality structure level there are three areas of sources from which stuttering may appear. One environmental source may be the parents—together or separately. Barbara (1954) identified them as overprotective and perfectionistic and unable to provide love and warmth at critical stages—and thus the environmental "soil" in stuttering is similar to other neuroses. Glauber (1958) considered the father to be passive and dependent and the mother as someone who has never separated from her own mother and who looks on speech as a symbol of separation. The mother as the source of "moral perfectionism" was noted by West (1958). The stutterer's own neurotic personality structure may be another basis from which stuttering grows (Glauber). Finally, the culture itself may demand the giving up of infantile pleasures and behaviors with fixation at or regression to earlier stages of personality development. The principal element in theories similar to those discussed is that a neurotic personality is created within the stutterer, with stuttering emerging as a symptom of this disturbed state.

Those who designate an organic basis for stuttering have nearly always assumed a condition in the child prior to the appearance of stuttering. West (1958) stressed a low threshold for seizures, while Eisenson (1958) felt that most stutterers are inclined to perseverate to a greater extent than most children. The psychoanalysts have stressed the ego defect of the stutterer but admit a possible somatic basis. Glauber (1958), for instance, considered that some stutterers may be hyperkinetic with lowered susceptibility to stimuli. Differences in conditionability, autonomic arousal, and behavioral activity level suggested to Brutten and Shoemaker (1967) that an organic condition may possibly have a bearing on the development of stuttering. Karlin (1947) theorized a delay in myelinization of cortical areas, and many others have called attention to some kind of neural irregularity or neuromuscular limitations as bases for stuttering. The organic theories concerned with causes antedating stuttering tend to concentrate on the neurological centers for speech.

With all theories, the student may well examine closely how the authorities relate the supposed "subsoil" to the emergence of the disordered speech, and the evidence on which this relationship is based. Some, for instance, infer predisposing causes from data obtained in examination of older stutterers and ignore the critical age level at which stuttering begins.

THE ONSET OF STUTTERING

As Bloodstein (1958) so aptly pointed out, anyone trying to explain the cause of stuttering must also clarify what he means by the beginning of stuttering—something which may prove difficult. He felt that the onset is a matter of relative potency of the amount of hesitancy the child exhibits and the degree of tolerance with which this hesitancy is reacted to—and thus producing blockages and other struggle reactions. A comprehensive theory of stuttering should probably give some attention to: a) what is happening inside the child and in his behavior as he changes from a "normal speaker" to a "stutterer"; b) how those persons around the child are feeling and acting; and c) what events seem to influence the process.

Probably the most detailed discussions of the onset of stuttering are provided by Johnson and his associates (1955, 1959, and 1967). He and others have identified the onset as an outgrowth of an interaction among three variables—normal disfluencies, the process of speaking, and the parents' attitudes. Bloodstein (1958, p. 31) agreed in principle but added that an essential condition is the child's belief that communication is a difficult process and that he must work hard at it. Eisenson (1958, p. 248) believed that in most instances stuttering grows out of the continued excessive perseveration which the speaker cannot prevent, but which he tries to stop. The stutterer mistakenly concludes that his struggle behavior is directly responsible for the release of the word.

At a somewhat deeper level of functioning, the primary stuttering symptoms, according to Sheehan (1958, p. 128), are prolongations and repetitions which probably represent the oscillations and fixations found in approach-avoidance conflict with regard to communication. Both Travis (1946) and Glauber (1958) saw stuttering as initiating from efforts to conceal repressed feeling and thoughts combined with a struggle to express oneself. Glauber also stressed the ego defect as a direct initiator of the muscular incoordination that causes stuttering. Although the hesitancies may first appear in response to parental prohibitions and restrictions, Barbara (1954) felt they may also be related to a basic difference in the stutterer's orientation to life and in his personality makeup. Eisenson (1958) also stated that the psychogenic stutterer as difficulty in "giving" himself as required in communicative, self-formulated language.

In the theories that denote an organic basis for stuttering, the repetitions or hesitations are considered as direct outgrowths of the constitutional deviation, but stuttering, as a communicative disorder, is usually precipitated by some kind of interaction involving personal or social stress. West (1958, p. 199) altered this pattern somewhat by his belief that the primary convulsions (producing repetitions in speech) are triggered by the *act* of communication, and the secondary activities are precipitated by *failure* of communication.

AFTER ONSET OF STUTTERING

There have been many descriptions of the process of the changes in stuttering after onset. Both maintaining and aggravating factors are presented in considerable detail in the literature. Perhaps writers have felt more confidence at this stage because this is when they see and work with stutterers and thus they have more experiential "data" to use as a basis for conclusions. The vicious circle of speech failures, attempts to "do something"—which in turn cause more frequent and disastrous failure—and the development of attitudes, feelings, and behaviors affecting total adjustment need not be repeated or summarized here. However, illustrations will be presented of differences along the depth continuum and in relation to predisposing or precipitating causes.

Bloodstein (1960) and Van Riper (1963) described four phases in the course of the development of stuttering, from an incipient or primary stage through advanced secondary stuttering.

Eisenson (1958) stated that both organic and nonorganic stutterers may develop similar traits, attitudes, and behaviors which are unreleated to the etiology or onset. Sheehan (1958) described five levels of conflict —word, situation, emotional, relationship, and egoprotective—which develop after stuttering is experienced. Johnson et al. (1967) and many others stressed the role of anxiety as a result of stuttering and as a maintaining factor. The variability in stuttering behavior has been studied extensively in relation to emotions, situations, and self-image. In some reports, secondary anxiety and guilt are noted at this stage, as contrasted with primary anxiety and guilt at the earlier stages.

Personality structure of the confirmed stutterer may both solidify and change. West (1958), for instance, talked about the characteristics of the "confirmed stutterer"—his perfectionism, ambivalence, and guilt—as basic in the personality. All adult stuttering is considered by him to be maintained due to the "psychoneurotic chain" because pyknolepsy (the organic basis) ceases at puberty. Barbara (1954) believed that there is further development of the neurotic structure of the personality as a result of stuttering.

In regard to the organic basis of stuttering, there are two opposing views: the original condition may cease to operate; the condition may continue into adulthood. As pointed out above, West definitely believed the cause of original repetitions disappears at puberty. Eisenson felt that this may be true in some cases. Karlin (1947) believed the condition ceases with completed myelinization. Glauber (1958), on the other hand, developed the idea that certain motor centers innervating the speech apparatus may ultimately be affected by the alteration in ego-structure.

In general, the theories agree descriptively but not as to the significance of some behaviors. There is general consistency with concepts concerning etiology, but there is also some acceptance of the idea that stuttering may come to represent a different entity as it develops and continues.

THERAPEUTIC PERIOD

Since this chapter is directed at a discussion of theories, the therapeutic stage may well be omitted except for some generalizations and some illustrations of the ways the therapy may be related to etiology.

In years past, it often appeared that although theories of etiology differed, the therapy suggested was remarkably in agreement. This characteristic is not as noticeable in recent writings. Therapy tends to be geared to the theoretical constructs and overlapping often reflects the areas of agreement. The ideas of Johnson for therapy (1967) showed his conviction that the evaluations of the listener and the resultant assumptions by the stutterer play a key role in the initiation of stuttering. Bloodstein (1958 and 1961) suggested differential treatment for the four phases of development and he concentrated on therapy for stuttering as an anticipatory struggle reaction. A further delineation of the approach was provided by Luper and Mulder (1964), who identified the four phases as incipient, transitional, confirmed, and advanced. Detailed therapeutic procedures for children (rather than adults) at each phase were provided without discussion of, or commitment to, any particular theoretical position. Van Riper (1963) proposed treatment designed to coincide with his multiple origin point of view. Brutten and Shoemaker (1967) designed clearly the therapeutic procedures in light of their learning theory concepts of stuttering. Sheehan (1958) aimed at reducing avoidance through a combination and interaction of speech therapy (by attacking word and situational fears directly) and psychotherapy (by reaching feelings, relationships, and defenses).

Those who see the stutterer as neurotic or with an ego-development deviation (such as Glauber, 1958) concentrate on a deep psychotherapy aimed at restructuring the total personality.

The organic basis for stuttering is not yet defined sufficiently for direct treatment (although some general attempts have been made with equivocal or poor success by the use of drugs and carbon dioxide). Treatment has thus been aimed at the factors which precipitate and maintain the stuttering, and on efforts to control the effects of the constitutional condition on the speech (West, 1958; Eisenson, 1958).

POST-THERAPY PERIOD

Many theories give little or no specific attention to this stage except as part of the therapeutic process. Few view it as a period with problems of its own if the therapy has been "successful."

Van Riper (1954 and 1963) expressed the need for continuing the conscious effort to cope with the problem—and thus the stutterer must become his own clinician. Johnson et al. (1967) described changes in attitudes toward stuttering, acceptance of stuttering, and improved word-fact relationships and other alterations in several dimensions, most of which involve conscious elements.

Sheehan (1958) is one of the few who has stressed the need for adjustment to fluency. He has also talked of getting acclimated to the new self-image, to feelings of strangeness and guilt for fluency, to disappointment in the discovery that not all problems disappear with fluency, and to problems that may be created by changes in behavior. Luper and Mulder (1964) discussed the post-therapeutic period from the standpoint of the clinician's obligations.

Personality structure may be altered. Glauber (1958) implied that after successful therapy the individual will act as a complete organism in all areas of behavior. Barbara (1954) also indicated that the individual will assume responsibility for his life, give up fictitious values, discard illusions, and have more realistic goals. West (1958, p. 187), however, believed that many will remain "stutterers" even after the blockings have disappeared—they may still retain the personality picture involving the moral perfectionism and guilt.

If the organic basis still remains, as in the perseverative theory of Eisenson (1958), the individual is faced with a continuing necessity to speak more slowly and in a manner consistent with the constitutional condition.

SUMMARY COMMENTS

An even cursory study of a few theories yields several conclusions. Not all theories give attention to the five stages of development. The framework reveals critical differences in the depth continuum and at various stages of development. Some theories give primary attention to personality structure as a source and as the focus for treatment of stuttering. Others concentrate on sources which are at the conscious level or which are unconscious but reasonably available for study and modification. Those who select a constitutional basis for the primary repetitions also recognize the role, at other levels, of many personal, social, and cultural factors in the development of stuttering. There are distinct differences at key points in developmental stages as illustrated by the Johnsonian concept of normal disfluencies (or "nonfluencies" in older writings) and Brutten's and Shoemaker's "fluency failure." This is noted at the *Before Stuttering* stage. Johnson and others look upon hesitations, repetitions, and other interruptions as normal. Brutten and Shoemaker feel that this leads to ignoring the disfluency (dysfluency) and to considering it devoid of meaning. Therefore, they prefer a term which identifies the event as evidence of some disruption in the functioning of the organism. At this same stage and in the onset stage, Van Riper and Wingate call attention to quantitative and qualitative differences in the disfluencies which they believe are significant. In the discussions of Travis and Glauber, on the other hand, the speech abnormality does not need to grow out of normal (or abnormal) disfluencies as such, but may be qualitatively something quite different—a direct expression of anxiety, conflict, and guilt.

III. What Contributions Toward Explaining the Phenomena of Stuttering Are Offered?

The statements above in regard to prestuttering and onset stages provide a general picture of the explanations for stuttering. However, attention has been directed to descriptions of *what* is happening; discussion in this section will concentrate on statements of *why* in reference to the depth continuum of the suggested framework. It will be noted that some theorists confine themselves to one depth level fairly consistently, while others present ideas that may be distributed at various levels. Understanding of the theories is further complicated by the fact that different level explanatory statements may occur with regard to the five stages of development. Most illustrations below will be limited to discussions of original or basic causes.

Several explanations involve primary elements which may be considered as conscious factors or which are readily available to consciousness. Johnson's et al. (1967) diagnosogenic (or semantogenic) theory identified the listener's reactions (particularly the parent) as the primary source of influencing the normally disfluent child to become a stutterer. Bloodstein (1958) saw stuttering as due to the relative potency of two factors: an unusual degree of disfluency from any source and an environment intolerant of disfluency. Van Riper (1963) suggested that in addition to parent reactions, the child by himself may become frustrated because of his need to communicate, but be blocked by fluency disruptors and thus develop the struggle behavior of stuttering.

At a somewhat "deeper" level, Sheehan (1958) saw the primary symptoms of stuttering (hesitations and prolongations) as the result of a double approach-avoidance conflict: an urge to speak and not to speak—and a desire to be silent and not be silent. This conflict may arise from many sources, but Sheehan considered primary guilt as lying behind the original appearance of stuttering. Secondary guilt contributes later in the development of stuttering. Also in the later stages, conflicts may be differentiated into Sheehan's five levels listed above. It is interesting to note that these five levels represent different levels of "depth"—from word fears (relatively conscious) to the ego-protective level (relatively deep in the unconscious). They represent immediate causes of the blocking rather than the original sources of the primary symptoms. Murphy and FitzSimons (1960) thought of stuttering as a reaction to anxiety which, in turn, may arise from five general sources, all of which comprise or produce a threat with which the child feels unable to cope.

At the personality structure level, the "psychoanalytic theories" go into extensive explanatory detail. The stuttering is viewed as a form of behavior growing out of basic drives and needs. Conflicts and anxiety are looked on as primary factors rather than something that emerges from reactions and situations surrounding the speech. The anxiety arises from the child's inability to express or gratify his subjective needs and, at the same time, adapt to parental expectations or standards. Stuttering is a compromise between seeking and inhibiting gratification. Authorities who consider stuttering as a neurotic symptom stress varied aspects of adjustment, and sometimes these aspects are viewed as beginning from different concepts of personality structure. Coriat (1931 and 1943) stressed the fixation at (or regression to) early pregenital stages of development as the source of stuttering and its symptoms. Glauber (1958) viewed the stutter as fixation and regression and as an attempt to defend against both. Travis (Chapter 40) draws similar conclusions but focuses more attention on the child's need to suppress strong unconscious tendencies toward enjoying culturally disavowed pleasures of sucking, eating, evacuating, and exploring. Barbara (1954) considered that the stutterer is like other neurotics in that he has lacked warmth, love, and respect, leading him to feel weak and insecure. There is excessive fear and concealed hostility toward himself and others with resultant guilt feelings.

In the late 1940's and throughout the 1950's there were relatively few studies which stressed the neurophysiological components that may be related to stuttering. This was in contrast to the period during and following the prominence of the cerebral dominance theory when literally hundreds of attempts were made to discover some physical attribute which could account for the speech behavior. Bryngelson (1942), for instance, reviewed 36 studies and concluded that they definitely supported the concept that stuttering is a symptom of an inner condition—dysphemia—which is an irregularity of neural integration in the portion of the central nervous system responsible for the speech musculature. Hill (1944a and 1944b), on the other hand, reviewed more studies of a similar nature and concluded that there were no true differences found between stutterers and nonstutterers in most cases. In researches where a constitutional variable was found, he felt that the differences could be accounted for by other means than to assume that they were indicative of a dysphemia. Throughout the years, however, there has been support for some sort of neurophysiological "subsoil" as being important in at least some cases of stuttering. Travis (1946) pointed out that the electroencephalographic findings of Freestone (1942), Knott and Tjossem (1943), and Douglas (1943) cannot be ignored. Although not all electroencephalographic studies have found differences between stutterers and nonstutterers, this point of view has further support from the study by Knott, Correll, and Shephard (1959) in which they found a difference in alpha band activity which seemed to follow the Ulett (anxiety-prone) group for one group of stutterers. Another group of stutterers did not show this difference. It is possible, as many have contended, that stutterers should not be studied or treated as a homogeneous group. As mentioned earlier, West (1958) held to a pyknolepsy concept as the basic origin of stuttering, and Eisenson (1958) advocated a basic tendency to perseverate. More recently interest in possible neurophysiological bases for stuttering has been raised by contributions in the area of servo theory and identifiable physiological differences which may relate to the learning of stuttering. Mysak (1960) viewed the disorder as a disturbance in reflexive and automatic mechanisms in various parts of the total linguistic circuitry. Stromsta (1959) related basic stuttering to distorted sidetone. This point of view offers a relatively precise active agent which directly produces blockages. Brutten and Shoemaker (1967) reported evidence of differences in conditionability, autonomic arousal, and behavioral activity which may have a possible relationship to fluency failures and the development of stuttering.

Those who propose a constitutional contribution to the complexity we call stuttering come closest to agreement in the idea that stuttering involves "something" at variance in the central nervous system—a variation in the neural flow which causes blocking of coordinated muscular activity. These findings do not seem to contradict the psychological or sociological determinants that have been found to be typical of stuttering, but they do offer additional explanatory material and are important to include in any integrated point of view.

COMPLETING THE INTEGRATION

The framework of basic questions to be answered in reference to levels on the depth continuum clearly provides a systematic procedure for simultaneous analysis of several theories. The selected theories are shown to have some fundamental differences that go beyond variation in emphasis and focus. At the risk of doing an injustice to some of the complexities and details of some theories, it is possible to note the following kinds of differences which discourage attempts at a single inclusive theory. (It should be repeated that the references are for purposes of illustration only and their inclusion does not imply that these are necessarily superior to some that are omitted.) First, there are the theories that look for an *active agent* which causes stuttering *within the child.* This may be constitutional or psychodynamic in nature. Constitutionally, the exact agent may lie in the relatively generalized cortical activity affecting the speech areas (West, 1958, and Eisenson, 1958); may involve relatively complex feedback circuits (Mysak, 1960); or may be a more precise auditory feedback disturbance (Stromsta, 1959). Psychodynamically, the interruption in neural flow may be triggered by a primary anxiety (Travis, Chapter 39). These theories are those which consider stuttering as growing out of what the individual *is*. They essentially say that "This is the kind of person he *is*, therefore he stutters." On the contrary, there are theories that seek this active agent *outside the child*—in the listener, in the immediate environment, or in the culture itself (Johnson et al. 1967). Some try to combine these and other possibilities in the "active agent" category—certain attitudes within the child plus factors in his environment (Bloodstein, 1958)—or constitutional elements plus social pressures (West, 1958).

Another quite different view is that the important aspects lie in the process by which the child learns to stutter. These theories do not necessarily ignore the somatic and personal dynamics but look on these as background that may vary considerably from stutterer to stutterer—but, the basic process by which the disorder develops is essentially similar. This point of view attempts to clarify relatively specifically and precisely the factors in this learning process (Brutten and Shoemaker, 1967).

Of course, there are some theories that attempt to bridge these two basically different approaches—psychodynamics plus the learning process (Sheehan, 1958). These, however, tend to be weighted in one direction or another. Furthermore, it becomes apparent that "learning" theories of stuttering may have fundamental differences.

Analysis, however, with differences becoming more apparent, is not the only outcome of the approach suggested here. Some synthesis is suggested. We find that there is often considerable basic agreement after the onset period. The factors influencing the complications of stuttering as it develops—personal, social, cultural—sound much the same in many theories. Differences are primarily on specifics, or the degree to which certain things are most critical, or on the relative importance of the original versus maintaining or complicating causes.

In our present state of ignorance, integration may need to stop at this point. There are still many intriguing unanswered questions. Is it not possible that the determinants actually vary in the degree to which they are precipitating, maintaining, aggravating, or complicating in different children? Just how may the balance of these factors alter as the child grows older and continues to stutter? Are the characteristics of the "stuttering" or "neurotic" stutters and of "normal" stutters different enough to dichotomize them? Why do certain children develop stuttering and not others who endure similar circumstances and biological background? Why do some stop stuttering under what would be thought of as adverse conditions? Why is there a 4:1 sex ratio of stutterers? Schuell (1946) proposed some thought-provoking conclusions, but recently Brutten and Shoemaker (1967) and others have taken direct issue with them. What combination of factors accounts for the radical, almost overnight change in the speech of stutterers? There are many other questions that need to be answered, but they do not materially affect the bringing together of what we already have, and there is no reason to expect that their answers could not find a place in this integration.

Even though some theories cannot at this time be easily reconciled, the integration method suggested here does provide a means for pointing up basic disagreements of definition, description, and explanation within the same framework. Nor is it necessary to "split up" a theory because parts of it fit in one category and parts in another. Practically, it means that in any argument or discussion of "stuttering" we have a way of making clear what "kind" of stuttering we are talking about; for it is not possible to think intelligently about "causes" unless we are aware of what is being caused and the process of development that the entity pursues.

Certain fundamental weaknesses of theories may become immediately apparent if they are placed in this framework. In this sense, the integrative structure is evaluative. Any theory which ignores the wealth of research on descriptive elements of stuttering, or bypasses the developmental characteristics during childhood, will be less likely to produce accurate and useful explanations. A theory which dwells on the essentially descriptive aspects and presents glib generalities for explanations is likewise suspect. Theorists who spend a great deal of time talking about the research and theories of others but who fail to show specific relationships to their ideas expressed on description, development, or explanation of stuttering may be expected to offer only random, accidental contributions of value.

An additional advantage of viewing theories in the pattern suggested here is that it allows for continual revision of integration as new theoretical concepts are found by the reader or experimenter. Thus by combining revisions with a standardized means for discovering differences in points of view in regard to each basic element of every theory, for systematizing essential contributions to stuttering theory, and for emphasizing weaknesses in information or construction, we come as close to integrating theories as seems possible at the present time.

BIBLIOGRAPHY

Adler, S. 1966. A clinician's guide to stuttering. Springfield, Ill.: Thomas.

Ainsworth, S. 1945. Integrating theories of stuttering. *J. Speech Disorders*, 10, 205–210.

———. 1957. Methods for integrating theories of stuttering. *In* Handbook of speech pathology. Travis, L., ed. New York: Appleton-Century-Crofts.

Barbara, D. 1954. Stuttering: a psychodynamic approach to its understanding and treatment. New York: Julian Press.

Berry, M., and Eisenson, J. 1942. The defective in speech. New York: Crofts.

———. 1956. Speech disorders. New York: Appleton-Century-Crofts.

Bloodstein, O. 1949. Conditions under which stuttering is reduced or absent: a review of the literature. *J. Speech Hearing Disorders*, 14, 295–302.

———. 1950. A rating scale study of conditions under which stuttering is reduced or absent. *J. Speech Hearing Disorders*, 15, 29–36.

———. 1958. Stuttering as an anticipatory struggle reaction. *In* Stuttering: a symposium. Eisenson, J., ed. New York: Harper.

———. 1960. The development of stuttering: II—developmental phases. *J. Speech Hearing Disorders*, 25, 366–376.

———. 1961. The development of stuttering: III—theoretical and clinical implications. *J. Speech Hearing Disorders*, 26, 67–81.

Brutten, E., and Shoemaker, D. 1967. The modification of stuttering. Englewood Cliffs, N.J.: Prentice-Hall.

Bryngelson, B. 1942. Investigations in the etiology and nature of dysphemia and its symptom, stuttering. *J. Speech Disorders*, 7, 15–27.

Cobb, S. 1943. Borderlands of psychiatry. Cambridge, Mass.: Harvard.

Coriat, I. 1931. The nature and analytical treatment of stammering. *Proc. Amer. Speech Correction Assn.*, 1, 151–156.

———. 1943. *In* Stuttering: significant theories and therapies, Hahn, E., ed. Stanford: Stanford.

Douglas, L. 1943. A study of bilaterally recorded electroencephalograms of adult stutterers. *J. exp. Psychol.*, 32, 247–265.

Eisenson, J., ed. 1958. A perseverative theory of stuttering. *In* Stuttering: a symposium. New York: Harper.

Fraser, M. ed. 1963. Stuttering words. Memphis: Speech Foundation of Amer.

Freestone, N. 1942. An electroencephalographic study on the moment of stuttering. *Speech Monogr.*, 9, 28–60.

Glauber, I. 1958. The psychoanalysis of stuttering. *In* Stuttering: a symposium. Eisenson, J., ed. New York: Harper.

Greene, J., and Wells, E. 1927. The cause and cure of speech disorders. New York: Macmillan.

Hill, H. 1944a. Stuttering: I. a critical review and evaluation of biochemical investigations. *J. Speech Disorders*, 9, 245–261.

———. 1944b. Stuttering: II. a review and integration of physiological data. *J. Speech Disorders*, 9, 289–324.

———. 1945. An interbehavioral analysis of several aspects of stuttering. *J. gen. Psychol.*, 32, 289–316.

Johnson, W., ed. 1955. Stuttering in children and adults. Minneapolis: Univ. Minn. Press.

———. 1957. Perceptual and evaluational factors in stuttering. *In* Handbook of speech pathology. Travis, L., ed. New York: Appleton-Century-Crofts.

———, 1958. Introduction: the six men and the stuttering. *In* Stuttering: a symposium. Eisenson, J., ed. New York: Harper.

———. et al. 1959. The onset of stuttering. Minneapolis: Univ. Minn. Press.

———, Brown, S., Curtis, J., Edney, C., and Keaster, J., 1967. Speech handicapped school children (3rd. ed.). New York: Harper & Row.

Karlin, I. 1947. A psychosomatic theory of stuttering. *J. Speech Disorders*, 12, 319–322.

Knott, J., Correll, R., and Shepherd, J. 1959. Frequency analysis of electroencephalograms of stutterers and nonstutterers. *J. Speech Hearing Res.*, 2, 74–80.

———, and Tjossem, T. 1943. Bilateral electroencephalograms from normal speakers and stutterers. *J. exp. Psychol.*, 32, 357–362.

Krausz, E. 1940. Is stuttering primarily a speech disorder? *J. Speech Disorders*, 5, 227–231.

Luper, H., and Mulder, R. 1964. Stuttering: therapy for children. Englewood Cliffs, N.J.: Prentice-Hall.

Murphy, A., and FitzSimons, R. 1960. Stuttering and personality dynamics. New York: Ronald.

Mysak, E. 1960. Servo theory and stuttering. *J. Speech Hearing Disorders*, 25, 188–195.

Robinson, F. 1964. Introduction to stuttering. Englewood Cliffs, N.J.: Prentice-Hall.

Schuell, H. 1946. Sex differences in relation to stuttering. *J. Speech Disorders*, 11, 277–298 (Part 1).

———. 1947. Sex differences in relation to stuttering. *J. Speech Disorders*, 12, 23–38 (Part 2).

Sheehan, J. 1953. Theory and treatment of stuttering as an approach-avoidance conflict. *J. Psychol.*, 36, 27–49.
———. 1958. Conflict theory of stuttering. *In* Stuttering: a symposium. Eisenson, J., ed. New York: Harper.
Steer, M. 1937. Symptomatologies of young stutterers. *J. Speech Disorders*, 2, 3–13.
Stromsta, C. 1959. Experimental blockage of phonation by distorted sidetone. *J. Speech Hearing Res.* 2, 286–301.
Travis, L. 1931. Speech pathology. New York: Appleton.
———. 1933. Speech pathology. *In* A handbook of child psychology (rev. ed.). Murchinson, C., ed. Worcester: Clark Univ. Press.
———. 1936. Studies in speech pathology. *Arch. Speech*, 1, No. 2 and No. 3, 7–247.
———. 1940. The need for stuttering. *J. Speech Disorders*, 5, 193–202.
———. 1946. My present thinking on stuttering. *West. Speech*, 10, 3–5.
Van Riper, C. 1939. Speech correction: principles and methods (1st. ed.). Englewood Cliffs, N.J.: Prentice-Hall.
———. 1947. Speech correction principles and methods (2nd. ed.). Englewood Cliffs, N.J.: Prentice-Hall.
———. 1954. Speech correction: principles and methods (3rd. ed.). Englewood Cliffs, N.J.: Prentice-Hall.
———. 1963. Speech correction: principles and methods (4th. ed.). Englewood Cliffs, N.J.: Prentice-Hall.
———, ed. 1966. Stuttering: training the therapist. Memphis: Speech Foundation of Amer.
West, R. 1958. An agnostic's speculations about stuttering. *In* Stuttering: a symposium. Eisenson, J., ed. New York: Harper.
Williams, D. 1957. A point of view about "stuttering." *J. Speech Hearing Disorders*, 22, 390–397.
Wingate, M. 1962. Evaluation and stuttering; speech characteristics of young children. *J. Speech Hearing Disorders*, 27, 106–115 (Part 1).
———. 1964. A standard definition of stuttering. *J. Speech Hearing Disorders*, 29, 484–489.

PART V

Language

43

Psycholinguistic Consideration in Language Development[1]

Harris Winitz

The year 1957, which marked the appearance of the "Handbook of Speech Pathology," signaled the beginning of a new age in linguistic theory. In that year Noam Chomsky's *Syntactic Structures*, a thin paperback of less than 120 pages, which in the next decade was to have a seismic impact on the many human disciplines, was published. Chomsky's intellectual influence has been so great that without it the discipline of language development would have continued as an uninteresting chronicle of developmental events whose only common feature was that the responses, events, or measures were described as vocal or verbal in kind.

Heralded by many as a Galileo or a Freud (Time, 1968) in his impact on linguistics, psychology, philosophy, and speech and hearing science, Chomsky's contribution has been twofold: 1. the derivation of a conceptual system, a generative or transformational grammar, to describe linguistic structures, whose many products have been 2. to question current behavioral approaches to higher order mental processes, and to arouse and stimulate those whose interest lies in resolving the fundamental questions of the theory and philosophy of human language.

"PROJECT GRAMMARAMA"

In a series of studies aimed to simulate the acquisition of a natural language, George Miller (1967) reports a number of fascinating findings under the title "Project Grammarama." Suppose a subject were placed before a typewriter, electronically tied to a computer, and told

TYPE A SERIES OF LETTERS USING ONLY THE "A" AND "B" KEYS AND THE SPACE BAR. WHEN THE SERIES IS COMPLETED THE COMPUTER WILL PRINT "RIGHT" OR "WRONG." TRY TO LEARN THE CORRECT SEQUENCES. WHEN FINISHED TYPE "STOP."

The subject decides to play the game and types:

```
AAABB
             WRONG
BABA
             WRONG
AAAA
             WRONG
        .
        .
        .
AAABBB
             RIGHT
BBBAA
             WRONG
AABB
             RIGHT
BBAA
             WRONG
AAAABBBB
             RIGHT
STOP
```

[1] Supported, in part, by U.S. Public Health Service (1-K4-HD-38, 907-01) and (HD-3571).

The subject stops typing. When questioned by the experimenter he is sometimes able to recite the grammatical rule for this miniature language: "Any number of "A's" followed by the same number of "B's."

How might a linguist characterize the subject's self-discovered rule? Perhaps by the following operation:

$$S \longrightarrow A(S)\,B \qquad (1)$$

Where S refers to sentence, $\longrightarrow$ to rewrite as, ( ) to an optional selection, and A and B to letters of this language.

Let us see how this rule evaluates "grammatical" strings.

A. Evaluate: AB
Derivation: AB (the optional rule is not used)
Representation by Tree Diagram:

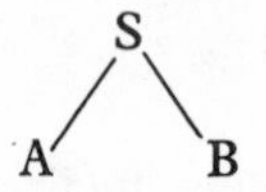

(2)

Decision: Accept as "grammatical."

B. Evaluate: AABB
Derivation: A(S)B (use rule with option)
AABB (use rule again without option)
Representation by Tree Diagram:

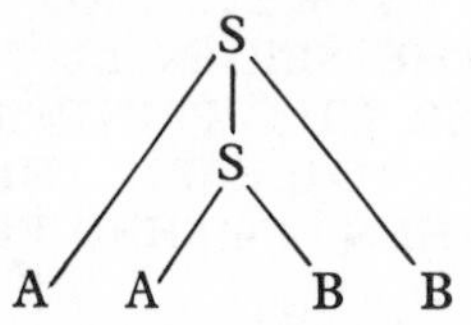

(3)

Decision: Accept as "grammatical."

C. Evaluate: ABAA (4)
Derivation: Impossible to obtain this string.
Decision: String not "grammatical" in this "language."

The above sets of letter-strings were evaluated by a set of rules which make use of a device called recursiveness. With Rule 1 we are able to generate, have as our output, an infinite number of strings beginning with any number of A's followed by the same number of B's, and only these. Strings in which the number of B's was less than the number of A's or strings which began with B, would be rejected by (1) as examplars of this miniature language.

Whenever we select S in (S), an infinite number of strings can be generated. All of the strings would, of course, take the form indicated above. The rewriting can go on forever because S is a constituent of S. Whenever an element to the left of the arrow appears to the right of the arrow the derivational process may go on indefinitely. This never-ending state of affairs, called recursiveness, is an important property of natural languages.

By using the mathematical operation of recursiveness there is no limit to the number of acceptable strings that can be generated by (1). Similarly, English, or any natural language, contains recursive devices, which accounts for the fact that the number of sentences of a natural language is infinite. Theoretically (but this is, of course, not the case) the sentences of English can be infinitely long in length. The well-known story of Jack's cat, "who ate the rat, that ate the malt . . ." is an example of recursiveness. It might be represented as follows:

the cat who ate the rat (S). (5)

Selection of S in (S) would result in an additional phrase.

Relative clauses are generated by using (S). For example, the sentence, "The car is old," can be expanded as follows:

The car (rel S) is old $\longrightarrow$ The car which I bought from Tom is old. (6)

Because the phrase "which I bought" is an inserted constituent of the primary sentence, "The car is old," it is called an imbedded phrase.

In everyday speech multiple instances of self-imbedding, phrases of the same type imbedded with each other, are characteristically avoided, presumably because discontinuities between subjects and predicates impose a heavy cognitive load on the speaker. Witness the difficulty in following this nontechnical sentence:

The car which Tom whom Mary loved
sold is parked on the corner. (7)

Although sentences like (7) are grammatical (because the grammatical rules of English have been applied correctly) they do not occur. Human factors, independent of the grammatical rules used to generate (4), curtail the occurrence of multiple self-imbedded phrases.

At first glance it may appear that (7) is ungrammatical, but note the following tree diagram:

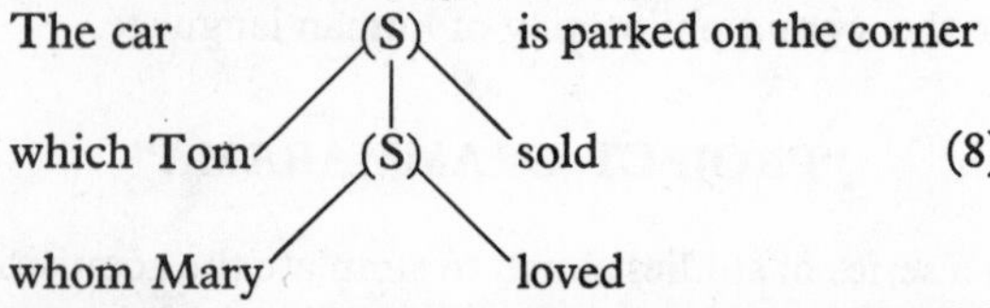

(8)

Sentence (7), as shown in (8), is similar to (6) with the exception that (7) has one more imbedded clause than (6).

Branches, Nodes, and Dominance

We can note some interesting relations provided by (2) and (3), reproduced below as (9) and (10), respectively:

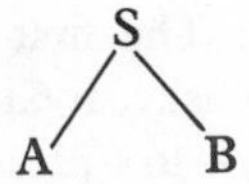

(9)

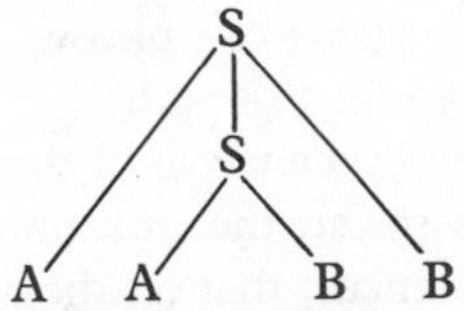

(10)

The trees have branches, represented by lines, and nodes highlighted by circles. The branches trace the history of each category symbol, the S's or A's or B's, while the nodes express the dominance of one symbol over another. Thus, in (10) the rightmost A comes from S, which itself comes from another S. The S-node which dominates the A also dominates the B; they are branches of the same basic stem.

Of psychological importance is the fact that the only observable items are the A's and B's, the terminal units of this miniature language. If one were to type strings of A's and B's which conform to Rule (1), an interested spectator would not observe the nodes, the S's, the ( )'s, and the branches. Yet these symbols are real. Later we shall learn that for the examples given above these symbols are items of linguistic competence, and that the symbols A and B are items of linguistic performance. A and B are terminal symbols because, according to Rule 1, they cannot be substituted by another symbol. And, although A and B are visible, their behavior is completely governed by linguistic abstracts.

Linguistic Competence

A speaker of a natural language has an unusual ability. He can produce sentences he has never heard before and interpret sentences he has never spoken. On every occasion his language behavior, as Roger Brown (1958) has remarked, is novel but appropriate. Can this ability be stated in some formal way? The generative grammarians presume it can and, therefore, take as their primary responsibility the grammatical representation of man's many sentences—those he has produced and those he has yet to produce. To do this the grammarian must first develop a formal device, a grammar, which operates according to established principles. The device, if it is working properly, will have as its output the sentences, presumably infinite in number, of the community language. Nonsentences will not be generated by this device. It is not enough, however, to have a device that operates simply as an input to a printout counter. Its mechanism will be faulty unless the "grammar-machine" has as its central goal the formal specification of the speaker-listener's knowledge of his language.

We can illustrate this process of grammatical generation by considering a miniature grammatical system, which utilizes noun phrases and verb phrases, the basic constituents of any sentence.

Once again an arrow (——→) will mean "rewrite as" or "become," and a plus mark (+) will indicate concatenation. Also the following grammatical categories and words will be used:

Grammatical Categories

S: Sentence
NP: Noun Phrase
VP: Verb Phrase
N: Noun (11)
V: Verb
Art: Article

Words

N: boy, girl, monkey
V: hits, loves, hates (12)
Art: the, a

Employing the symbols of (11) and (12), the grammatical rules are as follows:

S——→ NP+VP (1)
NP——→ Art+N (2)
VP——→ V+NP (3)
Art——→ a, the (4) (13)
N——→ girl, boy, monkey (5)
V——→ hits, loves, hates (6)

To derive a sentence we begin with that which is given, the category S. We then rewrite one symbol from left to right until rewriting is no longer possible. The procedure is as follows:

S
NP+VP (by rule 13.1)
Art+N+VP (by rule 13.2)
Art+N+V+NP (by rule 13.3)
the+N+V+NP (by rule 13.4)
the+boy+V+NP (by rule 13.5) (14)
the+boy+hits+NP (by rule 13.6)
the+boy+hits+Art+N (by rule 13.2)
the+boy+hits+the+N (by rule 13.4)
the+boy+hits+the+monkey (by rule 13.6)

The string "The boy hits the monkey" is called a terminal string, and the set of operations which began with S and ended with the terminal string is called a derivation. Categories, such as NP, VP, etc., are the basic grammatical components of a sentence. The grammatical relations which are expressed by these components, as a result of using the grammatical rules given in (13), is referred to as the deep structure of the sentence. Because we selected an impoverished grammatical system, the set of rules expressed in (14), the deep structure of "The boy hits the monkey," is obvious. It can be obtained by a simple parsing procedure, which first isolates the NP and the VP and then divides the NP into Art+N and the VP into V+NP, and so on. We might also apply names to some of the elements in the sentence, for example *hits* would be a transitive verb and *the monkey* might be called a complement. For the moment, however, we shall not be concerned with an analysis of this sort.

Using a tree diagram one can express the grammatical structure given in (14), as follows:

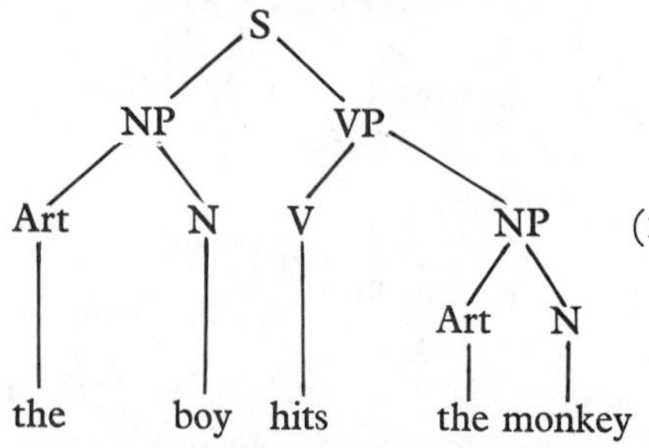

(15)

Or by using a bracketing system, the syntactic structure of (15) can be expressed as follows:

[(the) (boy)] [[(hits)] [(the) (monkey)]] (16)

The tree and labeled-bracketing diagrams show the basic constituents of the sentence as well as their interrelationships. Note that there is a direct and obvious correspondence between each item of the terminal string and its underlying structures. We shall soon see, however, that the deep structure of a sentence corresponds only infrequently with what would seem in some cases to be the obvious structure of the terminal or surface string. And, we shall soon realize that a sentence may have two structures, a deep structure and a surface structure. In the case of (14), the surface structure, represented by (15), a tree diagram, and (16), a labeled bracketing, is the same as the deep structure. In many instances, however, a surface analysis will lead to an incorrect accounting of the speaker-listener's linguistic competence; what he knows about his language—his tacit linguistic knowledge.

The difference between the surface structure and the deep structure of a sentence can best be explained by several examples which have gained notoriety in the past few years. The first example involves the sentence pairs (Chomsky, 1964):

John+is+easy+to+please (17.1)
John+is+eager+to+please (17.2) (17)
(NP+be+adj+to+verb)

where a grammatical analysis of the type given in (15) or (16) would associate the same phrase configurations to the two sentences, that is, their tree diagrams or labeled bracketing diagrams would be identical. Both sentences would be split into a NP and a VP. The NP would become John and the VP, at a certain point, would be rewritten as be+adj+to+verb. Finally the use of the rules adj ⟶ easy, eager, and verb ⟶ please, would fully mark the phrase constituents of the two sentences. This completed grammatical analysis, however, would not correspond to the speaker-hearer's linguistic knowledge of these two sentences. For having said *John is easy to please*, we can also say *it is easy to please John*, *to please John is easy*, and *what pleases John is easy*. Having uttered *John is eager to please* we would not construct the following sequences: *it is eager to please John*, *to please John is eager* and *what pleases John is eager*.

At the surface level the utterance pairs of (17) are identical in form, but at a deep and abstract level they are different. For in *John is easy to please*, "John" is the *direct object* of "please," which is not shown in a superficial (surface) analysis. In the case of *John is eager to please*, "John" is the *subject* of "please." The linguistic analysis should show that (17.1) and (17.2) are not comparable because they have a different linguistic history. The deep level will show this history or derivation; it will explain that "someone is pleasing John" when "easy" is the adjective, and "John is pleasing someone" when "eager" is the adjective. The underlying linguistic structure for *John is easy to please* will be represented at some point by *John is easy for someone to please*, while *John is eager to please* will have an underlying form that might look like *John is eager for John to please*.

We are in command of many grammatical relations such as this one. They should be represented in a formal way, written into a grammar; otherwise, the many linguistic abstractions, the linguistic code we utilize, will never be described adequately.

Stringing phrases together with "and" is a complex process. A maker of sentences must have a good degree of linguistic sophistication before he attempts conjunction. Consider the following two sentences:

John saw Mary.
Bill saw Mary. (18)

From these two sentences we can abstract some structural similarities. For example, we note that the VP is the same in both sentences. This permits the sentence:

John and Bill saw Mary (19)

In the following sentences the NP's are the same but the VP's are different:

Bill read a book.
Bill painted a picture (20)

Applying a conjunction transformation gives:

Bill read a book and painted a picture (21)

Similarity of surface form does not, however, always guarantee conjunction. Witness the impossibility of conjoining (22.1) and (22.2) to form (22.3).

Bill called up Mary. (22.1)
Bill called up stairs (22.2)
Bill called up Mary and up stairs. (22.3)

In (22.1) and (22.2) the grammatical representation of "called up" differs and, therefore, conjoining is disallowed. We may not have explicit knowledge of these rules, but nevertheless we make use of such rules. As we shall see below, a transformational analysis tries to express these abstract (deep) relationships.

One final example will be presented to demonstrate the complex character of grammatical rules, what we implicitly know about English grammar.

We can say:

A pleasing cigarette. (23.1)
A smoking cigarette. (23.2) (23)
A very pleasing cigarette. (23.3)

But we cannot say:

A very smoking cigarette. (23.4)

On the surface (23.1) and (23.2) appear to be similar, but a deep analysis reveals that "smoking" and "pleasing" have different underlying representations, the former is marked with the syntactic feature *verb*, the latter with *adjective* and, therefore, the rule *adj* ——→ *very adj* applies only to "pleasing."

For the moment let us reconsider the grammar of (13). A grammar which contains the rules exemplified by (13) is called a phrase structure grammar. Here each symbol is rewritten in a linear order and is given by the rule X ——→ Y. A more general form of this rule might be symbolized as WXZ ——→ WYZ, meaning X cannot become Y unless it is in the grammatical environment of W . . . Z. Restrictions can also be placed on W and Z, such as they may or may not be null, or they may or may not be identical. For example, a rule of this type might be used to distinguish between singular and plural verb forms and would look like the rules for C, rules (24.2) and (24.3) below:

Verb ——→ C+V (24.1)
C ——→ S when C follows a singular NP (24.2) (24)
C ——→ Ø (null) when C follows a plural NP (24.3)

Using a permutation rule (Chomsky, 1957) the S or Ø is placed after V, giving V+S or V+Ø, ultimately becoming hit+S or hit+Ø. Phonological rules would convert hit+S into hits and hit+Ø into hit.

Using a phrase structure grammar, well-formed utterances can be developed. For example, we can have by the grammar of (13) the following sentences:

the boy hits the girl (25.1)
the girl hits a boy (25.2)
the girl loves a monkey (25.3)

But not: (25)

the girl hits monkey the (25.4)
girl the monkey hates boy a (25.5)
the boy girl a loves (25.6)

The grammatical rules given in (13) will generate a number of well-formed English sentences and prevent the derivation of a large number of non-English sentences. However, a grammar limited to phrase structure rules will not only be clumsy and bulky, but will fail to express the many linguistic abstractions of which the speaker-listener makes use. (Chomsky, 1957, and Postal, 1964, for example). A phrase structure grammar which contains contextual restrictions is not entirely discounted by linguists if one's goal is simply to indicate structural regularity. Linguists, however, are interested in more than the kinds of structural regularity that can be expressed by phrase structure models. Models which list phrases and sentences and their constituent parts do not express precisely the many linguistic intuitions which speakers use. A level of achievement which seems to embody primarily taxonomic principles (segmentation and inclusion expressed by context-free or context-restricted phrase structure rules) is typed by Chomsky (1964) *observational adequacy*. Linguistic descriptions which terminate at this level fail to provide, as Postal (1964) has remarked, ". . . an account of all the grammatical information about a sentence which is in principle available to the native speaker." And so another "level of success for grammatical description" has been suggested by contemporary grammarians. This is called *descriptive adequacy* (Chomsky, 1964, 1965, 1966). A linguistic theory which is descriptively adequate will specify in a formal way the linguistic competence of a speaker. If obtained, this goal would be a monumental accomplishment for man, ranking closely to the major physical science achievements of this century.

Imagine specifying in complete detail a set of linguistic operations which describes what we know about what we say or hear. It would need to account for not only our syntactic structure but out phonological and semantic interpretations as well. In summary, then, for a linguistic theory to reach descriptive adequacy, it must contain a syntactic description and a semantic and phonetic representation giving each sentence a structural description which is in accord with the speaker-listener's linguistic competence. The linguists' responsibility is to select a grammar which best does the job.

How is a single grammar selected from a potential set of grammars? What form should these grammars take? We will face these problems shortly, but first an explanation of the semantic and phonological components seems essential.

The examples we have given above all pertain to the syntactic component (the rules of sentence analysis), but it is clear that sentences have semantic meaning and sentences have a phonological expression. All three systems, syntactic, semantic, and phonological, describe the grammatical competence of the speaker. Competence, therefore, is not restricted to the syntactic component, although most of our examples seem to suggest this view.

The syntactic component is viewed as the primary system on which the semantic and phonological systems rest. As developed by Chomsky (1957, 1964, 1965, and 1966), Katz and Fodor (1963), and Katz and Postal (1964), the semantic system operates on the deep structures of the syntactic component and the phonological system operates on the surface structures of the syntactic component. Chomsky (1964, p. 17) says, "The syntactic component generates SD's [syntactic descriptions] each of which contains a deep structure and a surface structure. The semantic component assigns a semantic interpretation to the deep structure and the phonological component assigns a phonetic interpretation to the surface structure."

We can think of a grammar, then, as having three components, syntactic, semantic, and phonological, with the syntactic component as primary. The input to the semantic component is the deep syntactic structure and the output is a semantic interpretation. The input to the phonological component is the surface syntactic structure and the output is the phonetic representation. Thus, syntactic descriptions pair phonetic signals with semantic interpretations.

Again, imagine a device which generates deep structures and then by a transformational process, to be explained below, generates a surface structure. Transformations which operate on deep structures do not alter the semantic meaning of the sentence. Assume that the sentences

Bill likes baseball (26.1)
Bill likes football (26.2) (26)

serve as the deep structure for,

Bill likes baseball and football (26.3)

The semantic interpretation of (26.3) is that which is given in (26.1) and (26.2). The "and" transformation serves, merely, to hook (26.1) to (26.2). Linguists have made no final statements as to how this process will be characterized, although a number of suggestions have been made (Chomsky, 1965; Katz and Fodor, 1963; Katz and Postal, 1964). What is of linguistic significance is the fact that steps have now been taken to assign to semantics a formal role in grammatical theory.

After the device has generated the surface structure of a sentence, phonetic rules will be invoked. For the purposes of this discussion we can think of the phonological component as applying to terminal strings, such as (26.1), giving [bll . . . b)l].

Since phonological rules assign a phonetic representation to surface structure, it is clear that two sentences which differ in deep structure but are similar in surface structure, will have identical phonetic representations. Each one of the sentences (27.1 and 27.2) will have two interpretations

Visiting professors can be boring. (27.1)
Fighting mobs can be dangerous (27.2) (27)

but only one phonetic transcription.

We can think of a grammar as having two meanings: the implicit linguistic knowledge of the speaker and the set of linguistic operations, syntactic, semantic, and phonological, which describe this knowledge. A grammar then, is a theory of language. And since language is a behavior of man, a grammar should describe in a formal way, man's linguistic expertise, his faculty of language. This singular achievement of man, as we have mentioned many times above, has been called by Chomsky *linguistic competence*. It would seem instructive to define competence in Chomsky's own words, as follows: ". . . a grammar mirrors the behavior of the speaker who, on the basis of a finite and accidental experience with language, can produce or understand an indefinite number of new sentences . . . We can test the adequacy of a given set of abstract linguistic levels by asking whether or not grammars formulated in terms of these levels enable us to provide a satisfactory analysis of the notion of 'understanding'." (Chomsky, 1957, pp. 15, 87).

"A distinction must be made between what the speaker of a language knows implicity (what we may call his *competence*) and what he does (his *performance*)" (Chomsky, 1966, pp. 9–10).

"It is obvious that sentences have an intrinsic meaning determined by linguistic rules and that a person with command of a language has in some way internalized the system of rules that determine both the phonetic shape of the sentence and its intrinsic semantic content he has developed . . . a specific linguistic competence" (Chomsky, 1967, p. 397).

How does a linguist select the grammar which best describes linguistic competence and is, therefore, descriptively adequate (that is, how does he select the most highly valued grammar)? This selection process is called *explanatory adequacy*. Some basis must be provided for this selection.

At least two considerations have been stressed (Chomsky, 1965, for example), only one of which has been stated explicitly above: 1. the speaker's linguistic competence of his native language and 2. man's faculty of language. The first principle is language dependent, the second language independent. The first pertains to the kind of grammar we select, when studying a single natural language, the second to the general grammatical principles that underlie all grammars, or stated in another way, man's faculty of language is a universal grammar which constrains the grammar of each natural language.

Transformations

The many linguistic abstractions of which we make use cannot be described adequately by a phrase structure grammar. Countless examples have been given which attest to this fact. (Chomsky, 1957, 1965; Postal, 1964, for example). A system which seems to handle this feature of language has its origins in symbolic logic and was introduced into linguistics by Chomsky (1955, 1957). It has the feature of analysis and in linguistic circles it is called transformational grammar, transformational-generative grammar, or simply generative grammar. The inclusive term at this time is probably generative grammar. As originally proposed, a generative grammar was most closely associated with the syntactic component and it had three properties: a phrase structure, a transformational structure, and a phonetic (morphophonemic) structure (Chomsky, 1957).

Using many of the facts but not the basic principles of the grammars that prevailed until the beginning of this present decade, Chomsky developed a procedure which best describes, at this time, the linguistic competence of the speaker. Its mechanism will become clear with several examples.

Examine the following sentence:

Dale likes Kansas City as much
as Betty (28.1)

It implies that,

Dale likes Kansas City as much
as Betty likes Kansas City. (28.2) (28)

but not

Dale likes Kansas City as much
as Betty likes St. Louis. (28.3)

The rule of analysis seems to be that when two NP compliments are identical, as in (28.1) and (28.2) above, the latter is deleted. It is called a deletion transformation, and can be stated with grammatical precision.

Consider the passive transformation which converts sentences like:

Richard defeated Hubert. (29.1)

into: (29)

Hubert was defeated by Richard. (29.2)

However, sentences like:

Richard is home. (30)

which do not have direct objects, cannot be converted into the passive.

In 1957 Chomsky proposed the following structural analysis for the passive:

$NP_1+Aux+V+NP_2$ (31.1)

which is changed into: (31)

$NP_2+Aux+be+en+V+by+NP_1$ (31.2)

The transformational rule which takes (31.1) into (31.2) is as follows:

$X_1+X_2+X_3+X_4 \longrightarrow X_4+X_2+be+en+X_3+by+X_1$ (31.3)

Two points, which may be puzzling at this time,

should be clarified. First, the auxiliary, abbreviated by Aux, is a necessary constituent in the underlying structure of the passive, although it may not be present in the surface structure. Thus sentences like:

The boy reads a book (32.1)

can be changed into: (32)

The book is being read by the boy (32.2)

by rule 31. The appearance of Aux in (31) can be understood easily by the student who wishes to give a little time to the study of generative grammar. Second, the arrow (———→) may be best defined as "becomes by structural change" (Chomsky, 1964). These two points of clarification, in reality, are significant ones and have consequences which are troublesome for psychological theories, which try to explain language acquisition. The principle point is this. There are structures which do not appear in the terminal strings of actives which are, nevertheless, critical for the derivation of passives. The invisible deep structures are "acted upon" prior to the derivation of the passive. The analysis takes place at a point high in the structural tree of the passive; it does not take place after the active sentence is derived. That is, (32.2) is not derived from (32.1), but from the underlying structure of (32.1) (actually the base structures which underlie all sentences).

Superficially, the derivation would look something like the following:

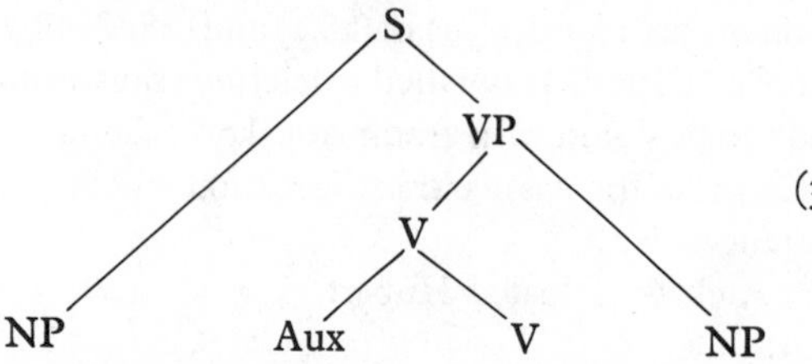

(33)

(Structural Analysis and Structural Change)

.
.
.

Passive Sentence

The structural analysis given in (31) does not represent fully our linguistic knowledge, as it permits constructions like:

Jennifer resembled Flora Sue (34.1)

to become: (34)

Flora Sue is resembled by Jennifer (34.2)

And so Chomsky (1965) recommended that manner adverbials be stated in the grammar of passive constructions. The deep structure, which governs the passive, was, therefore, altered to reflect this new fact about transitive verbs.

The deep structure of a relative clause transformation (Wh-transform) might look like the following (Chomsky, 1964):

$NP_1 + V + Wh + NP_2$ (35.1)

The structural change would be: (35)

$Wh + NP_2 + NP_1 + V$ (35.2)

Thus, from the underlying structure of:

Bill drove the car (36.1)

would be derived, in part: (36)

The car which Bill drove is nice (36.2)

One important step was neglected in the derivation of (36.2) from (36.1). We did not mention that relative clauses are embedded in NP's. Thus, using words to represent deep structures, a more accurate description of the derivation would be:

The car is nice (37.1)
Bill drove the car (37.2)
The car Bill drove the car is nice (37.3)
The car Bill drove Wh+the+car is nice (37.4) (37)
The car Bill drove which+car is nice (37.5)
The car which Bill drove is nice (37.6)

It is important to realize that, although in the above example "Bill drove the car" appears as a deep structure, it is never realized in the surface structure of (37.6). We would not say "Bill drove the car" (really the grammatical representation of this sentence) prior to uttering "The car which Bill drove is nice," yet the former sentence appears in the abstract representation of the latter sentence.

For purposes of this discussion we can think of transformations as having the properties of deletion, permutation, expansion, reduction, substitution, and so on. Expressions like substitution transformation and deletion transformation are common in the theory of linguistic transformations. The execution of such properties is specified precisely in transformational grammars. For example, an NP has been deleted in (28.1), because the NP's are considered to be identical. You can also think of transformations as corresponding roughly to the many sentence structures and types of which you are familiar, for example, passive, nominalization, relative clause, complement, question, negation, and so on. In any event, transformations, in an explicit and formal way, tell us about the linguistic history of every sentence. In contrast to the strict point by point substitutional (X——→Y) character common to phrase structure grammars, transformational grammars analyze structures and strings of structures, before a structural change is made. Whereas rules of phrase structure seem only to categorize events as they appear in a derivation (a sentence is composed of an NP+VP or S——→NP +VP, for example), transformational rules seem to express, by the method of analysis, the basic linguistic generalization of sentence formation.

Strict adoption of phrase structure rules will fail also to give grammatically permissible sentences for sentences which appear to display little abstract complexity, such as those generated by grammars similar to (13). We cannot generate sentences acceptable to native speakers of English which do not place restrictions on the part of speech which is inserted in a terminal string. Random insertion of lexical items would give unacceptable sentences such as:

sadness hates the man	(38.1)	
the man urged sad	(38.2)	
the ball knows John	(38.3)	
we escalate our enjoy	(38.4)	
grammars are happy	(38.5)	(38)
they persuaded	(38.6)	
the book likes me	(38.7)	
the John is nice	(38.8)	

Sentences (38.1, -3, 5, 7) seem to flow while sentences (38.2, -4, 6, 8) do not. In fact, if we reread the odd-numbered sentences several times they seem to make sense, perhaps as metaphorical expressions. No amount of imagination gives sense to the even-numbered sentences. They seem wrong or incomplete.

It is now clear that rules of the form given in grammars like (13), are not precise even for very simple sentences because they produce unacceptable sentences, such as those given immediately above. Additional rules need to be introduced, and they turn out to have the property of structural analysis which makes them more like transformational rules than phrase structure rules. In advanced theories of grammar (Chomsky, 1965) the odd-numbered sentences are said to violate certain syntactic markers for words which are placed into the correct grammatical slots. For example, the adjective *happy* in (38.5) is restricted to animate subjects and the verb *know* in (38.3) is to be used as a nonaction verb. The even-numbered sentences violate subcategorization principles which apply to parts of speech. Thus *urged* (38.2) is placed into a linking verb slot and *John* in (38.8) is placed into a common noun slot.

Phrase structure rules, therefore, are considered inadequate at the level of lexical insertion. To overcome this deficiency an analytical component has been added which applies to preterminal strings. For this reason, as well as for many others, transformations are regarded as basic to all sentence derivations. We shall no longer think of sentences which contain transformations and those which do not (actually those which contain obligatory and those which contain optional transformations); rather, we will think of a base component which begins with phrase structure rules but quickly utilizes transformational rules. No final decisions have been made as to the shape of the base component, but over the years (Chomsky, 1965, 1967) the base component has become rich in structure.

Explanatory Adequacy

Chomsky (1964, 1965) compares a child's acquisition of language with the procedures a linguist must use when he constructs a generative grammar of a language. What principles direct him to construct a descriptively adequate grammar? At the present time there are no such principles, only a sketch of some of the principles. That is, we know that the grammars of language will probably contain transformational rules, a syntactic component, a system for translating surface structure into strings of phones and the like. As descriptively adequate grammars are developed for the world's many languages some principles may emerge, perhaps at a deep structural level, which apply to all languages. Principles which have universal application will come most likely from the concerted efforts of linguists who use the exacting precision common to generative grammars. Explanatory adequacy, as a level of linguistic success, "aims to provide a principled basis, independent of any particular language, for the selection of the descriptively adequate grammar of each language" (Chomsky, 1964, p. 29).

Linguistic Universals

An explicit assumption of comparative psychology is that laws of learning will be discovered which are applicable in principle to all of this earth's animal species. Studying the simple forms of life, psychologists believe, will enhance their potential for the detection of variables which contribute importantly to the acquisition and retention of human responses. Similarly, linguists wish to discover universal principles of languages. Their search is for linguistic forms: linguistic substantives, and linguistic formals. Linguistic substantives are the elemental units of the grammatical system, such as phonetic (distinctive) features, noun as opposed to verb, plural as opposed to singular, etc. Linguistic formals are the rules of the grammatical system, such as transformational devices, phonetic organizational principles, lexical insertion rules, etc. Linguistic universals mirror man's faculty of language—man's set of linguistic abstractions which are said to govern the workings of all natural grammars.

A linguist searching for language universals is motivated by the belief that explanatory adequacy can be achieved. He assumes that although languages differ in certain details, all languages represent man's biological makeup. The biology of man assures a faculty of language; the biological unity of man assures one such faculty. Man is, thus, endowed with a selection procedure by which grammars are to be evaluated. This selection procedure, this faculty of language, Chomsky believes, has the form of an empirical constant.

Chomsky's Language Acquisition Device

The belief "that all languages share deep-seated properties of organization and structure" and that psychological theories "are intrinsically incapable of giving rise to the system of rules that underlies the normal use of language" (Chomsky, 1968, p. 68), leads the generative grammarian to the unavoidable conclusion that language acquisition contains a heavy nativistic component. Psychological theorizing as we know it today is not free from innate mechanisms invoked to explain behavior. Gradients of stimulus discrimination and generalization, deprivation states, fatigue factors, selector mechanisms, storage space for memory, and reflexes of all kinds are subjectlike mechanisms which play important roles in descriptions of human behavior. These attributes are considered by Chomsky, however, to be mechanisms by which knowledge is acquired and correctly belong to a theory of performance. Belief in linguistic universals presumes a faculty of language which possesses not mechanisms but ideas.

The distinction between mechanisms and ideas is not always clear. For example, depending on one's emphasis a mediational chain or a learning set may be considered either a mechanism or a structured event. Without entangling ourselves in a needless debate on the classificational nature of subjectlike properties in psychology, it seems Chomsky's emphasis is substantially correct. Psychologists have hoped to gain an understanding of the laws of learning by restricting themselves to simple events, like bar presses and mazes, and consequently little attention has been paid to the event which is to be learned. In his later years, Kenneth Spence (see Spence, 1956) often remarked to his students that much of his research would be restricted to a rat who runs a straight alley because laws of learning might be discovered initially from the study of relatively simple events. Perhaps for reasons such as this psychologists neglected the "what" when studying the "how" and the "why."

The central core of Chomsky's model of language acquisition, as would now be expected, is a biological faculty which predisposes a child to learn language. This biological faculty is his faculty of language, one of man's many intellectual faculties. This particular faculty may be thought of as a device which is capable of constructing a grammar, presumably a generative grammar, of a particular natural language. Stimulated by the utterances the child hears this device, because of its biological character, has the ability to construct a grammar. The input, resolution, and output of this process is diagrammed below:

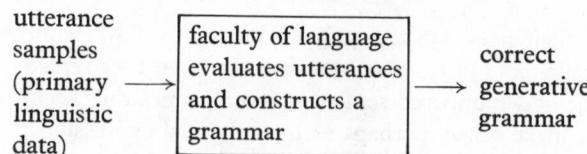

utterance samples (primary linguistic data)	→	faculty of language evaluates utterances and constructs a grammar	→	correct generative grammar

Having constructed a grammar the child has the ability to assign structural descriptions to the utterances he happens to hear or wishes to speak. Stated somewhat differently, the faculty of language has provided the child with an explanatorily adequate device, which predisposes him to select the most highly valued grammar for a particular language. In other words, he is guaranteed descriptive adequacy from the beginning. When it has been acquired the child cannot state these rules explicitly, but he has the requisite knowledge (a tacit grammar), which Chomsky calls linguistic competence. Although for Chomsky language stimulation is merely an energizer of an innate language mechanism (Chomsky, 1965, p. 34) as mother-neonate contact is a facilitating stimulus for a lamb's perception of space, he recognizes that language acquisition is not instantaneous. He and

Halle say (Chomsky and Halle, 1968), "A more realistic model of language acquisition would consider the order in which primary linguistic data are used by the child and the effects of preliminary "hypotheses" developed in the earlier stage of learning on the interpretation of new, often more complex data." This most recent statement is not unlike many found in the child development literature, but it is still a statement about competence as the context from which it was taken suggests, rather than an illusion to S–R variables.

Aside from the specific contributions of generative linguistics to the study of language acquisition, the implications of what Chomsky says for the discipline of child development and its "sub-disciplines," language acquisition, cognitive development, perceptual growth, for example, are, of course, extremely significant. But, such considerations have not been ignored in the past. Statements heard in a recent gathering of child psychologists echoed once again the general philosophical viewpoints of those who study child development. Particularly relevant to our discussion were the comments of Charles Spiker (1966, pp. 51–52):

> The student of the development of cognitive behavior and learning is concerned with the cognitive behavior of children that changes with age. He is also concerned with any processes of variables that he finds associated with changes in such behavior . . . we should certainly expect to find that there are physiological and anatomical accompaniments of cognitive behavioral changes, which accompaniments are largely independent of the organism's experience. . . . we should expect to find changes in cognitive behavior that are largely independent of the physiological changes that are not dependent on experience. . . . we should not be surprised if we find that an interaction between variables of experience and physiological factors is necessary to explain some, perhaps most, developmental changes in cognitive behavior We should not be surprised if any of these three statements turns out to be true since each statement is an empirical one; logic cannot settle the issues a priori.

It is interesting to note that the emphasis in speech pathology is largely nativistic, but it takes a different name and a somewhat different form. The principle is called maturation, and it is borrowed from the fields of child psychology and child physiology. Statements like the following are not uncommon by writers in speech pathology:

> Later, a few words, the most frequently used ones, become meaningful—then, of course, with maturation the entire vocabulary begins its development. (Wepman, 1960, p. 328.)

Perhaps for this reason experimental work in language acquisition, by those whose primary interest is language retraining, has been discouraged. Chomsky's model of language acquisition retains some of these same pessimistic overtones for psychologists wishing to investigate the acquisition of cognitive functioning within the general framework of S-R theories. It is also discouraging for psychologists with no theoretical attachments, who take the viewpoint that the environment contributes a significant but unknown quantity to the development of cognition. In any event, we will see that Chomsky's theorizing has provided the basis for recent proposals of language acquisition which are exclusively nativistic and have prompted statements like the following:

> The most obvious universal of language is simply that all normal children learn language merely by being exposed to it, without being taught it formally or conditioned to speak it . . . all languages have complex relationships among their words and sentences and other units. Children are not taught these relationships —they simply listen to language and figure it all out for themselves, the result being fluent speakers of a language. (Horton, 1968, pp. 248–249.)

Linguistic Performance

Although in psycholinguistic circles the term linguistic performance is in common contrast with the term linguistic competence, it is not easy to define. When Chomsky proposed these two concepts they seemed to have clear and clean operational properties. Competence was to refer to linguistic knowledge, performance to the acquisition, perception, and production of this knowledge. Competence, Chomsky assumes, is the central element about which performance models revolve, but performance will not determine the structure of competence. The mechanisms which govern language behavior are performance variables, like memory, attention, etc., and they can distort or make unacceptable speech utterances. An utterance like (7), repeated here as (39):

The car which Tom whom Mary loved
sold is parked on the corner. (39)

results from a straightforward application of the competence component (the grammatical rules which assign structural descriptions to sentences) of language use. Yet most speakers, including linguists, would reject (39) as a sentence. Since (39) does not qualify as a sentence, a structural description would not be tendered, on intuitive grounds; the identical operation linguists use to determine sentencehood (Bever, 1968). Although the generative linguists' strategy cannot be seriously questioned because of instances like (39), it is clear that such examples expose the abstract and complex relationship between performance and competence.

In 1966 two important conferences on psycholinguistics were held, one at Edinburgh University and one at the University of Kentucky. The Edinburgh conference (Lyons and Wales, 1966) focused primarily on the issues and relationships between competence and performance; the Kentucky conference (Dixon and Horton, 1968) contained several important papers on these topics as well as papers in related disciplines of verbal learning. What evolved from these conferences is the simple fact that the psychology of language is a tantalizing topic which tortures the minds of psychologists because they seem to have no general principles for handling abstract systems which make use of an orderly execution of rules. Crothers and Suppes (1967), in their text on the learning of Russian as a second language, believe that learning principles surely need to be extended if they are to handle complex language behavior, but they contend that there is no principled basis to exclude them from language behavior or even from the competence component.

What prevails now is a confusing picture of performance. Fodor and Garrett (1966) comment that many of the early studies in psycholinguistics conceived of competence as a distinct entity, a closed self-operating subsystem of the performance mechanism (see the perception model of Halle and Stevens, 1964, since it may have contributed to this conception). In fact, some psycholinguists took the linguistic distinction between competence and performance as a serious and confused psychological issue, stimulating Osgood (1968) to stress that one does not set up the grammatical rules and then begin to speak. That Chomsky had not this in mind is now most clear, when he recently said:

> It would be temping, but quite absurd, to regard it (competence) as a model of performance as well. Thus we might propose that to produce a sentence, the speaker goes through the successive steps of constructing a base-derivation, line by line from the initial symbol S, then inserting lexical items and applying grammatical transformations to form a surface structure, and finally applying the phonological rules. . . . In fact, in implying that the speaker selects the general properties and sentence structure before . . . deciding what he is going to talk about . . . seems counter to whatever vague intuitions one may have about the processes that underlie production.

That the competence-performance distinction must be rigorously obeyed in linguistic research is clearly obvious; confusion at this level would muddy attempts to develop grammatical principles. For models of language usage, performance will interact with competence at every mental turn to determine language behavior. The configuration of the competence component, when incorporated into a model of language usage, will retain its linguistic form, but it will seem disfigured beyond recognition. It is like playing a poker hand. Both the rules of the game, your own abilities and motivations, and your assessment of the skills of others, determine your next move. The knowledge of the rules of poker and the execution of such rules are a complex pairing throughout which your knowledge of the rules remains intact.

An obvious question, which may haunt you as it does me, is the psychological status of "the speaker's intent to say something." Certainly we would like a model of performance to account for the mechanisms which place the competence component or any mental or motor process into motion. Granted that in some instances, perhaps all if we extend our behavioristic definitions, stimulation and motivation initiate "what we are going to talk about." Yet how are these thoughts represented and how do they interact with grammatical competence? Such questions are unanswerable at this time and for many behaviorists are silly.

Can behavioristic models be used to explain language behavior? There are generally two answers to this question. Writers like Katz and Postal (1964), Weksel, Fodor, and Bever (1966), McNeill (1966), and Lenneberg (1967), braced by the transformational approach, say definitely not. Those like Jenkins (1966), Crothers and Suppes (1967), Osgood (1968), Kendler (1968), and Braine (1966), steeped in one form or another of behaviorism, say no to current behavioristic models, but believe that behaviorismlike models can be extended to include language behavior. All psycholinguists agree that Chomsky's conceptual contribution to the understanding of language acquisition and language perception, to say the least, has been significant. Not all concede that behaviorism should give way to a mental automaton.

The attack on behaviorism takes essentially two forms: 1. the inability of associative chains to explain syntactic principles, and 2. the inability of stimulus events to cause or contain linguistic abstractions. The first of these two purported weaknesses of behaviorism has not been mentioned up to now, simply because most behaviorists do not contend that left-right dependencies can be instituted as a serious model of syntactic functioning or of cognitive models in general (Bruner, Goodnow, and Austin, 1956, Kendler and Kendler, 1963, Osgood, 1968, for example). A model of this sort (Chomsky, 1957, Miller and Chomsky, 1963) has been called a finite-state grammar. In the simplest case it would consist of words strung together, their juxtapositioning determined by unit probabilities and transitional probabilities. This system would produce many strings that would be rejected by speakers as English sentences. For example, from:

Smoking accelerates cancer (40.1)

and:

The boy is smoking (40.2) (40)

one obtains:

The boy is smoking accelerates cancer (40.3)

Most importantly, however, this approach ignores the structural descriptions (deep and surface structures) of sentences, the very reason for the development of the transformational approach.

This criticism has also been leveled at mediational theories (Bever, Fodor, and Garret, 1968) as well, because the elements of mediational chains are superfluous, conceptual baggage, which when open to careful scrutiny turn out to be part of a linear chain, whose unobservables are, in fact, observables and therefore could not qualify as abstract entities of the sort found in current grammatical descriptions of language. Thus S-R behaviorism, according to some psycholinguists, is conceptually unequipped to forge a model of competence.

This attack largely confuses the issue, for S-R mediation models, in most instances, are performances models, not statements of competence. When S-R mediational "chains" are employed as models of competence, they seem to take on the same psychological "status" as deep structures of sentences. There is, of course, no formal equivalence between mediational models and linguistic abstracts (and mediational models are humble by comparison) but there are some similarities.

Consider the mediational model in verbal learning known as A-B, A-B′—A-B (Postman, 1959). This sequence denotes a retention schema. Here two lists of verbal associates are learned on one occasion and only the first list is tested for retention several hours or days later. The verbal pairs might look like the following:

Original Learning (A-B)	Interpolated Learning (A-B′)	Retention (A-B) (41)
3-table	3-chair	3-table
7-dress	7-suit	7-dress

In (41) the stimuli remain the same, but the responses change. B′ signifies that the response pairs of the interpolated list (the second list, denoted as A-B′) are common verbal associates to the corresponding response pairs of list A-B (the first list). That is, a common free associate to "table" is "chair" and to "dress" is "suit."

In paradigm (41) response pairs are recalled with considerable efficiency. Retention is far greater than would be the case if the responses of lists one and two were not verbal associates. Presumably subjects utilize a mediational chain when learning the second list, pictured as follows:

Stimulus		Implicit Response		Overt Response
3	- - -	(table)	- - -	chair (42)
7	- - -	(dress)	- - -	clothes

If verbal associates are not used as response pairs in the second list, response interference takes place and the recall scores for the first list are considerably reduced (retroactive interference).

The left-right chain of (42) expresses only a time-dependent relation. No doubt hierarchial relationships and structural analyses of a complex sort are taking place as the subject solves the paradigm represented in (41). No doubt it is far more complex than that depicted in (42). Even so (42) provides a schema which predicts, given the same experimental situation, but not the same words, retroactive facilitation.

When looked at closely, mediation models as models of language usage do not express left-right dependencies between elements in a chain of elements, but rather characterize, sometimes in mathematically rigorous ways, R as a function of S. And indeed vertical as well as horizontal processes are explicit dimensions of these cognitive models (see, for example, Kendler and Kendler, 1963). Jenkins (1965) has remarked that mediational models may be a stepping stone for the study of simple grammatical systems. He realizes that, as the models now stand, they are incapable of explaining the acquisition of language or conceptual systems less complex than language.

In summary it would seem that the potential contribution of mediational models is in the performance domain of language acquisition and usage. It is doubtful that competence models of language will be developed from mediational accounts. On the other hand, one cannot discount the possibility that mediational models will someday develop to the point where they can be used as final arbitrator in decisions of linguistic competence. For, if linguistic competence is to reflect a distinctly human function it should be psychologically real. And this is the direction in which psycholinguistic research seems to be bending (Wales and Marshall, 1966).

It now seems clear why Chomsky (1959) was so disenchanted with Skinner's (1957) *Verbal Behavior*. Skinner's paradigms, which made use of stimulus and reinforcement events, do not account for the development of the competence component. His behavioral system did not say how rules and abstract elements are learned. His performance paradigms were of no assistance in the development of linguistic competence. Although the bulk of Chomsky's review was a critique of Skinner's performance model of language usage—because he insists that behavioral terms were employed as "cover terms" for the many superficial accounts of language usage—it is evident that his annoyance lay with the fact that behavioral descriptions of language usage are conceptually too thin to wrestle with the complexities of grammatical competence.

Biological Considerations in the Development of Language

MATURATIONAL CONSIDERATIONS

Language learning cannot take place without maturational prerequisites. This point is made clearly by Lenneberg (1967) in his **Biological Foundations of Language.** Lenneberg's thesis is well documented and well expressed. He contends that the biological mechanisms which underlie the acquisition and use of language are specific to man. He does not deny that environmental effects may be sizeable, but he does seem to say that the balance of control lies within the brain. His text musters biological support for the mentalistic position—the environment triggers innate mechanisms which determine the form of all natural languages. Lenneberg's position is not disagreeable to learning theorists (see Spiker's comments above). However, probing into Lenneberg's bits of evidence uncovers areas of potential disagreement. For example, according to Lenneberg, the several language stages are acquired across languages and across cultures with uncanny regularity, although he recognizes that linguistic deprivation will result in language retardation. He notes that all normal and healthy children begin to utter their first words at about 12 months, two-word utterances at about 18 months, and so on. Psychologists of learning might ask why Ute and Cowichan children (Stewart, 1960) do not utter their first words until about 15 months and are considerably delayed in saying their first sentences. Possibly the environment is more structured than Lenneberg supposes. Possibly elementary skills must antedate complex skills. Possibly motivational factors, which may have a biological basis, relate in a complex way to language learning.

IMPRINTING

A curious bit of behavior, called imprinting, has fascinated the minds of ethologists and psychologists for almost a century (Sluckin, 1965). Presumably there is a short, fairly well-defined interval of time in the life of certain species, primarily young precocial birds, when approach and follow responses to a moving object are established. In the natural habitat the imprinted object is the parent of the newly hatched infant, but in the laboratory other species, geometric forms and even the hands of the experimenter have been stimulus sources for early attachments. It was generally believed that this "stamping in" process, called imprinting, took place during a critical period, perhaps the first few days of infancy, was irreversible, and although innate provided a foundation for early learning. Of late some of these general notions have been expanded and amplified (see Sluckin, 1965). For example, experimenters have observed that the stimulus need not be specific. It is as though the imprinting mechanism is a given avian universal which accepts any stimulus that impinges upon its sense organs.

Although the underlying mechanism of imprinting is no doubt innate, there is a wide range of stimulus conditions which show its effect. Attachments will vary with the kind of movement presented. Visual and auditory stimulation may vary in dominance for a given species. Early experiences such as socialization and isolation alter expected outcomes.

Can we develop any analogies between imprinting and language acquisition? Perhaps not, because the permanency of imprinting is not well known, information on human infants is fragmentary and incomplete, and the relation between imprinting and associative learning is only now being studied. Like the development of imprinted responses, language acquisition varies with the stimulus conditions, which are more elaborate than those which accompany "approaching and following" responses. Unlike imprinting, however, language acquisition occurs at a time when the human infant has developed many simple and complex responses which no doubt contribute to the language learning process. Whether one takes a strong or weak position on the relation between maturation and language development, it is unclear why acquired mechanisms and all that they imply might be excluded when a species-specific behavior as complex as language is about to be developed.

Syntactic Development

With the new developments in linguistics a style of data collection, familiar to three generations of speech pathologists, has ended. It began with McCarthy (1930) and terminated with Templin (1957). Characterized by precision and persistence it provided the background for many of the language tests developed by speech pathologists. To scorn (Tikofsky, 1968) these studies as simple counting exercises is to misunderstand the flow of scientific inquiry. Who could have predicted the elegance and balance of the transformational approach? Who could have guessed that when "structure" is interpreted as "competence" all of the linguistic parts seem to fall into place?

Within the classical tradition, length of response and structural completeness were the primary measures employed to describe the growth of syntax. Length of response refers to the number of words per sentence (or utterance). Since this metric is derived from a sample of sentences, usually 50 it is often called mean length of response. Structural completeness has been described in at least two ways: 1. the percentage of sentence types (e.g., functionally complete but structurally incomplete, simple sentence, and compound sentence) and 2. the mean of the structural complexity index, which is calculated by assigning weights to sentence types (e.g., 0 to functionally complete but structurally incomplete and 4 to complex sentences). Scores from measures like these have been correlated with a number of social and individual variables like sex, I.Q. and socioeconomic status (see Chapters 44 and 45).

Length of Response

At approximately 18 months the young child is uttering phrases almost a word and a half in length. By seven years his average utterance is seven and one-half words. This development is given in more detail below:

AGE (YEARS)	MEAN WORD-LENGTH OF RESPONSE (FROM MCCARTHY, 1930, AND TEMPLIN, 1957)
1.5	1.2
2.0	1.8
2.5	3.1
3.0	4.1
4.0	5.4
5.0	5.7
8.0	7.6

The above values should not be viewed as developmental constants, since the experimental setting may contribute a sizeable degree of variance not completely known at this time (Fischer, 1934, and Cowan, Weber, Hoddinott, and Klein, 1967). No doubt the above age increments reflect the increasing complexity of syntactic usage. Brown and Fraser (1964) have reported that sentence length in morpheme shows an increase of almost two units when children of about two and one-half years employ the "be" in progressive construction and the modals "will" and "can."

The structural complexity of sentences also increases with age. Below you can see that, as the child gains years, functionally complete but structurally incomplete sentences decrease, while simple sentences without a phrase and compound and complex sentences increase (other types omitted):

AGE	PERCENTAGE OF FUNCTIONALLY COMPLETE BUT STRUCTURALLY INCOMPLETE	PERCENTAGE OF SIMPLE SENTENCES WITHOUT A PHRASE	PERCENTAGE OF COMPLEX AND COMPOUND SENTENCES
1.5	78	10	0
2.0	54	17	1
2.5	35	38	2
3.0	28	32	3
5.0	17	36	9
8.0	9	32	15

(from McCarthy, 1930 and Templin, 1957)

Other structural measures were reported in great

detail in these studies. For example, Templin (1957) charts subject omissions and verb omissions, prepositional development, and slang responses, to name just a few. However, it is Menyuk (1963a, 1964b), influenced by the transformational approach, who gives the most complete account of the acquisition of sentence types. The earliest age group of Menyuk's two studies was about three years and the latest age group was about five and a half years. Although during this age interval children continue to acquire many of the sentence types (presumably the underlying transformational rules) children of three years of age use such complex structures as negation, question, relative clause, conjunction, *do*, pronominalization, and adjective (transformation). From three to four years many children use the passive, reflexive, *if* and *so*, and the auxiliary *have*. By five and a half years children compare favorably with the adults from whom they acquired or were stimulated to learn their language. Achievement of language skills continues beyond this age, but it seems that the bulk of syntactic learning (phonological and semantic as well) occurs from about two years to about five years, depending upon environmental and social factors.

A tantalizing if not the critical, consideration from the standpoint of psycholinguistic theory is that of the development of linguistic competence. All students of language development are concerned with this matter, since they focus on the mastery of language forms as a function of age. But only until recently have the issues become clear, the experimental method unclear.

Studies which will be reviewed shortly emphasize the emergence of grammatical rules. Heretofore the emphasis has been on the elimination of (grammatical) errors. Menyuk (1963a, 1963b, 1964a and 1964b) makes this point clear when she speculates that those utterances of children which adults regard as ungrammatical, are generated by alternate restricted rules (that is, rules restricted to children).

Pushing aside methodological considerations, such as whether or not many of the sentences analyzed by Menyuk were well formed, that is, revisions, false starts and stops, and isolated from semantic reference, we are confronted with a complex research problem. How do we characterize the development of competence? What abstract schemas allow the generation of those utterances we regard as "well formed" and those we regard as alternate forms in the specific way in which these matters are handled in the descriptions of "fully-developed" languages? For example, Menyuk (1964b) reports errors of inversion, such as "Crayons I want" and "I know who is he." It is clear from her report that children use permutation rules, but that they are not applied "correctly" in all instances. This finding suggests that studies of child language would need to show the acquisition of abstract schemas (like permutation and placement rules) which govern transformations, as well as an age-by-age description of their relation to the development of transformations. This last statement implies that competence descriptions of child language are regarded as far more complex than those for adult grammars, since the grammars would need to include (deep) syntactic rules and (deep) syntactic rules of language change. In a study by Brown (1968), to be discussed below, it is suggested that the alternate grammatical structures of children are intermediate forms which reflect the acquisition of internal structures. For example, an utterance "what his name?" could be classed as an alternate verbomission form. But we would not know whether the child's structure is "what is his name?" or "what his name is?" The latter sentence is, as we shall see below, an intermediate form which occurs prior to the development of the English question form. Brown and others (e.g., Bloom, 1967) contend that a close examination of the discourse patterns between child and parent may disclose, in part, the process by which a child learns transformations. A static analysis might obscure or wrongly interpret the child's early utterances.

The diachronic study of child language is further complicated by the fact that reference is usually made to the community language, hence Menyuk's reason for calling sentences which adults would not utter "alternate restricted forms." Terminology such as this implies that alternate forms are generated by changes in grammatical trees, some deep and some shallow, using the adult grammar as the primary system for analysis. As we shall see below, students of child language have begun to emphasize the regularity of language acquisition by recourse to universal laws of acquisition, a suggestion made by Jakobson (1941) many years ago. Within this context let us assume that certain grammatical forms do not appear in all languages, for example, certain verbs or articles, like *be* and *a*. These might be introduced into languages like English by an "introduction" transformation. Thus, in some instances, structures like verb and article omissions, might be regarded as basic forms not alternate forms. They would appear in the deep levels of the base component and, thus, would not be regarded as deletions. The implications of this approach would seem to be obvious.

Finally, we may ask whether or not it would seem propitious, from a performance point of view, to call underdeveloped grammatical forms errors. This view is not wholly unjustified, especially for one who wishes to examine the role of learning in sentence acquisition. Suppose we accept the premise that children change, in a series of steps, their language responses (really the underlying rules) until they are isomorphic to the language responses of the adults who surround them. Why? Because impoverished sentence forms are considered errors and errors result in no reinforcement? Because the cortical system is maturing and can only handle certain sentence types at certain age levels? Because the cortical system can handle all sentence types between the ages of two and three years, but the rules must be induced (given the cortical ability to do so), and that the induction process is roughly correlated with axiomized systems of grammatical competence in that base structures are acquired early, transformations later and recursions at some point in between?

A number of general experimental questions can be generated almost immediately. Two which quickly come to mind are: 1. can late-appearing sentence types be learned early if subjects are presented with a learning situation which demands their usage? and 2. can difficult grammatical structures be learned early if cognitive functions which are expressed by these structures are acquired early? Before we gain momentum in our speculations we should turn to those studies which describe the genesis of syntax.

Early Syntactic Development

Early writers of the discipline of child language were much aware of the creative aspect of language even though they did not have a "feeling" for the term "competence" as writers seem to have today. Carroll (1939), in a paper now generally forgotten, posed questions that are no different in character from those which have emerged in the past decade. With regard to the child's early two-word phrases Carroll (1939, p. 225) remarks:

> An element . . . is differentiated grammatically when it has a functional individuality independent of any phrases in which the element may occur. The concept of differentiation proposes to explain the detaching of "a" from "a doll," and its use in "a telephone" before the child has ever heard that phrase.

Carroll realized that phrase construction is a creative process, and he speculated that it involves differentiation of adult phrases into its constituent parts which can then be reconstructed to form novel phrases. More than 20 years elapsed, however, before investigators took up the problem in earnest. Their investigations were begun in those transitional years of the early 1960's when for the transformational school the sine curve of linguistic productivity was moving from 0° to 90° and in their hearts and minds linguistic knowledge was moving from just beyond zero to one.

At about 20 months of age, equipped with maturational prerequisites, as yet undefined (Lenneberg, 1967), many children begin putting two words together. These two-word assemblies signal the beginnings of a productive grammatical career. It is now realized that these "primitive" sentences display many of the complexities of adult sentences. Both high-frequency items (function words, such as *of*, *the*, *a*, *no*) and low-frequency items (content words, such as nouns, verbs, adjectives, and adverbs) can be found in the child's speech. The basic syntactic constructions of modifier-head, noun-verb, and verb-complement occur. As is true with most human skills, the language performance of children exhibits an expected measure of individuality, yet a degree of structural regularity is shared by all.

Braine (1963a) noted that the two-word utterances of his three subjects contained two classes of words, one subset included a small number of words frequent in occurrence, and another subset included a large number of words infrequent in occurrence. He called the former pivot words (P-words) and the latter class words (X-words). The pivot words fell into two groups, those occurring in the initial position of a phrase and those occurring in the final position. For example, one subject was observed to say:

see baby see pretty	shoe off shirt off water off
no mama no water	mail come mama come
other shoe other shirt other milk	

Braine called utterances, as instanced above, "pivotal constructions" because the underlying grammatical schema seemed to be that of a P-word operating on an X-word. He speculated that in most instances the phrase structure formulae might be:

$$S \longrightarrow P_1X \quad (43.1)$$
and
$$S \longrightarrow XP_2 \quad (43.2) \qquad (43)$$

The above rewrite rules suggest there are two parts of speech and that the grammatical distinction of the P-words is positional regularity. Realizing that there was not complete overlap within each of the two P-X constructions (e.g., P_1X = verb + pronoun, as in "push it" and "do it," and P_1X = adjective + noun, as in "big boat" and "big bus"), Braine acknowledged that although (43.1) and (43.2) are generative they may be insufficient descriptions of grammatical competence[2]. Using terminology introduced early in this chapter, (43.1) and (43.2) might be closer to the linguistic level of success called observational adequacy than that called descriptive adequacy. However, grammatical descriptions which fall short of descriptive adequacy will surely fail at the level of observational adequacy. But how does one begin to study grammatical competence with children?

Later, Braine (1963b) was able to demonstrate that in an experimental situation children can learn the absolute position and the relative position of nonsense items imbedded in short phrases. He called this learning "contextual generalization" and speculated that it might account for the beginnings of grammatical utterances. However, his position was questioned by Bever, Fodor, and Weksel (1965) because it seemed to deny the development of hierarchial (underlying) structures.

Proceeding along lines similar to Braine (1963a), Brown and Fraser (1964) and Brown, Fraser, and Bellugi (1964) offered grammatical descriptions which systemized utterances one, two, and three words in length. For example, using the symbol C with a subscript number to denote a word class, they expressed one child's utterances as follows:

$$\begin{array}{lll} S \longrightarrow (C_1)+(C_3)+C_2 & (44.1) & \\ C_1 \longrightarrow \text{see, that, two, etc.} & (44.2) & \\ C_2 \longrightarrow \text{bear, bird, block, etc.} & (44.3) & (44) \\ C_3 \longrightarrow \text{a, the, etc.} & (44.4) & \end{array}$$

The following trees can be generated with the grammar of (44):

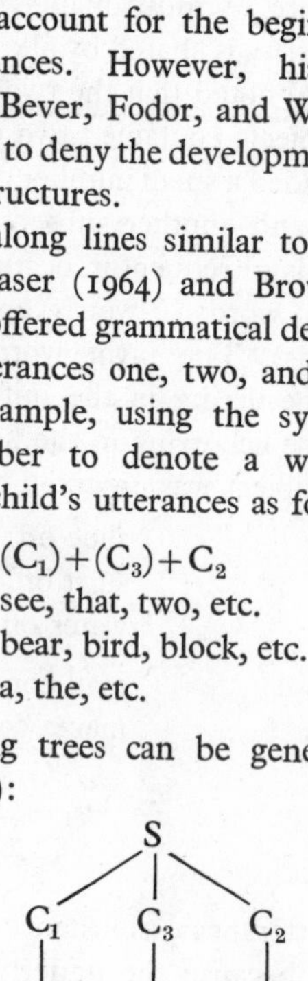

(45)

[2] See Bloom (1970) for an analysis of the theoretical limitations of P-X grammars.

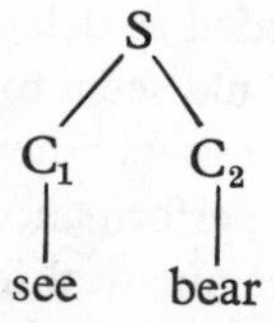

(46)

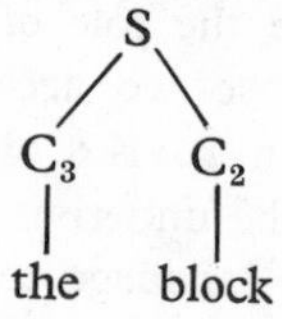

(47)

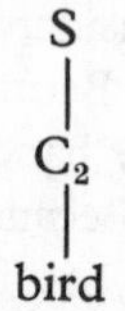

(48)

Not only did grammatical rules of this sort condense in an accurate way the utterances of the past, but they predicted almost precisely the many utterances of the immediate future (Brown, Fraser, and Bellugi, 1964). By isolating parts of speech and describing the rules which operate on them Brown and his colleagues achieved a level of linguistic sophistication for which students of child language are much indebted. A study by Miller and Ervin (1964), similar in some respects to those by Brown and his associates, and one by Klima and Bellugi (1966), on the development of the negative transformation are also valuable and should be read.

As is often the case in scientific inquiry, however, new data raise new questions. McNeill (1966), in an excellent review of the papers referred to above, takes issue with a suggestion by Brown and Bellugi (1966, p. 21) that "one major aspect of the development of general structure in child speech is a progressive differentiation in the usage of words and therefore a progressive differentiation of syntactic classes." McNeill (1966) summarizes well the contents of two-word constructions. He notes that they are generally of three types, denoted P-X, X-P, and X-X, with X usually taking the form of nouns and P usually taking the form of adjectives, articles, possessives, verbs, etc. How, McNeill asks, does a child learn to make the appropriate differentiations? Surely, he says, words belonging to a P-class could not have been randomly assigned, as this would nullify later attempts to subcategorize. For example, if P_1 contains verbs and function words and P_2 contains verbs and function words, and P_1 breaks up into verbs and P_2

into function words, what would be the basis for this differentiation?

There seems to be general agreement among students of child language that children's two-word utterances can be described as containing a content word and a word which operates on the content word, a pivot or a function word. It is also recognized that many of the adult grammatical distinctions are not present at this time. Possibly, word-class categories undergo abupt rather than progressive differentiations with maturation, as children acquire or make use of underlying linguistic schemata.

On the other hand, sentences with a limited number of word slots may represent syntactic classes falsely. Perhaps young children are making use of most adult syntactic classes but performance factors (such as memory and distortion of the speech signal) reduce in a systematic way (what Brown and Fraser, 1963, have called telegraphic speech) vocal output. Since understanding of syntax precedes correct verbal usage of syntactic forms (Fraser, Bellugi, and Brown, 1963), and since it would seem unwise to credit a child with two grammars—a perceptive grammar and a productive grammar—grammatical accounts which rest on speech output may be misleading. Descriptive accounts of the perception of grammar are difficult to obtain, however.

McNeill suggests another way to handle the differentiation of syntactic classes. If it is assumed, he contends, that an early grammatical category is a generic set, then, syntactic knowledge of the componential items must be known in advance. For example, if one class breaks up into articles and demonstratives and another class into adjectives and possessives, knowledge of an article, demonstrative, adjective, and possessives must be known prior to differentiation. It is as though "a child honors in advance some of the distinctions on which adult classes are based" (McNeill, 1966, p. 28).

Because empiricists (behaviorists) with their tools of learning seem unable to explain the development of syntactic classes and syntactic rules (the development of hierarchial structures), and because the theory of language universals is compelling, McNeill finds no alternative but to accept the fact that the innate "faculty of language," the guiding force behind the development of language, includes prescriptive categories. He suggests, for example, that linguistic substantives (such as NP, VP, modifiers, etc.) are available to the child from the beginning of his grammatical career. His position which cannot be covered in detail here, is that the child's early grammatical competence contains knowledge of the structure of sentences and that transformations develop somewhat later, although others (e.g., Fodor, 1966) disagree and consider that transformations of an abstract sort (language independent-rules) are initially available.

It should be pointed out that, however nativists, and this word is somewhat inappropriate because it applies to behaviorists as well, express their enthusiasm for innate mechanisms they agree (McNeill, 1966, and Lenneberg, 1967) that environmental factors weigh heavily in the acquisition of language. McNeill's point of view is that the environment is "directional" in that it assists the child in making decisions among grammatical choices that lie within the boundary of the given grammatical universals. Thus, for example, as the child is increasingly burdened with semantic interpretations and expressions he invokes or makes use of given abstract linguistic principles. Stated somewhat differently, the child brings to the language-learning situation a set of rules which ". . . would implicitly define the space of hypotheses through which . . . (he) . . . must search in order to arrive at the precisely correct syntactic analysis of this corpus" (Fodor, 1966, p. 115).

The child's path to grammatical success is rocky and rough, as observed by Miller and Ervin (1964, p. 28), who write "The linguistic system of a child is very unstable. . . . The formal patterns are not set, and the child frequently lapses back into older patterns. It takes a long time for the learned patterns to become automatic." Observations such as this one would suggest that principles of learning, tempered by maturational restrictions, are the obvious explanatory devices on which a theory of language acquisition should rest. But, it has been suggested that although language will not develop unless there is direction from (McNeill, 1966) and exposure to (Lenneberg, 1967) a natural language, the basic principles of learning do not apply. What, the nativists ask, is reinforced? What is shaped? What is programmed?

In 1958 Jean Berko, under the direction of Roger Brown, published a paper on the development of English morphology. This was an exciting development a decade or so ago because it outlined a general procedure by which children's construction rules could be tested and charted. For example, to test for the plural allomorph /-z/ the child would be shown a birdlike figure and told, "This is a wug, now there is another one. There are two of them. There are two ——." By using nonsense items such as this one Berko was able to separate imitative responses from rule-formed responses.

Berko's results indicated that the correct use of morphological markers increased with age, first-graders showing greater mastery than preschoolers. In some instances morphological constraints determined the rate of acquisition, as illustrated by the fact that /-əz/ was applied correctly more often as a possessive than as a plural. In other instances phonological constraints seemed to determine the rate of acquisition, as illustrated by the fact that the plural /-əz/ developed more slowly than either /-s/ or /-z/. It was later found (Miller and Ervin, 1964, and Ervin, 1964) that the correct extension of inflections, as tested by the use of nonsense items, postdated by several or more weeks the correct use of these forms in English words.

Even though morphological development resembles, on the surface, the acquisition of nonverbal responses, some (e.g., McNeill, 1966) have felt that its development represents an apparent contradiction to all known facts about learning. Using the systematic reports of Miller and Ervin (1964) and Ervin (1964) to corroborate a general observation by students of language development, McNeill (1966) asked why non-weak verbs are often used correctly when children begin to speak (e.g., "go," "do," and "come"), but after some experience weak verbs are uttered incorrectly (e.g., "goed," "doed," and "comed"). He adds, "the very difference in frequency that favored the appearance of the non-weak verbs means that highly practiced forms, the non-weak verbs, were so unstable as to be swept away by a few occurrences of the regular past tense inflection on weak verbs" (McNeill, 1966, p. 71). McNeill emphasizes that children seem to be responding to an adult pattern which can be expressed by a rule which itself is determined by universal linguistic constraints. There is nothing here that is inimicable to certain behavioral formulations except perhaps the way McNeill uses this evidence to suggest that performance factors like "rote learning" and "frequency of practice" and all that they imply are of minor significance in language learning. Without asking how the correct forms of non-weak verbs are recaptured, let's turn to an experiment by Palermo and Eberhart (1968) which seems to explain the anomaly described above.

Palermo and Eberhart (1968) summerized the known facts as follows: 1. there are more regular verbs than irregular verbs in English, 2. these irregular verbs are more frequent, 3. regularized inflections once learned are applied correctly to newly acquired weak verbs, and 4. the regularized inflections are applied to non-weak verbs with some degree of consistency. They wished to study the acquisition of irregular structures under controlled laboratory conditions. A miniature language system, after Esper (1925), was devised.

A matrix of 16 bigrams, partially represented below, was developed:

		Stimuli	
		1	2
Stimuli	6	VM* (DL)	VF
	7	HM	HF* (PC)

where * refers to omitted bigrams, and (DL) and (PC) to substituted bigrams, as explained below.

Using procedures common to the verbal behavior laboratory, college students were shown pairs of numbers and were to learn the appropriate bigram response. Consider the consistency of associations for the following pairs:

S	R
61	VM
62	VF
71	HM
72	HF

The numeral "6" is to be associated with the letter "V," "7" with "H," "1" with "M," and "2" with "F."

Tree diagrams of this miniature "linguistic system" for the stimuli "61" and "71" might look like the following:

Two basic manipulations were made by Palermo and Eberhart. First the pairs denoted with an asterisk were completely omitted in the training trials, but during the several test sessions the stimuli for these pairs, "61" and "72," in the example above, were given. First, it was found that subjects acquired the omitted pairs at about the same rate as the presented pairs. Second, the pairs denoted by an asterisk were omitted again, and the irregular pairs, those enclosed in parentheses, "DL" and "PC" in the example above, were presented equally often with all the other pairs. The irregular pairs were acquired at a faster rate. This finding might have been expected since the presentation rate of the irregular pairs was relatively more frequent (there were four irregular pairs and 12 regular pairs). Of considerable interest is the fact that the analysis revealed many errors of regularization for the irregular pairs after one errorless trial had been reached.

What evidence is there which suggests that formal instruction is critical in the language learning situation? One could cite evidence from several different sources that would seem to be relevant, but we shall limit our discussion to two investigations in which the data were garnered in the child's home and the subjects were the same three children.

Although some (e.g., Chomsky, 1965; McNeill, 1966; Lenneberg, 1967) regard the dialogue between a parent and a child as basically irrelevant to the language learning process, others (e.g., Fraser, 1966; Cazden, 1968; Brown, 1968) contend that it merits experimental considerations. Students of child language have often observed that parents repeat, modify, and reconstruct the utterances of their children presumably because they cannot understand their many demands and expressions. Called "expansions" by Brown and Bellugi (1964), these parental responses seem to display many of the elements of formal language instruction. Children seem to harass their parents by cries and disruptive behavior until some recognition, verbal or nonverbal, is made of their primitive language responses. I can recall that my two children between the ages of two and three years often cried and kicked until I repeated their tacts or responded to their mands. During this interval child and father made many verbal revisions. My children were not quieted with a "yes" or "no"; often the entire sentence, frequently unintelligible, had to be repeated. Sometimes the revisions were phonetic, but at other times they were syntactic. Colors were an early pivot word of my children, having learned these first as separate items, and thus "more [Ĩmb]" meaning "more meat" or "more milk" or perhaps "more eat" would be modified to "more white [Ĩmb]" for "milk" or "more brown [Ĩmb]" for "meat." There were some meals that involved more language instruction than eating!

Hattori (1965, p. 59), a Japanese linguist, remarks, ". . . little children begin to learn their mother tongue not by listening to natural, rapid conversations consisting of various sentences long and short, but by imitating words or very short sentences uttered clearly and repeatedly by their mothers and nurses who are eager to teach them to speak . . . my elder daughter learned very quickly the Japanese words which her grandmother taught her by pronouncing them clearly and repeatedly, whereas she was unable to learn the Tartar language although she was interested in the natural rapid conversation in Tartar between my wife and me."

The first (Cazden, 1968) of the two naturalistic studies to be reported below focused on noun and verb inflections, and the second (Brown, 1968) on the wh-question. The findings in these two investigations were derived from the parent-child dialogues of three children whose language responses were recorded at monthly intervals in the home. Transcripts were available from about the time each child began to utter two-word phrases. The interval for analysis stretched from the time each child uttered sentences of 1.75 morphemes until sentences of 4.0 morphemes were reached. For one child this interval was from about 19 to 28 months and for the other two children it was from about 28 to 45 months.

In Cazden's (1968) investigation an expansion was defined as a parental utterance which contained the appropriate inflection following an omitted or inappropriate inflection of the child. Acquisition of an inflection was defined as correct usage of an inflection in 90 percent of the contexts in which it was required, taking the first of three consecutive speech samples as the time of acquisition.

Cazden found that age of acquisition was unrelated to either the relative proportion or absolute number of parental expansions, even though the frequency of parental models (usage of the inflections by the parent) was about the same for all three children. When mean length of morpheme, rather than age, was used as a measure of maturity a relationship was also not found. At first glance, these findings might suggest that certain elements of learning theory have nothing to say for the process of language acquisition. However, frequency of occurrence as used in this study is not analogous to the way in which trials and acquisition are related in learning experiments. The variations reported above reflect individual differences (in trials to criterion), not parametric evaluations. Further, learning theorists would probably insist upon an analysis of correct responses as well as incorrect responses. Reinforcement of correct forms, whether verbal or nonverbal, is as critical to the learning process as is the modification of incorrect usage. It is also important to know whether expansions are related to sentence intelligibility, as an expansion of a particular linguistic segment may not be offered by a parent when the utterance, as a whole, is understood. Finally we should inquire about the parental behavior which accompanied the expansions. Possibly the incentive value of expansion is directly related to the accompanying pattern of reinforcement.

An analysis of the discourse patterns between child and parent may be "the richest data for the discovery of grammar," Roger Brown (1968) believes. The abstract manipulations of deep structures may develop as a result of certain instructional patterns imposed upon the child. Consider the transformational character of *wh*-questions. A superficial description of the underlying strings would involve the assignment of *wh* to the NP to be questioned, and permutation of *wh* to the front of the sentence, perhaps looking something like the following:

Erik dated Nancy (or someone)
Erik dated wh-Nancy
wh-Nancy Erik did date
whom did Erik date

A linguist interested in identifying language universals might wish to determine if operations such as "placement of *wh*" and "inversion of *wh*" are abstract principles which govern the question transformation, or a related set of transformations for all languages, and whether there are restrictions on the *wh*-operation (e.g., the number of times *wh* can replace an NP and the number of times *wh* can be inverted for a particular sentence type). A psychologist might ask, given certain linguistic constraints and knowing that knowledge of the deep structure is not represented directly in the surface structure, "How is the deep structure of a sentence type learned?" Possibly hints as to how mastery of internal structures is obtained can be gained by examining in detail the verbal exchanges between child and parent and relating these to linguistic abstracts.

We turn now to Roger Brown's (1968) study of the *wh*-question. Brown suggests that the occasional form of *wh*-questions may weigh heavily in the development of the abstract structures of the normal form of *wh*-questions. Observe the contrast between occasional and normal questions (the examples are from Brown, 1968):

Normal Question
what will John read
where will John read

Occasional Question
John will read what
John will read where

Linguistic theory suggests that normal questions are generated from occasional questions (actually, the underlying structures of these sentences), as in the example below:

Base:	John will read what
Preposing:	what John will read
Transposing:	what will John read

The occasional question is relatively frequent in mother-child conversations, Brown (1968) reports. It apparently clarifies children's solicitations most efficiently. Children's requests, possibly expressed as "I want milk" or "I want it," usually stimulate parental replies like "you want what." This verbal interchange seems to tell the child that "what" can replace specific instances as well as general instances of nouns (e.g., "what" for "milk" and "what" for "it"). Linguistic interchanges, such as those given above, probably account for the large number of coincident preposed (rather than transposed) sentences. Brown's subjects were heard to say sentences that were similar in form to "what I want milk" and "what I want it."

The many varieties of the occasional question seem to expose the underlying structures of surface strings. The preposed forms uttered by the child are externalized examples of the development of underlying structures. Probably much of what the child says represents intermediate linguistic forms. The study by Roger Brown illustrates a valuable experimental routine, since ". . . discourse patterns, . . . which are rich in structural information . . . may constitute the basis of a learning process" (Brown, 1968, p. 279).

Another approach to the study of child language would involve experimental manipulation of the child's linguistic environment. For example, a number of experiments could be tried during the time two-word constructions are frequent. One possibility would involve inversion of the words of some of the two-word phrases. Children might be placed in an experimental preschool in which a good share of their time would be spent in learning specialized linguistic phrases. Perhaps singular events would be expressed as P_1X and plural events as XP_1. Thus the children would hear phrases like "more candy" and "the boy" signifying singularity, and "candy more" and "boy the" signifying plurality. Could the children be taught to respond appropriately to inverted word order and would they begin to utter phrases which contain word inversions? What kind of linguistic errors would they make? Would learning word-inverted phrases indicate evidence of an underlying transformational device?

With older children one might teach a second plural. The phonological shape might be /-əm/, signifying three or more objects or events. Developmental psycholinguists might observe the conditions under which this response is acquired, the age level at which it develops, and whether special traning in numeration is required.

Semantic and Lexical Development

The recent advances in grammatical theory have sparked renewed interest in semantics (see Katz and Fodor, 1963; Katz and Postal, 1964; Chomsky, 1965). Because of the obvious complexity of this domain, however, only preliminary sketches have been put forward. With reference to language acquisition one point should be emphasized. However linguists describe the several grammatical systems and their relationship to each other, it does not imply that these systems function that way in language usage and language acquisition (Brown, 1957; Fodor, 1966). In language acquisition the relation between syntax and semantics may be symbiotic.

A study by Brown (1957) suggests that children use grammatical cues to detect semantic properties of word classes (defined earlier as selectional rules). Preschool subjects were shown several sets of pictures depicting a mass substance, a specific object, and an activity, as follows:

1. Mass noun: "Have you ever seen any sib? Now show me another picture of some sib."
2. Particular noun: "Do you know what a sib is? Now show me another picture of a sib."
3. Verb: "Do you know what it means to sib? In this picture you can see sibbing. Now show me another picture of sibbing."

The children were able to select, in most cases, the correct picture. Presumably they employed grammatical markers to decide among alternative pictures. Brown (1957, p. 5) hypothesizes that semantic correlates of the various form classes enable "the learner to use the part-of-speech membership of a new word as a first clue to its meaning."

The semantic system relates in a complex way to the acquisition of vocabulary items. We have no information as to how lexical items are acquired. However, an investigation by Smith (1926), now regarded as classic, charts the early development of vocabulary. Smith (1926) reported the results of a test designed to estimate the size of the spoken vocabulary of children. She selected every twentieth word from Thorndike's list of 10,000 most commonly used words in the English language, obtaining a total of 500 words. Of these she eliminated 297 which did not appear frequently in 77 published lists of children's vocabularies. The remaining 203 words were used as test items in the vocabulary test. Vocabulary responses were elicited through the use of pictures and questions. The following estimates of vocabulary size for children between the ages of two and six years were obtained:

Vocabulary Estimates (from Smith, 1926)

AGE	BOYS	GIRLS
2	304	743
3	822	920
4	1,571	1,576
5	2,181	2,058
6	2,606	1,964

Phonetic and Phonemic Development

In classical phonological theory the phoneme is regarded as the significant unit of the sound system of a language (Gleason, 1961). Linguists have long recognized that every natural language contains hundreds of sound-types (phones) which cluster in interesting ways to form a small number of functional sound-units called phonemes. For psychologists (Carroll, 1953; Berko and Brown, 1960; Fry, 1966) the phoneme is a superb example of a relatively complex nonlaboratory-learned cognitive event which seems to encompass, in a way not completely known (Winitz, 1969), stimulus sampling, stimulus selection, stimulus generalization, etc.

To appreciate the functional attributes of a phoneme, consider the following allophonic variations of the English /t/ phoneme:

[tʰ] — aspirated in "Tom"
[t¯] — unreleased in "cat"
[t] — unaspirated in "bit"
[ṙ] — r-flap in "better"
[t̪] — dentalized in "bathtub"

The above t-variants are five of many allophones of the American-English /t/ phoneme. They can be regarded as variations about a central tendency point called the /t/ phoneme. Similarly, the /k/ phoneme shows variation. The [k] of "key" is fronted while the [k] of "cool" is backed. Yet when word pairs are uttered these variations are not perceived as functionally significant.

Consider the following word contrasts:

1. [tʰæp] versus [kʰæp] "tap" versus "cap"
2. [bæt-] versus [bæk-] "bat" versus "back"
3. [bæt] versus [bæk-] "bat" versus "back"
4. [bæt] versus [bækʰ] "bat" versus "back"
5. (skeɪt] versus [steɪt] "skate" versus "state"

The above example seems to tell us that there are two functional stimuli, a /t/ and a /k/, at least when words are constrasted. However, there is no certainty that phonemic statements bear a one-to-one relation with psychological reality. Many experimental phonetic studies attest to this fact. For example, Lotz et al. (1960) found that when [s] is spliced away from /sp-/ clusters, the [p] is identified by listeners as a /b/. Unfortunately a number of other possible comparisons were not made, such as /sp-/ versus /sb-/ and /spʰ/ versus /sp-/ and /sb-/. Possibly English speakers would not regard the [p] and [b] stops as identical in phonetic contexts such as these.

The subjects in the Lotz et al. (1960) investigation may have been responding to a stimulus pattern that encompassed more than just the /p/ phoneme. That is, the lenis, unaspirated [p] in initial word clusters may be regarded as belonging to /b/ whenever the stimulus pattern in which [p] is usually imbedded is altered so as to reflect the stimulus pattern of an acoustically similar sound (such as the devoiced, lenis [b]). This conclusion follows from the fact that stimulus elements are not learned as isolated elements of a stimulus set (see Atkinson, Bowers, and Crothers, 1965; Spiker, 1963).

No doubt the model of classical phonemics is simply not equipped to handle the complex processes of speech perception. Indeed it was not developed for this purpose. The various models of speech perception and production (as well as the many interesting findings generated from these models) suggest that interpretations of the phonetic and phonemic acquisition process may be totally in error if the basic frame of reference is classical phonemics.

A number of examples can be given which illustrate the misgivings we have about phonetic and phonemic principles, as traditionally conceived, when these are used to explain the acquisition of sounds. We shall cite only two. First, it is now well known that for certain consonants a good degree of information is present in the vowel transitions, and in some instances the transitions for a particular consonant are not constant for a range of phonetic contexts (e.g., Liberman et al. 1967). Therefore, one could speculate that the primitive perceptual system of young children may have as its building blocks the steady-state portion of the vowel phonemes. Second, recent considerations of the articulation process (e.g., Öhman, 1966; Kozhevnikov and Chistovich, 1965) suggest that the basic physiological unit of sound production is not the phone or phoneme but an integrative or hierarchial mechanism (or mechanisms) which dominates the production, storage, and retrieval of phonemes. Restricting our attention to sounds, conceived of as elements of a linear sequence, may obscure a complex neurophysiological process.

The picture is further complicated by the fact that recent developments in linguistics suggest that the phonological component, as indicated above, is constrained by the syntactic component. Phonological competence involves the mapping of surface syntactic structures (morphemes) into phonetic (distinctive) features. Classical phonology regards the phonological component as primarily independent of the syntactic component, but this viewpoint is considered by generative linguists to be largely in error (see Chomsky, 1964; Halle, 1962; Chomsky and Halle, 1968). However, since research in children's phonology has its origins in classical phonemics, our discussion will be restricted to this approach.

The procedures of classical phonemics have been used to describe the phoneme systems of young children (Leopold, 1947, 1961; Velten, 1943; and Albright and Albright, 1956, 1958, for example). In one study (Albright and Albright, 1958) a child of one year in age was reported to have 41 phones, 27 vowels, and 14 consonants. His consonantal contrasts for manner of articulation were primarily oral-nasal and stop-continuant. For place of articulation four contrastive positions were observed. He possessed front, central, and back vowels and high and low vowels. His vowel and consonantal phonemes are shown below:

Vowel Phonemes

ɪ		ʊ
	ə	
ɛ		ɑ

Consonant Phonemes

	Labial	Apical	Velar	Glottal
Stop	b	d	g	
Fricative				h
Nasal	m	n		

Jakobson (1941) and later Jakobson and Halle (1956) proposed that phonemic acquisition proceeds from the simple or gross perceptual contrasts to the more complex contrasts. The first contrast is syntagmatic; vowels and consonants are contrasted. The second contrast involves a splitting of the consonantal phoneme into a nasal and an oral phoneme. As phonetic features are distinguished, phonemes continue to split until the phonemes of the community language are acquired. Jakobson (1941) and Jakobson and Halle (1956) hold the belief that this process is an orderly one among languages in that gross acoustic distinctions are learned early, while fine acoustic differences are learned late. Jakobson (1941) notes further that phonemic development shows an extraordinary parallel to the frequency of contrast usage of the world's many languages—contrasts which are frequent are acquired early while contrasts which are infrequent are acquired late. Because phonemic acquisition involves phonetic units which are common to all languages the process is considered to be a universal one.

Consider the following consonantal matrix:

	Bilabial	Labiodental
Nasal	L_1	L_2
Continuant	L_2	L_1
Stop	L_1	L_2

(49)

where L_1 and L_2 are two different languages.

Note that in (49) nasals, stops, and continuants, and bilabial and labiodental placement are common to L_1 and L_2. Assume now that the oral-nasal distinction, because of reasons mentioned above, is the first contrast to take place. The primordial consonant phoneme divides into a nasal and an oral phoneme as shown below:

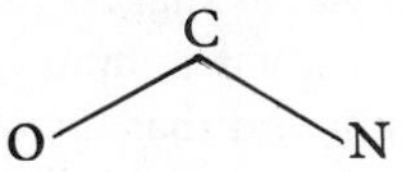

For language L_1 the contrast involves a bilabial-nasal versus an oral-continuant stop. For language L_2 the oral-nasal contrast involves a labiodental nasal versus an oral, continuant-stop. Yet, although the sound patterns (phonemes) are different, the contrasts—in this case oral-nasal—are constant, resulting in a universal pattern of development.

Employing all distinctive features of matrix (49) would give the following phonemes for L_1 and L_2:

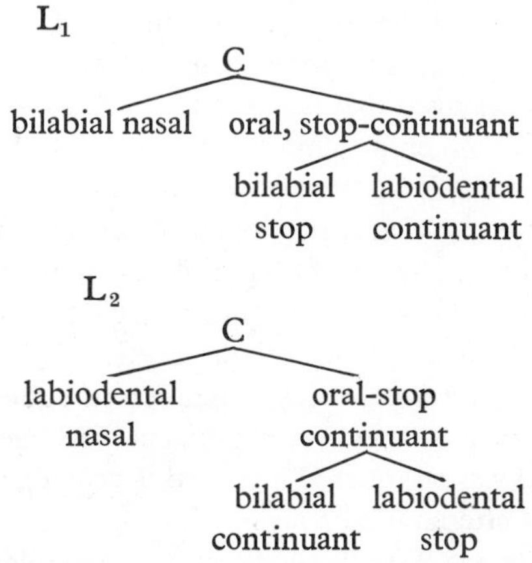

We should note again that universal regularity, as illustrated directly above, refers to the development of distinctive features and not to phonemes. The process is governed by the operation of distinctive features; the phonemes are outcomes of this process.

We would not expect perfect prediction of phoneme development from this model for many reasons, some of which are: 1. distinctive features are elements of a stimulus compound and discrimination of phonetic elements are without doubt affected by pattern differences (the way distinctive features are conjoined to form phonemes and the dimensions along which phonemes contrast); 2. frequency of distinctive features and patterns of distinctive features vary among languages; and 3. grammatical constraints vary among languages.

There are a number of studies (see Ervin-Trip, 1966) which seem to support the general outlines proposed by Jakobson (1941) and Jakobson and Halle (1956). However, as yet this model has not been shown to predict precisely the evolution of phonemic contrasts across languages. Indeed there is considerable variation among children for a particular natural language (see Albright and Albright, 1958; Ervin-Trip, 1966; Templin, 1957).

Of particular interest to American speech pathologists is the order of acquisition of English phonemes. The most recent account of phoneme development is reported by Templin (1957) and is shown below:

AGE (YEARS)	CONSONANTS
3	m n ŋ p f h w
3.5	j
4	k b d g r
4.5	s ʃ tʃ
6	t θ v l
7	ð z ʒ dʒ

There are a number of ways in which Templin's findings may be interpreted. First, however, it should be acknowledged that her results reflect most directly the age at which a sound is used correctly in words, since articulation protocols were used to assess sound productions. Yet it is possible that the developmental order given by Templin reflects phoneme-class learning, although the testing procedures were not those common to classical phonemics. We say this because she tested a large number of subjects and employed a stringent requirement for correctness (a sound was considered mastered if 75 percent of the subjects uttered it correctly).

Elsewhere (Winitz, 1969) we have speculated that articulation mastery is acquired prior to age three, often in nonfunctional units (traditionally called jargon). Yet it is doubtful that language behavior could develop at the pace it does with a phoneme system that is so underdeveloped, as Templin's (1957) findings seem to suggest. It would seem reasonable to conclude, then, that phonemic perception is acquired at an early date and that what is learned at later age levels is simply the integration of articulatory units in new lexical items and morphemic units. However, we say this haltingly because many studies (e.g., Templin, 1957) show that the discrimination of minimal pairs is a monotonic function of age. Also, one cannot shrug off allophonic variation as a random process. The assignment of allophones to phonemes suggests that a range of stimuli as well as a central tendency is being discriminated. We would have no quarrel with a discrimination hypothesis which rests on distinctive cues, if the relevant cues remain unorganized. As soon as we assume (as we do in Jakobson's treatment of phonemic mastery), however, that irrelevant cues are distributed according to some rule, then we must assume that allophones are discriminated in the same way phoneme contrasts are.

An example may help make the above point clear. Assume we develop a learning situation in which boxes are discriminated by color contrast, black versus white, for example, and boxes of all sizes, shapes, and weights are used. Children could be taught to learn the appropriate discrimination. This procedure is so common in learning experiments that there is no need to document it here. However, if children were asked to organize box size, shape, or weight according to some "distribution" principle, then clearly they must discriminate size, shape, and weight. Future research studies must look into this matter.

Babbling

Chapters on language development usually begin with babbling, but we have decided to end our description of language acquisition with a question or two about this process. Long recognized as fascinating but perplexing, much has been written and said about this topic (see Miller and Dollard, 1941, and Lewis, 1951). Until recently babbling was regarded as an interesting instance of secondary reinforcement. Babies babble because their utterances take on secondary reinforcing properties, suggests Mowrer (1952, 1958, 1960). A secondary reinforcer is any event or stimulus which takes on reinforcing properties by virtue of its association with a primary reinforcer. A mother's voice signals the advent of most events in the first half-year of an infant's life. And because the child's vocalizations are similar in acoustic quality to his mother's vocalizations, transference takes place, and the process of secondary reinforcement begins.

Only three studies of any significance have dealt with the conditioning of infant vocalizations (Rheingold et al., 1959; Weisberg, 1963; and Todd and Palmer, 1968). First, these studies have generally shown that the vocalizations of three-month-old infants can be increased by the application of conditioning procedures. Second, stimuli usually regarded as nonsocial (such as the sound of a door chime) do not increase vocalizations, at least for three-month-olds (Weisberg, 1963). However, social responses, smiles, and verbalizations (even prerecorded verbalizations) increase infant vocalizations (Weisberg, 1963; Todd and Palmer, 1968). Third, the mere presence of an unresponding adult will not increase vocalizations (Weisberg, 1963). Mowrer's theoretical position as well as the usual discrimination learning paradigm would suggest that infant vocalizations will increase when a human face is present. Actually Weisberg found that the operant vocal level was decreased, although not significantly for the subjects who did not see a human face. In addition, Todd and Palmer found that prerecorded verbalizations (such as "hello baby" and "pretty baby") increased vocalizations when experimenters were present. Possibly the presence of a human face serves to increase vocalizations, but the effect may not be strong at three months of age.

As yet there is no explanation for vocal drift (see Brown, 1958, pp. 198–202). Irwin (1947, 1948) found that the vocalizations of American infants are at first back consonants and front vowels. By about two years of age the frequency of the average child's vowels and consonants approximates those of his parents. Because Weir (1966) observed that Chinese infants show tonal variations over individual vowels, as is typical of their language at six months, but that Russian and American infants of the same age do not, we would guess phonemic drifting begins as early as the second half of the first year of life.

What is the reason for phonemic drifting? Differential reinforcement, as usually conceived, does not seem to be a likely explanation. For parents reinforce strings of phonemes and not individual phonemes in a string. It would be of interest to know whether infants who are reinforced for a range of responses would drift toward the conditioned (discriminative) stimulus. Charles Galloway, a student of mine, first suggested to me an experimental paradigm to handle this question. He asked whether subjects would drift toward a discriminative stimulus, say the sound of a bell, when any one of a number of motor responses, each one actuating a different auditory stimulus (e.g., bell, buzzer, vowel /a/, etc.) would be equally reinforced. Possibly the effect would not be forthcoming unless the task required two or more contrasting stimuli.

It may well be that babbling represents something very different from that which we have suggested above. Possibly babbling shows drifting because syntactic comprehension (and, of course, phonemic discrimination) of a primitive sort has begun.

Another consideration is the articulation unit during the babbling stage. In what way is articulation in the babbling stage similar to articulation in words? Although the syllables which the infant babbles on the surface may appear structurally similar to those uttered after words are acquired, basic articulatory arrangements may be absent (e.g., timing and co-articulation factors). Superficially the "articulatory units" in the prelinguistic and language stages show similarities. For example, Irwin's (1951) graphing of consonantal position reveals that by six months of age consonants in all three syllable positions are frequent, and Winitz (1961) noted that syllables of all varieties are common in infancy. Yet we know that many of the articulatory deviations of young children can be described (but not explained) under the rubric of assimilation, suggesting that phonemic and syntactic interpretations need to be supplemented by articulatory considerations.

Maturational precepts, strongly conceived, have penetrated the study of babbling. Lenneberg et al. (1965) propose that infant cooing responses are "not contingent upon specific, acoustic stimuli." Their premise is supported by the fact that the frequency of vocalizations was similar for infants of hearing and deaf parents, who were studied from about two weeks to three months in age. However, in the study by Lenneberg (1965) and his associates response frequency, but not response type was analyzed. Overall frequency, measured in time units, would not necessarily reflect consonantal type or frequency.

To call attention to the needs of the infants of the deaf parents a voice-operated relay had been installed in each child's bedroom and was operative during the time of this study. When actuated the relay flashed a light which signaled to the deaf parents that their child was crying or vocalizing. The light was clearly visible to the child, in some instances flashing in the child's face. The light may have served as an elicitor for or reinforcer of vocalizations.

Most importantly, however, the study terminated when the infants were three months of age, a point in time which most students of language behavior regard as infant vocalizations. Babbling is generally said to occur at about six months. Clearly babbling is tied to maturational prerequisites, but to deny at this time the effect of environmental contingencies seems premature.

CONCLUDING STATEMENT

In the past decade and a half the discipline of linguistics has experienced what some now regard as a revolution. Called generative grammar by Noam Chomsky, its innovator, the new linguistics shares little with the procedural methods and philosophical objectives of the linguistics of the past. Generative grammar was immediately attractive to psychologists because it displayed in a coherent and logical way that language, although awesomely complex, is the kind of symbolic system they should struggle to understand.

In the preceding pages we have described briefly the issues which the new linguistics has entertained, the confrontations of generative grammar with psychology, and the heavy burdens which now rest on the shoulders of those who study child language. No longer can language development be viewed as a chronicle of developmental events whose structural complexity increases with age. Rather it must be recognized as the acquisition of an abstract and complex process, the understanding of which may lead to remarkable discoveries of the human mind and its environment.

BIBLIOGRAPHY

Albright, R., and Albright, J. 1956. The phonology of a two-year-old child. *Word*, 12, 382–390.

———, and ———. 1958. Application of descriptive linguistics to child language. *J. Speech Hearing Res.*, 1, 257–261.

Atkinson, R., Bower, G., and Crothers, E. 1965. An introduction to mathematical learning theory. New York: Wiley.

Berko, J. 1958. The child's learning of English morphology, *Word*, 14, 150–177.

———, and Brown, R. 1960. Psycholinguistic research methods. *In* Handbook of research methods in child development. Mussen, P., ed. New York: Wiley.

Bever, T. 1968. Associations to stimulus-response theories of language. *In* Verbal behavior and general behavior theory. Dixon, T., and Horton, D., eds. Englewood Cliffs, N.J.: Prentice-Hall.

———, Fodor, J., and Garret, M. 1968. A formal limitation of associationism. *In* Verbal behavior and general behavior theory. Dixon, T., and Horton, D., eds. Englewood Cliffs, N.J.: Prentice-Hall.

———, ———, and Weksel, W. 1965. On the acquisition of syntax: a critique of "contextual generalization." *Psychol. Rev.*, 72, 467–482.

Bloom, L. 1967. A comment on Lee's "developmental sequence types: a method for comparing normal and deviant syntact development." *J. Speech Hearing Disorders*, 32, 293–296.

———. 1970. Language development; Form and function in emerging grammars. Cambridge, Mass.: M.I.T. Press.

Braine, M. 1963a. The ontogeny of English phrase structure: the first phase, *Language*, 39, 1–13.

———. 1963b. On learning the grammatical order of words. *Psychol. Rev.*, 70, 323–348.

———. 1965. On the basis of phrase structure: a reply to Bever, Fodor, and Weksel. *Psychol. Rev.*, 72, 483–492.

Brown, R. 1957. Linguistic determinism and the part of speech. *J. abnorm. soc. Psychol.*, 55, 1–5.

———. 1968. The development of wh questions in child speech. *J. verb. Learn. verb. Behav.*, 7, 279–290.

———, and Bellugi, U. 1966. Three processes in the child's acquisition of syntax. *In* Language and learning. Emig, J., Fleming, J., and Popp, J., eds. New York: Harcourt, Brace and World.

———, and Fraser, C. 1964. The acquisition of syntax. *Child Devel. Monog.*, 29, No. 92, 43–79.

———, ———, and Bellugi, U. 1964. Explorations in grammar evaluation. *Child Devel. Monog.*, 29, No. 92, 79–92.

Carroll, J. 1939. Determining and numerating adjectives in children's speech. *Child Develop.*, 10, 215–229.

———. 1953. The study of language. Cambridge: Harvard.

Cazden, C. 1968. The acquisition of noun and verb inflections. *Child Develop.*, 39, 433–448.

———. 1971. Chap, 45, this vol.

Cowan, P., Weber, J., Hoddinott, B., and Klein, J. 1967. Mean length of spoken response as a function of stimulus, experimenter, and subject. *Child Develop.*, 38, 191–205.

Chomsky, N. 1957. Syntactic structures. 's. Gravenhage: Mouton.

———. 1959. Review of verbal behavior by B.F. Skinner. *Language*, 35, 26–58.

———. 1964. Current issues in linguistic theory. The Hague: Mouton.

———. 1965. Aspects of the theory of syntax. Cambridge: M.I.T.

———. 1966. Topics in the theory of generative grammar. The Hague: Mouton.

———. 1967. The formal nature of language, (Appendix A). *In* Biological foundations of language. Lenneberg, E., ed. New York: Wiley.

———. 1968. Language and the mind. *Psychol. Today*, 1, 48–51, 66–68.

———, and Halle, M. 1968. The sound pattern of English. New York: Harper & Row.

Crothers, E., and Suppes, P. 1967. Experiments in second-language learning, New York: Academic Press.

Dixon, T., and Horton, D. eds., 1968. Verbal behavior and general behavior theory. Englewood Cliffs, N.J.: Prentice-Hall.

Ervin, S. 1964. Imitation and structural change in children's language, *In* New directions in the study of language. Lenneberg, E., ed. Cambridge: M.I.T.

Ervin-Tripp, S. 1966. Language development. *In* Review of child development research, 2. Hoffman, M., and Hoffman, L., eds. Ann Arbor: Univ. Mich. Press.

Esper, E. 1925. A technique for the experimental investigation of associative interference in artificial linguistic material. *Language Monogr.*, No. 1.

Fischer, M. 1934. Language patterns of preschool children. *Child Develop. Monog.*, No. 15.

Fodor, J. 1966. How to learn to talk: some simple ways. *In* The genesis of language. Smith, F., and Miller, G., eds. Cambridge: M.I.T.

———, and Garrett, M. 1966. Some reflections on competence and performance. *In* Psycholinguistic papers. Lyons, J., and Wales, R., eds. Edinburgh: Edinburgh Univ. Press.

Fraser, C. 1966. Discussion of the creation of language by children, by D. McNeill. *In* Psycholinguistic papers. Lyons, J., and Wales, R., eds. Edinburgh: Edinburgh Univ. Press.

———, Bellugi, U., and Brown, R. 1963. Control of grammar in imitation, comprehension, and production. *J. verb. Learn. verb. Behav.*, 2, 121–135.

Fry, D. 1966. The development of the phonological system in the normal and the deaf child. *In* The genesis of language. Smith, F., and Miller, G., eds. Cambridge: M.I.T.

Gleason, H. 1961. An introduction to descriptive linguistics (rev. ed.). New York: Holt, Rinehart and Winston.

Halle, M. 1962. Phonology in generative grammar. *Word*, 18, 54–72.

———, and Stevens, K. 1964. Speech recognition: a model and a program for research. *In* The structure of language. Fodor, J., and Katz, J., eds. Englewood Cliffs, N.J.: Prentice-Hall.

Hattori, S. 1965. The sound and meaning of language. *Foundations of Language*, 1, 95–111.

Horton, S. 1968. A diachronic examination of the linguistic universal. *Asha*, 10, 247–249.

Irwin, O. 1947. Infant speech: consonantal sounds according to place of articulation. *J. Speech Disorders*, 12, 397–401.

———. 1948. Infant speech: development of vowel sounds. *J. Speech Hearing Disorders*, 13, 31–34.

———. 1951. Infant speech: consonantal position. *J. Speech Hearing Disorders*, 16, 159–161.

Jakobson, R. 1941. Kindersprache, Aphasie und allgemeine Lautgesetze. Uppsala: Almqvist and Wiksell.

———, and Halle, M. 1956. Fundamentals of language, 's Gravenhage: Mouton.

Jenkins, J. 1965. Mediation theory and grammatical behavior. *In* Directions in psycholinguistics. Rosenberg, S., ed. New York: Macmillan.

———. 1966. Reflections on the conference. *In* The genesis of language. Smith, F., and Miller, G., eds. Cambridge: M.I.T.

Katz, J., and Fodor, J. 1963. The structure of a semantic theory. *Language*, 39, 170–210.

———, and Postal, P. 1964. An integrated theory of linguistic descriptions. Cambridge: M.I.T.

Kendler, H. Some specific reactions to general s-r theory. *In* Verbal behavior and general behavior theory. Dixon, T., and Horton, D., eds. Englewood Cliffs, N.J.: Prentice-Hall.

———, and Kendler, T. 1962. Vertical and horizontal processes in problem solving, *Psychol. Rev.*, 69, 1–16.

Klima, E., and Bellugi, U., 1966. Syntactic regularities in the speech of children. *In* Psycholinguistic papers. Lyons, J., and Wales, R., eds. Edinburgh: Edinburgh Univ. Press.

Kozhevnikov, V., and Chistovich, L. 1965. Speech: articulation and perception. U.S. Department of Commerce, Joint Publications Res. Service, No. 30543.

Lenneberg, E. 1967. Biological foundations of language, New York: Wiley.

———, Rebelsky, F., and Nichols, I. 1965. The vocalizations of infants born to deaf and to hearing parents, *Vita Humana*, 8, 23–37.

Leopold, W. 1947. Speech development of a bilingual child, 4 vol. Evanston: Northwestern Univ.

———. 1961. Patterning in children's language learning. *In* Psycholinguistics, a book of readings. Saporta, S., ed. New York: Holt, Rinehart and Winston. Pp. 350–358.

Lewis, M. 1951. Infant speech. New York: Humanities Press.

Liberman, A., Cooper, F., Shankweiler, D., and Studder-Kennedy, M. 1967. Perception of the speech code, *Psychol. Rev.*, 74, 431–461.

Lotz, J., Abramson, A., Gerstman, L., Ingemann, F., and Nemser, W. 1960. The perception of English stops by speakers of English, Spanish, Hungarian, and Thai: a tape cutting experiment. *Language and Speech*, 3, 71–77.

Lyons, J., and Wales, R., eds. 1966. Psycholinguistics papers. Edinburgh: Edinburgh Univ. Press.

McCarthy, D. 1930. The language development of the preschool child, *Institute of Child Welfare Monog. Ser.*, No. 4, Minneapolis: Univ. Minn. Press.

McNeill, D. 1966. Developmental psycholinguistics. *In* The genesis of language. Smith, F., and Miller, G., eds. Cambridge: M.I.T.

Menyuk, P. 1963a. Syntactic structures in the language of children, *Child Develop.*, 34, 407–422.

———. 1963b. A preliminary evaluation of grammatical capacity in children. *J. verb. Learn. verb Behav.*, 2, 429–439.

———. 1964a. Syntactic rules used by children from preschool through first grade. *Child Develop.*, 35, 533–546.

———. 1964b. Alteration of rules in children's grammar. *J. verb. Learn. verb. Behav.*, 3, 480–488.

Miller, G. 1967. The psychology of communication, New York: Basic Books.

Miller, N., and Dollard, J. 1941. Social learning and imitation. New Haven: Yale.

Miller, W., and Ervin, S. 1964. The development of grammar in child language. *Child Develop., Monog.*, No. 29, 9–34.

Mowrer, O. 1952. Speech development in the young child: 1. the autism theory of speech development and some clinical applications. *J. Speech Hearing Disorders*, 17, 263–268.

———. 1958. Hearing and speaking: an analysis of language learning. *J. Speech Hearing Disorders*, 23, 143–152.

———. 1960. Learning theory and the symbolic processes. New York: Wiley.

Öhman, S. 1966. Coarticulation in VCV utterances: spectrographic measurements. *J. Acoust. Soc. Amer.* 39, 151–168.

Osgood, C. 1968. Toward a wedding of insufficiencies. *In* Verbal behavior and general behavior theory. Dixon, T., and Horton, D., eds. Englewood Cliffs, N.J.: Prentice-Hall.

Palermo, D., and Eberhart, V. 1968. On the learning of morphological rules: an experimental analogy. *J. verb. Learn. verb. Behav.*, 7, 337–344.

Postal, P. 1964. Limitations of phrase structure grammars. *In* The structure of language. Fodor, J., and Katz, J., eds. Englewood Cliffs, N.J.: Prentice-Hall.

Postman, L. 1961. The present status of interference theory. *In* Verbal learning and verbal behavior. Cofer, C., ed. New York: McGraw-Hill.

Rheingold, H., Gewirtz, J., and Ross, H. 1959. Social conditioning of vocalizations in the infant. *J. comp. physiol. Psychol.*, 52, 68–73.

Shriner, T. 1971. Chap. 44, this vol.

Skinner, B. 1957. Verbal behavior. New York: Appleton-Century-Crofts.

Sluckin, W. 1965. Imprinting and early learning. Chicago: Aldine.

Smith, M. 1926. An investigation of the development of the sentence and the extent of vocabulary in young children. *Univ. Iowa Stud. Child Welf.*, 3, No. 5.

Spence, K. 1956. Behavior theory and conditioning. New Haven: Yale.

Spiker, C. C. 1963. The hypothesis of stimulus interaction and an explanation of stimulus compounding. *In* Advances in child development and behavior. Lipsett, L., and Spiker, C., eds. New York: Academic Press.

———. 1966. The concept of development: relevant and irrelevant issues. *Monog. Soc. Res. Child Develop.*, 31, No. 5, 40–54.

Stewart, J. 1960. The problem of stuttering in certain North American Indian societies. *J. Speech Hearing Disorders, Monog. Suppl.*, No. 6.

Templin, M. 1957. Certain language skills in children, their development and interrelationships. *Inst. Child Welf. Monogr. Ser.*, No. 26. Minneapolis: Univ. Minn. Press.

Tikofsky, R. 1968. Discussion of theories of language acquisition and practices in therapy by P. Menyuk. *In* Speech pathology: some principles underlying therapeutic practices. *Asha*, 10, 201–202.

Time Magazine. Feb. 16, 1968 (whole issue).

Todd, G., and Palmer, B. 1968. Social reinforcement of infant babbling. *Child Develop.*, 39, 591–596.

Velten, H. 1943. The growth of phonemic and lexical patterns in infant language. *Language*, 19, 281–292.

Wales, R., and Marshall, J. 1966. The organization of linguistic performance. *In* Psycholinguistic papers. Lyons, J., and Wales, R., eds. Edinburgh: Edinburgh Univ. Press.

Weir, R. 1966. Some questions on the child's learning of phonology. *In* The genesis of language. Smith, F., and Muller, G., eds. Cambridge: M.I.T.

Weisberg, P. 1963. Social and nonsocial conditioning of infant vocalizations. *Child Develop.*, 34, 377–388.

Wepman, J. 1960. Auditory discrimination, speech and reading. *The Elementary School*, 60, 325–333.

Winitz, H. 1961. Repetitions in the vocalizations and speech of children in the first two years of life. *J. Speech Hearing Disorders Monog. Suppl.*, No. 7, 55–62.

———. 1968. Articulatory acquisition and behavior. New York: Appleton-Century-Crofts.

44

Economically Deprived: Aspects of Language Skills[1]

Thomas H. Shriner

In the past decade, rapid changes have taken place in our economic and educational systems. With the positive aspects of change, of course, come the negative: we have experienced problems associated with increased ethnic, educational, and economic desegration. Educators, psychologists, linguists, sociologists, speech pathologists scientists, etc., highly aware of the negative aspects, have taken great strides to cope with existing differences brought to light by integration of the minority groups. One difference of paramount importance to this paper is that of speech and language.[2]

In 1965, the American Speech and Hearing Association at the request of federal agencies such as the Office of Education, Children's Bureau, and the Office of Economic Opportunity established a Committee on Language. While our profession has always played a significant role in the diagnosis and treatment of various language problems, little attention has been given to the language problems of the disadvantaged child. In a statement prepared by Michael Marge (1968), Chairman of the 1965 Committee on Language, and modified by John V. Irwin, President, for presentation before a meeting of a group of organizations concerned with language problems of the disadvantaged, it was felt that

> The language handicaps of the disadvantaged child were not originally of primary concern for speech pathology and audiology, in part, because we (the profession) were told that other professional groups were adequately serving the needs of these children, and in part, because the problem of language among the economically disadvantaged is only now receiving full recognition . . . In reaffirmation of its policy to serve the communicatively handicapped of our nation, the profession, through the American Speech and Hearing Association, has taken steps to define the problem of language management and to identify appropriate strategies for meeting this new responsibility.[3]

While the charge of the committee was much larger in scope, one aspect was to evaluate language training programs for school-age children who use a dialectal language form, such as Negro dialect.[4] Many other professions such as linguistics, psychology, departments of special education, etc., have also been concerned with the communication problems of the economically disadvantaged child.

The question of communication problems in the

[1] Supported by Public Health Service Research Grant NB 07346 from the National Institute of Mental Health.

[2] Various terms such as lower-class child, disadvantaged child, inner-city child, economically disadvantaged child are used throughout the chapter to refer to the same problem area. In reviewing the work of selected authors, I have tried to use the terms selected by them. The term *culturally* disadvantaged was not used, however, because all children do have a culture.

[3] Sponsored by the Speech Association of America and held on January 26, 1968, at the Statler Hilton Hotel, New York, N.Y.

[4] The recommendations of the Committee on Language will be published in ASHA (1969)—private communication, John J. O'Neill, President, American Speech and Hearing Association.

economically disadvantaged child merits serious study, and many more scientific contributions must be made by the various disciplines interested in communication before an adequate program of remedial instruction can be developed. With this viewpoint in mind, the author will review the salient, and what he considers the important, contributions of various investigators to the communications problems of the economically disadvantaged child.

One attribute of man, and probably his most important attribute, is his ability to communicate with his fellow man. Speech is far more than a means of communication, for it involves language. Speech is defined for purposes of this paper, as the expressive (oral) verbal output of man. Language is far more than a means of communication. While speech is an integral part of language, language has become one of the principal means of thought, memory, introspection, and problem solving, and is related to all other mental activities. Educated man, in particular, should be articulate or at least moderately articulate in the speech patterns of his community. If he fails to meet certain proficiencies or has certain deviations from socially accepted speech patterns, his speech may be or usually is referred to as odd or substandard, and he is placed into nonacceptable categories or thought to be unequal. Our economically deprived or minority groups find themselves facing a communication barrier and, regardless of their abilities or qualifications, they may be denied many opportunities because of their speech.

Obviously, variations in speech (articulation, prosodic patterns, and syntactical structures) exist both within and between different speech communities. The variations which exist within a speech community may or may not present themselves to be a problem. Spectrograms (energy vs. displays of visual frequency of sound) have shown that repetitions of the same phoneme by the same individual will reveal differences. These differences are referred to as allophonic variations of the same phoneme and, for our purposes, do not make a perceptual difference. When differences do occur within a speech community, that is, for example, one phoneme substitution for another phoneme substitution, then a speech problem is said to exist and a speech pathologist is consulted for remedy. The individuals who comprise a particular speech community and who do not have remedial speech problems usually communicate in a particular dialect. On a national level, for example, one only need recall the dialects of Presidents John F. Kennedy or Lyndon B. Johnson as compared with that of Richard M. Nixon. If one were to define "speech community" on a municipal level, differences also would exist. In our large cities, it is not uncommon to find a number of different dialects of general American speech such as the Spanish-American, Negro, etc.

Dialect pronunciations as regionally distributed variations (within) may or may not be "socially different" when contrasts are made among the various speech communities. One may contend that particular dialect patterns may have certain merits and advantages, such as the former example of our presidents, or the added example of the psychiatrist who deliberately learns to speak a Viennese dialect to function more effectively as a psychotherapist.

When comparisons are made among the various speech communities, in a sense when they become substandard or socially nonacceptable relative to general American speech, then a problem is said to exist. (There is considerable controversy as to whether this problem is simply a *difference* or a *deficit*.) In almost the same sense that speech problems can exist within a speech community, speech problems can also exist between speech communities. Our economically deprived or minority groups find themselves facing a communication barrier when taken from their immediate environments. This communication barrier is not only one of a speech problem but usually involves a language problem as well. Williams and Naremore (1967), in an extensive review of the literature on language and poverty, generalized that dialect and language difference have known associations with social stratifications, and they also state that it has been demonstrated that a person's dialect can be a reliable basis for classifying his social status. Thus substandard speech appears to be characteristic of the poor, or more formally, the economically disadvantaged. Hurst and Jones (1966) were concerned with a more precise definition of substandard speech, dialect, etc. They state that speech referred to under these headings involves such oral aberrations as phonemic and subphonemic replacements, segmental phonemes, phonetic distortion, defective syntax, misarticulations, mispronunciation, faulty phonology, and unintelligibility, which can be found singly or in combinations. To refer to the subvariables mentioned above, they prefer the term "dialectolalia." Their concern for a more precise definition of the communicative problems of the disadvantage points out the faulty interrelationship found between speech and language for this population. Although there is general awareness that low social status actually does have quantitatively depressing effects on certain forms of language production, there appears to be little agreement as to what the deficits are and what to do about them. Much has been written and many studies have been completed comparing the language of the disadvantaged child to that of his privileged peers. It is hoped that this review will shed more light on the problem.

As mentioned previously, the dialect variations which exist within and between various speech communities may reveal information about the social status of the speaker, his background or origin, and, depending on the training of the listener (linguist, speech pathologist, scientist), his particular speech community and personality (Markel, Eiseler, and Rees, 1967). In other words, sociolinguistic information is conveyed by certain features of a person's speech which has been acquired from interactions within his particular speech community.

If members of the American Speech and Hearing Association (as well as others interested in communication) are to be concerned with socially acceptable speech, then those aspects which convey patterns not thought to be socially acceptable by the listener(s) must be studied. It is important that information be obtained on which kinds of "corrections" are to be emphasized. It is important that we understand which phonological deviations (articulatory deficits), which syntactical "errors," or which lexical substitutions have the most negative effect on the listener. Moreover, implicit in the definition of dialectolalia by Hurst and Jones (1966) is the relationship between speech and language. The relationship between speech and language deficits (in particular—syntax) was recently reported for children with articulatory deficits by Shriner, Holloway, and Daniloff (1969). They reported that articulatory defective children performed significantly lower in the areas of grammatical usage and used shorter sentences. Specifically, with respect to the disadvantaged child, it must be remembered that any child's language is related not merely to the way he speaks but also to the way he thinks. Low-status dialect may hamper the child's social mobility, but a restricted language development may limit his intellectual potential as well (Gussow, 1965). The nature of the relationship between speech and language deficits has not been explored in specific detail for the disadvantaged child. We do not know which interferes the most with social mobility or educational opportunities or which kinds of standard speech, if any, we should teach. The emphasis on correct speech may appear questionable if there is no improvement in language behavior. If we assume that the listener has difficulty understanding the speech behavior of the disadvantaged child, the listener in all probability will respond accordingly (Rosenthal and Jacobson, 1968). The child will then alter his behavior in response to the listener. For dialect remediation we need to know what deviant aspects of the speech code have the most negative effects on the listener and how these deviances are reflected in language development. It is assumed, of course, that one wishes to learn the jargon of another speech community.

Many studies have been completed which emphasize the importance or influences of the listener in speech perception with respect to sociolinguistics (Harms, 1961; Aninsfeld, Bogo, and Lambert, 1962; Voiers, 1964; Hymes, 1964; Markel, Eisler, and Reese, 1967; Bryden, 1968). These studies emphasize the importance of phonological patterns in regional dialects as a significant factor in judging the personality of the speech. Probably the most comprehensive research to date is the recently completed study of Bryden (1968). His study was designed to focus specifically on the psychoacoustics of certain features believed to convey sociolinguistic information. His attempt was to specify acoustic, social, and personal variables which may constitute a basis for the quality judgment of speakers by listeners. Ninety-one adult subjects were speakers and 86 were listeners: of the 91 speakers 47 were Negroes and 44 were Whites, and of the 86 listeners 43 were Negroes and 43 were Whites. All subjects served as both listeners and speakers in groups of 15. The results demonstrated that the number of phonetic distortions was significant in predicting whether recorded speech samples were identified as spoken by Negroes or Whites. The number of phonetic distortions functioned significantly in cases in which White speakers were identified as being Negro speakers and in cases in which Negro speakers were thought to be White speakers. In all cases, phonetic distortions applied to vowel sounds, which means that significant cues for racial perception, according to Bryden, were related to vowel production. The socioeconomic status score of the speaker and the articulatory product score (Guttman, 1966) were also found to be significant in predicting the speech quality-rating received by the speaker from listeners. Other variables studied by Bryden such as age, sex, articulatory errors (omissions and substitutions), total numbers of misarticulated phonemes, and self-rating of speech proficiency were not found to function significantly in listener perception of racial identity and quality of speakers; also, no significant differences were found between formant frequencies for the vowels /i/ and /u/: relative amplitudes of Negro speakers were consistently lower on /i/ and /u/ than those of Whites, but were not found to be significant.

Bryden points out one limitation of his study: subjects were required to read a preselected passage under experimental conditions. It may be that they adjusted their speech patterns to meet the experimental conditions. It is not unreasonable to presume that adults can possess and reflect two levels of linguistic-phonological competence with respect to dialect deviations (see chapters 43 and 45). In a reading-experimental setting, subjects may be highly aware of their speech patterns, which would lead them to articulate more precisely the consonants of the language: this may not be true of the vowels, which would be more difficult to change. In a speaking situation, especially among peers in the same speech community, one might and usually does find different patterns of communications. As reported by Stewart (1967), pronunciation differences between a non-standard dialect and standard English can become unintelligible even though in grammar and vocabulary the dialect may be similar to the standard English equivalent. Illustrating his point, he states that

> . . . a non-standard version of "I don't know where they live" might in one dialect become cryptic to the standard speaking listener, merely because of its being pronounced something like *Ah 'own know wey 'ey lib.*

or another example from Stewart,

> . . . a listener may take a non-standard sentence *Dey ain't like dat* to mean "They aren't like that," when it really means "They didn't like that."

Stewart's examples do show that consonant omissions and substitution can occur in dialect patterns and that if they occur to a listener outside of that particular speech community, meaning can be lost.

Although much research has been completed in our large cities (see the proceedings of a conference, *Social Dialects and Language Learning*, Shuy, Davis, and Hogan, 1964), practically no studies on the specific phonological-dialectal deviations of disadvantaged children within speech communities to see which of these deviations have the most negative effect (loss of meaning) between speech communities. Perhaps it is asking too much of linguists to study in depth entire dialectal "systems" and to compare these systems to those of other dialects. This should involve more than vowel quality changes, unless these vowel quality changes interfere with changes in meaning. It also should involve study of phoneme substitutions and omissions, which would be of great benefit to the speech-language clinician. It is not uncommon, in fact, it is very common, to read phonological or morphological studies that were completed in one dialect area to have no particular application to another dialect area. For example, in a recent study by this writer and Miner on "Morphological Structures in the Language of Disadvantaged Children" (1968), we received letters from various sections of the country stating something to this effect: "Because you tested linguistic competence of disadvantaged midwestern, white children and found no significant differences when compared with control subjects who were not disadvantaged—I do not think you would get the same results, for example, on southern Negro children who commonly omit morphemes at the end of words." A statement of this nature also causes a problem in methodology that was discussed earlier. Subjects with dialect patterns may have control over their particular patterns in a testing situation; that is, competence (a speaker-listener's stored knowledge of his language) may be manifested in performance in more than one way or may reflect competence in two different dialects. Stewart (1964) seems to imply two different levels of competence when he suggests that we teach English as a foreign language to disadvantaged children. Teaching them English would give them another level of competence which then could be manifested in performance: performance defined as the expression of competence in speaking or listening, i.e., how we actually put it to use, realize, and express it.

Studying the phonological aspects of the disadvantaged child raises certain theoretical questions concerning diagnostic methodology. A study by Ringgaard (1965) reported on the unreliability of three fieldworkers who were trained phoneticians. He emphasizes that phoneticians must be able to liberate themselves from their native speech in studying dialectal variations. He reached the sad conclusion that the narrow transcriptions of the phoneticians do not tell us much about the actual dialectal realizations of the phonemes but tell us more about the fieldworkers themselves, about their native pronunciations, and about their confusion when coming to new regions. Probably more important for students of speech pathology are not the slight phonetic variations that exist within and between speech communities, but those of phoneme substitutions or omissions that make such a difference to warrant speech therapy.

Dialectal variations existing within speech communities, such as the example given earlier about our presidents, should not be sufficient to cause alarm to the speech pathologist (although it was not uncommon to hear from them comments about President Kennedy's New England dialect or the southern drawl of President Johnson). If a child moves from one local dialect setting to another, for example, from New England to the Midwest, the question immedately arises, should the speech pathologist enroll the child in therapy, or if a disadvantaged child is "bussed" from his local dialect group to another part of the city where he must mix with children of a different dialect, should the speech pathologist enroll this child in therapy? As this review has attempted to show thus far, little is known about the dialect patterns of individual speech communities and these effects on the listener(s) of other speech communities. The speech pathologist of a particular locale should use discretion, perform the proper phonemic tests, and make his diagnosis: there can be no hard-and-fast rule concerning dialectal problems. Probably the most significant problem that will be encountered by the speech pathologist will be that of changes in intonation, inflection, and vowel duration—problems that today's average speech pathologist is not well trained to treat clinically.

In diagnosing phonemic problems of the disadvantaged child, theoretical problems arise for the speech pathologist. Paraphrasing Chomsky (1964): the phonemic system, in effect, extracts all regularities from the acoustic system and, a priori, there is no reason to suppose that such a system exists psycholinguistically. He states, for example, that it is obvious that a child does not first construct a phonemic system and then proceed to take this phonemic system to build syntax and semantics. Curtis (1968) has also emphasized the same point of view. He states that to describe running speech analytically we encounter problems of segmentation, which naturally requires a decision of where to segment. A decision to segment involves units of some kind, which will have an inevitable effect on the nature of the relationship we deduce between the physiological events which produce the signal and the acoustical waveform that comprises the signal. The unit also will effect the classification system that we develop and the types of measurements that we consider fundamental to the speech models of perception and production. Curtis further states that

> For most of us any suggestion of segmenting the stream of speech into units immediately suggests the process of making a phonetic (or phonemic) transcription of an utterance. This is natural enough since most of us received our first real experience with observing speech analytically, and attempting to describe it with some degree of precision, when we learned to record what we heard in terms of a conventional system of phonetic or phonemic symbols. Thus we learned to segment speech into phone sized units. If we continued to study and work with speech, as linguists, phoneticians, speech pathologists, etc., we doubtless have practiced this type of auditory analysis and description until we have become highly skilled at it. However unnatural and forced such an analysis may have seemed at the beginning, as practice continued it doubtless came to seem more and more natural. The phone size segments (speech sounds, phonemes, etc.) that are assigned separate symbols in the transcription process also may have come to be regarded as *the natural units* of speech analysis, so much so, in fact, that it would be quite unlikely to occur to most of us that any other segmentation of the speech stream would be possible. In short, most of us have come to accept as axiomatic the fundamental assumption that the speech stream is, in point of fact, a linear sequency of discrete units each of which can be labelled and classified, and which can be considered to be independent and commutable. Moreover, not only has it apparently not occurred to many persons to question this assumption, but, further, it has been little realized that the validity of this assumption may be related to the particular purpose for which speech is being analytically studied, e.g., whether one is concerned with the description of language structure, the processes of speech production, the nature of speech perception, the acquisition of language by small children, or the learning of a foreign language by an adult. Presumably the same segmentation is assumed to be appropriate for all such purposes.

The fundamental purpose of the papers by Chomsky and Curtis was to call attention to and question the assumption of the phoneme as the basic unit of speech at the levels of physiological performance and of perceptual input. (The reader is referred to Liberman, Cooper, Shankweiler, and Studdert-Kennedy, 1967; Öhman, 1967; Kozhevnikov and Chistovich, 1965; and Daniloff and Moll, 1968, for further theoretical discussions of the relationship between speech production and speech perception.)

If the speech pathologist is concerned with speech

as learned motor behavior, then the philosophy expressed by Curtis and Chomsky should be taken into consideration. The characteristics of the model of the speech-production process that will be most relevant for speech pathologists still remains unanswered. Moreover, can the same model be used for both the disadvantaged child with a dialect problem and the child with an articulatory problem when the dialect problem is classified as an articulatory problem? Curtis has suggested exploration of models other than the present "phoneme model"; models that presumably could be based on the physiological (motor) aspects of the speech code. Support for his suggestion is based upon the recent research of Öhman (1967), Kozhevnikov and Chistovich (1965), and Daniloff and Moll (1968), which indicates that articulatory production involves possible articulatory units larger in size than the phoneme. These units may be syllabic, morphemic, or larger. Which unit to teach to the disadvantaged child with dialectal patterns remains obscure and unanswered. Moreover, a disadvantaged child with deviant dialect productions that are also classified as articulatory deficits may also have associated syntactical problems, such as the syntactical problems reported by Shriner, Holloway, and Daniloff (1969) with respect to speech-defective children. (As mentioned previously, this relationship is implied in the definition of dialectalalia by Hurst and Jones but has not been experimentally tested for disadvantaged children.)

Emphasis, however, on correct speech production for the disadvantaged child is questionable if the child has associated language problems. Gussow (1965) stated, appropriately,

> What is undoubtedly and unfortunately true is that a good deal more effort has been expended on modifying the pronunciation and syntax of lower-class speech than has been expended on improving language functioning for these children.

This suggests that we not only adopt a viewpoint which is concerned with dialectolalia per se, but that we also adopt a larger viewpoint which emphasizes the improvement of language functioning for these children. Language problems should be considered more fundamental than speech problems, and only after the child has made significant gains in language development should speech therapy be initiated.

Much has been written and many studies have been completed comparing the language of the disadvantaged child with his more privileged peers on such speech measures as sentence length and complexity, vocabulary, or on tasks of verbal comprehension and cognition. Accordingly such studies have indicated consistently the existence of a quantitative deficit among the disadvantaged, though the factors of sex, age, I.Q., and other variables such as the ethnic identity of the experimenter appear to affect the results significantly, and often unpredictably. Overall, though, the studies indicate that low social status actually does have a quantitatively depressing effect on certain forms of language production, that is, when comparisons are made between speech communities.

Baratz (1968), in one of her reviews of the literature, has stated that the language of the disadvantaged child can be described from several questionable viewpoints. Quoting Frazier (1964), the first viewpoint is "true verbal destitution," which means that the disadvantaged child has less or has really not acquired language when compared with the middle class child. The results of a number of studies have shown that these children are less verbal and know conventional names for fewer things, whether objects or actions; they have a more restricted grammatical range and produce simpler sentences (Gussow, 1964; Cazden, 1966; Deutsch, 1965; Raph, 1965; Williams and Naremore, 1967; Newton, 1965; Bernstein, 1967; and many others). It is mentioned that most of these studies used standard English to evaluate differences between the populations.

Language, however, as defined previously, is more than either verbal communication or countable, audible items, which bears directly on Baratz's second questionable viewpoint. It has been hypothesized that the difficulty of the disadvantaged child has been defined as due to an underdeveloped language system that does not allow language to function in aiding cognitive development. Highly relevant is the Whorfian hypothesis of linguistic relativity (1956) that all higher levels of thinking are dependent on language and that the structure of the language one habitually uses influences the manner in which one understands his environment. A low-status dialect may hamper the child's social mobility, but a restricted language development may limit his intellectual potential as well. Williams and Naremore (1967), in a review of the literature, generalized that a poverty environment has a socializing influence upon its population, an influence which manifests itself in distinctions of language and cognition, and these distinctions in turn serve in the definition and perception of the population of the poverty culture. They also state that the language of a poverty or disadvantaged class symptomizes a perceptual restriction to the nonabstract—to that which is directly, personally, and grossly experienced, and with only limited recognition of higher levels of conceptualization. Others, for example Bernstein (1961), John (1963), and Loban (1965), also are in general agreement that children from the lower class do not have the means to express abstractions, logical, spacial, and temporal relationships, generalizations, and individual feelings and differences. Cazden (1966), however, has approached the relationship between impoverishment of language and cognition more cautiously. She states, "Whether non-standard English is, in addition, a cognitive liability to the speaker is much harder to determine." In an excellent review of Bernstein's elaborated vs. restricted codes she also states, "Whether the use of a restricted code is an indication of limited ability or merely of preference in particular social settings has not been answered" (1968). Restricted code as defined by Bernstein (1965) is a code which inhibits (restricts) an orientation to symbolize intent in a verbally explicit form, while an elaborated code has just the opposite function. Cazden (1968) presents the well-taken argument that since the number of experimental situations is infinite, the experimenter should be cautious and well aware of whether use of a restricted code is an indication of limited ability or merely a result of that particular testing situation. Robinson (1965), for example, had 120 middle class and lower class 12- and 13-year-old children perform two writing assignments. The first task was to write a good friend news of the past few weeks, while the second task was to advise the governor of a school on how to spend money that he had donated. The first task presumably would evoke a restricted code while the second would evoke a more elaborated code. There were no significant differences between the two groups on the formal letter. However, differences were observed on lexical diversity (number of different nouns, etc.) for the informal letter. This led Robinson to suggest that lower class children have a less varied vocabulary rather than a distinctly different code. Cazden (1968) also suggests that where interests are strong and motivation is high, as in planning a strike, for example, lower class speakers may, in fact, use an elaborated code. The nature of the relationship(s) and an adequate developmental theory to explain the relationship between language, speech, and social structures for disadvantaged children as postulated by Bernstein waits the outcome of further research, most of which he is now conducting on a large scale.

Research directed, in a broad sense, toward the identification and description of cross-cultural and developmental differences in the conceptualization and linguistic expression of spatial, temporal, causal, and logical relationships was studied in depth by Brent and Katz (1967), Katz and Brent (1968), Brent and Klamer (1967), and more recently by Herder, Cazden, and Brown (1968). Because it is necessary to understand the cognitive processes that underlie a child's acquisition of language skills, their research findings will be reported in greater detail.

Brent and Katz (1967), and Katz and Brent (1968) were interested in analysis of different levels of language comprehension and the inferences that could be drawn about the nature of the underlying thought processes. Three methods were used to study connectives; 1. spontaneous speech; 2. paired sentence test and 3. explanation of connectives. To obtain spontaneous speech samples, the subject is simply shown a series of pictures and asked to tell a story about them. The authors presume that this method gets at the use of temporal, causal, and logical relationships on a spontaneous level, while the other two techniques measure his understanding in terms of deliberate, conscious level. First- and sixth-grade students from a predominantly White, working class neighborhood in Detroit were used as subjects in their first study. The subjects were shown a series of picture stories from the WISC Picture Arrangement Task and asked to tell a story about the pictures (narrative discourse task). Katz and Brent state that the critical difference between the two groups and college speakers of standard dialect was that the elementary school children preformed lower on their ability to explain the function of connectives in the sentences on the test. Brent and Katz also report the need to examine in detail the use of logical connectives to relate simple descriptive elements, the use of syntactically correct but semantically vague pronouns, and the over-explicit use of nouns where pronouns would do just as well. With respect to the over-explicit use of nouns, children frequently say "*the dog* saw the basket of food and *the dog* jumped up and ate the food." College speakers of standard dialect, in contrast, typically say "*The dog* saw the basket of food and *he* jumped up and ate the food." This example illustrates that children frequently use a noun where a relative pronoun would do equally as well. Their report is highly interesting when compared to findings of Bernstein's (et al). Middle class five- to seven-year-old children of high verbal ability score higher on most of the measures of form class usage, for example, number of different nouns, verbs, and adjectives:

> Not predicted by a simple developmental interpretation, but compatible with Bernstein's conceptualization of code differences is the finding that independent of the measured ability of the children, there was a broad tendency for the middle-class to use the *noun* and its associated forms more frequently while the working class made greater use of the pronoun.

Lower class children appear to differ from middle class children in pronoun usage. In private communication with Brent and Katz what seems likely or at least speculative at this point is that lower class children use fewer nouns and have more redundant pronoun usage than upper class children. The over-explicit use of nouns may be simply developmental or the use of vaguely referenced pronouns may also indicate developmental trends. The issued raised, however, seems to indicate lower levels of language functioning. More specifically, the largest difference between middle class and lower class children is in the greater usage of exophoric pronouns by lower class children (pronouns which refer outward to the situational context, e.g., *they're playing football and he kicks it*). No differences were reported between the groups in the use of anaphoric pronouns (pronouns which refer to previously mentioned nouns, e.g., *The boy kicked the ball and it broke the window*, Cazden, 1968). This difference (that lower class children use more exophoric pronouns) appears important because the lower class child appears to be tied to the context in which the language responses are evoked; the lower class child apparently assuming that the listener can see the pictures used to evoke the responses. Less use of exophoric pronouns at this level by the middle class child enables him to be understood outside of the immediate context without reference to the pictures displayed in front of him; that is, it apparently gives him the greater power of abstraction.

Brent and Katz (1967) tentatively explored pronoun usage in greater detail. They raised the question that since the subjects in their first study used a great deal of implicit depiction with respect to pronouns, what would their subjects do if the pictures were removed? Subjects were 39 children, four to six years old, enrolled in a summer Headstart program in a Detroit neighborhood. In this study each subject told a story with the pictures present, then the pictures were removed and he was asked to tell the same story again.

The tentative results of this study proved to be most interesting because a comparison of the stories with and without pictures revealed that the stories told without the pictures were superior to those told with the pictures. The authors state that without the pictures there was a dramatic improvement in the quality of language used to relate stories, greater connectedness of the ideas, and a marked increase in the amount of spontaneous speech. The authors argue that the actual presence of the pictures may interfere with the younger child's ability to form a temporally distributed and logically continuous story. When the pictures are removed, however, the subject is free to integrate into a more continuous story those aspects of the original content he is able to recall. "In this respect, it is interesting to note that the recall stories frequently include appropriate content not mentioned in the presence of the picture themselves." The child in the testing situation without pictures is given more freedom to use his power of abstraction.

Why is the disadvantaged child's language restricted in the presence of a picture and apparently the middle class child's is not? Why, if further detailed research does not find specific differences, should both groups be relatively equal when the picture is removed from the testing situation? Brent and Katz speculate that their youngest subjects exhibit a high degree of "nominalization"; that is, their verbalizations consist primarily of naming the various details in each picture. The author's personal experience with testing middle class as well as lower class children corroborates the findings of "nominalization" for lower class children, more so than for middle class children. Although I never thought to remove the picture and repeat the task as did Brent and Katz, I found it helpful to stop the child and to give additional directions in the form of "Tell me what's happening in the picture" or "Tell me a story about the picture." Nominalizations when they occur in our studies are not scored as part of the narrative discourse analysis. The responses that are evoked are, in part, a function of the directions given to the child. The directions given to the child should be considered important because Hess and Shipman (1965) reported that lower class Negro mothers used simple short sentences and gestures in teaching their children simple conceptual tasks while upper class mothers used more speech and more elaborate speech in the same task situation. Because the parents of middle class children use a more elaborate and abstract speech code as compared with lower class mothers with respect to their children, directions may have to be given differently for the two groups to evoke similar response patterns. Taking the picture away from the disadvantaged child may be putting him on par with the middle class child, which presumably would force him to use the same cognitive processes, although differences would be expected in vocabulary. It should also be emphasized that the child first saw the picture and then was asked to tell a story about it. The picture was then removed and he was again asked to tell a story. It may be that the child became more relaxed or less shy in the testing situation and more familiar with the experimenters, factors that operate to increase and enhance verbalizations. More thorough investigations are needed to answer the above questions.

The authors do not elaborate with respect to pronoun differences in their progress report but do mention that further studies on several groups of lower class children were underway. Their future results should be interesting with respect to exophoric pronouns. If their results do not agree (picture not present) with Bernstein's et al., this would mean that the disadvantaged child is limited by the testing situation; moreover, his language usage is a function of the situation and that, if given the opportunity, he may be able to use the same rules of language as his middle class counterpart. If their results do agree with Bernstein's et al., it would mean, at least with respect to pronoun usage, that disadvantaged children are impaired in their ability to use language as cognitive tool.

As mentioned previously, one result of the Katz and Brent study was the noted difference of logical connectives used to relate simple descriptive sentences. In this study, they reported that some of their subjects repeated the sentence of their choice spontaneously. The subjects' task, for example, was to choose between *Jimmy went to school, but he felt fine* and *Jimmie went to school, but he felt sick.* The subjects often altered markedly the conjunction which had been read to them, either substituting or adding new conjunctions, or omitting the conjunction altogether. The authors noted that many children who had been scored as endorsing the erroneous sentence (the first in the above-mentioned example) were actually saying *Jimmy went to school*, and *he felt fine*, *Jimmie went to school*, because *he felt fine*, which indicated that the children had knowledge of connectives because they changed the incorrect conjunction *but* to *and* and *because*. The authors are exploring these results in further detail, which again indicates that there may not be differences in the cognitive functioning of disadvantaged children, if their language is properly assessed and the results are not a function of the testing situation.

In the two-person communicative game Brent and Klamer (1967) focus on another aspect of cognitive functioning and language. While the narrative discourse technique evoked language samples in response to pictures with an "authority" (examiner) figure present, this second task involves two peers in a back-to-back situation in which the speaker and listener do not share the same concrete, perceptually grounded field of reference. The two subjects have four identical geometric patterns, with the exception that they differ in color, in front of them. The speaker is to get the listener to do something with his patterns, for example, to build a house. The subjects the authors selected for this task were 26 university freshmen, ages 17–19, and 32 Negroes, ages 16–18, from the Franklin Settlement House, which is located in the heart of the Negro section of inner-city Detroit. The authors did not place emphasis on the subjects' ability to solve the problems; emphasis was placed instead on the language used for solution. One interesting finding of the experiment was that *metaphoric* description was used by the inner-city subjects far more often than the college students, who used more of a geometric technique vocabulary. The inner-city subjects adopt but never really integrate the geometric technical description to the task. The college students use, but do not really integrate the metaphoric mode, rather, it "exists for them as a distinct mode, a kind of after thought, which is tacked on at the end but which does not enter as a functionally integral part of the problem solving."

The authors also state that the results of their two-part communication game bears directly on the Whorfian theory of linguistic relatively. The linguistic mode used by the college students was predominately of the form, "place —— so that ——," while this form was almost totally absent in the inner-city group. The predominant linguistic mode used by the inner-city group was the *placing* of one geometric pattern next to another. It appears as if the college students are forced by their syntactic form (place —— so that ——) into a more sophisticated kind of problem solving, "for not only is the placing of one piece instructed, but also the specific *relationship of that piece to another*."

> What seems to be happening is that college students are delivering an empty form. For them the problem demands a "place —— so that ——" syntax. This syntax is delivered first, there is then a long pause, then the cognitive processes needed to fill out the form proceed. Language is in this instance clearly prior to thought, the thinking out of the relationship between

the placed piece and the surfaces of the piece against which it is to be placed is dictated and partially determined by the deliverance of an initially empty syntactic structure.

That is, the structure of the language that the subject uses habitually in this situation determines his higher levels of thinking (Whorfian hypothesis). The following example was given.

Place the longest side of the third object *so that*—you know *so that* all these—uh—*so that* the—oh, uh—you're going to *place* the longest side against the side of the triangle.

The example indicates that the subject often initially delivering the form "place —— so that ——" finds that she cannot describe the relationship and proceeds to generate a different syntactic structure utilizing for example "against."

It should be noted that while the college subjects predominately used a geometric technical mode and the inner-city subjects used more of a metaphoric mode in problem solving, the solution times for both groups were about equal. If the metaphorical mode is considered to be part of nonstandard dialect, then, at least with respect to solving tasks, it is just as good a means of communication as standard English. Heider's, Cazden's, and Brown's (1968) study also found no evidence that children of one social class communicated more accurately with each other than with children from the other groups.

Brent and Katz also noticed that two distinct strategies were employed by their subjects. The inner-city group predominately began by describing to the listener what the final product would look like, that is, they gave the "whole" picture, referred to by the authors as synthetic strategy. College students used both a synthetic strategy and a linear-analytic strategy: linear-analytic strategy defined as how to place each block, one at a time in a serial position or a "part" by "part" approach. Their findings agree nicely with those of Heider (1968).

Heider found that lower class 10-year-old children gave predominately "wholistic inferential responses," for example, "He looks surprised" in response to pictures of male facial expressions, or in response to abstract figures (squiggles) they would give, "It looks like two snakes are fighting at each other." Middle class 10-year-old children, on the other hand, gave predominately part-descriptive statements, for example, "It's a figure which is even on both of its sides, and has an opening at the top and it is curved at the bottom," or, "He has his left eyebrow raised more than any of the other faces."

Differences are also reported between middle and lower class subjects with respect to children's part-whole coding abilities. The subjects in their first study were 143 10-year-old boys and girls, one-third White middle class, one-third White lower class, and one-third Negro lower class. In their first session, the child's task was to describe one abstract figure or face out of six items so that another child could pick out that item at a later time, which constituted their second session. The results were classified as part-whole, inferential-descriptive, whole-inferential, and part-descriptive. Part-whole was defined as whether the image referred to the whole stimulus or only to a part of it, and inferential-descriptive was defined as whether the image represented an inference going beyond the stimulus or simply described the stimulus. Another language style reported by them to be common of both classes was called whole-inferential, which described the whole picture in terms of what the picture looked like, for example, of a face, "He's mad," or of an abstract, "It's a flying saucer." These descriptions accounted for 80 percent of the lower class images but for only 33 percent of the middle class images. The middle class children also used language referred to as part-descriptive, which described a minute part of the picture in terms of physical description, for example, of a face it might be said that "one ear is dark," or of an abstract, "There's a tiny circle in the middle." This type of language accounted for 13 percent of the verbalizations from the lower class children and 53 percent of the verbalization of the middle class children.

In their second session, a child had to select one of the stimulus arrays from the verbalizations of another child. Communication effectiveness was measured by the accuracy of the decoders in identifying the intended pictures. The middle class children were better overall decoders than lower class children: middle class children were better decoders of both the wholistic as well as the analytic style, while lower class decoders were more successful with the wholistic encoding of middle class children than with their own.

The recent findings of Williams and Wood (1971) and Williams (1969) are in general agreement with those of Brent and Katz (1968), Heider (1968), and Heider, Cazden, and Brown (1968). To study decoding performance between lower class, junior high school girls and middle class, junior high school girls, Williams and Wood used Taylor's (1954) *cloze* technique. The cloze technique, briefly involves the deletion of words (usually every fifth word) from sentences, paragraphs, etc., then having a decoder attempt the replacement of the deleted item. To the extent the subjects in Williams' study were successful in making such replacements, the decoders would be closely approximating the language habits of the original encoders. Language samples were obtained from small group discussions about the students' problems and attitudes concerning school. Three encoder subjects and a fieldworker participated in each discusslon. The discussion topics were divided into segments where the fieldworker's probe was followed by at least 50 words of student speech. From this pool of segments, 16 transcripts were prepared by deleting every fifth word, assembled into test booklets of 16 pages each, and given to 15 decoder subjects in each of two lower class and middle class Negro schools. The results indicated that the middle class students could approximate the language of the middle and lower class samples, but the lower class students did significantly more poorly in approximating the language of the middle class students, although they performed as well as the middle class students in approximating language in samples from students of their same social class.

Williams (1969) also reported that when 16 middle class subjects were asked to talk about their favorite television programs, 15 responded by telling narratives and only one subject gave an isolated episode. In his lower class group, 11 children, by contrast, gave reports of isolated episodes and six gave narratives. Williams interpreted his results by stating that the stereotype advanced by the remarks of the lower class children was the "concrete and particularistic description of some visually emphasized action in a program, as compared with the H.S. (middle class) child's tendency to abstract the 'point' from such action to describe it within the story context of the program."

Williams further states that young children (he used fifth- and sixth-graders) will attend and respond to the type of stimulation found in their family environment and, as previously mentioned (Hess and Shipman, 1965), communication patterns of middle class mothers are different from those of lower class mothers. He hypothesizes that children from different environments would be expected to react differently to a given television program because lower class children seemed to be attuned to the concrete, the direct verbal and physical action level of the program. The middle class child is capable of responding to both

> . . . the concrete and to the more abstract—the verbal—levels of a program. It is on this higher level that the visual and concrete components of the programs may be combined by the verbal components into the 'reason' for the action, or the "story-line" of the program.

More specifically, Williams appears to be referring to higher level functioning where strong syntactic habits are operating. This could be interpreted as the representational level of the model used as the basis for the Illinois Test of Psycholinguistic Abilities (Kirk, McCarthy and Kirk, 1968). The representational level of the model is viewed as a more complex mediating process and uses symbols which carry meaning. Another level of the model, the automatic, is viewed as less complex and presumably accounts for the child's ability to perform less symbolic tasks; however, this level still requires habits that are highly organized and integrated but less voluntary. This level appears to account for Williams' statements about the lower class child being attuned to "the concrete, the direct verbal and physical action level of the program." It appears as if the middle class child is operating at a higher level, the representational, while the lower class child is operating less efficiently at the representational level or more so at the automatic level of cognitive function.

Through use of the Illinois Test of Psycholinguistic Abilities, a study was designed by Barritt, Semmel, and Weener (1968) to compare psycholinguistic functioning of educationally deprived and educationally advantaged children. Subjects were three groups of kindergarten and first-grade children. Sixty-four subjects, approximately 70 percent Negro, comprised the first group and are referred to by the authors as "The Unity School" sample. The Unity School is located in a "ghetto" of a midwestern city. The second sample (Diversity School) consisted of 65 children selected randomly from an area which borders the area of the Unity School with approximately 50 percent of the population being Negro. The third sample, 62 subjects, was chosen from schools in the suburban areas: approximately 3 percent of the population of these schools is Negro.

They reported that three subparts of the ITPA, Auditory-Decoding, Auditory-Vocal Automatic, and Auditory-Vocal associations, drew the lines of distinction most clearly among the three groups:

suburban schoolchildren significantly outperforming both the Unity and Diversity School groups. Briefly, Auditory Decoding (labeled Auditory Reception in the revised edition, 1968) assesses the child's ability to derive meaning from verbally presented material and is a test of the receptive process at the representational level of the ITPA model. The test contains 50 short, direct questions such as, "Do dogs eat?" or "Do carpenters kneel?" and with the child's responding by "yes" or "no" or even a nod or shake of the head. Auditory-Vocal Association tests the child's ability to relate concepts presented orally and is a test of the *organizing* process at the representational level. The child's task is to manipulate linguistic symbols in a meaningful way by verbal analogies, such as, "I cut with a saw; I pound with a ——" or "A dog has hair; a fish has ——." Auditory-Vocal Automatic assesses correct grammatical form and is a test of *clozure* at the automatic level of the model (revised considerably in the new edition). The child's task, for example, would be to complete "Here is a hat. Here are two ——." These three subtests of the ITPA distinguish the language functioning of the lower class from the middle class on a receptive vocabulary task, an organizing analogies task, and a task at the automatic level which apparently measures grammatical habits. The nature of these tasks require the subjects to draw upon past learning and experience to facilitate recall from long-term memory. On other subsets of the ITPA there were no differences between the groups on tasks which require sequential habits which are more dependent on the relatively fixed capacity of the child's short-term memory. These tasks, for example, are the Visual-Motor Sequencing Test (requiring the reproduction of a series of geometric forms), the Auditory-Vocal Sequencing (digit repetition), and the Vocal-Encoding Subtest (description of an object such as a ball and the subject is asked to "tell me all about this." The score is the number of discrete concepts enumerated).

Barritt et al (1968) report an interesting observation between tasks requiring sequential habits and an earlier study of the comparison between normal children and retarded subjects on a word-association task. They found that while normal children gave more responses of the same form class as the stimulus words, retarded subjects gave more responses to word-association stimuli which could occur sequentially in a sentence. Although they simply suggest the relationship between the results of their findings for lower class children, retarded children, and normal children on the sequential tasks, their suggestion is highly relevant to the findings of Entwisle (1967), Entwisle and Greenberger (1968), and Entwisle (1968a, 1968b).

Entwisle and her associates have provided normative word-association data for sizable groups of young children over the past eight years. Recently (1967) she began studying word association in children by residential locus, social class, or subcultural group membership. Several different groups of children from Grades 1, 3, and 5 from rural American children, both Amish-Pennsylvanian and a cross section of typical Maryland farm children, and some rural German children are represented in her research. She also used subjects from urban Baltimore of three different socioeconomic levels, upper middle class, blue collar, and slum. The association task consisted of 96 stimulus words, chosen to represent different form classes and, where possible, different degrees of rarity. The Throndike-Lorge count was used to estimate frequency (Throndike and Lorge, 1944). For nouns, adjectives, and verbs, stimuli are divided into three strata, one with frequency greater than 1000, a second with frequency 500 to 1000, and a third with frequency below 500. No frequency division was possible for adverbs and pronouns. The children are interviewed one at a time and instructed that each is going to play a word game: the interviewer says a word aloud and the child's task is to respond by saying aloud the first word he thinks of.

The results are prefaced by a definition and explanation of terminology. In general adult responses differ from those of children's on a word-association task. Adult responses are characterized as paradigmatic while children give more associations characterized as syntagmatic. Paradigmatic associations of the adult or older children are usually of the same form, for example, of noun to noun (man-woman, table-chair). Syntagmatic associations are heterogeneous with respect to part of speech. A child, for example, is likely to associate a noun with a verb (man-work, boy jumps). The label "syntagmatic" gives the impression that children's associations are guided by the grammar of their language (although Anisfeld, 1964, takes issue with this assumption).

Entwisle determined the percentage of paradigmatic responses in the various sample strata to study relative rates of linguistic development. Analyses of the comparisons of paradigmatic rates support the following conclusions by her:

1. There are negligible differences between suburban children from upper middle-class and blue collar heighborhoods.

2. Rural Maryland children tend to develop more slowly than the suburban children, especially those of middle or low IQ.

3. Amish children develop even more slowly than the rural Maryland children.

4. White slum children are *advanced* compared to suburban children at first-grade, but retarded at third-grade. Negro slum children are generally behind white slum children, but at first-grade the Negro slum children are on a par with white suburban children.

Entwisle's observations for first-grade American children of different social strata, with respect to her findings on word associations, would rank all children as follows: White slum children, Negro slum children, and suburban middle class and working class children of both socioeconomic levels, rural Maryland children, and Amish children residing in rural Pennsylvania. She states that her results are surprising in two respects:

1. Rural Maryland children develop more slowly than suburban Maryland even though the children are of the same age and the same tested intelligence, and are closely matched in terms of schools attended, father's educational level and general economic status.

2. First-grade white children living in the slums of Baltimore City are *accelerated* compared to first-grade white children living in suburbs and first-grade Negro children are *not behind* white suburban children . . . rural Amish children lag behind rural Maryland children—slum children being behind suburban children at third and fifth grades . . .

In a later, more elaborate study on *urban* slum groups, both Negro and White, she gives a breakdown of the paradigmatic responses by form class, i.e., responses to adjectives, verbs, and adverbs and pronouns. The analysis of variance for paradigmatic responses for adjectives revealed a highly significant triple interaction—grade level × low-high I.Q. × race of interviewer × race of child. Negro children performed noticeably lower than urban, White children in the average percentages of paradigmatic responses to adjectives. The third-grade children were most affected by race of interviewers. When races of interviewers and children are mixed, Negro interviewers elicit more paradigmatics from White children than White interviewers elicit from Negro children. (In another study, Entwisle, 1968a, states, "Both white and Negro children tend to give more paradigmatic responses, i.e., more mature behavior, when the race of the interviewer *differs* from their own.") Drawing upon her previous work with Baltimore suburban children who had similar I.Q.'s to the urban slum children used in the above-mentioned study, she reported that:

rates (paradigmatic responses to adjectives—developmentally) for first-grade slum children exceed rates for first-grade suburban children matched for IQ. The medium IQ slum children respond to adjectives much like the high IQ (over 130) suburban children, and although the Negro slum children are less advanced than the white slum children, those of average IQ are responding at rates close to 10 percent higher than either the high—low SES (social economic status) suburban white groups. The low IQ white slum children are responding at rates close to those for the medium IQ white suburban children, and the low IQ Negro slum children are about the same as low IQ white suburban children.

Different effects are reported by her for the third-grade children. The medium I.Q. slum children of both races *lag* behind suburban children; that is, at later grades, including fifth grade, the early advantage of slum children in terms of paradigmatic response rates to adjectives is lost.

For verbs, first-grade slum children are more advanced than first-grade suburban children at both I.Q. levels. The reversals that were noted with respect to adjectives also occurred in the paradigmatic responses for verbs for the third-grade children: the relative advantage of the slum children disappears at this level. "Generally the same patterns with age and the same relative position of slum children with respect to suburban children are seen whether adjectives *or* verbs are analyzed" (Entwisle, 1968b).

With respect to pronouns and adverbs, the finding of a superiority of first-grade lower class children and a falling behind at later grades is similar to those for adjectives and verbs. By the third grade, however, adverbs are noticeably depressed, especially for young Negro children. Pronouns by contrast are the least depressed (re: adverbs, verbs, adjectives) at third grade and seem to be the most highly developed of any form class for the lower class children. Entwisle states, "pronouns are the most frequent class in spoken conversation, and their relative frequency must be higher for simple short interchanges than for complex utterances. Adverbs, on the other hand, express much more subtle meanings."

Entwisle (1968b) also studied the frequency of primary responses to nouns of urban slum children.

Frequency of primary responses is defined as the single response with the highest frequency: "chair," for example, would evoke the response "table," which is more of an adult response, or it would be a more frequent response at age 10 than at age five. Frequency of primary, then, would be a measure of maturity that "is independent of other measures previously considered" (Entwisle, 1968b).

Responses that increase in frequency between grades one and three in the large suburban samples were arbitrarily defined by Entwisle as "mature" so that the prevalence of mature responses in grade-one slum and suburban groups could be compared. She reported, for example, that the response "pepper" to "salt" increases in frequency from 44 percent to 55 percent in suburban children between grades one and three. Grade-one slum children gave this response 50 percent of the time, and so in their primary response they are between grade-one and -three suburban children. With the exception of three responses, "fly, table, crayon," to the stimulus words "bird, chair, color" respectively, all other responses (13) increase in the suburban children between grades one and three. This means that grade-one slum children responses to the other stimuli are considered "mature."

Entwisle's research with both Negro and White, grade-one, slum children suggests that they are more advanced in linguistic development (via a word-association paradigm) than suburban children of the same intelligence level. A reversal then occurs at grade three, and continues at grade five with the surburban child outperforming the lower class child or, more simply, the suburban child responds with more mature (adultlike) word associations.

Of the several explanations offered by Entwisle (1968a; 1968b) to account for the lower class child's paradigmatic response superiority at the early levels and the reversals that occur at later levels, the following is thought to be relevant. She contends that "simple verbal concepts, the verbal interaction required to support language acquisition activities may be more favorable for the very young slum child than for the (young) suruban child." The research of Hess and Shipman (1965) is used to support her contention. Their work suggests that the verbal models presented to lower class children are relatively simple and uncomplicated. They studied the verbalizations presented to the Negro lower class child by his mother when the mother was teaching the child simple-conceptual tasks. They report that the lower class child was exposed almost entirely to short, straightforward sets of utterances and gestures. Lower-class mothers were more apt to limit the range of choices open to the child and the time required to make a choice. Entwisle argues that "such exposure could favor early development, and lead to an early appreciation of form class properties, particularly for very common words and for verbal concepts at a low level of abstraction."

The verbalizations of Negro mothers from three different social classes also were studied on the same tasks. Upper status mothers used more elaborate and abstract forms of speech, which provided a more complex verbal-cognitive environment. This more complex verbal-cognitive environment of the suburban preschooler might be a temporary handicap. "Hierarchial and abstract meanings, partially learned, would not be very evident in word association measures." Such specific modes of language instruction displayed by the Negro mothers from different social class levels (college educated to welfare) suggests how acquisition of early verbal skills could be aided at the expense of more sophisticated skills. She further states (1968a):

> As the child continues to develop and requires more elaborate verbal models to stimulate growth, however, the suburban youngster begins to profit from his rich environment whereas the slum child falls progressively behind and fails to redeem his early promise. The syntax that the slum child is not exposed to may hinder communication later in a most insidious way be depriving the child of the tools of thought. The plain talk that aids early development may lead to a conceptual poverty that is more than just a restriction in vocabulary.

The explanation offered by Entwisle is plausible and consistent with her results. It also emphasizes the effects of early environmental influences on language development for lower class youngsters; moreover, it highlights the importance of environmental influences on the maturational processes including the role of parental interactions in this process. Entwisle's research points out the early superiority of the urban lower class child with respect to word associations by advancing the argument that the slum child appears to be exposed almost entirely to a straightforward and redundant set of utterances. This type of exposure, however, appears to be detrimental to later stages of language development, which is supported by her findings (on the same task) that the slum child is behind the surburban child at grades one and three. She further states that the language environment of the slum child may deprive the child of the tools of thought and thus lead to a conceptual poverty that is more than a vocabulary restriction.

In general, as the lower class child matures, he begins to fall further and further behind his middle class peers, in language as well as academic skills. According to Minde and Werry (1967) and Hurst and Jones (1966), factors such as poor self-image, negative attitudes toward change, and undesirable personality characteristics begin to enter: factors that cannot be overlooked in considering special instruction.

Although research continues to identify specific areas and types of language patterns of disadvantaged children, certain factors emerge from this review which have specific implications for early, special, educational instruction. As stated earlier, phonetic distortions of vowels were reported by Bryden (1968) to be the significant factor in identifying the speech samples of Negroes or Whites. It also was pointed out that consonant omissions and substitutions can occur in dialect patterns (Stewart, 1967) and that meaning could be lost to a listener outside of a particular speech community. Curtis (1968) and Chomsky (1964) also questioned the assumption of the phoneme as the basic unit of speech at the levels of physiological performance and of perceptual input and suggested that we explore models other than the present "phoneme model": models that presumably could be based on the physiological (motor) aspects of the speech code.

Baratz (1968) also has expressed an interesting viewpoint with respect to dialectal variations. When certain phoneme omissions occur, for example, in consonant blends, she states:

> The omission of the final /d/ in "hand" by the dialect speaker does not indicate that the speaker has been incapable of learning to produce the final /d/, but rather that the /nd/ blend does not normally occur in his dialect, in the same way that the initial /ps/ does not occur in standard English (initial /ps/ is usually reduced to /s/ as in "psychology").

She goes on to state that our (speech pathologists') work with the disadvantaged child should be treated differently from our work with other language-deviant children, such as the mentally retarded. The question of what directions, if any, speech pathologists should take with respect to phonological variations of lower class children arises immediately. When a child is "within" his speech community he exhibits a language system which enables him to communicate with his particular peer group. The problem seems to arise when the child enters the middle class culture, where he is now expected to perform and compete with his middle class counterpart. Baratz is of the opinion that we must not try to obliterate the lower class child's "within-language" system, because it enables him to communicate outside of the middle class culture where the majority of his experiences occur. She presents the argument that the speech pathologist's

> job is to teach the child a second language system (dialect if you wish) without denying the legitimacy of his own system, and if possible, by using examples from his own system to teach the new system. For example, if in the child's language code 'he walk' and 'he walks' are in free variation, then just insisting upon the child's uttering "he walks" in school may not ever teach him the distinction that you wish to make, i.e. that "he walk" and "he walks" are not in free variation and that only 'he walks' is permissible in standard English.

She further states "that these children do not need to be 'remediated' in the traditional sense of the word, but rather that they need to be taught standard English." Bryden's finding of phonetic vowel distortion; Stewart's report that meaning can be lost "between" speech communities when certain phoneme omissions and substitutions occur; Curtis' and Chomsky's question of the "phoneme model"; Baratz's example of a morphological omission, "he walk" and "he walks," and her contention that standard English be taught to the disadvantaged child as more or less a second language, raise certain problems with respect to special instruction for the disadvantaged child.

Baratz rather presumptuously assumes that standard English can be superimposed over the disadvantaged child's code without devaluing the dialect. While this is possible in the teaching and learning of a foreign language, we must not assume carelessly that the child is so naive as not to recognize the differences (re: the middle class) of his language system, which could possibly lead to the psychosocial concomitants of substandard speech mentioned by Hurst and Jones (1966).

The question arises, "Is the speech pathologist sufficiently trained to handle the above-mentioned problems?" Baratz presumes that 1. Headstart programs will employ and 2. speech pathologists are trained to function as teachers of English of disadvantaged children. The speech pathologists should be trained sufficiently to act as team members or consultants on phonemic, morphemic, and syntactic problems. They also should have knowledge of various physiological-perceptual speech models which would enable them to plan and facilitate programs of instruction. Traditionally, they lack the training to function as classroom learning specialists and can at this time make their greatest contribution as team members or consultants in Headstart or instructional programs because of their expertise of the normal speech and hearing mechanism.

It was mentioned earlier in the review, however, that emphasis on correct phonemic production is not warranted when a child has an associated language problem. Language problems are considered more fundamental than speech problems, and only after significant gains in language development should speech therapy be initiated.

Generally accepted by a number of educators and/or investigators, is that children from the lower class do not have the language to express abstractions, logical, spacial, and temporal relationships, or to generalize about individual feelings and differences. The ongoing, excellent work of Brent and Katz, 1967, Heider, Cazden, and Brown, 1968, Williams, 1969, and Williams and Wood, 1971, have approached this generally accepted notion with caution and empiricism. Cazden presents the well-taken argument that since the number of experimental situations is infinite, examiners should be cautious about generalizing their findings from one environmental testing situation to another; that is, a lower class child may use a restricted code in one experimental situation but use a more elaborate code in another situation. "Whether non-standard English is, in addition, a cognitive liability to the speaker is much harder to determine" (Cazden, 1966). Research of the problem, however, has revealed certain consistent factors with implications for educational instruction.

Berstein and Entwisle are in agreement that lower class children differ from middle class children in pronoun usage. More specifically, this difference occurs in the lower class child's use of more exophoric pronouns—pronouns which indicate that his speech is therefore tied to the context in which it occurs. It appears that the lower class child is tied to the context in which the language responses are evoked; that is, the child appears to be stimulus bound. If the stimulus is removed, however, Brent and Katz tentatively report a dramatic improvement in the quality of language used to relate stories, greater connectedness of the ideas, and a marked increase in the amount of spontaneous speech. Further research is needed to resolve the issue of pronoun differences. It has mentioned that if Brent and Katz's future results do not agree (picture not present) with Bernstein et al., this would mean that the lower class child is limited by the testing situation and that if given the opportunity he may be able to use pronouns which enable him to be understood outside the immediate context. The issue remains, though, that differences were observed between lower class and middle class children on the usage of pronouns with the stimuli present. They may, however, function differently by shifting to more elaborate language if given freedom to use their power of abstraction.

Another interesting factor is the consistency of the findings with respect to wholistic vs. part-by-part description; that is, the majority of middle class children will respond (encoding) by using more descriptive types of language as opposed to lower-class children, who respond by using more wholistic language (Brent and Katz, 1967; Heider, Cazden, and Brown, 1968; Williams, 1969; Cazden, 1968). It appears that the middle class child notices and points out differences, while the lower class child ignores many differences and group similarities to arrive at a more wholistic response. Heider, Cazden, and Brown are conducting a more specific search into the differences in encoding styles between the two groups.

It also was reviewed that middle class children were better overall decoders than lower class children; middle class children were better decoders of both the wholistic as well as the part-by-part style, while lower class decoders were more successful with the wholistic encoding of middle class children. Williams also mentioned that lower class children seemed to be attuned to the concrete while middle class children were capable of responding to both the concrete and to a higher, more symbolic level of cognitive function. It may be that the more systems which are brought into play, such as syntax, semantics, and others, the easier it is for the middle class child to respond to situations (previous stimuli) not immediately present, thus facilitating more abstract recall. This would mean that the lower class child, shaped by the language of his environment, who is also deficient in any aspect of syntax, semantics, vocabulary, or other areas, would be less able to draw upon higher order cognitive processes. The lower class child is more or less bound by the immediate context when tested in certain situations or when required to use more abstract language because of semantics, syntax, vocabulary, etc., but this may not be so when placed in a situation more familiar to him. When the stimulus is removed his system may be more taxed, which requires him to draw upon partially or fully learned cognitive habits that apparently are not taxed when the stimulus is present. This explanation possibly accounts for Barritt's finding that Auditory-Decoding, Auditory-Vocal Automatic, and Auditory-Vocal associations, three subtests of the ITPA, drew the lines of distinction most clearly between lower class and middle class subjects. Auditory-Decoding and Auditory-Vocal association presumably test the representational level of the ITPA model. Representational level was defined as a more complex mediating process and uses symbols which carry meaning. The Auditory-Vocal Automatic presumably tests the automatic level of the ITPA model. The Automatic level was defined as a less complex level and presumably accounts for the child's ability to perform less symbolic tasks. Previously, for the Auditory-Vocal Automatic subtest, the example was given of "Here is a hat. Here are two ——" with the child's task to supply the missing *meaningful* word. The question of how a meaningful task vs. a nonmeaningful task, such as "Here is a teep. Here is another teep. Now there are two ——" with the child's task to supply the missing *nonmeaningful* word was explored by Shriner and Miner (1968). In the study two groups of preschool children, 25 disadvantaged and 25 advantaged, were matched by mental age and compared in their ability to apply receptive and expressive morphological rules to unfamiliar situations. A comparison of morphology scores between the disadvantaged and advantaged revealed no statistically significant differences on this meaningful task. In another study Shriner and Daniloff (1970) studied perception-resynthesis performance of 80 normal-speaking first- and third-grade children on meaningful vs. nonmeaningful consonant-vowel-consonant syllables. Nonmeaningful cvc syllables were much less easily resynthesized than meaningful syllables (resynthesization is defined as the child's ability to synthesize the separated phonemes of a syllable or word and to verbally produce the integrated whole). The large meaning vs. nonmeaning finding reported by Shriner and Daniloff was thought to bear directly on the ITPA model. Our results suggested that meaningful stimuli are processed at the representational level of the ITPA model where rules of syntax (deep structure) assist to facilitate resynthesis and *not* at the automatic level as Kirk et al. (1968) have postulated. We suggest that the more systems brought into play (such as, syntax, semantics, etc.) the easier the task becomes for the child which would facilitate short-term memory recall. This means that with the addition of the syntax-semantic components, the less complex the task of the mediating process at the representational level with respect to the automatic level: the automatic level, according to our results, apparently processing nonmeaningful stimuli. It can be argued that the meaningful task "Here is a hat. Here are two ——" is really a test of the representational level of the ITPA model. Shriner's and Miner's results then would be a test of the automatic level of the model. Since Williams reported that middle class children were capable of responding to both the concrete and to higher, more symbolic levels of cognitive function, middle class children would be able to perform equally well with lower class children on Shriner's and Miner's test of the nonmeaningful stimuli but lower class not as well on Barritt's et al. test of meaningful stimuli. This interpretation also is consistent with Barritt's et al. finding of no differences between the groups on tasks which require sequential habits (automatic level).

Another interesting result of this review is the findings of the systematic research of Entwisle. As stated earlier, she reports that inner-city first-grade children are more advanced in paradigmatic responses on a word-association task than suburban children. A reversal takes place at grade three and continues at grade five, with the suburban child outperforming the lower-class child, responding with more mature word associations. She contends that early parental exposure to simple verbal concepts and the verbal interaction required to support language acquisition activities may be more favorable for young inner-city children than for young suburban children. The lower class child apparently is exposed almost entirely to short, straightforward, redundant sets of utterances and gestures as opposed to the middle class child, who is exposed to more elaborate and abstract utterances. This early exposure appears to enhance the later cognitive-language development of middle class children. Lower class children, however, appear to be penalized in later cognitive-language development because of their early exposure to a different type of language system; apparently, this also may cause problems in pronoun usage, wholistic decoding, and encoding response characteristics and word-association problems—problems that may eventually lead to conceptual poverty as well as the psychosocial problems reported by Hurst and Jones (1966).

Instructional methods or programs are often initiated with little rationale before research has defined or established adequately specific patterns or avenues of approach. Educator or speech-language clinicians utilizing clinical intuition feel that something must be done: they then proceed without adequate models or guidelines to amend the existing problem. More often than not, what was once clinical intuition or an initial approach to meet the needs of a problem area now becomes and accepted truism or statement of fact. It is only the wholehearted who are willing to abandon the old and adopt the new and the foolhardy who are willing, always too readily, to adopt the new and abandon the old. This has been especially true with respect to the disadvantaged population.

Probably the most widespread and controversial program of instruction for disadvantaged children was created by Bereiter and Engelmann at the University of Illinois. Their instructional program, published in book form in 1966, has been reported to the public through newspapers (including *The New York Times*), popular magazines (*Saturday Review*), and national TV (CBS—Twenty-First Century). The authors refer to their cookbook (their term) as "supercharged," consisting of little rationale and much written "verbal bombardment" (again their terminology). Their cookbook approach also has been called most appropriately a "pressure-cooker approach" (*Sat. Rev.*, June 15, 1968). Basically, instruction consists of stressful, boisterous, repetitious drill of the form

"Teacher: (presents picture of rifle)
This is a ——.
Child B: Gun
Teacher: Good. It is a gun. Let's all say it: This is a gun. This is a gun. This is a gun. Let's say it one more time: This is an alligator.
Child D: It ain't neither. It is a gun.
Teacher: That's what I said. I said 'This is a bulldog'
Children (A, B, C, D, E): No, No. It ain't no bulldog. That a gun.
etc." (pg. 105).

The task being presented is that of classifying things as weapons or nonweapons. It would take a highly skilled teacher less than 10 seconds to present the above example to a group of disadvantaged children. Their rationale is to abandon the "whole child" approach because it amounts to dividing his time, which they state would do nothing more than give the child a "smattering of learning in many areas, but leaving him with all the deficiencies he had before, only to a lesser degree—The authors are convinced that there is a better choice" (pp. 12–13). Their strategy is to focus upon academic objectives by concentrating upon a small range and relegating all nonacademic objectives to a secondary position. At the time of their writing, they admit that their curricula was premature and that their methods had not been field-tested for long, but they nevertheless felt an immediate need to publish them.

Negative criticism of their approach is that instead of appealing to whatever cognitive-language processes and verbal behavior that the disadvantaged may possess, teachers attempt (quite successfully, I may add) to inject information by rote in such a way as to instill reflex responses of primitive Aristotolian-logical relations, and of specific recall of numbers and sentence formation. They assume that if material can be learned by rote and later recalled, then these children will eventually become equal to middle class elementary school children. The child is not taught to accept or be "responsible" for future learning; rather, he is considered an organism in which repetitous drills followed by ritualistic rewards mechanically fill his mind. While the method may or may not have short-term effects, long-term effects are generally thought to be more desirable in education.

In the review it was pointed out that lower class mothers limit the range of choice open to the child and also limit the time required for the child to make a choice. The mother tells him what to do rather than to think something through. Further, they use simple, short, straightforward, redundant sets of utterances much like the Bereiter-Engelmann method. It was pointed out that on a word-association task Negro and White inner-city children were ahead of suburban children at first grade, but gradually fell behind at grades three and five. The interpretation given was because of what may be early parental exposure to poor cognitive-language stimulation, again much like the Bereiter-Engelmann task. It was also pointed out that the lower class child appears to be stimulus bound or tied to the immediate context, a factor that the Bereiter-Engelmann approach enhances; what actually is needed is a method of instruction that will facilitate more abstract recall. The child should be started with the familiar (to him) syntax-semantic components to facilitate "representational" recall and not "automatic" recall as the Bereiter-Engelmann method teaches.

"There are undoubtedly class differences in dispositional and maturational variables, and there are undoubtedly class differences in cognitive abilities as well. One important problem in research as well as in education—is how not to get the two mixed up" (Heider, Cazden, and Brown). Probably what is needed is an approach similar to the one reported by Quay (1968) on the facets of educational exceptionality: a conceptual framework for assessment, grouping, and instruction. The framework offered by Quay consists of a set of functions and the relation of these functions to certain modalities of the learning parameters of input, response, and reinforcement. When specific language-learning patterns of the disadvantaged child are known more exactly, then the interaction of these three components provides a basis for a technology of instruction. Quay's conceptual framework can be used by the educator in classroom teaching or used by the speech-language clinician once specific language patterns are noted; that is, it is a framework aimed at improving those aspects of the learning process in which any child, especially the disadvantaged, may eventually require.

Perhaps the question of aspects of language skills in the economically deprived can best be summarized by another question: when does *any* individual break the language of his immediate environment which would permit him to extend himself beyond that to which he has been exposed?

BIBLIOGRAPHY

Anisfeld, M., Bogo, N., and Lambert, W. 1962. Evaluation reactions to accented English speech. *J. abnorm. soc. Psychol.*, 65, 223–231.

———. 1964. Language skills in the context of the child's cognitive development. *Project Literacy Reports*. No. 2. Ithaca: Cornell. 37–43.

Baratz, J. 1968. Language in the economically disadvantaged child: a perspective. *Asha*, 10, 143–145.

Barritt, L., Semmel, M., and Weener, P. 1968. A comparison of the psycholinguistic functioning of "educationally-deprived" and "educationally-advantaged" children. Univ. Mich., Center Res. Lang. Behan (unpublished report).

Bereiter, C., and Engelmann, S. 1966. Teaching disadvantaged children in the preschool. Englewood Cliffs, N.J.: Prentice-Hall.

Bernstein, B. 1961. Social class and linguistic development: a theory of social learning. *In* Education, economy and society. Halsey, A., Floud, J., and Anderson, C., eds. Glencoe, Ill.: Free Press.

———. 1965. A sociolinguistic approach to social learning. *In* Penguin survey of the social sciences. Gould, J., ed. Baltimore: Penguin.

———. 1967. Social structure, language and learning. *In* The psychology of language, thought and instruction. De Cecco, J., ed. New York: Holt, Rinehart and Winston.

Brent, S., and Katz, E. 1967. A study of language deviations and cognitive process. *Progress Report No. 3, O.E.O.* Job Corps Res. Contract 1209.

———, and Klamer, P. 1967. A study of language deviations and cognition. *Progress Report No. 2, O.E.O.* Job Corps. Res. Contract 1209.

Bryden, J. 1968. An acoustic and social dialect analysis of perceptual variables in listener identification and rating of negro speakers. Office Educ. Bur. Res., *Final Report No. 7-C-003*.

Cazden, C. 1966. Subcultural differences in child language: an interdisciplinary review. *Merrill-Palmer quart.*, 12, 185–219.

———. 1968. Three sociolinguistic views of the language and speech of lower-class children—with special attention to the work of Basil Bernstein. *Developm. Med. Child Neurol.*, 10, 600–612.

Chomsky, N. 1964. Comments for project literacy meeting. *Project Literacy Reports, No. 2.* Ithaca: Cornell. 1–8.

Curtis, J. 1968. Segmenting the stream of speech. Paper presented Lincoln Land Conference on Dialectology. Charleston, Ill.: Eastern Ill. Univ.

Daniloff, R., and Moll, K. 1968. Co-articulation of lip rounding. *J. Speech Hearing Res.*, 11, 707–720.

Deutsch, M. 1965. The role of social class in language development and cognition. *Amer. J. Orthopsychiat.*, 35, 24–25.

Entwisle, D. 1967. Subcultural differences in children's language development. *Report Proj. No.* 6-1610. Baltimore: Johns Hopkins Univ.

———. 1968a. Subcultural differences in children's language development. *Int. J. Psychol.* 3. 13–22.

———. 1968b. Developmental sociolinguistics: in inner-city children. *Amer. J. Sociology*. 74, 37–49.

———, and Greenberger, E. 1968. Differences in the language of negro and white grade-school children 1, 2. *Report Proj. No.* 61610-03-03. Baltimore: Johns Hopkins Univ.

Frazier, A. 1964. A research proposal to develop the language skills of children with poor backgrounds. *In* Improving english skills of culturally different youth. Jenett, A., Mersard, A., and Gunderson, D., eds., Washington, D.C.: U.S. Gov't. Printing Office.

Gussow, J. 1965. Language development in disadvantaged children. *IRCD Bull.*, 1, 5.

Guttman, W. 1966. Measurement of articulatory merit. *J. Speech Hearing Res.*, 9, 323–339.

Harms, L. 1961. Listener comprehension of speakers of three status groups. *Language and Speech*, 4, 109–112.

Heider, E., Cazden, C., and Brown R. 1968. Social class differences in the effectiveness and style of children's coding ability. *Project Literacy Reports*. Ithaca, N.Y.: Cornell.

Hess, R., and Shipman, V. 1965. Early experience and socialization of cognitive modes in children. *Child. Develop.*, 36, 869–886.

Hurst, C., and Jones, W. 1966. Psychosocial concommitants of sub-standard speech. *J. Negro Educ.*, 36, 409–421.

Hymes, D. 1964. Language in culture and society. New York: Harper & Row.

John, V. 1963. The intellectual development of slum children; some preliminary findings. *Amer. J. Orthopsychiat.*, 33, 13–22.

Katz, E., and Brent, S. 1968. Understanding connectives. *J. verb. Learn. verb Behav.*, 7, 501–509.

Kirk, S., McCarthy, J., and Kirk, W. 1968. Illinois test of psycholinguistic abilities (rev. ed.). Champaign-Urbana: Univ. Ill. Press.

Kozhevnikov, V., and Chistovich, L. 1965. Speech, articulation and perception. Eng. trans. from Russian. Washington, D.C.: U.S. Dep't. Commerce.

Liberman, A., Cooper, F., Shankweiler, D., and Studdert-Kennedy, M. 1967. Perception of the speech code. *Psychol. Rev.*, 74, 431–461.

Loban, W. 1965. A sustained program of language learning. *In* Language problems for the disadvantaged. Corbin, R., and Crosby, M., eds. Champaign, Ill.: Nat. Council Teachers, Eng.

Marge, M. 1968. The role of the profession of speech pathology and audiology in the management of language problems. *Asha*, 10, 221–222.

Markel, N., Eisler, R., and Reese, H. 1967. Judging personality from dialect. *J. verb. Learn. verb. Behav.*, 6, 33–35.

Minde, K., and Werry, J. 1967. The response of school children in low socioeconomic area to intensive psychiatric counseling of their teachers: a controlled evaluation. Paper presented to Annual Meeting of the Amer. Psychiat. Assn. Boston.

Newton, E. 1965. Planning for the language development of disadvantaged children and youth. *J. Negro Educ.*, 34, 167–177.

Öhman, S. 1967. Numerical model of co-articulation. *J. acoust. Soc. Amer.*, 41, 310–320.

Quay, H. 1968. The facets of educational expectionality: a conceptual framework for assessment, grouping and instruction. *Except. Children*, 25–31.

Raph, J. 1965. Language characteristics of culturally disadvantaged children: review and implications. *Rev. Educ. Res.*, 35, 373–400.

Ringgaard, K. 1965. The phonemes of a dialectal area, perceived by phoneticians and by speakers themselves. Proceedings 5th international congress phonetic sciences. The Hauge: Mouton. Pp. 495–501.

Robinson, W. 1965. The elaborated code in working-class language. *Lang. Speech*, 8, 241–244.

Rosenthal, R., and Jacobson, L. 1968. Teacher expectations for the disadvantaged. *Scientific Amer.* 218, 19–23.

Shriner, T., and Miner, L. 1968. Morphological structures in the language of disadvantaged and advantaged children. *J. Speech Hearing Res.*, 11, 605–610.

———, and Daniloff, R. 1970. Resynthesization of meaningful and non-meaningful CVC syllables by children. *J. Speech Hearing Res.*, 12, 319–325.

———, Holloway-Sayre, M., and Daniloff, R. 1969. The relationship between articulatory deficits and syntactical errors in speech defective children. *J. Speech Hearing Res.*, 12, 319–325.

Stewart, W. 1964. Urban negro speech: sociolinguistic factors affecting English teaching. Social dialects and language learning. Champaign, Ill.: Nat. Council Teachers Eng.

———. 1967. Sociolinguistic factors in the history of American Negro dialects. *The Florida FL Reporter*, 5, 2.

Shuy, R., Davis, A., and Hogan, R. 1964. Social dialects and language learning. Champaign, Ill.: Nat. Council Teachers Eng.

Taylor, W. 1954. Application of cloze and entropy measures to the study of contextual constraint in samples of continuous prose. Univ. Ill.: Ph.D. dissertation.

Thorndike, E., and Lorge, I. 1944. The teacher's word book of 30,000 words. New York: Bur. Pub., Teacher's Coll., Columbia Univ.

Voiers, W. 1964. Perceptual bases of speaker identity. *J. acoust. soc. Amer.*, 39, 736–740.

Whorf, B. 1956. Language, thought and reality. Carroll, J., ed. New York: Wiley.

Williams, F., and Naremore, R. 1967. Language and poverty: an annotated bibliography. Institute Res. on Poverty, Univ. Wis.

———. 1969. Social class differences in how children talk about television: some observations and speculations. Institute Res. on poverty. Univ. Wis. (unpublished report).

———, and Wood, B. 1971. Negro children's speech: some social class differences in word predictability. *J. Speech Hearing Disorders*, 34 (in press).

45

The Psychology of Language

Courtney B. Cazden

"Each language can be regarded as a particular relationship between sound and meaning" (Chomsky, 1958, p. 15). Any physical signal that is a spoken sentence expresses and communicates a particular meaning. How is this accomplished? When a person knows a language, what does he know? What does he have in his head, in the neurobiology of his brain? We can be certain that he does not have a set of sentences from which he makes a selection at the moment of speaking. Beyond conversational routines like "When will you be home?" and routinized statements like proverbs, each spoken sentence is constructed anew to express and communicate particular meanings to particular individuals. As speakers, we are able to construct an infinite number of such sentences—infinite because we can always insert another modifier like *very*, attach another clause with *and*, or contruct any number of other variations. As listeners, we can understand the potentially infinite number of sentences so constructed by others.

Such abilities exist only if what we know in common with other members of our language community is a finite set of rules. These rules express the relationships between sound and meaning in our language. They represent the ways in which an idea in the mind becomes a sequential structure of linguistic units.

> Subjectively, we seem to grasp meanings as integrated wholes, yet it is not often that we can express a whole thought by a single sound or a single word. Before they can be communicated, ideas must be analysed and represented by sequences of symbols. To map the simultaneous complexities of thought into a sequential flow of language requires an organism with considerable power and subtlety to symbolize and process information (Miller and Chomsky, 1963, p. 483).[1]

The rules of a language constitute powerful but implicit or tacit knowledge (Miller, 1964a, 1964b). We know the rules; we act on the basis of them in speaking and listening. We cannot state them, however, without serious linguistic study. Consider a simple example from English morphology. When asked to pluralize nonsense syllables such as *wuq*, *bik* and *gutch*, all adult speakers of English and many children as young as four years agree that the answers are *wuq/z/*, *bik/s/* and *gutch/əz/* (Berko, 1961). Yet few readers can state why this is so.

> By calling a rule implicit, we mean, among other things, that if it were formulated and offered for consideration to the persons concerned, they would accept it as codifying their previous practise, and that after such acceptance their behavior would not be substantially changed. (Black, 1962, p. 131.)

We also mean that when a rule of our language is violated, we have a general sense that something is

[1] In an important article originally published in 1951, Lashley (1961) discusses the relation between simultaneous thought and sequential speech as "the problem of serial order in behavior," and relates it to types of aphasia. See also Miller, Galanter and Pribram (1960) for provocative comments about the role of plans in many aspects of human behavior, including "plans for speaking."

amiss. Hearing a waitress ask, "Anybody wants any?" as she removes the basket of rolls, most readers would register a mismatch between their rules and her speech. It would be difficult to explain the discrepancy, but we would be aware of its existence. Or we may, for expressive purposes, utter the imperative, "Tell it like it is," and be aware in so doing that it comes from a dialect whose rules are different from our own and derives its special expressive value from that source.

A grammar is a description constructed by linguists of such a system of rules. Like all descriptions of natural phenomena, grammars are subject to continuous revision and correction. In the range of phenomena they explain, the most powerful grammars we have today are the transformational grammars being written by a group of linguists centering around Noam Chomsky (1957, 1965, 1968). While grammars are written by linguists, they constitute psychological theories about one aspect of the organization of human knowledge.

> At several levels the linguist is involved in the construction of explanatory theories, and at each level there is a clear psychological interpretation for his theoretical and descriptive work. At the level of particular grammar, he is attempting to characterize knowledge of a language, a certain cognitive system that has been developed—unconsciously, of course—by the normal speaker-hearer. At the level of universal grammar, he is trying to establish certain general properties of human intelligence. Linguistics, so characterized, is simply the subfield of psychology that deals with these aspects of mind. (Chomsky, 1968, p. 24.)

In addition to language there is speech. While language is knowledge in our heads, speech is the realization of that knowledge in behavior. Language exists even in moments of silence and sleep; speech exists only in moments of actual speaking or listening (including silent activization of language in thought). Because it is language (though not language alone) that makes speech possible, these contrasting phenomena have come to be called "competence" and "performance" in transformational grammar. "If language were a game, competence would be the rules of the game, while the actions of its players would constitute performance" (Blumenthal, 1966, p. 81). The contrasting pairs of labels line up as follows:

language	speech
knowledge	behavior
competence	performance
rules of the game	actions of the players.[2]

Descriptions of speech are also part of psychology, but they are far less advanced than descriptions of language. As yet we know little about the cognitive processes by which sentences are produced and comprehended. This is the field of psycholinguistics proper (Ervin-Tripp and Slobin, 1966; Miller and McNeill, 1969; Slobin, 1971). We also know little about the distribution of acts of speaking: who says what to whom, how, when, and to what purpose. This is the field of sociolinguistics (Ervin-Tripp, 1969). While psycholinguistics deals primarily with the processes of speaking and listening in an individual mind, sociolinguistics deals with the interactions of individuals in social settings. The two are related in important ways because any act of speaking involves decisions about function, topic, and form which are affected by characteristics of the speaker and listener(s) and the setting both are in. Similarly, any act of listening is affected by the expectations set up in the listener about what he is likely to hear from a particular person at a particular time.

After these introductory remarks, this chapter is

[2] I am grateful to Laura L. Lee for clarifying the difference between the use of the terms language and speech in this chapter and their traditional meanings in the field of Speech Pathology.

> Back in the 20's and 30's, when Speech Pathology first became a professional discipline, the reported research centered around disorders which were largely on the production side of communication: stuttering, voice, cleft palate, cerebral palsy, etc. While problems of speech reception were acknowledged and discussed, it was not until the field of Audiology began to develop in the 40's, that active research into speech comprehension, deafness, and hearing loss was expanded. It was about that time that the Association changed its name from the American Speech Correction Association to the American Speech and Hearing Association to unify these two areas of research under one title. But the emphasis of clinical training was still largely upon the production of intelligible "speech" with less consideration given to problems of concept development, vocabulary, and word meanings or to sentence formulations, syntax, and morphology. In the early 50's, both research and clinical methods began to focus upon these other considerations, and it was natural that we should try to differentiate them from the old "speech" category by using another name. That's when we began to use the word "language" to mean these other aspects of communication, not just articulation or production alone. Furthermore, we recognized two different kinds of language use, receptive and expressive, and this dichotomy has been helpful to us in describing types of adult aphasia and neurological impairment in children. Thus, historically, we have tended to use the word "speech" to mean "production" and "language" to mean "everything-else-that-is-not-production."
>
> Many of us are trying to break down this artificial speech-language dichotomy in our field, and the newer terminology of psycholinguistics is helpful in doing this. By placing the "rules" of phonology-semantics-syntax altogether under Competence and the "use of the rules", both receptively and expressively, under Performance, psycholinguists have given us a new perspective from which to view our own work. Using psycholinguistic terminology, we would no longer tend to label a case as "speech" or "language", and we might not make such a sharp distinction between "receptive" and "expressive" language skills. What we would tend to do is to determine whether a particular problem involves phonology and/or vocabulary and/or syntax, or to what extent each of these aspects of communication is involved. Whichever aspect the clinician selects to work on, he must be concerned with both Competence and Performance, with rules and their use (Personal communication, 1969).

divided into four sections: a discussion of the distinction between deep and surface structure in language, and introductions to the threefold division of a grammar: semantics, syntax, and phonology. Although chapter 44 is on sociolinguistics, I will occasionally raise sociolinguistic questions here as well in order to make the full scope of the issues clear. Since chapter 43 is on language development, I will deal only with the organization and use of structured language, not with its acquisition.

The chapter as a whole does not constitute a comprehensive survey of psycholinguistics; it is rather a selection of ideas of particular relevance as a background for understanding and diagnosing individual differences in language competence and performance.[3] While the phrase "individual differences" will be used hereafter, the discussion applies to group differences as well. They are simply individual differences whose distributions correlate with attributes of group membership such as I.Q., social class, or degree of physical or emotional impairment such as deafness or schizophrenia.

Before turning to these sections, however, let us be clear about how impressive the universal human accomplishments of language and speech really are. Computers which, as I am writing, have just guided and controlled man's first trip to the moon cannot translate natural language, and there is increasing reason to believe that they will never be able to do so.

> Consider the simple sentence "Time flies like an arrow."* . . . A grammar that pretends to describe English at all accurately must yield a structure for "Time flies like an arrow" in which "time" is the subject of the verb "flies" and "like an arrow" is an adverbial phrase modifying the verb. "Time" can also serve attributively, however, as in "time bomb," and "flies" of course can serve as a noun. Together with "like" interpreted as a verb, this yields a structure that becomes obvious only if one thinks of a kind of flies called "time flies" which happen to like an arrow, perhaps as a meal. Moreover, "time" as an imperative verb with "flies" as a noun also yields a structure that makes sense as an order to someone to take out his stopwatch and time flies with great dispatch, like an arrow.
>
> A little thought suggests many minor modifications of the grammar sufficient to rule out such fantasies. Unfortunately too much is then lost. . . . Anything ruling out the nonexisting species of time flies will also rule out the identical but legitimate structure of "Fruit flies like a banana."
>
> Semantics, the all too nebulous notion of what a sentence means, must be invoked to choose among the three structures syntax accepts for "Time flies like an arrow." No techniques now known can deal effectively with semantic problems of this kind. . . . We do not know how people understand language, and our machine procedures barely do child's work in an extraordinarily cumbersome way (Oettinger, 1966, pp. 168–169.)

[3] For other excellent introductions, see Chapters 6 and 7 in Brown (1965); Chapters 7–10 in Neisser (1967); and an appendix in McNeill (1970). See Jensen (1968) for a survey of social class differences (and by implication other individual differences) in the use of language in thought.

DEEP AND SURFACE STRUCTURES

The grammar of a language is a formal representation of the implicit knowledge of a native speaker. The first and probably most important attribute of that knowledge which the grammar must reflect is that it is not limited to the noises we speak and hear. We know that the subject of the imperative "Go home" is *you*. We know that the following three sentences say the same thing despite different physical forms:

(1a) The astronauts photographed the moon.
(1b) The moon was photographed by the astronauts.
(1c) It was the moon that the astronauts photographed.

And we know that a complex sentence like

(2) The man fed the dog that belonged to his son,

is a combination of at least two ideas: a boy had a dog, and his father fed that dog.

Such facts as these have led transformational grammarians to postulate two distinct structures for each sentence: a deep (underlying and abstract) structure, and a surface (superficial and perceptible) structure (Postal, 1966). The deep structure represents the basic relationships in the meaning being expressed—relationships of actor-action, action-object, and modification. The surface structure represents the grammatical relationships such as subject of verb and object of verb in the sentence as spoken. For any sentence, the deep structure and surface structure are related by a set of transformational rules which act to delete, permute, substitute, and combine elements.

Both deep and surface structures are hierarchical in nature, not linear. Try dividing sentence (1a) into its component parts. The sequence of divisions would look like this (after Brown, 1965, p. 283):

The astronauts photographed the moon.							Sentence
The astronauts			photographed the moon.				Subject-predicate
The astronauts			photographed		the moon.		Subject-verb-object
The	astronauts		photographed		the	moon.	Words
The	astronaut	s	photograph	ed	the	moon.	Morphemes

In the following quotation from Chomsky (1968) we can follow a description of one sentence. The symbols used are the following:

S—sentence

NP—noun phrase

VP—verb phrase.

I believe that the most appropriate general framework for the study of problems of language and mind is the system of ideas developed as part of the rationalist psychology of the seventeenth and eighteenth centuries, elaborated in important respects by the romantics and then largely forgotten as attention shifted to other matters. According to this traditional conception, a system of propositions expressing the meaning of a sentence is produced in the mind as the sentence is realized as a physical signal, the two being related by certain formal operations that, in current terminology, we may call *grammatical transformations*. Continuing with current terminology, we can thus distinguish the *surface structure* of the sentence, the organization into categories and phrases that is directly associated with the physical signal, from the underlying *deep structure*, also a system of categories and phrases, but with a more abstract character. Thus, the surface structure of the sentence "A wise man is honest" might analyze it into the subject "a wise man" and the predicate "is honest." The deep structure, however, will be rather different. It will, in particular, extract from the complex idea that constitutes the subject of the surface structure an underlying proposition with the subject "man" and the predicate "be wise." In fact, the deep structure, in the traditional view, is a system of two propositions, neither of which is asserted, but which interrelate in such a way as to express the meaning of the sentence "A wise man is honest." We might represent the deep structure in this sample case by formula 1, and the surface structure by formula 2, where paired brackets are labeled to show the category of phrase that they bound. (Many details are omitted.)

1 $$[_S\, [_{NP}\, \text{a man}\, [_S\, [_{NP}\, \text{man}\,]_{NP}\, [_{VP}\, \text{is wise}\,]_{VP}\,]_S\,]_{NP}\, [_{VP}\, \text{is honest}\,]_{VP}\,]_S$$

2 $$[_S\, [_{NP}\, \text{a wise man}\,]_{NP}\, [_{VP}\, \text{is honest}\,]_{VP}\,]_S$$

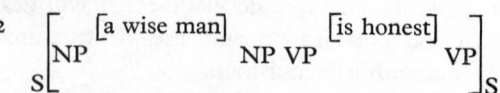

An alternative and equivalent notation, widely used, expresses the labeled bracketing of 1 and 2 in tree form, as 1′ and 2′ respectively:

1′

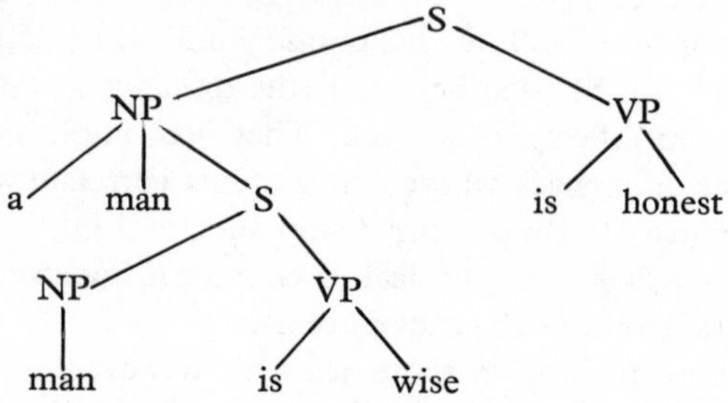

2′

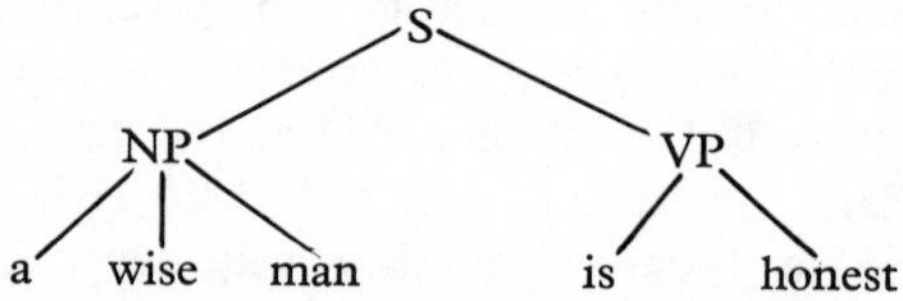

If we understand the relation "subject-of" to hold between a phrase of the category noun phrase (NP) and the sentence (S) that directly dominates it, and the relation "predicate-of" to hold between a phrase of the category verb phrase (VP) and the sentence that directly dominates it, then structures 1 and 2 (equivalently, 1′ and 2′) specify the grammatical functions of subject and predicate in the intended way. The grammatical functions of the deep structure (1) play a central role in determining the meaning of the sentence. The phrase structure indicated in 2, on the other hand, is closely related to its phonetic shape—specifically, it determines the intonation contour of the utterance represented.

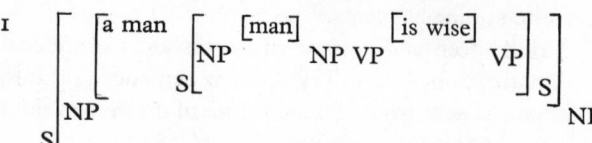

Knowledge of a language involves the ability to assign deep and surface structures to an infinite range of sentences, to relate these structures appropriately, and to assign a semantic interpretation and a phonetic interpretation to the paired deep and surface structures. This outline of the nature of grammar seems to be quite accurate as a first approximation to the characterization of "knowledge of a language."

How are the deep and surface structures related? Clearly, in the simple example given, we can form the surface structure from the deep structure by performing such operations as the following:

3 (a) assign the marker *wh-* to the most deeply embedded NP, "man"
(b) replace the NP so marked by "who"
(c) delete "who is"
(d) invert "man" and "wise."

Applying just operations (a) and (b), we derive the structure underlying the sentence "a man who is wise is honest," which is one possible realization of the underlying structure (1). If, furthermore, we apply the operation (c) (deriving "a man wise is honest"), we must, in English, also apply the subsidiary operation (d), deriving the surface structure (2), which can then be phonetically interpreted.

If this approach is correct in general, then a person who knows a specific language has control of a grammar that *generates* (that is, characterizes) the infinite set of potential deep structures, maps them onto associated surface structures, and determines the semantic and phonetic interpretations of these abstract objects. From the information now available, it seems accurate to propose that the surface structure determines the phonetic interpretation completely and that the deep structure expresses those grammatical functions that play a role in determining the semantic interpretation, although certain aspects of the surface structure may also participate in determining the meaning of the sentence in ways that I will not discuss here. A grammar of this sort will therefore define a certain infinite correlation of sound and meaning. It constitutes a first step toward explaining how a person can understand an arbitrary sentence of his language. (Chomsky, 1968a, pp. 25–27.)[4]

As further evidence for the surface structure-deep structure distinction, consider McNeill's discussion of three sentences (in press):

(3a) They are buying glasses.
(3b) They are drinking glasses.
(3c) They are drinking companions.

Despite the superficial similarities of these sentences, particularly in their written versions, they differ in important ways. Say them aloud and note the differences in where pauses can be placed.

[4] From LANGUAGE AND MIND by Noam Chomsky, © 1968 by Harcourt Brace Jovanovich, Inc, and reprinted with their permission.

With sentence (a), one might say *they—are buying—glasses*, but probably not *they—are—buying* glasses. It is the opposite with sentences (b) and (c). One could say *they—are—drinking companions* or *they—are—drinking glasses*, but not *they—are drinking—companions* or *they—are drinking—glasses* unless the reference was to cannibalism or suicide (McNeill, 1970).

A difference in where pauses can be placed in the sentences as pronounced means a difference in surface structure.

Now consider possible paraphrases, or synonomous statements of meaning, for (3b) and (3c).

Sentence (b) means "they are glasses to use for drinking," and sentence (c) means "they are companions that drink." Exchanging the form of the paraphrase between (b) and (c) leads to a nonparaphrase. Sentence (b) does not mean "they are glasses that drink" any more than sentence (c) means "they are companions to use for drinking" (McNeill, 1970).

A difference in possible paraphrases means a difference in the deep structure.

Following is a diagram of the parts of a person's knowledge of his language, and the parts of the grammar which describe the realationships between them:

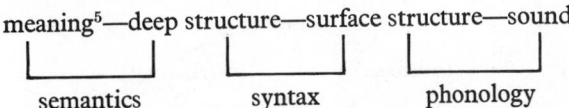

meaning[5]—deep structure—surface structure—sound

semantics syntax phonology

While it is true that speech production consists of the transformation of meaning into the spoken sentence, and speech comprehension consists of the reverse process, one cannot assume that production moves from left to right through the above diagram or that comprehension moves from right to left. The diagram shows the parts of linguistic competence; not the sequential processes involved in speech behavior (Blumenthal, 1966, p. 84).

We turn now to more detailed comments on semantics, syntax, and phonology in that order.

[5] Transformational grammarians have asserted that the meaning of a sentence is determined by the deep structure only. Currently, the effect on meaning of certain features of the surface structure is being explored. For instance, the stress on particular words is an aspect of surface structure. Yet the meaning of the following sentence changes when stress (signified by capital letters) is changed:

(14a) When he entered the room, Mary KISSED John. (*He* refers to *John*.)
(14b) When HE entered the room, Mary kissed JOHN. (*He* refers to someone other than *John*.)

SEMANTICS

Descriptions of the semantic component of English grammar are less advanced than descriptions of syntax or phonology. I will describe briefly one system proposed by Katz and Fodor (1964) and then suggest possible sources of individual differences in semantic competence.

The Meanings of Words

In order to understand a sentence, a person must have a mental dictionary which contains the words in that sentence and a set of rules for combining dictionary entries into the meaning of the sentence as a whole. In the mental dictionary, all that we know about the meaning of a word must be organized and represented in some economical form. Katz and Fodor (1964) suggest that each word has a set of markers or tags of various kinds.

Consider their example *bachelor*. Its meaning can be represented as follows (Katz and Fodor, 1964, p. 496):

bachelor
noun
(Human) (Animal)
(Male) (Male)
[who has never married] [young knight serving under the standard of another knight] [who has the first or lowest academic degree] [young fur seal when without a mate during the breeding time]

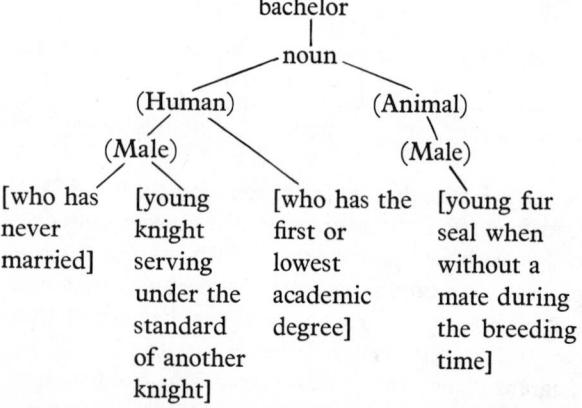

The unenclosed marker *noun* is a grammatical marker, in this case of the lexical category or part of speech to which the word belongs. This marker reflects knowledge of the slots in a sentence in which the word can appear. Markers of lexical subcategories such as *count noun* might have been added as a further specification that *bachelor* can appear in the slot *some* +——+ plural *s* which a mass noun like *rice* cannot. The markers enclosed in parentheses are semantic markers. Some of these, like human (or animate which could have been included), restrict the words with which *bachelor* can co-occur. For instance, as an animate noun *bachelor* can be the object of a verb like *frighten*, while an inanimate noun like *stone* cannot. Other semantic markers like *male* express part of the meaning of the word. Together the semantic markers exhibit the relations between different dictionary entries—e.g., between *bachelor* and *spinster* which would have identical entries except for the marker for sex. The items enclosed in brackets are distinguishers, each expressing an idiosyncratic meaning of the word. "The distinction between markers and distinguishers is meant to coincide with the distinction between that part of the meaning of a lexical item which is systematic in the language and that part of the meaning of the item which is not" (Katz and Fodor, 1964, p. 498).

The analysis of word meaning into semantic markers is similar to distinctive-feature analysis for speech sounds and componential analysis of kinship terms in anthropology. Fig. 45–1 diagrams these two analyses. Distinctive features represent universal potentialities of the human articulatory system from which a unique selection is used in each language; similarly, the dimensions of a componential analysis (or the semantic markers in transformational grammar) may represent universal ways of categorizing reality from which a unique selection is expressed in each culture.

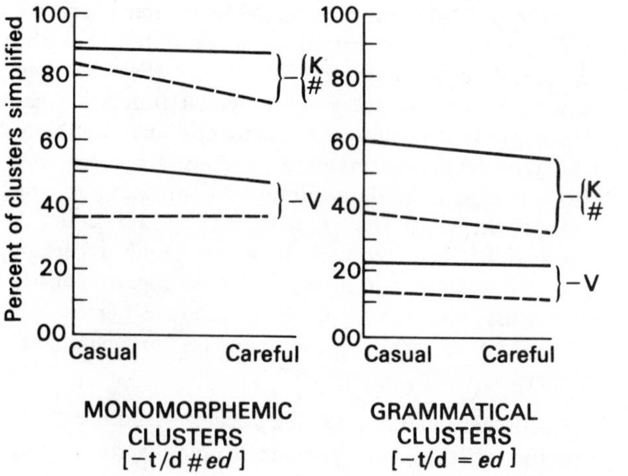

Fig. 45-1. The effects of style, class, grammatical status and phonetic environment on the simplification of consonant clusters ending in t/d; some preliminary data from adults in South Central Harlem. *From Labov & Cohen, 1967, p. 70.*

All the above aspects of meaning refer to the denotation of a word, the criterial or essential parts of a word's meaning which are shared by members of a given language community. Words also have connotations, aspects of meaning which are more idiosyncratic to individual persons. According to the semantic differential scale, the dimensions of connotative meaning can be reduced to three: evaluation (good-bad); potency (strong-weak); and activity (active-passive) (Osgood, Suci, and Tennenbaum, 1957). Connotative meanings reflect individual experience—whether dogs are loved or feared, whether the mention of spinach arouses anticipation or disgust.

The Meanings of Sentences

In addition to a knowledge of dictionary entries, people know rules for combining word meanings into a meaning for a sentence. Each word contributes to the sentence one of its meanings (a single path in the dictionary entry for *bachelor*); each word also contributes to the elimination of all but one of the possible paths for the other words in the sentence. For example, *man* can have a concrete meaning of an individual man, or it can have the abstract meaning of *mankind*. In the sentence

(5) The man hits the ball.

man must have the concrete meaning because *the* is marked for restriction to use with nouns that are concrete in this sense.

Note that the job which the computer could not do in interpreting "Time flies like an arrow" is similar, but here certain meanings of words are ruled out by our knowledge of the real world—that *like* cannot be a verb because then *time flies* would have to be a noun phrase with *adjective+noun* and no such flies exist. Katz and Fodor (1964) explicitly set out only to describe our ability to understand sentences apart from our knowledge of the settings in which they occur.

For a full description of human language ability, the notion of "interpret a sentence" must be expanded beyond the kind of literal interpretation which Katz and Fodor (1964) discuss. Consider the sentence "I am hungry" as spoken by a beggar at the door or by a child who hopes to delay bedtime. Clearly the meaning of the sentence is different in the two contexts.

Or consider two different messages conveyed by the utterance "Here are too few seats," depending upon which of two different nonlinguistic contexts constitutes its situational framework. The speaker is in either case a political candidate who has rented a room for a campaign meeting, and the utterance occurs shortly before the meeting starts. The hearer, however, is in one case the janitor who is standing in front of the closet where extra chairs are stored. In the other case, the utterance is made in response to a telephone call from the speaker's wife who is eager to know whether her husband has attracted a large crowd. . . .

The integration of the utterance in the situation may under such conditions be so perfect that the receiver can hardly tell which components of the message were mediated verbally and which were not. If we ask the janitor what the speaker said, he may very well respond: "He told me to bring more seats." The wife, on the other hand, may rush from the telephone and tell her children: "Daddy has attracted a large crowd tonight." And such spontaneous recodings of the same utterance suggest that transmission has been successful in both cases. The linguistic medium has brought about correspondence between intended and received message by virtue of its embeddedness in pre-established relationships between sender and receiver and other features of the communication setting (Rommetveit, 1968, p. 50).

In both these examples, a single sentence expresses two different communicative intents. The converse is also possible: a single communicative intent can be expressed in multiple forms which may not be synonomous in their literal meaning at all. For example:

(6a) Please turn on the lights.

(6b) We need the lights.

(6c) Are the lights on?

(6d) My, it's gotten dark in here.

Human ability to "interpret a sentence" frequently must go beyond recovery of the literal meaning ("beyond" in the sense of further removed from the actual perceptible sentence) to an inference about the intent of the speaker. The knowledge that makes this performance possible is not knowledge of language alone; in addition to linguistic rules, our tacit knowledge must include sociolinguistic rules which "specify linguistic output, or conversely, the interpretation of linguistic output, in terms of categories of social variables such as sex, age, relative rank, social situation (e.g., court session) and so on" (Ervin-Tripp, 1969). This more inclusive knowledge Hymes (in press) has called "communicative competence."

Individual Differences in Semantic Competence

Individual differences in the semantic component of linguistic competence can take several forms. Most obviously, mental dictionaries differ in their degree of completeness. Readers of this volume will be familiar with the two human meanings of *bachelor*, but few will also know the animal meaning. Differences exist not only in whether a word is known or not, but whether particular markers are present as part of the meaning. A child may understand that *father* is male, but not understand the generational relationship and so ask a grown woman if the man with her is her father. When a child asks his mother to "draw a letter" the listener can infer that the semantic marker is missing which restricts the use of *draw* to nonsymbols (except in the special case of calligraphy). Presumably, learning the word *write* will add the markers for this distinction to both words.

Alternate possible meanings for a single word (paths in the diagram for *bachelor*) probably acquire differential weightings for us depending on frequency of occurrence. In Webster's dictionary entries for a word are listed in historical order from archaic to contemporary slang. In mental dictionaries, however, they must be organized to reflect differential experience in the past and, as a result, differential expectations in the future. (Actually, the order of acquisition in any individual life history may reflect frequency of occurrence because the most frequent meaning will probably be learned first.) Depending on our experience, we may be more likely to think of a *bachelor* as an unmarried man or as a college graduate; depending on our experience we may think first of *father* as a label for a biological relationship or a role in a religious order. These weightings can facilitate or impede communication, depending on whether the speaker and his listener have shared or contrasting experience.

Finally, there are large differences among people in connotative meaning. *Cheap* may have a good connotation to people of limited means—synonymous with "not expensive;" it may have a bad connotation to the affluent—meaning sleazy or poorly made. The adjective *black* is undergoing an interesting (and deliberate) change at the present time. Instead of having a bad connotation—reinforced by the use of many expressions like "black magic"—now "black is beautiful." A recent study of word associations of first-, third-, and fifth-grade children in Baltimore found a significant racial difference in associations for *black*: "Differences between Negro and white responses to 'black' are particularly interesting. No responses that pertain to human beings are given by white children, whereas Negro children respond 'child', 'girls', 'hand', 'man', and even 'yes' to the stimulus word 'black'" (Entwisle and Greenberger, 1968, p. 11).

Of great interest is the behavior of such "rule-breakers as poets and schizophrenics" (Wales and Marshall, 1966, p. 75). Poetic violations of semantic restrictions can be distinguished from child speech only by an assumption that poets act deliberately and in full knowledge while children act out of ignorance. When the child says "Coffee dancing" as the cream swirls in his mother's cup, we assume he does not yet know that dancing properly takes an animate subject; when used by an adult, as in poetry, we call such rule-breaking metaphor. It is the difference between generalization before and after differentiation. But what about the language of schizophrenics? Wales and Marshall give some examples of schizophrenic speech and then raise interesting questions:

> *I find all the things that are Thursday; the colours of tradesmen are mostly dry as when the grass withers—red as when it burns away; I started with a sense that justice was next to the nebulous thing which no one can describe.* We do not, of course, claim that all schizophrenics talk like this, or even those who do, do so always. Many, however, sometimes do and would be described, for obvious reasons, as "thought-disordered." This fact may take us out of the realm of language studies as such; for, if the schizophrenic has disordered feelings, thoughts, beliefs, and so on, or is unwilling to disclose his thoughts except in code, then we would expect no more than that this would be reflected in his language. The paranoid patient who complains that "the prime minister and the archbishop are poisoning me with x-rays" may have a pathological belief system, but nothing is wrong with his language. However, when the patient's speech seems similar to certain types of poetic or mystical discourse we might expect that rigorous studies of "semi-sentences" may give some insight into the underlying "thought-disorder" or "communication-barrier." A theory of "semi-sentences" should help us to discover the "source" sentences which underlie the overt behavior. . . . One point at least is clear: if language studies are to be of any use in this area we must go well beyond counts of the relative frequency of *I* and *you*, abstract and concrete nouns, and so on. We must describe when and how specific rules of the semantic component are broken by individual patients (Wales and Marshall, 1966, pp. 75–76).

SYNTAX

The first section of this chapter introduced three central features of transformational grammars: a) the hierarchical arrangement of sentence constituents, b) the distinction between deep and surface structure, and c) the existence of transformational rules which state formally how the two are related. Since a transformational grammar presumes to be a formal description of the organization of our knowledge of language, some psycholinguistic experiments have been conducted to test the psychological validity of such grammatical constructs. Other experiments have attempted to define the nature of syntactic complexity. Following a brief review of a few representative experiments, I will explore sources of individual differences in syntactic competence and then report one linguistic description of what happens when hesitations occur and the verbal planning process is interrupted in the middle of a sentence.

Psycholinguistic Experiments on Syntax

Fodor and Bever (1965) presented subjects with a sentence in one ear and a simultaneous click at various positions in the sentence in the other ear. When asked where they had heard the click, the subjects tended to displace subjectively the click toward the major syntactic boundary (e.g. the break between *astronauts* and *photographed* in sentence (1a)). Mehler (1963) and Sachs (1967) showed that memory for the deep structure, or meaning of a sentence, is independent of (and easier than) recall of the particular transformation—e.g., active or passive sentence—that the subjects heard. Blumenthal (1967) and Blumenthal and Boakes (1967) showed that the success with which individual words prompt the recall of previously heard sentences varies with their grammatical relation in the deep structure of the sentence even when their position in the surface structure is identical; i.e., *tailors* is a more effective prompt for *Gloves are made by tailors* (where it is the underlying subject) than *hand* is for *Gloves are made by hand* (where it is only part of an adverbial phrase). Savin and Perchonock (1965) found that a sentence which contains three transformations (negative, passive, and emphatic) such as *The ball HASN'T been hit by the boy* is harder to remember than *The boy hit the ball* when memory load is measured by the number of unrelated individual words which can be remembered in addition to the sentence.

More recently, psycholinguistic studies and research on the acquisition of syntax by children have attempted to specify in more detail the nature of syntactical complexity. This is a question of considerable practical as well as theoretical importance. Theoretically, understanding which sentences are hard for people to comprehend will be one step toward understanding the processes involved in all sentence comprehension. Practically, once sentences can be differentiated in terms of their complexity, then people can be differentiated in terms of their ability to cope with syntax at particular levels of complexity.

What aspects of the structure of a sentence make it more or less easily understood? Length has been one traditional answer, and the assignment of sentences to age levels in the Stanford-Binet intelligence test seems to be made primarily on this basis.[6] While length and complexity are undoubtedly correlated, they are not related in any intrinsic way. For a while it seemed that the number of transformational rules in the description of a sentence would be a useful criterion of complexity (Miller, 1962). That generalization did not hold, however, outside of a small set of sentence types. For instance, according to grammatical descriptions, separation of the parts of a separable verb such as *put on* requires one more rule: the sentence, *Put your coat on* has one more rule in its description than the sentence, *Put on your coat.* Yet there is no evidence that the former sentence is more complex in any psychological sense. So this first approximation to a definition of complexity had to be revised.

Recent studies suggest that a more general and valid criterion may be the extent to which the basic relationships between words which are critical to meaning are revealed or masked in in the sentence as spoken—i.e., on the degree to which cues to the deep structure are present in the surface structure.

> We suggest that the complexity of a sentence is a function not (or not only) of the transformational distance from its base to its surface structure but also of the degree to which the arrangement of elements in the surface structure provides clues to the relations of elements in the deep structure. Insofar as increasing the number of transformations tends to increase complexity, we suggest that this is not because of the increasing transformational distance between base and surface structures per se but rather because of the consequent obliteration of the surface structure clues upon which the reconstruction of the deep structure depends (Fodor and Garrett, 1967, p. 289).

[6] As part of the study of "the imitation, comprehension and production of English syntax" my colleague Arthur McCaffrey is currently investigating the pattern of correct and incorrect imitations of Stanford-Binet test sentences. He is comparing the results with the order of difficulty assumed by Binet (which seems to be based primarily on length) and an order based on criteria of linguistic complexity.

Fodor and Garrett found, for example, that sentences with relative pronouns in the surface structure were easier to understand (as demonstrated by paraphrasing) than sentences in which those pronouns were omitted. Sentence (7a) is easier to understand than (7b):

(7a) The pen which the author whom the editor liked used was new.

(7b) The pen the author the editor liked used was new.

Presumably, the presence of the relative pronouns makes it easier for the listener to relate each noun to its appropriate verb.

Carol Chomsky suggests three further criteria of syntactical complexity:

1. A sentence is harder to understand if "The syntactic structure associated with a particular word is at variance with a general pattern in the language" (C. Chomsky, 1969). Consider the following two sentences:

(8a) John told Bill to leave.

(8b) John promised Bill to leave.

In both sentences the subject of the complement verb *leave* is not expressed and must be supplied by the listener. In (8a) the subject is Bill, the noun nearest to the verb, following what C. Chomsky calls the "Minimal Distance Principle," whereas in (8b) it is John. Since the majority of English verbs act like *told*, sentences with *promise* which constitute an exception should be more difficult for subjects to understand.

2. A sentence is harder to understand if "A conflict exists between two of the potential syntactic structures associated with a single verb" (C. Chomsky, 1969). Whereas the syntactic structure associated with *promise* always violates the Minimum Distance Principle, *ask* can take both kinds of structures:

(9a) I asked her to leave. (Subject of *leave* is *her*.)

(9b) I asked her what to draw. (Subject of *draw* is *I*.)

On this basis, learning to interpret *ask* correctly in all possible syntactic structures should be more difficult than learning to interpret *promise*.

3. A sentence is harder to understand if "Restrictions on a grammatical operation apply under certain limited conditions only" (C. Chomsky, 1969). In most sentences with both a pronoun and a noun phrase (e.g., 10a) the pronoun *he* can refer either to the noun phrase *John* or to someone else not mentioned in the sentence. In certain sentences, however, (e.g., 10b) a restriction is imposed on the pronoun's reference. In (10b) *he* must refer to someone else, not John.

(10a) John knew that he was going to win the race.

(10b) He knew that John was going to win the race.

Since this restriction on the pronoun is so rare, it should be a harder structure to learn to interpret correctly.

Whereas Fodor and Garrett verified their hypothesis about structural complexity by giving adults the task of providing paraphrases, Chomsky verified her hypotheses by studying the order of acquisition of the structures by children from five to 10 years. Presumably those structures learned later are more complex in psychological terms.

It is important to keep in mind that the syntactic complexity of sentences will never account completely for psychological complexity. In ways which we are only beginning to understand, the relation between the meaning of the sentence and aspects of its nonlinguistic context also plays a part. Three examples can be given. Huttenlocher (1968) asked children to create a pile of two blocks in response to a description like "The red block is on top of the green block." One of the two blocks was fixed on the middle rung of a ladder. The task was much easier when the block which was free for the child to manipulate was the grammatical subject of the sentence (above, the red block) than vice versa. Evidently in the reverse case children had to transform the statement to correspond to the extralinguistic situation. Wason (1965) found that negative statements can be differentiated according to the likelihood of the proposition being negated; given a pattern of one blue dot and seven red dots, it is more natural to say *One dot is not red* than to say *Seven dots are not blue*. And the more natural or plausible denial takes less time to interpret. Finally, Slobin and Welsh discovered one suggestive phenomenon when they were asking a two-and-a-half-year-old girl "Echo" to imitate sentences.

> Often Echo will spontaneously produce a fairly long and complex sentence [e.g., *If you finish your eggs all up, Daddy, you can have your coffee.*] and if this utterance is offered as a model immediately after its production, it will be (more or less) successfully imitated. However, if the very same utterance is presented to the child ten minutes later—i.e. the child's own utterance—she will often fail to imitate it fully or correctly. . . . It would seem that the child has "an intention to-say-so-and-so"—to use William James' phrase—and has encoded that intention into linguistic

form. If that linguistic form is presented for imitation while the intention is still operative, it can be fairly successfully imitated. Once the intention is gone, however, the utterance must be processed in linguistic terms alone—without its original intentional and contextual support. In the absence of such support, the task can strain the child's abilities, and reveal a more limited competence than may actually be present in spontaneous speech. Thus whatever we discover in systematic probes of imitation must be taken as a conservative estimate of the child's linguistic competence (Slobin and Welsh, 1967, pp. 6–7).

Individual Differences in Syntactic Competence

The question of individual differences in syntactic competence is really a set of four questions. The dimensions of qualitative vs. quantitative variation and intrapersonal vs. interpersonal variation combine as follows:

NATURE OF VARIATION	LOCUS OF VARIATION AMONG INDIVIDUALS	WITHIN INDIVIDUALS
Quantitative	1. Do some people control a reduced grammar of their language? Or are observed deficits in linguistic performance due instead to limited exploitation of the internalized grammar in performance?	2. Why can people comprehend more complex sentences than they produce? Does this imply the existence of separate comprehension and production grammars, or is the gap due to greater performance demands in production?
Qualitative	3. How do the dialects of English differ from each other?	4. Do individuals control more than one dialect? If so, how should this knowledge be included in descriptions of their linguistic competence?

Let us look in more detail at these four questions in turn.

1. Transformational grammarians assert frequently that individual differences in language, other than vocabulary, are a matter of performance only, not of underlying linguistic knowledge at all. For instance, Katz (1964, p. 415) states that "variation in performance with intelligence (in non-linguistic tasks) contrasts with the performance of speakers with respect to some purely linguistic skill, where no significant differences are found." Such assertions are derived from a theory that the acquisition of language is accomplished by the young child (approximately two to four years of age) in a remarkably short time because human beings are so neurologically preprogrammed with a "language acquisition device" that only a minimum of environmental exposure to language is necessary for the realization of innate potentiality. This minimum is almost universally available to the growing child (with the dramatic exception of deaf children), and shared competence is the result. (See Smith and Miller, 1966 for extensive discussion of this theory.)

One can separate stronger and weaker versions of the hypothesis of no significant individual differences in syntactic competence. According to the strong version, no individual differences in competence exist even during the developmental period. According to the weak version, no such differences are present among mature speakers. I doubt if linguists would stand by the strong version if pressed to defend it. It is not necessary for their theory and is directly contradicted by widespread empirical evidence (see Cazden, 1966, for further argument). Lenneberg (1966) discusses this evidence with particular attention to "the development of children with various abnormalities."

The status of the weaker version is much less clear. It is difficult to test this hypothesis experimentally because competence can only be tapped by some kind of performance test, and the claim can always be advanced that differences between subjects are due to differences in some ability required in the experimental task. For instance, Gleitman et al. (1965) found that graduate students were better able to give paraphrases for three-word compound nouns like *duck food man* than subjects who had not gone beyond high school or college. And Stolz (reported in Rommetveit, 1968) found differences within a group of college students in their ability to decode into three simple sentences a written sentence containing one relative clause embedded in another:

(11) The movie that the novel that the producer found made was applauded by the critics.

In both studies, the cause of the results may be individual differences in tacit linguistic knowledge, or the cause may be differences in metalinguistic strategies required by the particular experimental task. Getting subjects to demonstrate their linguistic knowledge without introducing confounding performance variables is extremely difficult. And, when subjects are patients with speech problems or members of any socially disadvantaged group, both the metalinguistic demands of the task and the interpersonal demands of the testing situation may cause significant interference with the realization of linguistic comptetence. Precisely because speech is so susceptible to situational influences, valid assessment is most difficult in this form of human behavior.

> The methodology of clinical tests is likewise an intricate and cardinal linguistic problem. What is obtained by such tests from the patient very often proves to be not his proper language but his so-called metalinguistic operations with language, his exercises in intralingual and interlingual translation. He works under constraint. Here we must heed Niels Bohr's wise warning: when we have to do with an observer and an object under observation, we must take into account the distortion of the object by the observer. We must measure and analyse such a distortion. And when an aphasic is being tested, the distortion may be quite high. . . . There can be no monopolizing solution which would eliminate the necessity of a qualitative linguistic analysis based primarily on the unconstrained speech of the patient (Jakobson, 1964, pp. 44–46).

The same caution applies to language assessment of disadvantaged children. Pasamanick and Knobloch (1955) and Resnick, Weld, and Lally (1969) report evidence that the verbal expressiveness of lower class Negro two-year-olds is artificially depressed in testing situations.

2. Most current psycholinguistic work assumes that speech production and comprehension are based on a single mental grammar. (See McNeill, 1968, on this issue.) It is not yet possible, however, to specify why the cognitive demands of the productive process are so much greater.

3. No language is spoken in exactly the same way by all its speakers. When members of a subgroup of a language community speak in ways which are like each other but different from other subgroups, we say they speak a dialect of the language. Standard English (SE) can be considered one dialect of English, simply the most prestigious one. Similarly, Negro speakers in northern ghettos speak a dialect of English (NNE for Negro Nonstandard English). And, if groups separable by some pathological condition all deviate in the same way, one could speak of the dialect of the deaf or the mentally retarded. When a language system is unique to an individual, we call it an idiolect. Considerable dialect research today is devoted to describing dialects of different socioeconomic and ethnic groups. We are beginning to be able to state how the rules of NNE differ from the rules of SE, and we are gaining significant insights into linguistic variation in general.[7]

The most extensive research on this question is linguist William Labov's study of the social stratification of English in New York City (Labov, 1966a, 1969; Labov and Cohen, 1967). We can only mention a few of Labov's findings here. First, he has identified a very few forms in NNE which probably indicate basic differences in the deep structure of the dialect, in the underlying meaning being expressed.

> One is the use of *be* to indicate generality, repeated action, or existential state in sentences such as *He be with us*; *They be fooling around*. We do not believe that there is any simple translation of standard rules which will produce these grammatical forms. Another such element is *done* to indicate an intensive or perfective meaning as in *The bullet done penetrated my body*; *I done got me a hat*. Both of these are part of an aspectual system which is plainly distinct from tense (Labov and Cohen, 1967, p. 76).

Second, given a certain idea to be expressed, NNE has different transformational rules governing its surface realization. One example is the deletion of the copula *be* in certain specified environments. The following are all samples of NNE (Labov, 1969):

Be deleted:	*Be* appears:
He fast in everything he do.	I was small.
You out the game.	I'm not no strong drinker.
They not caught.	Is he dead?
He gon' try to get up.	Allah *is* God. (emphasis)
	It always somebody tougher than you are.

[7] It is important to maintain a distinction between differences in linguistic rules and differences in matters of style (Ervin-Tripp, in press). We are here discussing only the former, with Labov's research as the best example. Most research on social class differences in speech deals with matters of style, the frequency with which optional linguistic structures are selected (for instance, pronouns versus nouns, active or passive clauses, simple versus complex sentences). The research of Basil Bernstein in London is an excellent example here. See Bernstein (1965) for an overview of his theory; Bernstein (1962) for an early experiment with adolescent boys; and Cazden (1968) for a review of his recent work on the speech patterns of children five to seven years old.

Labov has found that this alternation between the deletion and appearance of *be* is not simply random variation produced by dialect mixtures, but rather a highly structured system. Phonological influences can be specified; e.g., *is* and *are* are deleted where *'m* is not because

> there are phonological processes which operate upon final [z] and [r] in NNE, but not upon final [m] . . . But the most important suggestion . . . is the relation between contraction and deletion. We find that the following general principle holds without exception: *wherever SE can contract, NNE can delete is and are, and vice versa; wherever SE cannot contract, NNE cannot delete is and are, and vice versa* (Labov, 1969).

It turns out that the rules governing SE contraction, and thereby NNE deletion, follow the stress assignment rules provided by Chomsky and Halle (1968) and, as Labov points out, provide independent confirmation of the validity of their work.

Labov has also studied the relation of linguistic stratification to the attitudes of his informants toward the speech they speak and hear. He concludes that in a pluralistic urban society dialect differences are maintained not out of isolation and ignorance but because of "the need for self-identification with particular sub-groups in the social complex" (Labov, 1966a, p. 450).

4. Labov found that speakers of a language, at least from adolescence on, exhibit considerable internal variation in their own speech behavior, variation which also is structured and predictable. An example is the tendency (which all speakers of English share to some extent) to simplify final consonant clusters, e.g., to reduce *first* to *firs'*. It turns out that this tendency depends not only on the social class of the speaker, but also on the formality or informality of the social context, whether the sound represents a separate morpheme such as past tense (*walked*) or not (*first*), and whether the subsequent sound is a consonant (*first thing*) or a vowel (*first of all*). Labov's work contributes much to our understanding of the complexity of the rules which underly our speech behavior. Fig. 45-1 shows his graph of variation among individuals and within individuals for the simplification of *-t* or *-d*. Following is his discussion of it:

> The percentage of simplification is given for casual speech and careful speech, for clusters followed by words beginning with a consonant K or a juncture # or a vowel V. The solid lines represent the working class speakers; the dashed lines, the middle class speakers, all Negro. On the left, the diagram for monomorphemic clusters first shows small stylistic shift for working class speakers, with the same slope for clusters before consonants as for clusters before vowels. But the middle class line for clusters before consonants moves sharply upward, approximating the position of the working class in casual speech. Note, however, that there is no such phenomenon for the middle class use of clusters before vowels. Here the percentage of simplification is low and does not rise sharply; we can interpret this lack of parallelism by noting that a pattern of simplification before consonants but not before vowels preserves the underlying forms of the words. If we say *firs' thing* but *first of all*, there is no doubt that the underlying form is *first*.
>
> In the right half of the diagram where t/d = the past tense *-ed* the same general pattern can be observed, but at a much lower level. The grammatical status of *-ed* is obviously important to both groups, since the position is lower and the slope of the lines from casual to careful speech is greater than for monomorphemic words. Furthermore, the middle class groups show a sharper downward shift than the working class. There is less tendency for the middle class to shift upward in casual speech to approximate the working class norm; that is, even before consonants we find no sharp stylistic increase in simplification. We can argue here that the middle class has a general constraint against the dropping of the grammatical formative *-ed* as a stylistic indicator. In these respects, the middle class group approximates the behaviour of white speakers as indicated in other studies (Labov and Cohen, 1967, pp. 70–71).

Labov's work is of great theoretical and practical importance. Theoretically there is an important contrast between his view of language and that expressed by most other transformational grammarians. For instance, Katz states that "a necessary condition for something to be part of the subject matter of a linguistic theory is that each speaker be able to perform in that regard much as every other does" (Katz, 1964, p. 415). In Labov's (sociolinguistic) view, however, the multidimensional structure of variation across persons and across settings is an essential feature. Labov is interested primarily in language change and the factors influencing it. His goal is a "socially realistic linguistics"—a description of the structure of social and stylistic variation and an explanation of changes in that structure over time. The shift from the study of language as a homogeneous abstraction to the study of variability as an integral part of the linguistic system can be related to a corresponding contemporary shift in biological theory from typological to population models and concepts. To the typologist, differences among individuals are a kind of troublesome noise in the biological system. The populationist, on the contrary, regards diversity among individuals as the prime observable reality and the source of evolutionary possibilities (Dobzhansky, 1967).

Labov's work also has important implications for clinical work. To obtain a full picture of the language of any patient, diagnosis should include samples of both careful and casual behavior. Equally important, features of a child's language which are shared with mature speakers of his language community should be distinguished from evidence of developmental retardation on the one hand and individually deviant grammar or pronunciation on the other hand. See Baratz (1969) for further argument. Teachers or speech therapists may decide to help a child learn the patterns of SE regardless of the cause of his non-standard speech; that is a matter of values and educational goals not under discussion here. The curriculum, however, will not be the same in all cases. For example, in auditory discrimination programs instruction to a child to attend to sounds which he does in fact make will be different from instruction in the perception and production of contrasts which are not part of his dialect (e.g., *during* and *doing*, or *Ruth* and *roof*).[8]

Readers will note that all the above examples of individual differences in syntactic competence are from research on the dialects of social class or ethnic communities (Tyack, 1969; Williams, et al, 1970; Stolz and Seitz, 1971; Compton, in press; and Tervoort and Verberk, n.d.). Researchers are also beginning to provide more linguistically sophisticated descriptions of the language and speech of other groups (Menyuk, 1964, Lee, 1966, and Bloom, 1967). See Goehnour, 1965 for a generative grammar of sign language.

When Hesitations Occur

So far we have assumed that the process of verbal planning always ends in a fluent and well-formed utterance. We know from our own experience, however, that this is not so. We often start a sentence and then stop—to search for a word or phrase to express our intended meaning more aptly, or to edit and readjust our expression for a better fit to the informational requirements of our listener(s).

One result will be a pause, either silent, or filled with sounds like *uh* and *mmm* which hold our right to the speaker's role while verbal planning proceeds. Goldman-Eisler (1964) has studied the frequency of such pauses and their relation both to the situation in which the speech was elicited, and to the predictability of the words before and after the pause.

Often, we do not just stop and start again where we were; we back up and repeat or change one word or several. Labov (1966b) has analysed this aspect of everyday speech behavior and finds that it too is highly patterned and described by formal rules. While the frequency with which such hesitations occur is a matter of speech performance, the editing rules by which we both cope with them in our speech and interpret the interrupted speech of others must be part of our syntactic competence. Labov has identified three categories of rules: cancellation rules (12a) in which the material preceding the pause becomes syntactically irrelevant; stammering rules (12b) in which the same material occurs before and after the pause; and replacement rules (12c, 12d, 12e) in which material after the pause either replaces or is inserted into the material before the pause.

(12a) He don't—It leaves him kinda blank.
(12b) Anybody with any—any thought in mind . . .
(12c) I never—I can't recall seeing it.
(12d) I tried to get back into it—onto it.
(12e) I worked with them—with some of them.

Occasionally, we get into a maze and end up with a series of words which are nongrammatical—that is, they cannot be described by rules. According to Labov, however, this happens with surprising rarity. Excluding sentences in which the above editing rules apply, less than three percent of the utterances in one set of 3,000 utterances were ungrammatical (Labov, 1966b). Middle class speakers have more ungrammatical sentences than lower class speakers—not because they are less competent with syntax but because they are more ambitious in what they're trying to say.

PHONOLOGY

The preceding section on syntax included a discussion of Labov's research on the relation of pronunciation to a set of linguistic and social variables. More general

[8] The National Council of Teachers of English (1968) has published a pamphlet which describes NNE and suggests a curriculum for teaching SE. It was originally prepared for New York City teachers by a committee which included Labov. See also Cazden (1971) for extensive suggestions for evaluating the language of children three to eight years old.

questions of the phonological component of linguistic competence quickly become too technical to give in detail here. We should note, however, that with the publication of Chomsky's and Halle's *Sound Patterns of English* (1968), the field of phonology is probably at the beginning of a period of significant controversy and reconceptualization. I will only attempt to give a brief introduction to what the theoretical shift is about.

Until the recent work of the transformational linguists, analyses of speech sounds have been based on a unit called the phoneme. A phoneme is defined as a class of sounds which a native speaker considers functionally equivalent and discriminates from other classes of sounds. Just as the color spectrum can be divided at different points to yield different color categorizations (not just different labels), so the categorization of speech sounds can vary as well. "Bassa, a language of Liberia, makes a single major cut—*hui* is for the blue-green end of the spectrum and *ziza* is for the red-orange end" (Brown, 1965, p. 315). Similarly, "within the range of sounds that are perceived as 's' by English speakers, there is *one* phoneme in English, but there are *two* phonemes in Arabic" (Carroll, 1964, p. 13). Each phoneme is a simultaneous bundle of distinctive articulatory features as shown in Fig. 45-2.

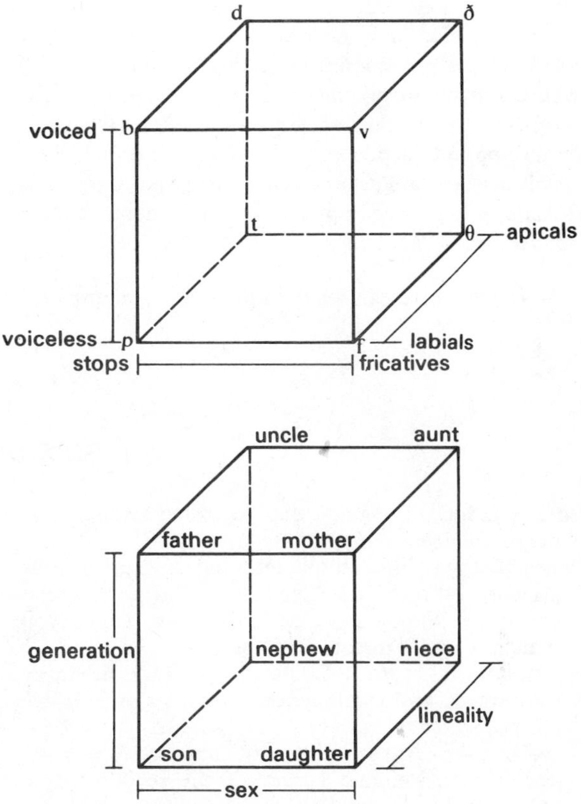

Fig. 45-2. Distinctive feature analysis of English consonants and componential analysis of eight kin terms. *After Brown, 1965, pp. 266, 307.*

The trouble with the phoneme is that it is a phenomenon of the surface realization of words only. As we noted earlier, our knowledge of language is not limited to the noises we speak and hear, and this generalization applies to our knowledge of the sound system of our language as well as to its syntactic structure. If our knowledge of the sounds of English words were limited to the phonemes present in words as spoken, all knowledge of morphemic relationships would be lost. That is, a phonemic system necessarily ignores sounds relationships among the following sets of words (Chomsky, 1970):

(13a) histor-y, histor-ical, histor-ian

(13b) anxi-ous, anxi-ety

(13c) courage, courage-ous

(13d) tele-graph, tele-graph-ic, tele-graph-y.

Yet the changes in pronunciation from one of these words to another is regular and can be formulated explicitly by rules.

The only way to account for this system of sound relationships is to postulate a deep and surface structure distinction for sounds as well as for syntax. The deep structure consists of a single and highly abstract "lexical representation" of each morpheme (a unit of meaning, whether "free" like *courage* or "bound" like *-ous*). This underlying representation, e.g., of *courage*, is related to the surface phonetic representation of the morpheme, in isolation or in combination, by a complex set of phonological rules. Chomsky and Halle (1968) provide a first description of these rules. (See Langacre, 1967 and O'Neil, 1969 for as readable introductions as the technicalities of the subject permit.)

Somehow this system of rules becomes part of the implicit linguistic knowledge of the native speaker, at least of the speaker of a rich version of spoken English.

Much of the evidence that determines, for the phonologist, the exact form of this underlying system is based on consideration of learned words and complex derivational patterns. This is clear from the examples presented earlier. . . . It is by no means obvious that a child of six has mastered this phonological system in full. He may not yet have been presented with the evidence that determines the general structure of this system. A similar question arises in the case of an adult who is not immersed in the literary culture. It would not be surprising to discover that the child's intuitive organization of the sound system continues to develop and deepen as his vocabulary is enriched and as his use of language extends to wider intellectual domains and more complex functions (Chomsky, 1970, pp. 16–17).

It is not yet clear what implications, if any, this reconceptualization of phonology will have for clinical practice. Chomsky (1970) provides a beginning discussion of the implications for reading. One striking fact about the abstract "lexical representations" is that, unlike the surface phonetic forms, they conform extremely well to standard English spelling. Because children usually learn to read before this abstract level is completely developed, however, its close relation to written orthography may not provide much help.

BIBLIOGRAPHY

Baratz, J. 1969. Language and cognitive assessment of negro children. *Asha*, 11, 87–91.

Berko, J. 1958. The child's learning of English morphology. *Word*, 14, 150–177. *Also in* Psycholinguistics. Saporta, S., ed. 1961. New York: Holt, Rinehart and Winston. Pp. 359–375.

Bernstein, B. 1962. Linguistic codes, hesitation phenomena and intelligence. *Language and Speech*, 5, 31–46.

———. 1965. A socio-linguistic approach to social learning. *In* Penguin survey of the social sciences 1965. Gould, J., ed. Baltimore: Penguin. Pp. 144–168.

Black, M. 1962. Words and metaphors. Ithaca, N.Y.: Cornell.

Bloom, L. 1967. A comment on Lee's developmental sentence types: a method for comparing normal and deviant syntactic development. *J. Speech Hearing Disorders*, 32, 294–296.

Blumenthal, A. 1966. Discussion. *In* Psycholinguistic papers. Lyons, J., and Wales, R., eds. Univ. of Edinburgh Press. Pp. 80–84.

———. 1967. Prompted recall of sentences. *J. verb. Learn. verb. Behav.*, 6, 203–206.

———, and Boakes, R. 1967. Prompted recall of sentences. *J. verb. Learn. verb. Behav.*, 6, 674–676.

Brown, R. 1965. Social psychology. New York: Free Press.

Carroll, J. 1964. Language and thought. Englewood Cliffs, N.J.: Prentice-Hall.

Cazden, C. 1967. On individual differences in language competence and performance. *J. spec. Educ.*, 1, 135–150.

———. 1968. Three sociolinguistic views of the language of lower-class children—with special attention to the work of Basil Bernstein. *Developm. Med. Child Neurol.*, 10, 600–612.

———. 1971. Evaluating language learning in early childhood education. *In* Formative and summative evaluation of student learning. Bloom, B., Hastings, T., and Madaus, G., eds. New York: McGraw-Hill. Pp. 345–398.

Chomsky, C. 1969. The acquisition of syntax in children from 5 to 10. Cambridge, Mass.: M.I.T. Press.

Chomsky, N. 1957. Syntactic structures. The Hague: Mouton.

———. 1965. Aspects of the theory of syntax. Cambridge: M.I.T.

———. 1968. Language and mind. New York: Harcourt, Brace and World.

———. 1970. Phonology and reading. *In* Basic studies on reading. New York: Harper and Row. Pp. 3–18.

———, and Halle, M. 1968. The sound patterns of English. New York: Harper and Row.

Compton, A. Generative studies of children's phonological disorders. *J. Speech Hearing Disorders* (in press).

Dobzhansky, T. 1967. Of flies and men. *Amer. Psychologist*, 22, 41–48.

Entwisle, D., and Greenberger, E. 1966. Differences in the language of negro and white grade-school children 1, 2. Baltimore: Johns Hopkins Univ.: The Center for the Study of Social Organization of Schools.

Ervin-Tripp, S. Discussion. *In* Mechanisms of language development. Huxley, R., and Ingram, E., eds. London: CIBA Foundation (in press).

———. 1969. Sociolinguistics. *In* Advances in experimental social psychology. Vol. 4. Berkowitz, L., ed. New York: Academic Press. Pp. 91–165.

———, and Slobin, D. 1966. Psycholinguistics. *Annual Rev. Psychol.*, 17, 435–474.

Fodor, J., and Bever, T. 1965. The psychological reality of linguistic segments. *J. verb. Learn. verb. Behav.*, 4, 414–420.

———, and Garrett, M. 1966. Some reflections on competence and performance. *In* Psycholinguistic papers. Lyons, J., and Wales, R., eds. Edinburgh: Univ. Edinburgh Press. Pp. 135–154.

———, and ———. 1967. Some syntactic determinants of sentential complexity. *Perception and Psychophysics*, 2, 289–296.

Gleitman, L., Shipley, E., and Smith, C. 1965. An experimental study of the use of compound nouns. Technical Report III. Eastern Penn. Psychiatric Inst.

Goehnour, E. 1965. A generative grammar of sign. Univ. Iowa: Master's thesis.

Goldman-Eisler, F. 1964. Discussion and further comments. *In* New directions in the study of language. Lenneberg, E., ed. Cambridge: M.I.T. Pp. 109–130.

Huttenlocher, J., and Strauss, S. 1968. Comprehension and a statement's relation to the situation it describes. *J. verb. Learn. verb. Behav.*, 7, 300–304.

Hymes, D. On communicative competence. *In* The mechanisms of language development. Huxley, R., and Ingram, E., eds. London: CIBA Foundation. (in press.)

Jakobson, R. 1964. Discussion: disorders of language. CIBA Foundation Syposium. Boston: Little, Brown. Pp. 42–46.

Jensen, A. R. 1968. Social class and verbal learning. *In* Social class, race and psychological development. Deutsch, M., Katz, J., and Jensen, A., eds. New York: Holt, Rinehart and Winston. Pp. 115–174.

Katz, J., 1964. Semi-sentences. *In* The structure of language. Katz, J., and Fodor, J., eds. Englewood Cliffs, N.J.: Prentice-Hall. Pp. 400–416.

———, and Fodor, J. 1964. The structure of a semantic theory. *In* The structure of language. Katz, J., and Fodor, J., eds. Englewood Cliffs, N.J.: Prentice-Hall. Pp. 479–518.

Labov, W. 1966a. The social stratification of English in New York City. Washington, D.C.: Center for Applied Linguistics.

———. 1966b. On the grammaticality of every-day speech. Paper given at the meeting of the Linguistics Society of America, New York.

———. 1969. Contraction, deletion, and inherent variability of the English copula. *Language*, 45, 715–762.

———, and Cohen, P. 1967. Systematic relations of standard and non-standard rules in the grammars of negro speakers. Project Literacy Reports No. 8. Ithaca, N.Y.: Cornell. Pp. 66–84.

Langacker, R. 1968. Language and its structure. New York: Harcourt, Brace and World.

Lashley, K. 1951. The problem of serial order in behavior. *In* Cerebral mechanisms in behavior. The Hixon symposium. Jeffress, L., ed. New York: Wiley. Pp. 112–136. *Reprinted in* Psycholinguistics. Saporta, S., ed. 1961. New York: Holt, Rinehart and Winston. Pp. 180–198.

Lee, L. 1966. Developmental sentence types: a method for comparing normal and deviant syntactic development. *J. Speech Hearing Disorders*, 31, 311–330.

Lenneberg, E. 1966. The natural history of language. *In* The genesis of language. Smith, F., and Miller, G., eds. Cambridge: M.I.T. Pp. 219–251.

McNeill, D. 1968. Production and perception: the view from language. *Ontario J. Educ. Res.*, 10, 181–185.

———. 1970. The development of language. *In* The manual of child psychology (3rd. ed.). Mussen, P., ed. New York: Wiley. Pp. 1061–1161.

Mehler, J. 1963. Some effects of grammatical transformations on the recall of English sentences. *J. verb. Learn. verb. Behav.*, 2, 346–351.

Menyuk, P. 1964. Comparison of grammar of children with functionally deviant and normal speech. *J. Speech Hearing Research*, 7, 109–121.

Miller, G. 1962. Some psychological studies of grammar. *Amer. Psychologist*, 17, 748–762.

———. 1964a. The psycholinguists. *Encounter*, 23, 29–37.

———. 1964b. Language and psychology. *In* New directions in the study of language. Lenneberg, E., ed. Cambridge: M.I.T. Pp. 89–108.

———, and Chomsky, N. 1963. Finitary models of language users. *In* Handbook of mathematical psychology. Vol. 3. Luce, R., Bush, R., and Galanter, E., eds. New York: Wiley. Pp. 419–491.

———, Galanter, E. and Pribram, K. 1960. Plans and the structure of behavior. New York: Holt, Rinehart and Winston.

———, and McNeill, D. 1969. Psycholinguistics. *In* The handbook of social psychology (2nd. ed.). Vol. 3. Lindzey, G., and Aronson, E., eds. Reading, Mass.: Addison-Wesley. Pp. 666–794.

National Council of Teachers of English. 1968. Non-standard dialect. Champaign, Ill.

Neisser, U. 1966. Cognitive psychology. New York: Appleton-Century-Crofts.

Oettinger, A. 1966. The uses of computers in science. *Scientific American*, 215, 161–172.

O'Neil, W. 1969. The spelling and pronunciation of English. *In* the American Heritage Dictionary of the English Language. Boston: Houghton-Mifflin. Pp. XXXV–XXXVII.

Osgood, C., Suci, G., and Tennenbaum, P. 1957. The measurement of meaning. Urbana, Ill.: Univ. of Ill. Press.

Pasamanick, B., and Knobloch, H. 1955. Early language behavior in negro children and the testing of intelligence. *J. abnor. soc. Psychol.*, 50, 401–402.

Postal, P. 1966. Underlying and superficial linguistic structure. *In* Language and learning. Emig, J., Flemming, J., and Popp, H., eds. New York: Harcourt, Brace and World. Pp. 153–175.

Resnick, M., Weld, G., and Lally, J. 1969. Verbalizations of environmentally deprived two-year olds as a function of the presence of a tester in a standardized test situation. Paper presented at the meeting of the Amer. Educ. Res. Assn., Los Angeles.

Rommetveit, R. 1968. Words, meanings, and messages. New York: Academic Press.

Sachs, J. 1967. Recognition memory for syntactic and semantic aspects of connected discourse. *Perception and Psychophysics*, 2, 437–442.

Savin, H., and Perchonock, E. 1965. Grammatical structure and the immediate recall of English sentences. *J. verb. Learn. verb. Behav.*, 4, 348–353.

Schlesinger, H., and Meadow, C. 1971. Deafness and mental health: developmental approach. San Francisco: Langley Porter Neuropsychiatric Institute, Mental Health Services for the Deaf, final report for research and demonstration grant No. 14-P-55270/9-013 (RD-2835-S).

Slobin, D., and Welsh, C. 1967. Elicited imitation as a research tool in developmental psycholinguistics. Univ. Calif., Berkeley: Dept. Psychol. (unpublished manuscript.)

———. 1971. Psycholinguistics. Glenview, Ill.: Sertt, Foresman.

Smith, F., and Miller, G., eds. 1966. The genesis of language. Cambridge: M.I.T.

Stolz, W., and Seitz, S. 1971. Word associations as indices of lexical growth in mentally retarded children. Interim report, Project No. 532163, U.S. Dept. Health, Education, Welfare, Office Educ. (April).

Trevoort, B., and Verberk, A. (no date). Analysis of communicative structure patterns in deaf children. Final report of Project No. RD-467-64-65, U.S. Dept. Health, Education, Welfare, Voc. Rehab. Admin.

Tyack, D. 1969. An analysis of the syntactic structures of a child with a language problem. Univ. Ill.: Unpublished masters thesis.

Wales, R., and Marshall, J. 1966. The organization of linguistic performance. *In* Psycholinguistic papers. Lyons, J., and Wales, R., eds. Edinburgh: Univ. of Edinburgh Press. Pp. 29–80.

Wason, P. 1965. The contexts of plausible denial. *J. verb. Learn. verb. Behav.*, 4, 7–11. *Reprinted in* Language. Oldfield, R., and Marshall, J., eds. Baltimore: Penguin. 1968. Pp. 246–253.

Williams, F. (ed.), Cairns, H., Cairns, C., and Blosser, D. 1970. Analysis of production errors in the phonetic performance of school-age Standard-English speaking children. Center for Communication Research: Univ. Texas. (Dec.).

46

Childhood Aphasia: An Evolving Concept

Helmer R. Myklebust

Study of children in relation to language behavior has a long history. Though it has been said that language disorders were observed in adults before they were recognized in children, this does not seem to be true. The first useful definition and discussion of aphasia in children may be the one presented by Gall (1825). This great forerunner of neurology described faulty memory for speech and clearly differentiated congenital aphasia from mental retardation and the speech of normal children.

Since publication of Gall's observations the concept of childhood aphasia has evolved immeasurably. Allen's (1952) study of the history of congenital auditory imperception revealed that there was considerable interest and discussion of aphasia in children prior to 1900. He cited a presentation in 1853 by Wilde, who noted that certain children did not acquire the spoken word though they were neither deaf nor mentally deficient. Further evidence was given by Broadbent (1872). He described an 11-year-old boy, whom he had observed for 12 months, as having a "congenital aphasia"; he was intelligent but unable to speak or read, even though he could do arithmetic; he clearly understood everything that was said to him but could not utter a connected sentence.

As in the case of adults (Nielsen, 1946), expressive aphasia was recognized in children earlier than its counterpart, receptive aphasia. Because he noted an inability to read, Broadbent (1872) also was one of the first to identify childhood dyslexia; more complete reports of this language disorder were made approximately 25 years later (Hinshelwood, 1895; Morgan, 1896). An unusually insightful discussion of the concept of aphasia in childhood was given by Ucherman (1891), who through excellent case illustrations distinguished among the conditions of aphasia, psychogenic deafness, and paralysis of the tongue. Only many years later did these critical insights again receive attention.

An early proponent of the concept of childhood aphasia was Bernhardt (1897). Because of differences of opinion concerning the real nature of this condition, he stated that "True phasia is not rare in childhood; it is a frequent symptom of infantile cerebral hemiplegia, mostly transient, rarely permanent. It is mostly motor in type" (Guttman, 1942).

Freud (1897, 1953) studied aphasia extensively, in both children and adults. He was concerned with the problem of definition and asserted that true aphasia in children was, 1. a disturbance of the speech faculty already acquired, and 2. a retarded development of speech in children who when they were taken ill had not yet acquired speech or were in the process of learning to speak.

Although generally unrecognized, Binet and Simon (1908) made significant investigations of childhood aphasia and the psychology of language. They also clearly distinguished between the mentally retarded and the aphasic. Moreover, Binet stated that "language does not represent a faculty unique, indivisible, moulded in a single piece, but is composed of a certain number of operations which are independent of each other, and each may be destroyed or conserved to the exclusion of others . . . according to the simplest and most schematic of these theories, language results from the four following operations: first, understanding; second, speaking; third, reading; fourth, writing; and each of these operations may be suppressed separately by a cerebral accident" (p. 162). One is impressed by these observations and their relevance to current psychoneurological constructs. Binet's understanding of language and the ways in which it might be altered by neurological disturbances is all but awesome. His emphasis throughout is reflected by the pronouncement, "Aphasia does not comprise a psychogenesis, this must not be forgotten" (p. 163).

During the same period that Binet was engaged in his studies, Guthrie (1907) in a book on nervous disorders in children included a chapter on disturbances of language. He described six cases of *idioglossia*, a term used to designate children with aphasia who also could not relate spoken sounds with letters of the alphabet.

McCall (1911) stressed language disability in relation to school success by presenting two cases, one who had "word-blindness" and one "word-deafness." In terms of an evolving concept it is noteworthy that McCall described an eight-year-old, who "when spoken to took no notice, and might easily be mistaken for a deaf child." He indicated that this child attempted to lip-read. This description is familiar to many teachers and clinicians because it characterizes children with marked disturbances of ability to comprehend.

One of the earliest references to the relationship of language disorders to delinquency was the report by Kerr (1917). His delineation of types through case illustration is impressive. McCready (1926) summarized many of the early contributions and presented a number of observations and additional case illustrations.

In contrast with child dyslexia, hereditary factors have been largely overlooked in childhood aphasia. An exception is the detailed report by Ley (1929), who made an extensive study of twins with congenital expressive aphasia; auditory comprehension was excellent, but utterance of speech was severely limited. Ley's conclusion was that expressive aphasia is a type of apraxia and may be hereditary. He carefully differentiated this condition from that of mental retardation, deafness, and other involvements which affect verbal functioning.

The work of Worster-Drought and Allen (1929) is outstanding in several respects. They raised various questions relative to terminology but, more importantly, they pointed the way for securing objective diagnostic information and outlined the implications for behavior and adjustment. Using Head's (1926) diagnostic techniques they established the level of function in several respects: auditory perception, visual perception, tactile perception, spoken language, writing, ability to imitate actions, and arithmetic. They emphasized that this approach is useful but should be modified when used with congenital aphasics.

A milestone is represented by the work of Ewing (1930). His studies showed the effects of moderate hearing loss in language development and clarified the need to distinguish receptive deficits in auditory language from deafness. Simultaneously Orton (1937), an indefatigable worker, was deeply involved with the problem of language disorders in children. His work remains a classic guide, emphasizing the necessity of obtaining both behavioral and neurological data in order to better understand childhood aphasia. This is an outstanding contribution to the concept of neurogenicity in relation to all types of verbal behavior.

During the decade of the 1940's much work was being accomplished. Guttman (1942) stressed the need for clarification and refined procedures in diagnosis. He presented one of the most extensive studies to date, 30 cases, and all but five were verified by operation or autopsy. He concluded that childhood aphasia is not rare, that intelligence remains at a high level, and that recovery is good in the motor type.

Eustis (1947) found a relationship between left-handedness, ambidexterity, clumsiness, and language disturbances. Moreover, he stated that "A family tree covering four generations illustrates the familial nature" of this relationship (p. 455).

Gesell and Amatruda (1947), whose renowned insights into child development continue to be inspiring, made many observations on handicapped children. They gave special attention to disorders of the central nervous system, and to language development in particular. In defining aphasia they stated, "We use the term *Infantile Aphasia* to designate a group of related symptoms in young children which are associated with language difficulties aside from hearing deficits, speech defects in the ordinary sense, and simple retardation in the acquisition of speech. These language difficulties have to do with comprehension of meaning of the heard word, verbal associations, the ability to call up the proper words and language forms to express meaning, and the ability to manipulate language easily" (p. 285). This definition and the techniques for evaluation of language development remain of great value and are a credit to this pioneering work.

Lefeure (1950), after giving an extensive review of the early studies, presented three cases in detail and compared his findings with those of Guttman and other investigators; he described characteristics associated with certain types of childhood aphasia. Karlin (1954), who had been studying aphasic children for a number of years, in summarizing his impressions emphasized the urgency for establishing the level of auditory acuity and stressed the usefulness of psychogalvanic audiometry. Instead of the term word deafness, he suggested *congenital verbal auditory agnosia*. However, in more recent work he stated, "Cognizant of the fact that there are differences between aphasia in the adult and aphasia in the child, for semantic reasons, I believe aphasia is a good generic term, since it denotes a cerebral form of language dysfunction. Finally, the term aphasia in children should not imply only a congenital disorder, for aphasia in children may have different etiologies" (p. 756).

Others who presented illustrative cases during this decade and discussed the significance of aphasic disorders in children include Subirana et al. (1950), Van Gelder et al. (1952), Morley et al. (1955), and Wolferman (1955). Morley et al. added to the concept through their presentation of a classification system and through refinement of terminology. For example, they stated that aphasia is a breakdown in the comprehension and formulation of words giving rise to disturbances of thought and language. Their studies revealed that aphasic children typically began using words at two years or later and phrases at four years or later. In some the condition was transient, with language usage developing well after four years of age. They emphasized the importance of history information and the determination of mental level, laterality, and emotional status. They concluded, "In spite of traditional objections, we favor the term developmental aphasia for children who are mentally normal, have good hearing, and no evidence of cerebral palsy or disease, but show considerable delay in the development of speech" (p. 467).

It was during this period that Myklebust (1953, 1954, 1955, 1956, 1956a) proposed the term *language pathology* to denote the area of effort pertaining to language disorders. He emphasized that although childhood aphasia may be congenital, as a condition it was similar to that found in adults; hence, the term aphasia was most suitable. He pointed out that aphasic children were characterized by behavioral patterns which varied from those who are deaf, mentally ill, or mentally retarded. He postulated that there were three primary types of auditory language disturbances; those predominantly affecting integrative functions (inner language), those resulting in deficits in receptive functions (receptive language), and those which disturb output (expressive language).

Extensive concern with the problems of language pathology, including childhood aphasia, can be seen in the present decade. A study by Landau, Goldstein, and Kleffner (1960) gave impetus to the concept that brain dysfunctions are determinable under certain circumstances. Moreover, contributions from interdisciplinary conferences are noteworthy (West, 1962; DeReuck and O'Connor, 1964; Rioch and Weinstein, 1964; Millikan and Darley, 1967; and Schiefelbusch, Copeland, and Smith, 1967).

THE EVOLVING CONCEPT

During the first century after Gall's work, from approximately 1825 to 1925, significant progress was made in understanding aphasia, this complex, unique human problem. Yet, the concern was mainly with terminology and description. Many case studies were made, some with remarkable precision and ingenuity. One might conclude that there were no great innovations or modifications of the concept of childhood aphasia; it evolved as would be anticipated. Those familiar with the history of mental retardation and mental illness in children see many similarities. Also, as would be expected, vestiges of the past remain, some helpful and some not so helpful. If we are to understand the present, it is necessary that we recognize the influences of the past.

As we approach the midpoint of the second century in the study of childhood aphasia, we note that a number of the original questions remain. Definitive evidence has not been forthcoming. However, certain advances are apparent. The concept always has entailed both physiological and behavioral facets; this is one reason for its being difficult. Fortunately, progress has been made physiologically and behaviorally. For example, Geschwind (1968, 1968a) has continued to search for anatomical evidence, a search that has been rewarding indeed. He has shown that the regions of the auditory cortex on the left hemisphere are not identical to those on the right. He states, "Our data show that this area is significantly larger on the left side, and the differences observed are easily of sufficient magnitude to be compatible with the known functional asymmetries" (1968a, p. 187). Surely this is one of the noteworthy contributions of this century. Understanding of the neurophysiological systems requisite for auditory language has been greatly enhanced; accordingly, the concept of childhood aphasia has been extended.

The studies by Geschwind and his associates serve as a background for interpretation of behavioral studies, such as those by Kimura (1968) and Milner, Taylor, and Sperry (1968). Kimura has shown that verbal (auditory) material is processed primarily on the left half of the brain, whereas melodic (nonverbal) patterns are processed primarily on the right. Using the same approach, Milner et al. have shown that the right ear and left hemisphere are substantially more consequential to auditory language processing than are the left ear and the right hemisphere.

It is in these terms that we consider childhood aphasia as an evolving concept. In this era we can look forward to highly refined scientific evidence. The trends, even guidelines, are obvious. Developmental deviations, sequelae from accidents or disease, may alter the natural relationships of one hemisphere to the other with the result that auditory processing is disturbed; a type of aphasia appears.

Pursuing these hypotheses further we have formulated a behavioral construct to indicate the levels at which such processing might be disturbed (Fig. 46-1). As suggested by this schema, auditory language processing deficiencies may be of five distinct types, or combinations of these. The disorder may be at the level of *perception*, the most basic aspect of learning and integration. Or, it may be in the processes for *storage*—information is perceived but cannot be processed for purposes of recall. Another possibility is that, though perceived and stored, it is not *integrated*. We are increasingly aware of the significance of this type of deficiency. Children may perceive and remember, yet be unable to generalize experientially. This too is a type of aphasia (see Case Illustrations in the next chapter). Memory is of various types and apparently is served by more than one neurophysiological system. As a minimum we must differentiate between the processes involved in storage and those requisite to *formulation* and recall; this distinction is made in the schematic construct.

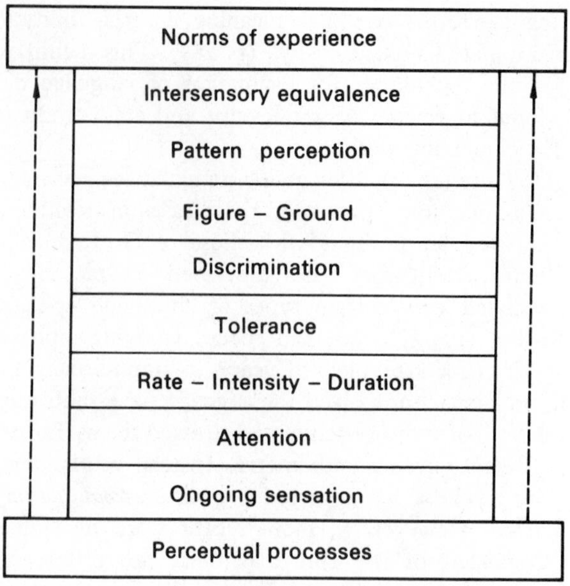

Fig. 46-1. Schema showing the processes involved in auditory perception and the disorders that might occur.

Lastly, for auditory language to be normally functional, it must be possible for the child to *utter the spoken word*. A deficit at this level is comprised classically in the designation of expressive aphasia.

Terminology

Though differences of opinion remain, it is evident that the term *aphasia* is most meaningful when it is delimited to refer specifically to disorders of auditory language. Designations such as articulatory defect or dysarthria do not implicate deficits in language learning. Likewise, aphasia does not connote defects in the production of speech. Further clarification entails use of the term aphasia to include disorders of read and written language. In the case of children this is confusing, inasmuch as auditory language involvements require diagnostic classification at an earlier age than those associated with reading and the written word. For both clinical and research purposes, it is suggested nosologically that the term aphasia refer only to disorders of auditory language.

Current Trends

A major trend has appeared during the past decade. Earlier, from the period when childhood aphasia was first recognized, the frame of reference and the terminology was essentially neurological; the model was that of neurological disease. More recently the trend is to employ a learning, behavioral model, albeit etiologically the role of the brain is accepted. Better understanding is reflected in a more refined depiction of this type of language disturbance. No longer can we refer to childhood aphasia only in terms of an inability to comprehend or to speak. Auditory symbolic behavior is the germain factor, but there is an array of subtleties that must be subsumed. Even the designations of auditory receptive, auditory expressive, input, output, and memory, must be further defined and delineated. Auditory receptive disturbances may be of various sorts or combinations. This is true also of deficits in expressive language, as well as of memory functions.

This trend can be seen in other ways. Stress now is given to the ways in which the child's total organismic integrities are reflected. An aphasia in childhood has implications for *all* learning, not only for facility with the spoken word. This language disorder has connotations for visual and tactile learning, for ego development, for total social adjustment, as well as for the development of intellectual functions. It is related directly to academic and vocational success as an adult. Experience has taught us that even though the onset of the handicap is in childhood, its significance in terms of years is far greater, with implications for programming in special education throughout a person's school life.

Despite the significance of the observations made in the past, and although these form the basis of more current work, the need for refinement seems obvious. Only in recent years have certain types of effort become possible, notably those that derive from computerized approaches and from use of biomedical engineering techniques. Such efforts reflect new discoveries in the neurosciences, comprising neurophysiology, biochemistry, neurosurgery, psychoneurology, and other interdisciplinary areas which impinge on the nature of learning (Quarton, Melnechuk, and Schmitt, 1967). As indicated above, unusually significant are the investigations of Milner, Taylor, and Sperry (1968) and Geschwind (1968a).

Especially relevant to many workers are developments in the field of learning disabilities. Childhood aphasia cannot be viewed as an isolated condition because it is one that is interrelated both with other language disorders and with certain types of nonlanguage disabilities (Doehring, 1960; McGrady, 1964; Myklebust, 1968). Although an aphasia might occur without significant complications, more commonly it is associated with other deficiencies in learning and development, directly or indirectly. The concomitant conditions may be *in addition* to the aphasia, or they may occur *as a result* of the basic inability to acquire facility with auditory language.

More precisely, childhood aphasia is one of the handicaps included in the field of learning disabilities; hence it is an important evolvement in the area of special education. Learning disabilities are a challenge of concern to various disciplines, the total population included being at least as large as any one of the other groups referred to as handicapped. Inasmuch as childhood aphasia is a type of learning disability requiring special education, it cannot be defined as a responsibility of speech pathology alone, but also as a responsibility of those workers whose major specialization is in the area of learning disabilities, and, more generally, of special education.

As a model, or construct, it is beneficial to view the problem of childhood aphasia within the framework of language pathology. McGrady's (1968) is a major contribution in this direction. He outlined the area of language pathology, reviewed the various language disorders, and related these deficits to the broader area of learning disabilities. During the past decade the trend has been to view language disorders not as an adjunct of any one discipline, but as an area entailing skills and knowledge from various areas of specialization. As a construct, it is in these terms that we consider the problem of aphasia in childhood.

An Evolving Definition

A notable development is the emergence of operational definitions not limited to a given discipline. It is recognized that a neurological criterion alone is inadequate, as is any single criterion. Presumptive evidence of organic dysfunctioning is admitted in studies of behavioral aberration. One of the difficulties has been the conflict involving terminology; new terminology is needed in order to better define this area of handicap. Luria (1963) introduced the term *neurodynamic*, referring to behavioral variations that assume shifting or modified neurological processes. Another of his terms, *psychoneurological*, also used by Myklebust (1964), provides new avenues for scientific investigation. This term stresses the obverse of neurodynamic. It highlights the shifts and modifications of *behavior* concomitant with dysfunctions in the brain. Hence, we might stress the psychoneurology of learning as encountered in childhood aphasia (Myklebust, 1968).

It is common for a discipline to define a given condition in terms of its own objectives and responsibilities; it is not necessary, and perhaps not desirable, to attempt definitions with the expectation that they serve all purposes. A more practical approach is to evolve specific criteria to serve the ends of the educator, of the physician, or of other groups.

Accordingly, in the definition of childhood aphasia we include the types of deficits discussed below. It must be emphasized that basically these deficits are not due to mental retardation, emotional disturbance, deafness, or motor paralysis. In other words, diagnosis and classification of childhood aphasia assumes integrity of intelligence, of emotional adjustment, of hearing, and of the motor system for speaking. It is clear that an aphasia might occur in a child who has an anarthria, who is mentally retarded, hearing-impaired, or emotionally disturbed. For purposes of definition, however, in and of themselves these conditions do not constitute an aphasia. Childhood aphasia must be differentiated from other types of disabilities. Only when it is so differentiated can it be properly defined and diagnosed; only then can the child's needs be adequately met.

It follows that the scientist-diagnostician is confronted with the question of how much intellectual deficit, how much emotional disturbance, how much hearing loss, how much motor involvement can be sustained without deleterious effects on use of auditory language. Because we have discussed this question elsewhere it is not considered here in detail (Myklebust, 1968). Nevertheless, its importance is underscored. Conceivably the learning quotient approach, a learning quotient for facility with auditory language, might be of advantage in this connection (see Illustrative Cases). Such a quantitative ratio of learning potential to physiological maturity, in relation to opportunity for learning, may provide the bases for delineating the degree of integrity (mental, physical, emotional) required for auditory language facility, as well as indicate the amount of deficit in auditory language that can occur without an actual aphasia being exhibited. In other words, definition of childhood aphasia assumes a degree of integrity that must be demonstrated, and the degree of deficit in auditory language that, in fact, constitutes a handicap, and therefore requires diagnosis and classification as an aphasia. Because measurement techniques have been slow to develop, much remains to be done before such objective guidelines can be established. However, an operational definition which we have found useful is:

Childhood aphasia refers to one or more significant deficits in essential processes as they relate to facility in use of auditory language. Children having this disability demonstrate a discrepancy between expected and actual achievement in one or more of the following functions: auditory perception, auditory memory, integration, comprehension, expression. The deficits referred to are not the result of sensory, motor, intellectual, or emotional impairment, nor to the lack of opportunity to learn. They are assumed to derive from dysfunctions in the brain, though the evidence for such dysfunctioning may be mainly behavioral, rather than neurological, in nature.

THEORETICAL CONSTRUCTS

In evolving a theoretical construct, it is useful to review the semiautonomous systems concept of brain function (Hebb, 1963). As a model it provides an excellent frame of reference from which to consider the problem of aphasia in childhood. It purports that the brain comprises systems which are semiautonomous one from another. For example, broadly conceived, there are input, integrative, and output systems, and no one of these is synonymous with the other; hence, we might encounter a predominantly receptive, or central, or expressive aphasia. From this point of view one might argue that there are many essentially independent systems, including those serving mainly auditory, visual, motor, memory, or other operations. Whatever our point of view, if we are to do justice to the concept of aphasia, we must assume that a dysfunction in the brain can occur without seriously debilitating the human being in other respects. If this were not the case, then the language deficit to which we refer would exist only in relation to a generalized debilitation and not as an entity in itself.

It is now rare to encounter the position that childhood aphasia does not exist. As in developmental dyslexia (Orton, 1937), it is generally acknowledged that a child can sustain a disorder of auditory language without having first acquired this verbal system; he might have an aphasia on a developmental, perhaps even genetic, basis. The evidence that dyslexia occurs on a familial, hereditary basis is all but incontrovertible (Hermann, 1959). Because of our lack of adequate objective criteria and measurement procedures, such evidence for childhood aphasia is less available. However, we are increasingly aware that aphasias sometime appear in more than one child of a given family, without accident or disease as probable causes. It is incumbent on all workers to be alert to this possibility because, etiologically, endogenous genetic factors are of more consequence than has been recognized.

A theoretical construct often interrelates with issues regarding causation. It is for this reason that we discuss etiological factors. An acceptable definition must encompass all types of aphasia in childhood, irrespective of age at onset or specific etiology. It seems clear that, accordingly, we must include the auditory language disorders that are developmental as well as those that are not. A critical factor related to this model is the age at which the deficit occurs. Developmental disorders are not the only disorders that may be congenital. Hence, *congenital* as a designation does not delimit the etiology in regard to exogeny or endogency. Neither, for that matter, does the term *developmental*. The aphasia may be caused by rubella, yet appear as a developmental anomaly. It is apparent, therefore, that adhering to criteria according to whether they are developmental or congenital is not advisable. The definition must encompass criteria which delineate the *condition*, not a specific type of etiology or a specific age of onset. On the other hand, it should include only the disorders that derive from dysfunctions in the brain, not those of other organic causation, nor those which result from other than organic factors or lack of opportunity.

An inclusive conceptualization of the disorders of auditory language entails broad appreciation of this verbal symbol system in comparison with man's other language systems. Man did not first acquire facility with the read and written word; he did not first learn to read and to write. The read and written forms evolved only in comparatively recent years (Diringer, 1962). The auditory form, facility with the spoken word, evolved millenia, ages, ago.

In considering the reasons for this phylogenetic pattern a fundamental factor is the varying nature of the two distance sense processes. Audition is permissive, even mandatory, whereas vision is directional and can be interrupted at will. Moreover, one can engage audition for language learning and communication without cessation of most ongoing preoccupations. For example, one can use the spoken word while carrying on a multitude of activities, such as wood-chopping, driving an automobile, and tying one's shoes. Reading and writing are possible only under marked restriction of one's activities.

This permissive nature of audition is crucial when viewing auditory language as more basic and primitive in comparison with the read and written forms, in comparison with the more visual forms. This permissiveness is never more apparent than when witnessed ontogenetically. The infant cannot avoid exposure to the spoken word. It impinges upon him from all directions—in the dark, as well as through walls, and from "around the mountain." Of major importance too is the fact that substantially less neurological, intellectual, maturational maturity is required for acquisition of the auditory form. Studies of the mentally retarded as well as ontogenetic developmental investigations clearly reveal that greater degrees of intellectual maturation are required for facility with the read and written forms (Goertzen, 1961; Jordan, 1966).

When we recognize this basic nature of auditory language we can appreciate the significance of childhood aphasia as a disability, as a handicap. In the discussion which follows we indicate the seriousness of this condition relative to total psychological development and adjustment. Here we emphasize that auditory language forms the basis of all verbal behavior. In other words, though not fully understood as a process, acquisition of the read and written forms assumes ability to superimpose these on the auditory form acquired first. As a group, children deaf from early life but having no visual handicap do not achieve average success in reading and writing (Myklebust, 1964a). Likewise, children with disturbances of the brain processes required for relating the auditory and read language forms have an auditory type of dyslexia (Myklebust and Johnson, 1962). Alphabetologists refer to the alphabet as man's greatest intellectual achievement (Gelb, 1963). The alphabet was evolved as a visual, graphic representation of the sounds produced while speaking. It is intriguing for the student of language behavior to note that for centuries such alphabetizing of the spoken word characterized only the western "phonetic" languages; currently, alphabetizing is becoming more prevalent in the Orient.

The basic nature of auditory language can be observed in other ways. Syntax, a feature of language systems, spoken, read, and written, derives from the spoken form. Our studies of written language, in which a Syntax Quotient was computed, clearly indicate that as soon as the child is capable of reading and writing he *has* essentially all of the syntax ability required for adult language usage (Myklebust, 1965). In other words, in learning to read and to use written language, he incorporates the syntax he has acquired auditorially.

AUDITORY PERCEPTION

There are a number of dimensions of auditory behavior, all of which must be operative at a minimum level of integrity if spoken language is to be acquired and used in a normal manner. To view the spoken word only in terms of ability to comprehend or to speak no longer suffices as a theoretical framework, nor as a construct for diagnostic and remedial efforts. In the study of handicapped children, especially those with learning disabilities, visual perceptual involvements often have been emphasized to the exclusion of auditory perception. Yet, in some respects, even in certain types of dyslexia, auditory perceptual disturbances are exceedingly consequential.

Auditory perception, one of the first facets of behavior to be studied psychologically, is an essential factor in understanding childhood aphasia. Therefore, it must be included in any theoretical formulation, in any model of auditory language and its disorders. More broadly, as a process auditory perception is basic to virtually all learning. Consequently, we postulated a hierarchy of experience and suggested the following levels: sensation, perception, imagery, symbolization, and conceptualization (Myklebust, 1954). Each of these experiential levels if disturbed brings about a characteristic imposition on learning. An imposition at the level of sensation results in sensory impairment such as deafness or blindness. If the deficit occurs at the level of perception, ability to structure the sensory environment is impaired. A deficiency in ability to engage in imagery results in disturbances of reauditorization and revisualization, in storage and retrieval operations. Symbolic deficiencies may be seen either as verbal language disorders or as disturbances of nonverbal representational behavior. Because of the nature of hierarchical relationships, a dysfunction may occur only at the higher cognitive level and be designated as a deficit in ability to conceptualize. The individual then cannot mentally organize units of experience having common values, which permits him to be identified categorically; he cannot engage in metaphorical reasoning.

Fundamental to this discussion is the position that, behaviorally, perception is one of man's most basic and primitive psychological functions. To some degree this level of behavior is found in virtually all forms of animal life. However, as suggested by the hierarchical structure of experience, disturbed perceptual processes in man result in malfunctioning at all of the higher levels. It is from this vantage point that we review the significance of auditory perceptual processes as they relate to childhood aphasia.

The Perceptual Process

Solley and Murphy's (1960) definitive statement indicates the progress made in understanding perceptual processes: "As a process, perception can best be conceptualized as an instrumental act which structures stimulation. As an act, it can be analyzed into stages, such as a preparatory stage, consisting of expectancy and attending, a sensory reception stage, a trial-and-check stage, and a final structuring stage. These stages do not exist as isolated units but merge and intertwine in the process" (p. 33). Allport (1955) also considered perception as a process and stressed other facets which are important to the study of language disorders. He differentiated between perception and cognition, emphasizing that in the study of perception we are observing the observer, studying how reality appears.

Cognizant of the contributions of these workers, and from experience with children who have learning disabilities, we evolved a construct to include these facets of perception which seem critical to developmental auditory behavior. These are shown schematically in Fig. 46-1 as they relate to auditory language and childhood aphasia.

Any analysis of perceptual processes is arbitrary insofar as this behavior is dissected into factors which appear basic to the "perceptual act." All authorities stress that simultaneity must be assumed, that perception is a complex but integrated process functioning as a whole. Nevertheless, as in other areas of science, we must segmentize the phenomenon so that we might better understand the total process. For example, we cannot dichotomize sensation and perception. Yet in the study of handicapped children it is of great advantage to consider them separately. It is apparent that a deaf child does not perceive sound because it is not delivered to the brain; hence, perception cannot occur. In contrast, the child with gross disorders of auditory perception clearly hears the sounds—he has sensation—but he cannot process these sensory stimuli so that they become intelligible.

Ongoing Sensation

Most workers agree that perception assumes sensation and that sensory stimuli might be taken as the basis or the beginning point in the analysis of perception. Though it is not necessarily a conventional position, we view perception as the process whereby ongoing sensations are meaningfully incorporated. It is the means through which significance is attributed to portions of the sensory environment. It is a primitive facet of behavior and is not limited to verbal symbols. However, the child who is grossly disturbed in this function cannot learn to associate significance with any auditory sensations, including the spoken word. This gross disability has been referred to as an auditory agnosia, and as congenital auditory imperception (Allen, 1952).

Arousal—Attention

Since the pioneering work of Moruzzi and Magoun (1949) neurophysiologists have pursued the phenomenon of attention, and the results have been unusually rewarding. Magoun (1963) indicated the significance of this work when he stated, "It now seems clear that ascending reticular influences upon the cerebral hemispheres are importantly concerned with initiating and modifying such states as arousal and wakefulness, as well as orientation and attention" (p. 74). The reticular formation serves as a "switching system" and makes it possible for an individual (or lower animal) to focus attention. Solley and Murphy (1960), among others, stressed the relationship between attention and perception. Presumably, unless arousal occurs and attention is alerted, ongoing sensations are ignored, hence perception is not possible.

We include this facet of the perceptual process, not only to stress the role of attention, but because the language pathologist often encounters the child who is unable to normally control his attentiveness. Pain level intensity may fail to bring about arousal, even though at other times while he engages in voluntary activities it can be shown that the deficit is not one of acuity. In some children of this type it is readily possible to stimulate arousal through vision and to then obtain normal scanning responses to sound. It is as though the activating system cannot be turned on through audition, but, after it has been aroused attention also can be focused on sound. If this deficit is present in infancy, these children do not learn to perceive auditorially (without remedial training); hence, they do not acquire language. As a group these children illustrate the role of attention if perception is to occur.

Rate—Intensity—Duration

Sensations can be described as having characteristic qualities which in themselves are intricately involved in the perceptual act. Sounds may occur at infrequent intervals or in rapid succession. Moreover, they may be loud or faint, of long or short duration. Each of these qualities contributes to or detracts from the ease with which the sensations might be perceived. Ability to perceive is impeded if the sounds are widely separated in time or if they occur too rapidly.

Similarly, whether the sensation is of short or long duration is an influential factor in perception. Unless the stimuli are of sufficient length, they cannot be recognized, and if the sequence is unduly long, again, it might not be perceived as a unit.

Intensity is another characteristic quality of sensations. Sounds may not be perceived because they are faint and cannot be differentiated from other sounds. Likewise, they may be of such great intensity that they are distorted and thus impede or preclude perception. A moderately amplified sound is more readily perceived, perhaps because making it louder assists in differentiating it from other sounds, or that amplification, per se, tends to structure the environmental field. Some children with disturbances of auditory perception benefit from the control of background sounds while amplifying those to which attention is being directed.

In studying children presumed to be aphasic, it is highly desirable to evaluate their auditory capacities relative to each of these qualities. Rate may be held constant while duration and loudness are varied; each factor is appraised independently of the others. A curious deficit is the inability to judge loudness; the child cannot perceive the quality of loudness and differentiate sounds accordingly. Ewing and Ewing (1947) emphasized that he often responds more successfully to "quiet" sounds than to those of high intensity. This type of perceptual disorder is often erroneously diagnosed as deafness.

Tolerance Levels

Miller (1964) demonstrated that the average individual's nervous system is capable of processing only a given amount of information (stimulation) at a given time; if it is overloaded the result is breakdown and confusion. This parameter is referred to as the tolerance level of the organism. Clinical teachers, and others in close contact with aphasic children, become aware of overloading and reduce stimulation. It is a common observation that tolerance levels are usually reduced by dysfunctions in the brain (Cruickshank, 1961). Clinically this is seen in many ways, including rejection of auditory sensation in favor of visual stimuli. To foster auditory perception it may be necessary to restrict input of other types of sensation, especially visual and tactile.

Tolerance disorders may be of various types. For example, the sensations received through one modality (e.g., visual) might impede perception of those received through other modalities (e.g., auditory). When two types of information are received simultaneously, instead of being processed normally a breakdown occurs, with one being obliterated. Inasmuch as most learning assumes simultaneous processing of more than one type of information, it is apparent that this type of perceptual disturbance may be seriously debilitating. But other factors might be involved. This type of disability is seen in those in whom a seizure is provoked if they are required to perform tasks such as reading aloud.

Discrimination—Differentiation

Included in the perceptual process is ability to differentiate among sounds according to their relative importance. This differentiation becomes markedly precise in connection with the spoken word. The child must discriminate the sounds of speech from other sounds, and also discriminate among the various speech sounds; *coal* and *cold* are not synonymous.

Ability to discriminate speech sounds has been extensively investigated by Wepman (1958) and Templin (1957). Templin demonstrated that this ability matures early in life, being well established by six to seven years of age. That this ability is related to childhood aphasia has been shown by McGrady (1964). He found aphasic children to be inferior as compared with normal children. Those with receptive aphasia were grossly disturbed in this facet of auditory perception.

Listening—Figure-Ground

The auditory world, like the visual, is conglomerate. Its significance is determined by the individual as he structures this conglomeration according to his needs and circumstances. This perceptual process relegates certain sounds into the background while selecting others for the focus of attention.

Auditory figure-ground behavior has been largely ignored, yet it is an essential facet of perception. In certain respects its importance can be highlighted by relating it to the act of listening. We have often stated that in working with children who have auditory language disorders, it is necessary to recognize that *many can hear but not listen.* Listening requires a concentration of attention, an attitude of anticipation, which is focused toward an expected type of auditory experience. Listening can be accomplished only when the sound field can be properly organized and structured. In other words, one cannot listen for all sounds simultaneously; it is difficult to listen for more than one sound at a given instant. Some children with auditory perceptual disturbances cannot normally engage in listening behavior. Inasmuch as virtually all tests of hearing assume ability to listen, these children may be classified erroneously as deaf. Moreover, this type of child frequently is distractible and unable to acquire language.

As a facet of perception, figure-ground behavior can be observed in the hard-of-hearing child, who because of his deficiency must treat all sound as being of equal importance—all sound is reacted to as *foreground.* Whenever it reaches his threshold of acuity it is responded to as being relevant.

It is not our intention to suggest that any one factor alone adequately explains the complex figure-ground process but, rather, to note that this facet of auditory perception is often disturbed in children who have receptive auditory language deficits. They cannot select speech sounds from the conglomerate auditory world or structure the flow of spoken language so that it becomes sequentialized into units which characterize it from other types of auditory experience. In a traditional sense, these children are not referred to as being aphasic because theirs is a listening, figure-ground disturbance, not a language disorder. If the sound field is properly structured, they may comprehend normally. This deficit causes a distortion of experience in general, rather than one which is directly related to verbal, symbolic learning.

However, because of its importance to language facility, it must be included in the concept of childhood aphasia.

Recognition—Identification

Auditory perception as a process cannot be viewed as a unitary phenomenon. It comprises several dimensions, some of which are understood better than others. One of these, ability to recognize and identify common sounds, was included by Spencer (1958) in an investigation of auditory perception in normal children. She found that the average child could identify everyday sounds when he was three to four years of age; this ability matures early in life.

We have indicated the basic scanning function which audition alone makes possible. Recognition and identification are related to perceptual awareness. This facet of the perceptual act is at the level at which meaning and significance are predominant. The individual is aware of the significance of the sensations, so he recognizes and identifies them according to their relative importance in meeting his needs at the moment. This dimension of perception is intriguing because of its importance in understanding childhood aphasia. Hence, we have developed an extensive battery of tests for its appraisal; the tests are delivered by electronic instrumentation (Myklebust, 1967). The child is required to identify both meaningful and meaningless sounds. Ability to recognize sounds and to identify them according to their usefulness is often disturbed in children with learning disabilities. Because this is a crucial factor in the development of normative experience auditorially, these children may have confusion in regard to various everyday life situations, although they acquire verbal facility.

Rhythm—Pattern Perception

Ability to perceive rhythm assumes facility in recognizing an auditory pattern in which there are regularly recurring elements or tones. These recurrences form groups within the body of the pattern so there is a clear time interval or sequence which characterizes the flow of the sounds. Normal persons vary in their facility to identify and follow rhythms. According to Spencer (1958) normal children below three years of age cannot perceive and recognize rhythmical patterns. This ability begins to mature by three and one-half years, with considerable facility having been achieved by six years of age. Research evidence of this type indicates that perception of rhythms is a dimension of perceptual behavior which falls at a higher level than certain other aspects of this behavioral process. Findings with lower animals support this presumption. Neff and Diamond (1958) have shown that after ablation of a given area of the auditory cortex the cat continues to discriminate pitch differences successfully but is unable to distinguish auditory patterns. Some aphasic children have great difficulty with this facet of auditory perception.

Rhythmical patterns characterize all spoken language forms. Not only basic comprehension but subtlety of meanings often is conveyed by the way an individual varies this component. In childhood aphasia this can be illustrated by contrasting jargon aphasia with echolalia. The jargon aphasic is incapable of pattern perception. He utters meaningless speech sounds because he is unable to perceive these sounds as meaningful units. In contrast the echolalic may function at a high level of auditory perception, including perception of rhythm; therefore, he utters speech sounds accurately. His disorder is not perceptual in nature but, rather, is one entailing integrative process; he perceives but cannot relate what he hears to units of experience. Disturbances of this type are seriously debilitating and have been referred to as central aphasia (Goldstein, 1948).

Intersensory Perceptual Equivalence

Studies of perception require distinction between *intra-* and *inter*-perceptual functioning. Though an oversimplification, it is beneficial to inquire into these processes when, to the extent possible, one modality is differentiated from the others, and when two or more functions are deliberately combined to evaluate the influence of one on the other. Myklebust and Brutten (1953) and Birch (1964), among others, have shown that a deficit in one modality (e.g., auditory) has implications for the development of other perceptual processes (e.g., visual). According to our hierarchy, auditory perceptual behavior attains its highest level of function only when it is enhanced by other perceptual functions. In other words, it is essential that the individual attain facility at the level of perceptual equivalence. What is perceived auditorially must be readily converted or transduced into visual, tactile, etc., equivalents. Although the brain is comprised of systems which function in a semi-autonomous manner, when presented with the sound of a motor the child automatically learns to relate it to the picture of an automobile.

Ability to identify perceptual equivalents often is disturbed in children who have childhood aphasia. This highly important process assumes integrity of function in the modality through which the information is to be converted. To illustrate, if perception of the sound of an auto horn is not properly perceived, it cannot be transduced into its visual equivalent. Intersensory perception is precluded by the deficit occurring in one of the sensory modalities involved.

A more subtle deficiency, less frequently recognized, is a disturbance in the transducing process itself. Auditory perception as well as visual and other forms may be intact. The deficiency consists of not being able to convert from one to the other. We have evolved a statistical procedure to assist in studying this aspect of psychoneurosensory behavior. Scores for perception of certain stimuli are determined by a battery of auditory tests and by a battery of visual tests. A child may score 90 percent correct on each of these. He is then given the test of perceptual equivalence; he must transduce from the auditory to the visual and from the visual to the auditory. His score for auditory to the visual may be only 70 percent correct. This is interpreted as a "conversion loss" of 20 percent. Such procedures are useful in diagnosis and provide a basis for clarification of the nature of the deficits found in children with disorders of auditory learning.

Meaning—Normative Auditory Experience

It is fortunate that psychologists are again focusing attention on the role of meaning in learning and behavior. It is gratifying also that in the study of language and its disorders, meaning as an area of interest and study has shown much growth. In general, authorities in the field of perception agree that a primary feature of this level of behavior is its role in the acquisition of meaning. In our hierarchy it is the result, the outcome, when the perceptual act is achieved normally. Certain investigators have made this the pivotal focus of their research. For example, Cantril (1950) demonstrated that individuals "knew" the size of an oak leaf without having had instruction; various other judgments were studied. It was shown that perceptual learning results in a *norm of experience*. This norm forms the basis of most relatively automatic judgments. Examples of these norms which determine much daily behavior include the judgment that a larger object is closer than a small one, even if in a given circumstance it might not be; normative experience becomes the basis for the decision. Likewise, the louder the sound, the closer it is assumed to be; again, in a given situation the judgment may be erroneous. These "sets of assumptions" derive from perceptual experience and constitute norms for many common judgments.

Perceptual norms are necessary so that each experience does not become a new judgment, but these norms may bring about a rigidity which in itself is a detriment, even a threat, to existence. However, our concern here is that children who have disturbances of auditory perception are deficient in the development of such norms; they are deficient in a type of behavior highly consequential to all adjustment. Because of this deficiency their norms of experience are constituted differently. Sometimes, even after comprehension is possible, they require educational remediation for deficiencies of *inner language*. Inner language, verbal and nonverbal, is basically dependent upon perceptual processes.

Summary

It has been our purpose to indicate the processes whereby an auditory sensation becomes a meaningful segment of experience, and in addition, to suggest that each of these processes which comprise the perceptual act is necessary for normal acquisition and use of the spoken word. As shown in the following chapter, the implication is that each dimension of perception must be appraised if we are to understand more fully the nature of a given child's aphasia. It has been our intent, also, to reveal the mammoth strides that have occurred in relation to childhood aphasia. The concept of this language disorder is not new, but it has evolved; it is still evolving.

VERBAL PROCESSES

Perception is the first step in the processes requisite for language learning. For auditory verbal behavior to ensue, however, that which is perceived must be remembered, integrated, recalled, and expressed in spoken form. Memory appears to be essential to all learning. Underwood (1965) stated that concept utilization occurs even in rote learning. In our construct of verbal processing, though we recognize the generalized as well as specific influence of memory, we subdivide this factor into storage and retrieval. Moreover, we hypothesize that retrieval can occur only after storage has been achieved—input precedes output. Jones and Wepman (1965) and Eisenson (1968) likewise differentiate between comprehension (input) and ability to reproduce (output).

Developmental levels or hierarchies have been stressed in child psychology. With respect to language these are reflected by observations such as, the child first acquires the spoken word—not the read or written. It is more difficult to indicate the exact levels of development that are requisite to acquisition of the spoken, read, or written word. Nevertheless, such models often are of value in the study of language pathology. We have found the formulation, shown schematically in Fig. 46-2, useful in understanding problems of childhood aphasia. As indicated, in addition to perception, for normal acquisition and usage of auditory language, the information (words) must be stored; it must be retained and preserved—it must be held in memory.

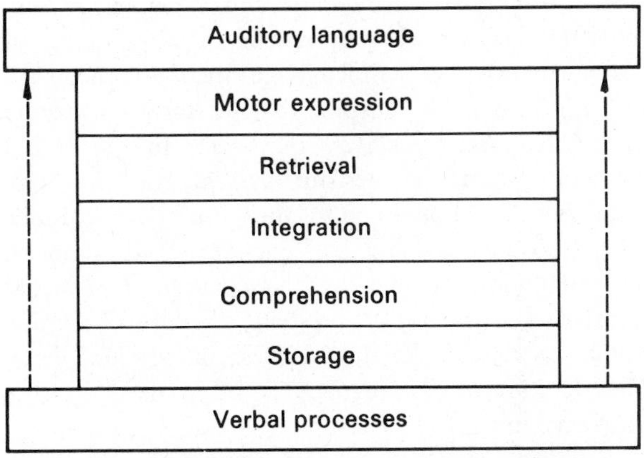

Fig. 46-2. Schema showing the functions requisite to auditory language and the disorders that might occur.

Retention of input, a reservoir of information, gradually makes comprehension possible. To understand is to be able to grasp, to recognize, and to know, which assumes a background of past experience. Comprehension is inextricably related to integration, however, albeit we cannot consider these processes as synonymous. In fact, at least to a degree, they may be made possible by different brain systems.

One might retain information, comprehend, and acquire meaning, yet be deficient in capacity to recall—retrieval is at a different level. On the other hand, some children have normal recollection but cannot activate the motor system for speaking. Though an oversimplification, as shown by Fig. 46-2, these five processes (storage, comprehension, integration, retrieval, motor expression) seem essential to acquisition and use of auditory language. We now consider each of these separately.

Storage and Sequencing Behavior

Memory distortions in relation to disorders of auditory language have been noted by various authorities (Nielsen, 1958; Weisenburg and McBride, 1964). Of critical interest is the work which has clarified the role of the hypocampi (Kimble and Pribram, 1963; Zangwill, 1963, 1964; Drachman and Arbit, 1966). Investigators have demonstrated that when the hypocampi are damaged immediate memory is disturbed. Immediate and delayed memory cannot be viewed as one and the same. One of the ways in which immediate memory has been studied is through the use of span or sequence tests. These investigations have assisted in evolving a concept of childhood aphasia.

Perhaps no aspect of learning has intrigued the psychologist more than sequencing, often referred to as memory span. Indeed, sequencing ability is critical to much mental functioning, including facility with auditory language. Binet and Simon (1916), whose work serves as the foundation for most current effort, measured memory span ability in various ways: digit span, word span, sentence span. One of the difficulties encountered in the study of memory is that as a behavioral attribute it is so all-inclusive. Guilford's (1967) studies may lead to significant progress in revealing more precisely the role of memory deficits in the language disorders of children (Kluever, 1971). So far as childhood aphasia is concerned, the auditory verbal system cannot be acquired unless storage processes are functioning adequately, unless the information (spoken word) can be stored both for immediate and for long-term (delayed) purposes.

Aphasic children are inferior in ability to repeat digits, words, and sentences (McGrady, 1964). It must be assumed that an auditory language disorder may comprise one of the following, or any combination of them: deficits in digit span, memory for word sequences, syllable sequences, or memory for sentences.

DIGIT SPAN

Ability to recall and repeat a series of numbers has been investigated extensively. Traditionally, digit span capacity has been studied (forwards and backwards), and various types of handicapped children deviate from the normal in this ability (Myklebust, 1964a). Clinical observation suggests that unless a child can retain a minimum of a sequence of three, he will not acquire facility with the spoken word. This deduction is supported by Binet's work to the effect that at two years the average child can retain a sequence of two digits, and at three, he has mastered a sequence of three digits.

WORD SPAN

Facility in retaining a series of digits seems not to be a direct assurance that the child is capable of normally recalling a series of related or unrelated words. This distinction may be related to Guilford's (1967) conception of differing memory functions according to the manner in which the information is embedded, or not embedded, in a given frame or structure.

SYLLABLE SEQUENCE

Although sequencing words and syllables may be correlated, these functions should not be viewed as identical. Aphasic children with receptive memory disturbances often cannot retain and sequentialize the syllables that make up words. They might be capable of reproducing words of one or two syllables but not words of more than three syllables. We use a syllable sequence test to reveal such deficiencies; the words are graduated in length from one syllable (bread) to six (conceptualization). When the length of the word exceeds the child's level of ability, typically he responds by giving only the first or the last syllable of the word. In using spoken language spontaneously, he produces words in which syllables have been erroneously sequenced or omitted.

SENTENCE SPAN

Ability to retain a sequence of words that express a thought or idea in grammatically correct syntax also serves as a guide to facility with auditory language. From Binet (Terman and Merrill, 1937) we learn that at five years of age the average child can retain and immediately reproduce a sentence of 10 words; at eight years, a sentence of 13 to 14 words; and as an adult, he can reproduce a sentence of 19 to 20 words. Sentence length, whether as a test of auditory memory or as a measure of facility with the written word, has proved to be a useful indicator of verbal capacities (Myklebust, 1965). Moreover, McGrady (1964) has demonstrated that both expressive and receptive aphasics fall below average on this facet of auditory memory.

Comprehension and Integration

Differentiation between comprehension deficits and disorders of integration and meaning remains a perplexing task for all disciplines. To comprehend is to integrate and to integrate is to comprehend, yet these processes are not identical. One cause of the perplexity is reflected by the term *central aphasia*, which implies that the deficit is limited to verbal processes when all integration is affected. Disturbances of auditory receptive language are more limited, mainly involving comprehension.

Terminology which defines inner language disorders clearly has not been evolved. Werner and Kaplan (1963) used the terms *inner* and *external speech*, as did Jackson (1926) much earlier. Goldstein (1948) used the terms *inner speech* and *central aphasia*, relating the two. He emphasized the importance of "abnormalities of nonlanguage mental processes" (p. 95). It is in this respect that the term *integration* is helpful. *Inner language* may refer to the verbal symbol system, the mediator system, used for self-reference or thought. On the other hand, inner language can be defined to encompass all symbolic representation, verbal and nonverbal. Nonverbal symbols (in art, music, religion, etc.) are of significance in relation to disorders of integration. As a designation, inner language is often used in this inclusive manner.

Receptive language, as contrasted with integrative disabilities, is functionally represented on the left hemisphere of the brain whereas nonverbal language is functionally represented on the right hemisphere. Accordingly, receptive aphasia results primarily from disturbances of the left, and nonverbal disabilities occur largely from dysfunction of the right hemisphere. Therefore, many children have excellent verbal facility but their verbalizations lack meaning. Normal language usage assumes integrity of both verbal and nonverbal processes—meaning, verbal representation, may be inadequate even though verbal input and output are at a high level. This type of disability should be included under the designation of inner language disorders.

Use of the terms inner speech and central and global aphasia, traditionally has not comprised the type of nonverbal language disorder referred to here —a significant type of disability indeed (Russell and Espir, 1961). These designations were intended to include the verbal deficits resulting from subcortical involvements. Penfield and Roberts (1959) focused attention on the nature of these disorders. They stated: "The centre-encephalic system is defined as that central system within the brain stem, which has been, or may be in the future, demonstrated as responsible for integration of the function of the hemispheres" (p. 21). It may be assumed that language serves the purposes of integration. Penfield and Roberts propose that "... the functions of all three cortical speech areas in man are coordinated by projections of each to parts of the thalamus, and that by means of these circuits the elaboration of speech is somehow carried out" (p. 208).

Inner language integrative disturbances may be classified as being of three types: 1) high verbal facility but significant deficiency in depth of meaning; left hemisphere intact, disturbances on the right; 2) inability to verbalize nonverbal meanings because of deficits in transcortical systems. These disorders differ from the first in that nonverbal meanings are acquired but cannot be related to the verbal system (Sperry, 1962); and 3) verbal and nonverbal integration is deficient because of subcortical dysfunctions; acquisition of meaning is deficient.

Inner language disorders can be contrasted with disturbance of comprehension. An auditory receptive involvement assumes integrity of nonverbal, transcortical, and centre-encephalic processes. In other words, disorders of comprehension are limited to disturbances of language reception; nonverbal meanings are acquired and can be related to words if comprehension can be developed—integration of nonverbal experience is not involved.

SYLLABLE BLENDING

Although not necessarily a measure of meaning, we have used auditory association tests to elucidate inner language functions. The child must draw upon the words he has learned, and these words usually reflect his inner language resources. Monroe (1932) was one of the first to recognize that auditory language facility includes ability to blend, to synthesize parts of words into wholes. Gates (1947) elaborated on this function and used it extensively in diagnosis of reading disabilities. McGrady (1964) devised a test of ability to synthesize syllables for use with young school-age children and demonstrated experimentally that speech-defective, aphasic, and normal children differed in their performances. The receptive aphasics were seriously deficient in ability to blend syllables auditorially.

A related type of facility is shown by the use of rhymes; e.g., the child is asked to think of a word that rhymes with *pan*; he is to make a judgment regarding words that sound alike. Because some children cannot mentally synthesize the syllables that form words, they cannot organize them on the basis of having a common ending. This capability is related to auditory inner language learning.

SCRAMBLED SENTENCES

Binet's (Terman and Merril, 1937) verbal absurdities and dissected sentences tests have proved to be excellent indicators of inner language functioning. Unless the child can abstract or generalize from the passage which reports an absurdity he cannot detect the "foolishness" which it conveys. Capacity to make such a deduction derives from generalization of meanings as acquired through auditory inner language.

Similarly, and perhaps more directly, ability to organize scrambled words into a sentence is unusually revealing of the child's inner language capacities; we combine verbal absurdities and scrambled sentences into a single task. One can unscramble words and form a sentence only after one has acquired considerable inner language facility, including how each word in a sentence relates to every other word. Various studies have revealed that syntax derives from the auditory form of language, not from the read or the written (Myklebust, 1965). Hence syntax, too, at least to a degree, is a manifestation of auditory integrative processes.

ORAL DIRECTIONS

We are indebted to Binet also for the suggestion that comprehension of directions given auditorially is a significant psychological function, revealing both language behavior and mental capacity. This ability is investigated by giving "three commissions" which are performed in the order given.

Executing oral directions involves recall of the commands as a sequence and relating this sequence to the appropriate actions. This ability appears to not be identical with facility in blending, repeating sentences, or memory span as measured by the digit test and apparently comprises greater capacity for mental organization of experience and verbal meaning. McGrady (1964) found receptive aphasics to be markedly inferior on oral directions. Though multiple causation is involved, children with deficits in comprehension often have disturbances of integrative processes.

PARAGRAPH MEANING

The "word-caller" has been recognized for some time. The child can read but he attaches no meaning to what he has read; integrative functions are deficient with respect to reading. The paragraph meaning test is useful in differentiating this child from children having other types of reading disabilities.

The psychologist and language pathologist concerened with childhood aphasia have shown less awareness of similar deficits in auditory language. To grasp the idea of a paragraph read to him, the child must hold the details in mind as they unfold and generalize the information to the idea expressed. This type of integrative processing seems not to be required for performance on the oral directions test, nor on tests of blending or memory span. In fact, currently as a measure of inner language, paragraph meaning is one of the most useful.

Many children show essentially average ability on other aspects of auditory language but fail on measures of paragraph meaning. Perhaps most children with learning disabilities, except those with expressive aphasia, suffer some deficiencies of integration. Apropos this possibility, studies using factor analysis and intercorrelation techniques have revealed that the intellectual abilities of these children are associated differently in comparison with normal children (McGrady, 1964; Myklebust and Boshes, 1964, 1969; Zigmond, 1966; Duff, 1968). They are of normal intelligence, but the "structure of their intellect" is aberrant. One can assume, therefore, that the psychology by which they learn also deviates from the average.

Inner language disorders are critical to this conceptualization because they reflect a disorganization of experience. It is our impression that paragraph comprehension reflects capacity to integrate at the abstract level—at the level of innuendo and metaphor, both of which are basic to acquiring abstract meaning. Unfortunately, our understanding of childhood aphasia is largely in terms of concrete language usage, comprehension, and utterance of words and sentences. Ability to function at this level does not assure competence at the more abstract, conceptual level. There is ample reason for thinking that many children fail academically even if they have no obvious disturbances of comprehension or of expression but because they have subtle, complex, disturbances of inner language.

Formulation and Retrieval

Before the child can use expressive language he must be able to recall words and to formulate mentally what it is he wants to say. These functions are psychoneurological in nature and in the brain there is a system largely concerned with such processing (Luria, 1963). Jackson (Taylor, 1958), a distinguished forerunner of psychoneurology, introduced the term *propositionalizing*, referring to those processes required for formulation of both the "propositions" to be expressed and the language through which they might best be uttered.

Others, notably Goldstein (1948), stressed the role of syntax and used the term *syntactical aphasia*. Perhaps ability to formulate and express ideas cannot be separated from considerations of syntax or from capacity to recall; we distinguish between use of syntax expressively and as a facet of inner language. However, formulation is not comprised merely of facility with syntax. Ability to recall and to mentally manipulate symbols are also involved. A facet of the retrieval process has been denoted as "word-finding ability". Typically this has referred to a specific disorder characterized by an inability to recall nouns and has been categorized as dysnomia. This raises the intriguing question of whether the brain actually codes and classifies in some manner relating to grammatical and syntactical construction.

Conceivably, two types of disorders are involved. In one the child, for purposes of expression, cannot recall the order in which words must be uttered (he cannot adhere to the rules of syntax) although he knows that his sentences are not spoken correctly; he cannot organize and sequentialize language syntactically. The second disorder more specifically entails processing of ideas for expression; he cannot organize and process the mental images and meanings that he has in mind.

THE TELL A STORY TEST

Until recently expressive language, spoken or written, could not be measured maturationally. Myklebust (1965) devised and standardized a test of written language, including scoring procedures for five types of language behavior: Total Words, Total Sentences, Words per Sentence, Syntax, and Abstract-Concrete (Meaning). The test consists of having children write a story about a picture.

McGrady (1964) used a similar procedure to study ability to formulate ideas and to use auditory language expressively. In comparing speech-defective, normal, and aphasic children he found those with receptive disorders to be inferior. Though less so, those with expressive disorders also fell below the normal. It has been well established that when input deficiencies are present we must expect deficits in inner language as well as in expressive; input precedes output. Integration and output are reciprocally affected by impairment of reception. However, McGrady's technique, as well as his findings, disclose that formulation and expression can be studied experimentally, and that these factors are of value in relation to childhood aphasia.

The retrieval aspect of expressive functions has been underlined by the problem of word-finding, or *amnesic aphasia* (Weisenburg and McBride, 1964). In amnesic aphasia, storage processes are not affected, but the individual cannot recall words normally. As suggested above, because of its obviousness in relation to nouns, this condition is often referred to as *dysnomia*. The individual cannot retrieve the correct word so he uses an incorrect one, but he is aware of his error. Because auditory monitoring processes are not involved, he recognizes the correct form. However, in the more severe form, he recognizes the correct word and repeats it correctly, but moments later he is unable to recall it.

For auditory language to be used effectively it must be available for expression at will. Unlike the child with deficits in motor processing who can recall the spoken form but not utter it, the amnesic can utter it but not recall it. This break in retrieval processes is an excellent example of the disturbances that occur as a result of dysfunctions in the brain. In addition, it recognizes that there are various types of childhood aphasia. In our model this deficit occurs at the level prior to innervation of the motor system for speaking.

Motor Processing

Historically, expressive aphasia was the first of the language disorders to be identified in both children and adults. In the case of adults, an individual with normal command of the spoken word was unable to utter words after a vascular illness. This observation fostered curiosity concerning brain function and led to greater understanding of this complex mechanism which makes learning possible. These initial clinical insights pertained directly to the condition which for decades has been denoted as an apraxia (Nielsen, 1946; Weisenburg and McBride, 1964). It is remarkable that we have not shown greater advancement in understanding this condition. Essentially we are at the level as when it was first observed by the pioneers.

The question is raised as to whether apraxia should be included as a type of language disorder. We view this deficit in motor processing as a type of aphasia, the assumption being that the child's motor processing otherwise is intact. His disability pertains only to utterance of the spoken word. According to the semiautonomous systems concept, it is not unusual for two systems to function normally when activated individually. The deficit is not in either system per se but in the processes involved in transducing from one to the other. The child cannot produce the motor equivalents for the verbal units he has in mind. He has no deficiencies of memory, he can formulate sentences, comprehend the spoken form, and detect the meaning of paragraphs. In this sense his disorder is not one of language. However, his motor disturbance relates only to utterance of words; he cannot innervate the motor system requisite for producing oral language. Thereby his disorder encompasses language usage; his motor system is not inactivated through paralysis, as in dysarthria and the cerebral palsies.

Unfortunately, as in various other aspects of language pathology, our knowledge is limited largely to gross involvement, to those children in whom ability to produce spoken language is highly deficient. The subtle, less obvious involvements are unrecognized.

Why the child cannot convert language units into motor impulses has been the subject of important investigations in recent years. Geschwind (1968a) states, "Broca's area is clearly a way station between Wernicke's area on the one hand and the neuron which sends axons to the motor nuclei of the speech organs on the other. But in keeping with our discussion above, it must be more than an intermediary step. It seems most likely that it contains the rules for turning the sounds of speech (this means not only single sounds but also many sequences) into motor acts. It might be called an auditory motor transducer" (p. 189). Therefore, this type of aphasia, this apraxia, apparently occurs when the neural mechanism referred to as Broca's area does not function normally. Such a dysfunction might occur developmentally, on an endogenous basis, or it may be the sequelae of disease and accident. Obviously, it may be present prenatally or sustained during or after birth.

Because this deficit in motor processing occurs at the last level of function (after reception and integration) it is much less debilitating than the other types of aphasia. Perceptual disturbances, disorders of storage, integration, or retrieval, all are more damaging both to intellectual, cognitive processes and to emotional, affective behavior. In fact, the generalized intactness and integrity in other respects than in production of speech is a useful diagnostic indicator for this type of disorder. Yet, as demonstrated by McGrady (1964), expressive aphasics as a group present important psychological and educational problems.

Other Variables

He who speaks more than one language often is struck by the fact that only a slight variation in accent, pitch, stress, or intonation determines whether the speaker makes himself understood or whether the "foreigner," whose native tongue he is distorting, looks quizzical and sympathetic without being able to comprehend what is being said. Such experiences have a profound impact on the student of aphasia. The normal listener, it is said, can tolerate much peak clipping and other modification of the language system without seriously disturbing comprehension. The language pathologist, on the other hand, is constantly being reminded that meanings are lost with minor deviations from the normal pattern. The differences in inflection and accent associated with geographic regions within a given country, even within the United States, often create problems of comprehension.

Here we emphasize that the concept of childhood aphasia must include a consideration of facets of auditory language other than comprehension or the utterance of words and sentences because *how* the spoken word is uttered is a basic factor as to what is meant by the speaker. The use of metaphor elucidates the nature of this problem. When one says, "Mighty oaks from little acorns grow," he is not referring mainly to the oak tree. Rather, he is conveying an abstraction to the effect that great things may have modest beginnings. But the problem is even more involved because how one utters any statement alters significantly the intended meaning. Thereby it is the task of every human infant to learn that words vary in meaning according to *how* they are used. In metaphorical usage, the words per se are not the critical factor; it is the peculiar reference to an abstraction. Likewise, because of the manner and circumstances under which it is uttered, a statement might mean the opposite from that when taken literally. The common expression, *It is a nice day*, might be used to convey the meaning, *Yeah! for ducks*. Studies in childhood aphasia rarely include these variables. Nevertheless, we must conclude that these are consequential facets of auditory language disorders.

CHILDHOOD APHASIA, READING, AND SPELLING

It is strange that the relationships among man's basic verbal systems are not emphasized more often because they are critical to all children, especially to those with language disorders. Our studies indicate that deficiencies in read and written language, as well as in spelling, frequently can be attributed to disturbed auditory processes (Myklebust, 1965). To learn to read the child must know what letters look like, but he must also learn the sounds associated with them.

The question arises as to whether a deficit in auditory learning which impedes acquisition of facility in reading or in spelling should be designated as an auditory type of dyslexia, or as an aphasia. Initially, we suggested that the term aphasia should be reserved for deficits in the spoken language form. However, we cannot overlook the fact that complex types of auditory disorders may be revealed *only* when the child is required to make associations with the read and written language forms.

So far as definition is concerned, the problem is analagous to that of motor processing discussed above. Should motor processing deficits be included in the concept of aphasia? We do so include them. Likewise, when the child cannot learn to read or spell because of deficits in auditory functioning, we classify this problem as being a type of aphasia.

CHILDHOOD APHASIA AND INTELLIGENCE

The psychologist, language pathologist, and other professional workers concerned with the role of verbal behavior in learning and adjustment cannot avoid the perplexing dilemma of the relationships between language and intellectual capacities. Through psychoneurology, neurophysiology, neurology, and electroencephalography, evidence is forthcoming which suggests that in some specific respects language and intelligence are interrelated and inseparable (Myklebust, 1968). Such knowledge is not construed to mean that without verbal language there is no thought; the cliché "no language, no thought" has been passé for some time. The basic issue is whether the child with a deficit which entails auditory processing of verbal information attains the same level of intellectual functioning, and, if so, is it qualitatively equivalent to that of the child without such disabilities.

Years of research will be necessary before definitive answers can be given. In the meantime, at least speculatively, we might gain from the work on the psychology of deafness (Myklebust, 1964a). Here we find that a sensory deprivation from early life does not basically impede development of most nonverbal intellectual processes. However, utilization of intellectual functions differs qualitatively from that of hearing children.

Findings for the deaf should not be applied directly to children who have childhood aphasia, but an aphasic involvement may be critical to facets of intelligence. In working with a large number of childhood aphasics, we have noted that those with input or integrative disorders are more handicapped than those with expressive deficits. When the problem is mainly receptive the brain area in which the dysfunction occurs usually is in the temporal lobe. That lesions in this area are seriously debilitating to behavior has been observed by various workers; it is the child with this type of neurological involvement who often manifests the syndrome propounded by Strauss and Lehtinen (1947)—children with other types of brain involvement usually do not.

The statement of Krieg (1955) to the effect that temporal lobe development may be taken as a rough indication of the psychic level of the specie is unusually pertinent to this discussion. A disturbance of the system for auditory processing as represented by the temporal lobe area may be one of the more basic types of dysfunctions sustained in childhood.

Also, when receptive disorders are present, there is a reciprocal impact on inner language. Inner language develops as a result of the sensory information received and integrated meaningfully; only when this occurs are mediation processes as conceived by the learning theorist possible (Mowrer, 1960). By their nature disturbances of auditory perceptive processes impede acquisition of meaningful experience, verbally and nonverbally; development of the *norm* of experience is affected, thus anticipatory behavior is impeded. A dysfunction which is mainly expressive in nature does not directly affect meaningful use of language for purposes of perception, conception, thought, and learning; in the hierarchy of reception-integration-expression it is only the last facet, expression, that is disturbed. The two more fundamental processes, input and integration, are available for purposes of learning and adjustment. As a result the pattern of intellectual development and function is not seriously impeded.

We do not infer that children with primary involvement of receptive auditory language, nor those with primary disturbances of integrative processes, necessarily have a concomitant mental retardation. Rather, the probabilities are greater that the child will experience difficulty in attaining average or above levels of mental capacity.

In a more general sense, man actualizes his true potential when language is not deficient. Though language and intellectual capacity are not one and the same, perhaps maximum development of intelligence is possible only when all verbal symbol systems function with complete integrity. This problem of interrelationships between childhood aphasia and mental capacity remains as one of the most difficult and challenging for investigators of the future.

BIBLIOGRAPHY

Allen, I. 1952. History of congenital auditory imperception. *N.Z. Med. J.*, 51, 239–247.

Allport, F. 1955. Theories of perception and a concept of structure. New York: Wiley.

Bernhardt, M. 1897. Die Erkrankungen der peripherischen Nerven. *In* Spezielle Pathologie und Therapie. (Vol. 2.) Nothnagel, H., editor. Vienna: A. Holder.

Binet, A., and Simon, Th. 1908. Langage et pensée. *Année Psychol.*, 14, 284–339.

———, and ———. 1916. The intelligence of the feebleminded. Baltimore: Williams & Wilkins.

Birch, H. 1964, editor. Brain damage in children—the biological and social aspects. Baltimore: Williams & Wilkins.

Broadbent, W. 1872. Cerebral mechanisms of speech and thought. *Medico Chir. Trans.*, 55, 145.

Cantril, H. 1950. The "why" of man's experience. New York: Macmillan.

Cruickshank, W. 1961. A training method for hyperactive children. Syracuse: Syracuse Univ. Press.

DeReuck, A., and O'Connor, M. 1964, eds. Disorders of language. London: J. & A. Churchill.

Diringer, D. 1962. Writing. New York: Frederick A. Praeger.

Doehring, D. 1960. Visual spatial memory in aphasic children. *J. Speech Hearing Research.*, 3, 138–149.

Drachman, D., and Arbit, J. 1966. Memory and the hippocampal complex. *Arch. Neurol.*, 15, 52–61.

———, and Ommaya, A. 1964. Memory and the hippocampal complex. *Arch. Neurol.*, 10, 411–425.

Duff, M. 1968. Language functions in children with learning disabilities. Northwestern Univ.: Ph.D. dissertation.

Eisenson, J. 1968. Developmental aphasia: A speculative view with therapeutic implications. *J. Speech Hearing Disorders*, 33, 3–13.

Eustis, R. 1947. The primary etiology of specific language disabilities. *J. Pediat.*, 31, 448.

Ewing, A. 1930. Aphasia in children. New York: Oxford Univ. Press.

Ewing, I., and Ewing, A. 1947. Opportunity and the deaf child. London: Univ. London Press.

Freud, S. 1897. Infantile Cerebrallhämung. Vienna.

———. 1953. On aphasia. New York: Int. Univ. Press.

Gall, F. 1825. On the function of the brain and each of its parts. Vol. 1–6. Phrenological Library. Boston: March, Capen & Lyon.

Gates, A. 1947. The improvement of reading: a program of diagnostic and remedial methods (3rd. ed.). New York: Macmillan.

Gelb, I. 1963. A study of writing. Chicago: Univ. Chicago Press.

Geschwind, N. 1968. Human brain: left-right asymmetrics in temporal speech region. *Science*, 161, 3837, 186–187.

———. 1968a. Neurological foundations of language. *In* Progress in learning disabilities, Vol. 1. Myklebust, H., ed. New York: Grune & Stratton.

Gesell, A., and Amatruda, C. 1947. Developmental diagnosis (2nd. ed.). New York: Hoeber.

Goertzen, S. 1961. Speech and the mentally retarded child. *In* Mental retardation. J. Rothstein, ed. New York: Holt, Rinehart and Winston.

Goldstein, K. 1948. Language and language disturbances. New York: Grune & Stratton.

Guilford, J. 1967. The nature of human intelligence. New York: McGraw-Hill.

Guthrie, L. 1907. Functional nervous disorders in childhood. London: H. Frowde.

Guttman, E. 1942. Aphasia in children. *Brain*, 65, 205–219.

Hardy, W. 1965. On language disorders in young children: a reorganization of thinking. *J. Speech Hearing Disorders*, 30, 3–16.

Head, H. 1926. Aphasia and kindred disorders of speech. New York: Cambridge Univer. Press.

Hebb, D. 1963. The semi-autonomous process: its nature and nurture. *Amer. Psychologist*, 18, 1, 16–27.

Hermann, K. 1959. Reading disability. Springfield, Ill.: Thomas.

Hinshelwood, J. 1895. Word-blindness and visual memory. *Lancet*, 2, 1564–1570.

Jackson, H. 1926. Hughlings Jackson on aphasia. Head, H., ed. *Brain*, 38, 8–10.

Johnson, D., and Myklebust, H. 1967. Learning disabilities: educational principles and practices. New York: Grune & Stratton.

Jones, L., and Wepman, J. 1965. Language: a perspective from the study of aphasia. *In* Directions in psycholinguistics. Rosenberg, S., ed. New York: MacMillan.

Jordan, T. 1966. Perspectives in mental retardation. Carbondale and Edwardsville, Illinois: Southern Illinois University Press.

Karlin, I. 1954. Aphasia in children. *Amer. J. dis. Child.*, 87, 752–767.

———, and Kennedy, L. 1936. Delay in the development of speech. *Amer. J. dis. Child.*, 31, 1138–1149.

Kerr, J. 1917. Congenital or developmental aphasia. *J. Delinquency*, 2, 6.

Kimble, D., and Pribram, K. 1963. Hippocampectomy and behavior sequences. *Science*, 139, 824–825.

Kimura, D., and Folb, S. 1968. Neural processing of backwards-speech sound. *Science*, 161, 3839, 395–396.

Kluever, R. 1971. Mental abilities and disorders of learning. *In* Progress in learning disabilities, Vol. II. Myklebust, H., ed. New York: Grune and Stratton.

Krieg, W. 1955. Brain mechanisms in diachrome. Evanston, Ill.: Brain Books.

Landau, W., Goldstein, R., and Kleffner, F. 1960. Congenital aphasia. *Neurology*, 10, 915–921.

Lefeure, A. 1950. Psychopathology of aphasia in children. *Arq. Neuropsiquiat.*, 8, 345–393.

Ley, J. 1929. Un cas d'audimutité idiopathique. Aphasie congenitale chez des jumeaux nonzygotes. *Enceph.*, 24, 121–165.

Luria, A. 1963. Restoration of function after brain injury. New York: Macmillan.

Magoun, H. 1963. The waking brain (2nd. ed.). Springfield, Ill.: Thomas.

McCall, E. 1911. Two cases of congenital aphasia in children. *British Med. J.*, I, 2628, 1105; 2632, 1407.

McCready, E. 1926–27. Defects in the zone of language (word-deafness and word-blindness) and their influence in education and behavior. *Amer. J. Psychiat.*, 83, 267–277.

McGrady, H. 1964. Verbal and nonverbal functions in school children with speech and language disorders. Northwestern Univ.: Ph.D. dissertation.

———. 1968. Language pathology and learning disabilities. *In* Progress in learning disabilities, Vol. 1. Myklebust, H. ed. New York: Grune & Stratton.

Miller, J. 1964. Adjusting to overloads in information. *In* Disorders of communication. Rioch, D., and Weinstein, E., eds. Baltimore: Williams & Wilkins.

Millikan, C., and Darley, F. 1967, eds. Brain mechanisms underlying speech and language. New York: Grune & Stratton.

Milner, B., Taylor, L., and Sperry, R. 1968. Lateralized suppression of dichotically presented digits after commissural section in man. *Science*, 161, 3837, 184–185.

Monroe, M. 1932. Children who cannot read. Chicago: Univ. Chicago Press.

Morgan, W. 1896. A case of congenital wordblindness. *British med. J.*, 2, 1378.

Morley, M., Court, D., Miller, H., and Garside, R. 1955. Delayed speech and developmental aphasia. *British med. J.*, 2, 4937, 463–467.

Moruzzi, G., and Magoun, H. 1949. Brain stem reticular formation and activation of the EEG. *EEG Clin. Neurophysiol.*, 1, 455–473.

Mowrer, O. 1960. Learning theory and the symbolic processes. New York: Wiley.

Myklebust, H. 1952. Aphasia in children. *J. except. Child.*, 1, 19, 9–14.

———. 1954. Auditory disorders in children: a manual for differential diagnosis. New York: Grune & Stratton.

———. 1955. Training aphasic children. Washington: Volta Bur. No. 660.

———. 1956a. Language training: a comparison between children with aphasia and those with deafness. *Amer. Annals Deaf*, 101, 2, 240–244.

———. 1956b. Some psychological considerations of the Rh child. *J. Speech Hearing Disorders*, 21, 423–425.

———. 1957. Babbling and echolalia in language theory. *J. Speech Hearing Disorders*, 22, 3, 356–360.

———. 1964a. Learning disorders: psychoneurological disturbances in childhood. *Rehab. Lit.*, 25, 12, 354–360.

———. 1964b. The psychology of deafness (2nd. ed.). New York: Grune & Stratton.

———. 1965. Development and disorders of written language (Vol. 1). Picture story language test. New York: Grune & Stratton.

———. 1967. Learning disabilities in psychoneurologically disturbed children. *In* Psychopathology of mental development. Zubin, J., and Jervis, G., eds. New York: Grune & Stratton.

———. 1968. Learning disabilities: definition and overview. *In* Progress in learning disabilities (Vol. 1). Myklebust, H., ed. New York: Grune & Stratton.

———, and Boshes, B. 1960. Psychoneurological learning disorders in children. *Arch. Pediat.*, 77, 6, 247–256.

———, and Boshes, B. 1969. Minimal brain damage in children. USPHS, Washington, D.C.

———, and Brutten, M. 1953. A study of the visual perception of deaf children. *Acta Oto-laryng.*, Supplementum 105.

———, and Johnson, D. 1962. Dyslexia in children. *J. except. Child.*, 29, 1, 14–25.

Neff, W., and Diamond, L. 1958. The neural basis of auditory discrimination. *In* Biological and biochemical bases of behavior. Harlow, H., and Woolsey, C., eds. Madison: Univ. Wis. Press.

Nielsen, J. 1946. Agnosia, apraxia, aphasia (2nd. ed.). New York: Hoeber.

———. 1958. Memory and amnesia. Los Angeles: San Lucas Press.

Orton, S. 1937. Reading, writing and speech problems in children. New York: Norton.

Penfield, W., and Roberts, L. 1959. Speech and brain mechanisms. Princeton: Princeton Univ. Press.

Quarton, G., Melnechuk, T., and Schmidtt, F., eds. 1967. The neurosciences: a study program. New York: Rockefeller Univ. Press.

Rioch, D., and Weinstein, E., eds. 1964. Disorders of communication. Baltimore: Williams & Wilkins.

Russell, W., and Espir, M. 1961. Traumatic aphasia. London: Oxford Univ. Press.

Schiefelbusch, R., Copeland, R., and Smith, J. eds. 1967. Language and mental retardation. New York: Holt, Rinehart and Winston.

Solley, C., and Murphy, G. 1960. Development of the perceptual world. New York: Basic Books.

Spencer, E. 1958. An investigation of the maturation of various factors of auditory perception in preschool children. Northwestern Univ.: Ph.D. dissertation.

Sperry, R. 1962. Some general aspects of interhemispheric integration. *In* Interhemispheric relations and cerebral dominance. Mountcaste, V., ed. Baltimore: Johns Hopkins Press.

Strauss, A., and Lehtinen, L. 1947. Psychopathology and education of the brain-injured child (Vol. 1). New York: Grune & Stratton.

Subirana, A., Corominas, J., and Oller-Daurella, L. 1950. Infantile congenital aphasias; clinical and electro-encephalographic study of 3 cases. *Actas Luso-esp. Neural.*, 9, 14–25.

Taylor, J., ed. 1958. Selected writings of John Hughlings Jackson (Vol. 2). New York: Basic Books.

Templin, M. 1957. Certain language skills in children. Minneapolis: Univ. Minn. Press.

Terman, L., and Merrill, M. 1937. Measuring intelligence. Boston: Houghton Mifflin.

Ucherman, V. 1891. The cases of dumbness (aphasia) without deafness, paralysis, or mental debility. *Arch. Otolaryng.*, 20, 321.

Underwood, B. 1965. The language repertoire and some problems in verbal learning. *In* Directions in psycholinguistics. Roseberg, S., ed. New York: Macmillan.

Van Gelder, D., Kennedy, L., and Lagauite, J. 1952. Congenital and infantile aphasia; review of literature and report of a case. *Pediatrics*, 9, 48–54.

Weisenburg, T., and McBride, K. 1964. Aphasia: a clinical and psychological study. New York: Hafner.

Wepman, J. 1958. Auditory discrimination test. Chicago: Language Research Associates.

Werner, H., and Kaplan, B. 1963. Symbol formation. New York: Wiley.

West, R., ed. 1962. Childhood aphasia. San Francisco: Calif. Soc. for Crippled Children.

Wolferman, A. 1955. Congenital auditory aphasia. *Arch. Otolaryng.*, 62, 509–514.

Wood, N. 1964. Delayed speech and language development. Englewood Cliffs, N.J.: Prentice-Hall.

Worster-Drought, C. 1952. Failure in normal language development of neurological origin. *Folia Phoniat.*, 5, 130–146.

———, and Allen, J. 1929. Congenital auditory imperception (congenital word deafness) with report of a case. *J. Neurol. Psychopath.*, 9, 192–208; 11, 289–319.

Zangwill, O. 1963. The cerebral localization of psychological function. *Advancement Sci.*, 64, 1–10.

———. 1964. Neurological studies of human behavior. *British med. Bull.*, 20, 43–48.

Zigmond, N. 1966. Intrasensory and intersensory processes in normal and dyslexic children. Northwestern Univ.: Ph.D. dissertation.

47

Childhood Aphasia: Identification, Diagnosis, Remediation

Helmer R. Myklebust

IDENTIFICATION OF APHASIC CHILDREN

Aphasic children must be identified before remediation programs for their special needs can be planned. The reasons for identifying children with auditory language disorders are threefold: medical, psychological, and educational.

Etiologically, childhood aphasia is a manifestation of dysfunctions in the brain. Hence, the implications for medical treatment and management are of the utmost importance; medical specialists must participate when evolving an overall plan for the child. Treatment for control of seizures, disinhibition, and hyperactivity may be prerequisite for optimal learning and adjustment (Giffin, 1968; Ong, 1968).

A significant relationship exists between aphasia and personal-social adjustment. Various investigators have found a correlation between this type of learning disability and other types of emotional disturbance. The specific nature of these relationships has not been clarified but, in addition to having an auditory language disorder, these children are often confused, disoriented, immature, disturbed in ego development, hostile, anxious, depressed, withdrawn, or otherwise emotionally and socially maladjusted. Physicians, psychologists, and educators are obligated to assist with identification in order that these psychic disorders, often more debilitating than the deficits in language, can be avoided. In general, we should assume that all aphasic children are in need of assistance with emotional development and adjustment.

A childhood aphasia, because of its basic relationship to learning, presents an educational problem of considerable magnitude. When the neurology of learning has been disturbed, a concomitant alteration occurs in the psychology of learning (Johnson and Myklebust, 1967; Myklebust, 1968). It is this modification which is of vital concern to the language pathologist and the special educator. The nature of the disability precludes the aphasic child from gaining maximum benefit through programs provided for the average child. Because the brain dysfunction affects not only auditory language behavior but the manner in which the child can best learn to read, write, tell time, understand maps, calculate, and in various other ways as well, special consideration is requisite to his total educational needs. When properly identified and evaluated medically, psychologically, and educationally the aphasic child can be assisted effectively in actualizing his true potential.

When to Identify

Because of the assumption that children with childhood aphasia will be discovered through speech clinics and hospitals, little attention has been given to screening procedures or to the most propitious age level for identification. However, this type of learning disability is not rare, screening procedures are applicable, and attention to identification must be forthcoming from a variety of disciplines.

If the child's disability is marked, severely influencing comprehension or utterance of the spoken word, parents will seek diagnostic assistance soon after the age at which ability to use speech is expected, usually between the ages of one to three years; comparatively, dyslexia is often not suspected until after the child is in the third or fourth grade. Auditory language is the first verbal system acquired, so deficits in this form frequently become troublesome in the prekindergarten years. It is common for parents to express concern as to their child's eligibility for school entrance because of his limitations with the spoken word. Use of auditory language, in fact, is an accepted "readiness" step for kindergarten and the first grade.

Perhaps the most critical time for identification is during the preschool years. It behooves all concerned to recognize the importance of discovering those with aphasia at this time; such awareness and planning includes participation of language pathologists, pediatricians, teachers, psychologists, social workers, psychiatrists, etc. Screening procedures that are useful even at this early age are gradually being developed.

It is unlikely that all children with childhood aphasia can be discovered before the age of school entrance, and case finding in early life is most successful with those who are severely involved. It is urgent that identification also be stressed upon school entrance, especially in relation to reading readiness. Children who have acute though moderate disturbances of auditory capacities often can be detected when it becomes necessary for them to combine auditory with visual learning. These functions entail complex psychoneurosensory processes, and the child with elusive deficiencies of auditory reception usually is identifiable at this time. Detection during this period of maturation and learning might prevent "overflow" involvements, such as emotional disturbance.

From the first to the fourth grade identification frequently involves underachievement, if not outright school failure. Again, the nature of the deficiency is related to the age at which recognition occurs; those with obvious disorders would have been discovered earlier. Auditory language deficits which affect reading, or more particularly spelling, are not recognized until this late age. Other types are complex disturbances of auditory perception, auditory memory, and formulation. In our language disorder clinics we frequently have children from 10 to 15 years of age with marked handicaps involving ability to remember directions (e.g., assignments), to tell stories, to formulate syntactically correct sentences, or to grasp the meaning of a paragraph that has been read to them. These too are disorders of auditory language.

Because only a few screening programs are in existence, many children remain to be identified up through the elementary grades and into high school. Though not specifically auditory in nature, tests of reading, spelling, and written language can be used for discovering some of these children (Myklebust, 1965).

The principle of "as early as possible" serves as the guide for when to identify. The age at which detection and diagnosis can be made varies, however, according to the nature and the extent of the disorder. As in other areas of handicap, the more elusive the disturbance the more difficult it is to recognize. Investigations are underway, some including large samples, so more reliable diagnostic procedures are becoming available for identification of all types of childhood aphasia (Myklebust, 1971).

Who Identifies

Discovering handicaps in children cannot be regarded as the responsibility of any single professional group. Because of the nature of auditory language disorders, if the involvement is severe the parents usually first consult their pediatrician. Hence, awareness of the problem on the part of these physicians is of paramount importance. Inasmuch as the deficit pertains directly to educational achievement, the "probables" frequently must be recognized first by the classroom teacher, who is in an excellent position to observe and to provide details concerning the child's use of auditory language; she can be of inestimable value in identifying aphasic children.

Direct observation is not necessarily the most effective approach, however, because some types of disturbances can be demonstrated only through use of objective tests. The clinical teacher, trained to teach children with childhood aphasia, should be competent in conducting surveys and in administering certain tests. Moreover, she can assist in interpretation of results so that those children requiring more intensive evaluation can be selected.

Children suspected of aphasia usually are evaluated by the language pathologist as well as by the psychologist. Ability and achievement levels must be determined. The diagnostic study should reveal discrepancies between potential for learning and actual performance in auditory language. These language, educational, and psycholgical evaluations comprise the basis for remedial education. Classification as an aphasia is essential whether or not further diagnostic study reveals disturbances of brain function. On the other hand, when behavioral evidence suggests an auditory language disorder, it is important to seek medical information. It may be desirable that the child be seen by a pediatrician, a neurologist, an electroencephalographer, and a psychiatrist. Final corroboration of a brain dysfunction most often is made through the neurological and electroencephalographic evaluations. Confirmation is complicated by the fact that certain types of neurological disturbances are difficult to demonstrate objectively. When such evidence is not forthcoming, the educator must proceed on the assumption that these disturbances are present, because only then does the child receive the advantages to which he is entitled and from which he will benefit most.

Diagnostic Programs

The objective of a screening program is comparable to that of the intensive evaluation—to reveal deficits in auditory processes. The tests and observations should include those children who reveal disturbances of auditory perception, comprehension, integration, and expression. In some instances the deficiency may be pervasive and entail several processes simultaneously. To illustrate, we saw Henry when he was three years of age. He was able to utter a few isolated words although comprehension appeared to be excellent, as did integration. He was given remedial assistance for three years, at which time he entered school. Two years later (eight years of age) the parents reported the following incident:

> The teacher gave Henry a reading test and he did very well except for auditory discrimination where the following item appeared: "Draw a line under the word that sounds like *goat*"; the words following were *boat* and *bed*. Henry insisted on underlining the word *bed* instead of *boat*. Being unable to convince him, the teacher asked his mother (also a teacher) to explain the correct response to Henry. However, he continued to underline *bed* even when the item was read to him over and over again. Finally the mother asked, "Henry, doesn't the word *boat* sound like *goat* to you?" Henry was amused and laughingly replied, "Mother, a *boat* can't make a noise like a goat."

Many deductions might be made; the initial diagnosis was an oversimplification—the problem was not merely one of expression. To Henry the word *sound* meant a noise. He could not get another meaning of the word, such as something *sounds like* something else—a sound meant a sound. Therefore, he had to look for a word that could *make a noise like a goat*, not one that *sounds like the word, goat*. Under these confusing circumstances, he found it more satisfactory to reject the word *boat* and select one less confusing

It is disconcerting to imagine the many times a day that children with auditory language disorders are confronted with their inability to comprehend a word, to associate proper meanings, to recognize multiple meanings, and to shift from one to another as usage dictates. We must be able to empathize with them in this bewilderment if we are to appreciate the disturbing and disintegrating consequences of aphasia. Moreover, we must be able to ascertain diagnostically the complex disorders that Henry reflected.

The nature of the diagnostic problem in childhood aphasia has been stated over and over again (Worster-Drought, 1952; de Hirsch, 1967). It must be shown that the child demonstrates integrities in certain respects, but despite these integrities he does not develop facility with auditory language. In addition, there must be evidence, presumptive or concrete, indicating that the lack of normal language can be attributed to dysfunctions in the brain. The integrities which must be demonstrated are: intellectual ability, hearing, emotional adjustment, and motor ability.

The question of the degree of integrity that must be shown in each of these areas is complex. Operationally defined criteria have been suggested, however (Myklebust, 1968). The basic principle is that there must be a discrepancy between the existing level of language and each of these integrities; the level of intelligence must be higher, and hearing, emotional adjustment, and motor ability must be adequate. In other words, it is necessary to show that intelligence falls at a level that does not preclude acquisition and effective use of auditory language; this criterion usually is met by applying nonverbal measures of mental ability. Integrity of hearing is demonstrated by standard pure-tone audiometry, or when necessary by EEG audiometry (Davis and Zerlin, 1966); when formal techniques are not applicable informal procedures often can be definitive (Myklebust, 1954).

Because of their verbal nature, tests of emotional adjustment usually cannot be used; nonverbal measures must be devised. The diagnostician, using history data and clinical observation arrives at a judgment concerning emotional aspects; often the language pathologist, psychiatrist, and psychologist render a combined decision. Psychogenicity should be considered inasmuch as auditory language behavior may be altered by emotional disturbance (Chess, 1944; Eisenberg, 1964). On the other hand, many aphasic children are more obviously characterized by their language disorder than by the symptomatology associated with psychogenic involvements; this may be true of children with reading disabilities (Connolly, 1971).

The area of motor behavior also presents difficulties in terms of objective criteria. Aphasic children may have ataxic involvements, as well as disturbances of laterality and other types of motor incoordination. The critical determination is whether the speech mechanism is intact for purposes of producing the spoken word. Anarthria, paralysis of this mechanism, does occur, as do cerebellar ataxic involvements. Moreover, these conditions may exist in addition to motor processing disorders of the apraxic type. Biomedical engineering techniques are being developed and may provide an objective basis for differentiation of these conditions (Myklebust, 1967). Meanwhile, the speech and language pathologist and the neurologist using clinical procedures must appraise the integrity of the speech motor system. Usually it can be shown that aphasic children have intactness in this respect and that the expressive deficits cannot be attributed to motor incapacities.

The Neurological Disturbance

Controversy has existed as to the type and extent of the neurological dysfunction that meet the criterion for diagnosis of aphasia (Sugar, 1952; Worster-Drought, 1952; Paine and Oppe, 1966). Again objective criteria have been difficult to obtain. But, pediatric neurology has indicated the type of examination and results that prove most fruitful (Boshes and Myklebust, 1964; Vukovich, 1968). Likewise, through studies which relate electrocortical disturbances to deficits in learning, electroencephalographers are providing results which may be crucial to substantiation of neurogenicity (Hughes, 1968). Moreover, indirect evidence of the type reported by Lawson (1968) should not be overlooked. His findings suggest that ophthalmological deficiencies correlate with neurogenic disturbances of language. Another type of indirect evidence is reported by Money (1962, 1966, Green and Perlman, 1971), who have disclosed an association between endocrinological diseases and impairment of verbal behavior.

DIFFERENTIAL DIAGNOSIS

Investigations of the relationships among disturbances of brain function, learning, and behavior now are voluminous; we can refer to only a few (Fessard, Gerard, and Konorski, 1961; Mountcastle, 1962; Millikan and Darley, 1967; Zubin and Jervis, 1967). That these works are relevant to the diagnosis of childhood aphasia is self-evident. Moreover, it is assumed that there are both medical and nonmedical facets when such a diagnosis is made; our discussion relates mainly to behavioral, nonmedical aspects.

In Chapter 46 we emphasized the importance of the type of work reported by Milner, Taylor, and Sperry (1968). Another approach holds promise for revealing associations between auditory language disorders and disturbances of electrocortical functions in the brain. Preprogrammed auditory and visual learning tasks are stored in a psychosensory, biomedical-engineering, computerized system. While the child responds to these tasks by pushing a button, his electroencephalogram is recorded (Myklebust, 1967). Then the EEG is summated by an analog computer and written out numerically by an automatic typewriter; the results represent the level of electrocortical output in microvolts.

This system was designed to investigate the verbal and nonverbal correlates of brain function especially with respect to the contingent negative variation in EEG (Cohen and Grey-Walter, 1966). The learning tasks were developed to include functions of a given modality (auditory and visual) and integrative functions (concept formation). Through a companion system these behaviors can be studied while the child is in the act of speaking, reading, or writing.

This approach to the study of children with language disorders represents a type of computerized procedure which makes greater precision possible. It is anticipated that more minute disorders of the brain can be revealed through these techniques. Also, it has the advantage of providing information on various psychoneurosensory processes simultaneously while the nervous system is engaged in a type of mental activity or problem solving. It seems that some dysfunctions can be evidenced only when the brain is activated in this manner. Such information is requisite for further understanding of children (or adults) who have seizures when required to speak or to read aloud. Though essentially at the level of research, this approach to differential diagnosis, to the study of behavioral correlates of brain function, is expected to be in common use within the next decade.

PERCEPTUAL PROCESSES

Capacity to perceive auditorially must be evaluated. The language pathologist and the psychologist carry major responsibility for this appraisal. As suggested in Chapter 46, perceptual processes cannot be separated definitively from other psychic processes, such as verbal comprehension and integration; differentiation becomes arbitrary. Nevertheless, in diagnosis of auditory language disorders demarcation of basic processes is propitious. Greater specificity and accuracy thereby is possible.

Attention

The psychopathology of perception has been the focus of much effort from a number of disciplines: neurobilogy, neurophysiology, psychiatry, psychology, etc. (Hoch and Zubin, 1965). It is increasingly apparent that electrocortical functions vary on the basis of attention and that approaches which utilize this rationale may be productive. The first step is to ascertain whether attention can be gained and sustained. The examiner presents sounds, verbal and nonverbal, keeping in mind the mental age of the child, and notes whether a scanning response can be elicited; this is sometimes referred to as the orientation reflex (Mark and Hardy, 1958). Myklebust (1954) has described attentional differences among certain types of handicapped children who show atypical patterns of auditory language.

Rate—Intensity—Duration

Objective standardized tests for determination of ability to function at different rates, levels of intensity, and for varying periods of time have not been developed. However, studies by Spencer (1958), McGrady (1964), Zigmond (1966), and Stambak (1960) are of value in providing techniques, as well as a frame of reference. The diagnostician usually evaluates the influence of rate by varying the presentation, from slow to average to fast.

It is necessary to determine whether the child's responses are altered by modifications of intensity, from faint to average to loud. Both verbal and nonverbal sounds should be used. Whenever possible it is revealing to have the child judge whether given combinations of sounds are of equal or unequal loudness. Duration, in terms of length, has been investigated more extensively, and as a facet of auditory behavior is interrelated with memory, especially with immediate recall ability. When appraised clinically various types of stimuli are presented: meaningful, nonmeaningful, verbal, nonverbal, rhythmical, nonrhythmical.

Tolerance Levels

Capacity to tolerate stimulation must be evaluated through clinical observation; history information suggests the extent and nature of the problem. As Johnson and Myklebust (1967) have shown, children with receptive auditory disturbances often reveal their tolerance deficits by becoming echolalic when the input exceeds their level of capacity for information processing. To elicit such behavior the clinician first presents simple language and gradually increases the level of complexity. The child responds meaningfully until the increased demand exceeds his tolerance level, at which point he becomes echolalic. Other indications of tolerance deficits are disinhibition, inattention, and, in rare instances, seizures. Another breakdown is that which occurs when two or more types of information are presented simultaneously, with one obliterating perception of the other, e.g., the child imitates a sound more successfully when he only hears it than when he hears it and looks at himself in a mirror.

Discrimination—Differentiation

Ability to discriminate sounds in relation to speech and language defects has been investigated by various workers (Travis and Rasmus, 1931; Hall, 1938; Kronvall and Diehl, 1954; Wepman, 1958; Wilson, Doehring, and Hirsch, 1960). Templin (1957) and Spencer (1958) have demonstrated that auditory discrimination ability in normal children progresses with age. Using the tests devised by these workers, McGrady (1964) found both expressive and receptive aphasics to be inferior in comparison with a normal control group. Discrimination ability should be evaluated when making a diagnosis of auditory language disorder.

Listening—Figure-Ground

It is remarkable that auditory figure-ground behavior rarely has been investigated. It is possible to do so with considerable accuracy using stereophonic dual-channel instrumentation. The clinician presents foreground sounds embedded in a background of conglomerate noise, using both verbal and nonverbal items. The child's task is to listen, recognize, and identify the foreground sounds. These tests can be administered either by a freefield technique or through earphones. It is of great value to present these tests using the procedure developed by Broadbent (1956), which provides diagnostic information relevant to capacities in auditory processing by the cerebral hemispheres.

It is sometimes necessary to demonstrate that the child can distinguish between the presence and absence of sound; until this distinction is made he cannot attend or listen. Because of the nature of their disorder some children can listen and engage in figure-ground behavior only after attention has been gained through other avenues, e.g., visual or tactile. In other words, to demonstrate this type of involvement the clinician may first present a sound (bell ringing) by having the child *see* it. When attention has been gained, an identical sound is produced out of sight of the child. Often he then recognizes it, scans, and localizes its source. Another procedure, helpful in distinguishing between ability to *listen* and ability to *look*, is to have the child close his eyes, present a sound, and have him point to its source without use of vision.

Recognition—Identification

Spencer's (1958) results reveal the importance of appraising ability to recognize and identify sounds. Her procedures are of value in that they are simple to administer and not time-consuming. Nonverbal sounds are recorded on tape and presented through a loudspeaker. The child has a set of toy noisemakers equivalent to those used in making the recording; each set of sounds is presented and, after a practice trial, the child selects the proper noisemaker and produces the sound that he has heard. Normal children learn to recognize common sounds early in life, but some with disturbances of auditory perception do not. Because ability to match experience with auditory information is critical to development of language, more diagnostic techniques to ascertain levels of capacity in this aspect of auditory perception must be developed; automated tests are being used experimentally (Myklebust, 1967).

Pattern Perception—Rhythm

We are indebted to Lewis (1936) for his classification of speech on the basis of 1. phonetic factors (succession of sounds) and 2. intonational aspects (patterns of rhythm, stress, and pitch). Travis and Davis (1926) showed differences in capacity to judge musical patterns in speech defectives as compared to normal speakers. Spencer's (1958) study indicated that judgment of pitch, rhythm, and melody varies consistently with chronological age. These judgments are maturationally dependent on complex interrelationships of auditory perceptual processes. A high correlation was found between perception of rhythms and memory span, as well as between rhythm and ability to synthesize auditorially. Zigmond (1966) showed dyslexics to be inferior on a rhythmical tapping test. It appears that disturbances of pattern perception may affect development of auditory language and also facility in reading.

Intersensory Perception

Those in close contact with children who have disturbances of brain function are increasingly aware that the scatter of abilities in these children is of importance in diagnosis, as well as in remediation. As Birch (1964), among others, has pointed out, the "interrelations among sensory modalities are not equally affected by damage to the nervous system" (p. 59); hence, developmental deviation of various processes should be expected. A crucial suggestion for diagnosticians, therefore, is that both intraperceptual and interperceptual functioning be evaluated. Many children with learning disabilities may not have deficiencies in auditory perception or in visual perception but show marked limitations in tasks requiring perceptual equivalence; that is, in intersensory perceptual processes (Zigmond, 1966; Duff, 1968).

It is advantageous to first establish the levels of

integrity present in intra-auditory perceptual behavior; this is accomplished by appraising the functions discussed above. Unless the child can attend adequately, distinguish rate-intensity-duration, discriminate, listen, identify, and perceive patterns, he should not be expected to normally engage in *inter*-perceptual functions.

Cross modal functions can be appraised in various ways. It is assumed that the intraintegrity of this motor system has been ascertained, a determination which establishes that the motor system per se is not significantly incapacitated. Diadochokinetic rate is basic because it requires intersensory perceptual processing, auditory to motor. Myklebust (1967) presented a method whereby the diadochokinetic rate can be automatically recorded and which permits computer analysis; correlations can be made with electrocortical functions, etc. Objective data can be obtained which make it possible to differentiate among disturbances due to cerebellar involvement, apraxic disturbances, and paralytic disorders of the dysarthric type.

McGrady (1964) compared speech-defective and aphasic children with a normal control group on both visual and auditory perception; the procedures are useful in making a differential diagnosis. The visual perception subtest of the Primary Mental Abilities Test (Thurstone, 1938) revealed that both experimental groups were inferior on auditory perception. The question of relationship between these findings has not yet been explored fully, but the significance of these functions has been documented. Comprehensive appraisal of children with disorders of auditory language requires that auditory perceptual processes be evaluated in detail, including both intra- and intersensory functions.

LANGUAGE PROCESSES

The previous discussion pertained to appraisal of perceptual processes. Verbal functions also must be evaluated inasmuch as language involvements are differentiated from disturbances of perception. In Chapter 46 we categorized the auditory language processes as verbal memory, comprehension, integration, formulation, and expression. This model assumes that the language disorder may be characterized by a deficit at any one of these levels, or it may comprise combinations of them. The diagnostic evaluation is planned accordingly.

Auditory Memory

Though it is often difficult, the diagnostician has no more important responsibility than to determine the integrity of those capacities requisite for storage of information. Inasmuch as a battery of tests designed for this purpose is unavailable, it is necessary to use subtest items from various sources. Diagnostic procedures and techniques that have proved of value can be demonstrated:

Jane was referred to our language disorders clinic because of school failure when she was nine years of age; verbal IQ of 96, nonverbal IQ of 104, total score of 100. Intensive evaluation of verbal functions revealed various deficits, including an auditory type of dyslexia. The learning quotient technique was used to ascertain the relationship between expectancy and actual achievement (expectancy age is derived by obtaining the average of mental age, chronological age, and grade age at the time of testing—the Learning Quotient (LQ) is the ratio of actual achievement to expectancy). Facets of auditory memory were measured by the Detroit Test of Learning Aptitude (Baker and Leland, 1959).

Learning Quotient Scores

Unrelated Words	90
Oral Directions	103
Sentence Span	63

These results indicate Jane's primary type of auditory memory disturbance. She can sequence a series of unrelated words and mentally organize and follow directions, but ability to sequence sentences is markedly deficient. We note that the first two memory tasks do not comprise syntax. Memory processing is disturbed precisely in the area of auditory sentence structure. Educational remediation must be planned in terms of this deficit.

Another type of auditory memory disorder is demonstrated by Joe, 16 years of age. Though of above average intelligence and an excellent reader, he could not reauditorize syllables and relate them to the written form; hence, he was an "atrocious" speller. When the clinical teacher dictated the word *container*, he wrote *conaner*. Recognizing the auditory nature of his disability, the teacher dictated the word one syllable at a time: *con—tain—er*. Joe then readily wrote any word correctly. He could not retain and auditorially sequence words of more than one syllable *while in the act of writing*.

Disorders of auditory memory may entail learning

the spoken sounds associated with the letters of the alphabet, as in the case of Fred, also 16 years of age. When asked to write words from dictation, he wrote:

table – tairl
paper – patpr
book – bobk

When given the names of the letters (e.g., t-a-b-l-e) he wrote the word. Until assisted through remedial education he could not "store" the sounds associated with the letters; words could not be phoneticized so auditory and visual equivalencies were impossible.

Other types of auditory memory disturbances are common. Using a test of ability to sequentialize syllables often reveals surprising results. A child eight years of age could repeat one-syllable words without error but when asked to repeat words of two syllables or more, she uttered fragments, like those produced in written form by the cases presented above. In appraising storage processes it is necessary to investigate memory span for digits, sentences, words, and ability to sequence syllables.

Comprehension and Integration

The diagnostician is confronted with a difficult circumstance when attempting to differentiate between receptive and inner language disorders; nevertheless such a distinction is of vast importance. The guiding principle is to determine the extent to which meaning in general is deficient. If ability to integrate verbally and nonverbally has been affected, the classification usually is in terms of deficits in inner language, whereas when limited to aspects of comprehension, classification is in the direction of receptive language disorders. A fundamental step is extensive appraisal of verbal and nonverbal intelligence. In the receptive aphasic the nonverbal score usually exceeds the verbal. When the deficit is one of inner language, the verbal scores often are higher. Diagnosticians should be cautious regarding use of a single test, e.g., the WISC (Wechsler, 1949). It is desirable to obtain corroborative evidence from other tests, e.g., Detroit Test of Learning Aptitude (Baker and Leland, 1959), E-G-Y Scales (Kent, 1946), Binet (Terman and Merrill, 1937), Nebraska Test of Learning Aptitude (Hiskey, 1966), The Leiter International Performance Scale (Leiter, 1940), and the Illinois Test of Psycholinguistic Abilities (Kirk, McCarthy, and Kirk, 1968).

COMPREHENSION

Auditory receptive language disorders are seriously disruptive of learning and adjustment. Jeff is no exception. When seen at the age of seven years and four months, he had a history of poor speech and development. In fact, his speech early in life consisted of jargon which inferentially appeared to be a reflection of marked inability to comprehend the spoken word. On the WISC his verbal IQ was 81 and his performance IQ was 114. On the Peabody Picture Vocabulary Test he earned an IQ of 85. Scores from the Detroit Tests of Learning Aptitude which showed disorders of auditory receptive language were auditory attention span (four years and three months) and sentence span (four years and six months). These results placed him at least three years below his age level. As was expected Jeff was experiencing great difficulty in learning to read.

Characteristic of children with disturbances of auditory verbal learning, Jeff has a severe disorder in ability to comprehend the spoken word. Typically auditory memory is involved, but it was not significantly inferior on either auditory or visual perception. His dysfunction is related to comprehension, a disability of the type commonly referred to as a receptive aphasia. The test results disclosed that Jeff had not sustained an involvement affecting general integration of meaning. Nonverbal "inner language" had been acquired at a level above his age group.

INTEGRATION

Deficiencies in the acquisition of meaning in a more general sense are usually included in the category of inner language disorders. It is in this connection that the experienced diagnostician notes the difference between intactness of nonverbal learning and experience and of pseudoverbal facility. Although some children with inner language deficits do not utter words, many of them do, but this is not the basic criterion. Rather, the critical factor is the extent to which meaning has been acquired, irrespective of the level of verbal facility. The language pathologist is struck by the relationship of nonverbal experience to meaningful use of language. The child who is deficient in acquisition of nonverbal meanings is more handicapped than the one who is unable to acquire use of words, such as Jeff, discussed above. Accordingly, clinical evidence can be secured through the Vineland Social Maturity Scale (Doll, 1953). Learning to care for oneself is more seriously limited when nonverbal integration is disturbed than when language, per se, is deficient. Words represent experience. When experience itself is not acquired normally, then facility in uttering words does not indicate proficiency in language behavior. Only when both verbal and nonverbal functions are intact is symbolic representational learning possible. The diagnostician must distinguish among these disorders. The following illustrates procedures and processes which have been found helpful:

John has a severe disturbance of auditory integration; he used no spoken language at three years of age but hummed tunes played on the piano. In early life he was variously thought to be mentally deficient, emotionally disturbed, and deaf. Our experience with John covers a period of six years; when last examined he was nine years and eight months of age. At that time his scores on the WISC were:

SCALED SCORES

Verbal		*Performance*	
Information	16	Picture Completion	11
Comprehension	5	Picture Arrangement	7
Arithmetic	10	Block Design	13
Similarities	16	Object Assembly	7
Vocabulary	9	Coding	7
Digit Span	13	Mazes	8
Verbal IQ	110	Performance IQ	92

Full Scale IQ—101

Children with disorders of auditory integration often score lowest on nonverbal measures of intelligence. John's verbal scores disclose that his problem is not of a generalized inability to comprehend, or of auditory memory as measured by the digit span. The Comprehension score reflects accurately a residual incapacity to abstract meaning; the findings for Picture Arrangement and Object Assembly reflect similar typical results.

Other manifestations of the nature of John's deficiencies are:

	Percent Correct
Memory for Unrelated Words	60
Oral Directions	81
Sentence Span	82
Paragraph Meaning (read to him)	86
Paragraph Meaning (read by himself)	70

These findings show that auditory memory processes also are involved, especially in sequencing of unrelated words. Paragraph meaning, an indicator of inner language functions, is inferior mainly when the material is read by himself. He is assisted with integration when the material is read to him, perhaps because intra-auditory processes have shown greatest improvement; reading by himself requires interrelating the heard and read language forms. John continues to be in need of highly specialized educational remediation in all respects, but the outlook is favorable.

Peter, who entered our language training program at four and one-half years of age, also illustrates a type of inner language disorder. Because of severe limitations of auditory integration and inattention, diagnosis of mental ability was deferred. He fell within average limits on selected visual-motor nonverbal tests. Auditory perceptual abilities were evaluated through use of everyday sounds; ability to identify was scattered and inferior, and disinhibition was marked. The clinical teacher's description was unusually revealing: "Peter shows severe disturbances of language; he has difficulty acquiring meaning from his experiences. He often demonstrates echolalia by merely repeating what he hears, but the echolalia predominates only when what is said to him is above his level of integration. If the language complexity is lowered, echolalia is reduced. When asked a 'why' question, and he begins to repeat it, the question should be reworded. He then answers it appropriately."

Various test results support the clinical teacher's observations. In a typical manner he continues to show deficits in auditory memory span: drum beats, three; unrelated words, three; simple commands, three; sentence word span, six; and Peabody Picture Vocabulary Test (Dunn, 1959), three and one-half years.

Retrieval Processes

Recognition and recall are not identical processes; both must be appraised. Standardized tests are not available for measuring capacity to reauditorize. By various objective procedures the diagnostician must determine levels of mental ability, memory, comprehension, and integration. When these fall higher than facility to recall words and to express in sentences, the diagnosis may be one of formulation deficits; motor processing disturbances also must be eliminated.

Dysnomia, a common form of "amnesic aphasia" is evaluated by having the child name common objects. Timing of the response adds information for appraising progress after remediation. However, one-word sentences, or the naming of objects alone, is inadequate as a measure of ability to reauditorize. Spontaneous use of expressive language should be explored. McGrady's (1964) technique of having a child tell a story is illustrative. In addition to the clinical information, various scores can be derived, as indicated by Myklebust (1965) for written language: number of words used in the story, number of sentences, words per sentence, accuracy (syntax), and meaningfulness (abstract-concrete). The child's story is tape-recorded and scored later. Though not directly comparable, as a measure of the expressive language "mean length of response" was used by Davis (1937), McCarthy (1954), and Templin (1957).

The following illustrates the pattern of results obtained when formulation ability is disturbed. Harry was seen in our language disorders clinic when he was nine years of age; he was referred for school failure, including a tendency to use mirror writing. His reading score was at the 10-year level but he often omitted short words and used wrong verb tenses. He could define words (Binet vocabulary) only with great effort and much encouragement. Digit span was at the average level but sentence span was inferior. His nonverbal mental abilities were not characteristic of inner language disturbance:

	Score Scaled
Picture Completion	15
Picture Arrangement	10
Block Design	11
Object Assembly	7
Coding	7
Mazes	10

The tell a story technique was used with Harry; his response was tape-recorded. Up to 20 and 30 seconds were required for recalling certain words:

Examiner: Harry, tell me about something you like to make.

Harry: Uh . . . well . . . well . . . models.

Examiner: What sort of models?

Harry: O, airplanes and ships.

Examiner: How do you do it?

Harry: Well, out of . . . um . . . out of . . . oh . . . what you . . . ma . . . call-ems . . . I can't uh . . . let's see . . . out of . . . plastic.

Examiner: How do you do it?

Harry: W . . . w . . . well, I paste . . . I past junk and stuff like that on it . . . the wings . . . and stuff like that.

Examiner: What else?

Harry: Well, I . . . um . . . oh . . . um . . . can't explain it . . . oh, I forget . . . let me see . . . hum . . . I can't remember.

Despite normal intelligence, good memory, and integrative functions, Harry has a severe disorder of auditory language. What he learns is not available for expression. He cannot formulate and recall the language required to relate experiences, and hence school success and emotional adjustment are tenuous. Our contact with him covers a decade—he is now almost 20 years of age. Recently we received this note: "Its come to a time when I must apply for college. One of the colleges I'm applying for request for a refference. I wonder if you wouldn't mind filling out this sheet and adding something about my learning disabilities. Every bit helps! Thank you very very much. Sincerly, Harry."

Motor Processing

The most commonly recognized type of auditory language disorder is that usually referred to as motor aphasia. Although identified many years ago, procedures for diagnosis have developed slowly. It has remained for workers in neuroanatomy (Geschwind, 1968), psychoneurology (Luria, 1966), psychophysiology (Young, 1964), and the psychology of learning (O'Connor and Hermelin, 1963; Lenneberg, 1967) to provide clues on the composition of this disorder of auditory language.

Diagnostically, the task is to ascertain whether the limitation is consequent to paralysis, to the incoordination resulting from ataxia, or whether the child cannot produce oral language despite integrity of the motor system requisite to speech. Luria's (1963) discernment in particular has provided additional insights into the nature of this condition, often designated as apraxia. He has shown that through controlling "verbal kinesthesia"—holding the tongue in a fixed position—it is possible to distinguish between deficits of inner language and deficiencies in motor processing.

Geschwind stresses that the character of expressive deficits should not be oversimplified. He emphasizes that the speech motor system repeats the messages received auditorially and that determination of expressive involvement assumes basic integrity of receptive capacities. He defined *conduction aphasia* as the lesion in neither the receptive nor the expressive systems but in the mechanisms which connect them. An attempt must be made to differentiate conduction aphasia from motor processing disorders.

Children who have motor expressive involvement are more intact psychologically than those with disorders of auditory language. Verbal and nonverbal mental test scores compare favorably with the average, and social maturity falls within normal limits. They are less deficient in ego development and in other aspects of emotional adjustment. They use gesture freely and compensate for their verbal inadequacies by using common sounds (meow, bow-bow) to convey ideas. Theirs is an inability to transduce speech sounds into motor equivalents, but otherwise they distinguish themselves by a pattern of generalized integrity.

Characteristically, the procedure in diagnosis is to make a comprehensive evaluation of intelligence, motor ability, social maturity, emotional adjustment, hearing, educational achievement, and language, and thereby demonstrate integrity in respects other than ability to produce the spoken word. A second step is to prove that the speech motor system is not impaired, that the disturbance is not one of dysarthria, ataxia, etc. A common error is to conclude that the motor processing system is not disturbed because the child can produce isolated speech sounds or words. Disturbances of motor speech production cannot be assumed to occur on an all-or-none basis. A wide range of deficits must be anticipated. As Luria has demonstrated, ability to utter isolated words does not assure competence in emitting fluent speech. Moreover, the disorder may be one of not being able to activate the motor system when attempting spontaneous discussion or when reading aloud, rather than when simply repeating what has been said; evaluation must include the influence of rate and duration. Some children can emit speech if permitted to do so at a reduced rate and if the production entails short sentences.

The following illustrates diagnostic procedures that have been applied successfully:

Dennis was seen for a diagnostic evaluation at the age of two years and 11 months. Except for a few words he was unable to speak. The history was negative for damage from disease or accident. However, both his mother and maternal grandmother had problems of articulation and speech fluency in childhood, but after eight to nine years of age their speech was not noticeably affected. Dennis was well adjusted emotionally, being friendly, outgoing, and socially responsive with children and adults. He made his wants known and presented no problem of discipline or home management. He was typical of children who have excellent generalized integrity but who cannot activate the speech motor system.

Children with auditory language disorders other than deficits in motor processing have been found to be inferior on the Social Maturity Scale (Doll, 1953). Moreover, Social Quotients correlate with neurological integrity (Boshes and Myklebust, 1964). Dennis' Social Quotient was 110, despite his inability to perform on items such as "talks in short sentences" and "relates experiences." Characteristic of children with this type of childhood aphasia, he had normal motor ability, competence in self-help (dressing himself, etc.). Nonverbal mental tests showed intelligence to be well within normal limits—block building, geometric designs, mannikin, figure drawing, etc. (Haeussermann, 1958; Taylor, 1959). Dennis' lack of speech could not be attributed to mental retardation.

The language evaluation focused on receptive and integrative verbal learning. Auditory perception was intact; he identified common social sounds, was able to discriminate among sounds, and even detected mispronunciations. Tests of receptive and inner language included obeying commands, recognition of body parts, pointing to objects in pictures, comprehension of prepositions, knowing what to do, information about things, and following directions (Gesell and Amatruda, 1947; Terman and Merrill, 1937; Anderson, 1940; Dunn, 1959). Through these measures it was determined that Dennis' comprehension and use of inner language fell at three years, average for his age.

Auditory memory (storage) and formulation (retrieval) also were evaluated. Use of receptive and inner language indicated that storage processes were functioning normally. In addition, he performed successfully in imitating nonverbal auditory sequences of three units (drum beats and nonverbal vocalizations), average for his age. He executed three unrelated commands, given as a single instruction. Ability to formulate sentences and use of syntax was appraised by having him indicate the correct use of subject, verb, and object construction. Though slightly dubious, it seemed that Dennis was capable of formulating sentences at the average level; specific tests for this purpose have not been devised. It was apparent that he could formulate sentences above the level at which he could utter them.

There remained the possibility that lack of speech was due to paralytic involvement or to ataxia of the speech mechanism. Examination revealed no difficulty with chewing, sucking, or swallowing. Moreover, he produced tongue-tip, back of the tongue, as well as lip sounds. He imitated the tongue movements of protrusion, up and down, and laterally. The rate and duration of his glossal functions were excellent. Motor integrity for speaking was well within normal limits.

When determining deficits in motor processing the diagnostic task is to obtain evidence on hearing acuity, auditory perception, storage processes, comprehension, integration, formulation, and speech motor functions. Dennis demonstrated intactness in all respects (including mental ability and emotional adjustment) except for motor processing; hence, he was classified as having this type of auditory language disorder. His program of remediation has extended over a period of nine months. This contact has confirmed the initial diagnostic classification and revealed a highly favorable outlook. It is our impression that Dennis' disorder is not due to brain damage but to an endogenous developmental dysfunction.

REMEDIATION

Remediation for childhood aphasia has been recommended since this condition was first recognized, but verifiable results have been slow to evolve. Advocates of specific programs often patterned their approaches on techniques used with adults (Froeschels, 1918; Hoffman, 1951). Remediation for aphasic involvements in general has been given an impetus by Luria (1963, 1966). His approach is psychoneurological, emphasizing the modification of brain processes that must occur if improvement is to be gained; he reported especially on his success with disturbances of "motor" aphasia. Luria's work was with adults, but he offers original insights and assists in formulating a conceptual model for remediation.

Perhaps the greatest distinction in remediation in children as compared with adults entails all aspects of learning (with the possible exception of those few in whom the only involvement is in motor processing). Because maturation and learning are continuing and are not at the adult level, the disorder tends to impede various facets of development, as shown by Behrens (1963) and McGrady (1964). All aspects—auditory, visual, tactile—may be affected. One of the most significant trends in the past decade is an increasing awareness that the needs of aphasic children cannot be met through programs of periodic therapy sessions. Instead, inclusive special education programs of the type planned for other handicapped children are necessary. It is from this frame of reference that we consider principle and guidelines for program development.

Educational Remediation

Programs of remediation should be planned according to the type of problem present, as defined by the diagnostic evaluation (Johnson and Myklebust, 1967). Strengths and weaknesses are shown by a profile analysis. This profile portrays residual capacities in perception, auditory memory, comprehension, integration, recall, and expression. Typically, combinations of these functions are affected. Consideration is given to both verbal and nonverbal functions, to the tolerance levels, and to the type and extent of the involvement. There is awareness that childhood aphasia is a multifaceted problem which requires remediation on a multidimensional basis and recognizes that the approach must be critically individualized.

Despite variations from child to child there are basic homogeneities. One of these concerns the nature of learning and development, i.e., *input precedes output*. To use the spoken word meaningfully, the child first must be able to comprehend it. Likewise, to express himself in writing, he first must be capable of reading. It is common to find teachers and clinicians who are not aware of these fundamental parameters. They might emphasize spoken utterances before the child is able to perceive the word, or to recognize what it is that he should say.

Another common assumption, usually erroneous, is that one should use every stimulation possible, that the multisensory approach be employed irrespective of other factors. Indiscriminate emphasis on multisensory stimulation may interfere with learning and be damaging. Overloading may be deliterious to attention, orientation, motivation, and in rare instances may cause severe fatigue, if not seizures. The knowledgeable clinical teacher uses multisensory stimulation by choice and with caution; she activates sensory modalities according to the diagnostic findings, on the basis of the child's capacity for stimulation.

Intra- and Interpsychoneurosensory Learning

A controversial principle is whether to teach to the integrities or to the deficits. This consideration includes much of what is known about the psychology of learning. Exceedingly relevant is the fact that research data consistently indicate that when brain functions are altered, learning processes also are altered. For example, children with neurogenic disorders cannot normally associate auditorially learned experiences with their visual equivalents, and vice versa. Teaching to the integrities does not assure that the deficits will be raised, nor can the opposite be assumed, i.e., if the deficits are raised, these gains will be generalized to other learning. The question is not only whether the deficits can be raised, but whether learning can be fostered *vertically and horizontally*. (Unfortunately, measures such as the WISC provide only slight information regarding horizontal learning on interpsychoneurosensory functions; therefore, many learning disabilities are not revealed by this type of test.) By implication it is necessary to consider both the *intra* and *inter* aspects of learning and to devise remediation approaches accordingly.

Studies of Remediation

Research studies designed to secure evidence on the affect of specific types of educational remediation are rare, especially in regard to childhood aphasia (McGinnis, 1963). McGrady's (1964) results make it clear that residuals affecting much of the educational experience are present long after the child enters school. Behrens (1963) evaluated the outcome of remediation, albeit with a selected sample of 41 children representing various types of language disorders. In his sample, the child was of average intelligence and had received remedial assistance for a period of six months or more; many had special instruction for more than two years. That auditory language learning was delayed is shown by the fact that 34 percent of the sample was 18 months of age before using their first word meaningfully, 33 months or older when two words were combined, and 36 months or older before using sentences of three words or more.

Behrens had initial and retest data covering the areas of intelligence, language, motor ability, social maturity, and electroencephalography. His findings showed a significant overall improvement in learning. Fifty-five percent of the sample showed normalization of the EEG. The profile of integrities and deficits remained essentially stable, with improvement occurring both in strengths and weaknesses. There was a trend for greater progress in verbal than in nonverbal areas. Advancement in learning was not correlated with chronological age, suggesting that positive results from remediation extended into high school age. However, the results indicated that the program of instruction was more successful in alleviating verbal deficits, inasmuch as social maturity remained at an inferior level.

Implications

There is an urgent need for developing programs of special education for aphasic children. Such programs should be broadly conceived with awareness of the influence of disorders of auditory language on all school learning. It must be recognized that when childhood aphasia is present, the psychology by which the child learns has been altered; different assumptions must be made in regard to the ways in which he learns most successfully. Not only are there deficits and integrities, but these functions are not interrelated and associated in the manner characteristic of normal children.

Childhood aphasia usually is present in early life, hence, the program of educational remediation should be concentrated at the preschool and early school years. Because of the basic nature of auditory language and its relationship to the read and written verbal systems, only when programs are provided early in life can the child be assured of actualizing his potential, of achieving success in learning and adjustment. Clinical teachers should be trained in special education and in the psychoneurology of learning, with a major in language pathology. Such training programs must be widely available if the needs of children with childhood aphasia are to be served. Much has been accomplished, but only then will the future be bright for this group of handicapped children.

BIBLIOGRAPHY

Anderson, J. et al. 1940. Minnesota Preschool Scale, Form A and B. Minneapolis: Educational Test Bureau.

Baker, H., and Leland, B. 1959. Detroit tests of learning aptitude. Indianapolis: Bobbs-Merrill.

Behrens, T. 1963. A study of psychological and electroencephalographic changes in children with learning disabilities. Northwestern Univ: Ph.D. dissertation.

Birch, H., ed. 1964. Brain damage in children—the biological and social aspects. Baltimore: Williams & Wilkins.

Boshes, B., and Myklebust, H. 1964. A neurological and behavioral study of children with learning disorders. *Neurology*, 14, 1, 7–11.

Broadbent, D. 1956. Successive response to simultaneous stimuli. *Quart. J. exp. Psychol.*, 8, 145–152.

Chess, S. 1944. Developmental language disability as a factor in personality distortion in childhood. *Am. J. Orthopsychiat.*, 14, 483–490.

Cohen, J., and Grey Walter, W. 1966. The interaction of responses in the brain to semantic stimuli. *Psychophysiology*, 2, 187–196.

Connolly, C. 1971. Learning disabilities—social and emotional factors: *In* Progress in learning disabilities, Vol. II. Myklebust, H., ed. New York: Grune and Stratton.

Davis, E. 1937. Mean sentence length compared with long and short sentences as a reliable measure of language development. *Child Develop.*, 8, 69–79.

Davis, H., and Zerlin, S. 1966. Acoustic relations of the human vertex potential. *J. acoust. soc. Amer.*, 39, 109–116.

de Hirsch, K. 1967. Differential diagnosis between aphasic and schizophrenic language in children. *J. Speech Hearing Disorders*, 32, 3–10.

Doll, E. 1953. The measurement of social competence: a manual for the Vineland social maturity scale. Minneapolis: Educ. Test Bur.

Duff, M., 1968. Language functions in children with learning disabilities. Northwestern Univ.: Ph.D. dissertation.

Dunn, L. 1959. Peabody picture vocabulary test. Minneapolis: Amer. Guidance Service.

Eisenberg, E. 1964. Behavioral manifestations of cerebral damage in childhood. *In* Brain damage in children. Birch, H., ed. Baltimore: Williams & Wilkins.

Fessard, A., Gerard, R., and Konorski, J., eds. 1961. Brain mechanisms and learning. Oxford: Blackwell Scientific Publications.

Froeschels, E. 1918. Kindersprache & Aphasie. Berlin: Verlag von S. Karger.

Geschwind, N. 1968. Neurological foundations of language. *In* Progress in learning disabilities Vol. 1, Myklebust, H., ed. New York: Grune & Stratton.

Gesell, A., and Amatruda, C. 1947. Developmental diagnosis (2nd. ed.). New York: Hoeber.

Giffin, M. 1968. The role of child psychiatry in learning disabilities. *In* Progress in learning disabilities Vol. 1, Myklebust, H., ed. New York: Grune & Stratton.

Goodenough, F., Maurer, K., and Van Wagenen, M. 1940. Minnesota pre-school scale, form a and b. Minneapolis: Educational Test Bureau.

Green, O., and Perlman, S. 1971. Endocrinology and disorders of learning. *In* Progress in learning disabilities, Vol. II, Myklebust, H., ed. New York: Grune and Stratton.

Haeussermann, E. 1958. Developmental potential of pre-school children. New York: Grune & Stratton.

Hall, M. 1938. Auditory factors in functional articulatory speech defects. *J. exp. Educ.*, 7, 110–132.

Hiskey, M. 1966. Nebraska test of learning aptitude. Lincoln, Neb.: Union College Press.

Hoch, P., and Zubin, J., eds. 1965. Psychopathology of perception. New York: Grune & Stratton.

Hoffman, J. 1951. Training of children with aphasic understanding. *Nervous Child*, 9, 85–88.

Hughes, J. 1968. Electroencephalography and learning. *In* Progress in learning disabilities (Vol. 1), Myklebust, H., ed. New York: Grune & Stratton.

Johnson, D., and Myklebust, H. 1967. Learning disabilities: educational principles and practices. New York: Grune & Stratton.

Kent, G. 1946. E-G-Y scales. New York: Psychological Corp.

Kimura, D., and Folb, S. 1968. Neural processing of backwards-speech sound. *Science*, 161, 3839, 395–396.

Kirk, S., McCarthy, J., and Kirk, W. 1968. The Illinois test of psycholinguistic abilities (rev. ed.). Urbana: Univ. Ill. Press.

Kronvall, E., and Diehl, C. 1954. The relationship of auditory discrimination to articulatory defects of children with no known organic impairment. *J. Speech Hearing Disorders*, 19, 335–338.

Lawson, L. 1968. Ophthalmological factors in learning disabilities. *In* Progress in learning disabilities (Vol. 1), Myklebust, H., ed. New York: Grune & Stratton.

Leiter, R. 1940. The Leiter international performance scale. Santa Barbara: State College Press.

Lenneberg, E. 1967. Biological foundations of language. New York: Wiley.

Lewis, M. 1936. Infant speech. London: Kegan Paul, Trench, Trubner.

Luria, A. 1963. Restoration of function after brain injury. New York: Macmillan.

———. 1966. Traumatic aphasia. The Hague: Mouton.

Mark, H., and Hardy, W. 1958. Orienting reflex disturbances in central auditory or language handicapped children. *J. Speech Hearing Disorders*, 23, 237–242.

McCarthy, D. 1954. Language development in children. *In* Manual of child psychology. Carmichael, L., ed. New York: Wiley.

McGinnis, M. 1963. Aphasic children. Washington: Volta Bur.

McGrady, H. 1964. Verbal and nonverbal functions in school children with speech and language disorders. Northwestern Univ.: Ph.D. dissertation.

Millikan, C., and Darley, F. 1967. Brain mechanisms underlying speech and language. New York: Grune & Stratton.

Milner, B., Taylor, L., and Sperry, R. 1968. Lateralized suppression of dichotically presented digits after commissural section in man. *Science*, 161, 3837, 184–185.

Money, J., ed. 1962. Reading disability. Baltimore: Johns Hopkins Press.

———, ed. 1966. Education of the dyslexic child. Baltimore: Johns Hopkins Press.

Mountcastle, V., ed. 1962. Interhemispheric relations and cerebral dominance. Baltimore: Johns Hopkins Press.

Myklebust, H. 1954. Auditory disorders in children: a manual for differential diagnosis. New York: Grune & Stratton.

———. 1965. Development and disorders of written language Vol. 1. Picture story language test. New York: Grune & Stratton.

———. 1967. Learning disabilities in psychoneurologically disturbed children. *In* Psychopathology of mental development. Zubin, J., and Jervis, G., eds. New York: Grune & Stratton.

———. 1968. Learning disabilities: definition and overview. *In* Progress in learning disabilities Vol. 1. Myklebust, H., ed. New York: Grune & Stratton.

———. 1971. The pupil rating scale. New York: Grune and Stratton.

O'Connor, N., and Hermelin, B. 1963. Speech and thought in severe subnormality. New York: Macmillan.

Ong, B. 1968. The pediatrician's role in learning disabilities. *In* Progress in learning disabilities Vol. 1. Myklebust, H., ed. New York: Grune & Stratton.

Paine, R., and Oppe, G. 1966. Neurological examination of children. London: Heineman.

Spencer, E. 1958. An investigation of the maturation of various factors of auditory perception in preschool children. Northwestern Univ.: Ph.D. dissertation.

Stambak, M. 1960. Trois épreuves de rhythme. *In* Manuel pour l'examen psycholojique de l'enfant. Suisse: Delachaux et Niestle.

Sugar, O. 1952. Congenital aphasia: an anatomical and physiological approach. *J. Speech Hearing Disorders*, 17, 301–304.

Taylor, E. 1959. Psychological appraisal of children with cerebral palsy. Cambridge: Harvard Univ. Press.

Templin, M. 1957. Certain language skills in children. Minneapolis: Univ. Minn. Press.

Terman, L., and Merrill, M., 1937. Measuring intelligence. Boston: Houghton Mifflin.

Thurstone, L. 1938. Primary mental abilities. *Psychometr. Monogr.* No. 1.

Travis, L., and Davis, M. 1926. The relationship between faulty speech and lack of certain musical talents. *Psychol. Monogr.*, 36, 71–81.

———, and Rasmus, B. 1931. The speech sound discrimination ability of cases with functional disorders of articulation. *Quart. J. Speech Educ.*, 17, 217–226.

Vuckovich, M. 1968. Pediatric neurology and learning disabilities. *In* Progress in learning disabilities (Vol. 1), Myklebust, H., ed. New York: Grune & Stratton.

Wechsler, D. 1949. Wechsler intelligence scale for children. New York: Psychological Corp.

Wepman, J. 1958. Auditory discrimination test. Chicago: Language Research Associates.

Wilson, L., Doehring, D., and Hirsch, I. 1960. Auditory discrimination learning by aphasic and non-aphasic children. *J. Speech Hearing Research*, 3, 130–137.

Wood, N. 1964. Delayed speech and language development. Englewood Cliffs, N.J.: Prentice-Hall.

Worster-Drought, C. 1952. Failure in normal language development of neurological origin. *Folia Phoniat.*, 5, 130–146.

Young, J. 1964. A model of the brain. Oxford: Clarendon Press.

Zigmond, N. 1966. Intrasensory and intersensory processes in normal and dyslexic children. Northwestern Univ.: Ph.D. dissertation.

Zubin, J., and Jervis, G., eds. 1967. Psychopathology of mental development. New York: Grune & Stratton.

48

Aphasia in Adults: Basic Considerations

Jon Eisenson

NATURE OF APHASIC INVOLVEMENTS

Considerations toward a definition:

Aphasia is a general impairment of language functioning associated with localized cerebral pathology. This concept (definition) of aphasia is consistent with that of Schuell, Jenkins, and Jiminez-Pabon (1964, p. 113), who consider aphasia to be "a general deficit that crosses all language modalities and may or may not be complicated by other sequelae of brain damage . . . the language deficit itself is characterized by reduction of available vocabulary, impaired verbal retention span, and impaired production of messages, perhaps secondary to impairment of the first two dimensions."

Implied in the opening statement on aphasia is that there are other pathologies of the central nervous system that are associated with language impairment. These may be temporary, as in the event of an episode of alcoholism, or more chronic, as in the effects of chronic alcoholism. We need also be mindful in distinguishing between the effects and implications of peripheral sensory impairments and impairments of the peripheral mechanisms for the production of language symbols—the oral-articulatory apparatus and the hand. Penfield and Roberts indicate their appreciation of the need to distinguish between central disturbances associated with localized cerebral pathology and more widespread pathology, as well as impairments associated with peripheral nerve involvements. Penfield and Roberts (1959, p. 92) define aphasia as "that state in which one has difficulty in speech, comprehension of speech, naming, reading, and writing, or any one or more of them; and it is associated with misuse and/or perseveration of words, but is not due to disturbance in the mechanism of articulation (as in pseudo-bulbar palsy) or involvement of peripheral nerves, nor due to general mental insufficiency".

Osgood and Miron (1963, p. 8), after reviewing several contemporary and historical definitions of aphasia, offer the following: "Aphasia is a nonfunctional impairment in the reception, manipulation, and/or expression of symbolic content whose basis is to be found in organic damage to relatively central brain structures. Such a definition would include all modalities and forms of linguistic signs, but would exclude such things as perceptual disorganization, disturbance in learning, in abstracting and problem-solving, and purely sensory or motor impairments—except as they specifically involve language symbols. This clinical distinction, of course, does not mean that aphasia should be studied without reference to simultaneous nonaphasic symptomatology or that language behavior is in any sense separable from behavior in general."

Without further laboring the matter of definition, the author would like to point out that agreement among aphasiologists and clinicians who have experience with aphasic patients in recognizing or identifying a person as aphasic, is likely to be much greater than their agreement as to definitions of aphasia or to the *essence* of aphasic involvement. So this author, based on his own experience, considers the following observations of primary importance:

1. At some stage in their involvement, persons designated as aphasic indicate impairment for intake of sequential verbal events as well as for verbal sequential output. Intake disturbances are often labeled as memory or attention span defects. Output sequential disturbances are manifest in syntactical defects for formulations that are appropriate and relatively specific to the situation.
2. On a probability basis, aphasic involvements are in general expressed in a reduced likelihood that a given linguistic formulation will be understood (appropriately evaluated), or produced (appropriately formulated) in kind and manner consistent with the situation (events associated with the linguistic formulation). In general, the more intellectual and abstract the expected linguistic reaction, the less likely it is that the reaction will occur.

Based on these fundamental observations about the verbal behavior of aphasic patients, we may then present the following as a restatement-definition of aphasic language disorders. *Aphasia is an impairment of language functioning of persons who have incurred localized cerebral damage that results in a reduced likelihood that an individual involved in a communicative situation will understand or produce appropriate verbal formulations.* The greater the degree of adjustment required on the part of the brain-damaged individual to determine the adequacy and appropriateness of the verbal formulation in the communicative interchange, the greater the likelihood that he will experience difficulty. Thus, verbal expressions of strong feeling, emotion, or any other *set linguistic formulation*—in general any established sequential utterance—are better retained and evoked than are those utterances which call for specific formulation and, not infrequently, reformulation according to the special demands of the communicative situation. Written language impairments (reading and writing) often parallel those for oral language. In addition, impairments in arithmetic processes may be present.

This expanded definition includes the concept of Henry Head (1926) that aphasia is a disturbance of "symbolic formulation and expression" and Hughlings Jackson's (1879) observation that subpropositional language (established word series as in counting statements of strong affect, etc.) tends to be better retained by aphasic patients than high-level, more "intellectual" propositional language—the language we use for our thinking and the expression of our thoughts.

The "localized cerebral pathology," to which several references have been made, will be considered in some detail in the chapter on Correlates of Aphasia in Adults. For the present, we wish merely to emphasize the need to distinguish between diffuse and bilateral damage associated with progressive brain disease and the person who is suffering from dementia and the localized cerebral pathology in the hemisphere dominant for language.[1] The latter pathology is associated with aphasia. The pathology of the dement is, we believe, associated with intellectual deterioration and so with modifications in language. We are mindful, however, that not all students of aphasia will accept this position and that the implications of the relationship between language and thinking—and the impairments of one as manifest in the impairments of the other—are deserving of long and sober consideration.

Aphasia and Aphasic Involvements: The Individual Aphasic

Up to this point we have discussed aphasia without emphasizing as we should that aphasic involvements happen to persons and are not disembodied impairments. We may, if we wish, try to separate the disturbances of language and thinking and the implications of such disturbances on the personality of the individual. However, we prefer to look upon the aphasic individual as one whose impairments are so interrelated that though we are mindful at some times of the manifestations of linguistic impairments, and at other times of the modifications in cerebration—the "crippled thinking"—and are impressed on still other occasions with the modifications in personality, we are nevertheless dealing with an individual with dynamics and processes that are complex, interrelated, and disturbed. The aphasic is what he is at the time we see and relate to him as a result of all that he was, and all that happened to him when and after he incurred this pathology. Thus, we must ever bear in mind that the involvements of aphasic persons can be understood only if we begin with the basic appreciation that aphasia constitutes a complexity of disturbances. The aphasic individual had habits,

[1] This is almost always the left hemisphere for right-handed persons as well as for about half the population of left-handed persons.

attitudes, and abilities, as well as capacities not yet translated into abilities, and a personality, before he became impaired. If the individual is an adult, he had learned and developed strategies for responding to illness, to incapacities, to frustration, and to the myriad of influences that human beings are exposed to, long before he became aphasic. How he is likely to respond to the immediate effects of aphasic involvements we believe will depend to a large extent on the kind of person he was before he became aphasic. Aphasic involvements are likely to bring about modifications in the patient's premorbid personality, almost never in the direction of improvement. They are not, however, likely to produce a new personality unrelated in any way to the individual's premorbid state and manner of behaving. A well-adjusted individual who becomes aphasic probably has a better chance of ultimate adjustment than a neurotic individual who becomes aphasic. The latter is likely to become a neurotic-aphasic with a reduced chance of recovery from either his neuroticism or his aphasic disturbances.

Some Basic Considerations and Definitions

It will help our understanding of the language impairments of aphasic persons if we review briefly some concepts in regard to the nature of language, and more generally, of human beings and their verbal (symbol) behavior. Man, as the philosopher Cassirer (1944) emphasized, is "*An animal symbolicum*". *Symbols* are arrangements of discernible stimuli (events) most frequently audible and/or visible, and less frequently tactile, which derive their meaning through a process of association. Thus White (1949, p. 25) held, "A symbol may be defined as a thing the value or meaning of which is bestowed upon it by those who use it. I say 'thing' because a symbol may have any kind of physical form, it may have the form of a material object, a color, a sound, an odor, a motion of an object, a taste."

Language consists of an arrangement (system) of symbols employed by beings who are capable of making associations between essentially arbitrary representations and events to express their thoughts and feelings. Until there is strong evidence to the contrary, we will assume that *only human beings* are capable of employing a linguistic sound system. Ordinarily, persons born with normal capacity for hearing of parents with normal hearing develop a spoken (aural-oral) language system. This system, regardless of what the particular language (national—cultural) may be, has design features which Brown (1965, p. 248) summarizes and generalizes as follows:

> Fewer than one hundred sounds which are individually meaningless are compounded, not in all possible ways, to produce some hundreds of thousands of meaningful morphemes, which have meanings that are arbitrarily assigned, and these morphemes are combined by rule to yield an infinite variety of sentences, having meanings that can be derived. All of the system of communication called language have these design features.

Speech and Language

Speech is a medium that employs a linguistic code, oral and/or visible, by which we are able to express feelings and communicate thoughts to others with comparable capacities. The linguistic code of speech is produced without need for mechanisms external to the human body. The code employed constitutes a language.

Critchley's (1967) definition that "Speech should be restricted to the *expression and reception of ideas and feelings by way of verbal symbols* (i.e., words, or any other verbal tools which we may come to regard as units of speech)" is acceptable to us, providing that the substitutes for verbal tools are limited to these visible symbols which do not require instruments external to the human body for their production.

Aphasic persons are defective in speech because they are impaired in language. They may also be defective in speaking because of neuropathologies which directly impair the oral-articulatory and respiratory mechanism for speaking. Deaf persons may become aphasic and be impaired in their ability for expression and communication through their visible code or codes; e.g., finger spelling and signs.

Propositional Speech

When linguistic symbols are used to *communicate* a specific idea or to elicit a specific response, we are dealing with *propositional speech.* The unit of linguistic content with which the individual produces specific symbol situations is termed the proposition. In a proposition, as the term was originally used by Hughlings Jackson, not only the words but the manner in which the words are related and refer to one another within the unit become important. A proposition, Jackson emphasized, implies both an internal and external relationship. The words are related to one another and to the situation in which they are used.

The aphasic individual's chief difficulty is in evaluating and in evoking propositional units. From the point of view of formulation and production of utterance, the aphasic is one who suffers from an impairment in his previously established ability to communicate meanings—to deal with propositions—more than he suffers from a loss of words per se. This is not to suggest that there is no diminution in the ability to understand and retrieve words, but rather to emphasize *that the ways words are used* are markedly different for the aphasic and the normal speaker, and for the person who has become aphasic, compared with his own premorbid abilities for language functioning.

Jackson directed attention to levels of speech and distinguished between *inferior* and *superior* speech. *Inferior* speech included the use of emotionally charged utterances, expletives, cliché "remarks," established verbal series (counting, alphabet, and verbal social gestures—terms of greeting). In general, they are utterances that are "triggered off" in set formulation that express a state of feeling (swearing, affectionate terms) and that require no special formulation (serial content) to be appropriate. In contrast, *superior* speech—the use of propositions—employs verbal formulations that are specific to a situation. Applying these distinctions to aphasia, we may generalize our observations to the effect that the aphasic individual can speak (express) his feelings through inferior, nonpropositional utterances much better than he can communicate his thoughts through superior, propositional utterances.

Words, Concepts, and Meanings

Concepts are generalizations about experiences. Concepts are the mental products which result from a succession of experiences with events which are considered by the respondent to be the same or similar in one or more essential respects. The *constellation of essential respects* constitutes the generalization which underlies the concept.[2] Concepts for normal persons are presumably subject to continued modification according to individual ongoing, direct or vicarious, experiences. Except for most proper names, vocabulary (lexicon) items are verbal representations of concepts. To the degree to which some proper names, e.g., Mary, Joe, Tom, Dick, Harry, Jonah, are likely to predispose or prejudice one's reactions to the utterance, these too may be said to have conceptual implication.

Though we may be able to form concepts without words, the words of our individual lexicons are the incorporations of concepts for which we have had associated verbal experiences. A single word (form) may stand for one or more concepts, which may or may not be related. Homonyms, such as *reign* and *rain*, *read* and *reed*, are examples of audible word forms which have different and unrelated meanings. Other single word forms, such as *board* and *race*, have both related and unrelated meanings. The word *water* is an example of one of many English words that have several meanings and concepts which, for the most part, are related to the most common or core meaning of the word. Other such English words are *run*, *head*, and *chief*. *Dry* may refer to things which are not sweet, or to degree of sweetness as well as to degree of wetness. Thus, a *dry* drink is one which, however wet, is relatively *not sweet*.

Except when a single word constitutes a complete utterance, the meaning of a word is determined by the utterance as a whole as well as the overall environment (circumstances) in which the utterance is produced. The meanings of single-word utterances are determined by the overall nonverbal circumstances and/or by the verbal circumstances of a preceding speaker. We may return to Jackson's postulation that we communicate in propositions, that the sentence rather than the word is the basic unit for the expression of our meanings when we are engaged in verbal behavior.

There is considerable research evidence to support the observation that aphasic patients, as a total population, show a reduction in vocabulary which is inversely related to the frequency of word usage. That is, the words most difficult to retrieve (available to the aphasic according to recognized lexical need) are those which occur least frequently in the language (Wepman, et al. 1956). We believe that the implication of this observation may be applied to the individual aphasic to the effect that word usages—the meaning and way a word was employed by the individual—are related to the reduction (available or retrievable "on demand") in inverse relationship to

[2] J. B. Carroll (Words, Meanings, and Concepts, *Harvard Educational Review*, 34, 1964, 178–190) considers a concept to be "the abstracted and often cognitively structured classes of 'mental' experiences learned by organisms in the course of their life histories."

his particular frequency of usage. Thus, the individual's most common (frequent) use of a word is more likely to be retained than the least frequent use of the word. So, presumably, for most speakers the use of *dry* for *not wet* is more apt to be retained than the use of *dry* for *not sweet*. However, it is conceivable that a given individual may provide an exception because he was and is *a given individual* and not a generalization of individuals.

We also have parallel evidence to support that reduction in comprehension is related to frequency of word usage along the same line as reduction for expression (Schuell et al., 1961). We believe that for comprehension, as well as for language production, that meaning is related to comprehension. The rarer the meaning and the more abstract the meaning, the greater the likelihood for failure of comprehension. We can project this for the individual on the basis of frequency of word and frequency of meaning for words with multiple meanings. We may, however, expect individual differences that will vary with the user's experience with the words, with his ways and the meanings of the words, in his receptive lexicon.[3]

Nonintellectual Use of Word Forms

Most intelligent human beings learn to use language with sufficient facility and proficiency to elicit specific responses or to express specific ideas according to the needs of varying situations. This is not all, however. Most human beings also learn to use language symbols without regard to specific ideas or without intention of eliciting specific responses. Words spoken under the influence of strong emotion, of anger, fear, and hate, as well as words of a more tender emotion, are *nonspecific* and *nonsymbolic*. The same word form, then, may have both abstract and specific (symbolic) meaning as well as nonabstract and nonsymbolic meaning. Some English words of Anglo-Saxon origin are rarely used except in nondenotative, nonsymbolic ways. It is possible, however, to utter any word, or any group of words, in a manner which makes them devoid of intellectual significance. This point is being emphasized because we regard an aphasic person as one for whom intellectual and abstract meanings are, in conventional communicative situations, considerably more impaired than the ability to express affect (feelings and emotions). As Jackson reminded us, the aphasic person is one who suffers impairment in his ability to communicate meanings more than he suffers loss of words.

Nonintellectual speech is not confined to emotional utterances. Other forms of nonintellectual speech are *automatic*, *serial-content*, and *social-gesture speech*. *Automatic speech* consists of linguistic material which has been so often repeated *in a given order* that the content has been memorized. Familiar verses, prayers, and songs are examples of speech content which initially may or may not have had intellectual significance but which became automatic and nonintellectual through repetition. Words of a song are usually automatic only when the melody as well as the words are produced. If the melody is intentionally inhibited, it will generally be found that voluntary effort is necessary to recall the words of the song.

Serial content speech consists of a series of words which have been learned and memorized in a given order. The alphabet, numerical sequences, and arithmetic tables are examples of serial-content speech. Automatic speech may become modified and require voluntary control when it becomes necessary to begin at other than the habitual starting point.

Social-gesture speech is another form of linguistic content in which individual words and their specific symbolic significance are relatively unimportant. In the use of such verbal social gestures as "How are you?" and "Pleased to meet you," we pay little attention to the specific symbolic or denotative meanings of the words. At best, these words have "area meanings." Social-gesture words are appropriate in broad ways to the situations in which they are used. In general, several possible choices may be equally appropriate to the same situation. For example, when two acquaintances meet it is not of great importance whether one greets the other with "Hello"; "How are you?"; or "How do you do?" It is usually equally unimportant whether the response to the greeting is "Fine, thank you"; or "How are you?"

Emotional utterance, automatic-content, serial-content, and social-gesture speech are examples of linguistic word forms and word usage which remain relatively intact for most aphasic patients. These, as we have indicated, are nonpropositional language utterances.

[3] For a discussion of the broad implications of the relationship of word-frequency to the concept of aphasia see D. Howes, Application of the word-frequency concept to aphasia, in A. V. S. De Reuck and M. O'Connor (editors) *Disorders of Language*, J. and A. Churchill, London, 1964.

Language and Thought

Is the aphasic person impaired in his thinking because of his impairments in language, or is he impaired in language because of a primary, adventitiously acquired deficit in thinking? Compared with his premorbid potential, is the aphasic an intellectually impaired person and so, at best, one who will continue to be linguistically impaired in that he will not recover fully his capacities for dealing with high-level abstract propositions? These are questions that we are raising without entertaining an aspiration that we will be able to supply definitive answers about thought without language or whether thinking is internal speech or self-talking.

We will make what may be an obvious assumption that even for those individuals for whom brain pathology seems to increase the flow of utterance, the quality of the utterances and of the related thinking is certainly impaired. We are for the present more concerned with the implications for intellectual functioning for aphasic persons who are reduced in their verbal output, who seem "lame" in communicative situations in which they once functioned with relatively good efficiency. Observations as to the "lameness" go back almost to the time when aphasia was first made as a differential diagnosis. Hughlings Jackson considered aphasia to be a disturbance in symbolic thinking and expression.[4]

Pierre Marie (1906) held that the *sine qua non* of aphasia were in deficits of intellect related to impairment in the use of language. Cole (1968), in a recent article, indicates that the intellectual deficit may be the same as that for comprehension of language. Marie's position was that true aphasia was basically one for impairment of language comprehension.

The relationship of aphasic impairment to intelligence, over and above the implication of verbal mediation for the aphasics, has been studied by De Renzi and his associates. In one study that involved identification and cognition of colors by aphasic patients, De Renzi and Spinnler (1967) concluded that the deficit found "on non-verbal association between colors and objects cannot be accounted for by the language disorders of these patients, and points to a more general involvement of mental abilities."

In an earlier article, De Renzi and Vignolo (1962) employed a test to determine to what extent the difficulty of aphasics for decoding messages can be attributed to an impairment in the capacity to apprehend the intellectual implications of the given task rather than to a difficulty in "decoding" per se. The patients were selected from aphasics who showed evidence of only minimal difficulty in language comprehension. The investigators concluded that the patients showed disturbances of speech comprehension related to impaired intellectual functioning which is not readily observable in conversation or through routine language testing.

Goldstein's (1942, 1948) position emphasized changes in the way an individual thought as a consequence of brain damage.[5] The aphasic individual was viewed as one whose behavior revealed a change from the ability to employ an *abstract attitude*—to perceive generalizations and deal in concepts, and to separate and project himself from the "demands" of the immediate present to broader and nonimmediate considerations—toward one of concretism. Such behavioral changes are expressed in language, but basically, according to Goldstein, are manifestations of intellectual change associated with cerebral damage *and* aphasia. The essence of the change is in a tendency towards concretism, so that the individual's "thinking and acting are directed by the immediate claims that one particular aspect of the object or situation in the environment makes."

DISTURBANCES FREQUENTLY RELATED TO APHASIA

Apraxia—Impairment of Voluntary Movement

The *concept of apraxia* was introduced by Liepmann (1900) to distinguish between motor disorders based on impairment of voluntary movement and those resulting from paralysis, ataxia, and pathologies affecting muscle tone. The term *apraxia* as we will use it will refer to impairment of voluntary and purposeful movements (acts) which cannot be accounted for on the basis of motor weakness. Apraxic patients often are able to execute an act on an "involuntary" basis which they seem unable to perform voluntarily. So, a patient may lick his lips on the basis of an inner urge, or even light and smoke a cigarette and yet not be able to imitate such acts or execute them

[4] See Head (1926, reprinted 1963, Vol. I, Ch. 3) for an appreciative review of Jackson's position on this point.

[5] K. Goldstein and M. Scheerer, Abstract and concrete behavior, *Psychol Monogr.*, 1941, 53, 2.

on direction or command by another person. We must, of course, make certain that a patient understands a command or direction before we attribute failure to an inability to execute purposive movements to accomplish an act.

We are, of course, primarily concerned with apraxic involvements that directly implicate language functions—the apraxias of the articulatory mechanism and for the movements in writing. Liepmann (1913) argued that some forms of motor, or so-called Broca's aphasia, have their etiology in a disturbance of the kinesthetic engrams (kinesthetic plans or "schemes" of movement) which form the mental framework or basis for each motor act. The patient who cannot produce words he seems able to understand may be suffering from a failure to recall the order of articulatory activity from an amnesia for verbal production, rather than from impairment of the inner formulation of the utterance.[6] Similarly, a patient may be unable to write because of an impairment for the plan or scheme for the movements to produce the sequence of letters he has in mind.

Although we shall not try to unravel the knot of where aphasic involvements begin and apraxia leaves off, we do wish to share the clinical impression that apraxic patients show greater impairment with propositional than with nonpropositional language. Impairments also increase as the patient needs to appreciate the *intention of another* person in the execution of an act.

The relationship of the propositional level of the act is emphasized by Denny-Brown (1958) in his concept of *ideational apraxia.*

"It is obvious that the more hypothetic the nature of the request, the more imaginary the circumstances, and the more the requested movement is a mimesis of the real thing, the more vulnerable it is to such disease. The patient is unable to *pretend* to drink from a glass of water, or even to pretend to drink from an empty glass, yet can perform without difficulty when presented with a glass with water in it. This is the distinction between the vulnerability of propositional performance versus spontaneous or emotional performance that Jackson pointed out in relation to disturbances of speech.

. . .

". . . in its highest elaboration, mimetic and propositional behavior is related to conceptual organization of space, objects and persons in the dominant hemisphere. Such behavior is more highly vulnerable to pathologic changes than is direct physiologic reaction to external events."

[6] See Luria (1966, Pp. 178–211) for a review of concepts of apraxia and the distinction between apraxias, dysarthrias, and aphasias.

Dysarthria

As defined by Schuell (1964), the term dysarthria refers to impairment of speech movements based on cerebral pathology "which occurs with or without aphasia, and is not correlated with reduction of language." Although our concept of dysarthria does not limit its etiology to cerebral pathology but includes lower motor neuron involvements, dysarthrias in aphasics are almost always related to cerebral damage. Functionally, we may accept Bay's concept that dysarthria is a nonlinguistic disorder which may or may not accompany aphasia. It is a primary motor disturbance of the articulary muscles which directly impair speech production (Bay, 1967). The dysarthric patient may slur individual sounds, or omit sounds, and may have difficulty in the production of contextual utterance. Unlike the apraxic patient, however, he does not suffer from an impairment of the plan or scheme of movements required for the production of an utterance.

Agnosias

Henry Head (1926) wrote, "before it is possible to determine the behavior of a supposed aphasic to tests which depend on reading or comprehension of spoken words, we must be certain that he is capable of appreciating the significance of sights and sounds." The term *agnosia* is attributed to Freud (1891). He applied the term to states in which the individual is able to receive sensory impressions but is unable to recognize (appreciate) their significance. Such impairments of perception have serious implications for language if they involve auditory or visual modalities or, in the case of blind persons, for the tactile modality. In assessing for agnosias we must make certain that due allowance is made for the possibility of sensory defect or limitation. Thus, hearing loss per se, or visual loss or defect, including that for visual field limitation, must be accounted for and considered before an assessment of agnosia is made. It is also essential that the patient being assessed is not in a state of confusion so severe that he does not know what behavior is expected of him. Most tests for *agnosias* call for some form of *matching to sample* through a single sensory modality at a time.

The artificiality of such an examining situation may serve to confuse patients with cerebral damage. They may, in fact, not believe that the examiner really expects the patient to perform a relatively simple task, and so fail to perform at all.

ACOUSTIC AGNOSIA

Acoustic agnosia, a disturbance of discriminative hearing, is regarded by Luria (1966, p. 107) as a fundamental source of speech disturbance. According to Luria, this disturbance arises because of impairment in the analytic-synthetic activity of the auditory cortex and is manifest in defective analysis of the speech-sound (phonemic) system of the language. The patient's errors for speech-sound discrimination increase as differences between sounds decrease. Thus more errors are likely to occur when discrimination needs to be made between sounds such as *t* and *p*, or *t* and *d*, than between *s* and *m*, or *k* and *r*. Luria considers acoustic agnosia to be the basis for auditory or temporal acoustic aphasia.

AUDITORY AGNOSIA

The term *auditory agnosia* is broader in its implications than is acoustic agnosia. Auditory agnosia refers to disturbances in the recognition of sounds or combinations of sounds without regard to the individual's ability to evaluate them. The disturbance may be for nonsymbolic (nonlanguage) sounds such as mechanical or animal noises; for human, nonlinguistic sounds (coughing, sneezing, hand clapping); or for sounds which are associated with spoken symbols (phonetic units, words, or groups of words). A patient who hears sounds which he cannot recognize will not be able to evaluate the auditory sensations. An individual with *auditory verbal agnosia* is not able to understand what he hears.

We may test for auditory agnosias by having a patient imitate sounds, or in some other way, as by pointing, indicate the source or origin of a sound. Verbal agnosias may be tested by repetitions of words or, on a higher level, by eliciting an appropriate motor response to a word or a group of words. A person who can point to the parts of his body when they are named reveals that he both recognizes and understands the words he hears.

A special form of auditory agnosia is *amusia*. Auditory musical agnosia (amusia) refers to a disturbance in a previously existing ability to recognize music. It is not to be confused with so-called tone-deafness, or with a lack of singing ability which is fairly common among nonaphasic persons. If amusia is actually found to exist in a patient, the disturbance may impair the person's ability to respond appropriately to inflectional and intonational changes in speech (dysprosody). On the whole, however, amusia is not one of the more important disturbances related to aphasia.

VISUAL AGNOSIA

This is disturbance of recognition of situations through the visual sense. The individual may sense that he is seeing something but may not be able to recognize what he sees. Visual agnosias may be specific for objects, representations, geometric forms, colors, letters, words, or other special configurations. It is unlikely, however, that an individual will have an agnosia for pictures and not for objects; for letters, and not for words; or for single words and not for words in context.

The importance of determining whether an individual has visual agnosia before deciding whether he has alexia is evident. If letters, or groups of letters, cannot be recognized they cannot be evaluated as symbols. It is essential, therefore, that a patient's ability to recognize visual configurations must be determined before a decision is made as to possible alexia.

TACTILE AGNOSIA

This disturbance is in the ability of an individual to recognize objects through the sense of touch. For the blind person, who has been trained in braille reading, tactile agnosia will impair reading ability. For other than the blind, there is little implication in this disturbance for language dysfunction.

Paraphasia

Freud (1891) defined paraphasia as a disorder of speech "in which the appropriate word is replaced by a less appropriate one, which, however, still retains a certain relationship to the correct word." Freud was mindful that the verbal behavior of the aphasic is not without its underlying psychodynamics and so compared the verbal errors of the aphasics with those made by many normal persons under conditions of stress, fatigue, and distraction (divided attention). Critchley (1967) defined *paraphasia* as "the evocation of an inappropriate sound in place of a desired sound or phrase." We consider paraphasia to be any error of commission modifying the individual word (sound and morpheme substitution) or of word substitution in the spoken or written production of a speaker or writer. Paraphasic errors are not limited to persons who are aphasic. For the aphasic, however, organic rather than psychodynamic factors are presumed to be primarily responsible for the linguistic distortions. The following are some samples of paraphasic errors in the spoken and written efforts of a 53-year-old male patient.

Paraphasic errors in oral sentence repetition:
(The car sped swiftly down the road)
The car would spit sweetly down the load
(Persistence is essential to success)
Mesastense is instans to sesatins
(Note perseverative nature of errors)

Oral Reading Errors:
(The crown and glory of a useful life is character)
The *crowd* and glory of a *ufless* life is *krakatic*

Errors in writing dictation:

(tell)	tale
(saw)	salt
(campaign)	parade
(occur)	concur
(was)	why

Neologism

When a speaker uses a neologism he has literally "invented" a new word. This form of verbal creativity is sometimes done for special effect by poets and frequently by writers of advertising copy. *Neologisms* may be regarded as a form of paraphasia in which an expected (conventional) word is replaced by a new one, the meaning of which is not apparent in the utterance. Some aphasics have "pet" neologisms, words, or phrases used frequently and without apparent differentiation as to possible referent. Other neologisms, however, may comprise combinations of words or of morphemes which do indicate intent and meaning. Thus the word "spork" may be evoked for *spoon* and *fork*. This type of neologism is likely to occur as a specific attempt at naming and not become part of an aphasic's habitual verbal behavior.

Jargon

Some aphasics produce a relatively free flow of unintelligible utterance. Critchley (1967) defined jargon-aphasia as "a type of speech impairment whereby the patient emits a profusion of utterance most of which is incomprehensible to the hearer, though perhaps not to the speaker." The key words in this definition are *profusion* and *incomprehensible*. It is our impression, however, that the apparent jargon is not devoid of underlying meaning. By analyzing a sample of jargon speech of an aphasic we were able to find some surprisingly "lawful" and regular sound and morpheme substitutions and so "break the code" of the jargon utterance.

Echolalia

The term *echolalia* refers to the tendency of an aphasic to repeat without modification (verbal transformation) an utterance addressed to him by another speaker. The echolalic product may constitute a complete sentence, or the final phrase or word of a sentence. Sometimes the echolalic product is repeated several times without evidence of comprehension. We consider echolalia to be a form of *verbal perseveration.*

Perseveration

The term perseveration refers broadly to any morbid tendency to maintain a mental set or to repeat an act not appropriate to the situation to which a response is required. When a perseverative response is overt an act is repeated which was originally organized by the respondent as a plan to meet a previous situation. The repeated act reflects an inability on the part of the responding individual to reorganize his behavior to meet the new situation or an inability to perceive that a new situation is present. Verbal perseveration is expressed in the production of utterances which may have been evoked as an appropriate response to a context other than the one to which the utterances continue to be made. Perseveration responses may also occur as original and maintained errors rather than as carry-overs from preceding situations. Such errors are most likely to be made when the aphasic is confronted with difficult new contexts, in states of fatigue, when situations change rapidly, and perhaps most generally in states of anxiety when the patient feels the need to say something despite his inability at the moment to say what is required. Under comparable conditions, a parallel phenomenon may be observed in the written products of the aphasic.

COMMON TERMINOLOGY FOR APHASIC DISORDERS

As we shall note in our discussion of classification of aphasic disorders, aphasiologists vary considerably in the terminology for language disorders.[7] In the following discussion we shall present and define terms for which there is fairly common acceptance by contemporary aphasiologists. Unless otherwise defined or explained, the definitions given will be the working ones for our later discussions. Despite an attempt of aphasiologists during the 1930's and 1940's to use the prefix *a-* for severe forms of aphasic disorders and *dys-* for moderate forms, the present practice is to use the single prefix *a-* for all degrees of disorder with modifying adjectives, *mild*, *moderate*, or *severe* to express degree. The term *dysprosody* seems to be an exception to the practice.

Auditory Aphasia

This refers specifically to disturbances in the comprehension of audible speech which normally is received and evaluated through hearing. Perhaps more often than we might suspect, auditory aphasic disturbances become apparent only as the quantity or complexity of speech is increased. Occasionally, it will become readily apparent only when the patient is fatigued. Sometimes a patient's difficulty in auditory comprehension is manifest only when there is a fairly rapid change in the nature or content of what he hears.

Anomia or Nominal Aphasia

This is probably the outstanding and most frequent subtype of productive disturbance. Anomia refers to the patient's difficulty in evoking an appropriate term *regardless of its part of speech.* The defect is most likely to be evident in the effort to evoke nouns (nominal words) only because nouns constitute the bulk of most vocabularies. As the patient recovers, anomia is most likely to be a residual disturbance. Most patients, unless they also have considerable evaluative difficulty, are able to recognize and repeat words readily which they cannot evoke easily. A patient with anomic difficulty, consciously or unconsciously, may learn to substitute a synonym or a phrase with approximate meaning for an elusive word, or he may engage in circumlocution, or use a gesture as a verbal substitute. This technique is not the special property of the aphasic patient. Normal speakers use it when, under some temporary pressure, they cannot readily find the most appropriate word to express an idea although, subjectively, the word seems to be at "the tip of the tongue." Typical anomic errors are the substitution of "in class" or "related" items for the term required for the situation. Thus a patient may refer to a knife as a fork, or use the term plate for cup. One patient's anomic errors shown below indicate that he probably understood the questions asked, but had difficulty in "zeroing in" for his answers.

(On what do you sleep ?)—Alarm clock, wake up.
(What's ink for ?)—To do with a pen.

Anomia may be tested by directing a patient to name objects or pictures, by having him supply words to complete sentences, by requiring the patient to supply a synonym for a word or a phrase, or by asking the patient to summarize in his own words content he has heard or read.

Alexia

This is a disturbance in the comprehension of written symbols. Alexic difficulties are difficulties in *silent reading*. These difficulties, as is the case with auditory aphasia, sometimes become obvious only when the patient is required to read comparatively difficult material or long, unbroken pages. Occasionally, the difficulty is apparent chiefly in the evaluation of "small words"—articles, prepositions, conjunctions, and others which are used semantically as connectives or to indicate relationships of words (ideas) within a sentence. Sometimes it will be found that the rate of reading is impaired. A once proficient reader may read accurately but laboriously, and with a feeling of insecurity about his ability. Alexic disturbances may be tested by presenting a patient with written material varying in length and complexity which he is directed to read silently. When he is finished reading, the patient is then required to answer questions or to carry out directions based on the reading.

Agraphia

Writing disturbances may be manifest in all writing, or in the writing of nominal words, as in anomia, or in faulty grammar, or by the omission of articles, prepositions, conjunctions, and other words which

[7] We accept Critchley's (1967) definition that "an aphasiologist is one who studies the pathology of language." From our point of view, aphasiologists may include speech pathologists, neurologists, psychologists, linguists, or a member of any other discipline concerned with the disorders of language *as they are manifest in the impaired verbal behavior of aphasic persons.*

serve as connectives or to indicate relationships of parts of a sentence. These errors may appear in writing to dictation, in spontaneous writing, and even in direct copying.

The following are examples of the writing errors of a 61-year-old patient who had suffered a spontaneous cerebral insult. We may note errors of spelling and substitutions and omissions of functional words.

Copying: (This month is August)
The month in Augrest.
(Mexico is south of the United States)
Macos is south Uinetest States.

In answer to the question, "What do you eat for breakfast?" the patient wrote:

I eggs and eat and drink coffee breakfast (agrammatism).

Agrammatism is defined by Critchely (1967) as "an aphasic disorder which impairs syntax rather than vocabulary." Critchley also observes that "agrammatism is naturally a more important feature in aphasics whose natural language comprises one of the highly inflected tongues, and in such the defect may entail considerable errors in the employment of prefixes and suffixes." We also find errors in functional words—articles, prepositions, and conjunctions—which serve to establish contextual relationships (grammatical context) of spoken and written content. In severe form, agrammatism may be expressed in *telegrammatism.*

Telegrammatism is defined by Critchley (1967) as "the type of speech which results after the sacrifice of the shorter terms which are less heavily charged with reference-function or 'meaning'." In written form, the product at best resembles an economically motivated form of expression voluntarily employed in writing a telegram.

Acalculia (Arithmetic Disturbances)

These disturbances may be present on a twofold basis: 1. because of actual difficulty on the part of the patient in dealing with arithmetic processes, or 2. because of related difficulty in the oral or written production of symbols involved in calculation. If the latter is the case, the difficulty is really one of word finding (anomia) rather than of acalculia.

Frequently we will find that an aphasic patient may do well in simple arithmetic computation, especially if he is permitted to write his responses. This apparently well-retained ability can probably be explained by the automaticity with which most of us do simple arithmetic. The arithmetic tables have become automatic for most adults, so that many of our computations are carried on without the need for quantitative conceptualization or reasoning. Despite this general finding, we occasionally come across an aphasic who cannot perform simple arithmetic operations accurately but who can do fairly well in numerical problem-solving situations.

Dysprosody

This term refers to changes of accent, cadence, rhythm, and intonation of speech (Monrad-Krohn, 1947). In English, dysprosody is likely to impair the expression of affect much more than the semantic or ideational content of the utterance. So, the expression of deep feeling may be impaired. On the ideational side, subtle changes or implications which are conveyed through inflection and intonation may be beyond the capacity of the aphasic with dysprosody. The patient with dysprosody may have difficulty, except for word order, in indicating and distinguishing between declarative and interrogative utterances. In languages such as Chinese, where inflection determines the basic meaning of the individual word, a speaker with dysprosody may be much more severely impaired than would one whose native language is English. We are inclined to accept the position of Bay (1964, p. 129) that dysprosody may be a component of *dysarthria* in so far as the prosodic components of speech are part of the motor aspects of articulatory production. In Chinese dialects, as well as in other East Asian languages, errors of "melody" might well be considered as anomias, in that they implicate the essential conceptual-semantic component of word selection.

Most patients with dysprosody—and many manifest this as a residual of aphasia—speak without the color normally provided by vocal inflection and intonation. Thus, they may sound as if they were speaking a second language for which they have a mastery of vocabulary and grammar, but not of intonation.

CLASSIFICATION OF LINGUISTIC DISTURBANCES

For reasons derived from clinical practice and surface logic, students of aphasia have tended to classify language disturbances according to whether the patient's intake (reception, evaluation, or *decoding*) is impaired or whether the manifest disturbance is in output (expression, production, or *encoding*). A problem recognized by aphasiologists is the need to assess intake by nonverbal production so that the patient's understanding of language can be demonstrated without the influence or contamination of possible productive errors.

Henry Head (1926; 1963, pp. 428–429) classified aphasic language disturbances (impairments of symbolic formulation and expression) into four broad categories. Because of their historic significance, we shall review them briefly at this time:

1. "*Verbal aphasia* consists of a difficulty in forming words for external or internal speech." The patient's ability to comprehend spoken or written content is usually considerably greater than is his ability for utterance or writing. "The disorder affects mainly verbal structure and words as integral parts of a phrase; their nominal value and significance remain relatively intact."

2. "*Syntactical aphasia* is essentially a disorder of balance and rhythm; syntax suffers greatly. . . . the patient has plenty of words, but their arrangement into coordinated phrases is defective. . . . Comprehension of the meaning of words, however, is always in excess of power to employ them in discourse."

3. "*Nominal aphasia* comprises loss of power to use names and want of comprehension of the significant value of words and other symbols . . . patients read with extreme difficulty, writing is grossly affected and they suffer from defective appreciation of single numbers or letters."

4. "*Semantic aphasia* consists in a want of recognition of the full significance of words and phrases apart from their direct verbal meaning . . . the patient may understand a word or a short phrase, but its ultimate significance escapes him and he fails to comprehend the final intention of some command imposed on him orally or in print."

Head's categories represented an attempt to avoid classification according to an intake-output dichotomy. In addition, they reveal Head's bias against the notion of discrete or single (pure) aphasic disorders. The categories were, however, too broad to differentiate clinically among aphasic patients. Too many subdifficulties are included under each category, and there is considerable overlap between categories. Despite these limitations, Head's classification system did influence the thinking of students of aphasia. The influence appears to be reflected clearly in the classification system of Weisenburg and McBride (1935).

Weisenburg and McBride, like Henry Head, developed a classification system that avoided a clear commitment to the intake-output dichotomy for aphasic disorders as well as the notion of pure or isolated language defects. They used the following classifications for aphasic linguistic disturbances:

Predominantly Receptive—The greatest amount of disturbance is in the individual's ability to comprehend spoken or written symbols.

Predominantly Expressive—The greatest amount of disturbance is in the individual's ability to express ideas in speech or in writing.

Amnesic—The patient's chief difficulty is in the evocation of appropriate words as names for objects, conditions, relationships, qualities, and so on. Amnesic disturbances are in effect a subtype of expressive disturbance.

Expressive-Receptive—Both receptive and expressive language functions are extremely disturbed. In early stages of aphasic involvements, this is likely to be true of a great many patients. Only a comparatively few patients continue to manifest equally severe disturbances of both reception and expression. Usually, receptive functions improve spontaneously to a greater degree than do expressive functions.

Essentially the same criticism we noted for the Head classifications may be directed to the Weisenburg and McBride categories. They are too broad, cover too many impairments under a single grouping, and do not serve to differentiate aphasic patients according to syndromes of impairment. The classifications probably represent a reaction against overclassification according to isolated linguistic symptoms and to discrete localization of cerebral pathology based on specific impairments. Despite the limitations of the Weisenburg and McBride classifications, they have served as a model for the development of aphasic inventories, such as *Examining for Aphasia* (Eisenson, 1954), which indicate awareness of the broad categories but have provided subcategories for differentiating aphasic disorders.

A. R. Luria (1964, 1966), a Russian neuropsychologist and aphasiologist, provides us with a classification system that has its basis in Pavlovian neurophysiology. Luria's system classifies aphasic impairments according to their underlying or primary disturbed function and the related defect in speech and language. The basic classifications follow:

1. *Sensory aphasia:* a disturbance in the analysis and synthesis of speech sounds (primary defect) resulting in defects in the comprehension of speech, defects in word production, and in writing which parallel those of speech.

2. *Acoustic-Amnestic aphasia:* a disturbance, often transitory, in the retention of audio-speech traces resulting in impairment that increases as the content —the amount of information the patient is required to process—is increased. Thus, a patient may be able to repeat or write a single word or a digit on direction, but have difficulty with a nonfixed series of verbal items. Patients often "find significant difficulty in developed speech and speech thought, which is greatly disturbed because of the instability of verbal traces" (Luria, 1964, p. 151).

3. *Afferent (kinesthetic) motor aphasia:* the basic disturbance is in the kinesthetic analysis of speech movements, "If the necessary afferent synthesis is impaired, the differential directional impulses, necessary for speech muscles, become impossible." The result of such underlying impairment is a disturbance in the production of the fundamental units of speech, the *articulemes.* In its most severe form, the patient may show a complete apraxia for articulation. In less severe form, the patient may repeat isolated sounds, or confuse sounds which are made by action of the lips (b, p, m) or by action of the tongue tip (l, d, n). Basically, the patient shows deficiency in using afferent stimulation as a control for articulatory production.

4. *Efferent (kinetic) motor aphasia:* the basic impairment is in the kinetic analysis for a *sequence or succession of speech movements.* The patient does not have difficulty with the production of the individual sound (articuleme) but with the sequential order of articulation required in oral linguistic production. Parallel defects are found in writing, so that patients may transpose letters, or repeat letters in their written effort, though they may have no difficulty in the correct writing of a single letter.

5. *Semantic aphasia:* the primary disturbance is in the simultaneous organization of the components of speech, the special significance a unit of language has by virtue of its context or verbal connections. This impairment is manifest in the patient's difficulty for the appreciation of the meaning of a verbal formulation, of the "logico-grammatical structure of speech" (Luria, 1964, p. 156).

6. *Dynamic aphasia:* "Fundamental to this dynamic aphasia is probably a disturbance of *inner speech* which . . . has a shortened structure, a predicative function, and serves as a fundamental means for the transformation of a fore-shortened idea into developed outer speech and for the change of developed speech into a fore-shortened scheme of thought" (Luria, 1964, pp. 159–160). Although Luria does not seem to be as certain as to the nature of the primary impairment for dynamic aphasia as he is for his other types, the patient's basic difficulty seems to be in a failure to transform self-talk into talk for others (to encode his thinking into verbal propositions) or transform (decode) another's propositions into self-thinking or "inner speech." The apparent defect is active propositionizing.

It is obvious that Luria's system of classification rejects any notion of dichotomy between intake and output defects, or of any discrete or pure aphasic disturbances. An underlying disorder (*primary defect*) as for phonemic analysis (sensory aphasia) may produce a variety of aphasic symptoms which include comprehension of speech, of naming, reading, and writing. How the individual learned language functions will in part determine his impairments. Thus a person who learned to read by "sounding out" will have more difficulty in reading in the event of sensory aphasia than will one who learned to read by the "whole word" or "word-picture" method and bypassed any sounding out of the visual (letter) representations.

Jakobson approaches the classification of aphasic language disorders from the position of a linguist on the premise that "the most striking symptoms of aphasia cannot be found without the guiding and vigilant assistance of linguistics" (1964, p. 21). Aphasic involvements, Jakobson believes, can be classified with two broad basic categories: *similarity disorders* and *contiguity disorders.* Similarity (selection) disorders are basic to errors in decoding; contiguity or combination disorders are basic to errors in encoding.

Jakobson reconciles his two broad categories with Luria's six types of aphasia. "Three types of aphasia —the so-called efferent, dynamic and afferent types are characterized by *contiguity* disorders with a deterioration of the context; whereas the three other types— . . . the sensory, semantic and amnestic— display *similarity* disorders with damage to the code. The same two groups, viewed in terms of verbal behavior, are opposed to each other as *encoding* and *decoding* disturbances (Jakobson, 1964, pp. 35–36).

Jakobson's emphasis on a dichotomy between decoding and encoding impairments seems to be moving in a direction away from Luria. We agree with Jakobson that the term *predominantly* should be the assumed prefix before each of the categories "since impairments in one of the two coding processes generally affect the opposite process also" (Jakobson, 1964, p. 26).

Wepman and Jones, in discussing their Language Modalities Test for Aphasia (1961 and 1966), present a fivefold classification for aphasic language disturbances. Three of the classifications, the pragmatic, semantic, and syntactic follow the model of the linguist, Charles Morris (1938), in his view of the language process. The Wepman and Jones classifications follow:

1. *Pragmatic aphasia*—defined as a disorder of symbol formulation in which the patient's impairment is in conceptualizing from a given stimulus. "In pragmatic aphasia there appears to be a disruption of the ability to obtain meaning from a stimulus and to use it as a basis for orderly symbol formulation" (Wepman and Jones, 1966, pp. 146–147). Patients so classified present the following defects in their speech: a) their utterances convey little meaning to a listener, b) their verbal output features high-frequency words and repetitive neologisms in place of substantive words (nouns, verbs, adjectives), c) they use inappropriate substantive words, and d) they show a lack of awareness of their errors.

On the positive side, pragmatic aphasics tend to mainatin appropriate pitch and intonation and, despite their restricted vocabularies, present a normal distribution of the various parts of speech.

2. *Semantic aphasia*—a disorder of symbol formulation in which the patient has difficulty in recalling and evoking an appropriate and meaningful verbal sign to a previously acquired concept. Patients with semantic aphasia present the following defects: a) except for very high-frequency generalized terms, the semantic aphasic has great difficulty in evoking once well-known proper names and substantive words, and b) circumlocutions and gestures may be substituted for words which cannot be recalled.[8]

Positive attributes of the semantic aphasic include the maintenance of appropriate grammatical forms and intonation and the high-frequency substantive words, as well as the function words (articles, prepositions, demonstratives, and pronouns).

3. *Syntactic aphasia*—defined as a disorder of symbol formulation characterized by impairment in the individual's previously established grammatical structure. Syntactic aphasic patients present the following defects: a) omission or misuse of function words and grammatical markers (inflectional endings) to indicate tense and numbers, b) except for automatic "set" phrases and sentences, e.g., "go away," there is a marked inability for producing conventional sentences; utterances become "telegraphic," consisting essentially of single substantive words, and c) pitch and intonation are absent though appropriate inflection may be used for single-word utterances.

4. *Jargon aphasia*—characterized by unintelligible sound combinations but by recognizable intonation. Significantly, though the utterances convey no meaning to a listener, the sounds and sound combinations used are consistent with the phonemic patterns of the patient's linguistic system.

We regard jargon aphasia as a transitory stage and not as a true aphasic classification.

5. *Global aphasia*—characterized by severe impairment in the production, and presumably in the comprehension of language. A patient's output may be limited to a single automatized word, phrase, or a neologism. The patient, if he attempts communication at all, is likely to do so by employing primitive gestures.

We regard global aphasia as a severe early state of disorder. If it is maintained, it is probably accompanied or is at least indistinguishable from intellectual deterioration. Wepman and Jones (1966, p. 146) regard the *pragmatic*, *semantic*, and *syntactic* aphasias as impairments of three specific linguistic processes which suggest that aphasia might be viewed "as a regressive psycholinguistic process phenomenon."

Schuell's (1964) classification systems differs from the others that we have discussed in that she is primarily concerned with the diagnostic and prognostic implications of the patients more than she is with categorizing the specific disturbances they present. Schuell rejects systems based on receptive-expressive dichotomies because she believes "no such dichotomy exists." She considers that the classical categories, such as amnesic and syntactic aphasia, offer no meaningful basis for classification because they are not mutually exclusive.

On the basis of her concept of aphasia as "a general language deficit that crosses all language modalities and may or may not be complicated by other sequelae of brain damage. . . . the language deficit itself is characterized by reduction of available vocabulary, impaired verbal retention span, and impaired perception and production of messages, perhaps secondary to impairment of the first two dimensions" (Schuell et al., 1964, p. 113). Schuell emphasizes that the aphasic's language impairment *is not modality specific*.

Schuell believes that almost all aphasic patients will fall into one of five major categories or groups (1964, pp. 190–191):

[8] We recognize, of course, that the Wepman-Jones classification of semantic aphasia fits into the traditional concept of *anomia*.

Group 1: Simple aphasia—the patient's functional language is characterized by decrements in all language modalities; the patient presents no specific perceptual, sensorimotor, or dysarthric components.

Group 2: The patient's aphasia is complicated by "central involvement of visual processes."

Group 3: The patient manifests "severe reduction of language in all modalities complicated by sensorimotor involvement."

Group 4: The patient has "aphasia with some residual language preserved, and scattered findings that usually include both visual involvement and dysarthria."

Group 5: The patient has "an irreversible aphasic syndrome characterized by almost complete loss of language skills."

The Schuell categories differ essentially in degree of severity of language disturbance and related central sensory or motor impairments.

SUMMARY OF CLASSIFICATIONS OF APHASIA

We could, of course, present other classification systems but prefer not to do so at this time. Other approaches to classification will be considered in our discussion of examination procedures and in our chapter on Correlates of Aphasia. Classifications depend upon how the individual aphasiologist, clinical or theoretic, views aphasic disturbances. Despite the apparent diversity of views, we think it is significant that over the past century, from Wernicke (1874) to the present, and despite differences in terminology, several basically common characteristics have been observed. These were summarized succinctly by the neurologist Geschwind in his discussion of the Wepman-Jones position (1966).

EXAMINATION PROCEDURES

The approach to testing of aphasic patients, and specific procedures consistent with the approach, depend upon the examiner's philosophy of the overall nature and implications of aphasic disturbances. If the individual's philosophy is one which looks upon the aphasic as a person who, because of brain damage, has undergone permanent intellectual changes and has evolved a "new" personality, then the testing should seek to evaluate the changes so that a therapeutic program consistent with the changes can be undertaken. For example, for the clinician who accepts the point of view of Kurt Goldstein (1948, Ch. IV) that the various dysfunctions of aphasia are the manifestations of a single basic disorder—the loss of ability to grasp the essential nature of a process—the approach should be one for determining the extent of the basic disorder. Assessment then would employ psychological techniques such as are used by Strauss and Lehtinen (1947) or by Goldstein and Scheerer (1941) in their test for abstract and concrete behavior, or by Weigl (1966). An aphasiologist such as Schuell (1964), who views aphasia as a unitary language disorder that "crosses all language modalities," approaches assessment differently from one such as Wepman (1961), who considers aphasic disturbances to be modality bound and, as we have already indicated, differentially classifiable. We shall review several of the published tests available and in current use in English-speaking countries as well as test inventories presently being developed. The problems inherent in test construction, as Benton (1967) observes, vary not only with how the author of the inventory views aphasia, but also of how he

TABLE 48-I
Nomenclature of the Aphasias[9]

CLASSICAL	WEPMAN	JAKOBSON	HEAD
Broca's, Motor, Expressive, Anterior	Syntactic	Contiguity	Verbal
Posterior Wernicke's sensory	Pragmatic	Similarity	Syntactic
Anomic Amnesic Amnestic	Semantic	Similarity	Nominal

[9] Dr. Norman Geschwind's tabulation, indicating essential similarities.

may view language or intelligence. We recommend the Benton essay on "Problems of Test Construction in the Field of Aphasia" (*Cortex*, III, 1, 1967) as required reading for students of aphasia.

EXAMINING FOR APHASIA (Eisenson, 1954) was devised as a clinical instrument to provide the examiner with a guided judgment for assessing the variety of language disturbances and disturbances related to language functions (agnosias and apraxias) which are considered to be common features of aphasic patients. It is avowedly a clinical instrument to provide a protocol of type and degree of severity of language and related deficits. Developmentally, the instrument and the general approach follows the lines of Weisenburg and McBride (1935). The various test items, some of which are taken directly or adapted from standardized educational achievement tests, are intended to reveal both the assets and liabilities of the patient at the time of testing. Much of the material is graded, so that level of ability within a given area of language function can be estimated. Although most of the items are scored on a pass-fail basis in terms of the actual examination stimulus material, the clinician is advised to consider any correct or near-correct responses offered by the patient. There are, in addition, open-ended test items intended to elicit responses which require individual evaluation. Test items are arranged to permit assessment for primarily receptive (evaluative) functions and for manifestly productive (expressive) functions. Receptive-evaluative items include visual, auditory, and tactile agnosias, auditory (verbal) aphasia, and silent reading (alexia). The manifestly productive (expressive) disturbances include nonverbal and verbal apraxias, subpropositional (automatic) speech, spelling, writing, naming (identification), word finding, and arithmetic processes. Two paragraphs for oral reading provide a basis for assessing paraphasic defects for nonspeaker-formulated content and an opportunity for comparing such content with the patient's spontaneous language.

Examining for Aphasia includes a manual of directions and a record entry form. The manual describes administrative procedures and scoring. It includes illustrative material used in the examination. A check sheet permits the clinician to make a profile of the patient's tested abilities.

The author has found the inventory useful as an initial examination for estimating the areas and approximate levels of linguistic abilities as well as a retest instrument for measuring patient improvement. The entire inventory takes from about 30 to 90 minutes to administer, depending upon the severity of involvement and the rate at which the patient is able to work. The examination need not be given at a single session if the patient demonstrates fatigue or frustration. If it is desired to use the inventory for rapid screening, then single items of each subtest may be administered.

THE LANGUAGE MODALITIES TEST FOR APHASIA (Wepman and Jones, 1961)

The authors view their test as an instrument to provide for a psycholinguistic analysis for an aphasic's language production. To highlight the difference between the Language Modalities Test and other inventories in current use, Wepman and Jones (1966, p. 142) observe: 1. that useful distinctions need to be made between responses to visual and auditory material, 2. that considerable information is obscured by testing according to a pass or fail dichotomy, and 3. often real differences become apparent in many patients in their comparative ability to respond to specific stimuli and their ability to communicate in relatively unstructured situations. As a result of these observations, Wepman and Jones developed a "differential psycholinguistic" method for the scoring of an examinee's responses to specific items related to input modality and an evaluation of the patient's free speech. Essentially, the Modalities Test assesses a patient's comprehension and functional use of language according to standardized procedures.

The overall content of the examination covers essentially the same areas as do older as well as other contemporary inventories. Test items which differ from those of the Eisenson inventory include the copying of geometric figures and the opportunity to produce "free speech" by a stimulus picture about which the patient is to make up a "story."

The basic psycholinguistic classifications arrived at by Wepman and Jones in their protocol analysis were discussed earlier. Their scoring system is summarized in Table 48-II.

MINNESOTA TEST FOR DIFFERENTIAL DIAGNOSIS OF APHASIS (H. Schuell, 1965)

Schuell says that her test inventory was "designed to permit the examiner to observe the level at which language performance breaks down in each of the principal language modalities, since this is what there is to observe in aphasia. . . . the Minnesota Test looks

TABLE 48-II
Language Modalities Test for Aphasia Scoring Summary (Wepman and Jones)[10]

	VISUAL STIMULI												AUDITORY STIMULI											
	ORAL RESPONSES						GRAPHIC RESPONSES						ORAL RESPONSES						GRAPHIC RESPONSES					
Scale value (s.v.)*	1	2	3	4	5	6	1	2	3	4	5	6	1	2	3	4	5	6	1	2	3	4	5	6
Stimulus type																								
Pictures				3	1	2				2	3	1												
Words	3			3									3				1	2	2	1		3		
Numbers	4			2									1			4		1						
Sentences	1		2	3										2		1	3							

* Scoring categories (s.v.) for all oral and graphic responses:
1: correct response
2: phonemic or orthographic response
3: syntatic errors
4. semantic errors
5: jargon or illegible
6: no response

[10] From *Brain Function,* Vol. III: Speech, Language, and Communication (E. C. Carterette, Ed.), University of California Press, 1966, p. 143.

at the language behavior of aphasic patients, and then proceeds to ask questions about the nature of the disruptions that occur" (Schuell, 1965, p. 3). Although Schuell's inventory assesses aphasia in the principal modalities, she nevertheless emphasizes that *aphasic disturbances cross all language modalities.* However, "the over-all pattern of involvement varies from patient to patient, and this variation makes differential diagnosis possible."

Schuell's major classifications of aphasia, based on an analysis of data derived from her inventory, were discussed earlier (pp. 1232–1233) in this chapter. Schuell views differential diagnosis as the basis for both description of the status of the patient and for prognosis relative to recovery from aphasia. "Careful description of aphasic impairment provides a guide for treatment, since therapy must deal with the disabilities that are present" (1965, p. 5).

The Minnesota Test is a long inventory that in depth and scope enables an examiner to assess the parameters of language and related sensory and motor involvements of aphasic persons. The major areas for assessment include: 1. auditory disturbances (items ranging from word recognition, discrimination to sentence and paragraph comprehension), 2. visual and reading disturbances (items include matching of forms to reading comprehension of paragraphs as well as oral reading of sentences), 3. speech and language disturbances (items include testing for articulatory movement to naming, word defining, picture description, and paragraph retelling), 4. visuomotor and writing disturbances (items include copying of forms and letters to writing to dictation and written sentence formulation), and 5. disturbances of numerical relationships and arithmetic processes (items include making change, clock setting, simple numerical combinations, and written problems).

The Minnesota Test takes considerably longer to administer than the other inventories we have discussed. A short version of the inventory, intended primarily as a screening test, is available (1957).

PORCH INDEX OF COMMUNICATIVE ABILITY (PICA)

Porch (1967) suggested that the two major requirements of an aphasia test are high reliability and a scoring system which specifies the nature of the patient's response in terms of multiple dimensions. He developed a test battery, the Porch Index of Communicative Ability (PICA), in an attempt to satisfy the clinical needs.

A multidimensional scoring system was designed for use with the PICA which describes a response in terms of several dimensions rather than limiting the description to the plus-minus dichotomy which ignores so much important information. This system includes the following dimensions:

Accuracy—the degree of correctness or rightness of a response.

Responsiveness—the ease with which the response is elicited, especially in terms of how much information the patient requires in order to complete the task.

Completeness—the degree to which the patient carries out the task in its entirety.

Promptness—the presence or absence of significant delay in making a response.

Efficiency—the degree of facility the patient demonstrates in performing the motoric aspects of the response.

The procedure for using the multidimensional scale is similar to that for using any rating scale. When the patient responds to a given test item, the scorer decides which of the 16 categories best describes the response and then records the score for that category.

The test battery is made up of 18 subtests, sampling gestural, verbal, and graphic abilities at various levels of difficulties. Each task revolves around 10 common objects placed before the patient, a method similar to the one suggested by Head (1926) in his serial tests. This method enables the tester to make some comparisons of results across modalities.

The PICA results are interpreted through the use of an Overall Score which is the mean response level for all test items, a mean response level for each modality, and a mean for each subtest. Additional test interpretation is provided by the use of profiles of subtest means plotted on graphs. These profiles, when compared with percentile contours based on aphasic patient norms, are useful in planning treatment and predicting degrees and rates of potential change in the patient's performance.

INTERNATIONAL TEST FOR APHASIA

Benton, Spreen, De Renzi, and Vignolo, a team of psychologists and neurologists, are presently constructing a test battery for aphasia that hopefully will be adaptable to languages throughout the world. At this writing, English and Italian versions are being developed at centers in the United States and Italy (Benton, 1967). The preliminary battery is based on the theoretic assumption that "the traditional associationist approach still possessed sufficient validity to warrant formulation of certain test procedures along these lines." The test battery includes the following (Benton, 1967, pp. 42–44):

1. *Visual naming* of common objects (10–40).

2. *Description of use*—the patient is directed to tell the use of 10–20 objects from the basic set of 40.

3–4. *Tactile naming*—on the basis of feeling alone, first with the right and then with the left hand, the patient is directed to name 10–20 objects of the basic set of 40.

5. *Sentence repetition*—the patient is instructed to repeat tape-recorded sentences.

6. *Digit repetitions*—the patient is instructed to repeat tape-recorded series of digits ranging in length from 3 to 9.

7. *Digit reversal*—the patient is instructed to repeat tape-recorded digit series ranging in length from 2–7.

8. *Word fluency*—the patient is instructed to say all the words he can recall beginning with a specific letter; three one-minute trials for three different letters (F, A, S).

9. *Sentence construction*—the patient is instructed to make up sentences from five (5) sets of 2 or 3 words.

10. *Object identification by name*—the patient is directed to point to objects named by the examiner. The objects are from the basic forty used in the inventory.

11. *Identification by sentence*—the patient's comprehension of language is assessed by observing disability to execute (perform) commands of progressively increasing complexity.

12. *Reading names orally*—the patient reads aloud the names of objects from the basic set of 40.

13. *Oral reading*—the patient is instructed to read twelve of the command sentences used in test 11.

14. *Silent reading of names*—the patient reads the written name of an object in a display of ten objects used in the test series.

15. *Reading sentence for meaning*—the patient is instructed to execute twelve written commands used in test 11.

16. *Visual-graphic naming*—the patient is required to write the names of ten objects presented visually. (In this subtest, performance is scored on ability (appropriateness) of naming and not for correctness of spelling.)

17. *Writing names*—essentially, a second scoring of test 16, this time for correctness of spelling. If a patient is not able to write the name of the object presented to him, he is told the name and asked to write it.

18. *Writing to dictation*—the patient is required to write sentences (2) presented to him orally. Performance is scored on the basis of spelling, punctuation, omissions, and duplications.

19. *Copying sentences*—the patient is presented with two short sentences and is instructed to copy them. Performance is scored as in test 18.

20. *Articulation*—the patient is instructed to repeat thirty (30) meaningful and eight (8) nonsense words presented from a tape recording. Performance is scored on the basis of the number of correctly articulated consonant sound and sound blends.

TABLE 48-III
Outline of Test Tasks
Porch Index of Communicative Ability*

TEST	OUTPUT	TASK
I	Verbal	To discuss each test object, differentiating its primary characteristics.
II	Gestural	To demonstrate the function of each object.
III	Gestural	To demonstrate the function of each object as it is handed to subject.
IV	Verbal	To name each object.
V	Gestural	To read each of ten cards and place it according to printed instructions near the object whose function is stated on the card.
VI	Gestural	To point to each object whose function is given verbally by the examiner.
VII	Gestural	To read each of ten cards and place it according to printed instructions near the object whose name is stated on the card.
VIII	Gestural	To match a picture of each object with the appropriate object.
IX	Verbal	To say the name of each object which completes a sentence about the object's function.
X	Gestural	To point to each object as it is named by the examiner.
XI	Gestural	To match identical objects with each object.
XII	Verbal	To imitate the name of each object.
A	Graphic	To write a sentence about the function of each object.
B	Graphic	To write the name of each object.
C	Graphic	To write each object's name spoken by the examiner.
D	Graphic	To write each object's name spelled by the examiner.
E	Graphic	To copy each object's name.
F	Graphic	To copy geometric forms.

* Reproduced by special permission from the PORCH INDEX OF COMMUNICATE ABILITY. By Bruce E. Porch, copyright 1967. Published by Consulting Psychologists Press, Inc.

Note. The test objects were selected according to the following criteria: 1. common to the experience of adults of both sexes. 2. capable of being demonstrated gesturally, 3. approximately equal in difficulty across all tests. The objects used in the present test are listed here in standard order, i.e., the order in which they are presented to the patient:

1. Toothbrush
2. Cigarette
3. Pen
4. Knife
5. Fork
6. Quarter
7. Pencil
8. Matches
9. Key
10. Comb

Benton and his collaborators do not consider that their test battery will provide in-depth protocols of aphasic patients. They view their inventory as an instrument to provide useful clinical information and serve as a valid research technique.[11]

Through the uniform application of a standard examination Benton hopes that aphasiologists may establish an *operational understanding* for scientific communication in the field of aphasia. Specific aims for the international (multilingual) battery include: 1. the development of standards for an examination that will assess quantitative and qualitative aspects of aphasic disorders, and 2. language performance that can be related to the nature of involvement, prognosis, and clinical procedures.

In final form, the International Test for Aphasia will be reduced to no more than 10 subtests that may be administered in an examination period not to exceed 50 minutes.

THE TOKEN TEST FOR RECEPTIVE DISTURBANCES IN APHASIA

E. De Renzi and L. A. Vignolo (1962) have developed a special test which they consider to be especially sensitive for the detection of receptive disturbances so slight that they are ordinarily overlooked during the course of a clinical evaluation. The test requires the patient to execute (perform) commands based on directions that involve an arrangement of tokens (forms) of two different shapes, two different sizes, and five different colors. The patient is given a series of oral commands which constitute progressively complex and nonredundant messages. In response to each command-message, the examinee is required to execute a simple manual act such as picking up, touching, or moving one or more of the token forms.

The Token Test (Fig. 48-1) is incorporated in the International Test for Aphasia. De Renzi and Vignolo view their test as "a practical clinical tool, endowed of great sensitivity and contaminated as little as possible by intellectual difficulties." They have, in fact, found that their inventory does detect receptive disturbances which, as already indicated, are not apparent in the usual clinical examination or in

[11] Report of A. L. Benton to World Federation of Neurology, Oct. 4, 1968.

The token test

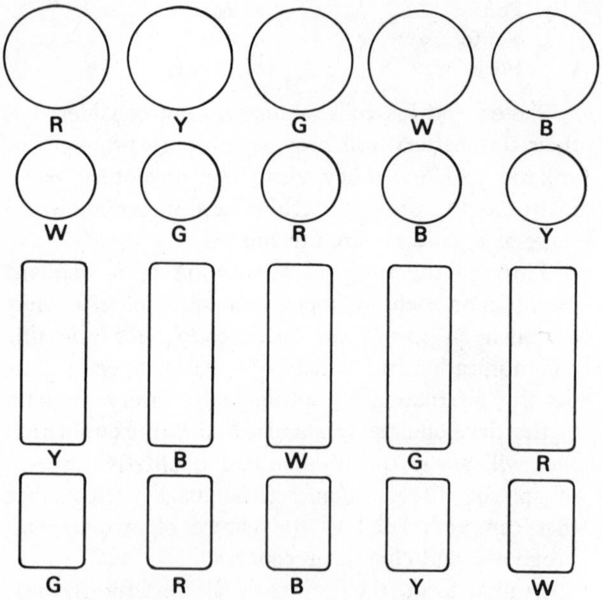

Fig. 48-1. R=red, B=blue, G=green, Y=yellow, W=white. Colors are distributed entirely at random. *By permission of E. de Renzi and L. A. Vignolo.*

conversation with a patient. We consider the Token Test to be an important clinical instrument for the assessment of verbal comprehension through non-verbal simple performance behavior. It is, therefore, as De Renzi and Vignolo indicate, a sensitive instrument for evaluating receptive verbal impairment which would not otherwise become apparent to clinicians. The sentence-directions translated by the authors from the original Italian follow:

1. Put the red circle on the green rectangle.
2. Put the white rectangle behind the yellow circle.
3. Touch the blue circle with the red rectangle.
4. Touch—with the blue circle—the red rectangle.
5. Touch the blue circle and the red rectangle.
6. Pick up the blue circle or the red rectangle.
7. Put the green rectangle away from the yellow rectangle.
8. Put the white circle before the blue rectangle.
9. If there is a black circle, pick up the red rectangle. (N.B. There is no black circle.)
10. Pick up the rectangles, except the yellow one.
11. When I touch the green circle, you take the white rectangle.
    (N.B. Wait a few seconds before touching the green circle.)
12. Put the green rectangle beside the red circle.
13. Touch the rectangles, slowly, and the circles, quickly.
14. Put the red circle between the yellow rectangle and the green rectangle.
15. Except for the green one, touch the circles.
16. Pick up the red circle—no!—the white rectangle.
17. Instead of the white rectangle, take the yellow circle.
18. Together with the yellow circle, take the blue circle.
19. After picking up the green rectangle, touch the white rectangle.
20. Put the blue circle under the white rectangle.
21. Before touching the yellow circle, pick up the red rectangle.[12]

OTHER TEST INVENTORIES AND APPROACHES

We do not pretend to have exhausted or even to have done justice to the numerous aphasia test inventories in current use. We are aware, of course, that many medical agencies and rehabilitation centers have their own inventories which serve them as useful clinical tools. We have concentrated on language test inventories that present divergent points of view as to the nature of aphasia and philosophy of assessment procedures. Approaches that emphasize the use of standardized tests of intelligence are described in the literature and may be found in the writings of Weisenburg and McBride (1935), Goldstein (1942 and 1948), and Goldstein and Scheerer (1941). More recent approaches may be found in the writings of Zangwill (1964), Weigl (1966), Bay (1962, 1964), and Luria (1964, 1965). This selection of references is by no means intended to be exhaustive or even fairly representative. At best, the references suggest the variety of philosophy and approaches to the assessment of changes of language and of intellect that are associated with cerebral pathology and aphasia.

[12] "It should be noted that the test has been originally designed for and applied to Italian patients. The orders presented here are the same, translated into English as accurately as possible; therefore, they should be considered merely as a demonstration of the degree of difficulty of the different items. It would be convenient, perhaps, to substitute or modify some of them, so as to make them convey, in English, differences of meaning comparable to those involved in the original Italian text" (De Renzi and Vignolo, *Brain*, 85, 1962, p. 671).

BIBLIOGRAPHY

Bay, E. 1962. Aphasia and non-verbal disorders of language. *Brain*, 85, B, 411-426.

———. 1967. The classification of disorders of speech. *Cortex*, III, 1, 26–31.

———. 1964. Principles of classification and their influence on our concepts of aphasia. *In* Disorders of language. De Reuck, A., and O'Connor, M., eds. London: Churchill. Pp. 122–142.

Benton, A. 1967. Problems in test construction in the field of aphasia. *Cortex*, III, 1, 32–58.

Brown, R. 1965. Social psychology. New York: Free Press.

Carroll, J. 1964. Words, meaning and concepts. *Harvard Educ. Rev.*, 34.

Cassirer, E. 1944. An essay on man. New York: Anchor Books.

Cole, M. 1968. The anatomical basis of aphasia as seen by Pierre Marie. *Cortex*, IV, 2, 172–183.

Critchley, M. 1967. Aphasiological nomenclature and definitions. *Cortex*, II, 1, 3–26.

Denny-Brown, D. 1958. The nature of apraxia. *J. nerv. ment. dis.*, 126, 9–32.

DeRenzi, E., and Spinnler, H. 1967. Impaired performance of color tasks in patients with hemispheric damage. *Cortex*, III, 2, 194–216.

———, and Vignolo, L. A. 1962. The token test: a sensitive test to detect receptive disturbances in aphasics. *Brain*, 85, 665–678.

DeReuck, A., and O'Connor, M., eds. 1964. Disorders of language. London: Churchill.

Eisenson, J. 1954. Examining for aphasia (rev. ed.), New York: Psychological Corp.

Freud, S. 1891. Zur Auffassung der Aphasien. *Trans. by* Stengel, E. New York: Internat. Univ. Press., 1953.

Goldstein, K. 1942. After effects of brain injury in war. New York: Grune & Stratton.

———. 1948. Language and language disturbances. New York: Grune & Stratton.

———, and Scheerer, M. 1941. Abstract and concrete behavior. *Psychol. Monogr.*, 53, 2.

Head, H. 1926. Aphasia and kindred disorders of speech. Cambridge Univ. Press and Macmillan. Reprinted by Hafner Pub. Co., New York, 1963.

Jackson, J. 1879. On affections of speech from disease of the brain. *In* Selected writings. Vol. 2. New York: Basic Books, 1958. Pp. 184–204.

Jakobson, R. 1964. Toward a linguistic typology of aphasic impairments. *In* Disorders of language. DeReuck, A., and O'Connor, M. eds. London: Churchill. Pp. 21–46.

Liepmann, H. 1900. Das Krankheitsbild der Apraxie. *Mschr. Psychiatr. Neurol.*, 8.

———. 1913. Motorische Aphasie und Apraxie. *Mschr. Psychiatr. Neurol.*, 34.

Luria, A. 1964. Factors and forms of aphasia. *In* Disorders of language. DeReuck, A., and O'Connor, M., eds. London: Churchill, Pp. 143–167.

———. 1966. Human brain and psychological processes. New York: Harper & Row.

———. 1966. Higher cortical functions in man. New York: Basic Books.

Marie, P. 1906. Troisieme circonvolution frontale gauche ne joue aucun role special dans la function du langage. *Semaine Medicale*, May 23. Reproduced in Marie, P. 1926. *Travaux et Memoires*, *Tome* I, Masson et Cie. Paris.

Monrad-Krohn, G. 1947. Dysprosody or disordered melody of speech. *Brain*, 70, 405–415.

Morris, C. 1938. Foundations of the theory of signs. International Encyclopedia of Unified Science. Chicago: Univ. Chicago Press.

Osgood, C., and Miron, M. 1963. Approaches to the study of aphasia. Univ. Ill. Press.

Penfield, W., and Roberts, L. 1959. Speech and brain mechanism. Princeton, N.J.: Princeton.

Porch, B. 1967. Porch index of communicative ability. Palo Alto, Calif.: Consulting Psychologists Press.

Schuell, H. 1957. A short examination for aphasia. *Neurology*, 7, 625–635.

———. 1965. Differential diagnosis of aphasia with the Minnesota test. Minneapolis: Univ. Minn. Press.

———, Jenkins, J., and Jiminez-Pabon, E. 1964. Aphasia in adults. New York: Hoeber Medical Division, Harper and Row.

———, ———, and Landis, L. 1961. Relationship between auditory comprehension and word frequency in aphasia. *J. Speech Hearing Res.*, 4, 30–36.

Stengel, E. 1953. *Aphasia: a critical study*. New York: International Press.

Weigl, E. 1966. On the construction of standard psychological tests in cases of brain damage. *J. neurol. Science*, 3, 123–127.

Weisenburg, T., and McBride, K. 1935. Aphasia. New York: Commonwealth Fund.

Wepman, J., Bock, R., Jones, L., and Van Pelt, D. 1956. Psycholinguistic study of aphasia: a revision of the concept of anomia. *J. Speech Hearing Disorders*, 21, 468–477.

———, and Jones, L. 1961. Studies in aphasia: an approach to testing. Chicago: Univ. Chicago: Education-Industry Service.

Wepman, J., and Jones, L. 1966. Studies in aphasia: a psycholinguistic method and case study. *In* Brain function, Vol. 3. Carterette, E., ed. Los Angeles: Univ. Calif. Press.

———, and ———. 1966. Speech, language and communication. UCLA *Forum Med. Sci.*, No. 4. Los Angeles: Univ. Calif. Press, 141–172.

White, L. 1949. The symbol: the origin and basis of human behavior. Reprinted from The science of culture, Ch. II, New York: Farrar, Straus and Cudahy.

Zangwill, O. 1964. Intelligence in aphasia: *In* Disorders of language. De Reuck, A., and O'Connor, M., eds. London: Churchill.

49

Correlates of Aphasia in Adults

Jon Eisenson

Etiology

Despite divergent points of view about the nature of aphasia, aphasiologists are in agreement that the underlying cause of aphasia is a physiological disturbance secondary to anatomical change resulting from brain damage of the dominant (usually left) hemisphere.[1] Although aphasic individuals all have incurred brain damage, this does not imply that all persons who have incurred brain damage even to the dominant hemisphere necessarily become manifestly aphasic.

The possible causes of cerebral damage with which aphasic disturbances are associated are many and varied. They include direct trauma by externally applied force, tumors, cerebral vascular lesions (embolisms, thromboses, aneurysms, hemorrhages), infectious diseases affecting brain tissue, and degenerative diseases invading the brain. Of the factors just enumerated, the vascular disturbances, embolisms, hemorrhages, and thromboses are the most frequent etiological associates. Brain damage resulting from head injuries, and brain penetrations from high-velocity missiles, are increased factors during war, both for the civilian and military population. For the most part, this cause of brain damage implicates a higher proportion of younger (below 30 years of age) than of older members of the population. As of now, it also implicates males considerably more than females.

Cerebral Dominance, Laterality, and Language Functions

We shall make no attempt to review the voluminous literature on the subject of localization of language function that has been accumulated over the past 100 years or more. We shall instead highlight some findings and observations since World War II that indicate considerable agreement as to hemisphere of involvement, the relation of involvement to handedness and, perhaps to a lesser degree, localization of function within the dominant hemisphere.

Penfield and Roberts (1959, p. 102) report on 522 patients who were operated on for treatment of focal cerebral seizure. These cases were reviewed for evidence of handedness and evidence of aphasia after surgery. They conclude that "With exclusion of cases of cerebral injury prior to the age of two years, there is no difference in the frequency of aphasia after operation on the left hemisphere between the left- and right-handed." Table 49-1, from Penfield and Roberts, summarizes the observations for patients whose injuries were incurred after two years of age.

On the basis of a study of 225 World War II patients with head-penetrating wounds which were associated with aphasia, Russell and Espir (1961, p. 170) concluded that with rare exception wounds causing aphasia are almost always of the *left* cerebral

[1] Later in this chapter we shall discuss the relationship of laterality preference and expression to cerebral dominance for language.

TABLE 49-I
Difference in Percentage of Patients Without Injury Before Two Years of Age and With Aphasia After Operation on the Left and Right Hemisphere

	LEFT HEMISPHERE			RIGHT HEMISPHERE			
HAND	TOTAL NO.	NO. WITH APHASIA	%	TOTAL NO.	NO. WITH APHASIA	%	SIGNIFICANCE OF DIFFERENCE
R[1]	157	115	73.2	196	1	0.5	<.001
L[2]	18	13	72.2	15	1	6.7	<.001
Total	175	128	73.1	211	2	0.9	<.001

(From Penfield and Roberts, 1959, p. 93.)

[1] Including predominantly right.
[2] Including predominantly left.

hemisphere. "Left cerebral dominance is therefore almost invariable, but the reasons for this are not clear."

Osgood and Miron (1964, p. 49) come to a similar conclusion. They say: "There now seems to be no question that there is 'localization' of language functions in the gross sense that one hemisphere, usually the left, is dominant. Aphasia is only rarely associated with lesions in the right hemisphere." Similar observations are reported by Goodglass and Quadfasel (1954), Ettlinger, Jackson, and Zangwill (1958), and Hecaen and Angelergues (1962). An excellent review of this subject may be found in the contribution by Milner, Branch, and Rasmussen (1964) in the Symposium on Disorders of Language. Table 49-II compares the Penfield and Roberts findings with those of Russell and Espir. The latter are for head-penetrating-wound patients.

The studies we have reviewed and cited are on varied populations relative to age, nature of cerebral insult, and language. It is clear that regardless of handedness, aphasic involvements are usually associated with left cerebral hemisphere damage. Nevertheless, we do find an incidence of up to 10 percent of aphasia in right-handed persons following right cerebral insult and perhaps 20 to 30 percent in left-handed patients (Milner, Branch, and Rasmussen, 1964, p. 204; Goodglass and Quadfasel, 1954).

Bilateral (ambidextrous) persons present a small but interesting population. Clinical observations strongly suggest that the *truly ambidextrous*, as distinguished from the ambinondextrous, may have bilateral representation for language functions. The possibility that most left-handed individuals are not too readily distinguished from the bilateral ambidextrous deserves serious consideration. Certainly, most left-handed (sinistral) individuals have more dexterity with their right hands than right-handed (dextral) individuals have with their left hands. In regard to aphasia, the evidence suggests that the ambidextrous may be considered as part of the population of the sinistrals. In general, we accept the conclusion of Milner et al. (1964, p. 205) that "This suggestion of a considerable margin of safety in the cerebral organization of left-handed and ambidextrous patients again accords well with the

TABLE 49-II
Incidence of Aphasia in Right- and Left-handed Persons With Lesions Limited to One Hemisphere

	LEFT HEMISPHERE			RIGHT HEMISPHERE LESION		
HANDEDNESS	NO.	NO. APHASIC	%	NO.	NO. APHASIC	%
Penfield and Roberts (Surgical Cases)						
R	157	115	78.2	196	1	0.5
L	18	13	72.2	15	1	6.7
Russell and Espir (Head penetrating wounds)						
R	288	186	64.6	221	3	1.4
L	24	9	37.5	24	4	16.7

notion of a more bilateral representation, and there may well be considerable individual differences in this respect which find no place in our all-or-none scoring."[2]

Cerebral Control (dominance) for Nonlanguage Functions

In our discussion thus far we have been careful to use the term cerebral dominance in relationship to the functions of language. We have intentionally avoided any suggestion that the left hemisphere, which is usually dominant for language, is also generally dominant for all functions under cerebral control. Similarly, we should not assume that persons who have right hemisphere dominance for language have overall right hemisphere dominance for cerebrally controlled functions. The position we take and recommend is that cerebral dominance or perhaps better, dominant cerebral control, is related to function. There are some functions, such as the appreciation of spatial relationships, which seem to be under right hemisphere control, at least as judged by the effects of damage to the right cerebral hemisphere (Hecaen, 1967). In broadest terms, we can accept the position that the right hemisphere is usually dominant for our nonverbal behavior and the left for verbal behavior. Thus, the kinds of functions that are assessed by the performance items of the Wechsler scales, e.g., The Wechsler Adult Intelligence Scale, are more likely to show impairment correlated with right hemisphere damage. Except for language functions, however, the difference in impairment of function is usually not as severe or as clear-cut in relationship to hemisphere of damage. Nevertheless, we can still accept the tentative conclusion of Meyer (1961) that "the most consistent claims are that patients with the left hemisphere lesions (dominant side) are relatively poor at verbal tasks, while those with rightsided lesions . . . are relatively poor at practical tasks. . . ." We need to appreciate that effects of brain damage are not invariable. The implications of brain damage are not manifest in precisely the same way in each individual. Assumptions that hold for experimental populations as a whole may not hold for all individuals within the population. Reitan's (1966) review of problems relating to psychological correlates of brain lesions is recommended reading for aphasiologists. Reitan (1955), Heilbrun (1956), Meyer (1961), Teuber (1962), and Weinstein (1962) have significant studies on interhemispheric differences in functions resulting from brain lesion.

Before concluding the discussion on the differential roles of the two cerebral hemispheres, we should like to direct attention to a study which suggests that right cerebral damage may have implications for language functioning when such functioning is related to high-level intellectual processes. Eisenson (1962) compared a population of right brain-damaged adults with a control adult group on a battery of language tests that included productive vocabulary (definition), multiple choice vocabulary, and a variety of sentence completion tasks. All of the test items were adopted from standardized tests of intelligence. The major finding was that right brain-damaged patients did not do so well as non-brain-damaged controls on the battery as a whole. The greatest differences were found in sentence completion items calling for the use of abstract words. The author interpreted this finding to "suggest that the right cerebral hemisphere might be involved with super- or extraordinary language functions particularly as this function calls upon the need of the individual to deal with relatively abstract established language formulations, to which he must adjust." An alternate interpretation is that, in a nonspecific way, the right hemisphere contributes to all intellectual functions. Damage impairs and reduces the level of contribution. Another possible intepretation is that any cerebral damage reduces intellectual functioning with implications for language in less specific and certainly less apparent ways than do aphasic involvements. The results tend to support Critchley's (1962) observations as a neurologist that closer attention needs to be paid "to the linguistic capacities and incapacities of right-handed victims of right brain disease." Critchley noted several functions which are affected by right brain damage. These include dysarthrias, creative literary work, word-finding difficulties, and difficulties in the full understanding of pictorial material.[3] So, we may conclude either that right brain-damaged persons may suffer from "latent aphasia" (Boller, 1968) or that right cerebral damage, in a nonspecific way, impairs language skills at a level

[2] Milner's conclusion is based on a population of patients with epileptogenic lesions for whom the sodium-amytal technique was used to determine cerebral dominance for language.

[3] Boller (1968) found that right brain-damaged adults were inferior to left brain-damaged nonaphasics and a control group in a word-production (object naming) task.

at which they are associated with higher abstract mental processes. Perhaps the most general and conservative conclusion is that despite man's billions of cortical cells, he really has few to spare if he is to function up to his full intellectual potential.

Anatomical Differences of the Hemispheres

It is clear from our discussion thus far that functionally, or perhaps better dysfunctionally, as far as language is concerned, man's two cerebral hemispheres are different. Are there any anatomical differences that may explain or at least be correlated with these functional differences? Von Bonin (1962, p. 6) sums up the available evidence by these observations:

> The left hemisphere has a slightly greater specific gravity than the right one. This would mean that there is a little more cortex on the left side. That fits in with the fact that the Sylvian fissure is a little bit longer, that the insula is longer and higher on the left side, that there is a doubling of the sulcus cinguli more frequently on the left side, and that the calcarine fissure has a hook more often on the left than on the right side.
>
> But all these morphological differences are, after all, quite small. How to correlate these with the astonishing differences in function, such as the speech function on the left side, is an entirely different question, and one that I am unable to answer.

Geschwind and Levitsky (1968) on the basis of postmortem findings of 100 adult brains report marked anatomical asymmetries between the upper surfaces of the human right and left temporal lobes. Of special significance to us is that the differences involve an area of the brain which include the primary auditory cortex and the auditory association cortex. Lesions in this area are etiologically associated with auditory (classical Wernicke's) aphasia.

Cerebral Localization for Language Functions

Information on cerebral localization for language functions has come to us by way of the pathology of dysfunction. Positive statements about localization are still assumptions and inferences. The underlying implications in the use of the term *localization of function* are that a healthy state, and so presumably normal functioning of a particular area of a brain, is essential to the execution of a particular function in a manner deemed normal. In regard to language, the assumption and implication for localization is that there are areas of the brain which are essential for particular functions; e.g., articulation, speech perception, reading, writing, etc.

We shall avoid any detailed presentation, except for a brief historical review, of positions relative to localization of function before World War II. There are still some "strict" or fine localizationists who accept the position exemplified by Nielsen (1947) as to specific correlations between relatively small areas of the brain and related functions. On the other hand, the position that all areas of the brain have equipotentiality for language function does not seem tenable.

Early Localizationists

Broca. Present-day localization theory relative to aphasic disturbances had its origin in the presentation by Paul Broca of two papers in Paris in 1861.[4] At first Broca postulated that a lesion in the second or third frontal convolution was associated with aphasia of the motor (expressive) type. Later, Broca fixed the third convolution as the site of the lesion associated with expressive (spoken) disturbances of language function. This is the area which is included in Brodmann area 44.[5]

Other names prominent among the early localizationists and "diagram-makers" are Bastian and Wernicke. Bastian (1880) went beyond Broca, and localized areas for auditory and visual functions. Wernicke (1874) located and described an auditory center in the temporal convolution.

Contemporary Localizationists

Nielsen. The name of Dr. J. M. Nielsen is foremost among contemporary exponents of localization theory. He is, however, not as rigid and pedantic a localizationist as Henschen. Nielsen (1941, p. 227), for example, admits that "Anatomy and physiology are still incompletely co-ordinated so far as the cerebral cortex is concerned." Though aware that ". . . logic would seem to stipulate that each area of a certain structure must have a function differing from that of

[4] An English translation of the original Broca article by J. Kann appeared in the *J. Speech Hearing Disorders*, 15, 1950, pp. 16–20.

[5] Brodmann divided and "diagrammed" the human cerebral cortex into areas according to cellular distribution. These have come to be known as Brodmann's cytoarchitectonic areas.

other areas with different structures . . . ," Nielsen (1941, p. 229) observes that certain areas of the brain (e.g., area 19 of Brodmann) ". . . [are] certainly divided physiologically." Nielsen (1941), Ch. 10) suggests several explanations for the apparent inconsistencies in localization theory. These include: 1. the possibility that ". . . even though the distribution of the cortical cells is the same throughout an anatomic area, the organization of the cells may be different in various portions of the same area"; 2. neurons establish different connections with use in order to subserve different purposes in the more minute and precise sense; and 3. an area can serve one purpose as a result of one method of training and another purpose as a result of different training.

Despite these reservations, Nielsen accepts localization theory in a comparatively strict sense both in his textbook (1941) and in his more specialized book on disturbances related to aphasia (1947). He lists and describes specific cortical areas and specific dysfunctions which are associated with lesions in these areas.

Henschen. Henschen, whose text on clinical pathology is referred to by Nielsen (1941, p. 306) as "a priceless classic," allowed for no leeway in his structural viewpoint. On the basis of 60 of his own cases and 1,500 taken from the literature, Henschen (1926) worked out what he considered to be unfailing one-to-one relationships between defective cortical area and linguistic disturbance. He also specified centers for arithmetic and music.

Opposition to Strict Localization

Hughlings Jackson. Opposition to the concept of strict localization of language function in specific cortical areas was not absent during the time of Broca and his followers. Hughlings Jackson, a chronological contemporary of Broca, was an early and outspoken oppositionist. Jackson emphasized the viewpoint that a knowledge of pathological conditions which disturb and impair language function does not per se provide information as to how the function is normally controlled in the healthy individual. Further, Jackson insisted that aphasic disturbances could not be understood without a knowledge of the patient who suffered the disturbances. He stressed the importance of observing the live aphasic patient rather than studying the autopsy findings of those who did not survive.

Jackson (1915 and 1931) did not deny that Broca's area was frequently damaged in patients who suffered from aphasic disturbances, especially when motor speech involvements were manifest. He refused, however, to localize language function in Broca's area alone, and stressed the notion that language was a psychological rather than physiological function. For language, as for other intellectual functions, the brain operates as a functional unit.

The concept that a destructive lesion can never be responsible for positive symptoms, and the much-quoted principle that "to locate the damage which destroys speech and to locate speech are two different things," were stressed by Jackson. Destruction, Jackson held, produces negative symptoms. Positive symptoms associated with destructions of cortical tissue are to be attributed to the effects of the released activity of the lower centers.

Among other contemporaries of Broca who opposed strict localization were Pierre Marie in France, Arnold Pick in Czechoslovakia, and W. R. Gowers in England. All three agreed with Jackson that while localized lesions could not be held responsible for language and speech disturbances, lesions in certain cortical areas can more readily disturb speech than do lesions in other areas.

Henry Head. The English neurologist Henry Head (1926) continued along the clinical, psychological paths of Hughlings Jackson. Head pointed out that the capacity to use language in any form is the result of physiological activities of certain parts of the brain cortex. All forms of language usage develop from the ". . . simple acts of speaking and comprehension of spoken words." Aphasia is defined as ". . . a disorder of symbolic fomulation and expression." Symbolic formulation and expression is characterized as a mode of behavior in which some verbal or nonverbal symbol plays a part between the initiation and the execution of the act. Destruction of brain tissue is likely to result in an interference of normal fulfilment of some specific forms of behavior. The reaction which follows is an expression of the organism as a whole to the new situation.

Although Head emphasized the function of the brain as a whole, he observed that, in the event of pathology, certain types of aphasic language dysfunction can probably be associated with lesions in broadly outlined areas of the brain. For example, impairments in the capacity to understand the deeper significance of words and the wider meaning of a sentence as a whole (semantic aphasia) seems to be associated with lesions of the supramarginal gyrus.

Similarly, Head postulated other likely areas of lesion associated with such subtypes of aphasia as the verbal, syntactical, and nominal. Head emphasized that aphasic disturbances are not discrete and noted that for the aphasic person there is a generalized defect in intellectual expression which requires symbolic formulation. The degree of defect is likely to be related directly to the propositional level of the expression.

"New" Localizationism

Psychological influences, especially Gestalt psychology, and the neuropsychology of Karl Lashly (1958) had considerable impact on concepts of cerebral function and cerebral localization. Of special importance to aphasiologists were Weisenburg and McBride, and Goldstein.

Weisenburg and McBride. As a result of their clinical and psychological study of aphasic patients, Weisenburg and McBride arrived at a comparatively moderate stand on the issue of localization of function. They accepted relatively fixed localization for such motor and sensory functions as motion, vision, hearing, and smell. In regard to intellectual functions such as language usage, however, they said (1935, p. 467):

> . . . it is impossible to localize language. In the majority of individuals language permeates the thought processes to such an extent that the one cannot be separated from the other; and for the present at least it is impossible to give an adequate explanation of intelligence, much less to localize it. That it is the result of the activity of the entire brain, however, there is no doubt.

Weisenburg and McBride do not deny that lesions in certain parts of the brain are more likely to be associated with aphasic disturbances than are lesions elsewhere. Although they avoid specific localization, they observe that (1935, p. 468):

> . . . in about 95 percent of the cases the lesion must be in the dominant hemisphere; and that it must implicate the anterior and to a less extent the posterior part of the brain within certain limits, including the lower portion of the pre-central convolution and probably the adjoining part of the frontal lobe, the lower portion of the parietal lobe, the upper part of the temporal lobe, and the anterior part of the occipital.

Weisenburg and McBride, as we have noted, divided their patients into four clinical types on the basis of predominant linguistic disturbances. For patients whose greatest difficulty is in expression, they found the lesion to be in the anterior or motor part of the brain; for patients with predominantly receptive (comprehension) difficulty, they found the posterior part of the brain more involved than in the expressive group, and a likelihood that the anterior part of the brain was also involved, but less severely than for the expressive patients. Patients with almost equal amounts of expressive and receptive difficulties were found to have more extensive and more permanent involvements of both anterior and posterior parts of the brain. Amnesic patients—those whose difficulty was in recall of names with relatively good ability to recognize the names not able to be recalled—were found to have no definitely localizable lesions.

Kurt Goldstein. Although Kurt Goldstein is likely to be regarded as an antilocalizationist, his clinical observations and many of his writings tend to contradict this opinion. Geschwind (1964), writing about Goldstein's position, observes, "His contribution as a localizer in the classical sense is in fact highly significant although rarely taught." Goldstein's position rejected narrow classification and the inadequacies of the rigid classical schemes. Among Goldstein's stated objections to classical (strict and rigid) localization theory are the following:

> The so-called classic theory of localization is based mainly on the material gained from postmortems. It should be observed that the objections against the theory stem first from a more careful consideration of the *pathologic-anatomic* data. There are so-called negative cases: on the one hand, absence of symptoms in a lesion affecting an area which was considered characteristic of this locality; on the other hand, appearance of symptoms without the presence of a correspondingly localized lesion (1948, p. 47).

Goldstein, however, does more than present a negative attitude toward localization. He discusses in his writings some of the positive factors which make strict localization theory difficult for him to entertain (1948, p. 48):

> It is very difficult, indeed, to evaluate the degree of damage; it is not only dependent on the direct destruction of the nerve cells but also on the condition of the glia, blood vessels, etc. Further, we have no idea of the relationship between a definite anatomic condition and a specific performance. *We are far from being able to decide whether the preserved tissue is still functioning sufficiently to allow for a certain performance or not.*

On the question of the inconsistency of symptoms as related to local brain injury, Goldstein holds (1948, p. 48):

> Whether certain symptoms will appear or not on account of a local injury certainly depends on many factors other than locality: i.e., on the nature of the disease process, on the damage of all or only some structures of the cortex, on the condition of the rest of the brain, on individual differences in co-operation of both hemispheres, . . . on the state of circulation in general, on the functional reactions of the organism to the defect . . . on the psycho-physical constitution of the personality, etc.

An important point relative to the effects of a lesion is made by Goldstein. He points out that "A lesion of a special locality in different cases may vary very much regarding the degree to which the substratum in general is affected, and particularly its different striata. Such a selective character of the process may be of paramount significance for the development of symptoms" (1948, pp. 47–48).

Goldstein's interpretation of localization is best understood in terms of Gestalt psychology, which emphasizes the function of the organism as a whole and the effects of a specific performance only as it is related to the organism functioning as a whole. With this in mind, it becomes possible to appreciate Goldstein's concept of cortical localization: ". . . *each performance is due to the function of the total organism in which the brain plays a particular role.* In each performance, the whole cortex is in activity, but the excitation in the cortex is not the same throughout (1948, p. 50).

From the above, it would appear that Goldstein did not reject cortical localization. Actually, he redefined localization in terms which were consistent with his own thinking. For Goldstein, localization is acceptable only insofar as an individual performance is considered. The role of a given cortical area is significant according to the particular influence it exerts on the excitation of the cortex as a whole, and so as to the total dynamic process which occurs as a result of the functioning of the entire nervous system.

With this concept of localization, Goldstein was able to accept and define symptom complexes as being related to definite areas. Indeed, for practical purposes, Goldstein and Weisenburg and McBride are in agreement. Goldstein accepts the likelihood that a motor (expressive) language disturbance will usually be correctly localized in the expanded Broca's region of the left hemisphere and that sensory (receptive) disturbances will usually be correctly located in the temporal lobes.

Luria's approach to localization of function, although rooted in Pavlovian neurophysiology, is often strikingly that of Kurt Goldstein's. In his Higher Cortical Functions of Man (1966, p. 35) Luria writes: "We therefore suggest that *the material basis of the higher nervous processes is the brain as a whole* but that *the brain is a highly differentiated system whose parts are responsible for different aspects of the unified whole.*" Luria is emphatic that his view of the organization of higher mental functions is opposed to both narrow localization and equipotentialism for brain function. He accepts Vygotsky's position that

> higher mental functions may exist only as a result of interaction between the highly differentiated brain structures and that individually these structures make their own specific contributions to the dynamic whole and play their own roles in the functional system. This hypothesis, intrinsically opposed to both narrow localization and diffuse equipotentialism is a thread running through the whole of this book (Luria, 1966, p. 36.)

Basic to the understanding of Luria's concept of localization of cortical function is the Pavlovian position that

> *sensation incorporates the process of analysis of signals while they are still in the first stages of arrival. . . .* According to this view, from the very beginning the sensory cortical divisions participate in the analysis and integration of complex, not elementary, signals. The units of any sensory process (including hearing) are not only acts of reception of individual signals, measurable in terms of thresholds of sensation, but also acts of complex analysis and integration of signals, measurable in units of comparison and discrimination. The sensory divisions of the cortex are the apparatuses responsible for this analysis, and indications of a lesion of these apparatuses are to be found, not so much in a lowering of the acuity of the sensations, as in a disturbance of the analytic-synthetic function (1966, pp. 97–98).

Fig. 49-1 gives Luria's conception of the cortical zones for the systems of analyzers.

The functions of the left temporal cortex and especially of the superior temporal gyrus (the secondary divisions of the auditory cortex), its contribution to the perception of sound as well as to the motor aspects of speech, and to aphasic involvements in the event of pathology, are explained by Luria as follows:

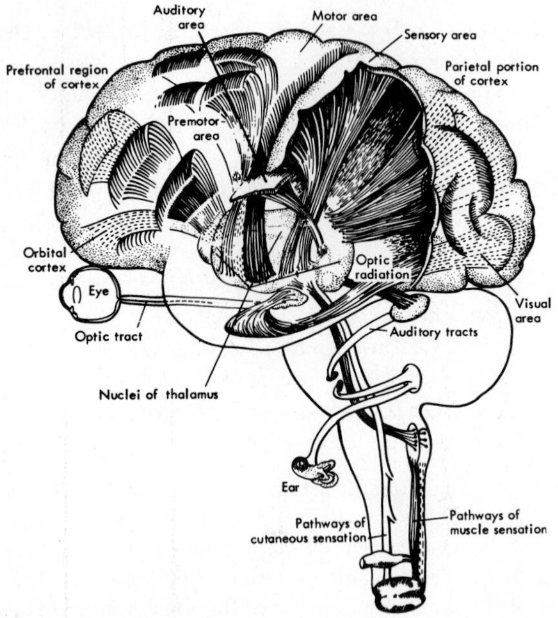

Fig. 49-1. Cortical zones of systems of analyzers. *From "Modern Data on the Structural Organization of the Cerebral Cortex" by G. I. Polyakov in HIGHER CORTICAL FUNCTIONS by A. R. Luria © 1966 Consultants Bureau Enterprises, Inc. and Basic Books, Inc. Publishers, New York, p. 45.*

All that has been said regarding the structure of the sounds of a language and regarding the hearing of speech is of decisive importance to the understanding of the nature of the work that must be done by the *secondary divisions of the auditory cortex of the left hemisphere*, those divisions that . . . are closely associated with the cortical apparatuses of kinesthetic (articulatory) analysis.

The work of these divisions consists of the *analysis* and *integration of the sound flow by identification of the phonemic signs of the objective system of the language.* This work must be carried out with the very close participation of articulatory acts which . . . constitute the efferent link for the perception of the sounds of speech. It consists of differentiating the significant, phonemic signs of the spoken sounds, inhibiting the unessential, nonphonemic signs, and comparing the perceived sound complexes on this phonemic basis (1966, p. 101).

The vulnerability of the left temporal cortex and its implications for aphasic involvement may be appreciated in Luria's statement that "A lesion of these cortical divisions, therefore, must cause, not the simple loss of acuity of hearing, but the disintegration of the whole complex structure of the analytic-synthetic activity underlying the process of the systematization of speech experience" (1966, p. 103).

The implication of lesions of the superior temporal region of the left hemisphere for aphasic involvements has been appreciated since Wernicke's time. The concept of impairment of phonemic analysis and the relationship of speech-sound discrimination to articulation is stressed by Luria as well as by investigators in the Haskins Laboratory (Liberman et al., 1963). Fig. 49-2 presents Luria's data on the site

TABLE 49-III
Classification of Types of Aphasia

APHASIA	DISTURBED FUNCTION	SPEECH DEFECT	BRAIN LESION*
1. Sensory	Acoustic Analysis	Phonemes	Posterior-Temporal
2. Amnestic	Retention of audio-speech traces	Repetition of series	Centro-Temporal
3. Afferent	Kinaesthetic analysis of speech movements	Articulemes	Posterior motor speech area
4. Efferent	Kinetic analysis of successive speech movements	Articulation	Anterior motor speech area
5. Semantic	Simultaneous organization of speech components	Logico-grammatical	Temporo-parietal
6. Dynamic	"Inner Speech"	Lack of spontaneity for active propositionalizing	Frontal

(From Luria, A. R., Factors and Forms of Aphasia, in DeReuck, A. V. S., and O'Connor, M. (1964), Disorders of Language. J. and A. Churchill, London, 143–167.)

* Each zone of the cerebral cortex makes a specific contribution; damage to any zone impairs functions of all zones and the brain cortex as a whole.

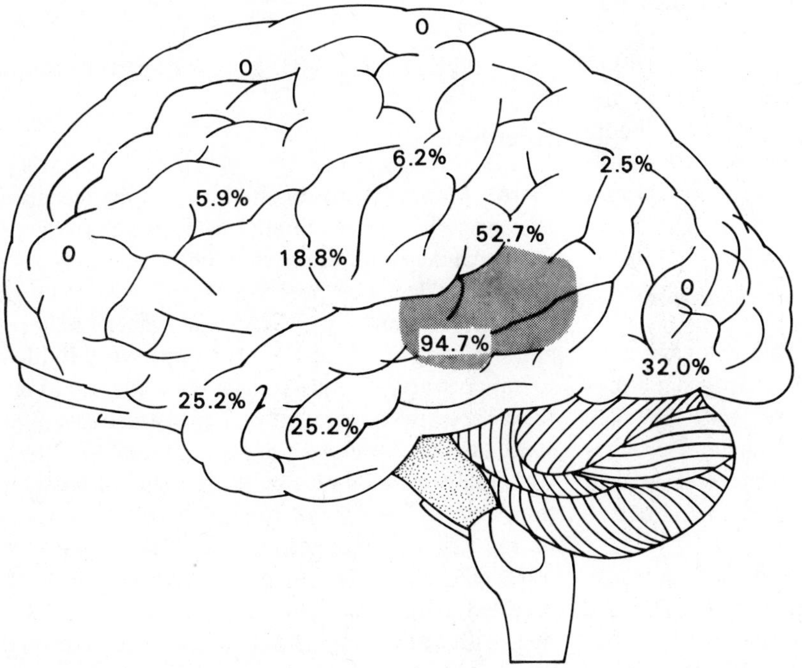

Fig. 49-2. Percentage distribution of cases with impaired phonemic perception related to site of cerebral lesion. Shaded region includes the auditory projection and association areas considered to be essential for normal phonemic perception. Note the relatively high incidence of impaired phonemic perception related to lesions in regions immediately adjacent to the shaded area. *After R. L. Masland, "Some Neurological Processes Underlying Language,"* Annals of Otology, Rhinology, and Laryngology, *77, 4, 1968, 787. Based on data from Luria, A. R. "Brain Disorders and Language Analysis,"* Language and Speech, ***1, 1,*** *1958, 14–34.*

of lesion for 800 patients who presented symptoms of impairment for phonemic discrimination.

A summary of Luria's concept of cortical localization for language functions, and for aphasic disturbances, is presented in Table 49-III.

Luria stresses the need to understand that superficially similar symptoms may have different causes and different dynamics. So, for example, "*disturbances of writing have very different structures in different localization* of cortical defect, and a careful neuropsychological analysis can single out *different factors underlying different forms of writing defects:* such *qualification of writing defects* makes it possible to use disturbances of writing as a means for topical diagnosis of brain injury" (1964).

Hécaen and Angelergues (1964) analyzed data based on observations of 214 right-handed patients who had incurred lesions of the left hemisphere. The lesions were varied but were predominantly of tumor and traumatic origin. All of the observations were verified either by postmortem examination or by surgery. Their data were analyzed for intensity of aphasic symptoms, type of symptoms, and site of lesion. They note that in relation to location and extent of lesion, "only isolated temporal lesions and, to a lesser degree, parietal lesions provoke a high average of aphasic symptoms." The greatest intensity of aphasic symptoms was attained in massive lesions involving the fronto-parietal-temporal and parieto-temporal-occipital regions. Fig. 49-3 presents a diagrammatic representation of type of aphasic disturbance in

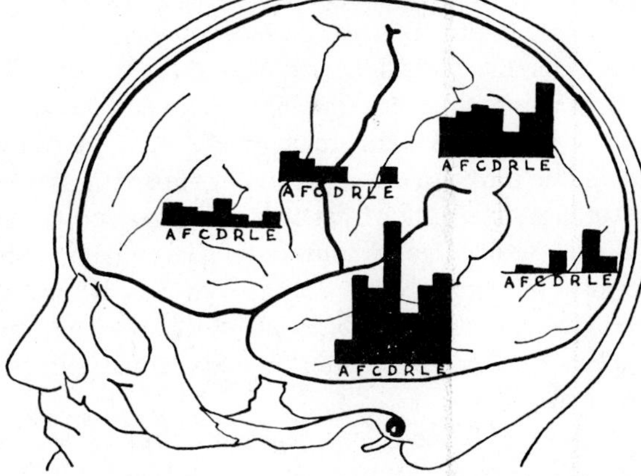

Fig. 49-3. Diagrammatic representation of the average degree of disturbance of various language modalities which occurs when there is an isolated lesion of various lobes (front, rolandic, parietal, temporal and occipital).

A: Articulatory disturbances.
B: Difficulties in the fluency of speech.
C: Disturbances of verbal comprehension.
D: Disturbances of naming.
R: Disturbances of repetition.
L: Disturbances in reading.
E: Disturbances of writing.

From Hecaen, N., and Angelergues (1964) in DISORDERS OF LANGUAGE, Ciba Fdn. Symp., London: Churchill.

relationship to site of lesion. It may be noted that with the exception of an absence of articulatory disturbances for lesions of posterior region, a variety of disturbances may be associated with lesions in the three crucial areas of the cortex. We should also note the high degree of disturbances for verbal comprehension associated with lesions of the temporal and parietal regions.

Toward a "New" and "Finer" Localization

From our discussion of Luria and Hécaen, it becomes apparent that cerebral localization for language functions has by no means been abandoned. The approaches represented by these investigators provide a basis for a new way to view and interpret aphasic symptoms and to correlate symptoms with determined lesions.

The investigations by Geschwind and his associates should be viewed in the light of the possibilities for "finer" localization than was the trend in the period immediately after World War II. Geschwind (1967) studied naming errors (anomia) which occurred on "confrontation," in situations in which a patient had difficulties in naming things shown to him rather than in free-flowing, spontaneous speech. On the basis of his observations Geschwind differentiated a group of patients with lesions in the region of the dominant angular gyrus who were characterized as having *classic anomia* (failure to produce a response, verbal paraphasias, circumlocutions, etc., but ability to choose correct name if presented to patient) from a second anomic group that was characterized by an inability to match a stimulus to its spoken name. The lesions for this group are those which isolate or produce *disconnections of sensory regions* from the speech area "probably from the left angular gyrus in particular."

Geschwind's study was selected as representative of the position of a contemporary neurologist who has available and makes use of new and sophisticated techniques for determining site of lesion, the nature of the language symptoms, as well as statistical procedures for the analysis of language data. Fortunately, the ready dissemination and sharing ot information by aphasiologists now makes it possible for findings to be checked throughout the world. From such studies may emerge new concepts of localization supported by hard data on live patients rather than on subjective observations and conjectures on patients no longer available for confirmatory assessment.

PSYCHOLOGICAL CORRELATES

Intelligence

Pierre Marie (1906) insisted that aphasics always showed some degree of impairment in comprehension and some degree of intellectual impairment associated with their language deficits. Marie also held that aphasia was a unitary disorder and that the only pure aphasia was the Wernicke (auditory) type. Evidence to support at least part of Marie's contention comes to us from post Word War II investigations. Weinstein (1964) compared the test results of 62 men with brain wounds on the Army General Classification Test (AGCT) with the scores of the same men on induction into the army. He found that the post test, taken approximately 10 years after injury, revealed a significant decline in score for almost all men with left parieto-temporal lesions. Interestingly, comparable deficits were shown by patients whose temporo-parietal lesions were not associated with aphasia. Weinstein concluded that "Thus, aphasia, per se, although frequently sufficient, is not necessary to produce intellectual impairment as we measured it."

Our own impression is that functionally, if not absolutely, aphasic persons, by virtue of their brain damage, are not able to work up to their intellectual potential *except under optimal conditions.* Since a testing situation is usually stressful and anxiety producing, it will in itself reduce the functional or immediately manifest expression of intelligence. More generally, we believe that brain damage is likely to result in modifications of personality and drive which further reduce the expression of intellectual potential. So, for practical purposes, we can accept both Marie's clinical observations and the findings of investigations such as Weinstein's. We will consider the implications of these observations in our chapter on Therapeutic Problems.

Personality Modifications

Goldstein (1948, p. 48) argued that whether certain symptoms will appear or not following a brain injury depends upon a number of factors, one of which is the "psycho-physical constitution of the personality." Unfortunately, Goldstein did not elaborate on the premorbid personality or behavioral characteristics of the aphasic. We believe that such traits as rigidity and tendencies toward concretism are premorbid characteristics of many, but not of all, persons who become aphasic. This observation is made as a result of conversations with parents, wives, and other relatives of young aphasic persons who suffered penetrating wounds in combat and became aphasic, and with relatives of older aphasics who suffered vascular brain insults. The so-called "organic personality" is not always a result of brain damage per se. Often it is the effect of brain damage on a person with premorbid tendencies to behave as he comes to behave. It is likely that prior to the onset of the effects of brain damage, the same tendencies were present. The individual, having some awareness of these tendencies, or at least of his being different from other persons in his environment, exercised special effort to make acceptable adjustments. The effect of the brain damage on the individual as a patient is probably to reduce his capacity to make the necessary adjustments, or to reduce his drive to overcome latent undesirable behavioral inclinations.

Rigidity and concretism, though frequently associated with withdrawal behavior, may also be discovered in aggressive and openly hostile persons. The general effect of brain damage is to make more readily apparent the extent of undesirable behavioral traits. Thus, tendencies become exaggerated and the latent becomes the actual. Essentially, then, the so-called "organic personality" is what it might have been in any event. Wepman (1951, p. 88), recognizing this in his aphasic patients, observes: "It also seems more and more apparent that the patient's reported on did not develop a so-called 'organic personality,' but rather seemed to possess and to project the same basic personalities they had in their premorbid condition. The major sign of change was not in their personality type but in the manner in which it was projected."

Critchley, in his closing remarks at a Symposium on Disorders of Language (1964, pp. 340–341), reminded his listeners that the patient's premorbid personality and his premorbid verbal equipment and literary attainment are "factors which may go some way, perhaps a long way, in determining the eventual aphasic picture. . . . Questions of natural eloquence, verbosity, size of vocabulary, literacy, pluralingualism, style, aesthetic delight in words for their own sake; and the sound, shape and colour of words; the choosing, matching, and combining of words in euphonious and pleasing patterns—however obsessional—these are surely most important when it comes to understanding the eventual picture of the victim who finds himself crippled in a linguistic sense."

In essence then, we should remember that an aphasic had a personality that is modified by the lesion and the impairments that become directly and indirectly associated with it. The pathology produces disruption and the need for reorganization. What the individual was before he became an aphasic patient determines considerably, if not objectively measurably, what he will become. We will consider these implications in our chapter on therapy.

BIBLIOGRAPHY

Boller, F. 1968. Latent aphasia: right and left "non-aphasic" patients compared. *Cortex*, XIV, 3, 245–256.

Critchley, M. 1964. Concluding remarks. *In* Language disorders. De Reuck, A., and O'Connor, M., eds. London: Churchill.

Eisenson, J. 1962. Language and intellectual modifications associated with right cerebral damage. *Language and Speech*, 5, 2, 49–53.

Ettlinger, G., Jackson, C., and Zangwill, O. 1956. Cerebral dominance in sinistrals. *Brain*, 79, 569–588.

Geschwind, N. 1964. The paradoxical position of K. Goldstein in the history of aphasia. *Cortex*, 1, 2, 214–224.

———. 1967. The varieties of naming errors. *Cortex*, III, 1, 97–112.

———, and Levitsky, W. 1968. Human brain: left-right asymmetries in temporal speech region. *Science*, 161, 186–187.

Goldstein, K. 1948. Language and language disturbances. New York: Grune & Stratton.

Goodglass, H., and Quadfasel, F. 1954. Language laterality in left-handed aphasics. *Brain*, 77, 521–548.

Head, H. 1926. Aphasia and kindred disorders of speech (2 vols.). New York: Macmillan. Reprinted by Hafner. New York. 1963.

Hecaen, H. 1967. Brain mechanisms suggested by studies of parietal lobes. *In* Brain mechanisms underlying speech and language. Millikan, C., and Darley, F., eds. New York: Grune & Stratton.

———, and Angelergues, R. 1964. Localization of symptoms in aphasia. *In* Language disorders. DeReuck, A., and O'Connor, M., eds. London: Churchill.

Hecaen, H. 1962. L'aphasie, l'apraxie, l'agnosie chez les gauchers. *Rev. Neurol.*, 106, 510–516.
Heilbrun, A. 1956. Psychological test performance as a function of lateral localization of cerebral lesion. *J. comp. Physiol. and Psychol.*, 49, 10–14.
Henschen, S. 1926. On the function of the right hemisphere of the brain in relation to the left in speech, music, and calculation. *Brain*, 49, 110–123.
Jackson, H. 1915. Selected writings of J. Hughlings Jackson. Head, H., ed. *Brain*, 38, 1–90.
———. 1931. Selected writings of John Hughlings Jackson. Taylor, G., ed. London: Hodder and Stoughton.
Lashley, K. 1958. Cerebral organization and behavior in the brain and human behavior. *Proc. Assn. Rev. Ment. Dis.*, 36, 1–18.
Liberman, A., Cooper, F., Harris, K., and MacNeilage, P., 1963. A motor theory of speech perception. *J. Acoust.*, 35, 1114.
Luria, A. 1966. Higher cortical functions in men. New York: Basic Books.
———. 1964. Neuropsychology in the local diagnosis of brain damage. *Cortex*, I, 1, 3–18.
———. 1964. Factors and forms of aphasia. *In* Disorders of language. DeReuck, A., and O'Connor, M., eds.
Marie, P. 1906. Revision de la question de l'aphasie. *Sem. Med. Paris*, 26, 241–247.
Meyer, V. 1961. Psychological effects of brain damage. *In* Handbook of abnormal psychology. Eysenck, W., ed. New York: Basic Books. Pp. 529–565.
Milner, B., Branch, C., and Rasmussen, T. 1964. Observations on cerebral dominance. *In* Disorders of language. DeReuck, A., and O'Connor, M., eds. Pp. 200–222.
Neilsen, J. 1941. A textbook of clinical neurology. New York: Paul Hoeber.
———. 1947. Agnosia, apraxia, aphasia (2nd. ed.). New York: Paul Hoeber.
Osgood, C., and Miron, M., eds. 1963. Approaches to the study of aphasia. Urbana: Univ. Ill. Press.
Penfield, W., and Roberts, L. 1959. Speech and brain mechanisms. Princeton N.J.: Princeton.
Reitan, R. 1955. Certain differential effects of left and right cerebral lesions in human adults. *J. comp. physiol. psychol.*, 6, 474–477.
———. 1966. Problems and prospects in studying the psychological correlates of brain lesions. *Cortex*, II, 1, 127–154.
Russell, W., and Espir, M. 1961. Traumatic aphasia. London: Oxford.
Teuber, H. 1962. Effects of brain wounds implicating right or left hemisphere in man. *In* Interhemispheric relations and cerebral dominance. Mountcastle, V., ed. Baltimore: Johns Hopkins Press.
Von Bonin, G. 1962. Anatomical asymmetries of the cerebral hemisphere. *In* Interhemispheric relations and cerebral dominance. Mountcastle, V., ed. Baltimore: Johns Hopkins Press.
Weinstein, S. 1962. Differences in effects of brain wounds implicating right or left hemisphere. *In* Interhemispheric relations and cerebral dominance. Mountcastle, V., ed. Baltimore: Johns Hopkins Press.
———. 1964. Deficits common with aphasia or lesions of either cerebral hemisphere. *Cortex*, I, 2, 154–169.
Weisenburg, T., and McBride, K. 1935. Aphasia. New York: Commonwealth Fund.
Wepman, J. 1951. Recovery from aphasia. New York: Ronald.

50

Therapeutic Problems and Approaches with Aphasic Adults

Jon Eisenson

Although direct therapy with aphasic patients was carried on by individual clinicians for many years, studies on therapeutic procedures, data on effectiveness, prognostic factors, and problems related to aphasia are post-World War II developments. The increase in our aging population and the survival rate for both traumatic and vascular origin aphasic patients have supplied both the impetus and the cases for investigation. The result has been the development of prognostic criteria and, fortunately, some hard data support for the value of therapy with aphasic adults. We are still a considerable distance from having all the answers we need as to when to begin therapy, and the values of specific direct and structured approaches compared with general stimulation and facilitation. We are not yet certain as to whether an aphasic relearns or reacquires language as a direct result of therapeutic efforts. We do, however, at least know that whichever it may be, the aphasic is more likely to progress in his language status if he has a therapeutic relationship identified with "language instruction" than if left alone for "spontaneous" recovery. We shall review some of the studies on the aforementioned points.

Aspects of Therapy

The objective of therapy for an adult aphasic is to restore him to as close to his premorbid status as circumstances will permit. For most adults this means that social, linguistic, and vocational readjustments need to be made. Wepman[1] refers to the "three faces of aphasia: the psychoneurological, the psycholinguistic, and the psychosocial." For some aphasics one aspect may need to be emphasized considerably more than the others. It may well be that an occasional aphasic may not be able to make any appreciable improvement in language and may yet be able to gain considerably from therapeutic efforts that emphasize psychosocial adjustments. This is a point stressed by Wepman in his personal communication to the author. Wepman wrote: "More recently, . . . I have begun to emphasize non-linguistic aspects of recovery using a more global attack upon the totality of the problem faced by the patient, where language is an important aspect but only an aspect and not the sole principle of the therapy." The ultimate goal of therapy is to help the aphasic to find a goal if not a purpose in the life that is ahead for him. In some instances this may well be a return, if he wishes, to his former position. In many instances, a modification of the position and role may be in order. The same kind of day in essentially the same setting, but a shorter and less strenuous one. In all too many instances the aphasic may not make sufficient gains either physically or linguistically for any such objective to be attained. Yet some of these patients may

[1] J. Wepman, personal communication.

also have some role in society other than that of completely dependent persons in a completely structured environment. Thus, we agree with Wepman that the need is for "the greatest emphasis being placed on the patient's role in life and reacceptance into society whether he talks or not."

What we have suggested relative to the aspects of therapy are not, of course, the sole responsibility of the language clinician. The family, the educational and vocational therapists, and the psychotherapist may need to be involved actively in the recovery of the aphasic. Most important, however, the aphasic must himself become as actively engaged as his physical condition permits. Recovery must necessarily be the concern of those professional persons identified as therapists, but must also become the primary concern of the individual identified as the patient.

Value of Direct Language Therapy

In the first edition of this Handbook we reported our impressions as to the positive value of direct language therapy and indicated that waiting for spontaneous recovery may be an injustice to the patient. We reported findings by Butfield and Zangwill (1946) and Wepman (1951, pp. 98–99) in support of the value of direct and early initiation of training. A retrospective study by Vignolo (1964) on 69 aphasic patients in answer to the key question: "Does specific language training and re-education have a decisive influence on the course and outcome of aphasia?" permits a positive affirmative answer. Vignolo concluded that "Re-education has a specific effect provided that it lasts more than six months. Its influence seems decisive in patients examined for the first time in the period between two and six months from onset."

When to Begin Training?

Our answer to the question above is "Just as soon as the patient is able to take notice of what is going on about him." Although it is true that the greatest amount of spontaneous recovery takes place during the first six months after the onset of the aphasic involvement, it has also been found that the period of two months after onset is crucial for the recovery process. Patients who were examined and had therapy initiated no later than two months after onset improved considerably more than patients for whom therapy was delayed beyond two months (Vignolo, 1964). Similar observations were made by Butfield and Zangwill (1946) on a group of British aphasic patients and by Eisenson (1949).

Even if there were no objective findings to support the recommendation for an early initiation of training, the following argument could be made. A delay in training permits aphasic patients to resort to and develop nonlinguistic methods of communication, or to reconcile themselves to being cut off from communication with their environment. For some patients, secondary gains from nonverbal communication might be established. Patients may expect that their needs and wishes will be anticipated, and so reduce their attempts at making their wants known. Once this attitude is assumed, its modification may be difficult.

Another approach to the problem is the need to appreciate that, except for physical therapy and reeducation, aphasic patients have little to occupy them. The psychological support afforded the patient by the therapist, the awareness that the patient is having something taking place in which he is an *active participant*, all undoubtedly help to accelerate improvement. Even if we should admit that the only real value of training is psychotherapeutic and arises out of a relationsip between the patient and the therapist, early reeducation is recommended. Wepman (1951, pp. 98–99) argues for early training with reasons which include the following: a failure to begin training may result either in the rejection of the patient, or in the patient becoming infantalized; patients who do not receive training may tend to become reconciled to their limitations and to withdraw from social intercourse; and later, they may resist attempts at assistance and evidence irritability or yield readily to catastrophic behavior reaction patterns if frustrated.

Prognostic Factors

An underlying danger in predicting recovery for aphasia patients is that the prediction may be self-fulfilling. If, for example, a clinician is persuaded that patients who do not show a fair amount of spontaneous improvement within six months after onset are not likely to make good ultimate recoveries, and so waits for six months to see what will happen, his prediction is likely to be fulfilled. Vignolo (1964) noted that "Time elapsed from onset is an important prognostic factor; two and six months from onset seem to be important milestones in the progress of aphasia." Further, "Reeducation has a specific effect provided it lasts more than six months. Its influence seems decisive in patients examined for the first time in the period between two and six months from onset."

What we have said is not intended to suggest that all aphasics have an equal chance in their recovery process. However differently they are stated, there are differences and predictive factors about which we have fairly good common agreement.

Eisenson (1949) summarized his observations of more than 100 aphasic patients ranging in age from 18 to above 60 years. "Prognosis would seem good for young aphasic patients whose disturbances are associated with traumatic causes, who have or had outgoing personalities, for whom a training program is started early, and who have a modest aspiration level. Prognosis appears less hopeful for older patients, for those for whom training is delayed, for those who have persistent euphoria, for patients whose personality picture reveals rigidity or psychopathic tendencies, and for those patients who develop great dependency on their clinicians."

Similar observations were made by Wepman (1951, pp. 68–82). Longerich and Bordeaux (1954) believe that expressive aphasics are more likely to recover than receptive aphasics. Vignolo (1964) observes that "there are hints that anarthria has a significant retarding effect on recovery from aphasia." Schuell's (1964, Ch. 9) prognostic factors are related to her test findings and are the basis for her classification of aphasic patients. Essentially, the findings indicate that the aphasic who does not have related perceptual, sensorimotor, or dysarthric components has a better outlook for recovery than one with such complications.

One prognostic factor that most clinicians accept as hopeful is the patient's ability for self correction. A negative implication is a patient's persistent failure to become aware of errors, or to correct an error when attention is directed to it.

The value of language training for the severe (global) aphasic seems doubtful. Sarno (1968, Research Brief)[2] reports that "Neither non-programmed nor programmed speech therapy enhanced language recovery in the severe aphasic subjects. . . ." This report agrees with that of Schuell who found, as we have indicated, that patients characterized by almost complete loss of functional language skills presented an irreversible aphasic syndrome." Schuell (1964, p. 199) observed, "We are therefore forced to the conclusion that there is a degree of cerebral damage that is incomparable with recovery of language skills."

We should note for the record that both Sarno and Schuell were limiting their observations to *recovery from language* skills. Nothing in their observation suggests that there should be no effort in the direction of social "skills." In fact, Sarno in her Research Brief is emphatic that "the rehabilitation emphasis for the severe expressive-receptive aphasic should be social and psychological in thrust."

We feel it important to add a precautionary note in regard to severe (global) aphasics. A conclusion that a patient has no functional speech should not be made on the basis of a single assessment or when the patient is severely ill. Judgment should be held for a period of two or three months after onset and made on the basis of two or three separate assessments at least a week apart.

SOME PROBLEMS RELATED TO THERAPY

Need For Motivation

The need for an aphasic patient to improve his linguistic ability is usually so strong that motivation for improvement may ordinarily be expected to come from the patient. This is generally so in the period immediately following awareness of the existence of impairment. Unless values become established that make linguistic improvement less worthwhile than the maintenance of these values, motivation for language rehabilitation may be assumed. Occasionally a patient may learn that it is possible to impose tyranny without words where tyranny with words could not previously be imposed. Such a patient may, for a short or an indefinite time, resist or reject reacquisition of language habits and will require external motivation to modify his attitude toward relearning. One of the advantages of early training is that the patient does not have an opportunity for realizing that there may be values in not using language, so that self-motivation rather than external motivation can function.

[2] Sarno, Martha T., 1968, Research Brief on Speech Therapy and Language Recovery in Severe Aphasia, Institute of Rehabilitation Medicine, N.Y. University School of Medicine.

As a rule, the problem of motivation, if it occurs at all, is one which begins to take place when the aphasic reaches his first plateau in learning. Then, having reacquired some language, and having improved to some extent in his comprehension and production of language and in his overall communicative ability, he may require urging to make the necessary effort for further progress. If effort has been great, and progress small, the discouraged patient may prefer not to try but to resort instead to wishful thinking that spontaneous improvement will occur, that tomorrow "things will be better." It is also possible that the patient may accept himself with or despite of his limitations and feel little need for further improvement. This attitude may in fact be nurtured by members of his family, or by his friends, who may overestimate gains, or who may begin to understand his nonlinguistic behavior or to anticipate his wants and so reduce the need for conventional language usage.

Degree and Direction of Motivation

Perhaps the most significant problem in regard to motivation is the problem of how much and to what degree. Should the highly educated patient be encouraged to believe that in a short time he may expect to be as linguistically proficient as once he was? Should the engineer, the mathematician, the lawyer, the teacher, or the physician be encouraged to believe that he will again have control of all he once knew and be able to return to his profession? No categorical answer can or should be given to these questions. At the present time we do not know how close to a premorbid level of verbal and intellectual proficiency a given patient can approximate. To promise too much may lead to disappointment and frustration. To promise too little may result in reduction of effort. The approach we recommend is to set up a series of short-term objectives which the patient can recognize, and to raise the sights and objectives as the individual patient's rate and amount of improvement warrant. To the patient's insistent question, "Will I be able to talk and read and write as well as I once could?" the safest and most honest answer is, "We'll see as we go along."

The goals and achievement objectives should be correlated with the overall training program planned for the patient. Questions about the patient's possible vocational training or retraining must be considered and answered. His sensory and motor limitations, if they are likely to be permanent, must necessarily be considered. His past interests, his hobbies, his avocations, must all be evaluated. If a patient, because of permanent motor or sensory disability, cannot possibly resume an occupation, even should complete linguistic recovery be possible, the new vocation, if any, should determine in large part the ultimate objective of the rehabilitative program, and so the degree and direction of motivation.

Level of Aspiration

It is understandable that most aphasic patients wish to become restored to a previous level of ability in the shortest possible time. Unfortunately, few if any normal persons ever know what level of ability they have. Normal persons may either underestimate or overestimate ability levels. So also may the aphasic patient. It is likely, however, that the aphasic may not appreciate how long it took him to achieve whatever premorbid level he thinks he had attained, and so he may become impatient to be restored to that level. A danger also exists that more often than not the patient will overestimate previously developed abilities and set himself too high an aspiration level for rehabilitation. In language performance this tendency may be expressed in the wish to speak in long sentences and in polysyllable, low-frequency terminology when short, simple sentences with high-frequency words could do as well.

The relationship between motivation and level of aspiration is apparent. The role of the therapist in helping the patient modify or reduce, *as an immediate objective*, a very high level of aspiration should be equally apparent.

Low Aspiration Level

Not infrequently a patient will become apparently satisfied with a relatively low level of achievement. There may be several possible reasons for this tendency. The patient may be one who in his premorbid state never tried particularly hard for any high level of achievement and was easily satisfied with what he could do readily. On the other hand, the patient may be one who reduced his level of aspiration to avoid frustration and repeated experiences of failure. His acceptance of a low-level achievement as an aphasic constitutes a continuation of a preinvolvement attitude and conduct pattern. A third possibility is that the aphasic patient has reevaluated his present assets and liabilities and has reached a decision as to how much language he needs to get along. In arriving at his evaluation, he has included the privileges and exemptions of the physically disabled. His aspiration level is a reflection both of what he expects of himself and what he expects others to do for and about him. Such a patient will require motivation to continue to make new evaluations in terms of amount of improvement. He must have his assets and his potentialities brought to his attention so that his low aspiration level does not become a persistent liability. The clinician should, however, be able to recognize that the acceptance of a low aspiration level may in effect constitute a patient's mechanism for avoiding future failure and frustration. With this awareness, he may be able to help the aphasic patient accept occasional failure in learning experience as a normal aspect of living as well as of the process of rehabilitation and training.

Concretism

Concretism, when it exists, is often an expression of the aphasic patient's attitude rather than an inherent aspect of his involvement. There is little question, however, that occasionally a patient does manifest concretism and indicates a strong preference to deal with situations that touch upon his immediate needs and experiences rather than to assume a more difficult attitude in which the needs and viewpoints of others require consideration. For the therapist, a patient's expression of concretism constitutes an additional challenge. Except with very old patients, and with patients who regardless of age were premorbidly so inclined, concretism as an attitude and as a mode of behavior can usually be modified in the course of therapy.

We have often been successful in modifying aphasic patients' tendencies and expressions of concretism by directing attention to its manifestations when they become apparent. If the patient has no appreciable difficulty in the understanding of speech, a frank discussion of the meaning and implications of concretism may be helpful. The patient can be helped by being given insights into the limitations imposed by concretism in reacquiring verbal behavior and especially in appreciating the intention of speakers as well as the literal or face meanings of their utterances.

The therapist should also be aware that concretism as a tendency may be developed by faulty training techniques. If, for example, a therapist working to build up an aphasic's vocabulary has the patient learn to identify and name objects such as a black pencil, a crayon pencil, and an automatic pencil, and fails to emphasize that despite the differences, all the objects are *kinds of pencils*, serve a common function, and are called *pencils*, an opportunity to abstract and generalize has been lost. Instead, a patient's tendency to be specific and concrete may be reinforced. In teaching names for objects, situations, or relationships, the therapist should emphasize the generic aspects of the names wherever and whenever the opportunity permits. Thus, a lesson on paper should include different kinds of paper, one on apples should include apples of different size, shape, and color, and so on. All this need not be accomplished in a single teaching session or in a given day. The therapist may confine the teaching to two or three members of a generic family, one during one learning period, and then begin a second period with a statement such as the following: "Yesterday you identified and named an apple when I showed you a red apple (presenting picture or actual apple). Today we have a green apple. It is shaped like the red one, and is about the same size, but it is green. Some apples are red, some are green, and others are yellow. In fact, apples may have several different colors or shades."

In reestablishing a patient's naming ability, the therapist should go out of his way to provide manifold stimulation for the name category. This means that the therapist's "bag of tricks" must be large, and the individual items must be changed frequently so that the associations the patient makes will not be limited to a single item under a general category. Specifically, not one comb but several combs of various sizes, shapes, and colors should be included to establish not only the *name* comb but the *concept* comb as well. So with other objects such as forks, books, brushes, and so on. The generic term should be taught as well as the specific term. It is the therapist's task to direct the patient's attention to why, *despite some differences, essential similarities make things belong to the same category and call for their having the same family name*.

Although the discussion above dealt with object naming, the principle is intended for naming in general. Relationships, representations, and situations in general which have either common or proper names can be similarly presented so that specific as well as generic names are learned at the earliest possible time. If this is done it is likely that a patient's tendency, if it exists, to be concrete-minded will be discouraged. Moreover, the therapist himself will avoid training the patient in a manner which might help to establish a concrete attitude that otherwise would not exist.

PERSEVERATION

Earlier it was indicated that the perseverating tendency was probably the most frequently found characteristic of persons with organic brain involvement. Perseveration was defined as the tendency for an act of behavior to persist or remount into consciousness spontaneously after it has once occurred. We can understand the significance of the perseverating tendency and will be better able to deal with it therapeutically if we have some insight into the dynamics of perseverations.

In general, perseveration may be thought of as a disturbance of volition. Perseveration becomes manifest when the usually potent tendencies for a given performance task are somehow blocked, diverted in some way by an inhibiting event or idea, or completely overcome by an interfering (previously performed or entertained) act or idea.

Normal persons tend to perseverate when they are fatigued; they also tend to perseverate under conditions which demand more rapid and more frequent change than they can achieve. Epileptic persons increase their frequency of perseveration after seizures. Perseveration, in general, may be the human mechanism's way of reacting to situations which demand adaptations and call for responses which the individual is not capable, momentarily or chronically, of making. If the failure to make the adaptation is momentary, the repetition of a previous act which requires little or no conscious effort affords the individual opportunity to select or to organize a new response which he hopes is appropriate. If, for organic or psychogenic reasons, the inability to make ready adaptations is chronic, the repetition of a response fills a void which would exist if no response were made. The individual, aware that some response is expected, repeats an old response to avoid the embarrassment of failing to make any response. In general, perseveration may be regarded as a manifestation of inadequacy on the part of the performer. When the aphasic patient perseverates, he is in effect saying, "I am not able to do what is expected, so I am doing something I have previously done which was appropriate. I hope it is better than doing nothing." Beyond this, however, he is saying something which is of greater significance to the therapist. He is signaling that the therapist's demands, at the given moment in the given situation, are excessive. It becomes the problem of the therapist to discover why the demands are excessive, and to modify them in keeping with the aphasic's present abilities.

The first recommended step for the therapist is to present a situation to the patient for which the perseverated act is appropriate. If, for example, a patient has named one of series of objects correctly and then, because of inability to name a new object, repeats the name of a previous one, that one should again be presented. The response then becomes appropriate. Then the therapist should review the series up to the point where perseveration had occurred. At this point the therapist should himself offer the name and ask for the patient to repeat it. If blocking or perseveration reoccurs, the therapist should again call for a previously successful naming performance and put aside for a later time the learning of the new object. It is then usually wise for the therapist to change the situation and the type of task required so that the patient's inadequacy will not be recalled and so interfere with new learning or relearning. In answer to my question, "What is the significance of perseveration in a learning situation?" a recovered aphasic replied, "It means that the therapist is not aware of what is going on with the patient. Good therapy avoids the need for perseveration. When it occurs, the therapist has failed to do a good job."

Although perseveration cannot always be avoided, awareness on the part of the therapist that his patient is showing signs of fatigue, irritability, or disinterest will go a long way to reducing its incidence. Moderation of pace, or a change of activity, frequently will be all that is needed to eliminate perseveration when it becomes evident, or to prevent the need for it to become evident.

THE CATASTROPHIC RESPONSE

The *catastrophic response* may be characterized as a "psychobiological breakdown" involving the organism as a whole in a situation where a successful performance does not seem possible. Vascular changes, irritability, evasiveness, or aggressiveness may precede or accompany the catastrophic response. An extreme catastrophic response may take the form of a loss of consciousness. The dynamics of the catastrophic response are comparable to those of perseverating behavior. The patient is revealing inadequacy and a wish to avoid the need to make a response. If a way out is not available and escape from the situation, psychological or physical, is not permitted, the catastrophic response may occur. Frequently, it will be preceded by perseverating behavior. Some patients resort to catastrophic behavior more immediately and more frequently than do others. We believe that many of these patients are ones who, prior to brain insult, were likely to resort to psychosomatic symptoms such as headache or fatigue to avoid difficult or demanding situations.

The significance of the catastrophic response for the therapist is essentially the same as that of perseveration. If it occurs during the course of therapy, the catastrophic response signifies that the therapist's demands, at the given moment, have exceeded the patient's ability in producing an appropriate response. Reduced demand or change of activity is indicated. It is best, of course, to avoid an extreme catastrophic response if this can be done. Alertness to signs of irritability, such as apparent disinterest, sweating, or excessive eyeblinking, should serve as cues to the therapist that the patient is finding the situation, or the changing situations, too difficult for his adaptive abilities. A brief recess in which a cigarette may be smoked, or a piece of candy eaten, or casual conversation undertaken, may be all that is needed to avoid pushing the patient into a catastrophic manifestation. Once the catastrophic response has been resorted to, a sensitive patient may need considerable time as an ego-saving measure. If he is not sensitive, there is danger that the patient will become consciously aware of a device he may use in the future to avoid difficult situations. In a large measure, the manifestation of the catastrophic response, as well as of perseveration, reveals failure on the part of the therapist to recognize the needs and abilities of his patient as well as inadequacy on the part of the patient to meet the needs of his situation.

PSYCHOTHERAPY

The Place of Psychotherapy

There is probably less question as to the aphasic patient's need for psychotherapy than there is as to whether and how this need can be met. It is fairly obvious that any individual whose thinking and communicative ability have been disturbed and who has awareness of these disturbances must reorient and readjust himself to the modifications which they impose. Any person deprived of a means of being economically self-supporting, or who is able to continue only with the help of others to whom he recognizes an obligation, can benefit from psychotherapy to assist him in making the necessary adjustments. If, in addition, an individual is suffering from varying and changing degrees of sensory and/or motor disability, there can be little doubt that psychotherapy, if it can be made available, is indicated. This includes most, if not all, aphasic patients. There is however, considerable doubt that psychotherapy can be made available to most aphasics. Nevertheless, we are concerned that in many instances more harm than good is accomplished through any direct attempt at psychotherapy. The basic reason for this concern is the appreciation that, despite the aphasic's need, language—the instrument for direct psychotherapy—is impaired. Without assurance that the patient is able to understand, to reveal the amount of his understanding or misunderstanding, direct psychotherapy is precarious. Certainly, direct psychotherapy should not be undertaken unless the aphasic patient has sufficient language ability to express himself and to understand what is being explained to him as well as the need for the explanation.

The therapist who undertakes to work directly and individually with an aphasic must not only be qualified in psychotherapy but must have specific experience with aphasic patients. He must be constantly aware that he cannot assume that the patient completely understands on even an intellectual level what he is trying to have him understand. The usual test of understanding—an appropriate verbalization—is not to be expected of the aphasic.

Beyond this precaution, there is another which should be observed. The aphasic patient should probably not be given direct psychotherapy if his problems, were he not an aphasic, would otherwise not come to the attention of a psychotherapist. An aphasic patient is entitled to a certain number of problems because he is a human being. As such, he, in common with other human beings, should be permitted to work his problems through himself. It is only when his problems are too severe, or too numerous, that psychotherapy should be considered.

An essential aspect of therapy for the aphasic, which can usually be worked out indirectly and without the intervention of an especially-trained psychotherapist, is the patient's necessary acceptance of himself as himself, disabilities included, on a temporary basis. The patient should be encouraged to postpone a "final assessment" and to make re-evaluations of his changing self as language, sensory, and motor improvements take place. The aphasic must be given time to adjust to his disabilities and limitations, and to the attitudes of his family, relatives, friends, and other members of his environment.

Dependency Relationships

Because of the aphasic's communicative, expressive, and frequent physical disabilities, there is a strong likelihood that he will quickly become dependent on the first person who understands him and apparently accepts him as he is. Frequently, such a person will be the language therapist. For the welfare of the aphasic patient, and to some degree for the therapist, it is important that dependency be avoided. There is grave danger that the aphasic who finds acceptance and understanding in the therapist will become satisfied with that relationship and so avoid others which may be less satisfactory. Having made one adjustment and worked out one relationship, he will not undertake the risks of other adjustments and relationships. Even in regard to language which is recovered, the aphasic patient may limit his verbal behavior to situations in which the therapist is involved. Doing so, he reduces the likelihood for disapproval, often more imagined than real, for communicative failure. Unfortunately, this limitation also restricts practice in expression and communication, with resultant undesirable effects for ultimate social adjustment as well as language improvement.

From the point of view of the therapist, a dependency relationship is also undesirable. The tendency for a therapist to become subjectively and personally involved in working with a handicapped individual is understandable. Frequently, such a relationship satisfies a need which the therapist may unconsciously have—a need to be needed. It is, however, difficult for effective therapy to be carried on when a patient's failure becomes one which the therapist shares. When the patient's moods, frustrations, successes, or defeats are felt by the therapist, he cannot do justice to the individual patient whose experience he is sharing subjectively. Nor, under the circumstances, can he work effectively with other patients with whom he has a different relationship.

The therapist must maintain objective interest and avoid subjective involvement. One way of doing this, if the rehabilitative program permits, is to have a team of therapists working with several aphasic patients individually, as well as in a group. If the therapist is in private practice, and does not have a group of aphasic patients, he must maintain objectivity though working individually. If he finds this too difficult, in fairness to the patient as well as himself, the patient should be referred to another therapist for treatment.

GROUP THERAPY

The question of whether aphasic patients should have the benefits of group therapy is one which cannot be decided solely on the basis of the values or of the shortcomings of group work per se. As a practical matter, few clinicians who do private work, and relatively few clinics, except those in large urban areas, are likely to have a sufficient number of aphasics in treatment at any one time to make the group approach possible.

We accept Schuell's position (1964, p. 343) "that individual therapy and group therapy are two entirely different classes of events, serve different purposes, and should not be confused." Group training cannot be justified on the basis of economy of effort or expense. It can be justified only as an adjunct to individual therapy providing the adjunctive values can be served better in a group of patients identified as aphasic rather than in some other community situation. Probably the greatest value of group therapy is that the patient becomes aware that his is not an isolated problem, that there are others "in the same boat." This very recognition, however, constitutes a basis for care in selection. If an aphasic assesses improvement in terms of how severe other patients' limitations may be after a period of training, rather than of how much progress may have been made, then a group experience may have negative effects for him. The decision as to whether a given patient is to participate in adjunctive group therapy must then be made on an individual basis, and often on a trial basis with the effects carefully observed and assessed by the responsible clinician.

Values of Group Therapy

Where feasible, group therapy for aphasics is recommended for the following assumed values:

1. Group training provides *an opportunity for socialization*. The aphasic because of his communicative handicap, cannot socialize with verbally normal

persons as an equal. As a member of a group of similarly handicapped persons, socialization becomes more possible. In setting up a group, it is essential that a relaxed attitude prevail. Blackman (1950) set up a group situation for aphasics and was able to report that the individual aphasic lost his feelings of isolation and apparently enjoyed the friendly competitiveness and social acceptance of the others. Activities that may successfully be included to increase socialization and group belongingness include: singing of both well-known and current popular songs; practicing "social-gesture" speech such as acknowledgements of greetings, introducing a new member to a group, and leave-taking from a group. These activities provide situations for the practice of linguistic units which most aphasic patients can evoke with relative facility.

In these group activities, the patient must be encouraged to do as well as he can. If he cannot sing with words, but can hum or whistle a tune, then the humming or whistling should be approved. One way of establishing group approval for nonverbal expression is to begin by setting up a music situation in which, initially, some individuals are asked to hum, some whistle, and some sing the words of the song. In response to a greeting, if the patient finds it difficult to respond with a "Fine, thank you" to a "How are you?" or "How do you do?" then a gesture or a simple "O.K." plus a gesture should be encouraged.

When the group has "jelled" and the members have built up an *esprit de corps*, then more ambitious projects such as skits, charades, and quiz programs may be included. With an advanced group, discussions of current problems may be introduced. Such discussions may be preceded by a reading of highlights of the day's news or a period of listening to or viewing a news broadcast. It is important to bear in mind that in the early stages of group work, participation and not accuracy of information is the objective. As the individuals of the group find participation becoming easier, other aspiration levels and objectives may be set.

2. Group training provides an opportunity for *motivation from peers* rather than from the superior clinician. It is easier for an aphasic to try to evoke a response, or read a phrase if another patient has tried, failed at first, and succeeded after a second or third attempt. The motivation of "You can do it, Joe. You saw me try and finally get it" coming from one aphasic is more readily acceptable to another than when it comes from a therapist who has no linguistic impairment.

3. The group approach provides a situation in which awareness of certain aphasic *speech "habits,"* such as telegraphic and agrammatical language structure, become apparent. The aphasic who uses telegraphic speech, who omits prepositions and conjunctions, will appreciate the difficulty of understanding such language when he hears it from others. Such appreciation should provide motivation for improvement. The verbalized "I don't know what you mean when you talk like that," or the implied failure of comprehension which one aphasic can read from the faces of others who are listening and trying to understand him, should stimulate an attempt at a more conventional language pattern so that "I-fish-Sunday" may be changed to "I'm going fishing next Sunday."

4. Group training provides an aphasic patient with an opportunity to observe the techniques of other aphasics for evoking speech and for getting speakers to make themselves understood. The individual patient also has in the group a ready-made and sympathetic audience for the testing of his own techniques for oral expression. The techniques which prove to be successful can then be used outside of the group. The unsuccessful techniques can be delayed for outside use until further testing indicates whether they are inappropriate for the given patient and should be put aside for others. In brief, the group provides an opportunity for vicarious as well as active learning. The aphasic can learn by observation without direct ego-involvement and risk of failure.

5. Still another advantage of group training is that it provides the aphasic with an opportunity in a learning situation to respond to more than one manner of speech and language usage. The clinician has habits of speaking which are peculiar to him. The aphasic whose learning is associated with the person becomes accustomed to the manner of this person. When others are introduced, learning is not limited to one speaker, and adjustments to others are not so difficult to make as they may become without group training.

6. The last of the advantages of the group approach to be considered is the opportunity it provides for *ventilation of feelings and an airing of grievances*. Aphasic patients, in common with most handicapped persons, develop feelings of hostility and aggression. Some of these are, undoubtedly, realistically justified; others are not. The expression of these feelings as

well as their evaluation can be accomplished in a group situation. The knowledge and assurance that an aphasic patient gains when he learns that others feel or have felt like him, and have to a large extent gotten over their feelings, is of invaluable help. This constitutes psychotherapy without imposition. With it, the aphasic is likely to feel less isolated, and in time, less hostile to the nonaphasics with whom he must live.

Shortcomings of Group Therapy

As we have indicated, the group approach is not without some possible disadvantages. For the most part, the disadvantages to be considered can all be overcome with skilled handling on the part of the clinician directing the group, or in individual sessions with the patient.

1. Withdrawn patients may find it difficult to attempt expression as members of a group. They may inhibit even the small amount of speech available to them rather than risk faulty expression before a group. Instead of attempting speech, as they may be encouraged to do in individual treatment, withdrawn patients may develop techniques of avoiding response, or may "hide behind" talkative ones and limit their own production to simple gestures of agreement or disagreement.

2. Group pressure may provoke some patients into talking about personal problems before they are entirely ready for such revelations. Patients not adequately able to define their problems may find their explanations misunderstood or improperly evaluated. The impact of such a reaction may set the patients back considerably in their rate of progress. Although an alert group therapist tries to avoid this situation, avoidance is not always possible.

3. The rate of a group is usually slower than the best member can manage and somewhat faster than the weakest member can progress. Patients who have made considerable improvement may be irked by having to slow down. Patients who are slow learners may find the pace uncomfortable, become confused, and cease trying to maintain the group's pace.

Despite these possible shortcomings, our experience with patients working in groups has been generally favorable. We cannot be too emphatic, however, that group training is recommended to supplement and not to replace individual training. If proper precautions are exercised, and no aphasic patient is introduced into a group until he has shown readiness for it, the advantages of group training will by far outweigh any possible disadvantages.

Learning Characteristics of Aphasics

Any generalization as to the learning capacities and characteristics of aphasics must be modified by the reservation that those who make a good and quick recovery are not likely to remain in settings where they can serve as subjects of experimental investigations. In effect, then, studies of hospitalized patients are likely to include subjects with *maintained aphasic involvements*, those which persist beyond six months or more after onset. Our references will be to studies that did not emphasize the use of language as a response mode or as a mediator for responses. We will present the findings of a few representative studies with no pretense of being exhaustive.

Tikofsky and Reynolds (1962) compared 15 aphasic subjects with 20 nonaphasics on a modification of Grant's Wisconsin Card Sorting Task. The results indicated that the learning rate of aphasics is slower than for nonaphasics. Perseverative errors appeared to be a major determinant of the aphasics' slower rate of learning. Carson, Carson, and Tikofsky (1968) studied 64 adult aphasics with a comparison group of 64 normals in a four experimental learning tasks. These included three which did not call for language responses (response uncertainty tasks, repeated digit symbol, and rule learning tasks) and one (rote serial learning) which did. The investigators concluded that the characteristics which distinguished the aphasics from the normals were slower speed and frequently lower level of attainment. The aphasics as a group did not indicate an inability to perform any of the difficult experimental tasks "despite the fact that aphasics demonstrated limited retention and transfer of learning in general, virtually every aphasic improved with practice in a specific stimulus-response situation." It is important to note that the experimental population was comprised of subjects who were all beyond the acute stage of illness (from six months to two years after the onset of their disturbances) and that they were engaged in an intensive therapeutic program which *selected out* both minimally impaired subjects and any that might evidence chronic deterioration.

Brookshire (1968) compared nine aphasics and eight nonaphasic hospital patients on a visual discrimination learning task in which the subjects had to learn a differential motor response to visual stimuli.

Brookshire concluded that the aphasic subjects as a group had more difficulty in learning the task than did the comparison group subjects. In addition, the aphasics showed greater variability of performance than did the control group.

LEARNING TECHNIQUES

The basic principles which govern the language learning of normal persons, adults as well as children, hold for aphasics. Associations are strengthened if they are rewarded. If information and insight can be added to or become an integral characteristic of the reward, learning progresses more smoothly and reliably than with noninformative, noninsightful rewards. Other things being equal, frequency of occurrence of an association helps to strengthen it. Learning situations which have an objective, meaningful, and significant goals for the patient, help to motivate and direct the relearning.

There are some essential similarities between an aphasic's relearning and the learning of a new (foreign) language by an adult without brain injury. There are, however, a few important differences which must be understood if a rehabilitative program with an aphasic adult is to be successful.

Differences Between Aphasic's Relearning and Normal Adult Language-Learning

1. The normal adult who learns a new—for him a foreign—language does so with unimpaired cortical association areas and with intact sensory and neuromotor mechanisms. For the aphasic, the association areas are, by definition, injured; and the sensory and neuromotor mechanisms may also be impaired.

2. The normal adult who learns a new language is not disturbed by remnants of what he once knew. He is aware that he is starting with a "clean slate." The aphasic in "relearning" is often hindered as well as helped by what he once knew. Residuals of established habits and old plans may interfere with the establishment of new strategies and techniques for learning.

3. The normal adult in a new learning enterprise cannot hope that patterns and associations will come to him spontaneously. He knows that he must apply himself to establish patterns and associations and to evolve rules for the new language. For the aphasic, some associations do come back spontaneously, and it is understandable that he will hope that spontaneous recovery will continue. This hope may, and frequently does, interfere with voluntary efforts at relearning.

Reinforcement Through Reward

The adult aphasic is susceptible to reward, but the rewards must not be too obviously made. The material or chocolate drop reward following an appropriate response may do very well for a child. For the adult, a more mature reward may consist in the information that he is "right." This information may come in the form of a verbal response, a gesture of approval, or the continuation of a conversation which incorporates the appropriate word in the therapist's response.[3] After a series of correct responses, a general type of reward might be given in the form of a drink, a snack, or some other pleasant break in the session. A break, however, should not be made if the patient is doing well and obviously enjoying his successes. It is better made when the patient shows first signs of fatigue, tension, or anxiety.

The severely aphasic patient from whom only limited and "approximate" responses may be anticipated may be helped by carefully planned "programmed" instruction. Such a program, described in general terms by Holland (1969), moves the patient in controlled small steps from a response the patient is able to emit toward closer approximations (shaping) of the response-objective determined by the clinician-teacher. A well-established program demands a series of continuing responses from the learner; at each step of the program an acceptable (correct or appropriate) response is differentially reinforced.

Intensification of Stimulation

Intensification of stimulation can be achieved through an actual increase in the size or loudness of the material presented, or through repetition of the material, or through both. If visual material is used, the print size, at least at the outset, should be relatively large. Type at least twice the size of the type of this book is recommended. If the material is audible, intensity may be increased simply through talking more loudly than for ordinary conversation. Care should be exercised, however, that increased loudness does *not suggest yelling*. If a patient seems embarrassed by the

[3] See Holland (1969) for a discussion of differential rewards following Skinnerian principles of learning and their application to language rehabilitation for aphasics.

raised level of the clinician's voice, an amplifying unit may be used. In early stages, especially for patients with auditory aphasia, increased loudness may help to break down the "barrier of auditory resistance." Some patients prefer to have the audible material personalized by listening through earphones. This technique serves as an ego-saving device. No outsider then becomes aware that loud sounds are being poured into the patient's ears when headset earphones are used.

Repetition of stimulation is most successful when it is not too obvious. The child may learn to read by being exposed to a sentence such as "Tim saw the rabbit go hop, hop, hop." The adult prefers to have his "hops" better distributed. More subtle distribution is recommended for all forms of presentation. If, for example, a "new" word is to be added to the patient's functional language inventory, the word should be incorporated in the therapist's responses several times during the course of a session rather than be successively repeated.

Negative Practice

The conscious and deliberate use of an inappropriate word or phrase—the technique of negative practice (Dunlap, 1928)—has for some time been recognized as an excellent technique for eliminating unintentional errors. This technique is described in some detail by Van Riper (1963) as a method of correcting articulatory defects. For the aphasic, a modification of the technique of negative practice along the following lines is suggested:

If a patient evokes a wrong response in answer to a question such as: "What do you use for cutting meat?" and says *spoon* instead of *knife*, the therapist should explain that "We use a spoon for eating soup. We use a *knife* for cutting meat." This should be followed by presenting the patient with an opportunity to use the word *spoon* as an *appropriate response*, and then by a second opportunity to use the word *knife* correctly. If the word *knife* still cannot be readily evoked, further opportunity for the appropriate use of *spoon*, or whatever other word tends to be evoked, should be offered the aphasic. Through this approach, even though the word *knife* is not forthcoming, the patient has been enabled to learn correct associations for the word *spoon*, and an appropriate association has been formed.

For the correction of dysarthric errors, the conventional approach to the use of negative practice is recommended. Attention is directed to the error which the patient is making. The patient is then directed to repeat his error as closely as he can with awareness of how the sound or sound combination is being produced. The correct sound or combination is then presented for imitation and for contrast with the defective articulatory product.

Negative practice for dysarthric errors provides practice in recognition of sounds, in the controlled production of sounds, and practice in the habitual formation of the desired sound combinations.

Determining the Original Approach

Learning for the aphasic will frequently be facilitated if the therapist can determine how the content or process was originally learned, and in what way the learning was symbolized or recorded. For example, if a patient learned manuscript writing before cursive writing, it may help considerably if the manuscript approach is used with the patient who has writing difficulty. If the patient learned to tell time by adding the minutes to the hour (6:40 (six-40), 7:10 (seven-10), and so on), he should be taught time-telling that way rather than to say 20 minutes to seven, or 10 minutes after seven. In writing numbers for division, some patients used the arrangement $X\overline{)XX}$ for both "short" and long division; others used $X\underline{)X}$ for "short" division and $XX\overline{)XXX}$ for long division; still others used $X\overline{)XX}$ for all division. Information about the habit of the patient can frequently be obtained from members of the family. If this information is not available, the age of the patient and his place of education may provide clues as to the likely approach to school learning. Most young patients probably learned to subtract by the additive process so that $\begin{array}{r}6\\ \underline{-2}\end{array}$ will be worked as "Two and what make six? Two and four make six." Older patients may have been taught to subtract by the "take-away" process—"Six minus two is four." If the patient has used the phrase "take-away" instead of "minus," then the therapist should use that term with him.

Essentially, it should be remembered, most aphasic learning is actually reawakening or reestablishing of associations. This can usually best be accomplished by determining how the old associations were formed in the first place rather than by imposing the therapist's own way of making associations on the patient.

Raising the Level of Response

Earlier it was pointed out that there is a considerable amount of speech which remains relatively intact for most aphasic patients. These forms include emotionally laden speech content, automatic and serial speech, and social-gesture speech. Use can be made of these "low-level propositions" for "higher level" speech purposes.

A patient who cannot evoke readily the name of a number can be trained to *count* serially until that number comes up in the sequence, and then to stop at it. Later, he can be taught to say the sequence quickly and silently, and then to utter aloud only the numeral which is appropriate. In this way, patients can learn to give their telephone numbers, their home addresses, the date, and other functionally useful number-phrases. Similarly, patients can be taught to evoke a particular day of the week, or months of the year.

Automatic content such as prayers, familiar verse, and songs, can be used to evoke significant words and phrase. *Good* and *morning* can be evoked separately through the relatively automatic gesture phrase, "Good morning." A physician, Dr. Rose (1948), who suffered a stroke and associated aphasic involvement described his own retraining through his recollection and memorization of familiar lines of poetry, psalms, and other material which, according to him, "At one time I could almost say it in my sleep." In the account of his recovery, Dr. Rose explained that he also memorized or near-memorized considerable amounts of "new poetry." He recommends "Read often aloud and you will come close to memorizing. . . ."

Where bodily action is customarily or frequently associated with given locutions, as is often the case with gesture-phrases, the patient should be encouraged to engage in such action as an aid in the evocation of the desired words. Terms of greeting, as well as the single-word responses *Yes* and *No* can frequently be evoked more readily when associated with bodily action than when attempted alone.

Other techniques for facilitation of responses are discussed by Kreindler and Fradis (1968, Ch. 9).

Handedness Change

For many aphasic patients the need for changing handedness, generally, from the right to the left hand, is an essential and inevitable procedure. If the paralysis of the preferred hand is severe, a shift in handedness must be accomplished if the patient is to relearn writing. For the patient with residual weakness, the desirability for effecting the change has not yet been experimentally proven.

The idea of handedness change is frequently resisted by patients who still have some amount of control of the preferred hand. It is probable that the patient's wish to be as much like his former self as possible is responsible for this resistance. We recommend change of handedness for patients with upper extremity paresis because it has become apparent that in most instances both motor control and legibility of writing are improved. To overcome resistance, we suggest to the patient that he write with the nonpreferred hand for a period of a month. If, at the end of the period, the patient wishes to resume writing with the original hand, no objection would be made. Almost all patients who agreed to the month's trial period continued, as a matter of choice, to write with the alternate hand. Some were pleased that they had become "ambidextrous." Several patients admitted that they began to feel more secure about what they were writing, that "things clicked right inside their heads" shortly after they attained some degree of skill with the nonpreferred hand.

The accomplishment of a shift in handedness seldom takes more than three or four weeks—providing that resistance to the change has been overcome. Gardner's (1945) manual for left-handed writing has been found most useful for establishing the new writing technique.

How to Begin Training

Training should begin with an evaluation of the patient's assets and limitations. These should include a knowledge of what the patient can do, as well as what he cannot do, at the time the evaluation is being made. This knowledge should go beyond estimating the patient's present linguistic and general "educational performance" level. The complete picture should include an assaying of the patient's health history, his premorbid manner of reacting to illness, to frustration, and to the need to exert intellectual effort. This information will determine, to a large measure, how the patient is likely to respond to his present limitations.

An evaluation of linguistic ability can be made

through the use of aphasia inventories, several of which were described earlier, and educational achievement tests. An estimate of premorbid tendencies should come through an interview with responsible members of the family. An evaluation of present behavioral tendencies should come from direct observation. When these areas of information are obtained, the therapist will know what the patient is presently able to do, as well as what kind of a patient he has for reeducation. The therapist will then be ready for the next question: How do I begin specific linguistic reeducation?"

Probably the best broad answer to the question is: begin in an area in which the patient can be stimulated. More particularly, the area will depend upon the individual patient's immediate needs as well as his ultimate objectives and the strength of inner motivation in arriving at the objectives. If these are not known to the therapist, and occasionally they may not even be known to the patient, a trial-and-error, or better, a "trial-until-success," period is indicated. A failure to elicit a favorable response may merely mean that the area or mode of stimulation, for the time being, is not an appropriate one. Another should then be tried.

Frequently, the obvious needs of the patient may serve as a guide. If the patient is still in the hospital, words such as *nurse*, *water*, *comb*, or better, phrase-sentences which include such words, might well become an immediate starting point. The patient who can call attention to his needs, and who can thereby save himself embarrassment, has been helped to rediscover how very functional language can be. He can rediscover the magical power of words! The patient who can acknowledge a greeting, who can thereby indicate that he is still a vital human being, will command some respect and will ward off injury to his ego. Language which will help to achieve this end is a good area in which to begin to stimulate a patient.

The patient's less immediate objectives will depend upon a number of factors. Among these are the type and amount of sensory and motor involvement, the degree to which these involvements are likely to be permanent, the effect of these upon his reemployability, and the language needs of the patient in the light of his vocational goal. If this goal is too remote as a basis for stimulation, then the patient's avocations and hobbies should be considered. A reservation, however, must be made in regard to this area. If the patient's physical disabilities are such that the avocations may forever need to be put aside, stimulation in this area should be avoided. Failure to do so may merely remind the patient of what was and can no longer be, and frustration rather than successful stimulation may be the result.

Some specific examples of what can be done may be of help. One patient with right hemiplegia who had been a golf enthusiast was stimulated to start language training after he was provided with a set of left-handed golf clubs, and received instruction in their use. He then was willing to learn to read a manual on how to play golf, to learn to spell and say such words as *hole*, *tee*, *fairway*, *par*, *birdie*, and to read numbers which approximated "average duffer" golf scores. Another patient wanted most to learn to read his young wife's letters and to be able to say in his own words "How much I love her." A middle-aged woman patient wanted to be taught "how to talk back" to her nurse.

The Pathway for Stimulation

In general, the best pathway for stimulation will be the sensory and motor avenues which are intact or relatively unimpaired. Which these will be will depend, of course, upon the individual patient and can usually be determined after an adequate physical and linguistic examination. The information provided by the neurologist as to sensory and motor abilities and disabilities is essential. Questions of hearing loss as well as auditory aphasia, apraxic involvements, and so on, must also be answered. With such information, the therapist can usually decide whether the sensory avenue should be through vision, hearing, or possibly through the tactual pathway. He should also be able to decide whether the primary motor expression or output should be through speaking, writing, or through the use of symbol-gestures. A selected "complete circuit" may, for an individual patient, be aural for reception and graphic for production; for another it might well be visual for reception and oral for production.

Unless the patient, for reasons which cannot always be determined, rejects the avenues selected on the basis of physical examination, the "circuit pathways" should be developed until the patient is able to achieve a fair degree of facility in revealing his moods, attitudes, and thoughts. If the patient rejects or resists the use of these avenues, then the therapist must accept those which the patient himself prefers. In any event, it should be made clear that other receptive and productive avenues are not to be ignored. As soon as possible, practice through other avenues should be provided so that multiple associations may be made.

Schuell (1964, p. 352) argues strongly that "Techniques for stimulating language are the backbone of aphasia therapy." The techniques "depend upon a barrage of controlled auditory stimulation and upon feedback processes from obtained responses." The method described by Schuell (1964, pp. 353–356) is essentially one which employs visual-auditory association, employing a set of two to three hundred basic vocabulary cards *for adults*. Such cards may be made and individualized for each patient, or may be commercially available published materials.[4]

The auditory-visual association is established by exposing the picture card to the patient who is directed to "Look at the picture, and look at the word, as I say it. Try to hear it, and try to think it. When you have it, let it come out, but do not force it." The clinician points first to the picture, and then to the printed word, "saying the word strongly and clearly each time, and using about twenty repetitions." It is important that the clinician wait long enough between repetitions to permit the patient to rehearse and evoke the word if it is available to him.

Picture identification by a single word is a first step for the more severely impaired aphasics. For the less impaired, and for those who succeed in this first step, Schuell recommends that visual-auditory representations intended to elicit phrases or sentences become the next step. This is exceedingly important so that the patient is not reinforced in the use of agrammatic utterances. So, on the second level, a picture may be associated with the question "What is this man doing?" with an acceptable answer, "He (the man) is driving a car."

We should like to note that although Schuell considers her approach basically one for auditory stimulation, we consider it to be a visual-auditory approach with oral (spoken) feedback response. If a patient evidenced oral apraxia, or a severe anomia, we would strongly recommend that he write, print, or select the appropriate response in a controlled multiple choice situation.

It should not be taken for granted that every aphasic patient is readily available for reeducation. Some patients require a considerable amount of stimulation in order to become available for therapy. Along this line, Wepman (1953) characterizes appropriate stimulation as "What is done externally to the patient which produces some heightening of his efforts. This includes . . . every possible form of persuasion."

SPECIFIC TECHNIQUES

It is not possible, and probably not desirable, to present numerous specific techniques for the rehabilitation of aphasic patients. The best techniques are those which are designed for the individual patient. The therapist will find some useful advice and information in texts and articles on the subject of remedial education. We should not, however, assume that teaching a person to *read again* presents the same problems as teaching a poor reader, or a slow-to-get-started-reader, how to read in the first place.

At all times, the therapist must bear in mind that his patient is going to relearn (reacquire) considerably more language than he can possibly be taught directly. The basic job of the therapist is to get the patient going, to help him to realize that he can relearn. Once the patient appreciates this, neither he nor the therapist will be surprised at the large amount of spontaneous linguistic recovery which takes place.

The literature on training approaches for aphasics has grown large since World War II. Much of what has been published should probably best be regarded as description of approaches that have been found to be helpful to individual patients which have been generalized to "types of patients" with comparable language impairments. Most clinical aphasiologists are by no means certain about the rationale for their approaches, except that what they recommend has been found to work. Exceptions, perhaps, are Soviet aphasiologists such as Luria (1948) and Beyn (1964) and others influenced by their position. They do seem confident about the relationship of their therapeutic principles and practices to their theoretic concepts of aphasia.

With these reservations in mind, we should like to emphasize that the approaches and technique about to be considered are to be regarded as suggestions and not as prescriptions.

[4] Among the published materials are the Taylor and Marks Rehabilitation and Therapy Kit (1959), the Longerich Aphasia Therapy Sets (1959), and the Picture-Word Series for the Language Master (Moore and Schuell, 1954). We recommend that published cards be adjuncts and that the basic word-picture cards, if at all possible, be made for the patient from magazine illustrations. A patient who is free of manual motor disability may be encouraged to make his own illustrations.

THERAPEUTIC TECHNIQUES FOR INTAKE DISTURBANCES

Agnosias

Visual agnosias, as we indicated earlier, must be determined if the patient manifests any reading disability or, more generally, a disability in responding appropriately to visual configurations. An agnosia for visual form may explain a patient's inability to read. Occasionally, a patient will fail because the size of the configuration is too small. In keeping with the principle of intensification of stimulation, it is recommended that larger configurations be tried. When recognition is established with the larger ones, then the therapist should introduce smaller configurations until ones approximating those most commonly found are used.

If the patient demonstrates an agnosia for flat representations of forms, and can recognize three-dimensional forms, he should be given practice in associating one with the other. Such practice might consist of his placing three-dimensional configurations on sheets which have two-dimensional ones. That is, he is directed to place a rectangular block on a rectangle, a triangular block on a triangle, and so on. When he succeeds in doing this, the process should be reversed, and the patient is asked to place a cutout of a two-dimensional figure on the actual object. A final step should be the appropriate and ready selection of the flat figure as it is named by the therapist.

Visual agnosia becomes a significant problem for aphasics if it involves *letter recognition.* In not all cases, however, are the two necessarily related. We have examined many patients who could recognize and read aloud whole words but who could apparently not recognize or at least identify individual letters of the words. It is possible that these patients learned to read by the word- or sentence-recognition method. For them, individual letters do not have the same significance as for persons who have learned to read by building up words from synthesizing letters and sounds. Because of this, the attitude of the patient may be such that he finds no reason for concerning himself with letter recognition. In effect, such persons manifest a disinclination rather than a disability in a recognition function.

For patients with actual *visual letter agnosia,* remedial procedures along the following lines may be tried. An alphabet book, or a series of alphabet cards, with pictures or pictures and words for each letter may be arranged. Children's alphabet books are not recommended because the representations are on a level which might cause ego insult. It is usually no great problem to get colored illustrations from magazine advertisements. Each picture should be edited so that the representation to be associated with the object is most readily evident. If possible, a single object representation should be used. So, a single picture of a book and the word *book* should be associated with the letter *B*. If it is possible to find common object-pictures the form of which suggests the letter, as, for example, a telegraph pole for the letter *T*, such pictures are especially worthwhile. The patient may be directed to copy these letters. If he cannot copy, then he should be asked to trace them, and later to copy them when tracing is easily accomplished. Again, the principle of intensification of stimulation may be used, with the ultimate objective of decreasing the intensity (size) of the letter to usual book-size print. The final step, of course, is for the patient to learn to write letters from dictation.

Some patients who were not readily able to learn to recognize words by the approach just described were helped through body pantomime. For example, a large letter *T* was attached to the corner of a large mirror before which the patient and therapist stood. The therapist stretched his arms out at shoulder height, said "*T*" and asked the patient to imitate the action he saw in the mirror. Later, the patient was able to respond with pantomime to the picture of the letter *T*. Finally, the patient learned to recognize the letter without resorting to pantomime.

These techniques, it is again emphasized, are suggestions. The therapist, using his own resources, should be able to invent suitable ones for his individual patients. Discussions of other successful techniques for dealing with the problem may be found in such texts as those of Goldstein (1932), Granich (1947), Wepman (1951), and Longerich and Bordeaux (1954).

Reading Disturbances (alexia)

Although some of the techniques of remedial reading for children may be employed with modification with adult aphasics, there are some fundamental differences between the reading disabilities of the child and the impaired reading of the adult. First, we must bear in mind that the aphasic, unless illiterate, was once able to read. If the aphasic was illiterate, then reading disability should not be considered part of his remedial problems. Reading impairment is rarely if ever the only difficulty presented by the aphasic. Other impairments are likely to be present which may compound the reading problem.

With these precautions in mind, the following approach to "remedial" reading is recommended:

1. Begin work at the patient's level of ability.
2. Build up sight identification of words, phrases, and short sentences.
3. Use the sound out (phonic) approach for words that are not easily read, *providing* that the patient has no dysarthria or inclination to paraphasic errors, or evidence of auditory aphasia.
4. Comprehension rather than oral style is the objective. Check comprehension by eliciting an oral or written response from the patient.
5. Secure interesting reading material at the patient's level of competence.
6. Upgrade the level of material as the patient progresses.
7. Make reading materials available that may be read by the patient *solely for enjoyment* and which will not become the content for instruction.

To begin at the patient's level of ability requires an evaluation of that ability. The usual standardized tests for reading achievement may be used for this purpose, with the recommended modification that the time allowance for testing be ignored.

Eisenson's Examining for Aphasia (1954) includes a series of reading items which are usually sufficient for preliminary purposes for moderately alexic disturbances and are sufficient for evaluating the reading level of severe alexic patients. Schuell (1964, p. 171) offers a series of questions to serve as a guide for assessing level of reading comprehension.

Building up of a readily functional sight vocabulary should be determined in part by the patient's needs and interests as an adult and in part by the provision of words selected from lists incorporating words and phrases most frequently found in the patient's language. The Thorndike-Lorge list (1944) has become a source for word selection for many books on reading. A list of spoken words (Jones and Wepman, 1966) based on responses to the Murray Thematic Apperception Cards, provides another source for vocabulary selection. We would like to reemphasize, however, that published lists can only suggest words the aphasic *should* know. In the final analysis, aphasics should be helped to recognize and read the words they *need* to know according to their situations and their objectives.

The use of a card with an "exposure slot" is helpful for many aphasic patients in the early stages of reading reeducation. Many patients become overwhelmed when confronted with large amounts of material. They tend to respond better when a small amount is presented at one time. The card serves the purpose of helping patients to believe that they are making progress, a little at a time, and reducing the size of the task. For some patients, pointing to each word as the word is read serves the same purpose. Ultimately, of course, the patient should be encouraged to try to do without this kind of an aid. It is well to remember that, for the aphasic, security and accuracy of comprehension are more important than speed of reading. As training progresses, speed of reading may be improved through the use of flash cards, or by having phrases or short sentences exposed for brief periods on a screen.

Many patients enjoy building up their own stock of reading cards. These may be prepared by the patient with illustrations cut from magazines. A sentence relating to the picture, with the most significant word or words underlined may be typed under, over, or to one side of the picture. A key word or phrase may be typed or written in one corner. If the patient is able to write, his own writing may appear under the printed material. The patient, in adding to his card list, may go over them by himself, or review them with a relative, friend, or another patient. Periodically, the stock may be separated into cards always read easily and correctly, ones usually read easily and accurately, and others "not yet" read easily and accurately. Through this device both the patient and the therapist can estimate improvement in single-sentence reading based on material selected by the patient.

Vocabulary-building cards such as the Dolch Sight Vocabulary Cards and Sight Phrase Cards can be used to considerable advantage. Although these sets of cards were prepared primarily for teaching children to read, their small size and general appearance make them suitable for adult use.

The development of comprehension cannot be taken for granted merely because a patient learns to read words and sequences of words aloud. It is essential—even more so than for children who do not read well—that comprehension be checked constantly. This may be done by having the patient indicate *in some form most readily availalbe to him* that he understands what he has read. The patient may retell the content in his own words, complete sentences with key words, or even use gestures to reveal his comprehension. As the patient improves, he may enjoy taking self-administered reading tests, such as are provided in many primers and in texts for teaching language to foreign-born persons. Considerable use can also be made of reading paragraphs and test materials of standardized reading scales.

Securing reading material at the present level of the aphasic is frequently a real problem. If the patient's alexia is severe, something comparable to a primer is needed. Primers, however, are infantile both in content and in format. The author undertook to "translate" a primer story for use with his patients. He found the task of using a simple vocabulary and casting the words and ideas into an adult form a much more difficult one than he anticipated. The results, however, were rewarding. In his "translation" he used black-line drawings and photographs to replace the multicolored pictures of the primer. The story including illustrations was then bound in hard covers. The aphasics did not suspect that they were reading a paraphrased primer story, and seemed pleased that they had a "book" especially prepared for them.

Probably the best type of initial reading material is that which is especially prepared for the individual patient. As patients improve, edited (rewritten) news reports are useful. They have the advantage of being timely, and so are usually of immediate interest.[5]

[5] We have found general acceptance by aphasics of specially prepared newspapers such as *Young America* (Eton Publishing Co., Silver Springs, Md.) and the special *Reading Skill Builder Series* (Reader's Digest Educational Service, Pleasantville, N.Y.). Among other books prepared for special groups of readers which we recommend as useful for aphasic patients are the following:

The *Everyreader Library Series* (Webster Publishing Co., St. Louis, Mo.) includes classics and biographies adapted by remedial reading experts for use with slow readers. A basic vocabulary and simple sentence structure are employed. Titles include *Ivanhoe*, *A Tale of Two Cities*, *The Gold Bug*, *Cases of Sherlock Holmes*, and *Simon Bolivar*.

The *Oxford English Course* (Oxford University Press, New York) consists of a graduated course intended for persons for whom English is a second language. The vocabulary for each course is based upon a selected list of essential words. The entire series includes language books for presenting basic vocabularies and teaching grammar. *Language*, Book One, Part One, introduces the alphabet arranged for reading and writing. The supplementary readers include simplified versions of the classics which employ limited (basic) vocabularies. Titles which employ vocabularies of from 1500 to 2000 words include *The Tempest* and *The Purloined Letter*.

AUDITORY DISTURBANCES

It is fortunate that most aphasic patients recover spontaneously considerable auditory comprehension in the early stages of their aphasic involvement. It is probably also true that patients and clinicians both tend to overestimate the amount of recovery which seems to have taken place. Much of what we say to patients in conversation, regardless of specific content, can frequently be answered by a single word, or a nod of the head. A patient who just has the merest hunch of what is said to him can frequently determine by observing the speaker's face whether a "Yes" or "No" is expected. Often the patient catches the rudiments of what is said, but if no specific response is expected of him he does not have any check or test of how much he really understood. Some patients stop listening, or become "functionally deaf," when they cannot readily understand what they hear. By doing this they avoid the challenge, the effort, and the possible frustration, of trying to comprehend. One of our patients, a highly social person, almost always took the initiative in conversational situations. He spoke with relevantly fluent circumlocutions and seldom permitted other persons in a conversational group to say much in response to him. By controlling the conversation, the patient seemed to understand conversational speech. When this patient's device of taking the initiative was evaluated for him, he accepted the evaluation and began to listen as well as to speak. By doing so, the first principle of training for a patient with auditory disturbances became established: *patients must learn to listen if they are to learn to understand what they hear*

Earlier, in our discussion of therapeutic problems and approaches, the technique of intensification of stimulation was considered. The auditory aphasic needs intensification. He also needs constant encouragement and reassurance that in time comprehension will come and two-way communication will be reestablished.

For the auditory aphasic, television observation is strongly recommended, especially for dramatic plays. The frequent close-ups permitting the patient to concentrate on the facial movements of speech, which may be associated with the total background situation, constitute excellent therapy as well as educational recreation. Newscasts, whether on television or radio, are also highly recommended. If possible, a discussion between patients and clinician should follow listening to news broadcasts. Such discussion, which should be held informally, will serve as a reinforcement of understanding. If a given newscast involves a matter about which there may be differences of opinion, then the patients may be encouraged to give their reactions or opinions about what was said.

For more formal teaching situations, Schuell (1953) offers a number of suggestions for determining whether a patient understands what he hears.[6] Schuell emphasizes that the only way to be certain whether an aphasic patient understands what he hears is to ask him to respond in some way. The nature and particular type of response which the patient should be encouraged to make will depend upon both the patient's productive abilities and the specific situation. Among the type of responses which may be elicited, Schuell suggests the following:

1. Identifying objects in a picture. This may be used in going over illustrations in magazines, books, or specially arranged cards.
2. Following directions.
3. Answering questions, formally or informally, in conversation with the therapist.
4. Completing sentences intentionally left incomplete by the therapist.
5. Answering specific questions presented by the therapist.
6. Identifying, by pointing, underlining, or naming specific words or sentences for a given context.
7. Paraphrasing in the patient's own words, or in words he recalls, what the patient heard.
8. Writing answers, especially if the patient can write more readily than he can use oral speech.
9. Presenting oral opposites of single words, phrases, or sentences: for example, high—low; come here—go away; it is early—it is late.

To this list, which is merely a list of suggestions, the therapist can and should add his own devices to insure the second basic principle of therapy for the training of a patient with auditory disturbances. The principle is that *the patient must understand what he hears.*

Auditory aphasics who show impairment in phonemic discrimination or *discriminative hearing* (Luria, 1966, pp. 103–113) present a special problem. Such patients, by virtue of their auditory disturbance, are likely to have difficulty in differentiating between words which have sounds not separated by wide distinctive features, e.g., *boat* and *coat*, *coal* and *goal*, *path* and *bath*. Such difficulties become apparent when contextual meanings do not bring out differences in word meaning. Fortunately, as Luria observes, patients with disturbances in phonemic hearing do not usually have any related disturbance in melodic hearing. This observation, plus "the characteristic of sensory (acoustic) aphasia is the fact that all functions not related to the defect of sound analysis and synthesis are usually preserved" (Luria, 1966, p. 112) provide the basis for therapy. The patient must direct his attention to the overall meaning of an utterance, to visual components of articulation, to the inflection, stress, and intonation to compensate for impairment in phonemic discrimination. As Luria points out, "Assistance from kinesthetic and visual-spatial analysis and synthesis may therefore be used for rehabilitation of patients in this group." More detailed rehabilitative writings on methods are outlined in Luria's writings on the rehabilitation of aphasics (Luria, 1948).

[6] Additional suggestions for determining how much the patient understands of what he hears are offered by Schuell (1964, pp. 170–171).

Therapeutic Techniques for Productive (Expressive) Disturbances

At the outset, it is well that productive disturbances as well as evaluative ones are seldom found as pure or isolated disabilities in the adult. Not infrequently, the patient's concern with one aspect of his disturbance may make him oblivious to other aspects. Without thorough examination, areas of productive defect may not become apparent to either the clinician or to the patient. This statement is not intended to imply that the clinician or therapist has an obligation to "reveal all" to the patient just as soon as "the all" is discovered. It is intended to imply that the ultimate object should be improvement, to whatever degree seems possible, in all areas of disturbance.

NONVERBAL APRAXIAS

The space limitations of this text do not permit any detailed discussion of this form of productive disturbance. It is obviously important, as indicated earlier, to determine whether a particular productive disturbance is one related to the symbol per se, or to the motor act per se. In the case of writing disturbance, it is essential to know whether the patient's basic difficulty is in knowing how to use a tool external to the body—a pen or pencil—intentionally and meaningfully, or to use the arm-hand-finger tools intentionally or meaningfully. For the most part, the speech therapist is not likely to be concerned with the patient's use of tools which are not part of the body. Such training is likely to be provided by other members of the therapeutic team. It may, however, become necessary to teach the patient how to handle writing equipment such as pencils, pens, chalk, the blackboard, and so forth.

Probably the best initial approach to the handling of tools is to have the patient imitate the therapist's act as a whole in a relatively simple movement. The first tool should be large, easy to grasp, and one that offers little resistance. Soft chalk and a large blackboard, soft black crayons and a large sheet of paper mounted on a blackboard, are good instruments for a start. If the patient cannot directly imitate the writing of a simple word outline such as *cat*, then the therapist may try placing the writing instrument in the patient's hand and moving the hand for the execution of the word outline. From soft chalk or crayon, the patient should progress to using a large, oversize pencil. If the patient finds it difficult to grasp a pencil, its width and tenability can be enhanced by tying multiple-strand string around the bottom of the pencil. If the notion of grasping itself needs to be established, the use of a half-filled bean bag or a sponge rubber ball is recommended. Other suggestions for this type of training may be found in some of the texts already referred to on aphasia therapy. The problem of the teaching of writing as an aphasic difficulty will be considered later.

ORAL APRAXIA

Control of articulatory activity may be enhanced by emphasis on the visual aspect of articulation. An approach we recommend requires imitation by the patient of simple articulatory movements made by the therapist. Imitation may be direct, with the patient observing the therapist, or may be mirror imitation, with the patient observing the therapist and himself in a large mirror. The use of photographs to enable the patient to imitate himself was also suggested.

From single sounds such as /i/ (ee), /u/ (oo), and /ɑ/ (ah), which, fortunately, have some word value in English, the patient should be helped to consonant-vowel combinations. To begin with, the readily visible consonants should be taught. The sound /p/ is a good one because of its distinctive lip movement and breath characteristics. It can be combined with each of the vowels mentioned above to constitute three word forms. The patient then is not only making sounds, but to a degree may be making sense. It is not recommended that the sound /m/ follow the teaching of /p/. The partial similarity in lip activity may confuse some patients. It is recommended instead that a sound differently produced, such as /t/ or /n/ be taught next. Fortunately, /t/ plus each of the three vowels adds at least two more word forms for most American speakers, and three word forms for American speakers who use Standard Eastern or British (London) dialect.

The concept of voiced and unvoiced sounds should be established after sound as such is appreciated. If the patient does not spontaneously vocalize sounds, the patient's hand may be placed at the therapist's larynx while the therapist produces voiced sounds. We have found that frequently all that is necessary for the patient to produce vocalized sound is to place his (the patient's) hand on his own larynx in imitation of the therapist. In this way, differences between cognate sounds are usually established readily.

The next step is to establish not readily visible speech sounds such as /s/, /z/, /r/, /k/, and /g/. These again may be taught in isolation and in combination with vowels in addition to the first three which have been suggested. Wherever possible, chosen combinations should be ones which are word forms rather than nonsense syllables. Word forms may be used, or recognized, in speech. For a patient with disturbances so severe as to include oral apraxia, the ability to use a few words may be a great morale booster.

It is a fairly common observation (Wepan, 1951, p. 218) that it is rarely necessary to teach a patient all sounds, or many combinations of sounds. Once the idea of articulatory activity is established, most apraxic patients progress by themselves in making additional sounds, and in going from sounds to attempts at words.

WRITING (AGRAPHIA)

We shall begin with the assumption that the patient has no external tool apraxia, or has overcome this form of disability and now must be trained to learn to form letters and to write words and sentences. The suggestion has already been made that, unless the patient shows resistance, a change of handedness is recommended. If the patient has a hemiplegia or a severe paresis which involves his preferred hand, a change of handedness is essential. The use of Gardner's manual for this purpose has already been indicated. Visual disturbances, especially those involving visual field, must also be considered. It is essential that the patient be able to see as well as feel the materials he is to use. If the material is to be copied, it should be placed so that it can be seen. If this can be accomplished, almost all aphasic patients can succeed in copying. Retraining might well begin with copying material on a blackboard. Next steps might include copying with a soft crayon on a large sheet of newsprint, copying with a pencil, and copying with a pen. Many patients are able to proceed directly from blackboard to pencil and paper. It is again emphasized that the therapist must assume the responsibility for the good working condition of the equipment. Mechanical difficulties should not be permitted to aggravate the patient's efforts at improvement.

If a patient cannot copy readily by looking at material above his writing space, he may be helped by placing letters underneath thin, transluscent paper, through which the letters underneath may be seen. The letters should be clear and simple in outline. If possible, they should be enlargements of the kind of writing the patient himself habitually used. Almost always, some specimen of the patient's own writing may be obtained from a member of his family.

Occasionally, a patient, for reasons not always apparent, has persistent difficulties with one or more letters. It frequently helps to personalize these letters. One patient learned to write the letter *I* by standing straight and tall, with his hands close to his sides, so that he looked like an *I*. Another, who was fond of smoking a pipe, associated the letter *P* with the picture of a pipe placed so that it suggested the letter *P*. The resourceful clinician may arrive at his own devices which meet the needs and interests, as well as the disabilities, of his particular patient. For further suggestive techniques, the clinician is referred to texts by Granich (1947) and Goldstein (1932), and to an article by Smith (1948).

Copying should be followed by writing from memory after visual presentation. The time period of stimulation-presentation should be reduced progressively to a brief period, sufficient only for the patient to read what is presented. Following this, the patient should be encouraged to write from dictation, beginning with single words and proceeding, as early as possible, to short phrases and short sentences. Eventually, short paragraphs should be used for dictation material.

In his attempts at writing, the patient should never be required to struggle for the letter or word he cannot evoke from memory. The elusive word should be made available to him so that he can copy what he cannot recall.

Spelling disability, in the sense that the appropriate sequence of letters cannot be recalled for a given word, is not an apraxic disturbance as the term *apraxia* has been used in this chapter. It is a higher level symbolic disturbance, and therefore is classified as agraphia. Many patients with writing disturbance have this form of difficulty. Some have both apraxic and spelling involvements. A few will have little difficulty with spelling as such once they overcome their apraxic disability.

For the patient with both forms of writing disturbance, practice in copying and writing from dictation has incidentally provided practice in spelling. Continued practice may be given in flash-card presentations, and in spontaneous writing with word lists available for copying when necessary. If it is determined, as is sometimes the case, that the patient's oral spelling is more accurate than his written efforts, then the oral approach should be emphasized. Similarly, if the patient seems to learn better through the auditory than through the visual avenue, the words should be spelled aloud for the patient, and he should practice writing while he spells aloud.

In teaching spelling, the selection of words to spell should be determined primarily by what the patient will need to write. The essential objective for spelling instruction, for aphasic adults as for children, is to equip them to write what they need and want to write. The needs of the mason and a lawyer are likely to be more divergent for the building of a writing vocabulary than for a speaking or reading vocabulary. This, however, should not overlook the possibility that some masons have avocations which include the need to write and spell to a greater degree than some lawyers.

Spelling lists serve as a guide to ultimate objectives. The lists previously suggested for basic reading vocabularies may obviously be used for spelling as well. These lists should be supplemented by special ones that are related to the patient's interests, and should include vocational and avocational vocabularies if the patient is likely to return to them.

It will frequently be found that many patients' spelling difficulties are similar to those usual with children. Devices such as enlarging the letters of the troublesome parts of the word, or writing the letter in colored ink or crayon, may be of help. The patient should be encouraged to keep his own list of troublesome words, written in a fashion best suited to help him learn the correct spelling of the words. In this regard it is hoped that the patient will pride himself on a list decreasing rather than increasing in size.

PARAPHASIA

Paraphasic errors—the errors of omission, substitution, or transposition of sounds or words—frequently constitute a final therapeutic problem for both the patient and the therapist. These, together with word-finding (anomic) difficulties, may persist as residuals of aphasic involvement. In some instances, there is little to do but to become resigned and adjusted to their continued presence, especially under conditions where intellectual vigilance is reduced.

Some patients evolve oral and written speech which is characteristically agrammatical. Their speech suggests the economical form of a message prepared as a telegraph or a cablegram. So-called "unessential" words—the connectives, prepositions, and conjunctions—are often omitted. A sentence such as "Let us go for a walk" may be reduced to "Go walk" or simply to "Walk." According to Goldstein (1932), many patients lose their attitude toward grammar and need to be reoriented to grammatical practices. This reorientation is not always possible, especially with a patient who has accepted his disabilities and the immunities associated with them. For such a patient, his new point of view seems to be "I am a patient, and I have many disabilities. It is up to others to make adjustments to me and to exert effort to figure out what I mean."

For patients who are motivated to make themselves understood, it is of some help to record their oral speech and to play it back. Then the patient may be asked to indicate what words he omitted that another speaker is likely to use to convey the same meaning. The patient is then encouraged to fill in the omitted words. The author has found that it may also be of help to reduce his own speech to telegraphic style when speaking to the patient, so that the patient can appreciate that such speech is difficult to understand. Where possible, this exercise should be given to a group of patients who may correct one another. Written speech may be corrected by having the therapist indicate the places within a sentence where words were omitted. The patient is then encouraged to fill in the omitted words. If he cannot do this, the words should be inserted for him, and the patient is then directed to rewrite the sentence with all words in conventional order.

Errors of sound reversal may be treated in a similar way. For some patients, the technique of negative practice may be used with success to create awareness of error. Fortunately, for most aphasics, severe paraphasic errors tend to disappear as general improvement takes place. If paraphasic errors are relatively infrequent, it may not always be worthwhile to correct them. It is well to remember that even normal nonaphasic persons sometimes commit paraphasia. We call them slips of the tongue. Their psychodynamics, from which aphasics are not free, are, as Freud indicates, a matter of the psychopathology of everyday life.

Word-finding difficulty (anomia)

Both logically and psychologically, the aphasic patient's language needs are greatest for oral speech, and training should, wherever possible, begin here. Unless he is an extremely withdrawn person, a patient can learn to get along without all other forms of productive language except oral speech. Word-finding difficulty is both the most common characteristic of the aphasic's disturbances and the most persistent even after considerable overall improvement has taken place. It is the form of difficulty most likely to return under conditions of tension, excitement, or fatigue. For many, and perhaps for most aphasics, it is to some degree a permanent residual problem. Sometimes, the substitute word may not readily suggest, in sound or meaning, the desired word. Some patients prefer to say something, in the remote hope that they may guess right, or because of an attitude that saying something—anything—is better than saying nothing. Most patients are able to recognize their errors and try to correct them. If, as indicated earlier, the word evoked in error is one which may be functionally useful, an attempt might be made to establish that word. If this is not the case, the therapist should return patiently to trying to establish the originally selected word.

In establishing a name of an object, the function of the object should be demonstrated, and the object should be named. The patient may then be asked to repeat the name after the therapist. If he can write, he should be asked to write and say the name, alone if possible, otherwise with or after the therapist. Finally, the patient should be given an opportunity at some later time in the therapeutic session to evoke the name by himself.

Once the naming process gets under way for descriptive action, as well as for nominal terms, progress may be accelerated and considerable spontaneous improvement may be expected. Improvement as a result of direct training may also be more rapid. Most patients, however, will continue to find that a few words are always elusive and will not be theirs for ready evocation. Some patients will learn to speak slowly, as if they are always hunting for words. Others will become adept in using synonymous terms and phrases. Still others will indulge in lengthy circumlocutions to suggest the meanings of the precise words which will not readily roll off their tongues.

As soon as possible, and at the very outset *if at all possible*, the patient should be urged to incorporate the words which have become established, or which are being established, into conventional oral sentence form. All too frequently patients become satisfied with naming as a sentence function. This device, though economical of effort, does not help the individual concerned, or others, to think of him as a recovered person rather than as a patient.

Arithmetic difficulty (acalculia)

Arithmetic disturbances may arise because of linguistic aspects per se, or because of the special processes involved in calculation and problem solving.

Fortunately, much of arithmetic effort is entirely automatic by the time the individual becomes an adult. Because of this, many aphasics can arrive at correct results without being able to name the numerals or tell what they did to arrive at their results. Speed of calculation can be enhanced by making the patient aware of automatic arithmetic series, and by showing him how he can make use of them. After relative automaticity is established, the patient may be shown the rationale of the various arithmetic tables. For example, the patient may be shown that the series 2, 4, 6, 8, . . . is arrived at by adding the amount 2 to each previous amount.

The need for reteaching arithmetic in a manner as close to the one in which the particular process was originally learned has already been discussed under Learning Techniques. Additional suggested approaches to calculation difficulties may be found in tests which deal with the teaching or the remedial teaching of arithmetic.

As with other symbolic functions, the amount and kind of calculation to be taught should be determined by the individual patient's immediate needs and later objectives. If the patient is ambulatory, counting sums for payment of purchases and making change should probably have priority.

PREVENTIVE APPROACHES

Earlier we discussed the value of undertaking treatment as soon after the onset of aphasia as possible as a preventive measure for aphasics. Another point of view in regard to prevention is described by Beyn and Shokhor-Trotskaya (1966). The basic principle of their approach is to anticipate what form of speech might recover in a patient's progress and "to reorganize the primary speech defect and thereby to prevent the emergence of secondary symptoms of speech disorders. . . . the characteristic feature of the preventive method of rehabilitation is its prophylactic nature." Specifically, as applied to a group of patients with motor aphasia, the investigators laid the foundation for the future development of a normal grammatical system in a group of patients who would be expected to develop agrammatisms by *regulating the content of the words* introduced into the patient's speech by external control.

> We took into consideration the well-known proposition of the psychology of speech that inner speech derives its content from external speech. Therefore, in contrast to the usual methods, in the early stages we *excluded* the communication from the outside of any nominative words, since these could only aggravate the pathology of inner speech peculiar to patients with motor aphasia (i.e., the disintegration of its predicative system). It seemed to us that only those words which were most closely connected with the utterance as a whole could successfully resist this pathological tendency. Our task, therefore, was to select for the speechless patients the simplest possible words which could function as a whole sentence.

In accordance with this theoretical position, the investigators started with words (first and second weeks) which were "partially verbs and partially interjections," such as "No," "There!" "Here," which served as predicatives and, with appropriate intonation and gesture, constituted "sentences." Pronouns were next introduced (third and fourth weeks) to constitute utterances such as "I want to stop," "I shall eat," followed by longer utterances such as "I am going for a walk" and "Give me a drink." We should note that up to this point, though nouns are used, they are in the objective and not in the nominative form. When nominative form words are first introduced, they are of generalized denotation, such as *man*, *woman*, *boy*, *girl*.

Beyn and Shokhor-Trotskaya report that none of 25 adults trained with the preventive approach employed telegraphic speech even though 16 of the group continued after considerable training to be unable to produce grammatically acceptable utterances. Nine of the group, interestingly, continued to have difficulties in the use of prepositions.

We do not know whether preventive training which implies the *control of utterances* will work with most patients. The basic notion, however, that *supplying a patient with a model for correct utterance before errors are produced, is consistent with learning principles.* We can certainly recommend reinforcing that which can be correctly evoked as a principle for aphasia therapy.

BIBLIOGRAPHY

Beyn, E. 1964. Aphasia and methods of its elimination. Leningrad: Meditsina.

———, and Shokhor-Troskaya, M. 1966. The preventive method of speech rehabilitation in aphasia. *Cortex*, II, 1, 96–108.

Blackman, N. 1950, Group psychotherapy with aphasics. *J. nerv. ment. Disorders*, 111, 154–163.

Brookshire, R. 1968. Visual discrimination and response reversal learning by aphasic subjects. *J. Speech Hearing Research*, 11, 4, 677–692.

Butfield, E., and Zangwill, O. 1946. Re-education in aphasia: a review of 70 cases. *J. Neurol. Neurosur. Psychiat.*, IX, New Series, 75–79.

Carson, D., Carson, F., and Tikofsky, R. 1968. On learning characteristics of the adult aphasic. *Cortex*, IV, 1, 92–112.

Dunlap, K. 1928. A revision of the fundamental law of habit. *Science*, 67, 370.

Eisenson, J. 1949. Prognostic factors related to language rehabilitation in aphasic patients. *J. Speech Hearing Disorders*, 14, 262–264.

Gardner, W. 1945. Left handed writing. Danville, Ill.: Interstate Press.

Goldstein, K. 1932. After effects of brain injuries in war. New York: Grune & Stratton.

Granich, L. 1947. Aphasia: a guide to retraining. New York: Grune & Stratton.

Holland, A. 1969. Some current trends in aphasia rehabilitation. *Asha*, 11, 1, 3–7.

Jones, L., and Wepman, J. 1966. A spoken word count. Chicago: Language Research Associates.

Kreindler, A., and Fradis, A. 1968. Performance in aphasia. Paris: Gauthier-Villars.

Longerich, M. 1959. Aphasia therapy sets. Los Angeles: Longerich.

———, and Bordeaux, J. 1954. Aphasia therapeutics. New York: Macmillan.

Luria, A. 1948. Rehabilitation of brain functioning after war traumas. Moscow: Acad. Science Press.

———. 1966. Higher cortical functions in man. New York: Basic Books.

Moore, P., and Schuell, H. 1954. The language master handbook for aphasia. New York: McGraw-Hill.

Schuell, H. 1953. Auditory impairment in aphasia: significance and retraining techniques. *J. Speech Hearing Disorders*, 18, 14–21.

———, Jenkins, J., and Jiminez-Pabon, E. 1964. Aphasia in adults. New York: Hoeber Med. Div., Harper and Row.

Smith, M. 1948. Teaching an aphasic how to write again. *J. clin. Psychol.*, 4, 419–423.

Taylor, M., and Marks, M. 1959. Aphasia rehabilitation and therapy kit. New York: Saxon.

Thorndike, E., and Lorge, I. 1944. Teachers word book of 30,000 words. New York: Bur. Pub., Teachers College, Columbia Univ.

Tikofsky, R., and Reynolds, G. 1962. Preliminary study: nonverbal learning and aphasia: *J. Speech Hearing Research*, 5, 2, 133–143.

Van Riper, C. 1963. Speech correction (4th. ed.). Englewood Cliffs, N.J.: Prentice-Hall. Pp. 296–298.

Vignolo, L. 1964. Evolution of aphasia and language rehabilitation: a retrospective exploratory study. *Cortex*, I, 344–367.

Wepman, J. 1951. Recovery from aphasia. New York: Ronald.

Author Index

Subject Index